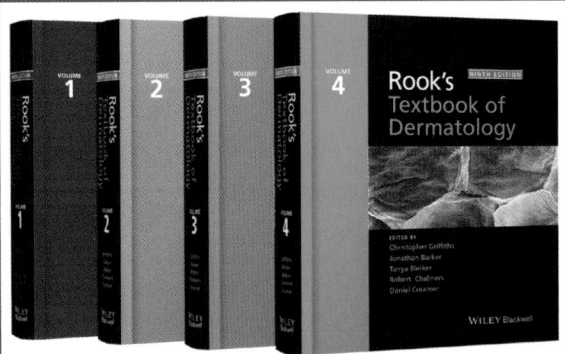
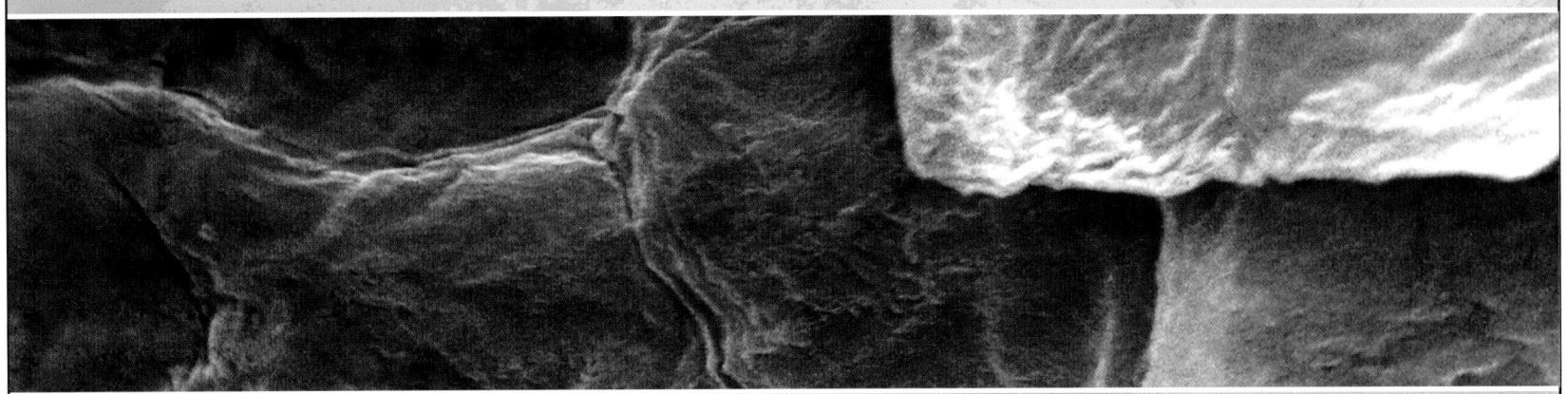

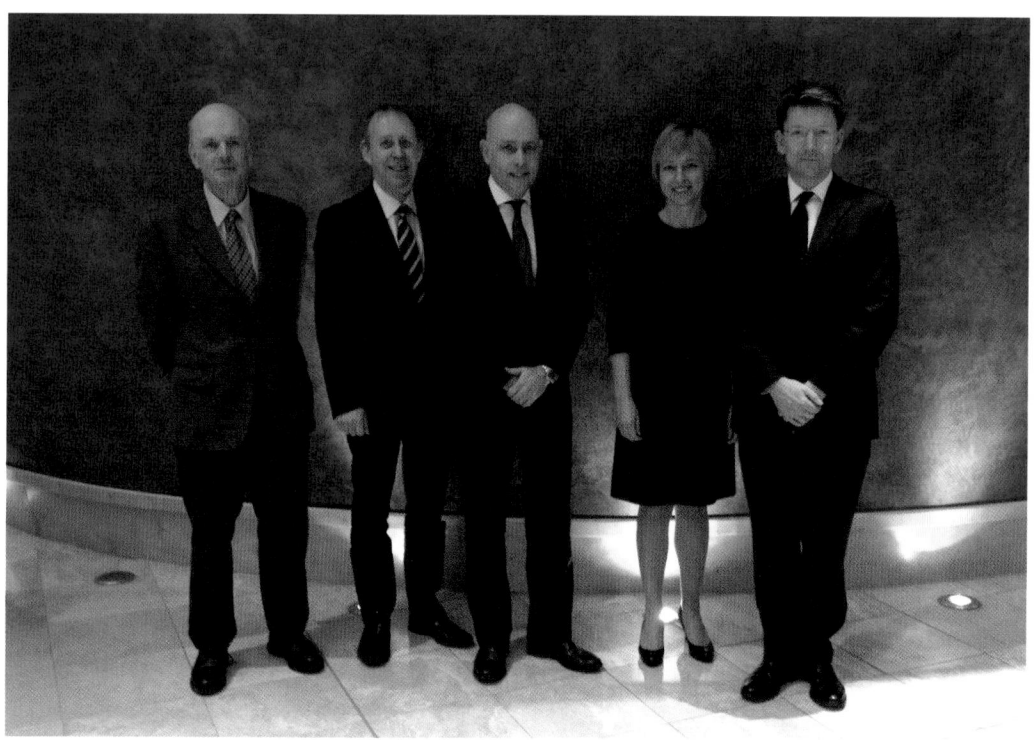

The Editors
From left to right: Robert Chalmers, Jonathan Barker, Christopher Griffiths, Tanya Bleiker, Daniel Creamer

Rook's Textbook of Dermatology

NINTH EDITION

EDITED BY

Christopher E. M. Griffiths MD, FRCP, FMedSci
Professor of Dermatology
The Dermatology Centre, Salford Royal NHS Foundation Trust
The University of Manchester
Manchester Academic Health Science Centre
Manchester, UK

Jonathan Barker MD, FRCP, FRCPath
Professor of Medical Dermatology
St John's Institute of Dermatology
Division of Genetics and Molecular Medicine
Faculty of Life Sciences and Medicine
King's College London
London, UK

Tanya Bleiker FRCP
Consultant Dermatologist
Derby Teaching Hospitals NHS Foundation Trust
Derby, UK

Robert Chalmers FRCP
Honorary Consultant Dermatologist
The Dermatology Centre, Salford Royal NHS Foundation Trust
Manchester Royal Infirmary
Manchester, UK

Daniel Creamer MD, FRCP
Consultant Dermatologist
King's College Hospital
London, UK

IN FOUR VOLUMES

VOLUME 3

WILEY Blackwell

ISBN: 9781118441190

A catalogue record for this book is available from the British Library and the Library of Congress.

Wiley also publishes its books in a variety of electronic formats. Some content that appears in print may not be available in electronic books.

Cover image: Getty Images/Science Photo Library

Set in 9.5/12pt Palatino LT Std by Aptara Inc., New Delhi, India
Printed and bound in Singapore by Markono Print Media Pte Ltd

1   2016

Contents

VOLUME 2

Part 4 Inflammatory Dermatoses

Part 5 Metabolic and Nutritional Disorders Affecting the Skin

Part 6 Genetic Disorders Involving the Skin

Part 7   Psychological, Sensory and Neurological Disorders and the Skin

VOLUME 3

Part 8   Skin Disorders Associated with Specific Cutaneous Structure

Part 9   Vascular Disorders Involving the Skin

Associate Editors

Anthony Bewley
BA(Hons), MB ChB, FRCP
Consultant Dermatologist, Department of
Dermatology, Barts Health NHS Trust, London; and
Senior Lecturer, Queen Mary College of Medicine,
University of London, London, UK

Eduardo Calonje
MD, DipRCPath
Consultant Dermatopathologist, St John's Institute
of Dermatology, Guy's and St Thomas' NHS
Foundation Trust, London, UK

Tamara Griffiths
MD, FRCP, FAAD
Consultant Dermatologist, The Dermatology Centre,
Salford Royal Hospital, Manchester, UK

Gregor B. E. Jemec
MD, DMSc
Professor and Clinical Lead, Department of
Dermatology, Roskilde Hospital; Health Sciences
Faculty, University of Copenhagen, Copenhagen,
Denmark

Nick J. Levell
MD, FRCP, MB ChB, MBA
Clinical Director of Dermatology, Norwich Medical
School, Norfolk and Norwich University Hospital,
Norwich; National Specialty Lead Dermatology,
National Institute for Health Research, London;
Clinical Vice-President, British Association of
Dermatologists, London, UK

John A. McGrath
MD, FRCP, FMedSci
Professor of Molecular Dermatology, St John's
Institute of Dermatology, Division of Genetics and
Molecular Medicine, Faculty of Life Sciences and
Medicine, King's College London, London, UK

Graham Ogg
DPhil, BM BCh, FRCP
Professor of Dermatology, MRC Human Immunology
Unit, Weatherall Institute of Molecular Medicine,
University of Oxford; and Consultant Dermatologist,
Oxford University Hospitals NHS Trust, Oxford, UK

Nick J. Reynolds
BSc, MB BS, MD, FRCP
Professor of Dermatology, Department of
Dermatology, Royal Victoria Infirmary and Institute
of Cellular Medicine, Newcastle University,
Newcastle upon Tyne, UK

Robert P. E. Sarkany
FRCP, MD
Consultant Dermatologist and Head of
Photodermatology, St John's Institute of
Dermatology, Guy's and St Thomas' NHS
Foundation Trust, London, UK

Eli Sprecher
MD, PhD
Professor and Chair, Department of Dermatology,
Tel Aviv Sourasky Medical Center; and Department
of Human Molecular Genetics and Biochemistry,
Sackler Medical School, Tel Aviv University, Tel Aviv,
Israel

Jane C. Sterling
MB BChir, MA, FRCP, PhD
Senior Lecturer and Honorary Consultant
Dermatologist, Department of Dermatology,
University of Cambridge, Addenbrooke's Hospital,
Cambridge, UK

Hensin Tsao
MD, PhD
Head, Skin Cancer Genetics Laboratory/Wellman
Center for Photomedicine; Director, MGH Melanoma
and Pigmented Lesion Center/Department of
Dermatology; Director, MGH Melanoma Genetics
Program/MGH Cancer Center Massachusetts
General Hospital, Boston, MA; Professor of
Dermatology, Harvard Medical School, Boston,
MA, USA

Contributors

Christina Antoniou
MD
Professor of Dermatology, Department of
Dermatology, University of Athens Medical School,
Andreas Sygros Hospital, Athens, Greece
Chapter 132

Michael R. Ardern-Jones
BSc, MB BS, DPhil, FRCP
Dermatoimmunology, University of Southampton,
Southampton General Hospital, Southampton, UK
Chapters 12, 41, 118

H. Ruth Ashbee
PhD
Principal Clinical Scientist, Mycology Reference Centre,
Leeds Teaching Hospitals NHS Trust, Leeds, UK
Chapter 32

Matthias Augustin
MD
Director and Professor of Dermatology and Health
Economics, Institute for Health Services Research
in Dermatology and Nursing, University Medical
Center Hamburg-Eppendorf, Hamburg, Germany
Chapter 6

Robert Baran
University of Franche-Comté, Nail Disease Centre,
Cannes, France
Chapter 95

Richard J. Barlow
MD, FRCP
Consultant Dermatologist, St John's Institute
of Dermatology, Guy's and St Thomas' NHS
Foundation Trust, London, UK
Chapter 23

Saqib J. Bashir
BSc(Hons), MB ChB, MD, FRCP
Consultant Dermatological Surgeon, King's College,
Hospital, London, UK
Chapters 123, 125

Tanya N. Basu
MA, PhD, MRCP
Consultant Dermatologist, King's College Hospital,
London, UK
Chapter 38

Jürgen C. Becker
MD, PhD
Head of Department, Translational Skin Cancer
Research (TSCR), German Cancer
Consortium (DKTK), University Clinic of Essen,
Essen, Germany
Chapter 145

Emma C. Benton
MB ChB, MRCP
Consultant Dermatologist, St John's Institute
of Dermatology, Guy's and St Thomas' NHS
Foundation Trust, London, UK
Chapter 4

John Berth-Jones
FRCP
Consultant Dermatologist, University Hospital,
Coventry, UK
Chapter 18

Anthony Bewley
BA(Hons), MB ChB, FRCP
Consultant Dermatologist, Department of
Dermatology, Barts Health NHS Trust, London; and
Senior Lecturer, Queen Mary College of Medicine,
University of London, London, UK
Chapters 84, 86

Balbir S. Bhogal
BMS, BSc, MSc
Head, Immunodermatology Laboratory, St John's
Institute of Dermatology, Guy's and St Thomas' NHS
Foundation Trust, London, UK
Chapter 3

Michael Bigby
MD, FAAD
Associate Professor of Dermatology,
Harvard Medical School and Beth Israel Deaconess
Medical Center, Boston, MA, USA
Chapter 17

Laurence M. Boon
MD, PhD
Coordinator, Center for Vascular Anomalies, Cliniques
Universitaires Saint-Luc; Professor, Division of Plastic
Surgery, Cliniques Universitaires Saint-Luc; Professor of
Human Genetics, Human Molecular Genetics, de Duve
Institute, Université catholique de Louvain, Brussels,
Belgium
Chapter 73

Elena Borzova
DMedSci
Associate Professor of Allergy, Russian Medical
Academy of Postgraduate Education, Moscow,
Russian Federation
Chapter 44

Johnny Bourke
MD, FRCPI
Consultant Dermatologist, South Infirmary-Victoria
University Hospital, Cork; Clinical Senior Lecturer,
University College, Cork, Ireland
Chapters 61, 64, 97

Stephen M. Breathnach
MA, MB BChir, MD, PhD, FRCP, DipDerm(USA)
Consultant Dermatologist, St John's Institute
of Dermatology, Guy's and St Thomas' NHS
Foundation Trust, London, UK
Chapter 37

Aparna Briggs
MA, MB BChir, MRCP, DipGUM, DFSRH, DipHIV
Specialist Registrar in Genitourinary Medicine,
Sheffield Teaching Hospitals NHS Foundation Trust,
Sheffield, UK
Chapter 30

Christine Bundy
PhD, CPsychol, AFBPS
Senior Lecturer in Behavioural Medicine and
Honorary Consultant Health Psychologist, Institute
of Inflammation and Repair, University of
Manchester, Manchester, UK
Chapter 11

Christopher B. Bunker
MA, MD, FRCP
Consultant Dermatologist, University College
London Hospitals and Chelsea & Westminster
Hospitals, London, UK; Professor of Dermatology,
University College and Imperial College, London,
UK
Chapters 31, 111

A. David Burden
MD, FRCP
Consultant Dermatologist, Western Infirmary,
Glasgow; Professor of Dermatology, University of
Glasgow, Glasgow, UK
Chapter 35

Nigel Burrows
MD, FRCP
Consultant Dermatologist, Department of
Dermatology, Addenbrooke's Hospital, Cambridge
University Hospitals NHS Foundation Trust,
Cambridge, UK
Chapter 72

Eduardo Calonje
MD, DipRCPath
Consultant Dermatopathologist, St John's Institute
of Dermatology, Guy's and St Thomas' NHS
Foundation Trust, London, UK
Chapters 3, 137, 138

Rino Cerio
BSc, MB BS, LRCP, MRCS, FRCP(Lond), FRCP(Edin),
FRCPath, DipRCPath, ICPath
Consultant Dermatologist and Director of
Dermatopathology, The Royal London Hospital,
Bart's Health NHS Trust, London; Queen Mary's
Medical and Dental School, University of London,
London, UK
Chapter 47

Kelly B. Cha
MD, PhD
Assistant Professor of Dermatology, Department of
Dermatology, University of Michigan Health System,
Ann Arbor, MI, USA
Chapter 143

Amy Y.-Y. Chen
MD, FAAD
Assistant Professor of Dermatology, Department of
Dermatology, University of Connecticut School of
Medicine, Canton, CT, USA
Chapter 100

Ai-Lean Chew
MB ChB, MRCP
Consultant Dermatologist, Guy's and St Thomas'
NHS Foundation Trust, London; King's College
Hospital, London, UK
Chapters 123, 125

Fiona Child
MD, FRCP
Consultant Dermatologist, St John's Institute
of Dermatology, Guy's and St Thomas' NHS
Foundation Trust, London, UK
Chapters 135, 140

Olivier Chosidow
MD, PhD
Professor and Chairman, UPEC-Université Paris-Est
Créteil Val de Marne, Department of Dermatology,
Hôpital Henri Mondor, Créteil, France
Chapter 34

Anthony C. Chu
FRCP
Professor of Dermatology, Hammersmith Hospital,
Imperial College Healthcare NHS Trust, London, UK
Chapters 36, 87

Derek H. Chu
MD
Resident, Department of Dermatology, Children's
Hospital of Philadelphia, Philadelphia, PA, USA
Chapter 63

Lis Cordingley
PhD, CPsychol
Senior Lecturer in Health Psychology, Institute of
Inflammation and Repair, University of Manchester,
Manchester, UK
Chapter 11

Ian H. Coulson
BSc, MB BS, FRCP
Consultant Dermatologist, Burnley General
Hospital, East Lancashire NHS Trust IHC, Burnley,
UK
Chapters 4, 94

Daniel Creamer
MD, FRCP
Consultant Dermatologist, Department of
Dermatology, King's College Hospital, London, UK
Chapters 53, 119, 121

Robert Dawe
MB ChB, MD, FRCPE
Consultant Dermatologist and Honorary Reader,
Photobiology Unit, University of Dundee, Ninewells
Hospital and Medical School, Dundee, UK
Chapter 127

David A. R. de Berker
BA, MB BS, MRCP
Consultant Dermatologist, Bristol Dermatology
Centre, Bristol Royal Infirmary, Bristol, UK
Chapters 89, 95

Pascal Delaunay
PharmD, PhD
Professor and Chairman, Department of
Parasitology-Mycology, Centre Hospitalier
Universitaire de Nice, Hôpital de l'Ardet, Nice,
France; INSERM, Centre Méditerranéen de Médecine
Moléculaire, Université de Nice-Sophia Antipolis,
Nice, France
Chapter 34

Christopher P. Denton
PhD, FRCP
Professor of Experimental Rheumatology, Division
of Medicine, University College London, London;
Consultant Rheumatologist, Royal Free London NHS
Foundation Trust, London, UK
Chapter 56

Nemesha Desai
MB BS(Hons), BSc(Hons), FRCP, PGCHE
Consultant, St John's Institute of Dermatology,
Guy's and St Thomas' NHS Foundation Trust,
London, UK
Chapter 92

Anne Dompmartin
MD, PhD
Coordinator, Consultation of Vascular Anomalies,
Université de Caen Basse Normandie, Caen;
Department of Dermatology, CHU Caen, Caen, France
Chapter 73

Christopher Downing
MD
Dermatologist, University of Texas Health Science
Center, Houston, TX, USA
Chapters 33, 131

Reinhard Dummer
MD
Professor, Department of Dermatology, University
Hospital Zurich, Zurich, Switzerland
Chapter 143

Alison B. Durham
MD
Assistant Professor of Dermatology, Department of
Dermatology, University of Michigan Health System,
Ann Arbor, MI, USA
Chapter 143

Jan Dutz
MD, FRCPC
Professor, Skin Care Centre, Vancouver General
Hospital, Vancouver, BC, Canada
Chapter 51

E. Anne Eady
PhD
Principal Research Fellow, Department of
Dermatology, Harrogate and District NHS
Foundation Trust, Harrogate, UK
Chapter 90

David J. Eedy
MD, FRCP
Consultant Dermatologist, Department of
Dermatology, Craigavon Area Hospital, Craigavon, UK
Chapter 85

Lennart Emtestam
MD, PhD
Professor, Department of Medicine Huddinge,
Karolinska Institutet, Stockholm; Department of
Dermatology, Karolinska University Hospital,
Stockholm, Sweden
Chapter 147

Robyn Evans
MD, CCFP
Director, Wound Healing Clinic, Women's College
Hospital; Lecturer, University of Toronto, Toronto,
Ontario, Canada
Chapter 124

Khaled Ezzedine
MD, PhD
Doctor and Consultant, Service de Dermatologie
et Dermatologie Pédiatrique, Hôpital St André,
Bordeaux, France
Chapter 70

Paul Farrant
MB BS, BSc(Hons), FRCP
Consultant Dermatologist, Brighton and Sussex
University Hospitals, Brighton, UK
Chapters 89, 107

Hiva Fassihi
MA, MD, MRCP
Consultant Dermatologist and Clinical Lead
for the National XP Service, St John's Institute
of Dermatology, Guy's and St Thomas' NHS
Foundation Trust, London, UK
Chapter 78

Louise Fearfield
MA, DM, FRCP
Consultant Dermatologist, Chelsea & Westminster
and The Royal Marsden Hospitals, London, UK
Chapter 120

Andrew Y. Finlay
CBE, FRCP(Lond, Glasg)
Professor of Dermatology, Department of
Dermatology and Wound Healing, Cardiff University
School of Medicine, Cardiff, UK
Chapter 16

Gary Fisher
PhD
Professor of Dermatology, University of Michigan
Medical Center, Ann Arbor, MI, USA
Chapter 155

Carsten Flohr
FRCP, FRCPCH, MA, MPhil, DLSHTM, MSc, PhD
Reader and Consultant, St John's Institute
of Dermatology, Guy's and St Thomas' NHS
Foundation Trust, London, UK
Chapter 41

Paul D. Flynn
PhD, FRCP
Consultant Physician, Acute and Metabolic Medicine,
Addenbrooke's Hospital, Cambridge; Associate
Lecturer, Department of Medicine, University of
Cambridge, Cambridge, UK
Chapter 62

John Frew
MB ChB, MRCP, FRCR
Consultant Clinical Oncologist, Northern Centre for
Cancer Care, Freeman Hospital, Newcastle upon
Tyne, UK
Chapter 24

Amit Garg
MD, FAAP
Associate Professor and Founding Chair, Department
of Dermatology, Hofstra NSLIJ School of Medicine,
Manhasset, NY, USA
Chapter 100

Caroline Gaudy-Marqueste
MD, PhD
Assistant Professor of Dermatology, Service de
Dermatologie et Cancérologie Cutanée, Hôpital de la
Timone, Marseille, France
Chapter 143

Andrew R. Gennery
MD, FRCPCH, MRCP
Reader in Paediatric Immunology and HSCT,
Institute of Cellular Medicine, Newcastle University,
Newcastle upon Tyne, UK
Chapter 82

Sam Gibbs
FRCP
Consultant Dermatologist, Great Western Hospital,
Swindon, UK
Chapter 15

Mary T. Glover
MA, FRCP, FRCPCH
Consultant Dermatologist, Great Ormond Street
Hospital for Children NHS Foundation Trust,
London, UK
Chapter 117

Robert Gniadecki
MD, PhD
Consultant and Clinical Professor of Dermatology,
Department of Dermatology, Bispebjerg Hospital and
University of Copenhagen, Copenhagen, Denmark;
and Division of Dermatology, University of Alberta,
Alberta, Canada
Chapter 148

Chee-Leok Goh
MD, MB BS, MRCP(UK), MMed, FRCPE
Senior Consultant Dermatologist and Clinical
Professor, National Skin Centre, National University
of Singapore, Singapore
Chapter 159

Simone M. Goldinger
MD
Senior Physician, Department of Dermatology,
University Hospital Zurich, Zurich, Switzerland
Chapter 143

Portia C. Goldsmith
MD, FRCP
Consultant Dermatologist, Barts Health and
Homerton University Hospital, London, UK
Chapter 103

Mark Goodfield
MD, FRCP
Professor and Consultant Dermatologist, Department
of Dermatology, Chapel Allerton Hospital, Leeds, UK
Chapters 51, 52, 54, 55

Kristiana Gordon
MB BS, MRCP, MD(Res)
Consultant in Dermatology and Lymphovascular
Medicine, St George's Hospital, London, UK
Chapter 105

Patrick Gordon
FRCP, PhD, MB BS
Consultant Rheumatologist and Honorary Senior
Lecturer, Department of Rheumatology, King's
College Hospital, London, UK
Chapter 53

Michael Gossop
BA, PhD
Emeritus Professor, National Addiction Centre,
King's College London, London, UK
Chapter 121

Clive E. H. Grattan
MA, MD, FRCP
Consultant Dermatologist, Norfolk and Norwich
University Hospital, Norwich; and St John's Institute
of Dermatology, Guy's and St Thomas' NHS
Foundation Trust, London, UK
Chapters 42, 43, 44, 45, 46

Malcolm Greaves
MD, PhD, FRCP
Emeritus Professor of Dermatology and Honorary
Consultant in Dermatology, Cutaneous Allergy
Clinic, St John's Institute of Dermatology, Guy's and
St Thomas' NHS Foundation Trust, London, UK
Chapter 83

Jean Jacques Grob
MD
Professor of Dermatology, Head of Dermatology and
Skin Cancers, Service de Dermatologie et Cancérologie
Cutanée, Hôpital de la Timone, Marseille, France
Chapter 143

Richard Groves
MB BS, FRCP
Head, Clinical Immunodermatology, St John's
Institute of Dermatology, Guy's and St Thomas' NHS
Foundation Trust, London, UK
Chapter 50

Girish Gupta
MB ChB, FRCP
Consultant Dermatologist and Skin Cancer Lead,
Department of Dermatology, Monklands Hospital,
Airdrie, UK
Chapter 142

Nadi K. Gupta
MB ChB, MRCP, DipGUM, DFFP, DipHIV
Honorary Senior Clinical Lecturer, University
of Sheffield, Sheffield; Consultant Physician in
Genitourinary Medicine, Sheffield Teaching Hospitals
NHS Foundation Trust, Sheffield; Rotherham
Hospital NHS Foundation Trust, Rotherham, UK
Chapter 30

Richard H. Guy
MA, PhD
Professor of Pharmaceutical Sciences, Department
of Pharmacy and Pharmacology, University of Bath,
Bath, UK
Chapter 13

Jürg Hafner
MD
Professor, Dermatologist, Angiologist and
Phlebologist (SIME/FMH) and Senior Staff,
Department of Dermatology, University Hospital of
Zurich, Zurich, Switzerland
Chapter 104

Philip J. Hampton
MB BS, BMedSci, PhD, FRCP
Consultant Dermatologist, Newcastle Hospitals NHS
Trust, Newcastle Upon Tyne, UK
Chapter 49

Catherine A. Harwood
MA, PhD, FRCP
Professor of Dermatology and Consultant
Dermatologist, Department of Dermatology,
The Royal London Hospital, London; Centre for
Cutaneous Research, Blizard Institute, Barts and the
London School of Medicine and Dentistry, Queen
Mary University of London, London, UK
Chapter 146

Roderick J. Hay
DM, FRCP, FRCPath, FMedSci
Professor of Cutaneous Infection, Dermatology
Department, King's College Hospital, London, UK
Chapters 26, 32, 93

Elisabeth M. Higgins
MA, FRCP
Consultant Dermatologist, King's College Hospital,
London, UK
Chapter 117

Colin A. Holden
BSc, MD, FRCP
Consultant Dermatologist, Department of
Dermatology, Epsom & St Helier NHS Trust,
St Helier Hospital, Carshalton, UK
Chapter 41

S. Walayat Hussain
BSc(Hons), MB ChB, MRCP(UK), FRACP, FACMS
Consultant Dermatological Surgeon, Leeds Centre
for Dermatology, Chapel Allerton Hospital, Leeds
Teaching Hospitals NHS Trust, Leeds, UK
Chapter 20

Sally Ibbotson
MB ChB, MD, FRCPE
Clinical Senior Lecturer in Photobiology and
Honorary Consultant Dermatologist, Photobiology
Unit, University of Dundee, Ninewells Hospital and
Medical School, Dundee, UK
Chapters 21, 22, 127

John R. Ingram
MA, MSc, DM, MRCP(Derm), FAcadMEd
Senior Lecturer and Consultant Dermatologist,
Department of Dermatology & Wound Healing,
Cardiff University, Cardiff, UK
Chapter 39

Alan D. Irvine
MD, FRCP, FRCPI
Consultant Dermatologist, Our Lady's Children's
Hospital, Crumlin; St. James's Hospital, Dublin; and
Trinity College, Dublin, Ireland
Chapters 76, 77, 79, 80

Peter Itin
MD
Professor for Dermatology and Venerology, Head
of Department of Dermatology, University Hospital
Basle, Basle, Switzerland
Chapter 67

Natalia Jaimes
MD
Attending Physician, Dermatology Service,
Universidad Pontificia Bolivariana and Aurora Skin
Cancer Center, Medellín, Colombia
Chapter 144

Gregor B. E. Jemec
MD, DMSc
Professor and Clinical Lead, Department of
Dermatology, Roskilde Hospital; Health Sciences
Faculty, University of Copenhagen, Copenhagen,
Denmark
Chapters 92, 93

Melinda V. Jen
MD
Assistant Professor, Department of Dermatology,
Children's Hospital of Philadelphia, Philadelphia,
PA, USA
Chapter 63

Marc G. Jeschke
MD, PhD, FACS, FCCM, FRCSC
Professor, Ross Tilley Burn Centre, Sunnybrook
Health Sciences Centre, Toronto; Department of
Surgery, Division of General Surgery, Plastic Surgery,
Department of Immunology, University of Toronto,
Toronto; Sunnybrook Research Institute, Toronto,
Ontario, Canada
Chapter 126

Timothy M. Johnson
MD
Lewis and Lillian Becker Professor of Dermatology,
Professor of Otolaryngology and Surgery (Division
of Plastic Surgery), Department of Dermatology,
University of Michigan Health System, Ann Arbor,
MI, USA
Chapter 143

Charles G. Kelly
MB ChB, MSc, FRCP, FRCR, FBIR, DMRT
Consultant Clinical Oncologist and Lead for
Radiotherapy, Northern Centre for Cancer Care,
Freeman Hospital, Newcastle upon Tyne; Deputy
Degree Program Director and Honorary Clinical Senior
Lecturer, Northern Institute for Cancer Research,
Newcastle University, Newcastle upon Tyne, UK
Chapter 24

Cameron Kennedy
MA, MB BChir, FRCP
Consultant Dermatologist, Bristol Royal Infirmary
and Bristol Royal Hospital for Children, Bristol;
Honorary Clinical Senior Lecturer, University of
Bristol, Bristol, UK
Chapter 108

Alexandra B. Kimball
MD, MPH, FAAD
Department of Dermatology, Massachusetts General
Hospital, Boston, MA, USA
Chapter 156

George R. Kinghorn
OBE, MD, FRCP
Honorary Professor and Consultant Physician in
Genitourinary Medicine, Sheffield Teaching Hospitals
NHS Foundation Trust, Sheffield, UK
Chapters 29, 30

Veronica A. Kinsler
MA, MB BChir, MRCPCH, PhD
Consultant Paediatric Dermatologist and Academic
Lead Clinician, Paediatric Dermatology, Great
Ormond Street Hospital for Children NHS
Foundation Trust, London, UK
Chapter 75

Brian Kirby
MD, FRCPI
Consultant Dermatologist, St Vincent's University
Hospital, Dublin, Associate Clinical Professor,
University College, Dublin, Ireland
Chapter 35

Eubee Koo
BS
Department of Dermatology, Massachusetts General
Hospital, Boston, MA, USA
Chapter 156

Magdalene Krensel
MSc
Project Manager in Health Economics, Institute
for Health Services Research in Dermatology and
Nursing, University Medical Center Hamburg-
Eppendorf, Hamburg, Germany
Chapter 6

Alison M. Layton
MB ChB, FRCP
Consultant Dermatologist, Department of
Dermatology, Harrogate and District NHS
Foundation Trust, Harrogate, UK
Chapter 90

John T. Lear
MD, FRCP
Consultant Dermatologist, Department of
Dermatology, Manchester Royal infirmary,
Manchester, UK
Chapters 133, 134, 141, 142

Laurence Le Cleach
MD
Consultant Dermatologist, Service de Dermatologie,
Satellite Français du Cochrane Skin Group, Hôpital
Henri Mondor, Créteil, France
Chapter 37

Haur Yueh Lee
MB BS, MRCP(UK), MMed(IntMed), FAMS(Derm)
Head of Department and Consultant Dermatologist,
Department of Dermatology, Singapore General
Hospital; Adjunct Assistant Professor, DUKE-NUS
Graduate Medical School, Singapore
Chapters 118, 119

Jonathan N. Leonard
BSc, MD, FRCP
Consultant Dermatologist, Department of
Dermatology, Imperial College Healthcare NHS
Trust, London, UK
Chapter 109

Tabi A. Leslie
BSc(Hons), MB BS(Hons), FRCP(Lond)
Consultant Dermatologist, Royal Free Hospital,
London, UK
Chapter 101

Nick J. Levell
MD, FRCP, MB ChB, MBA
Clinical Director of Dermatology, Norwich Medical
School, Norfolk and Norwich University Hospital,
Norwich; National Specialty Lead Dermatology,
National Institute for Health Research, London;
Clinical Vice-President, British Association of
Dermatologists, London, UK
Chapters 1, 102

Fiona Lewis
MD, FRCP
Consultant Dermatologist, Wexham Park Hospital,
Frimley Health; St John's Institute of Dermatology,
Guy's and St Thomas' NHS Foundation Trust,
London, UK
Chapter 112

Joyce Teng Ee Lim
MB BS, FRCPI, FAMS(Derm)
Senior Consultant Dermatologist, National Skin Centre,
National University of Singapore, Singapore
Chapter 159

Dan Lipsker
MD, PhD
Professor, Faculté de Medicine, Université de
Strasbourg, Strasbourg, France
Chapter 45

Diana N. J. Lockwood
BSc, MD, FRCP
Professor of Tropical Medicine, London School of
Hygiene & Tropical Medicine, London; Consultant
Leprologist, Hospital for Tropical Diseases,
University College Hospital NHS Trust, London, UK
Chapter 28

Christopher R. Lovell
MB ChB, MD, FRCP
Consultant Dermatologist, Department of
Dermatology, Royal United Hospital and Royal
National Hospital for Rheumatic Diseases, Bath, UK
Chapters 45, 96, 154

Nicholas J. Lowe
MB ChB, MD, FRCP, FACP, FAmAcadDerm
Consultant Dermatologist, The Cranley Clinic,
London, UK; Clinical Professor of Dermatology,
UCLA School of Medicine, Los Angeles, USA
Chapter 158

Calum Lyon
FRCP
Dermatologist and Honorary Clinical Lecturer, York
Hospital NHS Trust, York; Salford Royal Hospital
NHS Trust, Salford, UK
Chapter 114

Vishal Madan
MD, FRCP
Consultant Dermatologist, Laser and Mohs Surgeon,
Dermatology Centre, Salford Royal NHS Foundation
Trust, Salford, UK
Chapters 23, 133, 134, 141, 142

Eleanor Mallon
MB BS, MD, FRCP
Consultant Dermatologist, Croydon University
Hospital, Croydon; Honorary Senior Lecturer in
Dermatology, St John's Institute of Dermatology,
Guy's and St Thomas' NHS Foundation Trust,
London, UK
Chapter 113

Juan Mañá
MD, PhD
Associate Professor of Medicine and Internal
Medicine Clinical Chief, Department of Internal
Medicine, Bellvitge University Hospital, Barcelona
University, Barcelona, Spain
Chapter 98

Joaquim Marcoval
MD, PhD
Associate Professor and Consultant Dermatologist,
Department of Dermatology, Bellvitge University
Hospital, Barcelona University, Barcelona, Spain
Chapter 98

Ashfaq A. Marghoob
MD
Attending Physician, Dermatology Service, Memorial
Sloan-Kettering Cancer Center, New York, NY, USA
Chapter 144

Alexander M. Marsland
BSc(Hons), MB ChB, FRCP
Consultant Dermatologist and Honorary
Senior Lecturer, Salford Royal Foundation Trust and
University of Manchester, Manchester, UK
Chapter 42

Marcus Maurer
MD
Professor of Dermatology and Allergology, Charité,
Berlin, Germany
Chapter 43

Collette McCourt
MB, BCH
Clinical Fellow in Immunodermatology, Skin Care
Centre, Vancouver General Hospital, Vancouver, BC,
Canada
Chapter 51

John A. McGrath
MD, FRCP, FMedSci
Professor of Molecular Dermatology, St John's
Institute of Dermatology, Division of Genetics and
Molecular Medicine, Faculty of Life Sciences and
Medicine, King's College London, London, UK
Chapters 2, 7, 71

Jane M. McGregor
MA, MB BChir, MRCP, MD
Senior Lecturer and Consultant Dermatologist,
Department of Dermatology, The Royal London
Hospital, London; Centre for Cutaneous Research,
Blizard Institute, Barts and the London School of
Medicine and Dentistry, Queen Mary University of
London, London, UK
Chapter 146

Kevin McKenna
MD, FRCP
Consultant Dermatologist, Dermatology Department,
Belfast Trust, Belfast, UK
Chapters 21, 22

Jemima E. Mellerio
BSc, MD, FRCP
Consultant Dermatologist and Honorary Senior
Lecturer, St John's Institute of Dermatology, Guy's
and St Thomas' NHS Foundation Trust, London, UK
Chapters 76, 77, 79, 80

Andrew G. Messenger
MB BS, MD, FRCP
Professor of Dermatology, Department of
Dermatology, Royal Hallamshire Hospital, Sheffield,
UK
Chapter 89

Dieter Metze
MD
Professor, Department of Dermatology, University
Hospital Münster, Münster, Germany
Chapter 65

George W. M. Millington
PhD, FRCP
Consultant Dermatologist, Dermatology Department,
Norfolk and Norwich University Hospital,
Norwich, UK
Chapter 74

Sonja Molin
MD
Assistant Professor, Department of Dermatology and
Allergology, Ludwig Maximilian University,
Munich, Germany
Chapters 150, 151, 152, 153

Gentiane Monsel
MD
Professor and Chairman, UPEC-Université Paris-Est
Créteil Val de Marne, Department of Dermatology,
Hôpital Henri Mondor, Créteil, France
Chapter 34

Fanny Morice-Picard
MD, PhD
Doctor and Consultant, Service de Dermatologie
et Dermatologie Pédiatrique, Hôpital St André,
Bordeaux, France
Chapter 70

Andrew Morris
BM BCh, MA, PhD, FRCPCH
Consultant in Paediatric Metabolic Medicine,
Manchester Centre for Genomic Medicine, Central
Manchester University Hospitals NHS Foundation
Trust, Manchester, UK
Chapter 81

Rachael Morris-Jones
BSc, MB BS, MRCP, FRCP, PhD, PCME
Dermatology Consultant, Dermatology Department,
King's College Hospital, London, UK
Chapters 26, 93

Peter S. Mortimer
MD, FRCP
Professor of Dermatological Medicine, St George's
Hospital, London, UK
Chapter 105

Richard J. Motley
MA, MD, FRCP, FAcadMEd
Consultant in Dermatology and Cutaneous Surgery,
Welsh Institute of Dermatology, University Hospital
of Wales, Cardiff, UK
Chapter 20

Megan Mowbray
BSc(Hons), FRCP, MD
Consultant Dermatologist, Department of
Dermatology, Queen Margaret Hospital, NHS Fife,
Dunfermline, UK
Chapter 107

Chetan Mukhtyar
MB, MSc, MD, FRCP, FRCP(Edin)
Consultant Rheumatologist, Norwich Medical
School, Norfolk and Norwich University Hospital,
Norwich, UK
Chapter 102

Colin S. Munro
MD, FRCP(Glasg)
Honorary Consultant Dermatologist, Queen
Elizabeth University Hospital, Glasgow, UK
Chapter 66

Rabindranath Nambi
MD, DD, DNB
Consultant Dermatologist, Royal Derby Hospitals
Foundation NHS Trust, Derby, UK
Chapter 122

Janakan Natkunarajah
MRCP(Derm)
Consultant Dermatologist, Kingston Hospital,
London, UK
Chapter 120

Tim Niehues
MD
Professor of Paediatrics, Centre for Child Health and
Adolescence, HELIOS Klinikum, Krefeld; Academic
Hospital, RWTH, Aachen; Immunodeficiency and
Rheumatology Centre, Krefeld, Germany
Chapter 82

Síona Ní Raghallaigh
MRCPI, MD
Clinical Research Fellow in Dermatology, Charles
Institute of Dermatology, University College Dublin,
Dublin, Ireland
Chapter 106

Stephanie Ogden
MRCP, PhD
Consultant Dermatologist and Honorary Senior
Lecturer, Salford Royal Hospital, Greater Manchester,
UK
Chapter 4

Vinzenz Oji
MD
Private Lecturer, Department of Dermatology,
University Hospital Münster, Münster, Germany
Chapter 65

Rasha Omer
MB BS, MRCP, DTM&H, DipGUM, DipHIV
Specialist Registrar in Genitourinary Medicine,
Sheffield Teaching Hospitals NHS Foundation Trust,
Sheffield, UK
Chapter 29

Anthony D. Ormerod
MB ChB, FRCP(Edin), MD, FRCP(Lond)
Emeritus Professor of Dermatology, University of
Aberdeen, Foresterhill, Aberdeen, UK
Chapter 49

Catherine H. Orteu
MB BS, BSc, MD, FRCP
Consultant Dermatologist, Department of
Dermatology, Royal Free London NHS Foundation
Trust, London, UK
Chapters 56, 57

David Orton
BSc(Hons), MSc(Allergy), MB BS, FRCP
Consultant Dermatologist, Hillingdon Hospitals NHS
Foundation Trust, Uxbridge; Honorary Consultant
Dermatologist, Royal Free London NHS Foundation
Trust, London, UK
Chapter 128

Edel A. O'Toole
MB, PhD, FRCP
Professor of Molecular Dermatology and Honorary
Consultant Dermatologist, Centre for Cutaneous
Research, Barts and the London School of Medicine and
Dentistry and Barts Health NHS Trust, London, UK
Chapter 10

Carol Ott
MD, FRCPC
Physician, Wound Healing Clinic, Women's College
Hospital, Toronto; Geriatrics and Wound Care
Clinics, Baycrest Hospital, Toronto, Ontario, Canada
Chapter 124

David G. Paige
MB BS, MA, FRCP
Consultant Dermatologist, Department of
Dermatology, Barts Health NHS Trust, London, UK
Chapter 116

Amy S. Paller
MS, MD
Walter J. Hamlin Professor and Chair of Dermatology,
Professor of Pediatrics, Departments of Dermatology
and Pediatrics, Northwestern University,
Chicago, IL, USA
Chapter 69

Ralf Paus
MD, FRSB
Professor of Cutaneous Medicine and Director
of Research, Centre for Dermatology Research,
Institute of Inflammation and Repair, University
of Manchester, Manchester, UK; Head, Laboratory
of Hair Research and Regenerative Medicine,
Department of Dermatology, University of Münster,
Münster, Germany
Chapter 149

Vincent Piguet
MD, PhD, FRCP
Clinical Professor of Dermatology, Department
of Dermatology, Cardiff University; Consultant
Dermatologist, University Hospital of Wales,
Cardiff, UK
Chapters 31, 37

Elena Pope
MD, MSc, FRCP(C)
Staff Dermatologist and Associate Professor, Hospital
for Sick Children, Toronto, Ontario, Canada
Chapter 136

William M. Porter
BSc, MB BS, MRCP
Consultant Dermatologist, Gloucestershire Hospitals
NHS Foundation Trust, Gloucester, UK
Chapter 111

Frank C. Powell
FRCPI
Professor and Consultant, Charles Institute of
Dermatology, University College Dublin, Dublin,
Ireland
Chapters 91, 106

Charlotte M. Proby
MA, FRCP
Professor of Dermatology and Consultant
Dermatologist, Skin Tumour Laboratory, Division of
Cancer Research, Medical Research Institute, Jacqui
Wood Cancer Centre, Dundee, UK
Chapter 146

Deepti H. Radia
BSc(Hons), MRCPI, FRCPath, MSc(MedEd)
Haematology Consultant, St John's Institute of
Dermatology; Department of Haematology, Guy's
and St Thomas' NHS Foundation Trust, London, UK
Chapter 46

Madhuri Reddy
MD, MSc
Director, Wound Healing Program, Hebrew Senior
Life Instructor, Department of Medicine, Harvard
Medical School, Boston, MA, USA
Chapter 124

Luis Requena
MD, PhD
Chairman of Dermatology and Professor of
Dermatology, Department of Dermatology,
Fundación Jiménez Díaz, Madrid, Spain
Chapter 99

Nicole Revencu
MD, PhD
Consultant Clinical Geneticist, Center for Human
Genetics and Center for Vascular Anomalies,
Cliniques Universitaires Saint-Luc, Université
catholique de Louvain, Brussels, Belgium
Chapter 73

Nick J. Reynolds
BSc, MB BS, MD, FRCP
Professor of Dermatology, Department of
Dermatology, Royal Victoria Infirmary and Institute
of Cellular Medicine, Newcastle University,
Newcastle upon Tyne, UK
Chapter 41

Bertrand Richert
MD, PhD
Clinical Professor, Dermatology Department,
Brugmann – St Pierre and Children's University
Hospitals, Université Libre de Bruxelles, Brussels,
Belgium
Chapter 95

Franco Rongioletti
MD
Professor of Dermatology, Section of Dermatology,
Department of Health Sciences (DISSAL),
University of Genova, Genoa; Consultant in
Dermatopathology, University of Genova, Genoa, Italy
Chapter 59

Adam Rubin
MD
Assistant Professor of Dermatology, Pediatrics,
and Pathology and Laboratory Medicine, Hospital
of the University of Pennsylvania, the Children's
Hospital of Philadelphia and Perelman School
of Medicine at the University of Pennsylvania,
Philadelphia, PA, USA
Chapter 69

Malcolm Rustin
BSc, MD, FRCP
Consultant Dermatologist, Royal Free London NHS
Foundation Trust, London, UK
Chapter 47

Thomas Ruzicka
MD
Professor and Chairman, Department of
Dermatology and Allergology, Ludwig Maximilian
University, Munich, Germany
Chapters 150, 151, 152, 153

Berthold Rzany
MD, ScM
RZANY & HUND, Private Practice for Dermatology
and Aesthetic Medicine, Berlin, Germany
Chapter 157

Dana L. Sachs
MD
Professor of Dermatology, University of Michigan
Medical Center, Ann Arbor, MI, USA
Chapter 155

Nazanin Saedi
MD
Assistant Professor, Department of Dermatology and
Cutaneous Biology, Thomas Jefferson University,
Philadelphia, PA, USA
Chapter 160

Robert P. E. Sarkany
FRCP, MD
Consultant Dermatologist and Head of
Photodermatology, St John's Institute of
Dermatology, Guy's and St Thomas' NHS
Foundation Trust, London, UK
Chapter 60

Karin Sartorius
MD, PhD
Consultant Dermatologist, Department of Clinical
Sciences and Education, Karolinska Institutet,
Stockholm; Department of Dermatology,
Södersjukhuset, Stockholm, Sweden
Chapter 147

Valerie P. J. Saw
MB BS(Hons), FRANZCO, PhD
Consultant Ophthalmologist, Moorfields Eye
Hospital NHS Foundation Trust and UCL Institute of
Ophthalmology NIHR Biomedical Research Centre,
London, UK
Chapter 109

Enno Schmidt
MD, PhD
Consultant, Department of Dermatology, Lübeck
Institute of Experimental Dermatology, University of
Lübeck, Lübeck, Germany
Chapter 50

David Schrama
PhD
Group Leader, General Dermatology Department,
University Clinic of Würzburg, Würzburg, Germany
Chapter 145

Stephan Schreml
MD, PhD
Attending at the Department of Dermatology,
University Medical Centre Regensburg, Regensburg,
Germany
Chapter 58

Crispian Scully
CBE, MD, PhD, MDS, MRCS, BSc, FDSRCS,
FDSRCPS, FFDRCSI, FDSRCSE, FRCPath, FMedSci,
FHEA, FUCL, FSB, DSc, DChD, DMed(HC), Dr.h.c.
Co-Director, WHO Collaborating Centre for Oral
Health-General Health; Council Member and
Examiner, Royal College of Surgeons of Edinburgh;
and Emeritus Professor, University College London,
London, UK
Chapter 110

Neil J. Sebire
BSc, FRCPath, MD
Professor of Paediatric Pathology, Paediatric
Pathology Department, Great Ormond Street Hospital
for Children NHS Foundation Trust, London, UK
Chapter 75

Rodney D. Sinclair
MB BS, MD, FACD
Professor of Medicine (Dermatology), University of
Melbourne, Melbourne; Director of Dermatology,
Epworth Healthcare, Richmond, Victoria; Director,
Sinclair Dermatology, Research and Clinical Trials
Centre, Melbourne, Australia
Chapters 89, 107

Catherine H. Smith
MD, FRCP
Professor of Dermatology and Therapeutics and
Consultant Dermatologist, Skin Therapy Research
Unit, St John's Institute of Dermatology, Guy's and St
Thomas' NHS Foundation Trust, London, UK
Chapters 14, 19

Reinhart Speeckaert
MD, PhD
Dermatologist, Department of Dermatology, Ghent
University Hospital, Ghent, Belgium
Chapter 88

Eli Sprecher
MD, PhD
Professor and Chair, Department of Dermatology, Tel
Aviv Sourasky Medical Center; and Department of
Human Molecular Genetics and Biochemistry, Sackler
Medical School, Tel Aviv University, Tel Aviv, Israel
Chapter 68

Sonja Ständer
MD
Dermatologist and Dermatopathologist, Department
of Dermatology, University Hospital Münster,
Münster, Germany
Chapter 83

Irene Stefanaki
MD
Dermatologist, Department of Dermatology,
University of Athens Medical School, Andreas Sygros
Hospital, Athens, Greece
Chapter 132

Martin Steinhoff
MD, PhD, MSc
Professorial Chair, Department of Dermatology; and
Director, UCD Charles Institute of Dermatology,
University College Dublin, Dublin, Ireland
Chapter 8

Jane C. Sterling
MB BChir, MA, FRCP, PhD
Senior Lecturer and Honorary Consultant
Dermatologist, Department of Dermatology, University
of Cambridge, Addenbrooke's Hospital, Cambridge, UK
Chapter 25

Alexander Stratigos
MD
Professor of Dermatology, Department of
Dermatology, University of Athens Medical School,
Andreas Sygros Hospital, Athens, Greece
Chapter 132

Alain Taïeb
MD, PhD
Professor and Head of Department, Service de
Dermatologie et Dermatologie Pédiatrique, Hôpital
St André, Bordeaux, France
Chapter 70

Ruth E. Taylor
MRCPsych, PhD
Consultant Liaison Psychiatrist, Department of
Liaison Psychiatry, Barts Health NHS Trust, London;
and Senior Lecturer, Queen Mary College of
Medicine, University of London, London, UK
Chapter 86

Fernanda Teixeira
MD, PhD
Consultant Dermatologist, Imperial College
Healthcare Trust, London, UK
Chapter 87

Michael J. Tidman
MD, FRCP(Edin), FRCP(Lond)
Consultant Dermatologist, Department of Dermatology,
Royal Infirmary of Edinburgh, Edinburgh, UK
Chapter 19

Thai Hoa Tran
MD, FRCP(C), FAAP
Research Fellow, Hospital for Sick Children, Toronto,
Ontario, Canada
Chapter 136

Heiko Traupe
MD
Assistant Professor, Department of Dermatology,
University Hospital Münster, Münster, Germany
Chapter 65

Kenneth Y. Tsai
MD, PhD, FAAD
Assistant Professor, Departments of Dermatology
and Translational Molecular Pathology, University
of Texas MD Anderson Cancer Center, Houston, TX,
USA
Chapters 137, 139

Stephen Tyring
MD, PhD
Clinical Professor, University of Texas Health Science
Center, Houston, TX, USA
Chapters 33, 131

Jouni Uitto
MD, PhD
Professor and Chair of Department of Dermatology
and Cutaneous Biology, Thomas Jefferson University,
Philadelphia; Director, Jefferson Institute of
Molecular Medicine, Sidney Kimmel Medical
College, Thomas Jefferson University, Philadelphia,
PA, USA
Chapter 2

Hessel H. van der Zee
MD, PhD
Department of Dermatology, Erasmus Medical
Center, Rotterdam, the Netherlands
Chapter 92

Nanja van Geel
MD, PhD
Dermatologist, Department of Dermatology, Ghent
University Hospital, Ghent, Belgium
Chapter 88

Samantha Vaughan Jones
MD, FRCP
Consultant Dermatologist, Department of
Dermatology, St Peter's Hospital, Ashford; and
St Peter's Foundation Trust, Chertsey, UK
Chapter 115

Miikka Vikkula
MD, PhD
Coordinator, Center for Vascular Anomalies,
Cliniques Universitaires Saint-Luc; Professor of
Human Genetics, Human Molecular Genetics, de
Duve Institute; Principal Investigator, Walloon
Excellence in Lifesciences and Biotechnology
(WELBIO), Université catholique de Louvain,
Brussels, Belgium
Chapter 73

John J. Voorhees
MD, FRCP
Duncan and Ella Poth Distinguished Professor
of Dermatology and Chair of Department of
Dermatology, University of Michigan Medical Center,
Ann Arbor, MI, USA
Chapter 155

Shyamal Wahie
MB BS, MD, FRCP
Consultant Dermatologist, University Hospital of
North Durham, Durham, UK
Chapter 52

Sarah Wakelin
BSc, MB BS, FRCP
Consultant Dermatologist and Honorary Senior
Lecturer, Imperial College Healthcare Trust, London,
UK
Chapter 40

Stephen L. Walker
PhD, MRCP(UK), DTM&H
Clinical Lecturer, Faculty of Infectious and Tropical
Diseases, London School of Hygiene and Tropical
Medicine, London, UK
Chapter 27

Sarah Walsh
MB BCh, BAO, BMedSci, MRCP
Consultant Dermatologist and Clinical Lead,
Department of Dermatology, King's College Hospital,
London, UK
Chapter 119

Timothy S. Wang
MD
Associate Professor, Department of Dermatology, and
Director, Cutaneous Surgery Unit and Micrographic
Surgery and Dermatologic Oncology (Mohs)
Fellowship Program, Johns Hopkins Health System,
Baltimore, MD, USA
Chapter 20

Molly Wanner
MD, MBA, FAAD
Department of Dermatology, Massachusetts General
Hospital, Boston, MA, USA
Chapter 156

Sheila Weitzman
MB BCh, FCP(SA), FRCP(C)
Senior Staff Oncologist and Professor, Hospital for
Sick Children, Toronto, Ontario, Canada
Chapter 136

Jonathan M. L. White
BSc, MRCP(UK)
Consultant Dermatologist, Department of Cutaneous
Allergy, St John's Institute of Dermatology, Guy's and
St Thomas' NHS Foundation Trust, London, UK
Chapters 129, 130

Sean J. Whittaker
MD, FRCP
Professor of Cutaneous Oncology, Division of Genetics
and Molecular Medicine, King's College London,
London; St John's Institute of Dermatology, Guy's and
St Thomas' NHS Foundation Trust, London, UK
Chapters 135, 140

Mark Wilkinson
MD, FRCP
Consultant Dermatologist, Leeds Teaching Hospitals
NHS Trust, Leeds, UK
Chapter 128

Hywel C. Williams
DSc, FRCP, FMedSci
Professor of Dermato-Epidemiology and Director,
Centre of Evidence-Based Dermatology, Nottingham
University Hospitals NHS Trust, Nottingham, UK
Chapters 5, 17

Niall J. E. Wilson
BSc(Hons), MB ChB, FRCP, FRCPI
Consultant Dermatologist, Royal Liverpool and
Broadgreen University Hospitals, Liverpool, UK
Chapter 94

Albert C. Yan
MD, FAAP, FAAD
Section Chief, Associate Professor, Department of
Dermatology, Children's Hospital of Philadelphia,
Philadelphia, PA, USA
Chapter 63

Victoria M. Yates
MB ChB, FRCP, DTM&H
Honorary Consultant Dermatologist, Formerly at
The Dermatology Centre, Salford Royal NHS Trust,
Manchester, UK
Chapter 27

Antony R. Young
BSc, MSc, PhD
Professor of Experimental Photobiology, St John's
Institute of Dermatology, Division of Genetics and
Molecular Medicine, Faculty of Life Sciences and
Medicine, King's College London, London, UK
Chapter 9

Christopher B. Zachary
FRCP
Professor and Chairman, Department of
Dermatology, University of California, Irvine, Irvine,
CA, USA
Chapter 160

Joanna M. Zakrzewska
MD, FDSRCS, FFDRCSI, FFPMRCA
Consultant and Lead for Facial Pain, Facial Pain
Unit, University College London Hospitals NHS
Foundation Trust, London, UK
Chapter 84

Mozheh Zamiri
MD, MRCP
Consultant Dermatologist, Queen Elizabeth
University Hospital, Glasgow, UK
Chapter 66

Christos C. Zouboulis
Prof.Dr.med., Prof.h.c., Dr.h.c.
Director and Professor of Dermatology and
Venereology, Departments of Dermatology,
Venereology, Allergology and Immunology, Dessau
Medical Center, Dessau, Germany
Chapters 48, 90

Axel zur Hausen
MD
Chair, Department of Pathology, Maastricht
University Medical Center, Maastricht, the
Netherlands
Chapter 145

Preface to the Ninth Edition

The ninth edition of *Rook's Textbook of Dermatology*, or 'Rook book' as it is known affectionately, marks a significant change from its traditional structure and format. The editorial team has changed: due to the retirements of Tony Burns and Stephen Breathnach and the untimely, early death of Neil Cox, only Chris Griffiths remains from the previous team. The current editors wish to pay tribute to these three, all of whom dedicated significant energy and knowledge to the success of previous editions. Four editors were deemed to be insufficient for a textbook of the complexity and size of Rook and thus a team of five editors supported by 12 associate editors was established for the ninth edition. The content has been reorganized into 14 sections with a total of 160 chapters, more than double the number in the previous edition although the overall size of the book is little changed. The new opening section, Foundations of Dermatology, provides a comprehensive introduction to the subject and there is an expanded section on Aesthetic Dermatology. The authorship has also enlarged with a mixture of authors from previous editions and newcomers, many of whom are from outside the UK and have thus added an important international dimension to the essential 'Britishness' of Rook.

The major change and the one which has catalysed the aforementioned restructuring is the requirement to bring the book into the twenty-first-century publishing world by designing it as much for online use as for a traditional print book. The hierarchical templating required for this has necessitated a complete rewrite and reformatting. The hard copy textbook mirrors the online version, the main difference being that only selected key references are printed in the former, the full reference list being available online.

This has enabled us to increase the number of figures and images, all of which are downloadable as PowerPoint slides. We also listened to comments about the inconvenience of the index being printed in only one of the four volumes of the eighth edition and have ensured that it is available in each volume of the ninth.

We view our editorship of Rook as a privilege and are cognizant of our responsibilities as the current custodians of an institution of British dermatology. Thus, the changes we have wrought on the book have been undertaken with a sense of trepidation. Dermatology is at an important and exciting point in its evolution as a subject. The promise of translational research, whereby advances in the understanding of basic pathomechanisms of skin disease have resulted in higher quality patient care, is being realized, much as Arthur Rook, Darrell Wilkinson and John Ebling envisaged in their preface to the first edition of Rook in 1968. We have tried to encapsulate this approach in the ninth edition.

Our thanks go to the wonderful team of Jenny Seward, Catriona Cooper, Nick Morgan, Charlie Hamlyn, Oliver Walter and Martin Sugden at Wiley who have worked tirelessly to help us realize our vision for the new Rook, and to our outstanding project manager Lindsey Williams, and her indefatigable team of copy editors (Jane Andrew and Karen Stephenson), indexer (Jill Halliday) and artist (David Gardner).

Chris Griffiths
Jonathan Barker
Tanya Bleiker
Robert Chalmers
Daniel Creamer

Preface to the First Edition

No comprehensive reference book on dermatology has been published in the English language for ten years and none in England for over a quarter of a century. The recent literature of dermatology is rich in shorter texts and in specialist monographs but the English-speaking dermatologist has long felt the need for a substantial text for regular reference and as a guide to the immense monographic and periodical literature. The editors have therefore planned the present volume primarily for the dermatologist in practice or in training, but have also considered the requirements of the specialist in other fields of medicine and of the many research workers interested in the skin in relation to toxicology or cosmetic science.

An attempt has been made throughout the book to integrate our growing knowledge of the biology of skin and of fundamental pathological processes with practical clinical problems. Often the gap is still very wide but the trends of basic research at least indicate how it may eventually be bridged. In a clinical textbook the space devoted to the basic sciences must necessarily be restricted but a special effort has been made to ensure that the short accounts which open many chapters are easily understood by the physician whose interests and experience are exclusively clinical.

For the benefit of the student we have encouraged our contributors to make each chapter readable as an independent entity, and have accepted that this must involve the repetition of some material.

The classification employed is conventional and pragmatic. Until our knowledge of the mechanisms of disease is more profound no truly scientific classification is possible. In so many clinical syndromes multiple aetiological factors are implicated. To emphasize one at the expense of others is often misleading. Most diseases are to some extent influenced by genetic factors and a large proportion of common skin reactions are modified by the emotional state of the patient. Our knowledge is in no way advanced by classifying hundreds of diseases as genodermatoses and dozens as psychosomatic.

The true prevalence of a disease may throw light on its aetiology but reported incidence figures are often unreliable and incorrectly interpreted. The scientific approach to the evaluation of racial and environmental factors has therefore been considered in some detail.

The effectiveness of any physician in practice must ultimately depend on his ability to make an accurate clinical diagnosis. Clinical descriptions are detailed and differential diagnosis is fully discussed. Histopathology is here considered mainly as an aid to diagnosis but references to fuller accounts are provided.

The approach to treatment is critical but practical. Many empirical measures are of proven value and should not be abandoned merely because their efficacy cannot yet be scientifically explained. However, many familiar remedies old and new have been omitted either because properly controlled clinical trials have shown them to be of no value or because they have been supplanted by more effective and safer preparations.

There are over nine hundred photographs but no attempt has been made to provide an illustration of every disease. To have done so would have increased the bulk and price of the book without increasing proportionately its practical value. The conditions selected for illustrations are those in which a photograph significantly enhances the verbal description. There are a few conditions we wished to illustrate, but of which we could not obtain unpublished photographs of satisfactory quality.

The lists of references have been selected to provide a guide to the literature. Important articles now of largely historical interest have usually been omitted, except where a knowledge of the history of a disease simplifies the understanding of present concepts and terminology. Books and articles provided with a substantial bibliography are marked with an asterisk.

Many of the chapters have been read and criticized by several members of the team and by other colleagues. Professor Wilson Jones, Dr R.S. Wells and Dr W.E. Parish have given valuable assistance with histopathological, genetic and immunological problems respectively. Many advisers, whose services are acknowledged in the following pages, have helped us with individual chapters. Any errors which have not been eliminated are, however, the responsibility of the editors and authors.

The editors hope that this book will prove of value to all those who are interested in the skin either as physicians or as research workers. They will welcome readers' criticisms and suggestions which may help them to make the second edition the book they hope to produce.

Arthur Rook, Darrell Wilkinson and John Ebling

PART 8

Skin Disorders Associated with Specific Cutaneous Structure

CHAPTER 87

Acquired Disorders of Epidermal Keratinization

Anthony C. Chu[1] *and Fernanda Teixeira*[2]

[1]Hammersmith Hospital, Imperial College Healthcare NHS Trust, London, UK
[2]Imperial College Healthcare NHS Trust, London, UK

Acquired ichthyosis

Definition and nomenclature

Acquired ichthyosis is a condition that arises in adulthood but is clinically and histopathologically similar to hereditary ichthyosis vulgaris. It is rare, and should raise the suspicion of an associated internal disease, particularly malignancy, endocrinopathy, some infections, autoimmunity or a reaction to medication [1].

Synonyms and inclusions
- Ichthyosis acquisita

Introduction and general description

Acquired ichthyosis usually arises in adult life and clinically resembles hereditary ichthyosis. It is not, however, inherited but is associated with a systemic disorder.

Epidemiology

Incidence and prevalence

Acquired ichthyosis is a rare condition. There are no available data on prevalence.

Age

Acquired ichthyosis occurs mainly in adulthood but acquired ichthyosis in children with systemic disease has been reported [2].

Associated diseases
See Box 87.1.

Box 87.1 Disorders which have been associated with acquired ichthyosis

- Neoplasia: particularly Hodgkin disease, mycosis fungoides, multiple myeloma, Kaposi and other sarcomas, and carcinomas (lung, breast, ovary, cervix; see Chapter 147) [3,4,5–8]
- Medications: statins, nicotinic acid, cimetidine, clofazimine [9]
- Endocrinopathies: diabetes [10], thyroid disease [2], hyperparathyroidism [11] and hypopituitarism [12]
- Infections: leprosy, tuberculosis, HIV disease [13] and HTLV-1 associated myelopathy [14]
- Autoimmune conditions: dermatomyositis, systemic lupus erythematosus and scleroderma/lupus overlap syndrome [15–17]
- Chronic metabolic derangements: including malnutrition [18], malabsorption syndromes [19], essential fatty acid deficiency [20] and pancreatic insufficiency (Shwachman syndrome) [21]
- Anorexia nervosa
- Miscellaneous: sarcoidosis, bone marrow transplantation and chronic renal failure [22]

Pathophysiology

The pathogenesis of acquired ichthyosis is not fully understood; it differs according to the entity with which it is associated.

In cases associated with diabetes, it is supposed that the changes in the skin are due to structural abnormalities in proteins resulting from non-enzymatic glycosylation [23,24]. However, well-controlled diabetics can also show ichthyotic changes, and for these, an abnormal host immune response has been proposed, probably against components of the granular cell layer [10]. The same hypothesis has also been advanced to explain acquired ichthyosis associated with autoimmune disorders [17], whereas those

Rook's Textbook of Dermatology, Ninth Edition. Edited by Christopher Griffiths, Jonathan Barker, Tanya Bleiker, Robert Chalmers and Daniel Creamer.
© 2016 John Wiley & Sons, Ltd. Published 2016 by John Wiley & Sons, Ltd.
Companion website: www.rooksdermatology.com

cases associated with tumours seem to be due to secretion by neoplastic cells of transforming growth factor α (TGF-α), which may exert a mitogenic action on keratinocytes [25].

Pathology
Histologically, the epidermis shows compact hyperkeratosis with a thinned or absent granular cell layer.

Environmental factors
Living in a hot and humid climate may hide the clinical manifestations of filaggrin deficiency [26]. Severe xerosis mimicking acquired ichthyosis can be observed in atopic individuals who immigrate from very humid atmospheres such as South-East Asia to Europe. In their home country, xerosis is not evident but the low humidity in Europe may precipitate an ichthyotic change in the skin.

Clinical features

History
The onset of acquired ichthyosis is typically sudden with initial involvement of the lower limbs but it may then generalize.

Presentation
Symmetrical dark thick scaling appears on the legs in a pattern likened to the skin of lizards. The arms and trunk can also be involved, especially the back (Figure 87.1), but flexures are spared, due to the higher humidity in these areas. The face is unaffected in most cases, probably due to the size and number of its sebaceous glands, but the scalp shows abundant fine scales. Pruritus can be pronounced. There may be palmoplantar hyperkeratosis, with fissures that can become infected [1].

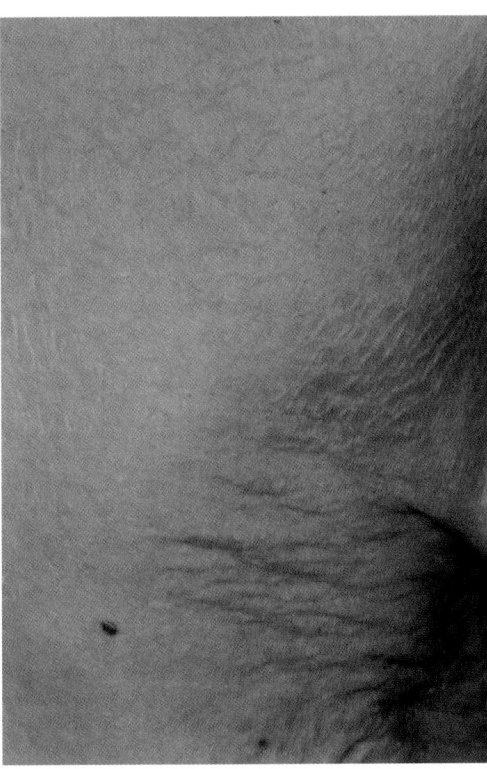

Figure 87.1 Acquired ichthyosis secondary to lymphoma.

Differential diagnosis
- Xeroderma.
- Asteatotic eczema.
- Atopic eczema.
- Drug eruptions.
- Hereditary ichthyoses.

Disease course and prognosis
Acquired ichthyosis may improve with successful treatment of the underlying disease or cessation of the responsible drug.

Investigations
The diagnosis of acquired ichthyosis is made clinically and confirmatory tests are unnecessary. Once the diagnosis has been made, a careful search for an underlying cause should be undertaken, with particular care not to overlook the possibility of occult malignancy, especially lymphoma. In addition to a full history, clinical examination, chest radiography and a detailed drug history should be obtained. Appropriate investigations should be performed to identify other potential causes.

Management
The primary aim in the management of acquired ichthyosis is to identify the underlying cause of the disorder. Its treatment can lead to improvement of the dermatosis.

Treatment of the acquired ichthyosis is symptomatic and involves the use of retinoids and keratolytic agents.

First line
Topical retinoids, particularly tretinoin and tazarotene, reduce the cohesiveness of keratinocytes [27].

Second line
Beta-hydroxyacids (salicylic acid) help to disaggregate the corneocytes.

Third line
Alpha-hydroxyacids (lactic or glycolic acids) produce loosening and desquamation of corneocytes, when applied twice daily. Urea 10–20% is an excellent humectant. Propylene glycol as a 20% preparation in aqueous cream hydrates the stratum corneum.

Acanthosis nigricans

Definition
Acanthosis nigricans (AN) is a dermatosis that manifests as asymptomatic and symmetrical darkening affecting the skin of intertriginous areas, in particular the axillae, groins, submammary folds and neck. The skin in those regions is thickened, has a velvety texture, and may be studded by skin tags. It is particularly associated with obesity and insulin resistance.

Introduction and general description
AN may present as an isolated skin condition but may be associated with a large range of conditions ranging from obesity to endocrinopathies to internal neoplasms.

PART 8: SPECIFIC CUTANEOUS STRUCTURE

Epidemiology

Incidence and prevalence

Benign AN is very common, and affects up to 20% of adults and 7% of children; this increases threefold if only overweight children are considered [1,2,3]. Malignant AN is rare.

Age

AN can occur at any age. The benign form is most common in adults but may be present at birth and is not uncommon in obese children. The malignant form, which is rare, usually arises in older age groups but has been observed in children with Wilms tumours and osteogenic sarcomas [3].

Sex

AN has an equal sex ratio.

Ethnicity

AN is more common in patients with darker skins. In one study AN was observed in 1% of white people, 5.5% in Latino populations and 13.3% in African American populations [4].

Associated diseases

Obesity is the most common association with AN (previously called pseudo-AN), and can regress with weight loss [5].

Many syndromes (Box 87.2) have been associated with AN; they usually involve the endocrine system or accompany autoimmune disorders.

Malignant AN (described in more detail in Chapter 147) has been associated with an extensive range of internal cancers, but over 90% have been seen in patients with gastrointestinal cancer, of which two-thirds are gastric [6,7,8]. Other tumours associated with AN are listed in Box 87.3. Malignant AN may be accompanied by other cutaneous paraneoplastic phenomena, particularly florid cutaneous papillomatosis in which there is a rapid development of numerous warty papules on the trunk and the extremities that are clinically indistinguishable from viral warts (see Chapter 147).

Pathophysiology

The most common associations with benign AN are obesity [2,9] and insulin resistance [1,10,11,12]. Insulin-derived growth factor (IGF-1) receptors are overexpressed in obese patients with hyperinsulinaemia and insulin resistance [13]. IGF-1 can stimulate the proliferation of keratinocytes and dermal fibroblasts. Epidermal growth factor receptors and fibroblast growth factor receptors (FGFR) are also implicated. In Beare–Stevenson syndrome, activating mutations of FGFR2 have been identified, and in Crouzon syndrome and thanatophoric dwarfism, mutations of FGFR3 have been found [14]. FGFR3 mutations have been identified in the familial form of AN [15].

Some drugs may contribute to AN development: FGFR activation can be produced by certain medications used in stem cell transplantation, such as palifermin [16], and insulin can provoke the development of AN at injection sites by activation of IGF receptors.

Box 87.2 Disorders associated with acanthosis nigricans

- Acromegaly and gigantism
- Alström telangiectasia
- Bloom syndrome
- Bartter syndrome
- Beare–Stevenson syndrome
- Benign encephalopathy
- Capozucca syndrome
- Chondrodystrophy with dwarfism
- Costello syndrome
- Crouzon syndrome [26,27]
- Dermatomyositis
- Diabetes
- Familial pineal body hypertrophy
- Gigantism
- HAIR-AN syndrome
- Hashimoto thyroiditis
- Hirschowitz syndrome
- Laurence–Moon–Bardet syndrome
- Lawrence-Seip syndrome
- Lipoatrophic diabetes
- Lupoid hepatitis
- Lupus erythematosus
- Motor tract degeneration
- Phenylketonuria
- Polycystic ovary syndrome
- Primary hypogonadism
- Pseudoacromegaly
- Prader–Willi syndrome
- Pyramidal tract degeneration
- Rud syndrome
- Systemic sclerosis
- Thanatophoric dwarfism
- Werner syndrome
- Wilson syndrome

Box 87.3 Internal malignancies associated with acanthosis nigricans

- **Gastric cancer**
- Gall bladder and bile duct cancer
- Bladder cancer
- Breast cancer
- Gynaecological cancer
- Hodgkin disease
- Kidney cancer
- Liver cancer
- Lung cancer
- Pancreatic cancer
- Prostatic cancer
- Testicular cancer
- Thyroid cancer
- Osteogenic sarcoma and Wilms tumour (in children)

In malignant AN, tumour-derived stimulating factors are produced, especially TGF-α, which is recognized by epidermal growth factor receptors. The levels of TGF decrease with tumour debulking, which may be followed by regression of the paraneoplastic phenomena [17].

Predisposing factors

AN is associated with a number of benign and malignant conditions with a common pathway of keratinocyte and fibroblast proliferation by circulating factors. Perspiration and/or friction are mechanical contributing factors which may be important in determining the characteristic distribution of AN in flexural areas.

Pathology

Despite its name, AN shows no or minimal acanthosis or hyperpigmentation microscopically. Histology shows hyperkeratosis and papillomatosis with finger-like upward projections of dermal papillae. Pigmentation is due to the hyperkeratosis; there is no increase in melanocyte numbers or in melanin production. Pseudo-horn cysts may be present. In mucosal lesions, parakeratosis may be observed [3].

Genetics

The familial form of AN is inherited in an autosomal dominant fashion. In familial AN, FGFR3 mutations have been identified [15].

Clinical features

History

AN usually starts as asymptomatic darkening of the skin of the neck, axillae and groins. With time, the patches become thicker and may develop skin tags in the affected areas. Pruritus is not common.

Presentation

AN presents as symmetrical velvety dark patches which are most commonly seen in the axillae, groins and on the back and sides of the neck (Figure 87.2). The back of the neck is the most common site in children. Skin tags (acrochordons) may be present in affected areas. AN may become widespread with delicate velvety furrowing of mucosal surfaces and involvement of the eyelids and conjunctivae. Associated nail changes include leukonychia and subungual hyperkeratosis.

Clinical variants

HAIR-AN is a familial syndrome, that manifests as *h*yperandrogenaemia, *i*nsulin *r*esistance and *a*canthosis *n*igricans. It typically affects young black girls, who develop polycystic ovaries, hirsutism, clitoral hypertrophy and frequently have high plasma testosterone levels. This condition, which is also known as type A insulin resistance syndrome, is described in more detail in Chapters 90 and 149.

Type B insulin resistance syndrome is characterized by the association of AN with diabetes and hyperandrogenism, or with an autoimmune disease (including systemic lupus erythematosus, systemic sclerosis, Hashimoto thyroiditis and Sjögren syndrome).

Familial AN is rare and transmitted as an autosomal dominant trait with variable penetrance. It manifests early in life and tends to stabilize in the teenage years. In some patients, it can improve with age.

Drug-induced AN has been associated with many different medications, particularly hormones, insulin, systemic corticosteroids, testosterone and exogenous oestrogens, including oral contraceptives [18,19]. One of the most common associations is with nicotinic acid. The dermatosis tends to resolve after discontinuation of the offending agent.

Generalized AN is very rare, and seen only in children. There is generalized hyperpigmenation and velvety thickening of the skin, and extensive investigation fails to show any associated systemic abnormality [20,21,22].

Acral AN is more common in skin phototypes 5 and 6. It is not associated with systemic disease, and manifests as a velvety

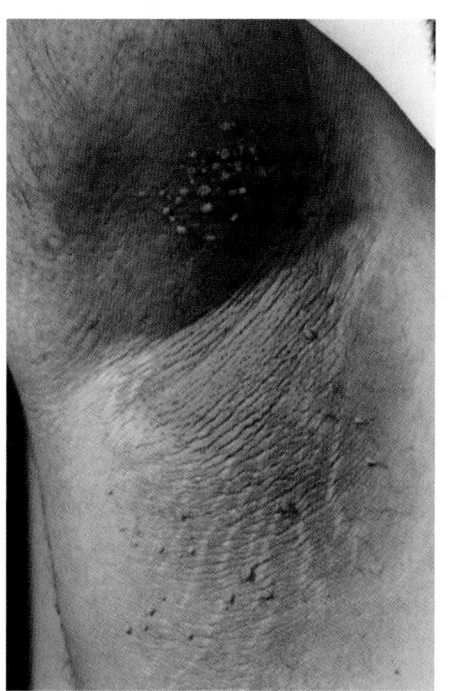

(a)

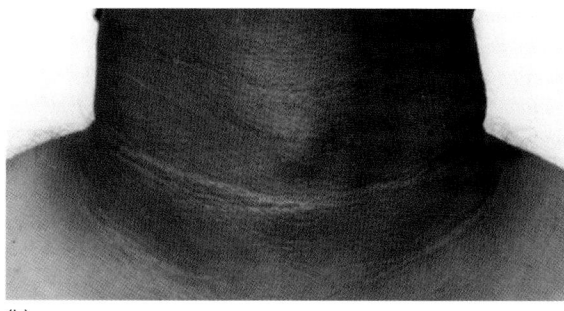

(b)

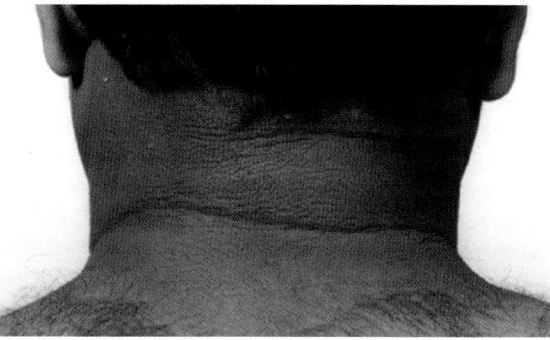

(c)

Figure 87.2 (a–c) Typical acanthosis nigricans in an obese 41-year-old man of South Asian descent with type II diabetes. Note associated striae and skin tags in the axilla (a), and darkening and velvety thickening of the skin around the root and nape of the neck (b,c).

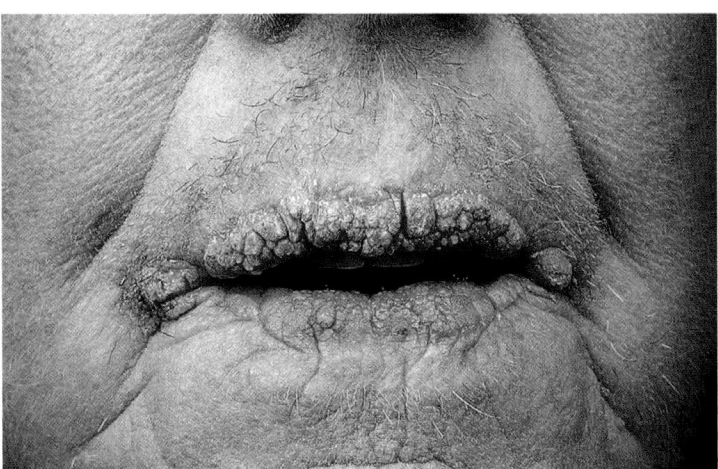

Figure 87.3 Malignant acanthosis nigricans: warty thickening of the oral margins in a patient with carcinoma of the breast.

thickening and hyperpigmentation of the skin on the dorsa of the hands and feet, especially the knuckles [23].

Unilateral AN (or naevoid AN) is very rare, and is assumed to arise from a somatic mutation during embryogenesis. It can appear in infancy, but not always, and cases have been reported with onset in childhood or adulthood. Clinically, it appears as a pigmented plaque, solitary or along a line of Blaschko, and resembles an epidermal naevus. Histopathologically, the typical changes of AN are seen. It has been described on the face and scalp, chest and abdomen, back and thighs [24].

Malignant or paraneoplastic AN (Figure 87.3) can be associated with an extensive range of internal cancers (see above and Box 87.3).

Differential diagnosis
The major differential diagnoses are as follows:
- Addison disease.
- Pellagra.
- Haemochromatosis.
  Fairly simple investigations will exclude these diagnoses.

Disease course and prognosis
Benign AN is not associated with systemic disease but generally persists and may be a significant cosmetic problem.

AN associated with metabolic abnormalities and insulin resistance may improve with treatment of the underlying condition. AN associated with obesity may improve with dietary restriction and weight loss.

The prognosis of patients with malignant AN is poor, with an average survival of only 2 years from diagnosis.

Investigations
In adult-onset AN, patients should be screened for underlying endocrinopathy or malignancy. A sensitive test for insulin resistance is serum insulin, the levels of which may be elevated before the onset of diabetes or elevation of glycosylated haemoglobin levels.

Management
Management of AN is the management of the underlying condition. In familial AN or AN not associated with an underlying condition, treatment is aimed at improving the cosmetic appearance of the condition.

Treatment ladder

First line
- Topical retinoids – may reduce the hyperkeratosis

Second line
- Topical α-hydroxyacids and keratolytics such as salicylic acid may improve appearance by reducing hyperkeratosis

Third line
- In extensive cases oral isotretinoin has been used with some success [25]

Confluent and reticulated papillomatosis

Definition and nomenclature
Confluent and reticulated papillomatosis (CARP) is an uncommon disorder of epidermal keratinization characterized by the development of hyperkeratotic papules which coalesce into confluent and, in places, reticulated plaques on truncal skin. An abnormal reaction to commensal microorganisms has been postulated to play an aetiological role.

Synonyms and inclusions
- Papillomatose pigmentée innominée
- Papillomatose pigmentée confluente et réticulée
- Gougerot–Carteaud syndrome

Introduction and general description
Gougerot and Carteaud first described this entity in 1927 [1]. It is a controversial disease and many had considered it to be a specific form of AN [2]. Diagnostic criteria have been established and it is now considered a specific form of cutaneous papillomatosis [3,4].

Epidemiology

Incidence and prevalence
CARP is a rare disease and there are no data on the prevalence of the disease.

Age
CARP is predominantly a disease of young adults. In one series of patients, the mean age at onset was 19 years [2].

Sex
It is likely that the sex incidence is equal but different reports have shown a predominance of women in white populations but a

predominance of men in Japan. A study from the Mayo Clinic [4] and a recent study from Lebanon shows an equal sex incidence [5].

Ethnicity
CARP has been reported in all ethnic groups.

Pathophysiology
The pathogenesis of CARP is poorly understood. It is thought that an abnormal host reaction to *Malassezia* organisms may be relevant in some patients [6,7] and it has also been suggested that actinomycete bacteria may play a role [8]. These hypotheses are discussed in more detail later. However, the anti-inflammatory properties of the antibiotics might be the true reason for the response.

Abnormal keratinocyte differentiation has been found on transmission electron microscopy and by immunohistochemical studies, which show an increased expression of involucrin, keratin 16 and Ki-67 [9]. These changes might explain the clustering of the condition in some families [10,11]. The number of Odland bodies is increased and this is associated with a higher turnover of epidermal keratinocytes as seen in psoriasis [12]. The role of metabolic abnormalities in the development of CARP is gaining supporters [2]. CARP has been associated with obesity and insulin resistance [13], as well as thyroid dysfunction and Cushing disease [14].

Pathology
There is hyperkeratosis and papillomatosis, with decrease in the thickness or disappearance of the granular cell layer. There may be increased melanin in the basal cell layer and in the stratum corneum, and this is reflected in the colour of the plaques. The dermis shows at most a mild non-specific inflammatory infiltrate [15].

Fungal stains frequently show *Malassezia* yeasts on the surface of the epidermis.

Causative organisms
A number of reports have demonstrated the presence of *Malassezia* organisms in CARP. This has led to speculation that CARP is due to an abnormal host reaction to *Malassezia*. Several studies have shown, however, that only about half of patients with CARP have significant yeast populations on affected skin [2,6,7]. Although some patients with CARP respond to topical imidazoles or other antifungal agents, about half of cases fail to respond [5,6,7] and in those cases only a few spores can be retrieved from the skin surface.

Some patients with CARP appear to respond to tetracycline and macrolide antibiotics, which has led to the suggestion that skin bacteria may be responsible for this disease. In 2005, a previously unknown actinomycete bacterium of the genus *Dietzia* was isolated from the skin of a patient with CARP. Sensitivity studies showed sensitivity to tetracycline and erythromycin and the patient cleared with tetracycline. The organism, which has subsequently been named *Dietzia papillomatosis*, has been implicated in a case of septicaemia but, to date, there have been no further reports linking it with CARP [8]. It has been suggested, however, that the response to antibiotics may be due to their anti-inflammatory rather than their antibacterial properties.

Genetics
Although familial forms of CARP have been reported [10,11] they are too rare to postulate a genetic inheritance.

Clinical features (Figure 87.4)

History
The patient is usually a young postpubertal individual. Plaques of CARP are located mainly on the trunk, especially on the presternal, interscapular and epigastric areas. They are generally asymptomatic.

Presentation
Patients first notice pigmented, 1–2 mm diameter hyperkeratotic papules on the trunk. These coalesce to form greyish-blue plaques which are confluent at the centre but become reticular towards the periphery of the plaques. Over weeks or months, the plaques spread to involve the lower abdomen and pubic areas [2]. The face and limbs may be affected. Localized forms affecting only the face

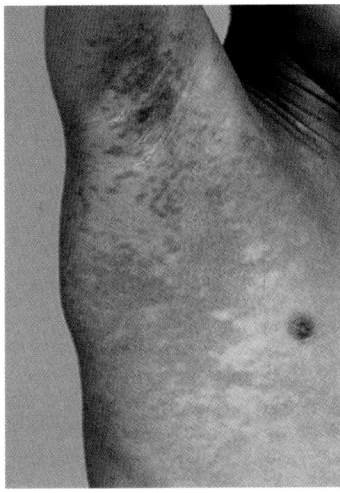
(a)

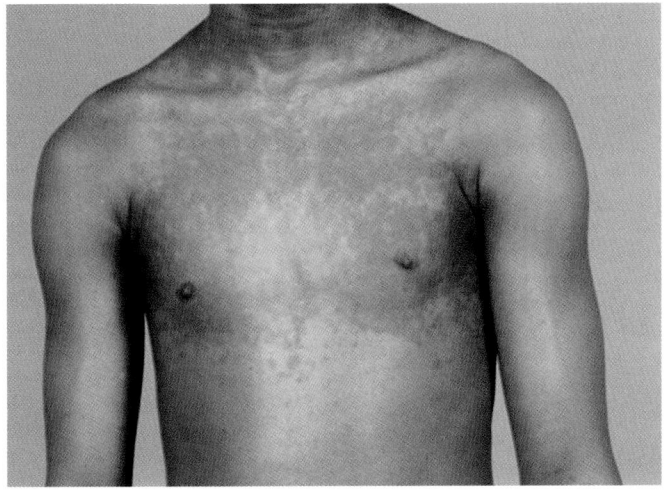
(b)

Figure 87.4 (a,b) Confluent and reticulate papillomatosis: an asymptomatic rash appeared 6 months earlier around the neck of this of 12-year-old boy before spreading to the axillae and upper torso. No response to antifungal medication.

or pubic area have been reported [16,17]. Mucous membranes are not involved. A number of different patterns of skin involvement have been described [18].

Differential diagnosis
The most common differential diagnoses proposed in cases of CARP include the following:
- Acanthosis nigricans.
- Macular amyloid.
- Darier disease.
- Epidermal naevus.
- Plane warts.
- Pityriasis versicolor.
- Seborrhoeic keratosis.
- Retention hyperkeratosis (deficient personal hygiene).

Disease course and prognosis
CARP is a chronic disease with remissions and exacerbations. If CARP responds to treatment, it often relapses when treatment is withdrawn.

Management
CARP is a chronic disease and is purely cosmetic, so no treatment is an option if the condition does not bother the patient. In overweight patients, weight reduction may result in improvement. In some women, CARP may improve during pregnancy or with the use of the oral contraceptive.

First line
A wide range of oral antibiotics have been found to be effective in CARP [21]: the most effective appears to be minocycline [4,19,20]. Topical mupirocin ointment has been of benefit in some cases [21].

Second line
Topical and systemic antifungal agents, including selenium sulphide shampoo, have been used with success in some patients [2, 22] but the results have been very variable. Topical retinoids and vitamin D analogues have been used with mixed results [23–25].

Third line
Both high- and low-dose isotretinoin have been used in the treatment of CARP with varying results [26,27].

Pityriasis rotunda

Definition and nomenclature
Pityriasis rotunda (PR) [1] is a dermatosis of unknown cause that presents as perfectly round, slightly erythematous or hyperpigmented plaques, with fine scaling, usually located on the trunk or buttocks, arms and legs.

Synonyms and inclusions
- Pityriasis circinata
- Acquired pseudo-ichthyosis

Introduction and general description
PR is a rare condition with very few reports in the literature. The most common form of PR is type 1 PR which is typically seen in older Asian or African individuals and is usually associated with underlying systemic disease or malignancy [2]: it may resolve with treatment of the underlying condition [2,3]. Type 2 PR is usually familial and presents in younger white patients: it is not associated with underlying disease.

Epidemiology

Incidence and prevalence
PR is rare with most reports coming from South Africa, Sardinia or Japan.

Age
Type 1 PR is usually seen in patients in their 60s. Type 2 PR is usually seen in patients in their forties.

Sex
PR has an equal sex incidence.

Ethnicity
Most case reports of PR have come from South Africa in black populations and the few reports from the UK have been in patients of African descent [4]. Type 1 disease is also seen in East Asian patients with most reports from Japan; it is rare in white populations [5]: type 2 PR has been reported principally from Sardinia.

Associated diseases
Type 1 PR has been associated with hepatocellular carcinoma. In a series of 10 black patients from South Africa with PR, 70% were associated with hepatocellular carcinoma [6]. In a further study from South Africa examining hepatocellular carcinoma, 15.9% of 63 patients had PR [7]. In the South African black population, PR has been associated with a number of systemic diseases listed in Box 87.4.

In Asian populations, PR is associated with underlying malignancy but not specifically with hepatocellular carcinoma [8].

Box 87.4 Diseases associated with pityriasis rotunda in black African populations
- Hepatocellular carcinoma
- Chronic myeloid leukaemia
- Squamous cell carcinoma of the hard palate
- Tuberculosis
- Liver disease
- Cardiac disease
- Nutritional disease
- Other malignancies
- Pulmonary disease
- Chronic renal failure
- Osteitis
- Chronic diarrhoea
- Systemic sclerosis

PART 8: SPECIFIC CUTANEOUS STRUCTURE

Pathophysiology

The aetiopathogenesis of PR is unknown. Histologically, it shares some characteristics with ichthyosis vulgaris and some authors feel it is a variant of this disease [9]. In South African patients it has been associated with malnutrition, but this is not generally accepted as a cause of the disease.

Pathology

Histological changes are restricted to the epidermis with hyperkeratosis and loss of the granular cell layer.

Genetics

Type 2 PR is inherited as an autosomal dominant trait [10].

Clinical features

History

PR is an asymptomatic condition and is often diagnosed incidentally in patients being investigated for other disease.

Presentation

PR presents as asymptomatic thin finely scaling plaques ranging from 0.5 to more than 20 cm in diameter located on the trunk, buttocks, arms and legs. The plaques, ranging in number from a few to more than 100, are sharply demarcated and can coalesce, forming polycyclic plaques. They are pink in lightly pigmented skin to dark brown in skin of phototypes 5 and 6 (Figure 87.5).

Clinical variants

PR types 1 and 2 are sporadic and familial, respectively (see earlier).

Differential diagnosis

Differential diagnosis includes post-inflammatory hyperpigmentation following fixed drug eruption, erythrasma, tinea corporis, pityriasis versicolor and psoriasis.

Disease course and prognosis

Once type 2 PR develops it usually persists lifelong. In type 1 PR associated with an underlying disease, treatment of the disease may result in resolution of the PR.

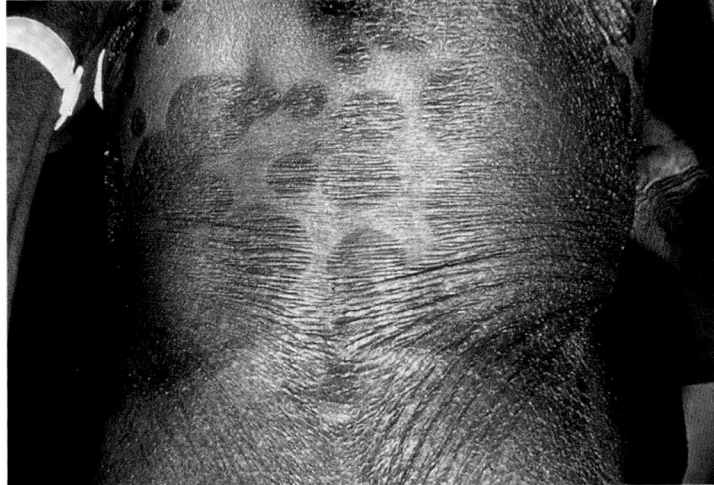

Figure 87.5 Pityriasis rotunda.

Investigations

A skin biopsy might be helpful to exclude other conditions, as the diagnosis of PR is one of exclusion.

Skin scraping and mycological examination will exclude dermatophytosis and pityriasis versicolor.

Management

Lesions of PR are notoriously resistant to therapy, but some improvement has been achieved with topical treatment.

Treatment ladder

First line
- Topical retinoids, such as tretinoin, isotretinoin or tazarotene

Second line
- Topical 10% lactic acid

Third line
- 5% salicylic acid ointment

Keratosis pilaris

Definition and nomenclature

Keratosis pilaris (KP) is an inherited abnormality of keratinization affecting the follicular orifices with varying degrees of keratotic follicular plugging, perifollicular erythema and follicular atrophy.

Synonyms and inclusions
- Follicular keratosis
- Lichen pilaris

Introduction and general description

KP [1,2] is a common skin condition, characterized by follicular keratotic papules and perifollicular erythema. Because up to half of the population present with the condition to some degree, it can be considered a variant of normal rather than a disease.

Epidemiology

Incidence and prevalence

KP is a very common condition affecting 50–80% of adolescents and about 40% of adults.

Age

KP often presents in the first decade of life and may worsen around puberty. In some patients, the disorder improves with age but any age group can be affected from childhood to old age.

Sex

Females appear to be more frequently affected than males.

Ethnicity

KP is not more prevalent in any racial group.

Associated diseases

KP may be associated with ichthyosis vulgaris and atopic eczema [3]. These conditions are, however, all common and the association may be coincidental. Some other reported associations are listed in Box 87.5. More recently, patients with *BRAF*-positive tumours under treatment with vemurafenib and sorafenib have been noted to develop KP as a side effect [4].

Pathophysiology

A plug of excess keratin is formed, possibly due to a defect of corneocyte adhesion at the follicular orifice, and this impedes the hair from emerging. The hair can become ingrown and result in an inflammatory response [18].

Pathology

Histology of KP shows hyperkeratosis, hypergranulosis and plugging of hair follicles. In the dermis, there is a mild perivascular lymphocytic infiltrate in the upper dermis.

Genetics

KP is inherited as an autosomal dominant trait with variable penetrance [18]. Reports have identified a partial monosomy in the short arm of chromosome 18 in patients with severe forms of KP and ulerythema ophryogenes [19].

Environmental factors

KP may show seasonal variation, improving in the summer [20].

Clinical features

History

KP generally starts in children, most commonly on the extensor surfaces of the upper arms, and can worsen around puberty.

Box 87.5 Disorders with which keratosis pilaris and follicular hyperkeratoses have been associated

- Ichthyosis vulgaris [3]
- Atopic eczema [3]
- Obesity [5]
- Insulin-dependent diabetes (seen in types 1 and 2) [5]
- Noonan syndrome [6]
- Cardio-facio-cutaneous syndrome [7]
- Prolidase deficiency [8]
- Down syndrome [9]
- Fairbanks syndrome [10]
- Olmsted syndrome [11]
- Renal failure and hypervitaminosis A [12]
- Monilethrix [13]
- Pachyonychia congenita [14]
- Ectodermal dysplasias [15]
- Systemic corticosteroids [16]
- Lithium [17]
- Vemurafenib and sorafenib [4]

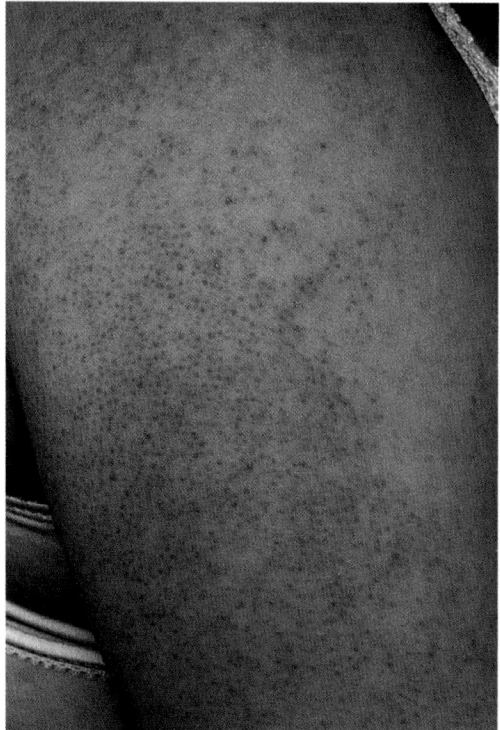

Figure 87.6 Keratosis pilaris on the extensor aspect of the upper arm.

Presentation

There are small, keratotic papules on the extensor aspects of the limbs, particularly the arms (Figure 87.6) and thighs [20]. The buttocks and the lumbar areas are also frequently affected. These areas acquire a 'goose-bump' appearance and rough texture. Lesions can become pustular with superficial pustules developing in affected follicles, precipitated by rubbing on clothing. On the buttock, deeper inflammatory lesions and nodules may develop.

Clinical variants

Erythromelanosis follicularis faciei et colli [21–23] is a condition that has been described as a subtype of KP and seen in India and other countries in the Far and Middle East. It manifests as follicular hyperkeratosis accompanied by erythema and hyperpigmentation, and affects, as the name indicates, the face, particularly the cheeks and neck (Figure 87.7).

KP atrophicans is a more inflammatory form of KP which results in follicular fibrosis and atrophy progressing to scarring alopecia. Three variants have been recognized as follows:
1 *KP atrophicans faciei*, also called ulerythema ophryogenes [24] or keratosis rubra pilaris faciei atrophicans, affects the cheeks and lateral eyebrows (Figure 87.8). There is fixed erythema, follicular plugging, pitted scarring and hair loss. It may be associated with common KP and may be inherited as an autosomal dominant trait [25].
2 *Keratosis follicularis spinulosa decalvans* has its onset in infancy, and affects the cheeks and nose [26]: follicular plugging results in follicular atrophy. The scalp may also be involved, resulting in scarring alopecia. It can be associated with palmoplantar hyperkeratosis.

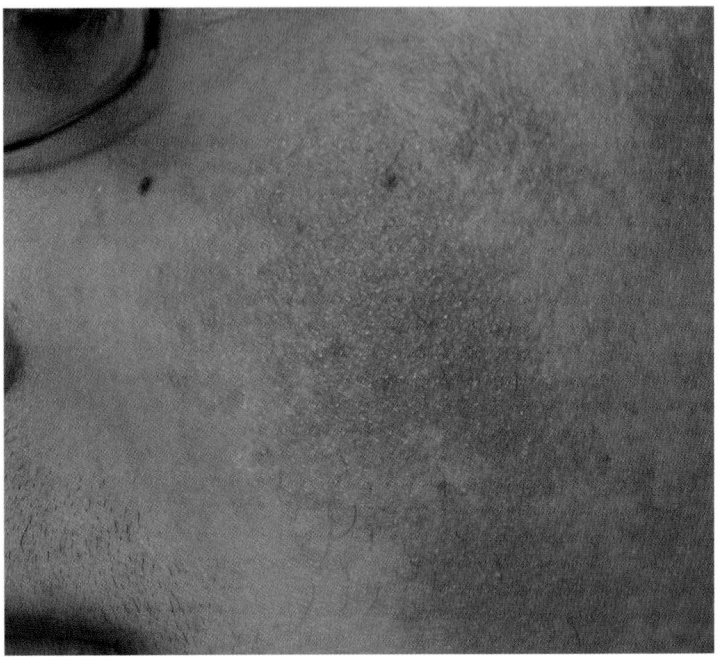

Figure 87.7 Erythromelanosis follicularis faciei et colli in a young Asian man.

3 *Atrophoderma vermiculatum* manifests in late childhood, and affects the cheeks and preauricular skin. The follicular plugging evolves towards reticulated atrophy of the skin (Figure 87.9) [27].

Differential diagnosis

KP may be confused with a large number of dermatoses including the following:

- Darier disease.
- Pityriasis rubra pilaris.
- Atopic eczema.
- Lichen nitidus.
- Eruptive vellous hair cysts.

If follicular lesions become inflamed KP may be confused with the following:

- Acne.
- Folliculitis.

KP atrophicans faciei may be confused with rosacea.

Disease course and prognosis

In the majority of patients KP is a mild cosmetic disorder which improves with age. Hypopigmentation, hyperpigmentation and scarring may occur.

Investigations

KP is a clinical diagnosis for which no tests are normally required.

Management

KP is principally a cosmetic problem and many people do not know they have it. If it does not bother the patient, treatment is unnecessary. Benefit from topical therapy is often limited and many patients will not persist with it.

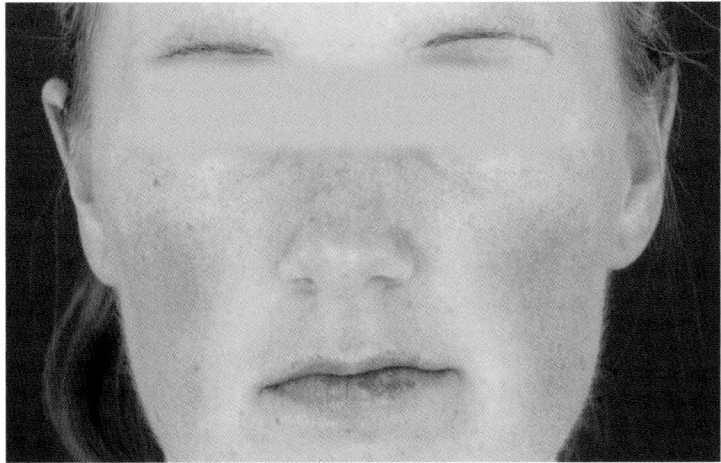

(a)

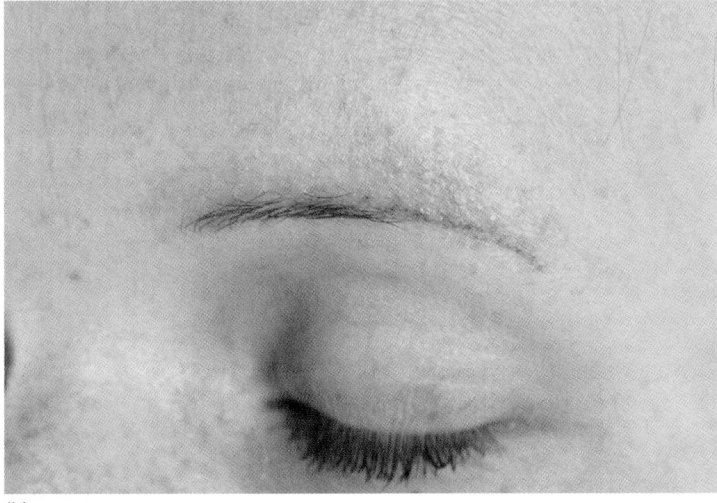

(b)

Figure 87.8 Keratosis pilaris atrophicans faciei (ulerythema ophryogenes): note well-defined symmetrical erythema on the cheeks and above sparse residual eyebrow hairs (a); the complete loss of hair from the lateral half of the eyebrows has been disguised by pencilling (b).

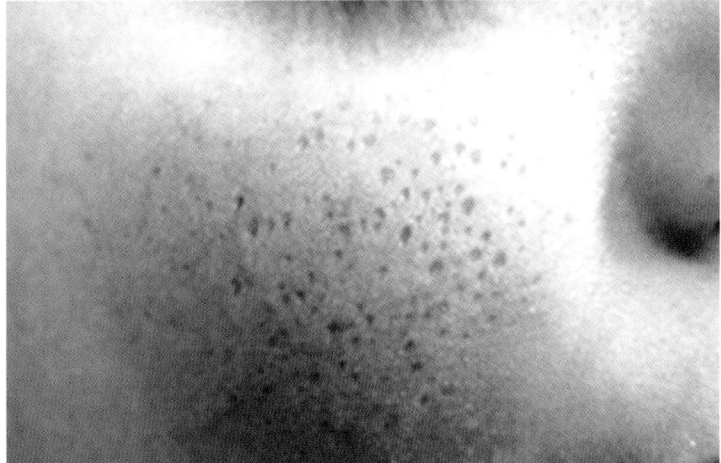

Figure 87.9 Atrophoderma vermiculatum the on the cheek of 10-year-old boy. (Source: http://www.ncbi.nlm.nih.gov/pmc/articles/PMC3163348/ from Apalla *et al. J Dermatol Case Rep* 2009 [32] copyright 2009 Specjalisci Dermatolodzy.)

First line

Keratolytics, particularly salicylic acid. Lactic and glycolic acid preparations also reduce roughness of the skin. Treatment may need to be continued for many years.

Second line

Topical retinoids may reduce hyperkeratosis and can be very successful when combined with 10% urea containing moisturisers. Topical retinoids are particularly useful for KP atrophicans faciei [28].

Third line

In severe KP, oral isotretinoin has been successfully used but relapse occurs on cessation [29].

Fourth line

Patients with severe fixed erythema from KP atrophicans faciei have been successfully treated with pulsed dye laser [30,31].

Lichen spinulosus

Definition and nomenclature

Lichen spinulosus (LS) [1,2,3] is a rare idiopathic condition, characterized by the appearance of hyperkeratotic follicular papules arranged into large plaques.

> **Synonyms and inclusions**
> • Keratosis spinulosa

Introduction and general description

LS was first described by Adamson in 1908 [4] as an acute eruption of grouped keratotic papules which form into plaques. They appear suddenly and are distributed symmetrically on the extensor surfaces of the limbs or on the trunk and neck [1,2,3]. They are coarse to the touch and typically measure 2–5 cm in diameter.

Epidemiology

Incidence and prevalence

LS is a rare disorder. From the first description [4], no further reports of the disease appeared in the literature until 1990, when Friedman described 35 patients in a survey of 7435 patients attending a dermatology clinic in the Philippines, accounting for 0.5% of patients surveyed [3].

Age

LS is a disease of children and young adults with an average age of onset of 16.2 + 10.1 years [3].

Sex

Case reports suggest an equal distribution of LS in males and females.

Ethnicity

There is no predilection of LS in any ethnic group.

Associated diseases

LS is not usually associated with any underlying systemic disease. There have been case reports of LS in HIV infection, Crohn disease and alcoholism, Hodgkin disease and syphilis [5–7]. Previously, LS has been associated with certain drugs including thallium, gold and diphtheria toxin.

Pathophysiology

The cause of LS is unknown. Some authors feel that LS is a variant of KP: the conditions share the same features on histology.

Pathology

Hair follicles are dilated by a thick keratinous plug, and surrounded by a mild to moderate chronic inflammatory infiltrate.

Clinical features

History

LS generally erupts acutely and is asymptomatic.

Presentation

Individual papules are follicular, measuring 2–3 mm in diameter and raised 1 mm above the surface of the skin with a pointed keratotic spine. Papules coalesce into plaques ranging from 2 to 5 cm in diameter. The patches are symmetrical and distributed on the trunk, buttocks (Figure 87.10), neck, knees and elbows. The face, hands and feet are usually spared. Plaques erupt in crops, grow rapidly and then remain stationary.

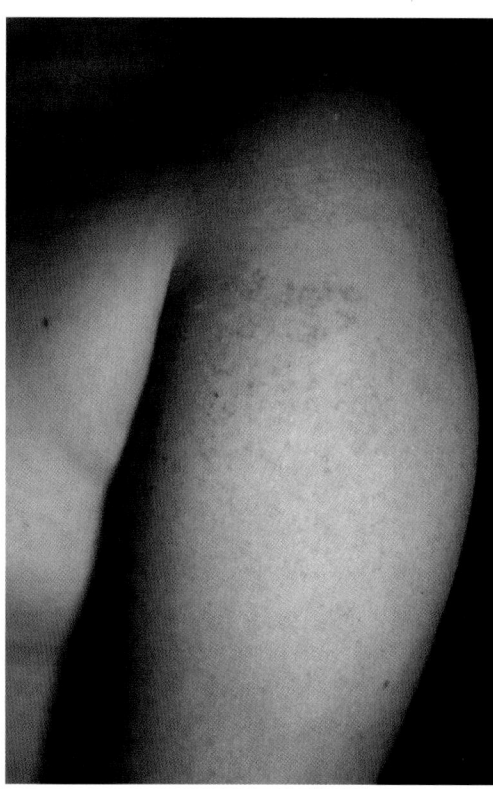

Figure 87.10 Lichen spinulosus present for 18 months as an asymptomatic eruption on the back, shoulder and upper arm of an 8-year-old girl.

PART 8: SPECIFIC CUTANEOUS STRUCTURE

Clinical variants
Spinulosis of the face, presenting with tiny keratotic spicules on the cheeks, may be a variant of LS.

Differential diagnosis
All other causes of follicular papules should be considered in the differential diagnosis, including KP, lichen nitidus, phrynoderma, and pityriasis rubra pilaris.

Disease course and prognosis
LS is a chronic but purely cosmetic disease. LS can persist for many years, but in most patients, it resolves spontaneously within 1–2 years.

Investigations
Diagnosis of LS is made clinically and can be supported by histology.

Management
Management of LS is aimed at improving the cosmetic appearance. The mainstays of treatment are topical retinoids and keratolytics [8].

Treatment ladder

First line
- Keratolyic agents including lactic acid (5–12%), salicylic acid (3–5%) and urea (10–20%) can be used

Second line
- Topical retinoids have been successfully used in LS [9]

Third line
- Successful use of topical tacalcitol in two children with an atypical presentation of submental LS has been reported [10]

Keratosis circumscripta

Definition
Keratosis circumscripta (KC) is a rare condition characterized by circumscribed areas of follicular hyperkeratosis.

Introduction and general description
KC was first described by Shrank in 1966 in 10 members of the Yoruba tribe in Nigeria [1]. It is rare and there remains controversy over its status as an individual dermatosis. In one report and review of the literature, the authors suggested that KC was in fact a form of psoriasis modified by environmental factors [2]. It has also been suggested that it is the same as type IV circumscribed juvenile-onset pityriasis rubra pilaris (see Chapter 36). Shrank's findings were, however, supported by a report of 10 patients from Kenya [3] and other authors have supported its recognition as an individual entity [4,5].

Epidemiology

Incidence and prevalence
KC is rare.

Age
KC first develops in childhood and is persistent thereafter.

Ethnicity
KC was first described in an African tribe and is more common in phototype 6 skin.

Pathophysiology
The aetiopathogenesis of KC is unknown.

Pathology
Histology shows follicular plugging and moderate hyperkeratosis. There is no involvement of the dermis.

Genetics
The condition appears to be sporadic but clustering of cases within a particular ethnic group would support a genetic predisposition.

Clinical features

History
KC normally starts at the age to 3–5 years with lesions developing quickly over a period of 2–3 weeks.

Presentation
The lesions of KC are well-defined areas of diffuse and follicular hyperkeratosis affecting the extensor surfaces of the arms and legs and the trunk (Figure 87.11). In his original report, Shrank described elbow and knee involvement in all his patients and 4–5 cm round discs of follicular hyperkeratosis on each hip. The dorsa of the hands and feet were occasionally involved but the palms and soles were rarely affected. Lesions may become thickened and hyperpigmented or violaceous in colour.

Differential diagnosis
A number of dermatoses can be confused with KC but can be clinically differentiated from this disease. These include the following:
- Type IV circumscribed juvenile pityriasis rubra pilaris (see Chapter 36).
- Lichen spinulosus.
- Psoriasis (see Chapter 35).

Disease course and prognosis
Once established, the condition persists. Patients tend not to develop new lesions but existing lesions may slowly increase in size and become more keratotic.

Management
KC is poorly responsive to treatment and generally does not improve with topical corticosteroids, topical retinoids or conventional keratolytics. 40% urea in white soft paraffin has been used successfully to improve the appearance of KC in one patient [3].

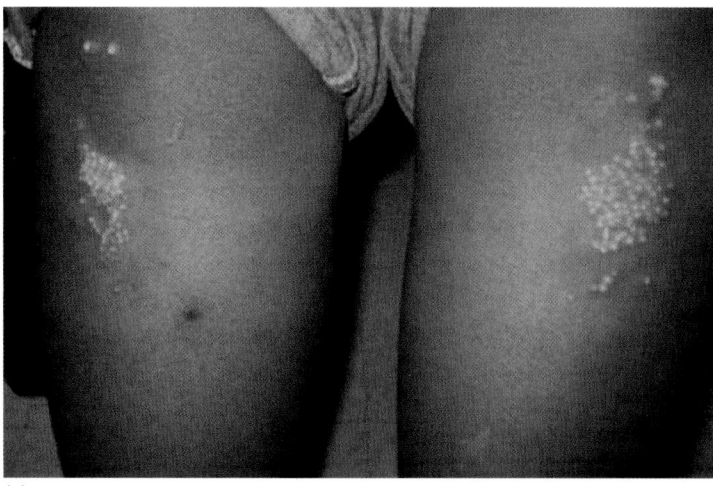

(a)

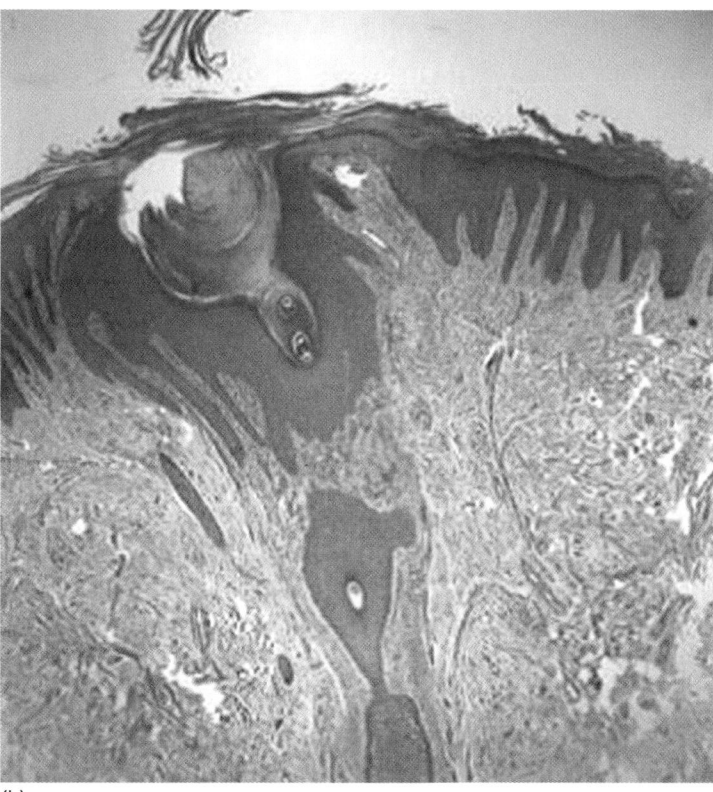

(b)

Figure 87.11 Keratosis circumscripta: coalescing hyperkeratotic papules on the thighs of 10-year-old African American girl (a); psoriasiform dermatitis with prominent follicular plugging but without neutrophils (b). (From Shams *et al.* 2011 [**5**] reproduced with permission from the copyright holder Wiley.)

Phrynoderma

Definition

Phrynoderma, which literally means toad skin, is one of the cutaneous manifestations of vitamin A deficiency but may also be associated with other nutritional deficiencies. It manifests as follicular hyperkeratosis. It is described in more detail in Chapter 63.

Introduction and general description

Phrynoderma was first described by Nicholls in 1933 in African labourers and was recognized as a manifestation of vitamin A deficiency [1]. It is usually seen in children living in economically deprived countries.

Epidemiology

Incidence and prevalence

Phrynoderma is more common in countries where malnutrition is prevalent, but can also be seen in Europe in individuals with liver cirrhosis, malabsorption syndromes or anorexia nervosa and in those who abuse alcohol or are homeless [2]. In economically deprived countries, it is seen in <5% of children and adolescents [3]. Recently, it has been recognized as a complication after bariatric surgery [4,5].

Age

Phrynoderma is commonest in children between the ages of 5 and 15 in economically deprived countries.

Sex

Sexes are equally affected.

Ethnicity

No data available.

Associated diseases

- Liver cirrhosis.
- Malabsorption syndromes.
- Anorexia nervosa.
- Alcohol abuse.
- Nutritional deficiency following bariatric surgery.

Pathophysiology

Phrynoderma was initially thought to be due purely to vitamin A deficiency. Vitamin A is essential for normal cellular growth and division, and maintenance of the immune response. Lack of this vitamin results in abnormal epidermal keratinization as well as immunosuppression [6–8]. Phrynoderma has now been described in patients with normal vitamin A levels and has been associated with other nutritional deficiencies including including B complex, riboflavin, vitamin C, vitamin E, essential fatty acids and malnutrition [1].

Pathology

Follicles are dilated with compact keratin and patchy parakeratosis with no dermal reaction.

Clinical features (Figure 87.12)

History

Phrynoderma starts gradually with mostly non-pruritic lesions on the elbows.

Presentation

Phrynoderma manifests as groups of papules, each one around 3–4 mm in diameter, with a central keratotic plug [9,10,11]. The papules have a follicular distribution and give the skin a rough

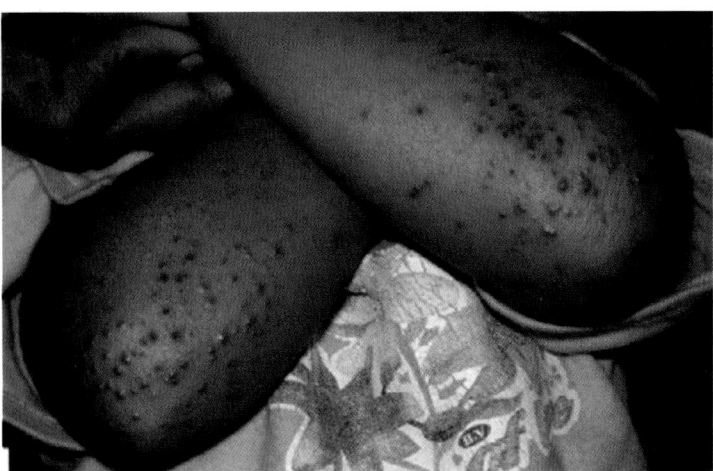

Figure 87.12 Phrynoderma: keratotic papules with intrafollicular plugging on extensor surfaces of the forearms of a 3-year-old Indian girl presenting with night blindness. Both conditions responded within 1 month to vitamin A supplementation. (From Murthy and Prabhakaran 2010 [14] http://www.ncbi.nlm.nih.gov/pmc/articles/PMC2854467/ last accessed October 2015 copyright of the *Indian Journal of Ophthalmology*.)

texture. The elbows and knees are the most commonly affected areas but the buttocks and extensor surfaces of the limbs may be affected. In generalized disease, the trunk and face may be affected. Papules are skin coloured or hyperpigmented. The condition is usually associated with ocular signs, such as night blindness, conjunctival xerosis and ulcerations [12].

Differential diagnosis
The differential diagnosis of phrynoderma includes the following:
- Keratosis pilaris.
- Lichen nitidus.
- Lichen spinulosus.
- Perforating disorders.
- Pityriasis rubra pilaris.

Complications and co-morbidities
Ocular involvement including the development of Bitot spots, conjunctival xerosis and blindness may be associated with phrynoderma.

Investigations
All patients with phrynoderma should have their vitamin A levels measured. Serum vitamin A levels lower than 35 μmol/dL indicate hypovitaminosis.

In some patients with nutritional deficiency, there will be concomitant hypoproteinaemia. In this circumstance, values of vitamin A can appear reduced despite adequate vitamin A stores.

Management
Treatment involves the correction of poor diet and administration of a multivitamin preparation containing vitamin A, since poor diet often results in other concurrent deficiencies. Oral administration is preferred over parenteral therapy. The dosage, in children aged 8 years or above and adults is 100 000 units daily for 3 days, followed by 50 000 units daily for 2 weeks, and then 10 000 units daily for 2 months, until liver storage is adequate [13].

Treatment ladder

First line
- Improved nutrition, vitamin supplementation and management of underlying disease

Trichodysplasia spinulosa

Definition and nomenclature
Trichodysplasia spinulosa is a rare and disfiguring condition caused by infection of the hair inner root sheath by a polyoma virus in immunocompromised patients.

Synonyms and inclusions
- Polyoma virus-associated trichodysplasia
- Trichodysplasia of immunosuppression

Introduction and general description
This is a rare condition first described in 1999 in immunocompromised patients [1]. It is due to a novel polyoma virus that appears to infect keratinocytes of the inner root sheath of the hair follicle.

Epidemiology

Incidence and prevalence
Trichodysplasia spinulosa is rare with only a small number of reported cases in the world literature.

Age
Trichodysplasia spinulosa has been reported in immunosuppressed patients of all age groups [2].

Ethnicity
All ethnic groups can be affected.

Associated diseases
Most patients with trichodysplasia spinulosa are immunosuppressed following organ transplantation [3]. The disease has been reported in a patient with lymphocytic leukaemia [4]. There have been rare reports of trichodysplasia spinulosa associated with systemic lupus erythematosus [5].

Pathophysiology

Predisposing factors
The trichodysplasia spinulosa polyoma virus (TSPyV) is an opportunistic virus: immunosuppression, whether caused by disease or medication, is a prerequisite for the development of trichodysplasia spinulosa.

Pathology
In affected areas, the hair follicles show abnormal maturation with dilation of the follicular infundibulum, which is plugged by

cornified eosinophilic keratinocytes containing large trichohyalin granules (see Chapter 89). Electromicroscopy shows 28 nm intracellular viral particles consistent with polyoma virus. Immunofluorescence studies using antibodies to trichohyalin and TSPyV VP1 protein have shown that the virus is restricted to the nuclei of inner root sheath cells [6]. However, virus has been identified using molecular techniques in the renal allograft of one affected patient [7].

Causative organisms

Trichodysplasia spinulosa is caused by TSPyV. TSPyV is a group I double-stranded DNA virus of the family Polyomaviridae and genus *Orthopolyomavirus* and is related to the Merkel cell polyoma virus. A study in the Netherlands [8] has shown that the virus is common in the general population with a seroprevalence of 70%; it only becomes symptomatic if a carrier is immunocompromised. In contrast to Merkel cell polyoma virus, TSPyV causes dysplasia rather than neoplasia.

Clinical features (Figure 87.13)

History

The original patient described by Haycox *et al.* [1] was a heart transplant recipient who developed alopecia of the eyebrows followed by the appearance of multiple painful follicular papules with spiny excrescences which then rapidly coalesced to form a leonine facies.

Presentation

Shiny follicular papules with central spiny keratotic spikes form on the facial skin. The condition progresses rapidly with multiple disfiguring lesions. Alopecia of the eyebrows and scalp may occur. The condition is usually asymptomatic but may be mildly pruritic.

Differential diagnosis

Trichodysplasia spinulosa is a very distinctive disease but in the early stages may be confused with other follicular keratotic dermatoses including the following:
- Keratosis pilaris.
- Lichen nitidus.
- Follicular mucinosis.

Complications and co-morbidities

All patients are immunocompromised.

Disease course and prognosis

Trichodysplasia spinulosa progesses unless specifically treated or unless immunosuppression is withdrawn. There have been no long-term reports of this disease so long-term prognosis is speculative.

Investigations

Skin biopsy shows characteristic changes in the hair follicle. The virus can be identified using molecular or immunofluorescence techniques.

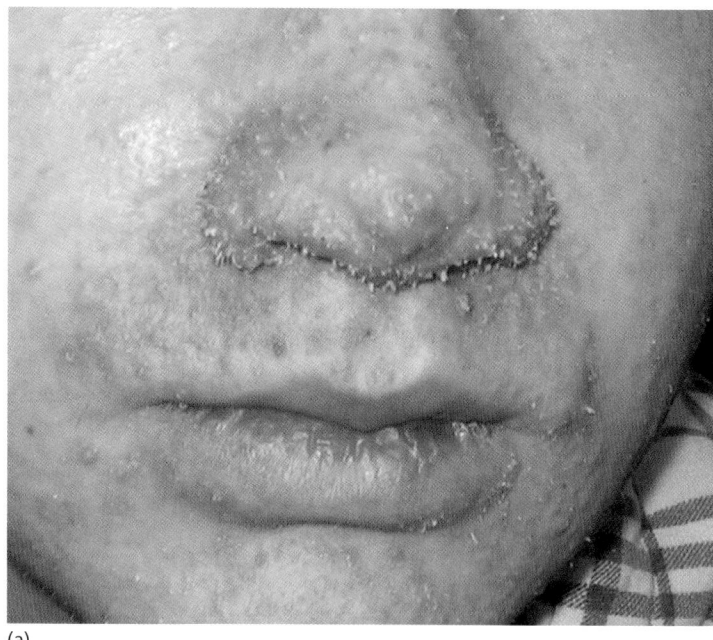

(a)

(b)

Figure 87.13 (a,b) Trichodysplasia spinulosa: multiple keratotic spicules on the nose of a heart transplant recipient. (Reproduced from *PLOS Pathogens* http://journals.plos.org/plospathogens/article?id=10.1371/journal.ppat.1001024 last accessed October 2015, courtesy and coyright of E. van der Meiden *et al.*, University of Michigan, USA © 2010 van der Meijden *et al.*)

Management

Trichodysplasia spinulosa is a persistent disease. In organ transplant recipients, reduction of immunosuppression has resulted in some improvement. Antiviral treatment has been successful in some patients [9,10] and one patient responded to surgery followed by topical tazarotene [11]. Firm guidance on management cannot be given due to the paucity of reports but oral antiviral therapy would appear to be the treatment of choice.

Treatment ladder

First line
- Reduction of immunosuppression: if feasible
- Oral valganciclovir: successful response has been reported in four patients
- Topical cidofovir: four of five patients who were treated improved [10]

Second line
- Topical tazarotene: one patient improved with topical tazarotene after skin lesions were shaved off under local anaesthesia [11]

Third line
- One patient treated with a topical compound of aciclovir, 2-deoxy-D-glucose, and epigallocatechin (green tea extract) showed improvement [12]

Flegel disease

Definition and nomenclature
Flegel disease (FD) is a rare dermatosis, first described by Flegel in 1958 [1]. It is characterized by the presence of flat keratotic papules on the lower legs and dorsa of the feet. It is a disease of the older adult, but it can be seen occasionally in younger persons.

Synonyms and inclusions
- Hyperkeratosis lenticularis perstans

Introduction and general description
FD is a rare dermatosis characterized by flat keratotic papules on the lower legs and dorsa of the feet. It is a disease of the older adult, but can appear occasionally in younger persons. Each papule measures 1–5 mm in diameter and is topped by a horny keratotic scale, the removal of which causes bleeding. Lesions are commonest on the dorsa of the feet and the lower legs, typically in older patients.

Epidemiology

Incidence and prevalence
FD is a rare disease and there are no prevalence data in the literature.

Age
FD is most commonly seen in mid to late adult life but cases in children have been reported [2].

Ethnicity
FD is seen in all racial groups but appears to be more common in white populations.

Associated diseases
A number of reports have suggested an association between endocrinopathies and FD [3], particularly diabetes.

Pathophysiology
The cause of FD is unknown. A number of hypotheses have been put forward. Some authors have suggested that UV light may play a role [4]. Electron microscopic studies have demonstrated a lack or paucity of Odland bodies in the stratum granulosum, suggesting a possible mechanism for localized hyperkeratosis [5,6]. Immunological studies have shown that the dermal infiltrate in FD is predominantly T cell and that these cells are activated, suggesting that the disease could be the result of a cell-mediated immune response to keratinocytes [7].

Pathology
Microscopic examination of a well-developed papule shows characteristic histological features. The stratum corneum is markedly thickened, eosinophilic and compact, and the underlying stratum spinosum is compressed. Patchy parakeratosis may be present. The intervening granular layer is thinned or absent. The surrounding epidermis can show papillomatosis. There is a lymphocytic dermal infiltrate in a band-like distribution beneath the affected epidermis [5].

Genetics
Both a familial and a non-familial variant have been recognized. At least in some cases, the disease is inherited as an autosomal dominant trait [8].

Environmental factors
Some authors suggest that exposure to the sun may be involved in the pathogenesis of FD.

Clinical features (Figure 87.14)

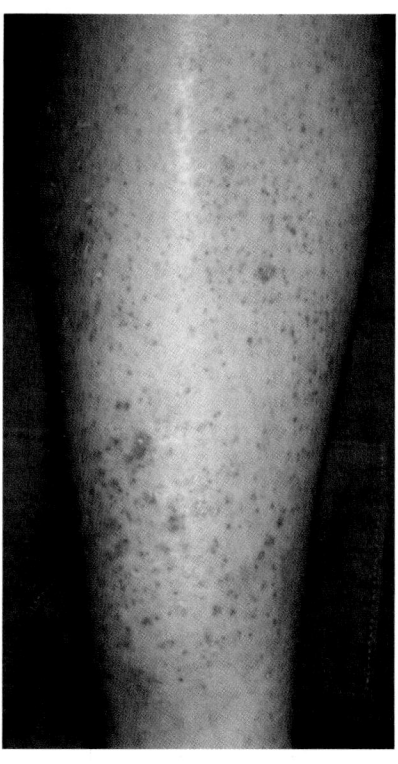

Figure 87.14 Flegel disease: multiple tiny thorn-like keratotic papules on the skin of the lower leg.

Box 87.6 Differential diagnosis of Flegel disease
- Actinic keratosis
- Arsenical keratosis
- Darier disease
- Acquired reactive perforating dermatosis (Kyrle disease)
- Porokeratosis
- Stucco keratosis

Synonyms and inclusions
- Multiple minute digitate hyperkeratoses
- Spiny hyperkeratosis
- Digitate keratoses
- Disseminated spiked hyperkeratosis
- Familial disseminated filiform hyperkeratosis
- Filiform keratoses
- Minute aggregated keratoses

History
Small keratotic papules develop on the lower legs in middle-aged to elderly patients and slowly spread up the legs. The lesions are asymptomatic.

Presentation
The lesions of FD are red/brown non-follicular keratotic papules measuring 1–5 mm in diameter. Rarely, the disease may affect the outer ear lobes, arms, palms, soles and oral mucosa [9]. If the scale is removed, the site is red and may have bleeding points. Involvement of the trunk is unusual but a generalized form of FD has been described [10].

Differential diagnosis
Diseases with localized areas of hyperkeratosis are considered in the differential diagnosis, as listed in Box 87.6.

Investigations
Skin biopsy will show the characteristic changes and will confirm a clinical diagnosis.

Management
FD is difficult to treat and medical treatment needs to continue for prolonged periods.

First line
The most consistent treatment results have been achieved with 5% fluorouracil, which needs to be continued for several months [11,12,**13**], dermabrasion and local excision [14].

Second line
Various systemic retinoids have been used with variable responses. Lesions tend to reform on cessation of treatment [15].

Third line
Treatment with topical vitamin D analogues have been reported with variable and inconsistent results [16,17]. Topical retinoids and keratolytics have been used with disappointing results [12].

Multiple minute digitate keratoses

Definition and nomenclature
The term multiple minute digitate keratoses (MMDK) describes a rare clinically distinctive but aetiologically heterogeneous disorder of epidermal keratinization occurring in adults.

Introduction and general description
Multiple minute digitate hyperkeratoses is a term introduced by Goldstein in 1967 [1] and more fully characterized by Ramselaar and Toonstra in 1999 [2] for a rare disorder of keratinization in which multiple tiny spiky cutaneous keratoses appear in adult life. The more appropriate label MMDK is preferred to define this disorder [3].

Epidemiology

Incidence and prevalence
MMDK is a rare disorder.

Age
The genetic form generally presents between the ages of 20 and 30 years. MMDK associated with malignancy or other systemic disease presents later in life, typically in the sixth decade of life [4].

Sex
MMDK shows a slight male preponderance [1].

Ethnicity
No racial predilection has been identified.

Associated diseases
Post-inflammatory/reactive cases of MMDK may be associated with solar damage, radiotherapy or may be related to drugs including acitretin, simvastatin and ciclosporin [5].

Sporadic cases of MMDK may be associated with systemic disease or may be paraneoplastic [1,6–8].

Pathophysiology
Three forms of MMDK have been proposed, although these divisions may not be real.

The genetic form appears to be inherited as an autosomal dominant trait and the disease becomes clinically apparent in the second and third decades of life.

MMDK has been associated with various drugs as well as following radiotherapy or chronic sun exposure.

Sporadic MMDK may be a paraneoplastic phenomenon but due to its rarity it is difficult to determine whether the associations with underlying neoplasms which have been noted are simply coincidental [6].

Pathology
Histologically, MMDK shows discrete columns of compact hyperkeratosis arising from acanthotic interfollicular epidermis. The

granular cell layer is intact. The dermis is uninvolved. Under the electron microscope keratohyalin bodies are smaller than normal but Odland bodies are present. The pattern of keratin is otherwise normal [9].

Genetics
The early-onset familial form is inherited in an autosomal dominant fashion.

Clinical features

History
Patients report the sudden appearance of asymptomatic tiny spiny keratoses on the skin.

Presentation
MMDK are typically located on the trunk and proximal limbs and may number in the hundreds (Figure 87.15). They are tiny flesh-coloured spikes that measure up to 2 mm in length and are non-follicular. Case reports have described patients with lesions restricted to the palms and soles [7,8].

Differential diagnosis
Other digitate keratoses including LS, phrynoderma, multiple filiform viral warts, trichodysplasia spinulosa and arsenical keratoses [10].

Investigations
In sporadic cases of MMDK, investigations for age-related underlying malignancy should be performed.

Management
There is no evidence for the treatment of MMDK. Reports have shown response to a number of treatments.

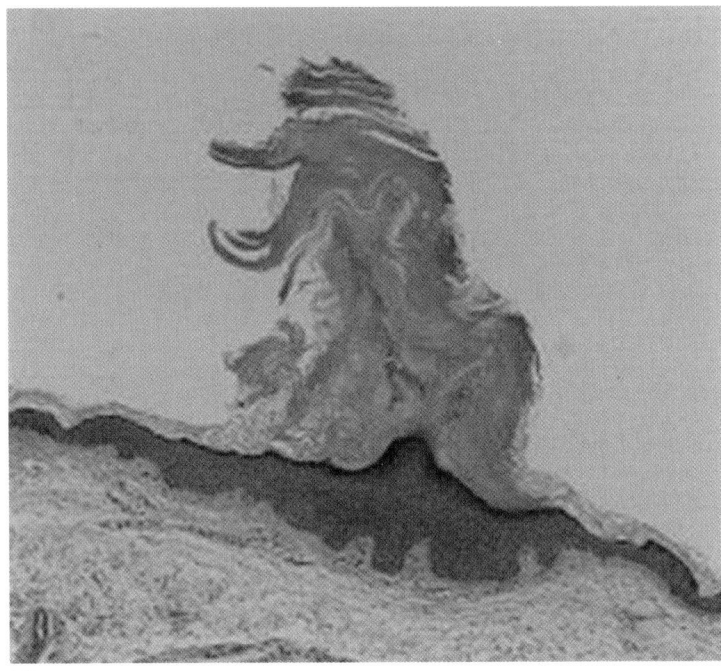

(a)

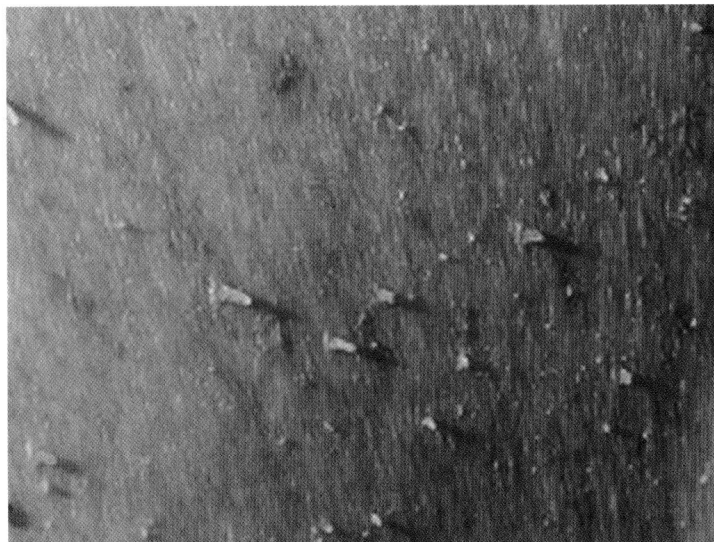

(b)

Figure 87.15 Multiple minute digitate keratoses: photomicrograph of hyperkeratotic spicule (a); close-up view of spicules on the back (b). (From Caccetta *et al.* 2012 [**10**] © 2010 American Academy of Dermatology, Inc. Published by Mosby, Inc. All rights reserved.)

Treatment ladder

First line
- Keratolytic agents, particularly salicylic acid and lactic acid, with emollients

Second line
- Topical retinoids in combination with emollients and urea-containing moisturizers

Third line
- Topical 5-fluorouracil

Porokeratoses

Definition and nomenclature
A porokeratosis is a clonal expansion of keratinocytes which differentiate abnormally but are not truly neoplastic. All forms of

porokeratosis show a thin column of parakeratosis, the cornoid lamella, representing the active border. Squamous cell carcinomas may develop within lesions.

Synonyms and inclusions
- Porokeratosis of Mibelli
- Disseminated superficial actinic porokeratosis (DSAP)
- Linear porokeratosis
- Punctate porokeratosis
- Disseminated actinic porokeratosis
- Disseminated palmoplantar porokeratosis

Introduction and general description

A porokeratosis is a clonal expansion of keratinocytes which differentiate abnormally but are not hyperproliferative. Porokeratoses may present as single or multiple lesions and may be localized or disseminated. All forms show a thin column of parakeratosis, the cornoid lamella, representing the active border [1,2].

Mibelli described the classical form which bears his name in 1893. This was followed by descriptions of superficial and disseminated forms of porokeratosis by Respighi in 1893, linear porokeratosis in 1918, DSAP by Chernosky in 1966, disseminated palmoplantar porokeratosis by Guss in 1971 and punctate porokeratosis by Rahbari in 1977.

A working clinical classification of porokeratoses is shown in Box 87.7 [1,2]. Lesions start as papules or plaques which develop into annular lesions with a thin, often thread-like elevated rim. Diagnosis is confirmed by finding the pathognomonic cornoid lamella on histological examination (Figure 87.16). It is likely that the different variants are related, as more than one type of porokeratosis has been reported in the same patient [3] and different types have been reported in different members of the same family [4]. Malignant change with development of squamous cell carcinoma may occur.

Epidemiology

Incidence and prevalence

Porokeratosis is listed as a rare disease and classified as such by Orphanet and the Office of Rare Diseases (ORD) of the National Institutes of Health. DSAP is the most common form [5].

Age

Classical porokeratosis of Mibelli and linear porokeratosis typically appear during infancy or childhood. Punctate palmoplantar porokeratosis and disseminated palmoplantar porokeratosis usually appear in adolescence while DSAP generally first manifest in adult life.

Sex

Porokeratosis of Mibelli, genital porokeratosis and punctate porokeratosis are more common in males whereas DSAP is more common in women. Linear porokeratosis has an equal sex ratio.

Box 87.7 Clinical classification of porokeratoses

Localized forms
- Porokeratosis of Mibelli
- Linear porokeratosis
- Punctate palmoplantar porokeratosis
- Genital porokeratosis
- Perianal porokeratosis

Disseminated forms
- Disseminated superficial actinic porokeratosis
- Disseminated superficial porokeratosis
- Systematized linear porokeratosis
- Disseminated palmoplantar porokeratosis

Adapted from Sertznig *et al.* 2012 [1] and Ferreira *et al.* 2013 [2].

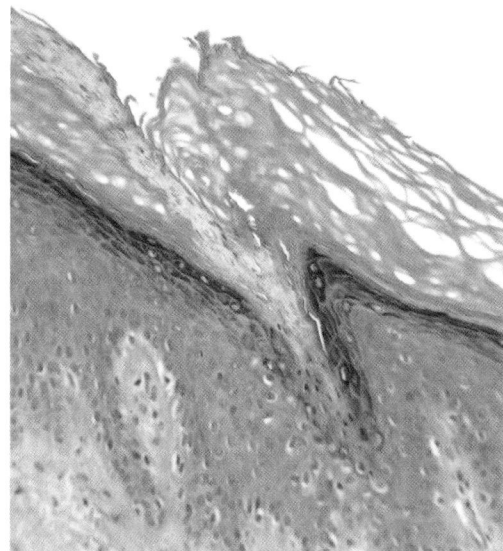

Figure 87.16 Cornoid lamella forming edge of a porokeratosis: a column of parakeratotic keratinocytes can be seen arising from invagination of the underlying epidermis.

Ethnicity

All forms of porokeratosis are seen predominantly in pale fair-skinned ethnic groups.

Associated diseases
- HIV infection [6].
- Crohn disease [7].
- Diabetes [8].
- Liver disease [9].
- Chronic renal failure [10].
- Haematological and solid tumours [11].

Pathophysiology

Porokeratosis represents a clonal expansion of keratinocytes [12] which show abnormal differentiation but are not hyperproliferative [13]. The cornoid lamella, which is the hallmark of porokeratosis, is composed of parakeratotic keratinocytes which result from either faulty maturation or an acceleration of epidermopoiesis. It has been shown that there is reduced keratinocyte loricrin and filaggrin expression and abnormal premature keratinocyte apoptosis underlying the cornoid lamella, indicating dysregulation of terminal differentiation [1]. Furthermore, abnormal DNA ploidy in keratinocytes has been demonstrated [14]. In DSAP mutations in the *SART3* and MeValonate Kinase (*MVK*) genes have been found [5]: *MVK* has a role in keratinocyte differentiation and may protect keratinocytes from apoptosis in response to damage from UV radiation [15].

Predisposing factors

Drug-induced immunosuppression in various diseases including organ transplantation may predispose to porokeratosis [16]. Natural or therapeutic exposure to UV radiation are recognized trigger factors for DSAP and porokeratosis of Mibelli.

Pathology

Identification of the cornoid lamella is essential for the diagnosis of porokeratosis. As this represents the peripheral thread-like border of the lesion it is essential that biopsy includes this border. Histologically, the cornoid lamella is a thin column of tightly packed parakeratotic keratinocytes within a keratin-filled invagination of the epidermis through the stratum corneum (see Figure 87.16) [1]. The underlying stratum granulosum may be absent or attenuated but is normal is other parts of the lesion. There is a perivascular or lichenoid lymphocytic infiltrate. Amyloid deposits have been reported in DSAP and in the intertriginous portion of perianal porokeratosis (porokeratosis ptychotropica). The central portion of a porokeratosis may show epidermal atrophy and areas of liquefaction degeneration.

Genetics

All forms of porokeratosis have been reported to have familial clusters with autosomal dominant patterns of inheritance but with variable penetration. A number of very different chromosomal loci have been identified in DSAP, including 12q23.2-24.1, 1p31.3-p31, 16q24.1-24.3 and 18p11.3 [17]. Linear porokeratosis follows the lines of Blaschko and may be systematized, indicating genetic mosaicism.

Environmental factors

Exposure to UV radiation is a factor in the induction of superficial actinic porokeratosis and porokeratosis of Mibelli.

Clinical features

History

Porokeratoses present with single or multiple papules or plaques which develop into annular lesions with a thin raised border. They are usually asymptomatic but may be pruritic and, if verrucous, may cause discomfort from pressure.

Presentation

Localized forms

Porokeratosis of Mibelli starts as a single or small group of keratotic papules which may be pigmented. These gradually grow over years to form one or more irregular plaques with a thin, keratotic and well-demarcated border. The central area may be atrophic, either hyper- or hypopigmented, hairless and anhidrotic (Figure 87.17). Lesions are generally distributed on the extremities but can occur anywhere on the body. Occasionally, giant and verrucous forms of the disease may occur [18].

Linear porokeratosis generally occurs in infancy as unilateral streaks or plaques of reddish-brown papules along limbs or the side of the trunk, head or neck following Blaschko lines, indicating underlying somatic mosaicism (Figure 87.18). There is a higher risk of malignant change in linear porokeratosis than in other forms of porokeratosis [19].

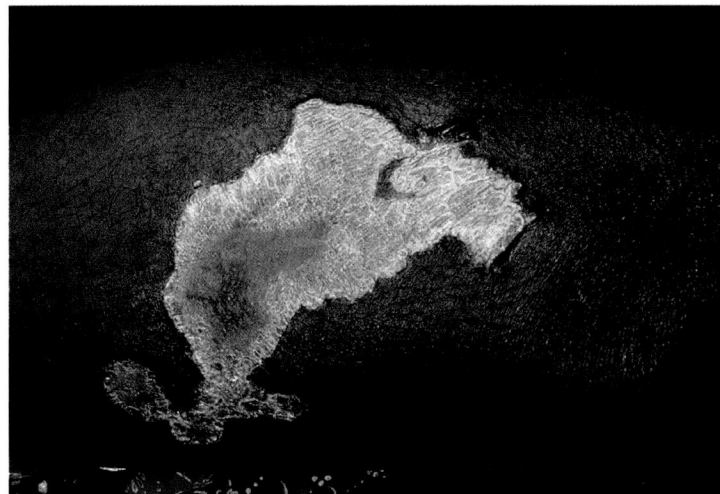

Figure 87.17 Porokeratosis of Mibelli.

Punctate palmoplantar porokeratosis is a rare type of porokeratosis in which seed-like punctate keratoses form on the palms and soles during adulthood [1].

Genital porokeratosis is a rare localized type which it is important to be aware of as it is frequently misdiagnosed clinically. It occurs almost exclusively in men, more often affecting the scrotum than the penis (Figure 87.19) [20]. Vulval porokeratosis is much rarer [21].

Perianal porokeratosis which has been termed porokeratosis ptychotropica [22], is another very rare type which may be very inflammatory and thus elude diagnosis until appropriate biopsies have been taken (Figure 87.20).

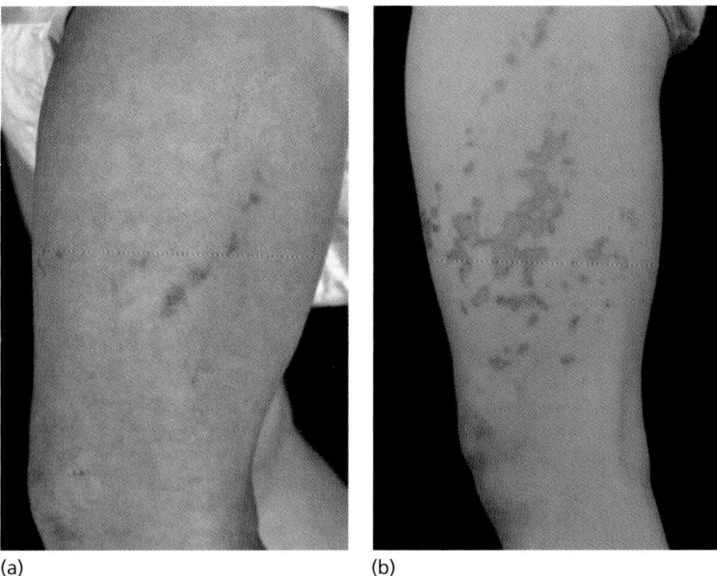

(a)   (b)

Figure 87.18 Linear porokeratosis: irregular linear and polygonal 'Chinese character' plaques developing in a blaschkoid distribution on the thigh, showing progression from 23 months to 5 years of age.

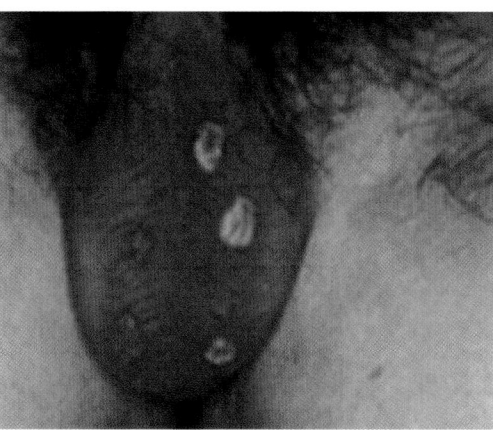

Figure 87.19 Genital porokeratosis: multiple lesions limited to the scrotum. (From Chen *et al.* 2006 [20]. Reproduced with permission from the copyright holder Wiley.)

Disseminated forms

DSAP is the most common form of porokeratosis [1,5], representing more than half of all cases. The condition is often overlooked as the lesions may be quite inconspicuous to the casual observer. Few or multiple flesh-coloured, pink or reddish-brown finely scaling macules with a thin but well-defined raised border start to appear in early adult life, predominantly on the lower legs and arms (Figure 87.21). Palms and soles are not affected. Lesions are generally small, <1 cm diameter and usually asymptomatic. Patients will often give a history of worsening of the condition following sun exposure.

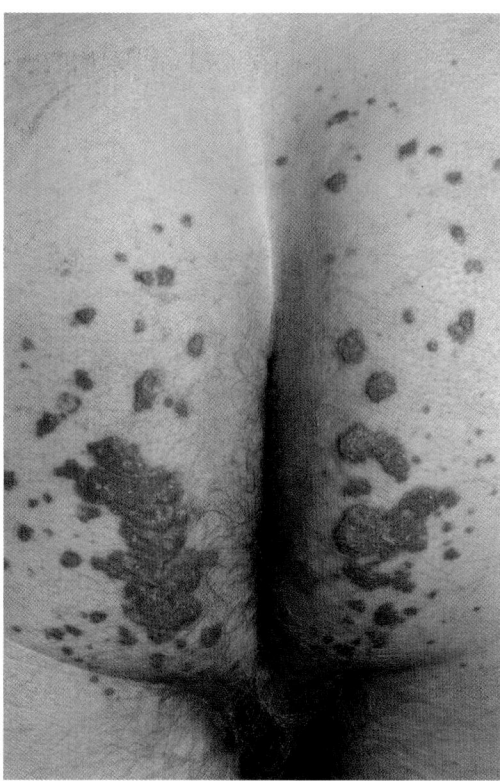

Figure 87.20 Perianal porokeratosis. (Courtesy of Dr P. Laws, Chapel Allerton Hospital, Leeds, UK.)

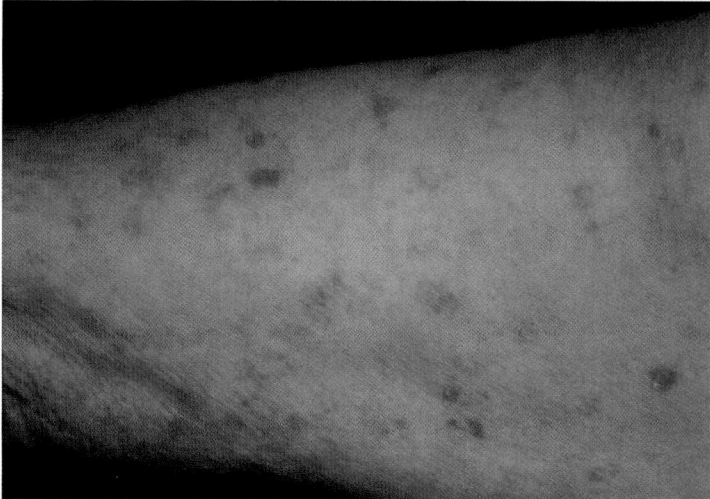

Figure 87.21 Disseminated superficial actinic porokeratosis: view of upper arm.

Disseminated superficial porokeratosis is not necessarily related to sun exposure and will then present in both sun-exposed and sun-protected sites, including sometimes oral mucosa and genitalia. It may be associated with immunodeficiency (e.g. organ transplantation, malignancy, HIV infection) or may develop sporadically during childhood [1].

Systematized linear porokeratosis is a disseminated variant of linear porokeratosis which may be unilateral or generalized and follows the lines of Blaschko [1,23].

Disseminated palmoplantar porokeratosis (porokeratosis palmaris et plantaris disseminata) is a rare generalized form of punctate palmoplantar porokeratosis in which palmoplantar lesions which first appear in the third decade of life are succeeded by multiple widely disseminated wart-like keratoses in both sun-exposed and sun-protected areas including oral mucosa and genitalia and often following Blaschko lines [1,24].

Clinical variants

CDAGS syndrome is a rare autosomal recessive disorder defined as *c*raniostenosis, *d*elayed closure of the fontanelles, cranial defects or deafness, *a*nal anomalies, *g*enitourinary abnormalities and *s*kin eruption, which is often porokeratosis [25].

Differential diagnosis

The main differential diagnosis of porokeratosis of Mibelli and disseminated palmoplantar porokeratosis is psoriasis. Disseminated superficial actinic porokeratosis may be confused with actinic keratosis or stucco keratoses. Differential diagnosis of linear porokeratosis includes linear verrucous epidermal naevus, lichen striatus and incontinentia pigmenti. Punctate palmoplantar porokeratosis may be mistaken for viral warts.

Complications and co-morbidities

Cutaneous malignancies, particularly squamous cell carcinoma may occur. This is most often seen in linear porokeratosis [19].

Regular monitoring of patients is needed to identify and treat skin malignancies, especially in immunosuppressed patients.

Disease course and prognosis
All forms of porokeratosis are chronic with no tendency for spontaneous resolution.

Investigations
Patients presenting with sudden onset of porokeratosis should be investigated for causes of immunosuppression including HIV and haematological malignancies.

Management
In many patients, regular monitoring for evolving skin cancer may be all that is needed. In patients with immunosuppression or in linear porokeratosis where the malignancy rate is increased or in those requesting treatment, there are principally two approaches as follows:
1 Target the underlying abnormal clone of cells using the same approach that is used for actinic keratosis.
2 Target the abnormal keratinization with topical or systemic retinoids.

First line
Cryotherapy, 5-fluorouracil [26], imiquimod [27], curettage and cautery, photodynamic therapy, carbon dioxide laser [28], topical diclofenac [29] and topical vitamin D analogues such as calcipotriol [30] have all been used to treat porokeratosis with varying degrees of success.

Second line
Oral retinoids including isotretinoin and acitretin have been advocated in patients with porokeratosis who are immunosuppressed or have the linear form of the disease in order to reduce the risk of malignant change [31].

Transient acantholytic dermatosis

Definition and nomenclature
Transient acantholytic dermatosis (TAD) is a relatively common transient or persistent monomorphous, papulovesicular eruption mainly affecting the trunk which may be pruritic or asymptomatic It was first described by Grover in 1970 [1].

Synonyms and inclusions
- Grover disease
- Papular acantholytic dermatosis

Introduction and general description
The term TAD is possibly misleading [2], for although it is self-limiting in some patients it may be very persistent in others. The physician needs a high index of suspicion to diagnose this disease, as clinically it resembles a number of inflammatory dermatoses and histologically is similar to several other dermatoses.

Epidemiology
TAD is a relatively common inflammatory dermatosis but there are no incidence data available. In a Swiss study [2], only 24 cases of TAD were found amongst 30 000 biopsies taken. Hospital studies of incidence in hospital referrals in the USA and France have shown an incidence of about 0.1% [3].

Age
TAD is a disease of older patients with a mean age at diagnosis of 61 years but may manifest throughout adult life [3].

Sex
The disease has a male predominance with a male to female ratio of 2.4 : 1 [3].

Ethnicity
TAD is commonest in white populations.

Associated diseases
TAD may be seen in conjunction with a number of other inflammatory dermatoses including psoriasis, asteatotic eczema, contact allergic dermatitis and contact irritant dermatitis. In one study, 11% of patients with TAD were found to have a concurrent inflammatory dermatosis [4].

TAD may also be associated with malignant disease including skin cancer and haematological malignancies [4].

Pathophysiology
The cause of TAD is unknown. A recent study has demonstrated autoantibodies against a number of proteins involved in keratinocyte development, activation, growth, adhesion and motility using proteomic microarrays to analyse immunoglobulin A (IgA) and IgG autoantibodies [5]. It is still unclear whether these autoantibodies are causative or are a reaction to the damage to keratinocytes seen in this disease.

Predisposing factors
TAD has been associated with exposure to natural UV radiation, heat and sweating, which has led to the hypotheses that the eccrine sweat glands are aetiologically involved. The disease has not, however been associated with artificial UV exposure and in some reports is more common in the winter [6]. A number of case series have reported the association of TAD with hospitalized and bedridden patients [7].

Pathology
The primary histological feature of TAD is the presence of small foci of acantholysis with dyskeratosis, intraepidermal clefting and sometimes vesicle formation (Figure 87.22). Five patterns of acantholysis have been described, present either singly or in combination. The incidence of these patterns observed in the three largest studies on TAD are: pemphigus vulgaris-like (47%), Darier-like (18%), spongiotic (9%), pemphigus foliaceus-like (9%) and Hailey–Hailey-like (8%) [2] (see Table 87.1).

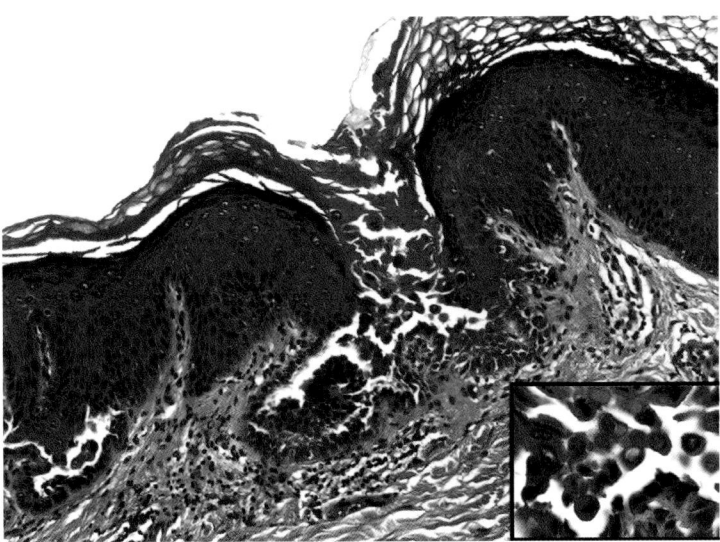

Figure 87.22 Transient acantholytic dermatosis: histopathological image of a papule demonstrating intraepidermal clefting and acantholytic cells (inset). (Reproduced courtesy and with permission of Professor Luis Requena, Universidad Autónoma de Madrid, Spain.)

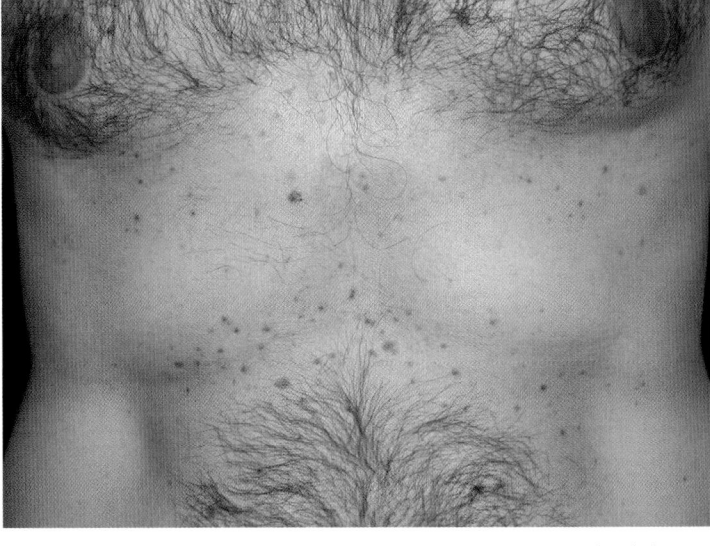

Figure 87.23 Transient acantholytic dermatosis: typical appearance on the abdomen. (Reproduced courtesy and with permission of Professor Luis Requena, Universidad Autónoma de Madrid, Spain.)

Within the dermis, there is usually a sparse lymphohistiocytic, perivascular infiltrate. Lichenoid change with basal vacuolization has been reported; eosinophils and neutrophils may be present [8].

Environmental factors
TAD is reported to be more common in the winter but may be exacerbated by UV exposure and sweating.

Clinical features

History
Patients usually give a history of the sudden onset of itchy papules on the trunk.

Presentation
The normal presentation is of a papulovesicular erythematous eruption on the trunk of a middle-aged or elderly white male. It starts with small papules and vesicles that quickly crust and develop keratotic erosions (Figure 87.23). The eruption is usually

very itchy and the patient presents with multiple excoriations, although in some patients there is no pruritus. In others, the distribution extends to cover the proximal limbs. In many patients, it may live up to its name and be transient, lasting 2–4 weeks; in some it may, however, persist for months or years or follow a chronic relapsing course.

Clinical variants
Some authors use the term 'persistent and recurrent acantholytic dermatosis' to encompass those cases which do not rapidly resolve.

Differential diagnosis
TAD has very characteristic clinical features and usually presents little problem in diagnosis. It may be confused with folliculitis, papular urticaria, scabies and herpes zoster. Galli–Galli disease, a rare acantholytic variant of Dowling–Degos disease occurs in a similar age group and may clinically resemble TAD but is usually more widespread, affecting the hands and groins and the reticulate pattern seen in Dowling–Degos disease may be present [9].

Complications and co-morbidities
TAD has been shown to be associated with skin cancer and in one study 8% of patients had a haematological malignancy [3].

Disease course and prognosis
TAD may resolve spontaneously after weeks or months or persist for years. There are no clinical or histological prognostic signs in this disease.

Investigations
Skin biopsy will confirm the clinical diagnosis. In view of the raised incidence of haematological malignancies seen in this disease, haematological work-up is advised.

Table 87.1 Histological patterns in transient acantholytic dermatosis [2].

Darier like	Suprabasal acantholysis with scattered dyskeratosis and apoptotic cells (corps ronds and grains) throughout the epidermis
Hailey–Hailey like	Acantholyisis throughout the stratum spinosum with more hyperplastic epidermis and no significant dyskeratosis
Pemphigus vulgaris like	Suprabasal acantholyisis often with large numbers of eosinophils present
Spongiotic	Epidermal oedema causing separation of keratinocytes and prominent desmosomes
Pemphigus foliaceus like	Superficial clefting in the superficial epidermis

Management

Patients should be advised to avoid sunlight exposure, strenuous exercise and heat, all of which may exacerbate the disease.

First line

In many patients, the disease resolves spontaneously after a few weeks and all that is needed is a potent topical corticosteroid for symptomatic relief. Topical vitamin D analogues and calcineurin inhibitors have been used. Systemic antihistamines can be used to control pruritus.

Second line

In more severe cases, short courses of systemic corticosteroids have been shown to give sustained improvement but rebound may occur. Systemic retinoids [10], phototherapy [11] and methotrexate have been used in more severe and refractory cases.

Third line

Recent case reports have claimed benefit from etanercept [12] and, in one patient with recalcitrant TAD, from photodynamic therapy [13].

Keratolysis exfoliativa

Definition and nomenclature

Keratolysis exfoliativa is a common disease of young adults in which discrete areas of superficial skin peeling occur on the palms, starting as air-filled blisters leading to a circinate or irregular annular pattern of scaling. This may be associated with localized hyperhidrosis.

Synonyms and inclusions
- Exfoliative keratolysis
- Dyshidrosis lamellosa sicca
- Focal palmar peeling
- Recurrent focal palmar peeling
- Desquamation en aires

Introduction and general description

Keratolysis exfoliativa represents an acquired form of non-inflammatory skin peeling. The condition was first described by Wende in 1919 [1].

Epidemiology

Incidence and prevalence

Keratolysis exfoliativa is a common condition but there are no epidemiological data available on it.

Age

Keratolysis exfoliativa typically affects young adults.

Sex

No sex predilection described.

Ethnicity

No data.

Associated diseases

Keratolysis exfoliativa may be associated with local hyperhidrosis.

Pathophysiology

The cause is unknown but a recent study suggests that premature corneodesmolysis is the main pathological mechanism [2]. This study showed no association with atopy and filaggrin mutations were not found.

Pathology

Histology and electron microscopy show cleavage and partially degraded corneodesmosomes within the stratum corneum [2]. There is no inflammatory infiltrate.

Environmental factors

Keratolysis exfoliativa often presents in the summer with warmer weather. It can be aggravated by detergents, solvents and irritants.

Clinical features (Figure 87.24)

History

Keratolysis exfoliativa starts as a sudden onset of discrete scaling on the palms of the hands.

Presentation

Keratolysis exfoliativa presents initially as small superficial blister-like air-filled pockets on the palms and palmar aspects of the fingers or occasionally the feet. These are formed as the result of focal separation of superficial layers of corneocytes from the stratum corneum. The roofs of the pockets rupture centrally as they expand centrifugally, leaving a ragged rim of residual scale surrounding an irregular superficial dry erosion. There is no irritation and vesicles are not present. Peeled areas of skin lack normal barrier function and may become dry and fissured, particularly on the fingertips.

Differential diagnosis

Keratolysis exfoliativa is a very distinctive disorder but may be confused with pompholyx, psoriasis, tinea manuum, epidermolysis bullosa simplex or acral skin peeling syndrome (see Chapter 65).

Complications and co-morbidities

Keratolysis exfoliativa may be associated with local hyperhidrosis.

Disease course and prognosis

Keratolysis exfoliativa is generally self-limiting but may recur each summer.

Investigations

No investigations are needed.

Management

Keratolysis exfoliativa is usually a self-limiting condition and treatment may not be needed. Patients should be advised to avoid contact with detergents and other irritants.

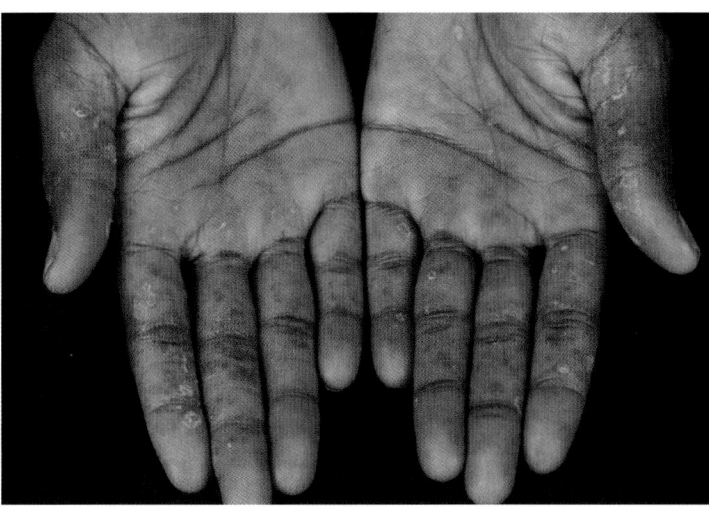

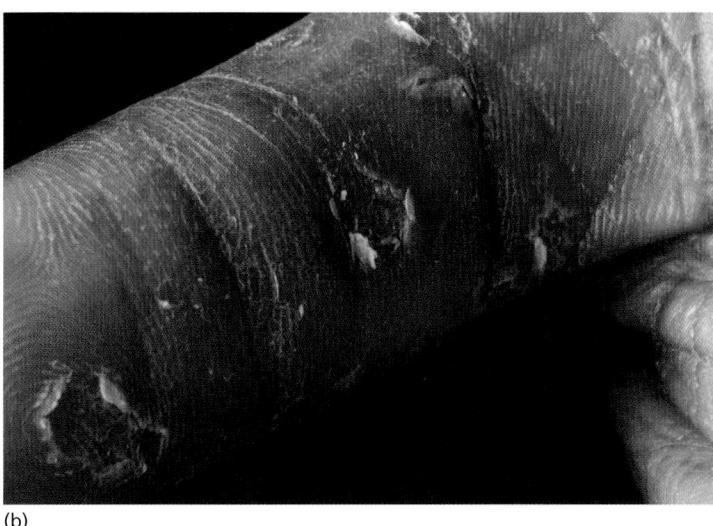

Figure 87.24 Keratolysis exfoliativa: view of the palms (a) with close-up of right index finger (b).

First line

Emollients and moisturisers, particularly moisturisers containing agents such as urea or salicylic acid. Topical steroids may exacerbate the condition by further drying the skin.

Xerosis cutis and asteatosis

Definition and nomenclature

Xerosis cutis (dry skin) and asteatosis (lacking in fat) are alternative terms used to describe an acquired abnormality of the skin which has lost its normal soft smooth surface and feels dry and rough to the touch. This may be the result of a range of endogenous and exogenous factors, especially ageing and low ambient humidity, and is associated with impaired epidermal barrier function. Xerosis cutis may be accompanied by pruritus (winter itch) and predisposes to eczematous inflammation (eczéma craquelé or asteatotic eczema).

Synonyms and inclusions
- Xeroderma
- Winter itch
- Dry skin

Introduction and general description

Xerosis cutis is very common and almost physiological in old age. Xerosis cutis (dry skin) and asteatosis (lacking in fat) are alternative terms used to describe an acquired abnormality of skin which has lost its normal soft smooth surface and feels dry and rough to the touch. The condition is associated with an impaired barrier function of the stratum corneum, as reflected by increased transepidermal water loss (TEWL) and reduced water content. Xerosis may however be more accurately assessed by clinical examination [1].

Xerosis is also a common component of eczematous skin diseases, e.g. atopic eczema (atopic xeroderma). This is discussed in detail in Chapter 41.

Epidemiology

Incidence and prevalence

Xerosis cutis is very common and almost universal in old age.

Age

It generally first manifests in the seventh decade of life and progresses with age.

Sex

It appears to be slightly more common in men.

Ethnicity

Xerosis cutis is universal in older age groups. In children, it is said to be more prevalent in sub-Saharan Africa, possibly due to frequent use of soap and high local temperatures: TEWL has been shown to be higher in phototype 6 skin compared to other skin types [2].

Associated diseases

It may be observed in association with marasmus, malnutrition, diabetes, renal failure and renal dialysis.

Pathophysiology

Xerosis cutis was initially thought to be due to reduced sebum production with age. The major factors in the development of dry skin, however, appear to be changes in stratum corneum function and lipids [3]. There is a deficiency of all stratum corneum lipids as well as premature expression of involucrin and persistence of corneodesmosomes [4,5,6,7]. Loricrin expression does not appear to be changed [5]. Dry skin also shows decreases in keratin 1 and 10 and an increase of keratin 5 and 14. In women, oestrogen substitution ameliorates dry skin, indicating a role for sex hormones [8].

Predisposing factors

More common in winter where humidity is low; central heating tends to aggravate the condition. Damage to the stratum corneum by excessive contact with soap or detergents or from frequent and prolonged bathing have each been proposed as additional

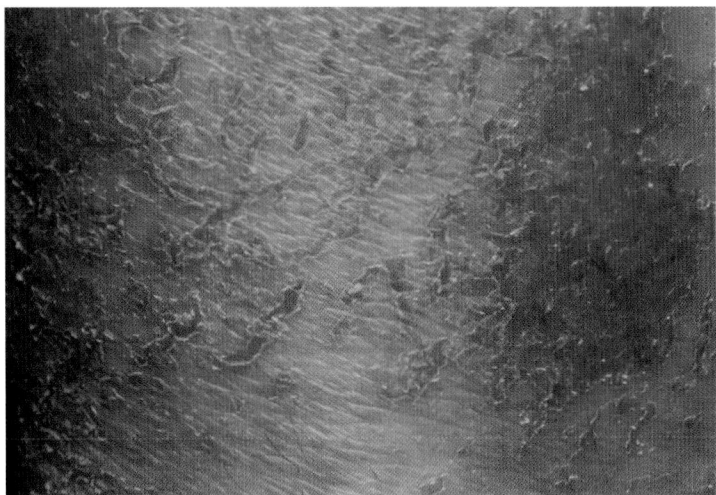

Figure 87.25 Xerosis cutis.

exacerbating factors, although one study found no difference in bathing habits between patients with widespread asteatotic eczema and controls, suggesting that other unknown factors may play a role [9]. Lack of oestrogen is thought to be a contributory factor in postmenopausal women [8].

Pathology
No histological abnormalities apart from slight irregularity in the stratum corneum.

Environmental factors
Low humidity in the winter and the drying effects of central heating exacerbate xerosis cutis. The generally dry atmosphere in hospital wards increases the risk in frail elderly patients confined to

hospital for prolonged periods. Targeted anticancer therapies may induce xerosis [10].

Clinical features

History
Dryness and scaliness of the skin is generally the first manifestation of the condition, followed by itching.

Presentation
Xerosis cutis most often affects the shins and may not affect any other area of the skin. It may become widespread but spares the face, neck, palms and soles. In elderly immobile hospitalized patients, it will frequently affect the abdomen and, in women, the anterior surfaces of the breasts, but spares the back and the undersurfaces of the breasts.

Affected skin looks dull, dry and covered with fine scale which sheds readily. The surface may become crazed with criss-cross superficial cracks in the stratum corneum giving the skin a crazy-paving look (Figure 87.25).

Clinical variants

Asteatotic eczema (eczéma craquelé). Xerosis cutis may progress to an eczematous inflammation in which the fissures in the skin surface become red, inflamed and itchy (Figure 87.26). Eczéma craquelé may sometimes be seen after episodes of acute distension of the skin, usually due to acute oedema (see Figure 87.28).

Differential diagnosis
Dry scaly skin is a component of many inflammatory skin diseases. These include atopic eczema (see Chapter 41), hereditary (see

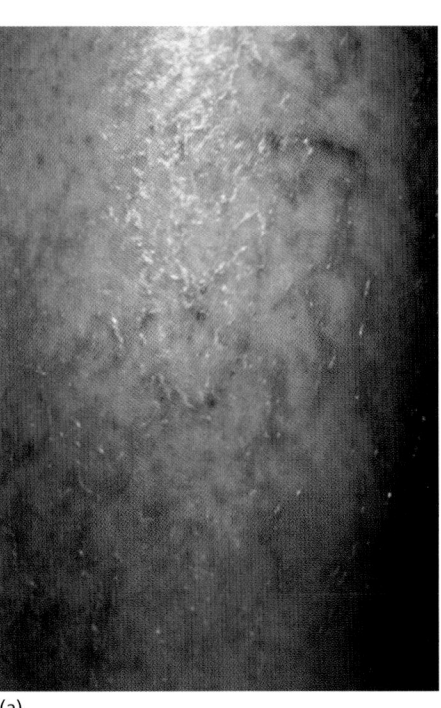
(a)
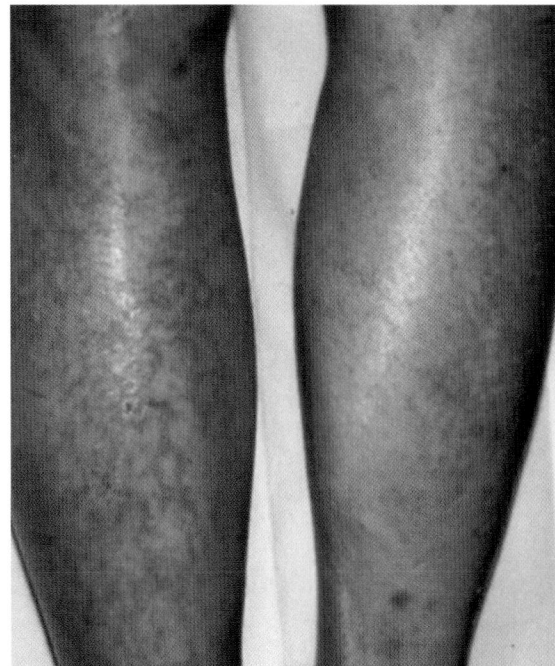
(b)

Figure 87.26 (a,b) Asteatotic eczema.

Chapter 65) and acquired ichthyosis (see earlier). Apart from the latter, these generally manifest at an early age.

Disease course and prognosis
Xerosis cutis is often seasonal, being worse or occurring only in the winter; it tends to worsen and become more persistent with age.

Management
Removal of precipitating factors: patients should be instructed to avoid applying potential irritants to the skin. Simple measures to increase the humidity of centrally heated rooms (e.g. placing a bowl of water close to radiators) may help.

First line
Emollients and moisturisers are the treatment of choice and usually result in rapid improvement.

Second line
If asteatotic eczema develops, anti-inflammatory treatment with a mild corticosteroid ointment may be necessary but long-term topical corticosteroids should be avoided, as these may further damage the skin barrier. Topical tacrolimus and pimecrolimus have also been advocated for the treatment of asteatotic eczema [11,12].

Acute epidermal distension and acute oedema blisters

Definition and nomenclature
There are certain situations where the epidermis is unable to withstand forces which would normally not affect its integrity. Acute distension of uninflamed skin in the absence of disordered epidermal integrity may at times result in epidermal separation or disruption. Most commonly, this is due to acute dependent oedema, as from acute congestive heart failure, and results in large bullae which may be mistaken for bullous pemphigoid. Alternatively, the distension may result in disruption of epidermal cohesion manifesting as eczéma craquelé.

> **Synonyms and inclusions**
> - Acute oedema blisters
> - Eczéma craquelé due to acute cutaneous distension

Introduction and general description
Subepidermal blistering is a well-recognized component of many skin disorders in which there are hereditary or acquired abnormalities affecting the normal adhesion of the epidermis to the dermis. It is also a normal reaction to excessive thermal or frictional trauma.

Bullae may also occur in otherwise normal skin as a consequence of the rapid onset of oedema. The speed of development of such acute oedema appears to be a more important risk factor than the degree of oedema. The blisters respond rapidly to reduction of oedema [1]. It has been described after attacks of angio-oedema as well as in the elderly following the sudden onset or exacerbation of oedema, e.g. after acute congestive heart failure [1,2,3,4].

Epidemiology

Incidence and prevalence
Reported only in case series, but no structured studies available.

Age
May appear in any person who develops oedema acutely, though the elderly appear to be more susceptible [2].

Pathophysiology
Little is known about the pathophysiology of this disease. Ultrasound studies of acute oedema suggests that fluids accumulate more superficially in the dermis than following lymphoedema or chronic stasis [5,6] which may sometimes be a contributory factor.

Pathology
Biopsies have shown marked epidermal spongiosis, and a slight lymphohistiocytic inflammatory infiltrate. Direct immunofluorescence was negative [2].

Clinical features

History
Acute onset of oedema without itching.

Presentation
Tense unilocular non-pruritic bullae appearing in areas of acute oedema (Figure 87.27).

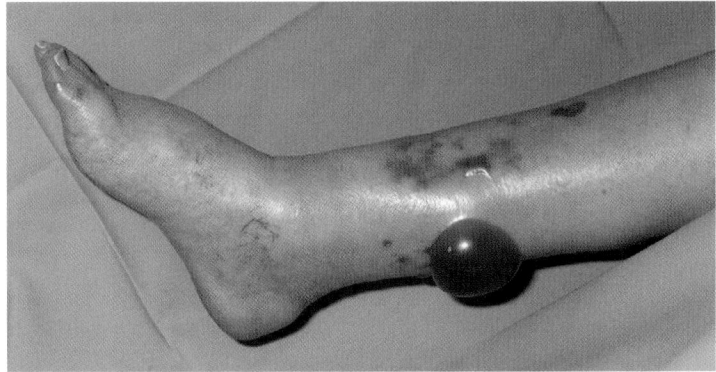

Figure 87.27 Acute oedema blisters in an elderly female: acute swelling of the lower limbs after withdrawal of diuretic therapy given for congestive heart failure (complicated by cellulitis which responded rapidly to antibiotics but left residual purpura).

PART 8: SPECIFIC CUTANEOUS STRUCTURE

Clinical variants

Acute cutaneous distension may alternatively result in disruption of the epidermis as seen in asteatotic eczema with crazing and fissuring of the epidermis and leakage of oedema fluid to the surface (Figure 87.28) [1,7,8].

Differential diagnosis

In the elderly population, autoimmune bullous diseases, particularly bullous pemphigoid, are an important differential diagnosis. The close temporal association with acute oedema, the absence of itching and the lack of spread to other areas of the body form important clues to the diagnosis.

Diabetic bullae (see Chapter 64) may resemble acute oedema blisters but are generally not so tense and they are not associated with acute oedema (Figure 87.29).

Disease course and prognosis

The lesions resolve rapidly as the oedema resolves, leaving no scars.

Investigations

This is a clinically defined disease without known pathognomonic tests. In some cases, the attending dermatologist may wish to rule out autoimmune bullous disorders through direct immunofluorescence or identification of circulating antibodies.

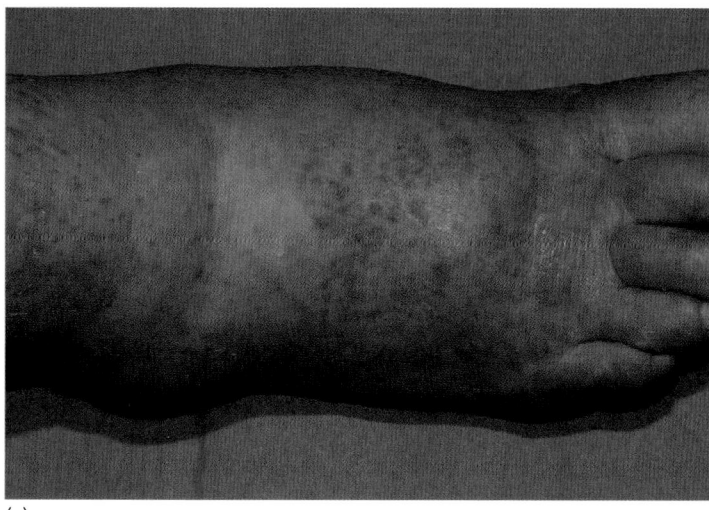

(a)

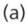

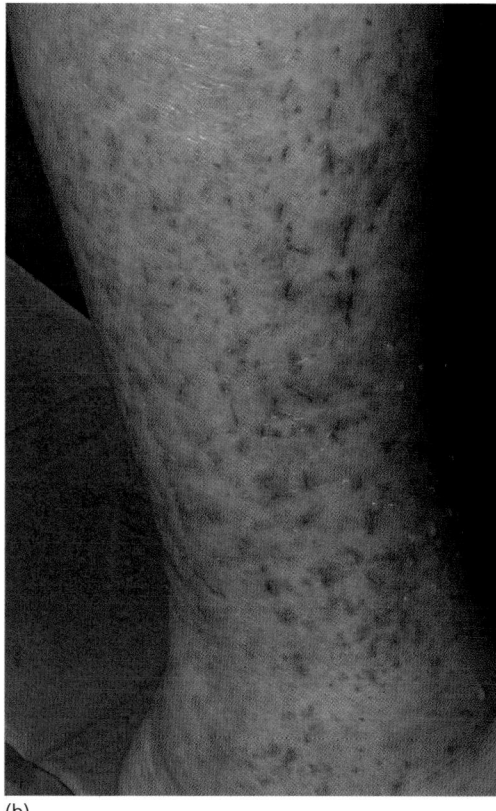

(b)

(c)

Figure 87.28 (a–c) Eczéma craquelé following acute onset of oedema due to congestive heart failure.

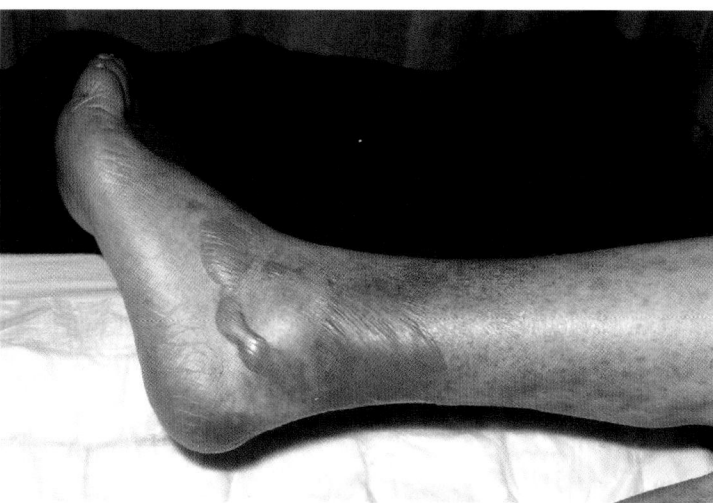

Figure 87.29 Diabetic bullae: recent development of extensive large bullae on the lower legs and feet in the absence of inflammation or oedema in a patient with longstanding diabetes: the bullae are less tense but more irregular in shape and there is no oedema.

Management

First line

Reduction of oedema through appropriate management of the underlying disease. Aseptic puncture of individual lesions to reduce risk of ulceration.

Key references

The full list of references can be found in the online version at www.rooksdermatology.com.

Acquired ichthyosis

1 Patel N, Spencer LA, English JC III, *et al*. Acquired ichthyosis. *J Am Acad Dermatol* 2006;55:647–56.
4 Berrady R, Baybay H, Khammar Z, *et al*. Acquired ichthyosis and haematological malignancies: five cases. *Ann Dermatol Vénéréol* 2012;139:9–14.
12 Dykes PJ, Marks R. Acquired ichthyosis: multiple causes for an acquired generalized disturbance in desquamation. *Br J Dermatol* 1977;97:327–34.
18 Kutting B, Traupe H. Acquired ichthyosis-like skin disease: a challenge for diagnostic evaluation. *Hautarzt* 1995;46:836–40.

Acanthosis nigricans

1 Brickman WJ, Binns HJ, Jovanovic BD, Kolesky S, Mancini AJ, Metzger BE. Acanthosis nigricans: a common finding in overweight youth. *Pediatr Dermatol* 2007;24:601–6.
2 Otto DE, Wang X, Garza V, Fuentes LA, Rodriguez MC, Sullivan P. Increasing body mass index, blood pressure, and acanthosis nigricans abnormalities in school-age children. *J Sch Nurs* 2013;29:442–51.
6 Krawczyk M, Mykala-Ciesla J, Kolodziej-Jaskula A. Acanthosis nigricans as a paraneoplastic syndrome. Case reports and review of literature. *Pol Arch Med Wewn* 2009;119:180–3.
10 Sadeghian G, Ziaie H, Amini M, *et al*. Evaluation of insulin reistance in obese women with and without acanthosis nigricans. *J Dermatol* 2009;36:209–12.
13 Cruz PDJ, Hud JA. Excess insulin binding to insulin like growth factor receptors: proposed mechanism for acanthosis nigricans. *J Invest Dermatol* 1992;98:82S–85S.
15 Berk DR, Spector EB, Bayliss SJ. Familial acanthosis nigricans due to K650T FGFR3 mutation. *Arch Dermatol* 2007;143:1153–6.

17 Koyama S, Ikeda K, Sato M, *et al*. Transforming growth factor alpha-producing gastric carcinoma with acanthosis nigricans: an endocrine effect of TGF alpha in the pathogenesis of cutaneous paraneoplastic syndrome and epithelial hyperplasia of the esophagus. *J Gastroenterol* 1997;32:71–7.
20 Piccolo V, Russo T, Picciocchi R, *et al*. Generalised idiopathic benign acanthosis nigricans in childhood. *Ann Dermatol* 2013;25:375–7.

Confluent and reticulated papillomatosis

2 Scheinfeld N. Confluent and reticulated papillomatosis: a review of the literature. *Am J Clin Dermatol* 2006;7:305–13.
4 Davis MD, Weenig RH, Camilleri MJ. Confluent and reticulate papillomatosis (Gougerot–Caryeaud syndrome): a minocycline-responsive dermatosis without evidence for yeast in pathogenesis. A study of 39 patients and a proposal of diagnostic criteria. *Br J Dermatol* 2006;154:287–93.
7 Yesudian P, Kamalam S, Razack A. Confluent and reticulated papillomatosis (Gougerot–Carteaud). An abnormal host reaction to *Malassezzia furfur*. *Acta Derm Venereol* 1973;53:381–4.
8 Natarajan S, Milne D, Jones AL, *et al*. *Dietzia* strain X: a newly described Actinomycete isolated from confluent and reticulated papillomatosis. *Br J Dermatol* 2005;153:825–7.
10 Inalöz HS, Patel G, Knight AG. Familial confluent and reticulated papillomatosis. *Arch Dermatol* 2002;138:276–7.
12 Jimbow M, Talpash O, Jimbow K. Confluent and reticulated papillomatosis: clinical, light and electron microscopic studies. *Int J Dermatol* 1992;31:480–3.

Pityriasis rotunda

1 Zur RL, Shapero J, Shapero H. Pityriasis rotunda diagnosed in Canada: case presentation and review of literature. *J Cutan Med Surg* 2013;17:426–8.
2 Findlay GH. Pityriasis rotunda in South African Bantu. *Br J Dermatol* 1965;77:63–4.
3 Grimalt R, Gelmetti C, Brusasco A, *et al*. Pityriasis rotunda: report of a familial occurrence and review of the literature. *J Am Acad Dermatol* 1994;31:866–71.
7 Berkowitz I, Hodkinson HJ, Kew MC, DiBisceglie AM. Pityriasis rotunda as a cutaneous marker of hepatocellular carcinoma: a comparison with its prevalence in other diseases. *Br J Dermatol* 1989;120:545–9.

Keratosis pilaris

1 Thomas M, Khopkar US. Keratosis pilaris revisited: is it more than just a follicular keratosis? *Int J Trichol* 2012;4:255–8.
2 Hwang S, Schwartz RA. Keratosis pilaris: a common follicular hyperkeratosis. *Cutis* 2008;82:177–80.
3 Mevorah B, Marazzi A, Frenk E. The prevalence of accentuated palmoplantar markings and keratosis pilaris in atopic dermatitis, autosomal dominant ichthyosis and control dermatological patients. *Br J Dermatol* 1985;112:679–85.
4 Wang CM, Fleming KF, Hsu S. A case of vemurafinib-induced keratosis pilaris like eruption. *Dermatol Online J* 2012;18:7.
20 Poskitt L, Wilkinson JD. Natural history of keratosis pilaris. *Br J Dermatol* 1994;130:711–13.
27 Luria RB, Conologue T. Atrophoderma vermiculatum: a case report and review of the literature on keratosis pilaris atrophicans. *Cutis* 2009;83:83–6.

Lichen spinulosus

1 Boyd AS. Lichen spinulosus: case report and overview. *Cutis* 1989;43:557–60.
3 Friedman SJ. Lichen spinulosus. Clinicopathologic review of thirty-five cases. *J Am Acad Dermatol* 1990;22:261–4.

Keratosis circumscripta

1 Shrank AB. Keratosis circumscripta. *Arch Dermatol* 1966;93:408–10.
4 Brumwell EP, Murphy SJ. Keratosis circumscripta revisited: a case report and review of the literature. *Cutis* 2007;79:363–6.
5 Shams M, Blalock TW, Davis LS. Keratosis circumscripta: a unique case and review of the literature. *Int J Dermatol* 2011;50:1259–61.

Phrynoderma

3 Ayyangar MC. Phrynoderma and nutritional deficiency. *Indian J Dermatol Venereol Leprol* 1967;33:13–24.
4 Ocón J, Cabrejas C, Altemir J, Moros M. Phrynoderma: a rare dermatologic complication of bariatric surgery. *J Parenter Enteral Nutr* 2012;36:361–4.

9 Ragunatha S, Kumar VJ, Murugesh SB. A clinical study of 125 patients with phrynoderma. *Indian J Dermatol* 2011;56:389–92.

11 Nakjang Y, Yuttanavivat T. Phrynoderma: a review of 105 cases. *J Dermatol* 1988;15:531–4.

Trichodysplasia spinulosa

1 Haycox CL, Kim S, Fleckman P, *et al*. Trichodysplasia spinulosa: a newly described folliculocentric viral infection in an immunocompromised host. *J Investig Dermatol Symp Proc* 1999;4:268–71.

2 Schwieger-Briel A, Balma-Mena A, Ngan B, *et al*. Trichodyplasia spinulosa: a rare complication in immunocompromised patients. *Pediatr Dermatol* 2010;27:509–13.

Flegel disease

1 Flegel H. Hyperkeratosis lenticularis perstans. *Dermatologica* 1958;9:362–4.

5 Kanitakis J, Hermier C, Hokayem D, *et al*. Hyperkeratosis lenticularis perstans (Flegel's disease). A light and electron microscope study of involved and uninvolved epidermis. *Dermatologica* 1987;174:96–101.

8 Bean S. Hyperkeratosis lenticularis perstans: a clinical, histopathologic, and genetic study. *Arch Dermatol* 1969;99:705–9.

9 Price ML, Wilson Jones E, MacDonald DM. A clinicopathological study of Flegel's disease (hyperkeratosis lenticularis perstans). *Br J Dermatol* 1987;116:681–91.

13 Pearson LH, Smith JG Jr, Chalker DK. Hyperkeratosis lenticularis perstans (Flegel's disease). Case report and literature review. *J Am Acad Dermatol* 1987;16:190–5.

Multiple minute digitate keratoses

1 Goldstein N. Multiple minute digitate hyperkeratoses. *Arch Dermatol* 1967;96:692–3.

2 Ramselaar C, Toonstra J. Multiple minute digitate hyperkeratoses: report of two cases with an updated review and proposal for a new classification. *Eur J Dermatol* 1999;9:460–5.

3 Wilkinson SM, Wilkinson N, Chalmers RJG. Multiple minute digitate keratoses: a transient, sporadic variant. *J Am Acad Dermatol* 1994;31:802–3.

9 Balus L, Donati P, Amantea A, *et al*. Multiple minute digitate hyperkeratosis. *J Am Acad Dermatol* 1988;18:431–6.

10 Caccetta TP, Dessauvagie B, McCallum D, Kumarasinghe SP. Multiple minute digitate hyperkeratosis: a proposed algorithm for the digitate keratoses. *J Am Acad Dermatol* 2012;67:e49–55.

Porokeratoses

1 Sertznig P, von Felbert V, Megahed M. Porokeratosis: present concepts. *J Eur Acad Dermatol Venereol* 2012;26:404–12.

2 Ferreira FR, Nogueira Santos LD, Nogueira Mendes Tagliarini FA, Lanzoni de Alvarenga Lira M. Porokeratosis of Mibelli: literature review and a case report. *An Bras Dermatol* 2013;88(6 Suppl. 1):179–82.

3 Dover JS, Phillips TJ, Burns DA. Disseminated superficial actinic porokeratosis: coexistence with other porokeratotic variants. *Arch Dermatol* 1986;122:887–9.

15 Zhang SQ, Jiang T, Li M, *et al*. Exome sequencing identifies MVK mutations in disseminated superficial actinic porokeratosis. *Nat Genet* 2012;44:1156–60.

17 Luan J, Niu Z, Zhang J, *et al*. A novel locus for disseminated superficial actinic porokeratosis maps to chromosome 16q24.1–24.3. *Hum Genet* 2011;129:329–34.

19 Happle R. Cancer proneness of linear porokeratosis may be explained by allelic loss. *Dermatology* 1997;195:20–5.

20 Chen TJ, Chou YC, Chen CH, Kuo TT, Hong HS. Genital porokeratosis: a series of 10 patients and review of the literature. *Br J Dermatol* 2006;155:325–9.

23 Hong J-B, Hsiao C-H, Chu C-Y. Systematized linear porokeratosis: a rare variant of diffuse porokeratosis with good response to systemic acitretin. *J Am Acad Dermatol* 2009;60:713–15.

25 Chouery E, Guissart C, Mégarbané H, *et al*. Craniosynostosis, anal anomalies and porokeratosis (CDAGS syndrome): case report and literature review. *Eur J Med Genet* 2013;56:674–7.

Transient acantholytic dermatosis

1 Grover RW. Transient acantholytic dermatosis. *Arch Dermatol* 1970;101:426–34.

2 Streit M, Paredes BE, Braathen LR, *et al*. [Transitory acantholytic dermatosis (Grover disease). An analysis of the clinical spectrum based on 21 histologically assessed cases.] *Hautarzt* 2000;51:244–9.

4 Davis MD, Dinneen AM, Landa N, *et al*. Grover's disease: clinicopathologic review of 72 cases. *Mayo Clin Proc* 1999;74:229–34.

5 Phillips C, Kalantari-Dehaghi M, Marchenko S, *et al*. Is Grover's disease an autoimmune dermatosis? *Exp Dermatol* 2013;22:781–4.

8 Fernandez-Figueras MT, Puig L, Cannata P, *et al*. Grover disease: a reappraisal of histopathological diagnostic criteria in 120 cases. *Am J Dermatopathol* 2010;32:541–9.

Keratolysis exfoliativa

1 Wende GW. Keratolysis exfoliativa. *J Cutan Dis* 1919;37:174.

2 Chang YY, van der Velden J, van der Wier G, *et al*. Keratolysis exfoliativa (dyshidrosis lamellose sicca): a distinct peeling entity. *Br J Dermatol* 2012;167:1076–84.

Xerosis cutis and asteatosis

1 Berry N, Charmeil C, Goujon C, *et al*. A clinical, biometrological and ultrastructural study of xerotic skin. *Int J Cosmet Sci* 1999;21:241–52.

3 Jensen JM, Förl M, Winoto-Morbach S, *et al*. Acid and neutral sphingomyelinase, ceramide synthase, and acid ceramidase activities in cutaneous aging. *Exp Dermatol* 2005;14:609–18.

5 Engelke M, Jensen JM, Ekanayake-Mudiyanselage S, Proksch E. Effects of xerosis and ageing on epidermal proliferation and differentiation. *Br J Dermatol* 1997;137:219–25.

Acute epidermal distension and acute oedema blisters

1 Cox NH, Chalmers RJG, Bhushan M. The acute edema/cutaneous distension syndrome. *Arch Dermatol* 2003;139:224–5.

2 Bhushan M, Chalmers RJ, Cox NH. Acute oedema blisters: a report of 13 cases. *Br J Dermatol* 2001;144:580–2.

CHAPTER 88

Acquired Pigmentary Disorders

Nanja van Geel and Reinhart Speeckaert

Department of Dermatology, Ghent University Hospital, Ghent, Belgium

PART 8: SPECIFIC CUTANEOUS STRUCTURE

SKIN PIGMENTATION AND THE MELANOCYTE

The colour of the skin [1, 2–7]

Normal skin colour is determined by a number of chromophores, the most important of which is melanin. Besides melanin, haemoglobin (in both the oxygenated and reduced state) and carotenoids both contribute significantly to skin colour. Racial and ethnic differences in skin colour are related to the number, size, shape, distribution and degradation of melanin-laden organelles called melanosomes. These are produced by melanocytes (Figure 88.1) and are transferred to the surrounding epidermal keratinocytes. Two types of melanin pigmentation occur in humans [1]. The first is *constitutive* skin colour, which is the amount of melanin pigmentation that is genetically determined in the absence of sun exposure

Rook's Textbook of Dermatology, Ninth Edition. Edited by Christopher Griffiths, Jonathan Barker, Tanya Bleiker, Robert Chalmers and Daniel Creamer.
© 2016 John Wiley & Sons, Ltd. Published 2016 by John Wiley & Sons, Ltd.
Companion website: www.rooksdermatology.com

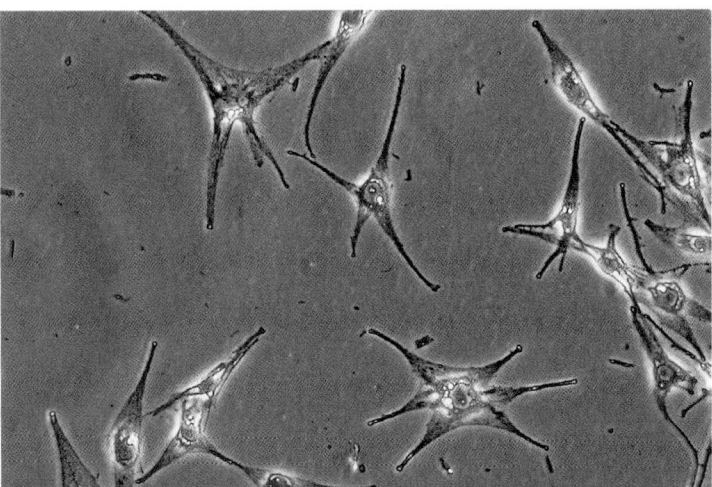

Figure 88.1 Melanocytes in culture.

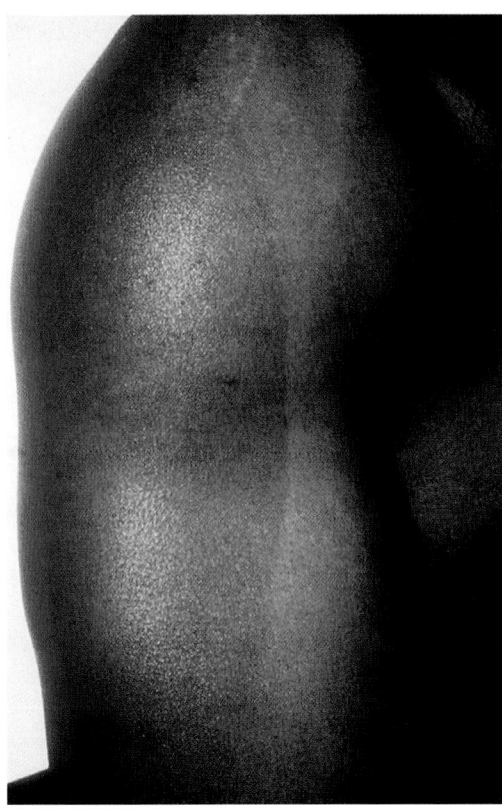

Figure 88.2 Voigt–Futcher lines. (Courtesy of the late Dr R. R. M. Harman, Bristol Royal Infirmary, Bristol, UK.)

and other influences. The other is *facultative* (inducible) skin colour or 'tan', which results from sun exposure. Increased pigmentation can also be due to endocrine, paracrine and autocrine factors [1,2].

The least pigmented human subjects are almost white and have a skin colour similar to that of an albino. In contrast, the most deeply pigmented human subjects are dark brown or black-brown in colour. Most peoples of the world fall between these two extremes and are moderate brown or yellow-brown in colour. The Caucasian peoples of Europe exhibit a light brown colour that can be enhanced by exposure to sunlight. The ability to tan is marked in Mediterranean and Middle Eastern peoples. In contrast, some people from the western parts of northern Europe have fair skin, red hair and a tendency to develop red-brown freckles after exposure to sunlight. The definitive method for the objective measurement of skin colour uses the recording spectrophotometer adapted for reflectance readings [3]. Application of reflectance chromameters in clinical practice includes the measurement of skin colour, the measurement of UV-induced pigmentation and the quantification of the bleaching effect of depigmenting agents [3].

In some ethnic groups, a sharply demarcated linear border is seen between more and less pigmented skin [4]. This has been studied most extensively in the Japanese and in black Americans, and is most frequently observed in darkly pigmented individuals (Figure 88.2). Six major forms (designated A–F) of natural pigmentary demarcation boundaries in the skin have been described [4]. These are summarized in Box 88.1.

A blue colour is seen in the congenital pigmentation termed 'Mongolian spot', a form of dermal melanocytosis that can occur on any part of the body, although it is most commonly found in the sacral region [5,6]. These patches fade after birth, but can persist in certain sites as in the naevus of Ota (see Chapter 132). Blue naevus is an example of acquired blue pigmentation of the skin. The blue coloration of the skin in both of these disorders is due to an optical effect that alters the perceived colour of brown pigment in the dermis. The melanin dispersed in the dermis absorbs incident visible light such that the diffuse reflectance in the longer (red) wavelengths is reduced, giving the pigmented sites a blue appearance.

Carotenoids are lipid-soluble yellow to orange-red pigments that are exogenously produced and can be obtained only from plants such as carrots and tomatoes in the diet. Carotenoids serve a photoprotective role in green plants, but their photoprotective effect in humans is small, even when taken in excess [7]. Carotenoids are found in the epidermis as well as the subcutaneous fat. When present in excess, carotenoids impart a yellowish hue to the skin which may sometimes be prominent [7].

The melanocyte [1–3]

Epidermal melanin unit

The estimated mass of all pigment cells within the body is about 1.5 g. Most of these are melanocytes within the epidermis [1].

Box 88.1 Pigmentary demarcation lines [4] **(designated A–F)**

- **A**: Located on the anterolateral portion of the upper arm (Voigt–Futcher line) (see Figure 88.2)
- **B**: Posteromedial portion of the leg
- **C**: Hypopigmented linear bands on the mid chest in the pre- or parasternal region
- **D**: A vertical line in the posteromedial area of the spine
- **E**: Hypopigmented macules located on the chest extending from the clavicle to the periareolar skin
- **F**: Lines on the face

The process of melanin production within these melanocytes is a three-stage process, which involves not only the production of melanosomes within the melanocyte, termed melanogenesis, but also the trafficking and transfer of these pigment granules via long arborizing dendrites to surrounding epidermal keratinocytes. Each epidermal melanocyte together with the epidermal cells that it serves, comprises an 'epidermal melanin unit', as first described by Fitzpatrick and Breathnach in 1963 [2,3]. Although the number of active epidermal melanin units varies considerably in the different regions of the body (Figure 88.3), the number of keratinocytes served by each melanocyte remains constant. It is estimated that a single melanocyte supplies melanosomes to a group of about 36 viable keratinocytes. The number of melanocytes in the skin varies according to the body location [4]. The intricate interface between melanocytes and their keratinocytes is essential for skin pigmentation. Adequate pigmentation of the skin is as dependent upon successful transport and transfer of melanosomes to keratinocytes as it is on the formation of the organelle itself.

Distribution of melanocytes [1–3]

Melanocytes are situated in the basal epidermis (Figure 88.4). The number of melanocytes within the skin shows little variation between different races or between the sexes. However, the

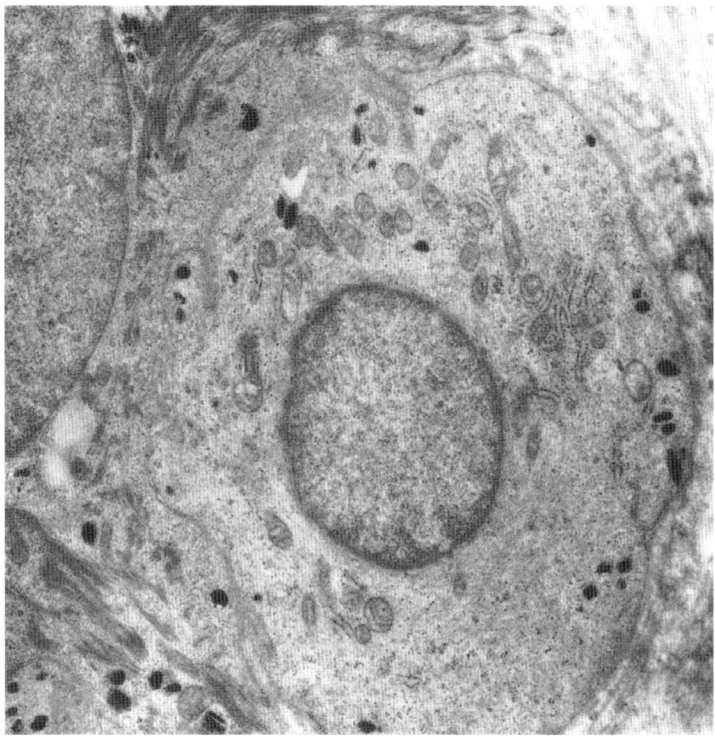

Figure 88.4 Melanocyte in the basal layer of the epidermis.

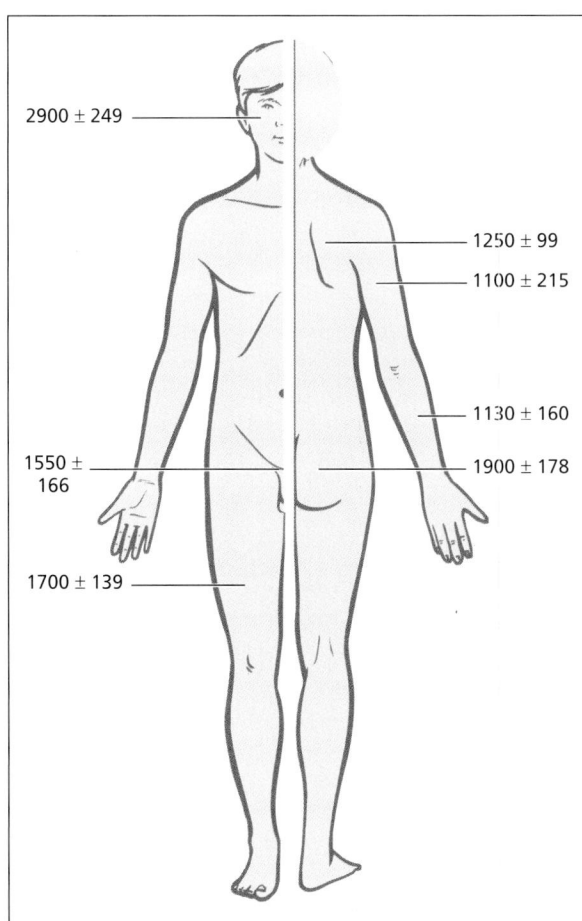

Figure 88.3 Regional variation in the distribution of epidermal melanocytes. The figures are mean values per mm² ± standard error of the mean. (From Rosdahl & Rorsman 1983 [1], reproduced with permission from the copyright holder Nature Publishing Group.)

In the figure: 2900 ± 249; 1250 ± 99; 1100 ± 215; 1130 ± 160; 1550 ± 166; 1900 ± 178; 1700 ± 139

capacity of melanocytes to synthesize melanin, both in the basal state (constitutive colour) and after stimulation (facultative colour) by sunlight, shows great variation. Melanocytes in those with dark skin or with the facility to tan darkly have a great capacity to synthesize melanin and to transfer it to surrounding keratinocytes. In contrast, those with fair skin and lack of tanning facility have very limited capacity. Melanocytes are found in nearly every tissue but are most numerous in the epidermis, hair follicles and the eye [1,2]. A reduction in the number of melanocytes occurs with ageing, with a decrease in melanocyte density of about 6–8% per decade [3]. The density of melanocytes is about two-fold higher in exposed than in non-exposed skin [2].

Melanoblast migration and differentiation

Pigment cells arise from the neural crest [1], a region of the embryonic ectoderm that originates from the margins of the neural plate at the time when it sinks in to form the tubular central nervous system. The developmental potential of neural crest cells has been studied by a variety of means including clonal analysis, cell grafting experiments and lineage-specific marker studies. Collectively, these studies indicate that most early neural crest cells are multipotent, and become fate-restricted over time [2–4]. Melanoblasts originate in the neural crest and migrate laterally, first to the dermis and then to the basal lamina of the epidermis. Immunocytochemical marker studies with the melanocyte-specific HMB-45 antibody have revealed that melanoblasts appear in the epidermis by 7 weeks' gestation, with a cell density of about 50% of that observed at birth [4]. Ultrastructural studies on early human embryos have demonstrated the presence of melanocytes containing melanosomes showing early melanization [5]. HMB-45 staining has revealed an approximately two-fold increase in melanocyte numbers between gestation weeks 10 and 14, possibly due to mitosis of cells already *in situ* rather than due to additional cell migration. Melanocytes associated with hair follicles arrive at their final location by following the downgrowth of epidermal cells in developing hair follicles [6].

Studies in mice have demonstrated that melanocyte lineage segregation starts early in neural crest development, with melanoblasts specified prior to or coincident with their emigration from the neural tube [7]. Initial segregation of melanocyte lineage involves the Wnt/β-catenin pathway [8]. The transcription factor *mi* is relatively specific for melanocytes differentiation, as was first identified in the microphthalmia (*mi*) mutant. *Mi* encodes the transcription factor Mitf, which regulates several melanocyte-specific genes [9,10]. In humans, mutations in *mi* are associated with Waardenburg syndrome type 2A, an autosomal dominant condition characterized by deafness and patchy abnormal pigmentation [11]. *Sox10* and *Pax3* are two other genes associated with Waardenburg syndrome, probably through regulation of expression of Mitf protein [12]. *Pax3* appears to prime cells for differentiation, whereas *Wnt* signalling allows cells to proceed along this route [13].

Much of our knowledge about melanocyte development in humans has been derived from studies on mouse pigment mutants [11]. To summarize this body of work in broad terms, mouse coat colour mutants arise from three main groups: those that affect the subcellular structure of melanocytes, those that disrupt the normal synthesis of melanin and those that alter development and differentiation of normal melanocytes. Where possible in this chapter, molecular and biochemical mechanisms for pigmentary abnormalities in humans with genetic disorders will be highlighted.

Melanosome transport [1–10]

The melanosomes are transported in melanocytes from the cell centre to the periphery. Melanosome transport depends upon effective dendrite formation by melanocytes. UV radiation and melanocyte-stimulating hormone are both known to stimulate this process [1]. Melanocyte dendrite formation requires actin polymerization, which in turn is controlled by the activity of the small guanosine triphosphate (GTP)-binding proteins Rac and Rho [2–4]. These are themselves controlled by regulatory associated proteins. Direct visualization of melanosome trafficking by video microscopy has revealed evidence to suggest that transfer of melanosomes along dendrites occurs on microtubules [5,6], a process driven by dynein (a minus end microtubule motor) and kinesin (a plus end microtubule motor) [7,8]. Dynein binds microtubules and adenosine triphosphate and produces forces which move the dynein and melanosome complex along the microtubule. Both dynein and kinesin remain bound to the melanosomes and their regulation modifies the direction of melanosome movement along the microtubules [9]. Once the melanosomes arrive at the cortical regions of the melanocyte, three individual proteins work together in the final stages of melanosome trafficking. One of these, myosin Va, functions to facilitate the 'capture' of melanosomes at the actin-rich tip of the dendrite [7]. Another, Rab protein, Rab27A, associates with the membrane of melanocytes and then forms a complex with myosin Va and a third protein, melanophylin. The

ability of melanophylin to bind actin, in addition to its ability to link with Rab27A and myosin Va, has led to the postulate that transfer of melanosomes from microtubules to actin filaments at the tip of melanocyte dendrites is the final part of the transport process prior to melanosome transfer [10]. The protein-protein interactions between the members of the Rab27a-Mlph-Myo5a tripartite complex have been extensively investigated and mutations in one of these genes result in genetic pigmentation disorders (e.g. Griscelli syndrome) [11,12].

Melanosome transfer to keratinocytes [1–7]

The successful synthesis of a melanosome, and its transport to the tip of a dendrite, is followed by transfer of the melanosome to the keratinocyte. Both UV radiation and the hormone melanocyte-stimulating hormone (MSH) stimulate this transfer, while niacinamide has been shown to suppress it [1]. However, the exact mechanism by which the melanosome is transferred to the keratinocyte remains unclear. One possibility is exocytosis of melanosomes from the tips of dendrites with subsequent keratinocyte uptake by endocytosis. In support of this, the exocytosis-associated proteins soluble N-ethylmaleimide-sensitive factor attachment protein receptor (SNARE) and Rab3a have both been identified on melanosomes [2–4]. Furthermore, *in vivo* high-resolution time-lapse digital images of this process have identified long dynamic filopedia arising from the melanocyte dendrite tips packed with melanosomes [4]. The filopedia have been observed to attach and detach from the keratinocyte membrane: melanocytes have been observed travelling in both directions within the filopedia [4]. Work from several groups has revealed that lectins and their glycosolated ligands may function as receptor-ligand pairs in these melanocyte–keratinocyte interactions [5–7]. Recently, electron microscopy analysis has provided additional evidence for exocytosis and endocytosis as the predominant mechanism of melanin transfer. Nonetheless, other hypotheses still exist [8]. In the theory of cytophagocytosis, melanosome-laden protrusions from the dendritic tips of the melanocyte breach the cell membrane of the keratinocyte. Subsequently, these protrusions are engulfed by the closure of the cell membrane of the keratinocyte. This results in the uptake of melanin granules by keratinocytes. The fusion hypothesis consists of the formation of connecting pores or channels between the membrane of melanocytes and keratinocytes facilitating the transport of melanosomes. A final theory suggests the formation of membrane vesicles containing melanosome globules which are released from the melanocytes [9]. This is followed by the fusion of these particles with the keratinocyte cell membrane or by phagocytosis. However, until now, none of these modes of transfer has been fully confirmed [10].

Melanocyte culture [1–8]

Melanocytes fail to grow and usually die in culture media used for skin fibroblasts or keratinocytes. In contrast to many other cell types, melanocytes do not produce any of the growth factors that are known to stimulate them [1]. Following an intensive search, the first highly effective natural melanocyte mitogen was identified as basic fibroblast growth factor (now termed FGF2) [2]. As more mitogens for melanocytes emerged, it was apparent that a combination of synergistic growth factors was required to stimulate quiescent or moribund melanocytes in culture [1,3]. Additional stimulatory peptides include mast cell growth factor/ stem cell factor (M/SCF, also known as Kit ligand and Steel factor), hepatocyte growth factor/scatter factor (HGF/SF), endothelins and, to a lesser degree, MSH. In the presence of FGF2, phorbol ester and cyclic adenosine monophosphate these peptides act synergistically on melanocytes in culture [1,4]. A more recent addition to the list of melanocyte mitogens is leukaemia inhibitory factor (LIF) [5]. With the exception of FGF2, most of these factors also promote melanocyte differentiation [6,7]. Endothelin 1 (ET1) can also sustain the viability of human melanocytes in the absence of other growth factors and stimulate the formation and elongation of dendrites [4,8].

Biochemistry of melanogenesis [1,2,3,4,5]

Melanins are usually classified into two main groups: the brown to black insoluble eumelanins, and the yellow to reddish-brown alkali-soluble phaeomelanins (Box 88.2). Both pigments are derived from dopaquinone, which is formed by the oxidation of the common amino acid L-tyrosine by tyrosinase. These two types of melanin are different in size, shape and packaging of their granules. Eumelanosomes have a more elliptical form, while phaeomelanin has a rounded contour. Whether eumelanin or phaeomelanin is produced is determined primarily by the melanocortin 1 receptor, which is itself under the control of α-MSH and agouti signal protein [1,2].

Eumelanin formation

Dopaquinone is a highly reactive intermediate and in the absence of sulfhydryl compounds it forms cyclodopa. The redox exchange between cyclodopa and dopaquinone then gives rise to the red intermediate, dopachrome, and dopa. Dopachrome then rearranges to 5,6-dihydroxyindole (DHI) and to a lesser extent to 5,6-dihydroxyindole carboxylic acid (DHICA). Finally, DHI and DHICA are oxidized and polymerized to produce eumelanins.

Box 88.2 Main types of epidermal melanin pigments. (Reproduced with permission from the copyright holder Wiley, courtesy of Prota 1988 [4].)

Eumelanins
- Brown or black nitrogenous pigments, insoluble in all solvents, which arise by oxidative polymerization of 5,6-dihydroxyindoles derived biogenetically from tyrosine

Phaeomelanins
- Alkali-soluble pigments, ranging from yellow to reddish-brown; most of them contain sulphur in addition to nitrogen and arise by oxidative polymerization of cysteinyl-dopa via 1,4-benzothiazine intermediates

Trichochromes
- A variety of sulphur-containing phaeomelanic pigments with a well-defined structure, characterized by a $\Delta^{2,2'}$-bi(1,4-benzothiazine) chromophore

---

Dopachrome tautomerase and Tryp1 (DHICA oxidase) are now both recognized as having a role alongside tyrosinase in the regulation and promotion of eumelanogenesis [3].

Phaeomelanin formation

In contrast to eumelanins, phaeomelanins contain sulphur in addition to nitrogen and are formed from cysteinyldopa (Figure 88.5). Further oxidation of the thiol adducts leads to the formation of phaeomelanin via benzothiazine intermediates. Most melanin pigments in skin are mixtures or copolymers of eumelanins and phaeomelanins. However, the situation is complicated by the fact that some phaeomelanin-like pigments may be structural variants of eumelanins [4]. Thus, in the presence of metal ions, black insoluble eumelanin may be oxidized chemically or photochemically to a soluble form (melanin-free acid), which is light in colour [5,6].

Trichochromes

A further complication is that red human hair contains, in addition to phaeomelanins, small amounts of intensely coloured pigments known as trichochromes [5,7]. Originally isolated from the red feathers of New Hampshire hens, trichochromes are sulphur-containing pigments of a well-defined structure, of which six variants have so far been identified (Figure 88.6).

Regulation of human pigmentation by UV light and by endocrine, paracrine and autocrine factors

Regulation of human melanocytes is complex: in addition to a direct stimulatory effect of UV radiation, there are also effects mediated by endocrine, paracrine and autocrine factors. Constitutive melanin content is determined by the rate of synthesis by melanocytes and by the rate and mode of melanosome delivery to keratinocytes. The response of cultured melanocytes to UV radiation involves growth arrest in conjunction with increased melanogenesis. A differential response is observed between melanocytes derived from individuals of skin types I or II and those from skin types V or IV, with the former showing more prolonged growth arrest, more cyclobutane pyrimidine dimers and less melanogenesis. Exposure of human skin to UV radiation induces a number of epidermal cytokines and growth factors which in turn induce proliferation of melanocytes and/or melanogenesis. Many devoted sun-worshippers know that by deliberately overdosing on sun exposure, the inflammatory sunburn that ensues is more effective at inducing tanning than a more patient, non-burning approach.

Melanocyte response to UV radiation

Skin exposed to sunlight is associated with an increased number of active melanocytes when compared with skin protected from the sun within the same individual. Friedmann and Gilchrest [1] were the first to demonstrate this direct responsiveness in cultured melanocytes by showing that irradiation with solar-simulated UV light resulted in a dose-dependent decrease in proliferation and an increase in pigment production. More recently, research using

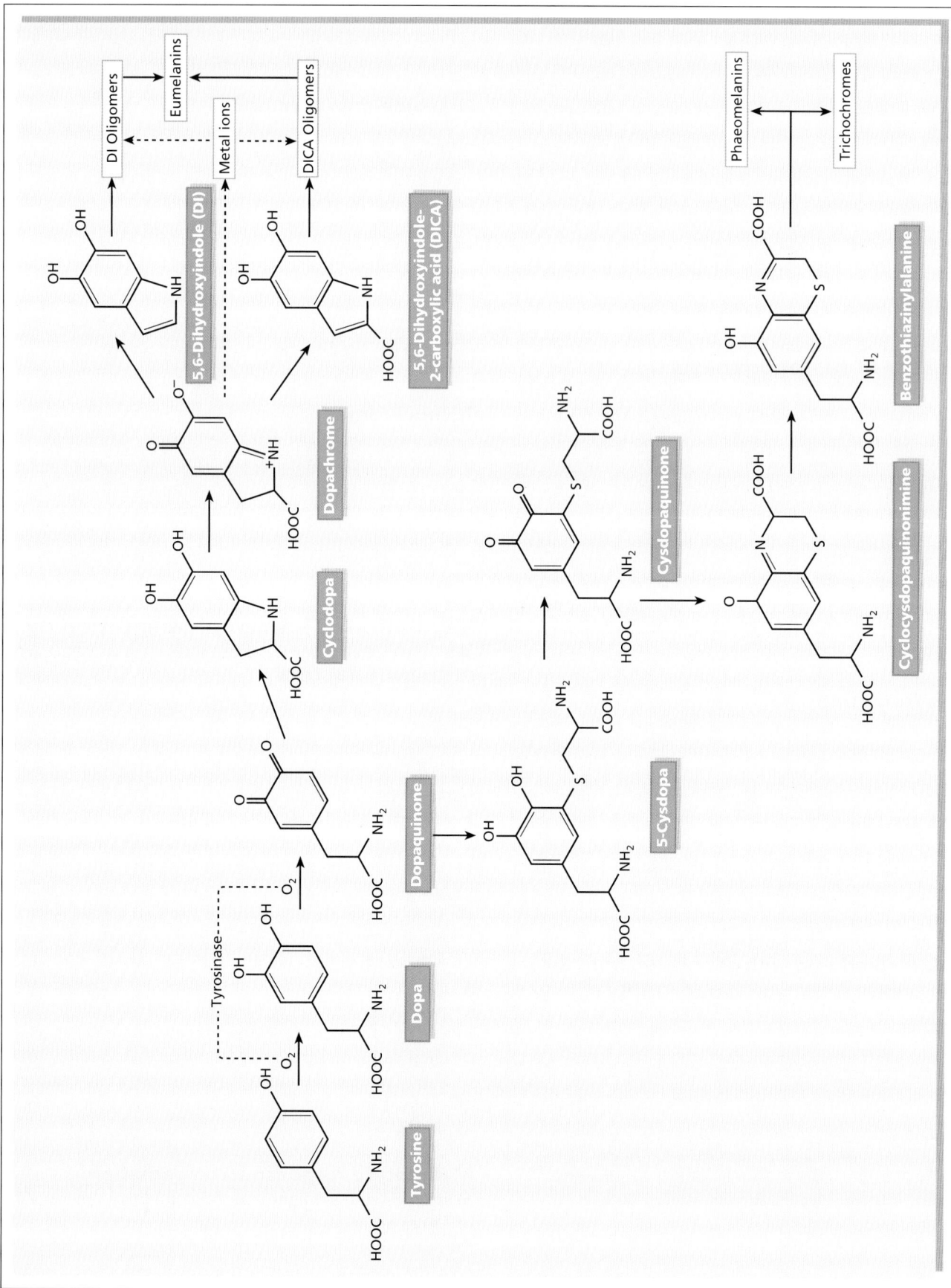

Figure 88.5 A simplified overview of the major metabolic pathways in the synthesis of melanins and trichochromes. (From Prota 1988 [4], with permission from the copyright holder Wiley.)

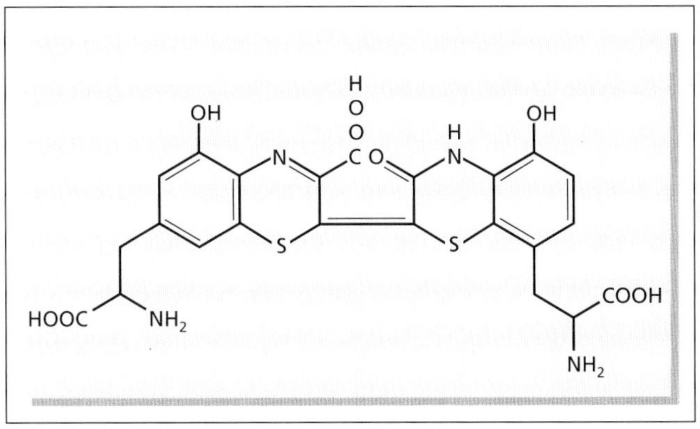

Figure 88.6 Structure of trichochrome B, one of six trichochromes so far identified.

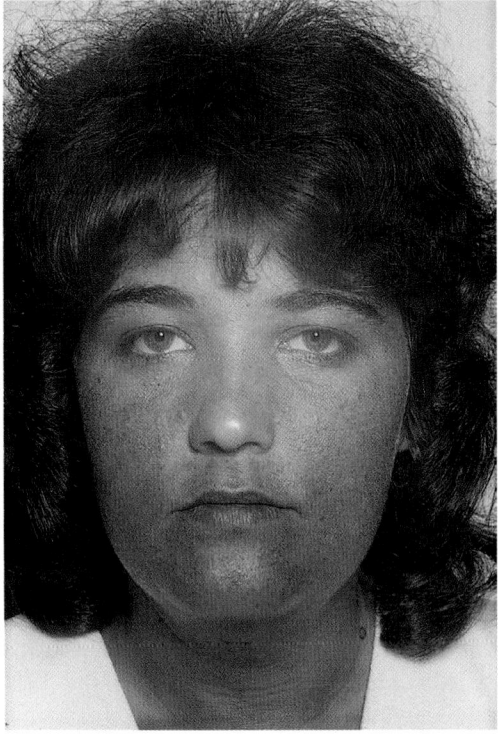

Figure 88.7 Diffuse hyperpigmentation with darkening of the hair and mucous membranes in a woman with Nelson syndrome following bilateral adrenalectomy.

sublethal doses of UVB showed inhibition of melanocyte proliferation as a result of arrest in G_2 phase of the cell cycle, and an increased tyrosinase activity and melanin content [2]. Melanocytes derived from different skin types all showed a similar pattern of response [2]. Subsequent research has confirmed that this UV-induced growth arrest of melanocytes is related to increased levels of the tumour suppressor gene product p53, with lightly pigmented melanocytes experiencing a more prolonged growth arrest and a more sustained increase in the p53 protein than occurs in darkly pigmented melanocytes [3]. Furthermore, lightly pigmented melanocytes show more cyclobutane pyrimidine dimers (a reliable marker for UV-induced DNA damage) after UV irradiation than occurs in heavily pigmented melanocytes [3]. In addition to increased activity of melanocyte tyrosinase, sun exposure leads to elongation and branching of melanocyte dendrites, and an increase in the number and size of melanosomes.

Melanocyte regulation by endocrine factors

The effects of oestrogens on cutaneous pigmentation have been recognized for more than 60 years [4,5]. High levels of oestrogens during pregnancy are implicated in the increased pigmentation that occurs on the face, areola, lower central abdomen and genitalia. Melanocytes express oestrogen receptors and increased levels of oestradiol stimulate enzymes involved in melanogenesis (e.g. tyrosinase, tyrosinase-related protein 1 and tyrosinase-related protein 2) [6].

In Addison disease, the diffuse brown hyperpigmentation results from the melanogenic action of melanocortins derived from the pituitary. The melanocortins are all derived from a precursor molecule, pro-opiomelanocortin. Other melanocortins released from the pituitary in increased quantities in Addison disease include adrenocorticotropin hormone (ACTH), β-lipotrophin, α-MSH, β-MSH and γ-MSH. These peptides all have a stimulatory effect on melanocytes [7], and, in the absence of negative feedback to inhibit their secretion, the hyperpigmentation produced is insidious and progressive (Figure 88.7) [8]. A similar mechanism takes place in Cushing syndrome, in which the hyperpigmentation is caused by an overproduction of ACTH from a corticotrophic adenoma or an ectopic non-pituitary tumour [9]. Human melanocytes express the melanocortin 1 receptor (MC1R) that binds α-MSH and ACTH with the same affinity [10]. α-MSH

causes a small rise in cyclic adenosine monophosphate (cAMP) but has no effect on basal or UV-stimulated melanogenesis in human melanocytes [11].

Melanocyte regulation by paracrine and autocrine factors

Post-inflammatory hyperpigmentation is believed to be mediated by immune inflammatory mediators including interleukin (IL)-1α, IL-1β, IL-6 and tumour necrosis factor (TNF)-α [12]. Human melanocytes have also been demonstrated to respond to and to synthesize IL-1α and IL-1β, which suggests an autocrine as well as a paracrine regulatory role [13]. Other inflammatory mediators that act on human melanocytes include eicosanoids, metabolites of arachidonic acid. Melanocytes respond to PGE_2 with increased melanogenesis and dendrite formation [14]. Scott *et al.* demonstrated an increase in dendricity of human melanocytes in response to PGE_2 and $PGF_{2\alpha}$ [15]. Prostaglandins, leukotrienes and thromboxanes are the main inducers of tyrosinase [16]. Basic fibroblast growth factor was the first paracrine factor for human melanocytes to be identified. It exerts its effect by binding to a tyrosine kinase receptor that is expressed on human melanocytes [17]. In contrast to IL-1α, IL-1β, IL-6 and TNF-α and the eicosanoids, basic fibroblast growth factor is not secreted by keratinocytes: direct contact between melanocytes and keratinocytes is required for its biological effects [18]. Additionally, leukotrienes C_4 and D_4 have been shown to act as potent mitogens on cultured human neonatal melanocytes [19].

Endothelins are a further important group of peptides that act upon melanocytes in a paracrine manner [20]. ET1 is both mitogenic and melanogenic for human melanocytes that express

ET1 receptors [21]. ET1 acts synergistically with α-MSH and basic fibroblast growth factor to stimulate human melanocytes proliferation [22]. ET3 has similar effects to ET1: both peptides bind the endothelin receptor on melanocytes with equal affinity [23]. Furthermore, endothelins appear to have a role in protecting melanocytes: Kadekaro *et al.* demonstrated that treatment of human melanocytes with ET1 reduced UVR-induced apoptosis and prolonged melanocyte survival [24].

Biological significance of melanin

The major biological function of melanin is generally assumed to be protection of the lower layers of the skin against UV light. If human pigment has such adaptive significance, we might expect to find that, among the races of the world, pigment is geographically distributed in relation to solar intensity. It appears to be generally true that pigmentation is greatest in the tropics and reduced in temperate zones, reappearing to some extent in northern races subjected to prolonged snow glare [1]. However, there are exceptions, for example Native Americans, whose skin colour varies little between polar and tropical regions, and Tasmanians, who are dark even though they live in a temperate climate.

The damaging role of UV light is well illustrated by the high incidence of epidermal carcinoma in Europeans exposed to excess sun. The evolutionary usefulness of pigmentation may be twofold. On the one hand, it protects against damage by sunburn. On the other, since it efficiently absorbs UV radiation and is readily activated to a free radical by incident light, it may serve to eliminate genetically damaged cells by a phototoxic mechanism.

Not all the effects of pigmentation are advantageous. Melanin has been demonstrated to react with DNA and produce reactive oxygen species after UVA radiation [2]. There is no doubt that pigmentation increases the heat load in hot climates, so that black people absorb 30% more heat from sunlight than Caucasian people, although this factor may be offset by more profuse sweating [3,4]. In addition, in cold climates, pale skin has the advantage that heat loss by radiation is reduced.

A further disadvantage of pigmentation is that it hinders synthesis of vitamin D, so that in areas where nutrition is poor and sun exposure limited black children are more liable to rickets than Caucasian children. Thus, loss of pigmentation may facilitate vitamin D synthesis in temperate climates. It might be presumed that the retention of pigment in Arctic latitudes, while providing a protection against snow glare, is only permitted by natural selection because of the high-fat diet in these regions.

Since pigmentation appears to be not entirely advantageous to life in the tropics, other hypotheses about its biological significance have been advanced. For example, Wassermann [5,6] suggested that the major adaptation of black people to tropical Africa is in the ability to survive malaria, multiple parasites and tropical diseases under the hazards of intense solar radiation and, more often than not, poor nutrition. He suggests that diseases, not climatic conditions, are the primary selective factors, and lists evidence that black Africans, in comparison with Caucasian people, show increased

reticuloendothelial activity and increased serum γ-globulin fractions. These features are inversely related to the size and activity of the adrenal cortex, suggesting that the increased secretion of MSH and ACTH by black people and the consequent enhanced melanogenesis and pigmentation might be secondary to a relative adrenocortical insufficiency.

Classification of disorders of melanin pigmentation

Disorders of melanin pigmentation can be divided on morphological grounds into two types. The first is hypermelanosis, where there is an increased amount of melanin in the skin. This excess may be confined to the epidermis, when the skin appears browner than normal, or it may be present in the dermis, producing a slaty-grey or blue appearance. The second type is hypomelanosis, where there is a lack of pigment in the skin, which therefore appears white or lighter than the normal colour. Amelanosis is the term applied when there is a total lack of melanin in the skin. Hypermelanosis and hypomelanosis can be generalized and diffuse, or may be localized and circumscribed. Sometimes, localized areas may have a segmental or dermatomal pattern. The term 'depigmentation' is used to describe a loss of pre-existing pigment from the skin. Leukoderma is a white skin that may be congenital or acquired and can be due to a variety of aetiological factors. Examination of the skin with a source of long-wave UV light, for example Wood's lamp, is often helpful in localizing abnormal variations in melanin pigmentation in the skin and as an aid to the diagnosis of various disorders [1].

Changes in pigmentation can arise in a number of ways and can be due to a variety of genetic and environmental factors. It is also pertinent to consider non-melanin pigmentation as a cause of cutaneous colour changes, as discussed at the end of this chapter.

Hypermelanosis similarly can be due to many factors, both genetic and acquired. It can be due to an increased number of melanocytes in the skin such as occurs in the dermal melanocytoses: the naevus of Ota, the naevus of Ito and the Mongolian spot. Many of the hypermelanotic disorders are due to an increase in melanogenesis due to genetic factors. Some may be induced by UV light, hormones and chemical compounds. Finally, the degradation of melanosomes may vary in different disorders of pigmentation.

Constitutive pigmentation, human pigmentation and the response to sun exposure

Genetic factors play the primary role in determining the degree of pigmentation that is normal for the individual. Variation in skin pigmentation is not due to differences in the number of melanocytes but is explained by differences in melanocyte structure and function; melanogenic activity, the size and number of melanosomes, the type of melanin deposited onto melanosomes, and the donation of mature melanosomes to adjacent keratinocytes all contribute to the resulting colour of the skin and are genetically determined [1]. Thus, constitutive skin colour, as well as how the colour changes in response to exposure to sunlight, are both genetically determined and show relatively little variation within different racial groups. There is, however, marked variation in human skin colour between the main racial groupings ranging from white (previously known as 'Caucasoid'), through lightly pigmented (Asian and Oriental) to black (previously known as 'Negroid' and 'Australoid' and some Asian races). Racial differences in melanocyte morphology and function are apparent, but there is little interracial variation in the density of melanocytes at a particular skin site. Ultrastructural studies have shown that melanosomes in white skin are small and tend to be in membrane-bound complexes of three or more within the keratinocyte [2]. The ellipsoidal melanosomes of Aboriginals and black people are larger, about 1 μm in length, and tend to be distributed as singlets rather than being aggregated. These larger melanosomes can be found intact in the stratum corneum. The melanosome complexes present in Caucasian people show degradative changes even in the basal layer of the epidermis and are presumably broken up by lysosomal enzymes [3]. Whether melanosomes are individually dispersed or aggregated in melanosomal complexes appears to depend on the size of the melanosome [2].

Melanin in the skin exerts its photoprotective effect by reducing the penetration of UV light through the epidermis and by quenching the reactive oxygen radicals that contribute to sun-induced DNA damage [4]. The superior photoprotection of the black epidermis is due not only to its increased melanin content but also to melanogenic activity, the size and number of melanosomes, the type of melanin deposited into melanosomes and the donation of mature melanosomes to adjacent keratinocytes. A classification of sun-reactive skin types based on sunburn and tanning history has been in widespread use since its introduction (Table 88.1) [5]. Two types of pigmentation of the skin in humans occur in response to sun exposure. The first is immediate pigment darkening (IPD), sometimes also referred to as the Meirowsky phenomenon. This is best observed in those with hyperpigmented skins and is most effectively induced by long-wave UV light (UVA). It is transient and, although rapidly induced, soon fades. The second is the increased pigmentation that follows the erythemal response. This is the delayed tanning reaction and can be seen 48–72 h after skin exposure to UV light.

Table 88.1 Classification of sun-reactive skin types.

Skin type	Sun sensitivity	Pigmentary response
I	Very sensitive, always burn easily	Little or no tan
II	Very sensitive, always burn	Minimal tan
III	Sensitive, burn moderately	Tan gradually (light brown)
IV	Moderately sensitive, burn minimally	Tan easily (brown)
V	Minimally sensitive, rarely burn	Tan darkly (dark brown)
VI	Insensitive, never burn	Deeply pigmented (black)

ACQUIRED HYPERMELANOSIS

Physiological hypermelanosis (tanning in response to UV radiation)

Introduction and general description

Tanning is the term used to describe the pigmentary response of the skin following exposure to UV radiation. Tanning occurs in three distinct phases: IPD, persistent pigment darkening (PPD) and delayed tanning. IPD occurs in response to low doses of UVA and manifests as grey-brown pigmentation. It appears within minutes of UV exposure and typically fades within 10–20 min. IPD is believed to result from oxidation and redistribution of pre-existing melanin. Higher doses of UVA induce PPD which persists for 2–24 h. This pigmentation is brown and is also caused by oxidation and redistribution of pre-existing melanin. Delayed tanning involves the formation of new melanin due to an increase in the number of melanocytes and increased melanocyte activity. Both UVA and UVB are able to induce delayed tanning, but UVB is more effective. Delayed tanning becomes visible about 72 h after UV exposure and persists for 1–2 weeks before gradually fading as keratinocytes are shed from the skin surface.

Tanning and DNA damage are closely associated. Repeated suberythemal doses of UV light induce tanning but have also been shown to induce DNA damage [1]. Tanning salon exposure has also been demonstrated to induce cyclobutane pyrimidine dimers and p53 protein expression in epidermal keratinocytes, changes linked with the early stages of cutaneous carcinogenesis [2]. It is widely believed by laypeople that a tan provides good protection against sunburn [3]. However, tanned skin has been shown to be less effective against formation of DNA photoproducts than constitutive pigmentation [3] and has a sun protection factor of 3–5 at best. Population-based surveys reveal that tanning remains popular, particularly with the young, and that episodes of sunburn remain common [4,5]. Disturbingly, newer sunbeds with a greater proportion of UVB are significantly more carcinogenic than the older lamps that emitted primarily UVA, with little UVB [6,7].

Facial melanoses

Hypermelanosis involving predominantly the face and neck is relatively common and often presents a complex diagnostic problem. Several more or less well-defined clinical syndromes can be recognized, but many transitional forms defy classification. The causes of the pigmentation are often obscure.

Genetic and racial factors are important, the increased pigmentation occurring more frequently in those with dark skins, especially those of Middle Eastern or Asian descent. Endocrine factors play a major role in melasma and are implicated to some degree in other melanoses. External agents (light and photodynamic chemicals) are essential factors in the occupational melanoses but are also implicated in photocontact dermatitis (Riehl melanosis), and

PART 8: SPECIFIC CUTANEOUS STRUCTURE

erythromelanosis and poikiloderma of Civatte. Other unknown factors are certainly involved, and wide individual variation in susceptibility must be postulated.

Cosmetics may occasionally cause facial melanosis. Facial melanosis is, of course, also a conspicuous feature of Addisonian pigmentation.

Melasma

Definition and nomenclature
Melasma is the most common cause of facial melanosis and is manifested by hyperpigmented macules on the face which become more pronounced after sun exposure (Figure 88.8a,b) [1,2].

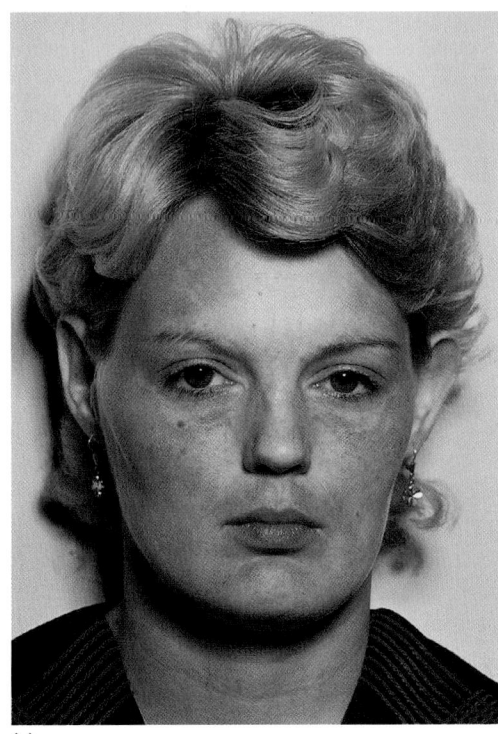

(a)

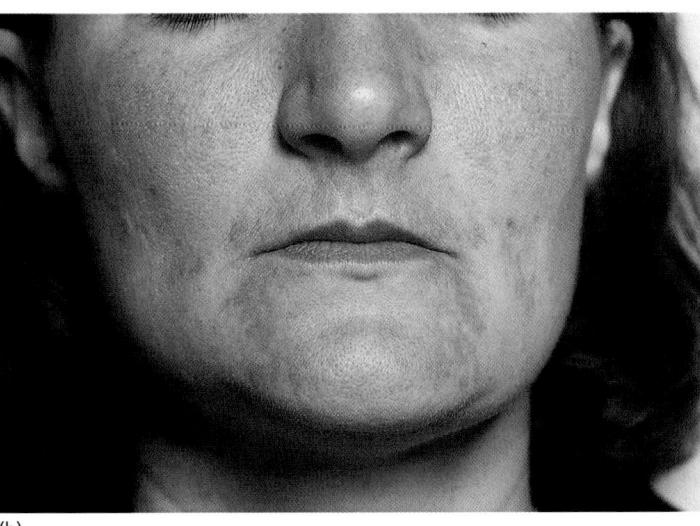

(b)

Figure 88.8 (a,b) Melasma in two female patients.

Synonyms and inclusions
- Mask of pregnancy
- Chloasma

Epidemiology

Incidence and prevalence
Common. Increased pigmentation is almost invariable in pregnancy and is most marked in brunettes. Melasma is frequently seen in women on oral contraceptives.

Age
Mostly starts between the ages of 20 and 40 years.
Dependent on pregnancy or use of oral contraceptives [3,4].

Sex
F > M.
Up to 10% of cases of melasma occur in men (Figure 88.9).

Ethnicity
More common in light brown skin types, particularly Latin Americans and those from the Middle East or Asia.

Pathophysiology

Predisposing factors
Several factors have been linked to melasma, among them UV exposure and hormonal factors appear to be the most significant. Local or diffuse hyperpigmentation can be seen in a subset of women, probably due to these hormonal factors. Pregnancy and oral contraceptives have been linked to increased skin pigmentation. It has been speculated that this is due to increased levels of oestrogen and progesterone stimulating the activity of melanocytes [5]. Melasma is common in the third trimester of pregnancy when levels of oestrogen, progesterone and MSH are elevated.

Many cases are attributed to pregnancy or the combined oral contraceptive pill [3,4]. In the context of pregnancy, melasma is regarded as a normal physiological change, along with darkening

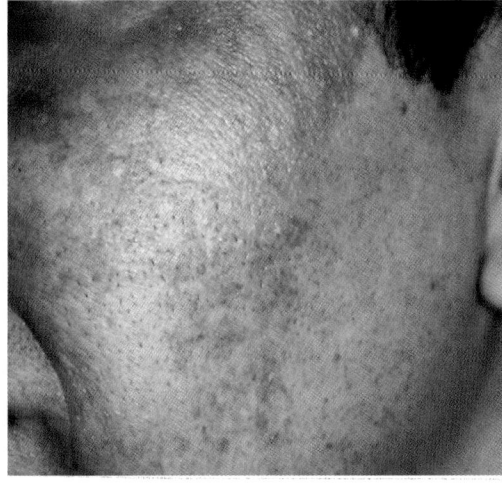

Figure 88.9 Melasma in an adult male from the Indian subcontinent.

of the nipples and linea nigra. It is not uncommon during the years of reproductive activity and has been attributed, without acceptable proof, to a variety of ovarian disorders. The rarity of melasma in postmenopausal women on oestrogen-containing hormone replacement therapy and the fact that men are occasionally affected suggests that oestrogen alone is not the causative agent.

Pathology

The mechanism is not fully elucidated, and although MSH may be involved, it plays a minor part. The plasma concentration of MSH is normal both in patients with idiopathic melasma [6] and in those with melasma attributable to oral contraceptives [7]. Oestrogens and progesterone are involved in the increased pigmentation but other factors are also implicated [8]. The number of melanocytes is not increased but they become enlarged and more dendritic, suggesting a hypermetabolic state. This is reflected by increased melanin deposition in the epidermis and dermis [8,9].

Despite light microscopic, ultrastructural and immunofluorescence studies, the condition remains an enigma [1]. An endocrine mechanism is postulated but the cause of melasma is unknown.

Genetics

No specific genes have as yet been identified but a family history is common (around 30%). The clinical manifestations are the same in sporadic and familial cases and is seen particularly in those who tan readily when exposed to bright sunlight [10].

Environmental factors

Exacerbated by sun exposure, combined oral contraceptives and other hormone treatments.

Clinical features

Presentation

Melasma is seen predominantly in women. Hypermelanosis affects mainly the upper lip, the malar regions, forehead and chin and may be associated with darkening of the nipples, the linea alba to form the linea nigra, and anogenital skin. Affected skin is brown in colour. The pigmentary changes are usually bilateral and are frequently symmetrical.

Differential diagnosis

See Box 88.3.

Classification of severity

Cosmetic problem.

Disease course and prognosis

Variable. The pigmentation usually fades after parturition but may persist for months or years. It is noted by some women to be more obvious just prior to menstruation [11]. The pigmentation takes a long time to fade after discontinuing oral contraception and, as after pregnancy, it may never fade completely.

Investigations

No investigations necessary.

Box 88.3 Differential diagnosis of acquired hyperpigmentation

(a) Acquired diffuse hyperpigmentation
- Endocrinopathies
- Metabolic conditions
- Metal-induced non-melanin pigmentation
- Neoplastic or tumoral conditions
- Nutritional conditions
- Physical agents
- Progressive systemic sclerosis
- Toxin- or drug-induced

(b) Acquired localized hyperpigmentation
- Circumscribed
  - Ephelides[a,b]
  - Erythromelanosis follicularis faciei et colli[a]
  - Exogenous ochronosis[a]
  - Fixed drug eruption[a]
  - Friction melanosis[a]
  - Iatrogenic[a]
  - Lentiginosis[a]
  - Melasma[a]
  - Poikiloderma of Civatte[a]
  - Riehl melanosis[a]
  - Secondary hyperpigmentation (post-infectious, post-inflammatory, post-traumatic)
    - Eczema[a,b]
    - Lichen planus[a,b]
    - Lupus erythematosus[a,b]
    - Macular amyloidosis[b]
    - Morphoea[a]
    - Erythema dyschronicum persistans[b]
    - Pityriasis versicolor[b]
- Disseminated
  - Endogenous ochronosis[a,b]
  - Idiopathic eruptive macular pigmentation[b]
  - Lichen planus pigmentosus[b]
  - Mastocytoses[a,b]
  - Phytophotodermatitis[a]

[a]Limited surface areas affected.
[b]Larger surface areas can be affected.

Wood's lamp examination can be helpful to identify the depth of the melanin pigmentation and determine the type of melasma (epidermal, dermal or mixed). Epidermal melasma normally appears light brown and shows enhanced colour contrast with Wood's lamp examination. Dermal melasma often appears slightly grey or bluish on gross examination and shows less colour contrast with Wood's lamp. Categorization of the type of melasma is useful because it may help guide treatment options and patient expectations since dermal melasma is generally less responsive to therapy, especially to topical modalities [1].

Management

Treatment of melasma can be difficult due to the refractory and recurrent nature of the condition.

PART 8: SPECIFIC CUTANEOUS STRUCTURE

Different skin depigmentation formulations can be used and contain one or several active compounds. Hydroquinone is the most extensively studied depigmenting agent for the treatment of melasma. It inhibits tyrosinase, an enzyme critical to the pigment-producing pathway in melanocyte. Topical retinoid therapy has also been used as monotherapy for melasma but with only moderate efficacy [12,**13**].

Triple combination therapy, comprised of hydroquinone, a retinoid and a corticosteroid, is a highly effective and safe treatment for melasma. A corticosteroid was introduced to this treatment to reduce inflammation as it is a side effect of both hydroquinone and tretinoin. In addition to this advantage, it also inhibits melanocyte metabolism [**13**].

Pregnancy-related melasma tends to improve spontaneously postpartum and treatment may not be necessary.

First line

A variety of topical treatments are effective at lightening melasma. Triple therapy with topical hydroquinone, tretinoin and corticosteroid (e.g. hydroquinone 4%, fluocinolone acetonide 0.01% and tretinoin 0.05%) is preferred [**13**,14]. Alternative, dual therapy (e.g. hydroquinone 2% plus glycolic acid 10%) may be used but can cause severe irritation [**13**]. Response to monotherapy is generally disappointing.

Treatment ladder

First line
- Sun protection/broad-spectrum sunscreen (SPF >30)
- Change oral contraceptive to an alternative low-oestrogen preparation, or change to a different form of contraception
- Avoidance of scented cosmetic products and phototoxic drugs
- Triple therapy with topical hydroquinone, tretinoin and corticosteroid compound cream

Second line
- Chemical peels, alone or in combination with topical treatment [15,16]
- Azelaic acid (15–20%) in monotherapy or combination of azelaic acid 20% and tretinoin 0.05% [17,18]

Third line
- Laser therapy [15]
- Intense pulsed light therapy, adjuvant to topical treatment
- Dermabrasion
- Topical liquiritin [19]
- Topical rucinol [20]
- Kojic acid, in monotherapy or in combination with hydroquinone [17,21]

Resources

Patient resources

Patient information leaflet http://www.bad.org.uk/for-the-public/patient-information-leaflets/melasma (last accessed November 2015).

Photocontact facial melanosis

Definition and nomenclature

Facial melanosis attributable to phototoxic reaction to skin contact with photoactive agents.

Synonyms and inclusions
- Riehl melanosis
- Melanodermatitis toxica
- Pigmented cosmetic dermatitis

Epidemiology

Age
Middle age.

Sex
The condition is more frequent in women.

Predisposing factors
Tar derivatives and fragrances are suspected to be the cause [1]. An outbreak of photocontact facial melanosis in Japan was attributed to contact dermatitis to cosmetic ingredients and prompted the term 'pigmented cosmetic dermatitis' for this condition [2].

Pathology
In the early stages, there is liquefaction degeneration of the basal layer of the epidermis and a perivascular or band-like dermal infiltrate with pigmentary incontinence. Later, the epidermis appears normal but many melanophages are present in the upper dermis [3]. Ultrastructural studies show intercellular and intracellular oedema of keratinocytes and a multilayered basal lamina, as well as many melanophages in the dermis [3].

Environmental factors
Cosmetic and textile materials.

Clinical features

History
A distinctive pattern of grey-brown facial pigmentation was first described by Riehl in Vienna between 1916 and 1920 [4]. Riehl attributed this pigmentation to contact with noxious substances or to wartime living conditions. It was subsequently seen in Europe and Asia during and after the Second World War and has also occurred in Argentina [5] and in the South African Bantu [6].

Presentation
Brownish-grey pigmentation develops quite rapidly over the greater part of the face but is more intense on the forehead and temples. Smaller pigmented macules, often perifollicular, lie beyond the indefinite margin. The pigmentation may extend to the chest, neck and scalp, and occasionally involves the hands and forearms. Horny plugs fill the follicles and there may be some scaling.

Differential diagnosis
See Box 88.3.

PART 8: SPECIFIC CUTANEOUS STRUCTURE

Disease course and prognosis
Gradual improvement if the causal substance is avoided.

Investigations
Patch testing.

Treatment ladder

First line
- Where a contact cause can be identified and avoided, there follows a slow improvement over many months
- Sun protection

Second line
- Slow improvement may be expected with the use of hydroquinone 2–5% plus tretinoin or glycolic acid [7]

Third line
- Intense pulsed light [8]

Poikiloderma of Civatte

Definition and nomenclature
Poikiloderma of Civatte presents as mottled pigmentation (atrophy, telangiectasia, hyper- and hypopigmentation) which typically appears on the sides of the face and neck and on the upper anterior chest after years of repeated UV exposure (Figure 88.10a,b) [1].

> **Synonyms and inclusions**
> - Erythromelanosis interfollicularis colli

Epidemiology

Incidence and prevalence
Unclear as mild cases are underreported.

Age
Age 30–50 years.

Sex
Female predominance.

Ethnicity
Predominance in fair-skinned individuals.

Predisposing factors
Exposure to light and photodynamic substances in cosmetics are influencing factors [2].

Pathology
Poikiloderma of Civatte is histopathologically characterized by thinning of the spinous layer, hydropic degeneration of the basal cell layer, presence of melanophages in the papillary dermis and

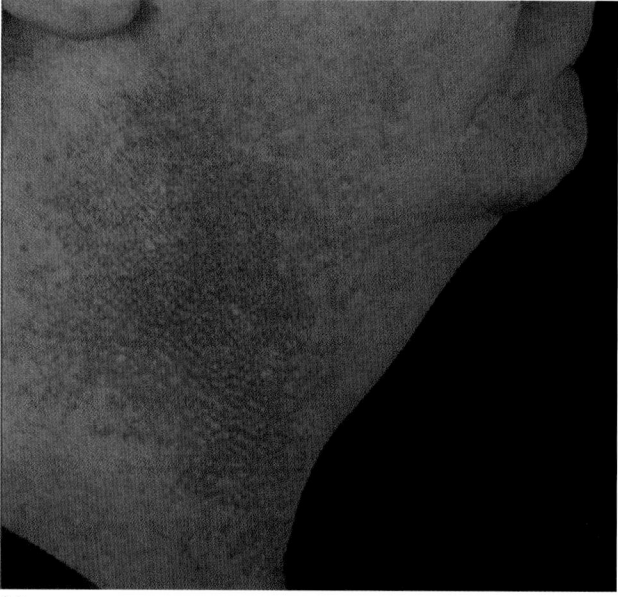

(a)

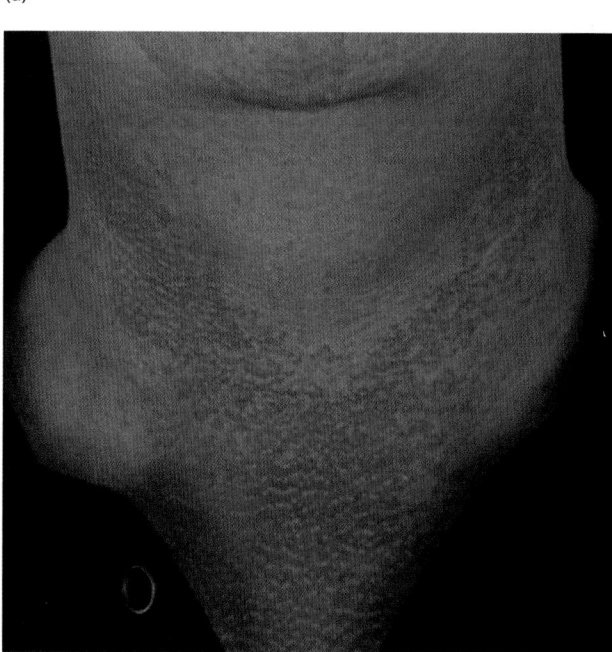

(b)

Figure 88.10 (a,b) Poikiloderma of Civatte: showing submental and submandibular sparing on the neck of a 43-year-old man.

dilatation of the papillary dermal capillaries. These findings are common to any case of poikiloderma [3].

Environmental factors
- Solar radiation.
- Phototoxic or photoallergic reactions to chemicals in fragrances or cosmetics.

Clinical features

History
This characteristic pattern of reticulate hyperpigmentation of the face and neck was first reported in 1923 by Civatte [1].

Presentation

Poikilodermatous changes develop symmetrically on the sides of the face, neck and upper aspect of the chest with hyperpigmentation, telangiectasia and dermal atrophy. The submandibular and submental areas are spared thus implicating sunlight in the pathogenesis of this condition (see Figure 88.10b). Milder forms are common and few patients seek medical advice. The condition is mostly asymptomatic, although some patients experience itching, burning and flushing.

Differential diagnosis

- Erythromelanosis follicularis faciei et colli.
- Melasma.

Classification of severity

Cosmetic problem.

Disease course and prognosis

Slowly progressive and irreversible.

Investigations

Patch testing can be useful if induction by allergen is suspected [3,4].

Treatment ladder

First line
- Photoprotection with a high SPF sunscreen
- Avoiding perfumes

Second line
- Intense pulsed light [5]
- Laser therapy with the tunable dye laser [6]

Erythromelanosis follicularis of the face and neck

Definition and nomenclature

Erythromelanosis follicularis of the face and neck presents with a reddish-brown discoloration affecting the preauricular and maxillary regions, in some cases spreading to the temples and lateral sides of the neck and trunk, with symmetrical distribution and sharp demarcation from normal skin.

Synonyms and inclusions
- Erythromelanosis follicularis faciei et colli

Epidemiology

Incidence and prevalence

Unclear as mild cases are underrecognized and underreported.

Age

Peak age of onset in the second decade of life.

Sex

Affects both sexes, but with male predominance.

Ethnicity

Affects all races, but more frequent in Asians.

Associated diseases

May be associated with keratosis pilaris.

Pathophysiology

Pathology

Histologically, there is slight hyperkeratosis and hyperpigmentation of the basal layer. The hair follicles are enlarged and contain lamellar horny masses. The sebaceous glands are also enlarged. The epidermis overlying the affected follicle is flattened and contains excess melanin. In the dermis, an inconspicuous lymphocytic infiltrate surrounds dilated vessels.

Genetics

Few familial reports.

Clinical features

History

This syndrome, of unknown origin, was originally described in Japan by Kitamura *et al.* in 1960 [1].

Presentation

The clinical picture is distinctive, characterized by a triad of hyperpigmentation, follicular plugging and erythema with or without telangiectasia, affecting the lateral aspects of the cheeks and in some cases the neck (Figure 88.11) [1–5]. It has been suggested that it is a subtype of keratosis pilaris [6]. A background of reddish-brown pigmentation and telangiectasia is studded with pale follicular papules. The hairs are lost from the majority of affected vellus hair follicles but terminal hair follicles of the scalp and beard are less conspicuously affected. The pigmentation involves the skin in front of, beneath and behind the ear, extending to the side of

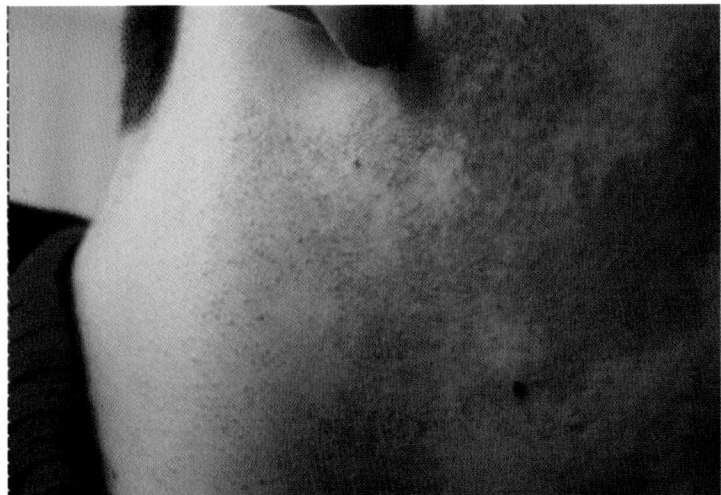

Figure 88.11 Erythromelanosis follicularis of the face and neck. (By permission of the copyright holder John Wiley and Sons, from Ermertcan *et al.* Erythromelanosis follicularis faciei et colli associated with keratosis pilaris in two brothers. *Pediatr Dermatol* 2006;23:31–4.)

the neck. It spreads slowly, is persistent and is not influenced by treatment. The distribution and lack of clinical follicular keratosis or scarring readily distinguish erythromelanosis from other forms of keratosis pilaris and from other facial melanoses.

Differential diagnosis
* Keratosis pilaris and its variants (see Chapter 87).
* Keratosis pilaris rubra.
* Melasma.
* Poikiloderma of Civatte.
* Corticosteroid-induced rosacea.
* Actinic telangiectasia.
* Response to therapy is generally poor and prone to relapse.

Treatment ladder

First line
* A variety of topical keratolytic therapeutics have been advocated, including urea cream (10–20%), ammonium lactate lotion (12%) and tretinoin cream (0.05–0.1%) [5,7]

Second line
* Salicylic acid peels and glycolic acid peels

Third line
* Isotretinoin (0.1–1 mg/kg/day)
* Laser treatment of the background erythema or hyperpigmentation

---

Peribuccal pigmentation of Brocq

Definition and nomenclature
Peribuccal pigmentation of Brocq is a diffuse brownish-red pigmentation around the mouth but sparing a narrow perioral ring [1–3].

Synonyms and inclusions
* Pigmented perioral erythema
* Erythrosis pigmentosa mediofacialis

Epidemiology

Age
Middle age.

Sex
This condition occurs predominantly in middle-aged women and has only rarely been reported in men.

Predisposing factors
A photodynamic substance in cosmetics is probably responsible.

Clinical features

History
It was Brocq in 1923 who first reported a case of perioral hyperpigmentation in a clinical pattern that now bears his name [1].

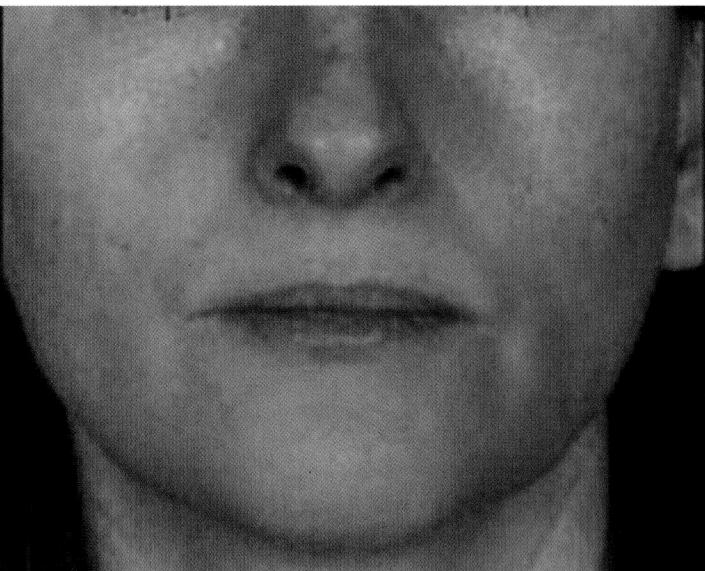

Figure 88.12 Peribuccal pigmentation of Brocq. (Courtesy and with permission of Dr Luciano Schiazza, Genoa, Italy.)

Presentation
Diffuse brownish-red pigmentation develops symmetrically around the mouth but spares a narrow perioral ring. It may extend up the centre of the face to the forehead and in some cases there are well-defined patches of pigmentation over the angles of the jaw and the temples (Figure 88.12).

Differential diagnosis
A similar post-inflammatory hyperpigmentation is seen in some patients with perioral dermatitis and may be the result of topical steroid therapy [2].

Classification of severity
Cosmetic problem.

Disease course and prognosis
The erythematous component, and hence the intensity of the pigmentation, may fluctuate over short periods. The pigmentation is usually persistent but tends to fade gradually if the cause is eliminated.

Ephelides

Synonyms and inclusions
* Freckles

Freckles or ephelides are very common and first appear at about the age of 5 years as light-brown pigmented macules on the light-exposed skin of fair-skinned individuals, typically of Celtic (Scottish, Irish, Welsh) origin with red or blond hair, fair skin and blue eyes (Figure 88.13a,b) [1]. Freckling is significantly associated with certain polymorphisms of the melanocortin 1 receptor gene [2,3] and is transmitted in an autosomal dominant fashion without

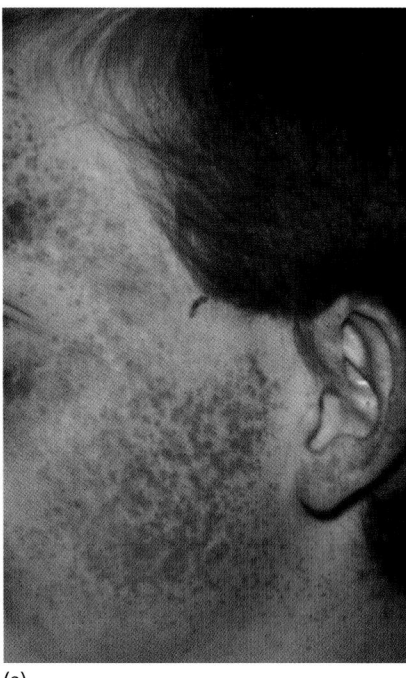

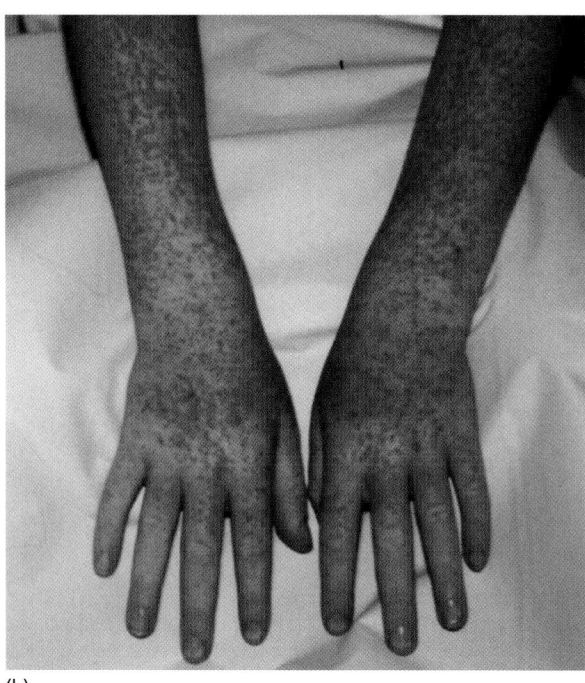

(a)   (b)

Figure 88.13 (a,b) Freckles in an 11-year-old boy.

associated abnormalities. Several pigmented skin disorders are, however, associated with freckles, including hereditary symmetrical dyschromatosis, xeroderma pigmentosum and cutaneous malignant melanoma [4].

Freckles are a feature of a number of inherited and acquired disorders. These include xeroderma pigmentosum [5], neurofibromatosis and progeria. The lesions in the various forms of lentiginosis (see later) must also be differentiated. Their distribution and the lack of relationship to light exposure should be noted. They are discussed in more detail in Chapter 132.

Treatment ladder

First line
• Broad spectrum sunscreen

Lentiginosis

The histological and clinical features of lentigo, together with other lesions in which the number of melanocytes is increased, are fully described in Chapter 132. A lentigo is a benign pigmented macule in which there is an increased number of melanocytes. The term 'lentiginosis' is applied either when lentigines are present in exceptionally large numbers or when they occur in a distinctive distribution. Genetic syndromes of which lentiginosis is a component are described in Chapter 70. The following isolated or sporadic forms of lentiginosis are recognized.

Generalized lentiginosis

Lentigines are commonly multiple but appear singly or in small crops at irregular intervals from infancy onwards. Their pathogenesis is unknown and in the great majority of cases no genetic factor is demonstrable.

Unilateral lentiginosis (zosteriform lentiginosis)

Lentigines may occur on one side of the body [1]. Cases have been reported with and without associated neurological abnormalities [2–4]. The lentigines can be zosteriform and occur in a dermatome-like or blaschko-linear distribution [5–8]. These cases are usually without central nervous system abnormalities and are naevoid. Lentigines have also been reported within naevoid hypopigmentation [8]. A case of unilateral lentiginosis with contralateral naevus depigmentosus has been reported [9].

Inherited patterned lentiginosis in black people [1]

O'Neill and James reported generalized lentiginosis in 10 adult black patients, with onset in childhood; seven showed familial clustering, suggesting autosomal dominant inheritance [1]. Distribution of the lentigines included the face, lips, extremities, buttocks, palms and soles, but not mucosal surfaces. The condition is extremely common in light-skinned black people, especially in combination with reddish-brown hair [2]. There are no known associated abnormalities.

Eruptive lentiginosis [1,2]

Widespread occurrence of very large numbers of lentigines that develop rapidly over the course of a few months to years is typical of eruptive lentiginosis (Figure 88.14). It is well recognized in adolescents and young adults who show no evidence of systemic abnormalities but has also been linked to treatment with cancer chemotherapeutic agents and to immunosuppression, particularly in transplant recipients. In 1956, Degos and Carteaud described telangiectatic papules that darkened and evolved into depressed

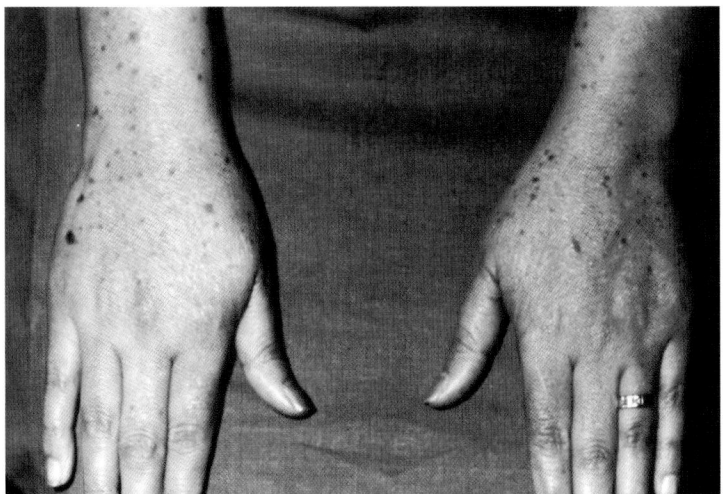

Figure 88.14 Eruptive lentiginosis: 4-month history of widespread eruption of lentigines over the neck, trunk and limbs in a healthy 49-year-old female. Note lentigines in different stages of evolution, particularly on the right wrist and the forearm.

scaly lentigines [1]. In spite of the misleading title of their report, Eady *et al.* reported two patients in whom very large numbers of lentigines developed over 2 years: histology and electron microscopy confirmed the diagnosis of eruptive lentiginosis [2].

PUVA lentigines [1–5]

These pigmented macules are a common complication of PUVA therapy occurring on treatment-exposed skin [1,2,3]. They are discussed in detail in Chapter 132. There is a dose effect with a tendency to a greater number of lentigines in those who have

had more therapy [3]. They vary in appearance and may be numerous in number and small in size. Occasionally, larger irregular lentigines are seen, some with a stellate configuration [3] (see Figure 132.7). PUVA lentigines are usually permanent and show little tendency to remit. A less common clinical pattern is localization of lentigines to sites previously affected by psoriasis, creating an appearance not unlike a naevus spilus [2]. The histology is that of a lentigo. The melanocytes are hypertrophic and some may be cytologically atypical [3]. Similar melanocytic macules have been reported following use of a sunbed [4]. PUVA lentigines can sometimes look quite alarming and should be differentiated from melanoma. Melanomas however tend to have more variation in colour density within the lesion than in lentigo. PUVA has also been reported to cause hyperpigmentation of the nails [5].

Hypermelanosis due to endocrine disorders

For a full discussion of the effects of endocrine disorders on the skin see Chapter 149. Endocrine disorders which may induce hypermelanosis are described briefly here.

Addison disease

Introduction and general description
Hyperpigmentation may be a cutaneous manifestation of Addison disease. The discoloration in Addison disease is typically diffuse with accentuation in sun-exposed areas (Figure 88.15) [1–4].

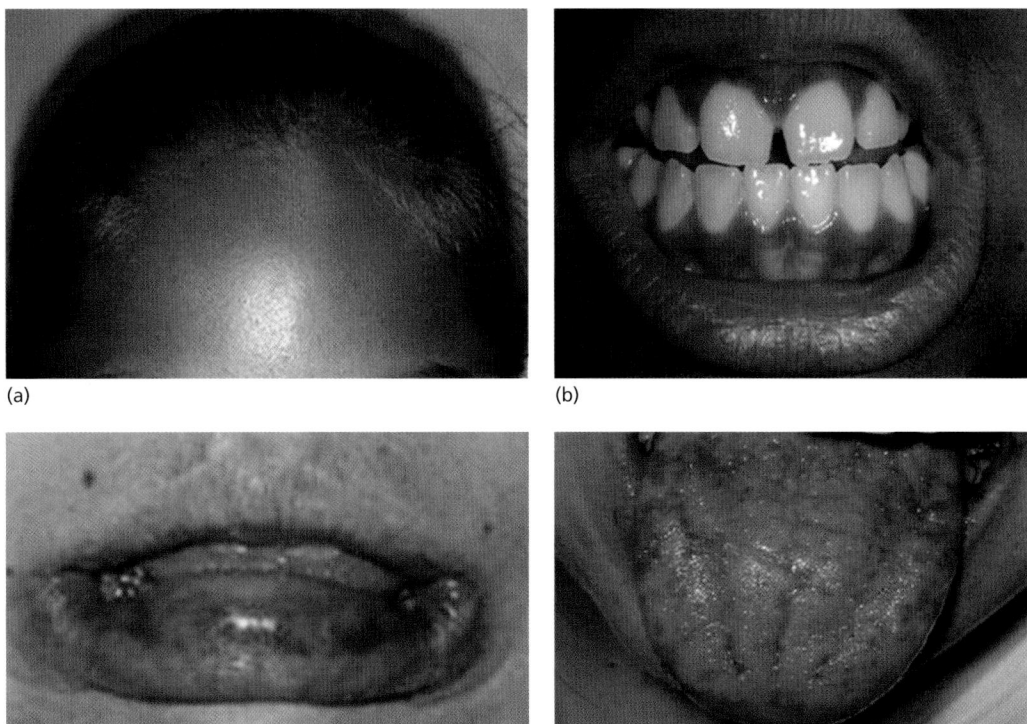

(a)

(b)

(c)

(d)

Figure 88.15 Addison disease: diffuse hypermelanosis of the skin (a) and gingivae (b) in a 13-year-old girl and of the labial mucosa (c) and tongue (d) of a 15-year-old girl. Both girls presented with fatigue, malaise, nausea and weight loss [7]. (Reproduced by permission of the copyright holder John Wiley and Son, Burk *et al.* Addison's disease, diffuse skin, and mucosal hyperpigmenation with subtle "flu-like" symptoms — a report of two cases. *Pediatr Dermatol* 2008;25:215–18.)

PART 8: SPECIFIC CUTANEOUS STRUCTURE

Pathophysiology

Pathology

The hypermelanosis is the result of increased secretion of melanotrophic hormones by the pituitary. Affected patients have elevated plasma levels of β-MSH-like immunoreactivity [5]. Absence of hypermelanosis in Addison disease was explained in a single case by a high degree of melanosome degradation in secondary lysosomes [1].

Clinical features

History

Addison disease was first described by Thomas Addison in 1855.

Presentation

Increased pigmentation is such a well-known feature of Addison disease that its absence may significantly delay diagnosis and endanger life [1,2]. When present, the hyperpigmentation of Addison disease is typically diffuse and is most intense on areas exposed to light [3]. It is also accentuated in the flexures, at sites of pressure and friction, and in the creases of palms and soles [3]. Normally pigmented areas, such as the nipples and genital skin, darken. Pigmentation of the buccal mucous membrane is often present, and the conjunctival and vaginal mucous membranes may also be involved [3]. However, less distinctive patterns of pigmentation are not exceptional and, in any unexplained cases of hypermelanosis, adrenal function should be carefully evaluated. Similarly, patients without hyperpigmentation but with other features suggesting Addison disease should have adrenal function assessed. Addison disease may be associated with generalized vitiligo [3,6].

Differential diagnosis

* Acquired diffuse hyperpigmentation: see Box 88.3a.
* Acquired pigmentary disorders of oral mucosa.
* Iatrogenic.
* Irritative (e.g. smokers' melanosis).
* Hyperplastic or neoplastic processes.

Resources

Patient resources

www.addisons.org.uk (last accessed October 2015).

Acromegaly

Definition

Acromegaly is an acquired condition caused by excessive growth hormone production leading to gradual body disfigurement.

Clinical features

Pigmentation of an addisonian pattern is present in some cases of acromegaly, and may be a striking feature [1,2].

Differential diagnosis

Acquired diffuse hyperpigmentation: see Box 88.3a.

Management

Cutaneous signs rapidly respond to hormonal control, with partial regression.

Topical therapy including tretinoin and adapalene creams can be used to ameliorate the cutaneous manifestations.

Resources

Patient resources

http://www.acromegalycommunity.com (last accessed October 2015).

Cushing syndrome

Definition

Cushing syndrome is caused by excessive amounts of cortisol leading to obesity, a moon-shaped face and increased fat deposition in the neck area. If due to endogenous hypersecretion of cortisol it is known as Cushing disease.

Pathophysiology

Pathology

Cushing syndrome is the overproduction of ACTH by a pituitary corticotrophic adenoma or an ectopic non-pituitary tumour.

Environmental factors

Excessive corticoid intake.

Clinical features

Presentation

Pigmentation of an addisonian pattern has been noted in about 10% of reported patients with Cushing syndrome. It is an indication of secretion of ACTH and β-MSH by the pituitary and suggests the presence of a pituitary tumour. After adrenalectomy, progressive hypermelanosis develops in a proportion of patients, about 10%, in spite of adequate hormone replacement therapy. Only in half of these patients is the sella turcica enlarged [1,2]. These patients with Nelson syndrome [3] show marked hypermelanosis (see Figures 88.7 and 88.16), with the mucous membranes also being involved. The hair is often darker and there are sometimes multiple lentigines and longitudinal pigmented bands in the nails. High levels of both β-MSH and ACTH are found in the plasma, with a degree of clinical hyperpigmentation correlating well with the quantity of β-MSH in the plasma [4].

Differential diagnosis

Acquired diffuse hyperpigmentation: see Box 88.3a.

ACTH administration

A small proportion of patients treated with ACTH in high dosages (120 units/day) develop pigmentation of addisonian pattern [1,2]. The pigmentation, which is accompanied by a combination of addisonian and cushingoid manifestations, fades when the dose is reduced. The incidence of melanosis appears to be rather higher in patients treated with tetracosactrin [2].

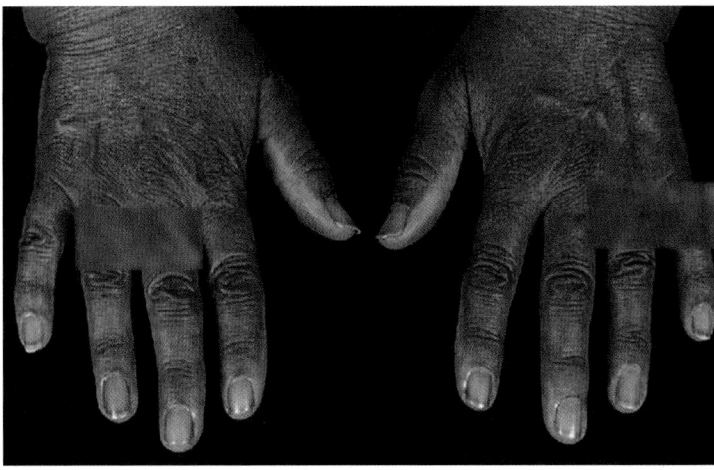

(a)

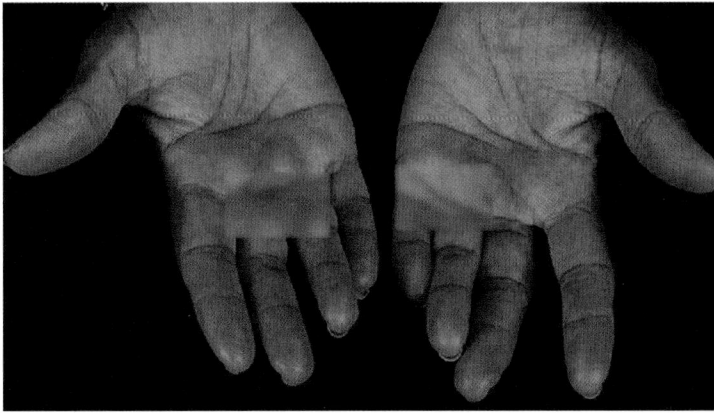

(b)

Figure 88.16 Nelson syndrome: hypermelanosis of the dorsa of the hands and of the palmar creases.

Hyperthyroidism

Definition
Hyperthyroidism is the excessive production of thyroid gland hormones.

Epidemiology

Incidence and prevalence
Pigmentation due to hyperthyroidism is present in 2–40% of patients with hyperthyroidism [1–3].

Pathophysiology

Pathology
It is speculated that the skin discoloration in hyperthyroidism may be due to increased release of pituitary adrenocorticotropic hormone, compensating for accelerated cortisol degradation [4].

Clinical features

Presentation
Pigmentation occurs in about 10% of patients with primary thyrotoxicosis [1]. It is usually diffuse and is broadly of addisonian pattern, although involvement of the mucous membranes is uncommon and pigmentation of the nipples and genital skin is less striking. The eyelids are occasionally conspicuously pigmented (the Jellinek sign). Some patients show melasma-like rather than diffuse pigmentation. The incidence of vitiligo is increased. Diffuse pigmentation was present at birth in the infant of a thyrotoxic mother [2]. Response of hyperpigmentation to therapy is poor.

Differential diagnosis
Acquired diffuse hyperpigmentation: see Box 88.3a.

Hypermelanosis in other systemic disorders

Neoplastic diseases

Definition
Increased pigmentation is an inconstant feature of a wide variety of systemic disorders and may be associated with malignant disease [1]. In most instances, the mechanism is obscure although, in some, elevated levels of β-MSH-like immunoreactivity are found. A genetic predisposition may be present in those affected. The hypermelanosis may be diffuse or localized. It may be confined to the epidermis, when the skin appears brown in colour, or it may be in the dermis, when often the skin is a slate-grey or blue colour. Pigments other than melanins may also be present.

Solid malignant tumours: ACTH-like peptides secreted typically from oat cell carcinoma of the bronchus may result in widespread hypermelanosis [2]. Diffuse cutaneous melanosis is a rare complication of metastatic melanoma [3–5].

Carcinoid syndrome: spectrum of neuroendocrine tumours, most frequently originating in the digestive tract. Symptoms of flushing, diarrhoea, heart failure and bronchoconstriction developing due to excessive secretion of hormones such as serotonin from carcinoid tumours (see Chapter 106) [6].

Lymphoma: spectrum of malignant neoplasms derived from mature B or T cells, B- or T-cell progenitors or natural killer cells (see Chapter 140).

Phaeochromocytoma: neuroendocrine tumour of the adrenal glands or extra-adrenal chromaffin tissue secreting high levels of catecholamines.

Epidemiology

Incidence and prevalence

Solid malignant neoplasms: rare.

Carcinoid tumour: see Chapter 106.

Lymphomas: pigmentation is an uncommon manifestation of lymphomas, occurring in 10% of cases of Hodgkin disease and in 1 or 2% of cases of non-Hodgkin lymphoma and lymphatic leukaemia.

Phaeochromocytomas: rare.

Pathophysiology

Pathology

Solid malignant neoplasms: the mechanism is uncertain. In ectopic ACTH syndrome, which may occur in patients with oat cell carcinoma of the bronchus, pigmentation is usual. The tumour has been shown to produce a distinct MSH-like compound [2]. Diffuse melanosis is a rare complication of metastatic melanoma and is usually associated with widespread visceral metastases. It is thought that free melanin is released into the circulation from the cytolytic breakdown of melanoma metastases and is deposited extracellularly around dermal blood vessels before being taken up by dermal melanophages [3].

Carcinoid syndrome: unknown.

Lymphoma: unknown.

Phaeochromocytoma: pigmentation possibly due to MSH-like activity of ectopic secretion of ACTH and its precursors. Release of α-MSH or analogues that bind on melanocortin 1 receptors.

Genetics:
About one-third of phaeochromocytomas arise as part of a genetic syndrome.

Clinical features

Presentation

Solid malignant neoplasms: in cachectic states, there may be diffuse hyperpigmentation of the skin as in Addison disease. In adults, acquired acanthosis nigricans may rarely be associated with internal malignancy, almost invariably an adenocarcinoma. The hypermelanosis affects the axillae, nipples and umbilicus, which also show a warty papillomatosis. These skin changes may later become generalized. The mucous membranes are frequently involved. A diffuse dermal melanosis, having a slaty-blue colour, can occur in patients with advanced melanoma and may be associated with melanuria [3,4,5].

Carcinoid syndrome: flushing of the face, neck and upper trunk frequently occurs. Diffuse hyperpigmentation of the skin has been noted in a number of patients with this syndrome [6]. A pellagra-like dermatitis on sun-exposed skin may also be observed.

Lymphomas: the pigmentation is of addisonian type, but allegedly without involvement of the mucous membranes. Malnutrition may be a factor and post-inflammatory pigmentation after scratching may modify the clinical pattern. Diffuse progressive hyperpigmentation can also be a manifestation of mycosis fungoides [7,8].

Phaeochromocytoma: pigmentation of addisonian pattern occurs in some cases of malignant phaeochromocytoma. Pallor of the face due to vasoconstriction may also occur. Hypertension, headaches, profuse sweating, palpitations and apprehension will suggest the diagnosis, which is established by the abnormal plasma catecholamines.

Differential diagnosis
Acquired diffuse hyperpigmentation: see Box 88.3a.

Hyperpigmentation in rheumatic diseases
(see Chapter 154)

Hypermelanosis is occasionally observed in rheumatoid arthritis and is a more frequent feature of Still disease. Most cases of hyperpigmentation in rheumatoid arthritis patients are however due to medications such as minocycline [1]. Hyperpigmentation has been reported with methotrexate in a patient with rheumatoid arthritis [2]. For differential diagnosis see Box 88.3a.

Systemic sclerosis and morphoea

Definition
Systemic sclerosis and morphoea (see Chapters 56 and 57) comprise a spectrum of autoimmune-mediated diseases of unknown aetiology affecting the connective tussue. Systemic sclerosis may also affect the internal organs, including the heart, lungs, kindneys and gastrointestinal tract.

Pathophysiology

Predisposing factors
Hyperpigmentation in systemic sclerosis is seen most commonly in patients with pigmented skin, and is less common in Caucasian people [1].

Pathology
Keratinocyte endothelin 1 production has been implicated as playing a central role in the pathogenesis of cutaneous hyperpigmentation in systemic sclerosis [2], as has local expression and systemic release of a stem cell factor [3]. Levels of soluble cell surface L-selectin are elevated in systemic sclerosis with diffuse hyperpigmentation [4].

Clinical features

Presentation
Generalized pigmentation in systemic sclerosis and morphoea may be intense and diffuse or of addisonian type, often with an accentuation in sun-exposed skin and areas of pressure, but without mucous membrane involvement. It may involve predominantly the face and limbs but is often far more extensive than the scleroderma itself (Figure 88.17). A mixture of hyper- and hypomelanosis may also occur in areas of chronic sclerosis.

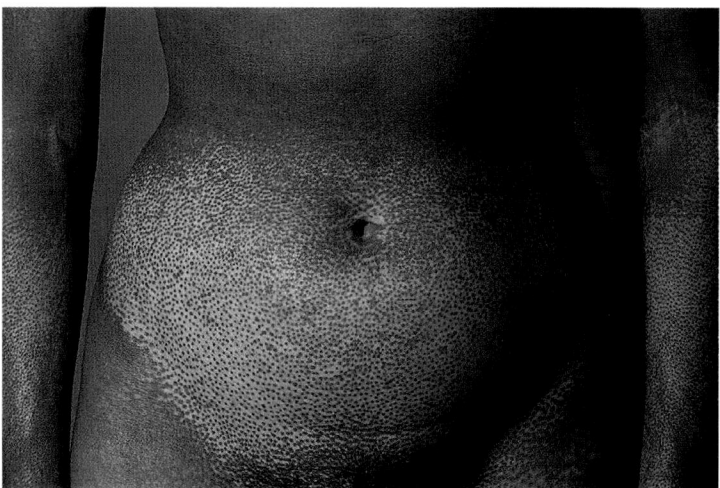

Figure 88.17 Generalized pigmentation in a woman aged 33 years with systemic sclerosis.

Pigmentation may also be a conspicuous feature of morphoea [5,6] and is occasionally the presenting symptom (Figure 88.18). Hyperpigmentation is sometimes a feature of atrophoderma of Pasini and Pierini [7], and has also been reported in the linear atrophoderma of Moulin [8].

Differential diagnosis
- Acquired diffuse hyperpigmentation: see Box 88.3a.
- Acquired localized hyperpigmentation: see Box 88.3b.

Dermatomyositis and lupus erythematosus

Definition

Dermatomyositis is an idiopathic inflammatory myopathy characterized by proximal muscle weakness and a cutaneous eruption.

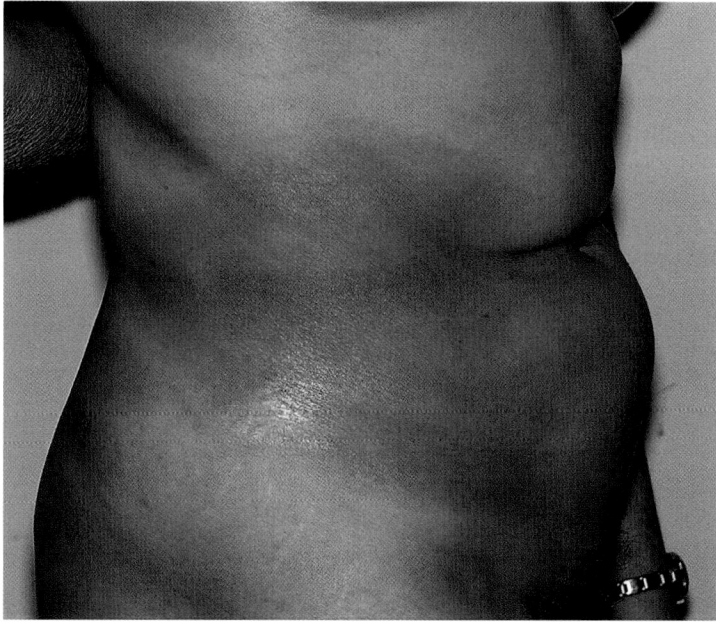

Figure 88.18 Morphoea. Hyperpigmentation was the presenting symptom.

Lupus erythematosus is a chronic idiopathic inflammatory disease affecting multiple organs including the skin.

Clinical features

Presentation
In both dermatomyositis and lupus erythematosus, diffuse pigmentation may accompany or follow the cutaneous lesions of dermatomyositis [1]. Acanthosis nigricans has also been reported in association with dermatomyositis [2]. In systemic lupus erythematosus, diffuse pigmentation of light-exposed skin occurs in about 10% of cases. Longitudinal melanonychia may occasionally be a feature of systemic lupus erythematosus [3]. Hyperpigmentation may also be secondary to treatment with antimalarials in systemic lupus erythematosus.

Differential diagnosis
Acquired diffuse hyperpigmentation: see Box 88.3a.

Disease course and prognosis
In systemic lupus erythematosus, the skin may gradually darken even though the disease is controlled by treatment.

Neurological disorders

Definition
Pigmentation, usually conforming to the addisonian pattern, occurs in some diseases of the nervous system, particularly those involving the diencephalon and the substantia nigra. Intense pigmentation is a feature of Schilder disease [1] but some increase in pigmentation is not uncommon in hepatolenticular degeneration [2] and in ependymomas. It is occasionally noted in chronic schizophrenia. In post-encephalitic parkinsonism, it may be diffuse but may be melasma-like. Pigmentation may sometimes develop after intense and prolonged emotional stress [3].

Clinical features

Presentation
Mostly diffuse hyperpigmentation conforming to the addisonian pattern.

Differential diagnosis
Acquired diffuse hyperpigmentation: see Box 88.3a.

Multiple organ failure, renal failure and primary biliary cirrhosis

Introduction and general description

Multiple organ failure: patients with multiple organ failure who survive for long periods are susceptible to hyperpigmentation. Renal failure, hepatic failure and polypharmacy may all contribute to this. An unusual case of intense green colour in a patient with multiple organ failure was attributed to dyes in the liquid tube feeds [1].

Renal failure: chronic renal disease with nitrogen retention is frequently accompanied by increased pigmentation of the skin. This hypermelanosis is diffuse and brown in colour. It is most intense on sun-exposed skin, including the hands and face. Hyperpigmented macules are common on the palms and soles [2].

Elevated levels of β-MSH are found in the plasma of these patients [1,3] and cause the excess production of melanin in the skin. The increased levels of β-MSH-like immunoreactivity are due to slow clearance by the kidneys rather than increased production by the pituitary. Lipochromes and carotenoids deposited in the skin may also play a part. Paradoxically, hypopigmentation with acquired lightening of the hair is sometimes a feature of chronic renal failure [4].

Primary biliary cirrhosis: a diffuse hypermelanosis is seen in patients with cirrhosis due to many aetiological factors, and is particularly striking in patients with primary biliary cirrhosis [1,2]. The hyperpigmentation is particularly striking on sun-exposed sites. The excess melanin is dispersed widely in the epidermis [1]. No significant difference from normal controls is observed in the levels of MSH-like peptides [1].

Disease course and prognosis
Dermatological manifestations increase with increasing duration and severity of renal disease.

Treatment ladder

First line
- Treatment of underlying cause
- Sun protection

Haemochromatosis

Definition
Haemochromatosis is a hereditary disorder due to excessive intestinal absorption of iron. The commonest and mildest form, accounting for some 90% of cases, is autosomal recessive and due to mutations in the *HFE* gene (*HFE*-related hereditary haemochromatosis). It manifests in the skin as diffuse pigmentation.

Introduction and general description
Haemochromatosis is a hereditary disorder due to excessive intestinal absorption of iron, resulting in gradual deposition of iron in the tissues throughout life [1,2]. The commonest and mildest form, accounting for some 90% of cases, is autosomal recessive and due to mutations in the *HFE* gene (*HFE*-related hereditary haemochromatosis) [3]. It is asymptomatic in 75% of cases, not usually presenting clinically until the fifth decade of life or later. It manifests in the skin as diffuse bronze pigmentation. Other clinical manifestations include hepatic cirrhosis, diabetes, cardiac failure, impotence and arthritis.

Epidemiology

Incidence and prevalence
It is estimated that 1 : 200 to 1 : 300 Caucasian people have homozygous *HFE* mutations [4], though only 50% of affected individuals show clinical features of the disease [4].

Age
Fifth decade onwards.

Sex
M > F.

Ethnicity
Most frequent in Caucasian people.

Associated diseases
Excessive alcohol consumption accelerates the development of hepatic cirrhosis [5].

Pathophysiology
The common form of haemochromatosis is due to mutations of the *HFE* gene [6].

Clinical features

History
The disease haemochromatosis was first described by Troisier, Hanot and Chauffard in 1865 [1]. The term 'haemochromatosis' was subsequently coined by von Recklinghausen in 1899 in recognition that the skin pigmentation originated from the blood [1].

Presentation
Pigmentation, bronzed or bluish-grey in colour, initially involves exposed sites but later becomes generalized (Figure 88.19) [7,8]. It is present in most cases [9], but may be subtle. Hyperpigmentation of mucous membranes and conjunctivae occur in 15–20%. The diagnosis should be suspected when pigmentation of this pattern occurs in middle-aged men in association with an enlarged liver and diabetes [10].

Differential diagnosis
Acquired diffuse hyperpigmentation: see Box 88.3a.

Investigations
Fasting transferrin saturation: if >45% arrange gene analysis for *HFE* mutations.

Management
Hyperpigmentation is reversible with phlebotomy [11].

Cutaneous amyloidosis

Definition
Cutaneous pigmentation is a common feature of cutaneous amyloidosis [1,2], which is discussed in detail in Chapter 58.

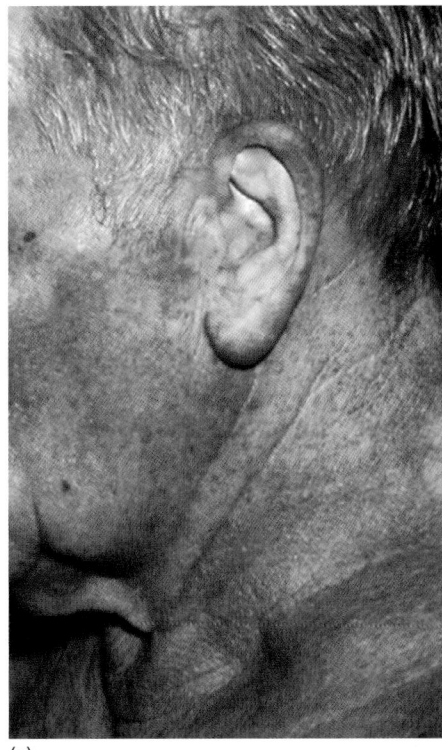
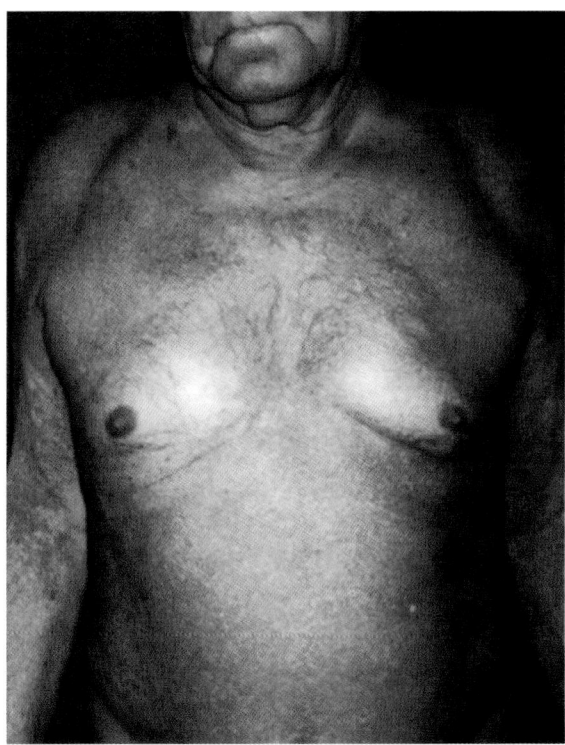

Figure 88.19 (a,b) Haemochromatosis: a 74-year-old male with gradual increase in skin pigmentation for 5 years. Extensive stippled skin pigmentation becoming confluent with marked iron deposition in addition to hypermelanosis on histology. Note gynaecomastia (b).

(a)

(b)

Pathophysiology

Pathology
Melanophages are found in the papillary dermis. The melanin contained in these dermal cells is derived from degenerating basal keratinocytes and melanocytes [1,3].

Clinical features

Presentation
Localized pigmentation, often symmetrical, and located on the upper back and anterior thighs and forearms, is seen in both lichen amyloidosis and macular amyloidosis [1,2].

Clinical variants
Macular amyloidosis is seen most commonly on the upper back (interscapular areas), chest, buttocks, forearms and shins.

Differential diagnosis
The macular type of amyloidosis may be mistaken for post-inflammatory hyperpigmentation, but the lesions usually have a distinctive 'ripple' pattern (Figure 88.20), and microscopic studies reveal the presence of amyloid (see Box 88.3a).

Nutritional deficiencies

Definition
The effects of nutritional deficiencies on the skin are addressed in detail in Chapter 63. Those that are associated with pigmentary change are briefly discussed here.

Malabsorption syndromes

Vitamin A deficiency: most frequently due to inadequate dietary intake.

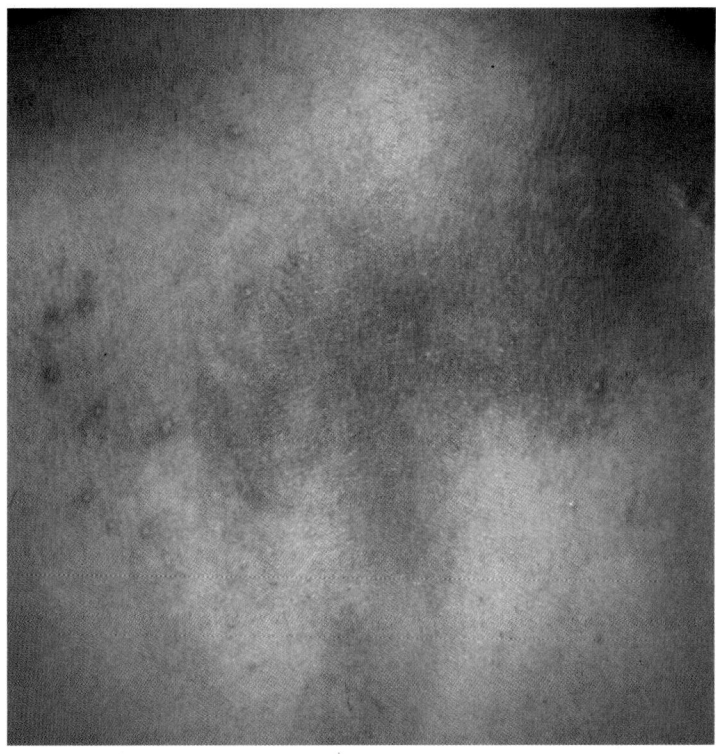

Figure 88.20 Macular amyloidosis: typical rippled hypermelanosis on the upper back of a 40-year-old Indian woman.

PART 8: SPECIFIC CUTANEOUS STRUCTURE

Vitamin B$_{12}$ deficiency: most frequently caused by inadequate absorption.

Folate deficiency: usually dietary with increased risk in pregnancy

Pellagra: the classical clinical manifestation of nicotinic acid (vitamin B$_3$) deficiency.

Vagabonds' disease: skin disorder typically occurring in older patients with poor diet, lack of personal hygiene and infestation with *Pediculus humanus*.

Epidemiology

Incidence and prevalence

In malabsorption syndromes, such as tropical sprue and Whipple disease (see Chapter 152), pigmentation is a common occurrence and may sometimes be prominent [1–3].

Pathophysiology

Vitamin B$_{12}$: the exact mechanism of hyperpigmentation in vitamin B$_{12}$ deficiency is still unknown. The lack of vitamin B$_{12}$ may lead to a lower intracellular reduced glutathione levels, causing a decrease in its inhibitory function on tyrosinase activity in melanogenesis, and inducing an increase in melanogenesis. Another hypothesis is that vitamin B$_{12}$ deficiency is associated with a defect in melanin transport and the incorporation of melanin into keratinocytes, causing incontinence of pigment [4].

Pellagra: is due to a cellular deficiency of niacin (vitamin B$_3$, nicotinic acid) from an inadequate dietary supply of tryptophan. It used to be endemic where diets were based on maize with little animal protein [5]. Although the condition has been recognized since the seventeenth century, it was not until the early twentieth century that it was recognized by Goldberger to be due to a nutritional deficiency [6], which was subsequently shown by Elvehjem to be niacin [7].

Vagabonds' disease: this classically occurs in those in whom poor diet is combined with lack of cleanliness, and heavy infestation with lice [8,9].

Presentation

General hyperpigmentation caused by nutritional deficiencies may be of addisonian type but without involvement of the mucous membranes, or may occur in well-defined patches on the face and neck and occasionally on the trunk [1]. The scaly inflammatory plaques that may develop in these syndromes are usually followed by intense pigmentation (see also Chapter 63).

Vitamin A deficiency: patients with severe vitamin A deficiency are often deficient in other vitamins as well. They have ocular and cutaneous abnormalities, of which xerophthalmia and phrynoderma (see Chapter 87) are the most characteristic, particularly in children: these may be associated with hyperpigmentation of the face and limbs. In adults, there is dryness and scaling of the skin with desquamation and generalized hyperpigmentation. Conjunctival pigmentation has been noted particularly in Oriental races and may be striking, especially in the lower fornix and bulbar conjunctiva.

Vitamin B$_{12}$ deficiency: the pigmentation seen in association with B$_{12}$ deficiency often has a rather dappled and mottled appearance; it particularly affects the face and the dorsum of the hands and feet [10–12] but may be limited to the fingertips and nails [13] or, rarely, may be generalized (Figure 88.21) [4,14,15]. Ill-defined hyperpigmentation of the mucosal surfaces and hypopigmentation of the hair may also occur.

Folate deficiency: a diffuse brown pigmentation is also seen occasionally in patients with megaloblastic anaemia due to folic acid deficiency, particularly during pregnancy [16,17].

Pellagra: affected skin becomes hard, dry and cracked and in extreme cases is black in colour [5]. The sites of involvement are the sun-exposed skin of the face, neck, dorsa of the hands and feet, and sometimes the forearms. Mucosal sites are also affected [18,19].

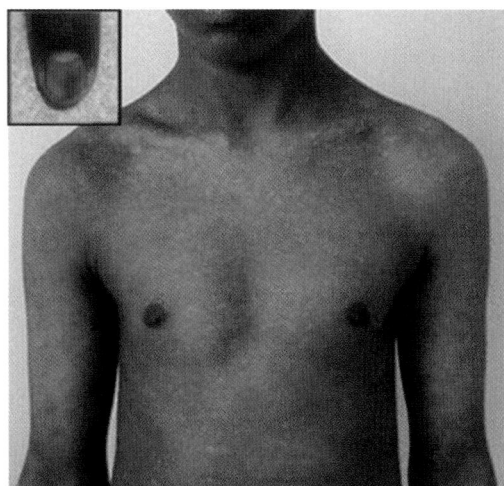
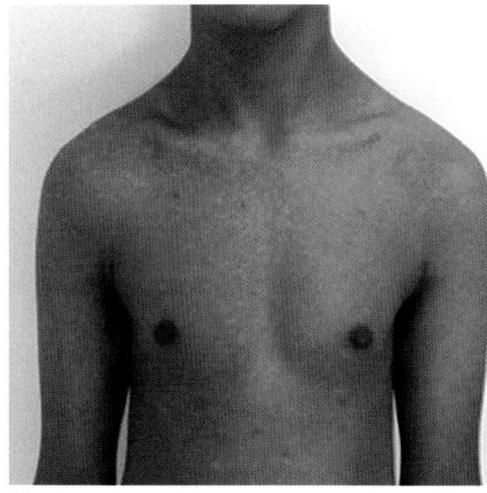

(a)   (b)

Figure 88.21 Vitamin B$_{12}$ deficiency: (a) generalized mottled hypermelanosis as presenting feature of pernicious anaemia in a 16-year-old boy with a 4-year history of progressive darkening of the skin and streaked pigmentation of the nails (inset); (b) marked reduction in pigmentation 9 months after initiation of vitamin B$_{12}$ therapy. (From Diamantino *et al.* 2012 [4]. Reproduced with permission of John Wiley & Sons Ltd.)

Vagabonds' disease: the pigmentation is basically of addisonian pattern and the mucous membranes may be involved. The pathogenesis is uncertain, but the hypermelanosis is probably post-inflammatory and related to the scratching from the pediculosis infestation. Areas of hypomelanosis occur and there is a decrease in the number of melanocytes that show degenerative changes [1]. Adrenal function is in most cases normal [8,9].

Differential diagnosis

Acquired diffuse hyperpigmentation: see Box 88.3a.

Acquired pigmentary disorders of oral mucosa: these include the following
- Iatrogenic.
- Irritative (e.g. smokers' melanosis).
- Hyperplastic or neoplastic processes.

Disease course and prognosis
Generally, normalization of pigmentation occurs with treatment of the deficiency.

POEMS syndrome

Definition
Hypermelanosis, along with acrocyanosis, hypertrichosis and skin thickening, is one of the cutaneous manifestations of this complex syndrome. The name POEMS syndrome derives from its principal characteristics, namely *p*olyneuropathy, *o*rganomegaly, *e*ndocrinopathy, *m*onoclonal gammopathy and *s*kin changes. It is discussed in detail in Chapter 148.

Presentation
Hyperpigmentation is reported to be a common cutaneous manifestation of POEMS syndrome, affecting the extremities, torso, areolae, head and neck. Hyperpigmentation may also be generalized [1].

Hypermelanosis of drug origin

Drug-induced hyperpigmentation

Definition
Localized or generalized hyperpigmentation can be caused by a wide range of medications and chemicals.

Introduction and general description
Skin pigmentation may be induced by a wide variety of drugs [1,2,3]. Several mechanisms are involved in drug-induced changes of pigmentation of the skin. These include increased melanin synthesis, increased lipofuscin synthesis, deposition of drug-related material and post-inflammatory hyperpigmentation. For example, the phenothiazines, particularly chlorpromazine, react with melanin to form drug–pigment complexes. In contrast to melanin, the chlorpromazine–melanin complexes are not metabolized by the

body. Many drugs induce hypermelanosis as a non-specific post-inflammatory change in predisposed subjects. The pigmentation following fixed drug eruptions is of this type. Other drugs induce pigmentation more directly; in the case of arsenic, it is believed that it combines avidly with sulphydryl groups in the epidermal cells and promotes the action of tyrosinase. A post-inflammatory hyperpigmentation of the skin is seen following the resolution of drug-induced lichenoid reactions. Oestrogens stimulate melanin production, and drug-induced hyperpigmentation may be seen with the combined oral contraceptive. Hyperpigmentation in AIDS patients may occur as a complication of drug therapy, most notably with zidovudine which causes pigmentation of the nail, skin and oral mucosa.

Amiodarone
Amiodarone is used in the treatment of ventricular and supraventricular tachycardia. Amiodarone has been reported to cause photosensitive and phototoxic reactions in more than 50% of patients [1–3]. Fewer than 5% of patients develop drug-induced discoloration of the skin, characterized by a slate-gray or purple discoloration of mainly the sun-exposed skin, especially the face, with prominent involvement of the nose and sometimes the ears (Figure 88.22a,b) [4–6]. Non-exposed skin may also be affected. The discoloration is caused by UV accumulation of amiodarone and lipofuscin in dermal macrophages. Skin type I patients are more prone to the development of this discoloration. The hyperpigmentation is related to the daily dosage (high risk with dosages >800 mg/day) and duration of treatment.

Antimalarial drugs
Chloroquine has been shown to have an affinity for dermal melanin [1]. A yellowish pigmentation of the skin is common with mepacrine [2]. Pigmentation appears to result from complexes of melanin, haemosiderin and mepacrine, in combination with sulphur [3]. Quinine and quinidine may also produce a generalized pigmentation [2,4].

Bluish-grey pigmentation appears mainly on sun-exposed areas, including the face, neck and anterior side of the legs and forearms (Figure 88.23). The nail beds may be affected diffusely or in transverse bands and the hard palate may be bluish-grey. The oral mucosa, especially the hard palate, may also be affected. Bleaching of the colour of the hair occurs and when associated with pigmentation of the skin should suggest the diagnosis [5]. The pigmentation manifests initially as isolated oval macules which then progressively spread and merge into large patches or diffuse pigmentation [2–5].

Clofazimine
This synthetic riminophenazine dye used in the treatment of leprosy produces an initial redness of the skin due to an accumulation of the drug. Later, with prolonged treatment, a violaceous brown colour develops that is most noticeable in lesional skin [1]. Reddish-blue pigmentation has been reported within scarred areas of lupus erythematosus in one patient [2]. Histochemical studies indicate a ceroid-lipofuscin pigment as well as clofazimine inside macrophage phagolysosomes [2,3].

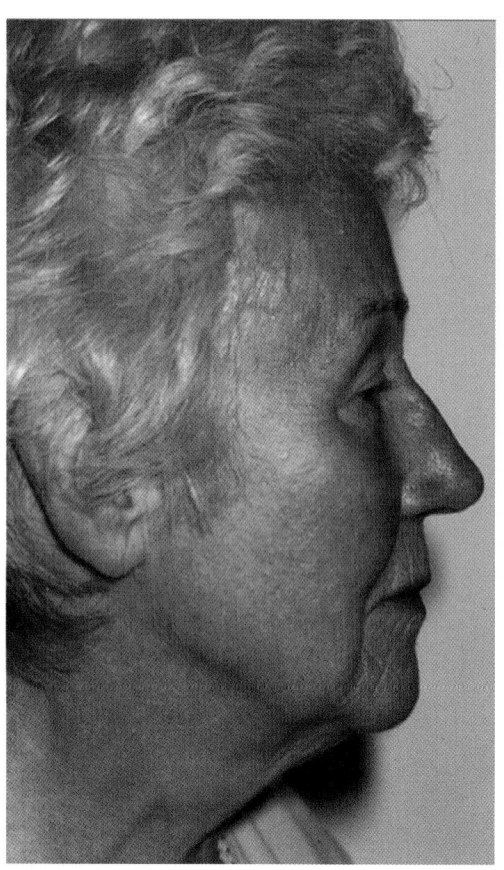

(a)

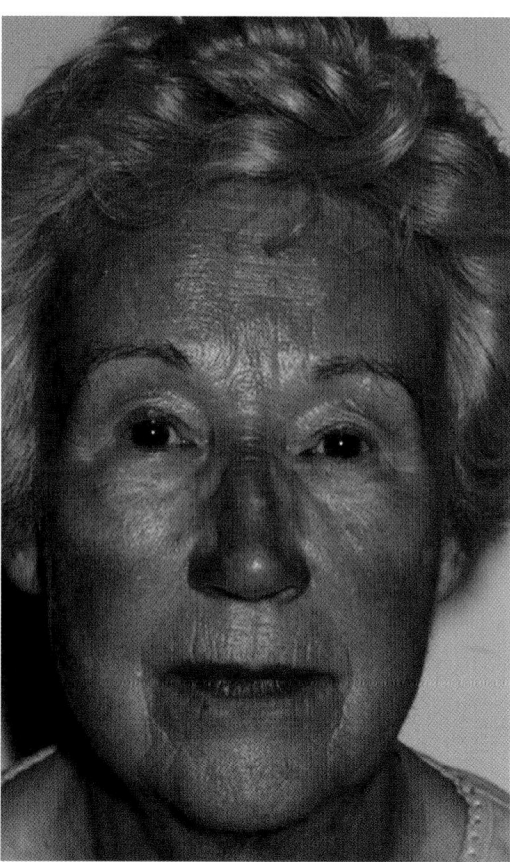

(b)

Figure 88.22 (a,b) Amiodarone pigmentation after 5 years of therapy: note slaty-blue dyspigmentation of the forehead, nose, cheeks and earlobe.

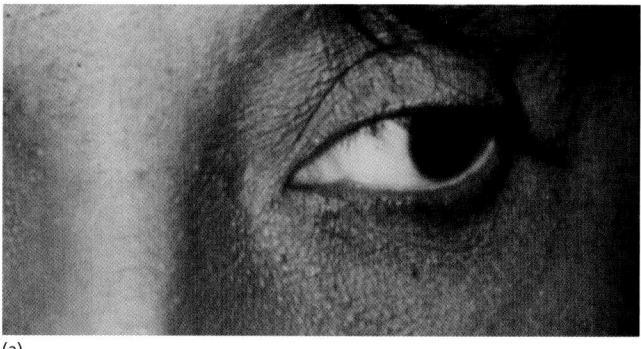

(a)

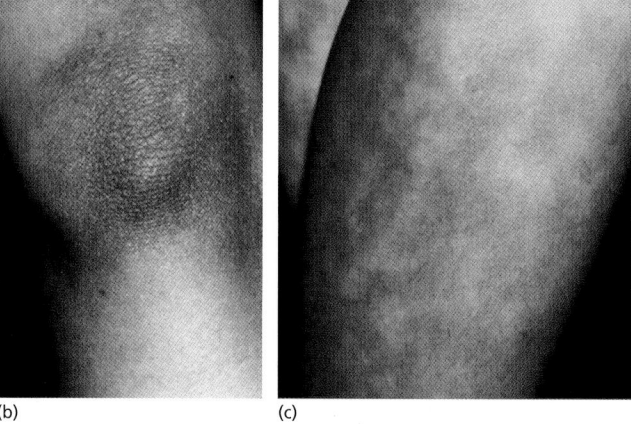

(b)   (c)

Figure 88.23 (a–c) Chloroquine pigmentation: patient received chloroquine for 9 years for rheumatoid arthritis and had developed increasing pigmentation of the periorbital skin and extremities for 4–5 years.

Cytotoxic drugs

Hyperpigmentation is a common side effect of antitumour agents used in cancer treatment. The skin discoloration may develop in a wide variable interval of time, ranging from 1 week to several months after initiation of the treatment. The hyperpigmentation can be either localized or diffuse, and may affect all parts of the tegument, including the mucous membranes, hair and nails [1].

Long-term administration of busulfan (busulphan) produces a diffuse brown pigmentation, particularly in non-Caucasian people with a dark complexion. Less commonly, Addison disease is simulated [2,3]. Light and electron microscopy studies suggest that busulfan has both a stimulatory and a toxic effect on melanocytes [4]. Both busulfan and doxorubicin cause mucous membrane pigmentation. Other cytostatic drugs that may produce hyperpigmentation of skin include cyclophosphamide, bleomycin, fluorouracil, hydroxyurea, daunorubicin, methotrexate, mithramycin, mitomycin, thiotepa and adriamycin [5,6]. Pigmentation of the nails can be caused by many cytotoxic agents, including cisplatin, doxorubicin, idarubicin, fluorouracil, bleomycin, docetaxel, dacarbazine and hydroxyurea. Topical cytostatic drugs that produce localized hyperpigmentation include carmustine, mechlorethamine and fluorouracil. Hair pigmentation may be induced by methotrexate, and pigmentation of the teeth may be seen with cyclophosphamide.

Hydantoin

Phenytoin (diphenylhydantoin) is the prototype of the hydantoin derivatives. It has been suggested that hydantoin exerts a direct action on the melanocytes inducing dispersion of melanin granules in the cutis, in addition to increased pigmentation of the basal epidermis. A patient on this drug developed pigmentation of addisonian type and other evidence of hypoadrenalism [1].

Anticonvulsants such as hydantoin, phenytoin and barbiturates may induce skin pigmentation with a pattern of melasma for hydantoins or a diffuse brown, post-exanthematous discoloration for barbiturates [1,2].

Psychotropic drugs (e.g. trifluoperazine, imipramine)

The mechanism is uncertain, but probably involves drug–melanin complexes. There is extensive deposition of melanin-like material throughout the reticuloendothelial system and in parenchymal cells of internal organs. The pigment found in the cells of the dermis stains as for melanin [1,2]. Electron microscopy studies [3] show increased melanin in the epidermis and perivascular macrophages in the dermis that contain electron-dense particles. Radioactively labelled chlorpromazine is found to localize in tissues containing melanin [4]. It is believed that this drug or some metabolite is bound to melanin in the tissues [5]. The level of immunoreactive β-MSH in the plasma of these patients is within the normal range [6]. A blue-grey pigmentation of the sun-exposed areas of the skin has also been reported with trifluoperazine and imipramine [7,8].

Blue-grey pigmentation of the sun-exposed areas of the skin is seen in a small percentage of patients receiving high doses of chlorpromazine for long periods (Figure 88.24) [1,2]. The pigmentation is cumulative and some develop a purplish tint. Related phenothiazines may cause a similar effect, but chlorpromazine is usually implicated [9]. Some of those affected also develop cataracts, corneal opacities and pigmentation of the conjunctivae [10]. The nail beds are also affected in severe cases [2].

Tetracyclines

The pathomechanisms of the discoloration is still uncertain. An isomorphic response with hyperproduction of melanin, particularly in inflammatory or sun-exposed zones, by a direct effect of the drug on melanocytes may be involved. Minocycline-induced hyperpigmentation types I and II are believed to be caused by minocycline-iron chelation products. Type III is believed to be caused by either minocycline-induced melanization or a minocycline–melanin complex, and type IV is due to either a calcium–minocycline or melanin–minocycline complex [1,2].

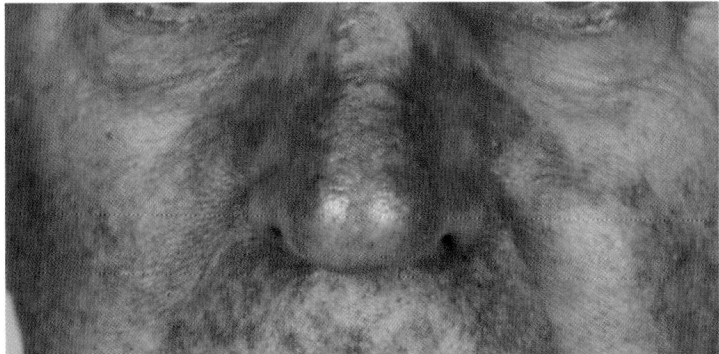

Figure 88.24 Chlorpromazine pigmentation: patchy bands of muddy pigmentation extending across the nose to the paranasal and preauricular skin in an elderly male receiving long-term therapy.

Tetracycline-induced skin discoloration although uncommon has been mainly reported with minocycline, and only rarely with doxycycline or first-generation molecules [1,2]. Minocycline-induced hyperpigmentation can affect various anatomical locations, including the skin, nails, oral cavity, sclera and conjunctiva, skeleton and cartilage, as well as viscera and body fluids. The risk of pigmentation is higher with longer duration of treatment or high cumulative dose (Figure 88.25), although cutaneous or oral pigmentation can occur regardless of dose or duration of therapy [3].

Four unique patterns of cutaneous minocycline-induced discoloration have been described [4–6]. They share a similar morphology, with well-circumscribed blue-grey macules located respectively in areas of acne scars (type I), at sites of previous inflammation distant from sites of inflammation or infection and mostly affecting sun-exposed areas including the shins, ankles and arms (type II), or on the vermilion of the lower lip (type IV). Type III is known as the 'muddy skin syndrome' and is characterized by diffuse symmetrical brown-grey discoloration with a tendency to photo-aggravation.

Electron microscopy reveals electron-dense material in dermal macrophages and X-ray microanalysis confirms the presence of iron [7]. Partial resolution of the pigmentation occurs after the drug is stopped [8]. Similar blue-black pigmentation of the legs has resulted from treatment with the 4-quinolone antibiotic pefloxacin [9] and the tetracycline antibiotic methacycline [10].

Epidemiology

Incidence and prevalence

Drug-induced hyperpigmentation accounts for 10–20% of all cases of acquired hyperpigmentation.

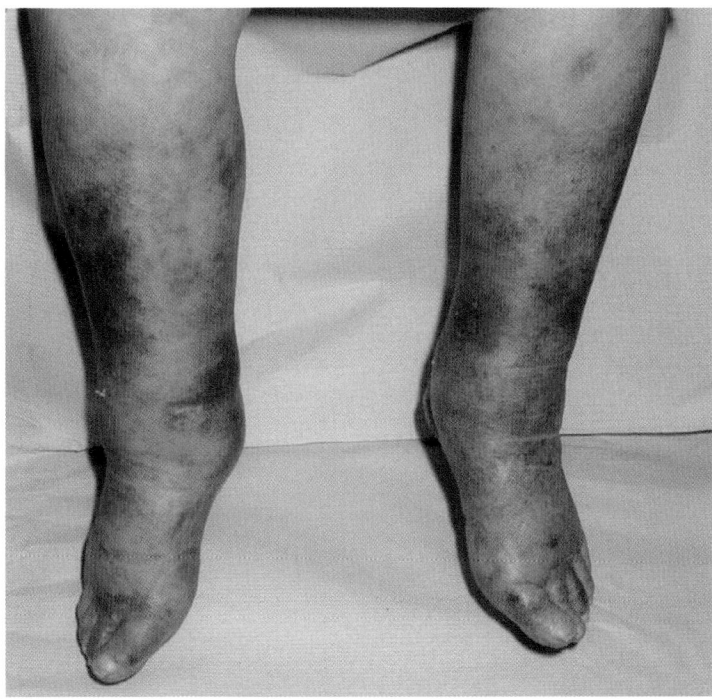

Figure 88.25 Minocycline pigmentation: marked dyspigmentation of the lower legs resulting from minocycline therapy commenced 2 years earlier as adjunctive therapy for control of bullous pemphigoid.

Antimalarial drugs: about 25% of patients receiving one of the four most commonly used antimalarials (chloroquine, hydroxy-chloroquine, mepacrine (quinacrine) and mefloquine) for at least 4 months will develop a discoloration of the skin.

Hydantoin: some 10% of patients receiving hydantoin preparations develop pigmentation of the face and neck, resembling chloasma, which fades in a few months when the drug is stopped.

Tetracyclines: minocycline-induced hyperpigmentation may affect up to 15% of patients receiving minocycline, particularly in long-duration treatments, with the bones of the oral cavity most frequently affected sites of pigmentation. Overall incidence is estimated between 3 and 5%.

Clinical features

Differential diagnosis
See Box 88.3a.

Disease course and prognosis
Discoloration is mostly reversible after discontinuation of the causative drug. In a small number of patients, the hyperpigmentation persist even after long-term discontinuation.

Amiodarone: in most cases, the pigmentation is slowly reversible and fades over months to years after discontinuation of the drug. Dose reduction or withdrawal of amiodarone can lead to complete disappearance of the pigmentation.

Antimalarial drugs: discoloration slowly fades after discontinuation of treatment, but may take several months to disappear, and rarely resolves completely. With continued therapy, the areas darken, particularly oval patches on the shins, which increase in size. A blue-black colour may develop. Also, these patches are more pigmented in light-exposed areas.

Cytotoxic drugs: after discontinuation of the causative agent, the pigmentation usually fades, at least partially, but may persist for a long time after discontinuation of the treatment (e.g. bleomycin). Rarely, hyperpigmentation can be irreversible.

Tetracyclines: complete resolution of minocycline-induced hyperpigmentation can be expected in types I and II, but can take several months to years after discontinuation of treatment. Types III and IV seem not to disappear over time.

Treatment ladder

First line
- Discontinuation of the causative drug (if possible)
- Sun avoidance/sun protection

Second line
- Laser therapy (e.g. Q-switched laser in minocycline-induced hyperpigmentation [1])

Fixed drug eruption

Definition
Fixed drug eruption is one of the most common forms of drug-induced exanthems. The acute eruption characteristically settles leaving residual hyperpigmentation, especially in those with darker skin types [1,2]. The topic is discussed in detail in Chapter 118.

Pathophysiology
Immunohistological findings suggest that the characteristic same-site recurrence may be induced by prolonged intercellular adhesion molecule 1 (ICAM-1) expression in the lesional keratinocytes correlated with the degree of residing epidermal T-suppressor cytotoxic cells. It is suggested that the eruption may be mediated by a type IV hypersensitivity, although the results of skin tests have been inconsistent and influenced by a range of factors including the causative drug [3].

Predisposing factors
Fixed eruptions are particularly frequent in black people.

Pathology
The slate-brown colour in fixed drug eruption is due to pigmentary incontinence with melanophages in the upper dermis [4].

Environmental factors
A great variety of causative drugs are known to be related with fixed drug eruptions. Most frequently reported drugs include tetracyclines, non-steroidal anti-inflammatory drugs, sulfonamides and sedatives.

Clinical features

Presentation
Well-circumscribed areas of slate-brown pigmentation commonly follow the erythematous and bullous stages of fixed eruptions (see Chapter 118) but almost universal brown pigmentation has followed the long-continued ingestion of phenolphthalein [5]. More or less symmetrical, discrete patches are usually seen but the melanosis may be diffuse or melasma-like, and the mucous membranes may be involved [6,7]. The genitalia and perianal area are often affected, although the eruption can appear anywhere on the skin surface. The characteristic course is recurrence of lesions at the same sites with development of new areas of involvement with repeated exposure to the causative agent.

Clinical variants
Rarely, fixed eruptions may be triggered by foods or UV light [8].

Differential diagnosis
See Box 88.3b.

Disease course and prognosis
The lesions may increase in size and/or number with continuation of the causative drug, leaving ever deeper residual pigmentation (Figure 88.26).

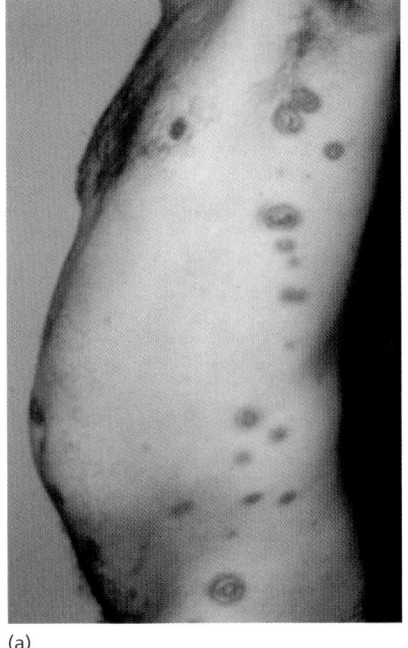

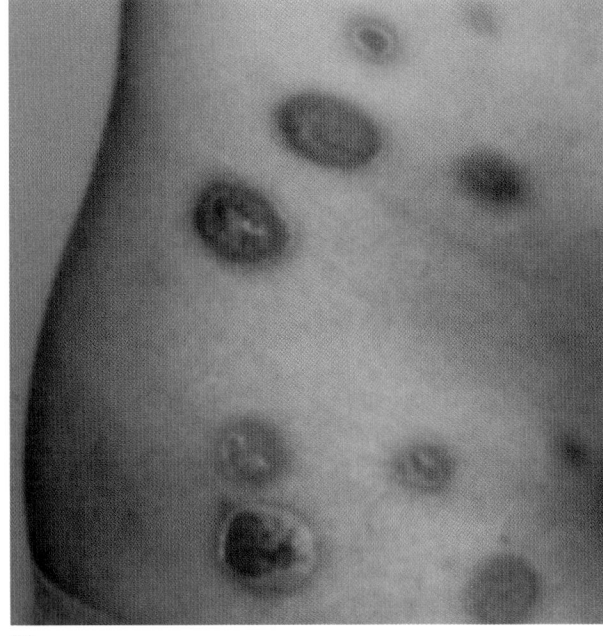

(a)   (b)

Figure 88.26 (a,b) Pigmented fixed drug eruption: extensive eruption following repeated courses of tetracycline.

Pigmentation resulting from acute photodynamic and phototoxic reactions

Definition and nomenclature

Drugs and other chemicals with photodynamic and phototoxic activity have the potential to induce skin hyperpigmentation (see Photocontact facial melanosis, p. 88.12). If the photodynamic agent is applied directly to the skin, the intensity of the pigmentary response is greatly enhanced as in the two conditions described here:

1 Phytophotodermatitis: an inflammatory and pigmentary reaction of the skin to light, potentiated by furocoumarins in plants (Figure 88.27) [1–5].

2 Berloque dermatitis: skin pigmentation due to phototoxic reaction to perfumes applied to the skin (Figure 88.28) [6–9].

Synonyms and inclusions
- Phytophotodermatitis: meadow dermatitis, strimmer dermatitis, weed-wacker dermatitis
- Berloque dermatitis: phototoxic reaction to fragrance

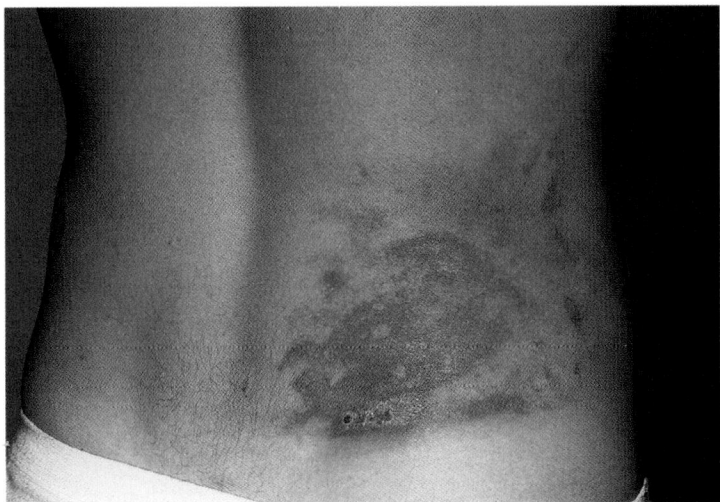

Figure 88.27 Phytophotodermatitis. Linear, streaky pigmentation following an acute blistering reaction caused by giant hogweed and sunlight.

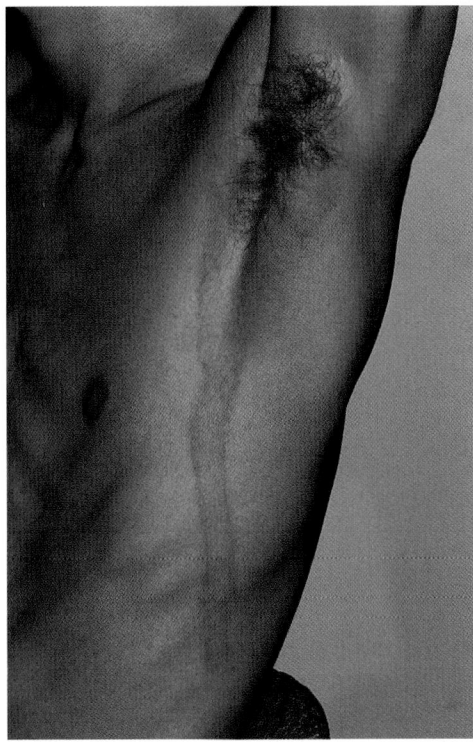

Figure 88.28 Berloque dermatitis.

Epidemiology

Incidence and prevalence
Not exactly established, although relatively common in the summer months.

Age
Any age.

Sex
M = F.

Ethnicity
No racial predominance.

Susceptibility

Phytophotodermatitis: there is some individual variation in susceptibility but with adequate exposure most will react [1,2].

Berloque dermatitis: there is wide variation in susceptibility, with the reaction occurring in only a small proportion of those exposed [6]. This variation depends on the readiness with which the bergapten is absorbed, the quantity applied, and the intensity and duration of exposure to UV light. Susceptibility is increased by stripping the horny layer. Hot humid conditions favour absorption. The pigmentation occurs in susceptible subjects who have been exposed to light after the application of perfume [7,8].

Pathophysiology

Phytophotodermatitis: all the plants reliably recorded as inducing this reaction in humans have been shown to contain furocoumarins: they include cow parsley (*Anthriscus sylvestris*) and giant hogweed (*Heracleum sphondylium*) [1,2]. The reaction occurs in those exposed to sunlight after skin contact with these plants, especially if they have been crushed.

Berloque dermatitis: Berloque dermatitis results from the potentiation of UV-stimulated melanogenesis by 5-methoxypsoralen (bergapten) in perfumes containing bergamot oil.

Clinical features

Presentation
Hypermelanosis may sometimes be heavy and persistent following photodynamic and phototoxic reactions. Phytophotodermatitis [1–5] and Berloque dermatitis [6–9] are two distinctive clinical syndromes. If the inflammatory phase is severe, bullae are formed [4,5]. Milder cases show pigmentary changes without inflammation.

Phytophotodermatitis: initially, intensely pruritic papulovesicular lesions with irregular shapes and criss-crossing linear streaks may be present. Multiple irregular large bullae may form (Figure 88.29). Typically, the lesions rapidly evolve into darkly pigmented macules (see Figure 88.27).

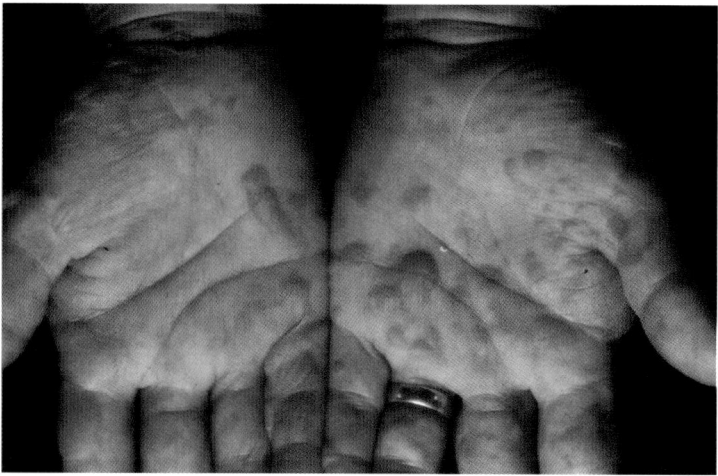

Figure 88.29 Phytophotodermatitis: acute irregular blisters across the palms after grasping giant hogweed.

Common clinical patterns for phytophotodermatitis include a bizarre network of pigmented streaks on the legs or arms (meadow dermatitis), and much finer spots and small streaks on the forearms and legs from contact with plant material during strimming (strimmer dermatitis). Squeezing limes outside when preparing cold drinks can cause blistering of the hands if carried out on sunny days. Handling celery either at harvest or when it is sold can cause phytophotodermatitis of the fingertips if it takes place in direct sunlight [4]. Handling giant hogweed in sunny weather is a particular hazard (see Figure 88.29).

Berloque dermatitis: the distribution of the lesions is therefore variable but their configuration is usually distinctive. Deep-brown pigmentation follows the pattern formed by the trickle of the droplets of perfume over the skin from their points of application (see Figure 88.28). The pigmentation fades after weeks or months. The condition is now much less frequent, although it is a continuing cosmetic problem [9].

Differential diagnosis (see Box 88.3b)
- Allergic photocontact dermatitis.
- Drug-induced phototoxicity – photosensitivity.

Disease course and prognosis
Favourable prognosis if the causing agent is avoided.

Investigations
Serial dilutions of psoralens may, in exceptional cases, be needed to distinguish photoallergy from phototoxicity [3].

Treatment ladder

First line
- Prevention: avoidance of photodynamic or phototoxic drugs, plants and perfumes
- Oral antihistamines
- Parenterally administered epinephrine in case of anaphylactic reactions

Post-inflammatory hypermelanosis

Definition
Post-inflammatory hypermelanosis is residual macular pigmentation resulting from prior skin inflammation.

Epidemiology

Incidence and prevalence
Common.

Age
Can develop at any age.

Sex
M = F.

Ethnicity
More common in deeply pigmented skin.

Pathophysiology

Predisposing factors
The intensity and persistence of the hypermelanosis are greater in dark-skinned subjects.

Pathology
Hypermelanosis commonly follows acute or chronic inflammatory processes in the skin. Disorders where there is disruption of the basal layer of the epidermis, such as in lichen planus or lupus erythematosus, frequently develop areas of slate-brown hypermelanosis. Similarly, in fixed drug eruptions, hyperpigmentation occurs due to damage of cells in the basal layer. There is pigmentary incontinence with melanophages in the upper dermis [1]. In the late phase of chronic graft-versus-host reaction, there is a poikilodermatous appearance with hyperpigmentation [2,3].

Hypermelanosis of the epidermis may also occur as a result of cutaneous inflammation, but more frequently there is reduced epidermal melanin pigmentation. This can be explained by an increased mitotic rate of keratinocytes, diminished transfer of melanosomes from the melanocyte to keratinocytes and a reduced transit time of the latter from the basal layer to the skin surface. Very frequently in inflammatory skin disease, hypermelanosis and hypomelanosis occur together, often with a slaty-blue colour due to the presence of melanophages in the upper dermis. There may be an associated loss of functional melanocytes in the skin [4].

The cause of the pigmentation is usually obvious, although the preceding lesions have sometimes not been noticed by the patient or have been transitory or clinically imperceptible.

Clinical features

Presentation
The pattern and distribution of the pigmentation will sometimes allow a retrospective diagnosis, as in lichen planus, herpes zoster, dermatitis herpetiformis and papular urticaria. Pigmentation is often conspicuous after lichenoid drug eruptions (Figure 88.30).

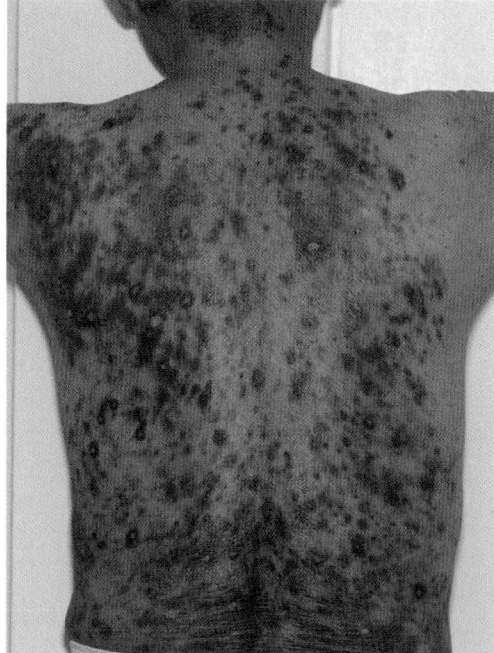

Figure 88.30 Post-inflammatory hypermelanosis on the back following propranolol-provoked lichenoid drug reaction.

The circumscribed nature and the location at the base of the scapula is characteristic of the pigmentation which typically accompanies notalgia paraesthetica, a sensory neuropathy of dorsal spinal nerves which presents as intense localized pruritus or paraesthesiae (see Chapter 85): the pigmentation may be due to chronic rubbing and scratching (Figure 88.31) [5]. Reticulate pigmentation corresponding to the underlying vascular network is seen in erythema ab igne (see Chapter 126), a more recently described cause of which is heat from laptop computers rather than open fires or hot water bottles [6]. Infective causes include late secondary syphilis, in which diffuse hypermelanosis of the sides and back of the neck and the shoulders may develop (leukoderma colli syphiliticum) (see Chapter 29) [7] and late pinta in which slaty-blue dyspigmentation may

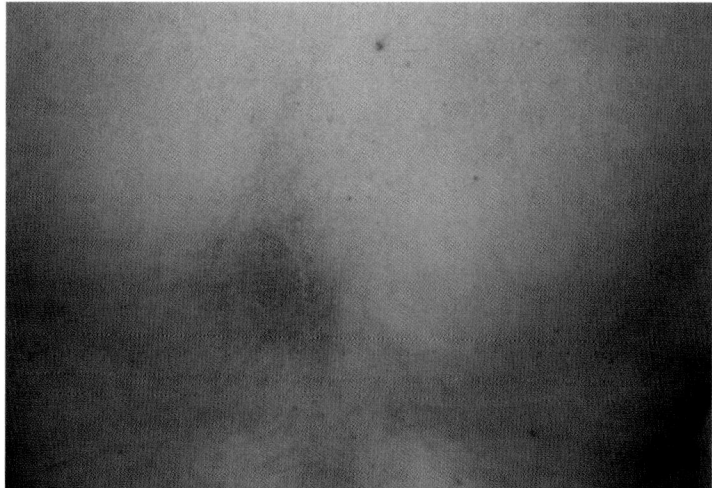

Figure 88.31 Notalgia paraesthetica: note the circumscribed area of hypermelanosis near the base of the left scapula.

be seen (see Chapter 26). Post-inflammatory hyperpigmentation may also occur following trauma to the skin, including procedures such as dermabrasion, particularly in darker skin types.

Differential diagnosis
• Acquired diffuse hyperpigmentation: see Box 88.3a.

Classification of severity
The degree of inflammation appears to be of less significance in determining the pigmentary response than the nature of the dermatosis, for it may be frequent and severe after some conditions and slight after others.

Disease course and prognosis
The skin lightens slowly over time spontaneously or with therapy. This is usually 6–12 months but may take several years.

Treatment ladder

First line
• Prevention of the inflammation, regardless of aetiology
• Treatment of underlying cause
• Sun protection

Second line
• A variety of topical treatments may be effective, including hydroquinone 2–4%, retinoids, azelaic acid and α-hydroxy acid, preferably in combination therapy

Third line
• Laser therapy (Q-switched ruby, alexandrite, Nd : YAG) but results are limited. Complete clearance of pigment is rare, and recurrence within 6–12 months is reported [8]

Ashy dermatosis and erythema dyschromicum perstans

Definition and nomenclature
A spectrum of cutaneous pigmentary disorders of uncertain aetiology characterized by the development of persistent grey-blue hypermelanotic cutaneous macules [1–5] for which no specific cause can be identified. It has been proposed that ashy dermatosis be used for all such cases but that erythema chronicum perstans be limited to those cases in which an inflammatory phase with erythema has been observed [1].

Synonyms and inclusions
• Ashy dermatosis of Ramirez
• Dermatosis cenicienta
• Erythema dyschromicum perstans
• Erythema chronicum figuratum melanodermicum
• Idiopathic eruptive macular pigmentation

Epidemiology

Incidence and prevalence
Dependent on the geographical region.

Age
From childhood to old age, most frequently in young adults.

Sex
It occurs in both sexes, but females more than males.

Ethnicity
Mainly observed in intermediate skin types. Most published cases have been from Central and South America or East Asia [4,5].

Pathophysiology
The underlying cause of ashy dermatosis is unknown and is likely to be heterogeneous. Those cases in which erythema is present share many features with lichen planus including lichenoid inflammation histopathologically with basement membrane zone damage and infiltration of T lymphocytes [6,7]. Exocytosis of cutaneous lymphocyte antigen (CLA)+ cells has been observed in areas of basement membrane zone damage, suggesting that response to antigenic stimulation may play a role in its development [7].

Pathology
The active border in cases of erythema chronicum perstans shows vacuolar degeneration of the basal cells. The epidermis contains much pigment and there is pigmentary incontinence; the dermal vessels are sleeved with an infiltrate of lymphocytes and histiocytes, and there are many melanophages [6]. Ultrastructural studies show vacuoles within the cytoplasm of basal and suprabasal keratinocytes that contain many melanosome complexes.

Genetics
In a Mexican population, HLA-DR4 has been associated with erythema dyschromicum perstans [8].

Clinical features

History
This clinical syndrome of unknown origin was first reported by Ramirez of El Salvador in 1957 under the term 'los cenicientos' (the ashy ones) due to the ashy discoloration of the skin. A further case series was reported by Convit, Kerdel-Vegas and Rodriguez from Venezuela in 1961 who commented on the presence of raised erythematous borders in the early stages and proposed the term 'erythema dyschromicum perstans' [3]. Initial inflammation is not, however, always apparent either clinically or histologically [1].

Presentation
Clinically, ashy dermatosis is characterized by numerous macules of varying shades of grey (Figure 88.32); there may initially be signs of inflammation with a red, slightly raised and palpably infiltrated margin (erythema dyschromicum perstans). In a recent review of 68 patients from Korea, less than a fifth were observed to have peripheral erythematous borders to their lesions [5]. In this

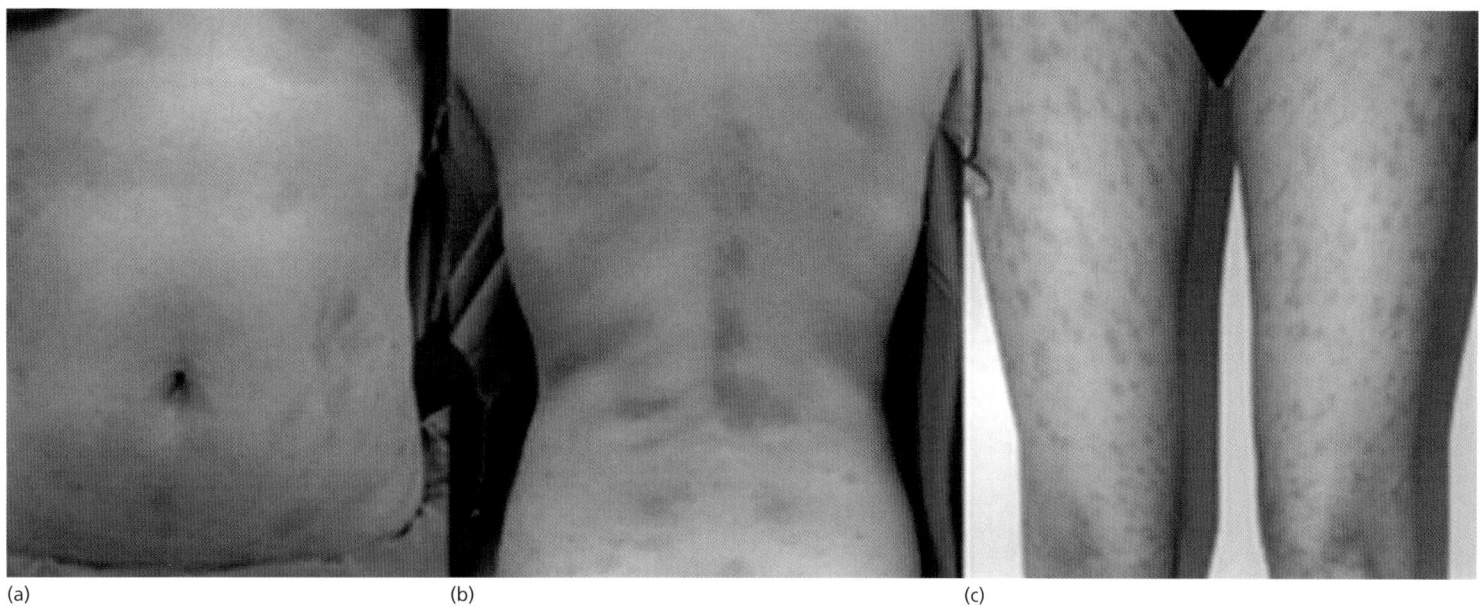

(a)   (b)   (c)

Figure 88.32 Ashy dermatosis: views of two females aged 31 years (a,b) and 15 years (c) with multiple muddy grey non-inflamed macules on the skin (From Chang *et al.* 2015 [5] .)

study, the trunk was affected in two-thirds and the face, neck and upper limbs each in just over one-third of patients; one-quarter had lower limb involvement. The macules vary in size and tend to coalesce over extensive areas of the trunk, limbs and face. Against the general greyish background are macules of hypomelanosis or hypermelanosis. The condition is persistent and slowly extends. The lesions are mostly asymptomatic, although some patients may experience mild pruritus. Mucous membranes are spared.

Differential diagnosis (see Box 88.3b)
- Lichen planus pigmentosus.
- Post-inflammatory hypermelanosis secondary to identifiable cause.
- Late pinta, which should be excluded in endemic areas.

Disease course and prognosis
The initial erythematous phase tends to settle after several months [1]. The pigmentation is persistent with a tendency to extend gradually over years.

Treatment ladder
- There is no consisently effective treatment.

First line
- Cosmetic: camouflage creams and make-up
- Clofazimine 100 mg/day for 3 months in inflammatory cases (response rate of 66–87%)

Second line
- Dapsone 100 mg/day for 3 months
- Oral corticosteroid therapy
- UV therapy

Treatment of hypermelanosis

Hypermelanosis, particularly affecting areas on the face, can be the cause of marked cosmetic disability and give rise to much mental distress. Treatment depends essentially on establishing the cause and if possible reversing the conditions that have given rise to the hypermelanosis. Because in many cases exposure to sunlight intensifies the pigmentation and lesions can be aggravated by UVA and UVB, a photoprotective preparation should be prescribed and applied during sunny weather. Cosmetic camouflage may also be indicated. In the majority of cases, topical therapy has no place, although some who are perturbed about their cosmetic disability will demand treatment with a skin-bleaching preparation.

A number of compounds have been used in skin-bleaching preparations. The most well-studied hypopigmenting agent used to treat melasma and other hypermelanotic conditions is hydroquinone. Topical hydroquinone is mostly used in a concentration of 4%, included in cold cream or a hydroalcoholic base. Acute side effects associated with hydroquinone include infrequent allergic reactions, post-inflammatory hyperpigmentation and transient hypopigmentation [1]. It can be applied alone or in the widely used triple combination cream consisting of hydroquinone 4%, a retinoid and a corticosteroid. Topical hydroquinone or this triple combination cream are highly effective and safe and can be considered as first line agents in the treatment of melasma. Because of concern about steroid-induced facial atrophy, telangiectasia and rosacea-like acneform eruptions, the use of triple combination cream has been limited to no more than twice daily for 6 months, disqualifying it as a maintenance therapy for melasma [1,2]. Topical hydroquinone and tretinoin are also effective in the treatment of post-inflammatory hyperpigmentation but require prolonged treatment [3]. The monobenzylether of hydroquinone has been used only to bleach away the remaining pigmented areas in patients with extensive vitiligo [4]. Several other substituted phenols, such as 4-isopropylcatechol, can produce cutaneous depigmentation; however, this compound and others are irritant and may sensitize [5].

In cases of pigmentary disorders such as melasma that are refractory to topical medication, combination with procedures such as peels or laser can be considered.

Chemical peels with glycolic acid or salicylic acid can be a useful adjunct to those topical treatments, although the therapeutic response is often unsatisfactory and a universally effective chemical peeling has not yet been discovered [1]. Due to the adverse effects associated with these chemical peels, such as burning, bleeding and an increased risk of hyperpigmentation, they are considered second line agents in the treatment of melasma and should be limited to cases refractory to topical treatment and used cautiously in dark-skinned patients who are at a higher risk of post-inflammatory hyperpigmentation [6].

Laser or light therapy for the treatment of melasma has become increasingly popular. As with chemical peels, they carry an increased risk of side effects due to direct damage to the skin. Despite the risks, some promising results are seen in randomized trials using laser or light therapy [3,7]. Serial treatments with intense pulsed light (IPL) therapy have been shown to be effective in the treatment of melasma and may be indicated in selected cases. Treatment of melasma with a Q-switched (QS) Nd : YAG laser has produced variable results and a high rate of relapse following treatment. The relatively limited experience and the common adverse effects of laser therapy call for more research to assess the safety and efficacy of this treatment. Lasers are considered third line agents for the treatment of melasma and should be used cautiously, especially in dark-skinned patients [2,6].

ACQUIRED HYPOMELANOSIS (Figure 88.33)

Vitiligo

Definition

Vitiligo is a common form of localized depigmentation. It is an acquired condition resulting from the progressive loss of melanocytes. It is characterized by milky-white sharply demarcated macules [1].

Vitiligo has in general been classified into two major forms: segmental vitiligo (typically unilateral maculae in a segmental/

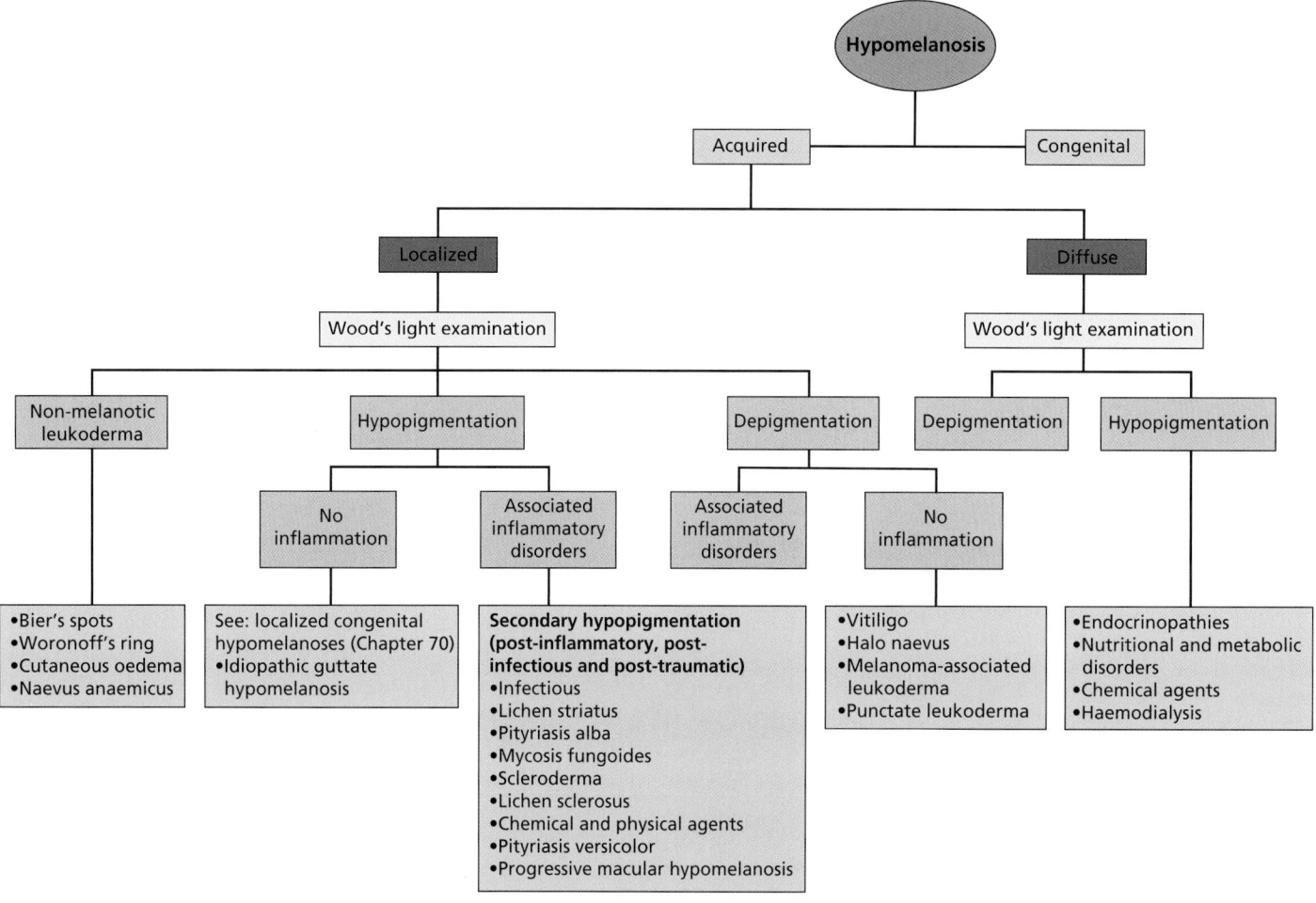

Figure 88.33 Algorithm for the differential diagnosis of hypomelanosis.

band-shaped distribution) and non-segmental vitiligo (bilateral maculae, often distributed in an acrofacial pattern or scattered symmetrically over the entire body). According to a recent Vitiligo Global Issue Consensus Conference, the term 'vitiligo' can be used as an umbrella term for all non-segmental forms of vitiligo (including several variants: acrofacial, mucosal, generalized, universal, mixed and rare variants of vitiligo) [2]. Segmental vitiligo (uni-, bi-, or plurisegmental) is classified separately. Focal lesions (small isolated depigmented lesions that are not segmentally distributed and have not evolved into non-segmental vitiligo after 1–2 years) and isolated mucosal lesions on one site are considered as undetermined/unclassified vitiligo.

Epidemiology

Incidence and prevalence
It is stated that vitiligo affects 0.5–1% of the world's population [2].

Age
Vitiligo can begin at any age but in the majority of cases becomes apparent between the age of 20 and 30 years.

Sex
The prevalence is most probably the same in both sexes [2], although in some series based on out-patient attendances a female preponderance was noted.

Ethnicity
Vitiligo affects all races.

Associated diseases
Conditions associated with vitiligo are listed in Box 88.4.

Amongst autoimmune diseases, the strongest association is with thyroid disease. The association between vitiligo and halo naevi is well established: several reports have documented the onset of vitiligo at the same time as or shortly after the appearance of a halo naevus and, in a recent study, halo naevi were present in 31.1% of all vitiligo patients [3]. Areas of depigmentation sometimes develop in patients with melanoma [3]: these may be local or distant. Vitiligo with uveitis, central nervous system involvement and premature greying of the hair occurs in the Vogt–Koyanagi–Harada syndrome (see later).

Pathophysiology

Pathology
Histochemical studies [4] show a lack of dopa-positive melanocytes in the basal layer of the epidermis (Figure 88.34). Immunohistochemical studies with a large panel of antibodies show only an occasional melanocyte in lesional skin [5]. Electron microscopy studies [6,7] confirm the loss of melanocytes. In the epidermis of areas around the margins of vitiligo abnormalities of keratinocytes [8,9] as well as degenerating melanocytes are reported. In inflammatory vitiligo, where there is a raised erythematous border, there is an infiltrate of lymphocytes and histiocytes. This infiltrate is also found in the marginal areas of some biopsies, mainly in an active stage of the disease [7].

Causative organisms
Various theories have been suggested for the aetiology of vitiligo; the same mechanism may not apply to all cases. Moreover, the loss of melanocytes in vitiligo may also be the result of different pathogenetic mechanisms working together ('convergence' or 'integrated' theory) [8,9].
- The autoimmune/autoinflammatory theory is currently the leading hypothesis and is supported by strong evidence. It is based on the clinical association of vitiligo with a number of disorders also considered to be autoimmune or autoinflammatory (see Box 88.4). The association with vitiligo has demonstrated a shared underlying genetic susceptibility to other autoimmune diseases [10].
- A combination of deregulated innate and adaptive immune responses has been proposed in vitiligo. Interestingly, several components of the innate immune system have been found to be associated with vitiligo (e.g. NLRP-1, XBP-1). Furthermore, an important role of heat shock protein 70 (hsp70) and

---

Box 88.4 Disorders associated with vitiligo

- Thyroid disease[a] (hyperthyroidism and hypothyroidism [7])
- Pernicious anaemia[a]
- Addison disease[a] [8]
- Diabetes[a] [9]
- Hypoparathyroidism[a]
- Myasthenia gravis[a]
- Alopecia areata
- Morphoea and lichen sclerosus
- Halo naevus[a]
- Malignant melanoma[a] [10]

[a]Autoantibodies demonstrable.

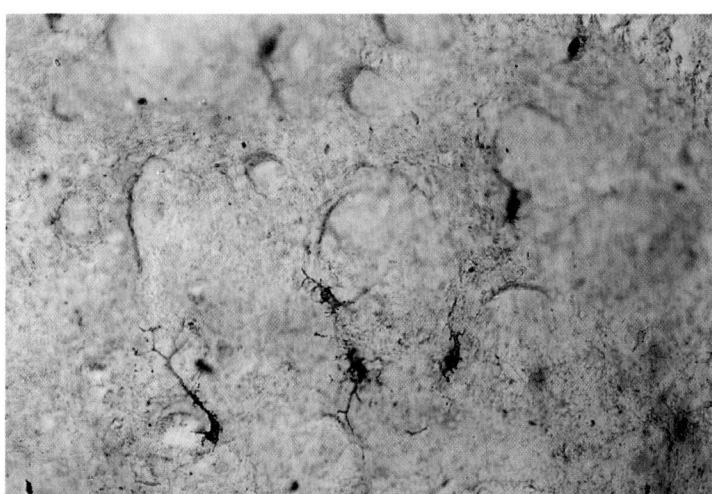

Figure 88.34 Vitiligo. Epidermal sheet of marginal depigmented area showing marked reduction in the number of melanocytes.

LL37 (which is released after cell injury) has been suggested [**11,12**,13].

- It has also been proposed that increased oxidative stress may trigger the process of 'haptenation' by increasing the levels of surrogate substrates of tyrosinase resulting in the formation of highly immunogenic neoantigens in vitiligo [14].
- Antibodies to normal human melanocytes have been detected using a specific immunoprecipitation assay [15,16], and may have a cytolytic effect on melanocytes [17]. The presence of these melanocyte antibodies has been linked to disease activity [18]. It is currently unclear if these antibodies play an initiating role in the development of vitiligo or are a secondary result of the disease [19].
- Accumulating evidence supports a major aetiological role for melanocyte-specific cytotoxic T cells in coordinating the targeted autoimmune tissue destruction of melanocytes in progressive vitiligo [20,21]. Both helper and cytotoxic T cells from progressing margins generate predominantly type 1 cytokines. This theory is supported by the fact that various effective treatment options in vitiligo have an immunosuppressive effect on the activation and maturation of T cells (e.g. local steroids and topical immunomodulators).

Many other hypotheses have been put forward. The self-destruction theory of Lerner suggested that melanocytes destroyed themselves due to a defect in a natural protective mechanism that removed toxic melanin precursors [22]. This hypothesis was based on the clinical features of vitiligo and on experimental studies of cutaneous depigmentation by chemical compounds that have a selective lethal effect on functional melanocytes [23]: these compounds can produce a leukoderma indistinguishable from idiopathic vitiligo. Other proposed mechanisms for vitiligo include defective keratinocyte metabolism with low catalase levels in the epidermis [24], defective tetrahydrobiopterin and catecholamine biosynthesis [25], and loss of melanocytes through inhibition of their adhesion to fibronectin by extracellular matrix molecules [26]. *In vivo*, repeated frictional trauma to perilesional skin in non-segmental vitiligo has been shown to induce detachment and death of melanocytes ('melanocytorrhagy') [27]. Additionally, a neurogenic mechanism has been suggested whereby it has been hypothesized that a compound released at peripheral nerve endings in the skin could have a toxic effect on melanocytes. Findings from a small number of studies on neuropeptide and neuronal markers in vitiligo suggest that neuropeptide Y may play a role [28]. So far there is, however, little support for this hypothesis.

Genetics

A genetic factor is undoubtedly involved in vitiligo. Inheritance has been suggested to be polygenic. Approximately 30% of patients have a positive family history [22] and vitiligo has been reported in monozygotic twins [29].

Genome-wide association studies have identified several susceptibility loci for generalized vitiligo, each responsible for a small part of the genetic risk. Nearly all of the genes identified at these loci encode components of the immune system. The exception is *TYR* [30], which encodes the enzyme tyrosinase, which is not a component of the immune system but catalyses melanin

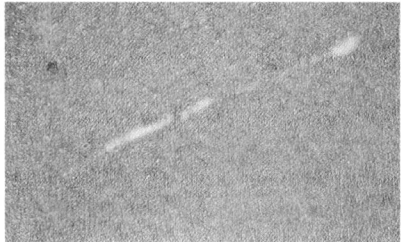

Figure 88.35 [Isomorphic or Koebner phenomenon at site of a scratch in a patient with vitiligo.

biosynthesis within the melanocyte and is a major autoantigen in generalized vitiligo.

Environmental factors

The Koebner phenomenon is a well-known phenomenon in vitiligo (also called isomorphic response) (Figure 88.35). It has been defined as the development of lesions at sites of trauma to uninvolved skin of patients with cutaneous diseases [31]. To create a universally acceptable specific system for the evaluation of Koebner phenomenon in vitiligo, the Vitiligo European Task Force (VETF) group introduced a new assessment and classification method for the evaluation of Koebner phenomenon in vitiligo [31]. It has been suggested that the Koebner phenomenon may function as a clinical parameter to assess and predict the clinical profile and course of vitiligo [32].

Clinical features

Presentation [22] (Figures 88.36 and 88.37)

The amelanotic macules in vitiligo are found particularly in areas of repeated friction, chonic pressure or trauma, for example the hips, dorsa of the hands/fingers, feet, elbows, knees and ankles [31]. The lesions are also prone to sunburn; rarely, itching may be present without previous sun exposure or sunburn. The distribution of the lesions is usually symmetrical, although in the

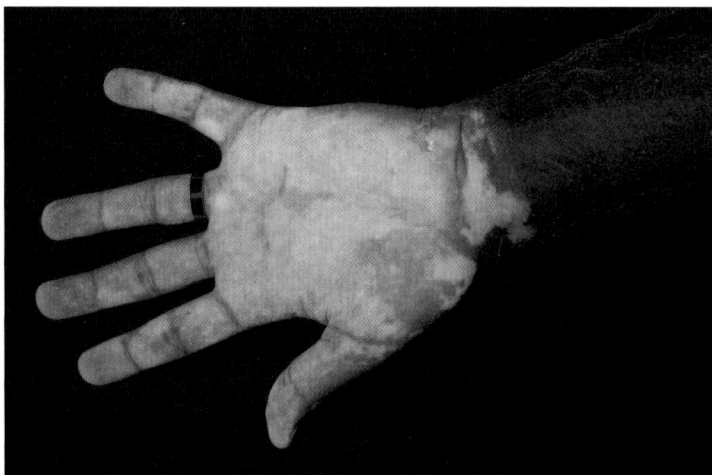

Figure 88.36 Typical distribution of vitiligo on the wrist and volar surface of the hand seen under Wood's light.

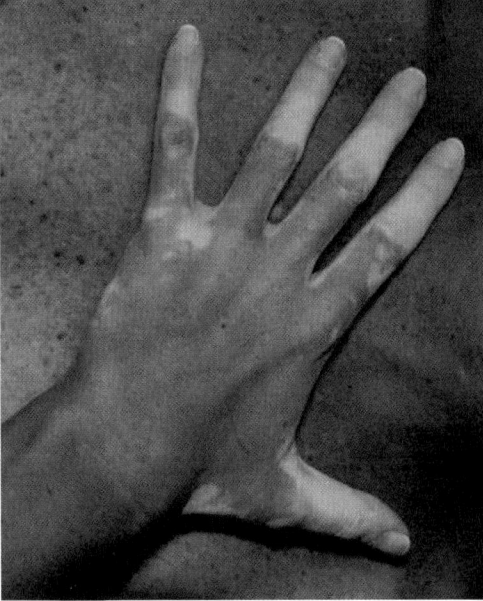
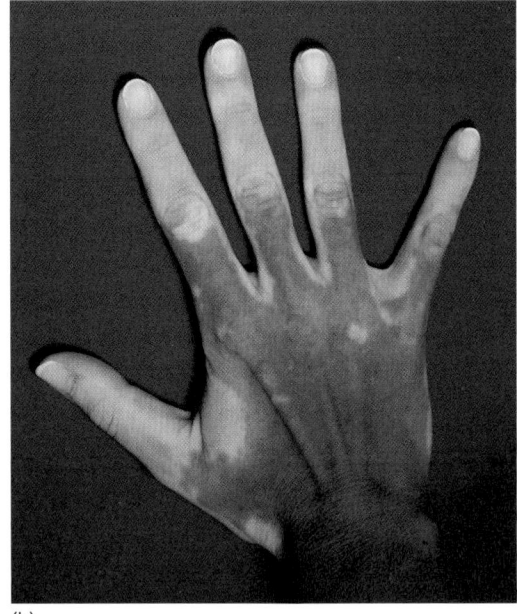

(a)   (b)

Figure 88.37 (a,b) Typical distribution of vitiligo on dorsum of the hand seen under Wood's light.

segmental subtype it is usually unilateral and band shaped (Figure 88.38). Rarely, there is complete vitiligo (universalis), although most often a few pigmented areas remain indefinitely (Figure 88.39). The pigment loss may be partial or complete, or both may occur in the same areas (trichrome vitiligo) (Figure 88.40). The macules usually have a convex outline, increase irregularly in size and fuse with neighbouring lesions to form complex patterns. The hairs in the patches can remain normally pigmented, but can also depigment after a certain period of time

(poliosis/leukotrichia). The margins of the lesions may become hyperpigmented. The main symptom is the cosmetic disability, although some patients present because of sunburn in the amelanotic areas. Vitiligo can also start in children, who are more likely to show segmental vitiligo [33].

Clinical variants

Mixed vitiligo: the coexistence of non-segmental and segmental vitiligo in one patient is called mixed vitiligo and is classified as a subgroup of vitiligo (NSV) [2].

Hypochromic vitiligo (vitiligo minor): a form of vitiligo (NSV) that seems to be limited to dark-sknined individuals [34]. The term 'minor' refers to the partial defect in pigmentation (Figure 88.41). The relation to true vitiligo is supported by pathological examination and its coexistence with conventional vitiligo macules. Repeated biopsies may be needed to exclude the early stages of cutaneous lymphoma as a differential diagnosis [2].

Halo naevi-associated leukoderma: a form of hypomelanosis analogous to melanoma-associated leukoderma, where discrete areas of depigmentation develop in skin distant from the halo naevi (see later), particularly in individuals with large numbers of them [35]. This phenomenon differs from classical vitiligo in that the depigmented macules are often more limited and not as clearly demarcated from normal skin as in vitiligo and often do not progress. The disorder probably results from a temporary autoimmune process directly linked to the halo phenomenon [35].

Differential diagnosis [36]
1 Halo naevi.
2 Naevus depigmentosus.
3 Naevus anaemicus.

Figure 88.38 Segmental vitiligo on the trunk seen under Wood's light. Note regressing congenital naevus in the centre of the affected area.

PART 8: SPECIFIC CUTANEOUS STRUCTURE

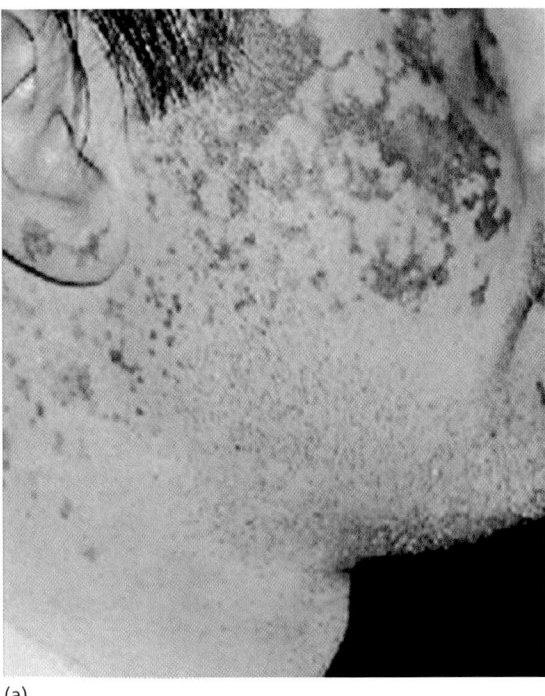
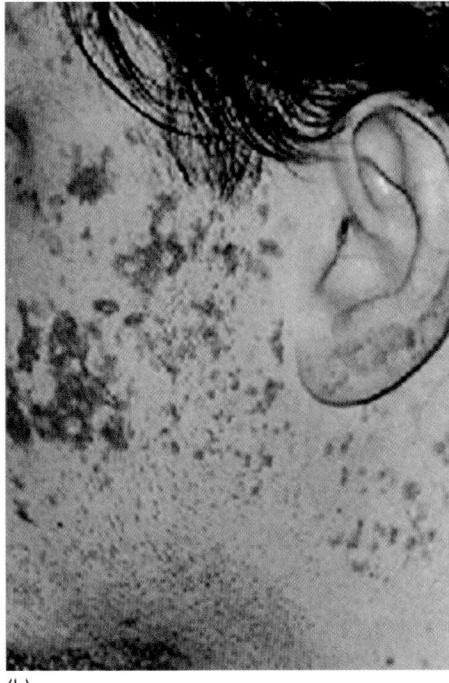

(a)   (b)

Figure 88.39 (a,b) Extensive vitiligo in a South Asian man: view of the sides of the face showing the convex expanding margins of the vitiliginous skin 'eating into' the few residual areas of normal pigmentation. Note that pigmentation of the scalp and beard hair is unaffected.

4 Inherited or genetically induced hypomelanosis (usually present at birth).
  • Piebaldism.
  • Waardenburg syndrome.
  • Tuberous sclerosis.
  • Pigmentary mosaicism (hypomelanosis of Ito).
5 Progressive macular hypomelanosis.
6 Secondary hypomelanosis.
  • Post-inflammatory hypomelanosis (e.g. pityriasis alba, lichen sclerosus, morphoea).
  • Post-traumatic hypomelanosis.

• Post-infectious hypomelanosis (e.g. pityriasis versicolor, leprosy).
• Cutaneous lymphoma.

Classification of severity
The affected body surface area is often used to score the severity of the disease.

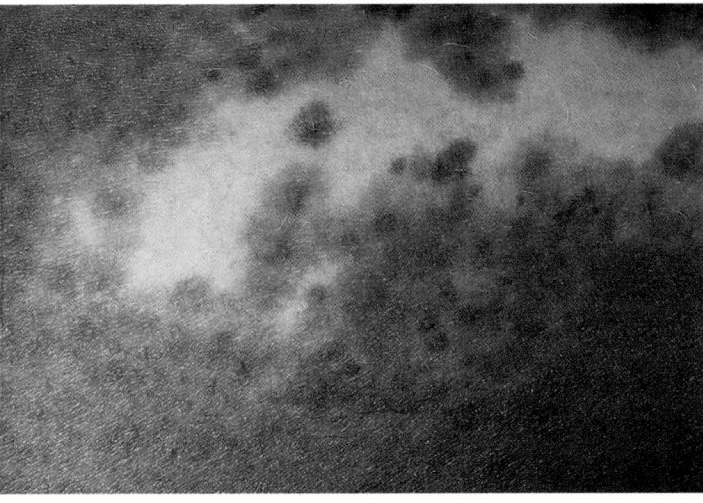

Figure 88.40 Trichrome vitiligo.

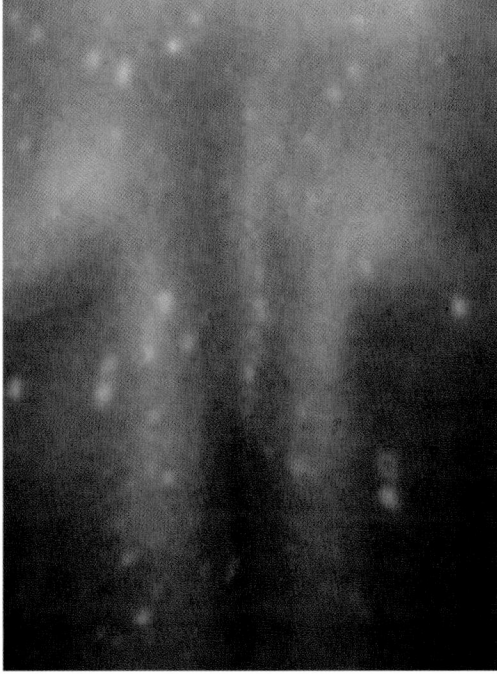

Figure 88.41 Hypochromic vitiligo affecting the back. (From Ezzedine *et al.* 2015 [44] reproduced with permission from the copyright holder Wiley.)

Complications and co-morbidities

See Associated diseases.

Disease course and prognosis

Most frequently, vitiligo is gradually progressive, sometimes extending rapidly over a period of several months and then remaining quiescent for many years. Spontaneous repigmentation can sometimes be noted in sun-exposed areas, and can have a typical perifollicular appearence [22]. Segmental vitiligo generally starts earlier in life than non-segmental vitiligo and often stabilizes within the first year of onset [33].

Investigations

The diagnosis of vitiligo is based essentially on clinical examination, because the lesions have a typical appearance. However, if the lesions are not distributed in the pattern of classical vitiligo, confusion with other hypomelanotic disorders can arise. Inspection with the aid of a Wood's light can then be helpful. The presence of a family history of vitiligo, the Koebner phenomenon, leukotrichia or associated autoimmune disorders such as thyroid disease can help to support a clinical diagnosis of vitiligo [36].

Management

Response to treatment of vitiligo varies between individuals but is often unsatisfactory, especially for acral lesions. Patients are best advised to seek effective cosmetic camouflage (Figure 88.42) and to use sunscreen. Furthermore, the risk of koebnerization resulting from everyday activities should be explained to patients. Some authors suggest that successful repigmentation is mostly the result of combinations of various interventions including light, indicating this is an effective, though not necessarily permanent treatment for generalized vitiligo. Providing ways of coping with vitiligo could also be of benefit to patients while this disease has no cure [37].

First line

In some patients, once-daily application of potent topical corticosteroid preparations (e.g. 0.1% betamethasone valerate or 0.05% clobetasol propionate) is effective at inducing repigmentation of areas of vitiligo. It is preferable to use an intermittent regimen (e.g. 15 days per month for 6 months) to avoid local side effects (skin atrophy, telangiectasia, striae, hypertrichosis and acneform eruptions) [38]. More recently, use of topical calcineurin inhibitors (pimecrolimus, tacrolimus) has been reported to be successful, mainly for lesions on the face and neck [38]: twice-daily applications are recommended, initially for 6 months.

Second line

Treatment with systemic psoralen photochemotherapy (PUVA) is effective in a proportion of cases [37]. Guidance on treatment regimens is given in Chapter 21 and in the European Dermatology Forum guidelines [36]. The use of topical applications of psoralens is more hazardous and may result in untoward blistering of the skin. Alternative photosensitizers including khellin have been advocated but there are concerns over hepatotoxicity and it has not been widely adopted [39].

UVB therapy can also be used selectively and localized targeted phototherapy devices (excimer lamp or lasers with a peak at 308 nm) [37]. There is no consensus as to the optimum treatment duration of phototherapy. Most often irradiation will be stopped if no repigmentation occurs within the first 3 months of treatment.

Third line

Grafting techniques [38,40]

Surgical methods have been proposed as a therapeutic option in patients with stable vitiligo (e.g. segmental vitiligo). These surgical techniques are based on a common basic principle: to transplant autologous melanocytes from a normal pigmented area to

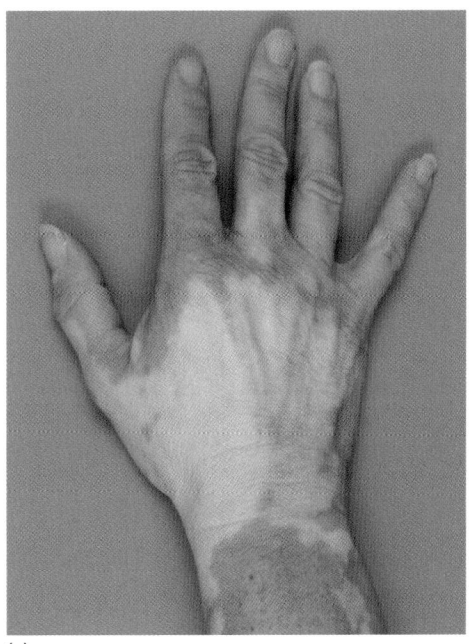
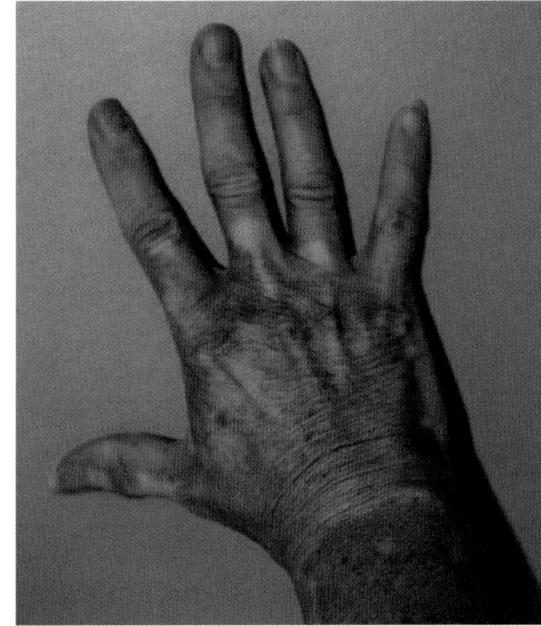

Figure 88.42 (a,b) Vitiligo: before and after camouflage of the hands.

(a)   (b)

the affected depigmented skin. Different surgical techniques for repigmenting vitiligo have been gradually devised and include tissue grafts (full-thickness punch grafts, split-thickness grafts, suction blister grafts) and cellular grafts (cultured melanocytes, cultured epithelial sheet grafts and non-cultured epidermal cellular grafts). Lately, the use of hair follicle outer root sheath cells has been introduced [41]. The three tissue grafting methods (full-thickness punch grafts, split-thickness grafts, suction blister grafts) seem to have comparable success rates in inducing repigmentation. Cellular grafting techniques were in general found to be nearly as effective, although the percentages of patients in whom repigmentation was achieved were slightly lower than with the tissue grafting techniques [42]. However, cellular grafting can be used to treat larger areas and has in general better cosmetic results compared to tissue grafts (Figure 88.43) [43]. Furthermore, adverse events seem to be less frequent with cellular grafts than with punch or split-skin grafts.

Depigmenting treatment

In those patients with extensive vitiligo and only a few residual areas of pigmentation, skin bleaching with laser therapy (e.g. Q-switched alexandrite 755 nm, Q-switched ruby 694 nm), cryotherapy or creams (e.g. 20% monobenzylether of hydroquinone), may be used [44].

Treatment ladder

First line
- Topical corticosteroids, topical calcineurin inhibitors [38]

Second line
- Phototherapy

Resources

Further information
Guidelines: references [38] and [42].

Patient resources
Vitiligo Society UK www.vitiligosociety.org.uk (last accessed October 2015).

Halo naevus

Synonyms and inclusions
- Sutton naevus
- Leukoderma acquisitum centrifugum

Introduction and general description
Leukoderma acquisitum centrifugum designates the development of a halo of hypomelanosis around a central cutaneous tumour [1–10]. This tumour is usually a benign melanocytic naevus but may be a neuroid naevus, blue naevus, neurofibroma, or primary or secondary malignant melanoma [1].

Epidemiology

Incidence and prevalence
The prevalence of halo naevi has been estimated to be approximately 1% in the white population [9].

Age
Halo naevi can be seen at all ages, but is usually seen in young people.

PART 8: SPECIFIC CUTANEOUS STRUCTURE

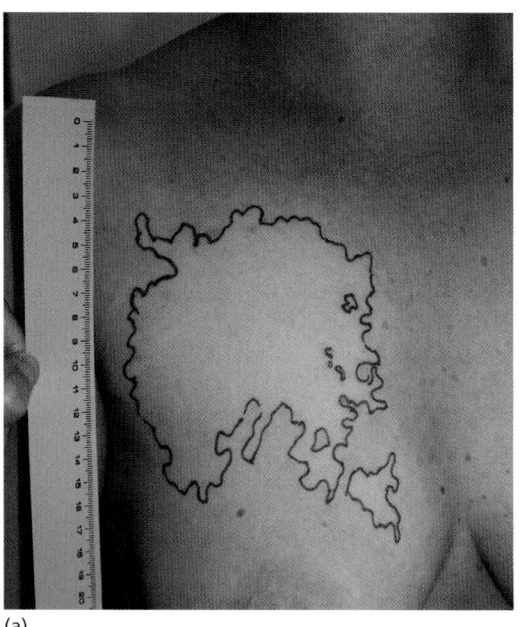

(a)

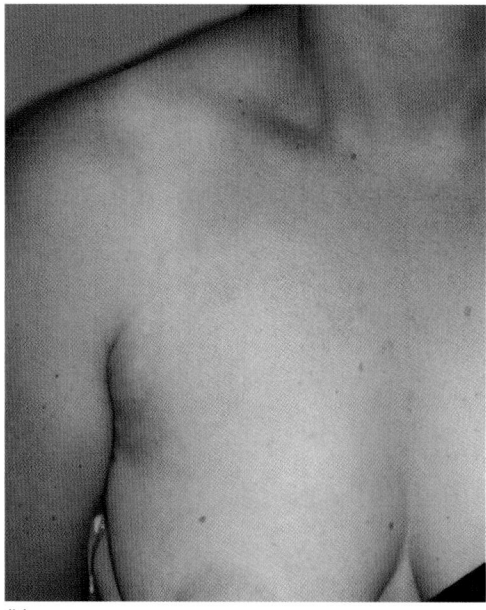

(b)

Figure 88.43 (a,b) Segmental vitiligo (a) before and (b) after treatment with non-cultured epidermal cell transplantation.

Sex
Either sex.

Ethnicity
Not known.

Associated diseases
Halo naevi occur with increased frequency in patients with vitiligo (see earlier) [9]. An immunological and clinical association of halo naevus with cutaneous malignant melanoma has been described. Antibodies against the cytoplasm of malignant melanoma cells are found in the serum of patients with halo naevi [3]. The prevalence of halo naevi was found to be 18% in a study of 72 patients with Turner syndrome compared with 1% in controls: the authors speculated that growth hormone therapy might have played a role [10].

Pathophysiology

Pathology
Most halo naevi are compound naevi, although a junctional or dermal naevoid pattern is also possible. Both congenital and acquired naevi can be affected. There is frequently a lymphocytic infiltration of the naevus and the constituent cells may show damage. Ultrastructural studies show the apposition of mononuclear cells with naevus cells that show cytotoxic changes [5]. In the depigmented halo, there is an absence of melanocytes, but Langerhans cells may be present [6]. Melanophages can be present in the dermis [1,7].

Causative organisms
Usually, no triggering factors are present, although the occurrence of halo naevi has occasionally been mentioned to be associated with sun exposure and sunburn. However, a causal relation has never been confirmed.

Genetics
Not known.

Clinical features

History
Vitiligo can be present in the personal or family history.

Presentation
Circular areas of hypomelanosis occur around pigmented naevi, particularly on the trunk, less commonly on the head and rarely on the limbs. Multiple lesions are common, the halos being about 0.5–2.0 cm wide and developing simultaneously or at intervals around several, but not all, naevi (Figure 88.44).

Clinical variants
A hypomelanotic halo may develop around a melanoma in a manner analogous to halo naevus (see Figure 88.44c).

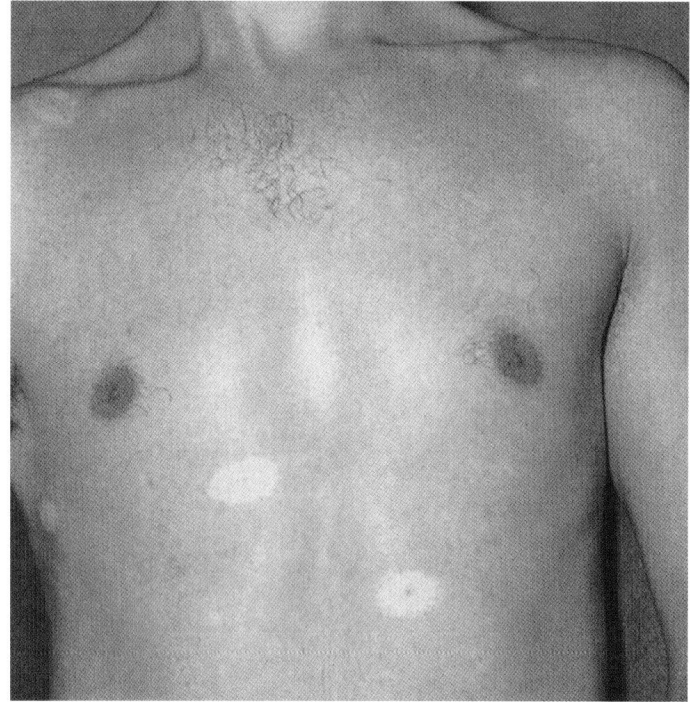

(a)

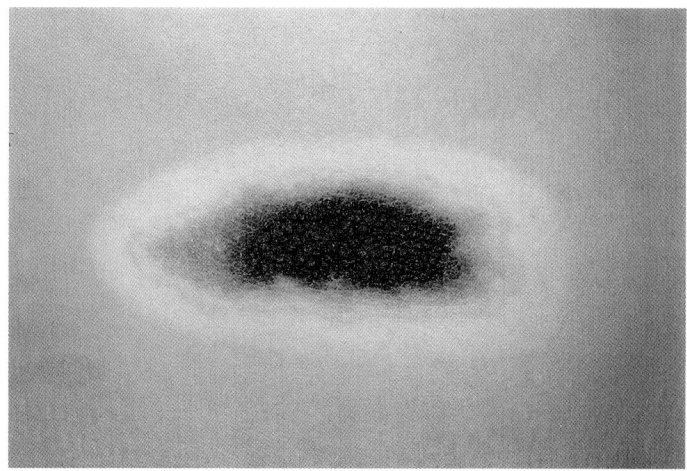

(b)

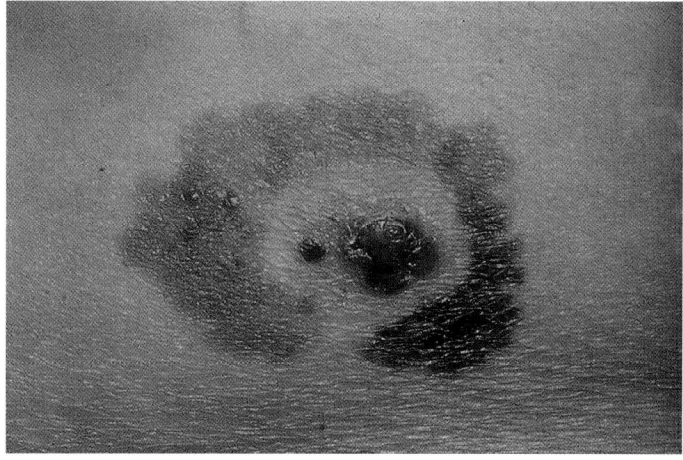

(c)

Figure 88.44 (a) Multiple halo naevi in a young man who also had vitiligo. (b) Unusually large halo naevus. (c) Halo phenomenon developing within a malignant melanoma that later proved fatal.

Box 88.5 Differential diagnosis of acquired hypo- and depigmentation

(a) Acquired diffuse hypo- or depigmentation
- Depigmentation
  - Vitiligo
- Hypopigmentation
  - Chemical-induced hypopigmentation
  - Endocrinopathies
  - Nutritional conditions
  - Post-inflammatory
- Non-melanotic leukoderma
  - Anaemia

(b) Acquired localized hypo- or depigmentation
- Depigmentation
  - Vitiligo[a,b]
  - Halo naevi[a]
  - Punctate leukoderma[b]
  - Melanoma-associated leukoderma[a,b]
- Hypopigmentation
  - Progressive macular hypomelanosis[b]

- Idiopathic guttate hypomelanosis[b]
- Secondary hypopigmentation (post-infectious, post-inflammatory, post-traumatic)
  - Lichen planus[a,b]
  - Lichen sclerosus[a]
  - Lichen striatus[a]
  - Lupus erythematosis[a,b]
  - Morphoea[a]
  - Pityriasis alba[a]
  - Pityriasis lichenoides chronica[b]
  - Pityriasis versicolor[a,b]
  - Psoriasis[a,b]
  - Sarcoidosis[a,b]
- Non-melanotic leukoderma
  - Bier spots[b]

[a]Limited surface areas affected.
[b]Larger surface areas can be affected

Differential diagnosis (see Box 88.5)
- Vitiligo.

Complications and co-morbidities
Halo naevi can be present with or without associated vitiligo lesions.

Disease course and prognosis
The naevus tends to flatten and may disappear completely (Figure 88.45). The depigmented areas often persist, but may pigment after many years.

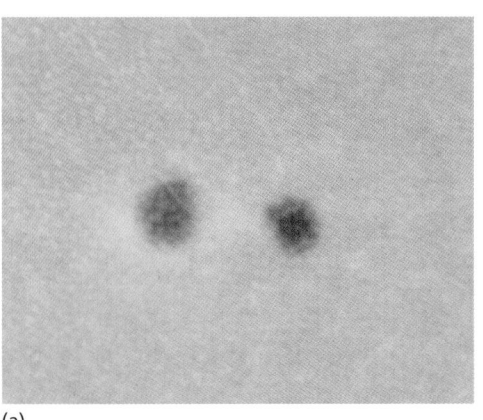

(a)

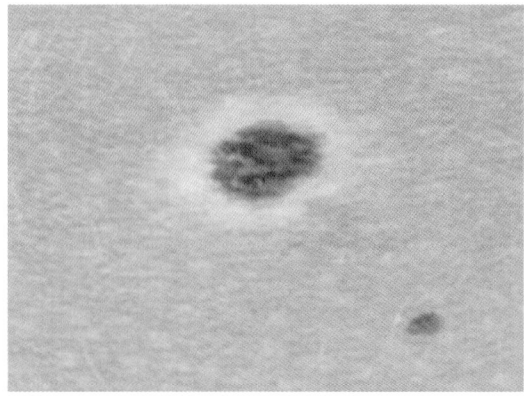

(b)

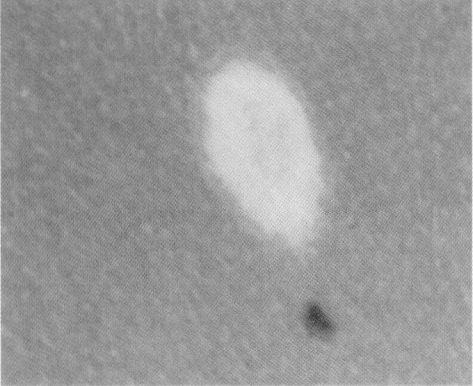

(c)

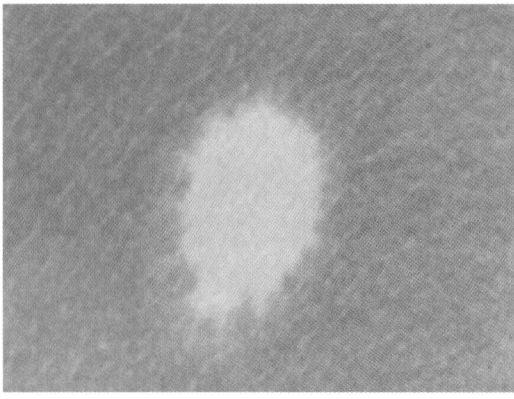

(d)

Figure 88.45 Halo naevi in different stages of evolution concurrently in a 13-year-old girl: (a) early depigmentation; (b) established halo naevus; (c) faint pink residuum of naevus just visible in the centre of the hypomelanotic macule; and (d) residual hypomelanotic macule following complete destruction of the naevus.

Investigations

Excision of the naevus may be indicated in case of doubt about its benign character.

Management

Normally none is required. The usual diagnostic criteria must be applied if there is any possibility that the central tumour is malignant. It should be remembered that a halo around a benign naevus is relatively common, whereas malignant melanoma is rare, and a melanoma surrounded by a halo is extremely rare. Mutilating surgery must never be undertaken without preliminary histological examination by an experienced pathologist.

Acquired syndromic hypomelanosis

Vogt–Koyanagi–Harada syndrome

In 1906, Vogt reported a patient with atraumatic, idiopathic uveitis, poliosis and alopecia, a syndrome that in time would be associated with his name [1]. In 1926, Harada reported five cases of bilateral posterior uveitis and retinal detachment [2]. In 1929, Koyanagi reported 16 patients with headache, fever, dysacousia, vitiligo, poliosis, alopecia, bilateral anterior uveitis with occasional exudative retinal detachment [3]. Various combinations of synonym have been used for this disorder, which is now generally referred to with the above three names, and abbreviated to VKHS.

Pathophysiology

The aetiology of VKHS has yet to be established. An abnormal response to a virus and immunological mechanisms have both been postulated.

Pathology

Electron microscopy of depigmented skin shows an absence of melanocytes as in vitiligo [4]. Colloid-amyloid bodies are also found at the dermal-epidermal junction [5]. Inflammatory skin lesions are characterized by a chronic mixed inflammatory cell infiltrate [6].

Clinical features [7,8]

VKHS mainly affects dark-skinned people or Caucasian people with dark pigmentation. It is rare but widely distributed. Most cases occur in the third and fourth decades but children may be affected. It affects the skin, eyes, inner ears and meninges.

Criteria for diagnosis are as follows:

- No history of ocular trauma or surgery preceding the initial onset of uveitis.
- No clinical or laboratory evidence suggestive of ocular disease entities.
- Bilateral ocular involvement: an early sign is diffuse choroiditis; a late sign is ocular depigmentation.
- Neurological and auditory findings: meningismus, tinnitus, cerebrospinal fluid pleocytosis.
- Skin and hair changes: alopecia, vitiligo, poliosis.

Typically, this condition is first diagnosed by ophthalmologists as the uveitis starts the march of symptoms and signs.

Diagnosis

The association of vitiligo with loss of pigment in the brows and lashes and with the residual ocular defects should clearly differentiate this syndrome from any other.

Alezzandrini syndrome [1–4]

Alezzandrini was involved in three papers describing the syndrome that now bears his name in the late 1950s and early 1960s [1–3].

Aetiology

The aetiology of this syndrome is unknown.

Clinical features

Alezzandrini syndrome has only been reported in a small number of cases [1–4]. It is characterized by unilateral, facial vitiligo associated with unilateral retinal degeneration, white hair, poliosis and deafness. There are similarities with the VKHS in which skin, eye and auditory changes are also observed.

Post-inflammatory hypomelanosis [1–17]

Synonyms and inclusions
- Post-inflammatory/secondary hypopigmentation

Introduction and general description

Hypomelanotic areas occur following the resolution of areas of eczema and psoriasis (Figure 88.46). Hypomelanosis is also seen in pityriasis lichenoides and cutaneous T-cell lymphoma [1].

The superficial eczema known as pityriasis alba (see Chapter 39) commonly presents with white, somewhat scaly, and not so

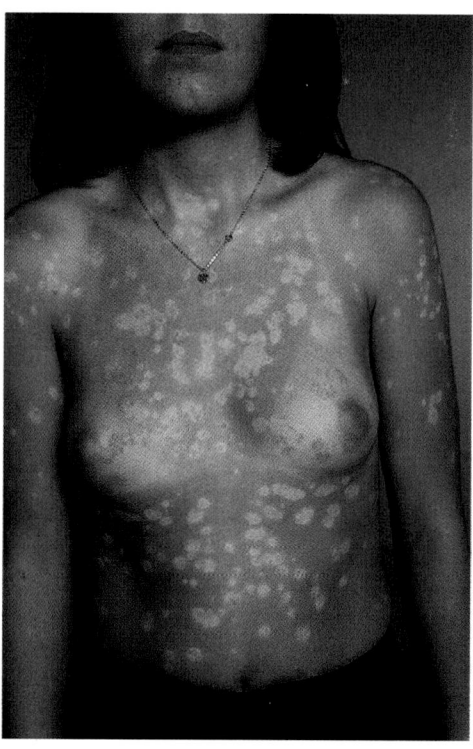

Figure 88.46 Hypopigmentation in a girl with resolving psoriasis.

PART 8: SPECIFIC CUTANEOUS STRUCTURE

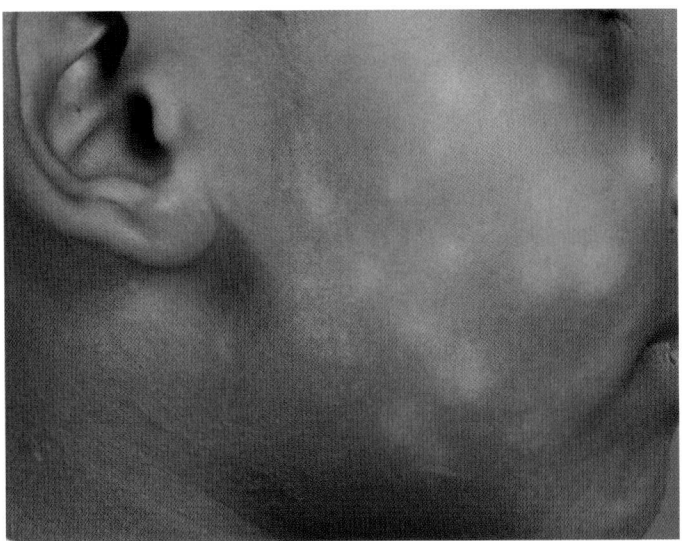

Figure 88.47 Pityriasis alba.

well-defined areas of skin, which are most noticeable on the cheeks of racially pigmented children (Figure 48.47).

Hypopigmented macules also occur in the superficial fungal infection pityriasis versicolor, a condition frequently mistaken for vitiligo (Figure 48.48). Hyperpigmented areas can also be present. In a number of other inflammatory disorders of the skin, there are areas of hypomelanosis and in these there may be a loss of functional melanocytes. This loss is seen in lupus erythematosus and lichen planus. Hypomelanosis is also seen in sarcoidosis [7,8], lichen stiatus, leprosy [9] and can occur in syphilis.

Epidemiology

Sex
Males and females are equally predisposed.

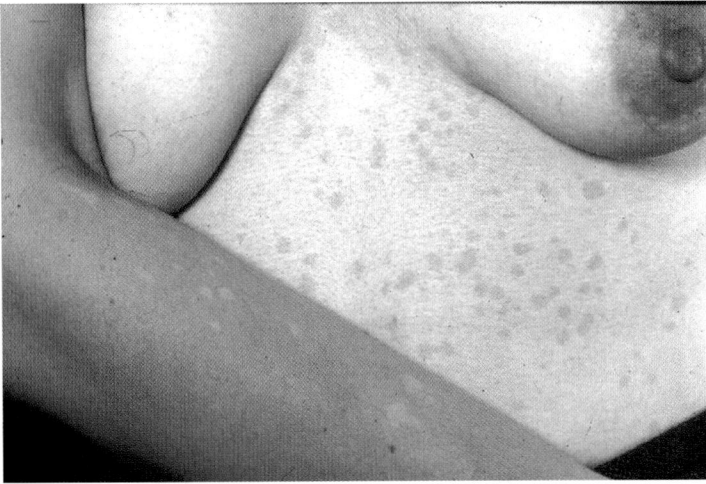

Figure 88.48 Hypomelanotic macules on a sun-exposed arm compared with tan-coloured macules on the trunk of the sun-protected abdominal skin of a woman with pityriasis versicolor.

Pathophysiology
The hypopigmentation can be a consequence of an impaired transfer of melanin to the keratinocytes secondary to the inflammatory process or the result of application of potent topical steroids. In a number of other inflammatory disorders of the skin, there may be a loss of functional melanocytes (e.g. lupus erythematosus and lichen planus) due to destruction of the epidermal basal layer.

Pityriasis versicolor is one of the most common yeast infections associated with pigmentary changes. It is caused by dimorphic, lipophilic organisms in the genus *Malassezia* [3,4]. Eleven species are recognized within this classification of yeasts, of which *Malassezia globosa*, *Malassezia sympodialis* and *Malassezia sloffiae* are the predominant species isolated in pityriasis versicolor [4]. These yeasts are part of the normal skin flora and seborrhoeic areas in humans (scalp, face, and the back and frontal aspect of the trunk) are always colonized by one or several species of this genus. They can cause disease when they convert to their pathogenic hyphal form. Factors that lead to this conversion include genetic predisposition, warm and humid environments, immunosuppression and malnutrition [4,5].

Environmental factors
See causative organisms.

Clinical features

Presentation
Post-inflammatory hypomelanosis usually presents as moderately to well-demarcated areas of pigment loss.

Pityriasis alba is characterized by hypopigmentation, presenting with pale white, well to moderately defined, very slightly scaling plaques. The lesions typically occur on the face and upper arms [1,2].

Cutaneous T-cell lymphoma may sometimes show prominent hypopigmentation. In poikilodermatous mycosis fungoides, clinical lesions are characterized by widespread poikiloderma rather than plaques or nodules. On clinical examination, there is alternating increase and decrease in pigmentation associated with epidermal atrophy. Hypopigmented mycosis fungoides tends to present in dark-skinned individuals: the areas of hypopigmentation are more prominent than in poikilodermatous mycosis fungoides [1,2].

Pityriasis versicolor. Well-demarcated finely scaling patches, hyper- or hypopigmentations are found on clinical examination.

Lichen striatus is an asymptomatic linear dermatosis and has been reported to follow the lines of Blaschko. The primary lesions (small, flat, skin-coloured to pink papules) can disappear spontaneously after several months or years, often leaving a linear macular hypopigmentation (post-inflammatory) [3].

Differential diagnosis
See Box 88.5b.

Complications and co-morbidities
These are related to the underlying cause.

Disease course and prognosis
Post-inflammatory hypomelanosis is in general reversible if melanin production and transfer to the keratinocytes can be restored.

Investigations
A skin biopsy can be helpful in investigating possible underlying causes, particularly if mycosis fungoides is suspected. In suspected pityriasis versicolor, demonstrating a yellow-green fluorescence on Wood's light may help confirm the diagnosis.

Progressive macular hypomelanosis

Definition
Progressive macular hypomelanosis (PMH) is a common acquired dermatosis characterized by ill-defined nummular macules, mainly affecting the trunk.

Epidemiology

Incidence and prevalence
The true prevalence of PMH is unknown, but it is a common skin disorder that is often misdiagnosed.

Age
Mostly in adolescents and young adults.

Ethnicity
Although PMH is described in people of mixed racial ancestry (known as 'Creole dyschromia'), it is seen in all races.

Pathophysiology

Causative organisms
It has been postulated that different subtypes of *Propionibacterium* species might be responsible for PMH [2,3].

Clinical features

Presentation
PMH is an entity that affects the trunk with ill-defined nummular hypopigmented non-scaly macules. The condition typically affects areas rich in sebaceous glands. The lesions often converge in and around the midline (Figure 48.49). Rarely, the proximal extremities, head and neck may be involved.

Differential diagnosis
See Box 88.5b.

Disease course and prognosis
PMH may be stable or slowely progressive over time. Spontaneous regression is rare, but possible.

Investigations
Wood's light examination: orange-red fluorescence.

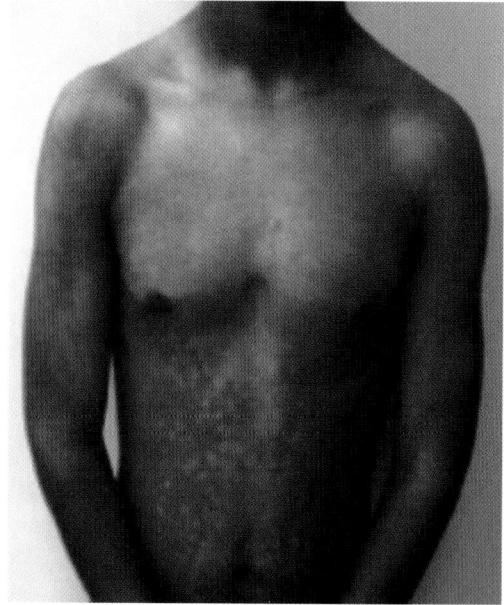

Figure 88.49 Progressive macular hypomelanosis in an 18-year-old man. (Reproduced with permission from the copyright holder Springer Publishing Company, from Relyveld *et al.* [5] Progressive macular hypomelanosis: an overview. *Am J Clin Dermatol* 2007;8:13–19.)

Management
In a recent study of 45 patients with intra-person comparison of two treatment strategies 5% benzoyl peroxide hydrogel/1% clindamycin lotion in combination with UVA irradiation versus 0.05% fluticasone propionate cream in combination with UVA irradiation, the antibacterial treatment was found to be superior (photometric measurements, patient assessment and dermatologist assessment) [3]. PUVA und UVB therapy was reported to achieve improvement [2,4], at least transiently, in a few cases. PMH may regress spontaneously within a few years.

Chemical depigmentation

A number of chemicals can produce cutaneous depigmentation when applied to the skin [1,2]. Several substituted phenols produce an occupational leukoderma in workers coming into contact with them (see also Chapter 130). Of these, *p*-tertiary-butylphenol is the most important [2,3,4]. Occupational leukoderma occurs in workers in contact with the monobenzylether of hydroquinone [5]; this compound is used in the treatment of hypermelanosis and can produce confetti-like areas of depigmentation in the treated areas [6] (Figure 88.50). The monomethylether of hydroquinone can induce a similar leukoderma [7]. Several phenolic germicidal preparations can produce depigmentation of the skin [4]. 4-Tertiary-butylcatechol is also a cause of occupational leukoderma [8], and this may follow contact sensitization [9]. The areas most likely to be affected in occupational leukoderma are the dorsa of the hands (Figure 88.51), but other areas may also be involved, not necessarily in contact with the chemicals. The depigmented areas frequently enlarge, and new ones appear even after the patient is no longer

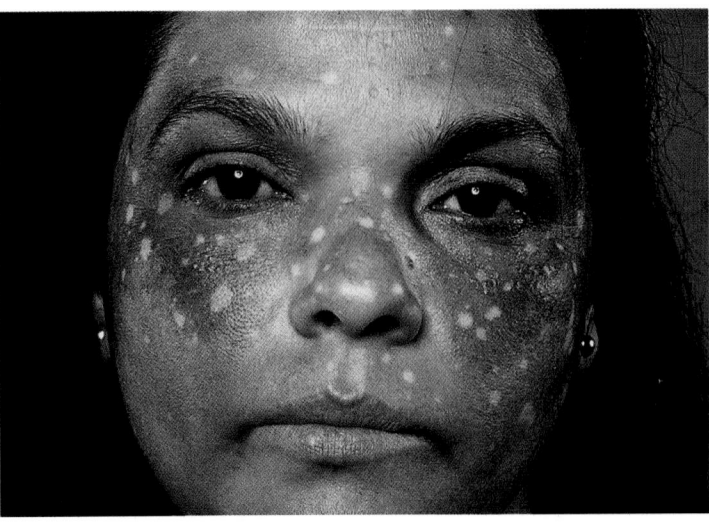

Figure 88.50 Depigmentation on the face following treatment of melasma with monobenzylether of hydroquinone. (Courtesy of St John's Dermatology Centre, London, UK.)

in contact. The areas may or may not repigment. Treatment with psoralens is usually ineffective. In the hypomelanotic and amelanotic areas, there is often an almost complete absence of melanocytes [3,4]. Experimental studies [1,10] indicate that these substituted phenols have a selective lethal effect on functional melanocytes.

Idiopathic guttate hypomelanosis

Definition and nomenclature
Idiopathic guttate hypomelanosis (IGH) is an acquired leukoderma with discrete round to oval porcelain-white macules approximately 2–5 mm diameter increasing in number with age [1–6].

Synonyms and inclusions
• Disseminate lenticular leukoderma

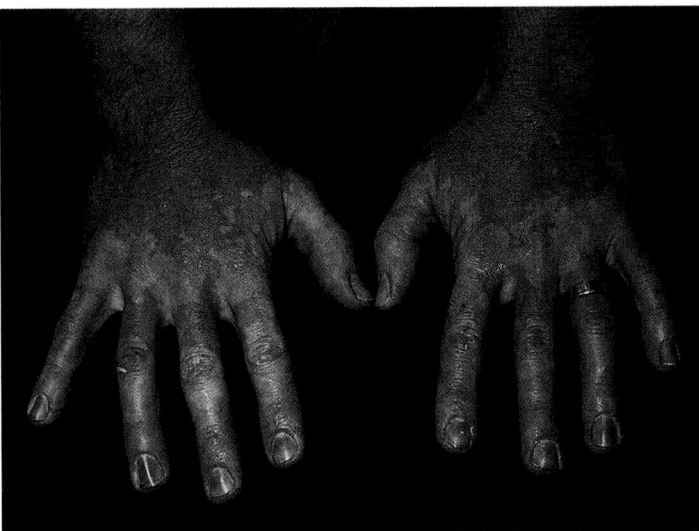

Figure 88.51 Occupational vitiligo due to tertiary-butylphenol.

Epidemiology

Incidence and prevalence
Common; seen in up to 80% of patients over the age of 70 years.

Age
Numbers increase with age.

Sex
F > M.
   Both sexes are most likely equally affected, but IGH may be more reported by women because of the subjective perception of cosmetic disfigurement.

Ethnicity
Most in people with light skin colour.

Pathophysiology

Pathology
Histologically, IGH lesions are characterized by slight basket-weave hyperkeratosis with epidermal atrophy and flattening of the rete pegs. Histochemical and ultrastructural studies show a decrease in melanocytes and melanin content of the affected epidermis and pigment granules are irregularly distributed [5,6].

Causative organisms
IGH has been hypothesized to be UV induced, although controversy exists. Some suggest that IGH may reflect the normal ageing or photoageing process.

Environmental factors
The lesions in Caucasian people most frequently occur in sun-exposed areas of the limbs. Solar damage is a factor in these cases.

Clinical features

Presentation
Clinically, the lesions are porcelain-white macules, usually 2–6 mm in size but sometimes much larger (Figure 88.52). The borders are sharply defined, often angular and irregular. The skin markings are normal.
   Susceptible locations include the pretibial side of the legs and the forearms. Other chronic sun-exposed sites, including the face, neck and shoulders may be affected. Non-actinic lesions occur in black people and may be located on the trunk in unexposed areas [1].

Differential diagnosis
See Box 88.5.

Complications and co-morbidities
These may be an indication of UV-damaged skin.

Disease course and prognosis
The number increases with age. No spontaneous repigmentation occurs.

Management
Treatment is not usually required. A variety of therapies have been advocated for IGH, including systemic and topical retinoids,

PART 8: SPECIFIC CUTANEOUS STRUCTURE

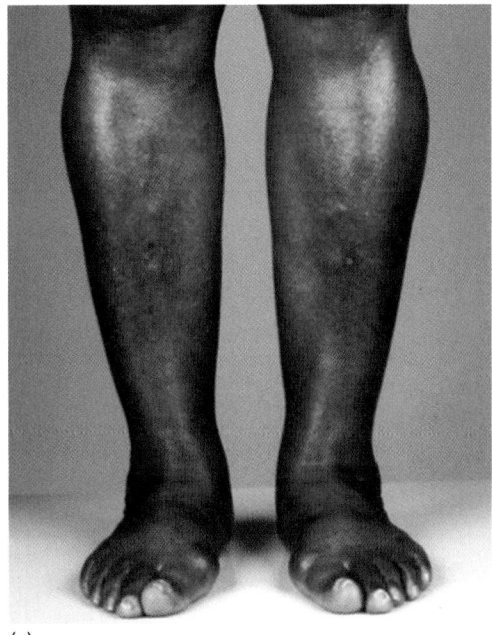 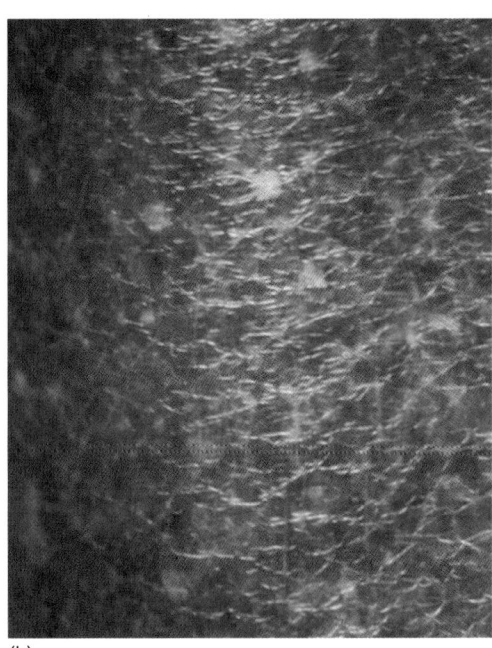

Figure 88.52 Typical appearances on the shins of a 57-year-old Afro-Caribbean woman (a) with close-up view illustrating discrete guttate hypomelanotic macules (b).

(a)

(b)

topical steroids, cryotherapy, topical tacrolimus and superficial dermabrasion (e.g. carbon dioxide laser). None are predictably successful [7–9].

Punctate leukoderma

Definition and nomenclature
Punctate leukoderma was first described in patients who developed multiple punctiform hypopigmented and achromic spots after several months of PUVA treatment [1]. Later, similar cases were described after UVB therapy for psoriasis and after topical and systemic PUVA for segmental vitiligo [2–4].

Synonyms and inclusions
- Leukoderma punctata
- Symmetrical progressive leukopathy

Epidemiology

Age
Punctate leukoderma develops in young adults.

Ethnicity
This has been reported from Japan and Brazil, where it is relatively common.

Pathophysiology

Pathology
Ultrastructurally, punctate leukoderma demonstrates slight to severe damage of keratinocytes and melanocytes not reported in IGH.

Causative organisms
It has been suggested that phototoxicity damage to keratinocytes and melanocytes is the aetiological factor.

Environmental factors
Sun exposure, UV therapy.

Clinical features

History
Leukoderma punctatum was first reported by Falabella *et al.* in 1988 [5].

Presentation
Multiple round or oval small sharply demarcated punctate macules measuring 0.5–1.5 mm in diameter are found symmetrically on the fronts of the shins and on the extensor aspects of the arms; less often they are also found on the abdomen and interscapular region. The macules are not related to hair follicles.

Differential diagnosis (see Box 88.5)
IGH: punctate leukoderma is considered to be distinct from IGH on the basis of its clinical and histological features – the macules are smaller and repigmentation may occur.

Disease course and prognosis
Persistent although spontaneous repigmentation has been observed [5].

NON-MELANIN PIGMENTATION

Endogenous non-melanin pigmentation

A variety of normal constituents of the body may give rise to alterations in skin colour, if present in excess or in an abnormal form or site. Substances formed as a result of metabolic defects may also produce pigmentary changes. Special stains of histological specimens, or techniques such as spectroscopy, may help to identify the nature of exogenous and other non-melanin pigments.

Cutaneous haemosiderosis

Definition and nomenclature
Brownish pigmentation resulting from deposition of the iron-containing pigment haemosiderin in the skin. Haemosiderin stimulates melanogenesis and much of the dyspigmentation associated with haemosiderosis may in fact be due to melanin rather than haemosiderin. The most common causes include repetitive minor trauma and venous insufficiency.

Synonyms and inclusions
• Haemosiderin pigmentation

Introduction and general description
Haemosiderin is a brown iron-binding pigment which is found predominantly within macrocytes. The deposition of haemosiderin is commonly the result of the local destruction of red blood cells, but also occurs in haemochromatosis (see earlier) [1]. The presence of haemosiderin stimulates melanogenesis. The accumulation of haemosiderin in the dermis and consequent hypermelanosis results in a brown or coppery discoloration of the skin. In addition to haemosiderin and epidermal melanin, the clinical picture may be due in part to dermal melanin resulting from pigment incontinence and even from dermal melanocytes [2].

Cutaneous haemosiderosis may arise through a number of different mechanisms of which the most important are as follows:
• Trauma: particularly repeated ecchymoses from minor trauma to the lower limbs (Figure 88.53).
• Hypostatic haemosiderosis: associated with chronic lower limb venous hypertension (Figure 88.54).
• Capillaritis (pigmented purpura) (Figure 88.55).
• Congenital haemolytic anaemias: this includes a variety of conditions associated with haemolysis, including sickle cell anaemia.
• Haemochromatosis: this may also be deposited in the skin as the result of repeated episodes of purpura from any other cause, e.g. following clothing- or drug-induced dermatitis.

Clinical features

Clinical variants

Hypostatic haemosiderosis (see Chapter 103)
In chronic venous hypertension, there is leakage of blood cells from small blood vessels into the tissues. Extravasated erythrocytes are broken down by tissue macrophages and the iron thus released is incorporated into haemosiderin, which remains predominantly intracellular within the macrocyte. Recently involved areas show grouped points of reddish pigment, but recurrent extravasation of red cells combined with increasing hypermelanosis soon produce a more or less uniform deep brown or coppery colour (see Figure 88.53).

The relative contributions of haemosiderin and melanin to the dyspigmentation seen in chronic venous insufficiency has been investigated by taking biopsies of pigmented and non-pigmented leg

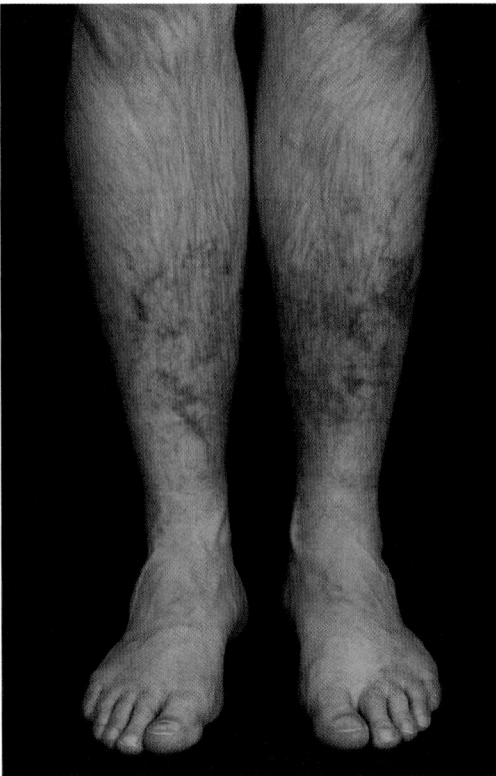

Figure 88.53 Haemosiderin staining on the shins of a 41-year-old rugby football player resulting from repeated minor trauma.

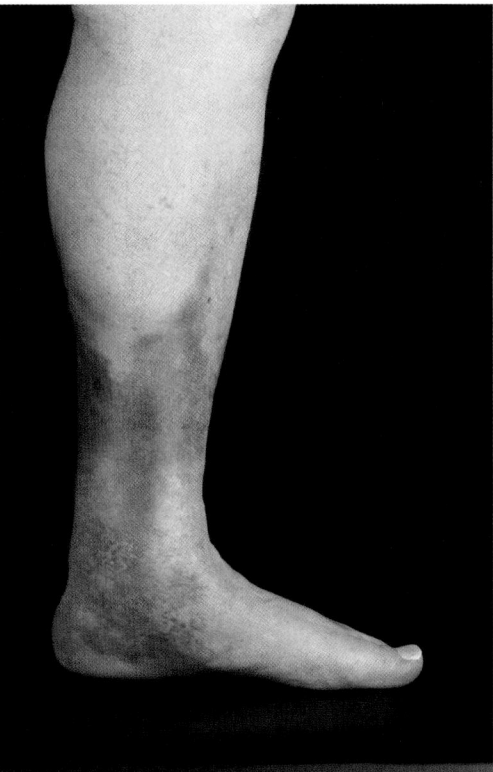

Figure 88.54 Haemosiderosis of the gaiter area in a 98-year-old man with longstanding venous insufficiency: note atrophie blanche above the medial malleolus.

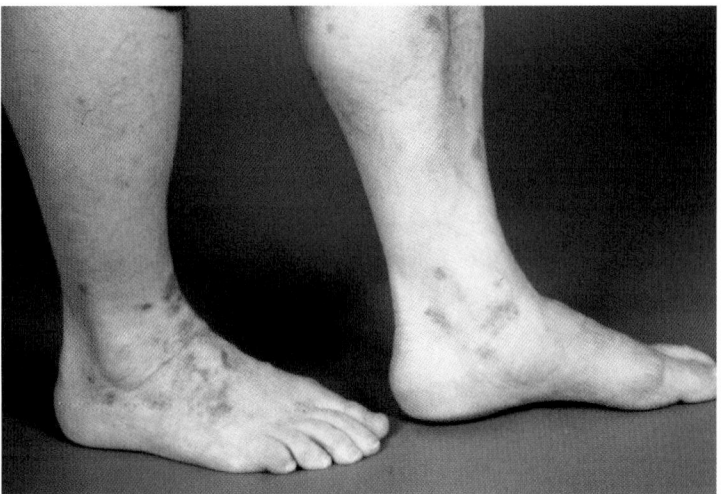

Figure 88.55 Haemosiderosis secondary to capillaritis which first erupted 6 months previously in a 57-year-old male.

skin from patients with venous hypertension undergoing varicose vein surgery. Control biopsies were taken from patients undergoing orthopaedic surgery. Unsurprisingly, all samples from pigmented skin showed a higher melanin content than those from unpigmented skin. Haemosiderin, however, was detected in only the most deeply pigmented skin. This suggests that hypermelanosis may be provoked by chronic venous insufficiency itself without the requirement for extravascular erythrocyte destruction and haemosiderin [3].

Interestingly, in a study of 46 patients with various types of leg ulcer it was shown that haemosiderin could be detected in skin biopsies from all patients but that urinary haemosiderin, which was absent from all patients with ischaemic ulcers, could be detected 22 of 24 patients with venous ulcers [4]. There was, however, no correlation between the amounts deposited in the skin and the amount detected in urine.

Capillaritis (pigmented purpura) (see Chapter 101)
Haemosiderosis without clinically evident hypermelanosis is seen in Schamberg capillaritis [4]. Reddish-brown plaques with cayenne-pepper points beyond their margins are present on the legs and thighs and sometimes on the arms (see Figure 88.55).

Congenital haemolytic anaemia
Conspicuous pigmentation of the lower leg in the third decade or earlier may develop in patients with sickle cell anaemia.

Haemochromatosis
The presence of haemosiderin stimulates melanogenesis, and hypermelanosis may dominate the clinical and histological picture, as in haemochromatosis (see earlier).

Dermatitis
Haemosiderosis of the trunk is a feature of some reactions to textiles. Small patches of haemosiderosis, most numerous on the lower legs but progressively involving the thighs and buttocks, are characteristic of drug reactions to anticonvulsants with a ureide structure, a property common to the majority of them.

Pathophysiology

Environmental factors
May occasionally be secondary to drug reactions or contact dermatitis due to clothing.

Clinical features

Presentation
The pigmentation is orange-red at first, later fading through ochre and tawny shades. It is distributed according to the underlying cause, i.e. either locally as in hydrostatic haemochromatosis or generally as in haemochromatosis.

Capillaritis initially presents with punctate bright red purpuric macules which may evolve into irregular plaques of orange or brown pigmentation. The lesions are chronic and persistent [3].

Differential diagnosis
See Box 88.3.

Disease course and prognosis

Hypostatic haemosiderosis
The pigmentation usually persists even if the venous insufficiency is relieved. In a single case report an IPL device was used apparently successfully to treat this condition [5].

Capillaritis
A chronic condition, this may clear spontaneously over a period from months to years, although recurrences are possible and not uncommon.

Haemochromatosis
See above.

Other
For other causes of secondary haemosiderin deposition, the prognosis depends on the successful management of the primary cause.

Management
Treatment of the underlying cause if possible.

Jaundice and bronze baby syndrome

Definition and nomenclature

Jaundice: yellowish discoloration of the skin, eyes and mucous membranes due to deposition of bile pigments [1].

Bronze baby syndrome: brown-bronze discoloration of the skin, mucous membranes and urine after phototherapy in children with clinical jaundice [2–4,5].

Synonyms and inclusions
- Jaundice: icterus

Pathophysiology

Pathology

Jaundice results from the deposition of bilirubin in the tissues. Clinically, it is often first noticed in the sclerae, because bilirubin has affinity for elastic tissue. The range of yellow shades produced by bilirubin may be modified by the presence of biliverdin, which adds a greenish hue. Bronzing is the effect of added melanin pigmentation and is often seen in jaundice of long duration.

Bronze baby syndrome: the nature and origin of the pigment are uncertain. The discoloration may be caused by an abnormal accumulation of a photoisomer of bilirubin, abnormal hepatic function leading to a copper–porphyrin complex which is photodestroyed or accumulation of biliverdin.

Clinical features

Presentation

Jaundice: range of yellow shades with a greenish hue.

Bronze baby syndrome: this striking grey-brown discoloration of the skin of neonates follows phototherapy for hyperbilirubinaemia and is often associated with evidence of liver dysfunction. The serum is also brownish.

Differential diagnosis (see Box 88.3a)
- Carotenaemia.
- Grey baby syndrome (after high doses of chloramphenicol)

Disease course and prognosis

Jaundice: outcome depends on the management of the underlying disease.

Bronze baby syndrome: the changes are reversible unless there is some chronic underlying liver disease.

Management
Treatment of underlying cause.

    Bronze baby syndrome: no treatment is required as pigmentation is reversible after discontinuation of phototherapy.

Treatment ladder

First line
- Neonatal jaundice is routinely treated with 460–490 nm visible light [6].

Carotenoderma

Definition and nomenclature
Carotenoderma is a benign yellowish coloration of the skin due to elevated blood carotene levels [1]. This may be primary due to diet, or secondary due to for example hepatic disease.

Synonyms and inclusions
- Hypercarotenaemia
- Carotenaemia

Pathophysiology

Predisposing factors
Primary carotenoderma is seen most obviously in food faddists who consume large quantities of oranges or carrots. However, it is now more commonly seen in young women drastically reducing their weight and eating foodstuffs with high carotene content [2,3].

    Iatrogenic hypercarotenaemia occurs in patients on oral supplements of β-carotene as a photoprotective agent in erythropoietic protoporphyria [4,5] with or without canthaxanthine. Carotenoderma typically occurs when β-carotene concentrations exceed 250 μg/dL or when daily ingestion exceeds 30 mg of β-carotene [6].

    In secondary hypercarotenaemia, some increased yellowness is seen in conditions with hyperlipaemia, diabetes, nephritis or hypothyroidism. It may also occur if conversion of carotene to vitamin A is impaired by an inborn metabolic error [7] or by hepatic disease.

Pathology
Carotene, a lipochrome, contributes a yellow component to the colour of normal skin. In the presence of excessive blood carotene levels, this yellow component is increased.

Clinical features

Presentation
The yellow colour is most conspicuous where the horny layer is thick on the palms and soles (Figure 88.56). The sclerae are not discoloured.

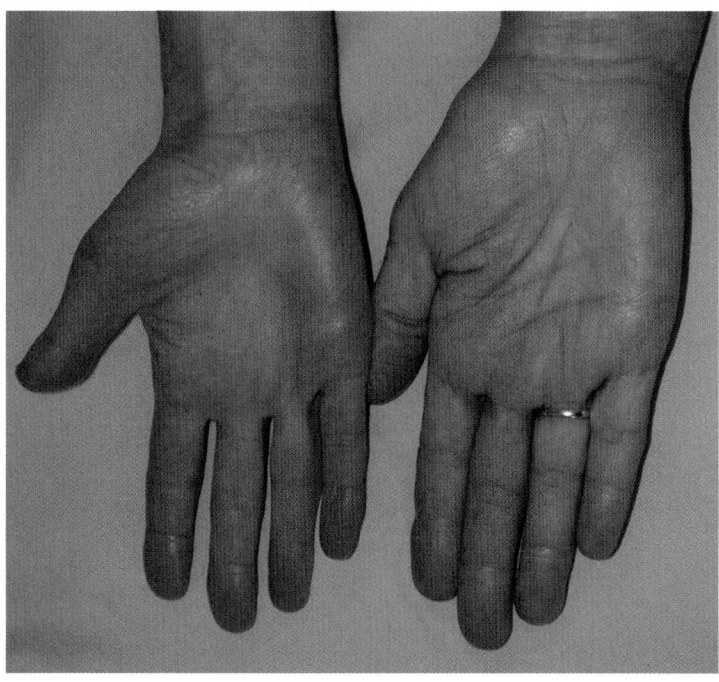

Figure 88.56 Carotenoderma: note yellowish hue of the palm on the right compared with the normal palm on the left. (Reproduced with permission and courtesy of the copyright holder Professor Barbara Leppard, University of Southampton, UK.)

Differential diagnosis
See Box 88.3a.

Disease course and prognosis
A diet low in carotene leads to resolution of the signs.

Treatment ladder

First line
- Treatment of underlying cause
- Diet low in carotene

Ochronosis

Definition

Endogenous ochronosis is the term used to describe the pigmentary changes that occur in connective tissue in patients with alkaptonuria [1].

Exogenous ochronosis: discoloration of the skin after topical use primarily of hydroquinone, but may also be caused by the use of phenol or resorcinol [2].

Epidemiology

Incidence and prevalence

Endogenous ochronosis is present in about 75% of patients with alkaptonuria (see Chapter 81).

Exogenous ochronosis: exact incidence is unknown.

Age
Alkaptonuria: congenital (see Chapter 81).

Sex
M = F.

Ethnicity

Alkaptonuria: all races, although more frequent in certain countries such as Slovakia and the Dominican Republic.

Exogenous ochronosis: seen in populations with widespread use of hydroquinine or phenol/resorcinol. High rates have been reported from South Africa.

Pathophysiology

Predisposing factors
- Exogenous ochronosis: often associated with the use of skin-lightening cosmetics.
- Most frequently reported in heavily pigmented skin, although it can occur in all phototypes.

Pathology
Histopathological examination of both endogenous and exogenous ochronosis is characterized by comma- or banana-shaped ochronotic collagen bundles. Histopathological differentiation between the two forms is not possible [2].

In alkaptonuria, a deficiency in homogentisic acid oxidase causes accumulation of homogentisic acid throughout the body [3].

In exogenous ochronosis, it may be caused by inhibition of homogentisic oxidase and accumulation of homogentisic acid (an intermediate in L-phenylalanine and L-tyrosine catabolism) which polymerizes to form ochre (brownish-yellow) pigment in the papillary dermis [2]. Microscopically, deposition of ochre-coloured pigment is seen [2].

Genetics
Alkaptonuria is an autosomal recessive disease.

Environmental factors
- Exogenous ochronosis: sun exposure
- Use of hydroquinone at concentrations higher than 3% for prolonged periods of time (>6 months). Discoloration is, however, also reported with the use of hydroquinone at concentrations of 2% and less.

Clinical features

History
The term was coined by Virchow in 1866 for the ochre-like (pale yellow) colour of the connective tissue when viewed down a microscope.

Presentation

Endogenous ochronosis: most frequent is darkening of the ear cartilages and of the sclerae and conjunctivae. Less often the axillary skin is pigmented and there is brown mottled pigmentation of the face (sometimes in a butterfly distribution), neck and trunk. Rarely, pigmentation of the palmar and plantar skin is seen [4].

Exogenous ochronosis: grey-brown or blue-black macules in the skin in contact with hydroquinone, normally the face, neck, back and the extensor surfaces of the limbs. No hyperpigmentation of cartilage, sclerae or conjunctivae occurs [2,5].

Differential diagnosis

Facial melanosis: as follows:
- Endocrinopathies: Addison disease, Cushing syndrome, hyperthyroidism.
- Metabolic conditions: porphyria cutanea tarda, haemochromatosis.
- Poikiloderma of Civatte.
- Post-inflammatory hyperpigmentation.
- Toxin- and drug-induced hyperpigmentation or discoloration (e.g. amiodarone, doxycycline).

Investigations
Alkaptonuria may be identified by urine organic acid analysis, whereas exogenous ochronosis is identified by the patient history.

Management

First line

Alkaptonuria

No definitive treatment exists; nitisinone, ascorbic acid 1 g/day in divided doses and a protein-restricted diet (1.3 g/kg/day) may be beneficial.

Exogenous ochronosis

Discontinuation of hydroquinone use; strict sun protection/avoidance.

Treatment of discoloration is difficult

The use of trichloroacetic acid and cryotherapy have been shown not to be helpful. Some improvement may occur with the use of retinoid acid, although transient hyperpigmentation may also occur. Topical low-potency corticosteroids may be of benefit in combination with photoprotection [2].

Second line

Exogenous ochronosis

Although results are not uniform, superficial dermabrasiom using carbon dioxide laser, glycolic acid peelings or Q-switched laser may improve the skin discoloration [2].

Exogenous pigmentation

A wide variety of chemicals, either from occupational or medicinal exposure, can produce discoloration of the skin. Some of these may not only produce an alteration of pigmentation by being deposited in the dermis but may also result in an increase in the amount of melanin in the skin. Of importance are the metals silver, gold, mercury and bismuth, which are cumulatively deposited in the dermis and can produce permanent disfiguring pigmentation. A number of drugs can discolour the skin. These include the antimalarials, the phenothiazines, clofazimine and minocycline. Of less importance is the transient staining of the skin produced by picric acid, dinitrophenol and chemical dyes.

Metals

Introduction and general description

Argyria

This may develop as a result of systemic absorption or from external contact with silver [1,2]. The silver may be deposited in the skin either as a result of medication containing silver salts [3,4,5] or from industrial exposure [2]. Localized argyria is most commonly caused by mechanical impregnation related to occupational exposure [2].

Most reported cases of generalized argyria occur following ingestion of colloidal silver, which is widely marketed as a folk remedy for various conditions, including diabetes, AIDS, cancers and infections: a cumulative dose of 4–5 g is required to produce clinical signs [6]. Light and electron microscopy studies [1,2,7–9] show silver granules in the dermis that are most numerous in relation to the basal lamina of the eccrine sweat glands, and in the dermal elastic fibres. Furthermore, silver particles may be seen lying free within the cell cytoplasm of epithelial cells of the secretory segment of eccrine sweat glands and in mast cells [9,10]. Silver granules are readily visible with dark-field illumination. X-ray-dispersive microanalysis confirms that the granules contain silver [2,10]. Silver is widely deposited in the tissues as well as in the skin. The diagnosis of argyria is established by skin biopsy.

The pigmentation is usually a slate-grey colour and may be clinically apparent after a few months, but usually takes many years to develop and depends on the degree of exposure. The hyperpigmentation is most apparent in sun-exposed areas of the skin, especially the forehead, nose and hands (Figure 88.57). In some patients, the entire skin has a slate blue-grey colour. The sclerae, nails and mucous membranes may additionally become hyperpigmented.

Blue macules have appeared at the sites of acupuncture needles [6]. Cases have followed the use of silver salts for the irrigation of nasal, oral and urethral mucous membranes and the excessive use of an oral smoking remedy containing silver acetate [1,10]. 'Food supplements' may also contain colloidal silver [8].

The pigmentation is usually permanent: treatment with depigmenting agents is not effective. Sun protection can limit further pigmentary changes [9].

Arsenic

Prolonged ingestion of inorganic arsenic may result in diffuse pigmentation, most intense on the trunk. The hyperpigmentation is characterized by macular areas of depigmentation within areas of hyperpigmentation produce the distinctive 'raindrop' appearance, diffuse dark brown spots or diffuse darkening of the skin on the

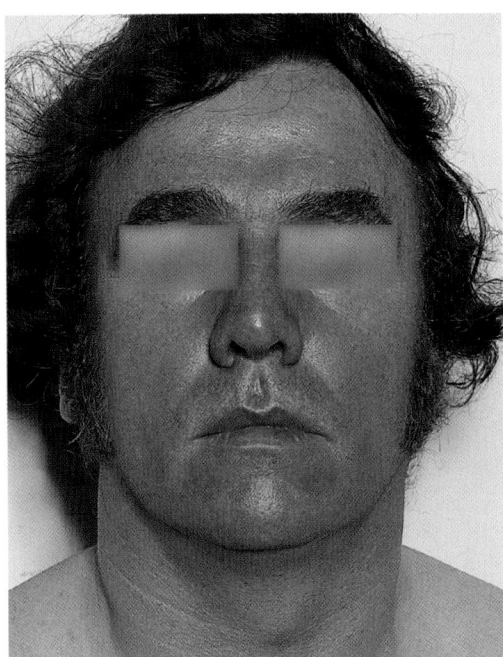

Figure 88.57 Occupational argyria.

limbs and trunk [1,2]. Many cases also show arsenical keratoses, usually appearing as bilateral thickening of the palms and soles. Nodular keratosis may also occur as multiple raised keratotic lesions in the palm and soles [2].

Bismuth

The administration of bismuth at regular intervals over a period of years has often been practised, yet generalized pigmentation is extremely rare. The diffuse grey pigmentation resembles that of argyria and involves also the sclera and the oral and sometimes the vaginal mucous membrane [1]. A distinctive blue-black line occurs at the gingival margin. This is due to deposition of bismuth that reacts with hydrogen sulphide formed by bacteria in the mouth [2].

Chrysiasis and chrysoderma

These are terms used to describe permanent pigmentation of the skin due to parenteral administration of gold salts.

Excessive administration of gold leads to its deposition in connective tissue. The diagnosis is confirmed histologically on microscopy with dark-field illumination and on electron microscopy with electron probe microanalysis [1]. The granules of gold are larger and more irregular than those of silver.

Chrysiasis has not been observed in any patient who has received less than 50 mg/kg of gold thiosulphate, and appears to be inevitable in any patient receiving more than 150 mg/kg. It may develop after a few months or after a longer latent period. The pigmentation is blue-grey or may show a purplish hue, and is limited to light-exposed skin and to the sclerae (Figure 88.58) [2]. The oral mucous membrane is not affected. The discoloration is permanent.

Mercury

Repeated applications of mercury-containing compounds can produce localized hyperpigmentation of the treated areas [1,2,3]. The pigment is observed in the upper dermis around capillaries and associated with collagen and elastic fibres. Electron microscopy

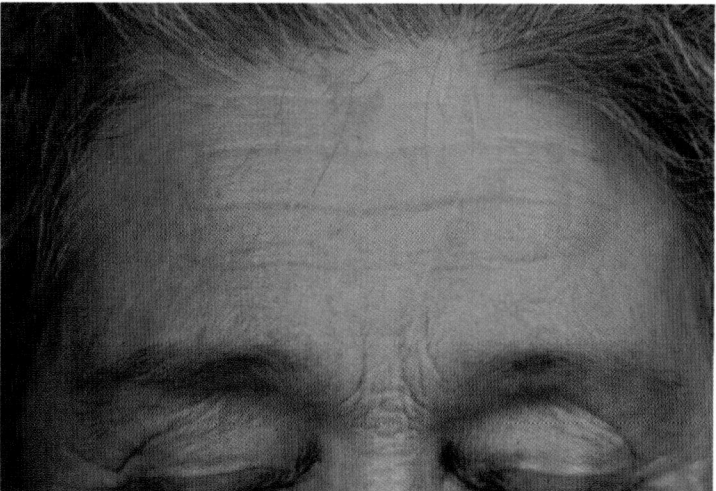

Figure 88.58 Chrysiasis: mild lilac discoloration on the forehead and eyelids contrasting with the yellow of the elastotic skin on the bridge of the nose and eyebrows in 64-year-old woman with rheumatoid arthritis who 8 years earlier had been treated with parenteral gold for over 2 years.

shows an increase in melanin pigmentation and the metal is present as granules in dermal macrophages [1,3].

Systemic administration of mercury results in gingival hyperpigmentation. A case report of homicidal subcutaneous injection of metallic mercury resulted in widespread skin lesions, remote from the radiologically visible mercury; these appeared at 40 days and began to clear at 6 months [4].

Differential diagnosis
See Box 88.3a.

Medication

See Drug-induced hyperpigmentation.

Tattoos

Accidental tattoos
Pigmented particles may be accidentally introduced as contaminants of wounds or may, at high velocity, penetrate previously intact skin.

Superficial abrasions contaminated with chemically inert particles may be followed by disfiguring tattoos. Such irregularly spattered pigmentation is quite commonly seen after road accidents and blast injuries. Some particles may eventually be extruded, but the disfigurement is often permanent. These tattoos often respond well to the Q-switched Nd : YAG laser (Figure 88.59) [1]. Small lesions may also be excised.

Colliers' stripes
These are a very distinctive occupational mark in coalminers [2]. The bluish grey, linear or angular stripes develop at the sites of abrasions. The commonest sites are the forehead, bridge of the nose, wrists and elbows. Histologically, particles of coal dust up to 100 µm in diameter are seen at all levels in the dermis. They tend to be grouped around blood vessels.

Therapeutic agents

Iron salts. The use of solutions of ferric sulphate and ferric chloride in the treatment of dermatitis has been followed by a reddish-brown tattoo [3,4]. The pigmentation may disappear after a few months or may persist indefinitely [5].

Occupational contact with iron salts [6] produced red-brown punctate perifollicular pigmentation of the forearms in a man employed in pickling metal in hydrochloric acid.

Crystal violet (gentian violet; hexamethyl pararosaniline chloride). This has, exceptionally, given rise to a tattoo when applied to a wound of the face [7].

Decorative tattoos (see also Chapters 23 and 123)

History and prevalence
From ancient times, the practice of tattooing has developed along more or less parallel lines in most cultures. Tattoos have traditionally been based on aesthetic considerations, i.e. to accentuate beauty, or as a permanent adornment in a more sociological or

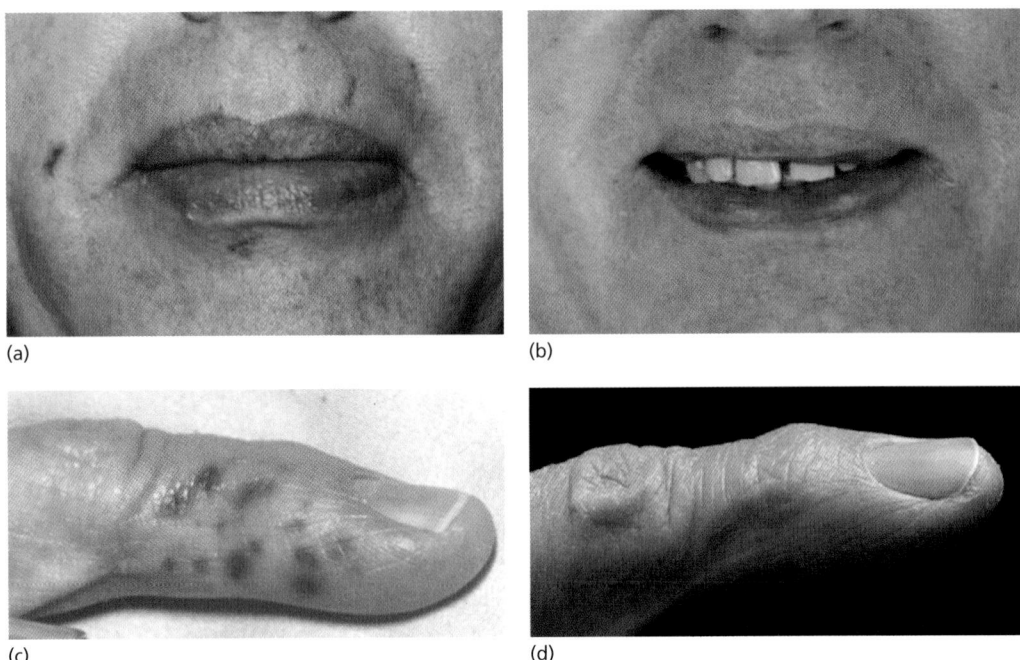

Figure 88.59 (a–d) Traumatic tattoo: accidental tattoo following explosion during school chemistry experiment; excellent response to Nd : YAG laser.

cultural context to make a statement. Occasionally, when used in a sociocultural context, tattoos serve to accentuate aggression or ugliness in order to make the wearer more intimidating. Tattoos with words or a name as a symbol of dedication or devotion have always been popular. Tattoos have also been used for more sinister motives. Tattoos were used as a means of identification by the Nazis in the Second World War for members of concentration and labour camps as well as for members of the SS. Formerly associated with religious ceremonies, fertility and marriage rites, tattooing in contemporary westernized civilizations thus fulfils a number of diverse functions and in so doing it survives and flourishes.

Contemporary life finds tattooing more popular than ever [8], even among the elite [9]. Tattoos are no longer the exclusive preserve of street gangs, prisoners and members of the armed forces [8,9]. Tattooing is viewed by many as an acceptable fashion accessory like any other, and is increasingly popular in Western societies with the young and with women, as well as the more traditional male stereotypes [8,9]. Tattooing and body piercing are now so common that health care workers are advised to maintain a non-judgemental attitude to tattoos [8], even in the face of the unexpected [10]. The decision to have a tattoo may be taken when an individual is in no position to make such a lifelong commitment, for example when intoxicated, under peer pressure or when mentally unwell [11,12]. Tattoos may also be a manifestation of deliberate self-harm [11,12].

Another contemporary trend is the use of temporary black henna 'tattoos' [13,14]. These are not true tattoos but represent application of a black dye to produce a tattoo-like appearance that lasts for a few days. Unfortunately, a high concentration of the well-known contact sensitizer *para*-phenylenediamine is usually present in these 'tattoos', which results in a risk of contact allergy [13,14].

Techniques and materials
The professional tattooist uses an electric needle to introduce particles of pigment into the dermis (see Chapter 23). The amateur, often a

child, pricks particles of soot or Indian ink into skin with any pointed object. The pigments commonly employed include the following:
- Blue-black (carbon).
- Red (cinnabar and vegetable dyes).
- Light blue (cobaltous aluminate).
- Green (chromic oxide or chromium sesquioxide).
- Yellow (cadmium sulphide).
- Brown (ochre, iron oxides).

Complications of tattoos
Infection, allergy to tattoo pigments (Figure 88.60) and koebnerization of other disorders, particularly sarcoidosis, to tattoos represent

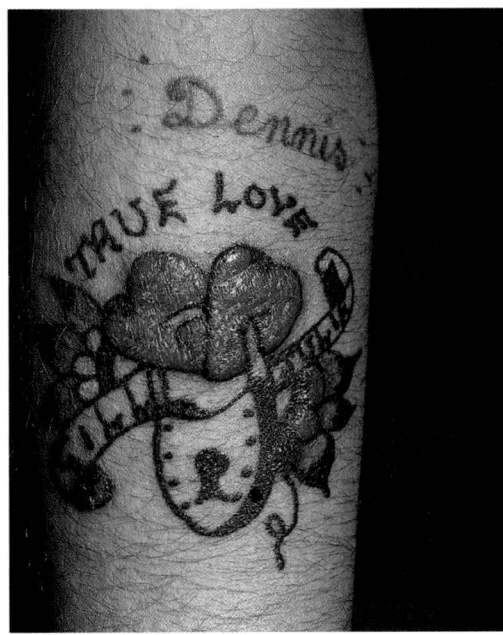

Figure 88.60 Lichenoid reaction in the red areas of a tattoo.

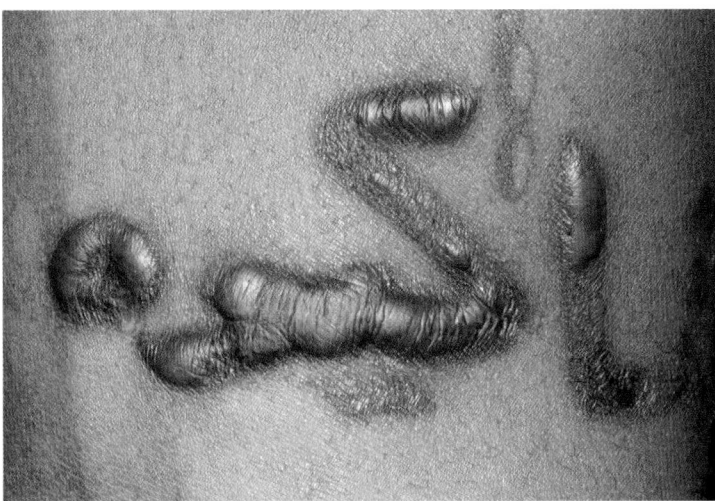

Figure 88.61 Keloid reaction to decorative tattoo: flattened areas have responded to the injection of triamcinolone.

the most common complications of tattoos. A sarcoidal granuloma in a tattoo may be the presenting manifestation of generalized sarcoidosis [15]. Foreign-body granulomas of sarcoid type are, however, extremely unusual after decorative tattoos, but have been reported in ochre tattoos, which have a high silica content [16]. Tattooing may also be complicated by keloids (Figure 88.61). Complications of tattoos are discussed in further detail in Chapter 123.

Removal of tattoos

Although most people who choose to have tattoos are satisfied with them, there are many who wish to have them removed [17]. In a recent study of 154 attendees with tattoos at a sexual health clinic in Denmark, 21 (13.6%) expressed regret about one or more of their tattoos [18]. Fortunately, the technology for removing them has improved greatly in recent years. Small tattoos may be amenable to removal by simple surgical techniques. Lasers are also widely used for tattoo removal. Their use is discussed in detail in Chapter 23.

Key references

The full list of references can be found in the online version at www.rooksdermatology.com.

Skin pigmentation and the melanocyte

The colour of the skin
1 Abdel-Malek Z, Kadekaro AL. Human pigmentation: its regulation by ultraviolet light and by endocrine, paracrine, and autocrine factors. In: Nordlund JJ, Boissy RE, Hearing VJ, et al., eds. *The Pigmentary System*, 2nd edn. Oxford: Blackwell Publishing, 2006:410–20.

The melanocyte
4 Brenner M, Hearing VJ. The protective role of melanin against UV damage in human skin. *Photochem Photobiol* 2008;84:539–49.

Biochemistry of melanogenesis
1 Hearing VJ. Determination of melanin synthetic pathways. *J Invest Dermatol* 2011;131:E8–11.

2 Rees JL. The genetics of human pigmentation disorders. *J Invest Dermatol* 2011;131:E12–13.
3 Hearing VJ. Invited editorial: unraveling the melanocytes. *Am J Hum Genet* 1993;52:1–7.

Constitutive pigmentation, human pigmentation and the response to sun exposure
5 Fitzpatrick TB. The validity and practicality of sun-reaction skin types I through VI. *Arch Dermatol* 1988;124:869–71.

Acquired hypermelanosis

Physiological hypermelanosis

Melasma
13 Gupta AK, Gover MD, Nouri K, Taylor S. The treatment of melasma: a review of clinical trials. *J Am Acad Dermatol* 2006;55:1048–65.
17 Picardo M, Carrera M. New and experimental treatments of cloasma and other hypermelanoses. *Dermatol Clin* 2007;25:353–62.

Photocontact facial melanosis
7   Pérez-Bernal A, Moñoz-Pérez MA, Camacho F. Management of facial hyperpigmentation. *Am J Clin Dermatol* 2000;1:261–8.

Poikiloderma of Civatte
2 Pérez-Bernal A, Moñoz-Pérez MA, Camacho F. Management of facial hyperpigmentation. *Am J Clin Dermatol* 2000;1:261–8.

Neoplastic diseases
1 Wright TS. Cutaneous manifestations of malignancy. *Curr Opin Pediatr* 2011;23:407–11.
3 Sebaratnam DF, Venugopal SS, Frew JW, et al. Diffuse melanosis cutis: a systematic review of the literature. *J Am Acad Dermatol* 2013; 68:482–8.
6   Bell HK, Poston GJ, Vora J, Wilson NJ. Cutaneous manifestations of the malignant carcinoid syndrome. *Br J Dermatol* 2005;152:71.

Hypermelanosis of drug origin

Drug-induced hyperpigmentation
1 Dereure O. Drug-induced skin pigmentation. Epidemiology, diagnosis and treatment. *Am J Clin Dermatol* 2001;2:253–62.
2 Lerner EA, Sober AJ. Chemical and pharmacologic agents that cause hyperpigmentation or hypopigmentation of the skin. *Dermatol Clin* 1988;6:327–37.

Tetracyclines
1 Dereure O. Drug-induced skin pigmentation. Epidemiology, diagnosis and treatment. *Am J Clin Dermatol* 2001;2:253–62.

Ashy dermatosis and erythema dyschromicum perstans
1 Zaynoun S, Rubeiz N, Kibbi A-G. Ashy dermatoses: a critical review of the literature and a proposed simplified clinical classification. *Int J Dermatol* 2008;47:542–4.

Treatment of hypermelanosis
1 Picardo M, Carrera M. New and experimental treatments of cloasma and other hypermelanoses. *Dermatol Clin* 2007;25:353–62.
3 Cestari TF, Dantas LP, Boza JC. Acquired hyperpigmentations. *An Bras Dermatol* 2014;89:11–25.

Vitiligo
1 Bologna J, Pawelek JM. Biology of hypopigmentation. *J Am Acad Dermatol* 1988;19:217–55.
2 Ezzedine K, Lim HW, Suzuki T, et al. Revised classification/nomenclature of vitiligo and related issues: the Vitiligo Global Issues Consensus Conference. *Pigment Cell Melanoma Res* 2012;25:E1–13.

11 van Geel N, Speeckaert R, Taieb A, *et al*. Koebner's phenomenon in vitiligo: European position paper. *Pigment Cell Melanoma Res* 2011;24:564–73.

12 Richmond JM, Frisoli ML, Harris JE. Innate immune mechanisms in vitiligo: danger from within. *Curr Opin Immunol* 2013;25:676–82.

31 van Geel N, Speeckaert R, Taieb A, *et al*. Koebner's phenomenon in vitiligo: European position paper. *Pigment Cell Melanoma Res* 2011;24:564–73.

33 van Geel N, Mollet I, Brochez L, *et al*. New insights in segmental vitiligo: case report and review of theories. *Br J Dermatol* 2012;166:240–6.

36 van Geel N, Speeckaert M, Chevolet I, *et al*. Hypomelanoses in children. *J Cutan Aesthet Surg* 2013;6:65–72.

37 Whitton ME, Pinart M, Batchelor J, *et al*. Interventions for vitiligo. *Cochrane Database Syst Rev* 2015;(2):CD003263.

38 Taieb A, Alomar A, Böhm M, *et al*. Guidelines for the management of vitiligo: the European Dermatology Forum consensus. *Br J Dermatol* 2013;168:5–19.

Chemical depigmentation

2 Lerner EA, Sober AJ. Chemical and pharmacologic agents that cause hyperpigmentation or hypopigmentation of the skin. *Dermatol Clin* 1988;6:327–37.

Non-melanin pigmentation

Endogenous non-melanin pigmentation

Cutaneous haemosiderosis

1 Jeghers H. Pigmentation of the skin. *N Engl J Med* 1944;231:88–100.

2 Kim D, Kang WH. Role of dermal melanocytes in cutaneous pigmentation of stasis dermatitis: a histopathological study of 20 cases. *J Korean Med Sci* 2002;17:648–54.

3 Caggiati A, Rosi C, Franceschini M, Innocenzi D. The nature of skin pigmentations in chronic venous insufficiency: a preliminary report. *Eur J Vasc Endovasc Surg* 2008;35:111–18.

5 Sardana K, Sarkar R, Sehgal VN. Pigmented purpuric dermatoses: an overview. *Int J Dermatol* 2004;43:482–8.

Jaundice and bronze baby syndrome

5 Kar S, Mohankar A, Krishnan A. Bronze baby syndrome. *Indian Pediatr* 2013;8:624.

6 Maisels MJ, McDonagh AD. Phototherapy for neonatal jaundice. *N Engl J Med* 2008;358:920–8.

Carotenoderma

6 Jen M, Yan AC. Syndromes associated with nutritional deficiency and excess. *Clin Dermatol* 2010;28:669–85.

Ochronosis

1 Lubics A, Schneider I, Sebok B, Havass Z. Extensive bluish gray skin pigmentation and severe arthropathy. Endogenous ochronosis (alkaptonuria). *Arch Dermatol* 2000;136:548–52.

2 Martins VM, Sousa AR, Portela N de C, *et al*. Exogenous ochronosis: case report and literature review. *An Bras Dermatol* 2012;87:633–6.

3 Turgay E, Canat D, Gurel MS, *et al*. Endogenous ochronosis. *Clin Exp Dermatol* 2009;34:865–8.

5 Jain A, Pai SB, Shenoi SD. Exogenous ochronosis. *Indian J Dermatol Venereol Leprol* 2013;79:522–3.

Exogenous pigmentation

Argyria

1 Pariser RJ. Generalized argyria. *Arch Dermatol* 1978;114:373–7.

2 Bleehen SS, Gould DJ, Harrington CI, *et al*. Occupational argyria: light and electron microscopic studies and X-ray microanalysis. *Br J Dermatol* 1981;104:19–26.

4 Marshall JP II, Schneider RP. Systemic argyria secondary to topical silver nitrate. *Arch Dermatol* 1977;113:1077–9.

6 Park SW, Shin HT, Lee KT, Lee DY. Medical concern for colloidal silver supplementation: argyria of the nail and face. *Ann Dermatol* 2013;25:111–12.

Arsenic

2 Majumdar KK, Guha Mazumder DN. Effect of drinking arsenic-contaminated water in children. *Indian J Public Health* 2012;56:223–6.

Bismuth

1 Dummett CO. Oral mucosal discolorations related to pharmacotherapeutics. *J Oral Ther* 1964;1:106–10.

2 Lueth HC, Sutton DC, McMullen CJ, *et al*. Generalized discoloration of skin resembling argyria following prolonged oral use of bismuth. *Arch Intern Med* 1936;57:1115–24.

Chrysiasis

1 Smith RW, Leppard B, Barnett NL, *et al*. Chrysiasis revisited: a clinical and pathological study. *Br J Dermatol* 1995;133:671–8.

2 Leonard PA, Moatamed F, Ward JR, *et al*. Chrysiasis: the role of sun exposure in dermal hyperpigmentation secondary to gold therapy. *J Rheumatol* 1986;13:58–64.

Mercury

2 Kennedy C, Molland EA, Henderson WJ, Whiteley AM. Mercury pigmentation from industrial exposure. *Br J Dermatol* 1977;96:367–74.

4 Burge KM, Winkelmann RK. Mercury pigmentation. *Arch Dermatol* 1970;102:51–61.

CHAPTER 89

Acquired Disorders of Hair

Andrew G. Messenger[1], Rodney D. Sinclair[2], Paul Farrant[3] and David A. R. de Berker[4]

[1]Department of Dermatology, Royal Hallamshire Hospital, Sheffield, UK
[2]University of Melbourne, Melbourne; Epworth Healthcare, Richmond, Victoria; and Sinclair Dermatology, Research and Clinical Trials Centre, Melbourne, Australia
[3]Brighton and Sussex University Hospitals, Brighton, UK
[4]Bristol Dermatology Centre, Bristol Royal Infirmary, Bristol, UK

PART 8: SPECIFIC CUTANEOUS STRUCTURE

Rook's Textbook of Dermatology, Ninth Edition. Edited by Christopher Griffiths, Jonathan Barker, Tanya Bleiker, Robert Chalmers and Daniel Creamer.
© 2016 John Wiley & Sons, Ltd. Published 2016 by John Wiley & Sons, Ltd.
Companion website: www.rooksdermatology.com

HAIR BIOLOGY

Andrew G. Messenger

Hair has no vital function in humans, yet its psychological functions are extremely important, as any clinical dermatologist or cosmetician can readily attest from routine daily practice. If the inevitability of scalp baldness makes it reluctantly tolerable to genetically predisposed men, in women loss of hair from the scalp is distressing, as is the growth of body or facial hair in excess of the culturally accepted norm.

Mammals probably evolved from Therapsid reptiles during the Late Triassic period over 200 million years ago (MyA). The earliest direct evidence of hair in mammals comes from fossilized casts and impressions in coprolites and pellets from the Late Palaeocene beds of Inner Mongolia [1]. Hairs from at least four extinct mammalian taxa have been identified, notably the multituberculate *Lambdopsalis bulla,* all showing striking preservation of the cuticular scale pattern. The three extant mammalian groups – monotremes, marsupials and placental mammals – all possess hair, indicating its presence prior to the divergence of therian mammals from monotremes, which probably took place between 170 and 230 MyA [2,3]. The multituberculate lineage extends back into the Triassic, suggesting that hair is a very ancient and possibly defining feature of mammals. Whatever its origin, it is clear that the warm-blooded mammals owe much of their evolutionary success to the properties of the hairy pelage as a heat insulator. Paradoxically, man's movement from the ancestral forest home to populate the globe is linked with a reversion to relative nudity and an ability to keep cool. Moreover, hair serves other purposes: in particular, it is concerned with sexual and social communication by constructing adornments such as the mane of the lion or the beard of the human male, or assisting in the dispersal of scents secreted by complexes of sebaceous or apocrine glands.

For these evolutionary reasons, hair follicles are not all under identical control mechanisms. To match the animal coat to seasonal changes in ambient temperature or environmental background requires moulting and replacement of the hairs. The process appears to involve an inherent follicular rhythm, modified by circulating hormones such as melatonin, prolactin, androgens or thyroxine, whose secretion is geared to environmental cues through the pineal gland, hypothalamus and pituitary.

The control of sexual hair growth must be differentiated from that of the moult cycle. The development of pubic, axillary and other body hair is delayed until puberty because it is dependent upon androgens in both sexes; that 'male' hormones are, in contrast, also a prerequisite for the manifestation of androgenetic alopecia still defies adequate explanation.

In all mammals, including humans but with the possible exception of merino sheep and the poodle dog, hair follicles show intermittent activity. Thus, each hair grows to a maximum length, is retained for a time without further growth, and is eventually shed and replaced.

Types of hair

Different types of hair may be produced by different kinds of follicle, and the type of hair produced in any particular follicle can change with age or under the influence of hormones. Animals characteristically have both an overcoat of stiff guard hairs and an undercoat of fine hairs [4]. Many species also have large vibrissae or sinus hairs, which are sensory and are produced from special follicles containing erectile tissue, but there are no such strictly comparable follicles in humans. In humans, a prenatal coat of fine, soft, unmedullated and usually unpigmented hair, known as lanugo, is normally shed *in utero* in the eighth to ninth month of gestation. Postnatal hair may be divided at the extreme into two kinds: vellus, which is soft, unmedullated, occasionally pigmented and seldom more than 2 cm long; and terminal hair, which is longer, coarser and often medullated and pigmented. However, there is a range of intermediate kinds. Before puberty, terminal hair is normally limited to the scalp, eyebrows and eyelashes. After puberty, secondary sexual 'terminal' hair is developed from vellus hair in response to androgens.

Development and distribution of hair follicles

Human hair follicles appear first in the regions of the eyebrows, upper lip and chin at about 9 weeks of embryonic development, and in other regions in the fourth month [5]. Hair over most of the scalp passes through a complete cycle and is shed *in utero*, and follicles in these regions have re-entered anagen by the time of birth. In the occipital scalp, telogen is delayed until after birth and this may give rise to a patch of hair loss in this region in the neonatal period. A fuller account of embryonic development is given in Chapter 2.

In humans, the full complement of hair follicles is probably established by the time of birth. Follicle density is highest in the fetus, when it may be similar across the skin surface. With growth there is a progressive reduction in follicle density, which continues until adult life, as skin surface area increases (Table 89.1).

Table 89.1 Hair follicle density in human fetal and adult skin. In adults, hair follicle density is highest on the head and is much lower on the trunk and limbs. At 24 weeks' gestational age hair follicle density is similar on the forehead and thigh skin. There is a pronounced reduction in thigh hair follicle density by adult life but only a small fall on the forehead.

	Fetal skin (follicles/cm²)				Adult (follicles/cm²)	
	24 weeks		Full term			
	Mean	± s.e.	Mean	± s.e.	Mean	± s.e.
Cheek					830	40
Forehead	1060		1060	110	765	20
Scalp					350	50
Forearm					95	15
Thigh	1010	250	480	40	55	5
Lower leg					45	10
Abdomen					70	15
Chest					75	25

s.e., standard error. Adapted from Szabo [6].

This occurs to a greater degree over the trunk and limbs than over the head so that the reduction in follicle density is less marked on the head than elsewhere [6]. The highest hair follicle densities, in the region of 800/cm², are found on the forehead and cheeks, with rather lower values for visible vellus hairs on the forehead in young adults of both sexes, and on the cheeks in women (400–450/cm²) [7]. Lower hair densities of 50–100/cm² are found on the chest and back in both sexes [7,8], and follicle densities of approximately 50/cm² on the thigh and leg [6]. Published values for average scalp hair density in white people vary between 250 and 320 hairs/cm² [9–12]. Scalp hair density shows a normal distribution in the population, with a wide range [12]. There is also racial variation in scalp hair density: average hair density in Africans (187/cm²) [13] and African Americans (171/cm²) [14] is lower than in white people, and it is lower still in Koreans (128/cm²) [15].

Anatomy of the hair follicle

Hair is the keratinized product of the hair follicle, a tube-like structure continuous with the epidermis at its upper end (Figure 89.1). The follicles are sloped in the dermis, and larger follicles extend into the subcutaneous layer. An oblique muscle, the arrector pili, runs from a point in the papillary dermis close to the dermal–epidermal junction to the mid-region of the follicle wall. Above the muscle, one or more sebaceous glands, and in some regions of the body an apocrine gland also, open into the follicle. The hair fibre is made up of three cell layers: an outer cuticle, the cortex (which forms the bulk of the fibre in most hair types) and a variable central medulla, all of which derive from highly proliferative cells in the hair bulb at the base of the follicle. Cells in the hair bulb also give rise to the inner root sheath that surrounds the hair fibre and which disintegrates before the hair emerges from the skin. The inner root sheath is itself enclosed by the outer root sheath, which forms a continuous structure extending from the hair bulb to the epidermis, although the functions and microscopic structure of the outer root sheath vary along the length of the follicle. The hair follicle also has a specialized dermal component, which includes the dermal or connective tissue sheath surrounding the follicle, and the dermal papilla, which invaginates the hair bulb.

The hair follicle is conventionally divided into two regions: the upper part consisting of the infundibulum and isthmus and the lower part comprising the hair bulb and suprabulbar region. The upper follicle is a relatively constant structure, whereas the lower follicle undergoes repeated episodes of regression and regeneration during the hair cycle. On the scalp, and some other regions of the skin, hair follicles are arranged in groups of three or more follicles known as follicular units (Figure 89.2). Several follicles within a follicular unit may coalesce so that hairs emerge through a common infundibulum.

Infundibulum. The infundibulum extends from the skin surface, where it merges with the epidermis, to the opening of the sebaceous duct at the junction with the isthmus. Infundibular epithelium differentiates in a similar manner to epidermis, producing a granular layer and stratum corneum, which desquamates into the follicular lumen.

Isthmus. The isthmus extends from the opening of the sebaceous gland duct to the insertion of the arrector pili muscle. It consists of a multilayered outer root sheath that is continuous with the infundibulum but differs in its structure. The innermost cells lack a granular layer and undergo a pattern of differentiation known as trichilemmal keratinization. The keratinized inner root sheath, which lies within the outer root sheath, disintegrates at or about the level of the sebaceous duct. The arrector muscle loops around the follicle in the manner of a sling [16]. Each follicular unit is supplied by a single arrector muscle, which splits to encircle each follicle within the follicular unit [17].

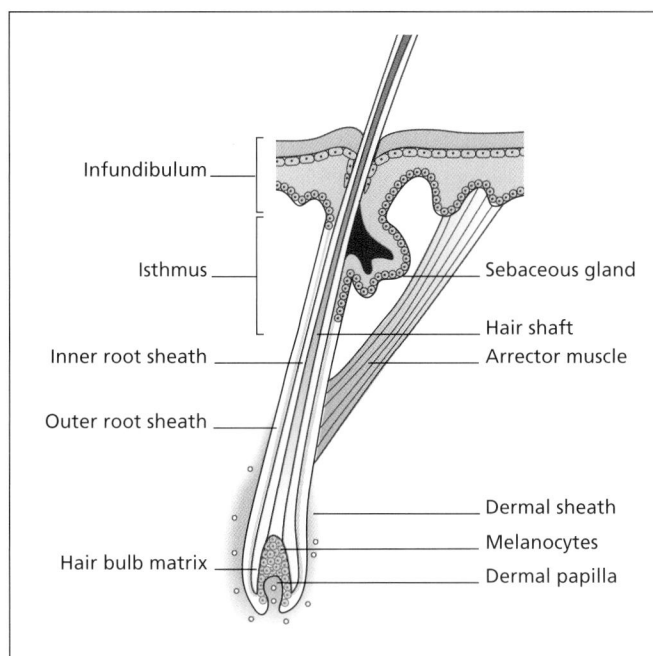

Figure 89.1 Diagram of an anagen hair follicle.

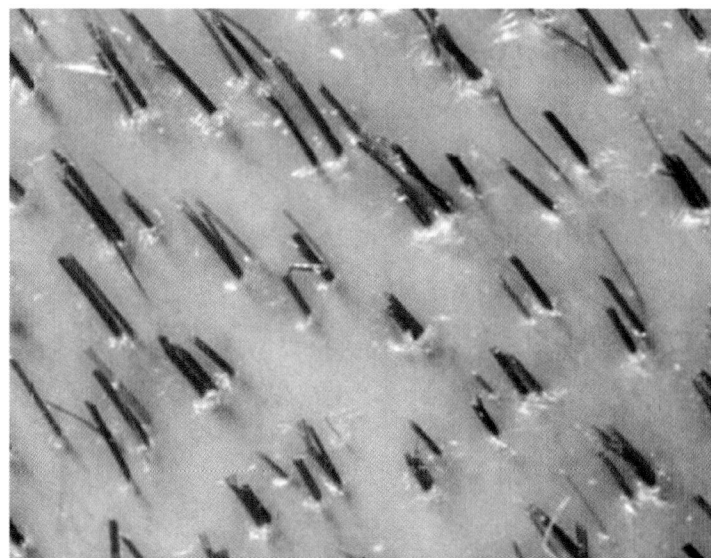

Figure 89.2 Grouping of hairs in follicular units on the human scalp. In some groups, multiple hairs emerge from a single follicular opening.

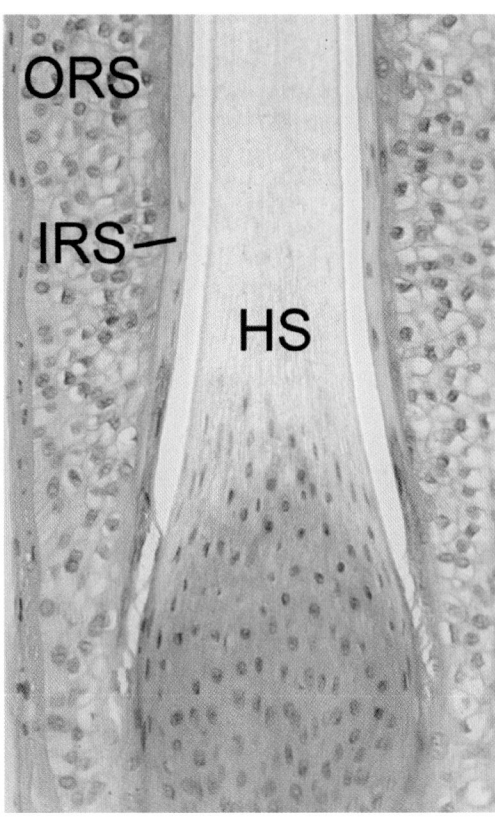

Figure 89.3 Longitudinal section through the suprabulbar region of an anagen follicle showing the keratogenous region of the hair shaft (HS). The inner root sheath (IRS) is keratinized at this level. ORS, outer root sheath.

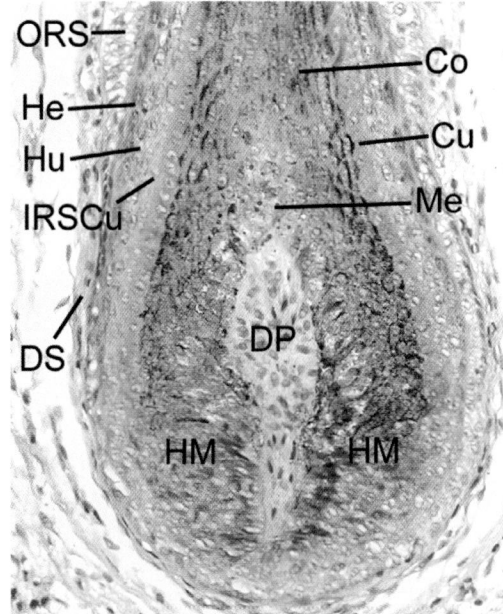

Figure 89.4 Anagen hair bulb. Co, hair cortex; Cu, hair cuticle; DP, dermal papilla; DS, dermal sheath; He, Henle layer; HM, hair matrix; Hu, Huxley layer; IRSCu, inner root sheath cuticle; Me, melanocyte; ORS, outer root sheath.

Hair follicle stem cells reside in the lower part of the isthmus, close to the insertion of the arrector muscle [18]. During embryogenesis, and in adult follicles in other species, this region shows a distinctive bulge, although a clearly defined bulge is often not seen in human adult hair follicles. Hair follicle stem cells show distinctive biochemical properties, they are slow cycling and proliferate only during the onset of anagen. Daughter cells, known as transient amplifying cells, input into the outer root sheath of the lower part of the hair follicle whence they migrate in a downward direction. On entering the hair bulb matrix, they proliferate and undergo terminal differentiation to form the hair shaft and inner root sheath [19]. The progeny of hair follicle stem cells may also migrate distally to form the sebaceous gland and, under certain circumstances such as wound healing, the epidermis.

Suprabulbar region. The suprabulbar region of the follicle, below the isthmus and above the hair bulb, is comprised of three layers (from outermost to innermost): the outer root sheath, inner root sheath and hair shaft (Figure 89.3). The outer root sheath is a multilayered epithelium enclosing the inner root sheath which, at this level, is a fully keratinized structure. Cells of the hair shaft, at the centre of the follicle, undergo terminal differentiation within the keratogenous zone in the middle part of the suprabulbar region. Keratinization of the inner root sheath precedes that of the hair shaft, suggesting that the inner root sheath has a role in 'moulding' the shape of the hair fibre.

Hair bulb. In large terminal follicles, the deepest part of the follicle, the hair bulb, is situated in the subcutaneous fat (Figure 89.4). The hair bulb is invaginated at its base by the dermal papilla, which is connected to the perifollicular dermal sheath by a narrow stalk. The hair shaft and the inner root sheath are derived from epithelial cells surrounding the dermal papilla, a region known as the hair bulb matrix or germinative epithelium. These cells have a high mitotic rate, with a rate of cell turnover similar to that in the bone marrow. Daughter cells migrate in an upward direction and differentiate in a highly ordered fashion to form the concentric layers of the inner root sheath and the hair shaft. The inner root sheath derives from cells in the lower, more lateral part of the matrix, whereas the hair shaft is formed from the upper, centrally situated cells. In pigmented hair follicles, highly melanized melanocytes are situated amongst cells destined to form the hair cortex. The outer root sheath surrounds the inner root sheath. At the level of the hair bulb it consists of a single layer of cells, which can be followed almost to the lower tip of the hair follicle.

Dermal papilla. In anagen follicles, the dermal papilla is a flask-shaped structure that invaginates the base of the hair follicle. It is made up of specialized fibroblast-like cells embedded in an extracellular matrix rich in basement-membrane proteins and proteoglycans, and in large follicles the dermal papilla often contains a loop of capillary blood vessels. It is connected to the dermal sheath surrounding the follicle by a narrow stalk. Both the dermal papilla and the dermal sheath are derived from a condensation of mesenchymal cells, which appears at an early stage in follicular embryogenesis. Tissue recombinant studies have shown that the dermal papilla plays an essential part in the induction and maintenance of follicular epithelial differentiation [20,21,22,23]. It is responsible for determining the follicle type, so that cultured dermal papilla cells derived from rat vibrissae follicles induce the formation of a vibrissa-like follicle when implanted into ear skin [24]. The volume of the dermal papilla may also be responsible for controlling the size of the hair follicle, and that of the hair fibre [25,26]. This is of particular relevance to androgen-dependent changes in human hair growth, as the dermal papilla is probably the primary target of androgen action in the hair follicle.

Dermal sheath. A collagenous layer known as the dermal or connective tissue sheath envelops the lower part of the hair follicle. Like dermal papilla cells, fibroblasts of the dermal sheath are specialized. In experimental circumstances, these cells can reconstitute the dermal papilla and induce the formation of new hair follicles in adult human skin [27]. As we move distally along the hair follicle, above the level of the arrector insertion, the dermal sheath becomes less distinct, both structurally and functionally, as it merges with the interfollicular dermis.

Inner root sheath. The inner root sheath consists of three layers (from outermost to innermost): the Henle layer, Huxley layer and inner root sheath cuticle. Inner root sheath cells accumulate filaments approximately 7 nm thick and, in contrast with the hair cortex, amorphous trichohyalin granules appear in the cytoplasm. As the cells move up the follicle towards the surface, the filaments become more abundant and the number and size of the granules increases. Each of the three layers of the inner root sheath undergoes abrupt keratinization. This occurs at different levels in each layer, although the patterns of change are identical. In the hardened cytoplasm, however, only filaments can be seen. The changes occur first in the outermost Henle layer, then in the innermost cuticle and lastly in the Huxley layer, which is situated between them. Cells of the inner root sheath cuticle become flattened and overlap, with their free edges pointing downwards to interdigitate with the upwards-pointing cells of the hair shaft cuticle, thus anchoring the hair shaft within the hair follicle. The inner root sheath hardens before the presumptive hair within it, and it is consequently thought to control the definitive shape of the hair shaft.

Outer root sheath. The outer root sheath forms the most peripheral layer of hair follicle epithelium, enclosing the inner root sheath. At the lower tip of the hair bulb it consists of a single layer of cuboidal cells, becoming multilayered in the region of the upper hair bulb. The cytoplasm of outer root sheath cells is rich in glycogen, giving a clear appearance with routine histological stains. In some follicles, particularly large beard follicles, there is a distinct single cell layer interposed between the outer and inner root sheaths, known as the companion layer [28]. Companion layer cells are flattened along the axis of the follicle and are relatively devoid of glycogen. They show numerous intercellular connections to the inner root sheath and are thought to migrate distally along with the inner root sheath to be lost in the isthmus region. The direction of movement of outer root sheath cells is unclear but they may migrate downwards towards the hair bulb, the companion layer forming the plane of slippage between the inner and outer root sheaths. The outer root sheath of the suprabulbar region merges imperceptibly with the isthmus where the innermost cells undergo tricholemmal keratinization.

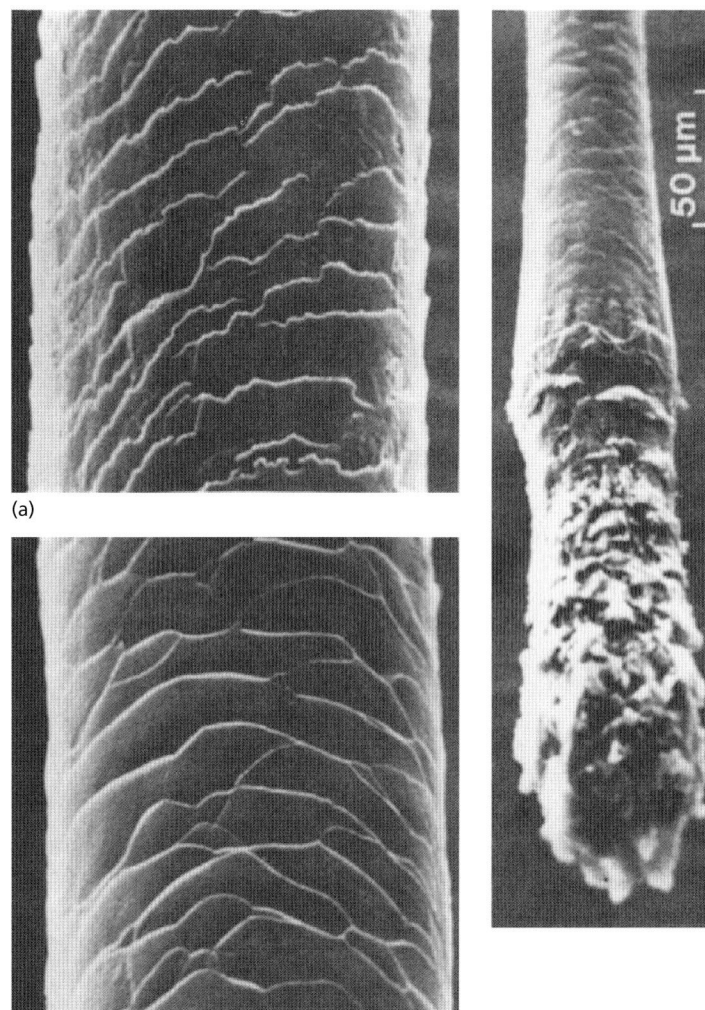

(a)

(b)

Figure 89.5 (a) Surface view of weathered cuticular scales in the distal portion of the hair shaft. (b) Surface view of undamaged cuticular scales in the proximal part of the hair shaft. (Courtesy of Dr D. Jackson, University of Sheffield, Sheffield, UK.)

Cuticle. The hair cuticle is formed initially as a single cell layer, but the cells become progressively imbricated (tile-like) as they move peripherally. The cells become flattened, first in a direction at right angles to the plane of the follicle, and then becoming progressively angulated so that the outer edges of the cells point in an upward direction. The flattened cells overlap, their free edges directed towards the tip (Figure 89.5) and interlocking with the cuticle of the surrounding inner root sheath. In the fully formed hair shaft, the cuticle consists of 5–10 overlapping cell layers, each 350–450 nm thick (Figure 89.6). The cuticle has important protective properties: it acts as a barrier to physical and chemical insults, and also maintains the integrity of the hair shaft. Wear and tear (e.g. from cosmetic procedures) leads to gradual degradation of the cuticle ('weathering'), with breaking and lifting of the free margins of the cuticular cells. Eventually this process may lead to exposure of the cortex and fracture of the hair shaft.

Cortex. Cells destined to form the cortex gradually become more fusiform in shape as they migrate upwards from the hair bulb. They develop a dense filamentous cytoskeleton in the upper hair bulb to become fully hyalinized in the suprabulbar region (the

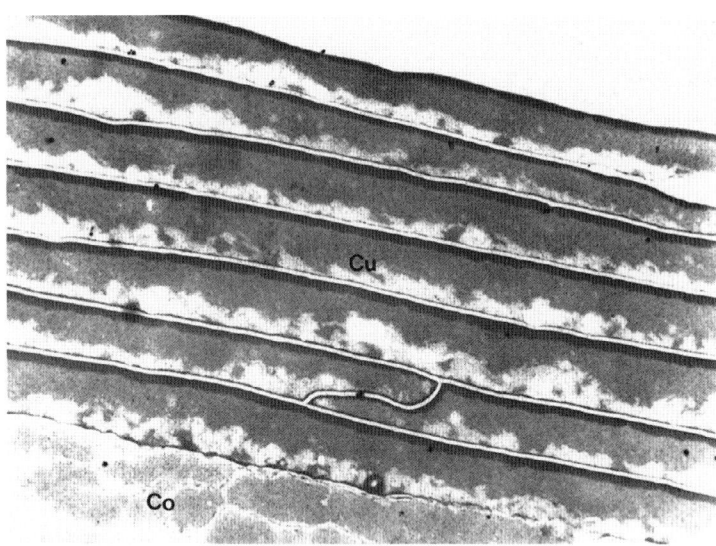

Figure 89.6 Cross-section through hair shaft showing cuticle layers (Cu) surrounding the central cortex (Co). Transmission electron micrograph, silver methenamine stain.

keratogenous zone) (Figure 89.7). The hard α-keratin intermediate filaments (α-KIF) are the major structural component of the mammalian hair cortex. The molecule in α-KIF is an obligate heteropolymer containing a type I and type II polypeptide chain [29,30,**31**], in which right-handed α-helices coil round one another in a left-handed manner to form a rod-like dimeric structure (a 'coiled coil') (Figure 89.8). The 8 nm keratin filaments (microfibrils) are formed from multiple α-KIF molecules, on average 16 molecules or 32 chains in cross-section [32]. Keratin filaments are cross-linked to keratin-associated proteins, which form a matrix between the filaments. More than 60 hair keratin-associated proteins have been found in various species. They are classified into three major families: high sulphur, ultra-high sulphur and high glycine–tyrosine proteins [33]. In some species, notably the sheep, the cortex can be divided into two regions: the orthocortex and paracortex, which differ in the arrangement of KIFs and the proportion of keratin-associated proteins. In humans, the hair cortex appears to contain mixtures of KIF arrangements within each cell [**34**].

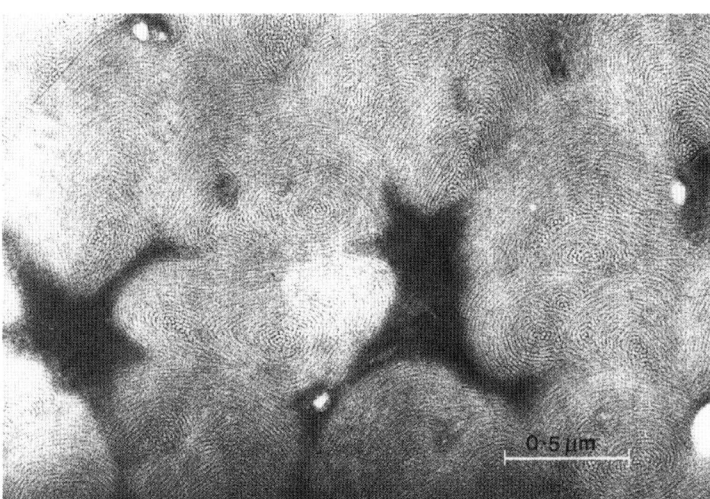

Figure 89.7 Cross-section of transformed cortical cells of human hair. The relatively translucent filaments, set in a more dense sulphur-rich matrix, appear as concentric lamellae (macrofibrils), giving a characteristic fingerprint pattern.

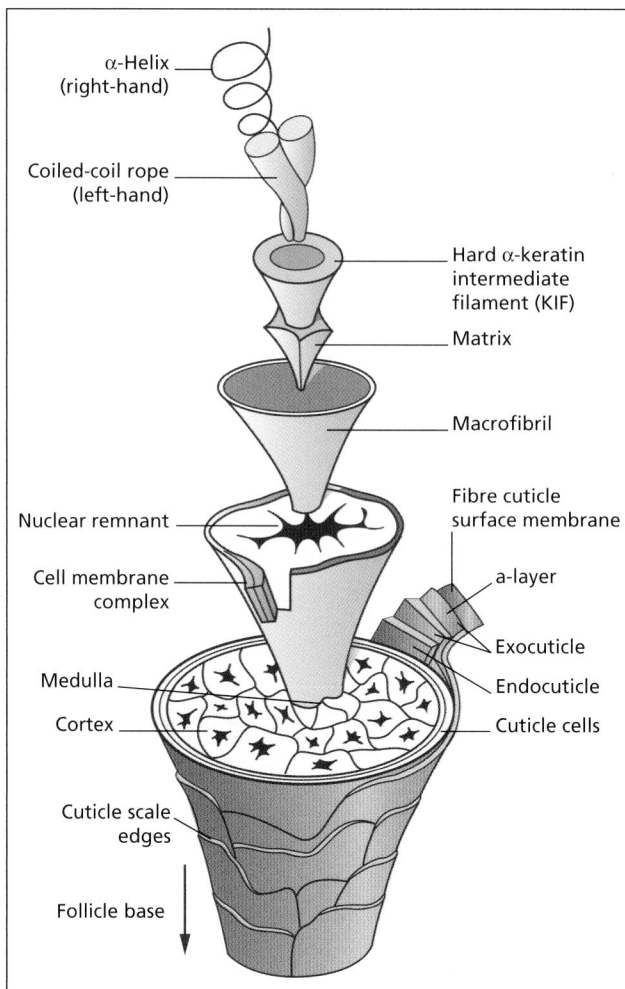

Figure 89.8 Exploded view of the major structural components comprising a human hair fibre. Pigment granules that are normally dispersed throughout the cortex are not included. (From Jones 2001 [**34**]. Reproduced with permission of Elsevier.)

Medulla. The medulla is a variable structure in human hairs, where it may be continuous, discontinuous or absent. Large-diameter hairs are more likely to contain a medulla, although the relationship between hair diameter and medullation is not clear-cut.

Hair follicle innervation. A plexus of longitudinally aligned sensory nerve fibres surrounds the isthmus region. Small nerve fibres may also be arranged in a circular fashion outside the longitudinal fibres. Several different types of nerve endings are found around human hair follicles, including free nerve endings, pilo-Ruffini nerve endings and Merkel nerve endings [35,36]. In other species, lamellated nerve endings are found in richly innervated sinus hair follicles (e.g. vibrissae follicles), which have specialized sensory function [36].

Hair cycle

Hair follicles undergo a repetitive sequence of growth and rest known as the hair cycle (Figure 89.9). The timing of the phases of the hair cycle and its overall duration varies between species, between follicles in different regions of the skin in the same species

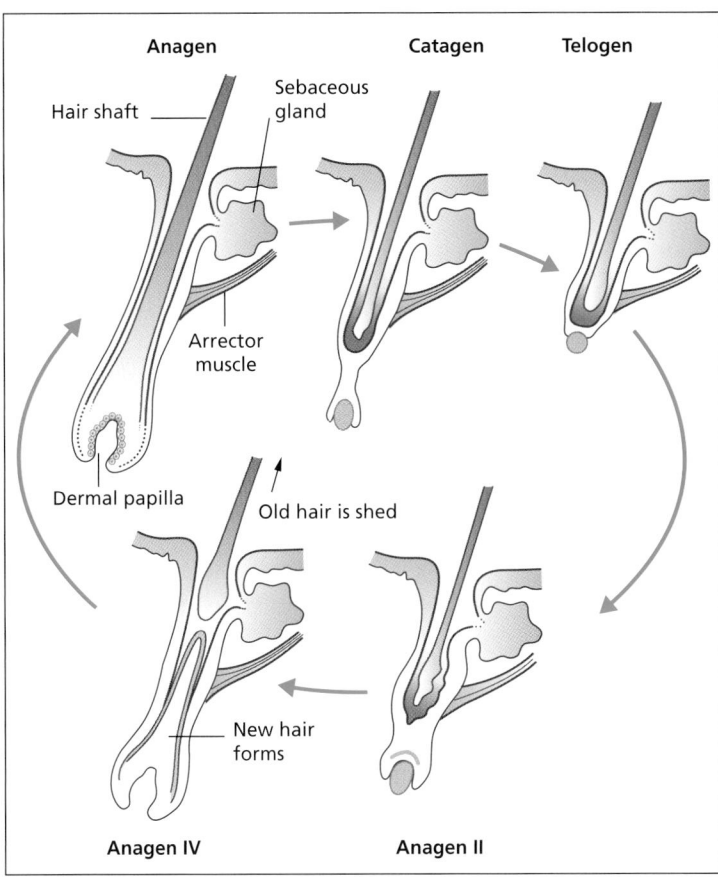

Figure 89.9 The hair cycle. (From Olsen 1994. Reproduced with permission of McGraw-Hill.)

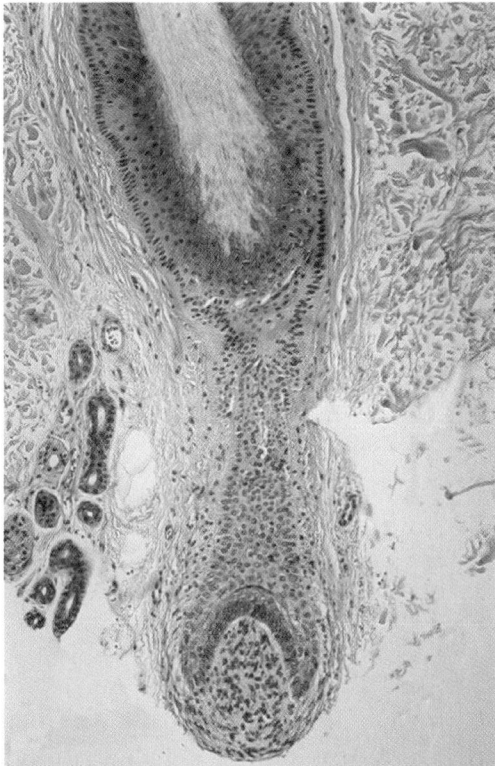

Figure 89.10 Scalp hair follicle in the anagen II stage of development. The club hair from the previous cycle is still present within the follicle. (Courtesy of Dr A. J. G. McDonagh, Royal Hallamshire Hospital, Sheffield, UK.)

and, in some animals, between different follicle types, such as guard hairs and underhairs, in the same region of the skin.

The period of active hair growth is known as *anagen* and the duration of this phase is responsible for determining the final length of the hair. In most hair follicles in most animals, anagen is relatively brief, lasting a few weeks at most. In some hair follicles, such as those on the human scalp, horse's tail and wool follicles in merino sheep, anagen may continue for several years, so that very long hairs are produced. Under normal circumstances, 80–90% of hair follicles on the human scalp are in anagen at any one time.

The entry of a resting hair follicle into anagen is heralded by the onset of mitotic activity in epithelial cells overlying the dermal papilla at the base of the follicle (the secondary epithelial germ). In most follicle types (vibrissae follicles are an exception), the lower part of the follicle elongates downwards along a preformed dermal tract (the stele). The developing hair bulb partly envelops the dermal papilla, and epithelial cells start to differentiate to form the inner root sheath and the hair shaft (Figure 89.10). The dermal papilla expands from a tightly packed ball of cells into a flask-shaped structure where the cells become separated by an extracellular matrix rich in proteoglycans and basement membrane proteins. A network of capillary blood vessels develops around the lengthening follicle, extending into the dermal papilla in larger follicles. In the fully developed anagen follicle, epithelial cells in the hair bulb undergo vigorous proliferative activity. Their progeny move distally and differentiate in an ordered fashion to form the layers of the inner root sheath and the hair shaft.

At the end of anagen, epithelial cell division declines and ceases, and the follicle enters an involutionary phase known as *catagen*. During catagen, the proximal end of the hair shaft keratinizes to form a club-shaped structure and the lower part of the follicle involutes by apoptosis (Figure 89.11). The basement membrane surrounding the follicle becomes thickened and corrugated to form the 'glassy membrane'. The base of the follicle, together with its dermal papilla, moves upwards, eventually to lie just below the level of the arrector insertion. The period between the completion of follicular regression and the onset of the next anagen phase is termed *telogen*. The club hair lies within an epithelial sac to which it is attached by tricholemmal keratin. The club hair is eventually shed through an active process termed *exogen*. In many species, follicles re-enter anagen prior to shedding of the club hair so that the old hair is not shed until the follicle is well into its next growth phase. This may also be seen in human follicles although it is unusual for a club hair to be retained much beyond the midstage of anagen development. In the human scalp, hair follicles may remain in a state of latency, also known as *kenogen*, for a prolonged period after the club hair is shed [37].

Control of the hair cycle

Hair cycling is controlled primarily within individual hair follicles but this intrinsic behaviour may be modulated by both local and systemic factors. In most newborn mammals, including humans, hair cycles are coordinated in a wave-like fashion (moult waves)

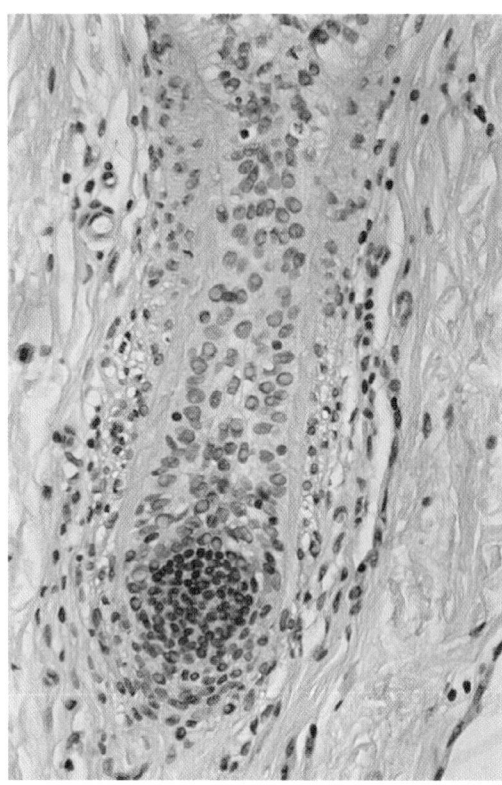

Figure 89.11 Human hair follicle in mid-catagen. There is a prominent glassy membrane surrounding the regressing epithelial column. The dermal papilla has rounded and condensed. (Courtesy of McGraw-Hill.)

across regions of the skin in the neonatal period. Moult waves are regulated within the skin and are accompanied by changes in other skin structures, such as epidermal and dermal thickness. In many mammals, living in their natural environment in temperate and higher latitudes, moult waves continue into adult life and occur on a seasonal basis. This allows adaptation of the thickness of the coat, and sometimes its colour, to different climatic conditions in summer and winter (Figure 89.12).

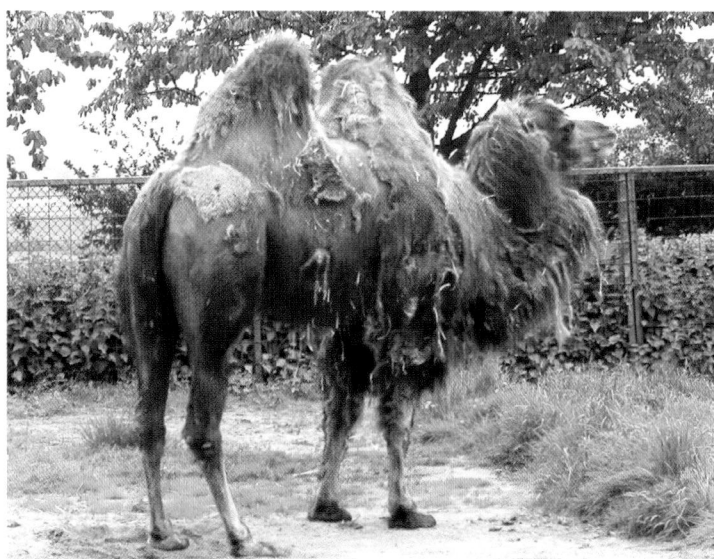

Figure 89.12 Bactrian camel in a spring moult.

Seasonal moulting is regulated by the endocrine system under the influence of environmental signals. The most important of these is change in day length (the photoperiod) [38,39]. The production of melatonin by the pineal gland, which transduces visual signals, and prolactin by the pituitary, play a key role in orchestrating endocrine control of seasonal hair growth [40–42]. Vestiges of seasonal variation in hair growth are present in humans [43], although the magnitude is seldom sufficient to be noticeable.

Although local and systemic factors modulate the hair cycle in some species, in adult humans and some other mammals hair cycling is asynchronous. Hair follicles in different regions of the skin may also cycle differently. In humans, for example, the duration of anagen on the scalp may last several years, whereas on the eyebrows anagen is very brief. Even in animals showing seasonal hair growth, hair cycles in different follicle types in the same skin region are not necessarily in phase. When scalp hair follicles are transplanted into other regions of the skin they retain the cyclical behaviour of the donor site, indicating that cycle control is determined within the follicle or its immediate tissue environment. Interactions between two key cell populations in the hair follicle – epithelial stem cells in the outer root sheath and mesenchymal cells in the dermal papilla and dermal sheath – are thought to underlie intrinsic control of hair cycling, and a large number of molecules have been implicated in this process [44]. Fluctuations in the inhibitory influence of bone morphogenetic proteins and the stimulatory Wnt/β-catenin pathway appear to play a key role in regulating stem cell activity during the hair cycle. A wide array of other signalling molecules with hair growth stimulatory (e.g. follistatin, transforming growth factor β2 (TGF-β2), fibroblast growth factor 7 (FGF-7), FGF-10) and inhibitory (e.g. Dkk1, FGF-18, 17-β-oestradiol) influences have also been implicated but, such is their complexity, a comprehensive model of hair cycle control has yet to be achieved [45].

Hair growth

Rate of hair growth

The rate of hair growth varies from species to species, and within one species from region to region, as well as with sex and age. Published rates of scalp hair growth in humans vary between 0.3 and 0.5 mm per day, slightly faster in adult women than men but greater in prepubertal boys than girls. Male beard growth has been recorded at 0.27–0.38 mm/day. Vellus hair growth is much slower: 0.03 mm/day on the forehead in one study [8].

Androgens and hair growth

Androgens influence hair growth in several ways. First, they participate in the endocrine control of moulting in animals that show seasonal hair growth [46]. Second, in some mammals, androgens stimulate the growth of hair follicles in certain regions of the skin following sexual maturity. Third, in humans and some other primates, androgens are necessary for the development of balding on the scalp.

Androgen-stimulated hair growth

The growth of obvious facial, trunk and extremity hair in the male, and of pubic and axillary hair in both sexes, is dependent on androgens. The development of such hair at puberty is, in broad terms and at least initially, in parallel with the rise in levels of androgen from testicular, adrenocortical and ovarian sources, which occurs in both sexes and is somewhat steeper in males. That testosterone from the interstitial cells of the testis is responsible for the growth of beard and body hair in male adolescence and that testicular activity is itself initiated by gonadotrophic hormones of the pituitary is unquestioned. However, the findings that growth hormone-deficient boys and girls are less than normally responsive to androgens, and that growth hormone is necessary as a synergistic factor to allow testosterone to be fully effective with respect to hair growth [47], as well as protein anabolism and growth promotion, suggest that hypophysial hormones also have a more direct role. Direct evidence of the role of testicular androgen is that castration reduces growth of the human beard [48], whereas testosterone stimulates it in eunuchs and elderly men. The role of androgen is further demonstrated in the treatment of hirsute women with the antiandrogen cyproterone acetate [49], which reduces the definitive length, rate of growth, diameter and extent of medullation of the thigh hairs [50].

At puberty, terminal hair gradually replaces vellus, starting in the pubic regions. In both sexes the first pubic hair is sparse, long, downy, slightly pigmented and almost straight. It later becomes darker, coarser, more curled and extends in area to form an inverse triangle. A British study showed that boys had the first recognizable pubic hair at an average age of 13.4 years, and the full adult 'male' pattern at 15.2 years, approximately 3.5 years after the start of pubertal development of the genitalia [51]. The corresponding mean ages for girls were considerably earlier, namely 11.7 years and 13.5 years [52]. In approximately 80% of men and 10% of women, the pubic hair continues spreading until the mid-twenties or later; there is no absolute distinction between male and female patterns, only one of degree.

Axillary hair first appears approximately 2 years after the start of pubic hair growth. The amount, as measured by the weight of the fully grown mass, continues to increase until the late twenties in males as well as in females, in whom, however, it is less at any age [48]. The mean amounts grown per day increase from late puberty until the mid-twenties and thereafter decrease steadily.

Facial hair in boys first appears at about the same time as the axillary hair, starting at the corners of the upper lip, and spreading medially to complete the moustache and then the cheeks and beard.

Terminal hair development is continued in regular sequence on the legs, thighs, forearms, abdomen, buttocks, back, arms and shoulders [53]. The extent of terminal hair tends to increase throughout the years of sexual maturity, but most patterns occur over a wide age range. The adult pattern is not achieved until the fourth decade, when the androgen levels are already somewhat lower than in early adult life. Moreover, aural hairs do not appear until late middle age, and a study of coarse sternal hair in men showed that the hairs continue to increase in length and number from puberty to the fifth or sixth decade.

There is considerable racial variability in androgen-dependent hair growth. The growth of facial and body hair is greater in European men than in Chinese men [48] and there is also variation within these broad racial categories – southern European men tend to be hairier than men from northern Europe [54].

Androgenetic alopecia
See section 'Androgenetic alopecia and pattern hair loss' later in this chapter.

Androgen synthesis and metabolism
Testosterone is the major circulating androgen, but in most body sites apart from the axillae and pubic region, the effect of testosterone on hair growth is mediated by its more potent metabolite 5α-dihydrotestosterone (DHT). The conversion of testosterone to DHT is catalysed by the enzyme 5α-reductase. There are three isoforms of 5α-reductase, which are encoded by different genes [55,56]. Type 1 5α-reductase is widely distributed in the skin, but expression of the type 2 isoform is restricted to androgen target tissues such as the prostate and epididymis. Evidence from studies in men with a genetic deficiency of 5α-reductase type 2, and from the response of androgenetic alopecia and female hirsutism to finasteride, an inhibitor of 5α-reductase type 2, indicates that this isoform plays the key role in regulating androgen-dependent hair growth. The type 3 isoform is widely expressed [57] but it is not yet known whether it regulates androgen responses in the skin.

Androgen receptor
The tissue effects of androgens are mediated through binding to the intracellular androgen receptor. The androgen receptor is a nuclear hormone receptor [58], and like other members of the nuclear hormone receptor superfamily it acts as a gene transcription factor following ligand binding. Mutations in the androgen receptor gene are responsible for the androgen insensitivity syndrome [59]. Individuals with the complete form of the syndrome, in which there is failure of functional androgen receptor expression, have intra-abdominal testes but female external genitalia, breast development and psychosocial development. After puberty, circulating testosterone is in the normal or elevated male range but pubic and axillary hair fail to develop and there is no beard growth and no balding.

Mechanism of androgen action on the hair follicle
The specificity of the response of hair follicles to androgens is determined within the skin. Hair follicles in occipital skin, a site that shows little or no response to androgens, retain their site-specific behaviour when transplanted into balding areas on the frontal scalp [60]. Conversely, hair follicles from a balding scalp continue to regress when transplanted into skin of the forearm [61]. The success of micrografting techniques, in which individual follicles are transplanted, shows that androgen responsiveness is determined at the level of the follicle or its immediate tissue environment. Three lines of evidence suggest that the dermal papilla is the primary target of androgen action in the hair follicle.
1 Androgen receptor expression in the lower part of the follicle is restricted to dermal papilla cells [62,63].
2 The size of the hair follicle is probably determined by the volume of the dermal papilla [25,64].
3 Dermal papillae express 5α-reductase type 2 whereas hair follicle epithelium expresses only 5α-reductase type 1 [65].

Androgens may act on hair growth by altering the number of cells in the dermal papilla and its extracellular matrix [64]. Cells cultured from dermal papillae of human beard hair follicles also release growth factors in response to androgens that stimulate the proliferation of keratinocytes [63,66], and the pattern of androgen metabolism by cultured and intact dermal papilla cells is consistent with that expected from their site of origin [67,68]. There is one report that dermal papilla cells grown from balding scalp follicles secrete TGF-β in the presence of testosterone [69]. TGF-β is a growth factor known to inhibit hair growth [70]. Hence the variable response of hair growth to androgens may reflect site-dependent differences in the types of growth factors produced by the dermal papilla.

APPROACH TO THE PATIENT WITH HAIR LOSS

Paul Farrant

Hair is an important cosmetic asset. It is also a means of social and sexual communication in many mammals including humans. Consequently, although few hair diseases produce physical disability, the disfigurement caused may lead to much distress in the patient and often in their family members. Particularly in view of the limited therapeutic options in many hair diseases, this aspect needs to be recognized and addressed by the practitioner.

History

Presenting complaint. Most adults presenting with a complaint of hair loss will complain of either gradual thinning of hair in a pattern over time or a rapid increase in the amount of hair being shed, with hair being evident in the shower, on pillows and carpets and hair coming out easily when brushed. Determining whether it is a thinning or shedding problem will help focus the history further on genetic and age-related changes or reasons why the hair cycle may be disturbed. These two complaints may coexist, as both are common. The hair cycle in genetic hair loss has a shorter growth phase and proportionally more hair will be in telogen phase at any given moment, so an increase in hair shedding can be expected. Hair loss in patches is likely to point to alopecia areata.

In addition to these complaints, a patient may be aware of hair breakage, focal areas of hair loss that are scar-like, recession of the hairline or loss of hair from other body sites such as the eyebrows. Symptoms such as itch, burning and pain should be noted as these are often associated with inflammation that can lead to scarring.

Background information. It is common for patients with gradual thinning to have a family history affecting either parent or extended family members of premature hair loss in either a male or female pattern. Female patients presenting with pattern hair loss may have hormonal disturbance and therefore one should enquire as to the regularity of menstrual periods, the presence of hirsutes or any other signs of androgenization. A contraceptive history should be recorded.

In patients complaining of hair shedding, likely to represent a telogen effluvium, the history should be directed to any particular life events or medications that began a few months before the onset of the shedding. Severe psychological stress, physical illness, new medications, dieting and weight loss may all be relevant. In acute telogen effluvium a trigger may be identified and the condition is usually self-limiting. If the hair shedding is more chronic or episodic it may be difficult to identify a specific trigger. With the exception of severe diets, eating disorders, inflammatory bowel disease or bowel surgery, profound nutritional deficiencies that result in hair loss are uncommon in the developed nations. Enquiries into normal diet, including whether adequate amounts of protein and iron are consumed may be appropriate, but the relationship between iron stores and hair loss remains controversial [1–4].

Associated symptoms. Most hair loss is asymptomatic. The presence of itch, burning or pain may point to inflammation which can be a feature of scarring hair loss. Pediculosis capitis and tinea capitis may both present with an itchy scalp.

Clinical examination

Clinical evaluation should include a visual assessment of the pattern and extent of hair loss. Does the patient have clinically evident hair loss? Is hair loss diffuse or patchy? Is it occurring in a distinctive distribution (such as seen in pattern hair loss or frontal fibrosing alopecia)? Hair colour, shine, texture and 'hair behaviour' may be altered by conditions affecting hair growth or the hair fibre characteristics. When dealing with patchy hair loss it is important to assess whether there are patent follicular ostia or whether these are lost – a key feature in scarring conditions [5].

The presence of scalp inflammation should be sought, which may include perifollicular erythema, follicular hyperkeratosis, plugged hair follicles, pustules or swellings.

Close inspection using magnification with a light source is often helpful to appreciate variation in hair fibre diameter, exclamation mark hairs, cadaverized hairs (black dots visible beneath the surface, representing hair remnants), abnormal scalp vessels or hair shaft abnormalities.

Hair pull test. A hair pull is a relatively crude test with high inter-operator variability that can be performed in the clinic to assess hair shedding in generalized hair loss and disease activity in focal conditions. A group of approximately 60 hairs is gathered between the thumb and forefinger of the non-dominant hand. With the dominant hand the strands of hair are loosely twisted to remove stray hairs and then the hairs are grasped between the dominant thumb and forefinger near the scalp. Gentle traction is applied in a smooth, gradual manner, away from the scalp. The number and type of hairs extracted may give clues to the underlying diagnosis. The test can be repeated from a number of sites on the scalp, avoiding the part lines (Table 89.2).

Grasping a few hairs from the edge of a focal area of hair loss may give an indication of disease activity. Telogen hairs may be extracted from the periphery of a patch of alopecia areata. Anagen hairs may be easily extracted from active areas of scarring hair loss.

A modified hair pull test can be used to assess hair breakage. With the non-dominant hand grasping a small group of hairs near

Table 89.2 Characteristic findings of the hair pull test in conditions presenting with hair loss.

Condition	Positive hair pull findings
Telogen effluvium	Increase in telogen hairs extracted from all areas
Alopecia areata	Increase in telogen hairs or dystrophic anagen hairs from affected areas
Primary cicatricial alopecias	Increase in anagen hairs extracted (pigmented bulb, ensheathed within root sheath)
Loose anagen syndrome	Painless extraction of dysplastic anagen hairs, often lacking root sheaths

to the scalp, the dominant hand pulls them as described above. If they break or snap, this may indicate brittleness and hair breakage that may typify a shaft abnormality.

Trichogram. A trichogram is a forced pluck of hair that includes the hair roots. A group of 60–80 hairs is clasped between rubber-armed forceps or needle holders, close to the scalp surface. The examiner holds the needle holders firmly and rapidly tugs the needle holders away from the scalp in a perpendicular direction to extract all the hairs in the sample. The hairs can then be analysed under a microscope to calculate the percentage of hairs in telogen and anagen phases. This technique has been used extensively in some countries, mainly to assess telogen effluvium and pattern hair loss, but it is time-consuming and of doubtful value.

Trichoscopy. Just as the examination of pigmented lesions has been transformed by the use of dermoscopy, the study of hair conditions has been enhanced by the use of magnified light sources. In the mainstay this confirms or highlights clinical signs, rather than demonstrating specific features characteristic of an individual disease. For example, exclamation mark hairs and cadaverized hairs are more easily visualized. Yellow dots, said to represent sebum in the empty follicular ostia, are a feature of active alopecia areata [6,7]. Examples of trichoscopic images are shown in Figure 89.13.

Although not a substitute for microscopy, a hand-held dermoscope can be used to identify some common hair shaft abnormalities.

Children with hair loss

Whilst conditions such as telogen effluvium and alopecia areata are relatively common in children, there are a number of other considerations in approaching the child presenting with hair loss, especially when hair loss is evident early in life. There is a much higher chance that the hair loss is part of a genetic syndrome, has an associated hair shaft abnormality or is associated with abnormal development of the ectoderm, with associated nail, teeth or sweating problems. The psychosocial aspects are also different from those in adults. Hair disorders may engender much anxiety in parents but young children are often unconcerned. Painful and potentially toxic treatments and repeated visits to dermatologists have the potential to change the child's attitude and are best avoided. In older children hair disorders may lead to teasing and bullying. Here, support from the school authorities and sometimes from a paediatric clinical psychologist may be needed.

The history should start with the pattern of hair at birth and how this changed during the first year of life, as hair may be normal initially and only when replaced with terminal hair towards the end of infancy does any problem become evident. A history of teeth and nail development should be recorded, as well as problems with heat intolerance that may represent anhidrosis, if an ectodermal dysplasia is suspected. A family history of any hair problems is more likely to be relevant in this age group. Failure of hair to grow beyond a certain length may indicate a hair shaft abnormality leading to breakage such as monilethrix, an increase in hair loss such as loose anagen syndrome, or a decreased growth phase such as short anagen syndrome.

Patches of hair loss present early in life may represent areas of absent hair follicle development such as aplasia cutis or the failure of terminal hairs to develop, leaving persistent vellus hairs such as triangular alopecia. Acquired patches of hair loss in children are far more likely to represent an infective cause such as tinea capitis, and hair samples should be routinely submitted for mycological analysis.

Clinical photography

It is impossible to remember one patient from the next over a period of time and to provide an objective opinion on the state of their hair without some form of photographic record. Ideally, photography should be standardized in terms of magnification, lighting and position of both the subject and their hairstyle. Stereotactic devices provide the optimum solution but are largely used for research only. Global photography of the vertex is useful in pattern hair loss. Recording patches of scarring hair loss is particularly tricky.

Microscopy

Light microscopy should be used for the investigation of possible hair shaft disorders. It is important to remember that hair shaft abnormalities may be focal, and sufficient hairs should be submitted for analysis to increase the detection rate. Hairs should be trimmed near their base and not plucked. Trichoscopy can be used to identify abnormal hairs to improve sampling and increase the yield. Polarization of hair shafts may be required to demonstrate some features such as the tiger-tail pattern of trichothiodystrophy, caused by a low sulphur content. Scanning electron microscopy provides incredibly detailed images of the hair shaft but availability, expense and expertise limit its use. Microscopy is also useful for demonstrating the typical 'ruffled cuticle' in the roots of plucked hairs in loose anagen syndrome.

Scalp biopsy

Histology is a useful tool in the evaluation of hair disease in certain circumstances. Important considerations include the biopsy technique, selection of biopsy sites, processing of the biopsies and access to a dermatopathologist skilled in the interpretation of hair pathology. Current practice is to take two 4 mm punch biopsies. In assessing a scarring alopecia one biopsy is sectioned vertically, and the second horizontally (Figure 89.14). In

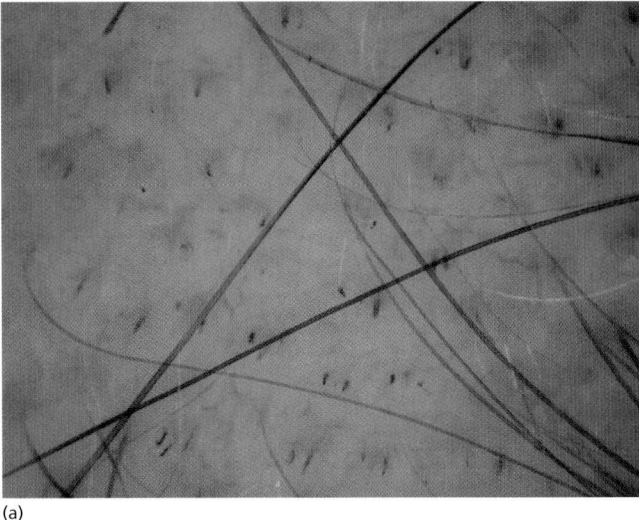

(a)

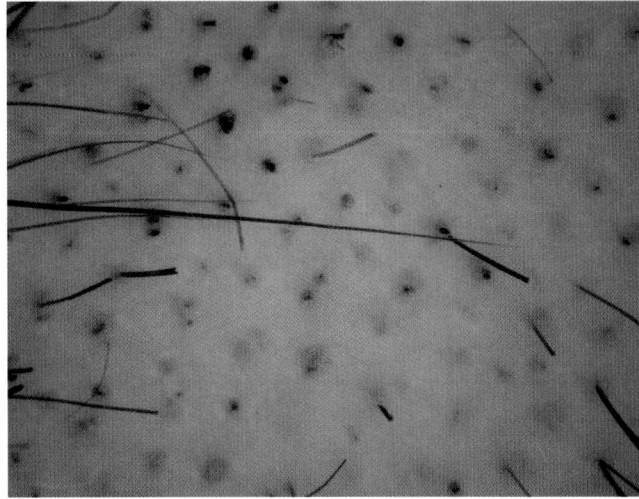

(b)

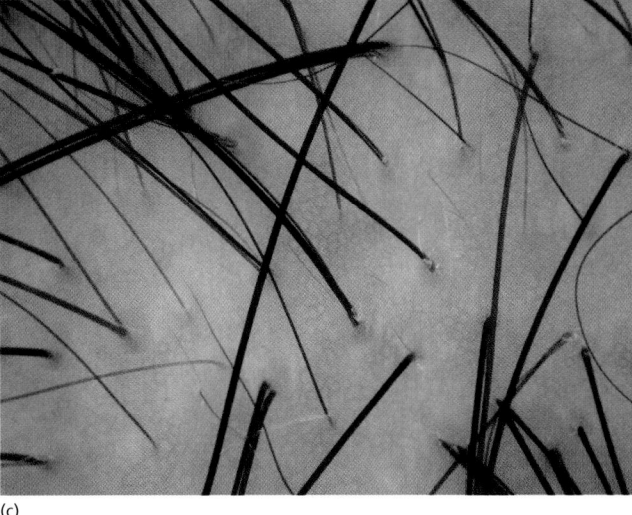

(c)

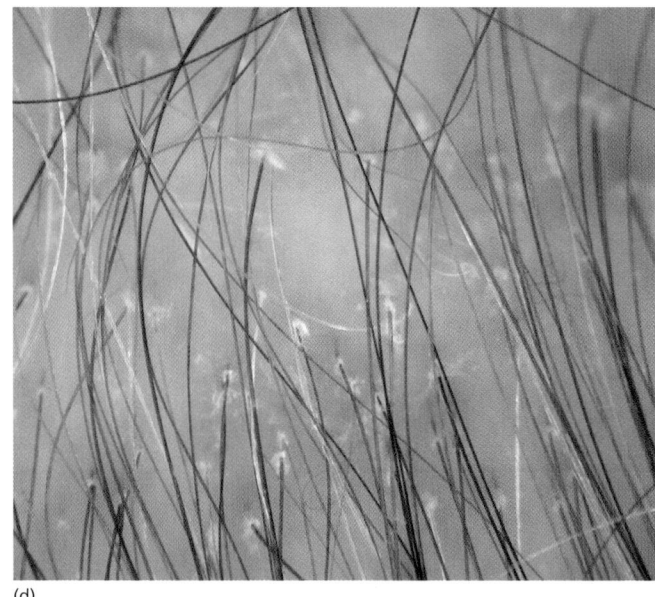

(d)

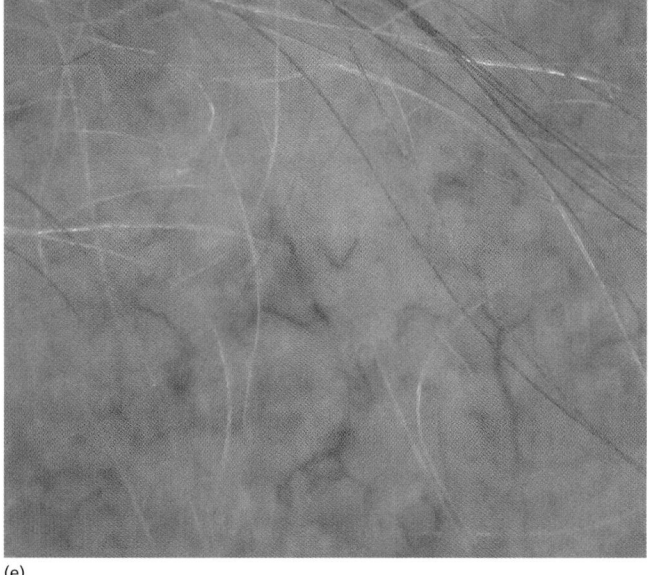

(e)

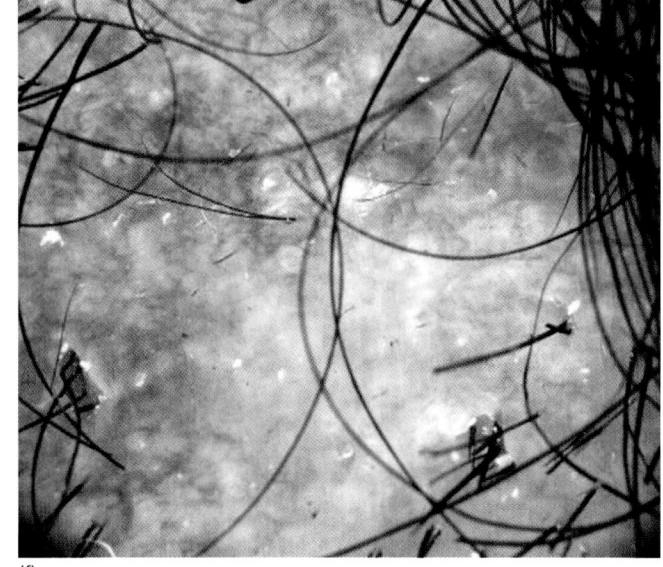

(f)

Figure 89.13 Trichoscopic images. (a) Yellow dots in alopecia areata. (b) Black dots and broken hairs in alopecia areata. (c) Variation in hair fibre diameter in female pattern hair loss. (d) Follicular hyperkeratosis in lichen plano-pilaris. (e) Arborizing vessels in discoid lupus erythematosus. (f) Tufting and inflammation in folliculitis decalvans.

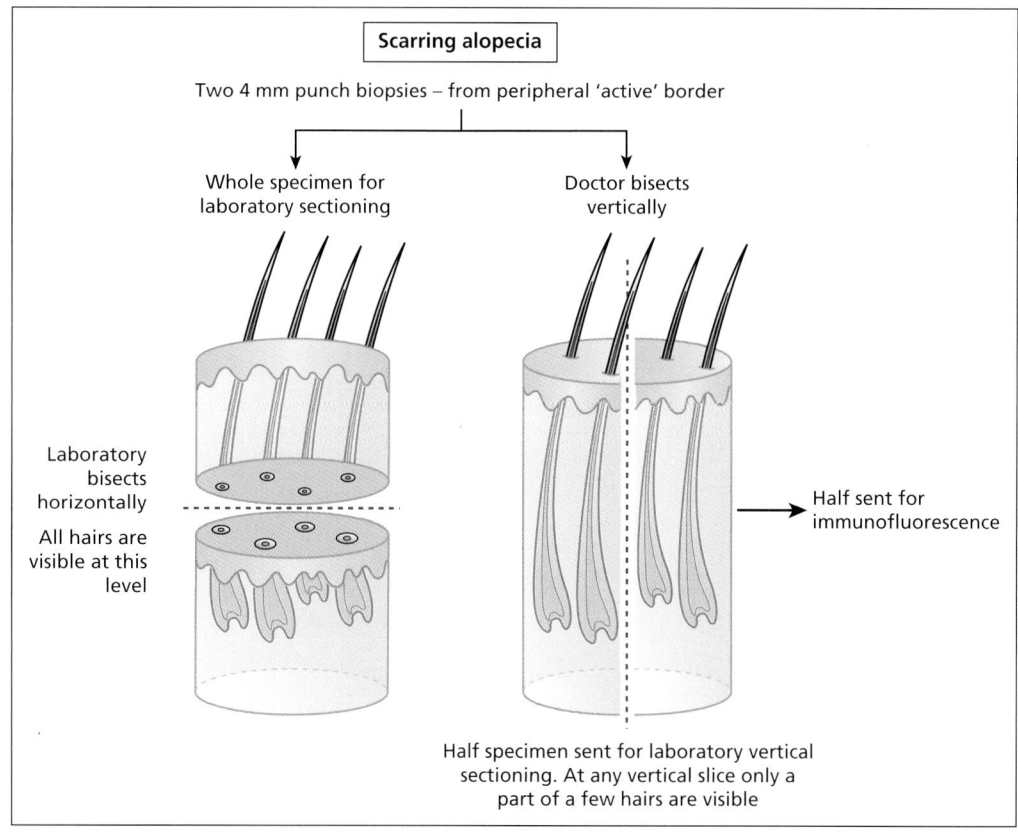

Figure 89.14 Biopsy – scarring alopecia protocol.

non-scarring conditions it is more useful for both biopsies to be sectioned horizontally (Figure 89.15). Processing a scalp biopsy in a horizontal fashion allows all the follicles in a given biopsy to be seen, typically 30–40 hairs per 4 mm punch. Sections can then be taken at different levels from the bulb to the isthmus and infundibulum, detecting conditions that focus on specific areas of the follicle [8]. Biopsies should be orientated in the direction of hair growth in order to minimize transection of follicles and should extend into the subcutaneous fat (Figure 89.16).

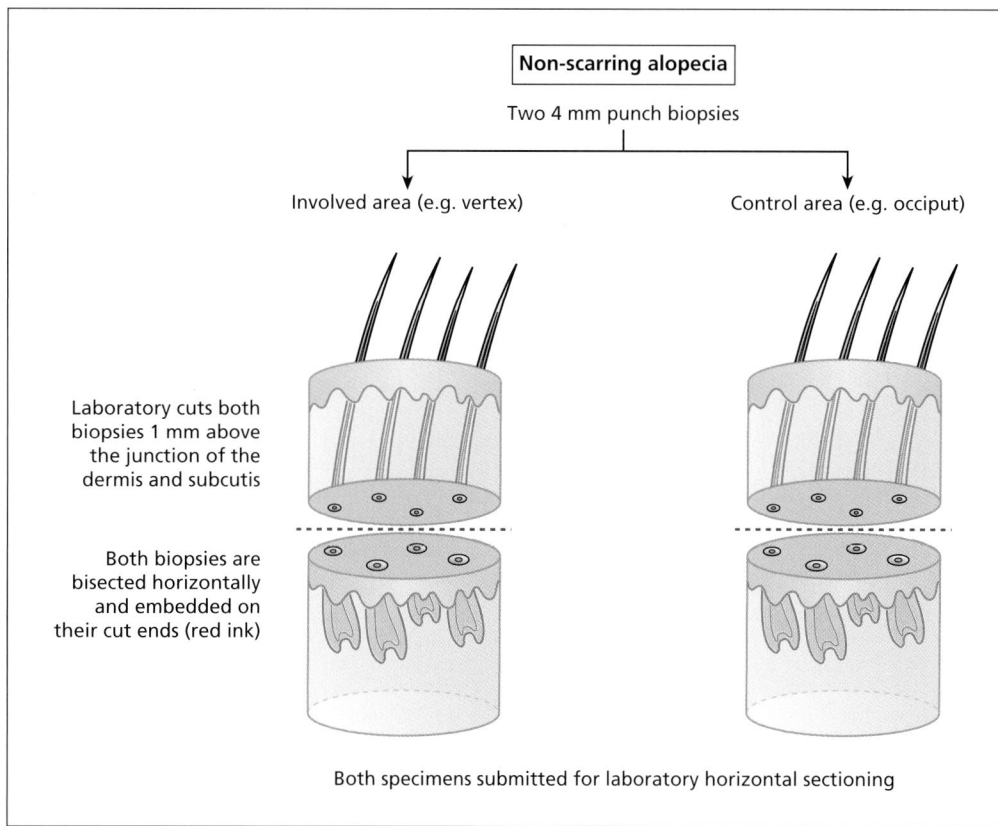

Figure 89.15 Biopsy – non-scarring alopecia protocol.

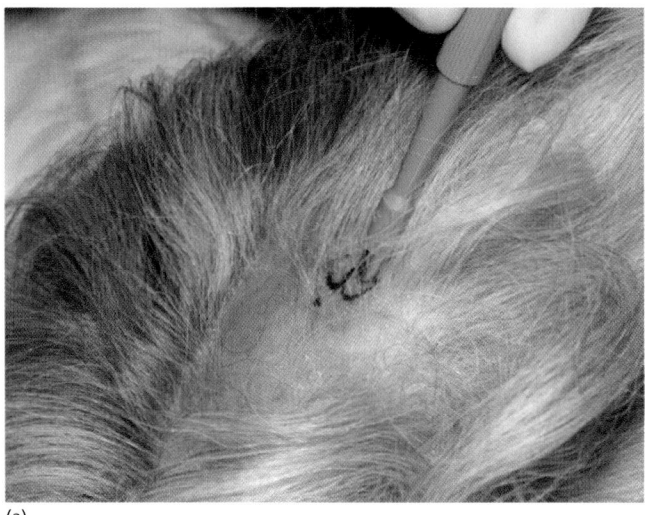

(a)

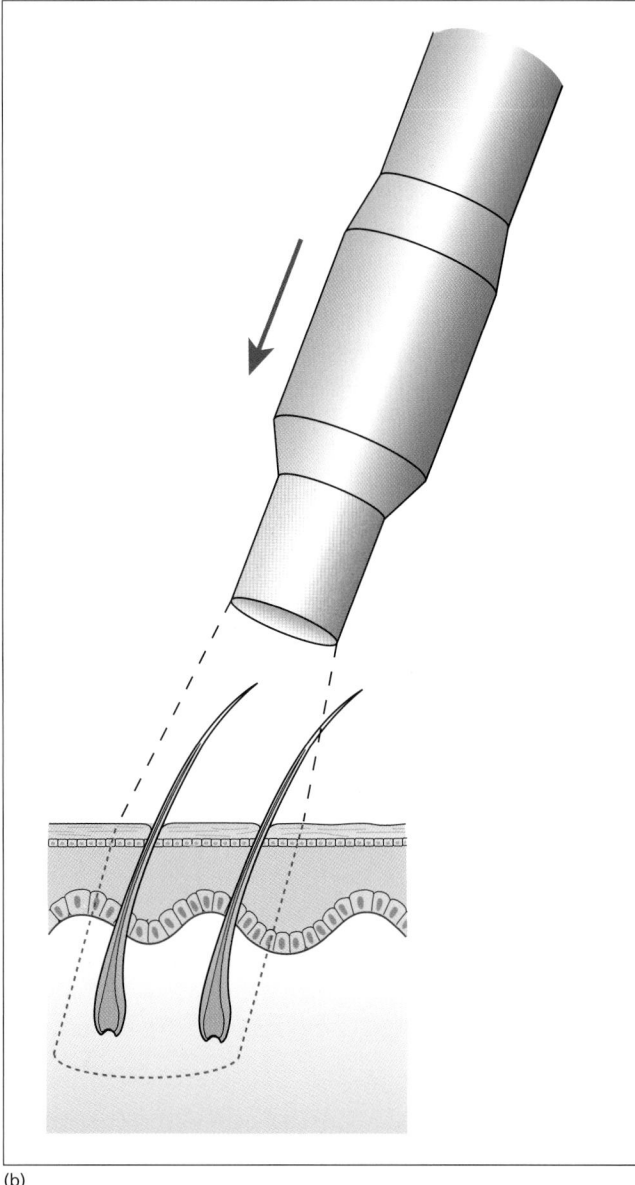

(b)

Figure 89.16 (a, b) Orientation of the punch biopsy in the direction of hair growth.

PART 8: SPECIFIC CUTANEOUS STRUCTURE

Biopsy site. To some extent the selection of the biopsy site depends on what information is needed. This is most important in scarring alopecias. Thus, a biopsy from the centre of a patch of putative scarring hair loss will confirm or deny whether hair follicles have been destroyed but will not demonstrate the causative pathology. Here, a biopsy from the active edge is more informative but could miss scarring. In alopecia areata a biopsy from the edge of a patch of hair loss may show the classic peribulbar inflammatory infiltrate, whereas the pathology in the centre can be subtle and require assessment of hair cycle status and the use of specific T-cell stains. In non-scarring conditions it is useful to sample the affected area and a control area, for example the vertex and occiput in suspected androgenetic hair loss.

A scalp biopsy is most useful in the following circumstances:
- In possible scarring alopecia to confirm the presence of hair follicle destruction and to distinguish between the major forms of primary scarring alopecia (i.e. discoid lupus erythematosus, lichen planopilaris and its variants, and neutrophil-rich forms).
- To distinguish between alopecia areata and trichotillomania.
- To assess for evidence of follicular miniaturization in patients presenting with excessive hair shedding but without clinical reduction in hair density (e.g. early pattern hair loss or telogen effluvium?).
- To diagnose diffuse hair loss of uncertain cause (e.g. alopecia areata, systemic lupus erythematosus).
- To diagnose rare causes of hair loss such as secondary syphilis, granulomatous disease, cutaneous lymphoma and other malignancies.

NON-SCARRING DISORDERS OF HAIR GROWTH

Androgenetic alopecia and pattern hair loss

Rodney D. Sinclair

Synonyms and inclusions
- Common balding
- Male pattern balding
- Male pattern hair loss
- Female pattern hair loss

Introduction and general description

The terms 'pattern hair loss' and 'common balding' describe a form of hair loss that occurs in a generally distinctive pattern and is characterized by a progressive decline in hair fibre production by scalp hair follicles and their eventual miniaturization. As the pattern of hair loss differs between men and women, the terms male pattern hair loss and female pattern hair loss are also used although the 'male' pattern may occur in women and vice versa [1]. Pattern hair loss in men is predominantly due to a combination of genetic predisposition and the effect of androgens, hence the term androgenetic alopecia (AGA) is often applied. Pattern hair loss in women has also long been referred to as female AGA. However, although similar endocrine and genetic factors may contribute to pattern hair loss in some women, their role in most women with pattern hair loss is less certain than in men. There is no universal agreement on the terminology – here we use the terms male balding or AGA and female pattern hair loss (FPHL).

Epidemiology

Incidence, prevalence and ethnicity
Almost all white men develop some recession of the frontal hairline at the temples during their teens. Deep frontal recession and/or vertex balding may also start shortly after puberty although in most men the onset is later. Hair loss progresses to a bald scalp in 50–60% of men by the age of 70 years. A small proportion of men (15–20%) do not show balding, apart from postpubertal temporal recession, even in old age. Some authorities have suggested that scalp hair loss in elderly men may develop independently of androgens (senescent alopecia) but this remains to be verified [2].

Balding is less common in East Asian men although there is quite wide variation in published frequencies. A Japanese study reported that male balding starts approximately one decade later in Japanese men than in white men and the prevalence is about 30% lower in each decade group [3]. In Korean men the frequency is also 20–40% lower than in white men in the 40–70-year age group although the difference becomes less pronounced with advancing age [4], and a large study in Chinese men reported that 41.4% of men aged over 70 had AGA [5]. Preservation of the frontal hairline was a common feature in the series reported from Korea: 11.1% of Korean men with AGA showed a 'female' pattern of hair loss, although this was less common (3.7%) in the Chinese study. There is less published information on the frequency of balding in African men. One older study reported that balding is a quarter as common in African American men as in white men [6].

The frequency and severity of pattern hair loss is lower in women than in men but it still affects a sizeable proportion of the population. Two studies in white women in the UK and USA reported prevalence rates of 3–6% in women aged under 30 years, increasing to 29–42% in women aged 70 and over [7,8]. As in East Asian men, pattern hair loss is less common and appears to start later in life in Asian women although nearly 25% of Korean women over 70 years of age show evidence of hair loss [4]. There are no published data on the prevalence in African women although clinical experience suggests that its frequency is similar to that in other racial groups.

Age
The age of onset of male balding is highly variable. If early balding is defined as Norwood–Hamilton stage II hair (Figure 89.17), then 40% begin to develop balding between the ages of 18 and 29 years, a further 24% first develop balding in their thirties, 3% in their for-

ties, 5% in their fifties, 9% in their sixties, 2% in their seventies and 1% at or beyond the age of 80 years [9].

There is wide individual variation in the rate of progression of hair loss in male balding. A small number of men achieve type V or VI hair loss in their twenties, indicating a very rapid rate of progression. In contrast, approximately 25% of balding men will show no visible progression of hair loss on standardized clinical photographs over a 5-year period [10]. Early-onset male balding progresses more rapidly. Men who develop balding in their twenties tend to advance one to two stages per decade, whereas men with late-onset AGA may take two decades to progress a single stage [9]. Not every man with AGA goes bald. Although 40% of men start losing their hair in their twenties, only 30% ever reach stage VI or VII. Hence, even for those with early-onset AGA, complete baldness is not inevitable.

Twin studies in males indicate that susceptibility, age of onset, pattern and rate of progression of AGA are all under genetic influence [11,12].

Sex
Patterned hair loss occurs in women, but the susceptibility, age of onset, rate of progression and pattern are different from men. Thirty-two per cent of women aged 80 years and above show no visible evidence of FPHL. The age of onset of FPHL is later than that seen in men. Only 3% first develop clinically detectable FPHL by age 29 years, a further 13% first develop it by age 49, a further 8% by age 69 and a further 6% after the age of 70 [7,13].

As many women wear their hair long, they are more aware of fluctuations in daily hair shedding. Women with FPHL-related hair shedding often present prior to the development of reduction in hair volume over the crown, making early diagnosis problematic.

Less than 1% of women progress to Hamilton–Norwood stage IV or above (equivalent to Ludwig stage III). Severe bitemporal recession (Hamilton–Norwood stage III) is uncommon and, as Ludwig pointed out, the most common pattern of hair loss seen in women is diffuse reduction of hair density over the crown, with complete or near complete preservation of the frontal hairline [14]. Olsen observed the so-called Christmas-tree pattern, with widening of the central parting line most noticeably in the mid-frontal scalp. Olsen also pointed out that the hair loss in women is often not confined to the crown but may extend ear to ear (Figures 89.18 and 89.19) [15].

Associated diseases
Trichodynia or scalp pain (see Chapter 107) may accompany AGA. It is most common in the context of increased hair shedding and may settle with treatment of the AGA.

Although a positive association between vertex balding and prostate cancer [16,17] has been identified, there is no clear association between male pattern balding and dense hair patterns on the trunk [18], virility [19] or number of children [20]. Men with male pattern baldness are considered to be less attractive and bald men have fewer lifetime sexual partners [19]. Several studies have reported an association between male balding and

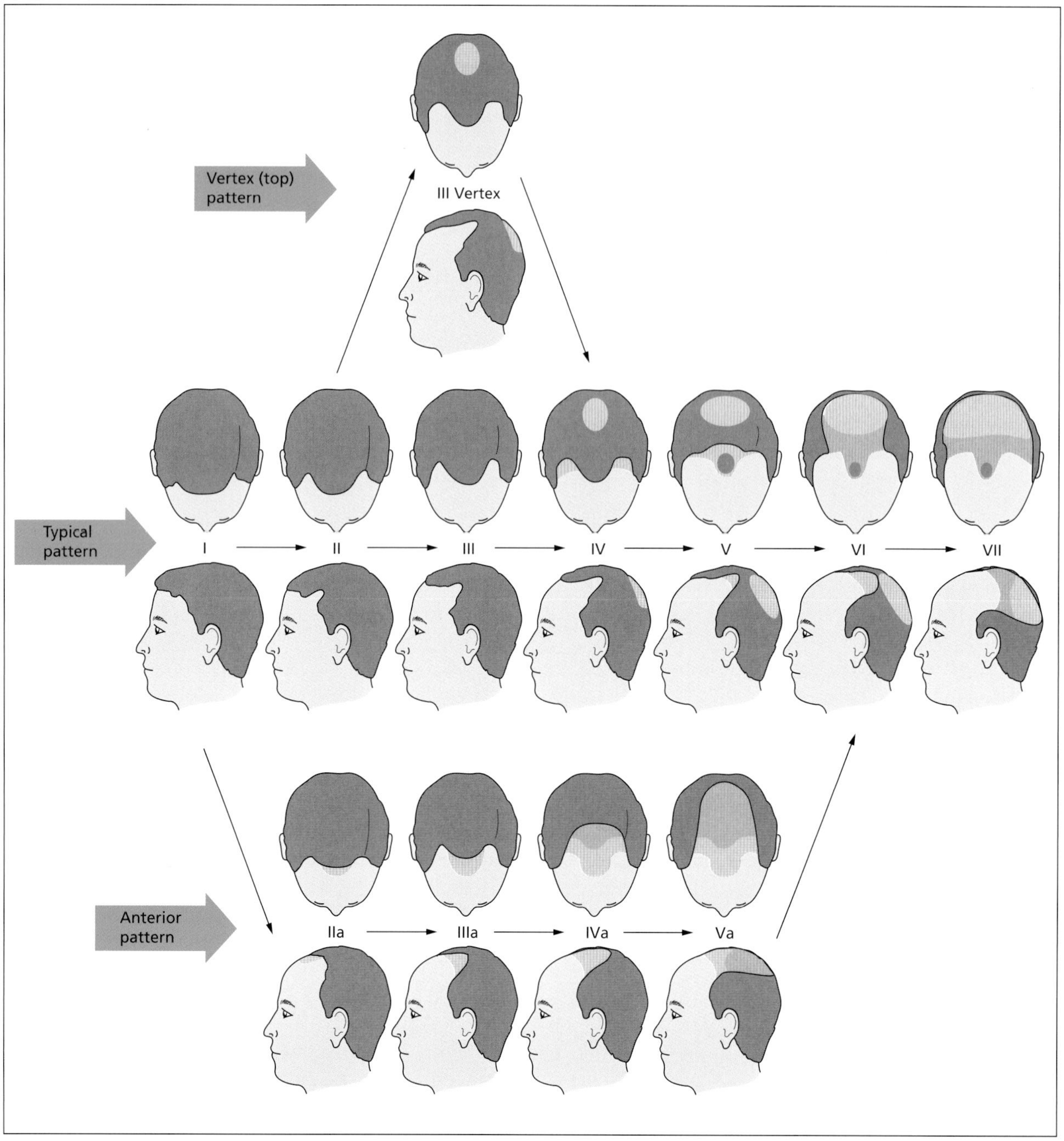

Figure 89.17 Hamilton–Norwood scale for grading male pattern hair loss (From Norwood 1975 [**9**]. Reproduced with permission of Wolters Kluwer Health.)

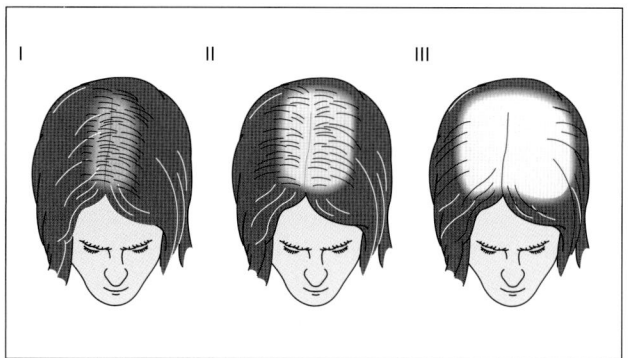

Figure 89.18 Ludwig scale for grading female pattern hair loss. (From Ludwig 1977 [**14**]. Reproduced with permission of John Wiley.)

coronary artery disease [21–23]. In the largest of these, a retrospective study conducted amongst 22 071 US male physicians, there was a weak association between coronary heart disease and vertex balding [22].

The neuromuscular disorder Kennedy disease (X-linked spinal and bulbar muscular atrophy), which is associated with a functional variant of the androgen receptor gene that causes partial androgen insensitivity, is associated with a reduced risk of AGA [24].

FPHL is associated with hyperaldosteronism, hypertension [25], hyperandrogenism and polycystic ovary disease. These women may also have elevated cholesterol and in increased risk of late-onset diabetes [26].

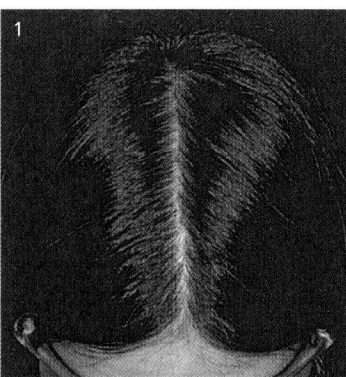
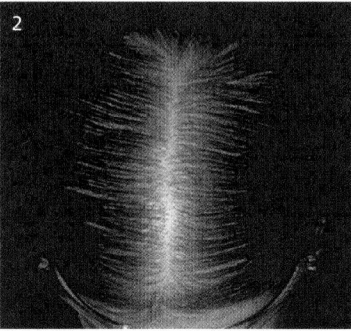
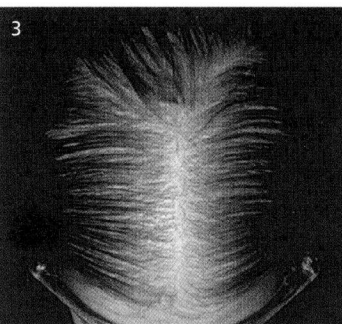
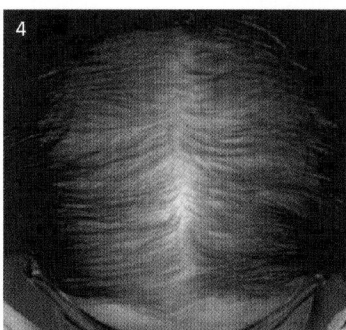
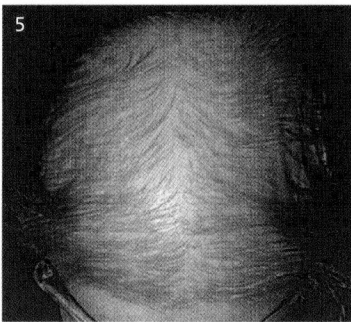

Figure 89.19 Pattern of frontal hair loss in women with androgenetic alopecia. Stage 1 is normal.

Pathophysiology

Pathogenesis

Hormonal influences

The key role of androgens in the pathogenesis of male balding was identified by the American anatomist James Hamilton, who noted that men castrated before puberty did not develop balding unless treated with testosterone [27]. Although testosterone is necessary for the development of male balding, its more potent androgenic metabolite dihydrotestosterone (DHT) is responsible for driving follicular regression. The conversion of testosterone to DHT is catalysed by the enzyme 5α-reductase. Men with a mutation in the gene for the type 2 isoform of 5α-reductase (pseudovaginal perineoscrotal hypospadias) do not develop male balding, have sparse beard and body hair growth and impaired genital development [28]. They show normal male levels of circulating testosterone but DHT levels are reduced by about 70% compared with normal. The expression of 5α-reductase type 2 is confined to androgen response tissues, including the genital tract and dermal papillae of hair follicles. The biological function of 5α-reductase type 1, which is encoded by a different gene, and which shows more widespread expression in the body, is unclear.

While the role of androgens is well established in the pathogenesis of male pattern hair loss, their role in FPHL has been questioned. On the one hand, scalp hair loss and hirsutism are undoubtedly features of hyperandrogenism in women; indeed, loss of hair was reported in women with androgen-secreting tumours prior to Hamilton's observations in men [29,30]. Several investigators have noted that women with hair loss are more likely to have elevated androgen levels, although usually of minor degree, or show an increased frequency of other features of androgen excess than women without hair loss [31–33]. On the other hand, several investigators have failed to find evidence of raised androgen levels in women with FPHL [34], and in all studies there is a variable proportion of women with hair loss who do not show clinical or biochemical signs of androgen excess. It is not yet known whether hair loss in this latter group relates to a high level of sensitivity of scalp hair follicles to normal female levels of androgens or is due to another, non-androgenic mechanism.

Local hormonal effects

Androgens do not affect all hairs equally. At puberty, body and facial hair growth is stimulated and scalp hair is lost whereas the eyebrows remain essentially unchanged. On the scalp there is a hierarchy of sensitivity, with the most anterior of the hairs at the temples being lost first, and subsequent hairs miniaturizing in a highly ordered fashion to produce patterned baldness. Similarly, in the male beard, hairs first appear on the upper lip at the lateral corners and then over the rest of the face in a highly ordered fashion. On the chest, hairs first appear centrally and then around the areolae before migrating across the rest of the torso.

In men, where circulating androgens are surplus to the requirements of the hair follicles for maximal stimulation, local factors determine individual susceptibility and severity of baldness. This intrinsic regulation is best demonstrated in hair transplantation experiments: occipital hairs maintain their resistance to AGA when transplanted to the vertex [35], and scalp hairs from the vertex transplanted to the forearm miniaturize at the same pace as hairs neighbouring the donor site [36].

Recently, prostaglandin D2 (PGD2), a known inhibitor of hair growth, has been shown to be elevated in the bald scalp of men with AGA [37]. PGD2 synthase has also been shown to be elevated at mRNA and protein levels in bald scalp compared with non-bald occipital scalp. PGD2 inhibits hair growth in explanted human hair follicles and when applied topically to mice. Hair growth inhibition requires the PGD2 receptor G protein (heterotrimeric guanine nucleotide) coupled receptor 44 (GPR44), but not the PGD2 receptor 1.

Hair cycle dynamics

In AGA, the duration of anagen decreases with each successive cycle, whereas the length of telogen remains constant or is prolonged. Prolongation of telogen occurs particularly in the latent phase of telogen (also known as kenogen) that follows the release of the club hair (exogen), leading to an increase in the proportion of empty hair follicles on the scalp, and further contributing to the balding process [38].

As the hair growth rate remains relatively constant, the duration of anagen growth determines hair length. Thus, with each successively foreshortened hair cycle, the length of each hair shaft is reduced. Ultimately, anagen duration becomes so short that the growing hair fails to achieve sufficient length to reach the surface of the skin, leaving an empty follicular pore.

Hair follicle miniaturization

The population density of hair follicles per unit area of the scalp does not change with balding. Rather, there is a gradual diminution in the size of follicles that results from the transformation of terminal follicles into vellus-type follicles. Hair follicle miniaturization leads to finer hair that is often lighter in colour. On the balding scalp, transitional indeterminate hairs represent the bridge between full-sized and miniaturized terminal hairs [1].

The dermal papilla is central to the maintenance and control of hair growth and is likely to be the target of androgen-mediated events leading to follicle miniaturization and hair cycle changes [39]. The constant geometrical relationship between the dermal papilla size and the size of the hair matrix suggests that the size of the dermal papilla determines the size of the hair bulb and ultimately the hair shaft produced [40,41].

The cross-sectional area of individual hair shafts remains constant throughout fully developed anagen indicating that the hair follicle, and its dermal papilla, remains the same size through each individual anagen stage of the cycle. Thus, miniaturization occurs between rather than within cycles. Follicular miniaturization has been traditionally thought to occur in a stepwise fashion although there have been suggestions that it occurs rapidly, possibly in the space of a single hair cycle [7].

Follicular miniaturization leaves behind stelae as dermal remnants of the full-sized follicle. These stelae, also known as fibrous tracts or streamers, extend from the subcutaneous tissue up the old follicular tract to the miniaturized hair and mark the formal position of the original terminal follicle. Arao–Perkins bodies may be seen with elastic stains within the follicular stelae. An Arao–Perkins body begins as a small cluster of elastic fibres in the neck of the dermal papilla. These clump in catagen and remain situated at the lowest point of origin of the follicular stelae. With the progressive shortening of anagen hair seen in AGA, multiple elastic clumps may be found in stelae, like the rungs of a ladder [42].

In contrast to hairs on the beard and body that emerge singularly from each pore, hairs on the scalp exist in groups known as follicular units. Hairs within follicular units may share a common infundibulum, emerging from a single pore. The diffuse hair loss pattern seen in FPHL is due to a reduction in the number of terminal hairs per follicular unit rather than miniaturization of entire follicular units [43]. Baldness occurs only when all the hairs within the follicular units are miniaturized and is a relatively early event in men and a late event in women. As a consequence, FPHL is generally less severe than male balding, occurs later and presents with diffuse thinning rather than a bald spot. This diffuse thinning that precedes baldness is also observed in men with early AGA, and can be readily identified on close examination of the scalp.

Pathology

The key elements of the histology of pattern hair loss in both sexes are a reduction in terminal hairs, an increase in secondary vellus hair with associated angiofibrotic streamers, a variable increase in telogen and catagen hairs, and a mild or moderate perifollicular lymphohistiocytic infiltrate, with or without concentric layers of perifollicular collagen deposition (Figure 89.20) [2].

A mild lymphohistiocytic infiltrate is found in approximately one-third of cases of male AGA and a similar number of controls, and is non-specific. In contrast, a moderate lymphohistiocytic inflammation is found in another one-third of cases of AGA, but in only 10% of controls [44]. Occasional eosinophils and mast cells can be seen. The cellular inflammatory changes also occur around lower follicles in some cases and occasionally involve follicular stelae. The diagnostic and prognostic significance of the degree of the inflammation is not known.

Many of these changes are best seen on horizontally sectioned scalp biopsies. Horizontal sections reveal pseudovellus hair follicles in the papillary dermis, reflecting a miniaturization process. In the majority of cases there is no genuine reduction in the number of follicles, and follicular fibrosis is seen in less than 10% of cases. The presence of arrector pili muscles and angiofibrotic streamers distinguishes them from true vellus hairs. There is a change in the ratio of terminal to vellus hairs from greater than 8 : 1 to less than 4 : 1. Also, the anagen to telogen hair ratio reduces from 12 : 1 to 5 : 1 [45]. The increased proportion of catagen and telogen hairs reflects the shortened duration of anagen and the relative increase in telogen hairs.

As the balding scalp loses its protective covering of hair, solar degenerative changes may be seen.

Genetics

Twin studies confirm the long-held belief that there is a genetic predisposition to male AGA [12,46]. Of the 54 father–son relationships in the Victorian Family Heart Study, 81.5% of balding sons had fathers who had cosmetically significant balding [47]. The high prevalence of balding in the male population, racial variation in the age-related prevalence of balding, the finding that baldness

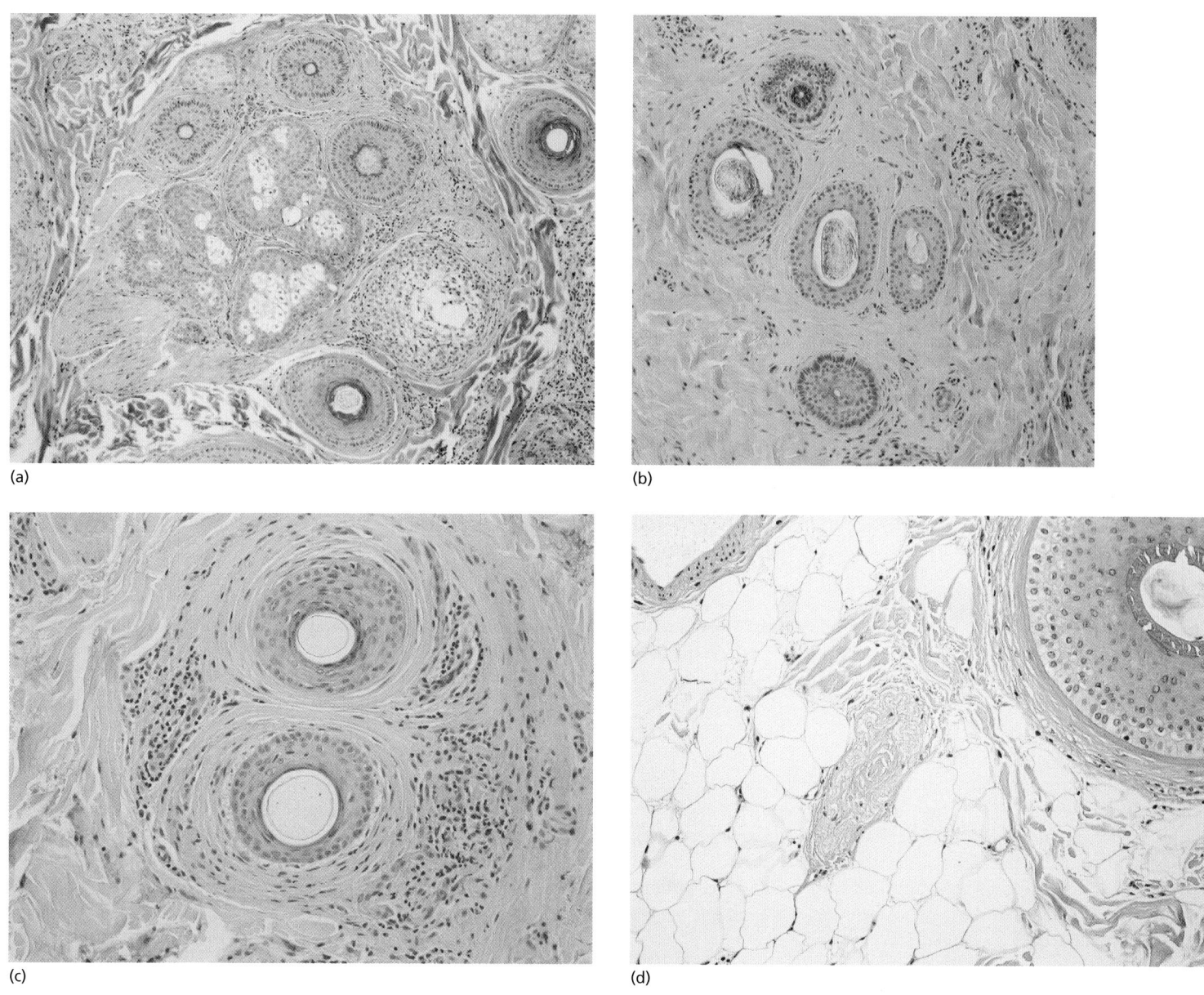

Figure 89.20 Histopathology of female pattern hair loss. (a) Increase in telogen forms – three of five follicles in a follicular unit are in telogen. (b) Follicular miniaturization – three of five follicles in a follicular unit are miniaturized. (c) 'Onion-skin' perfollicular fibrosis and mild inflammation at the infundibular level. (d) Fibrous tract adjacent to the terminal follicle.

risk increases with the number of affected family members, and the high frequency of baldness in the fathers of balding men can all be explained by polygenic inheritance [48].

Gene association and candidate gene studies comparing DNA from young bald men with that of old non-bald men have identified an X-chromosome locus containing the *androgen receptor (AR)* gene and the *ectodysplasin A2 receptor (EDA2R)* gene. Genetic variability at the *AR/EDA2R* locus is thought to enhance the effect of androgens by increasing the number of androgen receptors in affected scalp tissue [47,49]. *AR* genetic variation accounts for up to 40% of male AGA heritability, leaving up to 60% of its risk profile currently unaccounted for. Polymorphism at this locus appears to be necessary for the development of AGA, but its presence in non-bald men indicates that it is not sufficient for the development of AGA [50,51].

Two genome-wide association studies independently identified a second locus associated with male AGA at *20p11.22* [52,53]. In one of these studies, 14% of men had risk alleles at both the *AR* and *20p11* loci and this was associated with a sevenfold increase in risk of balding [52]. A further 10 loci scattered across the genome have subsequently been reported to associate with male balding, some of which may be involved in regulating WNT signalling [54,55].

In women, there is a weak association between *AR/EDA2R* locus and early-onset FHPL [56]. However, no association has been found between FPHL and any of the 11 other loci that confer susceptibility to male pattern baldness [56–58]. Two case–control studies have found a weak association with the oestrogen receptor gene *ESR2* [59,60], suggesting that oestrogens may be involved in the pathogenesis of FPHL. A twin study in older women found evidence of strong heritability for frontotemporal recession and greying but none for hair thinning, suggesting that the latter, at least in this age group, is determined mainly by non-genetic factors [61].

Environmental factors
Evidence for environmental influences on AGA remains slight. In one large study, no associations were found between pubertal growth spurt or acne, reports of adult body size at time of interview, urinary symptom score, marital status or current smoking status or duration of smoking and the risk of any form of AGA. The consumption of alcohol was associated with a significant increase in risk of frontal and vertex AGA but not full AGA. Previously reported or hypothesized associations with smoking and benign prostatic hypertrophy were not confirmed [21].

Clinical features
The essential clinical feature of balding in both sexes is patterned hair loss over the crown. Terminal hairs are progressively replaced by shorter, finer hairs which may also appear less pigmented. This process may begin at any age after the onset of adrenarche and may precede pubarche.

Male features
The clinical appearance of male balding is instantly recognizable in most cases. Hamilton defined the progressive pattern of male baldness and produced the first useful grading scale [62]. This classification was modified by Norwood [9], who added grades IIIa, III vertex, IVa and Va (see Figure 89.17). Although the grades are imprecise measures of the continuum of hair patterns that are seen in adult males, they are useful as diagnostic aids and in the classification of extent of hair loss in clinical investigations.

The posterior and lateral scalp margins are relatively spared, and only affected in the most advanced cases and with old age. Twin concordance studies indicate that variations in the pattern are governed, at least in part, by genetic factors, as is the rate of progression [46].

The main significance of hair relates to socialization – hair is an essential part of an individual's self-image. Thus, the consequences of AGA are predominantly psychological. Despite an identical libido, bald men are likely to have fewer lifetime sexual partners than non-bald men, reflecting reduced physical attractiveness to potential partners [21]. Several studies have shown that the negative self-perception of balding patients appears to be consistent between western [63,64] and East Asian cultures [65]. The negative impact of AGA is often trivialized or ignored by the non-bald [66]. However, there is evidence that perception by others may compound the psychological problems suffered by balding men. A Korean study of the perception of balding men by women and non-balding men found that their negative perception of men with AGA was similar to the psychosocial effects reported by the patients themselves [65]. Of note was that a perception of bald men looking less attractive was found in more than 90% of subjects surveyed. Importantly, this view was more common in women than non-balding men. Such negative perceptions may further impair the social functioning of balding men.

However, it is important to note that most affected men cope well with AGA, and it does not have significant impact on their psychosocial function. Thus, those who do seek help are likely to be in greater emotional distress and to have been dissatisfied with any treatment they have received. The most distressed balding men are those with more extensive hair loss, those who have very early onset, and those who regard their balding as progressive (often arising from observation of their father) and socially noticeable [63].

Female features
The clinical presentation of pattern hair loss in women differs from men. Women may present with either an episodic or continuous increase in hair shedding without any noticeable reduction in hair volume, increased hair shedding with loss of hair volume over the crown, or diffuse thinning over the crown with no history of hair shedding [67].

The most informative question to ask balding women is about the change in the thickness of their ponytail. This enables women to estimate their degree of hair loss. Loss of volume or thinning over the crown is best detected when the hair is parted centrally. Widening of the central parting may follow a Christmas-tree pattern and is used to score the hair loss [68].

The pattern of hair loss in women was first defined by Ludwig in 1977 [14]. FPHL presents with diffuse thinning (loss of hair volume) over the mid-frontal scalp with minimal or no bitemporal recession. Vertex baldness is rare. Ludwig illustrated the stages of progression of FPHL into three grades (see Figure 89.18). The Sinclair scale identified five visually distinct stages and can be used to monitor clinical severity and treatment response (see Figure 89.19) [69]. Stage 1 is normal hair density; stage 2 shows widening of the central part; stage 3 demonstrates additional thinning of the hair at the sides of the partline; stage 4 reflects the development of a bald patch distal to the anterior hairline; and stage 5 represents advanced hair loss.

Not all women who develop FPHL maintain their frontal hairline. Bitemporal recession occurs in 13% of premenopausal women and 37% of postmenopausal women [70]. In many women the hair loss is confined to the scalp vertex, but in a significant proportion hair loss also occurs diffusely over the parietal scalp. Generalized hair loss often precludes women from hair transplantation procedures because of a diminished donor population in the occipital region.

Most women who present with hair loss have no other evidence of virilization. However, if the hair loss is of sudden onset, rapidly progressive and advanced, a full medical history and examination, and endocrinological investigation, are desirable to exclude virilization, which can rarely be caused by a virilizing tumour. Investigation is also indicated in women with FPHL of gradual onset accompanied by menstrual disturbance, hirsutism or recrudescence of acne.

In contrast to the prevailing attitude to male balding, society generally regards it as abnormal for women to lose their hair and the adverse effect of hair loss on quality of life tends be more severe in women than in men. As a group, women seeking medical advice for their hair loss experience more negative body image feelings, more social anxiety and poorer self-esteem and psychosocial well-being than control subjects with non-visible skin disease, as well as dissatisfaction with their hair. In quality of life studies, individual responses were more related to self-perception of hair loss than to objective or clinical ratings and those women most distressed by hair loss were more poorly adjusted and had a greater investment in their appearance [71,72].

Differential diagnosis

The principal differential diagnosis of early FPHL is chronic telogen effluvium (CTE) [73]. Women with CTE present with chronic diffuse hair shedding without noticeable widening of the central parting. They may describe a loss in volume of the ponytail of up to one-third, and there is commonly mild bitemporal recession. Scalp biopsy of women who present in this fashion reveals pattern hair loss in approximately 60% of cases and CTE in 40% [69]. Scalp biopsy is not required in women who present with loss of hair volume either alone or associated with increased hair shedding.

Other potential differential diagnoses, albeit rare, include alopecia areata incognita and systemic lupus erythematosus.

Investigations

Diagnostic techniques

The hair pull test, hand-held epiluminescent microscopy and global photography are valuable in the diagnosis and management of this condition. The hair pull test (described earlier in this chapter) is usually used to assess a hair cycle disturbance, such as telogen effluvium, and may be normal in pattern hair loss. However, an increase in easily extracted telogen hairs may be found in active pattern hair loss.

Scalp dermoscopy in the early stages of pattern hair loss reveals contrasting hair density between the mid-frontal and occipital scalp. Over the occipital scalp it is common to see two or three terminal hairs of equal fibre diameter emerging from a single infundibulum. In comparison, the number of terminal hairs per infundibulum is reduced to one or sometimes two over the mid-frontal scalp and the total number of infudibuli also reduce over time. When two hairs emerge from a single infundibulum on the mid-frontal scalp, one is often noticeable thinner than the normal hairs indicating miniaturization of the follicle. This has been described as hair diameter diversity [74]. In advanced hair loss, dermoscopy is valuable in demonstrating the non-scarring nature of the process.

Investigations in men

Investigations are unnecessary in men with AGA unless there is diagnostic uncertainty.

Investigations in women

In the absence of clinical evidence of hyperandrogenism, extensive metabolic and endocrinological work-up is not routinely necessary. Women with a history of menstrual disturbance, impaired fertility or signs of androgen excess should be investigated for hyperandrogenism (e.g. polycystic ovary syndrome, androgen-secreting tumour). Women with FPHL may benefit from screening for hypertension, hypercholesterolaemia and late-onset diabetes (Box 89.1).

Box 89.1 Investigations in female pattern hair loss

- Full blood count
- Serum ferritin
- Thyroid function test
- Fasting lipids
- Fasting glucose

If there are signs of virilization or hirsutism:

- Serum testosterone
- DHEAS (morning sample on days 1–5 of cycle; make sure the patient is not on the oral contraceptive pill)
- 17-hydroxyprogesterone
- Androstenedione
- Ovarian ultrasound
- Adrenal imaging

DHEAS, dehydroepiandrosterone sulphate.

Scalp biopsy

Scalp biopsy is seldom required to diagnose pattern hair loss. It may be useful, however, in distinguishing between early FPHL and chronic telogen effluvium in women with excessive hair shedding and minimal reduction in hair density. The ratio of terminal to vellus hairs on a horizontally sectioned 4 mm punch biopsy is used to make the distinction – a ratio of <4 : 1 is diagnostic of FPHL, whereas a ratio of >8 : 1 is indicative of chronic telogen effluvium. Ratios in between these values are usually indeterminate [69]. A triple biopsy procedure performed on the vertex rather than a single horizontal biopsy increases the likelihood of reaching an accurate diagnosis.

Management

As pattern hair loss is not life-threatening and the morbidity is variable, most people do not seek treatment. Some patients simply attend for a diagnosis, and when the currently available therapies are discussed, decline treatment. Without therapy, pattern hair loss is progressive, although the rate of progression is extremely variable. Twenty-five per cent of men will have no visible progression after 5 years. Some will achieve Norwood–Hamilton stage VII within 5 years, whereas others may take 50 years.

Before a patient embarks on therapy he or she should be counselled carefully and made aware of the requirement for maintenance therapy for sustained effect. Many 'treatments' of unproven value are widely promoted and advertised, particularly through the internet, and patients should be advised to avoid such products.

Camouflage and wigs

Camouflage is the simplest, easiest and cheapest way of dealing with mild pattern hair loss. Balding becomes most noticeable when the scalp can be seen through the hair. Camouflage treatments involve either adding small fibres held in place electrostatically or dyeing the scalp the same colour as the hair to create the illusion of thicker hair. Numerous brands are available, each in a range of colours. Although many of the newer agents are water resistant, if the hair becomes wet in the rain the dye may still run.

Wigs are an alternative to scalp surgery. For many women, an alternative to a full wig is a smaller hairpiece that can either be interwoven with existing hair or worn over the top of existing hair. Because interwoven wigs lift as the hair beneath grows, they require periodic adjustment. Wig hair is composed of either synthetic acrylic fibre that withstands wear and tear very well, or natural fibre (usually Asian or European human hair). Natural fibre wigs look better, are easier to style and last longer, but are considerably more expensive. Wigs can be styled and washed, and modern wigs provide excellent coverage that looks natural. A drawback of wigs is that the head may be hot in the summer, and some patients find them difficult to wear for this reason.

Advice on wigs is available from alopecia patient support groups in the UK, USA and Australia.

Medical management

Established medical management for pattern hair loss consists of antiandrogens, 5α-reductase inhibitors and topical minoxidil. They may be used alone or in combination. Although improvement may be seen after as soon as 4 months, 1 year of treatment may be required before a clinical response is apparent. Maintenance therapy is required to sustain any benefit. Monitoring of clinical response can be problematic. Patients are often anxious about their hair and inspect it frequently. Subtle fluctuations are often overinterpreted, and patients' subjective assessment of hair density is commonly unreliable. Serial photography at 6–12-monthly intervals promotes patient adherence to treatment in the medium and long term [6].

Management of male pattern baldness

Minoxidil lotion. Minoxidil is a piperidinopyrimidine derivative and a potent vasodilator that is effective orally for severe hypertension. When applied topically in a lotion or foam vehicle, minoxidil increased terminal hair density in up to 30% of individuals [75,76]. Terminal hair appeared to regrow at the margins, but complete covering of the bald areas was seen in less than 10% of responders. De Villez [77] suggested that men who responded best to minoxidil were those in whom the balding process was at an early stage, with a maximum diameter of the bald area of less than 10 cm, and in whom the pre-treatment hair density was in excess of 20 hairs/cm^2. There is a slight increase in benefit if the concentration is increased to 5%. The benefit is most pronounced in the first 6 months of therapy and thereafter is marginal.

Topical minoxidil appears to be a safe therapy with side effects only of local irritation and hypertrichosis of the temples, and a low incidence of contact dermatitis [78]. If treatment is stopped, clinical regression occurs within 6 months to the state of baldness that would have existed if treatment had not been applied [79]. Patients should be warned that in order to maintain any beneficial effect, applications must continue once or preferably twice daily indefinitely.

Finasteride. Finasteride is a synthetic aza-steroid that is a potent and selective antagonist of 5α-reductase type 2, which inhibits the conversion of testosterone to DHT. A scalp biopsy study of patients with AGA found that after 12 months of finasteride treatment, terminal hair counts increase and vellus hair counts decrease, demonstrating the ability of finasteride to reverse the miniaturization process and to encourage the growth of terminal hairs [80].

An oral dosage of 1 mg/day reduces scalp DHT by 64% and serum DHT by 68% [81]. Clinical trial data showed that, after 1 year, patients who received finasteride had a 10% increase in the mean number of terminal hairs on their vertex scalp compared with baseline counts [82]. After 5 years of continuous therapy, vertex hair counts remained close to the 1-year level, whereas the counts in the placebo patients had dropped by 30%. Using global photography to assess scalp coverage, 48% of patients taking finasteride had increased vertex hair density compared with 7% of the placebo group at the end of 1 year. At 2 years, coverage continued to improve in the finasteride group, with 66% having increased density, whereas only 7% of the placebo subjects had increased coverage. By 5 years, 10% of treated patients had a lowered hair density, 42% had no change, and 22%, 21% and 5% were assessed as moderately, markedly and greatly improved, respectively [83]. In contrast, 19%, 31% and 25% of patients in the placebo group were greatly, markedly or moderately worse. Nevertheless, 25% of the patients in the placebo group showed no deterioration over the 5-year period, reflecting the variable rate of progression of balding among males. These data suggest that the finasteride-responsive follicles are all activated after 1 year, and the clinical improvement in scalp coverage results from increase in hair length, diameter and pigmentation.

Trial participants who received placebo for 12 months before receiving finasteride grew less hair than participants who received finasteride for 12 months before crossing over to placebo. This indicates that the potential for regrowth diminishes as the AGA progresses and suggest early initiation of therapy will achieve better results. Finasteride is also effective on the mid-frontal scalp, although the magnitude of regrowth appears less than on the vertex [84]. Finasteride may arrest bitemporal recession but does not reverse it.

Finasteride is generally well tolerated [82,83]. At a dosage of 1 mg daily, reduced libido is seen in 1.8% and erectile dysfunction in 1.3%. Similar events are also reported in the placebo group, albeit at lower frequencies of 1.3% and 0.7%, respectively. These events appeared to resolve on cessation of the drug and, in some cases, with continued treatment. It has been suggested that even these figures overstate the true incidence of sexual dysfunction [85]. Reports of persistent sexual dysfunction following discontinuation of therapy are difficult to interpret due to the high frequency of these events in the control group.

Older men on finasteride are likely to experience a 50% reduction in serum prostate-specific antigen levels, which could result in an underestimation of prostatic cancer risk. The value should be doubled to correct for the finasteride effect.

Finasteride has the potential to impair genital development in a male fetus. As the drug is secreted in the semen and can be absorbed through the vagina during intercourse, it was originally advocated that men taking finasteride should avoid unprotected intercourse with pregnant women. In practice, the concentration of finasteride in the semen is well below the minimum effect dosage, and no recommendations regarding the use of condoms are made in the product information leaflet. There are no reports of adverse pregnancy outcomes among women exposed to finasteride taken by their partners [86]. Finasteride has no effect on spermatogenesis or semen production [87].

Finasteride has now been in widespread use for over 10 years. Many recipients are elderly men taking 5 mg/day for prostate hyperplasia. Very few side effects have been observed [88].

Dutasteride is a combined type 1 and 2 5α-reductase inhibitor. It produces a dose-dependent reduction in serum and scalp DHT levels to a greater degree than that seen with finasteride, and is more effective than finasteride in stimulating hair regrowth in male pattern baldness [89]. Dutasteride is currently marketed at a 0.5 mg dosage for benign prostatic hypertrophy, but is also widely used off-label for treatment of AGA. Sexual side effects are more common with dutasteride than with finasteride, and are also dose related. Retrograte ejaculation is reported but appears to be reversible on cessation. Because of the long biological half-life, side effects may take many months to reverse.

Management of female pattern hair loss

Minoxidil lotion. Topical minoxidil arrests hair loss or induces mild to moderate hair regrowth in approximately 60% of women with FPHL [90]. A clinical trial comparing 5% and 2% topical formulations of minoxidil found mean increases in non-vellus hair counts after 48 weeks of 18% and 14%, respectively [91]. Treatment has to be continued to maintain the response.

Antiandrogens. Oral antiandrogen therapy with cyproterone acetate, spironolactone, finasteride or flutamide is widely used in the treatment of FPHL. However, there is little evidence of efficacy from good-quality controlled trials and their use is largely based on clinical experience and case reports.

Spironolactone is generally the best tolerated and easiest to use. Spironolactone is a synthetic steroid, structurally related to aldosterone, which acts by competitively blocking androgen receptors. It also weakly inhibits androgen biosynthesis. Its primary use is as a diuretic and antihypertensive, and many of its side effects and numerous drug interactions relate to this. There are no controlled trials in FPHL. There is one report that women treated for 1 year with spironolactone showed less hair loss than in an untreated group [92]. Dosage ranged from 50 to 300 mg/day. Side effects were dose-related and included menstrual irregularities, postmenopausal bleeding, breast tenderness or enlargement, and fatigue. Spironolactone has the potential to feminize a male fetus and women should not become pregnant while taking it. Concomitant use of oral contraceptives will reduce the hormonal side effects. The antialdosterone effect can result in an elevation of serum potassium and a slight reduction in blood pressure, although this is rarely significant in the absence of renal impairment. A large cohort study involving almost 1.3 million women aged 55 and over with a follow-up time of 8.4 million patient-years found no evidence of an increased incidence of breast cancer in women exposed to spironolactone [93].

Cyproterone acetate is an androgen receptor blocker and potent progestin. It also has an anti-gonadotrophic effect. In a study comparing cyproterone acetate with topical minoxidil lotion, hair density had declined after 1 year in the cyproterone acetate group but had improved in those using minoxidil [94]. However, subset analysis showed some increase in hair density in women with clinical evidence of androgen excess taking cyproterone acetate,

suggesting that antiandrogens may be more effective in women with hyperandrogenism. There are no dose-ranging studies, but most practitioners use cyproterone acetate 50–100 mg/day for the first 10 days of each menstrual cycle. For postmenopausal women, cyproterone acetate may be used continuously, with or without oestrogens. The side effects of cyproterone acetate are dose dependent and include lassitude, weight gain, breast tenderness, loss of libido, depression and nausea. Feminization of a male fetus may occur so patients should be advised to cease the medication before attempting conception. The combination of cyproterone acetate and oral oestrogen therapy provides effective contraception and stabilizes menstrual irregularities.

Flutamide is a non-steroidal antiandrogen that acts by inhibiting androgen uptake and by inhibiting nuclear binding of androgen within the target tissue. A small comparative study in hyperandrogenic women with FPHL reported improvement with flutamide but no response to finasteride or cyproterone acetate [95]. Rare but potentially fatal hepatotoxicity seen with high-dose flutamide limits the use of flutamide for this condition.

Finasteride used in a double-blind, placebo-controlled study involving almost 100 postmenopausal women with FPHL, at a dose of 1 mg, was found to be no better than placebo [96]. Subsequent case reports and a case series have reported benefits in both pre- and postmenopausal women, but teratogenicity remains a relative contraindication to use in premenopausal women [97,98].

Surgery

Surgical treatment of male balding involves the redistribution of terminal hair to cover the balding scalp – the number of terminal hair follicles on the scalp remains the same. In most cases this means transplanting hair follicles from the occipital scalp to the balding areas. Other techniques, such as excising the balding skin (scalp reduction) and rotational flaps are now less widely used. Surgical treatment can achieve very satisfactory results but careful patient selection and surgical skill allied to the aesthetics of scalp hair growth are essential. Key considerations include the following [99]:

- There should be an adequate donor area, i.e good hair density in the occipital scalp.
- Age – the predictive value for men aged <25 years is very uncertain. Surgery in young men may result in misplaced hairlines or an unnatural appearance 20–30 years later as balding progresses.
- The correction of established frontal hair loss is more effective than vertex balding, which tends to progress with time.
- Thicker hair shafts give better coverage than fine-calibre hair. In white people, fair hair gives a more natural appearance than dark hair (which exaggerates the contrast with the colour of the scalp skin).

Experienced surgical teams can give significant improvement after 1–2 sessions. The final results take 5–6 months to become apparent.

Complications of surgery include scalp erythema and crusting, and facial oedema. Less common problems include infection, postoperative bleeding, scarring and arteriovenous fistula formation.

Hair transplantation is less widely used in treating FPHL but can give good results in selected cases [99]. It is most appropriate in women with pronounced hair loss of limited extent who retain good hair density in the donor site. Those with a mild degree of hair loss are less suitable as are those with involvement of the occipital region.

Resources

Patient resources
Alopecia UK, Wigs: http://www.alopeciaonline.org.uk/wigs.asp.
Macmillan Cancer Support, Wigs and hairpieces:
http://www.macmillan.org.uk/information-and-support/coping/changes-to-appearance-and-body-image/dealing-with-hair-loss/wigs-and-hair-pieces.html.
NHS Choices, Wigs and fabric supports: http://www.nhs.uk/NHSEngland/Healthcosts/Pages/Wigsandfabricsupports.aspx. (All last accessed April 2015.)

Telogen effluvium

Rodney D. Sinclair

Definition and nomenclature

Telogen effluvium describes an increase in the shedding of telogen club hairs due to premature termination of the anagen phase of the hair cycle.

> **Synonyms and inclusions**
> • Telogen defluvium

Introduction and general description

The term telogen effluvium was coined by Kligman in 1961 [1]. It refers to the shedding of club (telogen) hair in disease states of the follicle. Kligman argued that whatever the cause of the hair loss, the follicle behaves in a similar way with the premature termination of anagen. 'The follicle is precipitated into catagen and transforms into a resting stage that mimics telogen.' The observation of increased telogen hair shedding does not infer a cause. To establish a cause, a history is required to identify known triggers, biochemical investigation to exclude endocrine, nutritional or autoimmune aetiologies and, in persistent cases, histology to determine if there is evidence of the earliest stages of androgenetic alopecia. The duration of the hair shedding at presentation helps predict those patients in whom further investigation will have the greatest yield.

In infancy, follicular cycling within anatomical regions is synchronous. Neighbouring hairs grow together, involute together and are shed together. Synchronous shedding produces a moult wave. Moult wave persists indefinitely in many mammals; however, in humans, synchronous hair growth disappears in childhood. Rather than episodically shedding all 100 000 scalp hairs over the course of a few months, adult humans tend to lose 100 or so hairs each day [2].

Scalp hair plucks reveals that an average of 86% of plucked hairs are in anagen, 1% in catagen and 13% in telogen. Data from the analysis of horizontal scalp biopsies puts these figures at 93% of follicles in anagen and 7% in telogen [3]. According to these biopsy data, if the average number of scalp hairs is 100 000, then 7000 hairs should be in telogen at any one time. As the approximate duration of telogen is 100 days, 70 hairs should be shed each day. However, most people are not aware of shedding this amount of hair each day and it still remains to be defined what amount of shed hair is normally noticed and how introspection might heightens one's powers of detection [4]. When people are concerned they are losing hair, they look harder and find more. In addition, hair length affects perception of hair loss.

Pathogenesis

Headington [5] described five functional types of telogen effluvium, based on different phases of the follicular cycle:

1 Immediate anagen release is a short-onset effluvium where follicles are stimulated to leave anagen and enter telogen prematurely, resulting in increased hair shedding at the end of telogen, approximately 2–3 months later. It is common after a physiological stress such as severe illness, and with drug-induced hair loss. Reversal is associated with resumption of the normal cycle.

2 Delayed anagen release is the cause of postpartum hair loss. During pregnancy, anagen duration is prolonged and hair cycling into telogen is reduced. Postpartum, a large number of follicles cycle into telogen together and increased shedding is noticed some months later.

3 Short anagen syndrome is caused by shortening of the duration of anagen and can cause a persistent telogen hair shedding in some individuals [5]. This is also seen in androgenetic alopecia where telogen effluvium commonly precedes visible balding of the scalp.

4 Immediate telogen release results from premature exogen. This may also be associated with a shortening of telogen duration. Exogen does not necessarily initiate the onset of anagen and telogen follicles may remain empty for weeks. An empty telogen follicle is called kenogen. Prolonged kenogen is seen in androgenetic alopecia. Drugs such as minoxidil can precipitate exogen, and this explains the temporary increase in hair shedding commonly noticed 4–6 weeks after commencement of minoxidil therapy for hair loss.

5 Delayed telogen release occurs after prolonged telogen followed by transition to anagen. It occurs in animals with synchronous hair cycles during shedding of their winter coats. It may occur seasonally in some humans.

Acute telogen effluvium

Acute telogen effluvium is an acute-onset scalp hair loss that occurs 2–3 months after a triggering event such as a high fever, surgical trauma, sudden starvation or haemorrhage [1,4,5,6]. In approximately a third of cases of acute telogen effluvium, no trigger can be identified. Acute telogen effluvium is commonly attributed to emotional stress, but the evidence for this is weak and there is no evidence that suggests the stresses of everyday life are sufficient to induce diffuse hair loss. The functional mechanism of shedding is immediate anagen release.

The patient may be particularly aware of increased loss on the brush or comb, or during shampooing. The daily loss ranges from under 100 to over 1000 hairs. If the lower rates of shedding are continued for only a short period there may be no obvious baldness, but if shedding occurs at higher rates, diffuse reduction in

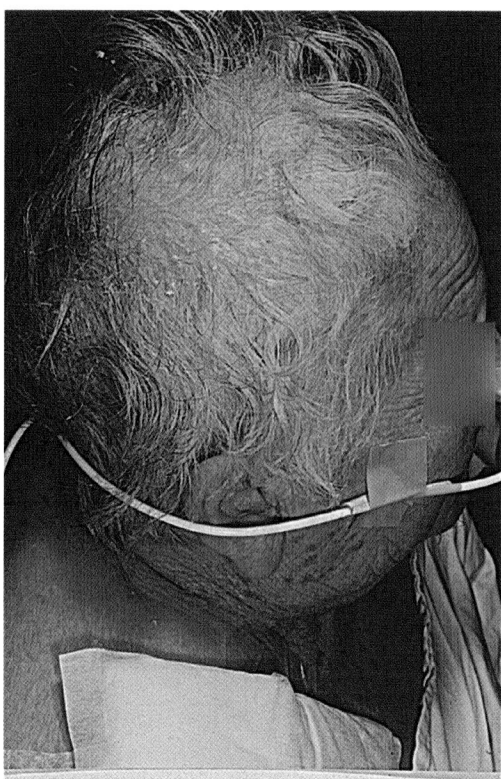

Figure 89.21 Acute telogen effluvium.

hair density is produced (Figure 89.21). Acute telogen effluvium does not produce total baldness.

Unless the trigger is repeated, spontaneous complete regrowth occurs within 3–6 months. The proportion of follicles affected, and hence the severity of the subsequent alopecia, depends partly on the duration and severity of the precipitating cause and partly on unexplained individual variations in susceptibility.

Telogen gravidarum

Telogen gravidarum refers to the telogen hair loss seen 2–3 months after childbirth [7,8]. It is an example of delayed anagen release. It is universal but variable in severity and is often subclinical. Most cases of telogen gravidarum resolve. However, a small proportion of women may experience persistent episodic shedding that may be diffuse or localized. It has been suggested that the pregnancy synchronizes hair growth and the subsequent hair shedding [9]. A similar state of synchronous hair growth may prevail with the use of oral contraceptives that leads to hair shedding when the contraceptive pill is subsequently discontinued [8,10].

Investigations

Abrupt-onset telogen effluvium is likely to be related to a specific event or trigger 6–12 weeks earlier. The hair pull test is positive, with normal club hairs. The hair loss is always diffuse and never total. Gradual onset or prolonged hair loss is more difficult to assess. Increased shedding of club hairs is a variable but often very obvious symptom of early AGA. Other differential diagnoses are discussed below under the heading of chronic diffuse telogen hair loss.

The hair pull test is notoriously difficult to interpret. In acute telogen effluvium, it is usually strongly positive for telogen hairs at the vertex and the scalp margins. However, a negative hair pull test does not exclude the diagnosis of telogen effluvium. The trichogram analysis of a hair pluck sample usually shows more than 25% of telogen hairs in acute telogen effluvium [1]. When an obvious explanation exists for recent-onset telogen effluvium, expectant management and observation is appropriate. Shedding can be expected to cease within 3–6 months and thereafter recovery should be complete. Histological examination shows no abnormality other than an increase in the proportion of follicles in telogen.

Chronic telogen effluvium

A short-lived insult usually produces a sudden-onset diffuse shedding 6–12 weeks later. If the insult is prolonged or repeated, shedding can develop insidiously. Chronic diffuse telogen hair loss refers to telogen hair shedding persisting for longer than 6 months. It can be a result of an idiopathic change in hair cycle dynamics (primary chronic telogen effluvium) or be secondary to a variety of causes including female pattern hair loss.

Before a potential trigger can be accepted as a true cause of chronic diffuse telogen hair loss, the relationship between the causative factor and the hair loss must fit chronologically. The hair loss should reverse when the causative factor is corrected and the hair shedding resume when the trigger is reintroduced. Other known causes of shedding, in particular androgenetic alopecia, also require exclusion.

Accepted causes of chronic diffuse telogen hair loss are thyroid disorders (Figure 89.22), profound iron deficiency anaemia, acrodermatitis enteropathica and malnutrition [6]. Both hyper- and hypothyroidism (including drug-induced hypothyroidism) may cause a diffuse telogen hair loss [11,12]. The mechanism of telogen hair shedding in thyroid disorders is unclear [13]. Hair loss is reversible when the euthyroid state is restored, except in longstanding cases. If replacement therapy fails to correct the hair loss, alternative causes such as androgenetic alopecia should be sought [14].

Profound iron deficiency anaemia can cause a diffuse telogen hair loss that is corrected by iron replacement. The relationship between iron deficiency with no anaemia or only mild anaemia and chronic diffuse hair loss is, however, more complex and controversial [15–17]. Depending on how it is defined, low iron stores are a common finding in women of child-bearing age. Pattern hair loss is also common in this age group and the shedding in the early stages of FPHL can be diffuse and episodic, and mimic a telogen effluvium. In patients with pattern hair loss the shedding tends to be chronic and relapsing, and recovery is generally incomplete. A punch biopsy from the mid-frontal scalp can usually clarify the diagnosis.

Acrodermatitis enteropathica and acquired zinc deficiency brought about by longstanding parenteral nutrition can lead to a severe telogen effluvium (Figure 89.23) [6,18]. However, low zinc levels found on routine blood biochemistry screening in patients being investigated for diffuse telogen hair loss are probably an incidental finding. Diffuse hair loss alone, with no other symptoms or signs, is never a result of dietary zinc deficiency [17].

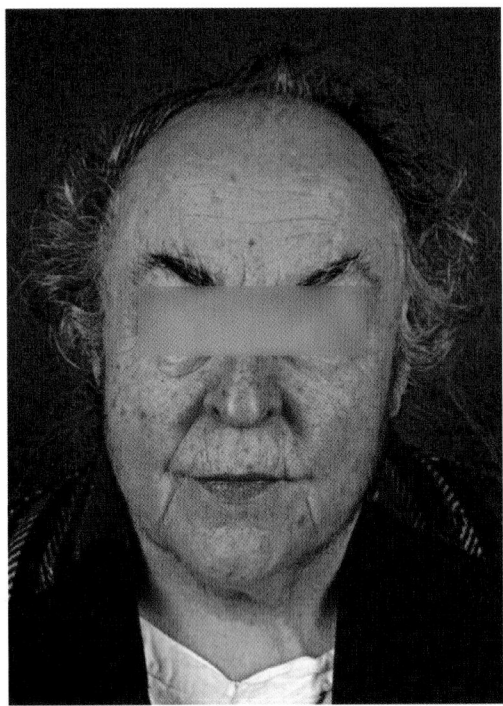

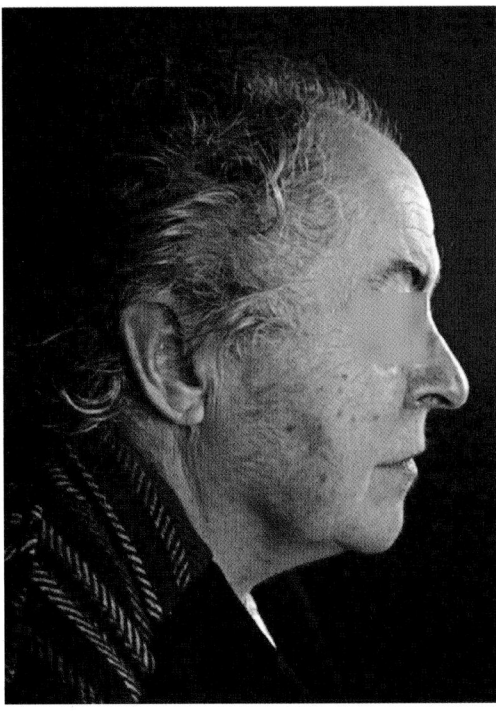

Figure 89.22 Diffuse alopecia in association with hypothyroidism.

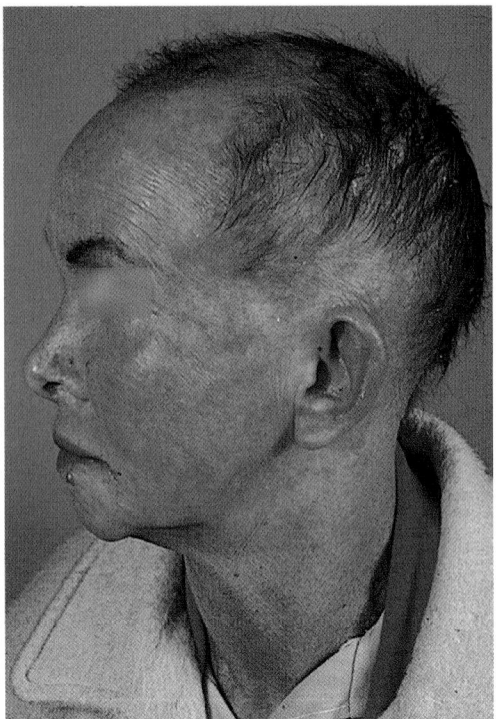

Figure 89.23 Acquired zinc deficiency resulting from prolonged parenteral feeding and inadequate zinc supplementation.

disease may be a result of hypoproteinaemia rather than the malignancy itself, but alopecia has occurred as an early sign of Hodgkin disease [26]. Systemic lupus erythematosus (Figure 89.24) and dermatomyositis can also cause telogen hair loss [27]. Diffuse hair loss may occur in secondary syphilis although the characteristic moth-eaten appearance is not always present [28].

Crash dieting with severe protein–calorie restriction can precipitate hair loss [19,20]. Chronic starvation, especially marasmus, causes a diffuse telogen hair loss, often accompanied by hair shaft abnormalities [21]. Hypoproteinaemia of metabolic as well as dietary origin can cause hair loss [6]. Pancreatic disease and other forms of malabsorption also cause a diffuse telogen hair loss [22], as do the essential fatty acid deficiencies seen in prolonged parenteral nutrition and hypervitaminosis A [23]. Metabolic disturbances such as liver disorders [6,24] and chronic renal failure can produce sparse scalp hair [25]. Hair loss in advanced malignant

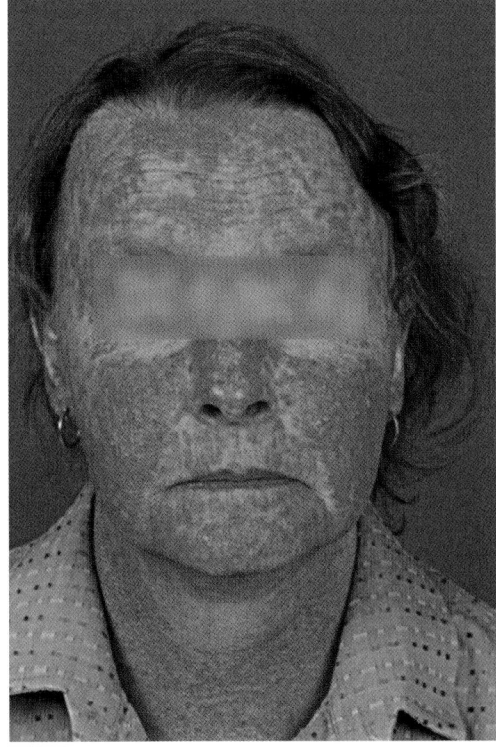

Figure 89.24 Hair loss and photosensitivity caused by systemic lupus erythematosus.

Diffuse hair loss occurs in Cronkhite–Canada syndrome, a rare idiopathic disease characterized by gastrointestinal polyposis, diarrhoea, protein-losing enteropathy and weight loss. Limited histological data indicate the hair pathology is non-inflammatory and that anagen–telogen conversion is the early event [29]. Follicular miniaturization has also been reported [30].

Drug-induced telogen effluvium

Drug-induced diffuse telogen hair loss usually starts 6–12 weeks after instigation of treatment and is progressive while the drug is continued [31,32]. It is most commonly a result of immediate anagen release [5]. The diagnosis of drug-induced telogen hair loss is made by demonstrating a compatible chronology of drug exposure and the onset of the hair loss, and exclusion of the other causes of alopecia. Shedding can recur with drugs that are chemically unrelated, suggesting that true cross-reactivity is rare, and individual susceptibility exists to drug-induced telogen effluvium. Chronic telogen effluvium and AGA are important differential diagnoses. If a particular drug is suspected, testing involves stopping it for at least 3 months. Regrowth following discontinuation and recurrence on re-exposure to the drug supports the conclusion that the drug caused the alopecia. Many drugs have been said to cause diffuse telogen hair loss but few have fulfilled the above criteria. Dose-related diffuse telogen hair loss is common with acitretin [33], but less common with isotretinoin. The retinoids appear to cause a telogen anchorage defect and reduce the duration of anagen. Patients who complain of continued retinoid-induced telogen effluvium, long after the retinoid has been stopped, often have coincidental AGA. Minoxidil causes a short-lived telogen shedding by immediate telogen release [34].

Management

Withdrawal of the trigger will arrest hair shedding within 3 months but a full recovery in hair density may take 6 months. Persisting hair shedding after 3 months, or incomplete recovery after 6 months, raises the possibility of coincidental, unrecognized androgenetic alopecia.

Primary chronic telogen effluvium

Primary chronic telogen effluvium (CTE) is an idiopathic and sometimes self-limiting condition affecting middle-aged women that is distinct from androgenetic hair loss and chronic diffuse telogen effluvium secondary to organic causes [3]. Women describe a sudden onset of increased hair shedding persisting for at least 6 months. There is no associated visible widening of the central parting line, and no miniaturization of hair follicles on scalp biopsy. CTE contrasts with the acute form by its prolonged fluctuating course and much less frequent occurrence. It occurs mainly in women aged between 30 and 50 years. Hair shedding is much less obvious in males with short hair, and for unknown reasons few males with long hair present with increased hair shedding [35]. Although some cases of CTE follow an acute telogen effluvium with an identified trigger, such as pregnancy or systemic illness, in most cases no trigger can be identified. Any of the functional types of telogen effluvium could account for CTE but it is believed to be related to a reduction in the variation of anagen duration without

any reduction in the mean duration of the anagen phase of the hair cycle [36].

Trichodynia or scalp dysthaesthesia may accompany CTE. The mechanism is unknown. Treatment is difficult, but many cases respond to measures to reduce hair shedding such as minoxidil [37].

Investigations

The diagnosis of CTE is made by exclusion of other causes of diffuse telogen hair loss. A thorough history is required, including a detailed drug and dietary history. A full clinical examination should be performed, including scalp examination and hair pull testing. The routine work-up includes full blood count and thyroid function tests. Syphilis serology, antinuclear antibody titre, serum zinc levels and other investigations of nutritional status should be performed if clinically warranted.

Affected women present with persistent severe shedding that runs a fluctuating course over several years (Figure 89.25) [5]. They often give a history of the ability to grow their hair very long in childhood, suggestive of a long anagen phase, and report a high hair density prior to the onset of hair loss [14,15]. They usually have a negative family history of AGA. Clinical examination reveals bitemporal recession but no widening of the central hair parting, which if present would support the diagnosis of AGA. However, these criteria are not absolute, and AGA can mimic this presentation. A positive hair pull test is common over the vertex and occipital scalp, and patients may describe a reduction in the thickness of their ponytail volume, stating it has decreased by up to 50% [5]. A negative hair pull test on any one given day does not exclude the diagnosis of CTE. Scalp dermoscopy does not reveal miniaturized hair fibres. and compound hair follicles with 2–3 fibres exiting from each pore is the norm.

The diagnosis of CTE can usually be suspected from the history and examination, but scalp biopsy may be required to differentiate

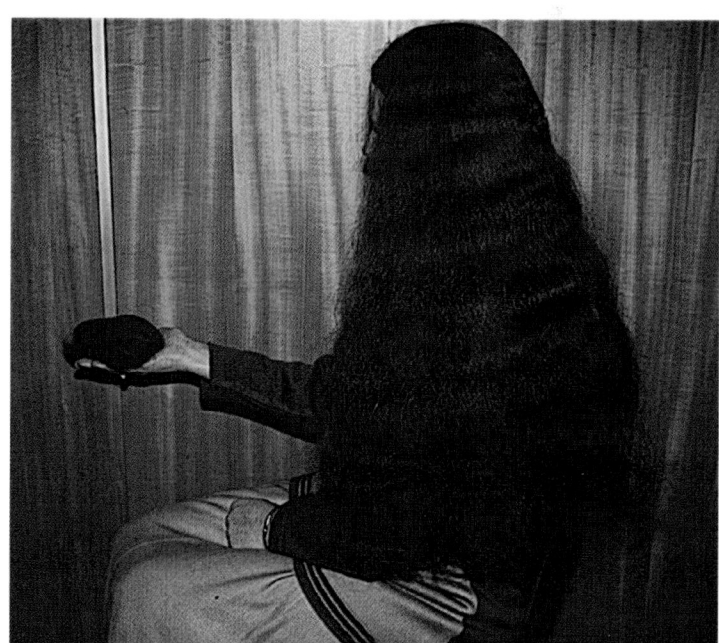

Figure 89.25 Idiopathic chronic telogen effluvium.

it from early androgenetic alopecia [3]. The optimal scalp biopsy is a 4 mm punch biopsy taken from the vertex of the scalp for horizontal embedding. A terminal to vellus ratio below 8 : 1 is suggestive of AGA.

Despite the assertion that CTE is a self-limiting process that does not evolve into AGA, its natural history remains poorly characterized, with only one published longitudinal study [38].

Chronic telogen effluvium has to be distinguished clinically from AGA as women with early AGA may present with periods of increased hair shedding without a discernible pattern to the loss. In an evaluation of 600 women presenting with chronic diffuse telogen hair shedding with little or no reduction of visible hair density, 60% were found on scalp biopsy to have hair miniaturization consistent with a diagnosis of AGA and 40% had CTE [39].

Management
No treatment is necessary as, while the hair continues to shed, it is replaced, and this condition does not lead to baldness. Antiandrogens have little effect on chronic telogen effluvium. Minoxidil can reduce hair shedding.

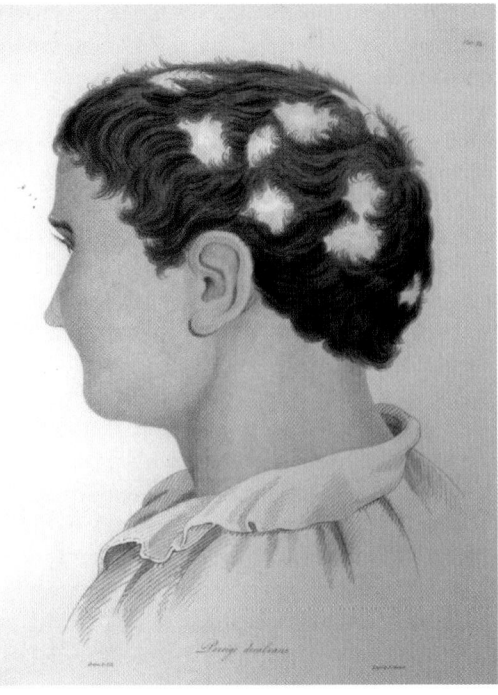

Figure 89.26 'Porrigo decalvans' (alopecia areata). Plate XL from Thomas Bateman's atlas *Practical Synopsis of Cutaneous Diseases*, 1819.

Alopecia areata

Andrew G. Messenger

Definition and nomenclature
Alopecia areata is a common, chronic, inflammatory disease that causes non-scarring hair loss. The severity ranges from small patches of hair loss, which usually recover spontaneously, to complete alopecia where the prognosis for hair regrowth is poor. The nails may also be affected. Current evidence indicates that alopecia areata is caused by a T-cell-mediated autoimmune mechanism occurring in genetically predisposed individuals. Environmental factors may be responsible for triggering the disease.

Synonyms and inclusions
• Alopecia totalis
• Alopecia universalis

Introduction and general description
The first description of alopecia areata is generally attributed to the Roman physician Celsus (*c.* 25 BC to AD 50). Under the heading 'areae' he described two types of hair loss; the first, known as 'alopecia' 'spreads in no certain form. It is found in the hair of the head, and in the beard.' The second type, called 'ophiasis', 'begins at the hinder part of the head … it creeps with two heads to the ears …'. The term alopecia areata was first used by Sauvages in 1763 (cited by Hebra and Kaposi [1]). In the English literature Robert Willan described alopecia areata under the title 'porrigo decalvans', illustrated in plate XL of Thomas Bateman's 1819 atlas (Figure 89.26). The first detailed account in more recent times was by Hebra and Kaposi [1] – many aspects of their description of the clinical features, the natural history and the response to treatment could appear in a modern textbook. Early ideas about the aetiology were numerous and included

infectious, metabolic, vascular, neuropathic and trophoneurotic theories. The current view, that alopecia areata is an autoimmune disease, was first suggested by Rothman in a discussion of a paper presented by Van Scott [2].

Epidemiology

Incidence and prevalence
In a population study of alopecia areata from Olmsted County, Minnesota, USA, the incidence rate was 0.1–0.2% with a projected lifetime risk of 1.7% [3]. As far as is known, alopecia areata occurs in all ethnic groups. Several large case series of alopecia areata have been reported from Europe [4], North America [5,6] and Asia [7,8], but these have generally been drawn from hospital clinic attenders and no accurate indication of variation in disease rates between populations is available.

Age
The onset of alopecia areata may occur at any age. However, in most affected individuals the first episode occurs before the age of 40, with the peak age of onset between the second and fourth decades.

Sex
The frequency of alopecia areata is probably the same in both sexes.

Ethnicity
Alopecia areata is common in all major ethnic groups although there are no studies that have assessed whether there is any difference in incidence between these groups.

Associated diseases

Alopecia areata is associated with several autoimmune diseases including thyroiditis, lupus erythematosus, vitiligo and psoriasis. The frequency of type 1 diabetes is not increased in patients with alopecia areata but diabetes is more common than expected in their relatives, suggesting a protective effect of the diabetes genotype. Atopic disease, especially atopic eczema, is also more common than expected in alopecia areata, and is associated with early onset and more severe forms of hair loss.

Pathophysiology

There is abundant evidence, albeit circumstantial, that alopecia areata is an autoimmune disease (reviewed in [9]):

- There is an increased frequency of other autoimmune diseases in patients with alopecia areata.
- There is an increased frequency of organ-specific autoantibodies in patients with alopecia areata. Serum antibodies to hair follicle tissue also occur with increased frequency in alopecia areata although these antibodies appear not to bind to hair follicles *in vivo* and their pathogenetic significance is not known.
- The pathology is characterized by infiltration of hair bulbs by activated T-lymphocytes.
- In animal models of alopecia areata, the depletion of CD4 and CD8 T cells results in hair regrowth [10].
- Alopecia areata shares genetic associations with several autoimmune diseases, particularly with genes of the major histocompatibility complex (MHC).

Immune privilege

There is a very low or absent expression of MHC class I proteins (HLA-A, -B, -C) in the lower part of the follicular epithelium. This has led to the concept that, like other tissues exhibiting this property such as the anterior chamber of the eye and the testis, the hair follicle is an immunologically privileged site where there is a reduced risk of attracting autoreactive cytotoxic CD8+ T cells that recognize antigen in association with MHC class I. Down-regulation of MHC class I may lead to attack by natural killer (NK) cells as NK cells are primed to eliminate MHC class I-negative cells. Hair follicles appear to protect from this event by down-regulating the expression of ligands that stimulate the activation of NK-cell receptors, and secreting molecules that inhibit NK-cell and T-cell activation. It has been proposed that, in individuals genetically predisposed to develop alopecia areata, pro-inflammatory signals such as interferon-γ (IFN-γ) upregulate the expression of MHC proteins and NK-cell-activating ligands, such as MICA and ULBP3, in the follicle. This leads to the collapse of immune privilege and attack by CD8+ cells [11].

Cytotoxic CD8+ NKG2D+ T cells are key players in the pathogenesis of alopecia areata and are the first intrafollicular lymphocytes to be observed. These CD8+ T cells produce IFN-γ that results in a release of interleukin 15 (IL-15) and IL-15Rα by follicular keratinocytes and promotes and sustains CD8+ T-cell autoreactivity. The involvement of IFN-γ and the γ-C cytokines (IL-2, IL-7, IL-15, IL-21) suggests downstream signalling via the Janus kinase (JAK) pathway. This idea is supported by the results of a study showing a positive effect on hair growth of JAK inhibitors in an animal model of alopecia areata and in a small clinical trial in humans [12].

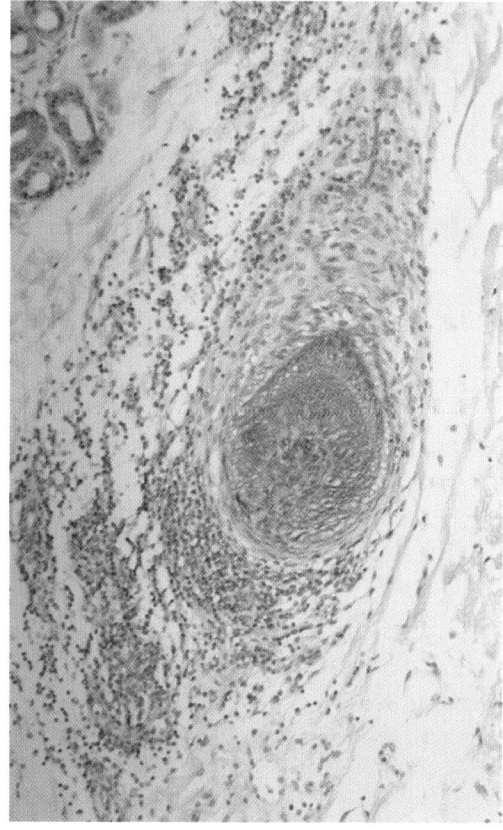

Figure 89.27 Lymphocytic inflammatory infiltrate surrounding an anagen hair bulb in alopecia areata.

Predisposing factors

The predisposition to alopecia areata is genetic.

Pathology

Anagen follicles at the margins of expanding patches of alopecia areata characteristically show a perifollicular and intrafollicular inflammatory cell infiltrate, concentrated in and around the hair bulb (Figure 89.27). The inflammatory infiltrate is composed mainly of activated T lymphocytes, with a preponderance of CD4 cells, and an admixture of macrophages, Langerhans cells and cells expressing NK cell markers [13,14,15]. In contrast to the inflammatory scarring alopecias, little or none of the inflammatory infiltrate is seen around the isthmus of the hair follicle, the site of hair follicle stem cells [16]. This may explain why follicles are not destroyed in alopecia areata. Lymphocytic infiltration of the dermal papilla and bulbar epithelium may be accompanied by increased expression of HLA class I and II antigens and of intercellular adhesion molecule-1 (ICAM-1) [17,18,19]. Normal numbers of follicles are found in established bald patches and in alopecia universalis. Both anagen and telogen follicles are found in these sites, with a higher proportion in telogen than in the normal scalp. Follicles are smaller than normal and anagen follicles do not develop beyond the anagen III–IV stage (see Figure 89.9), when the hair shaft starts to be formed [2]. The inflammatory infiltrate tends to be less pronounced than in early lesions and is associated mainly with anagen follicles.

Alopecia areata causes a disturbance in the normal dynamics of the hair cycle. Anagen follicles are precipitated into telogen.

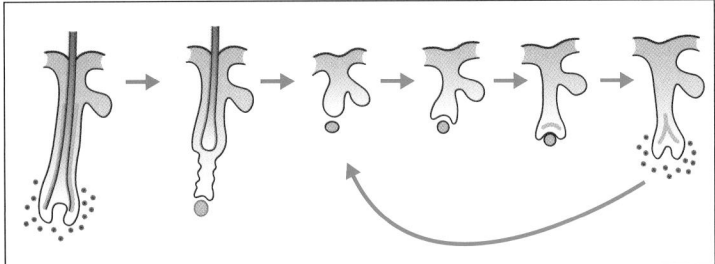

Figure 89.28 Proposed pathodynamic changes in alopecia areata. An inflammatory attack on anagen follicles precipitates follicles into telogen. Follicles re-enter anagen but development is halted in anagen stage III–IV and follicles return to telogen prematurely.

This may occur as a centrifugal wave, reminiscent of a moult wave [20]. Follicles are able to re-enter anagen but, whilst the disease is active, are unable to progress beyond the anagen III–IV stage [2]. It has been suggested that they then return prematurely to telogen and that these truncated cycles continue until disease activity wanes (Figure 89.28) [21].

Cells of several different types and differentiation pathways are found in the hair bulb, but which of these is the primary focus of the pathology is unknown. Trichocytes in the hair bulb matrix undergoing early cortical differentiation may show vacuolar degeneration (Figure 89.29) [22,23] and are also the predominant cell type showing aberrant MHC expression. However, it is pos-

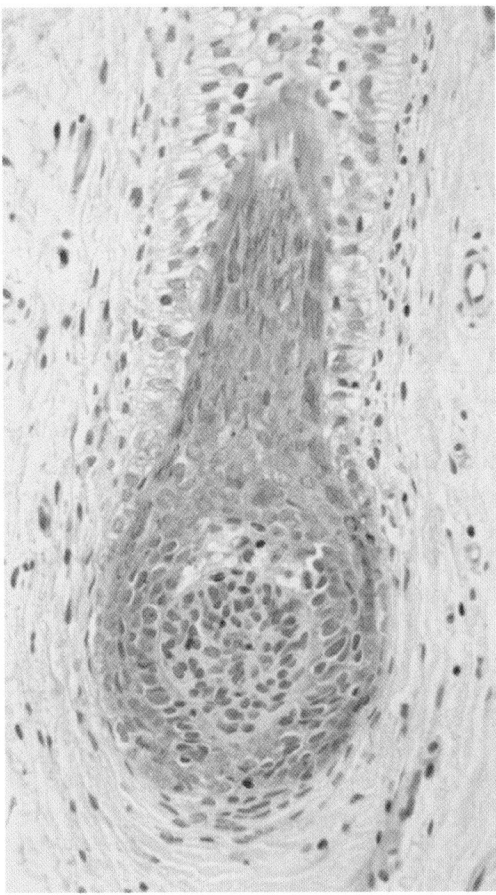

Figure 89.29 An early anagen follicle in alopecia totalis, showing vacuolation in the hair matrix epithelium around the upper pole of the dermal papilla.

sible that changes in the epithelial compartment of the hair follicle are secondary to dysfunction of the dermal papilla. The sparing of white hair sometimes seen in alopecia areata has also raised the possibility that alopecia areata is primarily a disease of hair bulb melanocytes. Alopecia areata may show other pigmentary features including reduced pigmentation in regrowing hairs and an association with vitiligo. However, the melanocyte hypothesis does not explain why sparing of white hair is often a relative phenomenon and is sometimes absent.

Genetics

The importance of genetic factors in alopecia areata is underlined by the high frequency of a positive family history in affected individuals [24]. In most reports, this ranges from 10% to 20% of cases, but mild cases are often overlooked or concealed and the true figure may be greater. The lifetime risk of alopecia areata in the children of a proband is approximately 6% [25,26]. A family history of alopecia areata is more common in those with disease onset before the age of 30 years (37% compared with 7.1% in patients with onset after 30 years). There are several case reports of alopecia areata in twins [27–29]. A small study in monozygotic and dizygotic pairs found a concordance rate of 55% for alopecia amongst monozygotic twins with no concordance among the dizygotic pairs [30]. Except in occasional families, alopecia areata is not inherited in a simple Mendelian fashion and the genetic basis appears to be multifactorial.

Gene associations. Case–control studies have reported associations between alopecia areata and a variety of genes involved in regulating immune and inflammatory responses (reviewed in [31]). The strongest associations to date have been with genes of the MHC, particularly the class II alleles *HLA-DQB1*0301* [32–34] and *HLA-DRB1*1104* [34,35]. A genome wide association study has confirmed the association with MHC genes and also identified several other genomic regions associated with alopecia areata. These included genes controlling the activation and proliferation of T-regulatory lymphocytes and some genes expressed in the hair follicle. There was a strong association with genes within the *ULBP* cluster coding for activating ligands of the NK cell receptor NKG2D, supporting a role for NK cells in the pathogenesis of the disease [**36**].

Environmental factors

The idea that alopecia areata is triggered by infection, either directly or as a consequence of a remote 'focus of infection', has a long history and still cannot be ruled out. It was the predominant aetiological theory until well into the twentieth century, and sporadic reports connecting alopecia areata with infective agents continue to appear. The 'external' factor most frequently implicated in triggering alopecia areata is psychological stress [37–39]. The significance of such an association is difficult to establish because of the problems in performing a controlled investigation. The published evidence is also conflicting, with some studies failing to show any relationship between stressful events and onset of hair loss [40,41], to the extent that no firm conclusion can be reached.

Despite the anecdotal nature of much of the evidence it is possible that environmental factors are responsible for triggering

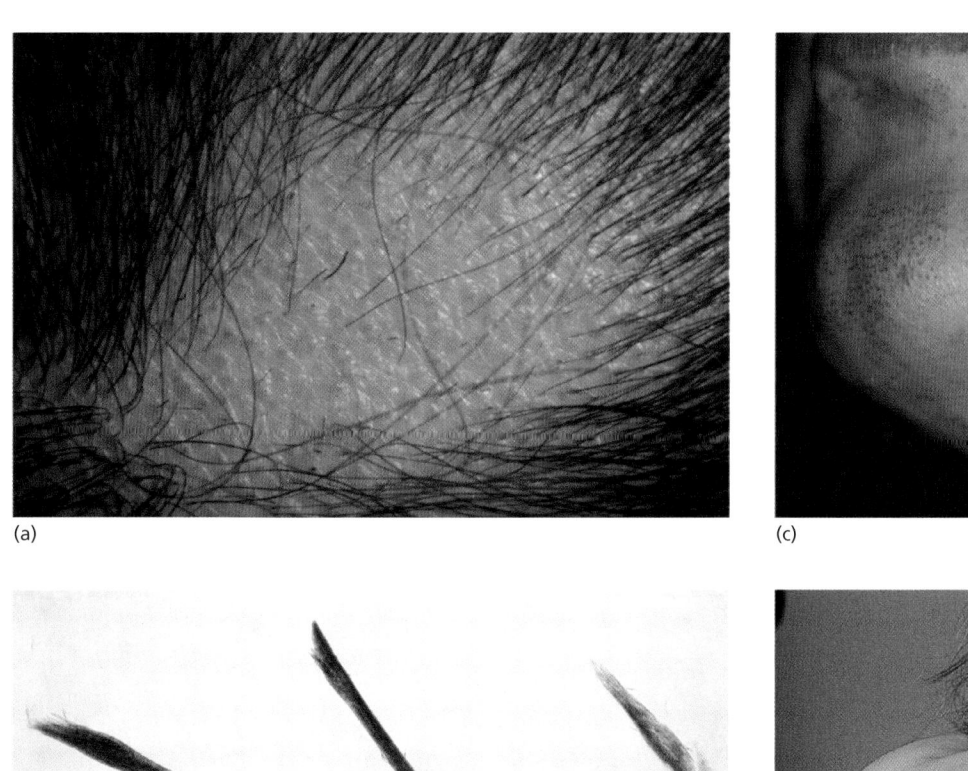

(a)

(c)

(b)

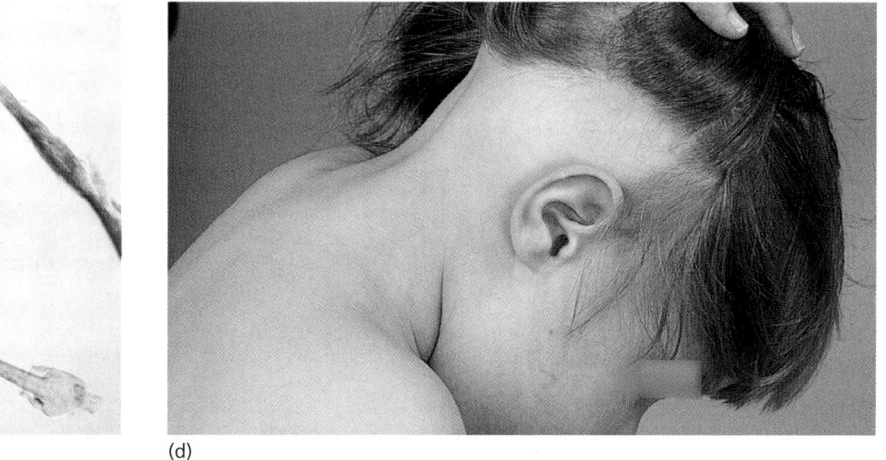

(d)

Figure 89.30 Alopecia areata. (a) Patch of alopecia areata showing broken 'exclamation mark hairs' towards the margins. (b) Close-up of exclamation mark hairs. (c) Alopecia areata affecting the beard. (d) The ophiasis pattern of alopecia areata.

alopecia areata in some patients. If so, it seems likely that a diversity of factors can operate in this way.

Clinical features

The characteristic initial lesion of alopecia areata is a circumscribed, hairless, smooth patch (Figure 89.30a). The skin within the bald patch appears normal or slightly reddened. Short, easily extractable broken hairs, known as exclamation mark hairs, are often seen at the margins of the bald patches during active phases of the disease (Figure 89.30b). The subsequent progress is unpredictable; the initial patch may regrow hair within a few months, or further patches may appear after varying intervals. A succession of discrete patches may coalesce to give large areas of hair loss. In some cases this progresses to a total loss of scalp hair (alopecia totalis) or a loss of all hair on the body (alopecia universalis). The initial hair loss is occasionally diffuse without the development of discrete bald areas. Regrowth is often at first fine and non-pigmented, but usually the hairs gradually resume their normal calibre and colour. Regrowth in one region of the scalp may occur while the alopecia is extending in others.

The scalp is the first affected site in most cases, but any hair-bearing skin can be affected. In dark-haired men, patches in the beard are conspicuous and in such individuals are often the first to be noticed (Figure 89.30c). The eyebrows and eyelashes are lost in many cases of alopecia areata and may be the only sites affected. The extension of alopecia along the back of the scalp is known as ophiasis (Figure 89.30d).

An intriguing feature of alopecia areata is the sparing of white hairs (Figure 89.31a). In patients with grey hair, which is an admixture of pigmented and non-pigmented hair, the disease process appears preferentially to affect pigmented hair, so that non-pigmented or white hair is spared. This may result in a dramatic change in hair colour if the alopecia progresses rapidly, and is probably the explanation for historical accounts of people 'going white overnight'. Sparing of white hair is a relative phenomenon and it is clear that the white hairs, although less susceptible to the disease, are not immune. During the regrowth phase hairs may be non- or hypopigmented (Figure 89.31b) but hair pigmentation usually recovers completely. In exceptional cases where regrowing hairs remain non-pigmented, the possibility of concurrent vitiligo should be considered.

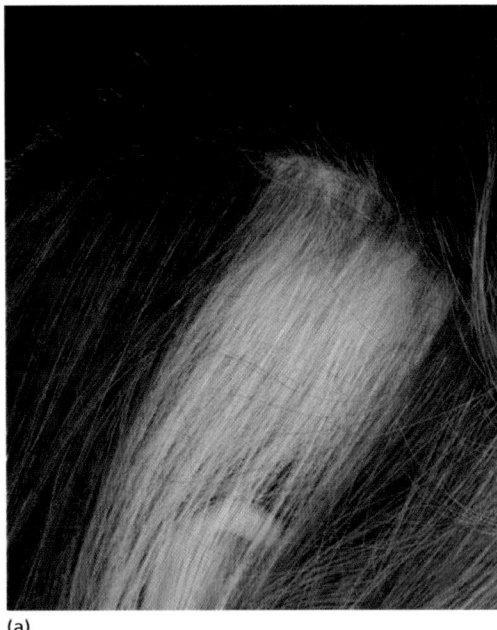

(a)

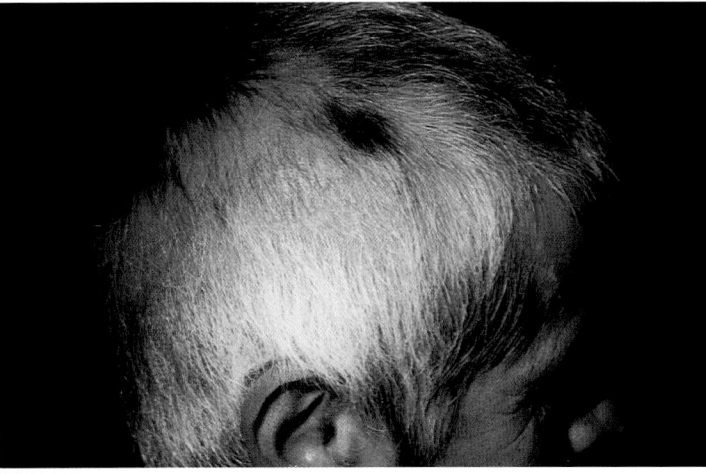

(b)

Figure 89.31 (a) Sparing of white hairs in a patch of alopecia areata.(b) Regrowth of hypopigmented hair in alopecia areata.

In 10–15% of cases referred for specialist opinion, alopecia areata also involves the nails, usually in the context of severe hair loss. Classically, alopecia areata causes fine stippled pitting of the nails (Figure 89.32), but some cases show less well-defined roughening of the nail plate (trachyonychia) or a non-specific atrophic dystrophy. For some patients, the latter problem is the most troublesome aspect of the disease.

Differential diagnosis
In children the main sources of difficulty are tinea capitis and trichotillomania. Tinea capitis should always be considered in children presenting with patchy hair loss. There is usually evidence of scalp inflammation but this may be limited to mild scaling. The hair loss in trichotillomania may be asymmetrical or occur in artificial shapes. Broken hairs are usually present across the areas of hair loss, giving a bristly texture, and, unlike exclamation mark hairs, are firmly anchored in the scalp. In most cases the true

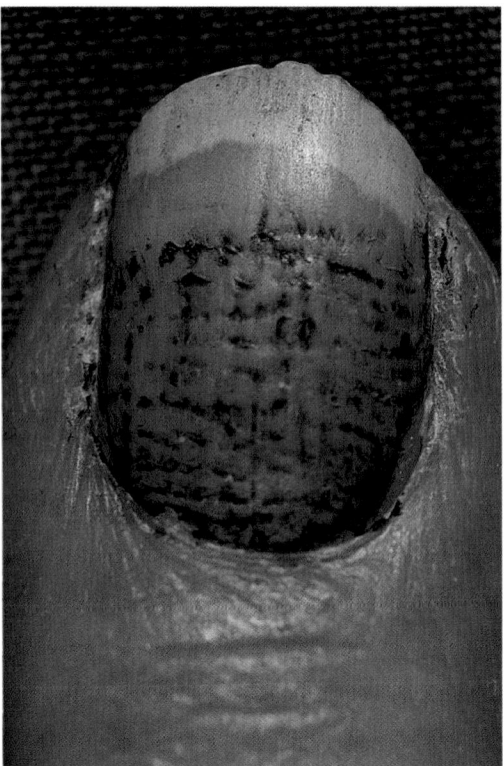

Figure 89.32 An organized pattern of pitting present on all fingernails 8 months prior to the onset of alopecia areata. The pits are highlighted with mascara.

diagnosis will become evident with time; a biopsy is useful when doubt remains. Occasionally, the early stages of scarring alopecia can resemble alopecia areata. The diffuse form of alopecia areata is perhaps the most difficult to identify. A history of previous episodes of hair loss, nail dystrophy and the usually rapid progression may provide clues, but other causes of diffuse hair loss, such as systemic lupus erythematosus, may need to be excluded by appropriate serological tests and a scalp biopsy. Secondary syphilis sometimes presents with diffuse or patchy hair loss.

Classification of severity
Alopecia areata is conventionally classified as patchy alopecia, alopecia totalis and alopecia universalis. In addition to these simple criteria a more detailed classification should include the disease duration and, with regard to patchy alopecia, the extent of the hair loss. Description of the pattern should include the presence of ophiasis, the involvement of sites on the trunk and limbs and the presence of nail disease. A scoring system, the Severity Alopecia Tool (SALT) has been devised [42].

Disease course and prognosis
Alopecia areata does not destroy hair follicles, and the potential for regrowth of hair is retained for many years and is possibly lifelong. In some patients, patches of hair loss occur at infrequent intervals interspersed with long periods of normal hair growth. In others, alopecia areata is more persistent, so that new patches of hair loss continue to develop at the same time as regrowth occurs elsewhere. In a relatively small number of patients, hair loss progresses to involve all of the scalp (alopecia totalis) or the entire

skin surface (alopecia universalis). In these cases, spontaneous recovery is the exception rather than the rule.

Data from secondary and tertiary referral centres indicate that 34–50% of patients will recover within 1 year, although almost all will experience more than one episode of the disease, and 14–25% progress to alopecia totalis or alopecia universalis, from which full recovery is unusual (less than 10%) [4,5,**43**]. One study from Japan reported that spontaneous remission within 1 year occurred in 80% of patients with a small number of circumscribed patches of hair loss [7]. The prognosis is less favourable when onset occurs during childhood [38,43] and in ophiasis [38]. The concurrence of atopic disease has been reported to be associated with a poor prognosis [7,38], but this was not found in a study from India [44].

Investigations

The diagnosis of alopecia areata is straightforward in most cases and investigations are usually not needed. If there is diagnostic uncertainty a biopsy may be necessary although the histological features may be subtle and require a pathologist experienced in the interpretation of hair pathology. Situations where a biopsy can be helpful include diffuse alopecia and possible early scarring alopecia. In selected cases other diagnostic tests may include the following:
- Fungal culture.
- Serology for lupus erythematosus.
- Serology for syphilis.

Unless relevant symptoms and signs are present it is debatable whether routine 'one-off' screening for other autoimmune diseases is appropriate as the risk is small and lifelong.

Management

General principles

A number of treatments can induce hair growth in alopecia areata, but none has been shown to alter the course of the disease, and the response rate in patients with extensive hair loss is low. Few treatments have been subjected to randomized controlled trials and there are few published data on long-term outcomes. These difficulties mean that counselling of the patient and, where relevant, of their family, are of paramount importance. This should include discussion of the nature of the disease and its natural history, the treatments available and their chances of success. Some patients have great difficulty coping with alopecia areata and require considerable support. Sources of support may include the physician, other patients, formal patient support groups and, in some circumstances, professional counselling services.

Leaving alopecia areata untreated is a legitimate option for many patients. Spontaneous remission occurs in up to 80% of patients with limited patchy hair loss of short duration (less than 1 year) [7]. Such patients may be managed by reassurance alone, with advice that regrowth cannot be expected within 3 months of the development of any individual patch. The prognosis in longstanding extensive alopecia is less favourable. However, all treatments have a high failure rate in this group and some patients prefer not to be treated, other than wearing a wig if appropriate.

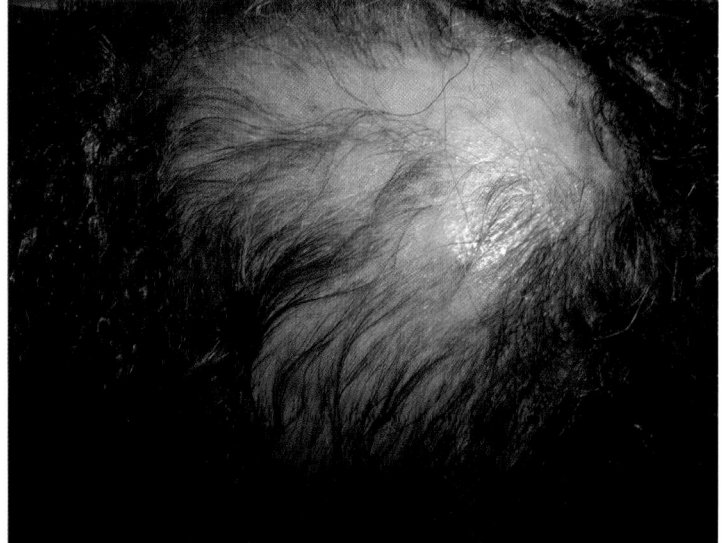

Figure 89.33 Alopecia areata showing regrowth of hair at sites of intralesional corticosteroid injection (triamcinolone acetonide).

First line

In limited patchy alopecia, a potent topical steroid (e.g. clobetasol), delivered in lotion, foam or shampoo formulation, may hasten the recovery of hair growth. Treatment should be continued for at least 3 months. Folliculitis is an occasional complication. Topical steroids are ineffective in alopecia totalis/universalis.

Intralesional steroids are probably the most effective treatment in patchy alopecia areata. A depot steroid (hydrocortisone acetate 25 mg/mL or triamcinolone acetonide 5–10 mg/mL), administered by fine needle injection into the upper subcutis or by a needleless device, will stimulate hair growth at the site of injection in some patients (Figure 89.33). Multiple injections are usually needed. Local atrophy is a common side effect but this recovers within a few months. Intralesional steroid will not prevent the development of alopecia at other sites and is not suitable for patients with rapidly progressive alopecia or alopecia totalis/universalis.

Various other treatments, such as topical minoxidil and anthralin (dithranol), have been advocated in patients with limited patchy alopecia but their benefits are uncertain.

Second line

In extensive and rapidly progressive alopecia areata, long-term daily treatment with oral corticosteroids will produce regrowth of hair in some patients. One small, partly controlled study reported that 30–47% of patients treated with a 6-week tapering course of oral prednisolone (starting at 40 mg/day) showed more than 25% hair regrowth [45]. Unfortunately, in most patients, continued treatment is needed to maintain hair growth and the response is usually insufficient to justify the risks. There are several case series reporting a favourable response to high-dose pulsed corticosteroid treatment using different oral and intravenous regimens [46–48]. In the only controlled trial, patients receiving prednisolone 200 mg once a week for 3 months showed better hair regrowth at 6 months than those taking placebo [49], but this was not statistically significant [50].

Third line

Contact immunotherapy is the most effective and best-documented treatment for alopecia areata. The patient is sensitized to a potent allergen by its application to a small area on the scalp and the same allergen is then applied to the scalp, usually at weekly intervals, in a concentration sufficient to induce a mild contact dermatitis. The contact allergens that have been used in the treatment of alopecia areata include dinitrochlorobenzene (DNCB), squaric acid dibutyl-ester (SADBE) and diphenylcyclopropenone (DPCP). Most centres now use DPCP [51]. A review of all the published studies of contact immunotherapy concluded that 50–60% of patients achieve a worthwhile response, but the range of response rates was very wide (9–87%) [52]. Patients with extensive hair loss are less likely to respond [53,54]. Other reported adverse prognostic features include the presence of nail changes, early onset and a positive family history [52]. In most studies treatment was discontinued after 6 months if no response was obtained. In one case series from Canada, clinically significant regrowth occurred in approximately 30% of patients after 6 months' treatment, but this increased to 78% after 32 months of treatment, suggesting that more prolonged treatment is worthwhile [55]. The response in patients with alopecia totalis and universalis was less favourable at 17% and this was not improved by treatment beyond 9 months. Relapses may occur following or during treatment. In the Canadian series, relapse following successful treatment occurred in 62% of patients. Two case report series of contact immunotherapy in children with alopecia areata reported response rates of 33% [56] and 32% [57]. A third study found a similar short-term response in children with severe alopecia areata, but less than 10% experienced sustained benefit [58].

Most patients will develop occipital and/or cervical lymphadenopathy during contact immunotherapy. This is usually temporary but may persist throughout the treatment period. Severe dermatitis is the most common adverse event, but the risk can be minimized by careful titration of the concentration. Uncommon adverse effects include urticaria [59] and vitiligo [60]. Cosmetically disabling pigmentary complications, both hyper- and hypopigmentation (including vitiligo), may occur if contact immunotherapy is used in patients with racially pigmented skin. Contact immunotherapy has been in use for 30 years and no long-term side effects have been reported. Sensitization of health professionals involved in delivering contact immunotherapy (doctors, nurses, pharmacy technicians) is a significant problem and they must take care to avoid skin contact with the allergen.

The mode of action of contact immunotherapy is unknown. Happle suggested that the contact allergen competes for CD4 cells, attracting them away from the perifollicular region ('antigenic competition') [61]. Other suggested mechanisms include the non-specific stimulation of a local T-suppressor-cell response [18] and increased expression of TGF-β in the skin, which acts to suppress the immune response [62].

There are several uncontrolled studies of photochemotherapy for alopecia areata, using all types of PUVA (oral or topical psoralen, local or whole-body UVA irradiation) [63–65], claiming success rates of up to 60–65%. Two retrospective reviews have reported low response rates [66] or suggested that the response was no better than the natural course of the disease [67], although these observations were also uncontrolled. The relapse rate following treatment is high and continued treatment is usually needed to maintain hair growth, which may lead to an unacceptably high cumulative UVA dose.

Non-medical treatments

Women with extensive alopecia will usually benefit from wearing a wig, hairpiece or bandana. A few brave patients prefer not to conceal their lack of hair. Men tend to shave their heads although some opt for a wig. The use of semipermanent tattooing can be helpful to disguise the loss of eyebrows.

Resources

Further information

Messenger AG, McKillop J, Farran P, McDonagh AJ, Sladden M. British Association of Dermatologists' guidelines for the management of alopecia areata. *Br J Dermatol* 2012;166:916–26. http://www.bad.org.uk/library-media%5Cdocuments%5CAlopecia_areata_guidelines_2012.pdf.

Patient resources

Alopecia UK: http://www.alopeciaonline.org.uk.
British Association of Dermatologists, patient information leaflet: http://www.bad.org.uk/shared/get-file.ashx?id=68&itemtype=document.
National Alopecia Areata Foundation: http://www.naaf.org. (All last accessed February 2015.)

SCARRING DISORDERS OF HAIR GROWTH

Rodney D. Sinclair

Cicatricial or scarring alopecia can result from many causes which are classified here into broad groups (Table 89.3) [1]. Some of the individual conditions are considered in this chapter in greater detail and many of the other causes and syndromes are discussed in other chapters where appropriate.

Acquired cicatricial alopecia

Definition and nomenclature

Cicatricial alopecia refers to patchy hair loss that follows the permanent destruction of hair follicles, either by a disease affecting the follicles themselves (primary cicatricial alopecia) or by an external process (secondary cicatricial alopecia). Any hair-bearing skin may be affected although cicatricial alopecia most commonly presents on the scalp.

Synonyms and inclusions
• Scarring alopecia

Introduction and general description

One of the earliest descriptions of cicatricial alopecia was by Brocq in 1885 [2]. He described what later became known eponymously as pseudopelade of Brocq [3], which is now regarded

Table 89.3 Classification of cicatricial alopecias.

	Cause	Condition		Cause	Condition
Primary cicatricial alopecia	Inflammatory:		**Secondary cicatricial alopecia** (Continued)	Infectious:	
	Lymphocytic	Chronic cutaneous lupus erythematosus		Bacterial	Folliculitis
		Lichen planopilaris (LPP):			Carbuncle/furuncle
		Classic LPP		Fungal	Kerion
		Graham–Little syndrome			Favus
		Frontal fibrosing alopecia			Tinea capitis (rarely scarring)
		Pseudopelade of Brocq		Viral	Shingles
		Central centrifugal cicatricial alopecia			Varicella
		Alopecia mucinosa			HIV
		Keratosis pilaris spinulosa decalvans		Protozoal	Leishmaniasis
	Neutrophilic	Folliculitis decalvans (including tufted folliculitis)		Treponemal	Syphilis
		Dissecting cellulitis/folliculitis		Mycobacterial	Tuberculosis
	Mixed	Acne keloidalis		Neoplastic:	
		Acne necrotica		Benign	Cylindroma
		Erosive pustular dermatosis			Other adnexal tumours
	Non-specific	Non-specific or end-stage cicatricial alopecia		Malignant, primary	Basal cell carcinoma
Secondary cicatricial alopecia	Traumatic	Radiodermatitis			Squamous cell carcinoma
		Mechanical trauma			Cutaneous T-cell lymphoma
		Postoperative (e.g. flap necrosis)		Malignant, secondary	Renal, breast, lung, gastrointestinal tumours
		Burns			Lymphoma, leukaemia
		Accidental alopecia	**Developmental defects and hereditary disorders**		Aplasia cutis
		Dermatitis artefacta			Facial hemiatrophy (Romberg's syndrome)
		Traction alopecia			Epidermal naevi
		Hot comb alopecia			Hair follicle hamartomas
	Sclerosing disorder	Morphoea			Incontinentia pigmenti
		Scleroderma			Focal dermal hypoplasia of Goltz
		Lichen sclerosus			Porokeratosis of Mibelli
		Sclerodermoid porphyria cutanea tarda			Ichthyosis
		Chronic graft-versus-host disease			Epidermolysis bullosa
	Granulomatous	Sarcoidosis			Polyostotic fibrous dysplasia
		Necrobiosis lipoidica			Conradi–Hünermann syndrome (chondrodysplasia punctata)
		Infectious granulomas			

as a syndrome in which the destruction of follicles leading to permanent patchy baldness is not accompanied by any clinically evident inflammatory pathology. Quinquaud [4] described folliculitis decalvans, a form of scarring alopecia in which pustular folliculitis of the advancing margin was a conspicuous feature.

In cicatricial alopecia, damage to the stem cell niche in the outer root sheath at the level of insertion of the arrector pili muscle (the bulge) destroys any potential for hair regrowth. Histologically, the follicles ultimately disappear or are replaced by fibrous stelae. Scar tissue is not seen on histology. Unlike patients with non-scarring alopecia who are generally asymptomatic, patients with cicatricial alopecia may complain of itching, burning, soreness, scaling or discharge. Primary cicatricial alopecia tends to run a chronic and progressive course and ultimately leads to disfigurement. The rate

of extension and the final severity are extremely variable and difficult to predict.

Cicatricial alopecia may result from a disease that affects the follicles primarily or a disease process external to the follicle that damages them secondarily. Secondary causes include trauma, as in burns or radiodermatitis, infections such as favus, tuberculosis or syphilis, or benign or malignant tumours. Chemicals used to straighten or curl hair may also cause a secondary cicatricial alopecia in susceptible persons. Inflammatory diseases such as scleroderma that do not specifically target hair follicles may also lead to a secondary cicatricial alopecia.

Classification of the primary causes of cicatricial alopecia is difficult because of changing clinical and histological features as these conditions evolve. The most common identifiable causes among people of European descent are lichen planopilaris (LPP), folliculitis decalvans and discoid lupus erythematosus. Among black people resident in North America and Europe, the most common cause is central centrifugal alopecia. Tumours, in particular metastatic nodules from renal, breast and lung carcinomas, should not be forgotten as a rare but important cause of cicatricial alopecia.

Epidemiology

Incidence and prevalence
Cicatricial alopecia is not rare. It represents approximately 7% of patients seen in specialist hair loss clinics [1].

Age, sex and ethnicity
The most common cause among people of European descent is LPP, while central centrifugal alopecia is more common than all other forms of cicatricial alopecia combined among people of African descent. White people are more commonly affected than dark-skinned people. Most cases of LPP are seen in women in aged 30–50 years. Discoid lupus erythematosus occurs twice as commonly in women than men, and is about three times more common in people of African descent than in white people. The incidence is approximately one in 2000. Familial cases occur in approximately 10%. The peak age of onset is around 40 years.

Central centrifugal alopecia develops in women of African descent in their mid-forties, with a female to male ratio of 3 : 1. Frontal fibrosing alopecia occurs almost exclusively in postmenopausal women. Folliculitis decalvans occurs equally in men and women from the age of 30. Dissecting cellulitis is most common in men in their twenties. Folliculitis keloidalis (acne keloidalis; see Chapter 93) tends to occur in black men of African descent in their early thirties. Erosive pustular dermatosis is most common in fair-skinned, balding European men and women in their seventies.

Associated diseases
Up to 40% of patients with scalp lichen planus and 30% of patients with discoid lupus of the scalp will have cutaneous disease elsewhere either at presentation or during follow-up. Although discoid lupus can be seen in patents with systemic lupus, very few patients with discoid lupus confined to the scalp will ever develop systemic lupus erythematosus. About 10% of patients with frontal fibrosing alopecia also have lichen planopilaris of the scalp. Linear morphoea may be associated with facial hematrophy. Dissecting cellulitis may be associated with the follicular occlusion tetrad. Keratosis pilaris spinulosa decalvans may be associated with keratosis pilaris elsewhere on the body. Follicular mucinosis may be associated with cutaneous T-cell lymphoma. Scalp metastases may be solitary or associated with widespread metastatic disease.

Investigations
Once the preliminary diagnosis of cicatricial alopecia has been made, the scalp should be examined for other clues as to the cause of the hair loss such as folliculitis, follicular plugging or broken hairs. Dermoscopy reveals a loss of follicular ostia. These signs may help to establish the cause of a cicatricial alopecia, but no single sign is pathognomonic for a particular disease, and clinicopathological correlation is usually needed to make a specific diagnosis. While pustules are strongly suggestive of folliculitis decalvans, they can also occur in lichen planopilaris and chronic cutaneous lupus. Hairs, even if grossly normal in appearance, should be extracted from the edge of the bald area for microscopy and culture. Any pustule should be swabbed and the fluid cultured. Careful examination of the skin, nails and oral mucosa should also be carried out: up to 40% of patients with scalp lichen planus and 30% of patients with discoid lupus of the scalp will have cutaneous disease elsewhere either at presentation or during follow-up.

In most cases, a diagnostic biopsy is indicated. The site for biopsy must be carefully selected: early lesions are likely to yield more information. Several punch biopsies are preferable to a single elliptical biopsy; in this way, the biopsies can be orientated along follicles, and different stages of the disease process can be investigated. Ideally, at least one 4 mm biopsy should be taken from a clinically active area, prepared for horizontal section and stained with haematoxylin and eosin. If vertical sections or immunofluorescence are desired, a second and third 4 mm biopsy specimen from an area of similar clinical activity should be obtained. Additional biopsies from the centre of a patch of alopecia to establish whether follicular loss has occurred or to assess potential regrowth may be desirable in some circumstances, as are further biopsies for special stains (e.g. elastin, mucin, periodic acid–Schiff (PAS)) [1].

Management
A number of treatments are used empirically; however, randomized controlled trial data are not available. The aim of treatment is to reduce symptoms and to slow or stop the progression of hair loss – it is not possible to restore hair growth where hair follicles have been lost. Early treatment is the key to minimizing the extent of permanent alopecia. However, inconsistent terminology, poorly defined clinical end points and a lack of good-quality clinical trials have long made management of these conditions very challenging [5].

Surgical correction with a combination of scalp reduction and hair transplantation is generally recommended for secondary cicatricial alopecia. Hair transplantation and scalp reduction surgery for primary cicatricial alopecia is more complicated due to the often progressive nature of the condition, lack of adequate donor population and the potential for graft rejection due to persisting inflammation in the recipient skin.

Attention to any associated hair loss disorders such as androgenetic alopecia is important, as the surrounding hair is required to conceal the patches of cicatricial alopecia. Camouflage powders and sprays as well as wigs are useful.

Despite multiple investigations a specific diagnosis is not always possible and a generic diagnosis of cicatricial alopecia is the best that can be offered. In such cases, a trial of oral steroids or antimalarials may be considered to assess the potential for regrowth. Surgical correction of small areas can be considered once the underlying disorder has burned out. This can be done either by follicle transplantation or excision of the area. Larger areas may require the prior use of tissue expanders [6].

Non-specific cicatricial alopecia

Epidemiology

This is by far the most common diagnosis made among patients presenting with cicatricial alopecia. In Whiting's series of 358 patients who were biopsied because of cicatricial alopecia, this was the diagnosis made in 32% of cases [7]. Although often called pseudopelade, this term is best avoided because of confusion with pseudopelade of Brocq, a specific and distinct clinical disease. This entity of non-specific cicatricial alopecia encompasses a range of idiopathic, non-inflammatory, irregular, permanent alopecias that are often slowly progressive. Many primary cicatricial alopecias ultimately burn out and the final common pathway is an irregular area of cicatricial hair loss of the scalp with no distinguishing clinical or histological features. Various authorities have estimated that between 15% and 90% of cases of non-specific cicatricial alopecia result from LPP, but there is no way of confirming this. That a small minority of patients initially diagnosed as having non-specific cicatricial alopecia later develop associated cutaneous lichen planus supports the existence of significant overlap between this condition and LPP.

Pathophysiology

The histology is variable and non-specific. Scalp biopsies taken from hairy skin at the edge of a scarred patch may be either completely normal or show a non-specific lymphocytic infiltrate around the follicular infundibulum and mid-follicle, with or without a light, superficial perivascular infiltrate. Follicles may be depleted and replaced by fibrous tracts, and sebaceous glands and follicular units may be disrupted. In the centre of areas of alopecia, follicles are absent or dramatically diminished in number and the epidermis is atrophic. Concentric lamellar fibrosis and follicular atrophy is seen around the residual follicles. The adjacent dermis is sclerotic. Follicle rupture can produce hair granulomas or pustules that may lead to an erroneous diagnosis of folliculitis decalvans.

Clinical features

The initial patch often occurs over the crown, but may occur anywhere on the scalp. The lesions tend to be oval, and several foci may coalesce to form irregular bald areas. There is usually no erythema and the patches are smooth, shiny and slightly depressed. Within any patch, a small number of terminal hairs may persist. These are often irregularly twisted and sometimes easily extracted. Folliculitis is rarely seen. The hairs at the edge of the patch of alopecia are also often irregularly twisted and easily extracted, even when in anagen, which indicates active extension of the alopecia.

Prognosis

The prognosis is extremely variable and unpredictable. Some patches extend almost imperceptibly over many years, whereas others enlarge rapidly. Whether this condition ever truly burns out, or merely extends too slowly to be noticed, is uncertain.

Management

Much has been tried empirically, but nothing has been shown to be effective.

Follicular lichen planus

Introduction and general description

Lichen planus is an idiopathic inflammatory disease that may affect the skin, hair and nails (see Chapter 37) and, in a minority of cases, has a follicular predilection, which, when it affects the scalp, tends to produce a cicatricial alopecia. The reasons why the hair follicle should become the target of inflammation are poorly understood.

Three variants of follicular lichen planus are recognized and each is discussed more fully below: classic lichen planopilaris (LPP), frontal fibrosing alopecia (FFA) and Graham-Little syndrome. All of them result in follicular scarring and hair loss.

By way of corollary, significant involvement of the scalp in lichen planus is relatively infrequent, with only 10 of 807 patients in one series [8]. The incidence is probably rather higher than such figures suggest, because they tend to exclude those patients in whom alopecia, classified as pseudopelade, was the only manifestation of the disease.

Lichen planopilaris

Introduction and general description

This is the commonest form of follicular lichen planus and typically presents with progressive scarring alopecia of the scalp. It is most commonly confined to the scalp but may affect other body areas with or without concomitant scalp involvement. See also Chapter 37.

Pathophysiology

Pathogenesis

Karnik *et al.* investigated the molecular basis for LPP using microarray analysis and identified a decreased expression of genes required for lipid metabolism and peroxisome biogenesis [9]. Immunohistochemical analysis of biopsies from LPP showed a progressive loss of peroxisomes, proinflammatory lipid accumulation and infiltration of inflammatory cells preceding the destruction of the pilosebaceous unit. The expression of peroxisome proliferator-activated receptor γ (PPAR-γ), a transcription factor that regulates these processes, was found to be significantly decreased in LPP. Targeted deletion of PPAR-γ in follicular stem cells in a murine model caused a skin and hair phenotype that emulated LPP. The investigators suggested that a loss of function of hair follicle PPAR-γ triggers LPP.

Pathology [9]

The initial abnormality is in the epidermis. Fibrillar changes in the basal cells lead to the formation of colloid bodies and at an early stage these, and macrophages containing pigment, may be seen in the dermis. By immunofluorescence, fibrin and immunoglobulin M (IgM) may be detected in the upper dermis, and various components of complement in the basement membrane zone. The damaged basal cells are continually replaced by the migration of cells from neighbouring normal epidermis. In the established lesion,

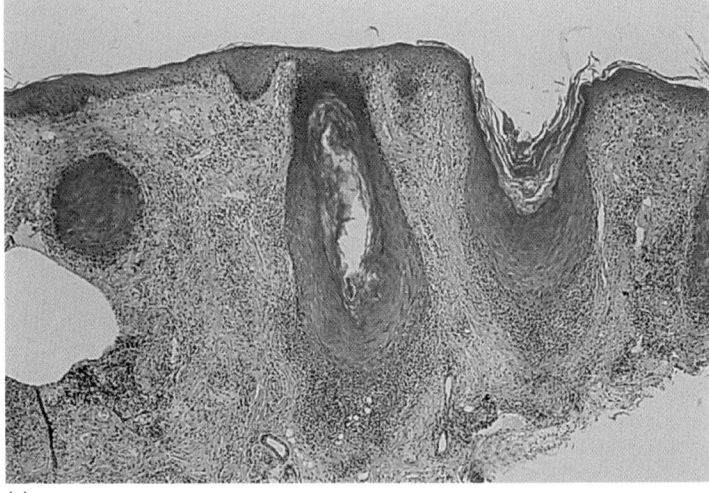

(a)

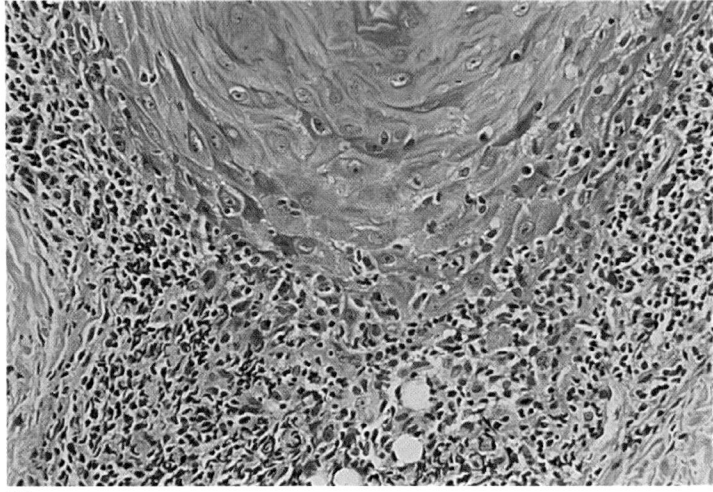

(b)

Figure 89.34 Lichen planopilaris. (a) Low-power photomicrograph showing follicular plugging and a periappendageal inflammatory infiltrate. (b) Base of the hair follicle showing hydropic degeneration of the basal layer and a lichenoid mononuclear cell infiltrate.

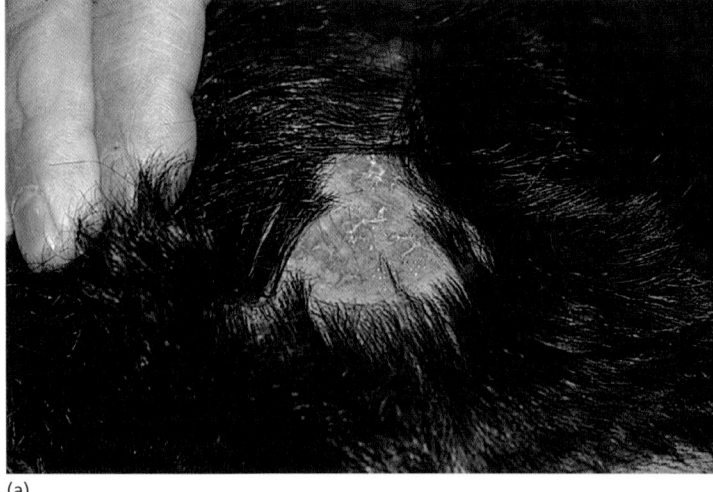

(a)

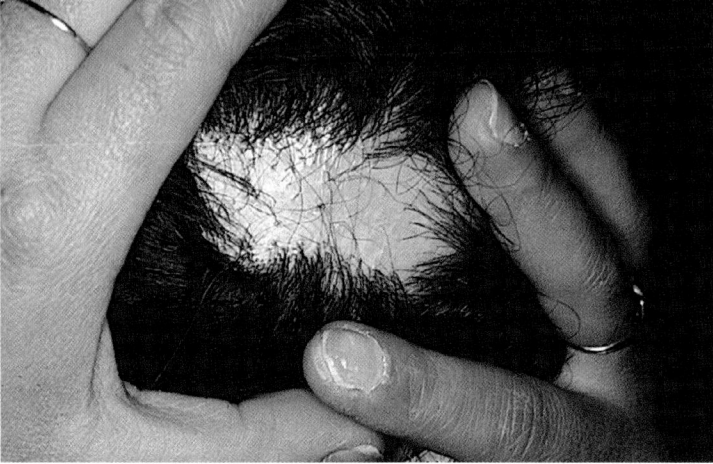

(b)

Figure 89.35 (a) Scarring alopecia caused by lichen planus showing active lesions. (b) More advanced lichen planus showing follicular plugs and scarring.

the horny layer and granular layer are thickened and there is irregular acanthosis. Flattening of the rete pegs gives rise to a saw-tooth configuration. There is liquefaction degeneration of the basal cells. Close up against the epidermis is a dense infiltrate of lymphocytes and some histiocytes. In many sections, colloid bodies can be seen. When the process involves hair follicles, the infiltrate extends around them and the hairs are replaced by keratin plugs. The follicles may ultimately be totally destroyed (Figure 89.34). Androgenetic alopecia with associated fibrosis may be confused histologically with patterned LPP, especially as mild to moderate lymphohistiocytic inflammation is commonly seen in AGA [10].

Clinical features [11]
Recent scalp lesions may show violaceous papules, erythema and scaling (Figure 89.35a). These papules are replaced quickly by follicular plugs and scarring (Figure 89.35b). Eventually, the plugs are shed from the scarred area, which remains white, smooth and atrophic. Follicular orifices are absent within the area of alopecia. If the patch is extending, horny plugs may still be present in fol-

licles around its margins, and the hair pull will be positive at the margins, with twisted anagen hairs being easily extracted by gentle traction.

Patients commonly present with pseudopelade-like patches of scarring that are non-specific. In these circumstances, the diagnosis of lichen planus can be made only in the presence of unquestionable lesions elsewhere and lichen planus histology. These may take the form of bullous lichen planus with shedding of the nails [12], of bullous lesions associated with typical lichen planus of the skin and mucous membranes, or of lichen planus of very limited extent involving, for example, the nails only.

Sites of predilection for LPP other than the scalp include the axillae, inguinal folds, sacrum and limb flexures. It manifests as grouped or disseminated follicular, flat, elevated or hemispherical erythematous papules or punctate keratoses [13]. Hair loss from such areas is less likely to be of concern to the patient than when the scalp is involved.

Prognosis
In some patients, the course of LPP of the scalp is slow and only a few inconspicuous patches are present after many years.

However, LPP may rapidly result in extensive and permanent baldness. Resolution of associated symptoms and the absence of visible inflammation do not automatically imply that hair loss has been arrested. Alopecia can progress insidiously over many years [5].

Management

A short course of systemic treatment with a corticosteroid may be desirable initially to stabilize the disease. In other cases, intralesional corticosteroids are helpful, but only at a stage when active inflammatory changes are still present [5]. Potent topical steroids such as clobetasol propionate ointment or shampoo once daily usually relieve associated symptoms such as itch or pain, and may slightly inhibit the process [14]. Hydroxychloroquine and acitretin have been tried with variable success. Ciclosporin is very effective for cutaneous lichen planus, and has been reported as useful in Graham-Little syndrome [15], as has thalidomide [16,17].

The lack of a clearly defined natural history, the permanency of the hair loss, the absence of any proven effective treatment to arrest disease progression, and the difficulty in monitoring clinical response, conspire to make treatment of this condition particularly frustrating for both patient and doctor. Specific PPAR-γ-targeted therapy with agents such as pioglitazone has, to date, proved disappointing [18].

Frontal fibrosing alopecia

Introduction and general description
This condition was first described by Kossard in 1994 [19]. It typically occurs in postmenopausal women, although it can occur earlier and in men. Familial cases have been reported [20], as has an association with discoid lupus erythematosus [21]. While once considered rare, it has been recognized increasingly commonly over the past 20 years. The explanation for this is unclear although an environmental cause has been postulated.

Pathophysiology
The histopathology is identical to that of LPP.

Clinical features
Recession of the frontal hairline is the cardinal feature of frontal fibrosing alopecia (Figure 89.36) [22]. In contrast to androgenetic alopecia, the frontal hairline recedes in a straight line rather than bitemporally and sideburns are commonly lost. There may also be some recession of the posterior hairline. Itch and pain may occur, but are often absent. Loss of eyebrows is an early and near universal finding. Body hair loss may also occur. On close inspection there is a loss of follicular orifices, and perifollicular erythema and hyperkeratosis at the marginal hairline. Small papules on the cheeks and temples due to involvement of vellus follicles are seen in some patients.

Prognosis
The natural history of frontal fibrosing alopecia is one of slow progression over many years [22,23]. Recession of the hairline eventually stops in most cases but this cannot be predicted and occasionally the hairline retreats as far as the scalp vertex.

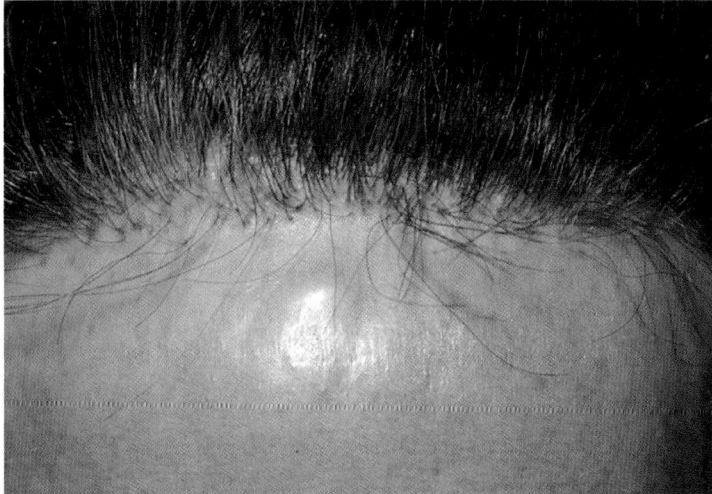

Figure 89.36 Frontal fibrosing alopecia showing scarring alopecia affecting the frontal hairline with follicular erythema and scale.

Management
A variety of treatments are used, including topical and intralesional corticosteroids, hydroxychloroquine, doxycycline and finasteride, but there is no convincing evidence that any is effective.

Graham-Little syndrome

Introduction and general description
In 1915, Graham-Little reported the case of a woman aged 55 years who had suffered for 10 years from slowly progressive cicatricial alopecia and for 5 months from groups of horny papules [24]. Since then many further cases have been reported. Whether this syndrome is or is not a form of lichen planus is still unresolved, although the immunofluorescence in typical cases strongly suggests lichen planus [25]. However, whatever its cause or causes, the syndrome is distinctive. It is known eponymously and variously as the Graham-Little, Lassueur–Graham-Little or Piccardi–Lassueur–Little syndrome.

Pathophysiology
In the scalp, the mouths of affected follicles are filled by horny plugs. The underlying follicle is progressively destroyed and eventually an atrophic epidermis covers sclerotic dermis. In the axillae and pubic region, the follicles are likewise destroyed, although the skin does not appear clinically to be atrophic.

Clinical features
Most patients are women between the ages of 30 and 70 years. The essential features of the syndrome are progressive cicatricial alopecia of the scalp, loss of pubic and axillary hair without clinically evident scarring, and the rapid development of keratosis pilaris [26].

In most patients, the earliest change has been patchy cicatricial alopecia of the scalp. In general, the scalp alopecia precedes the widespread keratosis pilaris by months or years [27]. In some patients, the alopecia and the keratosis pilaris appear to have developed more or less simultaneously, or the keratosis pilaris has preceded the discovery of the alopecia [28]. The scalp changes are commonly described simply as patches of cicatricial alopecia. Some authors specifically mention associated follicular plugging of the scalp [28]; others refer to 'scaly red patches'.

The keratosis pilaris is referred to in early case reports as lichen spinulosus, which emphasizes that the horny papules are prolonged into conspicuous spines. In most cases they have developed aggressively over a period of weeks or months and have been grouped into plaques, often on the trunk, or the trunk and limbs, but occasionally involving the eyebrows and the sides of the face. Pruritus is an inconstant symptom; it was noted in several reported cases [5]. Thinning and ultimately total loss of pubic and axillary hair has been noted in many cases.

Management

No treatment is universally effective. A short course of oral prednisolone is used to stabilize rapidly progressive disease. Ciclosporin was reported as useful in a single case [14]. Potent topical steroids, hydroxychloroquine and thalidomide have also been used.

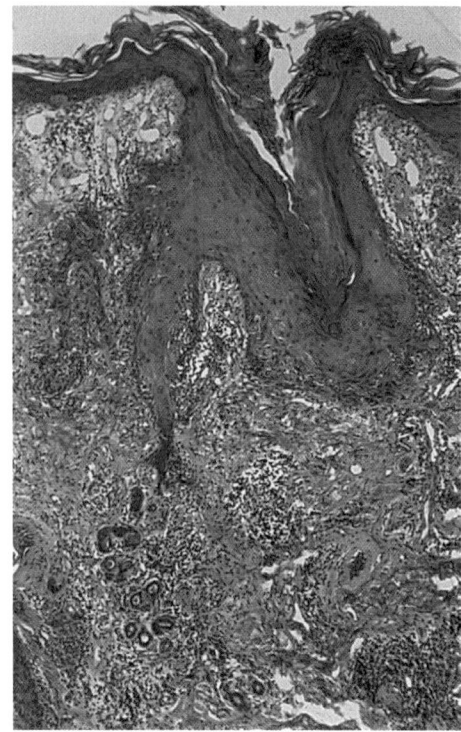

(a)

Chronic cutaneous lupus erythematosus

Synonyms and inclusions
• Discoid lupus erythematosus

Introduction and general description

Lupus erythematosus is an autoimmune, connective tissue disease characterized by the presence of circulating non-organ-specific autoantibodies to cell nuclear antigens (see Chapter 51). Three different forms are described: systemic lupus erythematosus (SLE), subacute cutaneous lupus erythematosus (SCLE) and chronic cutaneous lupus erythematosus (CCLE). However, only CCLE regularly produces cicatricial alopecia. Inflammation of the infundibular region of the hair follicle that contains the stem cells is thought to be the basis of the scarring alopecia that occurs in CCLE, but this does not explain why the identical pattern of inflammation seen in SLE does not scar. The diffuse hair shedding that accompanies SLE is believed to be an acute telogen effluvium.

Pathophysiology [7]

The histology of CCLE, in common with SLE, shows hyperkeratosis with follicular plugging, a perivascular and periadnexal lymphoid infiltrate – which may be sparse, moderate or heavy – and the essential feature of focal basal layer vacuolar degeneration (Figure 89.37). This may be associated with colloid body formation, pigmentary incontinence, papillary dermal oedema, thickening of the basement-membrane zone and exocytosis of lymphocytes into the epidermis and follicular epithelium. Mucin can be seen in the dermis as a faint blue tinge between widely separated collagen bundles. Scarring occurs only in CCLE and manifests as homogenized collagen fibres running parallel to the surface, a loss of appendages and lone arrector pili muscles. Staining for elastin shows that elastic fibres are absent from the scar.

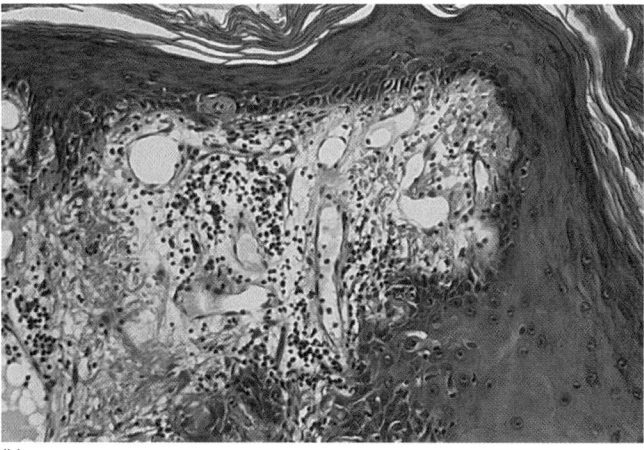

(b)

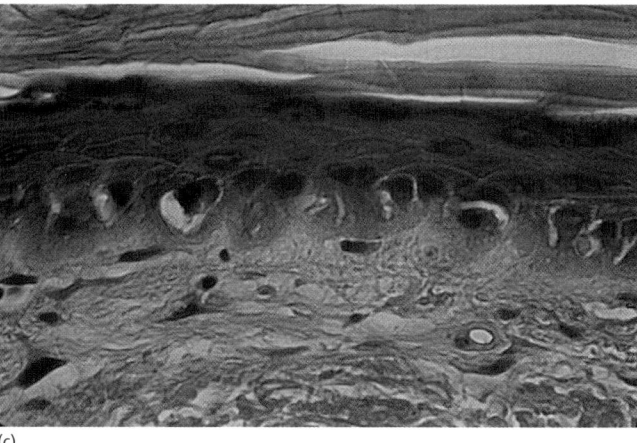

(c)

Figure 89.37 Discoid lupus erythematosus. (a) Low-power photomicrograph showing follicular plugging, superficial and deep perivascular and periappendageal lymphocytic infiltrate. (b) High-power photomicrograph showing the hydropic degeneration of the basal layer and the mononuclear cell infiltrate. (c) Higher-power photomicrograph showing the hydropic degeneration of the basal layer. (Courtesy of Dr G. Mason, Melbourne, Australia.)

PART 8: SPECIFIC CUTANEOUS STRUCTURE

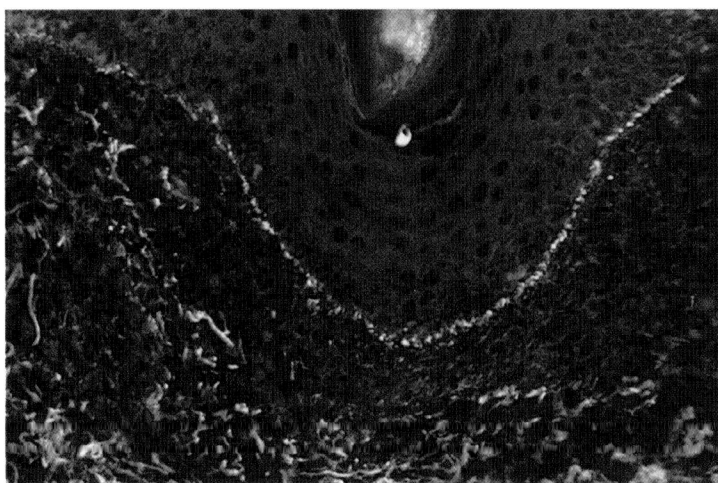

Figure 89.38 Positive linear immunofluorescence to IgG: the lupus band test. (Courtesy of Dr G. Mason, Melbourne, Australia.)

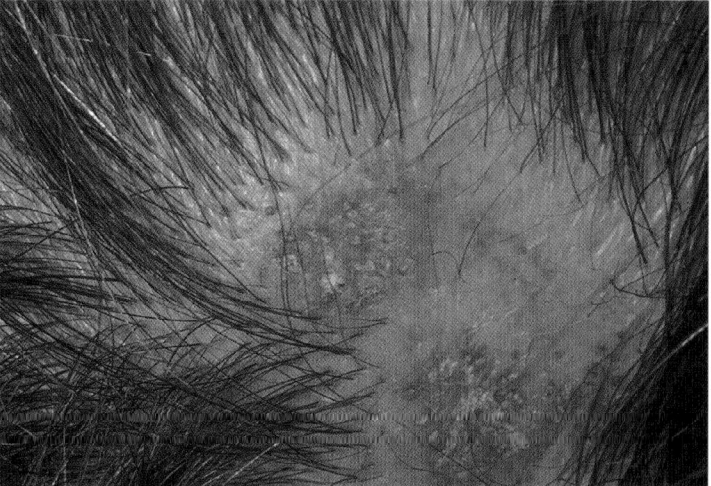

Figure 89.39 Discoid lupus erythematosus showing scarring alopecia with scalp erythema and follicular plugging.

Hypergranulosis, saw-toothed rete ridges, perifollicular fibrosis and clefts are not seen in lupus, and this helps to distinguish it from lichen planus. However, it is frequently not possible to separate these two conditions on routine histological examination and in such cases immunofluorescence may be decisive. There is linear staining of deposits of complement (C3), IgM and IgG on the basement membrane in more than 80% of cases of lupus erythematosus, but not in lichen planus. Direct immunofluorescence is also positive in non-lesional skin in approximately 50–75% of cases of SLE, depending on whether sun-exposed or non-exposed skin is chosen. Only approximately 20% of cases of CCLE will have positive immunofluorescence of uninvolved skin. A weak false positive immunofluorescence to IgM can occur on the head and neck and is a source of confusion. Only positivity to IgG or very strong positivity to IgM (Figure 89.38) should be used as supportive evidence of lupus on the scalp, as this only rarely occurs in the absence of lupus. In old, burnt-out lesions, the histology and immunofluorescence may be inconclusive, and in such cases a non-specific diagnosis such as scarring alopecia is all that can be made.

Clinical features [7]
Scarring alopecia occurs in 20% of men and 50% of women affected with CCLE, and the scalp is the only area affected in a significant number of patients. Patches on the scalp are often itchy. Areas of erythema and scaling with follicular plugging extend irregularly across the scalp and produce scarring (Figure 89.39). Symptoms may include pruritus, burning or scalp tenderness. Inflammatory activity is most pronounced centrally within the area of alopecia. Sometimes patches of scarring alopecia develop with little in the way of preceding inflammation, and then resemble pseudopelade of Brocq. Ultimately, large areas of alopecia may form. Some cases burn out after 1–2 years, but others continue to progress for many years.

Pigmentary disturbance, particularly in dark-skinned people, is common. Rarely, calcification occurs in the patches. Squamous cell carcinoma has been reported in chronic cicatricial lupus erythematosus of the scalp [29].

Antinuclear antibody (ANA) is positive in approximately 35% of patients with CCLE. Anti-Ro antibodies are found in 10%.

CCLE may occur on its own or associated with SLE. If the initial CCLE is confined to the head and neck, the risk is 1–2%, whereas if the lesions are generalized the risk is 22%. SLE first presents with CCLE in 10% of cases and CCLE can be found at some stage during the course of SLE in 33%.

Management [5]
As CCLE is often made worse by exposure to UV radiation, photoprotection with a hat or a broad-spectrum sunscreen should be used daily. Potent topical corticosteroids, intralesional triamcinolone and systemic prednisolone (1 mg/kg) may halt the progression of active CCLE. Antimalarials form the mainstay of treatment in chronic cases refractory to topical steroids. Hydroxychloroquine in a regimen of 200–400 mg/day produces a remission within 3 months in the majority and the dosage can then be tapered gradually. Scarring is permanent, but early treatment may produce a surprising amount of regrowth. Chloroquine may be used as an alternative antimalarial, however there is a greater risk of ocular toxicity. Oral retinoids such as acitretin have been investigated in randomized controlled trials and found to have similar efficacy to antimalarial treatment. Dapsone, thalidomide, vitamin E, oral gold, clofazamine, topical pimecrolimus or a combination of these medications may be useful in refractory cases. Cyclophosphamide, methotrexate and ciclosporin have also been used in severe, rapidly progressive cases where all other treatments have failed.

Pseudopelade of Brocq

Introduction and general description
Pseudopelade of Brocq is an idiopathic, chronic, slowly progressive, patchy cicatricial alopecia that occurs without any evidence of inflammation [3]. It is primarily an atrophy rather than an inflammatory folliculitis. The term pseudopelade was first used by Brocq to distinguish this condition from the 'pelade' of alopecia areata. The French term *pelade* had been in use at that time for more than 200 years and is derived from *pelage* – the fur, hair, wool, etc. of a mammal. In recent times, the term pseudopelade has been used to describe a generic

scarring alopecia, the end result of any number of different pathological processes, and the interchangeable use by some of 'pseudopelade' and 'pseudopelade of Brocq' has led to confusion in the literature.

Pathophysiology [30]

Early lesions may have a light lymphocytic infiltrate around the upper two-thirds of the hair follicle (including the hair bulge) that spares the epidermis and eccrine glands [31]. This infiltrate invades the walls of the follicles and sebaceous glands and eventually destroys the entire pilosebaceous unit. Single hairs may survive within a patch for many years.

Later patches are smooth, soft and slightly depressed, and histological examination reveals only a thin atrophic epidermis overlying a sclerotic dermis containing fibrotic streams extending into the subcutis. There are no inflammatory changes at this stage. These fibrotic streams are follicular 'ghosts'. Arrector pili muscles may be seen inserting into these fibrous remnants of hair follicles. Elastic stains are important in differentiating pseudopelade of Brocq from lichen planus, CCLE and other scarring alopecias. With an acid–alcohol orcein stain, elastic fibres are seen around the lower part of the follicle, whereas in all the other scarring alopecias the scar tissue consists of collagen devoid of elastin.

Clinical features

Pseudopelade of Brocq may occur in both sexes at any age. Most commonly, women over 40 years are affected. Childhood cases are rare. The aetiology and pathogenesis are unknown. The condition is almost always sporadic, but the occurrence in two brothers suggests a genetic factor may be important. There is no doubt that lichen planus can produce a very similar clinical picture and there are some authorities who maintain, on the basis of associated skin lesions and histopathological findings, that 90% of cases of 'pseudopelade' are caused by lichen planus [32].

The alopecia is asymptomatic and is often discovered by chance. It always remains confined to the scalp. The initial patch is often on the vertex but may occur anywhere (Figure 89.40). On examination, the affected patches are smooth, soft and slightly depressed. At an early stage in the development of any individual patch there may be some

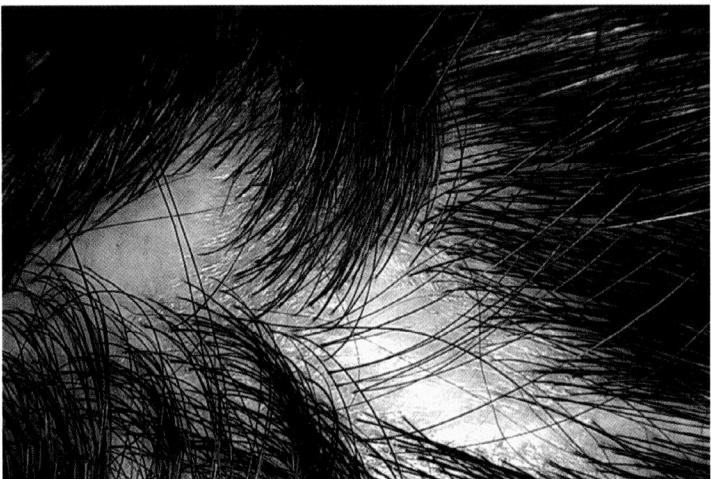

Figure 89.40 Pseudopelade of Brocq.

Box 89.2 Diagnostic criteria for pseudopelade of Brocq

Clinical criteria
- Irregularly defined and confluent patches of alopecia
- Moderate atrophy (late stage)
- Mild perifollicular erythema (early stage)
- Female : male ratio 3 : 1
- Long course (more than 2 years)
- Slow progression with spontaneous termination possible

Histological criteria
- Absence of marked inflammation
- Absence of widespread scarring (best seen with elastin stain)
- Absence of significant follicular plugging
- Absence, or at least a decrease, of sebaceous glands
- Presence of normal epidermis (only occasional atrophy)
- Fibrotic streams into the dermis

Direct immunofluorescence
- Negative (or only weak IgM on sun-exposed skin)

From Braun-Falco *et al*. 1986 [3].

---

erythema. The patches tend to be small and round or oval, but irregular bald patches may be formed by the confluence of many lesions. The hair in the uninvolved scalp is normal, but if the process is active the hairs at the edges of each patch are very easily extracted.

The course is extremely variable. Most often there is slow development over many years of small, round patches of alopecia that ultimately converge to produce larger irregular areas of hair loss. The hair in the uninvolved scalp is normal and the progression is sufficiently slow that even after 15–20 years patients may still be able to arrange their hair in such a way as to conceal the bald areas. The entire process can burn out spontaneously at any stage, leaving behind only relatively small areas of alopecia.

The diagnostic criteria of Braun-Falco *et al*. [3] shown in Box 89.2 and based on the histological criteria of Headington [33] should be fulfilled before this specific diagnosis is made. Cases that do not fulfil these criteria should be diagnosed generically as scarring alopecia.

Management

The alopecia is irreversible and does not respond to topical or intralesional corticosteroids. No treatment is known to arrest progression. If the disfigurement is considerable and no active inflammatory changes are present, autografting from unaffected to scarred scalp may be considered [34], or surgical 'expansion' techniques in severe cases.

Central centrifugal cicatricial alopecia

Synonyms and inclusions
- Follicular degeneration syndrome
- Hot comb alopecia
- Pseudopelade of the central scalp

Introduction and general description

Central centrifugal cicatricial alopecia (CCCA) is a form of scarring alopecia that mainly affects women of African ethnicity [35]. It begins as a single focus of cicatricial alopecia over the vertex of the scalp that gradually spreads outwards in a centrifugal pattern, but remains unifocal. The female to male ratio is approximately 3 : 1. The pathogenesis of CCCA is unknown, but is likely to be multifactorial, with both genetic and environmental factors playing a role. Traumatic hair care practices of various types have long been implicated, and it was originally called hot comb alopecia, but this idea has proved difficult to verify. The name 'follicular degeneration syndrome' was subsequently proposed, and this focuses attention on the histological identification of premature degeneration of the inner root sheath, which is variable and not entirely specific [7]. The current name central centrifugal cicatricial alopecia reflects the clinical appearance of the condition.

Pathophysiology

A superficial perivascular and perifollicular lymphocytic infiltrate is seen in active areas. There is no associated interface change. Sebaceous glands are lost early, but eccrine glands are spared. Premature disintegration of the inner root sheath epithelium has been emphasized, but is not always found. Hair follicle destruction is severe and widespread and leaves prominent concentric lamellar fibrosis. Release of hair fragments into the dermis results in granulomatous inflammation.

Clinical features

The alopecia is slowly progressive and symmetrical. It is predominately centred on the crown with forward progression. It follows a pattern similar to female pattern hair loss. There may be clinical evidence of inflammation at the advancing margin. Pustules and crusting may be found in a minority of patients with rapidly progressive disease or bacterial or fungal superinfection. Although usually asymptomatic, unusual sensations, such as pins and needles, itch or tenderness may occur. The skin is smooth, shiny and non-inflamed and often soft and supple to the touch. The alopecia is incomplete, with a number of hairs remaining within the area of scarring. The condition eventually burns-out spontaneously.

Management

Minimal hair grooming is recommended, but many patients find this difficult. Culture for occult tinea capitis is recommended. Potent topical corticosteroids may arrest progression and doxycycline or minocycline is useful in inflammatory cases with pustules. Olsen postulated an overlap between this condition and FPHL with fibrosis and advocated the use of topical minoxidil. Many patients resort to wearing a suitable hair piece [36].

Folliculitis decalvans and tufted folliculitis

Introduction and general description

Folliculitis decalvans is an uncommon, progressive purulent folliculitis that may involve any hair-bearing site, although it is most common on the vertex of the scalp [37]. Usually there is only a single focus of disease; however, additional foci may evolve over years.

Tufted folliculitis occurs when the infundibular epithelium of damaged follicles heal with the formation of a large, common infundibulum. Up to 30 hairs may emerge through a common dilated pore. Although tufting is most common in folliculitis decalvans, it can also be seen in other forms of cicatricial alopecia including central centrifugal alopecia and pemphigus vulgaris.

Epidemiology

The cause of folliculitis decalvans is still not fully understood. *Staphylococcus aureus* may be grown from the pustules. In the vast majority of people who develop a bacterial pustular folliculitis of the scalp it is transient, resolves with antibiotics and heals without scarring. In some, the folliculitis is more persistent, penetrates more deeply within the hair follicle, tends to recur in the same site after apparently successful treatment with antibiotics, and produces a scarring alopecia. Spread tends to be limited to neighbouring follicles so that the condition presents as a slowly enlarging solitary area of cicatricial alopecia. While additional patches of alopecia may develop over years, it is commonly unifocal.

Failure to confine the *S. aureus* to the infundibulim of the hair follicle and to eradicate it from the isthmus is postulated, possibly due to disruption by bacterial proteases of the protective barrier provided by the inner root sheath. No consistent defect in cell-mediated immunity or inner root sheath keratinization has been identified in patients with folliculitis decalvans.

Familial cases are extremely rare. Douwes *et al.* reported simultaneous occurrence in identical twins, with no identifiable immune abnormality [38].

Pathophysiology [7,33,37]

Histology reveals follicular abscesses, with a dense perifollicular polymorphonuclear infiltrate, and scattered eosinophils and plasma cells in the upper portion of the follicle with partial or complete epithelial disruption. Foreign-body granulomas occur in response to follicular disruption, which is succeeded by scarring. Eventually all that remains of the follicle is extensive fibrosis. Large dilated infundibula surrounded by a zone of fibrosis correspond to areas of polytrichia and tufting.

Clinical features [37]

Men may be affected from adolescence onwards, whereas women tend not to develop this condition until their thirties. It is characterized initially by painful follicular pustules that become crusted. A patch of alopecia then develops from an expanding zone of folliculitis, eventually resulting in a central area of scarring. Unlike CCLE and LPP the scar is indurated and boggy rather than atrophic, at least in the early stages. Multiple hair tufts may be found emerging from a common dilated follicular opening, giving the appearance of doll's hair.

In advanced cases there is usually one, but occasionally more, rounded patches of alopecia over the vertex of the scalp surrounded by crusting and a few follicular pustules. Successive crops of pustules appear and are followed by progressive destruction of the affected follicles and lateral expansion of the alopecia (Figure 89.41). In some cases the folliculitis spreads along the scalp margin in a coronal pattern. The severity of the inflammatory changes fluctuates, but the course is prolonged.

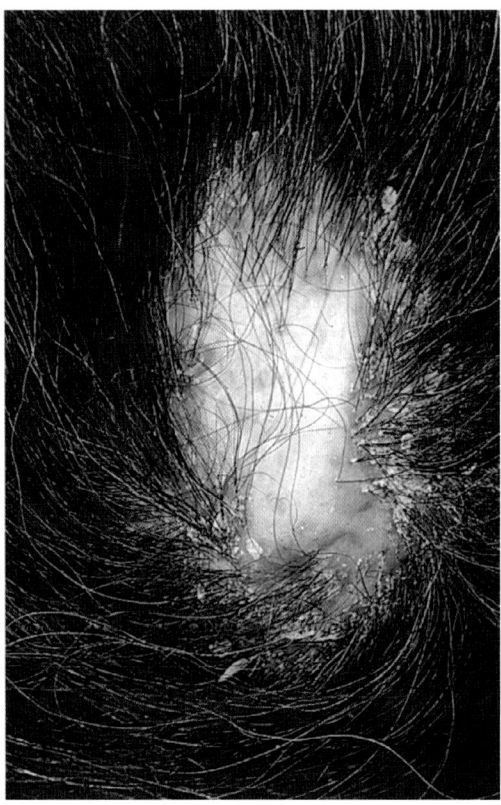

Figure 89.41 Folliculitis decalvans showing active pustulation and scarring.

Tufted folliculitis is a variant of folliculitis decalvans where circumscribed areas of scalp inflammation heal with scarring characterized by tufts of up to 30 hairs emerging from a single orifice (Figure 89.42) [39–41]. The tufts consist of a central anagen hair surrounded by telogen hairs, each arising from independent follicles, converging towards a common dilated follicular infundibulum. Cases in which the tufts were comprised of only anagen hairs have also been described. A scalp biopsy is required to confirm the diagnosis and swabs should be taken of any pustules. Investigation for an underlying defect in cell-mediated immunity is generally unrewarding, and only indicated when there is additional

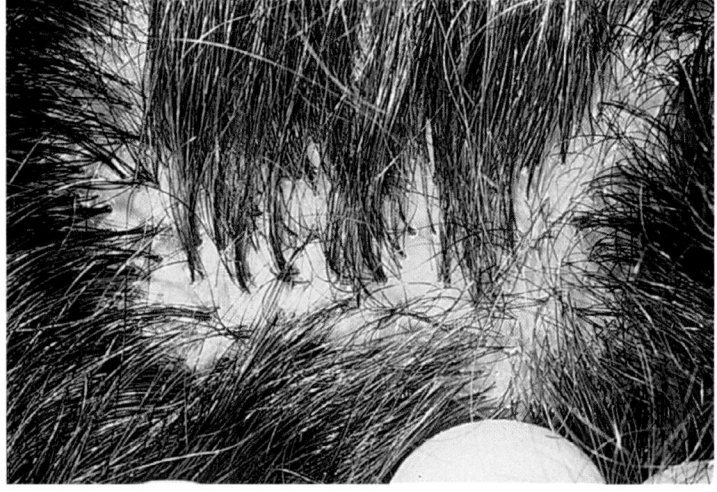

Figure 89.42 Tufted folliculitis.

evidence of impaired immunity. As fungal kerion may mimic folliculitis decalvans, hairs should be plucked for fungal culture and a PAS stain should be performed on the scalp biopsy.

Management [37]

Treatment is mainly aimed at eradicating *S. aureus* from the scalp. Antiseptic shampoos and topical clindamycin are sufficient for mild cases. Prolonged courses of dicloxacillin or flucloxacillin induce remission, but relapse occurs when the antibiotics are stopped. Tetracyclines are also commonly effective. Isotretinoin has been used to alter the follicular environment to make it less suitable for *S. aureus* colonization, but it may increase cutaneous carriage of this organism and make the condition worse. The only treatment shown to induce prolonged remission is rifampicin in a dosage of 300 mg twice daily [42]. This should be given in combination with other antibiotics to prevent the emergence of resistant organisms. Drugs commonly used in combination include clindamycin 300 mg twice daily, fusidic acid 150 mg three times daily, ciprofloxacin, doxycycline or clarithromycin.

Tufting may be reduced by measures directed at reducing the scale, such as the use of tar shampoos and topical keratolytics.

Other measures tried include oral dapsone, oral zinc, laser depilation and surgical excision [5].

Artefactual alopecia

David A. R. de Berker

Cosmetic alopecia

Cosmetic practices can be result in damage to the hair shaft or the scalp. The application of heat (e.g. from heated tongs) to damp hair may cause breakage due to the formation of bubbles in the hair shaft ('bubble hair') [1]. Fracture of hair shafts, which can be extensive, may also be caused by overuse of chemical treatments such as permanent waves and relaxers.

Traction alopecia

Traction alopecia is brought about by hairstyles that impose sustained pulling on the hair roots. The clinical features in the many variants of this syndrome include folliculitis, hair casts [2], reduction in hair density with vellus hairs and sometimes broken hairs in the affected areas, and eventually scarring alopecia. It can be associated with headache, relieved when the hair is loosened [3]. The pattern of the hair loss is often distinctive and reflects the distribution of the traction (Figure 89.43).

Traction alopecia is particularly common in African women. A population study from South Africa reported an incidence of traction alopecia in 17.1% of schoolgirls and 31.7% of adult women. It was more common in women with relaxed hair as well as traction hairstyles such as braiding [4,5]. The hair loss commonly begins in the temporal regions and in front of and above the ears, but may involve other parts of the scalp, particularly where 'corn row' patterns are adopted (Figure 89.43). Problems typically start in childhood, where they may initially be reversible [6]. A degree of temporal thinning may also be part of a genetic hair pattern seen in those with no traction.

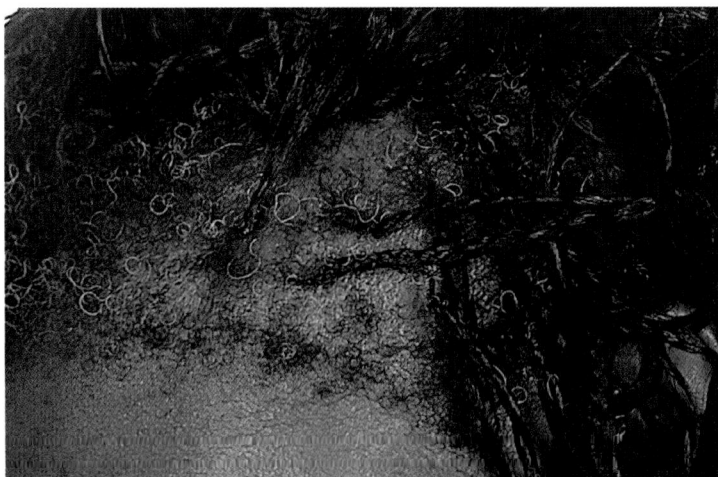

Figure 89.43 Traction alopecia from braiding.

Pony tails, hair twisting in Sikh boys (Figure 89.44) [7] and tight scarf styles can all result in hair loss [8].

Management

In its early stages traction alopecia may be reversible. The patient, or parents of affected children, need to be educated to adopt hairstyles that do not pull the hair tight [9]. Where there is inflammation, mild steroids can be helpful, but are not a substitute for a non-traction hairstyle. Once traction alopecia is established and follicles have been lost, the hair loss becomes permanent.

Medical trauma hair loss

There are instances where medical intervention may result in scalp trauma and be implicated in scarring alopecia. Scalp electrodes or infusion [10] or forceps delivery in the neonate can result in trauma. Uterine rings have also been reported as causes of infant scalp problems [11]. Marks from such interventions need to be distinguished from aplasia cutis which can sometimes be the underlying diagnosis [12].

Interventions in adulthood, directly through scalp and brain surgery or indirectly though local embolization procedures, can result in scarring. Adler *et al.* described a case in which ischaemic

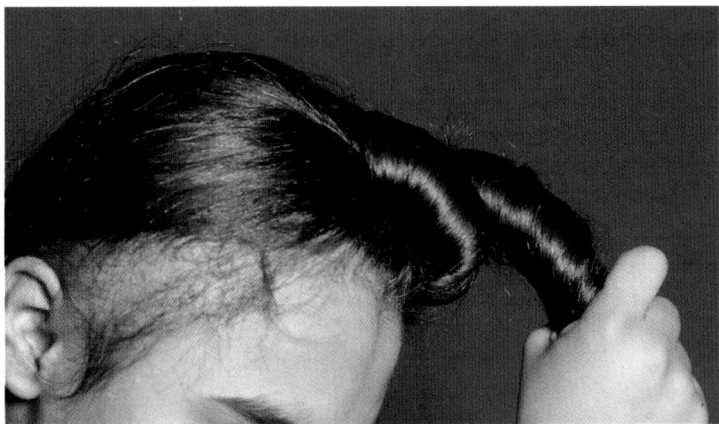

Figure 89.44 Traction alopecia in a Sikh boy.

necrosis of the occipital scalp occurred following embolization and surgery for a large convexity meningioma [13].

Pressure ischaemia can occur during intensive care or gynaecological surgery in the Trendelenburg position [14]. In one large clinic, over a period of 3 years, 60 cases of occipital pressure alopecia were observed after open-heart surgery [15]. In 29 of these cases, the hair loss was permanent. Temporary alopecia followed prolonged pressure on the scalp by a foam rubber ring used to prevent such an occurrence [16].

Trichotillomania

Introduction and general description

Trichotillomania is a behavioural disorder characterized by compulsive hair pulling. It presents as a pattern of hair loss, often bizarre, with no clear biological or overt traumatic explanation [1]. Compulsive hair rubbing (trichoteiromania [2]) and hair cutting (trichotemnomania [3]) fall into the same general category. See also Chapter 86.

Epidemiology and psychopathology

Trichotillomania occurs in two main forms. In infants and young children it is usually a habit akin to thumb-sucking and nail-biting. It seems slightly more common in boys and usually resolves spontaneously or with minimal treatment. Parents who have not noticed hair-pulling behaviour in their offspring may deny the diagnosis. In older age groups (adolescents and adults) trichotillomania is seen predominantly in females, with women outnumbering men by up to 7 : 1, and evidence of some form of psychological or behavioural stress is often apparent [4]. The American Psychiatric Association classifies trichotillomania as an impulse control disorder, in which there is an irresistible desire to pull out the hair. This process results in an instant release of tension and sense of relief. The diagnostic criteria are given in the fourth edition of the *Diagnostic and Statistical Manual of Mental Disorders* (DSM-IV), and are listed in Box 89.3, although not all patients with trichotillomania fit these criteria.

Trichotillomania shares some features of obsessive–compulsive disorder (OCD), but some authorities consider it may be the result of a number of psychopathologies including OCD, personality

---

Box 89.3 DSM-IV criteria for trichotillomania

- Recurrent pulling out of one's hair resulting in noticeable hair loss
- An increasing sense of tension immediately before pulling out the hair or when attempting to resist the behaviour
- Pleasure, gratification or relief when pulling out the hair
- The disturbance is not better accounted for by another mental disorder and is not due to a general medical condition (e.g. a dermatological condition)
- The disturbance causes clinically significant distress or impairment in social, occupational or other important areas of functioning

disorders, body dysmorphophobic disorders, mental retardation and psychosis. There is an extensive psychiatric literature on trichotillomania, but this may be biased because psychiatric help is likely to be sought only in those patients who accept that it is a self-inflicted problem. This is not true of all patients presenting to dermatologists.

Pathophysiology

Microscopy may be undertaken of the hair or of a scalp biopsy. Hairs may be of different length in an affected area. They may be broken, where trauma has snapped the shaft, or be tapered, where trauma is in the form of plucking. The scalp itself is usually clinically normal except in the instances where the trauma is rubbing or scratching. In these instances there are often scalp symptoms and the problem may present primarily as a scalp dermatosis – even if it is wholly artefactual. Rubbing can also lead to hair breakage or interfere with the normal anagen cycle without specifically altering the hair shaft.

Dermoscopy of the scalp may help differentiate between trichotillomania and alopecia areata, where follicular orifices may appear as yellow dots [5].

Scalp histology varies according to the severity and duration of the hair plucking. Numerous empty canals are the most consistent feature. Some follicles are severely damaged; there are clefts in the hair matrix, the follicular epithelium is separated from the connective tissue sheath, and there are intraepithelial and perifollicular haemorrhages and intrafollicular pigment casts (Figure 89.45) [6]. Injured follicles may form only soft twisted hairs – a process that has been described as a separate entity under the name of trichomalacia [7]. Many follicles are in catagen, with very few or no follicles in telogen. Some dilated follicular infundibula contain horny plugs [8].

Clinical features

In young children, the hair-pulling tic develops gradually and unconsciously. Hair is plucked most frequently from one frontopa-

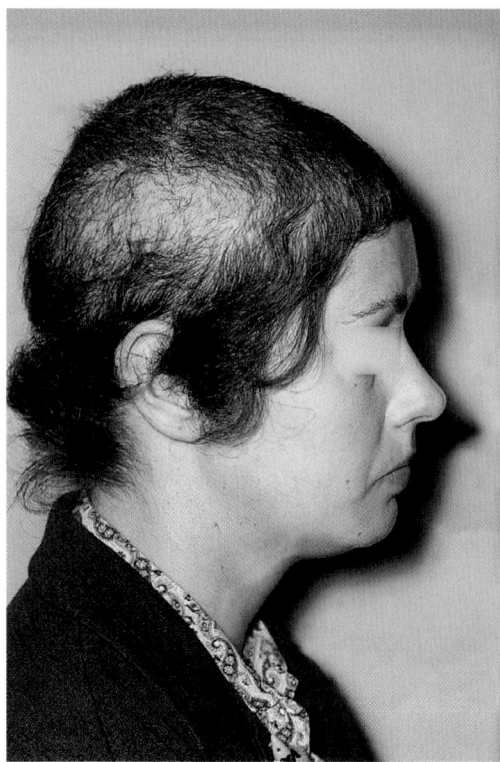

Figure 89.46 Trichotillomania showing a characteristic 'tonsure' pattern with the scalp margin hair spared.

rietal region. This results in a patch of hair loss, often in a bizarre or angular pattern, in which the hairs are twisted and broken at various distances from the clinically normal scalp. Older patients present with an area of scalp on which the hair has been reduced to coarse stubble uniformly, 2.5–3 mm long. The plucked area may be asymmetrical or cover the entire scalp apart from the margin (Figure 89.46). It is unusual for hair to be lost completely within the affected area (in contrast with alopecia areata). The scalp skin appears normal. Over time the extent of hair loss can vary, and hair growth may recover temporarily.

Hair in sites other than the scalp can also be affected, such as eyelashes, eyebrows and beard. Exceptionally, the patient may pluck hair also, or only, from other regions of the body, such as the mons pubis and perianal region.

A hairball (trichobezoar) is a rare accompaniment of trichotillomania in those who also eat the plucked hair (trichophagia) [9].

Differential diagnosis

The minor form in young children can be confused with ringworm or with alopecia areata. In ringworm, the texture of the infected hairs is abnormal and the scalp surface may be scaly. Alopecia areata may be difficult to exclude with certainty at the first examination, but the course of the condition usually establishes the correct diagnosis. Unlike alopecia areata, it is unusual for hair to be lost completely in trichotillomania and, in contrast with exclamation mark hairs, the broken hairs of trichotillomania are firmly anchored in the scalp. Where doubt remains dermoscopy [5] or a skin biopsy will usually establish the correct diagnosis. However, there are reports of the coexistence of alopecia areata and trichotillomania [4,10]. In rare cases, genetic disorders characterized by

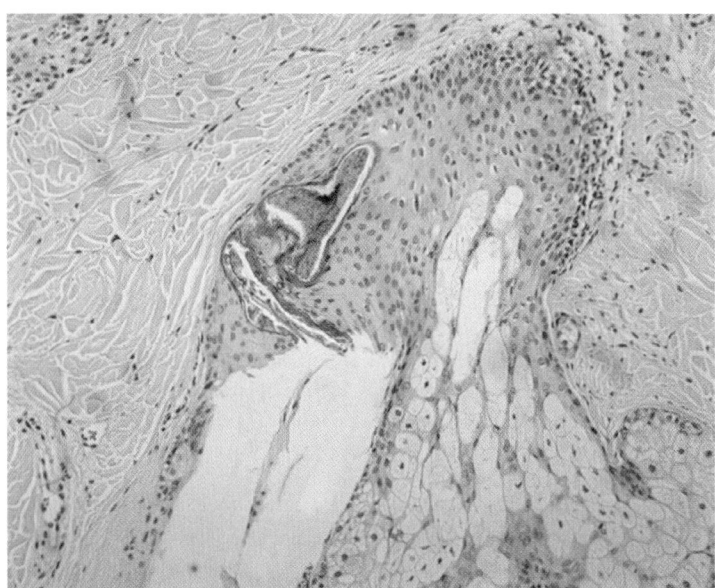

Figure 89.45 Histology of trichotillomania showing fragmentation of the hair shaft.

increased hair fragility, such as monilethrix, may resemble trichotillomania and should be excluded by hair microscopy.

Management

The establishment of a relationship between the physician and the patient, or with the parents of an affected child, is an important step in the management of trichotillomania. A confident diagnosis is essential, but this is not always easy and may require observation over time and sometimes a scalp biopsy. The habit tic in young children is often self-limiting, but input from a paediatric psychologist can be very helpful. Trichotillomania in adolescents and adults is a different proposition, and can be intractable [11]. Patients with insight should be referred to a psychiatrist or clinical psychologist. A number of psychotherapeutic approaches have been used, particularly behavioural therapy aimed at habit reversal, and pharmacotherapy using clomipramine or selective serotonin-reuptake inhibitors (SSRIs), but none is uniformly successful. A systematic review of published studies found that habit-reversal therapy is superior to drug treatment [12]. Clomipramine was more effective than placebo but there was no convincing benefit from treatment with SSRIs. A Cochrane review of pharmacotherapies reported than no particular medication class definitively demonstrated efficacy in trichotillomania but there was some evidence of a treatment effect from small trials for clomipramine, olanzapine and the glutaminergic agent *N*-acetylcysteine (NAC) [13]. A randomized controlled trial of NAC in adults with trichotillomania reported improvement in 56% of subjects taking NAC compared with 9% on placebo [14]. However, a trial of NAC in children with trichotillomania found no benefit [15].

Some patients are helped by contact with fellow sufferers, and there are several patient support groups and internet websites devoted to trichotillomania. Patients who fail to admit the self-inflicted nature of the hair loss present particular difficulties, as they are unlikely to accept psychiatric referral and, as with dermatitis artefacta, a confrontational approach will probably be unsuccessful. Management should be aimed at helping the patient recognize the cause for themselves. This can be a long and slow process requiring skill and empathy on the part of the physician.

Resources

Patient resources

NHS Choices, trichotiomania information sheet: http://www.nhs.uk/conditions/trichotillomania/Pages/introduction.aspx.

Trichotillomania Support Online: http://www.trichotillomania.co.uk. (Both last accessed April 2015.)

Infections

Andrew G. Messenger

Tinea capitis

See Chapter 32.

Infestations

See Chapter 34.

Syphilis

Hair loss occurs in approximately 4% of cases of secondary syphilis and may be the presenting feature [1,2]. The hair loss typically has a moth-eaten appearance but may be diffuse in nature [3]. Other features of secondary syphilis are present in most cases, particularly lymph node enlargement and hepatomegaly, but hair loss has been reported as the only sign of the disease [4]. Histological features include an increase in catagen and telogen forms, and a peribulbar lymphocytic infiltrate, similar to the changes seen in alopecia areata [3]. Additional features in syphilis include lymphocytic infiltration of the isthmus region, parabulbar lymphoid aggregates and the presence of plasma cells within the infiltrate.

The serpiginous nodulosquamous syphilide of tertiary syphilis may affect the scalp and the syphilitic gumma is a cause of scarring alopecia.

Human immunodeficiency virus infection

A variety of alterations in hair growth have been described in patients with HIV infection (see Chapter 31). Telogen effluvium is a common cause of hair loss [5]. Causes include chronic HIV-1 infection itself, secondary infections, nutritional deficiencies and drugs. Hair loss on the body as well as the scalp has been reported with several antiretroviral drugs, particularly indinavir [6] and other protease inhibitors. There are also reports of alopecia areata occurring in patients with HIV infection [7–9].

There are several reports of hypertrichosis of the eyelashes (eyelash trichomegaly) in HIV infection [9–11]. The cause of this striking and unusual feature is not known. It is usually associated with advanced disease and has been noted to regress with antiretroviral treatment [11].

Straightening of the hair is a common feature of HIV infection in black patients [12].

Various forms of folliculitis are seen in HIV infection, including acneform eruptions, staphylococcal folliculitis and eosinophilic pustular folliculitis.

Leprosy

A loss of eyebrow and body hair may occur in lepromatous leprosy but the scalp is rarely involved.

Trichodysplasia spinulosa

This rare disease is due to a novel human polyomavirus (13,14,15,16,17). It has been reported mainly in patients receiving immunosuppressive drugs. It has also been described in patients with HIV infection and in lupus erythematosus (see Chapter 87). It presents as small, skin-coloured, follicular papules. These occur most commonly on the nose and central face although other sites elsewhere on the skin may also be involved (Figure 89.47). The histopathology is distinctive, showing aberrant keratinization of the inner root sheath (Figure 89.48). Inner root sheath cells contain viral inclusions that are positive for polyomavirus on immunohistochemistry. The condition responds to treatment with topical cidofovir.

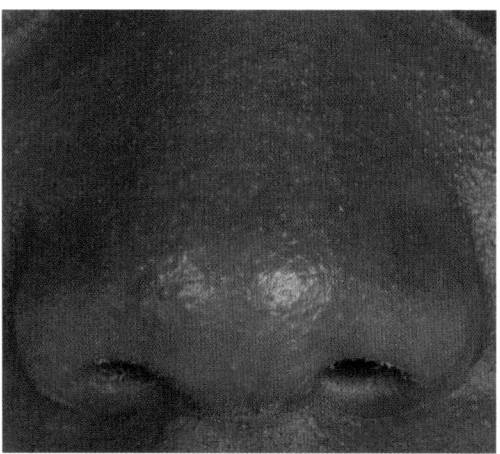

Figure 89.47 Trichodysplasia spinulosa.

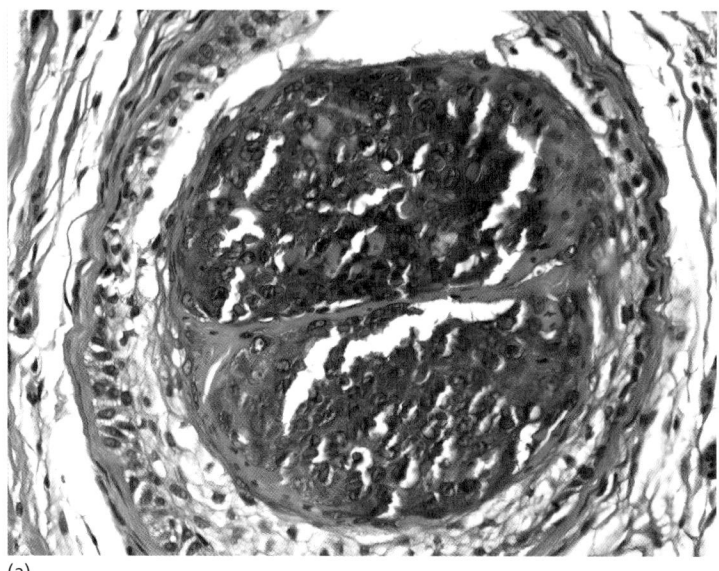

(a)

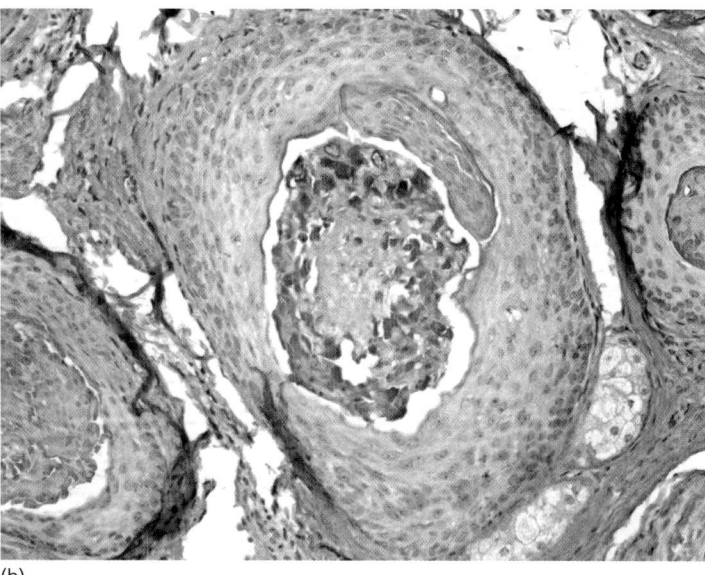

(b)

Figure 89.48 Trichodysplasia spinulosa histopathology. (a) Aberrant keratinization of the inner root sheath. (b) Positive immunohistochemical staining for polyomavirus in the inner root sheath. (Courtesy of Dr Misha Rosenbach and Dr Karolyn A. Wanat.)

OTHER DISORDERS OF HAIR GROWTH

Andrew G. Messenger

Chemotherapy alopecia

Introduction and general description
Alopecia is a common and often distressing complication of anti-mitotic chemotherapy. Hair shedding typically occurs within 1–3 weeks and is complete within 1–2 months after the initiation of chemotherapy. In most cases hair loss is temporary and recovers fully within a period of months following cessation of the causative insult [1]. A wide variety of anticancer drugs will cause hair loss with frequencies differing for the four major classes – more than 80% for antimicrotubule agents (e.g. paclitaxel), 60–100% for topoisomerase inhibitors (e.g.)doxorubicin), more than 60% for alkylating agents (e.g. cyclophosphamide) and 10–20% for antimetabolites (e.g. 5-fluorouracil) (Table 89.4). The risk of chemotherapy alopecia is also related to the particular therapeutic protocol and is greater if treatment combines two or more antimitotic agents [2].

Pathophysiology
The intense cell proliferation in the anagen hair bulb means that hair growth is particularly vulnerable to antimitotic medication. Anagen is abruptly terminated leading to shedding of dystrophic or broken hairs (anagen effluvium). Hairs that survive may show constrictions of the shaft [3]. A recent study has also shown an increase in telogen hairs, possibly indicating that the response of the follicle is determined by its stage in anagen at the time of the insult [1].

Clinical features
Hair loss is acute, diffuse and associated with a large increase in hair shedding. It varies in degree with different chemotherapy regimens and between patients receiving the same regimen.

Management
Various methods have been employed to prevent the development of chemotherapy alopecia. The most widely used is scalp cooling

Table 89.4 Drugs causing chemotherapy alopecia.

Agents that usually cause hair loss	Agents that sometimes cause hair loss	Agents that uncommonly cause hair loss
Cyclophosphamide	Amsacrine	Carboplatin
Daunorubicin	Bleomycin	Capecitabine
Docetaxel	Busulphan	Carmustine
Doxorubicin	Cytarabine	Cisplatin
Epirubicin	5-Fluorouracil	Fludarabine
Etoposide	Gemcitabine	Methotrexate
Ifosphamide	Lomustine	Mitomycin C
Irinotecan	Melphalan	Mitroxantrone
Paclitaxel	Thiotepa	Procarbazine
Topotecan	Vinblastine	Raltritrexate
Vindesine	Vincristine	6-Marcaptopurine
Vinorelbine		Streptozotocin

From Trueb 2007 [2].

using ice packs or custom-designed cooling caps. The results are variable but there is good evidence for efficacy in some patients [4]. Concern that scalp cooling increases the risk of scalp metastases is probably unfounded [5].

One small trial suggested that topical minoxidil hastens recovery from chemotherapy alopecia [6].

Wigs or other means of disguising hair loss may be needed if hair loss is extensive.

Permanent chemotherapy alopecia

Although chemotherapy alopecia is usually reversible this is not always the case. Persistent or permanent hair loss is particularly associated with conditioning regimens for bone marrow transplantation and with taxane therapy for breast cancer.

Bone marrow transplantation. Permanent alopecia following conditioning treatments for bone marrow transplantation most commonly affects scalp hair, but loss of eyelashes, eyebrows, axillary and pubic hair has been reported [7]. Regimens incorporating busulphan, a drug that is widely used in patients undergoing allogeneic or autologous bone marrow transplantation, seem most likely to cause permanent alopecia [7,8,9,10]. The extent of the alopecia appears to be dose related, but there is no clear threshold over which all patients treated with busulphan will develop permanent alopecia.

Incomplete scalp hair regrowth and permanent hair loss has also been reported in bone marrow transplant patients receiving high-dose chemotherapy with combination therapy of cyclophosphamide, carboplatin and thiotepa [11]. Permanent hair loss was associated with having had more than one course of treatment. Graft-versus-host disease may be a contributory factor [12].

Taxane therapy. Persistent hair loss may occur following treatment of breast cancer with taxane drugs (paclitaxel, docetaxel) [13]. Clinically and histologically this resembles severe female pattern hair loss [14,15].

Antioestrogen drugs

Hair loss is listed as a side effect of the oestrogen receptor antagonist tamoxifen and of aromatase inhibitors used in the treatment of breast cancer. A meta-analysis of trials of various endocrine therapies for cancer concluded that 6.4% of patients taking tamoxifen developed hair loss as a result of treatment [16]. However, a detailed phototrichogram study found no change in hair growth parameters in patients taking tamoxifen [1] and it is not yet clear whether hair loss is a genuine side effect of antioestrogen drugs or just reflects the relatively high frequency of diffuse hair loss that occurs naturally in the relevant age group.

Circumscribed alopecia of congenital origin

The differential diagnosis of circumscribed alopecia of congenital origin presents little difficulty if a reliable history is available [1,2]. Without it, alopecia areata and the acquired cicatricial alopecias must be considered.

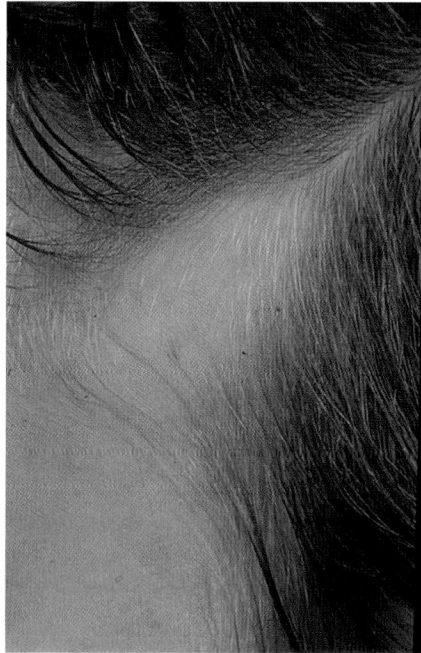

Figure 89.49 Triangular alopecia.

Sebaceous naevus (organoid naevus). Sebaceous naevus usually presents in childhood as a hairless patch on the scalp, often in a linear configuration. The affected skin may have a yellowish hue. See Chapter 75.

Aplasia cutis. Aplasia cutis is a heterogenous group of conditions characterized by the localized absence of a portion of skin at birth. It most commonly presents as a single patch on the scalp vertex but lesions may be multiple and other parts of the skin may be involved. At birth the affected skin may be superficially or deeply ulcerated or may have healed leaving an atrophic scar. Aplasia cutis is usually an isolated defect but it can be associated with a variety of malformation syndromes. See Chapter 75.

Sutural alopecia. Multiple patches of hair loss overlying the cranial sutures are a feature of the Hallermann–Streiff syndrome, in which dysmorphic facies, skeletal anomalies, microphthalmia, congenital cataract and hypodontia are also found.

Triangular alopecia. This usually presents during childhood – although often referred to as congenital it is often not noticed at birth [3,4,5]. In the usual form, a triangular area overlying the frontotemporal suture just inside the anterior hair line, and with its base directed forwards, is completely bald or covered by sparse vellus hairs (Figure 89.49). It may be unilateral or bilateral. The histology shows normal vellus follicles. Triangular alopecia can be treated surgically, either by simple excision or by hair transplantation.

ABNORMALITIES OF THE HAIR SHAFT

David A. R. de Berker

Structural defects of the hair shaft may be sufficient in degree to cause significant cosmetic disability, or they may render the hair abnormally susceptible to injury by minor degrees of trauma

Table 89.5 Terms used to define hair shaft pathology.

Term	Meaning	Associations
Trichorrhexis nodosa (Figure 89.56a)	A circumferential break in the hair cuticle, with cortical fibres extruding through the fracture	Physical and chemical trauma to the hair elicits this appearance at a threshold dependent upon the age and fragility of the hair; seen in normal hair
Brush end	When a trichorrhexis node breaks it leaves the proximal end looking like a chimney sweep's brush	As above
Trichoclasis	A 'greenstick' fracture of the hair, where the cuticle is partly stripped in continuity with the fracture	Trauma and moderate fragility
Trichoptilosis	Split ends – in continuity with the tip	Common outcome of cumulative brushing and chemical trauma
Circle hairs	Circle and spiral hairs on the thigh and abdomen; usually trapped beneath the stratum corneum; in males	Normal in more hirsute males; not the same as scurvy
Trichomalacia	Softened hair residue with keratin in open scalp follicular orifice	Trichotillomania
Trichoschisis	Clean transverse fracture across the hair	Typically associated with sulphur-deficient hair of trichothiodystrophy
Pohl–Pinkus constriction	Zone of constriction within the hair shaft, possibly due to transient physiological compromise of hair growth; comparable with a Beau line	Period of ill health or cytotoxic medication, where not sufficient to precipitate telogen effluvium or anagen effluvium
Tapered hairs	The tip of a hair that has been generated *de novo* at the commencement of anagen will be tapered	Characteristic of hair that is regrowing after shedding or of hair with a short anagen phase, e.g. eyebrow
Bayonet hair	Slight kink in hair within 1–2 mm of tapered tip	Variant of normal
Trichonodosis	Knots in hair	Usually a simple reef knot, seen where hair is rubbed or where the hair is markedly curly and predisposed to knotting; can contribute to fragility; most common in African hair
Bubble hair (Figure 89.64)	Bubbles within the hair shaft	Arises due to extreme heat or singeing of hair; attributed to leaning over a fire, or hot hair treatments where thermostatic controls are faulty
Hair casts	Keratin cylinders moving freely on the proximal hair shaft and arising from the upper part of the internal root sheath	May be associated with scaling scalp conditions or hair styling where there is tension on the hair; sometimes referred to as 'pseudonits'
Tiger tail (Figure 89.57)	Light and dark transverse stripes on a hair shaft when viewed with cross-polarization, preferably in histological medium	Sulphur-deficient hair has a weakened cortex that loses its longitudinal rigidity and tends to become wavy; this alters light polarization characteristics
Nit	The egg case of a head louse adherent to the shaft	The egg case may be empty or still contain the louse nymph; only nits proximal on the shaft are likely to represent active infestation, which needs to be confirmed by identification of a live head louse
Pili torti (Figure 89.52)	Twisting of hair through 180° within the long axis of the hair	Although this is a sign, it is sometimes used as a diagnosis; it is associated with the specific diagnosis of Menkes syndrome, but also presents as an isolated autosomal dominant condition

(excessive weathering). Hair microscopy can be a useful part of clinical assessment in some situations [1], including a range of hereditary or acquired metabolic disorders, where the hair shaft can sometimes provide clues to the diagnosis (Table 89.5) [2,3]. Dermoscopy (10×) [4] and videodermoscopy (20× to 160×) [5] may be useful screening tools within the clinic for scalp and hair shaft evaluation as a preliminary to hair sampling and formal microscopy. A measure of the rate and range of proteins enzymically eluted from hair has been suggested as a means of quantifying hair shaft damage both in cosmetic and genetically determined weathering [6]. It is common to classify hair shaft defects into those that are due to shaft fragility and those that are not. This classification will be used in this section.

STRUCTURAL DEFECTS WITH INCREASED FRAGILITY

Monilethrix

Synonyms and inclusions
• Beaded hair

Introduction and general description
Smith initially called this condition as 'a rare nodose condition of the hair' [7]. Radcliffe Crocker subsequently suggested the term monilethrix. Nevertheless, some early reports, and even some more recent ones, confuse monilethrix with other shaft defects (e.g. trichorrhexis nodosa) when 'weathering' is severe.

Pathophysiology
The hair shaft is beaded and breaks easily (Figure 89.50). Elliptical nodes 0.7–1 mm apart, are separated by narrower internodes with a form resembling the body and neck of a skittle. The widths of the nodes and the distances between them vary between the hairs of an individual and between members of the same family [8]. The nodes and some of the internodes show a normal imbricated scale pattern, but most internodes show longitudinal ridging. True monilethrix must be distinguished from pseudomonilethrix, an artefact produced by tweezers or compressing overlapping hairs between two glass slides.

Histologically, the follicle shows wide and narrow zones corresponding to the nodes and internodes. Attempts have been made to investigate the mechanism of node formation and to relate it to the diurnal rate of hair growth, but with no overall conclusion. Intermittent administration of an antimitotic agent can give rise to zones of constriction alternating with zones of normal diameter.

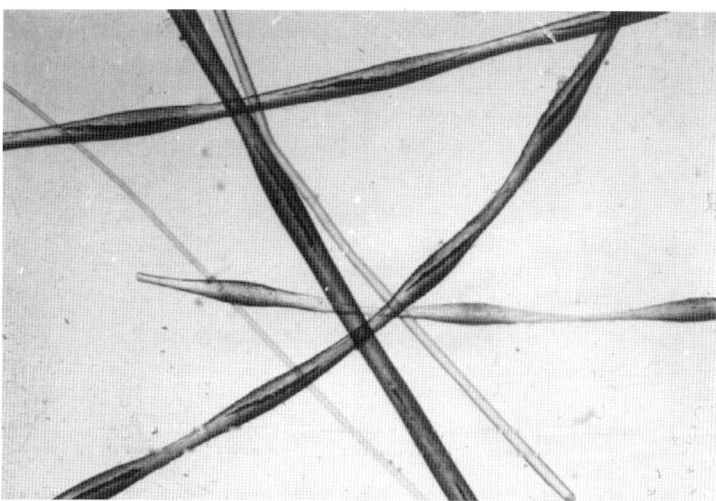

Figure 89.50 Monilethrix with swollen (node) and narrow (internode) fluctuations in the hair bore.

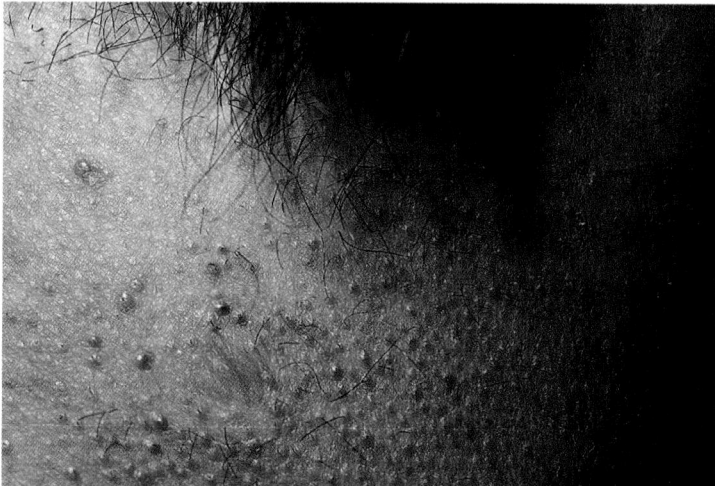

Figure 89.51 Monilethrix on the nape of the neck showing follicular keratoses and short, broken hairs.

Clinical features

Monilethrix shows considerable variation in age of onset, severity, expression within a family and course. Hair loss or broken hair is accompanied by follicular keratoses most commonly on the nape and occiput (Figure 89.51). In some cases, the eyebrows and eyelashes, pubic and axillary hair and general body hair may be affected.

In many patients, the condition persists with little change throughout life. Spontaneous improvement or complete recovery has occurred, including during pregnancy and with some medications.

Pili torti

Synonyms and inclusions
• Twisted hair

Introduction and general description

In pili torti the hairs are flattened and at irregular intervals completely rotated through 180° around their long axis (Figure 89.52a).

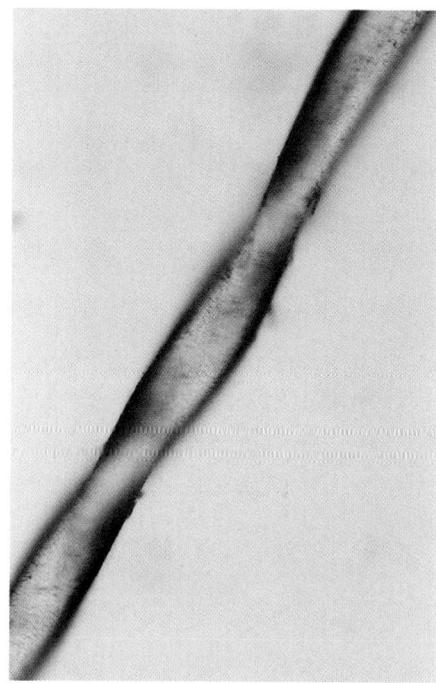

(a)

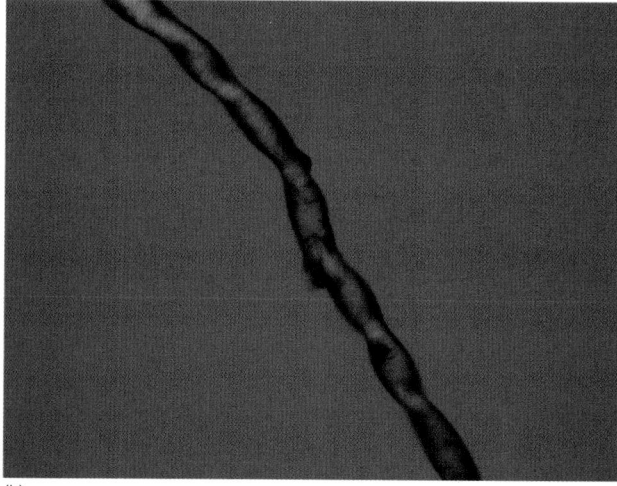

(b)

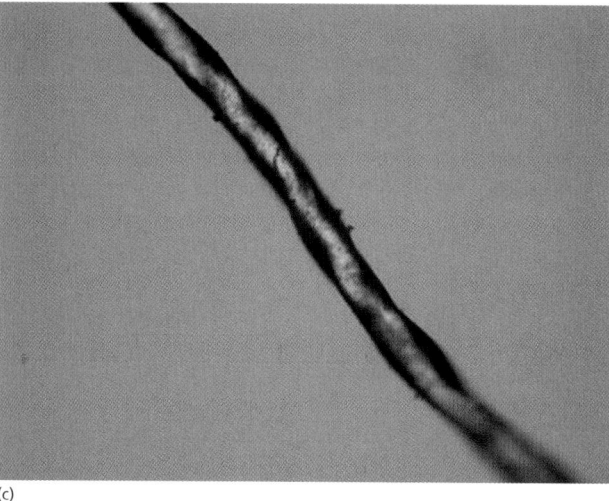

(c)

Figure 89.52 Pili torti. (a) Light micrograph showing 180° twists. (b) A 6-month-old boy with Menkes syndrome. (c) A 27-year-old woman with no personal or family history of associated disorders.

Table 89.6 Diseases where pili torti and other twisted hair abnormalities are found.

Name	Genetics	Mechanism	Features
Pili torti, isolated [9]	Both dominant and recessive reported	Not known	Pili torti, fragile hair, sometimes with hypoplastic dental enamel; could be female carrier of Menkes syndrome
Menkes syndrome [**10**]	X-linked recessive carried on Xq12-q13	Mutation in gene encoding the Cu^{2+}-transporting ATPase, α protein	Blond fine hair in boys, with poor neonatal development, evolving into status epilepticus and brain damage as cumulative copper metabolism damage progresses
Female carrier of Menkes syndrome	As above	As above	Pili torti in 43% of obligate female carriers
Björnstad syndrome [11,69]	Autosomal recessive disease due to mutation in *BC1SL* gene on 2q33	Altered function of mitochondrial respirasome protein, in turn affecting transmission of inner ear neurosensory hair responses	Neurosensory deafness with hypogonadism in some instances (Crandall syndrome)
Twisted hairs – poor evidence for true pili torti			
Bazex syndrome [70,71]	X-linked dominant Xq24-q27	Possible loss of efficacy of a DNA repair protein produced by the *UBE2A* gene	Hypotrichosis, follicular atrophoderma and multiple basal cell neoplasms; hypohidrosis also reported
Pseudomonilethrix [72]	Putative dominant inheritance	Probably an artefact in hair plucking or twisting	Intermittent nodes and internodes in hair shafts that mimic monilethrix, but may be in the form of a flattened spiral
Trichothiodystrophy [73]	Autosomal recessive 19q13.2-q13.3, 6p25.3, 2q21	Transcription syndrome with defects in transcription factors II H and possibly others	Multiple phenotypes and subtypes, with flattened fragile hair that can twist; common factor is sulphur deficiency in hair amino acid constituents
Anorexia nervosa [74]	Acquired	May be mediated through lack of vitamin C	Wiry hair
Retinoid hair [41,75]	Acquired	Secondary to systemic retinoid therapy	Wiry hair with hair loss and dry skin
Scarring alopecia [76]	Acquired	Secondary to scarring inflammation, most common with folliculitis decalvans	Wiry hair at the margins of active scarring folliculitis
Tuberous sclerosis complex [77]	Autosomal dominant	16p13.3, 12q14, 9q34	Corkscrew hairs, multiple hamartomas, renal cysts and epilepsy

This rotation runs for three to five twists before the shaft normalises [9]. True pili torti of Menkes syndrome and the isolated expression of the abnormality in an otherwise unaffected person, demonstrate the same distinct twisting (Figure 89.52b, c). Scanning electron microscopy has made it clear that twisted hairs occur in many different forms, and that not all twisted hairs are pili torti. Occasional twists of varying angles should not be taken to be this distinctive, genetically 'fixed' abnormality of pili torti – many dystrophies and distortions of the follicular zone of keratinization will vary the hair shaft 'bore', sometimes showing less than 180° irregular twists. Screening *in vivo* for abnormal hairs or where to sample scalp hair can be done with dermoscopy. However, in Menkes disease the hair is often so sparse as to be difficult to sample and is best assessed with light microscopy.

There are a number of syndromes in which twisted hair is a feature (Table 89.6) (see Chapter 68). Menkes syndrome, Björnstad syndrome with sensorineural deafness and Crandall syndrome are all associated with pili torti [10,11,12]. Other diagnoses found in the literature are probably erroneous and based on a loose interpretation of the term pili torti. The spiral is either too low-pitched, a single twist or around an axis that is not within the long axis of the hair and hence represents a helix. Twist and partial twists of this kind can be seen in a range of syndromes and as a side effect of oral retinoids.

Epidemiology
In those cases in which classic pili torti of early onset appears to have occurred as an isolated defect, examples suggesting autosomal dominant and recessive inheritance can be found.

Pathophysiology
The earlier reports emphasized that the affected hairs were flattened and twisted through 180° around their long axis at irregular intervals along the shaft. Hairs can manifest fragility with the shape making them more vulnerable to the effects of weathering.

Clinical features
The hair may be normal at birth and change in the first few months. There is a wide variation from case to case in the fragility of the hair, and hence in the clinical picture. Affected hairs are brittle and may break off at a length of 5 cm or less, or grow longer in areas of the scalp less subject to trauma. There may therefore be only short, coarse stubble over the whole scalp or there may be circumscribed baldness, irregularly patchy or occipital. Affected hairs have a spangled appearance in reflected light. The cosmetic appearance of isolated pili torti can improve greatly with transition from childhood to early adulthood.

Netherton syndrome

Synonyms and inclusions
• Bamboo hair

Introduction and general description
Netherton observed bamboo-like nodes in the fragile hairs of a girl with 'erythematous scaly dermatitis' [13]. Ichthyosis linearis circumflexa (ILC) and 'bamboo hairs' (trichorrhexis invaginata) (Figure 89.53) are two features of Netherton syndrome, which is characterized by these features coupled with atopy, recurrent skin infections and a predisposition to skin malignancy (see Chapter 65). Most cases of Netherton syndrome have had ILC but some have ichthyosis vulgaris or both conditions, or ichthyosiform erythroderma [14]. Features of ILC may be seen in variants of psoriasis. It is controversial as to whether it occurs as an isolated disease in the absence of Netherton syndrome, or whether it is the fluctuating prevalence of the hair shaft changes that leads to difficulty in detecting both characteristics at the same time in some patients.

Netherton syndrome results in fragile hair. Samples should be cut at the scalp surface, thus reducing the chance that the hair will break at the point of diagnostic interest and making diagnosis more difficult. Light microscopy is the best tool for detecting features of Netherton syndrome in hair. However, an individual may have multiple hairs with characteristic changes in one sample and then no features in another sample taken some months later.

Because of this it is important that samples of at least 100 hairs are carefully examined on several occasions before a definite negative is asserted. Alternatively, finding a single trichorrhexis invaginata node in a single hair is a conclusive positive (Figure 89.54).

To assess such large numbers of hairs it is necessary to use a light microscope, as electron microscopy will only allow assessment of small lengths of a small number of hairs. Detail of the surface features is enhanced using partially crossed polarizing filters; the cortical anatomy of the hair is revealed if the hair is prepared on a slide in histological mounting medium. Scanning electron microscopy of the hair shafts shows focal defects that predispose to the development of torsion nodules, invaginated nodules (trichorrhexis invaginata) and trichorrhexis nodosa.

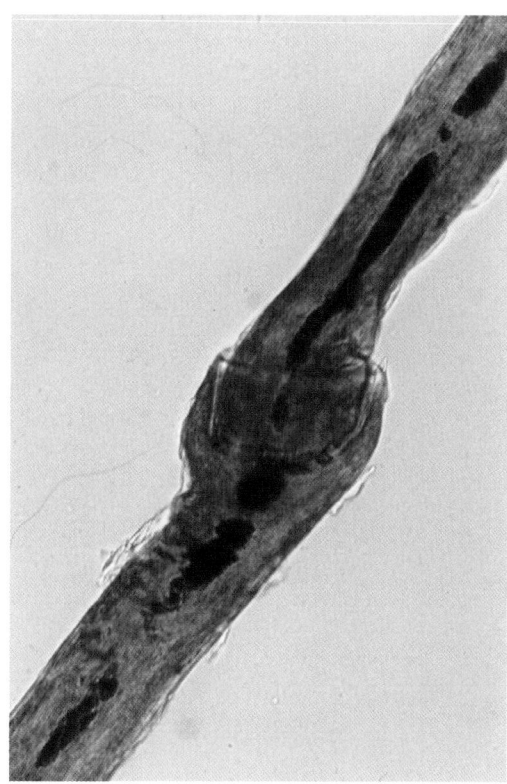

Figure 89.53 Trichorrhexis invaginata in Netherton syndrome.

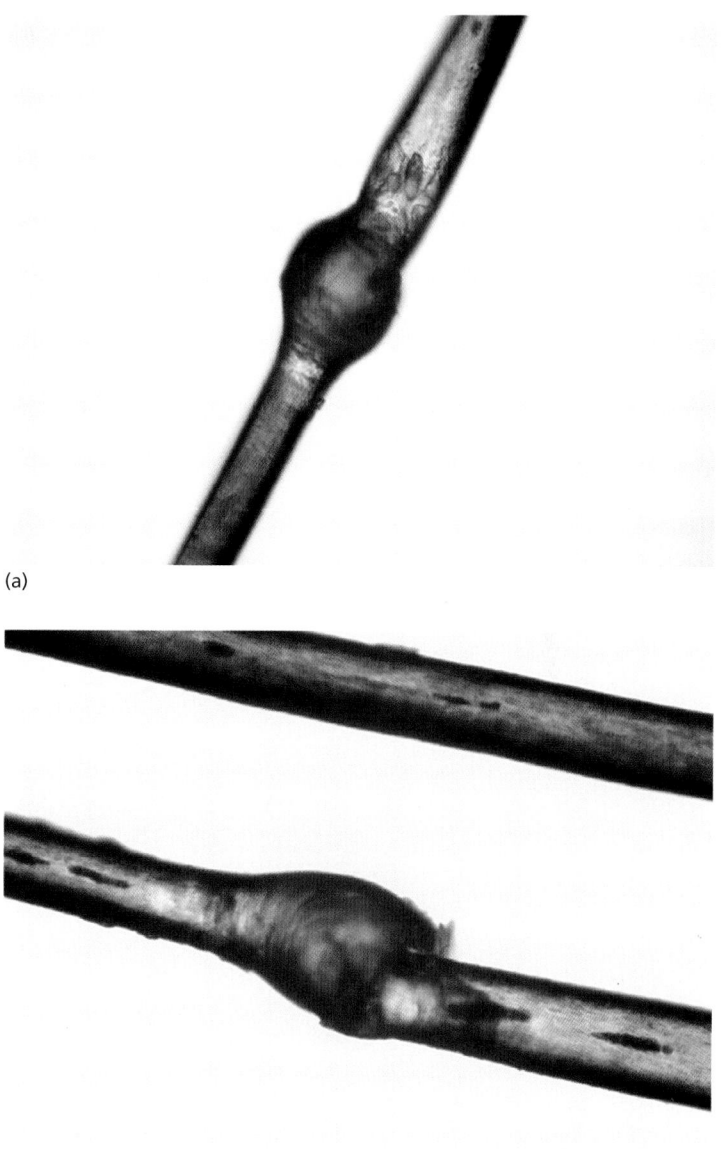

(a)

(b)

Figure 89.54 Netherton syndrome. (a) An invaginate node showing partial twisting of the hair at the upper pole. (b) An invaginate node acting as a point of weakness in the hair shaft.

Where diagnosis is difficult, sampling eyebrows hairs may provide confirmation. Alternatively, screening with dermoscopy or videodermoscopy may help [15,16]. With the magnification of dermoscopy at 10×, it is difficult to differentiate trichorrhexis invaginata from trichorrhexis nodosa; however, the proximal remnant of an invaginate node may resemble a golf tee and can allow diagnosis where classic nodes are absent.

Clinical features
The patient may present primarily either with cutaneous changes or complaining of sparse and fragile hair. Generalized scaling and erythema are present from birth or early infancy, but the degree, extent and persistence of the erythema are very variable. In some cases, it may be slight and transient. In many it has the characteristics of atopic eczema accompanied by an elevated IgE. On the trunk and limbs, the fine, dry scales are associated with a polycyclic and serpiginous eruption whose horny margin slowly changes its pattern.

The hair defects may be detected only if deliberately sought, but in most cases are readily apparent clinically. The hair is short, dry, lustreless and brittle, and the eyebrows and lashes are sparse or absent.

Management
Management of Netherton syndrome is discussed in Chapter 65. There is no specific treatment for the hair dystrophy other than avoidance of physical and chemical trauma.

Trichorrhexis nodosa

Introduction and general description
Trichorrhexis is best regarded as a distinctive response of the hair shaft to injury. If the degree or frequency of the injury is sufficient, it can be induced in normal hair, and this is probably the most common scenario. The cuticular cells become disrupted, allowing the cortical cells to splay out to form nodes [17]. If, however, the hair is abnormally fragile, trichorrhexis may follow relatively trivial injury. The trauma of hairdressing procedures has often been incriminated, such as with combing [18] or ceramic flat iron use in African hair. It may also follow hair follicle transplantation. Scratching may produce identical changes in pubic hairs. The cumulative effect of shampooing, brushing, sea bathing and sunlight has led to seasonal summer recurrences. Trichorrhexis nodosa is an extreme form of weathering (see Weathering of the hair shaft later in this chapter).

Congenital and hereditary defects of the hair shaft resulting in fragility can predispose to trichorrhexis nodosa.

Trichorrhexis nodosa is a feature of the rare metabolic defect argininosuccinic aciduria where there is a deficiency of the enzyme argininosuccinase, and in which it is associated with mental retardation [19]. The hair tends to be dry, brittle and lustreless and may show trichorrhexis nodosa, but it does not occur in all patients with this metabolic disorder. Biotinidase deficiency and the trichohepato-enteric syndrome can both present with trichorrhexis nodosa.

Trichorrhexis nodosa may occur in certain families as an apparently isolated defect of the hair: node formation and fracture are induced by minimal trauma and develop during the early months of life. Wolff *et al.* described as 'trichorrhexis congenita' the presence from birth of trichorrhexis nodosa confined to the scalp, with normal teeth and nails [20].

Localized autosomal recessive hypotrichosis
This disorder presents with brittle hair that fractures readily leading to extensive loss of hair [21]. The hair may appear unusually stiff. Hair microscopy shows trichorrhexis nodosa. Monilethrix-like beading may also be seen. Localized autosomal recessive hypotrichosis is due to mutations in the gene *dsg4* for the desmosomal protein desmoglein 4 (Figure 89.55).

Pathophysiology
In simple trichorrhexis nodosa, the shaft may appear normal with a light or electron microscope, except at the nodes; or the shaft, apart from the proximal 1 cm, may show signs of abnormal wear and tear. At the nodes, the cuticle bulges and is split by longitudinal fissures (Figure 89.56a). If fracture occurs transversely through a node (trichoclasis), the end of the hair resembles a small paintbrush.

Clinical features
In trichorrhexis nodosa complicating a congenital defect of the hair shaft, the hair breaks so easily that large or small portions of the scalp show only broken stumps and alopecia may be gross. However, the common situation is where trauma plays a major part and predisposition has a relatively minor role. In this setting there are three principal clinical presentations:
1 Distal trichorrhexis nodosa occurs in all races. Often it is discovered incidentally, and only a few whitish nodules are seen near

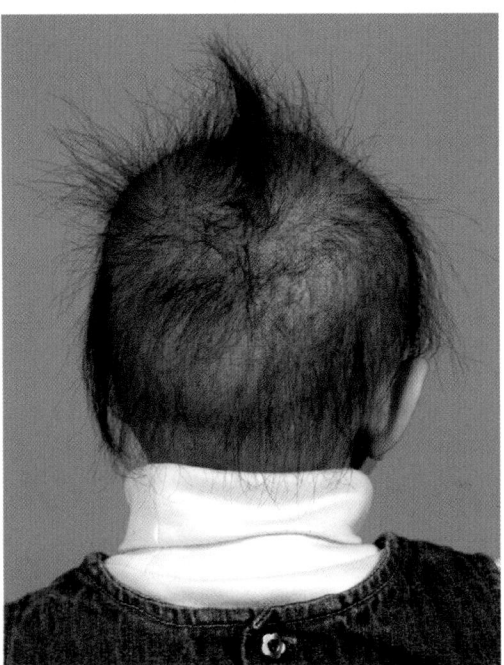

Figure 89.55 Localized autosomal recessive hypotrichosis due to a *dsg4* mutation.

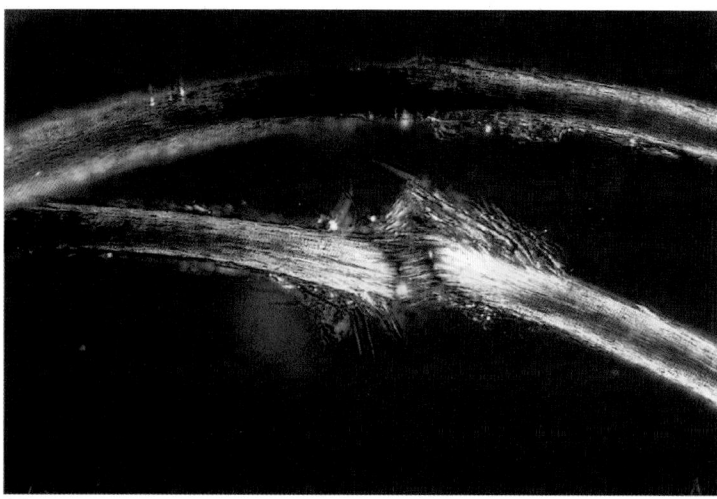

(a)

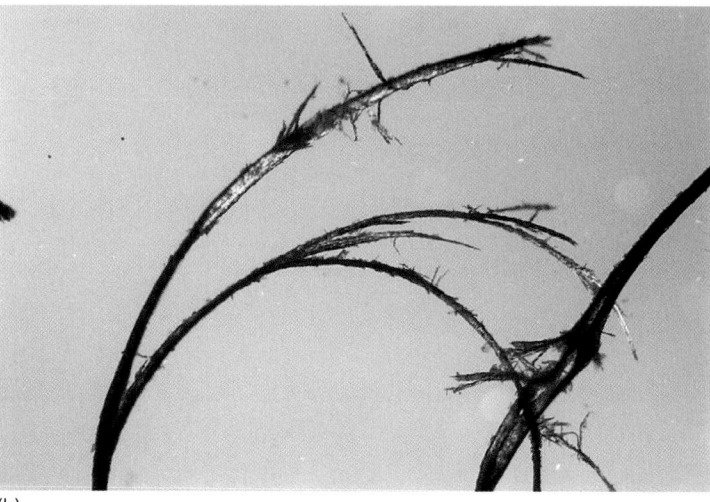

(b)

Figure 89.56 Trichorrhexis nodosa. (a) Polarized light examination demonstrates the splayed cortical fibres radiating from the transverse fracture in a trichorrhexis node. (b) Proximal trichorrhexis nodosa nodes and dramatic split ends (trichoptilosis) visible in the hair from an Afro-Caribbean woman.

the ends of scattered hairs. If many hairs are affected, the patient may complain that the hair is dry, dull or brittle. The longer the hair, the more likely it is to occur.

2 There is a generalized variant seen in Afro-Caribbean women called proximal trichorrhexis nodosa. The scalp hair is universally short and brittle and demonstrates severe weathering on light microscopic examination (Figure 89.56b). There may be an association with the follicular degeneration syndrome where there is a central scarring alopecia in the absence of an overt inflammatory process [22].

3 The third clinical form was well described by Sabouraud but it appears now to be rare [23]. In a localized area of scalp, moustache or beard, some hairs are broken and others show from one to five or six nodules.

Investigations

The congenital forms must be differentiated from other shaft defects. The distal acquired form may simulate dandruff or even pediculosis. In all cases, diagnosis depends on careful microscopy.

Excessive physical and chemical (cosmetic) trauma must be avoided, apart from shampooing.

Trichothiodystrophy

Introduction and general description

The term trichothiodystrophy (TTD) was coined to describe brittle hair with abnormally low sulphur content [24]. The term covers a range of phenotypes, with low-sulphur fragile hair representing the central defining criterion [25,26]. TTD can be classified according to the constellation of features that accompany the hair changes. It is one of a group of nucleotide excision repair disorders that have overlapping characteristics and aetiology. See also Chapter 68.

Pathophysiology

The hair is brittle and weathers readily [27], with abnormalities inversely proportional to the sulphur content. A similar pattern of change can be seen in distal segments of African hair subjected to chemical relaxers. Sulphur amino acid reduction is commensurate with clinical abnormality in the hair of those with associated autism. With trauma it may fracture with a clean transverse break (trichoschisis) or may form nodes resembling trichorrhexis nodosa. The hairs are flattened and can be twisted into various shapes – rather like a ribbon or shoelace. Details of these changes are clarified by scanning electron microscopy [28]. The shaft is irregular, with ridging and fluting, and the cuticular scales are patchily absent. Transmission electron microscopy demonstrates a decrease in high-sulphur protein staining in the hair shaft and a reduction of this protein in the exocuticular part of the cuticle cells.

Using crossed polarizing filters with a light microscope the hairs show alternating bright and dark zones (Figure 89.57). This feature is sensitive for TTD, but not specific [29]. It may occur in a range

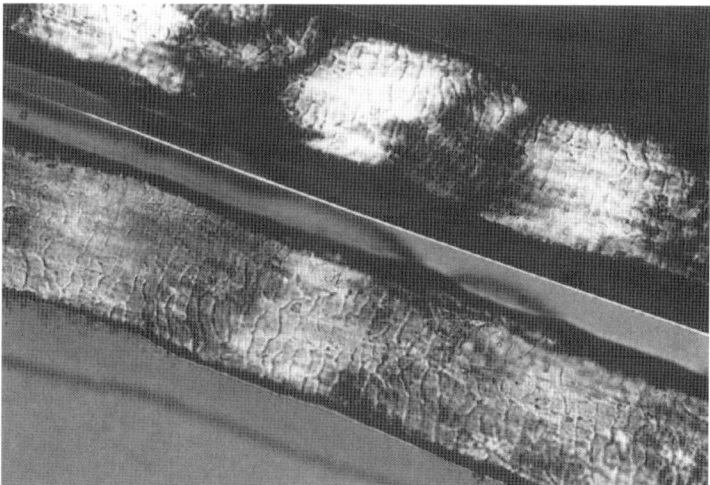

Figure 89.57 Trichothiodystrophy showing alternating bright and dark zones under a polarizing microscope. (Courtesy of D. Van Neste, Brussels.)

PART 8: SPECIFIC CUTANEOUS STRUCTURE

of genetic and acquired disorders where the longitudinal organization of cortical fibres within the hair is thrown into a sine wave pattern through loss of rigidity. As a sign, it may arise at different stages in infancy. In one instance it has been used prognostically when identified in a fetal eyebrow biopsy obtained *in utero*. Other cases illustrate that the sign may fail to develop until a few months of age.

Clinical features

There is a wide range of phenotypic characteristics, depending on the variant of TTD. The hair is sparse, short and brittle, but the degree of alopecia varies considerably. There may be lamellar ichthyosis. The nails may be dystrophic. Mental and physical development may be normal but one or both may be slightly, moderately or severely retarded. The central feature of altered hair remains the basis of diagnosis, but the mechanism linking the associated features requires further elucidation.

STRUCTURAL DEFECTS WITHOUT INCREASED FRAGILITY

Pili annulati

Synonyms and inclusions
• Ringed hair

Introduction and general description

This abnormality is characterized by hair showing alternate light and dark bands along its length [1,2]. In extreme cases there may be some additional fragility as the lighter areas seen with light microscopy represent a split in the hair cortex. The condition is inherited as an autosomal dominant, and although the molecular basis of the abnormality remains unknown, the genetic defect maps to chromosome 12q [30,31].

Pathophysiology

With the light microscope the abnormal dark bands alternating with normal light bands are reversed. The bright appearance of the abnormal bands in reflected light is caused by air spaces in the cortex (Figure 89.58) [32]. Detection of the cortical defect is made easier if the hair is mounted in histological mounting medium because this enhances the transmission of light through the hair. Although this illustrates that the pathology can result in structural weakness, it only rarely leads to a clinical complaint of fragility. Dermoscopy is not as reliable in pili annulati as it is in some other dystrophies because the perception is based largely on light transmission through the hair and not reflection [4].

Electron microscopic studies have shown that the clusters of air-filled cavities, which are randomly distributed throughout the cortex in the abnormal bands, lie partly within cortical cells and between macrofibrils or, in the case of larger cavities, appear to replace cortical cells [33,34].

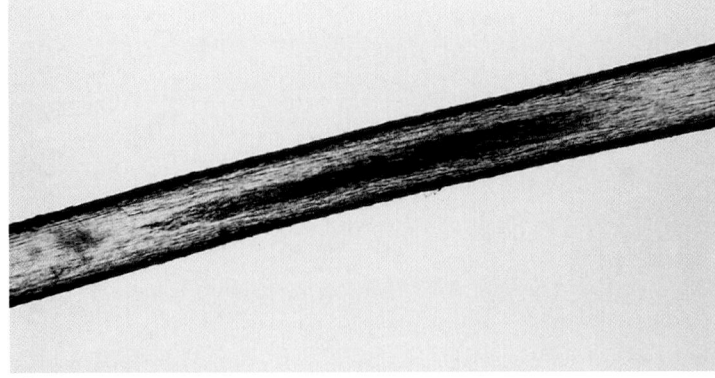

(a)

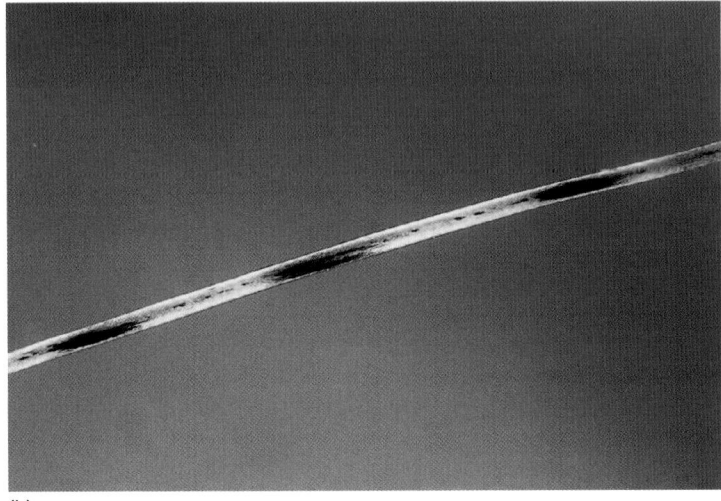

(b)

Figure 89.58 Pili annulati. (a) Hair shaft by transmitted light showing an abnormal dark band (central part) caused by multiple cortical air spaces. This corresponds to a bright region as seen by reflected light. (b) The abnormality is intermittent, causing a beaded or ringed appearance.

Clinical features

Pili annulati is normally diagnosed as a coincidental finding or as part of a pursuance of the unusual, but quite attractive, spangled appearance. The condition has been reported in association with alopecia areata on several occasions. It is uncertain whether this represents a genuine association or if medical scrutiny for the presenting disease reveals the otherwise subtle diagnosis of pili annulati. Fragility is occasionally a presenting feature and can be based on more severe expressions of the disease, where the longitudinal fracture in the hair cortex weakens the shaft and predisposes to fracture. Axillary hair is occasionally affected.

The diagnosis is readily established on microscopy of affected hair. A defect in which partially twisted shafts have an elliptical cross-section has been named pseudopili annulati because such hair may give an impression of alternating light and dark bands [35].

Prognosis

The prognosis is good in the sense that the severity of the defect does not increase with age.

Woolly hair

Woolly hair is more or less tightly coiled hair occurring over all or part of the scalp. In those of African origin, woolly hair is the norm. Tight coiling, knots and fractures are common. Woolly hair in non-African individuals may be generalized or localized. The generalized forms may be inherited. The investigation by Hutchinson *et al.* was important in delineating the clinical types [36].

Hair microscopy in all the woolly hair disorders reveals non-specific features that are consistent with a woolly, stiff hair phenotype. This usually arises in association with grooves, partial twists, irregularity of bore and sometimes features of trauma. When a hair shaft has an irregular shape and is stiffer, it is more prone to damage. The changes are often subtle, and are better appreciated on assessment of at least 20 and preferably 50 hairs or more. Isolated reports describing hair morphology often fall into the trap of describing individual hairs rather than the population of hairs as a whole. This mistake can be compounded by using scanning electron microscopy for the main assessment rather than as a supplementary tool. Although electron microscopy is excellent for revealing great detail in a small number of hairs, it is very poor at showing the characteristics of a population of hairs, which is the usual determinant of a phenotype.

Autosomal dominant woolly hair. See Chapter 68.

Autosomal recessive woolly hair. Naxos disease and Carvajal disease are characterized by woolly hair and other cutaneous and systemic features including cardiomyopathy (see Chapter 68).

Woolly hair naevus. Woolly hair naevus presents with a circumscribed patch of hair showing altered colour and texture (Figure 89.59). The hair may be fine in infancy, becoming coarser with age,

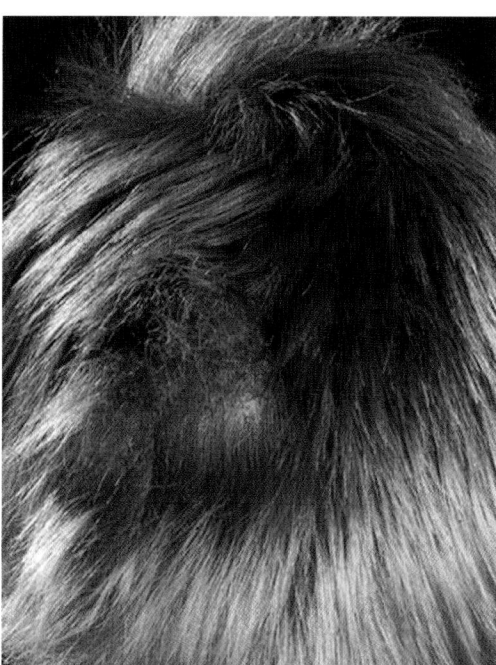

Figure 89.59 Woolly hair naevus.

especially at puberty. It is commonly associated with melanocytic or epidermal naevi elsewhere on the skin. Associated ocular and auditory defects, digital abnormalities and precocious puberty have been reported [37–39].

Acquired woolly hair. This is a heterogeneous group. It occurs most commonly in the context of patterned hair loss (acquired progressive kinking of hair) [40]. It may also be caused by drugs such as valproate and retinoids [41,42].

Uncombable hair syndrome

Synonyms and inclusions
- Spun-glass hair
- Cheveux incoiffables
- Pili trianguli et canaliculi

Introduction and general description
This is a combination of a striking clinical presentation and distinctive hair shaft defect [43] first described by Dupré and Bonafe [44]. Since then, many more cases have been reported, some of them under the name of 'spun-glass hair'. Others have preferred the term pili trianguli et canaliculi, with emphasis on the triangular cross-section and longitudinal groove that is commonly found on microscopy. The mode of inheritance is probably autosomal dominant [45].

Pathophysiology
Light microscopy reveals the features in a hair shaft that make it rigid: the triangular cross-section (Figure 89.60a) and longitudinal grooving (Figure 89.60b). Twisting can also be present and contributes to stiffness to a minor degree. Scanning electron microscopy of selected hairs can be helpful (Figure 89.60c). The pili canaliculi are present in all cases, pili trianguli in the majority and pili torti in a few.

Clinical features
The abnormality may first become obvious from 3 months to 12 years of age. The hair is normal in quantity and sometimes also in length, but the wild, disorderly appearance totally resists all efforts to control it with a brush or comb. In some cases, these efforts lead to the hair breaking, but increased fragility is not a constant feature [46]. The hair is often a silvery blonde colour. The eyebrows and eyelashes are normal. The appearance becomes less marked with time [47]. Some people with loose anagen syndrome may have a similar appearance and the condition has been reported in association with neurofibromatosis I in one instance.

With light microscopy the diagnosis is dependent upon the experience of the microscopist, as the three-dimensional aspect of the shaft changes can be difficult to establish. No treatment is known, although oral biotin therapy has been suggested. The features often diminish with adulthood. An acquired form can be seen following chemotherapy or in association with certain long-term medications such as sodium valproate [48].

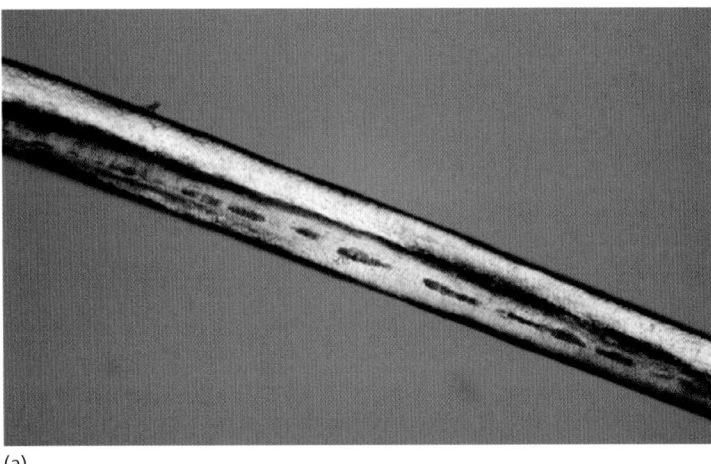

(a)

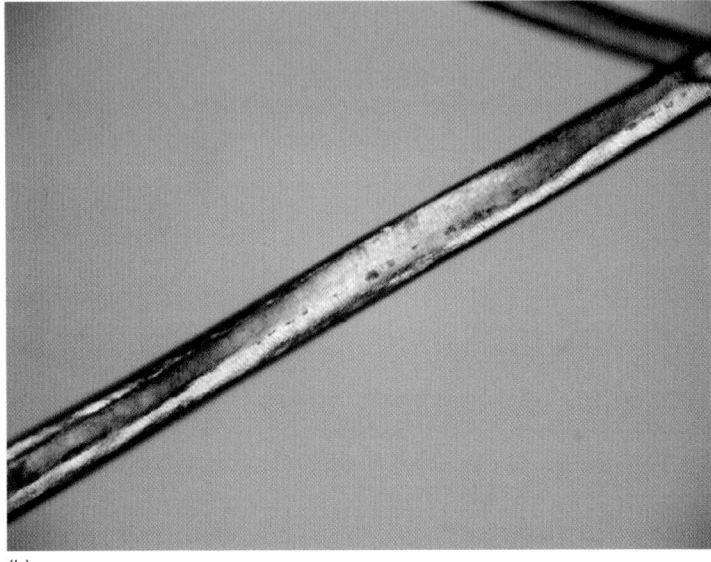

(b)

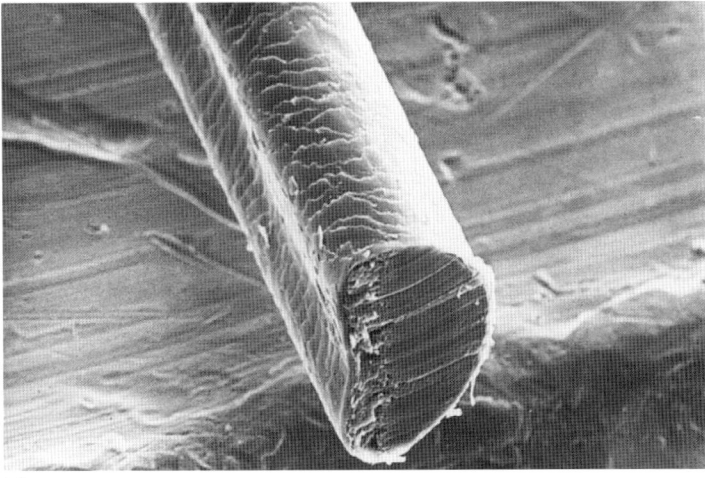

(c)

Figure 89.60 Uncombable hair syndrome. (a) The triangular cross-section of the hair contributes to its stiffness. (b) Light microscopy revealing grooving when using partially crossed polarizing filters.(c) Scanning electron micrograph showing a triangular cross-section and canalicular depression or gutter along one side.

Loose anagen hair syndrome

This condition features anagen hairs that are loosely anchored and easily pulled from the scalp [49,**50**,51]. The majority of cases are fair-haired children, aged 2–9 years, mostly girls, but it has also been reported from Egypt and India in children with darker skin and hair. The hair is typically slightly unruly, of uneven length and patchy in quality, with a history of not growing properly and never needing cutting. The clinical picture is, however, variable – with some complaining of stiff, uncombable hair and others of excessive shedding of hair. All three phenotypes may coexist within the same family. The children may present with patchy alopecia, leading to a misdiagnosis of alopecia areata, but which, in fact, represents modest hair pulling.

Hair is usually easily and painlessly plucked with the hair-pull test, although this is not a constant or specific finding. Microscopy of plucked hair may show ruffling of the cuticle adjacent to the anagen bulb, giving the appearance of a 'floppy sock' (Figure 89.61). The hair shaft may have twists and grooves, and be angular in cross-section. The root sheath is absent or there may be a small everted remnant. Scalp biopsy may show irregular keratinization

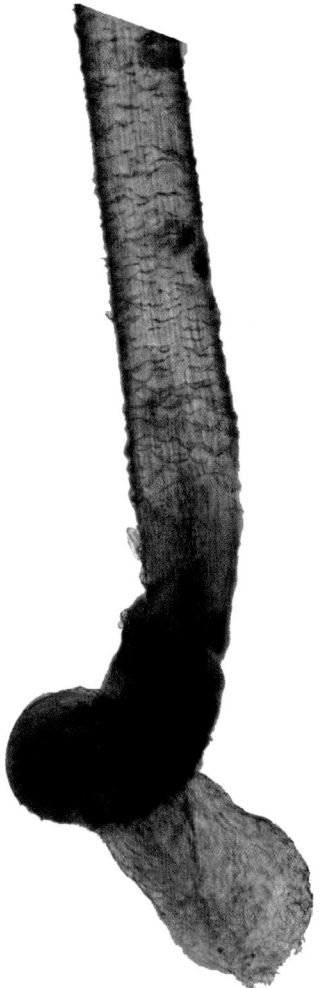

Figure 89.61 Plucked anagen hair in the loose anagen syndrome, showing a vestigial root sheath and a ruffled cuticle.

and dyskeratosis of the root sheath cuticle cells. But whatever tests are done, if the hair is not loose on the hair-pull test, the diagnosis can not be made. Conversely, if the hair is loose, the main differential diagnoses are telogen effluvium and alopecia areata.

Histological examination shows premature keratinization of the inner root sheath layers of Huxley and Henle. Trichograms show 98–100% anagen hairs. Keratin K6irs is an inner root sheath keratin proposed as a protein that might control manifestations of the disorder [52]. In one report, mutations in the gene coding for such a keratin supported this possibility [53].

The hair becomes more normal with age, although the pull test may still yield abnormally large numbers of hairs into adulthood. The child is well, and there are rarely any other abnormalities. There have been isolated reports of loose anagen syndrome associated with hypohidrotic ectodermal dysplasia, ocular coloboma, epidermolysis bullosa and the autosomal dominant condition, Noonan syndrome. Such children are characterized by facial dysmorphism, short stature and congenital heart defects.

Management involves advice on gentle hair grooming and reassurance that the defect usually resolves spontaneously with age.

Trichostasis spinulosa

Epidemiology
This is probably a normal, age-related phenomenon – easily overlooked – in which successive telogen hairs are retained in predominantly sebaceous follicles [54].

Trichostasis is found most commonly in the middle-aged or elderly and is said by most authors to occur particularly on the nose and face. Other sites were perhaps not always examined, for others have found it to be not uncommon on the trunk, limbs and interscapular area [55]. It has been reported in association with the use of topical minoxidil [56], topical steroids and in the clinical setting of facial pruritus, chronic renal failure and focal pathologies of syringoma and epidermoid cysts.

Pathophysiology
The affected follicles contain up to 50 vellus hairs embedded in a keratinous plug. A mild perifolliculitis is often present. The condition must be differentiated from the 'multiple hairs' of Flemming–Giovannini in which up to seven hairs grow from a composite papilla with a common outer root sheath. Follicles may contain *Malassezia* yeasts and *Propionibacterium acnes*.

Clinical features
It is reported at all adult ages, although it appears to be more common in the elderly. The lesions, which closely resemble comedones, may occur predominantly on the nose, forehead and cheeks, or the face may be spared and the nape, back, shoulders, upper arms and chest may be affected. The number of follicles affected varies greatly. Dermoscopy can help in assessing the extent: comedo-like lesions are prominent and in some cases a tuft of hairs may be seen projecting through the horny plug.

Management
Keratolytic preparations have often been recommended but we have found them of little value. The most effective treatment is topical retinoic acid, which should be used as in the treatment of acne [57]. Depilatory wax, specialized cleaning pads and a variety of laser treatments have been advocated [58].

Pili multigemini

Synonyms and inclusions
- Pili bifurcati

Introduction and general description
The term pili multigemini describes an uncommon developmental defect of hair follicles that fuse [59]. As a result multiple hairs from a composite follicular structure emerge through a single pilosebaceous canal. This is different from instances where separate follicular bulbs generate hairs that fuse in the infundibular region and also can emerge from a single opening. Numerous follicles showing this defect have been seen in a patient with cleidocranial dysostosis, and a naevoid pattern on the back has also been described [60].

Pathophysiology
From two to eight matrices and papillae, each with its internal root sheath, form hairs that are often flattened, ovoid or triangular in configuration and may be grooved. In the follicular canal, contiguous hairs may adhere, bifurcate and then re-adhere.

Clinical features
Multigeminate follicles occur mainly on the face, especially along the lines of the jaw [61]. Tufts of hair may be seen emerging from a few or many follicles. Their discovery is often a matter of chance, but the patient may complain of recurrent inflammatory nodules, leaving scars.

Weathering of the hair shaft (including trichoptilosis)

All hair fibres undergo some degree of cuticular damage and secondary cortical breakdown from root to tip before being shed during the telogen or early anagen phase of the hair cycle. The term 'weathering' has been used to describe this. *In vivo* and *in vitro* studies have shown the type of damage that combing, brushing, bleaching, UV radiation and permanent waving can cause [62]. Scalp hair, having a long anagen phase and being subject to more frictional damage and cosmetic treatment, shows more deep cuticular and cortical degeneration than fibres from other sites.

Weathering of scalp hair has been studied in greater detail than hair from other sites. At the root end, surface cuticle cells are closely apposed to deeper layers. Within a few centimetres of the scalp, the free margin of these cells lifts up and breaks irregularly. Increasing scale loss leads to surface

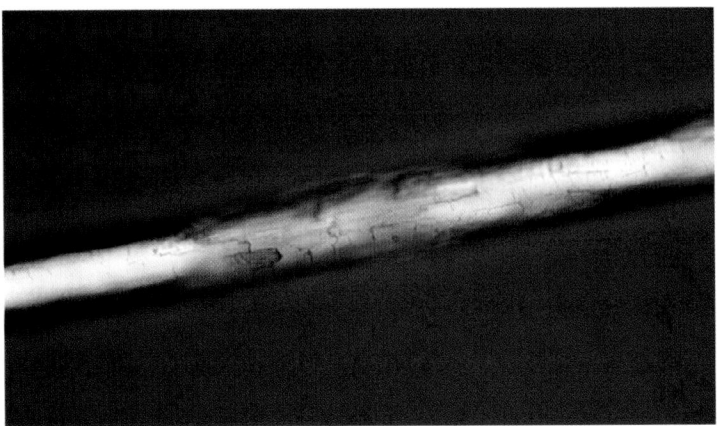

Figure 89.62 Focal loss of the cuticle in a weathered hair.

areas denuded of cuticle. Many fibres show a complete loss of overlapping scales well proximal to the tip (Figure 89.62). This is particularly common on long hair shafts, which frequently also have a frayed tip. Proximal to terminal fraying, longitudinal fissures may be present between exposed cortical cells. Hairs subjected to considerable friction damage may show transverse fissures and some nodes of the type seen in trichorrhexis nodosa [17]. Hair that has been bleached or permanently waved may show shaft distortion. The most severe changes in normal scalp hair are mostly seen near the distal part of the hair shaft. Hair knotting and braids are a significant source of hair shaft trauma, with loss of cuticle and damage to cortical fibres (Figure 89.63).

Trichoptilosis is a term for 'split ends', which is an inherent component of weathering. It is more common as hair gets longer and is usually only pathological if it is found in short hair, save for African hair, where it is common at all lengths and has a less clear association with weathering. Trichoptilosis can appear as whitish blurred ends to the hair shaft and be visible to the

naked eye or with dermoscopy. It has been reported in childhood in association with the use of hair gel, but normally it is seen in adults and most commonly seen with other features of hair weathering, particularly as related to styling or medicated treatments [63].

Trichorrhexis nodosa is the most severe form of weathering. Many of the changes seen in normal hair towards the tip are visible more proximally in congenitally weakened hair [64] and in trichorrhexis nodosa, caused by overuse of cosmetic treatments [65]. In some hair structure abnormalities, such as monilethrix and pili torti, specific weathering patterns may be seen.

Bubble hair

Bubble hair is a change caused by heat, where typically a faulty hairdryer or tongs at high temperature have caused focal damage (Figure 89.64) [66]. Although damp hair has been suggested as a contributory factor, it is not a requirement [67,68]. Bubble hair can be intentionally created on any hairs by the use of a naked flame or conducted heat. The damage has been assessed by light and electron microscopy with additional assessment to demonstrate that the bubbles are gas-filled rather than containing fluid. They are not well demonstrated by dermoscopy as transmission of light through the defect is needed to demonstrate the bubbles [4]. Conversely, assessment is enhanced by the use of DPX fluid slide mountant by diminishing reflection at the hair surface.

Management
Any appliances with hot components should be serviced or replaced. Affected hair needs to be trimmed to cut out of the affected areas and subsequent hair will be normal.

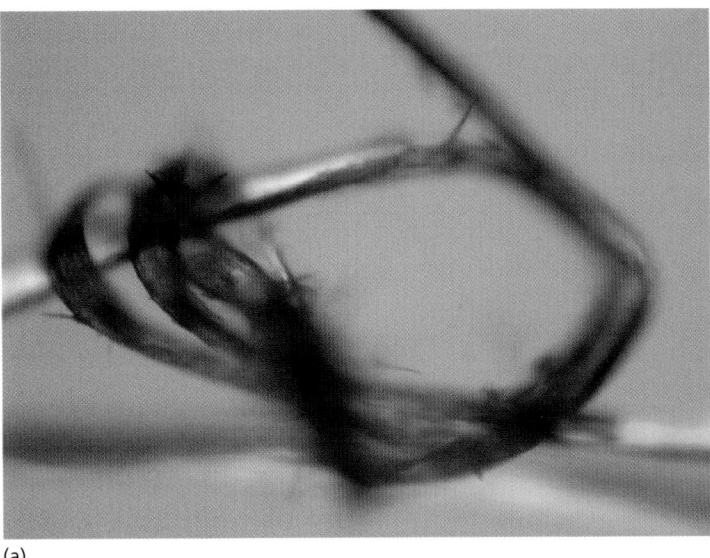

(a)

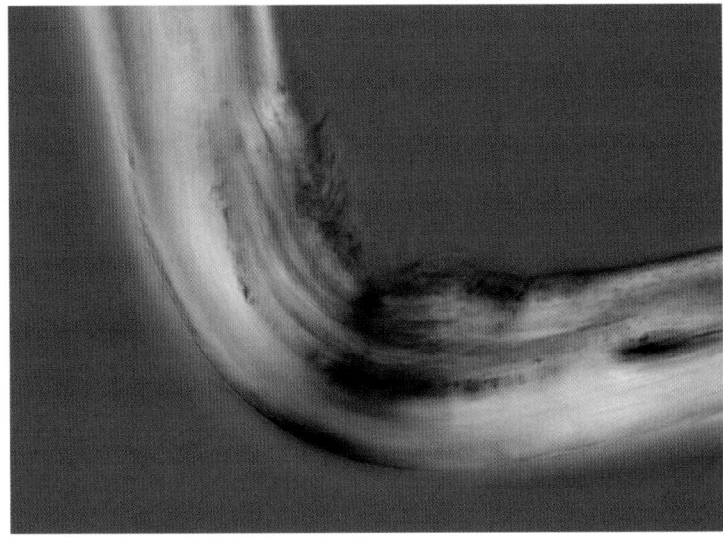

(b)

Figure 89.63 (a) Knotting of single and multiple hairs contributes to hair shaft trauma. (b) Braiding damages the hair shaft cuticle.

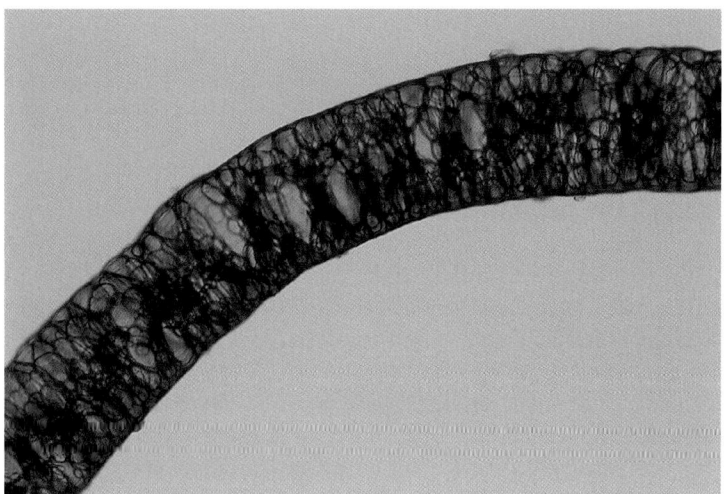

Figure 89.64 Appearance of normal scalp hair after exposure to a naked flame. Bubbles form within the cortex.

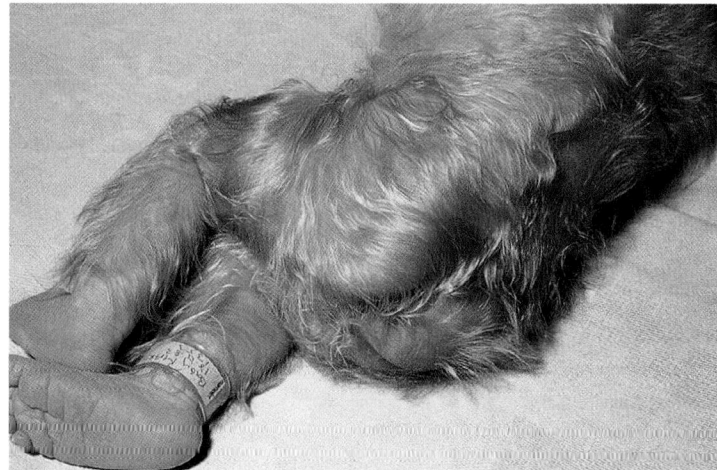

Figure 89.65 Congenital hypertrichosis lanuginosa. (Courtesy of Dr Partridge, Leamington, UK.)

EXCESSIVE GROWTH OF HAIR

Paul Farrant

Growth of hair that at any given site is coarser, longer or more profuse than is normal for the age, sex and race of the individual is regarded as excessive. The term hirsutism will be restricted to androgen-dependent hair patterns of, typically, terminal hair, and the term hypertrichosis will be applied to other patterns of excessive hair growth. Hypertrichosis can be classified as either localized or generalized, of congenital or acquired pattern where congenital is loosely interpreted as that seen in infancy.

Hypertrichosis

Congenital generalized hypertrichosis

Definition and nomenclature
In congenital generalized hypertrichosis, the fetal pelage is not replaced by vellus and terminal hair but persists, grows excessively and is constantly renewed throughout life (Figure 89.65). It is associated with a number of different genetic mutations and chromosomal aberrations. Some types are associated with gingival hyperplasia and other malformations. Congenital generalized hypertrichosis is discussed further in Chapter 68.

> **Synonyms and inclusions**
> • Hypertrichosis lanuginosa

Associated syndromes
Congenital hypertrichosis can be associated with other syndromes, which include the following.

Hurler syndrome and other mucopolysaccharidoses. Hypertrichosis is usually present from early infancy or early childhood on the face, trunk and limbs and may be a conspicuous feature. The eyebrows are often bushy and confluent. In abortive forms, the hair growth may first appear after puberty and be more limited in extent.

Cornelia de Lange syndrome. These mildly microcephalic, intellectually impaired children have a low hairline and profuse overgrowth of the eyebrows. The forehead is covered with long fine hair. Hypertrichosis is usually also conspicuous on the lower back, and may be generalized.

Winchester syndrome. This rare hereditary disorder is characterized by dwarfism, joint destruction and corneal opacities. The skin in many parts of the body becomes thickened, hyperpigmented and hypertrichotic [1,2].

Berardinelli syndrome. From early life, growth and maturation are accelerated and there is lipodystrophy with muscular hypertrophy. Enlargement of the liver and hyperlipidaemia are other constant features. The skin is coarse and often hypertrichotic [3].

Fetal alcohol syndrome. In this teratogenic syndrome, mental and physical retardation affects the infants of mothers with chronic alcoholism [4]. The cutaneous changes include hypertrichosis and capillary haemangiomatosis.

Congenital localized hypertrichosis

Definition and nomenclature
Congenital localized hypertrichosis refers to both areas of excess hair present at birth and hamartomas that may have a delayed clinical presentation. They may occur in isolation as an area of increased hair density or in association with congenital melanocytic naevi, Becker naevi, spinal dysraphism or neurofibromas.

> **Synonyms and inclusions**
> • Naevoid hypertrichosis

Congenital localized hypertrichosis of specific anatomical sites

There are a number of congenital conditions associated with increased hair growth in a specific anatomical site such as hypertrichosis cubiti or hairy elbow syndrome. In a number of these conditions there is a clear pattern of inheritance. Whilst hypertrichosis may be evident at birth, it may not become apparent until later in childhood or adolescence.

Naevoid hypertrichosis. Naevoid hypertrichosis refers to a localized area of hypertrichosis. This is usually well circumscribed. It can occur in a hair-bearing site such as the scalp with a localized area of marked increased density of terminal hair fibres or in areas normally lacking terminal hairs where it is more of a cosmetic issue. The lesions are usually solitary but multiple patches have been described. They can be of normal hair colour, grey or white and can be associated with premature greying [5].

Congenital melanocytic naevi and neurofibromas. Congenital melanocytic naevi are often associated with prominent terminal hairs. The hair may be present from infancy or may develop after puberty. Plexiform neurofibromas are also associated with hypertrichosis.

Lumbosacral hypertrichosis. Lumbosacral hypertrichosis or the faun tail sign is a tuft of hair in the lumbo-sacral region that is often associated with spina bifida or diastematomyelia (Figure 89.66).

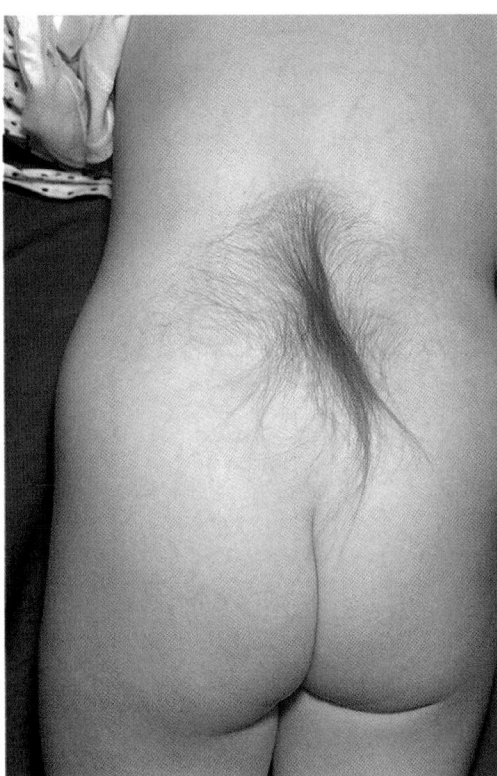

Figure 89.66 Lumbosacral hypertrichosis ('faun tail'), here associated with diastematomyelia.

Becker naevus. Becker naevus or pigmented hairy epidermal naevus is a hamartoma that usually presents with hyperpigmentation affecting the upper back, flanks or upper chest. It is frequently associated with the development of terminal hair from puberty. See also Chapter 75.

Malignant acquired generalized hypertrichosis

Definition and nomenclature

This is the sudden and generalized development of lanugo or non-androgen-dependent hair in adult life. This presentation is often a sign of underlying malignancy but can also be due to other factors including drugs. It is a rare sign most commonly associated with carcinomas of the gastrointestinal tract, lung or breast [6,7,8,9]. The hypertrichosis may precede the diagnosis of the neoplasm by several years.

Synonyms and inclusions
- Acquired hypertrichosis lanuginosa
- Acquired hypertrichosis lanuginosa associated with malignancy
- Paraneoplastic hypertrichosis lanuginosa
- Drug-induced hypertrichosis

Clinical features

In the milder forms ('malignant down'), hair is confined to the face, where it attracts attention by its appearance on the nose and eyelids, and other sites that normally are clinically hairless [10]. As the growth of hair continues, it may ultimately involve the entire body, apart from the palms and soles. Existing terminal hair of the scalp, beard and pubes may not be replaced, and may contrast in colour and texture with the very fine, white or blonde lanugo. Such hair may grow abundantly, even on a previously bald scalp. The hair may grow exceedingly rapidly, up to 2.5 cm/week, and may be more than 10 cm long.

Investigations

If the development of generalized lanugo hair precedes a known diagnosis of a neoplasm, then patients should be radiologically screened for cancer, concentrating on the lung and gastrointestinal tract.

Non-malignant acquired generalized hypertrichosis

Definition

Generalized hypertrichosis can occur as the consequence of systemic disease and medications. Generally, the hair is coarser and less profuse than the lanugo hair associated with malignancy.

Associated disorders

Drug-induced hypertrichosis. The most common cause of acquired hypertrichosis is systemic medications. Drug-induced hypertrichosis is a well known side effect of ciclosporin [11], phenytoin [12] and minoxidil [12,13], which has been turned to commercial benefit in the case of the latter. It has also been described with diazoxide [12] and psoralens [14] (Table 89.7)

Hypothyroidism. A profuse growth of hair on the back and the extensor aspects of the limbs develops in some children with hypothyroidism [15].

Table 89.7 Iatrogenic hypertrichosis.

Drug	Comment
Steroid – systemic, injected and topical [27]	Analogous to Cushing syndrome, with additional local effects with injection or topical use
Diphenylhydantoin [12]	Takes 2–3 months to be apparent
Psoralen [14]	Possibly linked to degree of photosensitization and only shortly outlasts treatment
Diazoxide [12]	
Minoxidil [12,**13**]	Systemic and topical effect; after only a few weeks; may affect forehead when applied to scalp
Ciclosporin [28,29]	Associated with sebaceous hyperplasia
Latanoprost and bimatoprost [**25**,26]	Increases growth of eyelashes and adjacent vellus hairs when used as eye drops; analogue of prostaglandin F2α

Eating disorders. An increased growth of fine downy hair on the face, trunk and arms, sometimes of severe degree, has been reported in 20–77% of adult cases of anorexia nervosa [16,17], and is also seen in children [18]. The prevalence of hypertrichosis in bulimia is reported to be half of that in anorexia, and both are associated with approximately 60% prevalence of scalp alopecia [16].

Dermatomyositis. Excessive hair growth has been noted mainly in children and principally on the forearms, legs and temples, but it may be more extensive [19].

Epidermolysis bullosa. Gross hypertrichosis of the face and limbs has occurred in association with epidermolysis bullosa of the dystrophic type, although this is rare (see Chapter 71).

Acquired localized hypertrichosis

Associated disorders

Porphyria (see Chapter 60). Hypertrichosis of exposed skin is a common feature of the very rare congenital erythropoietic porphyria. Appearing first on the forehead, it later extends to the cheeks and chin and, to a lesser degree, to other exposed areas. It is also present in some cases of the much more common erythropoietic protoporphyria [20].

Hypertrichosis is a common finding in porphyria cutanea tarda [**21**] and may be the presenting complaint. It typically affects the cheeks, eyebrows, hairline and forearms (Figure 89.67). It is usually accompanied by other cutaneous manifestations including hyperpigmentation, blistering and skin fragility on exposed sites. Similar hypertrichosis also occurs in variegate porphyria. Darkening of scalp hair in a subject with white hair at the onset of porphyria cutanea tarda has been reported [22].

The most extreme degree of hypertrichosis is seen in children with hepatic porphyria induced by hexachlorobenzene or other chemicals.

Topical medications. Localized hypertrichosis can be seen at sites of topical corticosteroid application. It has also been seen after sclerotherapy [23] and topical tacrolimus [24]. The prostaglandin analogues lanatoprost [**25**] and bimatoprost [26] cause increased growth of eyelashes when used in the treatment of glaucoma.

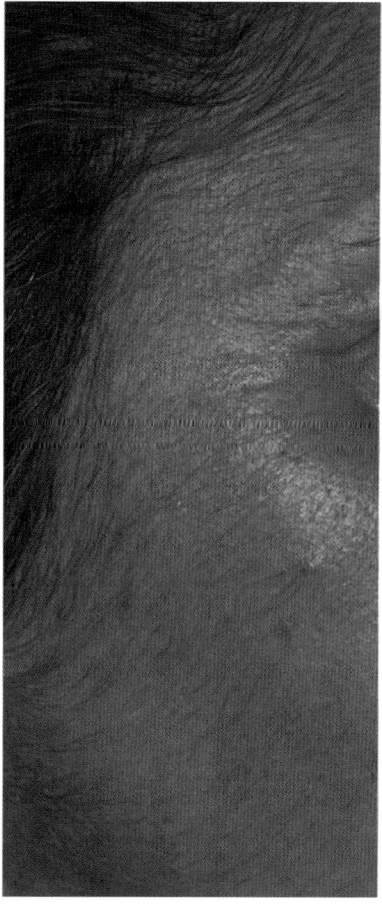

Figure 89.67 Facial hypertrichosis in porphyria cutanea tarda.

Graves disease. The growth of coarse terminal hairs is a common feature in plaques of pretibial myxoedema associated with Graves disease.

Miscellaneous. Localized hypertrichosis may occur at sites of chronic skin trauma, rubbing and around skin cancers (Figure 89.68).

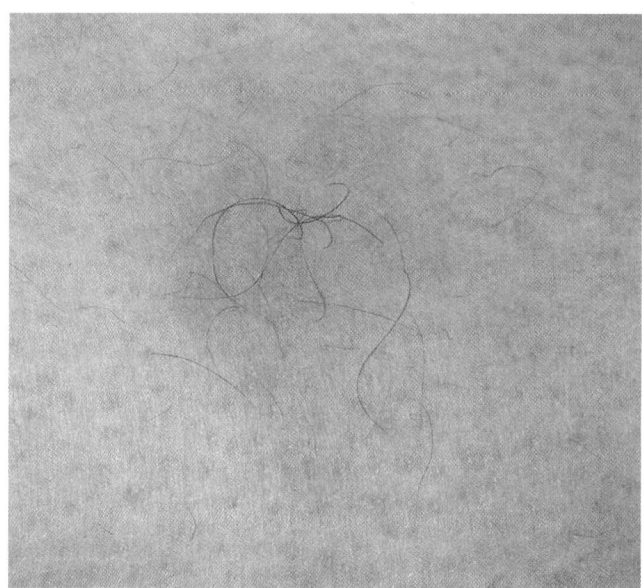

Figure 89.68 Localized hypertrichosis at the site of underlying panniculitis.

Hirsutism

Definition
Hirsutism refers to excess terminal hair in a woman that occurs in a male pattern involving areas such as the beard, moustache and chest. Hair at these sites in men is often under the influence of androgens and occurs after puberty. In women, hirsutism may occur with or without a detectable increase in androgens. See also Chapter 149.

Introduction and general description
The presence of terminal hair in a male pattern in women is referred to as hirsutism. Both the severity of the hirsutism and the degree of its acceptance depend on racial, cultural and social factors. The scheme employed in the study by Ferriman and Gallwey has become the standard grading system and defines hirsutism on quantitative grounds [1]. In clinical practice, it has often been suggested that 'real' hirsutism is simply that which the woman in question thinks is excessive. Studies of the psychological burden of hirsutism among women seeking medical treatment suggest that it has a significant impact and adversely affects quality of life [2].

Epidemiology

Incidence and prevalence
Because of different scales used to determine hirsutism and varying perception by patients based on race and social factors, it is difficult to state incidence accurately but it is estimated that it affects 5–10% of women.

Age
Hirsutism usually becomes apparent after the onset of puberty. In the presence of ectopic androgens it can occur at any age.

Sex
By definition, hirsutism is a condition that affects women.

Ethnicity
Facial and body hair is less commonly seen in Asian peoples, African peoples and indigenous Americans than in white people. Even among white people there are differences; hair growth is heavier in those of Mediterranean than those of Nordic ancestry. The pattern of hair growth in hirsutism within different racial groups is identical.

Associated diseases
Hirsutism is a feature of polycystic ovary syndrome (PCOS). It is also a feature of endocrine disturbance leading to androgen excess.

Pathophysiology
Terminal hair in a male pattern is governed by circulating androgens. In women, androgens originate from the ovaries and the adrenal glands. The first sign of androgen production in women occurs 2–3 years before the menarche and is caused by adrenal secretion. The major androgens secreted by the adrenals are androstenedione, dehydroepiandrosterone (DHEA) and DHEA sulphate (DHEAS). Ovarian androgen production begins under the influence of the pubertal secretion of luteinizing hormone (LH) and takes place in the theca cells. The predominant androgen secreted by the ovaries is androstenedione during the reproductive years, and testosterone after the menopause.

In normal women, the majority of testosterone production (50–70%) is derived from the peripheral conversion of androstenedione in the skin and other extrasplanchnic sites. The remaining proportion is secreted directly by the adrenals and ovaries.

In non-pregnant women, the majority of circulating androgens are bound to a high-affinity β-globulin, sex hormone-binding globulin (SHBG). A further 20–25% is transported loosely bound to albumin, and approximately 1% circulates freely. The free steroid is believed to be active, and the binding protein is therefore of paramount importance.

Whilst abnormal degrees of hair growth are often seen in endocrine disorders characterized by hyperandrogenism, many women with hirsutism will lie within the range of normal for their age and ethnic origin. For those objectively classified as hirsute, many will have underlying PCOS. Most of the others will have no detectable hormonal abnormality and are usually classified as having 'idiopathic' hirsutism. In addition to an increase in circulating androgens, an increased sensitivity to normal levels of androgens or metabolism of the end organ, the dermal papilla of the hair follicle, may well be relevant.

Clinical features

Presentation
Women present with terminal hair that is frequently coarse and pigmented in areas that are usually typical for men only (Figure 89.69). Seborrhoea, acne and female pattern hair loss may also be evident. Frequently, measures will be taken to deal with the hair, such as shaving, and therefore only stubble may be visible.

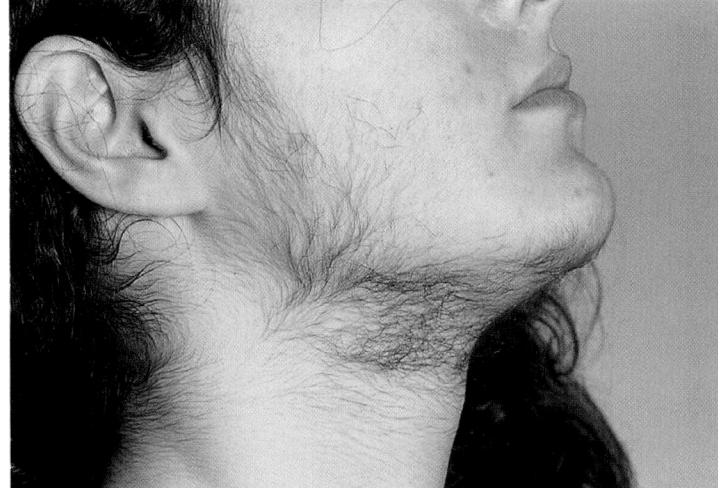

Figure 89.69 Facial hirsutism: in this case it was not associated with any systemic disease or detectable biochemical endocrine abnormality.

Clinical variants

SAHA syndrome. The term SAHA syndrome is used by some to describe the constellation of features that arise with cutaneous virilization. The acronym stands for seborrhoea, acne, hirsutism and androgenetic alopecia. The term does not suggest any specific aetiology; all the causes of hirsutism need to be considered and investigated where clinically indicated.

Polycystic ovary syndrome. The 2003 Rotterdam consensus [3] defined PCOS as having two out of the following criteria:
1 Clinical (acne or hirsutism) and/or biochemical hyperandrogenaemia (measured elevated androgen levels).
2 Menstrual irregularity.
3 Polycystic ovarian morphology on ultrasonography.
It is necessary to exclude other specific disorders, such as non-classic adrenal 21-hydroxylase deficiency, Cushing syndrome, hyperprolactinaemia and androgen-producing tumours.

Polycystic ovaries can occur in normal women or mildly polycystic ovaries in hirsute women with normal menses; women can have the metabolic syndrome of PCOS with normal ovaries on ultrasound. An estimated one-third of women in the UK have polycystic ovaries – defined as 10 or more follicles per ovary detected on ultrasound. One-third of these women will suffer from PCOS. The pattern of these features will depend upon the presenting complaint, be it dermatological, endocrinological or gynaecological. In a gynaecology service, Conway *et al.* [4] found the following clinical features in a series of 556 patients: hirsutism (61%), acne (24%), alopecia (8%), acanthosis nigricans (2%), obesity (35%), menorrhagia (1%), oligomenorrhoea (45%), amenorrhoea (26%) and infertility (>29%). However, those patients who present to a dermatologist almost invariably have acne and/or hirsutism.

Laboratory investigations in PCOS usually reveal an elevated level of LH, often with an increased LH to follicle-stimulating hormone ratio. Testosterone, androstenedione and oestradiol levels are also often raised [4], although these tests are neither sensitive nor specific.

In addition to the presence of elevated testosterone, 50% or more of patients will have hyperinsulinaemia of varying degrees. This appears to be the case for both the classically obese and the non-obese PCOS patient. Insulin acts to inhibit production of SHBG and stimulates ovarian testosterone production. Both effects amplify androgenic features in PCOS. Excess insulin production is related to the feedback loop of peripheral insulin resistance which increases in PCOS. This is characteristic of type 2 diabetes, which is a disease that is more common in PCOS. Consistent with this association, PCOS patients are also at higher risk of dyslipidaemias and coronary artery disease. Altered glucose tolerance, hyperinsulinaemia and hirsutism are all exacerbated by obesity.

Family studies of PCOS suggest there is a strong heritable component. However, to date 70 candidate genes have been evaluated with no conclusive result [5], possibly consistent with the multifactorial mechanism and variability of the disease.

Ovarian tumours. Hirsutism is an almost universal feature in virilizing ovarian tumours; however, functioning tumours that cause virilization represent only about 1% of ovarian tumours. Amenorrhoea or oligomenorrhoea develop in all premenopausal patients with such tumours, and alopecia, clitoromegaly, deepening of the voice and a male habitus develop in approximately half. The majority of patients with virilizing ovarian tumours have raised plasma testosterone levels. As a rule, these levels exceed double the upper limit of normal and combine with the more extreme and evolving clinical picture to distinguish these women from those with PCOS.

Congenital adrenal hyperplasia. Cholesterol is metabolized in the adrenal cortex, via a complex pathway, into aldosterone, cortisol, androgens and oestrogens. A defect in cortisol synthesis results in redistribution of the precursors to other pathways, which results in overproduction of the other hormones. In approximately 95% of cases, 21 hydroxylation is impaired so that 17-hydroxyprogesterone (17-OHP) is not converted to 11-deoxycortisol. Because of defective cortisol synthesis, adrenocorticotrophic hormone levels increase, resulting in overproduction and accumulation of cortisol precursors, particularly 17-OHP. This causes excessive production of androgens, resulting in virilization.

Congenital adrenal hyperplasia (CAH) is divided into four categories:
1 Salt-losing, which presents in infancy with dehydration.
2 Simple virilizing, in which children present with precocious puberty and short stature.
3 Non-classical, attenuated or acquired: it is this variant that is likely to present to the dermatologist with degrees of hirsutism in otherwise well women.
4 Cryptic.
The diagnosis of non-classical late-onset CAH (LO-CAH) cannot be made clinically, and dynamic endocrine investigations are required to differentiate between it, PCOS and idiopathic hirsutism. These women may have only mild degrees of hirsutism, normal physique, normal menses and no metabolic sequelae to the changes in cortisol pathways; however, approximately 80% will have polycystic ovaries. 21-Hydroxylase deficiency is the most common defect found with LO-CAH (>90%). As many as 3–6% of women presenting with hirsutism may be affected with this form.

Acquired adrenocortical disease. Adrenal carcinomas usually present with abdominal swelling or pain; however, 10% of both adenomas and carcinomas may present with isolated virilization. The combination of virilization and Cushing syndrome strongly suggests the presence of a carcinoma. The testosterone level is usually markedly raised in the latter.

Patients with Cushing syndrome are said to have both hypertrichosis, a generalized diffuse growth of fine hair resulting from hypercortisolaemia, and androgen-induced coarse hair in the usual male pattern.

Idiopathic hirsutism. Idiopathic hirsutism is the diagnostic label given to those hirsute women in whom no overt underlying endocrine disorder can be detected. Normal values for total testosterone are found in 25–60% of hirsute women and in 80% of those with regular menstrual cycles. This may be a result of the effect of SHBG or the wide fluctuations in plasma testosterone seen in hirsute women, or it may reflect the role of androgen receptor sensitivity. Although many women classified as having

Table 89.8 Ferriman–Gallwey score of hirsutism. Each site is assessed on a scale of 0 (no terminal hair growth) to 4 (extensive growth of terminal hair). A score of 8 or more is conventionally regarded as indicating significant hirsutism.

Area	Score
Moustache	0–4
Beard	0–4
Chest	0–4
Abdomen	0–4
Suprapubic – extending to umbilicus	0–4
Upper arms	0–4
Thighs	0–4
Upper back	0–4
Lower back	0–4
Total	X/36

idiopathic hirsutism may have subtle PCOS, others may be completely normal.

Classification of severity

Clinical severity can be assessed by examining the extent and distribution of hair, associated features (acne, seborrhoea, pattern hair loss), signs of virilization (clitoromegaly, deepening of voice) and assessing the impact on quality of life. The Ferriman–Gallwey system is the current standard for evaluating hirsutism, which records the presence and degree of hair at different body sites to produce a cumulative score. A score greater than 8 is regarded as diagnostic of hirsutism (Table 89.8).

Investigations

A short history with dramatic change should prompt investigation for an underlying androgen-secreting tumour (Table 89.9). Whilst a sudden change from regular to irregular menses is concerning, normal menses is typical of hirsutism without any endocrine disturbance. Lifelong irregular menses would be in keeping with PCOS.

The extent to which it is necessary for hirsute women without suspicious signs or history to be investigated is debatable. If the primary concern is to exclude an androgen-secreting tumour, a measure of serum testosterone is a good screening tool. It can be supplemented by measurement of DHEAS. Clarifying the diagnosis of PCOS may be appropriate or further investigation arranged in collaboration with a primary care physician, endocrinologist or gynaecologist.

Management

The treatment of hirsutism can be broadly divided into measures aimed at removing unwanted terminal hair and those that reduce the androgen drive to vellus–terminal conversion (Table 89.10). The management of patients with hirsutism may also entail addressing other issues, such as menstrual disturbance, infertility, cardiac risk, type 2 diabetes and obesity, that are generally beyond the scope of the dermatologist and will not be discussed here.

Physical methods of hair removal

There are a number of approaches to hair removal in hirsutism:

- The most widely used methods are shaving and plucking. Shaving the face is unpopular as it seen as a male activity. Various means of plucking hairs include the use of tweezers, waxing, sugaring and threading. Bleaching may help to disguise unwanted dark hair but may give it a yellow hue.
- Depilatory creams contain thioglycolates that dissolve sulphur bonds within the keratin molecules, making the hair gelatinous. They are irritant and require care in terms of strength of preparation and duration of exposure.
- Electroepilation ('electrolysis') is a more permanent method of hair removal. A fine wire is slid into the hair follicle, which is ablated by an electric current using galvanic electrolysis, thermolysis or a combination of the two ('blend'). Electroepilation is a slow method most suited to relatively small areas of hirsutism but good results can be obtained by skilled therapists.
- Laser thermolytic hair removal is now widely used. Although its long-term efficacy is not yet known, laser-assisted hair removal has been in use for sufficient time to allow a reasonable estimate of its efficacy and safety. A Cochrane review observed that the data to support laser and intense pulsed light (IPL) treatment were poor, but favoured alexandrite and diode lasers over

Table 89.9 Investigation of hirsutism.

Severity	Tests	Relevance
Mild hirsutism with normal menses	Debatable whether any tests are required	–
	Testosterone	Excludes an androgen-secreting tumour (if more than twice upper limit of normal, more extensive investigations as below should be considered; mildly elevated levels are common in PCOS)
Moderate hirsutism with or without menstrual irregularity	Luteinizing hormone (LH)	Best measured on days 1–3 of cycle
	Follicle-stimulating hormone (FSH)	Raised LH : FSH is suggestive of polycystic ovaries
	Pelvic ultrasonography	Ultrasound criteria for PCOS are 10 or more cysts, 2–8 mm in diameter
Severe hirsutism, rapid onset	Morning 17-hydroxyprogesterone	Late-onset congenital adrenal hyperplasia
Elevated testosterone	Dehydroepiandrosterone sulphate (DHEAS)	Marker of adrenal androgen secretion, especially in adrenal excess
	24 h urinary cortisol	Cushing syndrome
	Dexamethasone suppression test	Striae, central abdominal weight gain and moon face are likely to point to diagnosis
	Prolactin	Hyperprolactinaemia
	Ovarian and adrenal imaging	Identification of tumours

Table 89.10 Management of hirsutism.

Aim	Method	Cost	Comments and side effects
Camouflage	Bleaching	Low	Good for concealing modest amounts of hair but can give hair a yellow hue
Hair removal	Pluck	Low	Soreness; folliculitis
	Shave	Low	Folliculitis; stubble; needs to be repeated regularly, often daily
	Waxing, sugaring	Medium	Can treat larger areas, but then more soreness; have to wait for hair to grow longer before retreating
	Depilatory creams	Medium	Irritant dermatitis; needs care on sensitive areas
	Electrolysis	High	Long-term therapy; folliculitis and scarring
	Intense pulsed light (IPL)	High	Course of multiple treatments with top-ups in following years; can be painful, burn and cause pigmentation, especially in darker skin types
	Laser	High	As above; both IPL and laser target darkly pigmented terminal hairs and neither are effective for lighter hairs
Inhibition of hair growth	Eflornithine cream	Medium	Folliculitis; can be used in conjunction with laser or IPL therapy
Suppression of androgen secretion or action	Oral contraceptives (OCP)	Medium	Dianette® (ethinylestradiol 35 µg, cyproterone acetate 2 mg) has higher thromboembolic risk
	Antiandrogens: cyproterone acetate (50–100 mg on days 1–10 in combination with OCP, spironolactone (50–200 mg daily) and flutamide	Medium	Menstrual irregularities; gynaecomastia; breast tissue tenderness; liver toxicity; must not get pregnant as will feminize male fetus
	5α-reductase inhibitors	Medium	Not licensed; must not get pregnant as will feminize male fetus; decreased libido; breast tissue tenderness

others. Lack of follow-up data was a particular shortcoming [6]. Most practitioners will select patients with dark hair and light skin. This maximizes the absorption of laser energy by the hair and minimizes absorption by the skin. Nevertheless, it is still possible for soreness and crusting to occur following treatment. In darker skin this can be associated with post-inflammatory pigmentary changes. Treatments are usually administered as part of a course of at least three visits separated by intervals of several weeks. This reflects the biology of the follicle, which is most responsive to abalation when in anagen. The gap between treatments allows those hairs initially in telogen to move into anagen. Broad-band IPL represents a cheaper technology with less restriction on the licensing of those who use it. It is likely to achieve some of the benefits of laser therapy [7].

Topical medication

Topical eflornithine cream reduces the rate of hair growth by inhibiting the enzyme ornithine decarboxylase. Limited clinical trial evidence suggests around one-third of women are helped by using topical eflornithine and it achieves an average reduction in hair growth of about 20%. Treatment has to be continued to maintain the response [8]. There is some evidence that supplementing laser therapy with eflornithine cream results in a greater benefit sooner than with either treatment alone [9].

Oral drug therapy

The main systemic therapies for hirsutism are antiandrogens [10]. The benefits in terms of reversing existing terminal hair growth are relatively modest but it is logical to assume antiandrogens will help to prevent further conversion of vellus follicles to terminal ones. Any benefits are lost within months of stopping treatment [11]. Hence, the patient and the person with responsibility for prescribing need to be aware of the following parameters when medication is commenced:

- All medications have potential side effects and they may need monitoring by blood tests and other measures.
- Pregnancy is contraindicated with these drugs, and a pregnancy prevention plan is required for the duration of therapy – which may be long term.
- Not everyone will respond to treatment and therefore some semiobjective measure of efficacy and timescale for assessment need to be discussed, for example frequency of use of depilatory aids at the outset and at 6 months, or photographs.
- At what point is it envisaged that the treatment will be stopped?
- Who will take responsibility for long-term prescribing and monitoring, where medication is being used outside the licensed indication?

When a hirsute woman has PCOS, prescribing may cross boundaries with treatment of other aspects of the disease, requiring collaboration with other clinicians.

Cyproterone acetate. Cyproterone acetate (CPA) is a synthetic progestogen that acts as both an antiandrogen and an inhibitor of gonadotrophin secretion [12]. It reduces androgen production, increases the metabolic clearance of testosterone and binds to the androgen receptor. In addition, long-term therapy is associated with a reduction in the activity of cutaneous 5α-reductase. Although CPA is a potent progestogen it does not reliably inhibit ovulation. It is usually administered with cyclical oestrogens in order to maintain regular menstruation and to prevent conception in view of the risk of feminizing a male fetus.

A Cochrane review found that CPA has only poor-quality data to support its use, although subjective improvements are recorded [12]. Several regimens have been advocated. Low-dose therapy (Dianette®; Schering AG) is an oral contraceptive containing 35 µg ethinylestradiol and 2 mg CPA, taken daily for 21 in every 28 days. However, many of the dose-ranging and efficacy studies have been performed using a preparation that contained 50 µg ethinylestradiol;

this may be relevant, as only the higher dose of oestrogen increases SHBG. Current dosage recommendations for CPA usually advise that 50 or 100 mg CPA should be administered for 10 days per cycle (e.g. days 1–10 or 5–15). However, there have now been many dose-ranging studies that suggest that there is no dose effect. Objective studies comparing low-dose therapy with and without extra CPA found no difference in the reduction of overall hirsutism grades, although the rate of onset of benefit was faster with the additional cyproterone [13].

Side effects of CPA include weight gain, fatigue, loss of libido, breast tenderness, nausea, headaches and depression. All these side effects are more frequent with higher dosage. As with all medication for a cosmetic problem, safety can be a concern for those needing long-term treatment. Contraindications to its use are the same as for the contraceptive pill. Venous thromboembolism is the adverse effect of greatest medical significance. A case–control study indicated that the risk of this was four times greater in women taking an oral contraceptive containing CPA as the progestogen in comparison with those containing levonorgestrel [14].

One retrospective study of 188 women taking CPA 50–100 mg/day described side effects in 23%. Nine per cent of the total group stopped therapy because of these effects, but it is difficult to discern whether the problems were a result of the CPA or the ethinylestradiol that many also took. Most of the problems were related to mood, weight or menstrual disturbance. Within the group, 24 had been treated for 5 years or more, nine for 10 years or more and two for 15 years [15].

Spironolactone. Spironolactone is a popular and relatively safe treatment for hirsutism. Formal proof of its efficacy is not to the highest standards, although a Cochrane review concluded that it was of some value [16]. Spironolactone has several antiandrogenic pharmacological properties. It reduces the bioavailability of testosterone by interfering with its production and increases its metabolic clearance. It binds to the androgen receptor and, like CPA, long-term therapy is associated with a reduction in cutaneous 5α-reductase activity. Different regimens of spironolactone have been studied, varying between 50 and 200 mg taken either daily or cyclically (daily for 3 weeks in every 4 weeks). Within this dosage range, the one chosen will depend on the severity of the hirsutism. A 3 out of 4 week cycle will result in a withdrawal bleed in the fourth week, which is similar to that seen with oral contraceptives. However, spironolactone cannot be relied on as a contraceptive and care must be taken to avoid conception while taking the drug.

5α-reductase inhibitors. Finasteride inhibits the type 2 isoenzyme of 5α-reductase and has been assessed in small placebo-controlled trials, with some benefit after 6 months' therapy. This group of drugs feminizes a male fetus, which is a drawback in the therapy of women of child-bearing potential and has precluded a drug licence for the treatment of hirsutism.

Metformin. Metformin is a biguanide originally used in the treatment of type 2 diabetes. It has found a place in the treatment of hirsutism associated with hyperinsulinaemia and insulin resistance. In this setting, it can reduce levels of insulin, increase insulin sensitivity and, particularly when associated with a low-calorie diet,

result in weight loss. In many, this constellation of problems will be part of PCOS, and metformin has also been shown to assist in the normalization of menstruation and improvement in lipid profiles. These broader metabolic effects can make it a useful therapy where hirsutism is not the only problem; it is not a drug likely to be prescribed by a dermatologist.

Flutamide. This acts as a pure antiandrogen and works by binding to androgen receptors. However, it has no antigonadotrophic effect, and the result of binding to central androgen receptors is that it prevents the negative feedback effect of testosterone, and consequently androgen levels rise. Flutamide is potentially hepatotoxic and requires close monitoring to avoid liver complications. It is not used in the UK.

Weight loss
Polycystic ovary syndrome is often associated with obesity. Weight loss will help to reduce insulin resistance and circulating testosterone, and excessive hair growth.

HAIR PIGMENTATION

Andrew G. Messenger

Hair colour is one of the most striking of mammalian characteristics. In humans hair colour is determined by melanin incorporated into the hair shaft, the relative proportions of eumelanin (black-brown) and phaeomelanin (yellow-red) and the number and degree of melanization of melanosomes. Other structural factors, such as hair fibre diameter, medullation and cuticle integrity may also affect its visual perception [1,2,3].

Biology of hair pigmentation

Hair melanin is formed by melanocytes situated in the hair bulb epithelium around the upper half of the dermal papilla amongst cells destined to form the hair cortex. The pathway of melanogenesis is described in Chapter 88. Ultrastructurally, hair bulb melanocytes appear more melanogenic than epidermal melanocytes and their population density is much greater than in the epidermis (approximately one melanocyte to four basal keratinocytes in the upper hair bulb compared with a ratio of 1 : 25 in the basal layer of the epidermis) [4]. In humans, hair bulb melanocytes donate melanized melanosomes almost exclusively to cells undergoing early differentiation to form the hair cortex (Figure 89.70). Therefore there is a close spatial and functional relationship between hair bulb melanocytes and the cells that act as pigment receptors (cortical keratinocytes). No pigment is transferred to presumptive cuticular and inner root sheath cells, although pigment granules have been detected in the cuticle of human nostril hair and in the coats of many animals [5].

Melanocytes are also present in the basal layer of the infundibulum and in the outer root sheath where they are non-melanized but identifiable by their expression of the melanocyte marker

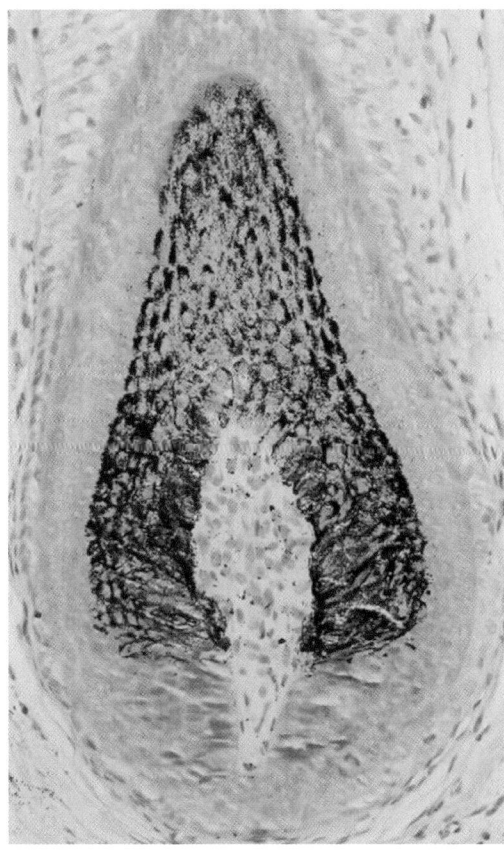

Figure 89.70 Human anagen follicle, showing pigment donation to the hair cortex. There is pigment incontinence in the dermal papilla. Masson–Fontana stain.

NK1beteb. A population of melanocytes with stem cell characteristics has been identified in the lower part of the permanent region of the follicle, in a similar distribution to follicular epithelial stem cells [6]. Like epithelial stem cells these are slow cycling and undergo proliferation only during early anagen, remaining quiescent through the rest of the hair cycle.

Melanogenic activity in the hair follicle is closely linked to the hair cycle. In early anagen, melanocyte stem cells are activated and their offspring migrate into the developing hair bulb. They congregate in the upper part of the anagen hair bulb amongst cells destined to form the hair cortex. Melanogenesis begins well after epithelial proliferation has started and coincides with the onset of morphological evidence of cortical differentiation. Tyrosinase activity becomes apparent in anagen 3 and pigment transfer to cortical epithelium begins in the anagen 4 stage of development [7,8]. In pigmented hair follicles, intense melanogenesis continues throughout the remainder of anagen (anagen 5 and 6) and then ceases with the onset of catagen. The close anatomical and functional association of hair bulb melanocytes with cells to which pigment is donated, cells destined to form the hair cortex, suggests that interaction between these two cell types has a key role in regulating pigmentary activity. The fate of hair bulb melanocytes during catagen is uncertain. Non-melanizing melanocytes have been observed in the regressing epithelial column in human catagen follicles [9] but apoptotic deletion of follicular melanocytes has also been described during this stage of the hair cycle [10].

Variation in human hair colour

Variations in human hair colour occur most commonly in European populations. In non-Europeans hair is predominantly dark brown to black in colour although pockets of lighter shades do exist in some parts of the world [4]. Hair colour, along with skin and eye colour, is determined by multiple genes, classified as SHEP genes by MIM (227220). These include *OCA2*, *MC1R* and *TYRP*. Polymorphisms in the *OCA2* gene are associated with blond and brown hair in Icelanders [11], and blond hair in a Melanesian population is associated with variation in the *TYRP1* gene [12]. The current catalogue of genes affecting human hair colour is undoubtedly far from complete – over 100 genes involved in regulating murine hair pigmentation have been documented.

Red hair
The incidence of red hair varies from 0.3% in northern Germany to as high as 11% in parts of Scotland. Phaeomelanin is the predominant pigment in some individuals with red hair or there may be a mix of eumelanin and phaeomelanin. Melanocytes in phaeomelanized hair follicles contain spherical melanosomes. In those showing mixed eu- and phaeomelanin, melanocytes contain either spherical melanosomes or ellipsoidal eumelanosomes [13].

In mice, the synthesis of eumelanin or phaeomelanin is determined by activation or blockade, respectively, of the melanocortin receptor-1 (MC1R). The receptor is activated by α-melanocyte-stimulating hormone and blocked by agouti signalling protein derived from the dermal papilla. It is not yet clear whether there is a human equivalent for agouti. However, variant regions within the highly polymorphic human *MC1R* gene confer reduced function of the receptor and are associated with red hair [14,15]. Most red-haired individuals are homozygous or compound heterozygous for these *MC1R* polymorphisms.

Greying of hair (canities)

Greying of hair is usually a manifestation of the ageing process. In white races, white hair first appears at the age of 34.2 ± 9.6 years, and by the age of 50 years 50% of the population have at least 50% grey hairs [16], although a more recent survey concluded that this is an overestimate [17]. The onset in black people is 43.9 ± 10.3 years, and in the Japanese between 30 and 34 years in men and between 35 and 39 years in women. The beard and moustache areas commonly become grey before the scalp or body hair. On the scalp, the temples usually show greying first, followed by a wave of greyness spreading to the crown and later to the occipital area. A twin study in women has suggested that hair greying is mainly determined by genetic factors [18].

The visual impression of greying is due to an admixture of pigmented and white hairs. Melanization of pigmented hairs on a grey scalp may be reduced compared with normally pigmented hairs but it is not clear if a decline in pigmentation occurs along the length of a hair shaft (i.e. during a single anagen cycle) or whether the level of reduced or absent pigmentation is established at the onset of an anagen cycle. Loss of hair pigmentation is associated with a decrease and eventual cessation of tyrosinase activity in the

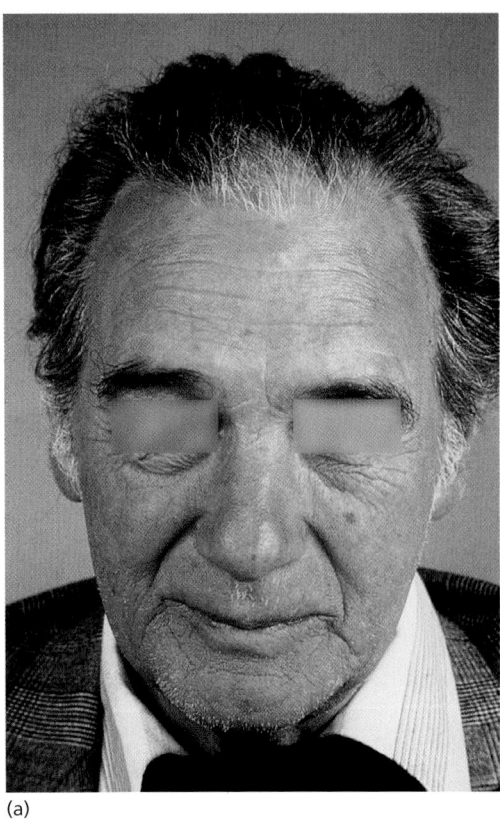
(a)

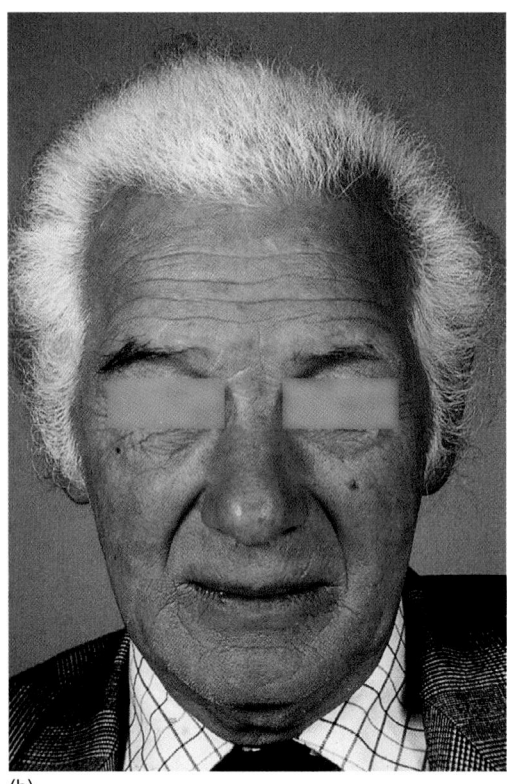
(b)

Figure 89.71 Rapid greying of the hair caused by alopecia areata. (a) A patient with slight greying of the hair, and (b) the same patient shown 1 week later. (Courtesy of Dr D. Fenton, St Thomas' Hospital, London, UK.)

lower bulb [19]. Melanocytes are absent from the bulbs of white hairs [20,21] although non-melanized melanocytes are still present in the outer root sheath [22]. The mechanism of hair greying has not been determined with certainty. It seems most likely to be due to exhaustion of the melanocyte stem cell reservoir. An alternative explanation is that melanocytes are depleted as a result of the accumulation of hydrogen peroxide in the hair follicle [23].

Rapid-onset, allegedly 'overnight', greying of the hair has excited the literary, medical and anthropological worlds for centuries [24]. Historical examples include Sir Thomas More and Marie Antoinette whose hair became grey over the night preceding their executions. The probable mechanism for rapid greying is the selective shedding of pigmented hairs in diffuse alopecia areata, with the non-pigmented hairs being retained (Figure 89.71).

In general, greying of the hair is progressive and permanent, but there are occasional reports of the repigmentation of previously non-pigmented hair [25–27].

Premature greying

The association between premature greying and certain organ-specific autoimmune diseases is well recognized although there are limited published data. In a controlled study of 125 patients with pernicious anaemia, 11% had premature greying, defined as onset before the age of 20, compared to 2% in the control group [28]. Premature greying is a feature in a number of genetic diseases. It occurs in the early ageing disorders the Werner and Rothmund–Thomson syndromes, which are due to defects in DNA helicases [29]. In progeria, premature greying is associated with

a marked loss of scalp hair as early as 2 years of age. In Böök syndrome, an autosomal dominant trait, premature greying is associated with premolar hypodontia and palmoplantar hyperhidrosis [30]. One-third of patients with chromosome 5p syndrome (cri du chat syndrome) have prematurely grey hair [31].

Poliosis

Poliosis is defined as the presence of a localized patch of white hair resulting from the absence or deficiency of melanin in a group of neighbouring follicles. Pigment absence can be congenital or acquired. In many cases of the former it is brought about by physically or functionally abnormal melanocytes from birth, or abnormal migration during embryogenesis. Such migratory defects may be restricted to the skin, but there can be associated abnormalities in other organs such as the ear or eye, where melanocytes or related neural crest cells have an important role.

Acquired forms of poliosis are due to vitiligo or to regrowth of non-pigmented hair following alopecia areata.

Hereditary pigmentary defects

These may affect hair colour; they are discussed in Chapter 88.
- Albinism.
- Piebaldism.
- Waardenburg syndrome
- Tuberous sclerosis: see Chapter 80.
- 'Silver hair' syndromes: see Chapter 68.

Acquired pigmentary defects

These are discussed in detail in Chapter 88.

In vitiligo, the white patches of skin may have white hairs within them. Scattered white hairs on the scalp may occur in children with vitiligo. In alopecia areata, regrowing hair is frequently white. It may remain so, although in most cases hair pigmentation recovers.

The Vogt–Koyanagi–Harada syndrome is a post-febrile condition comprising bilateral uveitis, labrynthine deafness, tinnitus and vitiligo, poliosis and alopecia areata [32,33]. It is likely to be an autoimmune disease, with the melanocyte, tyrosinase or tyrosinase-related protein as targets.

Alezzandrini syndrome, which shows some similarity to Vogt–Koyanagi–Harada syndrome, combines unilateral facial vitiligo, retinitis, hypoacusis and poliosis of the eyebrows and eyelashes [34].

Permanent loss of hair pigment may be induced by inflammatory processes that damage melanocytes (e.g. herpes zoster). X-irradiation often causes permanent hair loss but less intense treatment leads to hypopigmented and, rarely, hyperpigmented hair.

Colour changes induced by drugs and other chemicals

Some topical agents temporarily change hair colour. Dithranol and chrysarobin stain light-coloured or grey hair mahogany brown. Resorcin, formerly used a great deal in a variety of skin diseases, stains black or white hair a yellow or yellowish brown colour.

Chloroquine and hydroxychloroquine occasionally cause reversible bleaching of the hair. The tyrosine kinase inhibitor imatinib, which inhibits the c-KIT and platelet-derived growth factor receptors, has diverse effects on pigmentation, causing both skin hypopigmentation [35] and reversal of hair greying [36]. The prostaglandin growth factor 2α analogues, such as latanoprost, used in the treatment of glaucoma, cause darkening of the iris and the eyelashes [37].

Colour changes induced by nutritional deficiencies

Because specific dietary deficiencies are rare in humans, most clinical knowledge of their effects is derived from laboratory and animal studies. Copper deficiency in cattle causes achromotrichia because it is the prosthetic group of tyrosinase; loss of hair colour from this mechanism occurs in humans as Menkes kinky hair syndrome. In protein malnutrition, exemplified by kwashiorkor, hair colour changes are a prominent feature; normal black hair becomes brown or reddish, and brown hair becomes blond [38]. Intermittent protein malnutrition leads to the 'flag' sign of kwashiorkor (*signe de la bandera*). Alternating white (abnormal) and dark bands occur along individual hairs. Changes similar to those in kwashiorkor have been described in severe ulcerative colitis and after extensive bowel resection.

Hair colour in metabolic disorders

- Phenylketonuria: see Chapter 60.
- Homocystinuria: see Chapter 60.
- Porphyria: see Chapter 63.

Accidental hair discoloration

Hair avidly binds many inorganic elements and thus hair colour changes are occasionally seen after exposure to certain substances. Exposure to high concentrates of copper in industry or from inadvertently high concentrations in tap water [39] or in swimming pools may cause green hair, particularly visible in blond-haired subjects [40]. A yellowish hair colour is not uncommon in white- or grey-haired heavy smokers resulting from the tar in cigarette smoke. Yellow staining may also occur from picric acid and dithranol.

Hair colour resulting from physical phenomena

The whiteness of hair seen when melanin is absent is an optical effect resulting from reflection and refraction of incident light from various interfaces at which zones of different refractive indexes meet. Thus, in general, non-pigmented hair with a broad medulla appears paler than non-medullated hair. Normal 'weathering' of hair along its length may lead to the terminal part appearing lighter than the rest as a result of a similar mechanism – the cortex and cuticle become disrupted and form numerous interfaces from internal reflection and refraction of light. This also applies in trichorrhexis nodosa (excessive 'weathering'), in which patients often note a lightening in colour of the brittle hair, and in the white bands of pili annulati. Because these optical lightening effects are caused by reflection and refraction of incident light, when such hairs are viewed by transmitted light microscopy they appear dark. Findlay showed that the perceived colour is affected by the physical characteristics of the hair shaft and may bear little relationship to the true chromaticity of the shaft [41].

Hairs on exposed parts may be bleached by sunlight.

HAIR COSMETICS

David A. R. de Berker

People have always been concerned about their hair, and have sought to modify it by grooming, colouring and cutting and the use of wigs [1,2,3]. There are references in Egyptian papyruses to the importance of arranging the hair prior to seduction [4,5]. Now, hair care and hair cosmetics are big business and many of the advances have come from cosmetic science laboratories [6,7]. Some aspects of cosmetic management can lead to scalp and hair shaft problems.

Shampoos

A shampoo may be defined as a suitable detergent for washing hair that leaves the hair in good condition [8–13]. It must remove grease, as it is the latter that attracts dirt and other particulate matter. The polar group of a detergent achieves this by displacing oil from the hair surface. The evaluation of shampoo detergency is difficult and complicated. The consumer tends to equate detergency with foaming; in western society, few shampoos sell unless they possess good foaming power. In the evaluation of detergents as shampoos no single criterion can be used, although instrumental methods have been devised. Efficacy can be based only on the subjective impression of the consumer.

Shampoo formulations

These vary enormously, but the basic ingredients can be resolved into a few groups: water, detergent and fatty material. Soap shampoos are made from vegetable or animal fats and remove dirt and grease as efficiently as detergents; however, a scum forms with hard water. Most shampoos contain detergents as the principal washing ingredient; detergents are synthetic petroleum products. Shampoos contain the following:
- Principal surfactants for detergency and foaming power.
- Secondary surfactants to improve and 'condition' hair.
- Functional additives to control pH and viscosity, or ingredients such as tar or antifungal agents.
- Preservatives.
- Aesthetic additives such as colourants and fragrance.
- Silicone conditioning agents.

Shampoo safety

Shampoos must be non-toxic, and must not irritate either the skin or eyes at concentrations used by the consumer. New shampoo formulations are tested exhaustively prior to marketing, particularly to assess their propensity to cause eye irritation, scarring or corneal opacities. Skin irritation is not usually encountered from shampoos that have low eye irritancy potential. In general, the eye irritancy of detergents is greatest with cationics, followed by anionics, and least with non-anionics. There are exceptions to this, suggesting that shampoo irritancy may be caused by properties other than detergency, including surface activity, pH, wetting power, foaming power (Ross–Miles test), and wetting and foaming power together. Most shampoos are, in fact, irritant but not dangerously so. Allergic contact dermatitis resulting from aesthetic additives, preservatives or biocides does occur (see Chapter 128).

Conditioners

Dry hair lacks gloss and lustre and is difficult to style. This results from natural weathering and is worsened by chemical and physical processes applied to the hair. Conditioners have a range of characteristics that may contribute to shine, reduction of static electricity, protection from ultraviolet radiation and possibly increased hair strength. Conditioners comprise fatty acids and alcohols: natural triglycerides (e.g. almond, avocado, corn, olive oil); waxes (e.g. beeswax, jojoba oil, mink oil, lanolin); phospholipids (e.g. egg yolk, soya bean); vitamins A, B and E, protein hydrolysates of silk, collagen, keratin (horn and hoof), gelatine and other proteins; and cationic polymers. Conditioners are available in a variety of forms and are widely used. They provide lubrication and gloss, and render the hair easier to comb and style. The most commonly used are those combined with a shampoo as a 2-in-1 preparation. These cationic chemicals bind with the hair at the negatively charged surface and areas of weathering. In so doing they reduce static by electrically neutralizing the hair, and provide a physical coating to the areas of damaged hair shaft with materials such as dimethicone. Other forms of conditioner may be applied as a separate procedure, and can take the form of creams and emulsions applied for a few minutes after washing and then rinsed off. Deep conditioners are left on for up to 30 minutes, often with damp heat. Fluids, gels and aerosol foams aid styling. Hair oils are traditional conditioners. Men may use brilliantines, greases or oils to leave the hair glossy and sleek [10].

Where the hair is significantly dry or damaged, or the scalp is inflamed or eczematous, conditioner may be used as a shampoo substitute in the same manner that one might advocate an emollient as a soap substitute on the skin of someone with eczema. The conditioner will mix with water to remove surface dirt and odour, but will not subject the hair and scalp to the powerful solvent effects of the shampoo.

Cosmetic hair colouring

Since the days of the pharaohs, women in particular have used hair dyes to hide grey hair. Use has increased enormously during the past 50 years and now men are using hair dyes. Or perhaps they always did!

The penetration of dyes into hair depends on molecular size and the aqueous swelling of the hair at the time of application of the dye; basicity of the dye is also important. The most successful dyes are relatively small molecules [14]. The most common adverse effect of a hair dye is an allergic contact sensitivity, usually to *p*-phenylenediamine (PPD). Internationally, the prevalence of this among those with eczema who are patch tested is between 4% and 6% [15]. There is a concern that hair dye may predispose to a range of cancers, including bladder cancer, because of uncertain toxicities in dyes. The arylamine and amino nitrophenol components give rise to this worry, but systematic reviews have suggested that it is not a hazard to those using it on their hair [16], although it might be a risk for hairdressers [17]. An increase in the incidence of solid tumours [18] and aplastic anaemia [19] has been suggested and contested [20]. None of these reports is sufficiently conclusive to warrant the withdrawal of such dyes.

Excluding bleaches, hair-colouring materials can be divided into three groups: vegetable, metallic and synthetic organic dyes. Synthetic organic materials are thought to give more 'natural' colours than those obtained with vegetable and metallic hair colourants.

Vegetable dyes

Henna may be used to give reddish auburn shades. It is obtained from shrubs found in North Africa and the Middle East: *Lawsonia alba*, *L. spinosa* and *L. inermis*. The dye is produced from dried leaves, which are removed before the plant flowers. The active principle is an acidic naphthoquinone (lawsone). Traditionally, it is applied as a thick paste 'pack', which is left *in situ* for 5–60 min. The effects last for up to 10 weeks. This process is non-toxic but messy, and fingernails may become stained. Henna rinses are mixtures of henna and powdered indigo leaves that produce blue-black shades. A wide range of products containing compound henna exist [8].

Ground flower heads of a Roman or German chamomile yield a yellow dye, 1,3,4-trihydroxyflavone (apigenin). It stains only the cuticle and can be used to lighten or brighten hair. Other vegetable dyes include extracts from logwood and walnut shell, and these can be used by patients who are paraphenylenediamine sensitive. 'Black henna' contains traces of PPD and carries the usual risks of sensitization [21]. These products are obtainable at herbalists and beauty shops.

Metallic dyes

Traditionally, hair dyes for men have been of this type, as the colour changes occur less rapidly and are not as immediately obvious as with the oxidative dyes. Inorganic salts are used, which are altered by the hair and coat the surface as either oxides from the reduction of the metal salts by keratin, or sulphides from the action of sulphur in keratin on the metal. They all give a rather dull (metallic) appearance and may cause brittle or damaged hair if used too often.

Lead acetate, with precipitated sulphur or sodium thiosulphate, gives brown to black shades; grey hair may be changed through yellow to brown or black. Silver nitrate used alone produces a greenish black colour; pyrogallol is used as the developer. Colours from ash blond to black are possible by mixing silver nitrate variously with copper, cobalt or nickel; brownish black skin staining is the great disadvantage. Bismuth salts give shades of brown. Newer metallic dyes, containing a metal plus an organic ligand, are used on textile fibres and in some hair dye patents. Metallic dyes cannot be removed without hair damage, and should be left to grow out.

Synthetic organic dyes

This group has now been in use for more than 60 years. They are the most important type because of the comprehensive range of 'natural' colours that can be obtained. Most penetrate the hair cuticle and so are potentially permanent, but in recent years less permanent types have been introduced.

Synthetic organic colourants are of three types:

1 *Temporary*. These wash out with one shampoo and last no longer than 1 week. Many temporary rinses belong to this group, including fashionable unnatural colours used by avant-garde sects and groups. They are available in aerosol sprays by incorporation into transparent polymeric plastics such as polyvinylpyrrolidone (PVP); the disadvantage of such vehicles is their tendency to flake off on to clothing.

2 *Semipermanent*. In the UK, these have the widest appeal. They are used frequently at home and also in salons to brighten or subdue a natural colour, modify a permanent or bleached colour, or modify white or grey. They are of sufficiently small molecular size to penetrate the cortex. They are intrinsically coloured and no developing is required. They are relatively easy to wash out with shampoos containing ammonia; other shampoos must be used 6–10 times to remove them. Some semipermanent dyes have an affinity for thioglycolate-waved hair. Many are now used in colour shampoos.

3 *Permanent* (developed or oxidation dyes). These do not rely on the natural colour of a single chemical dye stuff, but require an oxidative developer – hydrogen peroxide – to produce the final colour:

Paraphenylenediamine (PPD) and/or paratoluenediamine (PTD)

+

Hydrogen peroxide

↓

Applied to hair

↓

Quinone diamine (small molecule)

↓

Penetrate hair (to cortex)

↓

Large molecules produced
(by diamine 'self'-condensation and modifiers, e.g. pyrogallol)

Other substances may be included in specific formulations to give greater intensity to the dye (e.g. resorcinol and polyhidric phenols).

Oxidative dyes are potentially hazardous. The need for hydrogen peroxide enables lighter shades to be obtained and is chiefly responsible for the structural damage to hair that may occur if care is not exercised. Additives such as pyrogallol and resorcinol are potential irritants. The greatest problem is the potential of PPD (less so with PTD) to cause allergic dermatitis. Up to 10% of users may develop type IV allergy [22]. All dyes in this group are therefore sold with instructions to carry out preliminary patch testing 24–48 h before the proposed dye is used. Thus, the dye system is applied to skin either behind one ear or on the forearm; any redness, swelling or blistering implies allergy and the dyeing should not therefore proceed. A negative patch test does not mean that subsequent allergy cannot develop, it simply shows the subject is not allergic at the time the test is carried out. If allergy is shown, it is not sufficient merely to stop all future use of oxidative dyes. Unfortunately, cross-sensitization also occurs with other aromatic benzenes (e.g. sulphonamides and some local anaesthetics), which must also be avoided for life. Modern formulations seem to cause less problems with allergy [23]. Permanent dyes last for several months and they must not be applied more frequently than every 2–3 weeks because hair damage will occur. Permanently dyed hair must therefore be allowed to grow out. However, if a light shade has been produced and the subject wants a darker shade, then temporary rinses may safely be used as these only coat the hair surface and have no propensity to cause structural damage.

PART 8: SPECIFIC CUTANEOUS STRUCTURE

Bleaches

Bleaching is used both to lighten hair and to prepare it to take up hair dyes [24,25]. Bleaching is an oxidative alkaline treatment that oxidizes and bleaches melanin. The hair lightens to reddish or yellow tones, depending on the underlying hair colour, and ultimately to platinum. Bleaching is very damaging to the hair, rendering it dry, porous and more prone to tangle. Overuse may cause disruption and fracture of the hair [26–28]. Thus, it is advisable to perform permanent waving before bleaching. Home bleaching is usually performed with 6% hydrogen peroxide (20 volumes) with ammonia to speed the reaction, which otherwise takes 12 h. Salons use more powerful bleaching creams, powders and pastes, which are much faster. They are often applied to individual strands of hair, others being left untreated to give highlights, which lessens the problem of darkened roots. Bleaching is terminated by shampooing or an acid rinse. The human eye perceives a more aesthetically acceptable blonde ('platinum' blonde) when the bleached hair is treated with a blue or lilac colourant.

Permanent waving

Permanent waving is often referred to as a 'perm'. It has been defined as the process of changing the shape of the hair so that the new shape persists through several shampoos [2,29]. This is done through restructuring the disulphide amino acid bonds within the hair [30]. During the last 70 years, increasing knowledge of keratin chemistry has enabled semipermanent chemical methods to be developed. Whatever the process used, three stages are involved in hair waving:
1 Physical or chemical softening of the hair.
2 Reshaping.
3 Hardening of fibres to retain the reshaped position.

Softening

Water can extend the hydrogen bonds between adjacent polypeptides in the keratin molecule, allowing temporary reshaping to be carried out – exposure to high humidity or rewetting immediately reverses the process. To obtain a more durable effect from water, steam may be used which, in a limited way, disrupts disulphide bonds. Heat and steam alone are rarely acceptable to modern women because their effects are temporary and the treatment is uncomfortable. Heat can be more effectively employed in conjunction with ammonium hydroxide and potassium bisulphite or triethanolamine as agents to reduce the disulphide bonds. Great skill is involved in this process as failure to judge the time of application of chemicals and heat may cause severe damage.

Since 1945, cold wave processes using substituted thiosulphates (thioglycolates) have largely superseded hot waving. Thioglycolates are potent reducers of disulphide bonds in the keratin molecule:

$$— S = S \rightarrow 2 —SH$$

A typical cold waving lotion contains thioglycolic acid plus ammonia or monoethanolamine.

Acid permanent waves have recently become popular for salon use. They contain glyceryl monothioglycolate and produce a softer curl, and can be used on damaged and bleached hair. Their disadvantage is the high frequency of sensitization in the hairdressers using the product and, occasionally, sensitization of the client [31].

Reshaping

The type of rollers or curlers used to reshape the softened hair depends on the training of the hairdresser and the fashion desired. The degree of curl or tightness of the permanent wave depends both on the diameter of the roller and the size of the strand wound round the roller. Increasing the time of exposure to the perming solution up to 20 min increases the curl, but longer times do not give a further increase. The strength of the solution used depends on the hair type, texture and previous bleaching. Home permanent waves are weaker and cannot achieve the same degree of curl. 'Tepid' waving involves using a weaker thioglycolate solution plus warm air. Neutralization is carried out initially with the curlers in place and again after they have been carefully removed. The reshaping stage is thus a test of hairdressing skill and experience.

Hardening (neutralizing or setting)

In general, this process involves a reversal of the softening (reduction) stages:

$$2 — SH \rightarrow — S = S —$$

It is important to note that a complete reversal to the presoftened 'strength' cannot occur because many free SH groups may not be in a position for oxidation to be effective, for example:

$$2 — SH \rightarrow — S — C— S— \quad (C = carbon)$$

$$2 — SH \rightarrow — S — Ba — S— \quad (Ba = barium)$$

Atmospheric oxidation may efficiently neutralize the waving process. This method is slow and rollers must be left in position for several hours overnight. Chemical oxidation is now the rule. Hairdressers generally use hydrogen peroxide, whereas most solutions for home use contain sodium perborate or percarbonate (in the UK), or sodium or potassium bromate (in the USA). This is why hair is lighter after permanent waving. Some neutralizers contain shellac, which may react with alcohol groups to cause hair discoloration.

Practical procedures

Hot waving

This four-stage procedure is almost never used:
1 Shampooing.
2 Hair is divided and the rollers or curlers applied under slight tension.
3 Waving solution is applied.
4 Heating.
Heating varies according to the solution used or the type of wave required. Electrical rollers or exothermic reactive chemicals may be used. The latter allow free head movement during the waving. The skill of this procedure lies in good hair sectioning, judging the

right amount of solution, correct winding tension and appropriate steaming time.

Cold waving

This also involves initial shampooing, hair division into locks, moistening with waving lotion and the application of croquignole curlers. Further solution may then be applied. The softening time is 10–20 min. Occasionally, mild heat is included, using exothermic chemicals or the natural heat from the head by enclosing the scalp in a plastic bag. These may add to the comfort of the process. Rinsing then takes place, followed by neutralization with the oxidizing solution for up to 10 min. After removing the curlers, further 'hardening' solution is usually applied. 'Loose' curl waves last for no more than a few weeks but 'tight' curl styles may persist for 4–12 months.

Hair straightening (relaxing)

In principle, the methods used to straighten hair are similar to those used in permanent waving [32,33]. The practice is used to straighten African hair and is also called relaxing. One survey found that relaxing formulations were used in 45% of African American women [34]. These practices are associated with a range of problems and ultimately may contribute to scarring alopecia [35].

Pomades

These are mostly used by men with relatively short hair. They are greasy and act by 'plastering' hair into position.

Hot-comb methods

Shampooing is carried out and the hair is towelled dry; oil is then applied (e.g. petroleum jelly, liquid paraffin), which acts as a heat-transferring agent. Heat pressing with hot combing is then used (64–126°C, 148–260°F), causing the breakage and reforming of disulphide bonds, allowing the hair to be moulded straight. Structural damage (and breakage) of hair is common with this process and scarring alopecia may occur as a result of hot waxes entering the follicles. Sweating and rain reverse this procedure.

Cold methods

The chemical methods employed use alkaline reducing agents (caustics), thioglycolates, ammonium carbonate or sodium bisulphite. Caustic soda preparations are usually creams and require the application of protective scalp oil or wax. They are combed through the hair and left for 15–20 min; the hair is combed and straightened again, then rinsed and neutralized. These preparations are limited to salon use because of their potential to cause irritant dermatitis and damage to the hair. Thioglycolate creams are the most common agents used. The cream is applied liberally to the hair, which is then combed until it is straight. The cream is then washed off and a neutralizer (oxidizing agent) applied. Other straighteners ('relaxers') do not contain thioglycolates (e.g. sodium bisulphite and ammonium carbonate, acidic ethylene glycol or 1,3-propylene glycol). Bisulphite straighteners are suitable for home use in combination with alkaline stabilizers.

Hair setting

Setting lotions have changed considerably in recent years [36]. The traditional semi-liquid gels based on water-soluble gums (e.g. tragacanth, karaya, acasia) have been replaced by various synthetic polymers in a bewildering array of forms – aerosol foams and sprays, liquids and gels. Most are based on PVP in a gelled aqueous solution and give an attractive glossy, non-greasy appearance [37]. Some preparations incorporate other ingredients to condition or to add antistatic action, lustre or sheen.

Key references

The full list of references can be found in the online version at www.rooksdermatology.com.

Hair biology

4 Dry FW. The coat of the mouse (*Mus musculus*). *J Genet* 1925;16:287–340.
5 Pinkus H. Embryology of hair. In: Montagna W, Ellis RA, eds. *The Biology of Hair Growth*. New York: Academic Press, 1958:1–32.
18 Cotsarelis G, Sun TT, Lavker RM. Label-retaining cells reside in the bulge area of pilosebaceous unit: implications for follicular stem cells, hair cycle, and skin carcinogenesis. *Cell* 1990;61:1329–37.
22 Oliver RF. The induction of hair follicle formation in the adult hooded rat by vibrissa dermal papillae. *J Embryol Exp Morphol* 1970;23:219–36.
23 Jahoda CA, Horne KA, Oliver RF. Induction of hair growth by implantation of cultured dermal papilla cells. *Nature* 1984;311:560–2.
24 Jahoda CA, Reynolds AJ, Oliver RF. Induction of hair growth in ear wounds by cultured dermal papilla cells. *J Invest Dermatol* 1993;101:584–90.
27 Reynolds AJ, Lawrence C, Cserhalmi-Friedman PB, Christiano AM, Jahoda CA. Trans-gender induction of hair follicles. *Nature* 1999;402:33–4.
31 Schweizer J, Langbein L, Rogers MA, Winter H. Hair follicle-specific keratins and their diseases. *Exp Cell Res* 2007;313:2010–20.
34 Jones LN. Hair structure anatomy and comparative anatomy. *Clin Dermatol* 2001;19:95–103.
37 Courtois M, Loussouarn G, Hourseau C. Aging and hair cycles. *Br J Dermatol* 1995;132:86–93.
46 Ebling FJ. The hormonal control of hair growth. In: Orfanos CE, Happle R, eds. *Hair and Hair Diseases*. Berlin: Springer Verlag, 1990:267–99.
48 Hamilton JB. Age, sex and genetic factors in the regulation of hair growth in men: a comparison of Caucasian and Japanese populations. In: Montagna W, Ellis RA, eds. *The Biology of Hair Growth*. New York: Academic Press, 1958:399.
55 Jenkins EP, Andersson S, Imperato McGinley J, Wilson JD, Russell DW. Genetic and pharmacological evidence for more than one human steroid 5-alpha-reductase. *J Clin Invest* 1992;89:293–300.
60 Orentreich N. Autografts in alopecias and other selected dermatological conditions. *Ann NY Acad Sci* 1959;83:463–79.

Approach to the patient with hair loss

7 Miteva M, Tosti A. Hair and scalp dermatoscopy. *J Am Acad Dermatol* 2012;67:1040–8.
8 Sperling L, Cowper S, Knopp E. *An Atlas of Hair Pathology with Clinical Correlations*, 2nd edn. London: Informa Healthcare, 2012.

Non-scarring disorders of hair growth

Androgenetic alopecia and pattern hair loss

1 Sinclair R. Male pattern androgenetic alopecia. *BMJ* 1998;317:865–9.
7 Birch MP, Messenger JF, Messenger AG. Hair density, hair diameter and the prevalence of female pattern hair loss. *Br J Dermatol* 2001;144(2):297–304.
9 Norwood OT. Male pattern baldness:classification and incidence. *South Med J* 1975;68:1359–65.
11 Nyholt DR, Gillespie NA, Heath AC, Martin NG. Genetic basis of male pattern baldness. *J Invest Dermatol* 2003;121:1561–4.

14 Ludwig E. Classification of the types of androgenetic alopecia (common baldness) occurring in the female sex. *Br J Dermatol* 1977;97:247–54.

27 Hamilton JB. Male hormone stimulation is prerequisite and an incitant in common baldness. *Am J Anat* 1942;71:451–80.

28 Imperato-McGinley J. 5alpha-reductase-2 deficiency and complete androgen insensitivity: lessons from nature. *Adv Exp Med Biol* 2002;511:121–31; discussion 31–4.

35 Orentreich N. Autografts in alopecias and other selected dermatological conditions. *Ann NY Acad Sci* 1959;83:463–79.

38 Courtois M, Loussouarn G, Hourseau C. Aging and hair cycles. *Br J Dermatol* 1995;132:86–93.

45 Whiting DA. Scalp biopsy as a diagnostic and prognostic tool in androgenetic alopecia. *Dermatolog Ther* 1998;8:24–33.

47 Ellis JA, Stebbing M, Harrap SB. Polymorphism of the androgen receptor gene is associated with male pattern baldness. *J Invest Dermatol* 2001;116:452–5.

73 Whiting DA. Chronic telogen effluvium: increased scalp hair shedding in middle-aged women. *J Am Acad Dermatol* 1996;35:899–906.

75 Rietschel RL, Duncan SH. Safety and efficacy of topical minoxidil in the management of androgenetic alopecia. *J Am Acad Dermatol* 1987;16:677–85.

82 Kaufman KD, Olsen EA, Whiting D,, et al. Finasteride in the treatment of men with androgenetic alopecia. *J Am Acad Dermatol* 1998;39:578–89.

91 Lucky AW, Piacquadio DJ, Ditre CM, et al. A randomized, placebo-controlled trial of 5% and 2% topical minoxidil solutions in the treatment of female pattern hair loss. *J Am Acad Dermatol* 2004;50:541–53.

Telogen effluvium

1 Kligman AM. Pathologic dynamics of human hair loss. I. Telogen effuvium *Arch Dermatol* 1961;83:175–98.

2 Kligman AM. The human hair cycle. *J Invest Dermatol* 1959;33:307–16.

5 Headington JT. Telogen effluvium. New concepts and review. *Arch Dermatol* 1993;129:356–63.

7 Schiff BL, Kern AB. Study of postpartum alopecia. *Arch Dermatol* 1963;87:609–11.

39 Sinclair R, Jolley D, Mallari R, Magee J. The reliability of horizontally sectioned scalp biopsies in the diagnosis of chronic diffuse telogen hair loss in women. *J Am Acad Dermatol* 2004;51:189–99.

Alopecia areata

3 Safavi KH, Muller SA, Suman VJ, Moshell AN, Melton LJ. Incidence of alopecia areata in Olmsted County, Minnesota, 1975 through 1989. *Mayo Clin Proc* 1995;70:628–33.

5 Walker SA, Rothman S. Alopecia areata: a statistical study and consideration of endocrine influences. *J Invest Dermatol* 1950;14:403–13.

11 Paus R, Bertolini M. The role of hair follicle immune privilege collapse in alopecia areata: status and perspectives. *J Investig Dermatol Symp Proc* 2013;16:S25–7.

15 Ito T, Ito N, Saatoff M, et al. Maintenance of hair follicle immune privilege is linked to prevention of NK cell attack. *J Invest Dermatol* 2008;128:1196–206.

17 Messenger AG, Bleehen SS. Expression of HLA-DR by anagen hair follicles in alopecia areata. *J Invest Dermatol* 1985;85:569–72.

21 Messenger AG, Slater DN, Bleehen SS. Alopecia areata: alterations in the hair growth cycle and correlation with the follicular pathology. *Br J Dermatol* 1986;114:337–47.

36 Petukhova L, Duvic M, Hordinsky M, et al. Genome-wide association study in alopecia areata implicates both innate and adaptive immunity. *Nature* 2010;466:113–17.

43 Tosti A, Bellavista S, Iorizzo M. Alopecia areata: a long term follow-up study of 191 patients. *J Am Acad Dermatol* 2006;55:438–41.

51 Happle R, Hausen BM, Wiesner-Menzel L. Diphencyprone in the treatment of alopecia areata. *Acta Derm Venereol* 1983;63:49–52.

52 Rokhsar CK, Shupack JL, Vafai JJ, Washenik K. Efficacy of topical sensitizers in the treatment of alopecia areata. *J Am Acad Dermatol* 1998;39:751–61.

Scarring disorders of hair growth

Acquired cicatricial alopecia, Non-specific cicatricial alopecia, Follicular lichen planus, Chronic cutaneous lupus erythematosus, Pseudopelade of Brocq, Central centrifugal cicatrical alopecia, Folliculitis decalvans and tufted folliculitis

1 Olsen EA, Bergfeld WF, Cotsarelis G, et al. Summary of North American Hair Research Society (NAHRS)-sponsored workshop on cicatricial alopecia, Duke University Medical Center, February 10 and 11, 2001. *J Am Acad Dermatol* 2003;48:103–10.

5 Harries MJ, Sinclair RD, Macdonald-Hull S, Whiting DA, Griffiths CE, Paus R. Management of primary cicatricial alopecias: options for treatment. *Br J Dermatol* 2008;159:1–22.

9 Karnik P, Tekeste Z, McCormick TS, et al. Hair follicle stem cell-specific PPAR-gamma deletion causes scarring alopecia. *J Invest Dermatol* 2009;129:1243–57.

11 Mehregan DA, Van Hale HM, Muller SA. Lichen planopilaris: clinical and pathologic study of forty-five patients. *J Am Acad Dermatol* 1992;27:935–42.

19 Kossard S. Postmenopausal frontal fibrosing alopecia. Scarring alopecia in a pattern distribution. *Arch Dermatol* 1994;130:770–4.

24 Graham-Little EG. Folliculitis decalvans et atrophicans. *Br J Dermatol* 1915;27:183–5.

35 Sperling LC, Sau P. The follicular degeneration syndrome in black patients. 'Hot comb alopecia' revisited and revised. *Arch Dermatol* 1992;128:68–74.

42 Powell J, Dawber RP. Successful treatment regime for folliculitis decalvans despite uncertainty of all aetiological factors. *Br J Dermatol* 2001;144:428–9.

Artefactual alopecia

1 Gummer CL. Bubble hair: a cosmetic abnormality caused by brief, focal heating of damp hair fibres. *Br J Dermatol* 1994;131(6):901–3.

4 Khumalo NP, Jessop S, Gumedze F, Ehrlich R. Hairdressing and the prevalence of scalp disease in African adults. *Br J Dermatol* 2007;157(5):981–8.

9 Wilborn WS. Disorders of hair growth in African Americans. In: Olsen E, ed. *Disorders of Hair Growth*, 2nd edn. New York: McGraw-Hill, 2003:497–518.

Trichotillomania

1 Hautmann G, Hercogova J, Lotti T. Trichotillomania. *J Am Acad Dermatol* 2002;46:807–21; quiz 22–6.

7 Muller SA. Trichotillomania: a histopathologic study in sixty-six patients. *J Am Acad Dermatol* 1990;23:56–62.

12 Bloch MH, Landeros-Weisenberger A, Dombrowski P, et al. Systematic review: pharmacological and behavioral treatment for trichotillomania. *Biol Psychiatry* 2007;62:839–46.

13 Rothbart R, Amos T, Siegfried N, et al. Pharmacotherapy for trichotillomania. *Cochrane Database Syst Rev* 2013;Issue 11:CD007662.

14 Grant JE, Odlaug BL, Kim SW. N-acetylcysteine, a glutamate modulator, in the treatment of trichotillomania: a double-blind, placebo-controlled study. *Arch Gen Psychiatry* 2009;66:756–63.

Infections

13 Haycox CL, Kim S, Fleckman P, et al. Trichodysplasia spinulosa – a newly described folliculocentric viral infection in an immunocompromised host. *J Investig Dermatol Symp Proc* 1999;4:268–71.

15 Van der Meijden E, Janssens RW, Lauber C, Bouwes Bavinck JN, Gorbalenya AE, Feltkamp MC. Discovery of a new human polyomavirus associated with trichodysplasia spinulosa in an immunocompromised patient. *PLOS Pathog* 2010;6:e1001024.

Other disorders of hair growth

Chemotherapy alopecia

1 Kanti V, Nuwayhid R, Lindner J, et al. Analysis of quantitative changes in hair growth during treatment with chemotherapy or tamoxifen in patients with breast cancer: a cohort study. *Br J Dermatol* 2014;170:643–50.

2 Trueb RM. Chemotherapy-induced alopecia. *Semin Cutan Med Surg* 2009;28:11–14.

3 Van Scott EJ, Reinertson RP, Steinmuller R. The growing hair roots of the human scalp and morphologic changes therein following amethopterin therapy. *J Invest Dermatol* 1957;29:197–204.

4 Grevelman EG, Breed WP. Prevention of chemotherapy-induced hair loss by scalp cooling. *Ann Oncol* 2005;16:352–8.

8 Baker BW, Wilson CL, Davis AL, et al. Busulphan/cyclophosphamide conditioning for bone marrow transplantation may lead to failure of hair regrowth. *Bone Marrow Transplant* 1991;7:43–7.

13 Prevezas C, Matard B, Pinquier L, Reygagne P. Irreversible and severe alopecia following docetaxel or paclitaxel cytotoxic therapy for breast cancer. *Br J Dermatol* 2009;160:883–5.

Circumscribed alopecia of congenital origin

5 Tosti A. Congenital triangular alopecia. Report of fourteen cases. *J Am Acad Dermatol* 1987;16:991–3.

Abnormalities of the hair shaft

1 Whiting DA, Dy LC. Office diagnosis of hair shaft defects. *Semin Cutan Med Surg* 2006;25:24–34.

3 Smith VV, Anderson G, Malone M, Sebire NJ. Light microscopic examination of scalp hair samples as an aid in the diagnosis of paediatric disorders: retrospective review of more than 300 cases from a single centre. *J Clin Pathol* 2005;58:1294–8.

5 Rakowska A, Slowinska M, Kowalska-Oledzka E, Rudnicka L. Trichoscopy in genetic hair shaft abnormalities. *J Dermatol Case Rep* 2008;2:14–20.

10 Menkes JH, Alter M, Steigleder GK, Weakley DR, Sung JH. A sex-linked recessive disorder with retardation of growth, peculiar hair, and focal cerebral and cerebellar degeneration. *Pediatrics* 1962;29:764–79.

13 Netherton EW. A unique case of trichorrhexis nodosa; bamboo hairs. *Arch Dermatol* 1958;78:483–7.

24 Price VH, Odom RB, Ward WH, Jones FT. Trichothiodystrophy: sulfur-deficient brittle hair as a marker for a neuroectodermal symptom complex. *Arch Dermatol* 1980;116:1375–84.

34 Price VH, Thomas RS, Jones FT. Pili annulati. Optical and electron microscopic studies. *Arch Dermatol* 1968;98:640–7.

36 Hutchinson PE, Cairns RJ, Wells RS. Woolly hair. Clinical and general aspects. *Trans St Johns Hosp Dermatol Soc* 1974;60(2):160–77.

40 Mortimer PS, Gummer C, English J, Dawber RP. Acquired progressive kinking of hair. Report of six cases and review of literature. *Arch Dermatol* 1985;121:1031–3.

50 Price VH, Gummer CL. *Loose anagen syndrome. J Am Acad Dermatol* 1989;20:249–56.

Excessive growth of hair

Hypertrichosis

7 Hensley GT, Glynn KP. Hypertrichosis lanuginosa as a sign of internal malignancy. *Cancer* 1969;24:1051–6.

13 Burton JL, Marshall A. Hypertrichosis due to minoxidil. *Br J Dermatol* 1979;101:593–5.

21 Grossman ME, Bickers DR, Poh-Fitzpatrick MB, Deleo VA, Harber LC. Porphyria cutanea tarda. Clinical features and laboratory findings in 40 patients. *Am J Med* 1979;67:277–86.

25 Demitsu T, Manabe M, Harima N, Sugiyama T, Yoneda K, Yamada N. Hypertrichosis induced by latanoprost. *J Am Acad Dermatol* 2001;44:721–3.

Hirsutism

1 Ferriman D, Gallwey JD. Clinical assessment of body hair growth in women. *J Clin Endocrinol Metab* 1961;21:1440–7.

3 Rotterdam ESHRE/ASRM Sponsored PCOS Consensus Workshop Group. Revised 2003 consensus on diagnostic criteria and long-term health risks related to polycystic ovary syndrome (PCOS). *Hum Reprod* 2004;19:41–7.

6 Haedersdal M, Wulf HC. Evidence-based review of hair removal using lasers and light sources. *J Eur Acad Dermatol Venereol* 2006;20:9–20.

8 Wolf JE, Jr, Shander D, Huber F,, *et al.* Randomized, double-blind clinical evaluation of the efficacy and safety of topical eflornithine HCl 13.9% cream in the treatment of women with facial hair. *Int J Dermatol* 2007;46:94–8.

12 Van der Spuy ZM, le Roux PA. Cyproterone acetate for hirsutism. *Cochrane Database Syst Rev* 2003;Issue 4:CD001125.

13 Barth JH, Cherry CA, Wojnarowska F, Dawber RP. Cyproterone acetate for severe hirsutism: results of a double-blind dose-ranging study. *Clin Endocrinol (Oxf)* 1991;35:5–10.

16 Farquhar C, Lee O, Toomath R, Jepson R. Spironolactone versus placebo or in combination with steroids for hirsutism and/or acne. *Cochrane Database Syst Rev* 2003;Issue 4:CD000194.

Hair pigmentation

1 Slominski A, Wortsman J, Plonka PM, Schallreuter KU, Paus R, Tobin DJ. Hair follicle pigmentation. *J Invest Dermatol* 2005;124:13–21.

6 Nishimura EK. Melanocyte stem cells: a melanocyte reservoir in hair follicles for hair and skin pigmentation. *Pigment Cell Melanoma Res* 2011;24:401–10.

7 Kukita A. Changes in tyrosinase activity during melanocyte proliferation in the hair growth cycle. *J Invest Dermatol* 1957;28:273–4.

11 Sulem P, Gudbjartsson DF, Stacey SN, *et al.* Genetic determinants of hair, eye and skin pigmentation in Europeans. *Nat Genet* 2007;39:1443–52.

13 Jimbow K, Ishida O, Ito S, Hori Y, Witkop CJ, King RA. Combined chemical and electron microscopic studies of pheomelanosomes in human red hair. *J Invest Dermatol* 1983;81:506–11.

14 Valverde P, Healy E, Jackson I, Rees JL, Thody AJ. Variants of the melanocyte-stimulating hormone receptor gene are associated with red hair and fair skin in humans. *Nat Genet* 1995;11:328–30.

16 Keogh EV, Walsh RJ. Rate of greying of human hair. *Nature* 1965;207:877–8.

18 Gunn DA, Rexbye H, Griffiths CE, *et al.* Why some women look young for their age. *PLOS One* 2009;4:e8021.

22 Commo S, Gaillard O, Bernard BA. Human hair greying is linked to a specific depletion of hair follicle melanocytes affecting both the bulb and the outer root sheath. *Br J Dermatol* 2004;150:435–43.

39 Goldschmidt H. Green hair. *Arch Dermatol* 1979;115:1288.

Hair cosmetics

1 Draelos ZD. The biology of hair care. *Dermatol Clin* 2000;18:651–8.

2 Bolduc C, Shapiro J. Hair care products: waving, straightening, conditioning, and coloring. *Clin Dermatol* 2001;19:431–6.

14 Morel OJ, Christie RM. Current trends in the chemistry of permanent hair dyeing. *Chem Rev* 2011;111:2537–61.

15 Thyssen JP, White JM; European Society of Contact Dermatitis. Epidemiological data on consumer allergy to p-phenylenediamine. *Contact Dermatitis* 2008;59:327–43.

35 Wilborn WS. Disorders of hair growth in African Americans. In: Olsen E, ed. *Disorders of Hair Growth*, 2nd edn. New York: McGraw-Hill, 2003:497–518.Classification links

CHAPTER 90

Acne

Alison M. Layton[1], E. Anne Eady[1] and Christos C. Zouboulis[2]

[1]Department of Dermatology, Harrogate and District NHS Foundation Trust, Harrogate, UK
[2]Departments of Dermatology, Venereology, Allergology and Immunology, Dessau Medical Center, Dessau, Germany

Acne vulgaris

Definition and nomenclature

Acne vulgaris is a chronic inflammatory disease of the pilosebaceous unit. The clinical lesions are non-inflammatory open and closed comedones (Figure 90.1) and/or papules, pustules and nodules of varying degree of inflammation and depth (Figure 90.2). The face, back and/or chest are the most frequently affected sites. Post-inflammatory macules, pigment changes (Figure 90.3) and scarring commonly occur (Figure 90.4a,b).

Synonyms and inclusions

- Acne (acne vulgaris)
- Comedonal acne (acne comedonica)
- Prepubertal acne
- Nodulocystic acne (acne conglobata, conglobate acne)
- Acne fulminans

Introduction and general description

Acne vulgaris is one of the most common skin diseases worldwide, affecting all ethnicities and races [1–3]. The highest prevalence

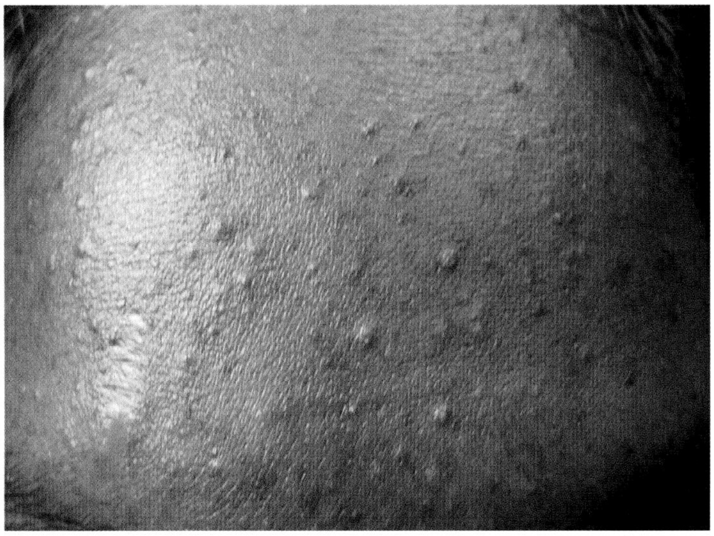

Figure 90.1 Predominantly comedonal acne. (Courtesy of Dr S. Chow, KL Skin Centre, Malaysia.)

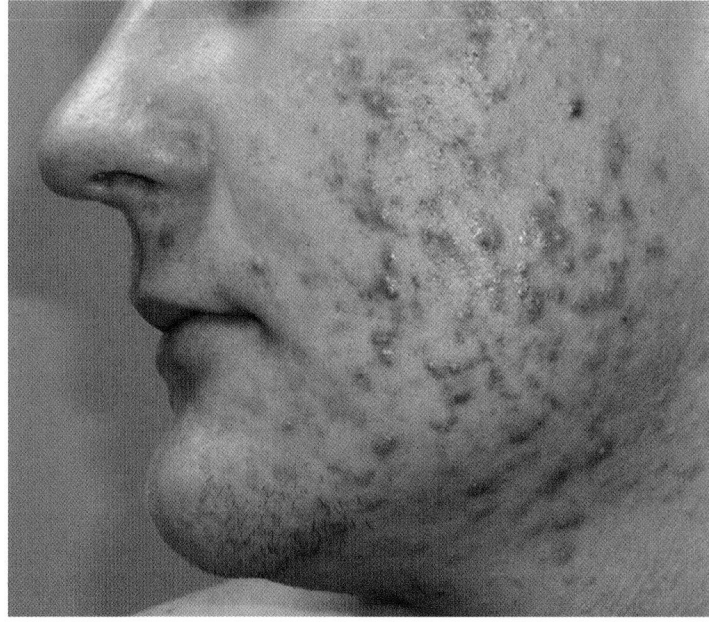

Figure 90.2 Moderate to severe inflammatory acne including a mixture of non-inflammatory and inflammatory lesions with seborrhoea.

PART 8: SPECIFIC CUTANEOUS STRUCTURE

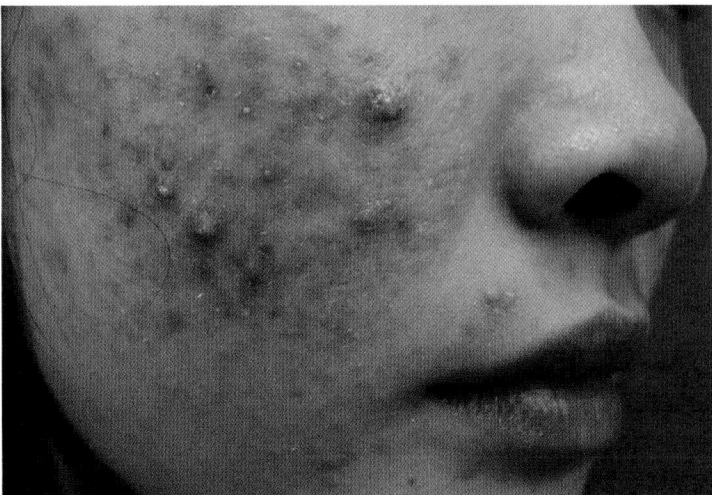

Figure 90.3 Post-inflammatory macules and pigment changes interspersed with inflammatory acne. (Courtesy of Dr S. Chow, KL Skin Centre, Malaysia.)

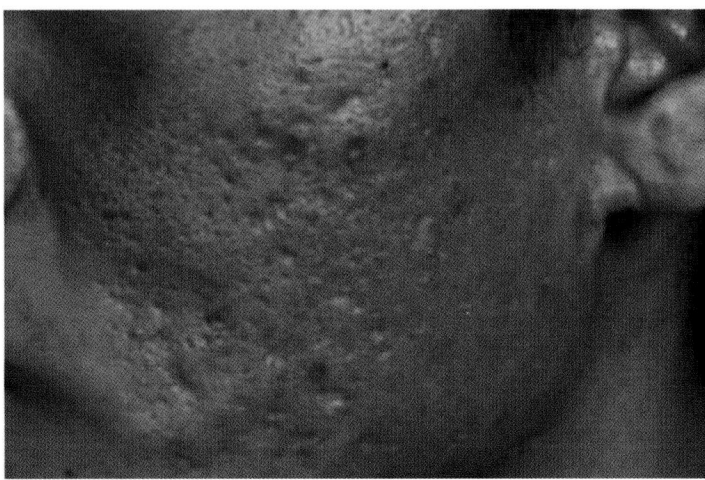

(a)

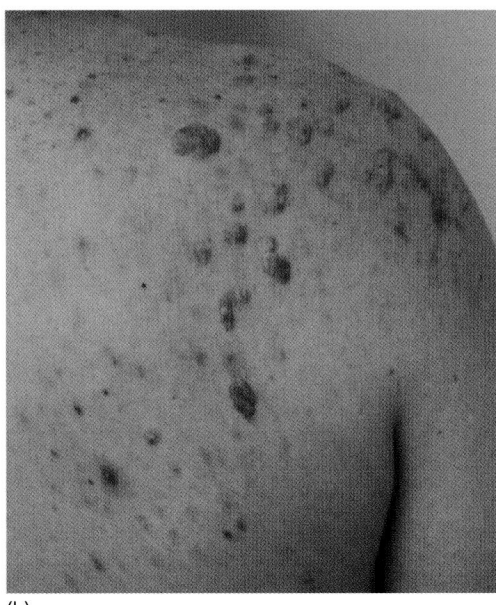

(b)

Figure 90.4 Acne scarring. (a) Atrophic scarring on the cheeks. (Courtesy of Dr C. L. Goh, National Skin Centre, Singapore.) (b) Hypertrophic keloid scarring of the trunk.

of acne occurs in adolescence where it may be diagnosed in 80% of all teenagers. The age of onset has changed over time, paralleling the earlier onset of puberty reported in recent years [4,5]. Acne commonly has a prolonged course, with acute or insidious relapse or recurrence over time. Clinical presentation includes non-inflammatory and/or inflammatory lesions extending over the face and/or trunk. Discomfort may be a significant manifestation of the inflammatory lesions. Seborrhoea of varying degree is usually present. The combined impacts of acne frequently result in psychosocial morbidity. Successful treatment correlates with improvement of psychological factors in many cases [**6**]. Acne scarring is more likely if treatment is delayed (Figure 90.5) hence early treatment is advocated [7]. Despite the reduced prevalence with age, the burden of acne remains high in adults [8].

Epidemiology

Age and gender

Once regarded as a transient disease of the teenage years, acne is now presenting earlier [9] and lasting longer [3,10]. Earlier development of acne has been linked with earlier onset of puberty, which may also relate to diet/obesity and other lifestyle factors [11,12]; however, earlier recognition may also lead to earlier presentation. Acne most commonly presents between the ages of 10 and 13 years in both sexes. Large community-based surveys and detailed smaller scale studies have shown that acne begins at a younger age in girls than boys aligning with earlier puberty [13–15].

Comedonal acne can be detected in some children before any overt signs of puberty [16,17]. This is consistent with the pathophysiology of acne in which rising adrenal dihydroepiandrosterone (DHEAS) output is the trigger for sebum production by androgen susceptible follicles in both girls and boys [17,18].

Early adrenarche in girls is a recognized risk factor for metabolic syndrome, polycystic ovary syndrome (PCOS) and insulin resistance [19]. The early development of comedonal acne in girls may be a predictor of more severe disease in later life. Post-adolescent

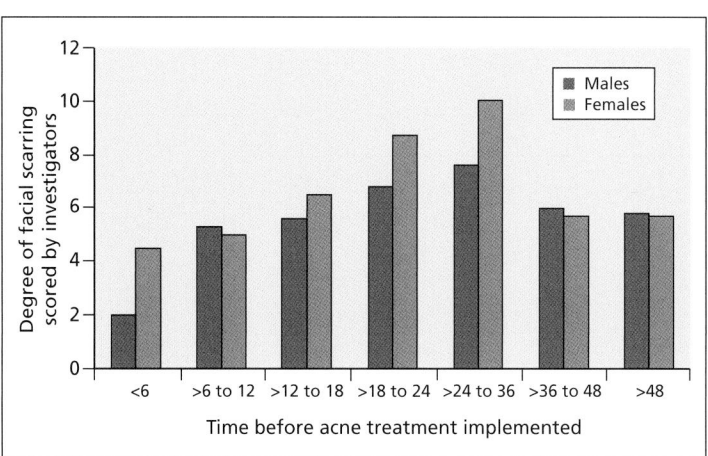

Figure 90.5 There is a correlation between acne scarring and duration of acne. Scarring is more likely to occur with delays in treatment. (Adapted from Layton *et al.* 1994 [7] with permission of Wiley.)

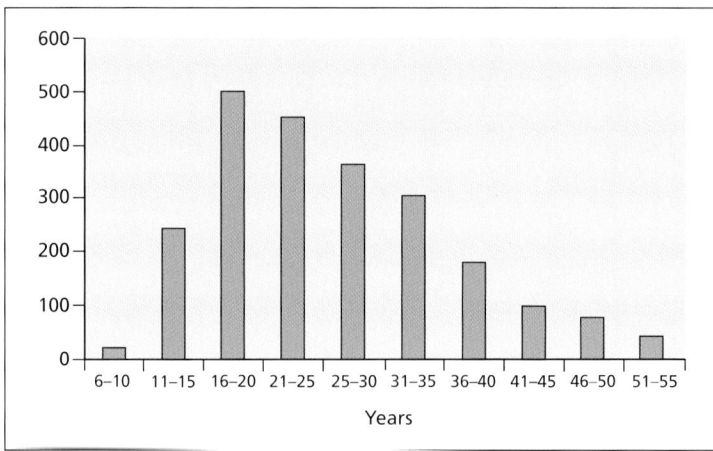

Figure 90.6 The age distribution of acne is widening in both sexes.

acne, both persistent and late onset, is more common in women than in men [15,20,21]. A large multinational cross-sectional study found that 26% of women aged 31–40 years and 12% of women aged 41–50 years had clinical acne (range 7–22%) depending on ethnicity [4,22]. Peak prevalence occurred between the ages of 15 and 20 years in all ethnic groups. Although data for females were not reported separately, the lower prevalence of post-adolescent acne 40 years ago is striking [16,17,23].

A historical review [13] identified a number of studies showing that males have more severe acne in late adolescence than girls. A similar observation has also been reported more recently [15,24–27]. Tracking changes in the epidemiology of acne over time is problematic; however, data indicate that the age distribution of acne is widening (Figure 90.6) and this is happening in both sexes but more prominently in women over the age of 40 years [17].

Ethnicity

Acne is now considered to be amongst the 10 most common diseases worldwide [28]. Epidemiological studies demonstrate how challenging it is to unravel the effects of ethnicity, socioeconomic and cultural factors. However, ethnic variation in the prevalence of acne does appear to exist even when socioeconomic and cultural differences are accounted for. In the USA, where prevalence data are collected by the National Ambulatory Medical Care Survey (NAMCS), acne is the commonest or second most common reason for visits to dermatologists by all racial groups including Asian Pacific islanders [29].

Associated diseases

Acne may be associated with a number of diseases in which there are underlying metabolic disturbances involving androgenic steroids, insulin resistance and increased growth factor receptor 2 (*FGFR2*) signalling, or in which there is a predisposition to inflammation. Table 90.1 summarizes medical conditions that may predispose to or protect against acne and highlights the abnormalities associated with each condition that may influence the course of acne.

Most acne patients have no underlying endocrinological abnormalities although, as an androgen-mediated dermatosis, acne is often a symptom of diseases in which androgen metabolism is abnormal [30,31]. The term 'endocrine' acne should be reserved for cases associated with clear signs and symptoms of endocrine disturbance such as PCOS, late-onset congenital adrenogenital syndrome and Cushing disease. Of these, PCOS is by far the commonest.

Polycystic ovary syndrome

PCOS is diagnosed according to the Rotterdam criteria [32] in which two of the following must be present:
- Overt symptoms of androgen excess (hirsutism, acne and/or alopecia).
- Ovulatory dysfunction (irregular or prolonged menstrual cycles).
- Polycystic ovaries.

In the US, the alternative National Institutes for Health (NIH) criteria continue to be used; see Table 90.2 for comparison. Using the Rotterdam criteria, between 5 and 10% of adult women are classified as having the syndrome. PCOS almost certainly encompasses a spectrum of related ovarian endocrinopathies; and subtypes are recognized (Table 90.3). Women with PCOS are frequently but not always overweight, have one or more raised serum androgen levels or a raised free androgen index and are insulin resistant, all of which predispose to acne. PCOS ovaries

Table 90.1 Medical conditions that may predispose to acne or in which acne prevalence is reduced. See text for abbreviations.

Condition	Abnormalities associated with this condition and relevant to acne	Effect/comments
PCOS	Raised serum DHEAS, total and/or free testosterone and androstenedione, reduced SHBG. Also raised luteinizing hormone, insulin, IGFBP-1 and IGF-1	Predisposes and/or worsens; effect on acne modified by BMI (or more correctly adiposity)
SAHA syndrome: subtype of PCOS	Serum androgens often but not always elevated. Subtypes can be characterized by which serum hormone levels are abnormal	Predisposes. According to Orfanos *et al.* [100], there are four types of SAHA: idiopathic, ovarian, adrenal and hyperprolactinaemic. Ovarian SAHA is associated with a more insulin-resistant profile
HAIR-AN syndrome: subtype of PCOS	Pronounced insulin resistance, with markedly raised serum insulin	Predisposes. May be a fifth subtype of SAHA syndrome. Insulin resistance is proportional to BMI. Onset usually during puberty/adolescence

(Continued)

Table 90.1 Medical conditions that may predispose to acne or in which acne prevalence is reduced. See text for abbreviations. (*Continued*)

Condition	Abnormalities associated with this condition and relevant to acne	Effect/comments
Premature adrenarche	Raised serum DHEA, DHEAS and androstenedione; often accompanied by insulin resistance	Much more common in girls than boys. Predisposes to earlier onset of acne and to PCOS. Rising insulin and IGF-1 appear to increase the adrenal sensitivity to ACTH, leading to overproduction of androgens
Premature puberty	Raised serum levels of gonadal androgens (highly variable depending on the cause)	Predisposes. Can be caused by premature adrenarche or tumours (of the pituitary or adrenal mainly)
Insulin resistance	Reduced IGF-1 and IGFBP-1	Predisposes
Hyperinsulinaemia	Raised serum insulin, IGF-1 and reduced IGFBP-3	Predisposes
Non-classical congenital adrenal hyperplasia associated with 21-hydroxylase deficiency (especially mild or heterozygous forms); more rarely 11β-hydroxylase or 3β-hydroxysteroid dehydrogenase deficiency	Elevated serum 17-OHP, progesterone, androstenedione, corticotrophin-releasing hormone and ACTH	Predisposes especially to early onset. May extend duration; reduces responsiveness to treatment
Apert syndrome	Associated with point mutations on *FGFR2*, which have been linked to acne	Predisposes to seborrhoea and an acne-like condition with involvement of the upper arms/forearms; responds to oral isotretinoin
Anorexia nervosa	Serum growth hormone raised, concomitantly IGF-1 is low	Predisposes
Turner syndrome	45,X. Rudimentary ovaries with reduced androgen synthesis leading to reduced serum levels of testosterone and androstenedione during puberty in affected girls	Only affects girls. Protects via reduced sebum production. Serum androgens are normal during adrenarche
Laron syndrome	Congenital deficiency of IGF-1	Protects
Mayer–Rokitansky–Küster–Hauser syndrome without *WNT4* mutation	Serum androgens are normal	?Protects. Lower prevalence of acne and PCOS but ovaries intact
Mayer–Rokitansky–Küster–Hauser syndrome with *WNT4* mutation (may be a distinct condition)	Raised serum testosterone	Predisposes via inability to repress ovarian androgen synthesis
Cushing syndrome (iatrogenic and endogenous)	Elevated serum cortisol, ACTH and corticotrophin-releasing hormone	Predisposes. Can cause acne in pre-adrenarchal children
Ectopic ACTH syndrome	Elevated serum ACTH	Predisposes. Can cause acne in pre-adrenarchal children
PAPA syndrome	Mutations in *PSTPIP1*. IL-1β and circulating neutrophil granule enzyme levels in serum are raised. Impaired production of IL-10 and increased production of GM-CSF	Acne is one of three diagnostic features of this syndrome; pyogenic sterile arthritis and pyoderma gangrenosum being the others
PASH syndrome	?Raised IL-1β (systemically or locally) or aberrant regulation of the function of this cytokine	Acne one of three diagnostic features, suppurative hidradenitis and pyoderma gangrenosum being the others
PASS syndrome	?Raised TNF-α (systemically or locally) or aberrant regulation of the function of this cytokine	As PASH but with axial spondyloarthritis
SAPHO syndrome	*P. acnes* sometimes recovered from bone samples	Acne one of five diagnostic features of this syndrome, synovitis, pustulosis, hyperostosis and osteitis being the others. Syndrome more likely to be associated with *P. acnes* than acne *per se*
Adrenal and ovarian tumours	Elevated serum androgens exclusively or with other raised hormones	Predisposes
Male pseudohermaphroditism	17β-hydroxysteroid dehydrogenase type 3 deficiency 5α-reductase type 2 deficiency	Normal pubertal development, normal levels of sebum and no altered risk of acne
Complete androgen insensitivity syndrome	Mutation in the androgen receptor	Protects. These patients produce no sebum and do not get acne
Exaggerated adrenarche	Specific elevation of adrenal hormones produced by the zona reticularis in adults; exaggerated DHEAS and androstenedione responses to ACTH stimulation test	Predisposes

Table 90.2 Criteria used to diagnose polycystic ovary syndrome.

Rotterdam diagnostic criteria – requires two of the following:	NIH diagnostic criteria
1 Oligo- or anovulation	**1** Oligo- or anovulation, and
2 Clinical and/or biochemical signs of hyperandrogenism	**2** Clinical and/or biochemical signs of hyperandrogenism
3 Polycystic ovaries	**Plus:** exclusion of other aetiologies such as congenital adrenal hyperplasia, androgen-secreting tumours and Cushing syndrome
Plus: exclusion of other aetiologies such has hyperthyroidism, hypoprolactinaemia, congenital adrenal hyperplasia, androgen-secreting tumours and Cushing syndrome	

appear more sensitive to insulin than non-PCOS ovaries resulting in excess androgen production. Hyperinsulinaemia is also associated with excess adrenal androgen synthesis. Data on the prevalence of acne among adult women with PCOS show considerable variation (Table 90.4). Overall, acne is a common finding; there is one striking exception: adult Pacific Island women with PCOS have little or no acne [61], which is consistent with the absence of acne in the island population as a whole. PCOS is increasingly being diagnosed in adolescents [62] and has been linked to the obesity epidemic [63–65]. In teenagers, the onset of PCOS overlaps with the traditional acne-prone years, during which transient insulin resistance is common, making it difficult to attribute individual cases of acne to PCOS as opposed to normal puberty [66]. Most investigators have studied the prevalence of acne in women with PCOS and shown a higher incidence [67–69] but others have examined the prevalence of PCOS or polycystic ovaries in female acne patients and demonstrated a higher prevalence of cystic ovaries in these patients [70,71]. Adult women with PCOS often have other signs of peripheral hyperandrogenism including androgenic alopecia and hirsutism (Figure 90.7).

Late-onset congenital adrenal hyperplasia

Non-classical or late-onset congenital adrenal hyperplasia (NCAH) is a relatively common autosomal recessive disorder

with an incidence reported as 1 : 500 to 1 : 1000 in white populations. NCAH arises due to mutations in the *CYP21A2* gene located at chromosome 6p21, which lead to 21-hydroxylase deficiency. 21-hydroxylase is a key enzyme in the synthesis of mineralocorticoids and glucocorticoids (including cortisol) from progesterone and 17α-hydroxyprogesterone (17-OHP). In deficiency, intermediates proximal to the enzyme accumulate; elevated 17-OHP, progesterone and androstenedione concentrations are typically found (Figure 90.8). Raised serum 17-OHP, basally or following an adrenocorticotropic hormone (ACTH) stimulation test, is a diagnostic marker for NCAH but is not 100% sensitive for carriers of mutations in *CYP21A2*. Table 90.5 outlines the clinical features of NCAH; acne is not a consistent feature. Reported prevalence in women with androgen excess ranges from 0.6% to 9% [72]. Higher prevalences are seen in some Jewish, Mediterranean, Middle-Eastern and Indian populations. The condition is most frequently diagnosed in late childhood or early adulthood but can present as precocious puberty. Severe, refractory or atypical forms of acne may represent late-onset congenital adrenal hyperplasia [73–77] (Figure 90.9a,b). If mild, it can go unnoticed until symptoms such as persistent acne, irregular menses or problems conceiving present. NCAH is a widely underdiagnosed disorder particularly in males [78]. Box 90.1 outlines suggested assessment in males.

For the treatment of acne associated with NCAH in male patients, oral glucocorticoids have been used. Systemic low-dose oral prednisolone (2.5–5 mg/day) or dexamethasone 0.25–0.75 mg/day) can be given although the latter may have a higher risk of adrenal suppression [79].

Hypercortisolism

This describes signs and symptoms associated with prolonged exposure to inappropriately high levels of cortisol or in consequence of Cushing disease.

Cushing disease

Cushing disease refers to hypercortisolism secondary to excess production of ACTH from a corticopituitary adenoma or investigations are indicated. ACTH levels are often lower in Cushing syndrome. For primary hypercortisolism, see Box 90.2 which outlines the symptoms and signs associated with Cushing disease.

Table 90.3 Subtypes of polycystic ovary syndrome (PCOS).

	Type I classical PCOS	Type II	Type III	Type IV
Hyperandrogenism	Present	Present	Normal	Present
Menstruation	Oligomenorrhoea	Irregular	Irregular	Regular
Ovarian cysts	Present	No cysts	Present	Present
Cardiovascular risk	High – metabolic syndrome 3× higher in these patients Relatively higher BMI Insulin resistance Dyslipidaemia with increased small dense LDL and lipoprotein		Lowest cardiovascular risk may be similar to those with no signs of PCOS	Lower BMI Lesser degree of hyperandrogenism Mildest degree of metabolic syndrome versus other subtypes Still at higher risk of CVD than those without PCOS

BMI, body mass index; CVD, cardiovascular disease; LDL, low-density lipoprotein.

Table 90.4 Prevalence of acne among women with polycystic ovary syndrome (PCOS).

Number of women, nationality	Age range; mean ± SD	Prevalence of acne (%)	Notes	References
87 British (47 South Asians, 40 Caucasians)	Asian 26 ± 4; Caucasian 30.1 ± 5	66 Asian, 30 Caucasian		[33]
716 Mexican	27.7 ± 7.3	15	Very low figure – article does not say how acne was defined	[34]
316 American	3 groups: 26.3 ± 6.9; 27.3 ± 6.9; 30 ± 7.8	19	Very low prevalence of acne for American women with PCOS	[35]
German	28	50	Versus 33% for women without PCOS	[36]
273 Chinese	24.83 ± 5.31	45		[37]
295 Taiwanese	14–40; 26.7 ± 5.4	48	Compared to 18% for age-matched women without PCOS	[38]
32 Tanzanian	29.3 ± 4.5	41	Compared to 17.6 for 68 women without PCOS	[39]
103 American	13–20	33		[40]
70 American	11–22; 16.2	70		[41]
49 Indian	12–19	67		[42]
51 Indian	15–32 22.2 ± 5.4	55		[43]
42 Indian	17–31 22.4 ± 5.53	54		[44]
62 Saudi-Arabian	29–43	39		[45]
115 Turkish	15–41	53	35% had seborrhoea	[46]
210 Iranian	17–18	27	Severe acne only	[47]
58 American	9–18	74	Five girls were premenarchal	[48]
318 Taiwanese	24.5 ± 5.0	39		[49]
74 Greek women				[50]
365 Croatian	26.1 ± 5.9	50		[51]
136 Indian girls; 49 with PCOS, 87 without	18.8 ± 8.5 PCOS; 19.8 ± 0.67 non-PCOS	33	Versus 14.9 in those without PCOS	[52]
100 Indian	20–38	13	Very low	[53]
133 Turkish	17–36	26 moderate or severe; 65 mild	Used Global Acne Grading System. Women with mild acne may be misclassified as no acne using a less stringent method	[54]
196 American	11–20; 15.7 ± 1.7	18 moderate or severe; 53 mild		[55]
10 Palestinian women	18–24	80	Versus 37.2% in those without PCOS	[56]
149 American (121 Caucasian, 28 Asian)	28 ± 5.4 Caucasian; 29.6 ± 5.9 Asian	68 Caucasian versus 74 Asian	Difference not significant	[57]
40 Korean	Two groups: 24.7 ± 5.1; 25.7 ± 8.2	95	Seborrhoea in 45%	[58]
254 American	Two groups 28.8 ± 5.67 27.8 ± 6.10	61		[59]
59 Turkish	21.49 ± 4.18	46		[60]

Acromegaly

Acromegaly, which relates to excess growth hormone production, has been associated with the development of acne [80]. Growth hormone and excess insulin-like growth factor 1 (IGF-1) can stimulate sebaceous gland differentiation and androgen-induced sebaceous lipogenesis [81–83]. Affected subjects may notice increased sebum production [83] and in some cases acne is the only presenting symptom [80].

Synovitis acne pustulosis hyperostosis osteitis syndrome (SAPHO)

This acronym, first described in 1987, represents a syndrome of pustular dermatoses together with aseptic osteoarticular lesions including synovitis, acne, pustulosis, hyperostosis and osteitis [84,85]. In the classical syndrome, patients present with sudden-onset haemorrhagic and ulcerative acne on the face and trunk, sterile pustular lesions on the palms and soles and pain especially

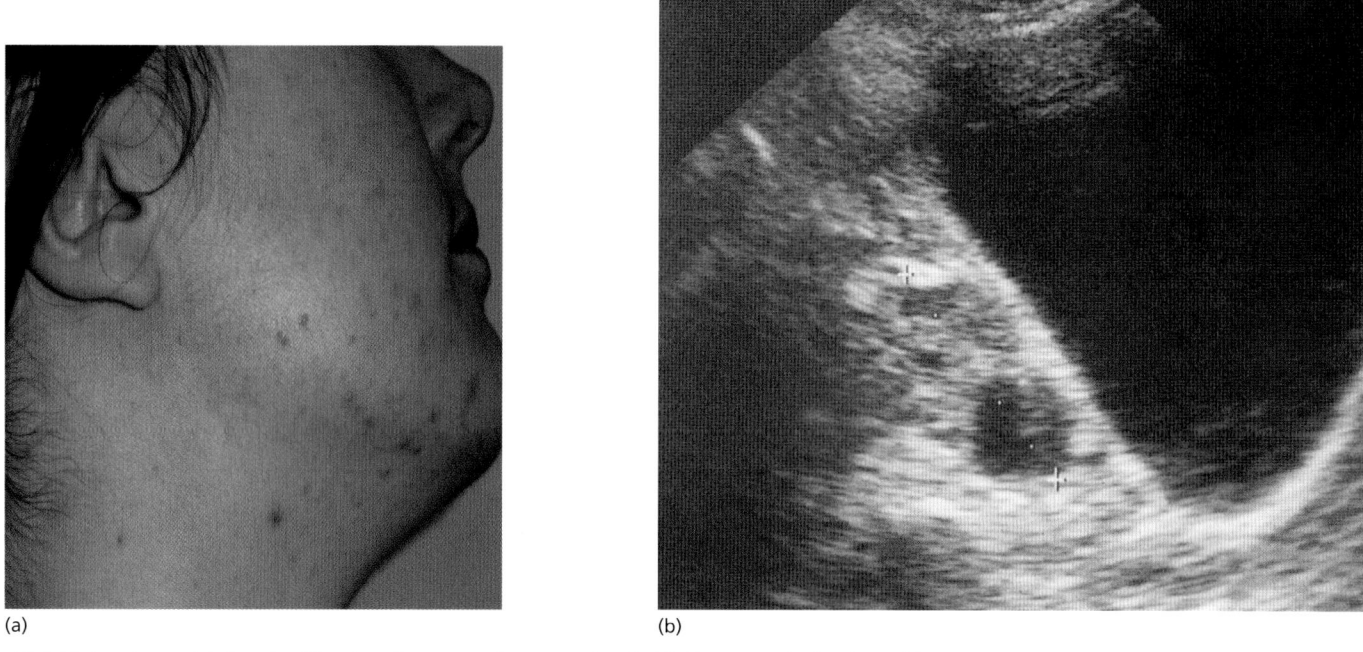

(a)   (b)

Figure 90.7 (a) Acne in an adult female with polycystic ovary syndrome associated with hirsutism and seborrhoea. (b) Ultrasound scan showing cysts (+) on the ovaries.

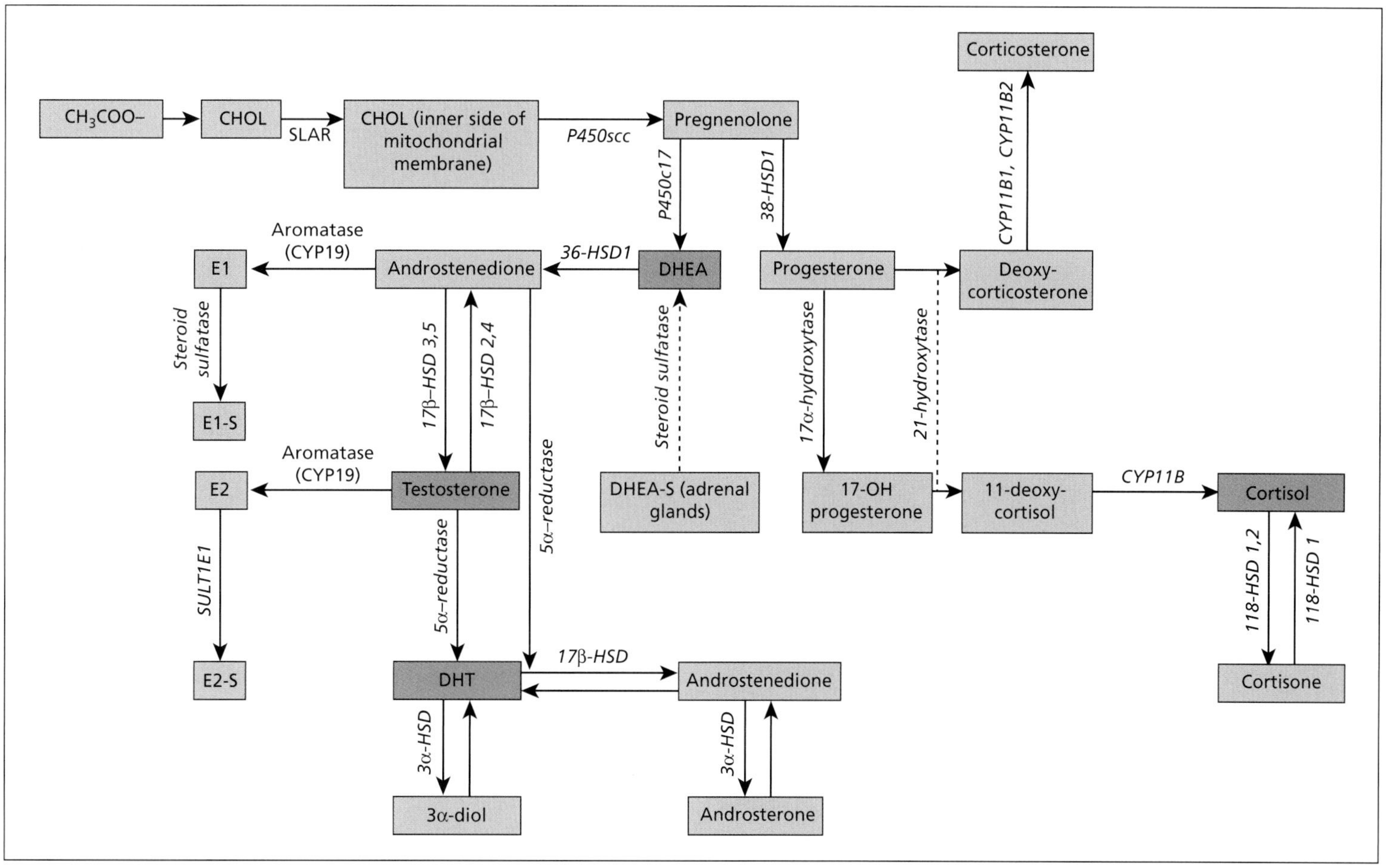

Figure 90.8 Schematic representation of the role of 21-hydroxylase in the adrenal steroid genesis pathway. See text for abbreviations.

Table 90.5 Clinical features of 21-OH non-classical adrenal hyperplasia.

Adulthood	Childhood
Short stature	Tall stature
Hirsutism	Pseudoprecocious puberty
Acne	Cystic acne
Testicular enlargement in boys	Premature pubarche
Oligospermia	
Menstrual irregularities	
Infertility both sexes	

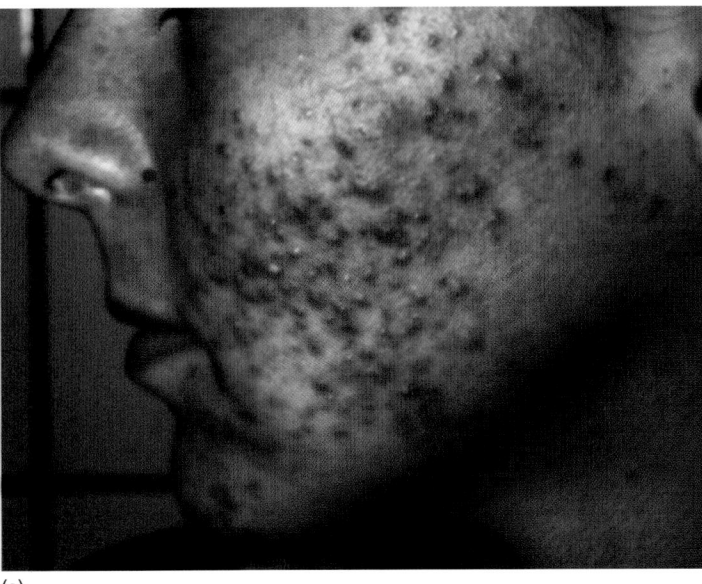

(a)

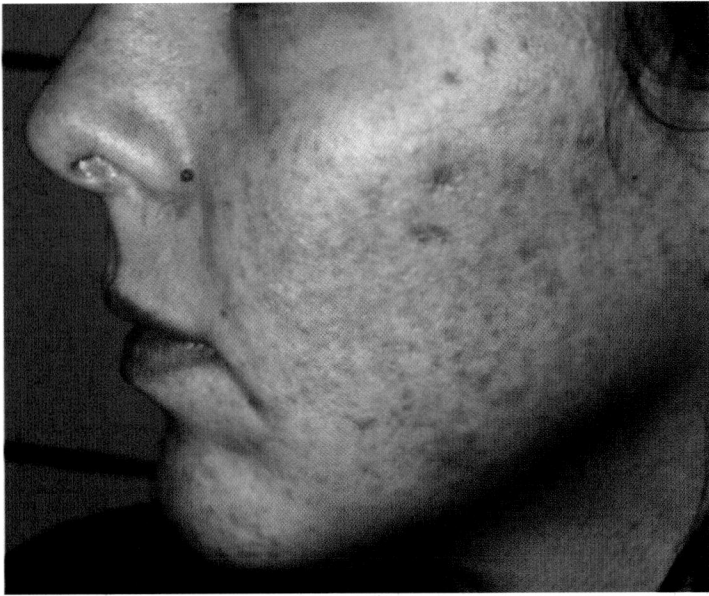

(b)

Figure 90.9 (a) Non-classical congenital adrenal hyperplasia in a 16 year old with oligomenorrhoea pretreatment. (b) Post-therapy with 2 mg oral prednisolone daily. (Courtesy of Dr P. Troielli, School of Medicine, University of Buenos Aires, Argentina.)

Box 90.1 Assessment of male patients with acne for congenital adrenal hyperplasia (CAH)

Medical history
- Acne/infertility

Physical examination
- Testicular examination

Biochemical investigations
- Basal level 17-hydroxyprogesterone (>6.1 nmol/L serves as a screening for non-classical adrenal hyperplasia)
- Adrenocorticotropic hormone stimulated plasma 17-hydroxyprogesterone (elevated basal levels or adrenocorticotropic hormone stimulated levels >260 ng/dL)
- Serum luteinizing hormone, follicle-stimulating hormone
- Testosterone, dehydroepiandrosterone sulphate, androstenedione 21-desoxycortisol

Testicular ultrasound

Semen analysis

Box 90.2 Symptoms and signs associated with Cushing syndrome

C – central obesity, collagen fibre weakness, comedones (acne)
U – urinary free cortisol and glucose intolerance
S – striae, suppressed immunity
H – hypercortisolism, hypertension, hyperglycaemia, hypercholesterolaemia
I – iatrogenic (increased administration of corticosteroids)
N – non-iatrogenic (neoplasms)
G – glucose intolerance, growth retardation

---

affecting the anterior chest wall. In mild cases, the condition is underdiagnosed. Skin manifestations are commoner in adults than in children and severe acneform skin disease, including acne fulminans, acne conglobata and/or hidradenitis suppurativa (HS), is seen predominantly in males. The disease may represent an immune reaction to an unspecified antigen. *Propionibacteria acnes* (*P. acnes*) have in some cases been isolated in osteitic bone lesions and the bony lesions fail to respond to antibiotics suggesting that they do not represent primary haematogenic spread [86]. Reports suggest that biphosphonates will improve bony lesions but they have no impact on the cutaneous manifestations [87,88]. Increased levels of tumour necrosis factor (TNF)-α have been identified. In isolated cases, benefit has been noted following treatment with infliximab [89] and ustekinumab [90]. Opposing effects on skin and osteoarticular symptoms may occur with TNF-α antibodies (articular improvement/cutaneous deterioration) as well as with isotretinoin (cutaneous improvement/articular deterioration) [91].

HAIR-AN syndrome

This syndrome consists of hyperandrogenism (HA), insulin resistance (IR) and acanthosis nigricans (AN) [92]. Patients present with typical signs of hyperandrogenism, hyperseborrhoea, hirsutism, acne, menstrual irregularities and androgenetic alopecia. They may also show other features including deepening voice, clitoromegaly and increased muscle mass [93]. Other autoimmune or endocrine diseases may be associated with HAIR-AN, including Graves disease, Hashimoto thyroiditis, Cushing syndrome, Cohen syndrome, acromegaly, congenital adrenal hyperplasia and insulinoma [93–95]. The primary abnormality is hyperinsulinaemia, elevated or upper limit levels of testosterone and androstenedione are frequent. The degree of excess insulin correlates directly to androgen levels [96]. The hyperinsulinaemia and hyperandrogenaemia stimulate epithelial proliferation and melanin accumulation resulting in the cutaneous changes seen. In some patients with HAIR-AN, a reduction in insulin receptors has been demonstrated and/or mutations in the receptor gene [97]. The binding of insulin to IGF receptors and insulin receptors on keratinocytes and fibroblasts leads to epidermal thickness which is thought to induce the changes seen in AN [93,98].

SAHA (seborrhoea, acne, hirsutism and androgenetic alopecia)

In 1982, the association of seborrhoea and acne with hirsutism and/or androgenetic alopecia in females was defined as SAHA (Figure 90.10) [99]. The syndrome is classified into idiopathic, ovarian, adrenal and hyperprolactinaemic types. All four major clinical signs are only present in about 20% of cases, seborrhoea is a consistent finding and acne is evident in around 10% of cases [100].

PAPA syndrome (pyogenic sterile arthritis, pyoderma gangrenosum and acne)

PAPA, first described in 1997, represents a rare autosomal dominant autoinflammatory disease caused by mutations in the gene for proline/serine/threonine phosphatase interacting protein 1 (PSTPIP1; also known as CD2BP1). PSTPIP1 is a cytoskeleton-associated adaptor protein expressed predominantly in haematopoietic cells and it modulates T-cell activation [101] and interleukin (IL)-1β release [102].

PAPA syndrome typically presents with recurrent sterile erosive arthritis in childhood occurring spontaneously after minor trauma, occasionally resulting in joint destruction. The joint problems tend to subside by puberty and there is a transition to cutaneous disease. Skin problems include pathergy, with abscesses developing at the sites of injections; severe nodulocystic acne appears in adolescence followed by recurrent sterile ulcers often diagnosed as pyoderma gangrenosum [103]. Pyoderma gangrenosum and acne may be present for several decades once present. Systemic or locally administered glucocoticosteroids are usually helpful for the inflammatory symptoms. TNF-α blockade has been shown to be effective in treating some of the cutaneous manifestions of PAPA syndrome [104].

Apert syndrome

Apert syndrome, also known as acrocephalosyndactyly, was first described in 1906 [105]. The prevalence is estimated at 15/1000 000 births based on a recent population-based study [106]. Apert syndrome is characterized by craniosynostosis and early epiphyseal closure which results in deformities of the skull, hands and feet. The characteristic facial abnormalities are hypertelorism, a flattened occiput, proptosis due to shallow orbits, prognathism, a parrot-beaked nose and fused shortened digits. Severely delayed tooth eruption, shovel-shaped incisors and malocclusion of teeth occurs. Abnormalities of the upper and lower respiratory tracts include cleft soft palate and bifid uvula [107]. Moderate to severe acne which generally presents early in puberty is a characteristic feature of Apert syndrome [108–110]. The acne typically presents on the trunk and face but also extends to unusual sites such as the forearms and buttocks (Figures 90.11 and 90.12) [111].

Early epiphyseal closure is an androgen-mediated event. No difference in the androgen receptor expression has been demonstrated suggesting that the underlying problem in Apert syndrome relates to abnormal sensitivity to normal circulating levels of androgens [112–114]. Other cutaneous changes reported in Apert syndrome include seborrhoea, hyperhidrosis, nail dystrophy, hyperkeratosis of the plantar surfaces and ocular and cutaneous

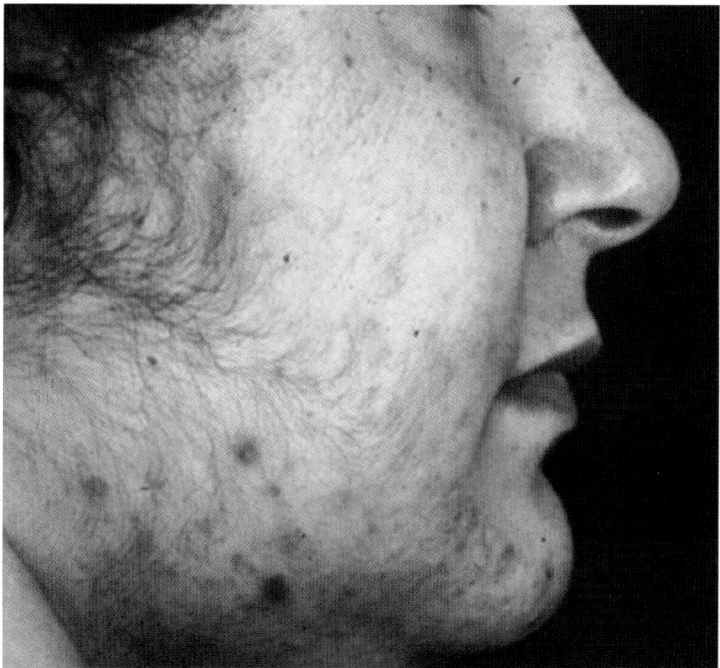

Figure 90.10 Seborrhoea, acne, hirsutism and/or androgenic alopecia (SAHA) syndrome.

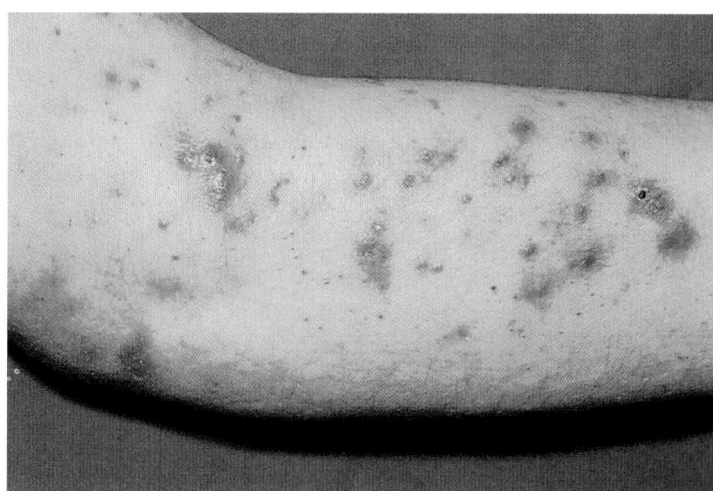

Figure 90.11 The unusual extent of acne in a patient with Apert syndrome.

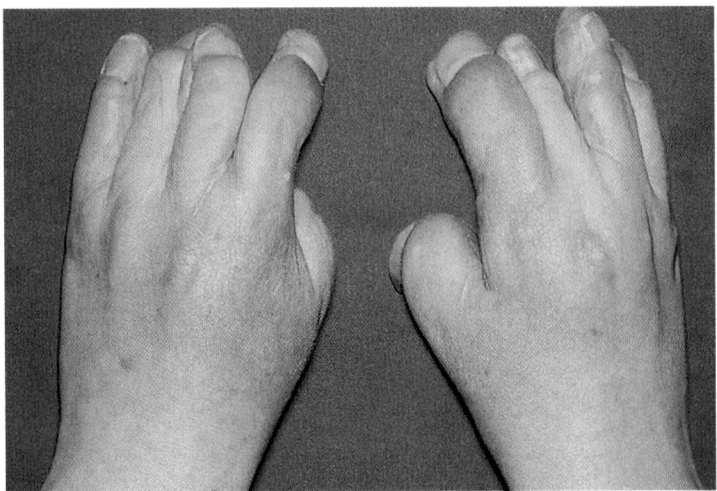

Figure 90.12 The typical appearance of the fingers of a patient with Apert syndrome.

hypopigmentation [115]. Apert syndrome may be inherited as an autosomal dominant or may be due to a new mutation of paternal origin. Two specific heterozygous missense germ line mutations of the *FGFR2* gene have been identified. The mutations of adjacent amino acid residues of *FGFR2*, either S252W or P253R, are localized in the linker region between D2- and D3-immunogolobulins-like regions of the *FGFR2*-ligand binding domain. Two major isoforms of *FGFR2* are formed. *FGFR2b* is exclusively expressed on epithelial cells, whereas *FGFR2c* is expressed only on dermal and mesenchymal cells. Both receptor isoforms and their specific ligands are involved in mesenchymal epithelial signalling [86] leading to downstream effects of activated *FGFR2* signalling on follicular keratinocytes proliferation, sebaceous lipogenesis and inflammatory cytokine response [116]. The acne in Apert syndrome frequently requires oral isotretinoin [117,118]. Etretinate has also been effective in refractory cases [119].

Drug-induced acne

Some drugs may cause acneform reactions; these account for about 1% of all drug-induced skin eruptions. Drug-induced acne embraces monomorphic inflammatory lesions with an absence of comedones, often presenting acutely on sites not commonly affected by acne. The face and upper trunk are most frequently affected. The interval between the onset of the acneform eruption and the start of the drug implicated depends very much on the agent provoking the response. Several reviews provide lists of drugs associated with acne or acneform rashes [**120**,121,122]. Table 90.6 identifies drugs that have been implicated in acneform eruptions.

Corticosteroids

Corticosteroids may provoke an acneform reaction regardless of their route of administration [123–128] (Figure 90.13). The precise mechanism is uncertain. Steroid acne is usually more monomorphic than true acne vulgaris; however, both inflammatory and non-inflammatory lesions may be present on the face, back and chest [129]. Abuse of androgenic anabolic steroids (AAS), synthetic

Table 90.6 Drug classes and types of medication that may exacerbate or cause acne.

Drug class or type	Examples
Corticosteroid	
Topical	Betamethasone
Oral	Prednisolone
Inhaled	Budesonide
ACTH	ACTH, synthetic ACTH
Anabolic steroid/synthetic androgen	Danazol, nandrolone, stanozolol
Anticonvulsant	Carbamazepine, phenytoin, phenobarbitone, troxidone, gabapentin, topiramate
Antidepressant	Lithium, sertraline
Other neuroleptic/ antipsychotic	Pimozide, risperidone
Antitubercular	Isoniazid, pyrazinamide
Antineoplastic/EGFR antagonists	Dactinomycin, pentostatin, cetuximab
Antiviral	Ritonavir, ganciclovir
Calcium antagonist	Nilvadipine, nimodipine
Halogen	Sodium fluoride, potassium iodine
Human growth hormone	Genetically engineered human growth hormone
Vitamins	Vitamin B_{12}, possibly other B vitamins
Miscellaneous	Buserelin, cabergoline, ciclosporin, sirolimus, tacrolimus, clofazimine, dantrolene, disulfuram, famotidine, follitropin alfa, isosorbide mononitrate, medroxyprogesterone, mesalazine, quinine, ramipril, sulphur, thiouracil, thiourea

ACTH, adrenocorticotropic hormone; EGFR, epidermal growth factor receptor.

derivatives of testosterone and testosterone salts, can exacerbate acne vulgaris (Figure 90.14) and induce acne fulminans or acne conglobata [130]. Acne induction is partly due to androgen receptor binding leading to hypertrophy of the sebaceous glands with consequent increased sebum output and a concomitant increase in the population density of *P. acnes*. However, not all AAS bind

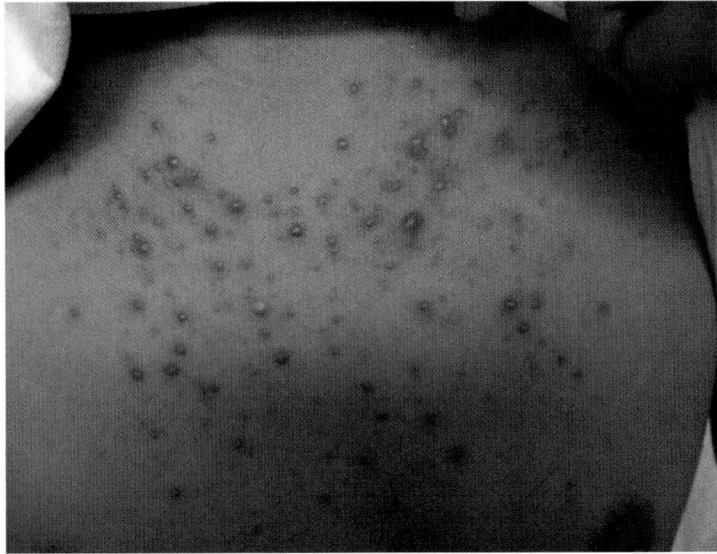

Figure 90.13 Monomorphic inflammatory papules and pustules associated with corticosteroid use. (Courtesy of Dr S. Chow, KL Skin Centre, Malaysia.)

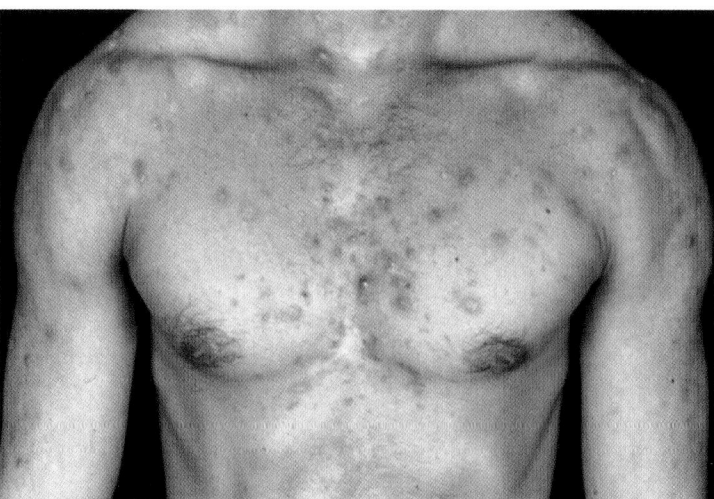

Figure 90.14 Severe acne vulgaris in a male body builder.

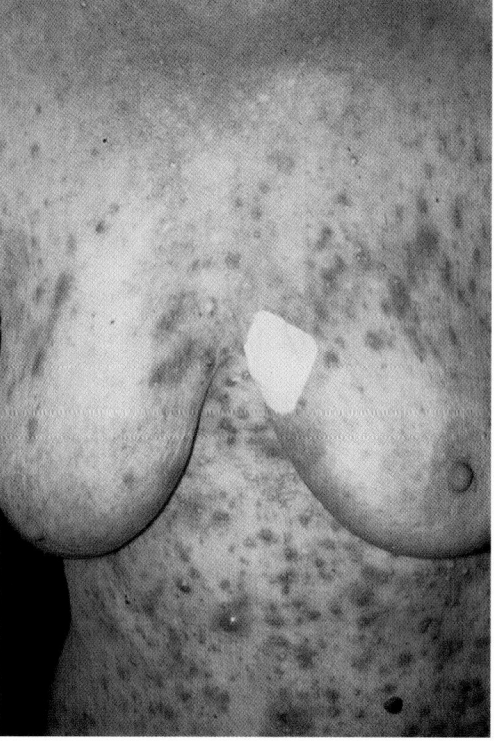

Figure 90.15 Lithium-induced acne. (Courtesy of Dr V. M. Yates, Royal Bolton Hospital, UK.)

to the androgen receptor suggesting that acne must be induced via other mechanisms [131,132]. Estimates suggest that as many as 43% of users have acne as a side effect [133].

Immunosuppressive drugs
Ciclosporin has been associated with induction of comedonal lesions 2–3 months after initiation of treatment and independent of dose. An acne-like eruption is seen as a consequence of immuno-suppressive drugs used in transplant patients in up to 25% of cases [134]. The reaction may extend beyond the face and trunk and a nodular component is common. Scalp folliculitis has been reported to occur within a few weeks of starting sirolimus [135]. Acne in this context can impact on quality of life (QoL) and may deter patients from taking their medication, particularly adolescent females [136]. Oral tacrolimus appears less likely to produce acneform reactions presumably due to the low accumulation in the skin. Localized acne has been reported in a patient using topical tacrolimus for vitiligo after 3 months of use [137]. Conventional acne therapies should be employed but if the acne is severe and refractory modification of immunosuppressant therapy may be required.

Psychotropic drugs
Some psychoactive drugs including lithium (Figure 90.15) and amineptine can induce acne [138–141]. Acne presents 2–3 months after starting therapy and severe forms such as acne conglobata have been described [142]. Male patients appear to be more susceptible to dermatological problems [143]. Lithium-induced acne is thought to occur through neutrophil chemotaxis and degranulation inducing an inflammatory cascade alongside a direct effect on follicular keratinocytes leading to follicular plugging. Discontinuation of the lithium is recommended if possible. Tetracyclines can increase levels of lithium.

Most cases of amineptine-induced acne have involved adult females. Comedonal lesions are the most frequently seen lesions and inflammatory lesions are usually sparse. The mechanism has been postulated to be via selective decrease in the uptake of dopamine followed by an inhibitory effect of elevated dopamine on prolactin with subsequent increase in testosterone output. Once

'acne' has been triggered, the drug should be withdrawn; response is variable and systemic therapy and physical treatment of the comedones may be required.

Progestins
Different progestins have varying androgenic effect (Box 90.3). The levonorgestrel-releasing intrauterine system, implants or mini-pills are all capable of exacerbating acne [144].

Isoniazid
Slow inactivators of isoniazid may develop an acneform rash [145].

Box 90.3 The relative androgenic effect of progestins in commonly used combined oral contraceptives

Generic name	Androgenic effect
Desogestrel	
Norgestimate	
Norethindrone	Increasing androgen effect ↓
Ethynodiol diacetate	
Levonorgestrel	
Norgestrel	
Norethindrone	

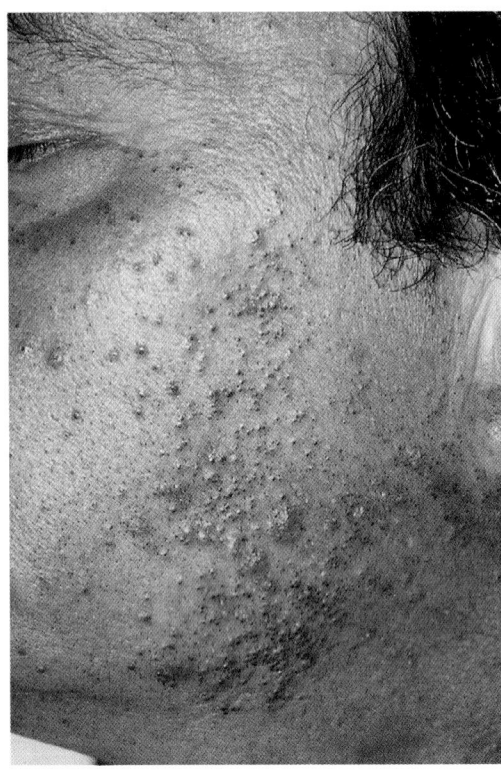

Figure 90.16 Chloracne – multiple comedonal lesions on the face.

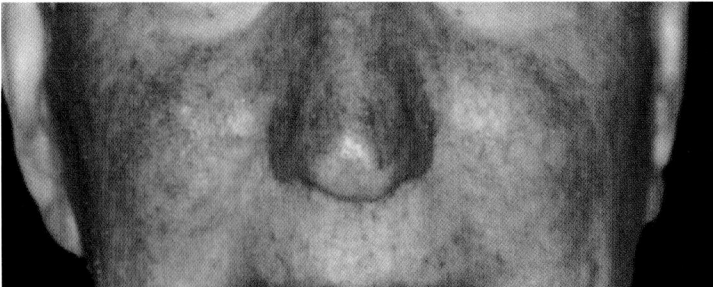

Figure 90.17 Epidermal growth factor receptor inhibitor producing follicular acneform eruption on the face of a patient receiving treatment for colonic cancer.

epidermal growth factor receptor (EGFR) inhibitors (Figure 90.17) [150,151]. Follicular papules and sterile pustules on the face and upper trunk occur and in severe cases the limbs may be affected. Comedones are not seen [152]. Histological examination of the lesions has found a superficial dermal inflammatory cell infiltrate surrounding a dilated follicular infundibulum. A direct correlation between efficacy to cancer therapy and severity of acneform reaction has been reported. Most reports suggest that topical acne therapies, oral tetracyclines and topical or oral corticosteroids are effective. Oral isotretinoin has also been used successfully [153].

Table 90.7 provides an aid for diagnosing acne associated with medications.

Predisposing factors

Genetic factors

Twin studies show that inherited factors influence the acne phenotype in monozygotic and to a lesser extent dizygotic twins [154]. Large cohort studies show that the risk of acne in a first-degree relative of someone who has had acne is approximately four to five times higher than in relatives of unaffected individuals [155–157]. A similar odds ratio has been found for the risk of adult (persistent or late-onset) acne in first-degree relatives of patients with acne aged 25 years or over [158]. A number of other studies have found adolescent and adult acne to be present in first- and second-degree relatives of acne patients at higher rates than in relatives of people without acne [21,156,159,160]. Heritability or susceptibility to adolescent acne seems to be more strongly linked to the maternal than the paternal line and risk increases as more family members are

Antiepileptic drugs

Acne triggered by antiepileptic drugs has been reported but a study of hospitalized patients with severe epilepsy receiving different anticonvulsants, including phenytoin, showed no increased risk of acne compared to matched controls in the general population [146].

Iodides and bromides.

Iodides and bromides commonly and rapidly cause follicular pustules [129,147]. Iodides may be found in non-prescription preparations for asthma, expectorants, kelp and teas. Sedatives and cold remedies often contain bromides. Chloracne (Figure 90.16) is a condition due to systemic poisoning most frequently found in occupational settings (see section on Occupational acne later).

Vitamins B_2, B_6 and B_{12}

A monomorphic eruption consisting of small follicular inflammatory lesions on the forehead and chin, upper arms and trunk has been described with B_{12} doses of 5–10 mg/day [148]. Women are almost exclusively affected and the onset of acne develops within the first 2 weeks post-injection. The acne-inducing dose of vitamin B_6 has not been established. A recent publication revealed that vitamin B_{12} supplementation in *P. acnes* cultures promoted the production of porphyrins, which have been shown to induce inflammation in acne, providing a potential mechanism for this reaction [149]. Conventional acne therapies are usually unsuccessful but withdrawal of the drug results in resolution of the acneform rash within 10 days.

Epidermal growth factor receptor inhibitors

A follicular acneform eruption often within a few weeks of therapy has been reported in more than 50% of cancer patients treated with

Table 90.7 Diagnosing drug-related acneform skin disease.

History	Secure a detailed history to include:
	• Onset of drug treatment
	• Dosage regime
	• Duration of treatment
Exacerbating factors	Exclude triggers:
	• Hormonal therapy
	• Occupation
	• Cosmetics
	• Environmental factors
Temporal relationship of the treatment	Establish the relationship between:
	• The start of the drug and the clinical signs
	• Improvement on withdrawal of the drug

Table 90.8 Heritable traits which may predispose to acne.

Factor	Effect
Sebum excretion rate (SER)	High SER predisposes – numerous genetic loci affecting sebaceous gland size and lipogenesis have been identified
Sebum composition	Poorly understood and may also be modulated by diet
Innate and acquired immune responses	Poorly understood – a number of candidate genes identified
Sex	Adolescent acne begins earlier in girls but tends to be more severe in males; being female is a risk factor for postadolescent acne
Ethnicity	Poorly understood; acne may be uncommon in all racial groups which have not adopted a Western/urban lifestyle

affected [27,159,161]. Studies in different settings have confirmed that acne occurs earlier in patients with a positive family history and may affect clinical presentation and treatment outcomes [159,162–164].

There are a number of heritable traits that might predispose to acne Table 90.8. Walton *et al.* [165] found greater concordance between sebum excretion rates (SER) in monozygotic than dizygotic twins. A recent study identified three genome-wide associations in patients with severe acne compared to controls. Results identified three loci 11q13.1, 5q11.2 and 1q41; these loci contain genes linked to transforming growth factor (TGF)-β cell signalling pathway, namely OVOL1, follistatin (FST) and TGF-β2. These data support a key role for the dysregulation of TGF-β-mediated signalling in susceptibitlity to acne [166].

Lifestyle and environmental factors

A plethora of lifestyle and environmental factors which predispose to acne or modulate its course have been reported although data are frequently contradictory (Table 90.9). Confounding factors are multiple and frequently not controlled for. The impact of diet is stimulating most debate. In most countries, it is rare to find families of any racial background with no acne. In contrast, acne is absent in some ethnic groups living in remote communities, e.g. the Kitavan Islanders of Papua New Guinea and the Aché hunter-gatherers of Paraguay do not suffer from acne in their native com-

Table 90.9 Lifestyle and environmental factors that may predispose to acne.

Factor	Strength of evidence
Diet	Moderate for glycaemic index and milk/milk products, low for other foodstuffs
Body mass index	Low
Smoking	High for comedonal acne in mature women with a history of chronic smoking; otherwise low
Alcohol consumption	Low
Psychological stress	Low
Cosmetics	Low
Prescription medicines	High for some drugs, low for others
Anabolic and androgenic steroids	High
Seasonal factors	High
Sunlight	Low
Lack of sleep/insomnia	Low

munities. Canadian Inuit only began to develop acne and other diseases of Western civilization following the urbanization of their communities [167,168]. Leading epidemiologists have speculated that this is attributable to diet rather than race. Diet in these communities is characterized by local production, constancy, as well as low consumption of milk, meat and processed carbohydrates. Academic interest has focused on milk, dairy produce and high glycaemic index foods as potential triggers for acne.

Diet

Many acne sufferers believe that diet modulates their skin condition [169–172] and unhealthy foods in particular are considered to make acne worse [173–175]. Some cross-sectional studies appear to support this [156,160,172,175,176] whereas others found no link between diet and acne [15]. Like many other Western diseases, acne is now also being linked to the obesity epidemic and to the rising prevalence of insulin resistance and hyperinsulinaemia [177].

There has been, a paucity of randomized controlled trials (RCTs) examining the link between diet and acne due to numerous possible confounding variables. Several investigators have used case–control, prospective cohort or cross-sectional studies to examine the link between current diet and acne and have adjusted odds ratios to take account of potential confounders. Table 90.10 excludes studies prior to 1990 which do not meet current quality standards [175]. Trends and inconsistencies have begun to emerge. Five studies have shown that a link between a high glycaemic load (GL) diet and acne [160,172,175,196,197]; in contrast, two studies found no association between GL and acne [150,151]. The trial by Smith *et al.* is weakened because participants on the low glycaemic index (GI) diet lost weight whereas those on the control diet did not. Investigations of serum markers were conducted in several studies on the effects of a low GI diet [196,198–200]. Findings are contradictory. Three studies from the same group consistently found that milk intake increased the risk of acne (see Table 90.10). However, it is unclear whether the risk is the same for whole and skimmed milk. Three further studies have also shown increased milk consumption in people with acne [157,160,175]; one of these implicated both whole and skimmed milk [157]. Any link with dairy products such as yoghurt, cheese and chocolate remains unproven. Some believe that the anti-inflammatory effects of diet are important protective factors in acne mediated via the effects of dietary components on the gut microbiota [201]. Non-food components are rarely considered in studies examining the impact of diet. Modern foodstuffs contain many ingredients; many of these are biologically active. Whilst many foods are considered acnegenic, others are under scrutiny because they may protect against acne. To date, most interest has been in healthy diets (e.g. Mediterranean, Paleolithic), fish/fish oils/polyunsaturated fatty acids [157,172,175,202–204] and probiotics [201,205–207]. A small randomized dietary intervention study, Ω-3 fatty acid and γ-linoleic acid supplementation were independently shown to reduce acne severity and the amount of IL-8 around acne lesions [208].

Body mass index

Numerous studies have examined the relationship between acne and body mass index (BMI), especially in adult women as acne and obesity coexist as symptoms of PCOS (Table 90.11). Taken

PART 8: SPECIFIC CUTANEOUS STRUCTURE

Table 90.10 Key findings from pivotal studies on acne and diet.

Type of study	Main findings	Strength of evidence and reason	References
2 arm investigator blind RCT comparing low GI and normal diet over 12 weeks	Low GI diet significantly reduced acne severity, fasting insulin, DHEAS and FAI, increased SHBG and IGFBP-1	**Low.** Low GI and normal diet differed in several other respects. Changes could be partly associated with weight loss in low GI group	[178]
RCT (subset of 2007)	No change in the amount of sebum produced on low GI diet. Ratio of saturated fatty acids to mono-unsaturated fatty acids increased significantly in low GI group and correlated with decrease in total lesion count	Strong evidence that diet affects sebum composition but not (in this case) sebum output. Cannot attribute change to GI though	[179]
Case–control study in young adults with and without acne	Significantly lower IGF-1 and markedly raised IGFBP-3 in acne patients but no difference in GI or GL. No insulin resistance associated with acne	**Low.** Dietary information unreliable; GI estimated by questionnaire. Calculation of GI and GL flawed by exclusion of numerous CHO-containing foods	[180]
7 day controlled feeding trial comparing high and low GI diet in 12 males with acne	Fasting insulin and HOMA-IR index significantly reduced in low GI group. FAI markedly increased in high GI group. IGFBP-1 and IGFBP-3 rose in low GI group compared to baseline	Some preliminary evidence from this study that the LGL diet improved insulin sensitivity but small sample size and males only	[181]
Case–control study in 47 355 US nurses	Milk (but not chocolate or chips) especially skimmed milk intake associated with severe acne. Positive correlations also found for total and supplemental vitamin D	**Low.** Acne status (except severe – verified by physician) and milk consumption during adolescence based on recall. Associations of acne and dietary components were weak. All grades less than severe acne included in control group	[182]
Prospective cohort studies in 6094 girls and 4273 boys aged 9–15 years in US	Found greater milk consumption was associated with acne in girls and boys. No association with vitamin D	**Low.** Annual questionnaire study in which acne and diet were self-assessed. In girls, association was for all types of milk, in boys for skimmed milk only. Adjusted odds ratios all 1.2 or less	[183] [184]
Cross-sectional study in 1002 Iranian students	Regular consumption of sweets, nuts, chocolates, and oily foods, were associated with increased acne severity	**Low.** Incomplete dietary information collected but acne was clinically assessed	[185]
Cross sectional study in 18 and 19 year olds in Oslo	No association of acne with consumption of sugary soft drinks or fatty fish. In males, significant associations were found with chocolate/sweets and crisps. In females, the only dietary association was with low intake of raw vegetables	**Low.** Acne self-reported and prevalence lower than expected in both sexes. Dietary associations differed between the sexes. In adjusted models, only the link with raw vegetables remained	[186]
Case–control study in 1245 Koreans (783 with acne)	Consumption of vegetable and fish significantly lower in those with acne. Consumption of selected meats, junk food, nuts, fizzy drinks and high GL foods higher in the acne group. Irregular dietary patterns also more prevalent in the acne group. Serum IGF-1 raised in subgroup who thought their acne was aggravated by food	**Moderate.** Acne was clinically assessed	[187]
Comparison of high and low GI diets over 8 weeks in adolescent males	Acne improved slightly on both diets – no significant difference between the groups. IGFBP-1 fell significantly on the low GI diet versus the high GI diet. IGF-1, IGFBP-3, SHBG, DHEAS and HOMA-IR unchanged.	**Low.** Not random allocation. Underpowered. Finding inconsistent with those of Smith *et al.* Other dietary components more balanced in this study. Can infer from discussion there was no weight loss on low GI diet	[188]
Case–control study in Italians aged 10–24 years	Cases drank significantly more milk (whole and skimmed) and ate less fish than controls	**Moderate.** Control group included mild acne. Acne was physician assessed from photos. Major foods (e.g. cereals, rice, yoghurt) omitted from questionnaire	[189]
Case–control study in Malayans aged 18–30 years	GL and consumption of milk and ice-cream significantly higher in cases than controls. BMI same in both groups. No difference in consumption of chocolate, nuts or yoghurt. Adjusted odds ratios for GL lost significance except for GL >175, for which the risk of acne was increased 25-fold	**Moderate.** Diet assessed from 3-day food diaries	[190]
Investigator blind RCT comparing low glycaemic load diet and a calorie-adjusted control diet over 10 weeks	Low GL diet reduced global acne severity, inflamed and non-inflamed lesion counts at 10 weeks; inflamed lesion count also reduced at week 5. Although significant, reductions were modest. Reduced sebaceous gland size and less IL-8 observed in skin of the low GI group	**Moderate.** Small sample size (*n* = 32). No change in BMI in either group	[191]
Case–control study in Italian adolescents investigating the effect of a Mediterranean diet on acne	Adherence to a Mediterranean diet, characterized by high intake of vegetables, fruit, nuts, cereals, fish and olive oil and low intake of dairy products and meat, was significantly less in group with acne. Score of ≥6 is protective.	**Moderate.** Examined patterns of consumption over a long period. Collected data on intake of specific food items but did not report these. Adherence to the diet was categorized as low (score 0–2), moderate (3–6) or high (7–9).	[192]

Type of study	Main findings	Strength of evidence and reason	References
Cross-sectional study in 248 young adults aged 18–25 years in the US	Participants with moderate to severe acne reported significantly greater dietary GI, added sugar, total sugar, number of milk servings per day, saturated fat and transfatty acids, and fewer servings of fish per day compared to those with no or mild acne	**Moderate.** Used a validated food frequency questionnaire. Acne self-assessed against given set of criteria	[193]
Pilot open study in 10 American males who consumed increasing amounts of 100% chocolate bars	Total number of acne lesions increased on day 4 and day 7. Good correlation between the amount of chocolate consumed and the number of lesions	**Low.** Open study. Risk of expectation bias	[194]
Double-blind, placebo controlled RCT in 13 American males aged 18–35 years with minimal acne comparing a single exposure to increasing amounts of unsweetened 100% cocoa versus hydrolysed gelatin	Significant exacerbation of acne (total lesions and comedones) noted on day 4 and day 7 post consumption of cocoa. Inflamed lesions increased on day 4 only. Low correlation with dose of cocoa consumed	**Low.** Only two subjects studied per dose. Data for all doses combined to generate means	[195]

CHO, carbohydrate; DHEAS, dihydroepinandrosterone; FAI, free androgen index; GL, glycaemic load; HOMA-IR, insulin resistance; IGF, insulin-like growth factor; IL, interleukin; LGL, low glycaemic load; RCT, randomized controlled trial; SHBG, sex hormone binding globulin.

Table 90.11 Studies which have examined the relationship between body mass index (BMI) and acne.

Reduced risk of acne	Increased risk of acne	No change in risk or severity of acne	Study population	References
Reduced risk of moderate to severe disease in subjects aged 10–24 years who are underweight (BMI <18.5); trend stronger in males than females		Risk not increased in subjects of either sex who were overweight (BMI >23)	Dermatology out-patients in Italy	[209]
Reduced risk of acne (any grade) in children aged 6–11 years with low BMI	Increased risk in children of both sexes who were overweight		Schoolchildren in Taiwan	[210]
Trend for reduced risk with low BMI (both sexes combined data)	Increased risk in children aged 9–16 years who were overweight. No separate analysis by sex		Schoolchildren in Ghana	[211]
	Increased acne prevalence in children aged 7–19 years who were overweight. No separate analysis by sex		Lithuanian schoolchildren	[212]
	Increased risk in girls aged 18 or 19 years who were overweight or obese	No effect of BMI on risk of acne in boys aged 18 or 19 years	Final year schoolchildren in Norway	[213]
	Men with acne had higher mean BMI than age-matched controls		Italian males with and without acne	[214]
		No difference in BMI between subjects aged 18–30 years with acne versus age- and sex-matched controls	Acne patients in tertiary care and students or staff of local university in Malaysia	[215]
Women with acne were more likely to be overweight or obese than controls. There was a positive correlation between BMI and acne severity			Turkish women with acne	[216]
Obese women had a lower prevalence of acne than non-obese women			Taiwanese women of reproductive age	[217]
Lower prevalence of acne in overweight/obese (BMI >25) versus non-obese women with PCOS			Female out-patients with PCOS in Taiwan	[218]

(Continued)

Table 90.11 Studies which have examined the relationship between body mass index (BMI) and acne. (*Continued*)

Reduced risk of acne	Increased risk of acne	No change in risk or severity of acne	Study population	References
Adult women with PCOS but no acne had higher mean BMI than those with PCOS and acne)			Female out-patients attending reproductive endocrinology clinic in Taiwan	[219]
Lower prevalence of acne in obese versus non-obese women with PCOS			Female outpatients with PCOS in Croatia	[220]
Reduced acne severity in women with PCOS who were overweight or obese (BMI ≥27)			Female out-patients with PCOS in Turkish hospital	[221]
	Acne strongly associated with obesity in women with PCOS		Female out-patients with PCOS in Saudi Arabia	[222]
	Acne more common in overweight than normal weight women with PCOS			[223]
		Prevalence of acne similar in normal (63%) and overweight (73%) girls with PCOS	Female adolescent out-patients with PCOS in the US	[224]
Trend for less acne with lower BMI (<23, NS)			Indian women with PCOS	[225]
Trend for less acne with increase in BMI (NS)			Indian women with PCOS	[226]

NS, not significant; PCOS, polycystic ovary syndrome.

together, studies to date suggest the risk of having acne and the severity appear to increase with age-adjusted BMI in adolescents. Paradoxically, acne may be less prevalent in overweight adult women with PCOS.

Smoking
The weight of evidence suggests smoking has little, if any, effect on the prevalence or severity of acne in teenagers and young adults. Mature women, who are persistent smokers, seem to be susceptible to a particular type of non-inflammatory acne, characterized by numerous comedones and macrocomedones [227]. Heavy smoking may exert some protective effect against inflammatory acne, possibly via the actions of nicotine [228]. Maternal cigarette smoking has been found to be associated with earlier onset of acne but not of puberty in sons [229].

Alcohol
No conclusions can be drawn about alcohol as a risk factor for acne at any age. Two cross-sectional studies [15,162] suggest that alcohol consumption and acne are related whereas another found no association between acne and drinking alcohol [161]. No link between acne and alcohol consumption was found in the Glasgow Alumni Cohort Study [230].

Menstrual cycle
It is documented that about 70% of women complain of a flare of acne 2–7 days before the onset of menstruation [13,16,231,232]. This appears to affect all ethnic groups but perhaps not equally (Table 90.12).

Stress and sleep deprivation
Few studies have examined the effect of psychological stress on acne. A small study in university students during exams found changes in stress scores significantly and highly correlated with changes in acne severity when confounding variables had been adjusted for [245]. In support of this observation, a study in students found more acne prior to exams (high stress) than during the summer vacation (low stress) but this only reached statistical significance in males [246]. Some investigators have found that acne sufferers report stress as an aggravator [162,173,247–250] or have

Table 90.12 Proportion of women experiencing a premenstrual flare.

Nationality	Number studied	Age range (or mean age), years	Per cent with premenstrual flare	References
American	100	NA	72	[233]
American	400	12–52	44	[234]
French	3305	25–40	78	[235]
Saudi-Arabian	200	Mean age 14.8	9.8	[236]
Jordanian	83	13–34	98	[237]
Indian	137	13–45	57.7	[238]
			35.5	[239]
Korean	NA	Mean age 24	60.1	[240]
French	591	10–25	55	[241]
Korean	756	10–56	61.3	[242]
Indian	230	Over 25	11.7	[243]
Thai	392	?<20?	>50	[244]

NA, not applicable.

shown that stress is a risk factor for more severe acne [156,159,251]. Stronger evidence of the link between acne and stress comes from data on the role of elements of the hypothalamopituitary–adrenal axis (HPA) on sebaceous gland function [252–254]. Weak evidence is available to show that sleep deprivation or insomnia are associated with both adolescent and post-adolescent acne [255].

Cosmetics

Acne cosmetica represents an acne variant associated with chronic use of cosmetics containing potentially comedogenic substances. Cited agents include lanolin, petrolatum, certain vegetable oils, butylstearate, lauryl alcohol and oleic acid. Skin bleaching agents containing steroids can cause or exacerbate acne in dark-skinned women [256,257]. Of note, some women believe cosmetics worsen acne and others over-zealously use skin care products leading to exacerbations of otherwise mild acne. Ingredients may be less important than how preparations are used.

Pomade acne. Pomades are greasy preparations used to defrizz curly hair. They can trigger non-inflammatory acne (Figure 90.18) [258]. Restriction of the pomades and treatment with topical retinoids achieves resolution.

Detergent acne. This uncommon form of acne develops in patients who wash many times each day in the mistaken hope of improving their existing acne. Trauma and the alkalinity of soap are likely to be involved in the mechanism. Inflammatory lesions are most noticeable [259]. Several bacteriostatic soaps contain weak acnegenic compounds, such as hexachlorophene.

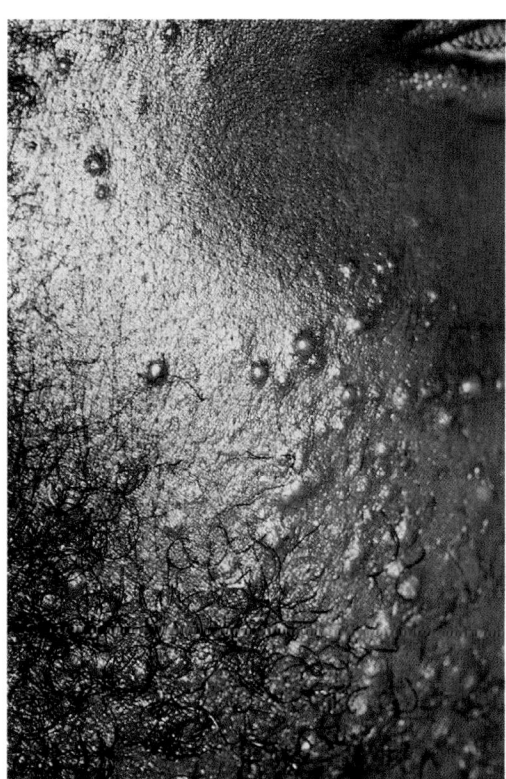

Figure 90.18 Pomade acne.

UV radiation

The assumed beneficial effect of UVR was questioned when 139 people in Munich were asked what happened to their acne during the summer months [260]. One third said it improved, one third said it worsened and one third said it stayed the same. A number of studies have shown seasonal variation with less patients seeking treatment in the summer months [261–264]. Workers in a hot humid environment, e.g. troops in the Second World War suffered badly when posted to the Far East [265]. Hence, high temperatures and humidity may negate any beneficial effects of sunlight. An acne variant, acne aestivalis or Mallorcan acne, has been reported in patients exposed to sunshine on vacation. Small follicular papules appear, especially on the upper trunk, during or after a holiday in a hot humid environment. A small number of patients receiving psoralens UVA (PUVA) treatment have been reported to develop a perioral dermatitis and/or an acneform eruption on the face [266,267]. Squalene monohydroperoxide is formed from squalene exposed to UVA and this compound appears to be responsible for comedogenicity [268]. UVR exposure has also been shown to alter the content of both pro- and anti-inflammatory cytokines in comedones *in vivo* [269]. Thus, evidence would support the fact that UVR may promote acne on sun-exposed skin in susceptible individuals not using adequate photoprotection.

Pregnancy

Among 415 Scottish women, 57.5% thought their acne improved during pregnancy and just 5.4% reported a deterioration [270]. In comparison, 75% of women thought their acne improved after giving birth and only 12% said it worsened. In South Korea [162], 28.4% of 756 women experienced a worsening of acne during pregnancy whereas 10% observed an improvement.

Birth weight

A large study conducted amongst Turkish schoolgirls found that acne was more common amongst those with a birth weight at term of less than 2500 g [271]. Low birth weight has also been linked to acne associated with an increased risk of insulin resistance and other features of PCOS [272]. It is well known that low birth weight is a risk factor for PCOS [273].

Miscellaneous factors

Lifestyle factors that have been proposed to modulate the risk of acne but for which there is virtually no evidence are hygiene/frequency of washing, touching the skin, mood, pollution, physical activity, use of recreational drugs, drinking water and sex [248].

Summary

Whilst the effects of some dietary components are becoming clearer, there is not enough evidence to inform treatment guidelines. It is not certain that being overweight predisposes to acne or that drinking alcohol has any effect. In some women with PCOS, being overweight seems to reduce the risk of acne. The relationship between smoking and acne appears complex; a variant of acne in adult women appears to be linked to habitual smoking over a long period whilst smoking might be protective in the early stages of inflammatory acne. It is virtually impossible to disentangle the impact of ethnicity and cultural factors, although it looks like a range of

PART 8: SPECIFIC CUTANEOUS STRUCTURE

lifestyle factors including what we put on our skin, the medicines/supplements we take and the recreational activities we pursue may all play a part. Whilst many people are convinced psychological stress makes their acne worse, the scientific evidence available is weak. The best advice to give patients who believe a lifestyle factor exacerbates their acne is almost certainly to avoid it for a while and keep a diary of how their skin reacts over a minimum period of several weeks. The exception is diet for which the best advice currently would be to eat healthily with everything in moderation and nothing in excess. There is reasonably good evidence that the presence of acne before puberty is a prognostic factor for more severe disease.

Pathophysiology

The classical concept is that acne results from the combination of increased sebaceous gland activity with seborrhoea, abnormal follicular differentiation with increased keratinization, microbial hypercolonization of the follicular canal and increased inflammation primarily through activation of the adaptive immune system. New research results have led to a modification of this classical explanation as more primary pathophysiological factors have been identified. Along with a genetic predisposition, other major factors include androgens, pro-inflammatory lipids such as ligands of sebocyte peroxisome proliferator-activated receptors (PPAR) and other inflammatory pathways. In addition, neuroendocrine regulatory mechanisms, diet and exogenous factors all may contribute to this multifactorial process [274,275,**276**].

Inflammation

Recently, there has been a debate as to whether hyperkeratinization of the follicular duct precedes the influx of inflammatory cells or vice versa (Figure 90.19) [277]. Recent studies support the latter hypothesis by demonstrating that an increase in IL-1 activity occurs before the hyperproliferation around uninvolved follicles and this triggers the activation of the keratinocytes [278,279]. Expression profiling of acne-involved and uninvolved skin from acne patients and from subjects without acne via cDNA microarrays have provided a better insight into the aetiological factors giving

rise to acne [280]. In inflammatory acne lesions, the majority of the up-regulated genes are involved in inflammatory processes. These include matrix metalloproteinases, human β-defensin (HBD) 4, IL-8 and granulysin. Nuclear factor kappa B (NF-κB), a transcription factor critical for up-regulation of many pro-inflammatory cytokine genes, has been shown to be activated in acne lesions [281]. NF-κB-regulated cytokine mRNA levels of TNF-α, IL-1ß, IL-8 and IL-10 are significantly up-regulated in acne-involved skin compared to uninvolved normal adjacent skin. Choi *et al.* showed that TNF-α induces lipogenesis in SZ95 sebocytes through the JNK and PI3K/Akt pathways [282]. IL-1β mRNA and the active processed form of IL-1β are abundant in inflammatory acne lesions [283].

Elevated expression of the chemokine IL-8 is able to attract inflammatory cells into the skin. Indeed, in early acne lesions (closed comedones), there is a marked increase in the presence of polymorphonuclear leukocytes (PMNs), as compared to the uninvolved skin whereas lymphocytes are prominently visible in papules, pustules and nodules as compared to normal controls [281]. Kelhala *et al.* illustrated the presence of IL-17A positive T cells and the activation of Th17-related cytokines in acne lesions, indicating that the Th17 pathway is activated and may play a pivotal role in the disease process. However, additional studies are needed to assess the clinical relevance of IL-17 in acne [284]. Inflammation is further characterized by the action of active lipid mediators, such as leukotrienes, prostaglandins and 15-hydroxyeicosatetraenoic acids. These molecules are synthesized from arachidonic acid (AA) or linolenic acid by the enzymes lipoxygenases (LOX) and cyclooxygenase (COX), respectively. Both COX isozymes, COX-1 and COX-2, are expressed in human sebocytes *in vitro*, in particular COX-2 expression is selectively up-regulated in acne involved sebaceous glands *in vivo* [285]. Activation of the platelet-activating factor signalling pathway (PAF; 1-*O*-alkyl-2-acetyl-*sn*-glycero-3-phosphocholine), which consists of a group of phosphocholines with various biological effects, including modulation of keratinocyte function and skin inflammation, can regulate the expression of inflammatory mediators, e.g. COX-2 and PGE$_2$, as well as IL-8 in

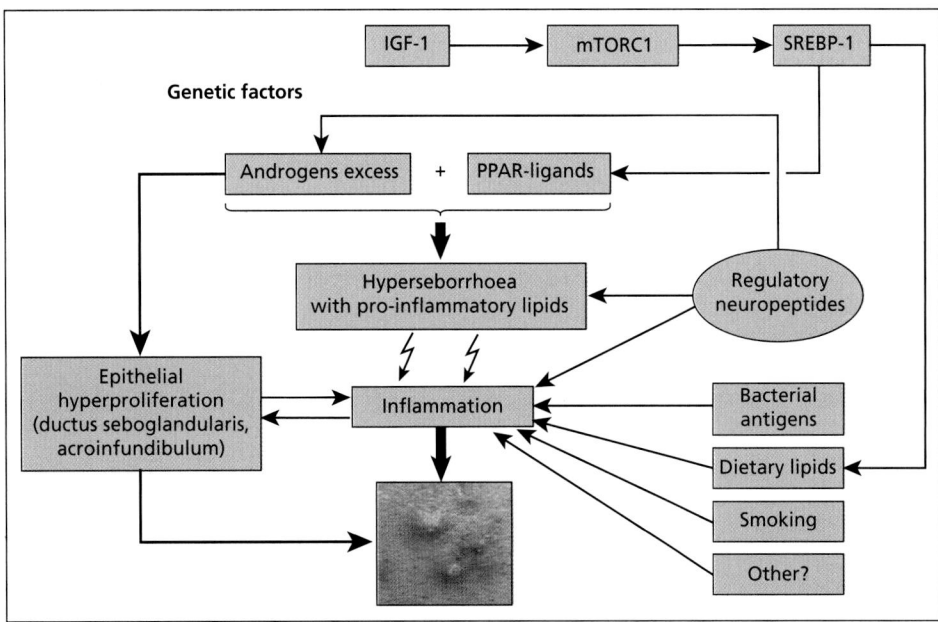

Figure 90.19 Inflammatory cascades involved in acne pathogenesis. SREBP-1, sterol response element-binding protein 1. (Modified from Zouboulis *et al.* 2005 [2].)

SZ95 sebocytes [286]. Transgenic keratin 5 promoter driven over-expression of COX-2 in the basal compartment of the epidermis of the mouse and increased PGE_2 levels have been documented to cause sebaceous gland hyperplasia and overshooting sebum production pointing to a role of COX-2-mediated PGE_2 synthesis in this process [287]. Activation of PPAR-γ by UVB irradiation and the potent lipid-soluble oxidant *tert*-butylhydroperoxide (TBH) induces COX-2 expression in SZ95 sebocytes and this inding indicates a PPAR-γ/COX-2-mediated pathway regulating sebocyte proliferation and/or lipogenesis [288]. Conversely, leukotrienes are potent pro-inflammatory mediators and neutrophil attractants produced from AA by 5-LOX. Human sebocytes express all necessary enzymes for a functional leukotriene pathway. The enzymes 5 LOX and LTA_4 hydrolase are expressed in SZ95 sebocytes at protein and mRNA level. These enzymes are essential for the formation of LTB_4. However, 15-LOX expression shows a weak expression in SZ95 sebocytes, indicating that sebocytes do not play a significant role in the biosynthesis of the anti-inflammatory 15-HETE. Treatment of SZ95 sebocytes with AA stimulates 5-LOX expression and induces LTB_4 synthesis [285]. In addition, AA induces the expression of the IL-6 and IL-8 cytokines. 5-LOX and LTA_4 hydrolase show a stronger expression in acne lesions than in normal skin and in uninvolved skin of acne patients. The involvement of 5-LOX in the pathogenesis of acne has led to new therapeutic strategies to deal with the disease, such as the 5-LOX inhibitor Zileuton [289].

Neurophysiology

Human skin and in particular the human sebaceous gland has been shown to express functional receptors for neuropeptides (Figure 90.20) such as corticotropin-releasing hormone (CRH) [253,290,291] the most proximal element of the HPA axis, melanocortins [252,278,292–296], β-endorphin, vasoactive intestinal polypeptide, neuropeptide Y and calcitonin gene-related peptide [254].

These receptors modulate the production of inflammatory cytokines, proliferation, differentiation, lipogenesis and androgen metabolism in human sebocytes [290–292,297]. Substance P, which can be elicited by stress, may promote the development of cytoplasmic organelles in sebaceous cells, stimulate sebaceous germinative cells and induce significant increases in the area of sebaceous glands. It also increases the size of individual sebaceous cells and the number of sebum vacuoles for each differentiated sebaceous cell, all of which suggests that substance P promotes both the proliferation and the differentiation of sebaceous gland cells. Facial skin from acne patients is characterized by rich innervation, by increased numbers of substance P-containing nerves and mast cells, and by strong expression of neutral endopeptidase, a potent neuropeptide-degrading enzyme, in sebaceous glands and E-selectin in venules around sebaceous glands, compared with normal skin [298]. These findings are attributed to local substance P activity. Recently, the ectopeptidases dipeptidyl peptidase IV (DP IV or CD26) and aminopeptidase N (APN or CD13), which have been shown to be involved in the degradation of several neuropeptides, especially substance P, have been found to be highly expressed in human sebocytes *in vivo* and *in vitro*. Further studies have shown unexpectedly that inhibitors of DP IV and APN can suppress proliferation and slightly decrease neutral lipids, but can also enhance terminal differentiation in SZ95 sebocytes. This suggests that ectopeptidases may be new targets to modulate certain sebocyte functions, and that ectopeptidase inhibitors may have potential therapeutic roles in acne pathogenesis [299].

Causative organisms: *Propionibacterium acnes*

Fitz-Gibbon *et al.* compared the skin microbiome at the strain level and genome level of *P. acnes* (Figure 90.21) between 49 acne patients and 52 healthy individuals by sampling the pilosebaceous units on their noses. Metagenomic analysis demonstrated that although the relative abundances of *P. acnes* were similar, the strain population

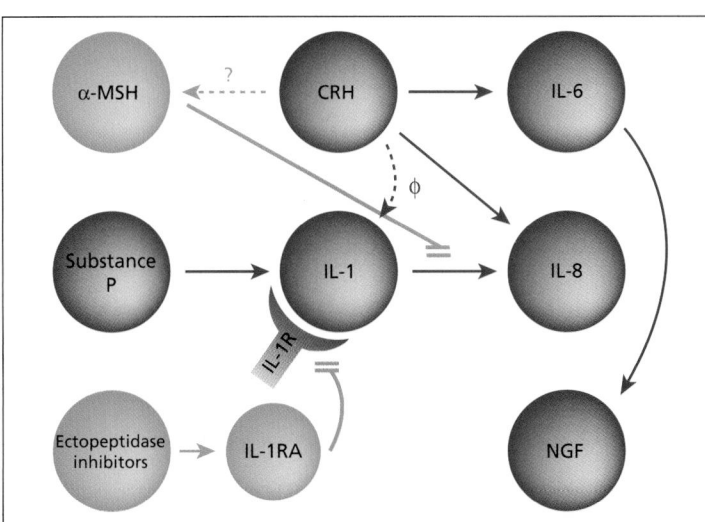

Figure 90.20 Neuropeptide–cytokine/chemokine signalling in human sebaceous glands and human sebocytes. Red: promoter of inflammation. Green: inhibition of inflammation. α-MSH, α-melanocyte-stimulating hormone; CRH, corticotrophin-releasing hormone; IL, interleukin; IL-1RA, IL-1 receptor antagonist; NGF, neural growth factor; Ø, no influence; ?, unknown regulation in sebocytes; =, inhibition. (From Zouboulis CC. Acne vulgaris and rosacea. In: Granstein RD, Luger T (eds) *Neuroimmunology of the Skin – Basic Science to Clinical Practice.* Berlin, Germany: Springer, 2009:219–32.)

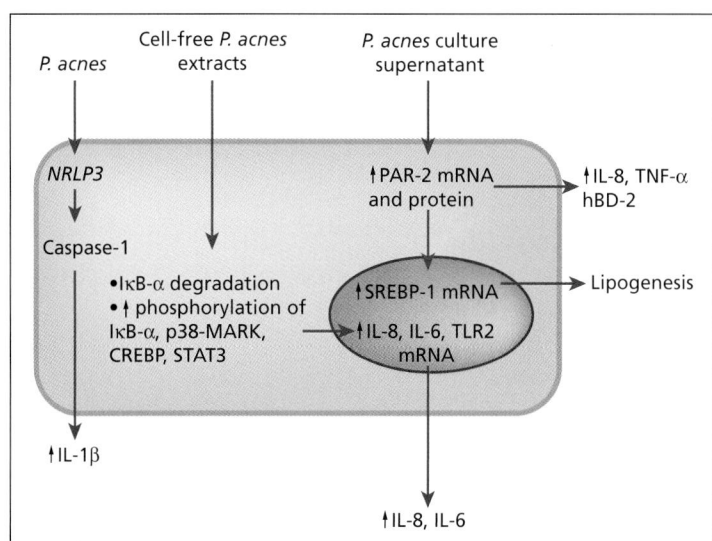

Figure 90.21 Effects of *P. acnes* extracts on human sebocytes. CREBP, cAMP response element-binding protein; hBD-2, human β-defensin 2; IL, interleukin; p38-MAPK, p38 mitogen-activated protein kinase; PAR-2, protease-activated receptor 2; SREBP-1, sterol response element-binding protein 1; STAT3, signal transducer and activator of transcription 3; TLR2, Toll-like receptor 2; TNF, tumour necrosis factor. (Courtesy of Lee *et al.* 2015 [781], Huang *et al.* 2015 [782] and Li *et al.* 2014 [308].)

structures were significantly different in the two cohorts. Certain strains were highly associated with acne, and other strains were enriched in healthy skin highlighting the importance of strain-level analysis of the human microbiome [300]. *P. acnes* strains modulate the expression of immune markers differently both at gene and at protein levels. *P. acnes* type III shows the highest pro-inflammatory potential by up-regulating the expression of PAR-2, TNF-α, matrix metalloproteinase 13 and tissue inhibitor of matrix metalloproteinase [301]. Treatment of cultured sebocytes with *P. acnes* and bacterial antigens (lipopolysaccharides (LPS)) significantly up-regulates the expression of pro-inflammatory cytokines [302]. However, there is a difference in the cytokine production curve over time after treatment between *P. acnes* and LPS. While LPS stimulates CXCL8, TNF-α and IL-1α, *P. acnes* only stimulates CXCL8 and TNF-α. *P. acnes* has no effect on IL-1α. Furthermore, viable *P. acnes* and not heat-killed organisms can stimulate the release of cytokines such as IL-1β, granulocyte–macrophage colony-stimulating factor (GM-CSF) and IL-8 [303,304]. New reports suggest that *P. acnes* induces IL-17 expression in peripheral blood mononuclear cells and present evidence that IL-17+ cells are found in the perifollicular infiltrate of comedones indicating that acne might be a T-helper type 17 (Th17)-mediated disease [305]. In accordance with this, Kistowska *et al.* show that, in addition to IL-17A, both Th1 and Th17 effector cytokines, transcription factors and chemokine receptors are strongly up-regulated in acne lesions. *P. acnes* can promote mixed Th17/Th1 responses by inducing the concomitant secretion of IL-17A and interferon (IFN)-γ from specific CD4+ T cells *in vitro* [306]. *P. acnes* also triggers monocyte–macrophage and sebocyte NACHT, LRR and PYD domain-containing protein 3 (NLRP3)-inflammasome activation [307].

Knocking down the expression of NLRP3 abolishes *P. acnes*-induced IL-1β production in sebocytes. The activation of the NLRP3 inflammasome by *P. acnes* is dependent on protease activity and reactive oxygen species generation [308]. Keratinocytes and sebocytes may act as immune cells capable of pathogen recognition and abnormal lipid presentation. Both cell types can be activated by *P. acnes* via Toll-like receptors (TLR), CD14 and CD1 molecules [309–311]. TLR2 is expressed in basal and infundibular keratinocytes, and sebaceous glands, and its activation provokes the release of IL-1α from primary human keratinocytes *in vitro* [312]. Bakry *et al.* documented statistically significant differences between acne-involved skin and normal skin and between acne-involved and non-involved skin regarding TLR2 expression intensity in pilosebaceous units and dermal inflammatory infiltrate [313]. Qin *et al.* showed that *P. acnes* induces robust IL-1β secretion in monocytes by triggering the activation of the NLRP3 inflammasome. *In vivo*, the encounter of *P. acnes* and macrophages in the perifollicular dermis could locally result in the release of substantial amounts of IL-1β and therefore exacerbate inflammation [307].

Human sebaceous glands may contribute to the skin immune defence by releasing antimicrobial peptides. For example, psoriasin, human β-defensins and cathelicidin are expressed in human pilosebaceous units, their expression is up-regulated in acne lesions [314] and the levels are up-regulated in the presence of *P. acnes* [302,315]. Each *P. acnes* strain has been shown to influence sebocyte viability and differentiation differentially which raises

the possibility that certain *P. acnes* strains may be responsible for opportunistic infections worsening acne lesions [302,315,316].

A description of phylogenetically distinct *P. acnes* clusters has been already undertaken [317]. The monounsaturated fatty acids (MUFA), mainly palmitoleic acid (C16:1) and oleic acid (C18:1), both of which are bactericidal against Gram-positive organisms [318], and stearoyl coenzyme A desaturase (SCD) 1, an enzyme responsible for the biosynthesis of MUFA are also produced by the sebaceous glands [319]. The TLR-2 ligand macrophage-activating lipopeptide 2 stimulates both SCD and fatty acid desaturase 2 mRNA expression in SZ95 sebocytes [318]. Lauric acid (C12:0), one of the sebum free fatty acids (FFAs), has strong antimicrobial activity *in vitro* against skin bacteria, including *P. acnes*. Topical application or intradermal injection of lauric acid *in vivo* shows remarkable therapeutic effectiveness against *P. acnes*-induced inflammation and significant reduction in the number of bacteria [320]. Furthermore, lauric acid, palmitic acid (16:0) and oleic acid (C18:1, *cis*-9), which are the typical FFAs found in human sebum, enhanced the hBD-2 expression and antimicrobial activity of human sebocytes against *P. acnes* [321], indicating that sebum FFAs are involved in the disinfecting activity of the human skin both through their direct antimicrobial characteristics and by inducing the expression of antimicrobial peptides in human sebocytes to enhance their innate immune defence ability [320].

Clinical features

History
Acne is predominantly a chronic disease of adolescence lasting on average 7 years. However, acne may present as young as 6 years depending on the onset of adrenarche and adults may develop acne *de novo* or as a continuum of their adolescent problems. Despite a better understanding of acne pathogenesis over the last decade reasons for these age differences remain unclear.

Presentation
Acne is a polymorphic inflammatory disease of the skin which occurs most commonly on the face (in 99% of cases; Figure 90.22)

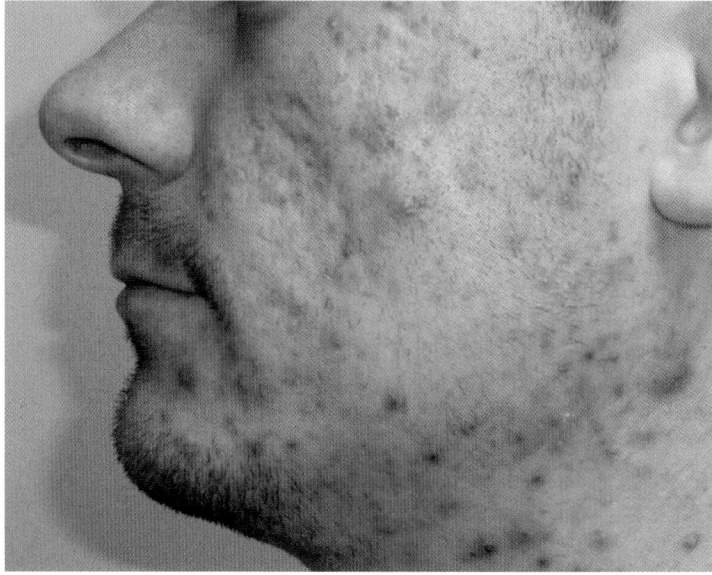

Figure 90.22 Moderate to severe inflammatory acne on the face.

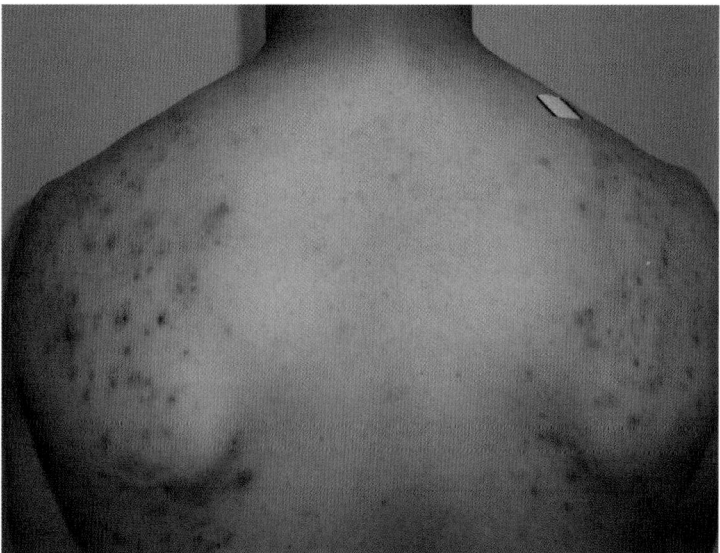

Figure 90.23 Acne on the back showing sparing of the central back.

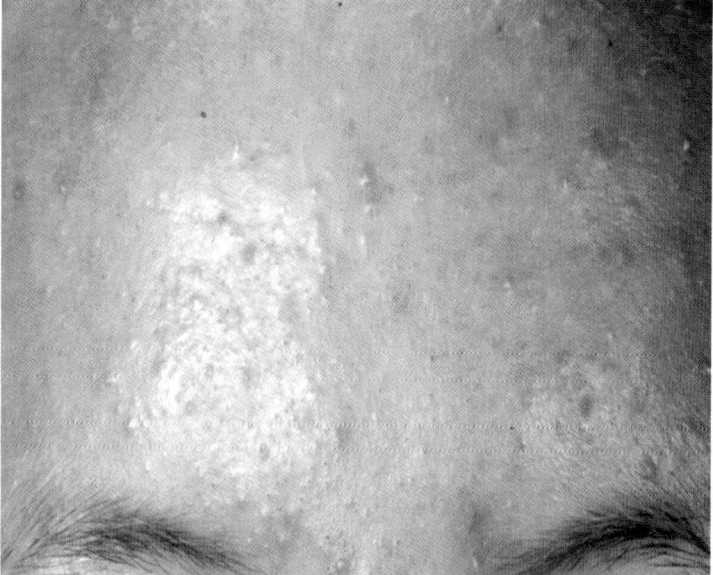

Figure 90.25 Comedonal acne with mid-facial distribution. This distribution is associated with poor prognosis.

and to a lesser extent on the back (60%) and chest (15%). The reasons for this varied distribution and extent are not clear (Figure 90.23). Seborrhoea along with scarring and post-inflammatory erythema and/or pigment changes (Figure 90.24) are common features. These may all contribute to significant physical and psychosocial impact.

The clinical picture can vary from very mild comedonal acne, with or without sparse inflammatory lesions, to aggressive fulminant disease with associated systemic upset. Non-inflamed lesions are the earliest lesions to develop in younger patients and embrace both open (blackheads) and closed comedones (whiteheads). Open comedones frequently appear in a mid-facial distribution (Figure 90.25), and when evident early they indicate poor prognosis [18]. Closed comedones are generally 1 mm in diameter, skin coloured and have no visible follicular opening. These lesions are often inconspicuous and require adequate

lighting and stretching of the skin to be seen. Most patients have a mixture of lesions.

Several subtle subtypes of comedones have been described.
- 'Sandpaper' comedones consist of multiple very small whiteheads, frequently distributed on the forehead (Figure 90.26), which produce a roughened, gritty feel to the skin.
- 'Macrocomedones' (Figure 90.27) are large whiteheads greater than 1 mm in diameter. Both macrocomedones and sandpaper comedones respond poorly to conventional topical treatments.
- 'Submarine' comedones (Figure 90.28) are large comedonal structures greater than 0.5 cm in diameter and reside more deeply in the skin; they are frequently associated with recurrent inflammatory nodular lesions.

Inflammatory lesions arise from the microcomedo or non-inflammatory lesions and can remain superficial or deep in nature. Lesions

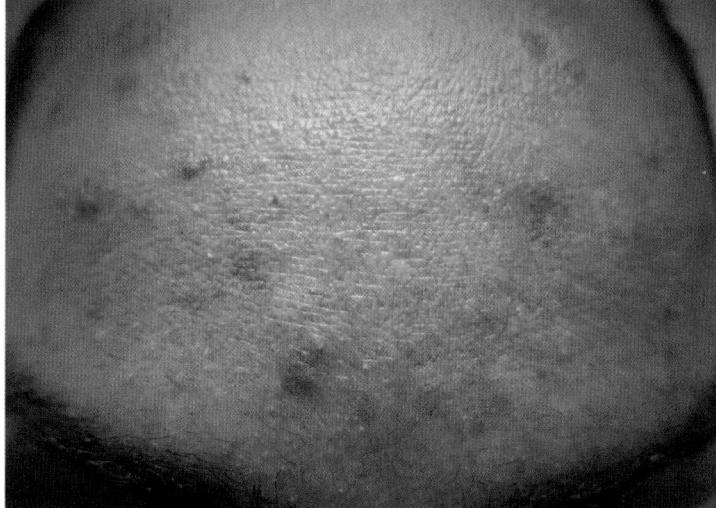

Figure 90.24 Post-inflammatory erythema and pigment changes on the forehead. (Courtesy of Dr J. Del Rosso, Las Vegas Skin & Cancer Clinic, Las Vegas, Nevada, USA.)

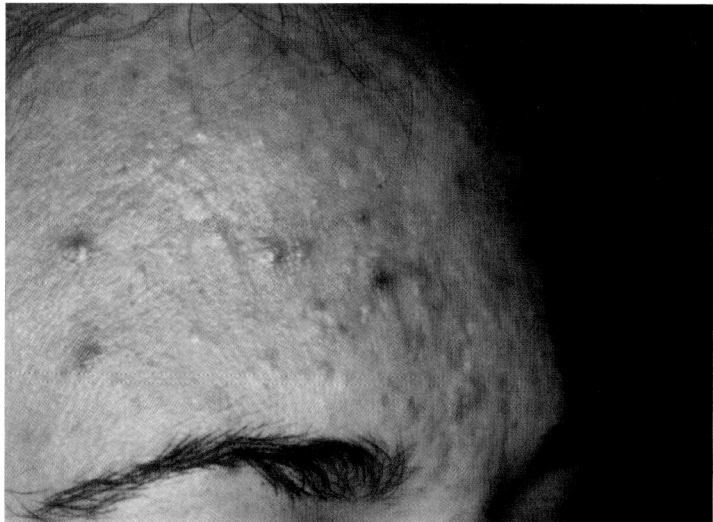

Figure 90.26 Sandpaper comedones on the forehead.

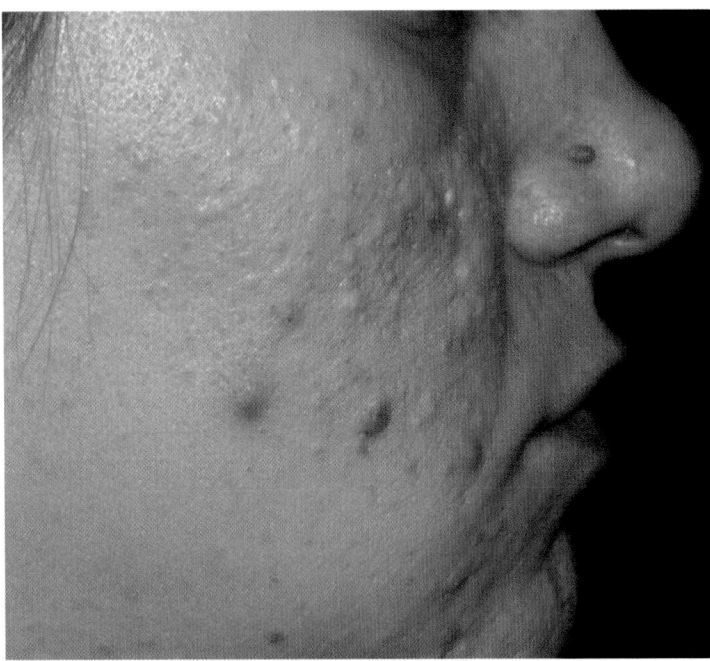

Figure 90.27 Multiple macrocomedones interspersed with some inflammatory lesions on the cheeks of a female patient with acne. (Courtesy of Professor M. Jackson, University of Louisville, Kentucky, USA.)

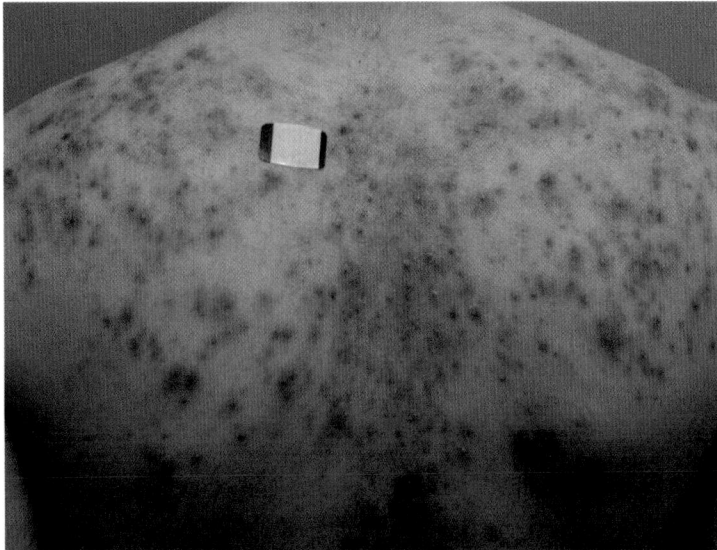

Figure 90.29 Severe acne of the back with many inflammatory papules and pustules.

embrace papules and pustules (5 mm or less in diameter) and can be extensively distributed on the face and/or back (Figure 90.29), deep-seated pustules and nodules (>5 mm) may also occur (Figure 90.30). Sinus tracts may develop between nodules and/or deep pustules leading to inevitable scarring (Figure 90.31). These lesions are frequently very tender, chronic and more resistant to treatment.

Itching is a rare symptom of acne and possibly relates to the release of histamine-like compounds from *P. acnes*.

Inflammatory macules represent regressing lesions that may persist for many weeks and contribute markedly to the general inflammatory appearance seen in acne (Figure 90.32).

Scarring is commonly seen as a consequence of acne and can present as atrophic scarring (Figure 90.33) due to loss of tissue or conversely excessive tissue can arise in hypertrophic and keloid scarring (Figure 90.34a,b).

Clinical variants
A number of variants of acne are recognized as follows:
1 Severe forms (see sections on Acne fulminans and Acne conglobata).
2 Drug-induced (see section on Predisposing factors).
3 Cosmetic acne (see section on Predisposing factors).
4 Occupational acne (see section on Occupational acne).

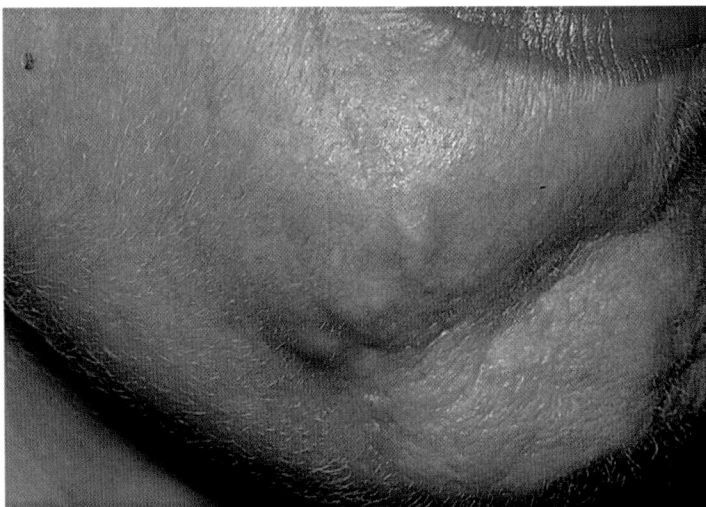

Figure 90.28 Submarine comedones. This patient required stretching of the skin in order for them to be seen.

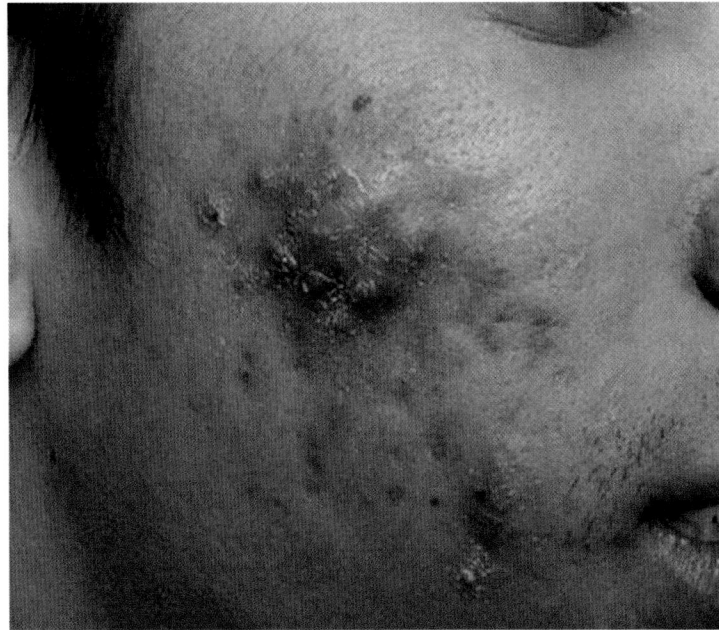

Figure 90.30 Nodular acne of the right cheek with scars. (Courtesy of Dr S. Chow, KL Skin Centre, Malaysia.)

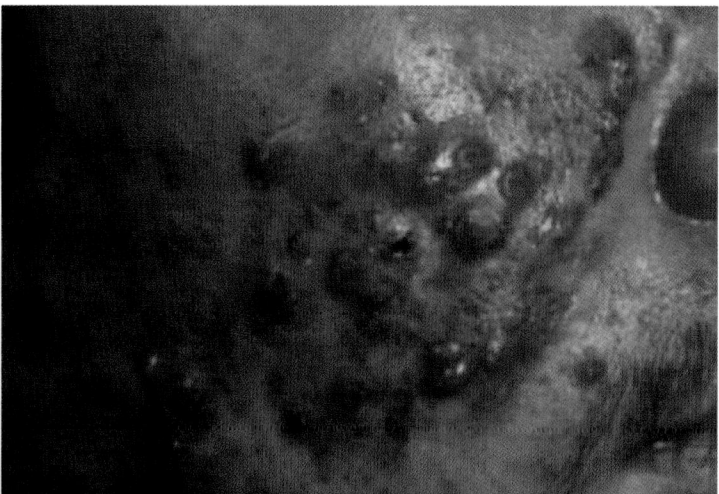

Figure 90.31 Nodular/conglobate acne with sinus tracts. (Courtesy of Dr C. L. Goh, National Skin Centre, Singapore.)

5 Acne associated with psychological problems:
  • Acné excoriée.
  • Body dysmorphic disorder (BDD).
  • Eating disorders.
6 Granulomatous acne.
7 Acne mechanica.

Acne associated with psychological problems

Acné excoriée (synonyms: excoriated acne, picker's acne). Acné excoriée is seen predominantly in adolescent girls (Figure 90.35) although the incidence is increasing in mature females and is

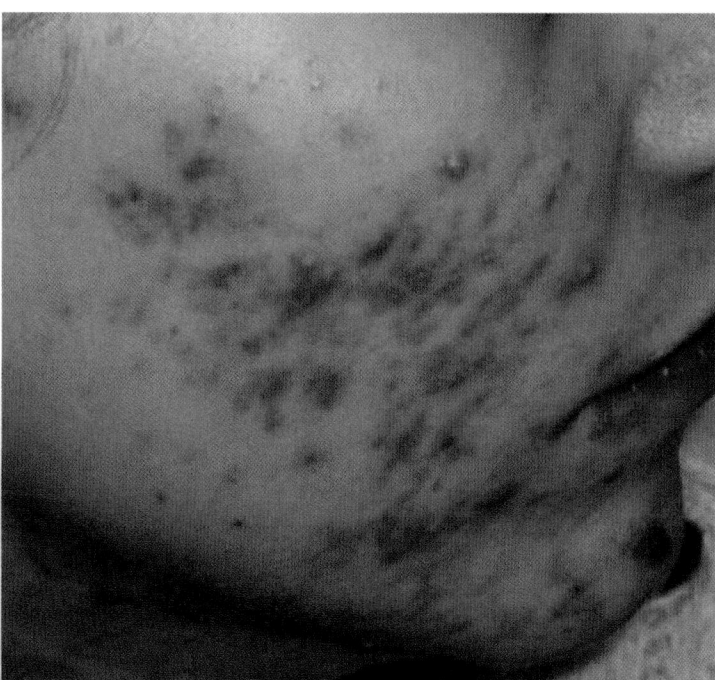

Figure 90.32 Inflammatory macules contribute to the erythema seen in acne.

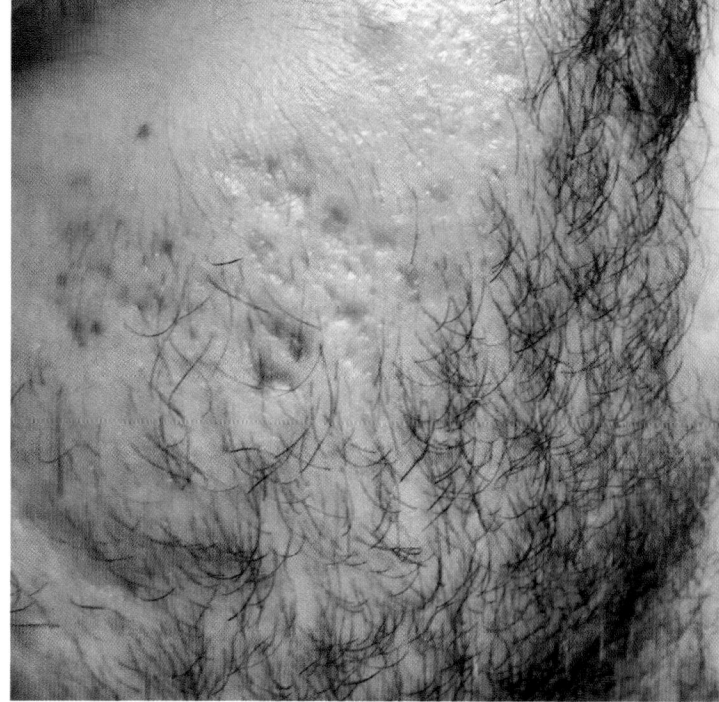

Figure 90.33 Atrophic scarring with associated inflammatory change. (Courtesy of J. Del Rosso Las Vegas Skin & Cancer Clinic, Las Vegas, Nevada, USA.)

frequently associated with stress. Acné excoriée is regarded as a self-inflicted skin condition in which the sufferer compulsively picks real or imagined acne lesions predominantly on the face. A personality or psychological problem often underlies the condition including obsessive compulsive disorder and bodily focused anxiety. BDD may be associated and contribute to the pathophysiology [322,323]. Evidence of linear erosions is suggestive of self-mutilation and underlying psychiatric disease should be suspected [324]. An atopic background may be evident. A contact dermatitis should be considered and excluded [325]. The persistent trauma frequently results in significant scarring.

Treatment is challenging; acne should be treated but topical treatments have a tendency to irritate. Some patients with acné excoriée may just need to break the habit of picking whilst others may have a compulsive skin picking disorder which may require psychological therapy or psychotropic drug treatments [326]. Hypnosis and cognitive behavioural therapy using habit reversal techniques may be effective [327,328]. Selective serotonin reuptake inhibitors including fluoxetine, paroxetine, sertraline and fluvoxamine are treatments of choice and are frequently employed alongside psychotherapy. Treatment for facial scarring and ulceration resulting from acné excoriée has been improved using the 585-nm pulsed dye laser along with cognitive psychotherapy [329].

BDD and acne. A small number of patients with BDD have acne as their prime symptom [330]. The perceived acne is out of proportion to physical signs. Patients require significant support; they are often depressed or have obsessional compulsive behaviours or anxiety. A significant risk of suicide has been reported [331]. Patients with BDD require dermatological and psychiatric management as many have global mental disorders. Some patients with BDD as the only

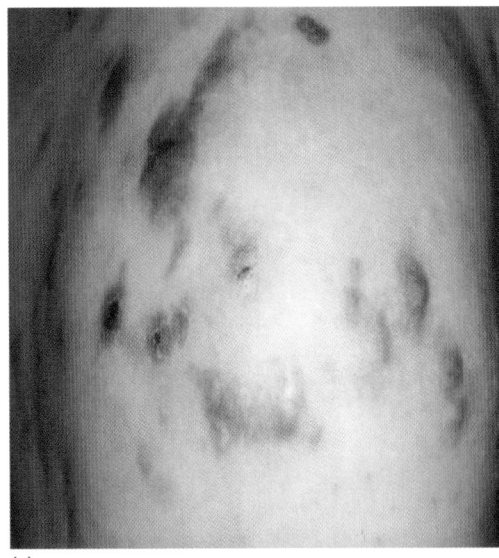

(a)

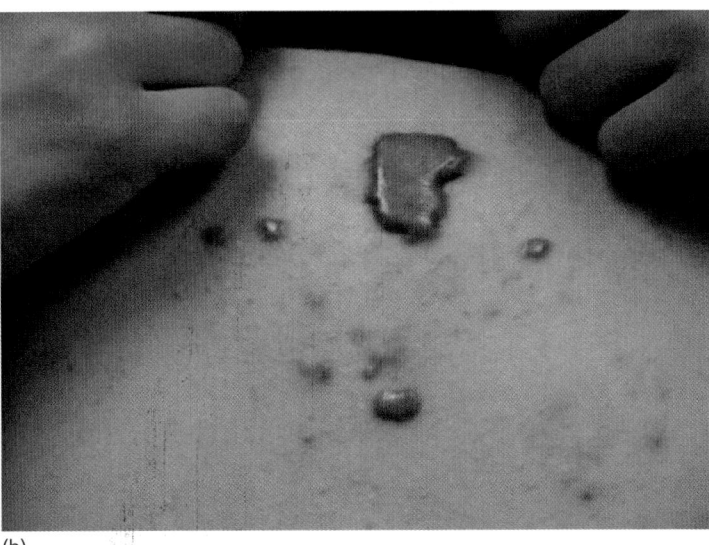

(b)

Figure 90.34 (a) Hypertrophic scarring of the shoulders in the context of moderate to severe acne. (b) Keloid scarring on the trunk associated with mild acne. (Courtesy of Dr S. Chow, KL Skin Centre, Malaysia.)

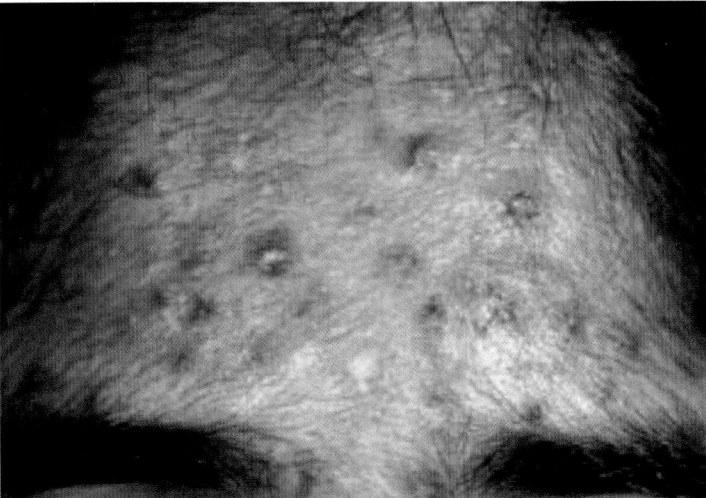

Figure 90.35 Acné excoriée on the forehead of a female. (Courtesy of Dr C. L. Goh, National Skin Centre, Singapore.)

behavioural symptom may gain relief by treating their mild acne aggressively. Isotretinoin has been prescribed in this context but 'relapse', either real or perceived, is common and further requests for isotretinoin frequent [332] (see Chapter 86).

Acne and eating disorders. Acne has been reported in anorexia nervosa. Acne itself may be a predisposing factor for anorexia in vulnerable teenaged age groups who adopt a diet in an attempt to control their acne [333]. Serum growth hormone has been shown to be raised in anorexia nervosa and concomitantly IGF-1 is low.

Granulomatous acne
The precise mechanism producing localized granulomatous acne is not known. The clinical picture is usually that of deep well-demarcated lesion(s), especially on the cheeks (Figure 90.36). Response to therapy is slow and often unsatisfactory; antibiotics and isotretinoin are of limited benefit; oral steroids are often required.

Mechanical acne (synonym: acne mechanica)
This term describes acne that occurs at the site of repeated mechanical trauma and/or frictional obstruction of the pilosebaceous outlet resulting in comedo formation [334–336].

Examples include 'fiddler's neck', which may occur on the neck of violin players, and is characterized by well-defined plaques with the presence of comedones, lichenification and pigmentation. Headbands, tight bra straps, suspenders and collars as well as turtleneck sweaters may cause localized acne in the frictional sites [335]. This has also been reported in amputees [337]. Treatment should include elimination of the causative force(s) as well as management of non-inflammatory and inflammatory lesions.

Differential diagnosis
A number of conditions may be considered in the differential diagnosis of acne vulgaris.

Milia
Closed comedones may be confused with milia. Milia represent intraepidermal keratin cysts predominantly infraorbital in distribution (Figure 90.37).

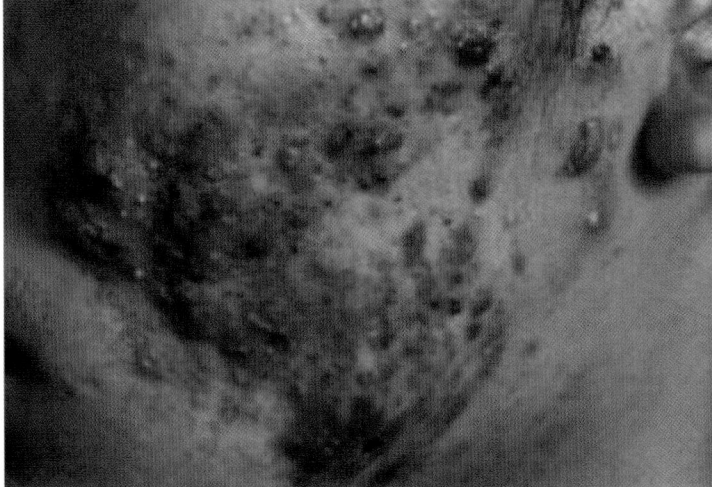

Figure 90.36 Granulomatous acne of the face. (Courtesy of Dr C. L. Goh, National Skin Centre, Singapore.)

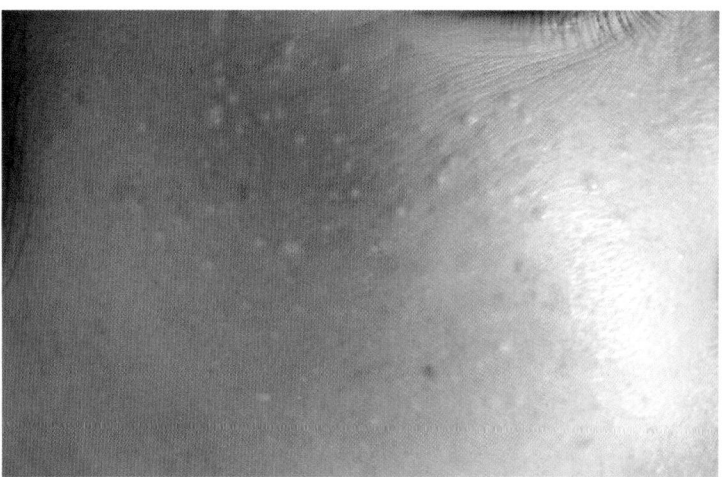

Figure 90.37 Multiple milia on the upper cheek. (Courtesy of Dr J. Del Rosso, Las Vegas Skin & Cancer Clinic, Las Vegas, Nevada, USA.)

Syringomas

Syringomas are non-inflammatory papules that occur primarily around the eyelids and upper cheeks. They are seen more frequently in Japanese women. Histology demonstrates a dense fibrous stroma with dilated cystic spaces that have small comma like tails resembling tadpoles (see Chapter 138).

Fibrofolliculomas

Fibrofolliculomas are 2–4 mm dome-shaped papules seen most commonly on the face (Figure 90.38) neck and upper trunk. They are characteristically seen in Birt–Hogg–Dube (BHD) syndrome. This is rare autosomal dominant inherited condition characterized by the development of benign tumours on the face and upper body including fibrofilloculomas, trichodiscomas and acrochordon. People with this syndrome are at increased risk of colon or kidney cancer as well as spontaneous pneumothorax due to pulmonary cysts. BHD syndrome is due to mutation in the BHD gene on chromosome 17p12-q11.2 encoding folliculin. If positive for the

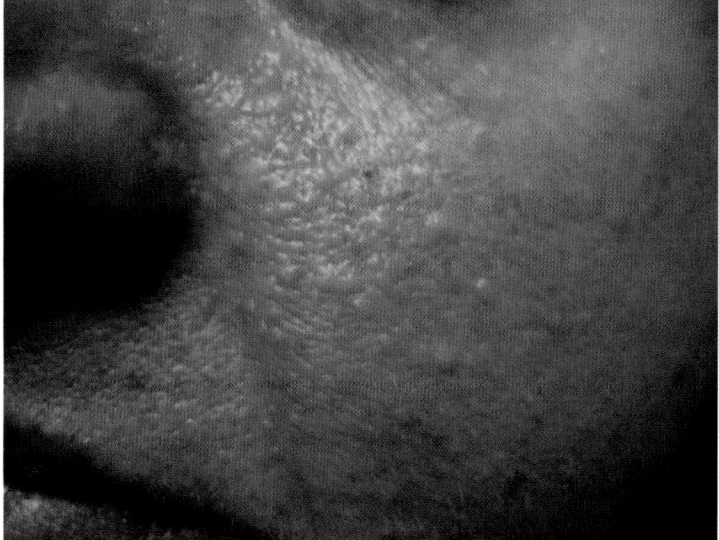

Figure 90.38 Fibrofolliculomas: Birt–Hogg–Dube syndrome. (Courtesy of Dr J. Del Rosso, Las Vegas Skin & Cancer Clinic, Las Vegas, Nevada, USA.)

gene, patients with BHD should undergo renal ultrasound and/or abdominal CT/MRI, chest X-ray and colonoscopy to determine any associated malignancies (see Chapter 138).

Ectopic sebaceous glands (synonym: Fordyce spots)

Fordyce spots are heterotopic sebaceous glands that can occur around the vermilion border of the lips or within the oral mucosa (see also Chapter 93). They are commonly multiple, and appear as symmetrical discrete yellow papules [338]. They are present in 25% of the population over the age of 35 years and are usually asymptomatic but can be disfiguring. Oral isotretinoin has been used with some success for extensive lesions [339]. Carbon dioxide ablative laser therapy has also been used with good effect [340]. Lesions may occur on the penile shaft and may become inflamed and a cause for concern. The areolar of the breast is another site occasionally affected [341].

Pilosebaceous naevoid disorders

Some of these disorders are only tenuously linked with the pilosebaceous system.

Acneform naevi

Symmetrical areas of normal skin set in the midst of severe acne on the back [342], or acne localized to one side of the back have been described. Reduced sebum excretion and surface bacteria have been demonstrated in the normal-looking areas.

Comedo naevus (synonyms: naevus comedonicus, naevus follicularis, naevus unilateralis comedonicus)

This uncommon naevus is usually a developmental defect of the hair follicles [343–349]. The associated sebaceous glands may be normal, hypoplastic or hyperplastic. Lesions usually occur on the scalp, face and trunk, and occasionally at unusual sites such as the genitalia. The individual lesions consist of keratin-filled pits, often grouped or linear in arrangement (Figure 90.39). Occasionally, inflammatory acne lesions may be found. Although usually present at birth, they often become more prominent at puberty [349]. *FGFR2* mutations have been identified in a comedonal naevus but not in the adjacent normal skin [350]. The somatic heterozygous Ser252Trp-FGFR2 mutation has been confirmed within the affected skin lesions of a male patient presenting with a unilateral acneform naevus [351]. An association with epidermolytic hyperkeratosis has also been reported [348]. Treatment is usually of only limited success. Topical retinoids and 12% aqueous ammonium lactate solution have been reported to benefit. Gentle cautery may help less severe cases [349].

Familial comedones

This uncommon genetic disorder presents with single comedonal lesions, but later the face may become extensively involved with gouped comedones and cysts; scarring may ensue. New lesions may continue into middle age.

Sebaceous naevus (synonym: naevus sebaceus of Jadassohn)

This is an organoid naevus, consisting of a mixture of relatively normal-looking epidermis, dermis, sweat and sebaceous glands. It usually presents on the scalp as an area of alopecia [352–356]. At puberty, the sebaceous glands enlarge and the epidermis becomes

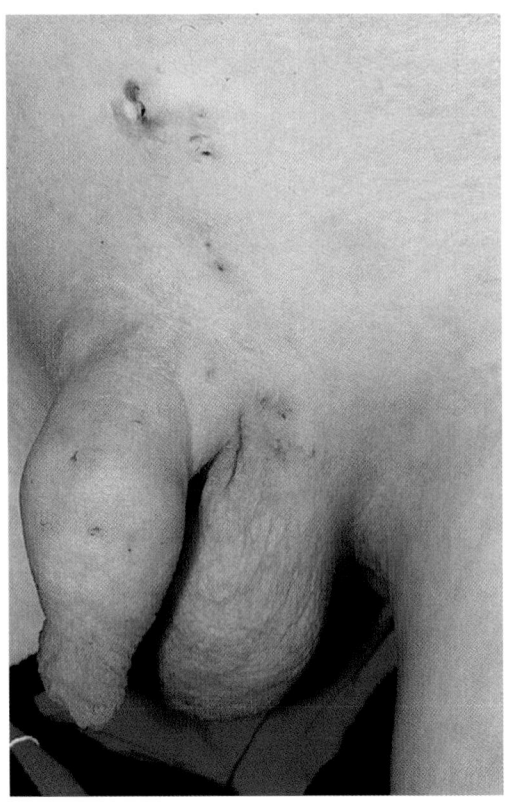

Figure 90.39 A patient with comedo naevus (naevus comedonicus) predominantly consisting of blackheads on the lower abdomen.

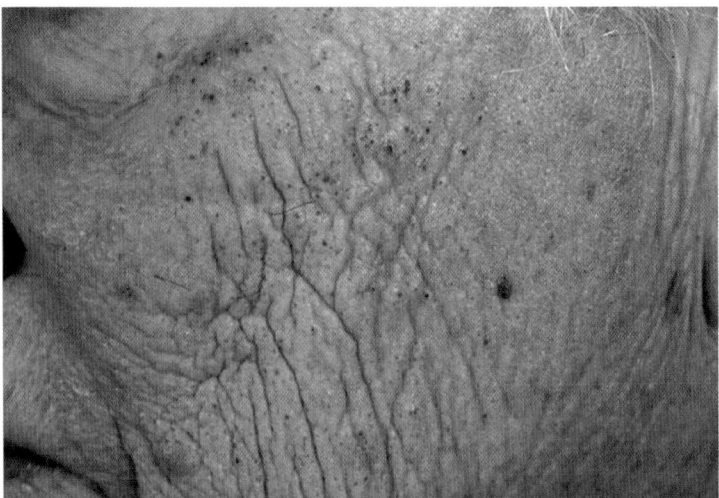

Figure 90.40 Favre–Racouchot syndrome (senile comedones). (Courtesy of Dr J. Del Rosso, Las Vegas Skin & Cancer Clinic, Las Vegas, Nevada, USA.)

verrucous. Co-occurrence with aplasia cutis has been reported [353]. Trichoepithelioma and eccrine syringoadenoma have been noted in naevus sebaceous [355]. An unusual haematopoietic proliferation at birth that spontaneously resolved at 4 months has been documented [356]. Excision is usually recommended because of potential to develop a squamous or basal cell carcinoma with a lifetime risk reported between 5 and 22% [354].

Favre–Racouchot syndrome (synonymous with senile comedones and solar comedones)

Multiple open and closed comedones occur on periorbital and malar areas of elderly people in the context of chronic sun exposure (Figure 90.40) (see also Chapter 96). UVR results in solar damage to the supporting dermis causing the pilosebaceous duct to become distended with impacted corneocytes. Occasionally lesions are unilateral. Histology demonstrates increased elastic tissue with thickened and tortuous fibres in the upper and mid dermis [357]. Similar change may be seen in pseudoxanthoma elasticum or post radiotherapy. A comedo extractor will remove lesions but they frequenty recur. Topical retinoids and electrocautery may be of benefit.

Sebaceous gland hyperplasia, adenoma and carcinoma

Sebaceous gland hyperplasia represents a benign proliferation of the sebaceous gland (Figure 90.41) producing yellow/pink lesions 1–3 mm in diameter on the face (see also Chapter 93). They may also present on the light-exposed skin of renal transplant patients receiving ciclosporin [358]. Treatment is rarely requested but gentle cautery, cryotherapy, trichloroacetic acid, carbon dioxide and pulsed dye lasers may help [359,360]. Lesions are occasionally diffuse,

producing a yellowish hue to the skin. Oral isotretinoin has benefited some cases [361]. Co-cyprindiol (Dianette® and Estelle-35®), with or without additional oral cyproterone actetate will also produce regression of sebaceous hyperplasia in some females. Photodynamic therapy using aminolaevulinic acid has also been shown to be successful in reducing sebaceous hyperplasia [362].

Adenoma sebaceum (synonym: angiofibromas)

Adenoma sebaceum are small translucent waxy-looking papules symmetrically distributed over the central face. Multiple lesions are associated with tuberous sclerosis. Histology of lesions demonstrates dermal fibrosis and vascular proliferation and dilatation.

Sebaceous gland tumours

These are uncommon but may be associated with internal malignancy and systemic disease.

Sebaceous adenoma

This is a benign tumour composed of incompletely differentiated sebaceous cells. It occurs in both sexes, predominantly in

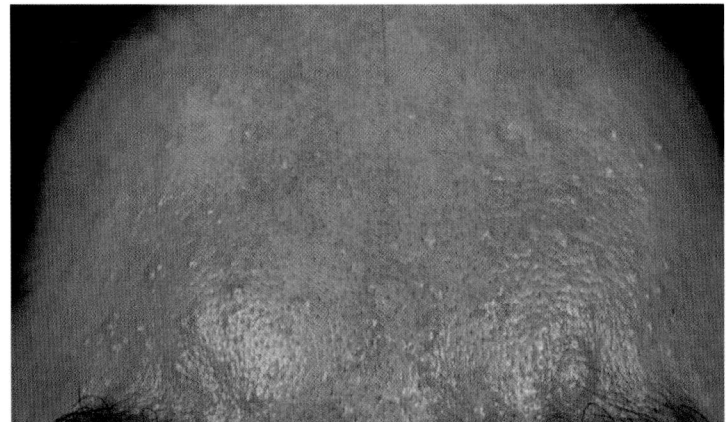

Figure 90.41 Sebaceous gland hyperplasia on the forehead. (From Zouboulis CC, Boschnakow A. Chronological ageing and photoageing of the human sebaceous gland. *Clin Exp Dermatol* 2001;26:600–7.)

the elderly on the face or scalp [363]. The waxy pink/yellow tumours are usually 10 mm or less in size and may form ulcerative plaques. Excision is recommended but they are radiosensitive. Rarely sebaceous gland adenomas can be associated with multiple visceral carcinomas, which present relatively early (45 years). This association is referred to as the Muir–Torré syndrome (MTS) (see Chapter 138). MTS is a rare genodermatosis defined clinically by the occurrence of a sebaceous neoplasm (adenoma, epithelioma or carcinoma) and at least one internal malignancy in the absence of other predisposing factors. Most patients present with sebaceous adenomas but cystic sebaceous neoplasms have been reported as specific markers of MTS. Gastrointestinal and genitourinary malignancies are the most commonly reported with colorectal cancers presenting at or proximal to the splenic flexure contrary to most sporadic colorectal cancers [364,365]. MTS is most frequently found as a variant of the autosomal dominant hereditary disorder non-polyposis colorectal cancer (HNPCC) [366], with tumours demonstrating microsatellite instability and germline mutations in the DNA mismatch repair genes Muts homologue *MSH2* and *MLH1*. However, the distribution of gene mutations in patients with MTS is slightly different from that seen in all patients with HNPCC and some cases of MTS arise spontaneously [367]. Clinicians should consider a diagnosis of MTS in patients presenting with sebaceous neoplasms and immunohistochemical examination of tumours for MSH2 and MLH1 protein can be used as a screening test for MTS. The neoplasms of MTS tend to follow a more indolent course than the sporadic cases which can be quite aggressive. Careful follow-up and active treatment are required for both familial and sporadic cases. Evidence suggests that patients with MTS and HNPCC should undergo colonoscopy every 1–2 years from the age of 25 years or at an age 10 years younger than the family member who originally presented with the disease. Others recommend annual history, physical examination including thorough review of the skin, and urinalysis as well as endometrial sampling and transvaginal ultrasound for females.

Sebaceous carcinoma

This is a rare malignant tumour arising from the sebaceous glands (see Chapter 142). It is commoner in men over the age of 40 years and presents as a firm solitary yellow-orange lesion usually on the face and scalp. Sebaceous carcinomas have a well-recognized association with MTS. The tumour grows slowly, but those arising in the eyelid (from the Meibomian glands) are more likely to metastasize [368]. Treatment is by excision or radiotherapy [369]. A tumour diameter of 10 mm or greater and/or tumours classified as T4 on the T classification of the tumour/node/metastasis staging system are linked to a poor prognosis [370].

Sebaceous (epidermoid) cysts and steatocystoma multiplex

The classical 'sebaceous' cyst is an epidermal structure; strictly, it should be referred to as an epidermoid cyst, and is discussed in Chapter 134. However, true sebaceous cysts occur as so-called steatocystoma multiplex (SM), a naevoid condition that histologically shows a mixture of a keratinizing epithelium and sebaceous lobules attached to the epidermis by a thin epidermal strand [371–373]. A clinical and histological study examined 64 sporadic

cases with an average age of onset of 26 years. They confirmed the presence of multiple smooth yellow dermal swellings varying from a few millimetres to 20 mm in size distributed on the arms, chest, neck and axillae and appearing and/or enlarging at puberty (Figure 90.42a,b). When extensive these can produce the so-called SM suppurativa, which mimics acne conglobata. SM shares many clinical features and may show overlapping histopathological features with eruptive vellus hair cysts (EVHC). In a case series, all exhibited eosinophilia and lack of granular layer, and 17–42% displayed vellus hair, hair follicles, keratin and smooth muscle components within the cavity, in the wall or adjacent to it. The results of this study suggest that SM is a hamartomatous condition and that SM and EVHC are variants which originate in the pilosebaceous duct [374]. SM is rare and is occasionally associated with type 2 pachyonychia congenita (PC-2 or Jackson–Lawler syndrome), in which natal teeth are also a feature [375–379]. Histologically, the cysts in PC-2 may be true steatocysts, EVHCs or keratinous cysts, even in the same family or in an individual [380–382]. To date, mutations in the Ia

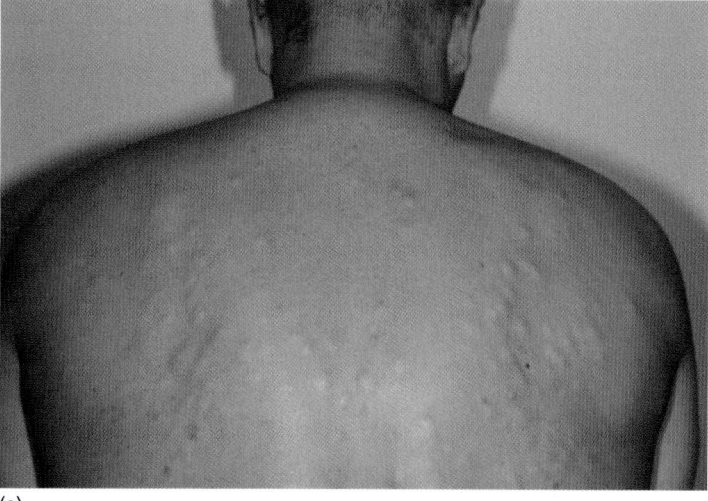

(a)

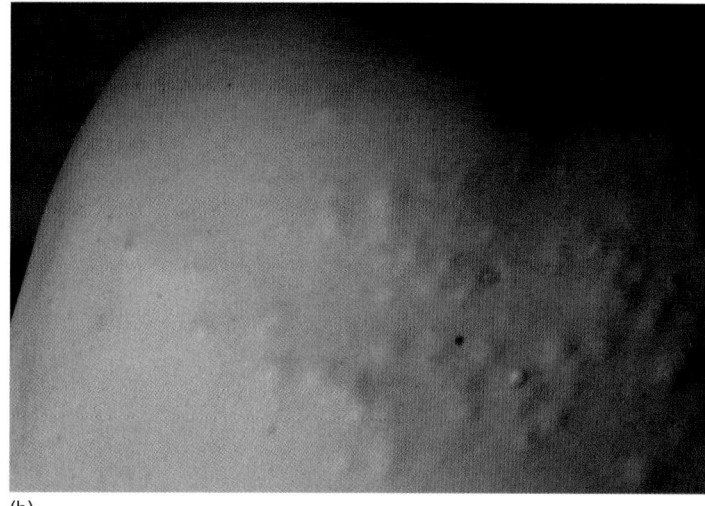

(b)

Figure 90.42 (a) Steatocystoma multiplex of the back. (b) Steatocystoma close-up of the multiple cystic lesions. (Courtesy of Dr N. Veien, the Dermatology Clinic, Aalborg, Denmark.)

domain of keratin 17 (K17) have been found in all cases [382,383]. In some families with clinically and histologically typical SM, mutations in the *K17* gene are also found [384]. Close inspection demonstrates that some members have nail changes which are usually but not always milder than those of PC. Familial SM has also been associated with natal teeth in the absence of nail dystrophy [384] and it seems likely that these cases are also due to keratin gene mutations. However, in a case of SM/EVHC and in another of EVHC, mutations in *K17* were not found along the Ia domain [383]; this would suggest that SM is genetically heterogeneous. Treatment is challenging [371]; excision of the larger cysts is possible but total removal of all cysts is impractical. Successful treatment employing a vein hook to locally extract cysts has been reported [385]. One study has also utilized the carbon dioxide laser with some improvement [386]. Topical therapy is of limited benefit. Systemic antibiotics may reduce inflammation and/or suppuration and oral isotretinoin reduces inflammation but does not affect the primary disease process.

Granulomatous rosacea (synonym: lupus miliaris disseminatus faciei, acne agminata)

Other diseases that may produce diagnostic difficulties include granulomatous rosacea (Figure 90.43; see Chapter 91).

Keratosis pilaris

Occasionally, inflammatory keratosis pilaris may masquerade as acne. Keratosis pilaris is most commonly seen on the proximal extremities (Figure 90.44a,b), and is characterized by follicular keratotic papules in hair-bearing areas which may or may not be associated with erythema (see Chapter 87). It has a familial tendency and is reported in the context of genetic syndromes such as chromosome 18p depletion in which there may be prominent and extensive keratosis pilaris [387–390]. One study suggests that the presence of moderate to severe keratosis pilaris on the arms

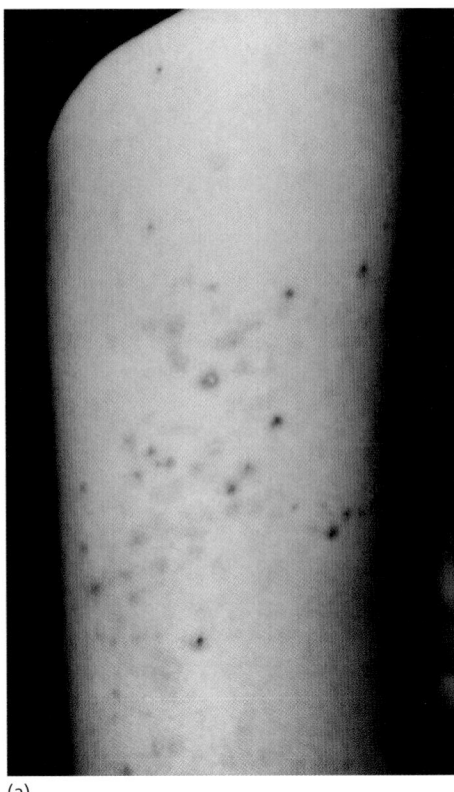

(a)

(b)

Figure 90.44 (a) Keratosis pilaris of the upper arms associated with some inflammation and excoriation. (b) A close-up view of keratosis pilaris.

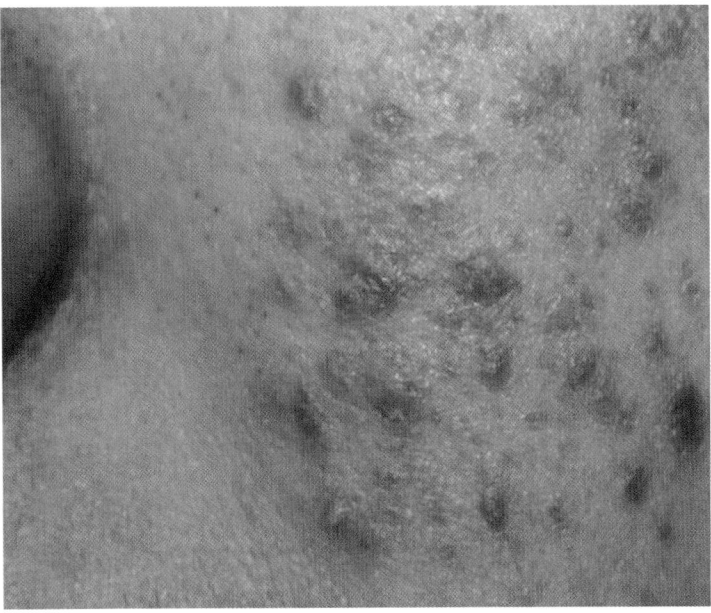

Figure 90.43 Granulomatous rosacea synonymous with acne agminata seen on the cheek.

is associated with a lower prevalence of acne vulgaris and lower severity of facial lesions in adolescents and young adults [391].

Rosacea

Rosacea may be mistaken for inflammatory acne. Rosacea usually occurs in an older age group of patients, i.e. 30–50 years of age, and lacks comedones or scarring and rarely affects the trunk (Figure 90.45).

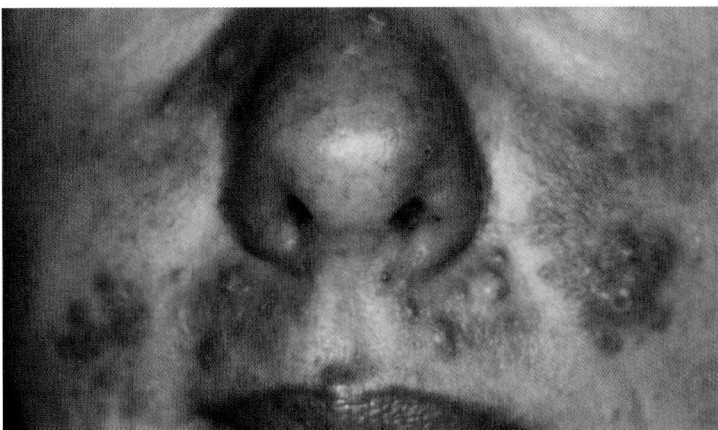

Figure 90.45 Rosacea on the mid-face with periorbital sparing.

The presence of facial flushing and specific triggers, including heat, spicy food or alcohol, are more in keeping with a diagnosis of rosacea. Rosacea patients may also have ocular involvement. Some patients have features of both diseases and clinical acne may evolve into more typical rosacea later in life (see Chapter 91).

Pyoderma faciale

Synonymous with rosacea fulminans (see Chapter 91), pyoderma faciale usually presents very acutely on the face in adult females (Figure 90.46). The lesions are deeply inflamed. Nodules, cysts and occasionally sinus tracts may form. Histology demonstrates a mixed inflammatory infiltrate in the upper and mid dermis with extravasation of red blood cells and haemosiderin deposition.

Perioral dermatitis

In perioral dermatitis, the papules and pustules present on an ery-thematous and/or scaling base localized symmetrically around the mouth with a clear zone around the vermillion border. Lesions

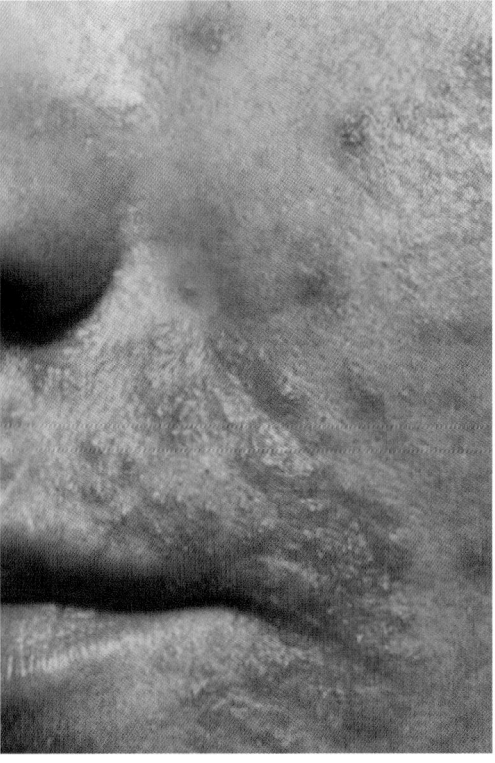

Figure 90.47 Perioral dermatitis demonstrating small papules on an erythematous base.

frequently itch in perioral dermatitis and no comedones are evi-dent (Figure 90.47) (see also Chapter 91).

Folliculitis

Gram-negative folliculitis due to Gram-negative organisms can occur as a complication of long-term oral or, less frequently, top-ical antibiotic therapy used to treat acne [392–394]. It has also been reported in HIV-positive patients and after hot tub immersion. Clinical features include a sudden eruption of multiple small follic-ular pustules or occasionally nodular lesions, most frequently local-ized around the perioral or perinasal skin (Figure 90.48). This results from overgrowth of Gram-negative organisms including *Klebsiella*,

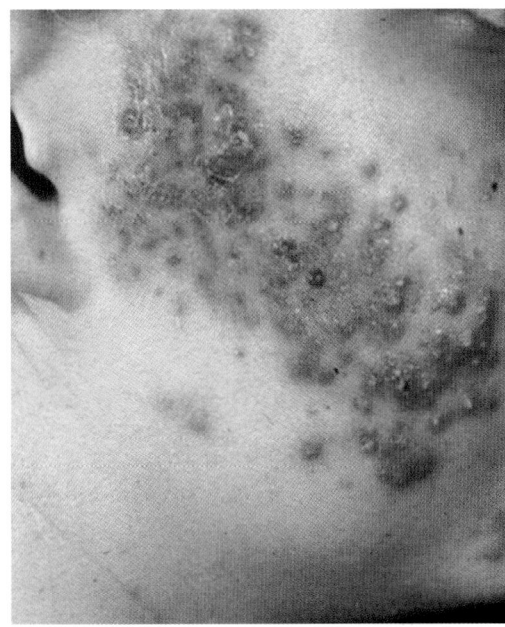

Figure 90.46 Rosacea fulminans (synonymous with pyoderma faciale).

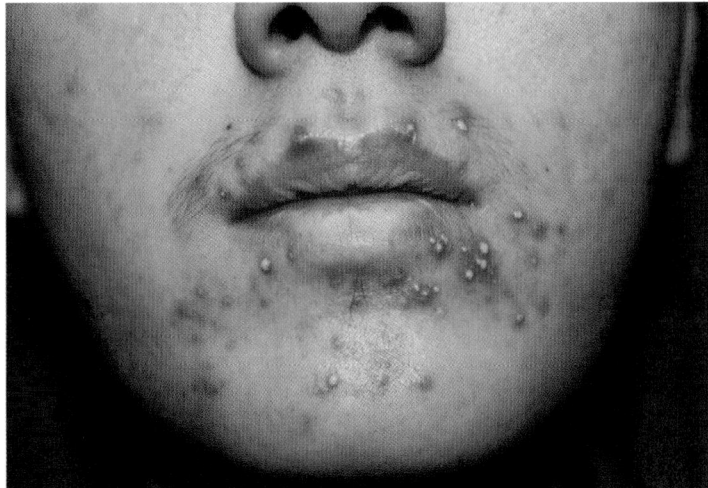

Figure 90.48 Gram-negative folliculitis after long-term antibiotic use showing multiple pustules. (Courtesy of Dr S. Chow, KL Skin Centre, Malaysia.)

Escherichia coli, Serratia marescens, Proteus mirabilis or *Pseudomonas aeruginosa*. These organisms replace the Gram-positive flora of the facial skin and mucous membranes. The current antibiotic should be discontinued replacing it with either ampicillin (250 mg four times a day) or trimethoprim (600 mg/day). However, response may be slow and relapse is common. Isotretinoin is now considered the treatment of choice as this results in lower relapse rates [395–397].

Malassezia *folliculitis (synonym: pityrosporum folliculitis)*

Malassezia folliculitis is due to proliferation of the yeast within the hair follicles. It presents most frequently on the upper trunk as a monomorphic acne like eruption with many papules or pustules which may itch (Figure 90.49). Topical or oral antifungal agents are generally helpful. In some cases oral isotretinoin to reduce the seborrhoea is beneficial [398,399].

Scalp folliculitis (synonym: acne necrotica miliaris, proprionibacteria folliculitis)

Scalp folliculitis is an inflammatory disorder of the hair follicles characterized by small itchy pustules on the scalp often around the hairline resulting from an inflammatory reaction to microorganisms including bacteria (*P. acnes, Staphylococcus aureus*), yeasts (*Malassezia* spp.) and mites (*Demodex folliculorum*) (see also Chapter 93). Patients receiving oral isotretinoin may develop scalp folliculitis due to *S. aureus* infection which responds well to oral flucloxacillin. A persistent scalp folliculitis has been recorded in patients with cyclical neutropenia [400].

Folliculitis keloidalis (synonym: acne cheloidalis nuchae, acne keloidalis)

Folliculitis keloidalis (Figure 90.50) represents an unusual chronic form of folliculitis affecting the nape of the neck and associated with

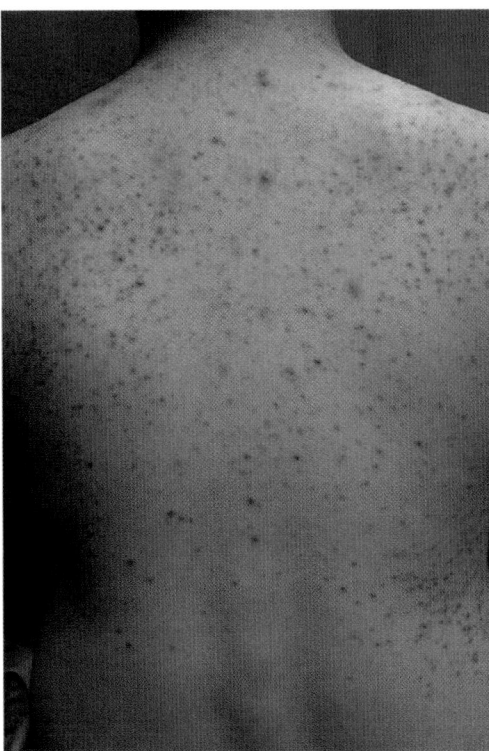

Figure 90.49 Pityrosporum folliculitis in an immunocompromised male. (Courtesy of Dr S. Chow, KL Skin Centre, Malaysia.)

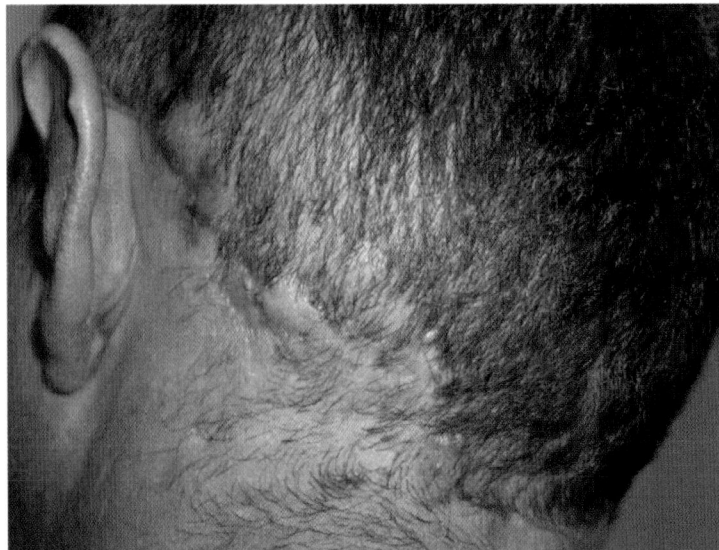

Figure 90.50 Folliculitis keloidalis affecting the nape of the neck and hairline resulting in cicatricial alopecia.

cicatricial alopecia (see Chapter 93). Folliculitis keloidalis is more common in black males. The lesions present as small itchy raised papules within or close to hair-bearing areas of the occiput, secondary infection with *Staphylococcus aureus* can ensue. The chronic process results in hairless scarring. Tufted hairs may be present representing multiple hair shafts emerging from single follicular openings. The cause is unknown but proposals include trauma following close shaving, ingrowing hairs which irritate the wall of the hair follicle and an association with obesity and metabolic syndrome has been noted. Treatment is challenging and includes avoiding friction from clothes and close haircuts, antimicrobial washes, topical steroids for small papules and intralesional steroids for large papules and nodules. Oral tetracyclines as anti-inflammatories or clindamycin and rifampicin have been used successfully. Laser and hair removal have also been shown to be of benefit. Optimum results occur if treatment is started early before significant scarring has occurred. Surgery, laser vaporization [401] or excision have been used to remove large nodules and plaques. Systemic isotretinoin has also been used with some success as has radiotherapy [402].

Folliculitis decalvans (synonym: tufted folliculitis)

Folliculitis decalvans is a chronic disorder of the hair-bearing areas on the scalp that leads to scarring, alopecia and atrophy [403–405] (see also Chapter 89). Areas of tufted folliculitis have been identified in cases of folliculitis decalvans and the histological features include hyperkeratosis, follicular plugging and perifollicular inflammation. The aetiology is unknown and treatment is difficult. It has been suggested that folliculitis decalvans may be the result of an abnormal host response to toxins from *S. aureus*. If *S. aureus* is identified systemic antibiotics are required; oral clindamycin or rifampicin may help by offering better tissue penetration; one case report suggests added benefit by also using topical mupirocin [406]. An isolated case report advocates the use of oral clindamycin in combination with oral isotretinoin and steroids [407].

Topical fusidic acid and oral zinc have also been used with some success in one series [408]. Radiation therapy and treatment with dapsone have also been reported in isolated cases [409,410].

Dissecting cellulitis of the scalp (synonym: perifolliculitis capitis abscedens et suffodiens)

This condition is predominantly seen in black males in their second to fourth decade. It is an uncommon chronic suppurative disorder of the scalp of unknown aetiology [411–415] (see also Chapter 107). Together with acne conglobata, HS and pilonidal cysts it is a component of the 'follicular occlusion tetrad'. Patients present with multiple tender inflammatory nodules and abscesses most commonly on the vertex and occiput of the scalp. Lesions frequently coalesce into sinus tracts. Scarring alopecia frequently results from the chronic suppurative changes. Follicular hyperkeratosis appears to be the primary feature in pathogenesis but secondary bacterial infection frequently occurs. Histology demonstrates a neutrophilic perifolliculitis with follicular destruction, granulomas and fibrosis. Lesions characteristically last for many years and are cosmetically disfiguring, painful and malodorous. It has been reported to occur with marginal keratitis [411] and squamous cell carcinoma may result in chronic cases [416]. Three cases of keratitis, ichthyosis and deafness (KID syndrome) have been reported in association with the follicular occlusion triad [417]. Response to therapy is poor. Options include high-dose systemic antibiotics used for acne (minocycline 100 mg twice daily or trimethoprim 300 mg twice daily). Success with oral zinc sulphate, 135 mg three times a day [412] and topical isotretinoin [413] have been reported. Oral isotretinoin is advocated as the most effective treatment [414]. Other treatment options include potent topical, intralesional and systemic steroids and widespread surgical excision with skin grafting [415]. One case of dissecting cellulitis associated with KID syndrome responded well to alitretinoin [417].

Hidradenitis suppurativa

HS is described in more detail in Chapter 92; it may be associated with severe nodular/conglobate acne. There is often a family history and the onset is usually in late adolescence; the disease prevalence gradually decreases with increasing age [418–421].

HS is a chronic disease that affects the axillae, breasts, genital and perianal areas (Figure 90.51a,b), and may sometimes spread extensively onto the buttocks and lower back. There is clinical evidence of open comedones (often polyporous), deep nodules, large abscesses, sinus tracts and scarring. The inflammatory lesions are frequently deep seated, exudative, painful and malodorous, resulting in significant compromise of daily activities and a high degree of morbidity [419]. It is primarily a disorder of follicular occlusion. Aetiological factors such as obesity, smoking and local irritation (e.g. from excessive sitting) may be relevant aggravating factors.

Miscellaneous causes of papular facial rashes

Papular facial rashes may be mistaken for acne. Rarely, dermatitis herpetiformis may present as a vesicular pustular facial eruption, but it is usually very itchy unlike acne. Linear immunoglobulin A (IgA) disease can also rarely present as a papular facial rash without comedones. Biopsy, including immunofluorescence studies, is essential to confirm the diagnosis. Facial lesions in micropapular sarcoid (see Chapter 98) are relatively monomorphic papules, often skin coloured or with a brownish appearance but if inflamed may be mistaken for inflammatory acne lesions [422]. A dental sinus can be confused with a persistent facial acne nodule (Figure 90.52). Epidermoid cysts may become inflamed and be

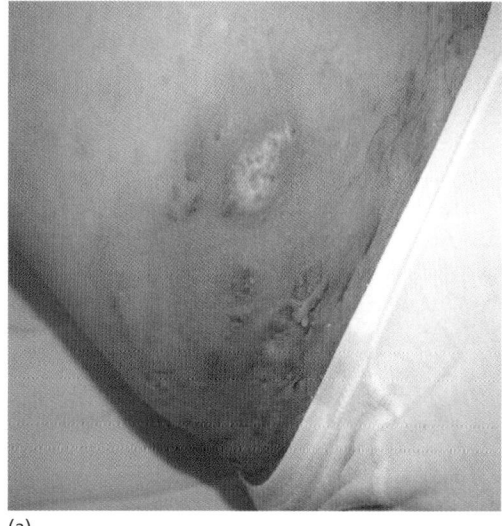
(a)

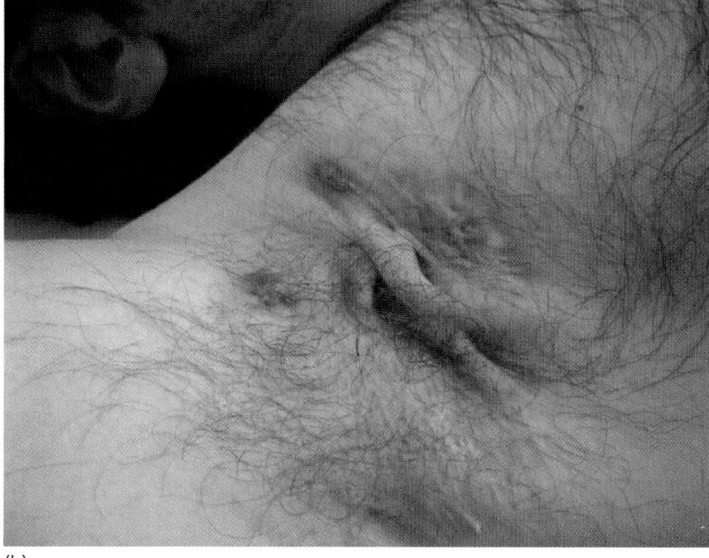
(b)

Figure 90.51 (a) Hidradenitis suppurativa of the groin showing inflammation, comedonal lesions and cribriform scarring. (b) Hidradenitis suppurativa of the right axilla. (Courtesy of Professor V. Bettolli, University of Ferrara, Ferrara, Italy.)

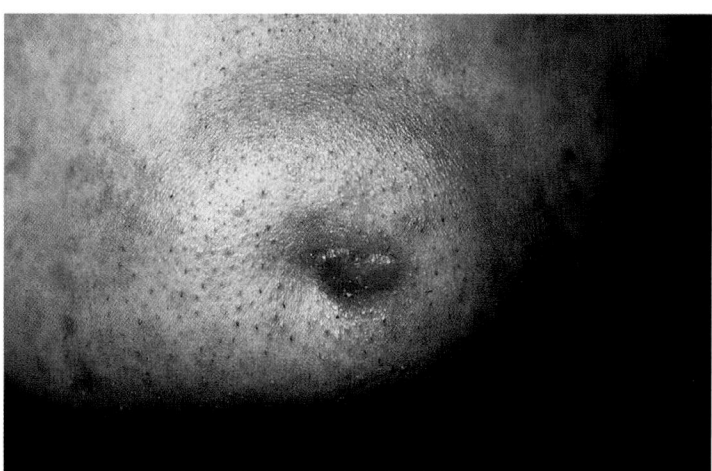

Figure 90.52 Dental sinus confused with persistent facial acne nodule.

PART 8: SPECIFIC CUTANEOUS STRUCTURE

mistaken for acne nodules. The severe papulopustular eruption associated with zinc deficiency can be mistaken for marked acne, and several cases have been reported after prolonged intravenous feeding without zinc supplementation [423].

Mimics of acne scarring

Scarring due to hydroa vacciniforme (Chapter 127), ulerythema ophryogenes (Chapter 89), folliculitis keloidalis (Chapter 93), varioliform atrophy and porphyria cutanea tarda (Chapter 60) can all masquerade as acne scarring. Acne necrotica varioliformis (necrotizing lymphocytic folliculitis; see Chapter 93) is associated with itching and smallpox-like scars, particularly around the scalp margin [424]. It can be mistaken for severe acné excoriée. Response to isotretinoin has been reported to be excellent [425].

Assessment

A medical assessment should include personal and family history, a record of present and previous therapies including response, careful physical examination and a psychosocial review.

Clinical severity

Accurately assessing outcome measures in acne is notoriously challenging. Many different approaches have been adopted but few are validated challenging the interpretation of results from clinical trials [**426**]. In clinical practice, severity of acne is assessed visually according to the extent of disease and number of lesions and frequently described as mild, moderate or severe. Outcome measures utilized to date can be divided into grading or counting. The evaluation can be further divided into: (i) overall or 'global' assessment; (ii) separate evaluations of individual lesions; and (iii) evaluation according to the predominant lesion type. Mechanisms to assess acne lesions using multimodal imaging are being evaluated [427] and patient-reported outcomes are now being considered as an important part of assessment [428].

The Leeds photometric grading scale (Figure 90.53) is the most commonly used global grading system. The acne is graded according to a scale of 0 to 10 on the face, back and chest [429]. However, this system does not adequately differentiate those with milder acne. The comprehensive acne severity system

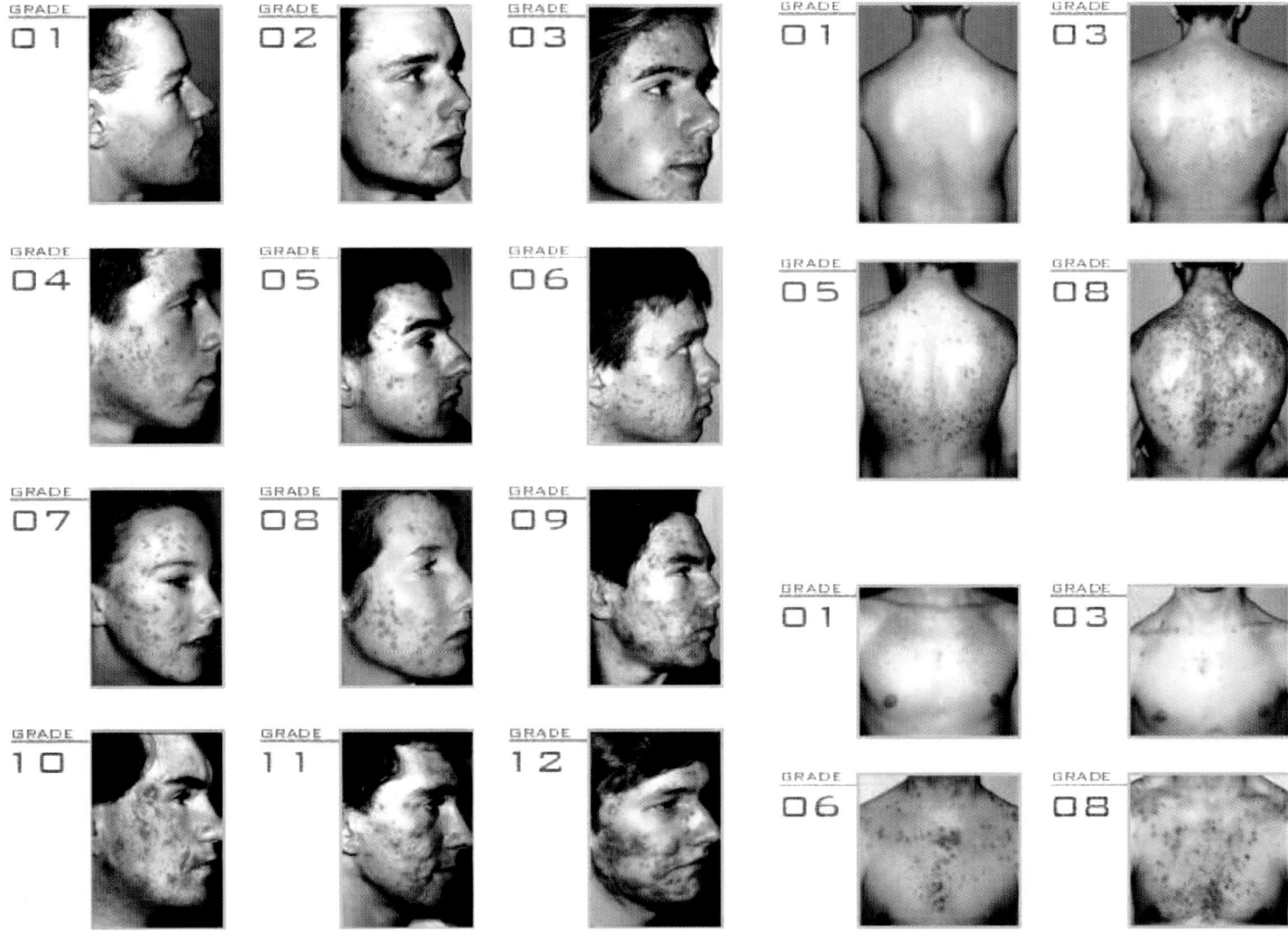

Figure 90.53 The Leeds photometric acne grading scale used to assess the face and trunk. (Reproduced from O'Brien *et al.* 1998 [429] with permission from the Leeds Foundation for Dermatological Research, Leeds, UK.)

(CASS) was developed by application of a pre-existing six-category facial investigator global assessment scale ranging from clear through to very severe grading (Table 90.13) to include the chest and back [430]. This has been validated and provides a global system that includes a restricted number of categories to allow for a practical and comprehensive approach when assessing treatment outcomes.

Lesion counts are essential for clinical trials as this offers a reliability not evident in global systems; however, counting remains impractical for use in the day-to-day clinic [431]. Other important outcome measures that should be considered when assessing the impact of therapy should include patient satisfaction, adherence to a therapeutic regime, speed of action of treatment, tolerability and adverse effects of therapy, evidence of scarring and impact on quality of life (QoL).

The use of QoL measures captures the impact of acne and treatment on the patient's life and helps to identify those vulnerable to psychological complications. Adopting a QoL measure as an integral part of acne management is recommended.

Several simple questionnaires including combinations of generic and dermatology-specific questionnaires are available (Box 90.4). Generic tools allow comparison between different diseases. Disease-specific questionnaires that relate specifically to acne include the Cardiff Acne Disability Index (CADI), the Assessment of the Psychosocial Effects of Acne (APSEA), the Acne Quality of Life Scale (Acne-QOL) and the Acne Quality of life four-item index (Acne-Q4) [430,432,433].

Acne also affects functional abilities. Patients are prone to embarrassment and social withdrawal, depression, anxiety and anger. The combined use of QoL and psychosocial questionnaires (see Complications) is essential to adequately understand just how severely the disease is affecting a patient, and can aid in assessing the efficacy of therapy. Acne scarring should also be included in the assessment of acne severity. Scars can produce significant disfigurement and psychosocial impairment in their own right. The difficulty in the evaluation of acne scars is manifold and there is currently no one simple clinically reproducible tool for evaluating the extent or volume deficiency of acne scars.

Box 90.4 Measurements available to assess the impact of acne on quality of life

Generic measures
- Euro-QoL (EQ-5D)
- SF-36

General Health Questionnaire (GHQ)
- UK Sickness Impact Profile (UK SIP)
- Preference-based measures of utility

Dermatology-specific measures
- Dermatology Life Quality Index (DLQI)
- Skindex
- Dermatology Quality of Life Scales (DQOLS)
- Dermatology-specific Quality of Life Instrument (DSQL)
- Children's Dermatology Life Quality Index (CDLQI)

Acne-specific quality of life instruments
- Acne/Cardiff Acne Disability Index (CADI)
- Acne-specific Quality of Life Questionnaire (Acne-QoL)
- Acne Quality of Life scale
- Acne Quality of Life Index (Acne-QOLI)
- Assessments of the Psychological and Social Effects of Acne (APSEA)

Investigations

Investigations may be required as part of monitoring or to exclude an underlying endrocrinopathy. Box 90.5 summarizes the signs and symptoms that may indicate an underlying endocrinopathy [434]. Table 90.14 outlines hormonal investigations required to identify an endocrine problem. Although not routinely done, quantifying sebum excretion may support the selection of therapy as those with higher sebum production respond less well to antibiotics. Assessment of sebum in the clinic can easily be performed using a microporous hydrophobic polymer film, i.e. Sebufix® or Sebutape®. The Sebutape measures the active follicle distribution

Box 90.5 Signs and symptoms that may indicate an underlying endocrinopathy suggesting the need for investigation

1 Signs of hyperandrogenism alongside acne
- Seborrhoea
- Hirsutism
- Androgenic alopecia
- Cushingoid features
- Increased libido
- Deepening of voice
- Clitoromegaly
- Acanthosis nigricans

2 Acne reported to be
- Therapy-resistant acne
- Rapidly relapsing
- Very severe
- Marked seborrhoea
- Sudden onset particularly in the context of other signs of hyperandrogenism

Table 90.13 The Comprehensive Acne Severity System (CASS).

Grade	Description	Face	Back	Chest
Clear	No lesions to barely noticeable ones. Very few scattered comedones and papules			
Almost clear	Hardly visible from 2.5 m away. A few scattered comedones, a few small papules and very few pustules			
Mild	Easily recognizable, less than half the affected area involved. Many comedones, papules and pustules			
Moderate	More than half the affected area involved. Numerous comedones, papules and pustules			
Severe	Entire area affected. Covered with comedones, papules and pustules and a few nodules and cysts			
Very severe	Highly inflammatory acne covering the affected area, with nodules and cysts present			

Table 90.14 Hormonal investigations required to identify endocrine problems (see text for abbreviations).

Suspected clinical diagnosis	Hormonal evaluation
PCOS	Luteinizing hormone
	FSH
PCOS	Total free testosterone
PCOS	Prolactin
CAH	DHEAS
CAH	17-hydroxyl progesterone
CAH	ACTH stimulation test
NCAH	TSH
Ovarian tumour	Free testosterone
Adrenal tomour	DHEAS

Table 90.15 The impact of acne on quality of life compared to other medical conditions using the Quality of Life SF-36.

	Social functioning	Role fulfilment for emotional reasons	Mental health	Energy and vitality
Acne	**11.1**	**7.4**	**13.4**	**7.0**
Asthma	5.9	6.3	4.2	6.0
Diabetes	8.7	9.5	5.9	9.1
Back pain	8.9	6.9	4.1	8.5
Epilepsy	7.4	5.3	3.4	5.9

but cannot measure the amount of sebum directly. After cleaning the skin with an alcohol wipe the tape is applied to the skin. The Sebufix shows the distribution of sebum with the aid of a UV light camera and calculates the sebum secretion area from the area evaluated [435]. Figure 90.54 shows in part (a) Sebutape on the forehead of a patient and comparison of two Sebutapes demonstrating the difference between patients with and without acne; in part (b) a patient with very low sebum production; and in part (c) a patient with high sebum production showing actively secreting sebaceous follicles and heterogeneity. Gravimetric assessments of sebum can also quantify the sebum output but these are labour intensive and not viable for use in the clinic.

Investigating for antibiotic-resistant strains of *P. acnes* may be of interest as there is a correlation between the presence of these strains and poor clinical response to antibiotics in some cases. Other investigations that should be considered in acne management relate to the treatment prescribed (see under specific treatments for acne).

Complications and co-morbidities

The main complications from acne relate to psychosocial and physical scarring. Post-inflammatory erythema or pigment changes may occur and solid facial oedema, and osteoma cutis have been reported. Pyogenic granulomas may occur in severe disease or result from treatment with isotretinoin. Seborrhoea may be a significant issue in some patients.

Psychosocial effects of acne

There have been many studies over the years investigating the specific psychological effects produced by acne using different measures.

Impact on QoL and perception

Studies have shown that many acne patients experience shame (70%), embarrassment and anxiety (63%), lack of confidence (67%), impaired social contact (57%) as well as problems with unemployment [436,437]. Severe acne may be related to increased anger and anxiety [438]. When compared to other serious organic diseases, acne patients describe levels of social, psychological and emotional problems as great as those reported with chronic disabling diseases such as asthma, epilepsy, back pain, arthritis and diabetes [439] (Table 90.15). Research has confirmed that physically attractive strangers attribute more positive qualities such as friendliness, intelligence and higher social skill levels to each other, compared with physically unattractive strangers [440]. Studies assessing independent reactions to photographs of patients with acne and acne scarring versus no acne and acne scarring have identified that those suffering disease are perceived more negatively.

Anxiety, depression and suicide

Clinical depression has been demonstrated in acne patients and this does not necessarily correlate with the clinical severity of disease. Suicide in acne patients has been reported in the literature [331] and the depressed acne patient should be assessed for suicide risk. Acne patients compared to other skin patients using a depression test inventory may have depression levels reaching

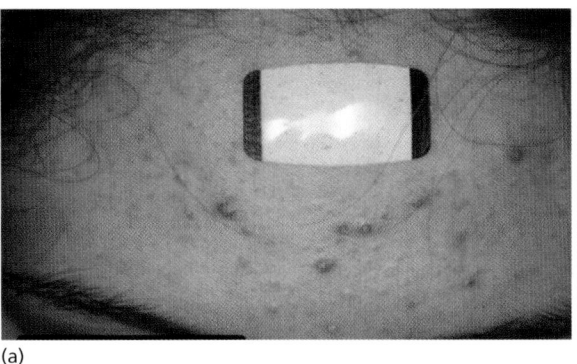
(a)

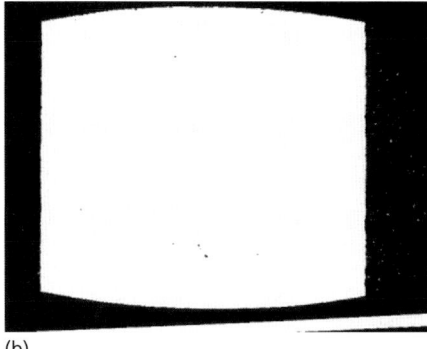
(b)

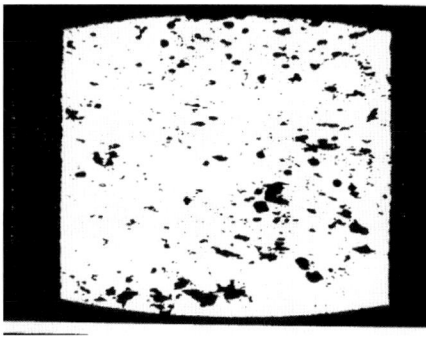
(c)

Figure 90.54 Sebutape analysis. Comparison of two Sebutapes demonstrating the difference between patients with and without acne. (a) Sebutape assessment of sebum. (b) Acne patient with very few secreting follicles. (c) Acne patient with high sebum production, actively secreting follicles and heterogeneity.

those identified from patients hospitalized with psoriasis [441]. Higher anxiety using the State-Trait Anxiety Inventory (STAI) has also been identified in acne patients versus controls [442].

Acne scarring

This is a common consequence of acne and may occur, albeit mild in most instances, in up to 90% of patients as a result of acne lesions [443]. The duration of inflammation relates to scar production hence a delay in appropriate management is more likely to result in significant scarring [430,444]. A cell-mediated immune response has been found to be involved in the inflammatory events in acne. Holland *et al.* [445] investigated the differences in cell-mediated immune responses in developing and resolving inflamed lesions between those acne patients who were prone to scarring and those with the same degree of inflammatory acne not prone to scarring. Clear differences in the cellular infiltrate were identified. In acne patients not prone to scar, the time course was typical of a type IV delayed hypersensitivity response, effective resolution occurred by both non-specific/innate and adaptive immune mechanisms. In lesions from acne patients who were prone to scar, a predominantly adaptive immune response was present, which was persistent and up-regulated in resolving lesions (Figure 90.55). This suggests that effective management of inflammation during the development and resolution stages of acne may help to control scarring. Scars may show increased collagen (hypertrophic scars and keloids) or be associated with loss of collagen (i.e. atrophic scars). Keloids by definition extend beyond the extent of original inflammation and are most prevalent on the trunk. Hypertrophic scars in contrast to keloids do not extend beyond the extent of the original inflammation. Limited morphological classification of scarring has been described and to date there is poor consensus and clinical assessment of scars demonstrates significant variation between assessors [446]. The lack of an accepted standardized objective quantification or qualitative scoring to estimate the global severity and burden of disease makes comparisons of treatments for scarring challenging. Atrophic scars are frequently multiple, they may be soft and distensible or fibrotic (Figure 90.56a,b). They often retain a vascular hue for many months before becoming less conspicuous. Perifollicular elastolysis is commonly found

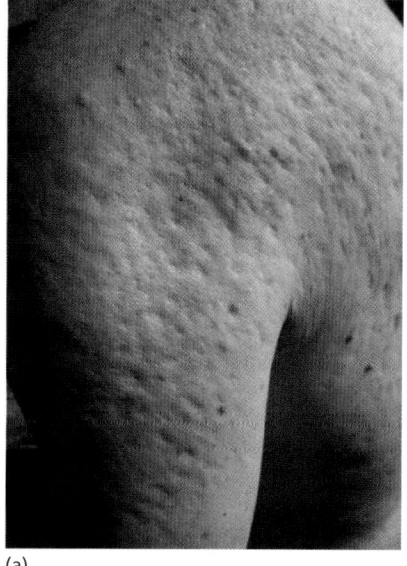
(a)

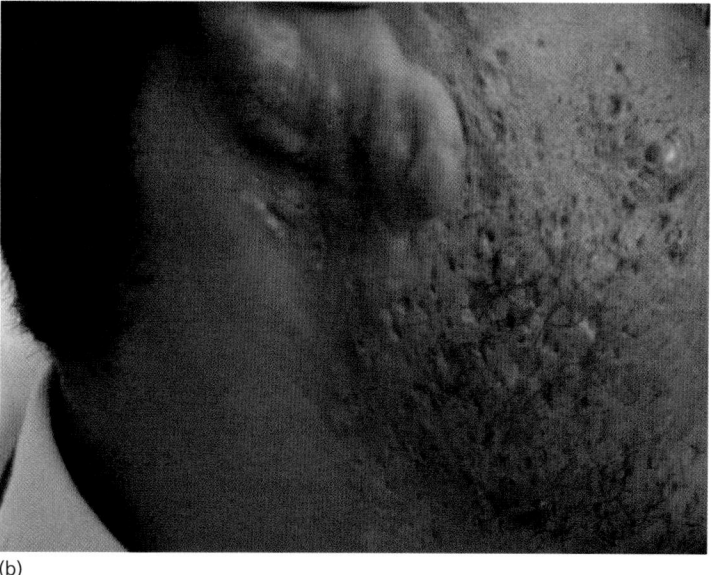
(b)

Figure 90.56 (a) Severe scarring of the arms and back showing soft distensible scars as a result of acne. (Courtesy of Dr S. Chow, KL Skin Centre, Malaysia.) (b) Fibrotic atrophic acne scars of the face.

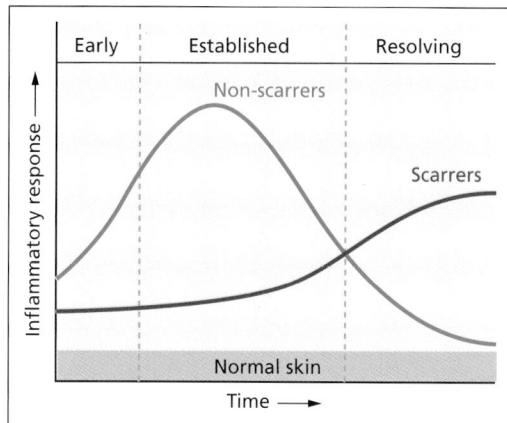

Figure 90.55 Immune responses vary between scarring and non-scarring acne patients.

on the trunk and consists of multiple follicular atrophic-looking lesions, sometimes seen without evidence of acne [447]. Calcification is a rare complication of scarring [448,449]. Persistent post-inflammatory hyperpigmentation, seen most frequently in pigmented skin (Figure 90.57) and post-inflammatory erythema are both common and cosmetically disfiguring. The pigmentary change can take many months to resolve or may persist.

Solid facial oedema (Morbihan disease)

This is a rare and disfiguring complication of acne [450] that has been reported in twins [451]. It is also reported as a consequence of rosacea [452] (see Chapter 91) and in Melkersson–Rosenthal syndrome. Thickened woody facial oedema leads to significant distortion of the midline face and cheeks due to soft-tissue swelling most likely due to pre-existing hypoplastic lymphatics. The

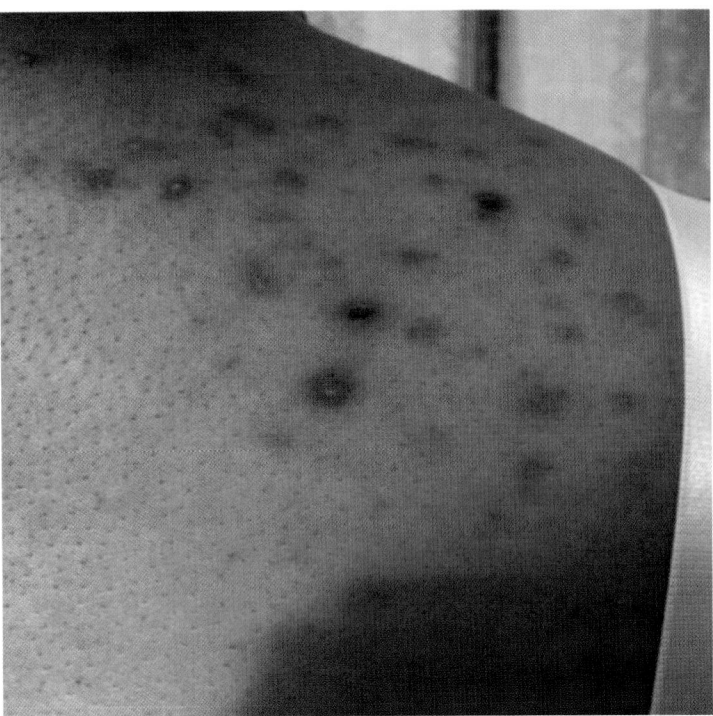

Figure 90.57 Post-inflammatory hyperpigmentation in Fitzpatrick type IV skin.

disorder is frequently progressive, and the associated acne must be treated aggressively to prevent permanent swelling. Successful treatment with oral isotretinoin alone or in combination with clofazamine or ketotifen has been reported [453–455]. Short or intermittent courses of oral steroids may also help the inflammatory component.

Osteoma cutis

This represents focal ossifications in the subcutaneous and dermal tissue. This uncommon complication of acne is described more commonly in women with longstanding inflammatory acne and usually needs no treatment [449,456,457]. The calcification presents as small 2–4 mm persistent papules which are firm to the touch [458]. Histology confirms calcified trabecular bone formation surrounded by a perivascular proliferation, often with increased fibrous tissue formation. Treatment modalities are limited. Topical tretinoin may promote transepidermal elimination of osteomas in small superficial lesions [459,460].

Surgical ablative therapy is most effective, techniques reported include combined dermabrasion and punch biopsy, scalpel incisions and curettage, extirpation of the small bone fragments after microdissection and laser therapies. The Erbium : YAG laser is said to be associated with minimal thermal injury with better cosmetic results than the carbon dioxide laser [461–465].

Pyogenic granulomas in acne

Pyogenic granulomas are occasionally seen on the trunk [466,467] in patients with very severe acne (Figure 90.58). They can also rarely (<1 : 10 000) be precipitated during treatment with oral isotretinoin and may be a feature of acne fulminans. Lesions may respond to clobetasol propionate cream applied topically twice daily and carefully to the lesions over a 2–3-week period.

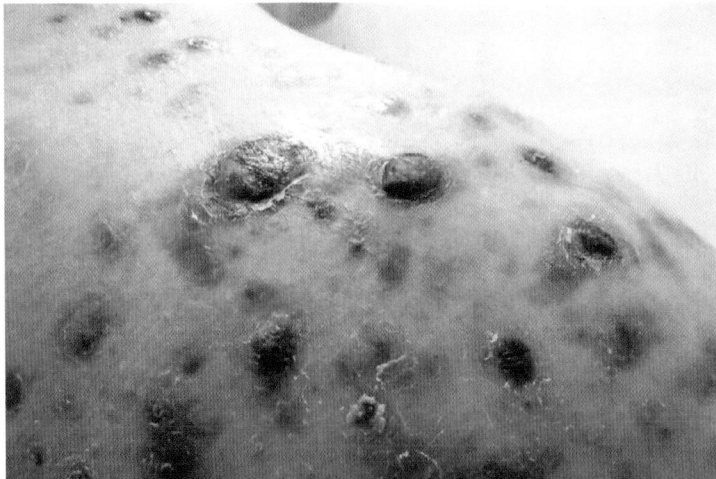

Figure 90.58 Pyogenic granulomas in severe acne.

Seborrhoea

Excessive sebum production may impact on QoL and can persist after the acne has regressed [468]. Underlying systemic causes such as acromegaly or parkinsonism should be considered. Justification for the use of systemic isotretinoin or anti-androgen therapy in females should be considered carefully as their use in this context is outside the recognized product license.

Disease course and prognosis

Although acne may be considered as a 'rite of passage' during the teenage years, a significant number of people suffer acne for many years. According to World Health Organization criteria, acne can be defined as a chronic disease [469]. Predisposing factors for developing acne are discussed elsewhere; certain factors link to severity of acne and risk of relapse (Table 90.16).

Table 90.16 Summary of factors associated with acne severity and relapse.

Specific factor	Impact
Positive family history	Linked to • Earlier occurrence of acne • Increased retentional lesions • Increased relapses
Early onset	Infantile acne shown to link to • Resurgence of acne in teenage years • More severe acne in teenage years • More frequent relapse in teenage years Mid-facial comedonal lesions prepuberty linked to more severe disease Earlier onset of acne relative to menarche related to more severe disease
Duration of acne	Prolonged duration of disease associated with reduced efficacy A family history of acne >25 years associated with more adult acne in relatives
Seborrhoea	High sebum production correlates with more severe acne High sebum production relates to reduced response to systemic antibiotics
Extent, location and nature of lesions	Truncal acne associated with reduced efficacy to systemic therapy when compared to acne on the face

Box 90.6 Aims of acne management

- Alleviate symptoms
- Clear existing lesions
- Limit disease activity by preventing new lesions forming as well as scars developing
- Avoid negative impact on quality of life

Management

General principles of acne management

Aims of acne management are summarized in Box 90.6. Patient information leaflets are valuable and a *British Medical Journal* patient decision aid for acne is available to support decision making (http://sdm.rightcare.nhs.uk/pda/acne/). Patients should be reassured that effective treatments are available but should be informed that response is slow and resolution is directly linked to good adherence [470–472]. Therapy is largely determined by the severity and extent of the disease but should be tempered by other factors such as duration, response to previous treatments, predisposition to scarring, post-inflammatory erythema and pigmentation, as well as patient preference, lifestyle and treatment cost [472]. Treatment algorithms exist, the Global Alliance algorithm is the most cited; this was developed with the implicit aim of improving outcomes in acne (Table 90.17). European Evidence-based S3 acne guidelines also provide recommendations [473]. Table 90.18 clarifies the definition used for determining acne severity in these guidelines.

First line therapy for mild, moderate and severe disease

Indications for topical therapy include mild acne, moderate to severe acne in conjunction with systemic treatment and as potential maintenance therapy. Systemic antibiotics alongside topical treatment is advocated for more moderate to severe disease but oral isotretinoin should be considered earlier in patients demonstrating poor prognostic factors as outlined in Table 90.16 [474]. Figures 90.59, 90.60 and 90.61 outline first, second and third line management based on evidence and expert opinion according to lesion type and severity.

Table 90.17 Global Alliance algorithm for improving outcomes in acne.

| | Mild | | Moderate | | Severe |
	Comedonal	Papular/pustular	Papular/pustular	Nodular[b]	Nodular/conglobate
First choice	Topical retinoid	Topical retinoid + topical antimicrobial	Oral antibiotic + topical retinoid ± BPO	Oral antibiotic + topical retinoid ± BPO	Oral isotretinoin[c]
Alternatives[a]	Alt. topical retinoid or azelaic acid[d] or salicylic acid	Alt. topical antimicrobial + alt. topical retinoid or azelaic acid[d]	Alt. oral antibiotic + alt. topical retinoid ± BPO	Oral isotretinoin or Alt. oral antibiotic + alt. topical retinoid ± BPO/azelaic[d] acid	High-dose oral antibiotic + topical retinoid + BPO
Alternatives for females	See first choice	See first choice	Oral antiandrogen + topical retinoid/azelaic acid[d] ± topical antimicrobial	Oral antiandrogen + topical retinoid ± oral antibiotic ± alt. antimicrobial	High-dose oral antiandrogen + topical retinoid ± alt. topical antimicrobial
Maintenance therapy	Topical retinoid	Topical retinoid ± BPO			

Adapted from Gollnick *et al*. 2003 [559].
[a]Consider physical removal of comedones.
[b]With small nodules (>0.5–1 cm).
[c]Second course in case of relapse.
[d]There was no consensus on this alternative recommendation; however, in some countries, azelaic acid prescribing is appropriate practice.
Alt., alternative; BPO, benzoyl peroxide.

Table 90.18 Defining the severity of acne according to lesion type and extent.

Type of acne	Descriptive of clinical lesions
Comedonal acne	Non-inflamed lesions embracing both open (blackheads) and closed (whiteheads) comedones
	Comedones arise from the microcomedo seen at a histological level early in the course of the disease development
Mild acne	Mixed but fairly localized inflamed and non-inflamed lesions. Superficial inflammatory lesions usually <5 mm diameter
Mild to moderate papulopustular acne	More extensive papulopustular lesions frequently in association with non-inflammatory lesion
Severe acne	Inflammatory lesions frequently deep seated and may evolve into nodules and deep pustules. Small nodules are defined as firm inflammatory lesions >5 mm; large nodules are >1 cm
	Large nodules extend over large areas and frequently result in painful lesions, exudative sinus tracts and disfiguring tissue destruction and scarring
	Acne conglabata includes multiple grouped comedones, interspersed with papules, tender inflammatory nodules of varying sizes some of which are suppurative and coalesce to form sinus tracts. Extensive scarring is a frequent outcome

PART 8: SPECIFIC CUTANEOUS STRUCTURE

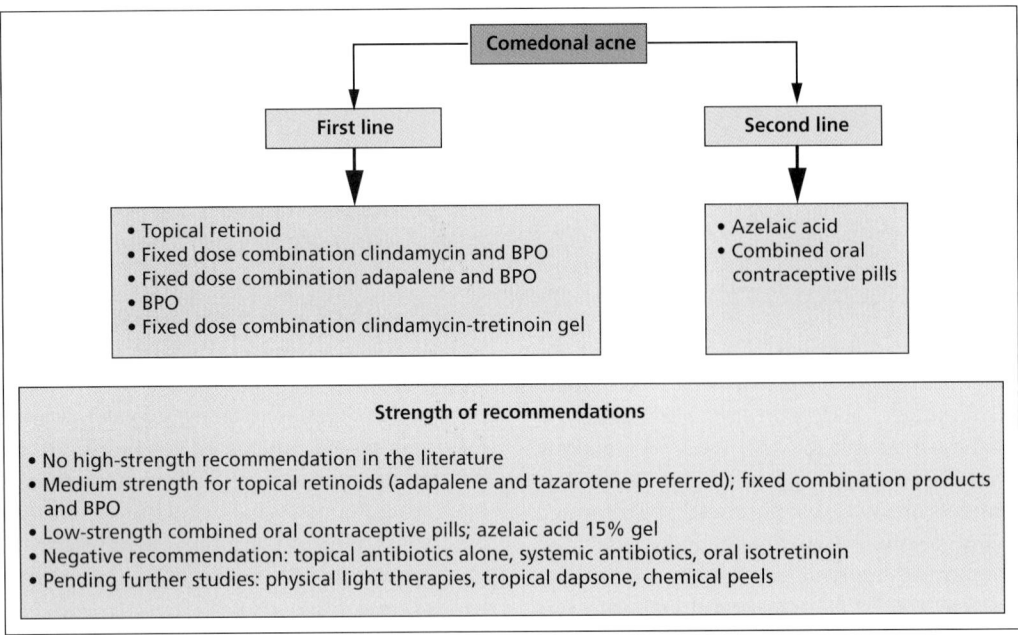

Figure 90.59 Treatment algorithm for comedonal acne. BPO, benzoyl peroxide.

Topical therapy should be applied to all areas of affected skin as histology of normal-looking skin from an acne-prone site demonstrates microcomedones as the precursors of all clinical lesions. Topical retinoids target microcomedones and are frequently considered in an acne regimen as a means of preventing progression of the microcomedo to active visible lesions. To enhance treatment success, a combination of agents should be employed to impact multiple aetiological factors. Combination products are more convenient for patients to use and aid adherence [472].

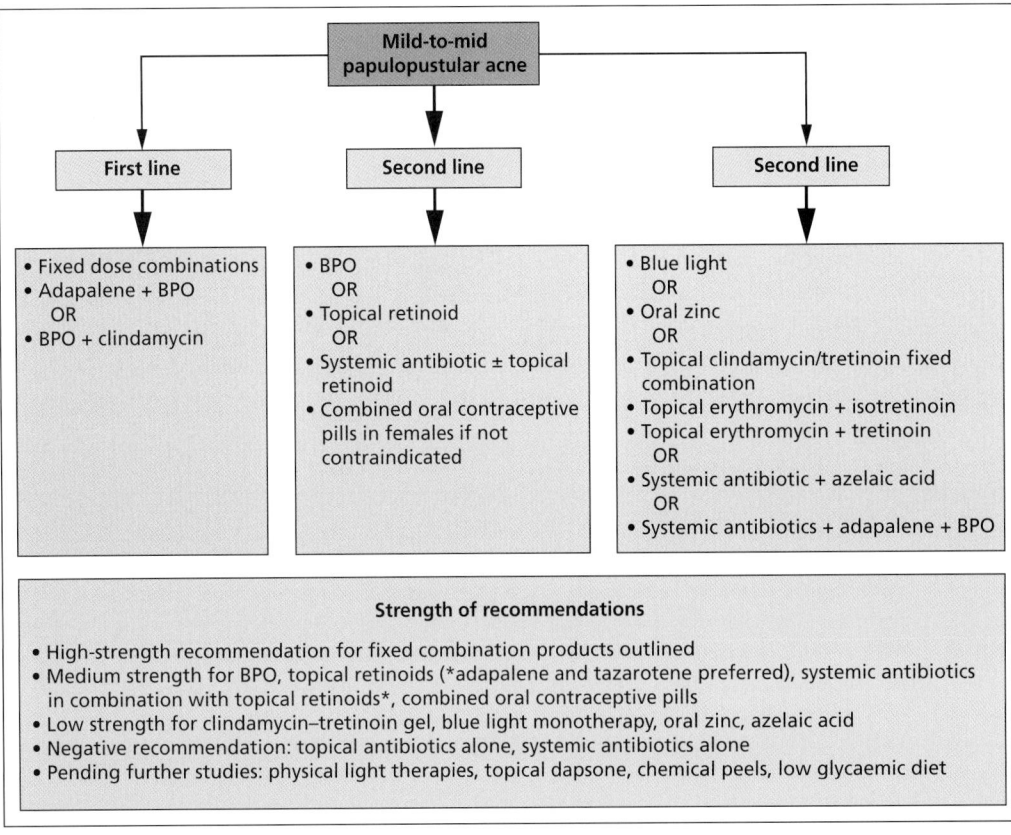

Figure 90.60 Treatment algorithm for mild to moderate inflammatory acne. BPO, benzoyl peroxide.

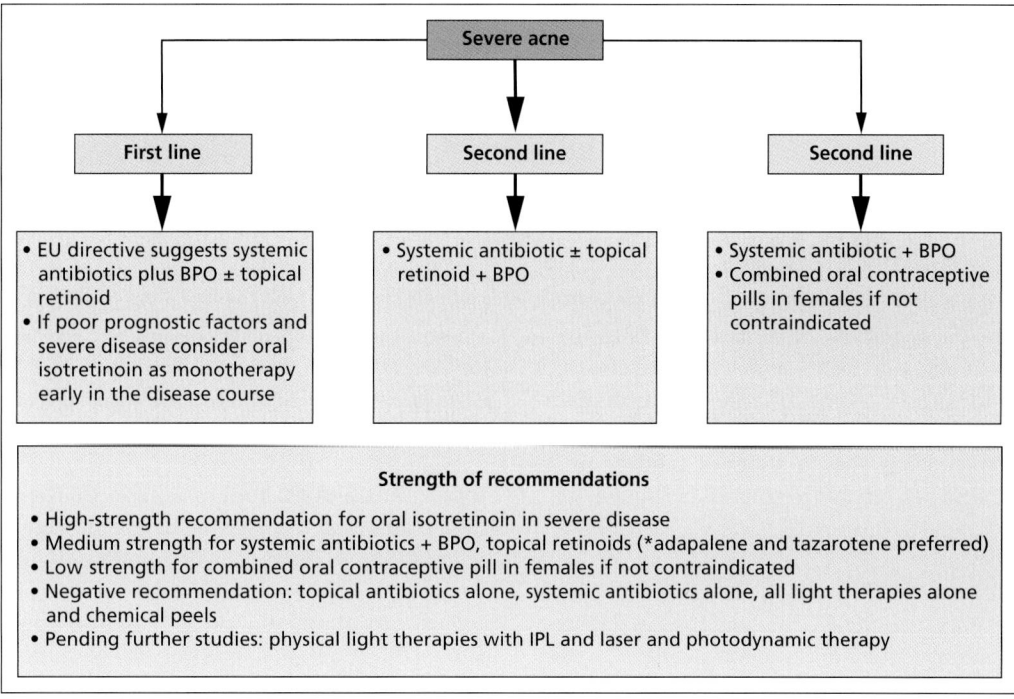

Figure 90.61 Treatment algorithm for severe acne. BPO, benzoyl peroxide.

Comedonal acne

There are a paucity of clinical trials addressing comedonal disease as it rarely exists as a single entity. Figure 90.59 summarizes the treatment for comedonal lesions.

Topical retinoids

All-*trans* retinoic acid (tretinoin; vitamin A acid) is available in 0.01 up to 0.05% concentrations as either a gel or a cream. Newer formulations, microsponge or polymer formulations are reportedly less irritant than original formulations. Isotretinoin 0.05% gel is a second-generation retinoid. The third-generation retinoid, adapalene 0.1% cream or gel, has significant and rapid anti-inflammatory action and has a greater benefit/risk ratio than tretinoin. In the US and a few other countries, the fourth-generation retinoid tazarotene is available for acne on prescription [475,476]. Retinoids reduce abnormal growth and development of keratinocytes within the pilosebaceous duct. The reversal of hypercornification within the follicular canal as well as the induction of the follicular epithelium helps to 'unplug' the follicle [477]. This also inhibits the development of the microcomedo and non-inflamed lesions resulting in less anaerobic conditions with fewer *P. acnes*, making the microenvironment less favourable for the development of inflammation. In addition, some of the novel retinoids reduce rupture of the comedones into surrounding skin which results in less inflammation [478–480].

In vitro, adapalene and tretinoin down-regulate TLR2 expression and function, which in turn influences the production of pro-inflammatory cytokines [481–485]. Topical retinoids have been shown to be superior to placebo for comedones and when used as monotherapy reduce the formation of microcomedones. Adapalene and tazarotene have the strongest evidence for efficacy and are more efficacious than tretinoin. Tretinoin has superior efficacy to azelaic acid and equivalent/superior efficacy to benzoyl peroxide (BPO). Topical retinoids are recommended for comedonal acne [473].

Benzoyl peroxide

BPO is currently available in a number of different formulations and concentrations (2.5%, 5% and 10%), some of which are available over the counter. BPO is a powerful antimicrobial [486,487] and rapidly destroys both surface and ductal *P. acnes* and yeasts [487]. The lipophilic nature of BPO allows it to penetrate the pilosebaceous duct. Once applied to the skin it decomposes in the sebaceous follicles to release free oxygen radicals with potent bactericidal and anti-inflammatory activity [484,487]. BPO has some comedolytic activity and has been shown in RCTs to reduce the number of non-inflamed lesions by decreasing follicular hyperkeratosis [488]. Like other topical agents it does not impact on sebum production. There is no evidence to support a dose–response effect of BPO but potential adverse effects, including irritancy and bleaching, are increased with the 10% concentration [489]. Allergic contact dermatitis has been reported with BPO but is rare with other topical agents. BPO bleaches clothes and hair and the patient must be informed of these inconvenient side effects.

Topical BPO has been noted to be superior to placebo and topical antibiotics (clindamycin and erythromycin) and equivalent to adapalene for the treatment of comedonal acne [**473**].

Topical antibiotics

Topical clindamycin has been shown to be superior to placebo when compared to vehicle for comedones but inferior to tretinoin. BPO has been shown to be superior to all topical antibiotics when used as monotherapy for treating comedonal lesions [473]. Topical antibiotics as monotherapy are not advocated for the treatment of comedones as there are superior therapies available and when used alone they have the potential to drive selection of antibiotic-resistant bacteria.

Fixed combination therapy

Fixed combination clindamycin–BPO is equivalent to BPO alone and superior to clindamycin alone for the treatment of comedonal acne. Fixed-dose adapalene–BPO is superior or equivalent to BPO and adapalene alone for the treatment of comedones. Both fixed combination products adapalene–BPO and clindamycin–BPO have similar efficacy and receive a medium strength recommendation for comedonal acne [473]. A fixed combination clindamycin–tretinoin recently introduced has shown superior efficacy to its component monotherapies with respect to comedonal acne.

Topical dapsone

There are insufficient data to recommend topical dapsone for comedonal acne. One study analysing two RCTs using topical dapsone in acne reported an 8% improvement in comedones after 12 weeks [490]; however, this is unlikely to be of clinical significance.

Azelaic acid

Azelaic acid reduces comedones by normalizing the disturbed terminal differentiation of keratinocytes in the follicle infundibulum [491]; 20% azelaic acid cream has shown superiority to placebo in the treatment of comedonal acne. In one study 20% azelaic acid cream had similar activity to 0.05% topical isotretinoin with approximately 80% reduction in comedonal lesion counts at 6 months [492].

However, based on available data this was given a low level recommendation for comedonal disease in the European S3 guidelines [473].

Mild to moderate papulopustular acne

Topical therapy

Contrary to popular belief, studies have demonstrated that topical acne treatments can be as efficacious as oral antibiotics [473]. No single topical agent is able to impact on the main aetiological factors implicated in acne pathogenesis and no topical agents have significant sebosuppressive effect. Recent evidence-based guidelines have advocated combination regimens in order to target as many aetiological factors as possible (see Figure 90.60).

Topical retinoids. All topical retinoids assessed in the European S3 Guidelines [473] were found to be superior to placebo or vehicle in the treatment of papulopustular acne. The efficacy of adapalene was found to be equivalent to BPO and tretinoin for the treatment of inflammatory lesions. Tazarotene has been noted to be superior to vehicle for inflammatory lesions and superior to or equivalent to adapalene and tretinoin for the treatment of inflammatory lesions. A medium strength recommendation for topical retinoids in the treatment of mild to moderate papulopustular acne is suggested. The novel topical retinoids are less irritant than some of the older established retinoids such as tretinoin and less likely to produce

an early treatment flare [493–495]; and the newer formulations of tretinoin (microsponge or polymer based) are said to be less irritating than the early formulations [496–498]. Retinoids are associated with teratogenicity but significant absorption of topical retinoids has not been demonstrated [499,500].

Benzoyl peroxide. BPO is more efficacious than vehicle in the treatment of papulopustular acne. It is equivalent to adapalene and conflicting evidence exists regarding its equivalence to tretinoin for the treatment of inflammatory lesions [473]. BPO receives a medium strength recommendation for mild to moderate papulopustular acne. Certain antibiotic/BPO combinations are less irritating than BPO alone [501], possibly explained by the anti-inflammatory action of the antibiotic.

Topical antibiotics. Topical antibiotics demonstrate superior efficacy compared to placebo in the management of inflammatory acne; however, their use as monotherapy in acne is not advocated due to the risk of emerging bacterial resistance, they receive a negative recommendation as monotherapy in the management of acne [473]. A detailed analysis of 144 clinical trials of topical antimicrobial therapy rejected over 50% because of poor trial design [502]. Adequate conclusions could not be drawn from the remaining data because of the different protocols, but BPO emerged as a successful treatment and appeared similar in effectiveness to topical erythromycin and clindamycin. Two systematic reviews examining acne management have identified comparative data on the use of oral versus topical antibiotics [484,503]. As oral antibiotics have a delayed onset of activity, shorter studies may bias the study in favour of the topical agent [504].

Fixed-dose combination topical therapy. Fixed-dose clindamycin–BPO is more efficacious than BPO alone for papulopustular acne. Both clindamycin–BPO and adapalene–BPO are superior to adapalene monotherapy and have been shown to be equivalent in efficacy for the treatment of papulopustular acne [473]. These agents have received a high strength of recommendation for mild to moderate papulopustular acne. Fixed-dose clindamycin–tretinoin gel is efficacious for inflammatory acne and superior to vehicle, topical 1.2% clindamycin and topical tretinoin 0.025% alone. There is also some evidence to suggest that clindamycin–tretinoin gel is superior to once-nightly 0.025% tretinoin gel [505]. As clindamycin resistance has not been assessed in studies conducted for longer than 12 weeks, fixed-dose clindamycin–tretinoin gel is currently given a moderate strength recommendation for mild to moderate papulopustular acne and not currently advocated for longer than 12 weeks.

Topical dapsone. Topical dapsone 5% gel has been shown in two placebo-controlled trials to improve acne severity more than vehicle [506–508]. This is not deemed clinically significant against criteria used in the European S3 guidelines and there are no comparative studies against other active agents to assess the potential benefit of this novel preparation.

Azelaic acid. Azelaic acid (1 : 2 heptanedicarboxylic acid) is available as a 20% cream for acne. It is not sebosuppressive but has been reported to reduce the numbers and function of *P. acnes* [509,510]. A number of RCTs have compared azelaic acid to placebo, vehicle, BPO, tretinoin and 2% erythromycin. In mild to moderate papulopustular acne, the studies would suggest that 20% azelaic acid has equivalent efficacy to 5% BPO, 0.05% tretinoin, adapalene and 2% topical erythromycin at 5–6 months but inferior efficacy to systemic tetracycline. The European S3 guideline gives azelaic acid a moderate strength recommendation for mild to moderate papulopustular acne [**473**].

General side effects of topical treatments

The most common side effect of topical acne products is a primary irritant dermatitis which often subsides with time and can be managed by reducing the frequency of application, using emollients and if severe short-term application of a type I potency topical corticosteroid [511,512].

Systemic therapy for papulopustular acne.

Systemic therapy is generally advocated when there is a significant inflammatory component and/or the acne is extensive rendering topical applications impractical.

Systemic therapy for the treatment of mild papulopustular acne includes antibiotics, hormonal options, zinc, oral isotretinoin and/or steroids for unresponsive disease [513]. Other drugs such as dapsone [514], clofazimine and vitamin A acid (10–20 mg/day) [515] are occasionally used but evidence to support their effectiveness is limited.

Systemic antibiotics in papulopustular acne.

Oral antibiotics are the most widely prescribed agents in acne and are indicated for severe acne, moderate facial acne not responding to topical therapies and/or extensive truncal acne. Response to systemic antibiotics varies. Young males with marked seborrhoea and truncal acne respond less well than females with purely facial acne [516].

Cyclines (tetracycline, oxytetracycline, doxycycline, lymecycline, minocycline) are the antibiotics of choice; however, there is insufficient evidence to support one agent or dose. The second-generation cyclines may aid adherence and of these lymecycline and doxycycline should be used in preference to minocycline [**474**]. Due to reports of potential serious adverse effects, minocycline is not recommended as first line therapy [503,517,518]. Adverse effects with minocycline include drug hypersensitivity syndrome (DHS) occurring within 3 months of treatment initiation characterized by fever, malaise, arthralgia and a diffuse exanthematous skin eruption. Systemic involvement may include pulmonary eosinophilia and hepatitis. Early recognition and withdrawal of the agent is essential, repeat exposure may result in recurrence of DHS within a few days [519]. A lupus-like reaction has also been reported occurring after 6–48 months of treatment. Patients are usually female and present with fever, malaise and polyarthralgia. A cutaneous rash is not always evident but urticaria, vasculitis and non-specific erythema have all been reported. Some patients have concomitant liver disease, which may occur in the absence of joint symptoms. Serology for lupus is evident with a positive antinuclear antibody (ANA), along with positive perinuclear antineutrophilic cytoplasmic antibodies (pANCA) and raised C-reactive protein. Severely deranged hepatic enzymes

and rarely liver damage requiring liver transplantation have also been reported [520,521]. Positive antihistone antibodies are rarely identified. The lupus-like reaction is reversible if the drug is withdrawn but abnormal serology may persist. Minocycline should be avoided in patients with a personal or family history of systemic lupus erythematosus. Before embarking on long-term minocycline it is advisable to check hepatic function and ANA at baseline and to repeat hepatic function, ANA and pANCA every 3–6 months.

A large RCT conducted in UK community practice demonstrated that oral minocycline and oral tetracycline were of similar efficacy to each other and comparable in terms of efficacy to topical BPO [521].

This same study, which compared five antimicrobial regimes for mild to moderate facial acne in the community, suggested that maximum improvement was reached at 6 weeks with both oral antibiotics and topical BPO [521].

Macrolides (erythromycin, clindamycin or azithromycin) prescribing for acne has increasingly fallen out of favour due to the emergence of antibiotic-resistant strains of *P. acnes* and though limited there is evidence showing tetracycline to be equivalent or superior in efficacy to erythromycin [374,522]. If antibiotic therapy is required in pregnancy, oral erythromycin is thought to be safe although there are no data available evaluating chronic use over prolonged periods in pregnancy [523]. The safest therapies in pregnancy are therefore topical BPO and/or topical erythromycin [524]. Erythromycin remains the preferred option in children (8–12 years depending on national licenses) as tetracylines are contraindicated due to potential musculoskeletal problems and discoloration of permanent teeth.

Clindamycin is highly lipophilic and very effective in acne but adverse effects, including diarrhoea seen in 5–20% of cases, and potential pseudomembranous colitis from overgrowth of *Clostridium difficile* has discouraged use [525,526].

Oral azithromycin using intermittent dosing schedules (250 mg three times a week) due to the long half-life of 68 h has been reported to be effective for acne in four open and two investigator-blinded trials [523,527].

Trimethoprim may also be helpful in acne management at a dose of 400–600 mg/day [528–530]; but has lower evidence of efficacy compared to tetracycline [531]. Adverse effects with trimethoprim include haematological reactions such as agranulocytosis, thrombocytopenia and pancytopenia. Risk of these developing is linked to higher dose regimens and those with folic acid deficiency and/or megaloblastic haematopoiesis [528,532]. It is advisable to take a baseline full blood count prior to starting any extended courses of trimethoprim and to repeat this if patients remain on treatment for more than a month. DHS has also rarely been reported with trimethoprim [519].

Despite reports of efficacy in acne, the use of azithromycin, trimethoprim and other antibiotics including cephalosporins and fluoroquinolones should be discouraged as they are commonly used to treat a variety of systemic infections [523]. Exceptions to this rule may include short-term use for extremely refractory disease and/or evidence of Gram-negative folliculitis where other agents are not acceptable and in cases where tetracyclines are contraindicated.

Table 90.19 outlines dosage regimens for systemic antibiotics recommended for the treatment of acne and considers potential adverse effects.

Table 90.19 Systemic antibiotics in the treatment of acne vulgaris: dosage and adverse effects.

Antibiotic tetracyclines	Dosage	Adverse effects
Oxytetracycline	500 mg twice daily, 30 min before food and not with milk; makes adherence to medication problematic for some	Common: gastrointestinal upset Rare: onycholysis, photosensitivity, benign intracranial hypertension
Lymecycline (not available in the US)	300–600 mg daily	As oxytetracycline but tolerated better
Doxycycline	100–200 mg daily	As oxytetracycline Photosensitivity (dose dependent)
Minocycline	100–200 mg daily	Rare but serious: headaches and dizziness associated with benign intracranial hypertension, pigmentary changes, autoimmune hepatitis/ lupus erythematosus-like syndrome
Erythromycin	500 mg twice daily	Common: gastrointestinal upset, nausea, diarrhoea
Trimethoprim	200–300 mg twice daily	Maculopapular rash Rare: hepatic/renal toxicity/ agranulocytosis

Table 90.20 Antibiotic prescribing policies.

Strategy to avoid propionibacterial resistance emerging	Comments
Avoid inappropriate use of topical and systemic antibiotics	Use oral antibiotics for 3 months in the first instance and only continue if clinical improvement continues
If extending the duration of oral antibiotics, utilize combination therapy	Combine with an agent that reduces the likelihood of promoting antibiotic propionibacterial resistance. e.g. benzoyl peroxide
If repeated courses of antibiotics are required and the initial clinical response was favourable, reuse the same drug	This will avoid multiple resistant strains emerging
Avoid prescribing different oral and topical antibiotics concomitantly	This will avoid multiple resistant strains emerging
Consider using topical retinoids and non-antibiotic antimicrobials wherever possible	These do not promote resistant isolates and when used with antibiotics may achieve more rapid efficacy and so reduce the duration of the antibiotic course
Topical benzoyl peroxide (BPO) can be used for 7 days between antibiotic courses	BPO is fully active against sensitive and resistant strains of *P. acnes* and able to eradicate resistant isolates
Remember to check medical adherence	Poor adherence to antibiotic therapies promotes resistance

Interactions of antibiotics with oral contraceptives

There is concern that combined oral contraceptive (COC) efficacy may be impaired when used alongside antibiotics based on the hypothesis that broad spectrum antibiotics reduce bacterial flora in the gut and thus may interfere with oestrogen absorption. However, pharmacokinetic studies have demonstrated that serum levels of oestrogen are unaffected by tetracycline and doxycycline. The failure rate of COCs when used with tetracycline resulting in pregnancy is reported as 1.2–1.4 pregnancies per 100 woman-years of oral contraceptive use which is no greater than background failure rate of COCs. The only antibiotic which has been shown to reduce COC efficacy is rifampicin [533–536].

General side effects of oral antibiotics

All oral antibiotics for acne can produce mild adverse effects (see Table 90.19). Several studies have confirmed that the use of antibiotics for acne drives bacterial resistance [521,537]. The presence of antibiotic-resistant *P. acnes* may correlate with poor clinical response to antibiotics [538]. The concentration of ductal antibiotics varies considerably and may fall below the mininimal inhibitory concentration for *P. acnes*. A low tissue drug concentration will encourage the acquisition of antibiotic-resistant *P. acnes*. [539]. Poor adherence to therapy will potentially reduce drug availability, and a high sebum excretion is likely to dilute an effective drug concentration [540].

A number of publications have proposed how antibiotics should be administered to achieve optimal therapeutic response whilst avoiding antibiotic resistance and produced antibiotic prescribing policies (Table 90.20) [474]. Suggestions include restricting the duration of antibiotics, use of combination regimens from the onset of therapy to expedite response and reduce duration of antibiotic courses, utilization of BPO either to reduce the emergence of or to treat antibiotic-resistant strains of *P. acnes* and avoidance of using chemically dissimilar antibiotics and regular switching of antibiotics. Table 90.21 summarizes possible factors that might indicate the presence of antibiotic-resistant *P. acnes*. Resistance is not the only reason for poor response to treatment (Table 90.22).

Hormonal therapy in papulopustular acne

Systemic hormone preparations are available for acne in female patients. Indications for use include the following:

1 Failed standard antibiotic/combination regimens.
2 Menstrual control and/or contraception required alongside acne therapy.
3 When oral isotretinoin is inappropriate or not available.

Table 90.21 Reasons to suspect poor response relates to resistance to antibiotic therapies.

Reasons to suspect possible antibiotic-resistant *P. acnes*	Comments
Failure to respond to antibiotic therapy	Confirm good adherence to therapy
Deterioration in acne despite continuing antibiotic therapy	Patients often confirm initial good results
History of poor adherence	This is thought to lend itself to resistance emerging
Multiple courses of oral and topical antibiotics	Particularly when used as monotherapy

Table 90.22 Reasons to suspect poor response to treatment.

Reason for poor response to therapy	Comments
Need for improved education of doctor or patient	Understanding of how to use therapies is mandatory for successful treatment
Poor adherence to therapy	Steadily diminishing adherence may lead to relapse
Presence of relevant antibiotic resistant *P. acnes* in patient complying to therapy	Colonization with resistant isolates from the start results in poor response, subsequent colonization leads to relapse
Development of Gram-negative folliculitis	See section on Differential diagnosis
Incorrect diagnosis	See section on Differential diagnosis
Presence of macrocomedones prior to starting isotretinoin	This can result in significant flare of acne
Refractory subtypes of acne	See section on Unusual cases
Intolerance to or side effects of treatment	See section on Adverse effects
Inadequate dose of antibiotics	Patients of high body weight or marked seborrhoea may require a higher dose

Topical therapy can be prescribed in conjunction with hormonal regimens. Potential hormonal treatments for acne include inhibitors of androgen production by the ovary (oral contraceptives) or adrenal gland (low-dose corticosteroids), androgen receptor blockers, and antiandrogens that block the effect of androgens on the sebaceous gland. Figure 90.62 outlines the mechanisms of action.

Oestrogens and progestins

COCs generally contain oestrogen (most commonly ethinyl oestradiol) and a progestin. Oestrogens increase the synthesis of sex hormone binding globulin (SHBG) leading to increased binding of testosterone and reduced levels of free circulating testosterone. Hence all oral contraceptives potentially improve acne. In addition, oral contraceptives suppress ovulation by inhibiting the production of ovarian androgens which results in reduced serum androgens and lower sebum production. Progestins in COCs include estranes and gonanes, which are derivatives of

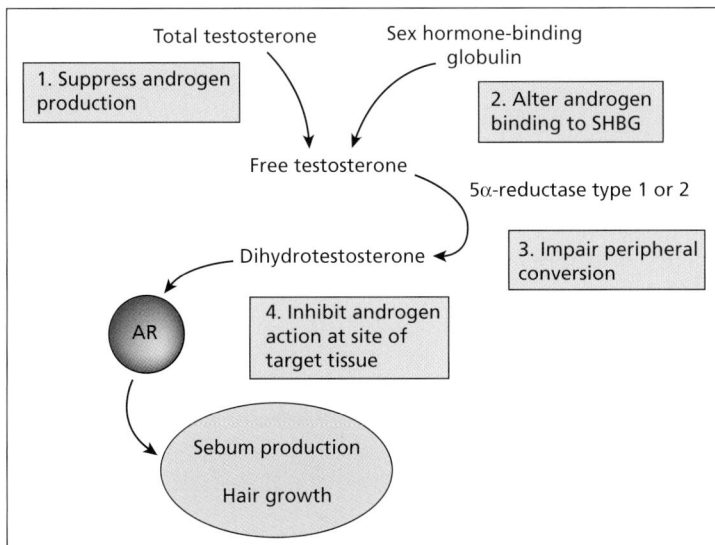

Figure 90.62 Potential mechanism of action(s) using antiandrogens in the management of acne. AR, androgen receptor; SHBG, sex hormone binding globulin.

19-nortestosterone, cyproterone acetate (CPA) and drosperinone. The third-generation progestins (gestodene, desogestrel, norgestimate) are less selective for the androgen and more selective for the progesterone receptor. Drosperinone is a novel progestin derived from 17α-spironolactone and has antiandrogenic activity, making it potentially helpful in acne. Yasmin® contains drospirenone 3 mg combined with ethinyl oestradiol 30 μg and Yaz® contains the same dose of drospirenone with 20 μg of ethinyl oestradiol. Box 90.3 outlines the androgenic effect of progestins in COCs.

A Cochrane systematic review determining the effectiveness of COCs for the treatment of facial acne compared to placebo or other active therapies confirmed that COCs reduced acne lesion counts, severity grades and self-assessed acne compared to placebo. Limited data suggested that chlormadinone or CPA achieved better efficacy than levonogestrel, and a COC containing CPA may produce better outcomes than one containing desogestrel. Limited data were available comparing COCs with other therapies [541].

Androgen receptor blockers

Androgen receptor blockers suppress sebum so offer potential for the treatment of acne. The antiandrogen CPA is licensed for acne in most European countries, but not in the US. It directly inhibits the androgen receptor. Co-cyprindiol (Dianette and Estelle-35) is an oral contraceptive that ameliorates acne. It is as effective as oral tetracycline 1 g/day given over a 6-month period, although slower in action [542]. CPA 2 mg with ethinyl oestradiol (35 μg) has a greater risk of deep venous thrombosis embolism (VTE) than first and second COCs [543]; as a result the current recommendation is that once the acne is under control co-cyprindiol formulations should be replaced by a COC containing a lower dose of oestrogen. In summary, COCs receive a medium strength recommendation for the treatment of mild to moderate papulopustuar acne in women being mindful of the fact there are associated risks which need to be explained to patients and that these agents are not necessarily licensed for acne.

Spironolactone in acne management

Spironolactone is reported in the literature as an effective treatment for acne. It is usually prescribed at a dose of 50–100 mg daily with meals, but many women with sporadic outbreaks do well with doses as low as 25 mg daily [544]. Although spironolactone is used in this context with clinical success there are a paucity of studies to confirm evidence of its effectiveness due to very small sample populations studied and poor trial design [545]. The main side effects are menstrual irregularity, breast tenderness, occasional fluid retention and, rarely, melasma. Pregnancy should be avoided due to potential abnormalities to the male fetus and serum electrolytes should be monitored due to potential risk of hyperkalaemia. All hormonal regimens should be combined with appropriate topical therapies.

Comparative effectiveness of hormonal treatment with other approaches

There are few good studies comparing hormonal approaches to antibiotics and isotretinoin. Isotretinoin has been shown to be more effective than co-cyprindiol for acne patients [546]. One systematic review assessed mean weighted effects across different reported variables. Isotretinoin scored 85±10% improvement compared with baseline, whereas tetracyclines and hormonal treatments were less effective, scoring 54±3%, and CPA plus ethinyl oestradiol 65±4% improvement compared with baseline levels [547].

Oral isotretinoin in papulopustular acne

Systemic isotretinoin is considered the most potent therapy for acne, but the effect has been shown to be comparable to minocycline plus azelaic in one study [548], comparable to high-dose doxycycline (200 mg daily |) plus BPO–adapalene in another and superior to tetracycline plus adapalene in a third study [549]. Conventional doses of isotretinoin aiming for 1 mg/kg/day are extremely efficacious in most cases of acne. However, due to the adverse side effect profile, national and international guidelines recommend isotretinoin should be reserved for those with severe disease and/or those who have failed to respond to other treatments. Two studies examining isotretinoin dose regimens found that lower doses of 0.25 mg/kg/day or 20 mg on alternate days were as efficacious as higher doses in the management of papulopustular disease [550,551]. See the section on the use of oral isotretinoin in severe disease.

Oral zinc in papulopustular acne

Two double-blind studies showed a significant benefit on inflammatory lesions, particularly with zinc gluconate (200 mg/day). Comparison with minocycline 100 mg/day demonstrated the antibiotic improved acne by 63% in contrast to 32% with 30 mg/day of elemental zinc after 3 months, no placebo was included in the study. The S3 European guidelines give zinc a low level strength of recommendation for mild to moderate papulopustualr acne [473].

Severe acne

Clinical evidence for the treatment of severe acne is limited. Figure 90.61 outlines a suggested algorithm for the treatment of severe acne. Oral isotretinoin is regarded as the treatment of choice for severe acne. However, if contraindicated or not acceptable, topical adapalene or fixed-dose BPO–adapalene may be used in combination with systemic antibiotics with the best evidence in support of doxycycline.

Systemic antibiotics

A combination of systemic antibiotic combined with BPO with or without adapalene has been given a medium strength recommendation for severe acne [473]. Given the concerns about antibiotic resistance, monotherapy with systemic antibiotics is not recommended.

Hormonal therapy

Evidence for the use of hormonal therapy in severe acne is lacking. In the UK, ethinyloestradiol/CPA is officially indicated for the treatment of severe acne unresponsive to systemic antibiotics and other available treatments.

Oral isotretinoin

Oral isotretinoin (13-*cis*-retinoic acid) is a synthetic vitamin A analogue which was first approved by the US Food and Drug Administration (FDA) in 1982 for the treatment of severe recalcitrant acne. Isotretinoin remains the most clinically effective acne therapy, producing long-term remission or significant improvement in many patients. It is licensed for the treatment of severe acne that has failed to respond to conventional antibiotic therapies. The European S3 guidelines recommend isotretinoin for the treatment of severe recalcitrant acne or moderate acne that has failed to respond to conventional antibiotic therapies [473]. Most patients who receive oral isotretinoin will be free of acne after 4–6 months of treatment depending on the dose used. Clinical experience suggests that the long-term cure rate may be lower than initially thought. Isotretinoin is now being used to treat patients with less severe acne than previously; the initial cohorts treated had severe disease and may have been less concerned by the resurgence of a few pustules and papules. Furthermore, some early reported 'cures' may have occurred in line with the acne spontaneously resolving as initial treatments were often commenced later in the course of the disease. There is evidence to suggest that younger patients relapse more frequently than older ones. Over the years, isotretinoin has been used to treat many different and difficult cases of acne with varying degrees of success, as outlined in Table 90.23.

The European Directive (ED) on prescribing of isotretinoin was introduced to ensure that generic prescribing was harmonized throughout the European Union and to minimize the risk of adverse effects including pregnancy [552]. Table 90.24 summarizes the recommendations which include monitoring of laboratory parameters to include primarily fasting lipids, and liver function tests at baseline, 1 month after starting therapy and if stable 12 weekly thereafter [553] (http://www.ema.europa.eu/docs/en_GB/document_library/Referrals_document/Isotretinoin_29/WC500010881.pdf). There has been much debate as to whether

Table 90.23 Relative success of isotretinoin in various acne and other clinical conditions.

Diagnosis	Excellent response	Moderate response	Limited response
Severe acne	×	–	–
Moderate acne[a]	×	–	–
Mild acne[a]	×	–	–
Acne fulminans[a,b]	×	–	–
Rosacea	×	–	–
Rosacea fulminans[a,b]	×	–	–
Acne conglobate	–	–	×
Gram-negative folliculitis	–	×	–
Solid facial oedema	–	–	×
Hidradenitis suppurativa	–	–	×
Vasculitic acne	–	–	×
Dissecting scalp cellulitis	–	–	×
Steatocystoma multiplex	–	–	×
Seborrhoea	–	×	–
Fordyce disease	–	×	–
Chemoprophylaxis of skin cancer	–	×	–
• Basal cell naevus syndrome			
• Xeroderma pigmentosum			
• Eruptive keratoacanthomas			

[a]Especially if associated with scarring and/or psychological problems.
[b]Also needs pre-isotretinoin therapy with oral steroids.

Table 90.24 Recommendations from the European Directive on isotretinoin prescribing.

	Pre directive	Post directive
Dosage	0.5–1.0 mg/kg/day	Start 0.5 mg/kg/day
Indications for use	Isotretinoin recommended as first line therapy for severe acne (nodular and conglobata) as well as acne not responding to 3 months' systemic antibiotics in combination with topical therapy	The new recommendations suggest isotretinoin should only be used in severe acne (nodular, conglobata) that has or is not responding to appropriate antibiotics and topical therapy; the inference of this being that it should now not be used at all as first line therapy
Age	Previously no age limit	Not indicated in children <12 years
Monitoring	Liver enzymes and lipids should be checked before treatment and 1 month after the maximum dosage has been used	Baseline investigations as before but at 1 month and 3 monthly throughout the course of treatment

liver function tests and blood lipids should be monitored during therapy. Elevated levels unrelated to any clinical significance are common and rapidly return to pretreatment levels after therapy has been discontinued [554,555]. Some authors only advocate repeat testing post-baseline in at-risk groups such as those with diabes and patients with known familial hypertriglyceridaemia [554]. However, as there is no good evidence when to taper dosage regimes or to discontinue therapy in the context of abnormal results and the absence of a laboratory abnormality does not preclude an adverse clinical outome [556], it would seem prudent to follow the ED and to interpret results aligned to the individual on treatment.

Reductions in haematological parameters including thrombocytopenia and neutropenia have been reported whist taking oral isotretinoin for acne but a large population-based study showed very few haematological abnormalities during treatment [556]. There are no explicit recommendations for the assessment of haematological parameters but the American Academy of Dermatology advises full blood counts alongside triglycerides, cholesterol and transaminases.

Regulatory authorities in each country have approved a Pregnancy Prevention Programme (PPP). This programme includes advice on education, therapy management and control of the distribution of oral isotretinoin.

Education – both patients and prescribers must be fully aware of teratogenicity. The patient should acknowledge the problem by signing a consent form and should accept detailed counselling by the clinician prior to and during treatment.

Therapy management includes medically supervised pregnancy testing before, during and 5 weeks after a course of therapy and provides advice on contraception.

Distribution control of isotretinoin suggests that only 30 days of oral isotretinoin can be supplied at one time to a female patient and the prescription will only be valid for 7 days.

The scope of the PPP suggests that it should include all females of childbearing potential. Clinicians can exercise clinical judgment if they establish that the patient is not currently sexually active, but it is mandatory that clinicians check carefully at each 4-week follow-up visit and record as well as act on any change in circumstance.

Pregnancy testing is recommended pre- and 5 weeks posttherapy. It has been suggested that the initial test can be done up to 2 weeks prior to the start of treatment provided contraception is used in those who require it. In addition, monthly pregnancy testing is recommended throughout the treatment period. The treatment should ideally start on day 3 of the menstrual cycle. The programme suggests that where possible patients should agree to at least one, and preferably two, complementary methods of effective contraception, including a barrier method, before therapy is initiated.

Dispensing restrictions do not apply to males as the process is aimed at ensuring that females do not receive extended periods of treatment without pregnancy tests being performed. The responsibility for the assessment of pregnancy tests and the administration of further prescriptions lies with the clinician. Clinical problems relating to the implementation of this approach include difficulties in females with irregular menses, potential lack of continuity of treatment due to potential unavailability of patient and/or health care workers as well as forgotten tests. Given the potential side effects of oral contraceptives, it may not always be appropriate to insist on all patients using specific contraceptives especially those not sexually active.

The USA has adopted a more rigid programme for pregnancy prevention and monitoring. In 2005, the FDA mandated that all male and female users of Accutane® (oral isotretinoin) would have to enrol into the National Registry 'iPLEDGE'. If not done, patients are no longer able to receive the drug. Women of childbearing age now have to provide two negative pregnancy tests before their initial prescription, show proof of another negative pregnancy test before each monthly repeat prescription, and use two forms of contraception throughout therapy and for 30 days after treatment. They must record the contraception used in the registry. All patients sign a document confirming that they are aware of potential adverse effects including depression and suicidal thoughts.

Current recommendations suggest that isotretinoin should no longer be used as first line therapy and/or should not be used below the age of 12 years. There are many publications advocating the use of isotretinoin for severe acne and scarring acne in the literature, hence delaying this effective therapy in certain cases and may go against best and evidence-based practice. Use of the drug has been expanded worldwide to include less severely affected patients who have responded unsatisfactorily to alternative treatments [557–561].

The ED recommendation is to start isotretinoin at 0.5 mg/kg/day and to titrate the dose as tolerated. The half-life is 22 h and the bioavailability is 25%. Absorption of isotretinoin is markedly affected by the presence of fat and pharmacokinetic studies show that absorption can be doubled by taking isotretinoin with or after a meal compared with the fasting state [562]. It is therefore advisable to take the capsules with fatty food at the same time of day. However, the amount of fat required is high and it is unlikely that patients ingest enough fat to optimize absorption. A novel lipid formulation is now available in some countries; the bioavailability of the drug is not fat dependent.

To date, the duration of therapy varies according to the dose administered over the course of the treatment period. Post-therapy relapse is said to be minimized by treatment courses that amount to a total of least 120–150 mg/kg [563]. However, there is not an a priori pharmacokinetic reason to support the concept of accumulation of drug or a cumulative dose effect and recent publications suggest that the dose should be tailored to the tolerability of the drug as well as the clinical response and have demonstrated that the cumulative doses previously recommended may not be necessary in all patients. The duration of therapy should be adjusted to give at least 90% clearance of acne based upon initial clinical acne grade scoring techniques followed by 4–8 weeks of consolidation.

Demographic factors, such as age, sex and duration of acne, may all govern the rate of response and relapse. Males with extensive truncal acne, more severe acne and/or suffering from acne for less than 7 years, fail to respond as well as, and relapse more quickly than, female patients with predominantly facial acne of a less severe grade.

A number of studies have been published using different dosing regimes of isotretinoin [473]. A study examining four different dosing regimens demonstrated that although lower doses appear to be efficacious in mild to moderate papulopustular acne the more conventional dose of 1 mg/kg/day was superior in treating more severe acne when compared to lower doses or intermittent regimes. Low-dose courses of isotretinoin have been used successfully in mature adults with persistent and late-onset acne [564,565]. A typical approach consists of 0.5 mg/kg/day taken 1 week out of 4 for a period of 6 months. Ninety-one per cent will be clear of acne using this regimen [566] but relapse is frequent. Furthermore, some patients will not accept even minimal disease and become very dependent on small doses, expecting to stay on the drug for many years. It is not clear whether this approach will result in long-term adverse effects and it is important to clarify with the patient that although nothing untoward has been reported to date this approach lies outside recommended guidelines and the current product license.

The physical and psychological severity of acne will play a role in the decision whether to prescribe isotretinoin. Some patients may require repeated courses of therapy. There are no reports of cumulative toxicity from using repeat courses and tachyphylaxis has not been noted.

Although the ED suggests isotretinoin should not be used in patients under 12 years of age, up to 0.5 mg/kg/day has been used successfully in a number of neonates or juveniles with acne who have not responded to all appropriate topical or oral therapies [567,568,569]. Oral isotretinoin should be considered for paediatric acne patients if there are sufficient clinical indications [570] (see section on Prepubertal acne). Apert syndrome is a rare disorder associated with a hyperresponse of the epiphyses (see earlier) and sebaceous glands to androgens, which results in premature epiphyseal fusion, and acne. These patients frequently respond well to oral isotretinoin [571].

Side effects of isotretinoin

Isotretinoin has many side effects but most are predictable and rarely interfere with patient management. Tables 90.25, 90.26,

Table 90.25 Adverse effects of isotretinoin: very common.

Type of disorder	Very common (≥1/10)
Blood and lymphatic system	• Anaemia • Increased red blood cell sedimentation rate • Thrombocytopenia • Thrombocytosis
Eye	• Blepharitis • Conjunctivitis • Dry eyes • Eye irritation
Hepatobiliary	• Increased transaminase
Skin and sebcutaneous tissues	• Cheilitis • Dermatitis • Dry skin • Localized exfoliation • Pruritus • Erythematous • Skin fragility
Musculoskeletal and connective tissue	• Arthralgia • Myalgia • Back pain
Investigation	• Increased triglycerides • Decreased high-density lipoprotein

90.27 and 90.28 outline the potential side effects and relative risk of occurrence. The common mucocutaneous side effects are dose dependent and are managed by modification of the dose and/or regular use of emollients or false tears. Occasionally, retinoid dermatitis (Figure 90.63), a severe retinoid cheilitis (Figure 90.64) or conjunctivitis complicated by secondary S. aureus (Figure 90.65) may occur. These patients may need treatment with an intermediate-strength corticosteroid ointment combined with an antiseptic or oral antistaphylococcal therapy such as flucloxacillin and/or topical mupirocin 2% ointment [572]. Teratogenicity is well recognized and regarded as one of the most serious potential adverse effects of isotretinoin [573]. Fifty per cent of pregnancies spontaneously abort, and of the remainder about half of the infants are born with cardiovascular or skeletal deformities.

Mood changes including depression are common among adolescents and have been reported in acne patients treated with isotretinoin. Two studies for the FDA in the US that looked at spontaneous reports of side effects [574,575] found little or no

Table 90.26 Adverse effects of isotretinoin: common.

Type of disorder	Common (≥1/100, <1/10)
Blood and lymphatic system	• Neutropenia
Nervous system	• Headache
Respiratory, thoracic and mediastinal	• Epistaxis • Nasal dryness • Nasopharyngitis
Investigation	• Increased blood cholesterol • Increased blood glucose • Haematuria • Proteinuria

Table 90.27 Adverse effects of isotretinoin: rare.

Type of disorder	Rare (≥1/10 000, <1/1000)
Immune system	• Allergic skin reaction • Anaphylactic reactions • Hypersensitivity
Psychiatric	• Depression • Aggravated depression • Aggressive tendencies • Anxiety • Mood alterations
Skin and subcutaneous tissues	• Alopecia

Table 90.28 Adverse effects of isotretinoin: very rare.

Type of disorder	Very rare (≥1/10 000)
Infection	• Gram-positive (mucocutaneous) bacterial infection
Blood and lymphatic system	• Lymphadenopathy
Metabolism	• Diabetes • Hyperuricaemia
Psychiatric	• Abnormal behaviour • Psychotic disorder • Suicidal ideation • Suicide attempt • Suicide
Nervous system	• Benign intracranial hypertension • Convulsions • Drowsiness • Dizziness
Eye	• Blurred vision • Cataract • Colour blindness • Contact lens intolerance • Corneal opacity • Decreased night vision • Keratitis • Papilloedema • Photophobia • Visual disturbances
Ear	• Impaired hearing
Vascular	• Vasculitis (i.e. granulomatosis with polyangiitis, allergic vasculitis)
Gastrointestinal	• Colitis • Ileitis • Dry throat • Gastrointestinal haemorrhage • Haemorrhagic diarrhoea • Inflammatory bowel disease • Nausea • Pancreatitis
Hepatobiliary	• Hepatitis
Skin and subcutaneous tissues	• Acne fulminans • Aggravated acne (acne flare) • Erythema (facial) • Exanthema • Hair disorders • Hirsutism • Nail dystrophy • Paronychia • Photosensitivity reaction • Pyogenic granuloma • Skin hyperpigmentation • Increased swelling
Musculo-skeletal and connective tissue	• Arthritis • Calcinosis (calcification of ligaments and tendons) • Premature epiphyseal fusion • Exostosis • Hyperostosis • Osteopenia • Tendonitis
Renal and urinary	• Glomerulonephritis
General	• Increased formation of granulation tissue • Malaise
Investigation	• Increased creatine phosphokinase

increase in psychiatric disease including depression and suicide over the background prevalence in the adolescent population. A further study of general practice databases in Canada and the UK showed similar findings [576] as have subsequent studies [577]. A more recent controlled case cross-over study suggested a relative risk for depression of 2.68 (95% CI = 1.03–3.89) for acne patients exposed to oral isotretinoin [578]. On the basis of contradictory reports, clinicians are advised of a potential rare idiosyncratic reaction in some young vulnerable patients which could lead to mood changes and clinical depression during treatment with isotretinoin. Specific enquiry about mood change and depression are recommended at each clinic visit. If significant depression is identified, a psychiatric referral is indicated. Increased aggression has been identified in some male patients and the FDA has advised clinicians to warn about this possible side effect. If there is any doubt, the drug must be withdrawn.

Significant systemic effects are uncommon; headaches may uncommonly be an early feature of benign intracranial hypertension and arthralgia is seen most frequently in those patients participating in regular and heavy exercise. Tetracyclines, including doxycycline and minocycline, must not be prescribed with isotretinoin, as both drugs may produce benign intracranial hypertension [579].

An acute flare of acne early in a course of isotretinoin is a recognized problem in about 6% of cases and is clinically significant in half of these [580]. The physician should inform patients accordingly and provide rapid access if this occurs as these flares can be aggressive producing physical and psychological sequelae. If the acne is very inflammatory, a lower dose of isotretinoin alongside oral corticosteroids may be required (e.g. 0.5–1.0 mg/kg/day for 2–3 weeks). Predisposing risk factors for a flare include the presence of macrocomedones and nodules [580]. If macrocomedones are present, light cautery or hyfrecation should be done prior to starting the isotretinoin. A local anaesthetic cream should be applied to the lesions beneath an occlusive dressing prior to starting the isotretinoin [581] (Figure 90.66). If a severe flare occurs, 0.5–1.0 mg/kg/day oral prednisolone is needed over a period of 2–3 weeks followed by a tapering of dose the following 6 weeks. The isotretinoin should either be stopped or reduced. If stopped, the drug can be slowly reintroduced at a dose of 0.25 mg/kg/day, and then increased or decreased as response dictates.

Reduced efficacy has been noted when isotretinoin is taken with heavy alcohol intake [582]. Isotretinoin is metabolized by cytochrome P450 enzymes, inducible by ethanol and inhibited

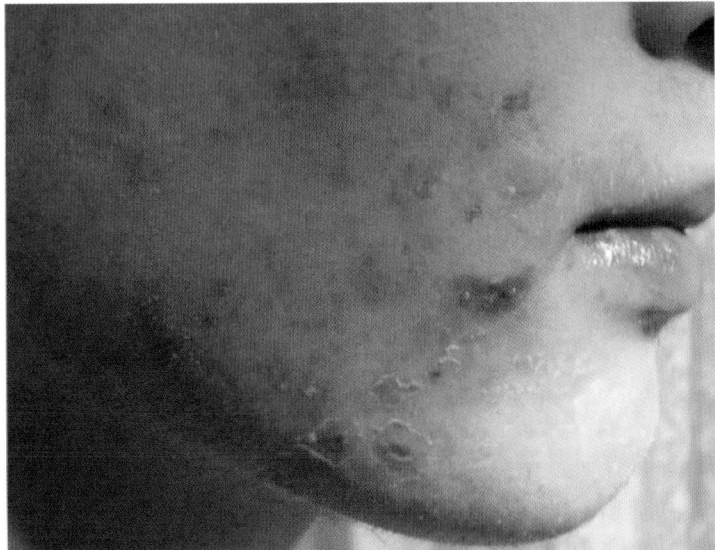

Figure 90.63 Retinoid dermatitis as a result of oral retinoids.

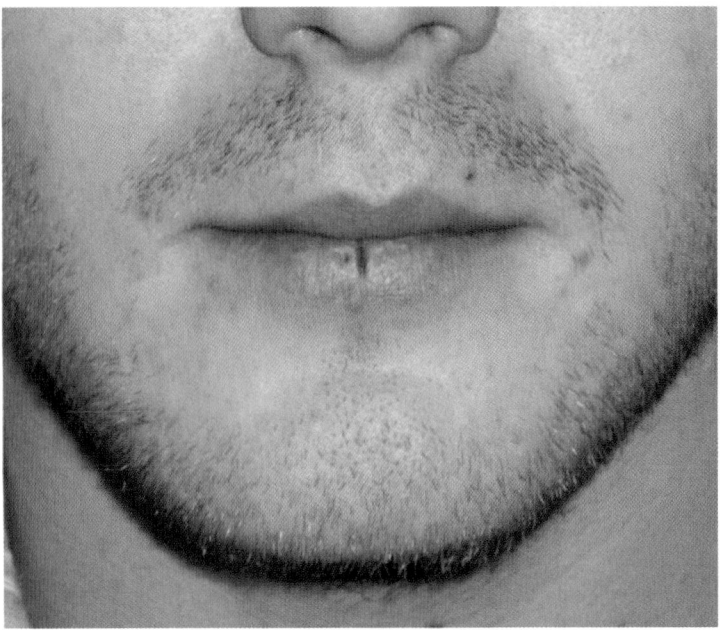

Figure 90.64 Cheilitis and fissure of the lower lip induced by oral retinoids.

by some drugs, for example ketoconazole. Hence, increased drug levels of isotretinoin may occur if combined with imidazole fungistatics. Salicylic acid and indometacin represent acidic drugs with a high affinity for albumin. If present in the blood in high therapeutic concentrations, they may displace isotretinoin from protein binding sites, resulting in an increase in the unbound concentration of the drug [583]. Carbamazepine plasma levels decrease when concurrent isotretinoin is taken, hence careful monitoring should be considered in epileptics on carbamazepine if requiring isotretinoin [584]. Vitamin supplements containing vitamin A should be avoided alongside isotretinoin, as additive toxic effects could ensue.

Other therapies for acne

Topical therapies
The efficacy of other topical treatments has not been established by controlled studies.

Topical nicotinamide
Topical nicotinamide 4% has anti-inflammatory actions and does not induce *P. acnes* resistance [585,586]. Double-blind studies have shown it to be better than vehicle alone against inflamed lesions, although the improvement with the placebo was also considerable

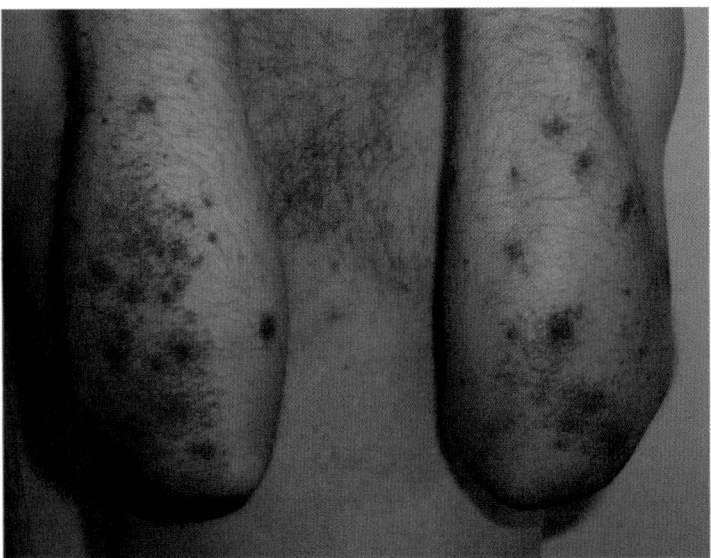

Figure 90.65 *Staphylococcus aureus* colonizing discoid eczema induced by oral retinoids.

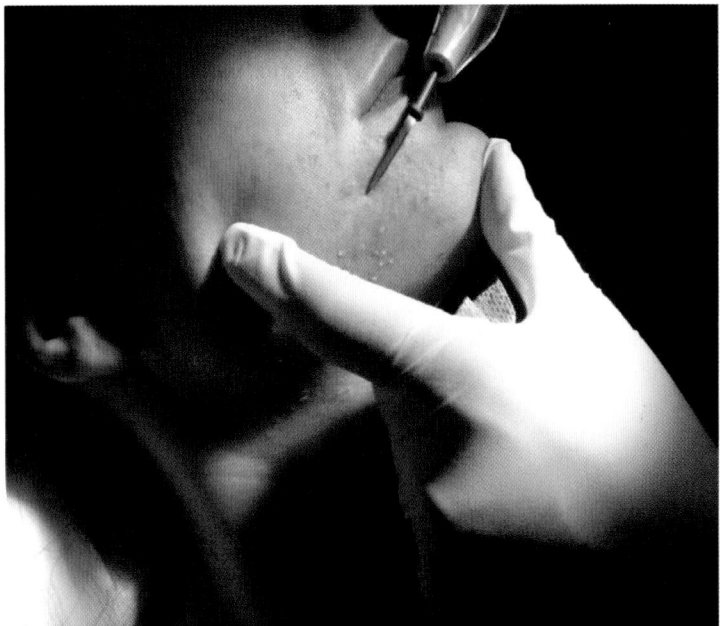

Figure 90.66 Hyfrecation of macrocomedones.

(32–76%) [587]. A comparison of 4% nicotinamide gel demonstrated it to be similar in efficiency to 1% clindamycin gel [588].

Salicyclic acid

Salicylic acid 2% has been shown to be more effective in reducing non-inflammatory and inflammatory acne lesions than alcoholic vehicle at 12 weeks in an RCT [589,590].

Sulphur

A longstanding antiacne therapy, which may be both comedogenic and comedolytic [591–593], sulphur is unpopular because of its smell, and is rarely used.

Corticosteroids

A few topical preparations contain weak corticosteroids but proof of their efficacy is lacking. Potent steroids such as clobetasol propionate applied twice a day for 5 days can dramatically reduce the inflammation in an active inflammatory nodule [594].

Complementary therapies

Data have been published on the potential value of traditional 'herbal' medicines in particular plant alkaloids. So far no clinical benefits have been established [595]. A systematic review of RCTs examining tea tree oil (TTO) in dermatological conditions, including acne, showed there were some promising data suggesting that TTO might be effective for acne and further investigation was advocated [596]. A further review examined the empirical evidence for the efficacy of complementary therapies in acne and concluded that many of the therapies were biologically plausible but in general poor methodology had been used in the studies. The authors concluded that further rigorously conducted trials were required to define efficacy and adverse effect profiles of currently used complementary therapies for acne [597]. The use of green tea for acne has recently been evaluated [598]. Further validation for safety and efficacy against standard medicines is required.

Devices and physical modalities for treating active acne

There are a variety of specially shaped tools available for black-head macrocomedo removal (Figure 90.67) Light cautery or hyfrecation has been shown to help patients with multiple macrocomedones; these are usually whiteheads but occasionally blackheads (up to 1.5 mm diameter), and chloracne can be improved [599,600]. A topical anaesthetic preparation is applied beneath an occlusive dressing. The cautery or hyfrecation should be set as low as possible to produce little or no pain. The aim is to produce very low-grade thermal damage. The treatment of each lesion takes seconds and is associated with very little scarring or

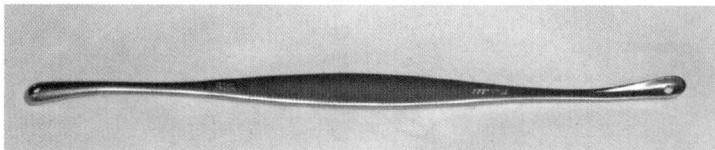

Figure 90.67 Comedo extractor.

Visible light

One study examining the combination of red-blue light phototherapy demonstrated superiority with this modality when compared to BPO for mild to moderate papulopustular acne [395]. Blue light reduced inflammatory lesions compared to the control and was superior to no treatment in reducing acne [602,603]. A more recent controlled study demonstrated that blue light improved inflammatory lesions by 76% compared with BPO, which resulted in a 60% improvement, this suggested the benefits of light therapy were only marginal [604]. Blue light has been given a low strength recommendation in the management of mild to moderate papulopustular acne.

Lasers and photodynamic therapy

There has been increased interest in the use of lasers and light-based devices for acne over the last few years. Light therapy destroys propionibacteria by targeting porphyrins produced by these bacteria. These regimens also suppress a range of pro-inflammatory cytokines [605,606]. To date, the evidence in support of the use of lasers and light devices is poor. A significant number of RCTs embracing light of diverse wavelengths have been conducted, but results from these studies have been contradictory. Many of the studies include small numbers, short follow-up periods and have adopted non-standardized regimes. They have also not compared these therapies to conventional treatments used for acne. Outcome measures have also been very variable, making comparison between trials and meta-analysis difficult.

A systematic review assessing lasers, light sources and photodynamic therapy for acne in 16 RCTs and three controlled studies confirmed most light sources do help inflammatory lesions in the short term, with photodynamic therapy showing the most consistent results (up to 68% improvement, aminolaevulinic acid, methyl aminolevulinate and red light) [607]. No robust studies are available to support the use of lasers or photodynamic therapy for comedonal acne.

A well-conducted RCT of infrared laser therapy versus placebo treatment showed no difference between the laser and placebo for acne, but there was a transient improvement in open comedones or blackheads [608]. An RCT comparing intense pulsed light versus BPO in Asian women found that both treatments improved acne, but there was no statistically significant difference between the two treatments [609]. A small randomized controlled trial of intense pulsed light–photodynamic therapy versus intense pulsed light versus control [610] with all subjects using adapalene 0.1% gel at night, showed no significant difference in improvements in acne lesions between the groups, but a statistically significant improvement in comedones in the light treatment groups. However, the confidence intervals for the results were large reflecting the small numbers of subjects and no definite conclusions could be drawn from this. Laser therapy with the NLite® laser, which emits light at 585 nm, has been reported in a small RCT to produce a 50% improvement in acne grade and lesion counts by 12 weeks after a single treatment [611]. One study reported complete remission after photodynamic therapy with aminolaevulinic acid activated by long-pulsed pulsed dye laser in patients who had failed oral isotretinoin [612].

Light therapy may cause pain, erythema, crusting, oedema, pigmentary changes and pustular eruptions. The intensity of these problems is more likely when aminolaevulinic acid or methyl aminolevulinate are employed in the treatment, and frequently leads to the patient not pursuing further therapy. The other concern relates to long-term safety, as sebocytes are necessary for the immune function of the skin and may be permanently damaged by photodynamic therapy. Topical amino laevulinic acid plus broadband visible light (550–700 nm) has been shown to produce acute damage to the sebaceous glands, resulting in significant sebum suppression for up to 20 weeks post-therapy; this was associated with a significant decrease in *P. acnes* for many weeks [613]. Patients should be informed of the existing evidence, which indicates that optical treatments are not currently included among first line treatments for acne but remain of interest and under investigation.

Chemical peels

Chemical peels are believed to promote desquamation which reduces corneocyte cohesion and keratinocyte plugging, so enabling the extrusion of inflammatory contents. Peeling agents include α-hydroxy acids (glycolic acid), salicylic acid and trichloroacetic acid. Guidelines and evidence for their use have been considered in a Japanese review [614]. A recent review of the efficacy of a variety of chemical peels for acne showed an average reduction in comedones by 35%; however, published studies are limited by sample size and design [615]. Evidence for the use of chemical peels in the treatment of acne is therefore lacking but they are relatively safe and inexpensive and many dermatologists worldwide use light chemical peels with the aim of helping to remove comedones as well as superficial scarring and hyperpigmentation.

Resources

Further information

Nast A, Dréno B, Bettoli V, *et al*. European Evidence-based (S3) Guidelines for the Treatment of Acne. *JEADV* 2012;26(S1):1–29 http://onlinelibrary.wiley.com/doi/10.1111/j.1468-3083.2011.04374.x/pdf

NICE clinical knowledge summary http://cks.nice.org.uk/acne-vulgaris

Primary Care Dermatology Society http://www.pcds.org.uk/

Thiboutot D, Gollnick, H, Bettoli V, *et al*. New insights into the management of acne – an update from the Global Alliance to Improve Outcomes in Acne Group. *JAAD* 2009;60(5):S1:S1–S50 http://www.sciencedirect.com/science/article/pii/S0190962209000826

Zouboulis C, Katsambas A, Klingman A. *Pathogenesis and Treatment of Acne and Rosacea*. Berlin: Springer: 2014.

All last accessed October 2015.

Patient resources

Acne Academy UK http://acneacademy.org/

Acne Patient Decision Aid (BMJ) http://sdm.rightcare.nhs.uk/pda/acne/

British Association of Dermatologists: patient information http://www.bad.org.uk/for-the-public/patient-information-leaflets

Embarrassing Bodies http://www.channel4embarrassingillnesses.com/

NHS Choices http://www.nhs.uk/Pages/HomePage.aspx

Talk Health http://www.talkhealthpartnership.com/

All last accessed October 2015.

Acne fulminans

Definition and nomenclature

Acne fulminans is a rare and severe destructive form of acne presenting primarily in adolescent males. It most frequently affects the trunk but can affect the face and presents acutely in association with systemic symptoms.

> **Synonyms and inclusions**
> - Acne fulminans
> - Acne maligna
> - Sine fulminans

Introduction and general description

Acne fulminans was first described in 1959 as acne conglobata with septicaemia [616]. The disease was later distinguished from acne conglobata by Plewig and Kligman in 1975 [617] they emphasized the characteristic features of sudden onset and severity of systemic upset as distinct features. It is a rare form of acne and the incidence appears to be diminishing, possibly due to more effective and earlier use of treatments [618]. A subset of patients with no systemic symptoms but with severe acne comparable to that seen in acne fulminans has been described as 'sine fulminans' [619].

Epidemiology

Age and gender

Acne fulminans is predominantly seen in young white males aged between 13 and 22 years [620] although there have been rare cases reported in females [621].

Ethnicity

The frequency and severity of acne fulminans is notably greater in patients of Northern European descent compared with those from East-Asian origin [622,623].

Associated diseases

Acne fulminans has been found in association with SAPHO syndrome (see earlier section on associated diseases). This suggests that systemic inflammatory cytokinaemia might be responsible. This proposal is supported by the fact that infliximab has been used to treat acne fulminans associated with SAPHO syndrome [89].

Acne fulminans has also been reported at the onset of Crohn disease but the significance of this association remains unclear [624]. There is just one case report of acne fulminans and ulcerative colitis in a 19-year-old Japanese male patient suggesting any association is very rare [625]. In a further single case report, a male with a leukaemoid reaction also developed posterior scleritis of his eyes and a pyoderma–gangrenosum eruption on the legs suggesting an autoimmune mechanism [626].

PAPA syndrome and acne fulminans

PAPA syndrome was described in 1997; it affects mainly the skin and joints, and the acne may present as acne fulminans or conglobata. The susceptibility gene is CD2-binding protein 1 (*CD2BP1*) gene. The CD2BP1 protein interacts with pyrin and a mutation in the protein may increase its ability to bind to pyrin, then reducing the inhibitory effect of the IL-1β pathway and innate immunity resulting in autoinflammatory reactions [627].

Pathophysiology

The pathophysiology of acne fulminans remains unclear. Infection, genetic predisposition and immunological causes have all been suggested. One theory suggests acne fulminans is an autoimmune complex disease, in favour of this is the rapid response to systemic steroids, increased levels of γ-globulins and decrease in complement levels seen in a number of patients. Immune complexes are found predominantly in patients with musculoskeletal problems. The association with autoinflammatory disorders described above has led to the hypothesis that abnormal innate immunity, such as in the IL-1 pathway, may be involved in the pathogenesis of acne fulminans.

Predisposing factors

Acne fulminans is seen most frequently in young males and there is some evidence to suggest that elevated blood levels of testosterone may play a role [628]. The increase in physiological levels of testosterone in males at puberty may explain this predisposition. There are reports of patients developing acne fulminans after receiving high-dose testosterone for the treatments of excessively tall stature, Klinefelter and Marfan syndrome [629–632]. One case of acne fulminans has also been reported in a young man with androgen excess as a result of late-onset congenital adrenal hyperplasia [633].

A number of case reports have cited anabolic-androgenic steroids as a trigger for acne fulminans [618,634–636]. As derivatives of the hormone testosterone, anabolic steroids lead to hypertrophy of the sebaceous glands, increased sebum production and as a result of this an increased density of P. acnes [637].

Paradoxically, another predisposing factor is the use of isotretinoin. In some patients, mild cystic acne rapidly evolves with ulcerative and necrotic lesions. In these patients, the dose of isotretinoin is usually 0.5–1.0 mg/kg/day and the treatment had been administered for an average of 3 weeks (range 1–7 weeks) before deterioration occurred [618]. Kellet et al. reported circulating immune complexes in two cases with a flare of acne fulminans apparently triggered by isotretinoin [638].

Pathology

Causative organisms

The presence in some patients of microscopic haematuria, erythema nodosum, increased response to P. acnes antigen on skin tests and depressed response to intradermal purified protein derivatives are in favour of an abnormal immunological response. Skin tests with P. acnes demonstrate a very extensive, immediate and delayed reaction, the immunohistology of which reveals a type III or type IV hypersensitivity reaction [639].

Isotretinoin can cause a significant flare of acne fulminans in some patients. Hypotheses to explain this suggest that the isotretinoin induced fragility of the pilosebaceous duct epithelium allows significant exposure of P. acnes antigens and/or P. acnes chem-

oattractants to the immune system. An exaggerated response to intradermal injection of P. acnes suspended in saline has been demonstrated in a case of acne fulminans and erythema nodosum suggesting P. acnes may act as an antigen in this context [638]. Another theory is that genetically determined changes in neutrophil activity/hyperreactivity to chemoattractants may result in reduced phagocytosis of P. acnes. Authors have suggested that P. acnes destruction results in increased neutrophil chemotaxis which may be responsible for the isotretinoin flares seen when patients start treatment. It has been suggested that patients who develop very severe flares of acne after starting isotretinoin may have an exaggeration of this response [640].

Genetics

Hereditary factors may play a role, acne fulminans has been reported in identical monozygotic twins who presented at the same age with identical clinical presentation [641,642]. Two siblings presenting with acne fulminans were noted to have identical human leucocyte antigen (HLA) phenotypes [643]. A genetic predisposition associated with HLA-Cw6 gene has been described [620]. A genetically determined change in neutrophil activity has also been proposed as a determinant.

Environmental factors

Infection as a trigger for acne fulminans has been reported. One case report indicates an association 2 weeks after a measles infection implying that the virus may trigger a transient release of inflammatory cytokines, resulting in acne fulminans in a predisposed individual [644]. An acne fulminans-like picture has been reported in association with Epstein–Barr virus infection [645].

Clinical features

History

Most patient with acne fulminans describe mild to moderate acne for 0.5–5 years (mean 2 years) before a sudden onset of febrile ulcerative necrotic acne lesions alongside arthralgia, fever and various systemic inflammatory signs and symptoms [618]. Patients typically fail to respond to antibacterial therapy.

Presentation

Patients present with numerous, inflammatory tender and ulcerative nodules covered with haemorrhagic crusts Figures 90.68 and 90.69. These are predominantly distributed on the upper chest, back and shoulders [646] and pyogenic granulomatous-like lesions may be present. The face may also be involved and the lesions undergo rapid degeneration resulting in ulcerations filled with necrotic debris. Comedonal lesions are rare.

Systemic signs and symptoms are present in the majority of patients and include malaise, arthralgia, joint swellings, polyarthritis, myalgia, fever, and anorexia and weight loss. A marked leucocytosis which may be leukaemoid is frequent; patients may also demonstrate anaemia (Table 90.29).

Painful splenomegaly [647], erythema nodosum [648,649] and bone pain due to aseptic osteolysis have also been reported [650]. Bone involvement is common [651]; in a series of 24 patients, 48% had lytic bone lesions on X-ray and 67% showed increased

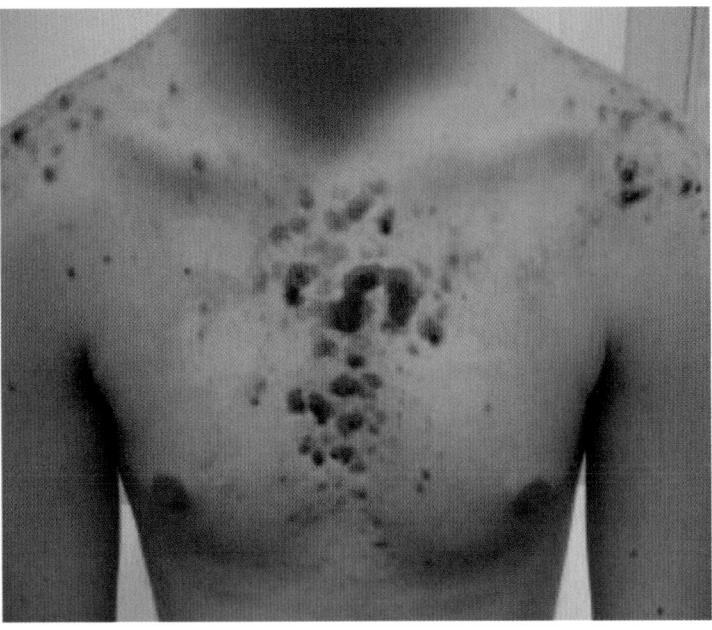

Figure 90.68 Acne fulminans in a young male.

radiolabel uptake; 25% showed destructive lesions resembling osteomyelitis [651,652]. The sites of predilection for bone lesions include the anterior chest, particularly the clavicles and sternum, but osteolytic lesions have also been reported in the ankles, hips and humerus. Sacroileitis has also been described.

Clinical variants
Acne fulminans may occur in the context of SAPHO syndrome and is considered by some as a spectrum of this autoinflammatory disorder [653,654].

Differential diagnosis
The main differential diagnosis is severe acne conglobata (see later). The latter is seen in both men and women and has a more

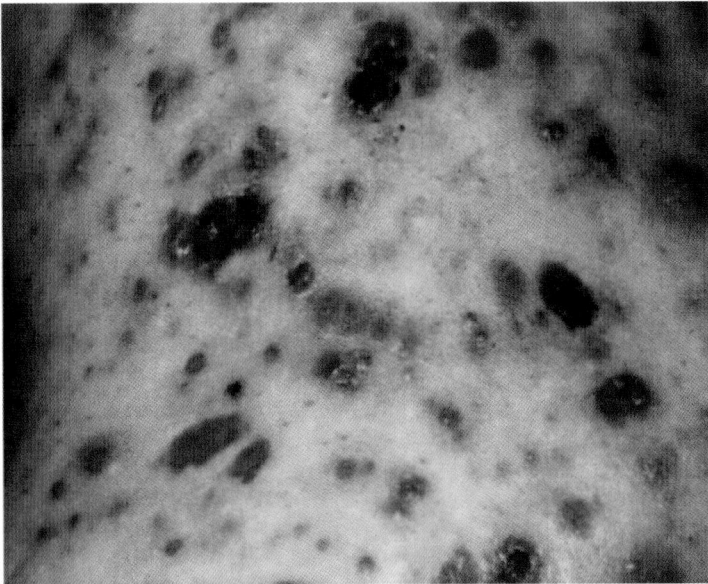

Figure 90.69 Erosive crusting lesions on the back of a young male with acne fulminans.

Table 90.29 The main features of acne fulminans.

Gender	Male gender dominant
Age	13–22 years
Pathogenesis	Unclear
Onset	Acute and sudden
Localization	Upper chest and back, shoulders, face
Clinical picture	Ulcerative lesions covered with haemorrhagic crusts healing with scarring
Laboratory findings	Leucocytosis, increased erythrocyte sedimentation rate, anaemia, proteinuria, microscopic haematuria
Response to conventional antibiotic therapy	Poor
Treatments of choice	Systemic corticosteroids combined with isotretinoin

insidious onset, whereas acne fulminans is generally very acute and rarely seen in females. Patients present with acne conglobata at an older average age and the condition has a protracted and more chronic course than acne fulminans with little or much less systemic symptoms. Comedonal lesions are generally much more florid in acne conglobata (Table 90.30).

Assessment
Acne fulminans always presents as a severe cutaneous inflammatory process with varying systemic signs and symptoms.

Investigations
There are no consistent laboratory abnormalities in acne fulminans. Bacterial cultures from blood, joint fluid and skin are generally sterile. There is one report describing a patient with acne fulminans and a lytic bone lesion from which *P. acnes* was cultured [655]. This contrasts with another report in which a patient had osteomyelitis and acne fulminans but cultures from bone were negative for *P. acnes* although red fluorescence in the affected bone characteristic of *P. acnes* was noted [656]. Abnormal laboratory findings may include an increased erythrocyte sedimentation rate (ESR), elevated C-reactive protein and thrombocytosis, together with a normochromic and normocytic anaemia. Characteristically, a leucocytosis is found sometimes with an associated leukaemoid reaction. There are a couple of reports in the literature in which 0.5–1.5% myeloblasts, promyelocytes and myelocytes were found in the peripheral blood [622,657]. Elevated liver enzymes and microscopic haematuria, proteinuria and other kidney abnormalities may be identified. Circulating immune complexes have been

Table 90.30 Differential diagnosis of acne fulminans and acne conglobata.

	Acne fulminans	**Acne conglobata**
Gender	Men	Men
Age	Adolescence (13–16 years)	20–25 years
Onset	Sudden	Slow
Location	Face, neck, chest and back	Trunk and upper limbs, facial lesions are rare
Clinical features	Haemorrhagic ulcerations	Nodules, inflammatory cysts, grouped comedones
Systemic symptoms	Very common	None

identified in some patients with acne fulminans and erythema nodosum [648,656]. Bone involvement is common and approximately 50% of patients have lytic bone lesions demonstrated by radiographs and 70% show increased uptake using technetium scintigraphy. Destructive lesions resembling osteomyelitis are demonstrated on radiographs in 25% of patient [658]. When present, bone biopsies have been performed to rule out malignancy; the histology usually reveals reactive changes only but a neutrophilic infiltrate with mononuclear cells and granulation tissue can mimic osteomyelitis. Patients with osteolytic lesions may have elevated serum alkaline phosphatase [659].

Complications

Radiographic changes such as hyperostosis and sclerosis may persist but rarely the symptoms and signs associated with any bony changes typically resolve with treatment. Mild musculoskeletal discomfort has been reported as a persistent symptom following the acute episode. The most common complication is significant and disfiguring scarring.

Disease course and prognosis

The prognosis for patients treated effectively with corticosteroids and isotretinoin is extremely good. Recurrent acne fulminans is very rare [651]. Relapse may occur as corticosteroid therapy is reduced but the risk reduces over time and is unusual after a year.

Management

The acute myalgia, arthralgia and fever can be treated with oral salicylates or non-steroidal anti-inflammatory drugs and gradu-ated physical exercise. Crusts should be removed by soaking the skin with emollient oil and this should be followed by the use of a potent steroid/antimicrobial cream for 2–3 weeks.

First line therapy

Oral prednisolone therapy should be commenced first line (0.5–1.0 mg/kg/day) and decreased slowly over 2–3 months. Low-dose oral isotretinoin (0.25–0.5 mg/kg/day) should be cautiously introduced either after 3–4 weeks of systemic steroid therapy [660–662] or parallelly with corticosteroids [663] and then gradually increased as tolerated and according to clinical response. Oral isotretinoin should be used with caution as paradoxically it has been reported to induce acne fulminans in some patients [664].

Alternative therapies

Clofazimine 200 mg three times a week has been shown to improve acne fulminans [665]. Pulsed intravenous corticosteroids administered alongside isotretinoin have been used to control the disease in a 16-year-old male with good effect [666]. Isotretinoin in combination with dapsone has been used successfully to treat acne fulminans associated with erythema nodosum [664]. Combining systemic steroids with azathioprine or ciclosporin has been shown to avoid relapses on withdrawal of steroids [647–670].

In cases of acne fulminans which appear in the context of auto-inflammatory disease, the effective use of biologicals has been described in some cases but others have noted improvement in the musculoskeletal symptoms without much impact or in some cases a deterioration in the cutaneous problems. Table 90.31 outlines systemic treatment options reported in the literature.

Table 90.31 Systemic treatments used for acne fulminans.

Treatment recommendation	Duration/outcome number of case	References
0.5–1 mg/kg/day prednisolone for 4–6 weeks reducing thereafter	Assessment of 25 cases treated over 25 years	[671]
Commence oral isotretinoin week 4 at 0.5 mg/kg/day and gradually increase until clearance	Continued isotretinoin until clear	
Low-dose/cautious introduction of oral isotretinoin. 4 weeks post start of systemic steroids at doses ranging 0.2 to 0.5 mg/kg/day	Repeat isotretinoin may be required in many cases	[672]
Systemic steroids plus 0.5–1 mg/kg/day isotretinoin	3–5 months, resolution	[673]
Oral prednisolone first line (0.5–1.0 mg/kg/day) and decreased slowly over 2–3 months.	Continued isotretinoin until clear	[662]
Low-dose oral isotretinoin (0.25–0.5 mg/kg/day) cautiously introduced after 3–4 weeks of systemic steroid therapy		
Systemic steroids plus azathioprine	Poor response to steroid resolution after addition of azathioprine over months	[668]
Isotretinoin in combination with dapsone	No steroids required, one case report	[665]
Infliximab	Acne fulminans presenting in the context of the autoinflammatory condition SAPHO	[89]
Systemic steroids plus ciclosporin A (5 mg/kg/day)	Addition of ciclosporin avoided relapse on withdrawal of steroids. Case report in a patient developing acne fulminans in the context of the autoinflammatory disorder PAPA	[669]
Systemic steroids plus dapsone 50–150 mg daily	Dapsone is an alternative to isotretinoin if not available. Case report useful if erythema no dose	[674]
Initial prednisolone 60 mg daily followed by	Case report	[670]
Isotretinoin 30 mg/day	Ciclosporin discontinued at 4 months as lesions resolved	
Followed by ciclosporin 5 mg/kg in place of prednisolone	Isotretinoin 100 mg/kg given over the 4 months	
Clofazimine (200 mg three times a week) has been shown to improve acne fulminans	Case report	[666]
0.5 mg/kg/day isotretinoin in combination with 30 mg/day prednisolone	Predisonole tapering and discontinuation at 1 month or longer	[663]

PART 8: SPECIFIC CUTANEOUS STRUCTURE

PART 8: SPECIFIC
CUTANEOUS STRUCTURE

Acne conglobata

Definition
Acne conglobata represents a rare and severe form of acne characterized by multiple and extensive inflammatory papules, tender nodules and abscesses which commonly coalesce to form malodorous draining sinus tracts. Multiple polyporous, grouped comedones are typical and extensive disfiguring hypertrophic and atrophic scars are also common features [675].

Introduction and general description
Acne congolobata has a chronic and persistent course, it may occur in the context of existing papulopustular acne or may present as a recrudescence of acne that has been in abeyance for many years. Lesions typically occur on the trunk and upper limbs but frequently extend to the buttocks. In contrast to acne fulminans, systemic features are generally not a feature. The malodorous, discharging sinus tracts and significant scarring frequently result in psychological impairment.

Epidemiology
Acne conglobata is a rare disease.

Age and sex
Acne conglobata usually presents in the second to third decade and may persist into the forties and fifties. Males are more frequently affected than females.

Ethnicity
There are no studies to indicate that acne conglobata is seen more frequently in different ethnic groups.

Associated diseases
Acne conglobata may occur in the context of a number of inflammatory disorders.

Hidradenitis suppuritiva. Acne conglobata is described in association with HS and in these cases the HS may involve the perineal and gluteal regions extensively [676]. HS and folliculitis decalvans have also been described in association with acne conglobata [677], as have pilonidal cysts.

Arthritis. The association of acne conglobata and arthritis is rare but has been reported in a number of case reports [**678**,679,680]. Spondyloarthritis associated with acne conglobata, HS and dissecting folliculitis of the scalp is also recognized [681].

Pyoderma gangrenosum. Acne conglobata has been described in association with pyoderma gangrenosum [682].

A number of autoinflammatory syndromes cite acne conglobata as a possible clinical presentation within the context of the syndrome; these are described in more detail in Chapter 49.

SAPHO syndrome: representing synovitis, acne conglobata, pustulosis, hyperostosis and osteitis [683].

PAPA syndrome: severe acne conglobata with sterile pyogenic arthritis and pyoderma gangrenosum has been reported as part of a related group of inflammatory disorders including psoriasis, uveitis and inflammatory bowel disease [103].

PASH syndrome: PAPA syndrome is also related to the triad of pyoderma gangrenosum, acne conglobata and suppurative hidradentitis, known as PASH syndrome [684].

PASS syndrome: a new linkage designated PASS syndrome has also been described; this includes pyoderma gangrenosum, acne conglobata, suppurative hidradenitis and seronegative spondyloarthritis [685].

Pathophysiology
The primary cause of acne conglobata remains unknown.

Predisposing factors
Acne conglobata, like acne fulminans, can be triggered by testosterone and may be induced by anabolic steroid abuse and can occasionally occur after withdrawal of testosterone [687]. Although rare, patients should be advised of this risk. Acne conglobata may also occur in the context of an androgen-secreting tumour and has been described following exposure to aromatic hydrocarbons or ingestion of halogens (see Occupational acne).

Causative organisms
No causative organisms have been implicated in the pathophysiology of acne conglobata. Gram-positive bacteria are often found secondarily infecting active lesions. *Mycobacterium chelonae* I infection has been described as a mimic of acne conglobata in an immunocompetent host [687].

Genetics
Familial cases have been reported with linkage to chromosome 15q24-26 in the region of IL-16 and *CRABPI* genes [688]. Chromosomal defects in the XYY karyotype of Klinefelter syndrome is believed to exclude from severe acne; however, there is one case report in the literature with the unusual combination of Klinefelter syndrome and acne conglobata [689]. PAPA syndrome has been mapped onto the long arm of chromosome 15 and it has been suggested that the distinct clinical entities seen in PAPA may share the same genetic aetiology [688].

The association with specific HLA phenotypes has been studied but antigen frequencies in one cohort of 65 patients with acne conglobata were found to be normal. A further group of patients with both HS and acne conglobata were studied: four of six patients had cross-reacting antigens and all had HLA-DRw4 [690]. PAPA was originally reported in a three-generation kindred with autosomal dominant transmission.

Environmental factors
Exposure to halogenated aromatic hydrocarbons or ingestion of halogens should be considered (see Occupational acne).

Clinical features

History
Acne conglobata (Figure 90.70) may develop in the setting of acne vulgaris that has been quiescent for a number of years but frequently the onset is insidious with a chronic and unremitting course. It is more common in males. Active inflammatory lesions

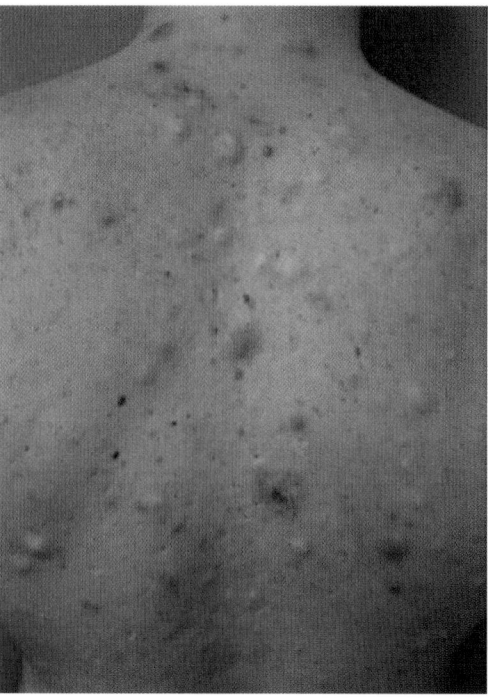

Figure 90.70 Acne conglobata of the back with multiple inflammatory lesions, grouped comedones, cysts and scarring.

may persist for many years and typically continue until the fourth decade of life. The healing of lesions is slow and associated with significant discomfort and disfiguring scarring. Patients typically fail to respond to antibacterial therapy.

Presentation
Patients with acne conglobata present with multiple comedones often in groups (Figure 90.71) and demonstrate highly inflammatory

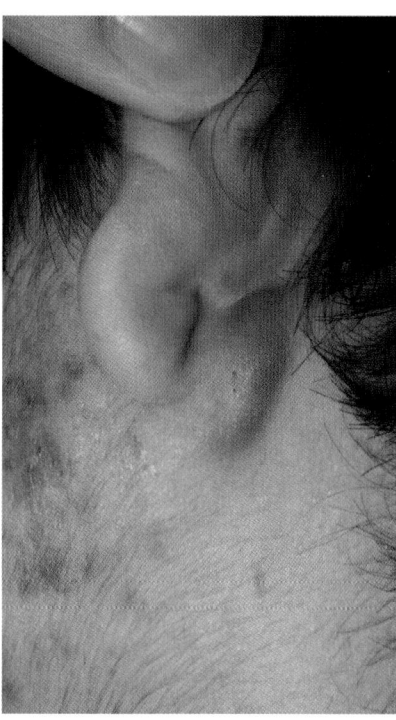

Figure 90.71 Patients with acne conglobata present with grouped comedones and deep-seated inflammatory lesions.

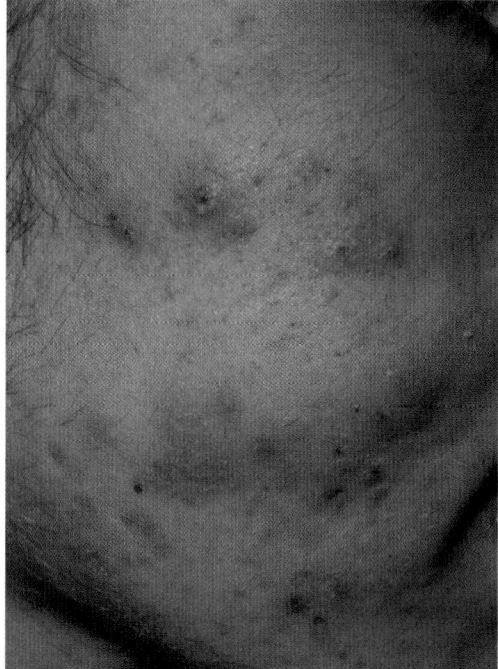

Figure 90.72 Patient with acne conglobata present with abscesses and cysts, causing interconnecting sinus tracts.

papules, pustules, tender nodules, interconnecting abscesses and draining sinus tracts. The nodules characteristically increase in size and deep ulcers may develop beneath the nodules which interconnect and produce draining sinus tracts (Figure 90.72). Hypertrophic and atrophic scars are frequently present (Table 90.32).

Clinical variants
As outlined earlier, acne conglobata may either be part of a number of collective inflammatory conditions or present as a distinct clinical entity.

Table 90.32 The main features of acne conglobata.

Sex	Males affected more frequently than females
Age	18–30 years
Pathogenesis	Unclear
Onset	May be an insidious onset with a chronic course on the background of previous acne or an acute deterioration of existing inflammatory acne
Localisation	Face, trunk and limbs extending to the buttocks
Clinical picture	Deep-seated inflammatory lesions, abscesses and cysts, causing interconnecting sinus tracts. Polyporous grouped comedones and, significant scarring
Laboratory findings	Gram-positive bacteria producing secondary infection
Response to conventional antibiotic therapy	Poor
Treatments of choice	Oral isotretinoin alongside systemic corticosteroids to reduce inflammation Systemic antibiotics to treat secondary infection and reduce inflammation

PART 8: SPECIFIC CUTANEOUS STRUCTURE

Differential diagnosis

The main differentials are severe inflammatory acne or acne fulminans. The latter has an acute onset and is rarely seen in females. Patients present with acne conglobata at an older average age and the condition has a protracted and more chronic course than acne fulminans with fewer systemic symptoms (see section on Acne fulminans; see Table 90.30). Comedonal lesions are generally much more florid in acne conglobata and present in a characteristic grouped manner. Severe acne vulgaris, occupational acne and drug-induced acne should be considered in the differential diagnosis.

Classification of severity

Acne conglobata always presents as a severe cutaneous inflammatory process with significant scarring resulting in disfigurement in most cases. Psychosocial sequelae as a result of the disease process and resultant scarring are very common [691].

Disease course and prognosis

The disease course is insidious and chronic. It leads to significant psychosocial morbidity as a result of extensive scarring and discomfort and malodour associated with the inflammatory lesions.

Assessment

No consistent laboratory abnormalities are identified in acne conglobata. Bacterial cultures from the skin are generally sterile but in some cases lesions are secondarily infected with Gram-positive bacteria. In cases where there is malodour, assessing cultures and treating with appropriate antibiotics may be helpful. An IgA gammopathy has been observed in a patient with pyoderma and acne conglobate [692].

Complications

The most common complication is extensive and disfiguring scarring. Psychosocial impairment including anxiety and depression are frequent. Renal amyloidosis has been reported with acne conglobata [693]. Malignancy has also been reported in chronic scars attributed to acne conglobata.

Management

Therapy is challenging. Treatment should aim to reduce the morbidity associated with discomfort and malodour with the use of appropriate analgesia alongside antiseptic washes and if necessary antibiotics. Treatment should also aim to prevent complications by reducing inflammation associated with resultant scarring. Large nodules may be aspirated and injection with intralesional triamcinolone or cryotherapy may be beneficial [694]. More extensive surgical excision of interconnecting nodules and laying open of sinus tracts my also prove helpful [695]. There are reports of benefit with laser therapy and modern external beam radiation [696,697]. A combination of medical and surgical approaches may be required to manage this refractory condition [698]. Recent reports have also indicated that some of the novel biologicals may be helpful in this challenging condition.

First line

Oral isotretinoin (0.5–1 mg/kg/day) for 4–6 months is the treatment of choice [618,699]. Isotretinoin may need to be combined with oral antibiotics such as erythromycin or trimethoprim. Concomitant use of systemic steroids such as prednisolone 1 mg/kg/day for 2–4 weeks may also provide benefit to control the inflammatory component of the disease at initial onset and intermittently during acute exacerbations [**700**]. Surgery may be required to lay open abscesses and sinus tracts [675,698]. Resultant scarring may be improved with the fractional laser postsurgical intervention [696].

Second line

Tetracycline antibiotics are frequently prescribed to reduce the inflammation but are notoriously ineffective. Dapsone has also been used with some success [698].

Alternative therapies

Alternative options for the management of acne conglobata include long-term high-dose antibiotics, dapsone with isotretinoin [701], ciclosporin and/or colchicine in conjunction with topical retinoids and antimicrobial therapy [698]. One case report has demonstrated the benefit of carbon dioxide laser in combination with tretinoin to open up cysts and to prevent the emergence of new lesions [696]. In addition, infliximab, an anti-TNF inhibitor, has proved helpful in isolated case reports [685,702,703], as has etanercept [704,705] and adalimumab [706]. Other case reports indicate improvement with electron beam therapy [684,697]. There are very few clinical trials assessing treatment in this refractory condition but one small study examining photodynamic therapy using 5% aminolaevulinic acid and red light demonstrated some advantage to control therapy [707]. Potential treatments for acne conglobata as reported in the literature are outlined in Table 90.33.

Histopathology

Draining sinuses are characteristic of acne conglobata. Histologically, they consist of elaborate, epithelialized galleries connected to the skin surface at multiple points. The draining sinus contains corneocytes, hairs, bacteria, serum, inflammatory cells and epithelioid granulomas [713].

Occupational acne

Definition and nomenclature

Occupational acne is a group of disorders characterized by the formation of acne-like lesions in previously acne non-prone patients after exposure to occupational agents, in most cases chemical compounds.

Synonyms and inclusions
- Chemically induced acne
- Occupational acne
- Chloracne

Introduction and general description

Environmental pollution can result in an acneform dermatosis imitating acne, which was first described in 1887 by Von Bettman and later by Herxheimer in 1899 [714].

Herxheimer suggested that the disorder was caused by chlorine exposure and hence called it 'chloracne' based on the similarity of its clinical features with acne vulgaris. Occupational acne can be

Table 90.33 Treatment options for acne conglobata.

Number of cases	Treatment employed	Duration/outcome of treatment	References
	Oral isotretinoin (0.5–1 mg/kg/day) 4–6 months. With or without systemic steroids	Reduction in some inflammatory lesions and better control of disease but not clearance in many	[708,709]
1 patient	Etanercept	Successful treatment	[704]
64-year-old male	Infliximab 3 mg/kg. Week 0, 2 and 6. Alternate months thereafter. Isotretinoin 0.8 mg/kg/day used in conjunction with infliximab – failed to control the acne conglobate prior to infliximab	Reduction of lesions at week 6 No new lesions after week 6 Isotretinoin tapered off Control maintained with infliximab	[702]
	Infliximab infusion	Successful treatment of acne with infliximab	[703]
	Vaporization of covering cyst wall with CO_2 laser, topical tretinoin	Clinical improvement with laser, maintained with tretinoin	[710]
	Isotretinoin and dapsone	Successful treatment achieved	[711]
53-year-old male	8 treatments of modern beam radiation over 2 weeks localized to the bilateral mandible cheeks	3 weeks postradiation reduced cyst size, absent drainage, reduced pain and improved self-esteem	[697]
1 male	Infliximab infusion	All dermatologocal and rheumatological manifestations reported to regress with infliximab. Previously failed on etanercept	[685]
	Interleukin 1-β blockade		[684]
18-year-old male	Adalimumab 80 mg loading dose followed by 40 mg twice monthly	Marked decrease in size and degree of inflammation of nodular lesions by 4 weeks at 12 weeks full resolution of nodular lesions. At 12 months on treatment sustained efficacy	[710]
42-year-old male	Etanercept 25 mg twice a week and isotretinoin 20 mg weekly for 3 months. Etanercept then tapered to once a week for 1 month then alternate weeks for 2 months and isotretinoin reduced to 10 mg daily	Reduction in lesions and activity of the disease	[712]

induced by diverse environmental agents and can, therefore, be classified in acne venenata/acne cosmetica, tropical acne/hydration acne, oil acne/pomade acne, coal-tar acne, detergens acne and chloracne [715,716,**717**] (Table 90.34).

Chloracne is caused by certain polyhalogenated organic (aromatic) compounds containing naphthalenes, biphenyls and phenols (herbicides and herbicide intermediates) and is considered to be one of the most sensitive indicators of systemic poisoning by these compounds [**718**] (Box 90.7).

Table 90.34 Differential diagnosis of occupational and environmental acne.

	Aetiology	Location	Lesions
Acne venenata/acne cosmetic	Cosmetics	Face	Closed comedones
Tropical acne/ hydration acne	Heat/humidity	Back, neck, buttocks, proximal extremities	Nodules, cysts
Oil acne/pomade acne	Oil	Arms, thighs, buttocks	Erythematous papules, pustules
Detergens acne	Alcalic soaps, detergens	Hands, face	Erythematous papules, pustules
Coal-tar acne	Tar/pitch	Exposed facial areas, esp. malar	Open comedones
Chloracne	Polyhalogenated organic (aromatic) compounds	Malar, retroauricular, mandibular	Comedones, straw-coloured cysts (0.1–1 cm)

Modified from McDonnell and Taylor 2000 [**718**] copyright Springer.

Box 90.7 Chloracne-inducing chemicals

Polyhalogenated naphthalenes[a]
- Polychloronaphthalenes
- Polybromonaphthalenes[b,c]

Polyhalogenated biphenyls
- Polychlorobiphenyls (PCB)
- Polybromobiphenyls
- Polychalogenated dibenzofurans[a]
  - (a) Polychlorodibenzofurans, esp. tri-, tetra-, penta-, and hexachlorodibenzofuran
  - (b) Polybromodibenzofurans, esp. tetrabromodibenzofuran

Contaminants of polychlorophenol compounds, esp. herbicides (2,4,5-trichlorophenol and pentachlorophenol) and herbicide intermediates (2,4,5-trichlorophenol)
- 2,3,7,8-tetrachlorodibenzo-p-doxin (TCDD)
- Hexachlorodibenzo-p-dioxin
- Tetrachlorodibenzofuran

Contaminants of 3,4-dichloroaniline and related herbicides
- 3,4,3′,4′-tetrachoroazoxybenzene (TCAOB)
- 3,4,3′,4′-tetrachoroazobenzene (TCAB)

Other
- Dihydrotrifluoromythylphenylbenzothiopyrazolone
- 1,2,3,4-tetrachlorobenzene (experimental)
- Dichlobenil (herbicide, clinical)
- Crude trichloronezene (DDT)[c]

[a]May occur as contaminants in some PCBs
[b]May occur as contaminants in some PBBs
[c]Not confirmed as chloracnegens

Table 90.35 Large single dioxin accidents in post-war history.

Year of outbreak	Country/city (references)	No. of registered victims	Pollutants	Occurrence	Long-term follow-up of chloracne prevalence (survey year)
1953	Germany/Ludwigshafen (Zober et al. 1990 [721])	248	TCP/TCDD	Leakage of byproducts of TCP production from a chemical reactor	10.1% (1989)
1963	Netherlands/Amsterdam (Dalderup and Zellenrath 1983 [722])	145	TCDD	Explosion of a factory producing crop-protection agents	48.9% (1983)
1976	Italy/Seveso (Pesatori et al. 2003 [723])	193 [a]	TCP/TCDD	Explosion of a TCP reactor	1 of 193 (1989)

Modified from Ju et al. 2012 [**716**] copyright Elsevier.
[a] 193 detected cases with chloracne (170 younger than 15 years of age).
TCDD, 2,3,7,8-tetrachlorodibenzo-p-dioxin; TCP, trichlorophenol.

Dioxins, a large family of halogenated aromatic hydrocarbons, are the most potent environmental chloracnegen. The most potent environmental chloracnegen of this group is 2,3,7,8-tetrachlorodibenzo-p-dioxin (TCDD) [719]. The chloracnegens are structurally similar, containing two benzene rings with halogen atoms occupying at least three of the lateral ring positions (75 isomers).

Epidemiology

Most cases of chloracne have resulted from occupational and non-occupational exposures. Non-occupational chloracne mainly resulted from contaminated industrial wastes and contaminated food products. The identification of dioxin as an elicitor of occupational acne was made with the cooperation of the dermatologists K. H. Schulz and J. Kimmig with the chemist G. Sorge in Hamburg, Germany, who investigated patients with atypical acne in a chemical plant [720].

Since then, there have been several large accidents caused by occupational exposures or food contaminations. After the Second World War, several episodes of large-scale dioxin poisoning (in Ludwigshafen, Germany; Amsterdam, the Netherlands; Seveso, Italy) were reported after industrial work explosions each with more than 100 victims [716,721–723] (Table 90.35).

Massive intoxication has so far happened twice through ingestion of contaminated oils, 'Yusho' in the Fukuoka Prefecture, Kyushu, Japan; in 1968 and 'Yu-Cheng' in Changhua,Taiwan, in 1979; both terms meaning 'oil syndrome' [716,724] (Table 90.36). The real prevalence of chloracne among Vietnamese civilians and American soldiers caused by Agent Orange (containing phenoxyl herbicide contaminated with dioxins) during the Vietnam War (1962–1971) is unknown [725]. The most recent sensational case report of chloracne incident was the TCDD poisoning of Viktor Yushchenko, a former president of Ukraine, in late December 2004 [726].

Associated diseases

Due to its extensive long-term developmental and neurological toxicity, hormonal and immunological disruption as well as cancer promotion, the production of polychlorinated biphenyls has been prohibited by the Stockholm Treaty on Persistent Organic Pollutants made effective from 2004.

Clinical features

Chloracne can be diagnosed by the history of exposure to chloracnegens, characteristic clinical manifestations such as acutely emerging comedones, papules, nodules and cysts followed by scars and specifically the detection of high serum concentration of chloracne (see Figure 90.16). A history of exposure to chloracnegens, progressively emerging comedones, papules, nodules and cysts followed by scars, skin xerosis and decreased sebogenesis, and high serum concentration of chloracnegens (Table 90.37) differentiates chloracne from acne vulgaris.

Investigations

As the assessment of chloracnegens in serum can only be carried out in specialized laboratories and the serum titres of dioxins are usually within the normal range, histopathological changes also offer important clues in the diagnosis of chloracne [726,727] as follows:
- Epidermal hyperplasia.
- Follicular hyperplasia – replacement by keratinizing epidermal cells.
- Sebaceous glands disappear and are replaced by keratinizing epidermal cells.

Table 90.36 Massive intoxication through ingestion of contaminated oils in postwar history.

Year of outbreak	Country/city (references)	No. of registered victims	Pollutants	Occurrence	Long-term follow-up of chloracne prevalence (survey year)
1968	Japan/Kyushu (Fukuoka, Nagasaki) (Yoshimura 2003 [724])	1684	PCB/PCDF	Contamination of PCB in rice bran oil	7.8% (1993)
1979	Taiwan/Changhua, Taichung (Lü and Wu 1985 [725])	2061	PCB	Contamination of PCB in rice bran oil	17% (1993)

Modified from Ju et al. 2012 [**716**] copyright Elsevier.
PCB, polychlorinated biphenyls; PCDD, polychlorinated dibenzofurans.

Table 90.37 Differential signs of chloracne versus acne vulgaris.

Clinical signs	Chloracne	Acne vulgaris
Usual age	Any	Adolescent
Comedones	Many (essential sign)	Present
Inflammatory papules and cysts	Uncommon	Common
Straw-coloured cysts	Pathognomonic	Rare
Temporal comedones	Diagnostic	Rare
Retroauricular involvement	Common	Uncommon
Nose involvement	Often spared	Involved
Associated systemic findings	Common	Rare

Modified from McDonnell and Taylor 2000 [**718**] copyright Springer.

- Sebaceous gland involution after a complete loss of structure. The remaining sebocytes appear normal. Sebaceous gland involution is due to cessation of sebocyte replenishment.

Management
The aim of treatment is to lower or to eliminate the accumulated dioxins in the body at the very beginning of intoxication, e.g. by using dioxin-chelating substances such as synthetic dietary fat substitutes. The problem of dioxin contamination and its potential health hazards should be taken seriously during the current wave of industrial globalization. Management is as follows:
- Olestra potato chips (Pringles® fat-free potato chips, 10 g olestra/28 g potato chips) over 38 days, using five different dosing regimens (from 15 to 66 g olestra daily) lasting 7 days each [726].
- Topical tretinoin over 1 year.

Prepubertal acne

Definition and nomenclature
Acne before the onset of puberty is uncommon. Descriptive terms used for acne in pre-adolescent children are generally based on age and include neonatal, infantile, mid-childhood and prepubertal or pre-adolescent acne. A recent classification of acne in children based on expert consensus included five subtypes according to age, i.e. neonatal, infantile, mid childhood, pre-adolescent and adolescent. However, the distinction between pre-adolescence and adolescence by age can be challenging; the term prepubertal acne has been adopted for use in this text.

Synonyms and inclusions
- Neonatal
- Infantile
- Mid-childhood acne

Introduction and general description
Prepubertal acne includes a number of clinical presentations and may be misdiagnosed. The definition by age does not necessarily identify children that are at risk of treatable forms of virilization and a focused history and examination should be adopted to ensure underlying hormonal abnormalities, adrenal or gonadal tumours are identified.

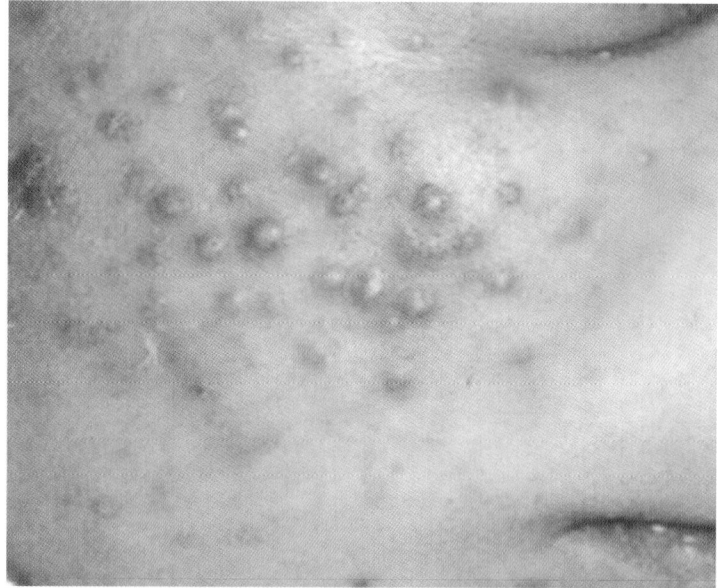

Figure 90.73 Neonatal cephalic pustulosis.

A broad range of treatment options are available but some medications used in the management of adult acne are contraindicated in children [729].

Epidemiology

Incidence

Neonatal acne defined as the presence of even a small number of comedones may affect up to 20% of neonates; however, this may reflect an overestimate as papulopustular conditions may masquerade as neonatal acne [730]. The most well recognized is neonatal cephalic pustulosis an acneform eruption thought to be caused by *Malassezia* (Figure 90.73) [731].

Infantile and mid-childhood. Infantile acne is less common than neonatal acne and mid-childhood acne is very rare [732,733].

Prepubertal acne. Prepubertal acne is defined as acne that commences before the onset of puberty. Acne has been reported in 60–71.3% of premenarchal females [16]. A mid-facial comedonal distribution is associated with poor prognosis (Figure 90.74).

Age and gender
Based on recent consensus [**569**] prepubertal acne can be defined as acne according to age as outlined in Table 90.38.

Neonatal acne. A neonate is defined as a newborn up to 35 days of age. Neonatal acne presents at birth through to the age of 4–6 weeks and is seen more frequently in boys (5 : 1) [734–737].

Infantile acne typically presents between 3 and 12 months but may occur as late as 16 months [738]. It shows a male predominance [732] (Figure 90.75).

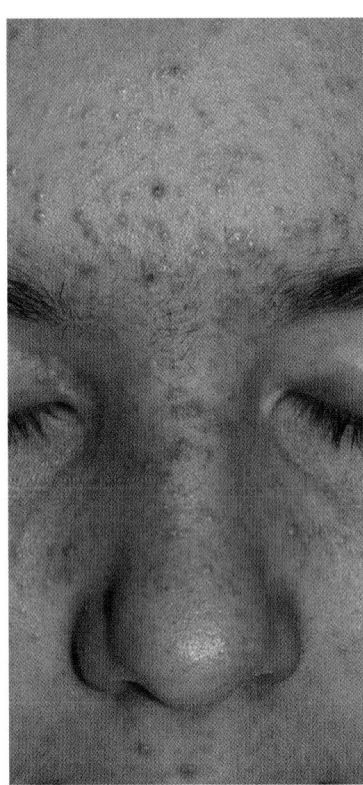

Figure 90.74 Mid-facial comedones are associated with poor prognosis.

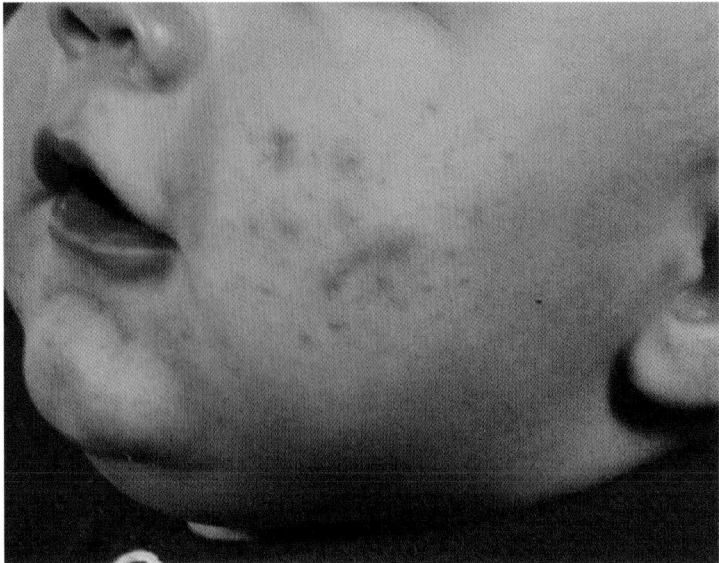

Figure 90.75 Infantile acne on the cheek. (Courtesy of Dr J. Ravenscroft, Queens Medical Centre, Nottingham, UK.)

Mid-childhood acne occurs from age 1 to 7 years.

Prepubertal acne presents before true puberty. Adrenarche represents maturation of the adrenal glands with adrenal production and increase in the return of the zona reticularis and acquisition of enzymes that facilitate synthesis of androgens from cholesterol. Adrenarche occurs at the age of 6–7 years in females and 7–8 years in boys. Prepubertal acne may occur from age 7 to 11 years [735,736]. However, depending on the age of puberty this will vary. Girls may present with acne as young as 8 years of age.

Ethnicity
There are no good studies comparing ethnicity in prepubertal acne but slight variation in the onset of puberty may influence the age of onset. The mean age of puberty in white girls is 10.2 years compared with 9.6 years in African Americans [739].

Associated diseases
Prepubertal acne may be associated with underlying endocrinopathies and virilizing tumours. SAPHO syndrome has been reported in childhood. Chronic cutaneous lesions were identified in 80% of

Table 90.38 Prepubertal acne defined according to age.

Acne description	Age of onset
Neonatal	Birth to 4–6 weeks
Infantile	6 weeks up to 1 year
Mid-childhood	1–7 years
Pre-adolescent	7 years up to 12 years or menarche in girls
Adolescent	12 years up to 19 years or after menarche in girls

children with SAPHO at follow-up visits at the University Children's Hospitals in Bern and Zurich and of 260 cases reported in the literature 25% had inflammatory skin problems with 6% of these presenting with severe acne [740]. There are other medical conditions in which acne is either absent or very mild. This includes Turner syndrome [741]. There appears to be a reduction of peripheral androgen production in these patients and the use of conventional hormonal replacement therapy that further decreases testosterone and dihydrotestosterone may explain the absence of moderate to severe acne in Turner syndrome.

Pathophysiology
The underlying pathogenesis of neonatal acne is not clearly understood but thought to relate to hyperactivity of the sebaceous glands stimulated by neonatal androgens from the testes in boys and adrenals in girls and boys [742]. Maternal androgens are thought to be transferred transplacentally and the hyperactive neonatal adrenal glands in both sexes result in an increased production of DHEA and the sulphated form DHEAS. During the neonatal period and for approximately 1 year afterwards, the adrenals secrete androgens. This restarts in mid-childhood, around 7 years of age, at which time the zona reticularis produces androgens again.

From birth through 6–12 months, there are pubertal levels of luteinizing hormone; in boys, this results in additional testosterone production as a result of the high levels of luteinizing hormone stimulating the testes. This may explain the increased incidence of neonatal acne in boys [743]. Increased sebum production in the first few months returns to normal at about 6 months.

The aetiology of infantile acne also remains poorly understood. Similar to neonatal acne, it may be associated with increased levels of androgens produced by adrenal glands in both sexes and by the testes in boys. DHEA from the adrenal glands stimulates sebum production for up to a year of age or until the DHEA levels drop at about 6–12 months [732].

Box 90.8 Examination and investigations that should be considered to rule out an endocrinopathy in prepubertal acne

History and examination
- Age of menarche in girls
- Tanner stage
- Telarche (palpable breast tissue below the areolae in girls, testicular enlargement in boys
- Pubarche (presence of pubic hair)
- Growth chart
- Height, weight, body mass index
- Bone age (left hand and wrist X-ray for those with high growth parameters)

Endocrine work-up
- Free and total testosterone
- DHEAS, luteinizing hormone, follicle-stimulating hormone
- Prolactin
- 17 hydroxy-progesterone (to rule out congenital adrenal hyperplasia)

During adrenarche, the secretion of androgens DHEA and DHEAS by the adrenal gland starts to increase resulting in androgen-mediated sebum production. DHEAS levels have been reported to be significantly higher in prepubertal girls with acne when compared to controls [16,744]. Gonadal secretions of androgens are very low at this stage. The development of mid-facial comedonal acne is considered a predictor acne severity [745].

Acute onset, persistent or severe acne particularly in the presence of virilization between 1 and 7 years of age should always raise the possibility of an underlying endocrinopathy. Infantile acne has been reported as an initial sign of an adrenocortical tumour in a 23-month-old boy with accelerated growth and signs of virilization [746]. In females, ovarian androgen excess is most commonly related to PCOS but rarely may be a consequence of benign or malignant ovarian tumours [747]. In boys, recalcitrant or severe acne may be a presenting sign of non-classical congenital adrenal hyperplasia [748].

A focused history and examination for signs of accelerated growth, precocious puberty and hirsutism or other signs of hyperandrogenism should be employed. Box 90.8 outlines a suggested approach. Referral to a paediatric endocrinologist should be considered.

Predisposing factors
See main section on acne vulgaris.

Causative organisms
Propionibacterium acnes is implicated in the pathophysiology of acne (see section on the pathophysiology of acne vulgaris).

The onset of sebum production triggers the expansion of *P. acnes* and this occurs earlier in children who develop acne than in those who do not [749].

In the case of neonatal cephalic pustulosis, a relationship has been suggested between the clinical presentation and *Malasezzia furfur*, *Malasezzia sympodialis* and other species [750] but not others [751].

Genetics
See genetic factors in the acne vulgaris section.

Environmental factors
Certain medications may be implicated in prepubertal acne as identified in the section on drug-induced acne. Maternal ingestion of phenytoin has been implicated [752]. Exposure to certain substances including greasy emollients, hair gels, occlusive topical agents as well as aromatic hydrocarbons and halogenides may be a trigger.

Clinical features
In the neonatal period, acne may present at birth or shortly afterwards up to 28 days [753]. It is a self-limiting benign process and does not generally result in any scarring.

Infantile acne is said to be seen more rarely than neonatal acne but is often misdiagnosed [754]. Neonatal acne typically presents after 6 months and most cases resolve by the age of 5 years but occasionally some remain as a continuum until puberty [743]. A history of a sibling with infantile acne may be notable and a family history of severe acne is not uncommon [755].

Mid-childhood acne presenting between the ages of 1 and 7 years is extremely rare. Production of androgens from the neonatal adrenal glands ceases around 1 year of life until the onset of adrenarche around the age of 7 years. As outlined previously, causes of hyperandrogenism should be ruled out if acne presents in this age group.

Presentation

Neonatal acne presents at or shortly after birth with erythematous papulopustular lesions commonly distributed on the cheeks, chin and forehead (Figure 90.76). Occasionally, these extend to the neck, scalp and upper trunk.

Infantile acne starts later than neonatal acne from 3 up to 16 months of age. The central cheeks are frequently affected [754] with a combination of inflamed papules and pustules with open

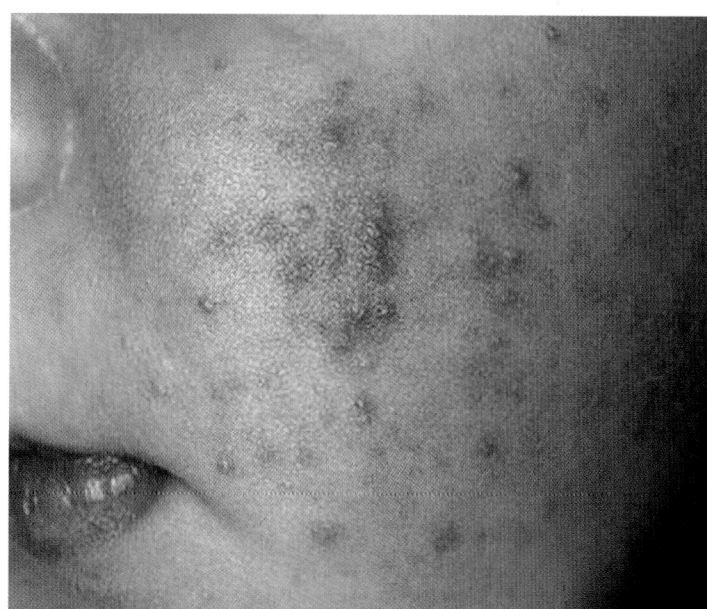

Figure 90.76 Neonatal acne presenting in the first few weeks of life.

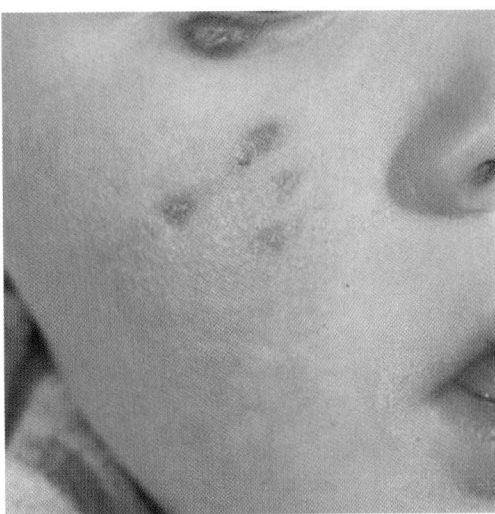

Figure 90.77 Infantile acne may involve cystic lesions and scarring. (Courtesy of Dr J. Ravenscroft, Queens Medical Centre, University of Nottingham, UK.)

and closed comedones. The presentation is usually more widespread than neonatal acne [755].

A study of 29 patients with infantile/juvenile acne seen in a specialist centre over a period of 25 years [755] demonstrated the median age of onset was 9 months; the disease was mild in 24%, moderate in 62% and severe in 14%. In 59%, the acne was predominantly inflammatory. Five patients (17%) were left with scarring.

Acne conglobata can present in infants resulting in severe inflammatory cystic lesions, sinus tract formation and significant scarring [729] (Figure 90.77).

Mid-childhood acne. Acne developing at an early age should always raise the suspicion of androgen excess.

Prepubertal acne. Acne in prepubertal children usually presents with comedonal lesions with or without some inflammatory papules. Lesions are frequently located in a mid-facial distribution and may precede any other signs of maturation [756]. Mid-facial comedonal acne (see Figure 90.74) can be the first sign of pubertal maturation in females, preceding areolar development, pubic hair and the menarche [16]. The development of acne in childhood along with premature adrenarche may be an initial sign of PCOS or metabolic syndrome [757,758]. Follow-up and anticipatory guidance is indicated in these children.

Clinical variants

Neonatal cephalic pustulosis has been considered by some as synonymous with neonatal acne but others consider it a separate entity as there are more inflammatory papules, significant pustules and a lack of comedonal lesions.

Acne conglobata is a severe variant of acne that can present in infants resulting in severe inflammatory cystic lesions, sinus tract formation and significant scarring [729].

Differential diagnosis

Neonatal acne. The differential diagnosis for neonatal acne [626] is outlined in Box 90.9.

Box 90.9 Differential diagnosis of acne in the neonate

Infections
- Bacterial
- *Staphylococcus aureus* (bullous impetigo)
- *Streptococcus* (β-haemolytic group B)
- *Pseudomonas aeruginosa*
- *Haemophilus influenzae*
- *Listeria monocytogenes*
- Fungal
- Candidiasis
- *Pityrosporum folliculitis*
- Viral
  - Herpes simplex
  - Varicella–zoster
  - Cytomegalovirus
- Parasitic
  - Scabies
  - Non-infectious
  - Erythema toxicum neonatorum
  - Infantile acropustulosis
  - Transient neonatal pustular melanosis

Other
- Milia
- Sebaceous gland hyperplasia
- Pustular miliariasis
- Eosinophilic pustular folliculitis of infancy
- Acneform eruptions
- Acne venenata infantum
- Acneform drug eruptions (steroids, lithium, hydantoin)
- Chloracne

Neonatal cephalic pustulosis was first described in 1991 [759] and historically referred to as neonatal acne [731]. This usually presents in the first 3 weeks of life (see Figure 90.76), and prevalence varies between 10 and 66% of newborns in the literature. It is characterized by erythematous papular/pustular lesions especially on the cheeks but also on the chin, eyelids, neck and upper chest. Comedonal lesions are not usually seen. It has been postulated that neonatal cephalic pustulosis develops in association with *Malassezia sympodialis* and *Malassezia globosa*; however, the exact aetiological role of *Malassezia* is uncertain, as the organism is part of the normal flora of neonatal skin, and up to 38% of cases had negative smears in one study [760]. Another explanation is that neonatal cephalic pustulosis relates to an overgrowth of lipophilic yeasts at birth that results in an inflammatory reaction leading to monomorphic papules and pustules in predisposed neonates with more sebum production.

Treatment is usually not required for neonatal cephalic pustulosis as it is a self-limiting disorder which usually heals without scarring in 1–3 months. If the condition does persist beyond this time and/or is widespread and unsightly, topical ketoconazole cream expedites recovery [732,761].

Infantile acne. The differential diagnosis of infantile acne includes neonatal acne, acne venenata infantum, chloracne and hyperandrogenism.

Mid-childhood acne. The differential diagnosis of mid-childhood acne includes keratosis pilaris and milia alongside endocrinopathies and conditions relating to hyperandrogenism as outlined in Box 90.9.

Prepubertal acne. The differential diagnosis of prepubertal acne includes childhood granulomatous periorifacial dermatitis, lupus miliaris disseminatus faciei and childhood granulomatous rosacea alongside endocrinopathies and disorders associated with an androgen excess as outlined in Box 90.9.

Classification of severity

Unlike adult acne, there is no recognized or validated grading system for prepubertal acne [755]. Severity is assessed as mild, moderate or severe and the persistence or appearance of scarring should be considered as a less favourable prognostic factors.

Investigations

It is important to consider underlying endocrinopathies and investigate accordingly with the support of a paediatric endocrinologist (see Box 90.8). A recent study indicated that there is a relatively low risk of true endocrinopathy in pre-adolescent children in the context of no other symptoms or signs of androgen excess [762].

Complications and co-morbidities

Acne scarring can result from acne lesions as in adult acne. In one study examining cases of infantile acne, secondary scarring affected 17% of the cases [755]. Acne conglobata is rarely seen in infants but the incidence of scarring is high in these patients [732–754]. Patients with infantile acne may develop a resurgence of their acne as teenagers and the likelihood of developing acne in adolescence is greater in these patients than in their peers [743].

Infantile acne is very rarely associated with other clinical features of androgen excess such as hirsutism or premature closure of the epiphyses; very occasionally, there may be transient or more persistent high plasma levels of testosterone, luteinizing hormone and follicle-stimulating hormone.

Disease course and prognosis

Neonatal acne usually settles spontaneously and leaves little scarring.

Infantile acne has a more persistent and variable course than neonatal acne and although most cases resolve by 5 years of age others may persist until puberty. Scarring from the deep-seated inflammatory lesions may ensue [755]. Patients with infantile acne may develop a resurgence of their acne as teenagers and parents should be advised accordingly [729,732,743,755,763,764].

Predictive factors for severity and persistence include a high number of comedones, mid-facial distribution, early development of comedones and high of normal levels of DHEAS, free and total testosterone and earlier menarche in females.

Management

General principles

The principles of treating acne in children involve adopting simple regimens that target the clinical lesions and pathophysiological factors implicated in acne whilst avoiding adverse effects. Most acne therapies are approved for children of 12 years and older. The exceptions include erythromycin, tetracycline derivatives approved for children 8 years and older by the FDA, adapalene/BPO gel approved for patients 9 years and older and tretinoin approved for patients 10 years and older. Apart from tetracycline antibiotics that should not be prescribed below 12 years of age in the UK because of the risk of damage to developing bones and permanent discoloration of dentition, most acne treatments are not contraindicated in younger children but they may be used off license. It is important to ensure parents are appropriately informed.

For mild disease, topical therapies such as topical retinoids and/or topical antimicrobials are recommended. For moderate disease, a topical retinoid and/or BPO combined with a systemic antibiotic such as erythromycin (as ethyl succinate, 125 mg three times a day) should be adopted. Systemic trimethoprim has also been used (100 mg twice daily) [755]. If prescribing an antibiotic, topical BPO should be used alongside the agent to reduce the likelihood of bacterial resistance emerging in *P. acnes*.

Deep nodules can be injected with a low concentration of intralesional triamcinolone acetonide (2.5 mg/mL). Infantile acne may take several months to resolve – the more inflammatory the disease, the longer the duration [755].

Isotretinoin is rarely needed, and only for severe non-responding cases. Successful treatment with isotretinoin has been reported in the literature using doses of 0.36–2 mg/kg/day for 4–6 months in children younger than 5 years [756–767]. Topical retinoids may provide maintenance following successful therapy [739].

In most cases of neonatal acne, daily cleansing is all that is needed; however, if more extensive topical agents aimed at treating comedonal and/or apparent inflammatory lesions should be employed.

First line

Neonatal acne: if lesions are causing concern or are more moderate to severe in nature an approach as outlined in Table 90.39 should be adopted for acne pre-adrenarche.

Table 90.39 Algorithm of therapeutic options for neonatal, infantile, mid-childhood and prepubertal acne.

Acne category	Treatment options
Neonatal	Gentle cleaners, oil-free emollients
	If marked pustules topical azole cream
Infantile	**First line**
Prepubertal	Benzoyl peroxide or topical retinoid (if primarily comedonal)
	Fixed combination products if mixed lesions all indicated from 12 years with the exception of 0.1% adapalene/2.5% BPO which is indicated from 9 years
	Second line for more severe disease
	Oral erythromycin (oral trimethoprim if allergic to macrolides) combined with benzoyl peroxide to avoid emergence of antibiotic-resistant *P. acnes* ± topical retinoid
	Third line
	Severe recalcitrant scarring acne, exclude underlying hyperandrogenism
	Consider oral isotretinoin
Mid-childhood	Exclude underlying pathology and treat as infantile and prepubertal

Table 90.40 Dosage regimens for isotretinoin in childhood acne.

Sex	Onset age of acne (months)	Isotretinoin dosage (mg/kg/day)	Duration (months)	Side effects	References
Female	18	0.5–1	5	Reduced hair growth, mood changes, high lactate dehydrogenase	[769]
Male	2 (comedones) 10 (cystic)	0.36–0.67	5	High serum glutamic-pyruvic transaminase and glutamic-oxaloacetic transaminase	[770]
Male	12	1	4	Mild eczema on neck	[771]
Male	6	0.5	4	None	[772]
Female	20	1 then 2 (+ prednisolone)	6 5	Transient umbilical granulation	[773]
Male	?	0.5	4	?	[774]
Female	20	0.5–0.6	7	None	[775]
Female	6	0.2–1.5	14	None	**[776]**
Female	7	0.5	5	None	
Male	9	?	–	None	[777]
Male	6	?		None	
Male	0	0.5	12	Transient perioral exanthema, diarrhoea 3 weeks	[778]
Male	4	0.5	4	None	[779]
Male	5	0.5–1	6	Slight lip desquamation	[780]

Second line

If oral antibiotics are required for more moderate to severe disease erythromycin is the treatment of choice [742]. Of note, oral tetracycline is contraindicated in children of less than 8 years of age in the US and 12 years in Europe as they can cause damage to developing dentitian and bones [756].

Third line

Clinicians face a dilemma when a patient presents with severe recalcitrant acne that is causing scarring and cosmetic sequelae where treatment with oral isotretinoin could be beneficial. Currently, oral isotretinoin is approved by the FDA and European Commission for the treatments of nodulocystic recalcitrant acne in children over 12 years of age [555,768].

However, there are reports in the literature confirming the safe and successful use of oral isotretinoin in patients ranging from 5 to 20 months of age. All patients had recalcitrant scarring acne that had failed to respond to topical and oral medications usually used for acne. The ideal dose of isotretinoin is not defined but Table 90.40 summarizes the dosage regimes used and the outcomes. Published reports suggest a dose range from 0.2 to 2 mg/kg/day divided in doses with food or milk to maximize absorption.

Administering capsules can be challenging in children of this age, isotretinoin is highly light sensitive and oxygen labile so splitting capsules may reduce potential efficacy if not conducted in dim light. Although mixing with food has been advocated this may affect the stability of the drug [767]. Freezing the capsule to a solid constituency enables it to be divided into halves or quarters to deliver the desired dose. This prevents drug wastage, minimizes degradation of the drug and masks any unacceptable taste [756].

Given that the use of isotretinoin is an off license indication in this context, clinicians should ensure parents are well informed if using oral isotretinoin for acne in this age group.

Resources

Further information

Eichenfield LF, Krakowski AC, Piggot C, *et al.* Evidence based recommendations for the diagnosis and treatment of paediatric acne. Paediatrics 2013;131:S163–86.

Key references

The full list of references can be found in the online version at www.rooksdermatology.com.

6 Thiboutot D, Gollnick H, Bettolli V, *et al.* New insights into the management of acne: an update from the Global Alliance to Improve Outcomes in Acne Group. *J Am Acad Dermatol* 2009;60(5 Suppl.):S1–50.

120 Momin SB, Peterson A, Del Rosso JQ. A status report on drug-associated acne and acneiform eruptions. *J Drugs Dermatol* 2010;9:627–36.

276 Kurokawa I, Danby FW, Ju Q, *et al.* New developments in our understanding of acne pathogenesis and treatment. *Exp Dermatol* 2009;18:821–32.

426 Barratt H, Hamilton F, Car J, *et al.* Outcome measures in acne vulgaris: systematic review. *Br J Dermatol* 2009;160:132–6.

473 Nast A, Dréno B, Bettoli V, *et al.* European evidence-based (S3) guidelines for the treatment of acne. *J Eur Acad Dermatol Venereol* 2012;26(Suppl. 1):1–29.

474 Dreno B, Bettoli V, Ochsendorf F, *et al.* An expert view on the treatment of acne with systemic antibiotics and/or oral isotretinoin in the light of the new European recommendations. *Eur J Dermatol* 2006;15:565–71.

562 Eady EA, Jones CE, Tipper JL, *et al.* Antibiotic resistant propionibacteria in acne: need for policies to modify usage. *BMJ* 1993;306:555–6.

568 Miller IM, Echeverría B, Torrelo A, Jemec GB. Infantile acne treated with oral isotretinoin. *Pediatr Dermatol* 2013;3:513–18.

569 Eichenfield LF, Krakowski AC, Piggot C, *et al*. Evidence based recommendations for the diagnosis and treatment of pediatric acne. *Pediatrics* 2013;131(Suppl. 3): S163–86.

664 Jansen T, Plewig G. Acne fulminans. *Int J Dermatol* 1998;37:254–7.

671 Seukeran DC, Cunliffe WJ. The treatment of acne fulminans: a review of 25 cases. *Br J Dermatol* 1999;141:307–9.

678 Ehrenfeld M, Samra Y, Kaplinsky N, *et al*. Acne conglobata and arthritis: report of a case and review of the literature. *Clin Exp Rheumatol* 1986;5:407–9.

700 Schwartz RA. Acne conglobata treatment and management http://emedicine. medscape.com/article/1072716-treatment (last accessed November 2015).

716 Ju Q, Yiang K, Zouboulis CC, Ring J, Chen W. Chloracne: from clinic to research. *Dermatol Sinica* 2012;30:2–6.

717 Ju Q, Zouboulis CC, Xia L. Environmental pollution and acne-chloracne. *Dermatoendocrinology* 2009;1:125–8.

718 McDonnell JK, Taylor JS. Occupational and environmental acne. In: Kanerva L, Elsner P, Wahlberg JE, Maibach HI, eds. *Handbook of Occupational Dermatology*. Berlin: Springer-Verlag, 2000:225–33.

776 Barnes CJ, Eichenfield LF, Lee J, *et al*. A practical approach for the use of isotretinoin for infantile acne. *Pediatr Dermatol* 2005;22:166–9.

**PART 8: SPECIFIC
CUTANEOUS STRUCTURE**

CHAPTER 91

Rosacea

Frank C. Powell

Charles Institute of Dermatology, University College Dublin, Dublin, Ireland

Definition and nomenclature

The definition of what constitutes the skin disorder rosacea has changed over time. Originally the term acne rosacea was used for this condition, and this equates to the condition currently referred to as papulopustular rosacea. The term rosacea has since been applied by dermatologists to a constellation of clinical features that present in patients who have in common a chronic disorder that primarily affects their face with a tendency to facial erythema and, in a significant number of cases, their eyes.

Synonyms and inclusions
- Acne rosacea
- Rosacea acuminate
- Gutta rosea
- Bacchia rosacea
- Couperose (French)
- Kupferrose (German)
- Rhinophyma has also been called brandy nose, copper nose and bulbous nose

Classification and grading of severity

Because the pathogenesis of rosacea is poorly understood, it is useful to classify rosacea into one of four subtypes based on the clinical features that predominate in each patient [1]. While this is a useful guide it has limitations. In clinical practice there is an overlap of clinical features between the different subtypes and individual patients may have more than one subtype at any given time. The subtypes are listed below and described in Table 91.1 together with guidelines on grading the severity of disease:
- Subtype 1: Erythematotelangiectatic rosacea (ETTR).
- Subtype 2: Papulopustular rosacea (PPR).
- Subtype 3: Phymatous rosacea (PR).
- Subtype 4: Ocular rosacea (OR).

Evolution of one subtype into another is not implied in this classification (i.e. subtypes are not equivalent to stages of progression).

To help monitor a patient's progress with therapy, the subtype with which they present should be graded 1 to 3 according to the severity of the clinical symptoms and signs (where grade 1 denotes mild disease, grade 2 moderate, and grade 3 severe disease). The impact of the disorder on the patient (psychological/social/occupational) should be included in the evaluation of severity [2].

Introduction and general description

The term 'rosacea' encompasses a spectrum of changes that occur mainly in the facial skin but may also involve the eyes.

Rook's Textbook of Dermatology, Ninth Edition. Edited by Christopher Griffiths, Jonathan Barker, Tanya Bleiker, Robert Chalmers and Daniel Creamer.
© 2016 John Wiley & Sons, Ltd. Published 2016 by John Wiley & Sons, Ltd.
Companion website: www.rooksdermatology.com

Table 91.1 Rosacea subtypes: clinical features and severity grading.

Subtype	Clinical features

Subtype 1: erythematotelangiectatic rosacea (ETTR)
Mild (grade 1):
  Occasional flushing
  Mild erythema
Moderate (grade 2):
  Frequent flushing
  Moderate erythema
  Telangiectases present
Severe (grade 3):
  Severe flushing
  Marked erythema
  Many telangiectases
	• Individuals usually have skin type 1 or 2
	• Facial erythema present usually with telangiectases
	• Facial vascular hyperreactivity and a tendency to flushing with environmental temperature change and some dietary components (hot liquids, etc.)
	• Skin sensitivity and dryness – easily irritated skin, frequent burning and stinging sensation
	• Intolerance of sunlight/harsh winds

Subtype 2: papulopustular rosacea (PPR)
Mild (grade 1):
  Few papules/pustules (<5)
  Mild perilesional erythema
  Little tendency to flush
Moderate (grade 2):
  Several papules/pustules (>5 but <10)
  Significant coalescing erythema around lesions
  Tendency to temperature intolerance and flushing
Severe (grade 3):
  Many papules/pustules (>10)
  Plaques of coalescing erythema
  Oedema may be present
  Scaling and dermatitic changes may be present
  Marked intolerance of temperature change (cold to heat) with resultant flushing
	• Erythema (mainly centrofacial) mostly related to inflammatory lesions (perilesional erythema)
	• Telangiectases may be present
	• Dome-shaped erythematous papules and papulopustules (small areas of apical pustulation is usual) mainly on the central face but can occur elsewhere (scalp/behind ears)
	• Flushing and skin sensitivity may be present but not as prominent as in ETTR
	• Dryness/dermatitis may be present in severe cases

Subtype 3: phymatous rosacea (PR)
For rhinophyma:
Mild (grade 1):
  Puffiness of nose
  Prominent follicular openings (patulous follicles)
  No change in nasal contour
Moderate (grade 2):
  Bulbous nasal swelling
  Change in nasal contour without nodular distortion
Severe (grade 3):
  Marked nasal swelling
  Nasal distortion with nodular component
	Rhinophyma:
	• Thickened, nodular skin
	• Patulous follicles (early disease)
	• Bulbous, distorted features (advanced disease)
	• Most commonly affects the nose but can also affect the chin, forehead (frontophyma), ears (otophyma) and eyelids
	• May be associated with other features of rosacea, occur in isolation, or be due to other causes (e.g. actinic damage)
	• Perinasal telangiectases sometimes prominent
	• Flushing not a common association

Subtype 4: ocular rosacea (OR)
Mild (grade1):
  Mild itch/gritty feeling
  Mild scaling/erythema of lid margins
  Mild conjunctival injection
Moderate (grade 2):
  Burning/stinging sensation
  Crusting/marked erythema of lid margins
  Collarettes and sleeves of keratin on the lash shafts
  Conjunctival injection
  Hordeolum/chalazion formation
Severe (grade3):
  Pain/photosensitivity
  Blurred vision
  Loss of eyelashes (madarosis)
  Corneal changes
  Scleral involvement
	• Usually bilateral but severity in each eye may vary
	• Dry, gritty sensation, sometimes itch
	• Watering of eyes
	• Conjunctival telangiectasia
	• Collarettes of scale around base of the eyelashes
	• Blepharitis with crusting
	• Swelling and erythema of eyelids
	• Chalazia (painless) and hordeola (painful)
	• Conjunctivitis/keratitis, episcleritis, scleritis, iritis (rare)

A common feature in the majority of patients with rosacea is the presence of facial erythema variably associated with the following:

- Facial vascular changes: subtype 1 (erythematotelangiectatic rosacea).
- Inflammatory lesions: subtype 2 (papulopustular rosacea).
- Hypertrophic changes: subtype 3 (phymatous rosacea).
- Ocular involvement: subtype 4 (ocular rosacea).

Rosacea is a chronic disorder with fluctuating severity. It is at least as common as psoriasis and affects predominantly fair-skinned individuals in middle age.

In the past it was assumed that rosacea was a single entity and a disorder that evolved progressively through stages, beginning with flushing and terminating in phymatous changes. However, the evidence for such progression through stages is lacking in individual patients and it may be that several closely related disorders are included in the subtype classification under the umbrella term rosacea.

The cause of rosacea is unknown. It is doubtful that any single aetiological factor is responsible for the diverse features that comprise this disorder. It appears that each of the different subtypes of rosacea has its own distinct pathogenetic pathway that is responsible for its particular clinical manifestations. The approach to treatment of a patient with rosacea is therefore strongly influenced by each patient's individual subtype. Thus, laser treatment may be indicated for subtype 1 (ETTR), antibiotic therapy (topical or systemic) for subtype 2 (PPR), surgery for subtype 3 (PR), and referral to an ophthalmologist for severe subtype 4 (OR) [2].

Epidemiology

Incidence and prevalence

Because the term rosacea is used to include such a broad spectrum of clinical features, many of which are not exclusive or specific for rosacea, the prevalence of rosacea in the population has been difficult to estimate accurately. Determination of the prevalence of the various subtypes of rosacea in the population is therefore likely to give more meaningful information.

A review of population studies of rosacea [3] has shown a prevalence ranging from 0.09% (Faroe Islands) to 2.3% (Germany) to 10% in Sweden and 22% in Estonia. While there is likely to be some genetically determined variation in prevalence in different countries, this marked difference in northern and central European studies more probably reflects the lack of a commonly accepted clear definition of rosacea and its subtypes. Those studies of subtype prevalence that have been carried out [4,5] and our own unpublished observations, have consistently shown that subtype 1 rosacea (ETTR) is by far the commonest subtype and is about four times more prevalent than subtype 2 (PPR).

Actinic damage in fair-skinned individuals can produce facial skin changes that are indistinguishable from those found in ETTR – facial erythema, facial vascular instability with temperature-related flushing and a propensity to the development of telangiectasia. Thus evaluating the prevalence of ETTR accurately in the general population is difficult if not impossible, particularly as there is as yet no specific diagnostic test for rosacea. With the above reservation, individuals who have clinical findings that satisfy the criteria for ETTR were found in 14% of the Irish population (unpublished observations [5]), 75% of whom have been shown to have skin types 1 or 2 [6].

Subtype 2 (PPR) is a well-defined clinical entity and the population studies of this subtype have been fairly consistent and have shown a prevalence of approximately 2% in northern European populations [3,5].

Individuals with subtype 3 (PR) are rarely identified in population studies. Those who are recorded almost always have rhinophyma. A study from Estonia stated that phymatous subtypes constituted 1% of all rosacea patients seen [4], and this probably reflects the experience of most clinicians who frequently see patients with rosacea. Of 1000 unselected Irish adults examined [5], only one individual was identified with rhinophyma, equating to a 0.1% prevalence in this population (unpublished observation).

The prevalence of subtype 4 (OR) is unknown because of the lack of specificity of the clinical features. Ocular features were associated with cutaneous changes of rosacea in 33% of 100 patients with cutaneous rosacea in Greece [7]. The incidence of rosacea in the UK has been reported to be 1.65 per 1000 person-years [8]; however the validity of this figure is open to question since the diagnostic criteria used to identify patients with rosacea in this retrospective database analysis were not established before collection of the data.

Age

Rosacea is predominantly a disease with onset in middle-aged adults (30–50 years old). Occasional cases of PPR and some cases of OR have been reported in children. The disorder appears to be less prevalent in the elderly. The age of onset of rosacea may be earlier in females than males [3].

Sex

Some population studies report a slight predominance of males affected by rosacea [5], while others (mainly hospital-based studies) suggest females are more frequently affected [8]. The different figures may reflect the varying age of onset of the condition and the age profile of the particular population studied, or possibly the increased likelihood of female patients presenting to their dermatologist for treatment. Male patients are said to develop more severe rosacea than women and are much more likely to develop rhinophyma than females.

Ethnicity

Rosacea is a disorder that predominantly affects fair, pale-skinned, sun-sensitive individuals: those of Celtic origin seem to be most susceptible (sometimes referred to as the 'curse of the Celts' for this reason). This is reflected in the much higher frequency with which rosacea is diagnosed in dermatology clinics in northern Europe as opposed to those in southern African countries with darker skin-type populations [9]. Rosacea also appears to be less common in individuals with an Asian skin type than with white skin.

Associated diseases

Patients who present with rosacea sometimes have associated facial seborrhoeic dermatitis. This can contribute to the facial erythema and skin sensitivity and needs to be treated separately for optimal results (see Chapter 40).

Migraine, depression and carcinoid syndrome have been suggested as occurring in association with rosacea but convincing evidence of a link between these conditions and rosacea is lacking.

An association between the cutaneous lesions of rosacea and gastrointestinal disturbance has long been considered, and in the past dietary measures (including hydrochloric acid dietary supplementation) have been recommended for treating rosacea. The possible role of *Helicobacter pylori* infection of the stomach causing vasoactive neuropeptide release was raised but subsequent studies suggest that such an association is unlikely. A recent report indicated that more than 50% of rosacea patients (mostly patients with ETTR) who were evaluated with a lactulose breath test showed evidence of small intestine bacterial infection. Treatment with rifaxin (a non-absorbed antibiotic acting locally within the intestine) resulted in significant improvement of the rosacea in the majority of these patients [10]. This study again suggests that a possible link between rosacea and gastrointestinal abnormalities should be re-evaluated.

Pathophysiology

The pathophysiology of rosacea is unknown. It is unlikely that a single pathophysiological pathway is responsible for the diverse clinical features seen in patients with the different subtypes of rosacea.

The role of *ultraviolet light* in the causation of rosacea has been repeatedly suggested and is supported by the facial distribution (mainly on the convexities) and its occurrence on the bald (exposed) scalp of male patients. Actinic elastosis is a prominent finding in facial skin biopsies from patients with rosacea, but whether this reflects the expected degree of change in middle-aged patients with skin types 1 or 2 or if this relates directly to the pathogenesis of rosacea is unclear.

It may be that ultraviolet light exposure is a subset-specific aetiological factor. Patients with ETTR consistently identify exposure to sunlight as well as wind and adverse weather conditions as factors that exacerbate their skin disorder. The degree of sun exposure was correlated with the severity of ETTR but not PPR in a Korean study [11]. In an Irish population study comparing PPR with individuals without rosacea, no significant relationship was shown between PPR and UV exposure or signs of actinic damage [5]. Indeed, some patients with PPR report an improvement in their skin condition after exposure to sunlight [12].

The extension of inflammatory PPR lesions onto the bald scalp of individuals with androgenetic alopecia might suggest that UV light is a causative factor. However, alteration in the follicles in androgenetic alopecia from terminal to vellus may also be significant and has to be considered as an alternative explanation.

The *innate immune response* in rosacea appears to be altered. Increased Toll-like receptor 2 (TLR2) activity, increased protease activity and cathelicidin production (LL-37) have been shown to occur in rosacea with the potential to increase angiogenesis, leukocyte chemotaxis production and extracellular matrix production. This pathophysiological mechanism is most likely to apply to patients with PPR [13].

Demodex mite proliferation in the pilosebaceous follicles of the face has also been suggested as a possible aetiological factor in the cutaneous and ocular inflammation seen in patients with PPR (see Chapter 34) [14]. These mites may also play a role in the modulation of the host innate immune system described above, as has been shown by other microorganisms in the skin microbiome [15]. Evidence to support the role of *Demodex* in the pathogenesis of rosacea include the following observations: (i) 1% ivermectin cream (which has been shown to reduce *Demodex* mite numbers) was significantly more effective than the cream vehicle in reducing numbers of inflammatory skin lesions in two large studies of PPR [16]; (ii) the use of topical calcineurin antagonists and systemic epidermal growth factor (EGF) inhibitor medications have been reported to result in rosacea-like dermatoses and an increased *Demodex* mite population (see section on causative organisms) [17].

Alterations in the cutaneous microenvironment in patients with rosacea such as changes in lipid profile, cutaneous pH or skin barrier function [18] may facilitate an overgrowth of commensal organisms, which may then trigger a host immune reaction once a critical level is reached.

It has been suggested that the phymatous changes of PR may be brought about by the up-regulation of fibrosis-promoting *matrix metalloproteinases* as a result of increased mast cell numbers and keratinocyte and macrophage activation [19]. The fact that some patients with rhinophyma do not record previous severe inflammatory PPR skin changes and the reason why rhinophyma occurs far more frequently in men than women (by a factor of up to 20) has yet to be explained by this hypothesis.

The pathogenesis of OR seems to be closely associated with *meibomian gland dysfunction*. A consistent finding is a reduced tear break-up time in patients with rosacea as a result of inadequate lipid components of the tear film. Meibomian cysts (usually painless), representing chronic inflammation of the meibomian glands, may appear in crops. It has been suggested that *Demodex* mite infestation may play a role in the initiation of inflammatory ocular changes that occur in these modified sebaceous glands of the eyelid. This hypothesis is supported by the presence of mites in the collarettes and sleeves of keratin at the bases of the lashes, indicating a possible common aetiological link between cutaneous and ocular rosacea [20].

Predisposing factors

Up to 25% of patients with rosacea have a family history of the condition, indicating a significant genetic predisposition in some individuals [21]. These patients may develop rosacea at an earlier age than those without a family history of the disorder. Studies have consistently shown that people with skin types 1 or 2 are more prone to developing rosacea than those with darker skin. It has been suggested that patients with the carcinoid syndrome who flush frequently are predisposed to developing rosacea, but convincing evidence for susceptibility to rosacea in this uncommon disease is lacking.

Pathology

The pathological findings in skin biopsies taken from patients with different subtypes of rosacea can differ significantly. A common finding is the histological evidence of chronic actinic damage, which is present in most biopsies, as might be expected in a predominantly sun-sensitive middle-aged population.

The histopathology of ETTR is characterized by the presence of enlarged and dilated bizarre-shaped capillaries and venules in the upper part of the dermis. A mild perivascular and interstitial lymphocytic infiltrate with frequent plasma cells is commonly seen in this subtype. Occasional *Demodex* mites may be present within the follicles. Solar elastosis (as mentioned earlier) is a prominent finding in ETTR patients.

The inflammatory infiltrate is much more conspicuous in PPR. While there is often a perivascular infiltrate of lymphocytes, the most marked changes involve the follicles, with numerous neutrophils, plasma cells and less commonly eosinophils. Increased numbers of mast cells have been reported in the lesional skin of rosacea patients and these may participate in the induction of inflammation and the recruitment of neutrophils. A correlation between the degree of follicular infestation with *Demodex* mites and the up-regulation of pro-inflammatory genes has been shown. Ruptured follicles with granulomatous changes may be present in florid cases. Sometimes *Demodex* mite remnants are seen within these granulomas or abscesses [22,23].

Sebaceous gland hyperplasia (which is marked in severe rhinophyma) with striking dermal fibrotic changes and a variable degree of perivascular lymphocytic/neutrophilic infiltration are the histological features of PR.

The histological findings of OR are non-specific. Blepharitis in rosacea mainly involves the posterior meibomian glands (posterior blepharitis). There is an inflammatory infiltrate (lymphocytic/histiocytic/neutrophilic) that varies according to the severity of the condition.

Some degree of granulomatous inflammation may be seen in biopsies from patients with all cutaneous forms of rosacea [24]. The term granulomatous rosacea (lupus miliaris disseminatus faciei, acnitis, acne agminata) is, however, best reserved for an uncommon variant which is discussed in further detail later in the chapter. In this condition sarcoidal or tuberculoid granulomas with or without abscess formation, were observed in biopsies from 25 patients with perifollicular fibrosis evident in some late lesions [25].

Causative organisms

The potential role of microorganisms in the pathogenesis of rosacea is supported by the up-regulation of TLR2 receptors in PPR and increased cathelicidin expression and leukocyte activity. A recent review of the microorganisms that might potentially induce rosacea has identified several possible candidates including *Staphylococcus epidermidis*, *Chlamydophila pneumoniae* and the *Demodex*-associated bacterium *Bacillus oleronius* [26]. Several studies have documented an increased population of *Demodex* mites in the facial skin of patients with rosacea [27,28]. A systematic review of case–control studies (with 28 527 participants) has shown a significant association between the degree of *Demodex* infestation and the presence of rosacea [29].

The biological significance and possible pathogenic potential of these ubiquitous mites is unknown [30]. Since they are present in the facial pilosebaceous follicles of adult humans with normal-appearing skin without causing any clinical or histological evidence of an inflammatory reaction, it is clear that in normal circumstances they excite no host immune reaction. However, they have the potential to induce inflammatory reactivity *in vitro* in cell culture environments (keratinocytes/sebocytes) and *Demodex* mites in histology sections of skin biopsy samples of PPR often show inflammatory changes located around the follicular infundibulum where the mites are found [20]. This suggests a possible pathogenetic role of these mites in this subtype. Their pathogenic potential may relate specifically to the size of the mite population (which is markedly increased in PPR patients) rather than simply their presence in the follicles.

Bacillus oleronius, isolated from a mite retrieved from a patient with rosacea, triggered a proliferative response in peripheral blood mononuclear cells of 73% of patients with PPR but only 29% of controls [31], indicating a prior sensitization in PPR patients. In another study the sera of 83% of a cohort of 75 patients with ETTR reacted to *B. oleronius* proteins on western blotting compared with only 27% of control sera. Reactivity was associated with reduced sebum secretion and a higher density of *Demodex* mites in facial skin (Figure 91.1) [32]. An increased interest in the potential role of this organism in skin disorders is indicated by a recently proposed classification of *Demodex*-related human dermatoses [33].

Genetics

Although up to 25% of patients with rosacea have a positive family history, no rosacea-specific genes have yet been identified. Transcriptome profiling analysis shows distinct gene profiles for each rosacea subtype (with certain genes overlapping between subtypes) [34]. This might suggest a 'developmental march' from an early inflammatory rosacea subtype to a more advanced fibrotic form, or alternatively support the hypothesis that each subtype represents a phenotype with clinical features

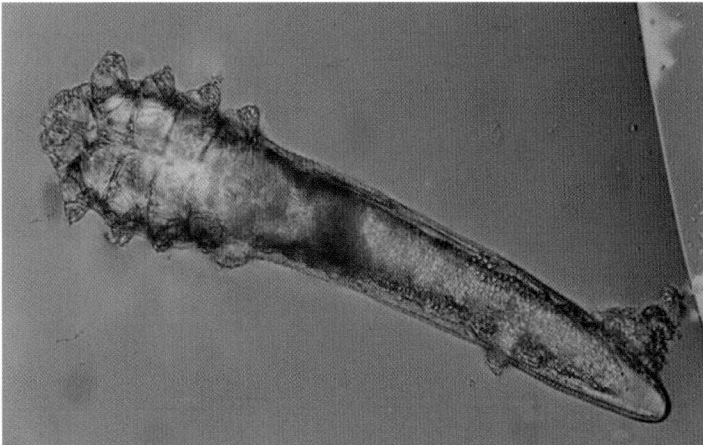

Figure 91.1 *Demodex folliculorum* mite showing its elongated worm-like posterior body (opistostoma) and four sets of short legs on the upper body (podostoma). The mouth parts (gnathostoma) are at the front of the podostoma. Magnification 100×.

that overlap with other subtypes but that there is a separate pathogenetic process in each subtype with different genes being up-regulated.

Environmental factors

Increased environmental temperature and dietary factors (ingesting hot liquids, spicy foods, large meals, alcohol, etc.) are often cited as potentially exacerbating rosacea. These elements may cause a transient increase in facial erythema and exacerbate a flushing tendency (predominantly in ETTR), but there is no evidence that they worsen the inflammatory lesions of PPR or the phymatous or ocular changes of PR and OR, respectively. In a UK retrospective database review, smokers were shown to be at a lower risk of developing rosacea than non-smokers, but caution in the interpretation of these results is necessary as the diagnostic criteria for rosacea in this and other retrospective reviews of large databases were not clearly defined before collection of the information.

Clinical features

Rosacea is a disorder that usually presents in middle age (peak onset between 35 and 50 years). Patients with rosacea present a spectrum of clinical features that differ according to each subtype.

History and presentation

Erythematotelangiectatic rosacea

Patients with ETTR usually complain of a gradual increase in facial redness. This affects the central face but is not confined to this region, with the lateral cheeks, the ears and sometimes the sides of the neck also being affected (Figure 91.2a). As the condition progresses patients note the onset of 'broken blood vessels' (telangiectases) (Figure 91.2b) and a tendency to a rapid-onset transient increase in facial redness (flushing) with environmental temperature change. Certain dietary constituents (hot liquids, spicy foods, alcohol, etc.) may also provoke flushing.

Many patients with ETTR, and to a lesser extent PPR, remark that their facial skin has become more sensitive and is easily irritated with skincare products that they formerly tolerated well, such as soaps, aftershave lotions, perfumed products, astringents, etc. Some patients complain of an unpleasant burning or stinging sensation in the skin; this is often exacerbated by sunlight and wind exposure. There is frequently other evidence of actinic damage (actinic keratoses, actinic lentigines, etc.) elsewhere on the face, ears or scalp in ETTR patients.

Papulopustular rosacea

Patients with PPR give a history of developing groups of 'spots, red bumps or pimples' that are located principally on the proximal cheeks, central chin, nose and central forehead (Figure 91.3a). The appearance of these inflammatory lesions is emphasized by the prominent perilesional erythema that in severe cases coalesces into plaques of inflammatory erythema (Figure 91.3b). There may also be mild facial oedema, most noticeable if there are widespread inflammatory lesions.

Individual lesions may be slightly tender but there are no associated symptoms such as pain, itch or discomfort. Some of these small dome-shaped papules (usually the minority) may have a tiny area of pustulation at the apex (Figure 91.3c).

Larger pustules occasionally occur in patients with PPR, but all lesions are relatively superficial and nodules and cysts are not a feature of PPR. Papules often appear to be in different stages of evolution and untreated lesions wax and wane spontaneously over a course of weeks. Lesions that resolve typically heal without scarring but may leave persistent post-inflammatory erythema. If scarring is present in a patient with PPR, it usually represents the result of previous acne vulgaris, which can be confirmed by an accurate history from the patient.

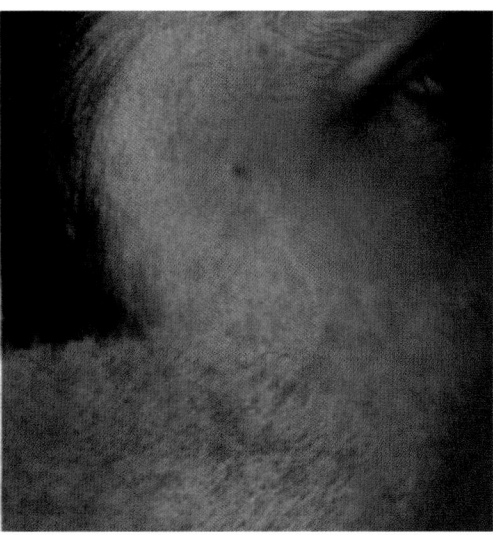
(a)

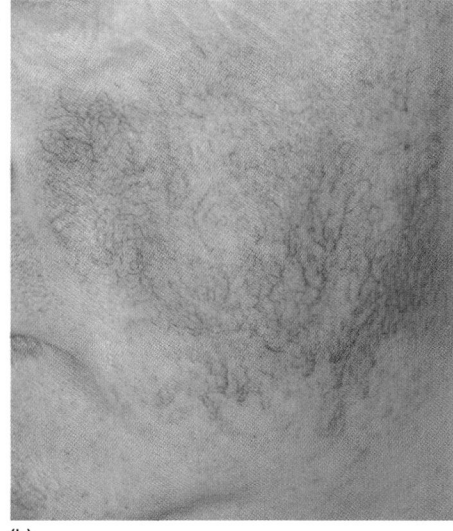
(b)

Figure 91.2 Erythematotelangiectatic rosacea (ETTR). (a) Facial erythema in moderate ETTR. (b) Prominent telangiectatic vessels on the lateral cheeks.

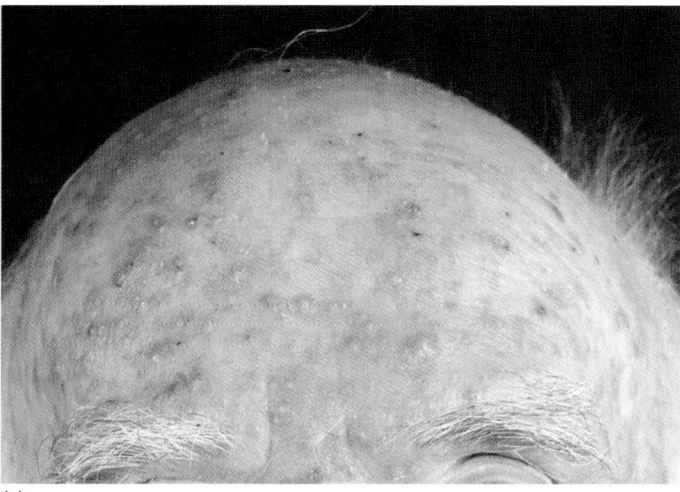

(a)

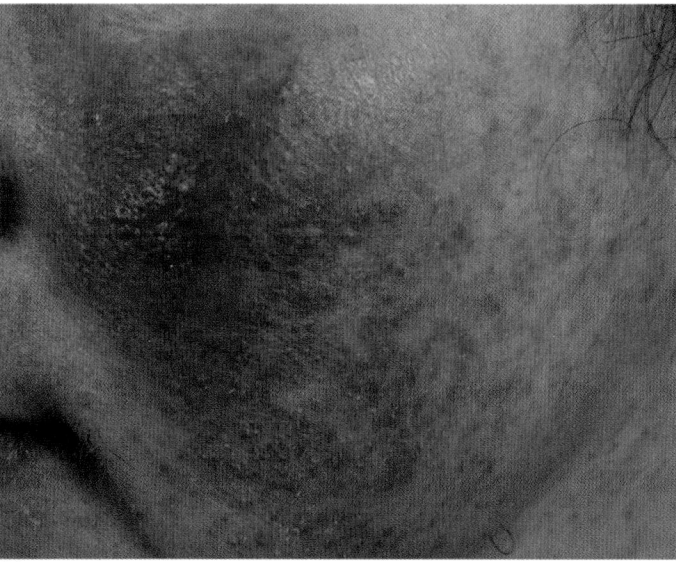

(b)

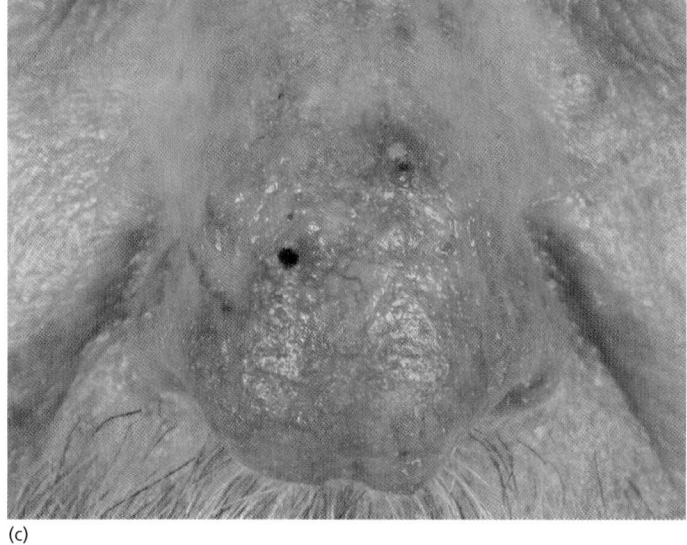

(c)

Figure 91.3 Papulopustular rosacea (PPR). (a) Papules and pustules on the forehead of a patient with PPR. (b) Erythema of the medial cheek area in a patient with grade 3 PPR who had several inflammatory lesions coalescing into a plaque in this area. (c) Small areas of pustulation are visible on the apex of some papules in this patient with grade 2 PPR on the bridge of his nose.

Phymatous rosacea

Rhinophyma (the commonest form of PR and seen typically in male patients) may appear *de novo* (without preceding inflammatory changes) or occur in a patient with pre-existing PPR. Rhinophyma has also been reported to follow actinic damage and to occur in patients with acne vulgaris. Patients with early rhinophyma generally complain of a thickening of the skin of their distal nose with increased prominence of the 'pores' (follicular openings). As the disorder progresses, patients remark that their nose is increasing in size and that the distal end is becoming bulbous. In severe rhinophyma, patients are only too well aware of the distortion in shape of their noses (Figure 91.4).

There is no associated pain or discomfort with these progressive nasal skin changes but the patient may note an unpleasant oiliness of the skin surface of the nose and malodorous greasy material may be discharged on squeezing the skin of the nose. The visual

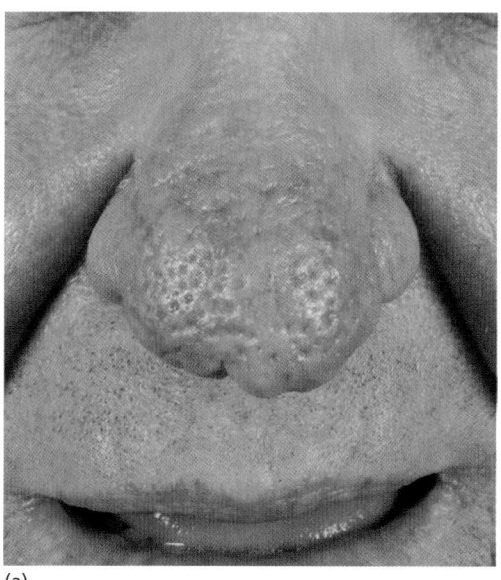

(a)

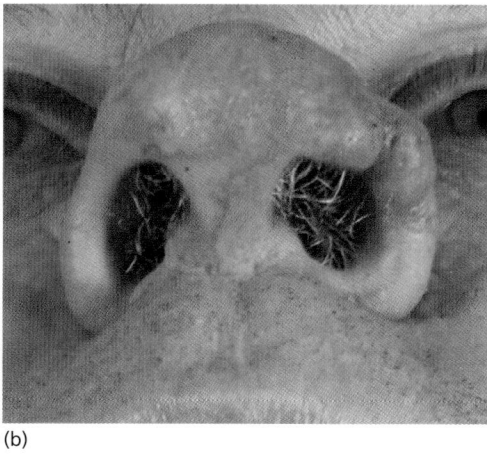

(b)

Figure 91.4 (a) Moderate to severe rhinophyma showing nasal distortion with a peau d'orange appearance of the prominent nasal follicles. (b) Swelling and distortion of the left ala nasi due to rhinophyma. Sometimes these changes are best visualized (as in this case) by viewing the nose from below.

impact of the condition (for themselves as well as for others) is usually the primary concern of patients presenting with rhinophyma. Skin surface biopsy to evaluate the contents of the dilated follicles in rhinophyma often reveals the presence of trichostasis as well as *Demodex* mites.

Enlargement of the ears (otophyma) is often overlooked in patients with longstanding rosacea, while thickening of the skin of the forehead (metophyma) sometimes with the formation of deep sulci creating a 'leonine' appearance can rarely be seen in rosacea patients.

Ocular rosacea

Patients who develop OR frequently complain of a sensation of dryness with slight itch or a 'gritty' feeling of the eyes in early-stage disease [20]. Patients who are in the habit of wearing contact lenses may complain of newly acquired intolerance to these. Paradoxically, some patients complain of 'watering' of their eyes (possibly reflecting the inadequate lipid contribution to the tear film from the meibomian glands with compensatory hypersecretion of the aqueous component from the lacrimal glands). With more advanced ocular involvement, rosacea patients complain of a burning/stinging sensation and there may be scaling or crusting of the eyelashes (blepharitis) and the development of styes at the lid margins (hordeolum and chalazion) and/or cysts in the eyelids (Figure 91.5).

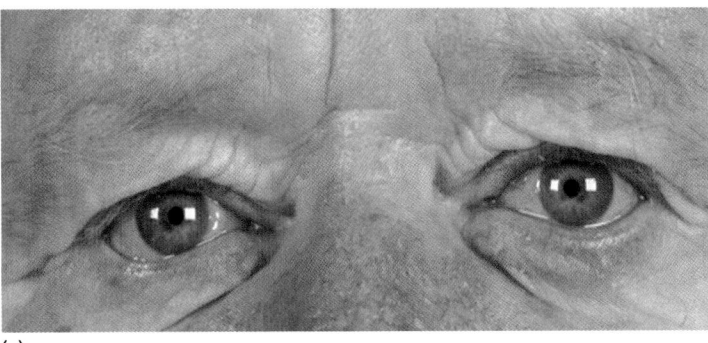

(a)

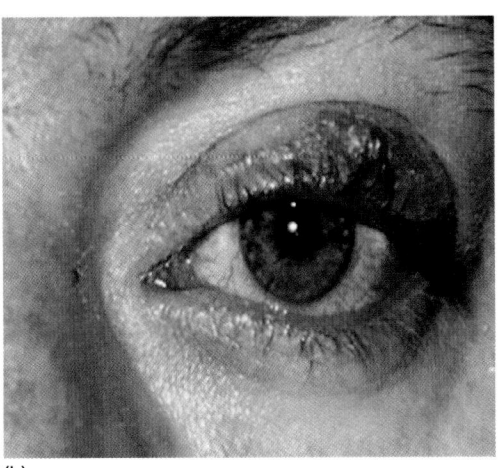

(b)

Figure 91.5 Ocular rosacea (OR). (a) Moderate (grade 2) OR with bilateral involvement, particularly of the lower eyelids. (b) More severe (grade 3) OR in this patient with chalazion of the upper lid and conjunctival injection.

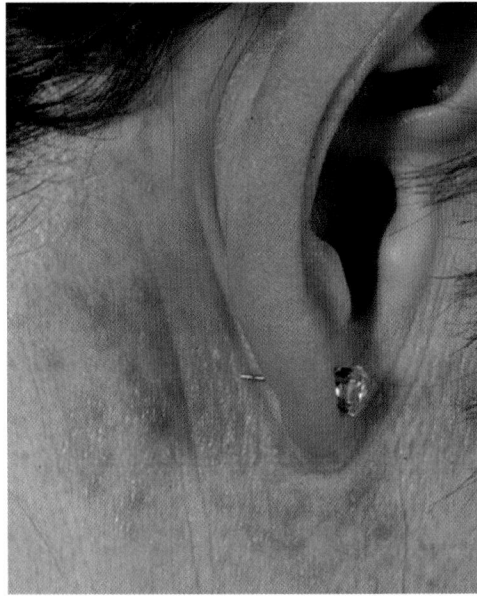

Figure 91.6 Grouped papules behind the ear of a patient with moderate papulopustular rosacea. This is a commonly overlooked location of inflammatory lesions.

Redness of the eyes (conjunctival hyperaemia), photophobia, pain and blurred vision are uncommon complaints and are indicative of a more advanced form of the disorder, as is telangiectasia of the eyelid margins and capping of the meibomian gland orifices. Conjunctival fibrosis and keratitis are rare and indicative of severe ocular rosacea. Scleral involvement in OR has been reported but appears to be very rare. OR is usually bilateral but may be more severe in one eye than the other.

Clinical variants

Atypical distribution

Papulopustular rosacea may be asymmetrical or may involve areas away from the usual centrofacial locations (periocular and post-auricular) (Figure 91.6).

Male patients with PPR and androgenetic alopecia frequently develop similar inflammatory lesions on their bald scalp (see section on pathogenesis). These lesions respond to the topical and systemic medications as prescribed for the facial lesions.

Phymatous rosacea may rarely occur in unusual locations. Metophyma, gnathophyma and otophyma refer to phymatous changes of the forehead, jaw and ears, respectively. Blepharophyma is the term used to describe swelling of the eyelids that is sometimes seen in patients with rosacea.

Granulomatous rosacea

Synonyms and inclusions
- Acne agminata
- Acnitis
- Lupus miliaris disseminatus faciei
- Lupoid rosacea of Lewandowsky

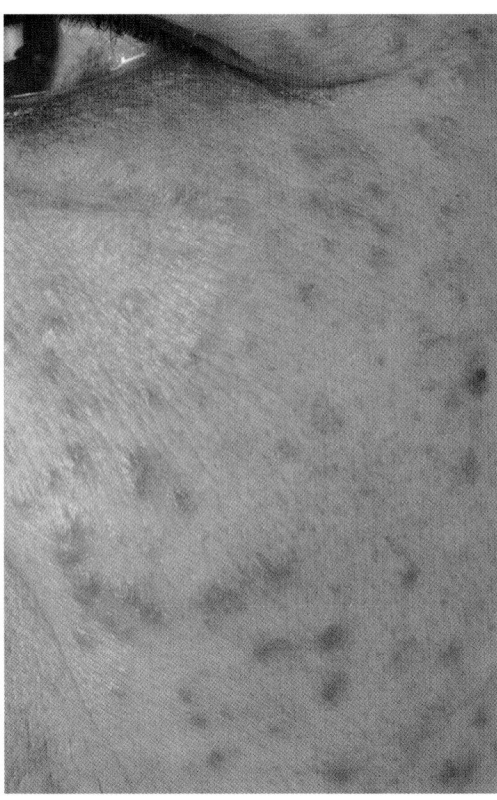

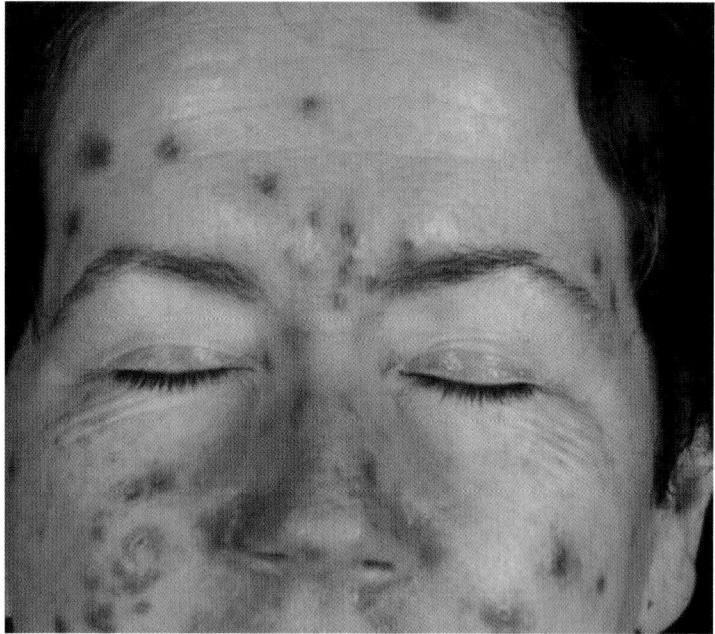

Figure 91.8 This woman was referred for management of 'treatment-resistant rosacea'. A skin biopsy showed non-caseating granulomas. Investigations revealed her to have pulmonary and ocular involvement making a diagnosis of sarcoidosis rather than granulomatous rosacea.

Figure 91.7 Granulomatous rosacea in a 55-year-old woman with a sudden onset of asymptomatic facial rash 4 months earlier. There is a profuse eruption of small, firm, monomorphic, plum-red, dome-shaped papules on the chin and cheeks and around the eyes. Histology showed multiple dermal granulomas.

Granulomas can sometimes be found histologically in all four common subtypes of rosacea. There is, however, an uncommon clinicopathological entity in which persistent, firm, non-tender, red to brown papules or nodules arise on otherwise normal-appearing skin around the mouth and eyes and on the cheeks (Figure 91.7). Its precise nosology is uncertain but it has been accepted by the National Rosacea Society Expert Committee as a variant of rosacea [1,35]. The appearance of the skin lesions is monomorphic in each individual. When they resolve there may be significant scarring. Histological evaluation of lesions shows granulomatous changes (sometimes clearly related to follicular rupture) and often foci of caseation necrosis [24]. Because of the granulomatous changes, this uncommon treatment-resistant condition was once thought to be linked to cutaneous tuberculosis (lupus miliaris disseminatus faciei) and its precise nosology is currently uncertain. It has also been termed lupoid rosacea of Lewandowsky or acne agminata. It is generally regarded as a rosacea 'variant' [1,36]. This condition has to be distinguished from cutaneous sarcoid, which it can resemble clinically and histologically (Figure 91.8).

Differential diagnosis
The differential diagnosis of the different rosacea subtypes is outlined in Table 91.2.

Erythematotelangiectatic rosacea

Chronic photodamage. Damage to facial skin from long-term exposure to sunlight, cold and damp may produce changes in fair-skinned individuals that are indistinguishable from ETTR. Larger and more laterally distributed telangiectases are often cited as being characteristic of the former condition, but in clinical practice this does not always hold true.

Seborrhoeic dermatitis. This may occasionally mimic ETTR or can accompany rosacea (typically PPR). Its characteristic orange-red appearance with adherent large scales and its distribution (alae nasi, eyebrows, scalp, etc.) help to make the diagnosis.

Contact dermatitis of the face. This can sometimes be difficult to distinguish from ETTR but a careful history and patch testing should clarify the diagnosis.

Lupus erythematosus. Lupus erythematosus (systemic and subacute) and dermatomyositis may present with photodistributed facial erythema and should be considered in a patient with systemic symptoms. Involvement of the neck and other exposed areas point towards the correct diagnosis and appropriate serological screening should be carried out.

Ulerythema ophryogenes. This may also present with facial erythema, but the presence of follicular keratoses and loss of the lateral eyebrow hair should point towards this diagnosis. Trichostasis spinulosa is a rare condition that may present with redness of the nose and prominent follicular openings with plugging.

Table 91.2 Differential diagnosis of rosacea subtypes.

Subtype	Differential diagnosis
Subtype 1: erythematotelangiectatic rosacea (ETTR)	• Chronic photodamage (difficult to distinguish) • Seborrhoeic dermatitis (characteristic distribution and scale) and may accompany several subtypes of rosacea • Facial contact dermatitis (demarcation and history) • Flushing/blushing due to other causes (see Chapter 106) • Lupus erythematosus (both systemic and subacute) • Dermatomyositis (systemic symptoms and serology) • Ulerythema ophryogenes (presence of follicular keratoses) • Trichostasis spinulosa
Subtype 2: papulopustular rosacea (PPR)	• Acne vulgaris (see Figure 91.8) • Granulomatous rosacea (lupus miliaris disseminatus faciei) (see Figure 91.7) • Perioral dermatitis (distribution and morphology differ) • Tinea faciei (skin scrapings) • Jessner's lymphocytic infiltrate (skin biopsy necessary for diagnosis) (see Chapter 105) • Pityriasis folliculorum (demodicosis: characteristic follicular scale; multiple *Demodex* mites on skin scraping) • Rosacea-like dermatoses due to medications (topical calcineurin inhibitors, epidermal growth factor receptor inhibitors, topical or systemic steroids) (see Figure 91.17) • Granuloma faciale (may mimic rhinophyma) • Lymphocytoma cutis (biopsy necessary for diagnosis)
Subtype 3: phymatous rosacea (PR)	• Solid facial lymphoedema (see Figures 91.12 and 91.16) • Infection (cutaneous tuberculosis) • Sarcoid (lupus pernio) (see Figure 91.11) • Chronic cutaneous lupus erythematosus of the nose • Granuloma faciale (may mimic rhinophyma) • Malignancy (squamous carcinoma/lymphoma/other)
Subtype 4: ocular rosacea (OR)	• Other causes of chronic blepharitis, dry eye syndrome, etc. (see Chapter 109)

Papulopustular rosacea

Acne vulgaris. Acne vulgaris in adult patients (particularly if associated with facial erythema) can be difficult to distinguish from PPR (Figure 91.9). The presence of oily skin, open and closed comedones, cystic lesions and scarring are all features supporting the diagnosis of acne vulgaris. Some patients do, however, appear to have both diseases concomitantly and some patients with acne vulgaris in early life may subsequently develop rosacea.

Rosacea-like dermatoses. This is a term used to encapsulate skin conditions that may mimic rosacea (usually PPR). Some drugs,

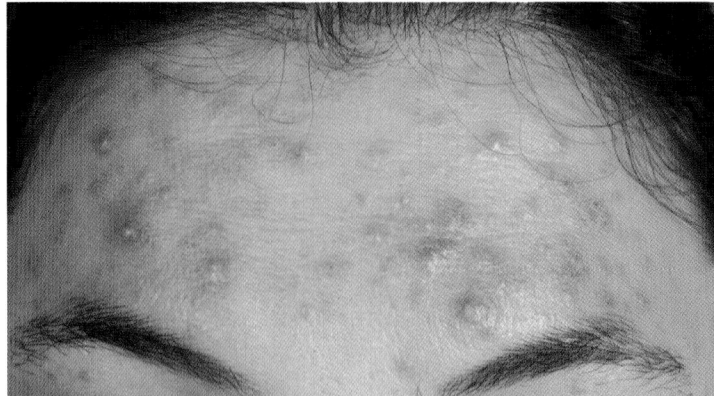

Figure 91.9 This patient with acne vulgaris has lesions that superficially resemble those of papulopustular rosacea (PPR). However, the lesions are larger and deeper than the superficial papules and pustules of PPR, the skin appears greasy and comedones are present.

especially EGF receptor and tyrosine kinase inhibitors such as cetuximab or erlotinib, can cause a florid facial acneform eruption with erythema that has a superficial resemblance to rosacea [34]. The history of sudden onset and the more acute inflammatory nature of the lesions are suggestive. Frequent application of a fluorinated topical steroid preparation to facial skin can also produce a rosacea-like eruption.

Pityriasis folliculorum. Pityriasis folliculorum (caused by a profound *Demodex* infestation of facial hair follicles) may be seen in some PPR patients or may occur in isolation with mild facial erythema without significant inflammatory lesions. The skin surface in such patients has a glazed or frosty appearance with multiple, fine, follicular scales (Figure 91.10). There is often mild

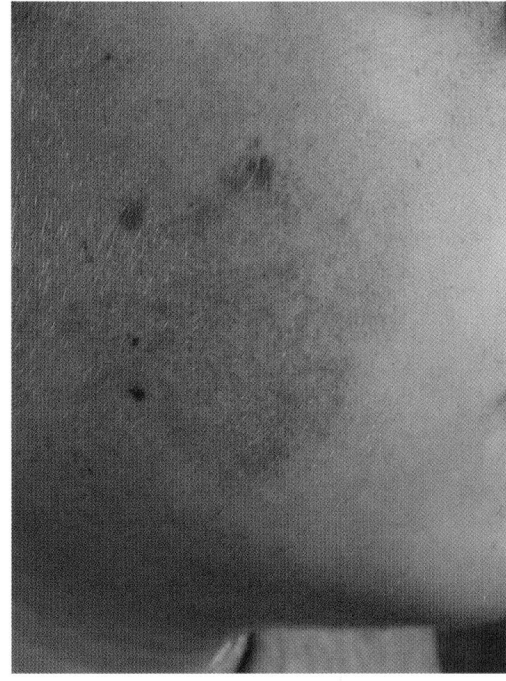

Figure 91.10 Pityriasis folliculorum in a young patient with localized area of erythema and fine scale.

accompanying itch and occasional papules and pustules may be present. Dermoscopy will reveal many follicles with fine projecting keratinous material that represent the opisthosomas of several *Demodex* mites inhabiting that follicle.

Perioral dermatitis. This has a different morphology (monomorphic small papulovesicles) from PPR and occurs in a characteristic perioral distribution. A periocular distribution is sometimes seen that can be more difficult to distinguish from rosacea. Topical or inhaled corticosteroid use may predispose to the development of perioral dermatitis (see separate section on periorificial facial dermatitis).

Jessner's lymphocytic infiltrate. This can present with persistent facial erythematous papules. Lesions tend to larger than the papules of PPR and no pustules are present. The condition is resistant to the usual rosacea therapies and can lead to scarring. A biopsy can establish the characteristic histological findings that make the diagnosis clear.

Tinea faciei. Tinea faciei can mimic rosacea with the presence of papules and pustules. Usually the distribution is asymmetrical and there is evidence of a peripheral scale at the border of the eruption. The patient typically complains of facial itch and a progressive enlargement of the area of inflammation.

Phymatous rosacea

Lupus pernio. Lupus pernio (cutaneous sarcoid of the nose) can mimic the presentation of rhinophyma although the follicular openings are not prominent (unlike PR where patulous follicles are a characteristic feature). Palpation reveals a firm, indurated quality to the affected skin, unlike the soft fleshy texture of PR (Figure 91.11).

Granuloma faciale. Granuloma faciale (see Chapter 102) is a rare condition characterized by indurated facial plaques (with

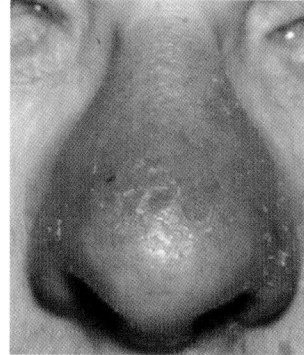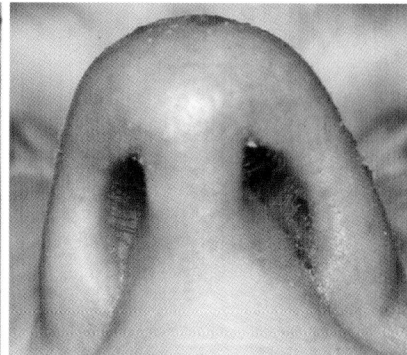

Figure 91.12 Solid facial lymphoedema involving predominantly the nose and mimicking rhinophyma. Note narrowing of the nares.

a predilection for the nose) and a chronic course that is often treatment resistant. A skin biopsy shows characteristic histopathological inflammatory changes enabling the diagnosis to be confirmed.

Lymphocytoma cutis. Lymphocytoma cutis (see Chapter 140) is another rare condition that may present with papules or nodules on the face and ears. A skin biopsy enables the diagnosis to be established with confidence in most cases.

Solid facial lymphoedema. Solid facial lymphoedema (Morbihan disease; see below) can be associated with facial erythema. It may be difficult to differentiate from rosacea and is believed by some to be a variant of rosacea (lymphoedematous rosacea) in which lymphatic drainage from the face is defective. The facial swelling may also involve the nose, mimicking rhinophyma (Figure 91.12).

Basal cell carcinomas, squamous cell carcinomas and lymphomas. These can all involve the nose and have been confused with rhinophyma. The clinician should not hesitate to take a biopsy if the condition appears atypical, progressive or unresponsive to adequate therapy.

Ocular rosacea

The clinical presentation of ocular rosacea is not specific and other causes of blepharitis and inflammatory ocular changes need to be considered, especially if accompanying skin lesions of rosacea are not present.

Complications and co-morbidities

In general, patients with rosacea do not suffer physical complications of their skin condition although a recent study has suggested that patients with rosacea may be more prone to cardiovascular disease than age- and gender-matched control subjects [37]. Rosacea can have a significant social impact, particularly in patients with flushing, in female patients and in patients with rhinophyma. Unlike acne vulgaris, scarring is not a feature of rosacea.

OR may inhibit the wearing of contact lenses due to dryness and has been reported rarely to cause severe inflammatory changes with visual impairment.

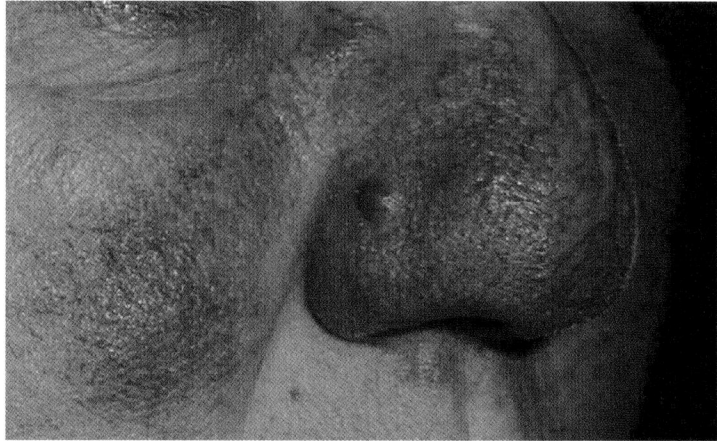

Figure 91.11 This patient with lupus pernio has skin changes that superficially resemble rosacea. Note the cyanotic hue more typical of sarcoid and the absence of patulous follicles. A skin biopsy showed the characteristic non-caseating granulomas of sarcoid.

PART 8: SPECIFIC CUTANEOUS STRUCTURE

Basal cell carcinoma may be obscured by phymatous tissue in patients with rhinophyma and the possibility of coexistent neoplasia should not be overlooked in the evaluation of patients with this subtype of rosacea.

As outlined already, seborrhoeic dermatitis may coexist with rosacea and its treatment should not be overlooked, as results will otherwise be suboptimal.

Migraine has been reported to occur more commonly in patients with rosacea. The presence of rosacea does not exclude the possibility of carcinoid syndrome and this needs to be considered in patients with paroxysmal flushing and rosacea. Further evaluation of patients with severe or generalized flushing is warranted, especially if accompanied by other symptoms (see Chapter 106).

Disease course and prognosis

Rosacea is a chronic condition and its course is characterized by episodes of partial remission and repeated relapse. Different subtypes tend to have different patterns of clinical behaviour.

Untreated ETTR patients develop persistent facial redness over time, often with prominent malar telangiectasia and increasingly sensitive facial skin (burning/stinging sensation) and intolerance of temperature changes or adverse climatic conditions (cold winds, etc.). Facial flushing becomes progressively more problematic. Dietary triggers of flushing can be identified in some patients.

The course of PPR is characterized by recurrent episodic crops of inflammatory lesions (mainly papules and some papulopustules) occurring usually in groups in the centrofacial region. Perilesional erythema that persists after the inflammatory lesions fade contributes to the overall facial erythema. PPR is less frequently seen in elderly patients suggesting that it may 'burn itself out' in this older age group.

Rhinophyma tends to be progressive through enlargement to distortion of the shape of the nose unless treated. Not all patients will develop the same degree of nasal deformity.

OR has a chronic course with episodes of exacerbation. Dryness tends to be a constant feature, while inflammatory lesions (hordeola, chalazia) occur intermittently. Without treatment the dry eyes of rosacea patients are susceptible to secondary bacterial, mainly staphylococcal infection. More serious complications including conjunctival fibrosis, punctate keratitis and corneal neovascularization have been reported in patients with OR but appear to occur rarely.

Investigations

Investigations are not required for patients who present with the typical clinical features of rosacea. In patients with atypical presentations or those with unusual symptoms, alternative diagnoses should be considered. There is no specific serological or histopathological test that will confirm the diagnosis of either cutaneous or ocular rosacea.

Management

The approach to the management of rosacea differs according to the principal subtype manifest in each patient [2]. However, some

aspects of skin care are common to the management of all forms of rosacea. Because most patients with rosacea are fair-skinned (skin types 1 or 2) they should be advised to avoid undue sun exposure and use sun-protective measures (apply daily sun block cream all year round and wear a hat) as chronic UV damage will contribute to facial erythema, especially in patients with ETTR. Physical sunscreens based on zinc or titanium are best tolerated. Wind and exposure to cold, which contribute to the development of facial telangiectasia and vascular instability, should also be avoided when possible.

Many patients with rosacea have dry, easily irritated skin. Daily application of a moisturizing cream is important for such patients. Cosmetic cover (with light liquid foundation preparations) and particular focus on the masking of erythema should be advised to lessen the social impact of the disorder. Avoidance of potential irritants (abrasive soaps, astringents, perfumes, aftershave lotions and skin-peeling preparations) is important as they tend to aggravate the facial erythema and the burning or stinging sensation, especially in patients with ETTR. Skin-peeling agents can exacerbate the facial dryness as well and should be avoided.

The use of topical corticosteroids should be avoided on the face of patients with rosacea except in particular circumstances. Patients with a tendency to flushing (mainly those with ETTR) should avoid agents that provoke flushing such as hot drinks, spicy foods, alcohol and some drugs. Some such patients find it helpful to keep a diary of flushing events to try to identify other precipitating or exacerbating factors (e.g. stress, temperature).

The approach to the general management of the skin in patients with rosacea is summarized in Box 91.1.

Box 91.1 Skincare management

- Use sunscreens with both UVA and UVB protection, and a UVB protection factor of 15 or greater. Sun-blocking creams containing the physical barriers titanium dioxide or zinc oxide are usually well tolerated
- Use soap-free, pH-balanced synthetic detergents ('syndets') and lukewarm water to wash the face
- Use cosmetics and sunscreens that contain protective silicones
- Water-soluble make-up containing inert green pigment helps neutralize the perception of erythema. Camouflage make-up may also be useful
- Moisturizers containing humectants (e.g. glycerine) and occlusives (e.g. petrolatum) may assist in restoring impaired epidermal barrier function
- Avoid astringents, toners and abrasive exfoliators, and procedures such as dermabrasion
- Avoid waterproof cosmetics and heavy foundations that are difficult to remove without irritating solvents or physical scrubbing
- Avoid cosmetics that contain alcohol, menthols, camphor, witch hazel, fragrance, peppermint and eucalyptus oil
- Avoid environments that may overheat and/or dry the skin such as saunas, heater fans in cars and open fireplaces

First line management

Erythematotelangiectatic rosacea. Sun avoidance and protection measures should be followed as outlined above. Use soap-free cleansers and apply a non-scented, colour-free moisturizer daily. Use cosmetic cover if needed. Identify and avoid factors that provoke flushing. Treat erythema with topical α-receptor agonists such as brimonidine or oxymetazoline [38]. These agents appear to be effective in diminishing the facial erythema temporarily, but have to be used repeatedly for sustained effect.

Papulopustular rosacea. Sun avoidance, sun protection, moisturizing and cosmetic cover should be undertaken as for ETTR. For active inflammatory lesions select topical agent such as metronidazole 0.75% gel or cream, azelaic acid 15% gel, ivermectin 1% cream or sodium sulfacetamide 10% and sulphur 5% preparations. Cream preparations are generally better tolerated if the skin is acutely inflamed. In the initial clearing phase, the selected preparation should be applied before use of a moisturizer twice daily for 6–8 weeks. As inflammatory lesions clear, once-daily application (usually preferred by patients in the evening) may be sufficient. If the skin remains clear after 3–4 months, treatment can be discontinued and replaced by regular daily use of a moisturizer. If flares occur the patient should be instructed to recommence topical treatment twice daily. Topical α-receptor agonists such as brimonidine and oxymetazoline may reduce perilesional erythema in patients with PPR but do not appear to have an effect on papule and pustule formation.

Phymatous rosacea. Treat accompanying inflammatory lesions, if present, as for PPR. Consider nasal application of a skin-peeling agent if there are large occluded follicles (sometimes due to trichostasis) and oily skin. Ablate perinasal telangiectatic vessels with electrocautery or laser. Discuss the possibility of isotretinoin therapy if the condition is progressive.

Ocular rosacea. Daily lid hygiene can be helpful for patients with early blepharitis and lid crusting. Instruct patients to dilute several drops of baby shampoo in warm water in an eggcup and apply the solution to the lid margins with a cotton bud (lid scrubs). Warm compresses used before the scrubs help to liquefy the solidifying secretion from the meibomian glands and facilitate its removal. Oily, tear substitute, lubricating eye drops/aqueous gels are important for all stages of OR and should be prescribed as first line therapy.

Second line management

Erythematotelangiectatic rosacea. Laser therapy (using pulse dye, intense pulsed light, 532 nm green light or combination devices, e.g. 595 nm neodymium:yttrium-aluminium-garnet (Nd:YAG) lasers) can eliminate malar telangiectatic vessels and reduce facial erythema significantly (see Chapter 23). This also tends to stabilize facial vascular reactivity in these patients. Improvement can persist for years but relapse eventually occurs. Laser treatment does not appear to have any effect on the subsequent development of papules and pustules.

Low-dose β-blocking medications (propranolol, nadolol, carvedilol) should be considered for those patients who are troubled by a persistent flushing tendency. Psychological counselling, group therapy sessions and development of biofeedback techniques can all be helpful for patients dealing with psychosocial exacerbation of flushing tendencies.

Papulopustular rosacea. A systematic review of rosacea treatments emphasized the need for additional studies in this area of therapy [39]. Traditionally, systemic antibiotic therapy (tetracycline, doxycycline, erythromycin, minocycline, trimethoprim) given in full dosage (as for patients with acne vulgaris) but for a shorter period (6–8 weeks as opposed to several months), either prescribed alone or in combination with one of the topical agents mentioned above, have been used and appear to be effective in clearing even florid PPR.

Doxycycline given in a subantimicrobial dose of 40 mg daily is as effective as the standard regimen (100 mg daily) but causes fewer adverse effects and less bacterial resistance. The facial erythema associated with florid PPR often subsides significantly when the inflammatory lesions clear but may persist in a lesser form for some weeks.

Phymatous rosacea. Low-dose isotretinoin therapy (10–20 mg daily) taken over a period of 2–6 months has been reported to reduce the degree of rhinophyma in some patients with PR (Figure 91.13). However, the effect may not be prolonged and the nasal enlargement may increase when the medication is discontinued. Appropriate patient monitoring is required.

Ocular rosacea. Consider careful lid massage to express the contents of blocked meibomian glands in addition to warm compresses and lid scrubs as described above. Add topical medication such as topical metronidazole gel, which appears to be well tolerated when applied on the eyelid margins with the eyes closed. Sodium sulfacetamide ophthalmic ointment and ciclosporin ointment have also been reported to be effective for OR. Fusidic acid ointment or erythromycin ophthalmic ointment applied twice daily to the lid margins can be helpful if secondary bacterial infection, which is usually staphylococcal, is suspected.

It has been suggested that topical tea tree (*Melaleuca alternifolia*) oil preparations may help ocular rosacea through anti-*Demodex* effects but, as for many other interventions listed above, this recommendation is based more on anecdote than firm evidence. Contact dermatitis (irritant or allergic) is a possible consequence of using this agent so caution is advised. Omega-3 fatty acids have been reported to be beneficial for some patients with rosacea-related blepharitis when taken orally.

The use of topical corticosteroids in blepharitis is controversial and is best avoided. If symptoms persist in spite of the above recommendations, the patient should be referred to an ophthalmologist.

PART 8: SPECIFIC CUTANEOUS STRUCTURE

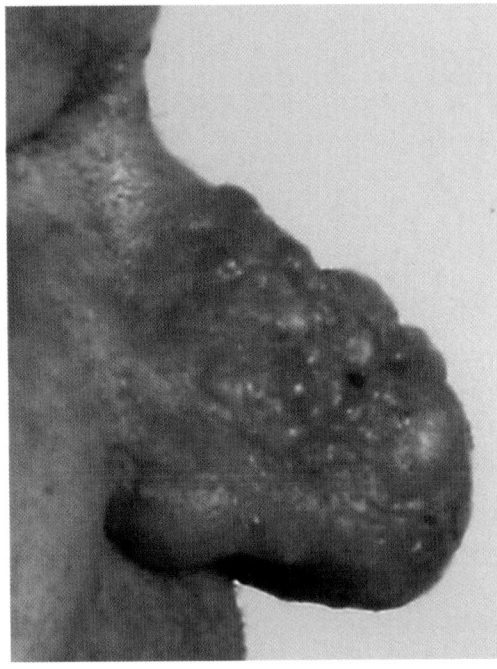
(a)

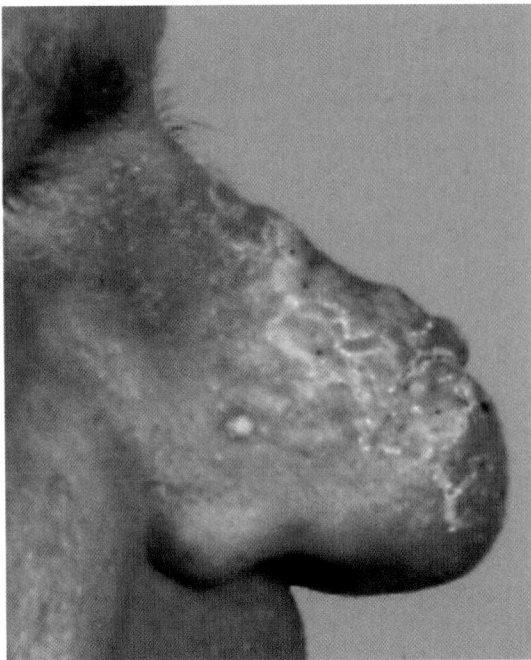
(b)

Figure 91.13 Rhinophyma before (a) and after (b) 4 months' treatment with isotretinoin.

Third line management

Erythematotelangiectatic rosacea. Botulinum toxin injections have been reported to be helpful for some patients with recalcitrant flushing reactions. Consider highly selective sympathectomy only in disabling cases because of the risk of serious side effects (see Chapter 94).

Papulopustular rosacea. In PPR patients resistant to conventional antibiotic therapy consider systemic metronidazole or isotretinoin low-dose therapy (as above) to gain control of the disorder. Careful monitoring for side effects is mandatory. Inflammation will tend to recur when these therapies are discontinued, so an alternative longer term treatment will need to be introduced when control is achieved.

If *Demodex* proliferation is considered to be relevant in a particular patient, the use of a topical acaricide such as crotamiton or permethrin can help to reduce the facial mite population. Some of these preparations can be irritating so caution is advised.

Phymatous rosacea. Rhinophymatous tissue ablation with carbon dioxide laser (see Chapter 23) or surgical electrosection of excessive nasal tissue with remodelling of the shape of the nose (see Chapter 20) are the treatments of choice for advanced rhinophyma. Results are often excellent and sustained in the long term.

Ocular rosacea. Systemic tetracycline, doxycycline and minocycline in a dose and for a similar duration as used for PPR often improve refractory ocular symptoms. Erythromycin is preferable for children and during pregnancy. Prompt referral to an ophthalmologist for specialist care is indicated if the patient complains of pain or photophobia or if improvement is not evident at an early stage of severe OR.

Treatment ladder

Erythematotelangiectatic rosacea

First line
- Sun avoidance and protection
- Non-scented, colour-free moisturizer
- Soap-free cleansers
- Cosmetic cover
- Avoid factors that provoke flushing
- Topical α-receptor agonists such as brimonidine or oxymetazoline

Second line
- Laser therapy for facial erythema and telangiectasia (see Chapter 23)
- Low-dose β-blocking medications (propranolol, nadolol, carvedilol)
- Psychological counselling and group therapy sessions

Third line
- Botulinum toxin
- Highly selective sympathectomy in disabling cases

Papulopustular rosacea

First line
- Sun avoidance, sun protection, moisturizing and cosmetic cover as for ETTR
- Topical metronidazole, azelaic acid, ivermectin or sodium sulfacetamide and sulphur for active inflammatory lesions
- Topical α-receptor agonists such as brimonidine and oxymetazoline for perilesional erythema

Second line

- Systemic antibiotic therapy with tetracyclines, erythromycin or trimethoprim

Third line

- Systemic metronidazole
- Isotretinoin low-dose therapy
- Topical acaricide (ivermectin, crotamiton, permethrin) if *Demodex* proliferation is relevant

Phymatous rosacea

First line

- As for PPR for accompanying inflammatory lesions
- Topical skin-peeling agent if there are large occluded follicles
- Electrocautery or laser for telangiectases

Second line

- Low-dose isotretinoin therapy

Third line

- Ablation of phymatous tissue with carbon dioxide laser
- Surgical remodelling of nose

Ocular rosacea

First line

- Daily lid hygiene
- Oily tear-substitute lubricating eye drops or aqueous gels

Second line

- Careful lid massage
- Topical metronidazole, sodium sulfacetamide or ciclosporin
- Fusidic acid or erythromycin ophthalmic ointment if secondary bacterial infection is suspected
- Topical tea tree (*Melaleuca alternifolia*) oil preparations

Third line

- Systemic tetracyclines or erythromycin
- Referral to ophthalmologist for specialist care

Resources

Further information

American Academy of Dermatology: http://www.aad.org/for-the-public/home.
British Association of Dermatology: http://www.bad.org.uk.
European Academy of Dermatology and Venereology leaflets: http://www.eadv.org/patient-corner/leaflets.
National Rosacea Society, USA: http://www.rosacea.org.
UCD Charles Institute of Dermatology, video and patient information: www.ucd.ie/charles.
(All last accessed September 2015.)

FACIAL DERMATOSES WITH AN UNCERTAIN NOSOLOGICAL RELATIONSHIP TO ROSACEA

There is a range of facial dermatoses that share some features with rosacea but for which there is currently no consensus as to their nosological relationship with rosacea. These are described below.

Idiopathic facial aseptic granuloma

Synonyms and inclusions
- Pyodermite froide du visage

Idiopathic facial aseptic granuloma (IFAG) was first reported as an entity under the name pyodermite froide du visage in 1999 [1]. It may not be uncommon in children. IFAG typically presents between 8 months and 13 years of age as a solitary inflammatory nodule on the cheek or eyelid superficially resembling an insect bite (Figure 91.14). The nodules are asymptomatic, usually red or purple in colour and soft to palpation. They may attain a diameter of 2–3 cm before spontaneously involuting after several months [2,3].

Rosacea conglobata and rosacea fulminans

Synonyms and inclusions
- Pyoderma faciale

Rosacea conglobata describes a rare rosacea-like eruption that has a gradual onset, mainly in young women. It is characterized by marked facial erythema with nodular abscesses and indurated haemorrhagic plaques that can result in significant scarring. Unlike acne conglobata, comedones are not a feature and the trunk is spared [5]. A similar more acute inflammatory facial eruption, which probably represents a severe variant of rosacea conglobata, has previously been called pyoderma faciale and, in more recent

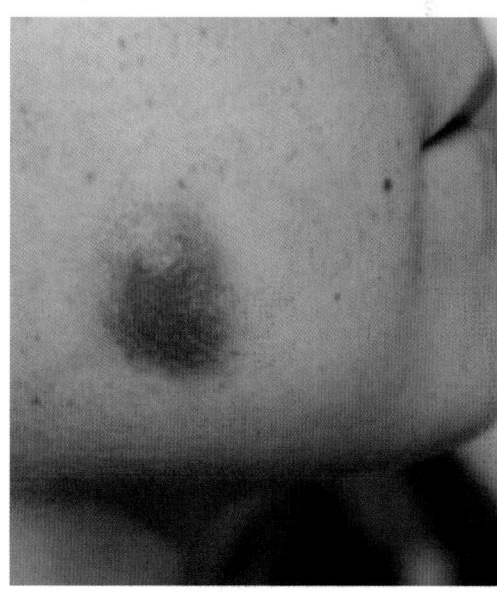

Figure 91.14 Idiopathic facial aseptic granuloma showing a well-defined plum-coloured nodule on the face of a 7-year-old boy. (From González Rodríguez *et al.* 2015 [3]. Reproduced with permission of Wiley.)

PART 8: SPECIFIC CUTANEOUS STRUCTURE

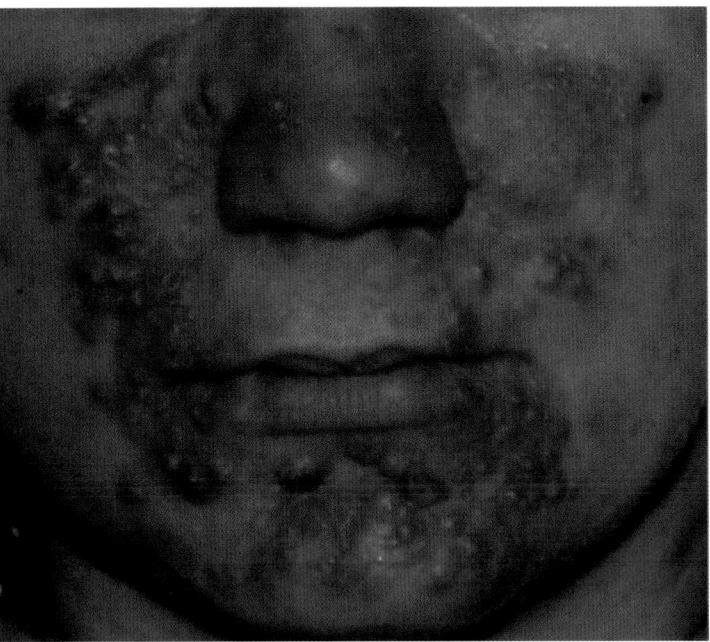

Figure 91.15 Rosacea fulminans showing an abrupt onset of severe inflammation with extensive pustule formation in a young woman.

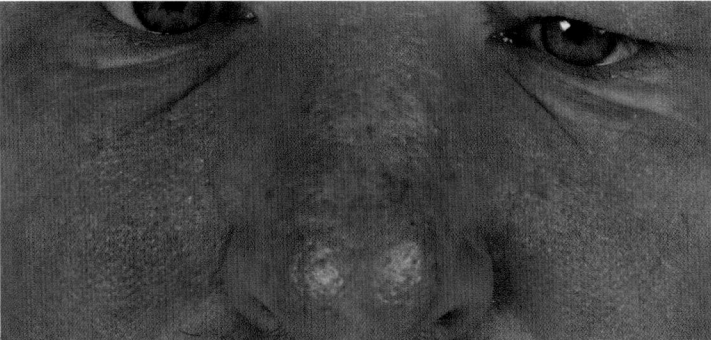

Figure 91.16 Solid facial lymphoedema is characterized by the presence of persistent, non-tender, firm, upper facial swelling. Note the creases under the eyes in this patient indicating the presence of this unusual type of facial erythema and swelling.

times, rosacea fulminans. This may affect either sex but typically presents in young women with oily skin, often during or immediately following pregnancy [6]. It may arise *de novo* but may also develop in patients with pre-existing rosacea [7]. Inflammatory haemorrhagic plaques surmounted by pustules erupt abruptly (Figure 91.15). It can be complicated by acute OR with conjunctivitis and severe keratitis [7]. It is sometimes difficult to distinguish rosacea conglobata from inflammatory variants of acne vulgaris, as which some forms were originally categorized. It can lead to major scarring.

Solid facial lymphoedema

Synonyms and inclusions
- Lymphoedematous rosacea
- Solid facial oedema
- Morbihan disease

Introduction and general description

A variable degree of facial oedema may be present in some patients with rosacea and accompany or follow the other clinical features, particularly severe PPR. Facial oedema may also be seen in inflammatory acne (see Chapter 90).

Rarely, however, patients may present with a much more pronounced, firm, upper facial, non-pitting oedema with erythema. In cases where this has not been preceded by a history of rosacea it has been termed by some solid facial oedema and by others lymphoedematous rosacea; it is also known as Morbihan disease (Figure 91.16) [8].

Pathophysiology

The factors underlying the development of this condition are poorly understood. It has been postulated that there is inadequate lymphatic drainage to cope with increased demand. The condition is characterized histologically by dermal oedema, perifollicular fibrosis and perivascular and perifollicular infiltration of lymphocytes, and mast cells [9]. It has been hypothesized that recurrent inflammation results in structural damage to the draining lymphatic vessels, and epithelioid granulomas next to obstructed lymphatics have been observed histologically [10]. The rapid response to systemic corticosteroids in one recent report would support this hypothesis [11], but this is by no means a uniform response in patients with this disorder. In many patients there is no clinical evidence of preceding or concomitant rosacea or of other inflammatory dermatosis. For additional information regarding reactive lymphatic disorders see Chapter 105 [8,9].

Clinical features

Solid facial lymphoedema is characterized clinically by persistent erythema and firm non-pitting oedema of the upper two-thirds of the face, affecting especially the eyelids, cheeks, nose and glabella. It is, however, a diagnosis of exclusion and other possibilities such as dermatomyositis, chronic actinic dermatitis and chronic allergic contact dermatitis need to be considered [9].

Management

Management is difficult. Antihistamines may be of some help but the best results have been obtained with long-term isotretinoin [9,12]. In a report of five patients treated with doses of 40–80 mg daily for up to 24 months, substantial improvement was not seen until at least 6 months after initiation of therapy [9]. Thalidomide has also been advocated [8].

Corticosteroid-induced rosacea-like facial dermatosis

Introduction and general description

The use of potent topical corticosteroids on the face often results in a papulopustular eruption accompanied by erythema that

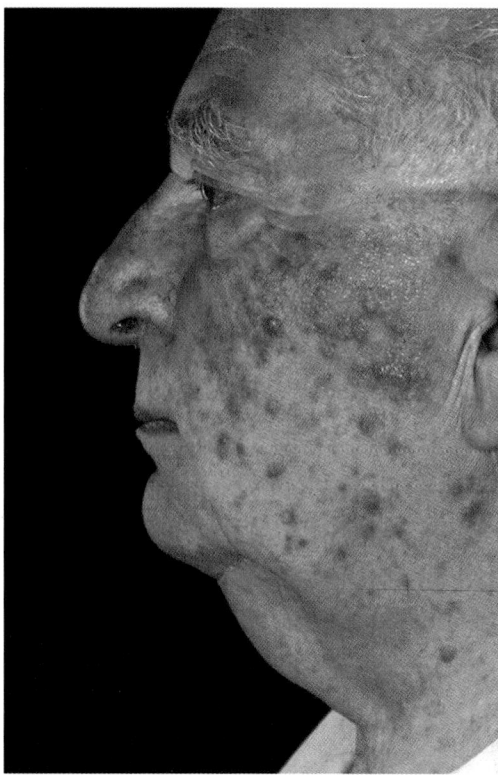

Figure 91.17 Corticosteroid-induced rosacea-like facial dermatosis.

may closely resemble rosacea (Figure 91.17) [13,14]. Patients of all age groups and either sex are susceptible although it is far commoner in women than men [15,16]. If application of the steroid continues, fixed erythema and telangiectasia develop, further increasing the similarity to idiopathic rosacea. It probably occurs with greater frequency in areas of the world where fluorinated corticosteroid preparations are cheap and readily available [15,16].

Pathophysiology
The precise mechanism by which topical corticosteroids can trigger a rosacea-like eruption is not well understood but alterations in the skin microbiome and their effect on the skin's innate immune system are likely to be involved [17].

Clinical features
Patients experience marked sensitivity of the involved skin to the slightest irritant; itching, burning and intense redness being major complaints. Whenever the treatment is discontinued, the eruption flares, leading to a state of dependence. Patients affected by steroid rosacea often fail to recognize the causal link between the treatment and the rash. On the contrary, the application of the steroid usually produces prompt, if transient, improvement in the symptoms, creating the illusion of significant benefit.

On occasions, even topical hydrocortisone 1% may provoke a rosacea-like eruption in children [18]. The use of corticosteroid nasal sprays has also been implicated [19]. A similar eruption has been described following use of topical tacrolimus 0.1% ointment [20].

Management
The first and most important step is withdrawal of the causative topical corticosteroid. Patients must be advised to anticipate a flare of the rosacea at this stage. In order to reduce the severity of this flare it is often necessary initially to introduce a less potent steroid. Topical or systemic antibiotic therapy as used for idiopathic rosacea may help suppress flares in the early stages of steroid withdrawal. Topical tacrolimus [21] or pimecrolimus [22,23] have both been advocated, although a rosacea-like eruption has also been reported to arise or worsen as a side effect of these agents.

Corticosteroid-induced rosacea-like facial dermatosis may take several weeks or even months to subside but eventually complete resolution occurs if topical corticosteroids are avoided.

Periorificial facial dermatitis

Synonyms and inclusions
- Perioral dermatitis
- Periocular dermatitis
- Periorbital dermatitis

Introduction and general description
Periorificial dermatitis is a term covering two erythematous and papulopustular facial dermatoses that are strongly linked to prolonged potent topical corticosteroid use, namely perioral dermatitis and periocular dermatitis. First described in the late 1950s and 1960s, perioral dermatitis became a commonplace diagnosis by the 1970s [24]. With increased awareness of the hazards of using potent topical corticosteroids on the face, it has become less common. It bears similarities to corticosteroid-induced rosacea but has a different clinical distribution.

Pathophysiology
As with corticosteroid-induced rosacea-like dermatosis it is likely that perturbation of the skin microbiome is relevant [25,26]. Topical steroid therapy is known to be an important aetiological factor. There appear to be associations with atopic eczema and with the use of potentially irritant products on the skin: impairment of the skin barrier has been postulated as a further aetiological factor [26].

There is a mild spongiotic dermatitis with perifollicular inflammation and pustules. Granulomas and *Demodex* mites are not normally found [27,28].

Clinical features

History
The preparation responsible may have been prescribed, possibly for a completely different indication, or may have been 'borrowed' for treating trivial facial blemishes. Most medical practitioners are now fully aware of the hazards of prolonged potent topical steroid use on the face.

Presentation
A patchy erythema with tiny papules and pustules forms on the lower face and chin, usually leaving a small border of

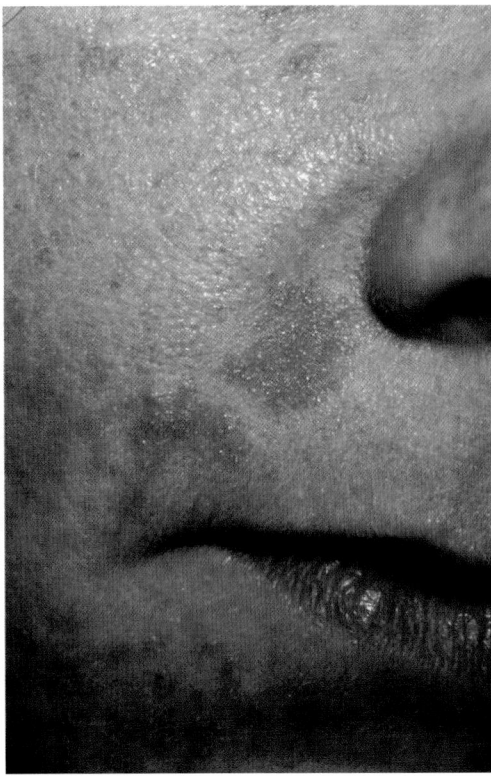

Figure 91.18 Perioral dermatitis.

unaffected skin around the mouth (Figure 91.18) [29]. The more potent the steroid, the more likely it is to result in perioral dermatitis, although it has also been reported with hydrocortisone [30]. Steroids from asthma inhalers and nebulizers have also been implicated [31].

Periocular dermatitis is similar to perioral dermatitis and affects the eyelids and periorbital skin. It usually results from the use of steroid-containing ophthalmic preparations (Figure 91.19) [32].

Differential diagnosis

The clinical picture is distinctive; important differential diagnoses are shown in Box 91.2.

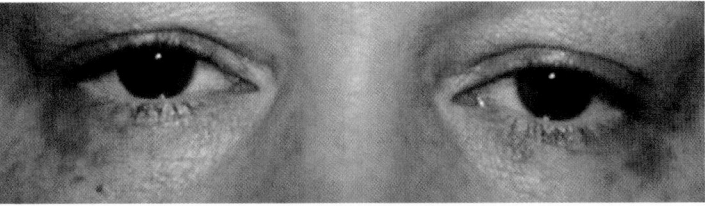
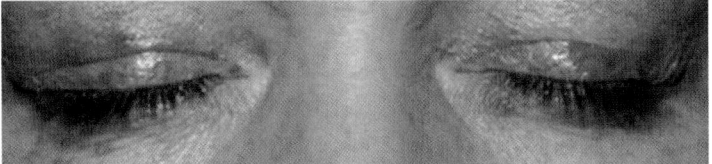

Figure 91.19 Periocular dermatitis.

> **Box 91.2 Important differential diagnoses for periorificial dermatitis (PD)**
>
> Rosacea
> • Usually no telangiectasia or flushing in PD
> Granulomatous rosacea
> • Generally firmer, larger papules than in PD
> • Often less background erythema than in PD
> • Granulomatous histology
> Granulomatous perioral dermatitis in children
> • Does not spare perilabial skin
> • No pustules
> • Predominantly in males
> Seborrhoeic dermatitis
> • Affects the naso-labial area, but is not usually circumoral
> • Scalp, ears and eyebrows are commonly involved
> Allergic contact dermatitis
> • Does not usually spare the immediate perioral area as in PD
> Late-onset acne vulgaris
> • Larger papules than in PD, with comedones and cysts

Disease course and prognosis

Most patients experience permanent remission after a fairly short course of broad-spectrum antibiotics [33]. Relapses occur in a small minority [34]. However, if untreated and especially if the provoking topical steroids are continued, perioral dermatitis can persist for years [35].

Management

The most important measure is to discontinue application of topical corticosteroids. As with other corticosteroid-induced skin disorders, the substitution of a milder version of topical corticosteroid will diminish the subsequent flare when the more potent preparation is stopped. Other applications, including cosmetics, should be avoided. The patient must be warned that an initial flare is to be expected. A 4-week course of an oral tetracycline, topical erythromycin or topical metronidazole are commonly used and are normally effective [**25**].

Childhood granulomatous periorificial dermatitis

Synonyms and inclusions
• Facial Afro-Caribbean childhood eruption

This rare dermatosis of children is of unknown aetiology and has been reported principally in prepubertal children of African descent [**25,36**]. It manifests as an eruption of asymptomatic, flesh-coloured, dome-shaped papules (Figure 91.20). As with periorificial dermatitis in adults, it affects principally perioral and periocular skin but can affect other parts of the head and neck. Its granulomatous nature can be confirmed by diascopy. Biopsy shows non-caseating epithelioid granulomas and a perivascular inflammatory infiltrate.

It resolves spontaneously within a few months to about 3 years without treatment but may leave milia or small pitted scars.

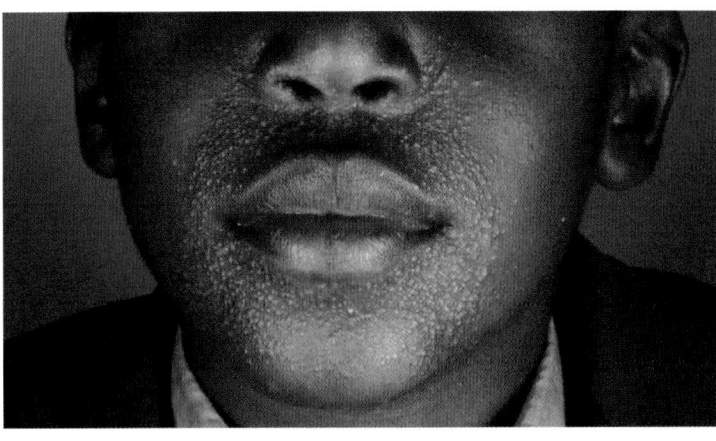

Figure 91.20 Childhood granulomatous periorificial dermatitis. (Courtesy of Professor Hywel Williams, University of Nottingham, UK.)

Key references

The full list of references can be found in the online version at www.rooksdermatology.com.

Rosacea

6 Gibson GE, Codd MB, Murphy GM. Skin distribution and skin disease in Ireland. *Ir J Med Sci* 1997;166:72–4.

15 Grice EA, Segre JA. The skin microbiome. *Nat Rev Microbiol* 2011;9:244–53.

24 Sánchez JL, Berlingeri-Ramos AC, Dueño DV. Granulomatous rosacea. *Am J Dermatopathol* 2008;30:6–9.

25 el Darouti M, Zaher H. Lupus miliaris disseminatus faciei: pathologic study of early, fully developed, and late lesions. *Int J Dermatol* 1993;32:508–11.

32 Jarmuda S, McMahon F, Zaba R, *et al.* Correlation between serum reactivity to *Demodex*-associated *Bacillus oleronius* proteins, and altered sebum levels and Demodex populations in erythematotelangiectatic rosacea patients. *J Med Microbiol* 2014;63:258–62.

33 Chen W, Plewig G. Human demodicosis: revisit and a proposed classification. *Br J Dermatol* 2014;170:1219–25.

37 Lee GL, Zirwas MJ. Granulomatous rosacea and periorificial dermatitis: controversies and review of management and treatment. *Dermatol Clin* 2015;33:447–55.

Facial dermatoses with an uncertain nosological relationship to rosacea

2 Neri I, Raone B, Dondi A, Misciali C, Patrizi A. Should idiopathic facial aseptic granuloma be considered granulomatous rosacea? Report of three pediatric cases. *Pediatr Dermatol* 2013;30:109–11.

3 González Rodríguez AJ, Jordá Cuevas E. Idiopathic facial aseptic granuloma. *Clin Exp Dermatol* 2015;40:298–300.

5 Jansen T, Plewig G, Kligman AM. Diagnosis and treatment of rosacea fulminans. *Dermatology* 1994;188:251–4.

6 Ferahbas A, Utas S, Mistik S, Uksal U, Peker D. Rosacea fulminans in pregnancy: case report and review of the literature. *Am J Clin Dermatol* 2006;7:141–4.

7 Kim TG, Noh SM, Do JE, Lee MG, Oh SH. Rosacea fulminans with ocular involvement. *Br J Dermatol* 2010;163:877–9.

9 Smith LA, Cohen DA. Successful long-term use of oral isotretinoin for the management of Morbihan disease: a case series report and review of the literature. *Arch Dermatol* 2012;148:1395–8.

10 Nagasaka T, Koyama T, Matsumura K, Chen KR. Persistent lymphoedema in Morbihan disease: formation of perilymphatic epithelioid cell granulomas as a possible pathogenesis. *Clin Exp Dermatol* 2008;33:764–7.

14 Ljubojevic S, Basta-Juzbasic A, Lipozencic J. Steroid dermatitis resembling rosacea: aetiopathogenesis and treatment. *J Eur Acad Dermatol Venereol* 2002;16:121–6.

25 Dessinioti C, Antoniou C, Katsambas A. Acneiform eruptions. *Clin Dermatol* 2014;32:24–34.

26 Lee GL, Zirwas MJ. Granulomatous rosacea and periorificial dermatitis: controversies and review of management and treatment. *Dermatol Clin* 2015;33:447–55.

36 Knautz MA, Lesher JL. Childhood granulomatous periorificial dermatitis. *Pediatr Dermatol* 1996;13:131–4.

CHAPTER 92

Hidradenitis Suppurativa

Nemesha Desai[1], Hessel H. van der Zee[2] and Gregor B. E. Jemec[3]

[1]St John's Institute of Dermatology, Guy's and St Thomas' NHS Foundation Trust, London, UK
[2]Department of Dermatology, Erasmus Medical Center, Rotterdam, the Netherlands
[3]Department of Dermatology, Roskilde Hospital; Health Sciences Faculty, University of Copenhagen, Copenhagen, Denmark

Definition and nomenclature

Hidradenitis suppurativa is a chronic, inflammatory, recurrent, debilitating, follicular disease that usually presents after puberty. There are painful, deep-seated inflamed lesions in the apocrine gland-bearing areas of the body, most commonly the axillary, inguinal and ano-genital regions. This definition is based on the San Francisco modification of the Dessau criteria [1].

The following three criteria must be met for the diagnosis to be made:

1 Typical lesions, that is deep-seated, painful nodules: 'blind boils' in early lesions; abscesses, draining sinuses, bridged scars and paired or multiheaded open pseudocomedones in secondary lesions.
2 Typical topography: axillae, groin, perineal and perianal region, buttocks and infra- and intermammary folds.
3 Chronicity and recurrence of lesions.

> **Synonyms and inclusions**
> • Acne inversa
> • Verneuil disease
> • Velpeau disease
> • Pyoderma fistulans significa
> • Ectopic acne

Introduction and general description

Velpeau was the first to describe the condition of recurrent, painful, inflammatory abscesses of the axillae and groin in 1839 [2]. Verneuil later coined the term hidradenitis suppurativa (HS), a misnomer derived from the historical hypothesis that the disorder related to inflammation of the sweat glands [3]. Current evidence demonstrates that HS is a primary disorder of the hair follicle.

HS is a chronic, inflammatory, follicular disorder characterized by recurrent painful nodules, abscesses, draining sinus tracts and scarring. It localizes to areas of apocrine gland-bearing skin, predominantly the axillae, groin and ano-genital sites. Severity is defined by Hurley stage, which is often used to direct therapy [4]. Management is challenging and requires a combined medical and surgical approach. Complications of severe disease include contractures, anaemia, lymphoedema and squamous cell carcinoma. The psychosocial impact is significant [5]. The impact on quality of life is higher on average than for other inflammatory dermatoses [6].

Epidemiology

Incidence and prevalence

An annual incidence of six per 100 000 person-years is reported in a US insurance-based study; the incidence was highest amongst young women aged 20–29 years (18.4 per 100 000). The incidence may be rising [7].

The estimated prevalence in large European population studies is 1–2% [8]. Reported rates vary from 0.00033% to 4%, relating to differences in study population, diagnostic criteria and use of self-reporting [7,8,9,10,11]. A prevalence of 4% was observed in young adults attending a sexually transmitted disease clinic [9].

PART 8: SPECIFIC CUTANEOUS STRUCTURE

Rook's Textbook of Dermatology, Ninth Edition. Edited by Christopher Griffiths, Jonathan Barker, Tanya Bleiker, Robert Chalmers and Daniel Creamer.
© 2016 John Wiley & Sons, Ltd. Published 2016 by John Wiley & Sons, Ltd.
Companion website: www.rooksdermatology.com

Age

The average age of sufferers is 24.2 years (± 12 years) [12]. HS typically presents after puberty; the average age of onset is between the second and third decade, with a sharp decline after the fifth decade. Onset after menopause is uncommon. There are rare cases of prepubertal onset associated with premature adrenarche.

Sex

Women are more frequently affected than men, in a ratio of 2.7 : 1 [12]. Topographical distribution of lesions can vary between sexes. For example, perianal and gluteal disease more commonly affects males; females are more likely to have genito-femoral and sub-mammary lesions [13].

Ethnicity

There are no formal studies of ethnic variation.

Associated diseases

Diseases associated with HS include disorders of the follicular occlusion tetrad, systemic inflammatory disorders and genodermatoses [14].

Follicular occlusion tetrad. Acne conglobata (see Chapter 90), dissecting cellulitis of the scalp (see Chapter 107) and pilonidal sinus (see Chapter 113) can coexist with HS; together they comprise the 'follicular occlusion tetrad'. Typical acne vulgaris occurs at a rate equivalent to the general population, although severe acne at atypical sites is more common in male patients with HS [12].

Inflammatory disorders. One inflammatory disorder associated with HS is Crohn disease (see Chapter 97), which shares epidemiological, histological and therapeutic features with HS. Seventeen per cent of patients with Crohn disease were considered likely to have had coexistent HS in one study [15]. An inflammatory spondyloarthropathy of axial and appendicular joints, which isHLA-B27- and rheumatoid factor-negative, is well described with HS. A temporal relationship is seen between flares of joint and skin disease [14]. Other associated inflammatory disorders include pyoderma gangrenosum and the syndromes SAPHO (synovitis, acne, pustulosis, hyperostosis and osteitis), PAPA (pyogenic arthritis, pyoderma gangrenosum and acne), PASH (pyoderma gangrenosum, acne conglobata and suppurative hidradenitis) and PAPASH (pyogenic arthritis, pyoderma gangrenosum, acne and suppurative hidradenitis) (see Chapters 45, 49 and 90) [14]. Furthermore, peripheral ulcerative keratitis (Mooren-type corneal ulceration) has been described in patients with HS [16].

Genodermatoses. Genodermatoses associated with HS or HS-like lesions include keratosis ichthyosis deafness syndrome, pachyonychia congenita (see Chapter 69), steatocystoma multiplex (see Chapter 134) and Dowling–Degos disease (see Chapter 70) [14].

Pathophysiology

Early studies implicated apocrine gland occlusion as a primary pathogenic event. However, histopathological observations have since demonstrated that follicular involvement is central to pathogenesis. The following sequence of events has been suggested: infundibular hyperkeratosis, follicular dilatation/cyst formation, follicular rupture with subsequent inflammation, and fistula formation by epidermal strands [17].

Predisposing factors

Obesity and smoking

Obesity and smoking are the two main factors associated with HS. Obesity is implicated as a risk factor and correlates with disease severity: 69–77% of patients are either overweight or obese [18]. An increase of $1\,kg/m^2$ body mass index was associated with a mean increase of 0.84 Sartorius score units in one study [19]. In addition to cases describing the beneficial effect on HS of weight loss, bariatric surgery and weight loss reduces self-reported HS in the morbidly obese [20]. Increased pro-inflammatory cytokine release from visceral fat, physical occlusion and epidermal barrier stress at intertriginous skin sites may all play a role [17]. There is an increased prevalence of smoking amongst patients with HS compared with controls (89% versus 46% in one study) [21]; 63–93.7% of patients are current or ex-smokers [18]. A temporal or dose effect of smoking is not consistently demonstrated. It is not known if smoking cessation improves the course of disease.

Hormonal influences

Hormonal influences are documented and supported by a female preponderance, observed perimenstrual disease flares and improvement during pregnancy [13]. Clinical signs of virilization are, however, usually absent, circulating androgen levels are typically normal and no differences in androgen metabolism have been observed in large case series [22].

Host defence

Alterations of the innate immune system are thought to underlie disease pathogenesis. No major immune abnormalities have been found. In one study no abnormalities in granulocyte function or serum immunoglobulin levels could be detected [23]. However, some aberrant immune functions have been reported in small studies. These include an enhanced production of free oxygen radicals by stimulated neutrophil granulocytes; an impaired secretion of tumour necrosis factor a (TNF-α) and interleukin 6 (IL-6) upon stimulation of monocytes by bacterial compounds; and a diminished percentage of natural killer cells in the blood [24].

In addition, several inflammatory and anti-inflammatory cytokines levels are elevated in HS lesions. Highly up-regulated cytokines include IL-1β, TNF-α and IL-10. On the other hand, IL-2, IL-4, IL-5 and interferon γ (INF-γ) are hardly detectable in HS lesions [25,26]. The IL-23/Th17 pathway seems to be activated, reflected by enhanced expression of IL-17A, IL-12 and IL-23 in HS skin [27].

There are also changes in the expression of innate immune system peptides. Significantly decreased expression of Toll-like receptors and a relative deficiency of a range of antimicrobial peptides have been reported in HS lesions [28–33]. In addition, the mRNA expression levels of regulators and inducers of

Table 92.1 Changes in protein levels of cytokines, Toll-like receptors and antimicrobial peptides and/or their mRNA in hidradenitis suppurativa.

Molecule	Change compared with healty skin	Change compared with psoriasis	Protein or mRNA	Reference
Cytokines				
IL-1β	Increased	Increased	Protein and mRNA	**25**,26,30,32
TNF-α	Increased	Increased	Protein	**25**,26,29
IL-6	Decreased/increased		Protein and mRNA	29,32
IL-8	Increased		mRNA	32
IL-10	Increased	Increased	Protein and mRNA	**25**,26,29,32
TGF-β	Decreased		Protein	29
CXCL9	Increased		Protein	26
Monokine induced by IFN-γ (MIG)	Increased		Protein	26
IL-11	Increased		Protein	26
B-lymphocyte chemoattractant (BLC)	Increased		Protein	26
IL-17A	Increased		Protein and mRNA	26,27
IL-12	Increased		Protein and mRNA	27
IL-23	Increased		Protein and mRNA	27
IL-20	Increased	Decreased	Protein and mRNA	30
IL-22	Increased	Decreased	Protein and mRNA	30
IL-24	Increased	Increased	mRNA	30
IL-26	Increased		mRNA	30
ICAM-1	Decreased		Protein	29
α-MSH	Decreased		Protein	29
IGF-1	Decreased		Protein	29
IFN-γ	Normal/Increased		mRNA	**25**,30
Matrix metalloproteinase 1 (MMP-1)	Increased		mRNA	32
Toll-like receptors (TLRs)				
TLR-2	Increased/decreased		Protein and mRNA	28,29
TLR-3	Decreased		Protein	29
TLR-4	Decreased		Protein	29
TLR-7	Decreased		Protein	29
TLR-9	Decreased		Protein	29
Antimicrobial peptides (AMPs)				
Human β-defensin-1 (HBD1)	Decreased			30
Human β-defensin-2 (HBD2)	Increased	Decreased	Protein and mRNA	29,30,31,32
Human β-defensin-3 (HBD3)	Increased	Decreased	Protein and mRNA	30,33
Ribonuclease 7	Decreased			33
S100A7 (psoriasin)	Increased/no change	Decreased	Protein and mRNA	30,31,33
S100A8	Increased	Decreased	mRNA	30
S100A9	Increased	Decreased	mRNA	30
Cathelicidin (LL-37)	Increased		mRNA	32

CXCL, chemokine(C-X-C motif); ICAM, intercellular adhesion molecule; IFN, interferon; IGF, insulin-like growth factor; IL, interleukin; MSH, melanocyte-stimulating hormone; TNF, tumour necrosis factor.

antimicrobial peptides (AMPs) such as IL-22 and IL-20 have been found to be reduced compared with psoriasis and atopic eczema [30]. Further details of all these changes are given in Table 92.1.

Medications

An exacerbation or onset of disease has been reported following lithium and sirolimus therapy [34,35].

Pathology

Histopathological changes vary with disease stage. Early changes, which precede clinically evident lesions, are character-ized by a sparse lymphocytic infiltrate of the terminal follicular unit and sebaceous gland atrophy [36,37]. Follicular hyperplasia, perifollicular lymphocytic inflammatory infiltration, interfollicular psoriasiform hyperplasia and dilatation of the follicular lumen follow in developed lesions [36]. Cysts lined by stratified squamous epithelium containing lammellated keratin and free hair shafts appear [36]. During flares, abscess formation and ruptured follicular units are seen, associated with a dense, dermal, mixed, inflammatory infiltrate including histiocytes and giant cells that extends to interfollicular apocrine and eccrine structures and deep into the subcutis. Sinus tract formation and fibrosis follows [36].

PART 8: SPECIFIC CUTANEOUS STRUCTURE

Histopathological variations less frequently seen include isolated inflammation of the apocrine gland (apocrinitis in 5%), sebaceous gland necrosis, epithelioid granulomas and B-cell pseudofollicles [36].

Causative organisms

The role of bacteria remains to be clarified. HS is currently regarded as a primary inflammatory disorder without a defined infectious trigger. Microbiology from superficial and deep sampling often demonstrates negative culture or only normal skin flora with multiple non-pathogenic bacterial species in the majority of cultures. The most common bacterial isolates are *Staphylococcus epidermidis* and *S. aureus*, followed by *Peptostreptococcus* species and *Propionibacterium acnes* [38–40]. Streptococcal antibodies are usually not found.

Genetics

Approximately one-third of patients have a family member with HS [12]. HS does not appear to be linked to specific human leukocyte antigen (HLA) types [41]. In some cases an autosomal pattern of inheritance can be found [42]. Loss-of-function mutations in the γ-secretase genes *Nicastrin*, *Presenilin-1* and *Presenilin enhancer-2* are probably responsible for a small number of familial cases. Gamma-secretase regulates notch signalling, which plays a role in epidermal and terminal hair follicle differentiation, immune cell development and immune functions. Deficient notch signalling in mice has been shown to be associated with the conversion of hair follicles to keratin-enriched epidermal cysts as a result of changes to the outer root sheath cells [43,44].

Environmental factors

Mechanical irritation and shear forces are potential contributory factors. There is no evidence that poor hygiene, variation in routine depilatory techniques or use of antiperspirant are relevant to HS.

Clinical features

All three diagnostic criteria shown in Box 92.1 must be met for a diagnosis of HS to be made.

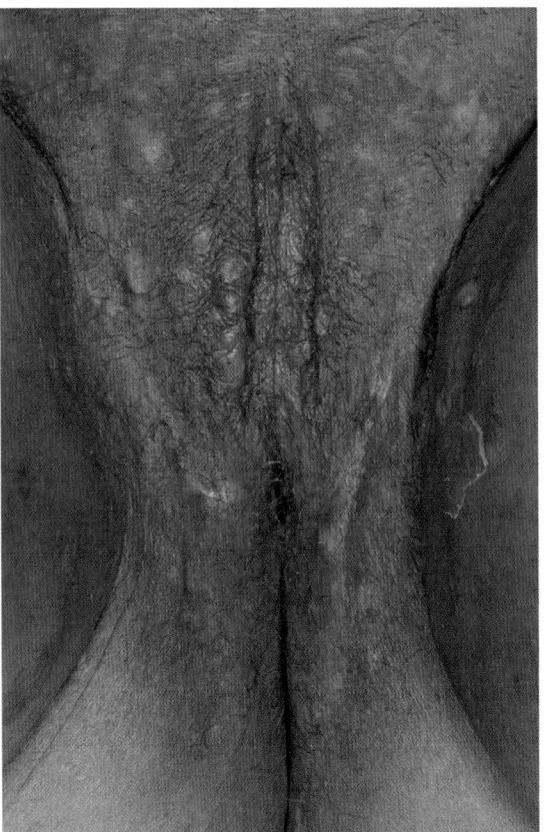

Figure 92.1 Multiple non-inflamed nodules in a patient with Hurley stage II disease of the genital area.

Box 92.1 Essential criteria for a diagnosis of hidradenitis suppurativa to be made

1 Typical lesions	Deep-seated painful nodules, abscesses, draining sinuses, bridged scars and paired or multiheaded open pseudocomedones
2 Typical topography	Axillae, groin, perineal and perianal region, buttocks, infra- and intermammary folds
3 Presence and recurrence of lesions	

History

A history of typical lesions at typical sites with recurrence and chronicity is required for diagnosis (Box 92.1). Typical index lesions consist of painful subcutaneous nodules or abscesses that persist for a mean duration of 7–15 days. This is followed by spontaneous regression, partial regression (to form non-inflammatory, asymptomatic nodules) or progression to abscess formation with the rupture and release of purulent malodorous discharges. Typical sites are the axillae; the inguino-genital, perineal, perianal and gluteal areas; and infra- and inter-mammary skin.

Recurrence takes the form of acute intermittent or continuous disease, involving new skin sites or pre-existing non-inflammatory nodules. Acute intermittent flares consist of solitary or multiple lesions, which are localized or disseminated across regions. Periods of remission (characterized by normal skin or persistent non-inflammatory nodules) may last for weeks to months. Continuous active disease can lead to the formation of coalescing nodules and sinus tracts associated with chronic, daily, purulent discharge and pain.

Presentation

Index lesions include inflamed and non-inflamed dermal and subcutaneous nodules (Figure 92.1), which may be evident on palpation alone; rounded (as opposed to 'pointing') abscesses (Figure 92.2); and draining or non-draining sinus tracts (Figures 92.3 and 92.4). Scarring is typically bridged or 'rope-like', it can be hypertrophic or

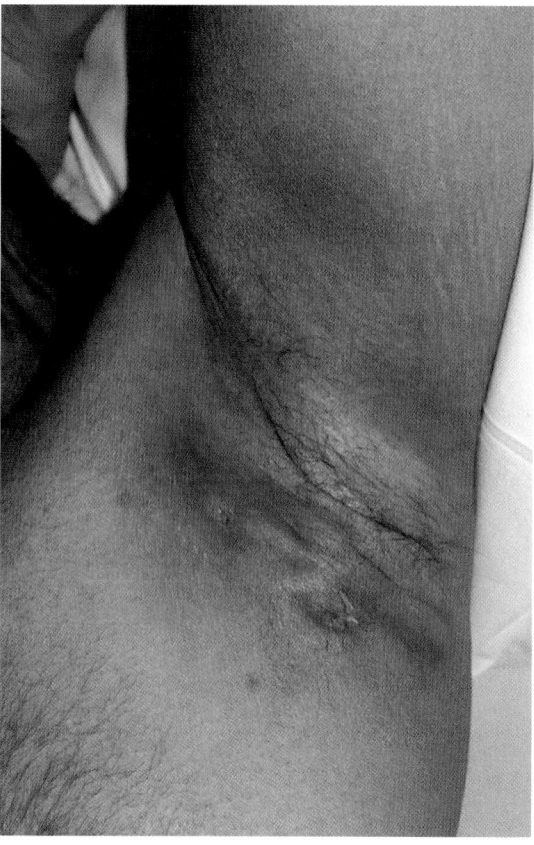

Figure 92.2 Classical axillary abscess as seen in hidradenitis suppurativa.

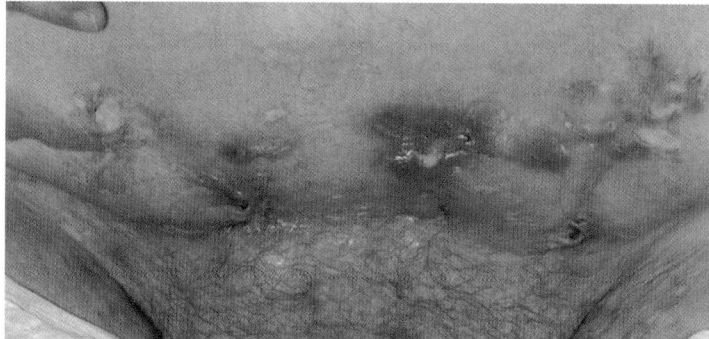

Figure 92.4 Multiple inflamed nodules and draining sinuses in active Hurley stage II disease of the mons pubis.

atrophic, producing depressions especially on the buttocks, and may be associated with contractures (Figure 92.5). Pseudo- (secondary) comedones are often seen, typically paired, polyporous and grouped (Figure 92.6). Closed comedones are not seen.

Associated lesions include follicular papules and pustules, pyogenic granulomas at sinus tract openings and indurated plaques. Epidermoid cysts are seen in some patients on external genitalia, the face and the thorax. Regional lymphadenopathy is not routinely seen.

Lesions are localized to inverse (flexural) areas. The commonest sites are the axillae and inguinal and ano-genital regions, including the external genitalia and the perineal, perianal and gluteal

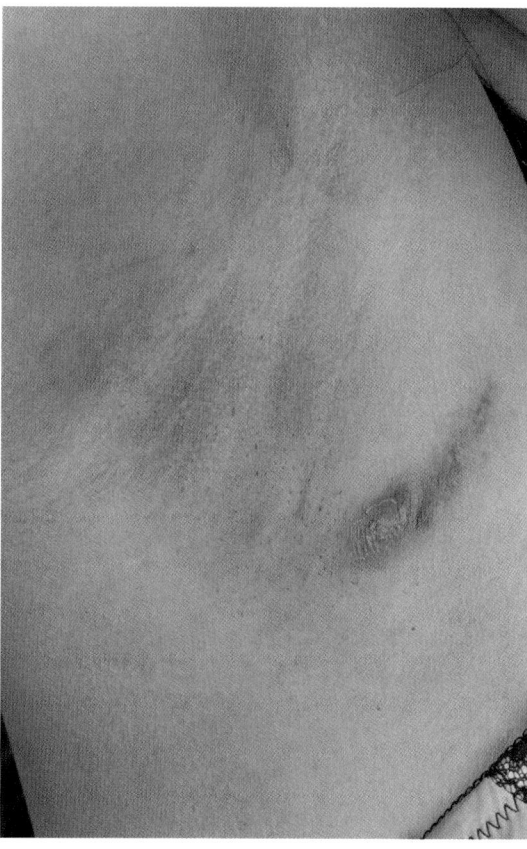

Figure 92.3 Non-draining sinus, recognized by the palpable oblong shape.

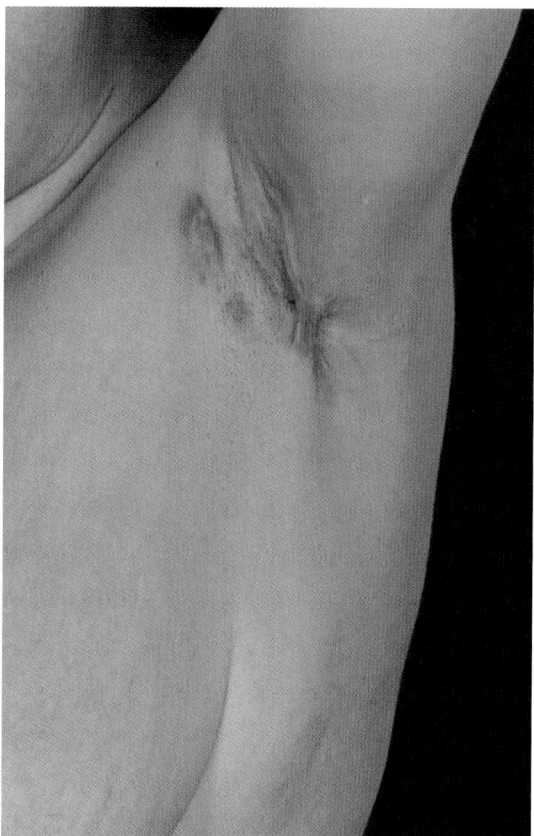

Figure 92.5 Scar: rope-like band formed by fibrotic tissue, most often seen in the axillae.

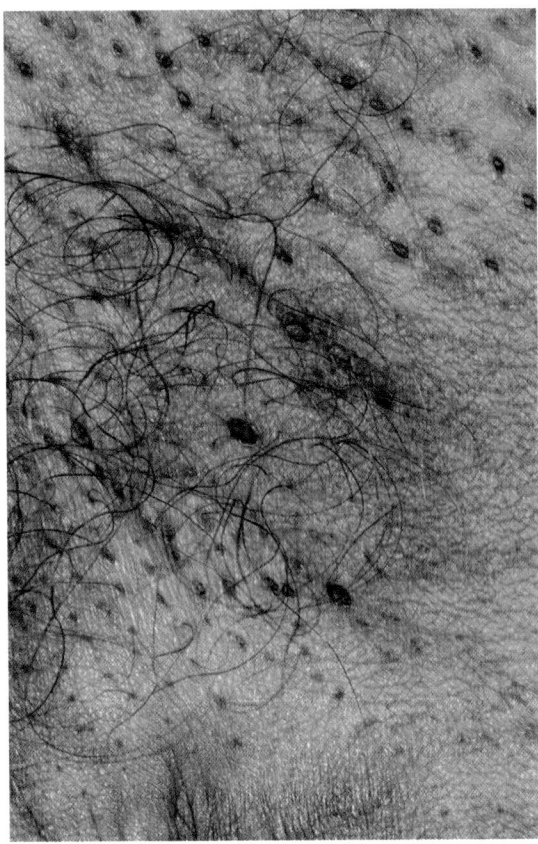

Figure 92.6 Tombstone comedones in the axilla.

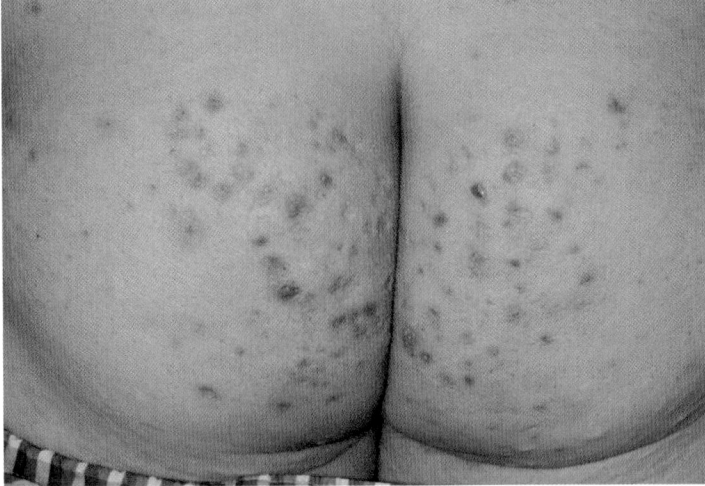

Figure 92.8 Follicular pattern involving the buttocks.

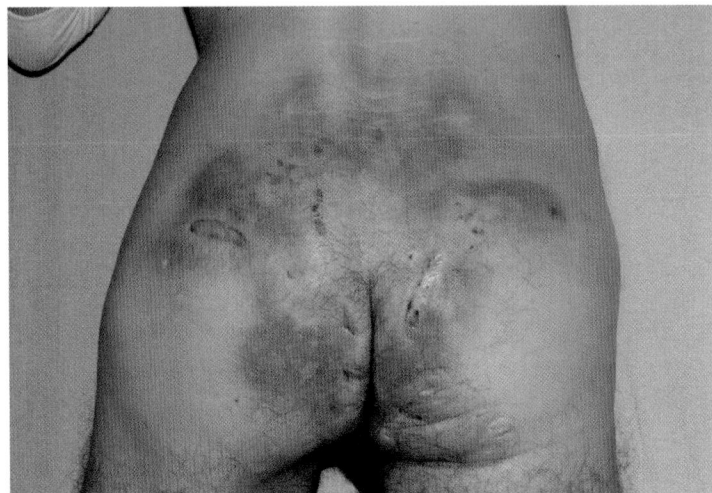

Figure 92.9 Nodules and sinus tracts involving the buttocks.

skin (Figures 92.7, 92.8 and 92.9). Sub- and intermammary skin can also be affected, as can, less commonly, retroauricular, preauricular and occipital skin (Figure 92.10). Truncal variants are also reported (Figure 92.11).

The clinical presentation varies with respect to the number of anatomical regions affected, the extent of the lesions and the types of lesions within a single region. The spectrum ranges from mild disease consisting of solitary nodules to severe disease comprising

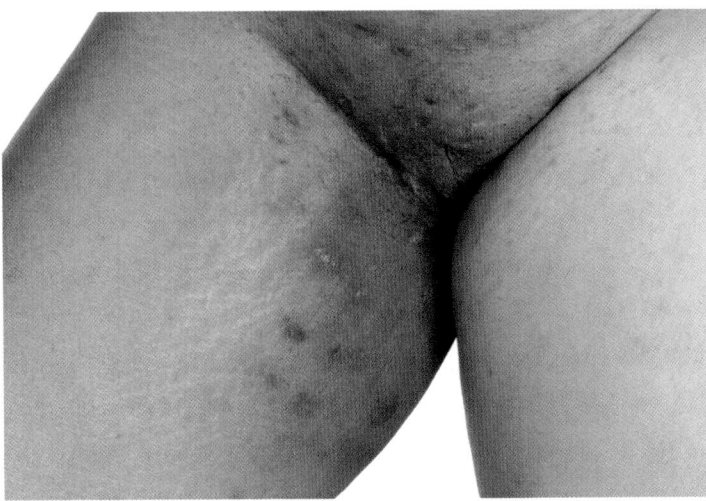

Figure 92.7 Follicular pattern involving the genito-femoral area showing non-active disease.

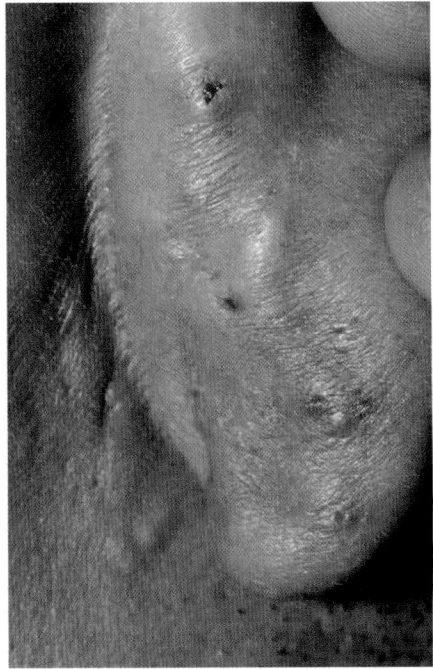

Figure 92.10 Ectopic disease with retroauricular involvement.

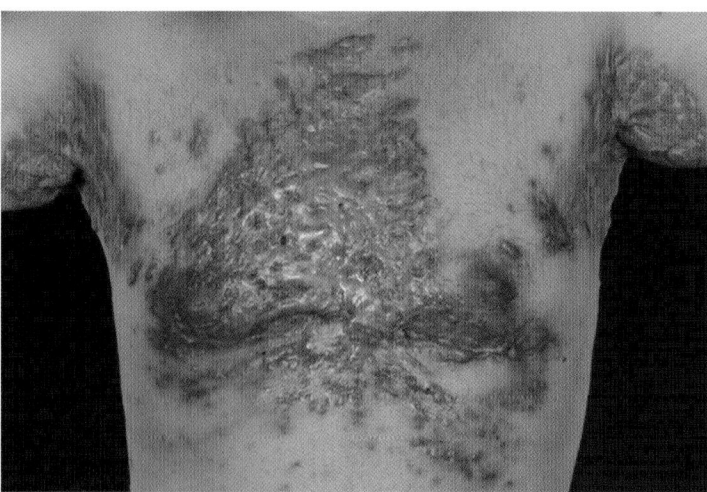

Figure 92.11 Ectopic plaque on the chest of a patient. Notice the classical involvement seen in the axillae.

extensive inflamed confluent nodules, sinus tracts and scarring filling an entire anatomical region.

Clinical variants

Hidradenitis suppurativa is a heterogeneous disorder. Epidemiological studies indicate that multiple phenotypic subtypes are likely to exist, grouped by topographical predilection and lesion subtype. Three clinical variants have been suggested, although their clinical significance has not been studied [45].

- The classical variant, characterized by scarring lesions in the axillae and under the breasts, occurs most often in women and often includes lesions in the ano-genital area.
- A second variant is characterized by the additional involvement of the ears, chest, back or legs, with pilonidal sinuses, comedones, severe acne and a family history of HS, which may be a part of the follicular occlusion triad (see Chapter 90).
- A third variant is characterized by gluteal involvement, papules and folliculitis and may be more common in men.

Differential diagnosis

The differential diagnosis of HS is extensive. Index lesions should be differentiated from abscesses, carbuncles or furunculosis associated with primary cutaneous bacterial infection (typically staphylococcal or streptococcal) or secondary infection of cystic structures (e.g. epidermoid cysts and Bartholin glands). Crohn disease can result in inflammatory abscesses and sinus tracts at ano-genital sites. However, in Crohn disease, fistulae are usually intersphincteric, whereas in HS they do not involve the gastrointestinal tract. Clinical and histological overlap results in diagnostic challenge. Rare infections, including tuberculosis, sporotrichosis, actinomycosis and lymphogranuloma venereum, can present with both abscesses and sinus tracts. Steatocystoma multiplex and neoplastic diseases such as Langerhans cell histiocytosis should also be considered in the differential diagnosis.

Classification of severity

The Hurley staging system refers to three stages based on the presence and extent of sinus tracts and scarring (Table 92.2) [4]. Hurley

Table 92.2 Definition of the three Hurley stages in hidradenitis suppurativa.

Stage	Features
I (Figure 92.12)	Recurrent abscess formation without sinus tracts and cicatrization
II (Figure 92.13)	Recurrent abscesses with widely separated sinus tracts and cicatrization
III (Figure 92.14)	Multiple interconnected abscesses, sinus tracts and cicatrization diffusely involving an entire region

staging allows stratification of therapy but is not useful for assessing response to therapy.

The hidradenitis severity score (HSS; or modified Sartorius score) is a more detailed, validated and dynamic score, which can be used to assess both severity and treatment response [46]. The HSS was originally developed to assess the results of surgery, but has been modified to include inflammatory elements. It correlates with the Hurley score but is more precisely defined and responsive to change [46]. The HSS incorporates assessment of the number of anatomical regions affected, lesions (counts of inflamed and non-inflamed nodules and sinus tracts), the extent of area involved and the presence of normal skin between lesions to give a regional and total score. The utility of the score is limited in severe disease where the presence of confluent nodules and sinus tracts reduces the accuracy of individual lesion counts.

The hidradenitis suppurativa clinical response (HiSCR) has been suggested as an outcome measure when studying treatments [47]. It is defined as a ≥50% reduction from baseline in the number of inflamed lesions (abscesses or inflamed nodules), without a concomitant increase in the number of draining fistulae. The HiSCR has been validated against Hurley stage, the HSS, the HS physician's global assessment (PGA) system and patient-reported outcomes (visual analogue pain scale, dermatology life quality index and work productivity and activity impairment questionnaire) [47]. Patients who achieve an HiSCR appear to have meaningful improvement of their disease.

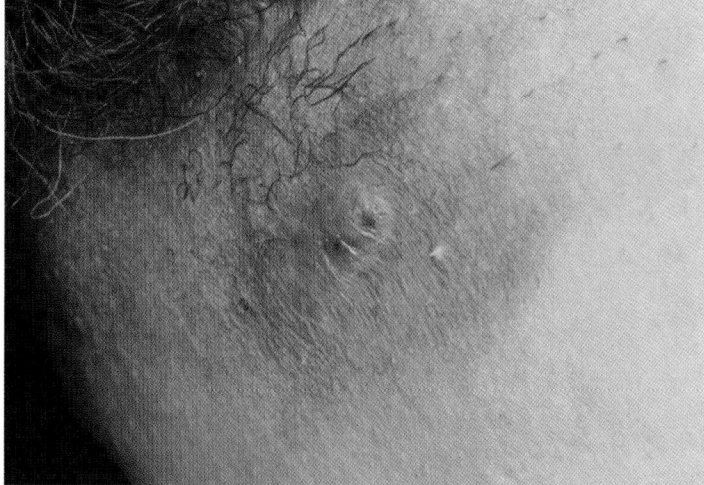

Figure 92.12 Hurley stage I disease of the genito-femoral area showing a solitary nodule. Notice the normal-looking surrounding skin and perilesional halo of discoloration indicating a recent episode of inflammation.

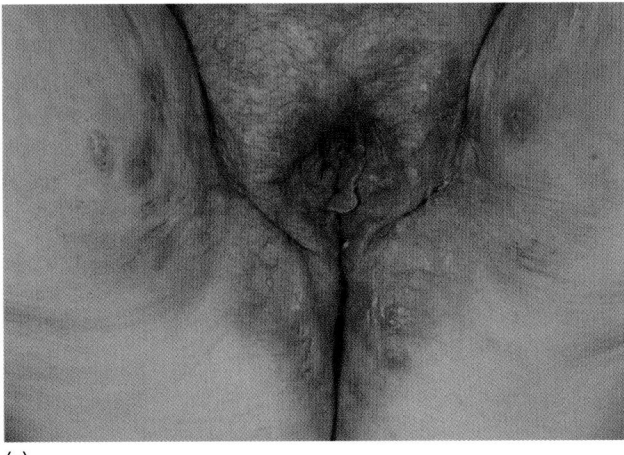

(a)

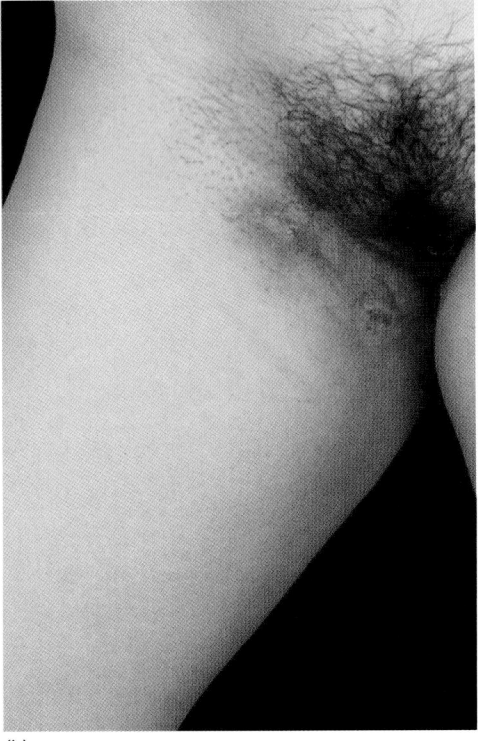

(b)

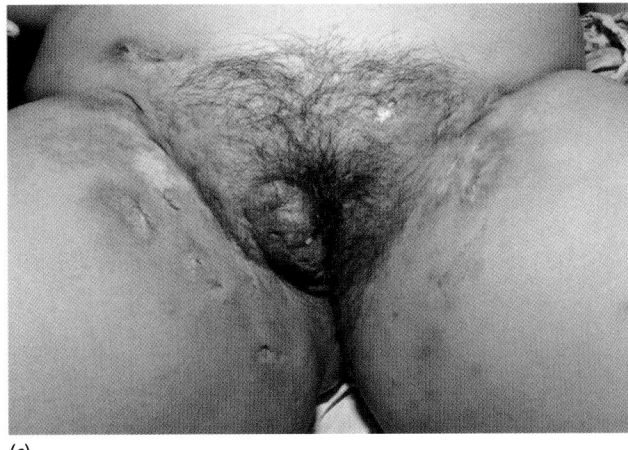

(c)

Figure 92.13 Hurley stage II disease of the genito-femoral area. (a) Hurley stage II is a broad category which may involve more severe disease as shown here. (b) Inactive, mild disease. (c) Severe, active, multifocal disease. Notice the areas of normal-looking skin separating the lesions.

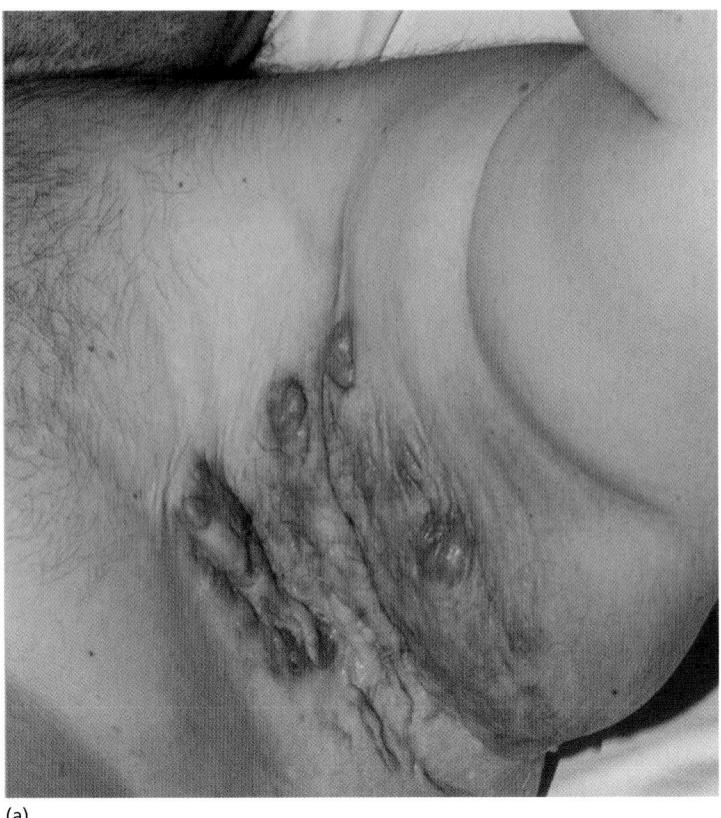

(a)

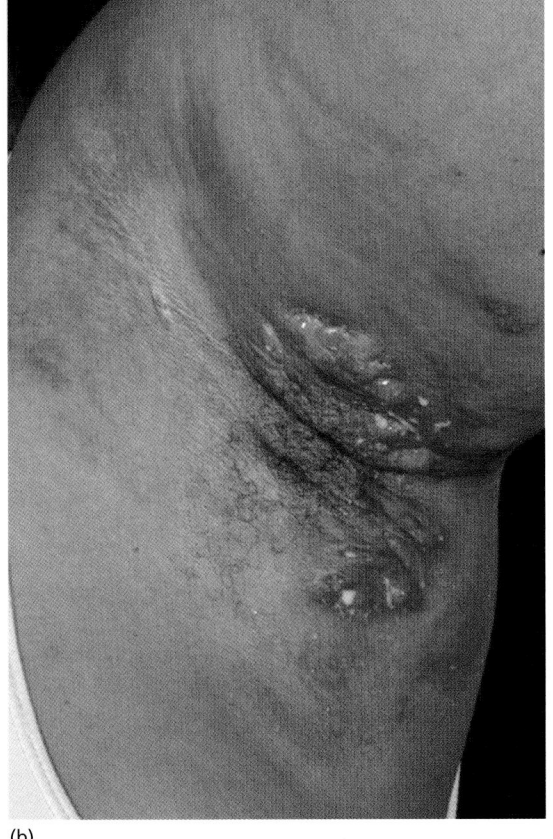

(b)

Figure 92.14 Hurley stage III disease. (a) Non-draining, confluent, chronic lesions involving the entire axilla. (b) Active draining lesions in the axilla.

Other quantitative outcomes used to support the assessment of disease severity include the HS PGA, pain scales (visual analogue or numerical) and validated quality of life questionnaires (e.g. DLQI, Skindex). The frequency of flares may play a role in the assessment of intermittent disease, and should be assessed over a minimum period of 3 months.

Complications and co-morbidities

Superinfection constitutes a curable complication, and should be suspected when flares are preceded by stinging or smarting pain or associated with the development of pustules and other superficial lesions. Structural complications of longstanding disease include lymphatic obstruction leading to clinical lymphoedema. The ano-genital sites are most severely affected and progression to scrotal elephantiasis can occur. Fistula formation to the gastrointestinal tract (anal canal and rectum), genito-urinary tract (urethra, bladder and vagina) and peritoneum are extremely rarely described, and when seen should trigger examination for Crohn disease. Cutaneous squamous cell carcinoma (SCC) can complicate chronic ano-genital disease, most commonly the gluteal skin of male patients, and carries a poor prognosis; it has been reported more often in men than in women [18]. There are no reports of SCC complicating axillary disease to date. Other complications of chronic disease include anaemia (multifactorial), hypoalbuminaemia, hypergammaglobulinaemia and rarely amyloidosis and sacral bacterial osteomyelitis [18].

A profound impact on quality of life complicates disease at all stages of severity. Significant psychological, social and economic impact appears more commonly than in many other chronic inflammatory dermatoses [6]. Depression is frequent, with one study suggesting 40% of patients have a concomitant diagnosis of depression [48].

Disease course and prognosis

Chronicity is the hallmark. The mean duration is 18.8 years [49]. Milder forms (Hurley stage I) are more frequent and reported to affect approximately two-thirds of patients, with intermediate disease (Hurley stage II) affecting one-quarter and severe disease (Hurley stage III) about one-fifth of patients [49]. Both intermittent and continuous disease can be seen at each stage. The natural course of progression between stages is not defined. In patients older than 50 years, the disease is progressively rarer with increasing age suggesting that spontaneous remission may occur over time. A long-term follow-up study has reported that this is seen in approximately 40% of HS patients after a median follow-up period of 22 years [50].

Investigations

Microbiology (swabs, purulent exudate and tissue) and histopathology are indicated for refractory or atypical cases to exclude flare secondary to superinfection and to consider relevant differentials. Imaging (both ultrasound and magnetic resonance imaging) defines subclinical extension, complications of severe disease and informs preoperative planning. Routine bloods in severe disease (Hurley stage III) may reveal anaemia (multifactorial), hypoalbuminaemia, polyclonal hypergammaglobulinaemia and elevated C-reactive protein or other less commonly used inflammatory markers that can serve as an adjunct for monitoring severe disease.

Management

Treatment strategy should be individually based and take the following into account:
1 The need for patient empowerment.
2 The recognition that the disease is multifocal from the onset and that generalized medical treatment is therefore as appropriate as in other inflammatory dermatoses.
3 The recognition that once scarring occurs, surgical removal of affected areas is the only curative therapeutic option.

A management flow chart for HS according to the Hurley stage is shown in Figure 92.15.

Adjuvant treatment

Hidradenitis suppurativa is a disease that significantly impacts on quality of life; self-care may help patients cope with day-to-day routine as well as with the disease itself. Patients should be encouraged and supported to lose weight. Tobacco abstinence should be encouraged. Patients should also be shown how to bandage suppurating lesions and recommended to wear loose fitting clothes [1].

Analgesics

Hidradenitis suppurativa is painful and patients should be offered appropriate analgesic therapy, including non-steroidal anti-inflammatory therapy and paracetamol. In selected cases centrally acting analgesics are indicated [1].

Topical therapy

Topical clindamycin lotion 0.1% may be beneficial and appears to offer control of milder lesions [51]. For patients with localized, recalcitrant, established lesions (Hurley stage II), topical resorcinol 15% in a suitable ointment appears to offer improved disease control [52]. The benefits of antiseptics such as chlorhexidine washes or benzoyl peroxide remain unproven.

Systemic antibiotics

Tetracycline and the combination of clindamycin and rifampicin have been used in the largest reported series. Oral tetracycline 500 mg b.d. for 3 months appears to be useful in mild but widespread disease [53]. Longer term treatment may be considered if the treatment is effective. For more advanced cases, combined treatment with clindamycin 300 mg b.d. and rifampicin 300 mg b.d. given for 10 weeks appears to be effective in a large proportion of cases [54,55]. This regimen reduced disease severity by an average of 50% as measured by HSS in one case series [54]. There are no formal studies of longer term treatment, but responders may require repeated treatments for recurrences.

A range of other antibiotics have been reported to be effective in smaller series, including the combination of rifampicin,

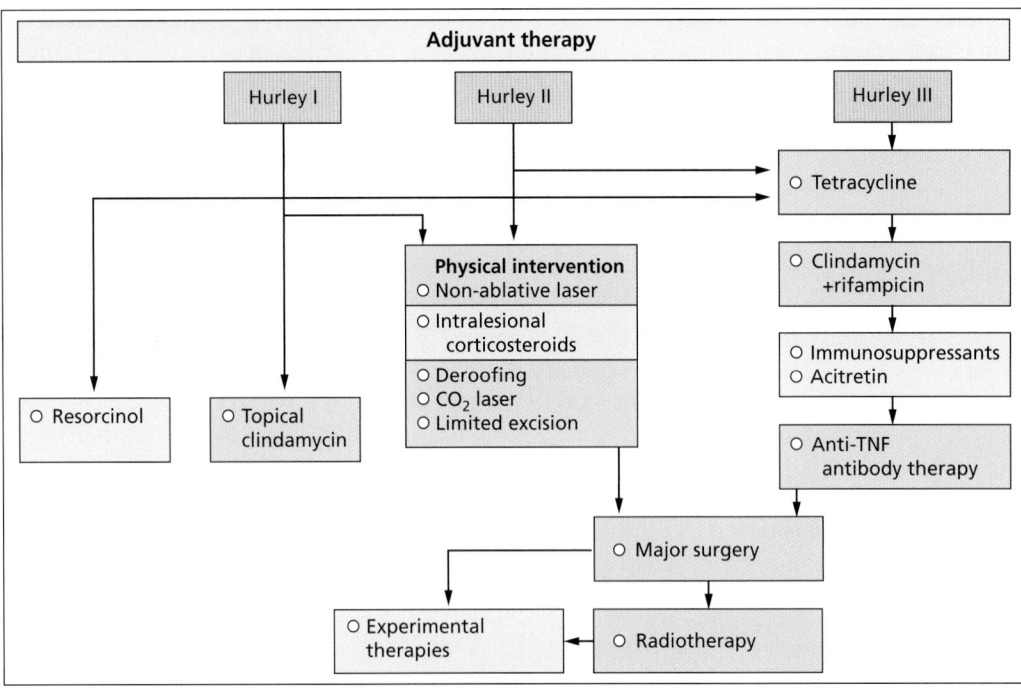

Figure 92.15 Management flow chart for the initial treatment of hidradenitis suppurativa according to the Hurley stage. Arrows indicate the recommended sequence of initial choice but, on failure to respond, secondary choices can be made freely from any treatment. Colour coding reflects the evidence level supporting the recommendations: blue, expert opinion; green, case series with 30+ patients or randomized controlled trial. TNF, tumour necrosis factor.

metronidazole and moxifloxacin [56]. On suspicion of super-infection, antibiotic therapy should be started based on prior microbial susceptibility testing.

Anti-inflammatory treatment

For single lesions, intralesional triamcinolone (3–5 mg) often ameliorates symptoms rapidly. For more severe disease, systemic therapy is often necessary. A variety of drugs may be used for this; short-term systemic prednisolone (0.5–1.0 mg/kg body weight) or ciclosporin (3–5 mg/kg body weight), or longer term treatment using dapsone (100 mg daily), have all been reported to be useful for disease control [57].

Biological agents

Tumour necrosis factor-α antibodies appear to have a beneficial effect in moderate to severe HS [57]. Three randomized controlled trials (RCTs) have been conducted with adalimumab. They indicated that approximately twice as many patients treated actively achieved a significant effect (as defined by HiSCR) using a dosing regimen similar to that used for inflammatory bowel disease (a loading dose of 160 mg at week 0 and 80 mg at week 2, followed at week 4 by 40 mg every week, for a total of 12 weeks) as compared with patients not treated actively (58.9% versus 27.6% respectively) [58,59]. An RCT of standard infliximab failed to reach its primary end point, but a *post hoc* analysis of the results indicated significant improvement in actively treated patients [60]. For etanercept, an RCT failed to confirm the initially promising results of open studies [61]. There have been anecdotal reports of benefit from ustekinumab and from anti-IL-1 agents but these have not as yet been systematically evaluated.

Retinoids

Isotretinoin is rarely effective in HS and its use is not encouraged. In contrast, case series suggest that acitretin (50 mg or more daily)

may be effective in a significant proportion of patients and in some cases offers long-term remissions [57].

Experimental therapies

Zinc gluconate (90 mg/day) has been advocated as maintenance therapy or in combination with other therapies [62]. Other treatments that have been reported to be effective in cases or small series include intramuscular immunoglobulin, metformin and botulinum toxin [63–65].

Surgery

Several lesion-directed therapies have been described as useful in the management of HS.

Incision and drainage. Classical incision and drainage is useful only when frank fluctuating abscesses appear. The inflamed nodules of HS only respond with additional scarring. Incisions carry a 100% recurrence rate and should only be used if manifest fluctuation is found [66].

Deroofing. Deroofing is a tissue-saving technique, whereby the 'roof' of an abscess or sinus tract is surgically removed either through electrosurgery (using a loop) or conventional surgery [67]. A blunt probe is inserted in sinus openings discharging purulent exudate. If an opening cannot be identified, a small incision can be made to introduce a probe into the lesions. The full extent of the lesion is explored systematically with the probe, and the roof of the lesion surgically removed using the probe as a guide, leaving the partly epithelialized/granulating floor of the lesion exposed. The ensuing defect is left open to heal by secondary intention.

Localized surgery. Single lesions can be surgically excised; this results in a lower recurrence rate than after incision and drainage [68]. Generally, complete surgical removal of the lesion is required, suggesting that wider excisions have a better result than more limited exision. Whether or not the defect should be closed is a matter of debate. Patients with few, clinically stable, non-inflamed lesions (nodules or sinus tracts) are most suitable for localized surgery.

Ablative lasers and electrosurgery. Removal of all involved tissue appears to be necessary for successful surgical treatment of HS. CO_2 laser evaporation provides a method whereby all visibly affected tissue can be vaporized using a scanner in a manner akin to macroscopic Mohs' surgery (i.e. systematically evaporating abnormal tissue under visual guidance until healthy tissue is reached everywhere) [69]. The technique offers radical treatment whilst still being tissue-sparing. Postsurgical defects are usually left to heal by secondary intention. They normally heal sufficiently for resumption of work after 2–3 weeks, but it can take 8–10 weeks for the tissues to re-epithelialize fully. Patient satisfaction with the technique is high [70].

Extensive surgery. In severe disease when entire sites are involved with multiple interconnecting sinus tracts, the only curative method is excision of the entire area involved. The margins of excision in the reported case series range from 1 cm up to the excision of all hair-bearing skin of the affected region. For extensive ano-genital disease, this may therefore require multidisciplinary collaboration with plastic surgery and, where a temporary colostomy may be required, with colorectal surgery. The often large defects can be left to heal by secondary intent. Particular attention should, however, be paid to mobilization of the affected areas in order to avoid the development of postoperative strictures, especially in the axillae. The defects can also be closed by split-skin graft or flaps [71].

Non-ablative lasers/intense pulsed light
Hair removal using light-based therapies appears to have a beneficial effect in HS. Studies have found significant improvement following monthly treatments with both neodymium:yttrium-aluminium-garnet (Nd:YAG) laser as well as intense pulsed light (IPL) [72,73].

Radiotherapy
In selected patients with particularly recalcitrant disease, radiotherapy may be considered. Fractionated radiotherapy has been described as effective in the older literature. Total doses of up to 12 Gy have been administered as single doses of 0.5–1.0 Gy given 4–12 times [72].

Key references

The full list of references can be found in the online version at www.rooksdermatology.com.

1 Zouboulis CC, Desai N, Emtestam L, *et al.* European S1 guideline for the treatment of hidradenitis suppurativa/acne inversa. *J Eur Acad Dermatol Venereol* 2015;29:619.

6 Matusiak L, Bieniek A, Szepietowski JC. Psychophysical aspects of hidradenitis suppurativa. *Acta Derm Venereol* 2010;90:264–8.

9 Jemec GB, Heidenheim M, Nielsen NH. The prevalence of hidradenitis suppurativa and its potential precursor lesions. *J Am Acad Dermatol* 1996;35:191–4.

17 Van der Zee HH, Laman JD, Boer J, *et al.* Hidradenitis suppurativa: viewpoint on clinical phenotyping, pathogenesis and novel treatments. *Exp Dermatol* 2012;21:735–9.

25 Van der Zee HH, de Ruiter L, van den Broecke DG, *et al.* Elevated levels of tumour necrosis factor (TNF)-alpha, interleukin (IL)-1beta and IL-10 in hidradenitis suppurativa skin: a rationale for targeting TNF-alpha and IL-1beta. *Br J Dermatol* 2011;164:1292–8.

43 Pink AE, Simpson MA, Desai N, *et al.* Gamma-secretase mutations in hidradenitis suppurativa: new insights into disease pathogenesis. *J Invest Dermatol* 2013;133:601–7.

48 Onderdijk AJ, van der Zee HH, Esmann S, *et al.* Depression in patients with hidradenitis suppurativa. *J Eur Acad Dermatol Venereol* 2013;27:473–8.

55 Gener G, Canoui-Poitrine F, Revuz JE, *et al.* Combination therapy with clindamycin and rifampicin for hidradenitis suppurativa: a series of 116 consecutive patients. *Dermatology* 2009;219:148–54.

66 Ritz JP, Runkel N, Haier J, *et al.* Extent of surgery and recurrence rate of hidradenitis suppurativa. *Int J Colorectal Dis* 1998;13:164–8.

69 Lapins J, Marcusson JA, Emtestam L. Surgical treatment of chronic hidradenitis suppurativa: CO2 laser stripping-secondary intention technique. *Br J Dermatol* 1994;131:551–6.

CHAPTER 93

Other Acquired Disorders of the Pilosebaceous Unit

Roderick J. Hay[1], Rachael Morris-Jones[1] and Gregor B. E. Jemec[2]

[1]Dermatology Department, King's College Hospital, London, UK
[2]Department of Dermatology, Roskilde Hospital; and Health Sciences Faculty, University of Copenhagen, Copenhagen, Denmark

Pseudofolliculitis

Definition and nomenclature
Pseudofolliculitis is an inflammatory follicular and perifollicular foreign-body reaction.

Synonyms and inclusions
- Pili incarnati
- Ingrowing hairs
- Pseudofolliculitis barbae

Introduction and general description
Pseudofolliculitis is an inflammatory follicular and perifollicular foreign-body reaction to hair trapped beneath the skin surface as may occur from penetration or retraction of the cut ends of hair into the skin following shaving or as the result of disturbed hair growth following plucking or waxing. Areas particularly affected are those most frequently shaved including the beard, pubic areas and lower legs.

Epidemiology

Incidence and prevalence
Pseudofolliculitis of the beard area is very common, with reportedly up to 80% of African males being affected.

Age
After puberty.

Sex
Males are most commonly affected.

Ethnicity
Men of African descent are particularly predisposed.

Pathophysiology

Predisposing factors
Inflammation results either from the hair being cut too short, so that it may retract into the follicle and then directly penetrate the follicle wall, or from hair left to grow for a few days after being cut or shaved, such that the hairs curve backwards and penetrate adjacent skin [1,2]. Curly hair is more liable to both of these aberrations, so that the condition is very common and more severe in those with tightly coiled hair [2]. Genetic predisposition is an important factor [3].

Skin folds or irregularities due to scarring may allow ingrowth of straight hairs. Any shaved surface in either sex may be affected, but the male beard area is naturally the most common. Both plucking [4] and waxing [5] of hair, particularly on the limbs in women, commonly lead to pseudofolliculitis. Cut nasal hairs may act similarly [6]. Pseudofolliculitis is particularly troublesome in the Armed Forces, where strict grooming standards demand clean shaving [2]. The exact prevalence is not known, although between 45% and 83% of African American men are thought to be affected [2]. Pseudofolliculitis has also been reported as an adverse drug reaction to oral minoxidil [7].

Pathology
Penetration of aberrant cut ends of the hair into the follicle or surrounding tissue results in acute inflammation, microabscesses and foreign-body giant cell granuloma formation.

Rook's Textbook of Dermatology, Ninth Edition. Edited by Christopher Griffiths, Jonathan Barker, Tanya Bleiker, Robert Chalmers and Daniel Creamer.
© 2016 John Wiley & Sons, Ltd. Published 2016 by John Wiley & Sons, Ltd.
Companion website: www.rooksdermatology.com

PART 8: SPECIFIC CUTANEOUS STRUCTURE

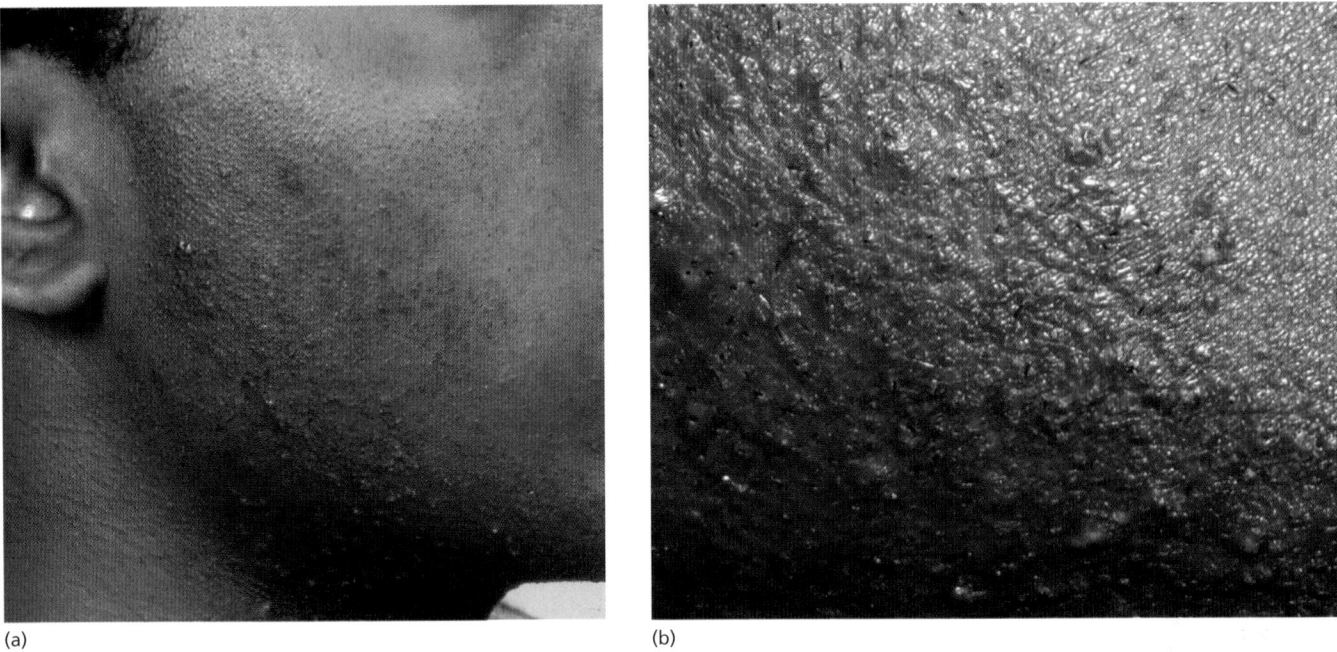

(a)   (b)

Figure 93.1 (a,b) Pseudofolliculitis barbae showing typical distribution (a) and close-up view (b).

Causative organisms

Coagulase-negative staphylococci may sometimes be grown from the lesions but the condition is not primarily infective but rather a foreign-body inflammatory reaction.

Clinical features

Presentation

The condition typically manifests as multiple small papules and pustules on shaven skin, particularly in the beard area. The skin of the neck and over the jaw is most commonly affected, although the cheeks may also be involved (Figure 93.1a,b). Papules may be large and may scar; keloid formation and hyperpigmentation may ensue. It is generally possible to identify some penetrating hairs but they may not be visible in all cases. Where there is clinical doubt, it is sometimes possible to extract a coiled hair using the tip of a sterile needle. The clinical appearance may lead to significant distress. The diagnosis is usually obvious. In cases where sites other than the beard area are affected, a history of shaving, plucking or waxing should help to clinch the diagnosis.

Differential diagnosis

Bacterial folliculitis including sycosis barbae and dermatophytosis.

Complications and co-morbidities

Pseudofolliculitis, particularly of the beard area, can result in hypertrophic or keloid scarring.

Disease course and prognosis

Pseudofolliculitis is a chronic condition with a relapsing and remitting course. Avoiding shaving can allow the skin to recover, otherwise intermittent treatment may be required. Permanent hair removal at high-risk sites may be appropriate in selected cases.

Management

The only certain cure is to stop shaving/waxing for a minimum of 4–6 weeks, to allow the inflammation to settle and allow the hairs to grow sufficiently long that ingrowth will not occur. Resumption of shaving or waxing will often, however, lead to relapse [2]. Studies examining the frequency of shaving have demonstrated that shaving 2–3 times per week rather than daily reduced papule and ingrowing hair numbers [7]. Lifting out re-entrant hairs with a needle is helpful but tedious: brushing with an abrasive sponge or toothbrush to 'release' the hair is less effective but quicker. Hair should be left about 1 mm long. This may be achieved by adjustment of individual shaving technique, or by specially designed razors [8] or electric clippers. Plucking should be avoided. Some relief is possible with topical steroid–antimicrobial combinations combined with intensive use of emollients. Hair removal with chemical depilatories or topical eflornithine hydrochloride cream may be helpful for some patients, and there is evidence that the combination of eflornithine and laser is better than laser epilation alone [9].

Treatment ladder

First line
- Stop shaving the affected area for 6 weeks and apply topical combination steroid/antibacterial cream

Second line
- Shave hair two or three times per week rather than daily
- Use chemical depilatories rather than physical hair removal

Third line
- Laser hair removal in the affected area

Folliculitis keloidalis

Definition and nomenclature
Folliculitis keloidalis is a chronic inflammatory process involving principally the hair follicles of the nape of the neck and leading to hypertrophic scarring in papules and plaques.

> **Synonyms and inclusions**
> • Folliculitis keloidalis nuchae
> • Acne keloidalis nuchae

Introduction and general description
Although this relatively common chronic follicular inflammatory dermatosis characteristically involves the nape of the neck (Latin: *nucha*), it may extend into the scalp; for this reason, the term folliculitis keloidalis is preferred to folliculitis keloidalis nuchae; in order to avoid confusion with keloid formation in association with acne vulgaris, the term folliculitis keloidalis is preferred to acne keloidalis.

Epidemiology

Age
Folliculitis keloidalis occurs in males after puberty and is most frequent between the ages of 14 and 25 years.

Sex
Males are most commonly affected.

Ethnicity
Most common in individuals of African descent.

Pathophysiology

Predisposing factors
This chronic inflammatory condition mainly occurs in black males. A study from Nigeria reported that 9.4% of all patients attending a dermatology out-patient department had folliculitis keloidalis [1]. Many patients have or have had significant acne, and a patient with previous hidradenitis has been reported [2]. No specific organism has been firmly implicated in the aetiology but *Staphylococcus aureus* may commonly be isolated from swabs from affected skin [3]. Although friction from the collar is often incriminated, the evidence is unconvincing [3]. An association between frequent haircuts (at <2 week intervals) has been documented in older boys attending high school [4]. This finding and the observation of foreign-body granulomas surrounding fragments of hair has led to the suggestion that the process begins with penetration of cut hair into the skin as in pseudofolliculitis. However, no evidence of this was found on a detailed histological examination [5]. Associated keloids in other sites seem not to have been reported, and the process is regarded more as hypertrophic scarring than as true keloid formation.

Pathology
The most frequent histological findings include chronic perifollicular inflammation, disappearance of sebaceous glands, destroyed follicles, lamellar fibroplasia and acute inflammation around degenerating follicular components. Serial sections may show a foreign-body reaction to hair and follicular remnants. The pathological findings seen in early lesions, perilesional skin and clinically normal skin suggest that antigens from follicular organisms such as *Demodex*, bacteria or other skin flora stimulate an inflammatory reaction which then destroys the sebaceous glands and follicles with resultant scarring [5].

Causative organisms
Staphylococcus aureus may be isolated from skin swabs but it is uncertain whether this organism can be implicated as a primary pathogen.

Clinical features

Presentation
Follicular papules or pustules, often in irregularly linear groups, develop on the nape of the neck just below and within the hair line (Figure 93.2). Less often, they extend upwards into the scalp. The early inflammatory stage may be inconspicuous, and the patient may be unaware of the condition until hard keloidal papules develop at the sites of follicular inflammation. The papules may remain discrete or may fuse into horizontal bands or irregular plaques. In other cases, the inflammatory changes are persistent and troublesome, with undermined abscesses and discharging sinuses. The condition is extremely chronic and new lesions may continue to form at intervals for years.

Disease course and prognosis
The condition usually becomes chronic with permanent keloidal scarring.

Investigations
Skin swabs can be taken if bacterial infection is suspected.

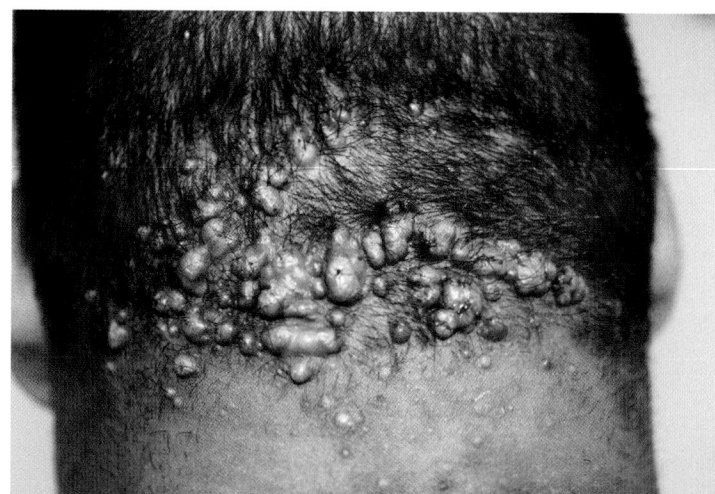

Figure 93.2 Folliculitis keloidalis of the nape of the neck. (Courtesy of Dr Ian Coulson, Burnley General Hospital, Burnley, Lancashire, UK.)

PART 8: SPECIFIC CUTANEOUS STRUCTURE

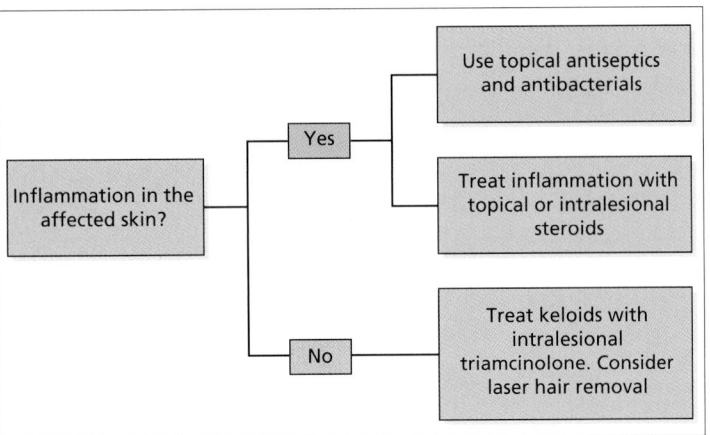

Figure 93.3 Treatment algorithm for folliculitis keloidalis.

Management

Bacterial infection should be treated if present; antiseptics may reduce further or secondary infection. No evidence-based reviews of therapy options are available. Close shaving of the hair on the nape of the neck and occipital scalp should be avoided. Intralesional or potent topical corticosteroids may reduce scarring and inflammation [5]. Oral corticosteroids prescribed for another condition helped in one severe case but long-term treatment is unlikely to be justified [2]. In general medical treatment is disappointing and, in troublesome cases, the affected area may be excised and grafted or excised and allowed to heal by secondary intention. Laser-assisted hair removal with the long-pulsed Nd:YAG laser led to significant improvement after five treatments in 16 patients with acne keloidalis [6]. The laser causes miniaturization of the hair shafts, which is thought to reduce subsequent inflammatory episodes. See Figure 93.3 for an approach to managing the individual patient.

Necrotizing lymphocytic folliculitis of the scalp margin

Definition and nomenclature

Necrotizing lymphocytic folliculitis is a rare and poorly understood chronic scarring follicular dermatosis characterized by necrotizing inflammation of follicles close to the scalp margins and resulting in multiple small round varioliform scars [1]. It has historically been termed acne necrotica varioliformis.

Synonyms and inclusions
• Acne necrotica varioliformis

Introduction and general description

This uncommon condition is characterized by a necrotizing folliculitis which appears in crops primarily along the frontal hairline and which is responsive to acne treatment.

Epidemiology

Incidence and prevalence
It is rare.

Pathophysiology

Pathology
Early lesions are characterized by a dyskeratotic follicular epithelium with associated spongiosis. A prominent lymphocytic perifollicular and perivascular lymphocytic infiltrate is also seen. As the lesions progress, more widespread necrosis appears involving the follicular epithelium, epidermis and dermis, and often containing fragments of hair. Bacteria are often seen in the stratum corneum.

Causative organisms
Staphylococcus aureus and *Propionibacterium acnes* have both been implicated but their role, if any, is uncertain. *Staphylococcus aureus* can sometimes be cultured from more advanced lesions.

Environmental factors
Aggravation in summer has been reported [1].

Clinical features

Presentation
Some patients experience mild pruritus but usually the disease onset is insidious with the appearance of papules in the frontal hairline or, more rarely, the seborrhoeic areas of the skin. Some soreness may be associated with the evolving reddish-brown papules which gradually umbilicate, developing focal areas of necrosis with crusting over the course of weeks, ultimately leaving depressed varioliform scars (Figure 93.4).

Differential diagnosis and co-morbidities
Emotional disturbance has been described as associated.

Investigations
Careful culturing to establish whether *S. aureus* is present.

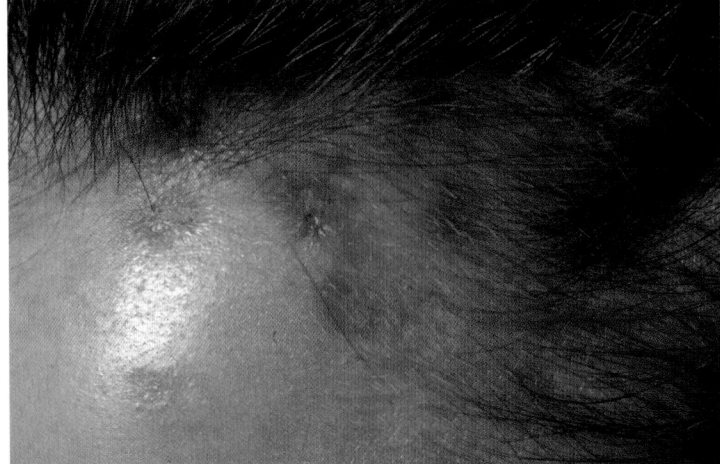

Figure 93.4 Varioliform scars at the scalp margin secondary to necrotizing lymphocytic folliculitis.

Management

Papulonecrotic tuberculid (see Chapter 27) and tertiary syphilis (see Chapter 29) should be excluded. Other potential differential diagnoses include repetitive excoriation, folliculitis decalvans, eczema herpeticum, pyogenic bacterial folliculitis and molluscum contagiosum [2–4].

In scalp folliculitis, the lesions are typically distributed throughout the scalp, and are smaller, usually more numerous, non-scarring and more pruritic (see later).

Treatment ladder

First line
- If *S. aureus* is found, antistaphylococcal therapy is recommended according to susceptibility, along with treatment of possible concomitant nasal carriage
- If *S. aureus* is not found, tetracyclines are recommended in acne dosing
- Antibacterial shampoos are also recommended

Second line
- Anti-inflammatory treatment with topical or intralesional corticosteroids

Third line
- Isotretinoin

Scalp folliculitis

Definition and nomenclature

A non-scarring chronic superficial folliculitis of the scalp that is typically characterized by multiple minute, very itchy pustules distributed throughout the scalp and which has been attributed to a reaction to the presence of microorganisms, in particular *Propionibacterium acnes*.

Synonyms and inclusions
- Chronic non-scarring folliculitis of the scalp
- *Propionibacterium acnes* folliculitis of the scalp

Introduction and general description

Scalp folliculitis is a relatively common chronic relapsing complaint in which multiple minute itchy pustules form in the scalp. Because of the itch, secondary excoriation and crusting is common (Figure 93.5). It has received very little recent attention by researchers. The best description comes from a report by Hersle *et al.* in which they presented their findings in 40 patients (30 males), whom they re-examined a mean of 8.3 years after they had first presented with scalp folliculitis [1]. Histologically, there was a neutrophilic folliculitis without necrosis; bacteriologically only the usual resident microflora of the scalp were detected, with *P. acnes*

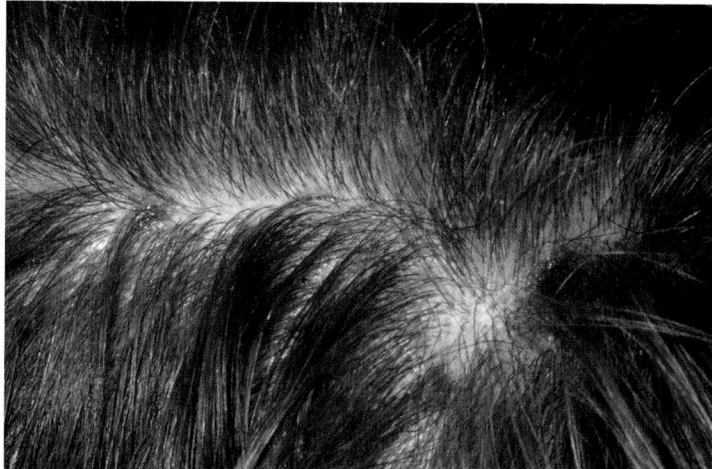

Figure 93.5 Scalp folliculitis with secondary excoriation.

being the most frequently isolated organism. They found *P. acnes* within the pustules but not on the overlying skin surface of three patients whom they investigated.

Very similar reports had been made previously by Montgomery and by Maibach [2,3]. Montgomery described a virtually identical clinical picture in 25 patients with up to 100 pustules confined (except in one case) to the scalp. He unfortunately used the term acne miliaris necrotica to describe these patients, even though necrosis is not seen; confusingly, others have used the latter term as an alternative for mild acne necrotica varioliformis (necrotizing lymphocytic folliculitis, see earlier), which has a different distribution and results in scarring. For these reasons, these terms are best abandoned. Maibach recognized the entity in 1967 and attributed it to *P. acnes* (formerly called *Corynebacterium acnes*), as have other authorities since.

Epidemiology

Incidence and prevalence
Unknown but relatively common.

Age
Onset in third and fourth decades.

Sex
Male to female ratio 3 : 1.

Pathophysiology

Pathology
Neutrophilic folliculitis without necrosis.

Causative organisms
Putative role of *P. acnes*.

Disease course and prognosis

In all 40 patients reported by Hersle *et al.*, there was still an active, recurring non-scarring folliculitis a mean of 8.3 years after first presentation, although seven had had temporary remissions [1].

Management

There is little information on whether topical preparations such as tar shampoos might be of benefit. Low-dose tetracycline appears to be of some benefit but topical corticosteroids do not help [1].

Actinic folliculitis

Definition and nomenclature

Actinic folliculitis is a rare photodermatosis of unknown aetiology characterized by the development of pruritic monomorphic follicular papules and pustules appearing on photo-exposed sites several hours to days after sunlight exposure.

Synonyms and inclusions
- Actinic superficial folliculitis
- Acne aestivalis

Introduction and general description

Actinic folliculitis is a rare photodermatosis of unknown aetiology characterized by the development of pruritic monomorphic follicular papules and pustules appearing on the face, neck, arms and/or upper trunk several hours to days after sunlight exposure. It normally resolves within 10–14 days. Cultures for microorganisms are negative. Histologically, there is a superficial neutrophilic folliculitis with an admixture of lymphocytes [1].

Epidemiology

Age

Actinic folliculitis has been described in young to middle-aged adults of both sexes.

Sex

Males and females are equally affected.

Pathophysiology

Environmental factors

Exposure to sunlight.

Clinical features

Presentation

Monomorphic follicular papules and pustules erupt over the face, neck, upper arms, shoulders and/or upper chest following as little a few hours of sun exposure [2]. A recent report describes lesions on the back, upper chest and shoulders occurring annually after the first sun exposure of the year [3], confirmed with provocative phototesting. There may be a burning sensation or pruritus at the onset, resolving within 10 days [4,5]. Another report describes itchy pustules and papules on the lower face resolving within 4 days [6]. The mechanism is unknown.

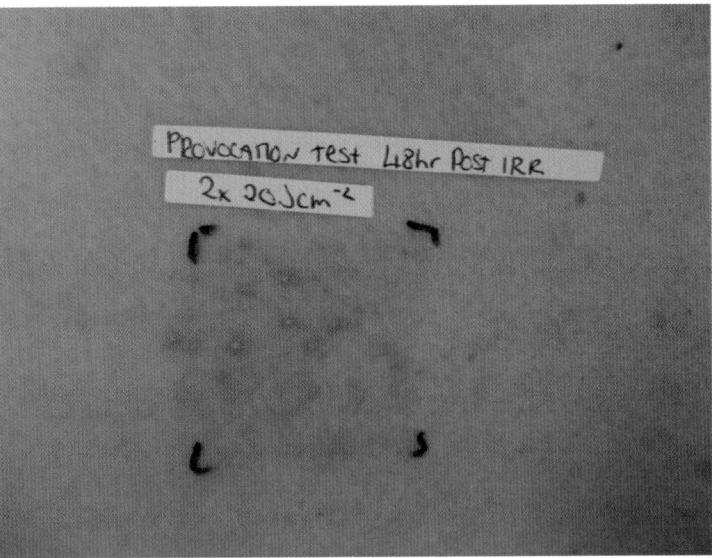

Figure 93.6 Follicular pustules on the anterior chest 48 h after irradiation with broadband UVA in a patient with actinic folliculitis.

Differential diagnosis

Polymorphic light eruption, miliaria, papulopustular rosacea, photoaggravated acne vulgaris.

Disease course and prognosis

It may recur annually over many years and is usually worse at the beginning of the summer.

Investigations

A follicular provocation test can be performed to support the diagnosis (Figure 93.6).

Management

Photoprotection with behavioural modification, hats, clothing and high factor sunscreen may be beneficial. Standard acne therapy is ineffective, but severe cases may respond to isotretinoin [2,6]. UVB phototherapy may provide useful desensitization.

Disseminate and recurrent infundibulofolliculitis

Definition

Disseminate and recurrent infundibulofolliculitis is a dermatosis of poorly understood aetiology affecting principally the chest, shoulders and upper arms of young black men. It is characterized by a disseminated low-grade spongiotic dermatitis involving the infundibula of multiple adjacent follicles. It manifests clinically as sheets of small monomorphic pruritic papules [1].

Epidemiology

Age

Begins in childhood or in adult life.

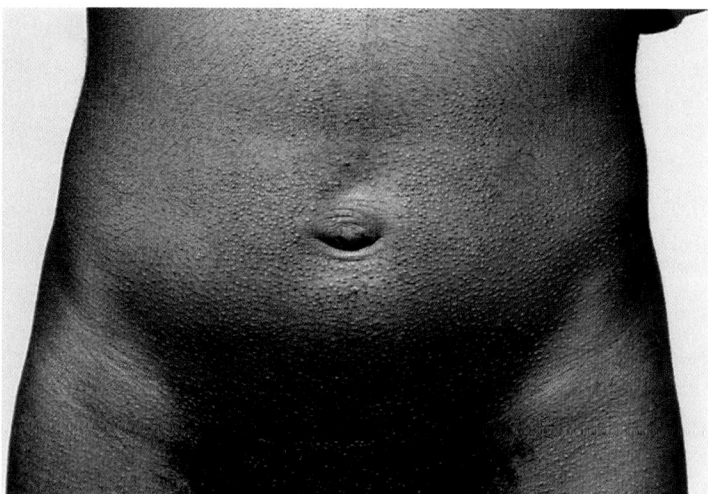

Figure 93.7 Disseminate and recurrent infundibulofolliculitis.

Sex
Mainly males.

Ethnicity
Mainly patients with black skin.

Pathophysiology

Pathology
Histologically, inflammatory changes are confined to the infundibular portion of the follicles with spongiosis and a mixed inflammatory infiltrate.

Causative organisms
No infective agent has been identified.

Clinical features

Presentation
A widespread eruption of small monomorphic follicular papules on the trunk and limbs sparing the flexures (Figure 93.7). Itch is often but not always present. Occasionally pustules develop. It tends to be persistent or may relapse periodically.

Management
It is generally poorly responsive to treatment including potent topical corticosteroids [2]. Psoralen photochemotherapy [3] and isotretinoin [4] have each been reported to be helpful in individual case reports.

Eosinophilic pustular folliculitis

Definition
Eosinophilic pustular folliculitis is an uncommon cutaneous reaction pattern characterized by infiltration of the pilosebaceous follicles by large numbers of eosinophils. Three different forms

are recognized: classical, immunosuppression-associated and infantile.

Introduction and general description
Eosinophilic pustular folliculitis is an uncommon inflammatory cutaneous reaction pattern of poorly understood aetiology, which is characterized by infiltration of the pilosebaceous follicles by large numbers of eosinophils. The classical adult form, Ofuji disease, is predominantly facial and is reported principally from Japan [1,2]. Immunosuppression-associated eosinophilic pustular folliculitis is strongly associated with HIV infection and is more often extrafacial [3]. Infantile eosinophilic pustular folliculitis, which has also been termed infantile eosinophilic pustulosis, would seem to have little in common with the adult forms and is described separately later.

Epidemiology

Age
Classical and immunosuppression-associated disease typically occur in young adults.

Sex
It is seen five times more frequently in men than in women.

Ethnicity
The majority of classical eosinophilic pustular folliculitis patients have been reported from Japan.

Pathophysiology
The cause of the immune dysregulation in eosinophilic pustular folliculitis is not understood. Immaturity or suppression of the immune system appear to be important, although this has not been demonstrated in the classical adult form. A large number of hypotheses including hypersensitivity reactions to *Malassezia* spp., *Demodex* spp. or sebaceous gland derived lipids have been proposed [1]. Various chemotactic factors have been detected in the fluid of the pustules, which are sterile, and it has been suggested that they may serve to localize excessive circulating eosinophils [4].

There are several reports of the condition erupting during pregnancy [5–7].

Pathology
The follicular inflammation is characterized by heavy infiltration of the outer root sheath and sebaceous gland by eosinophils accompanied by scattered mononuclear cells and neutrophils (Figure 93.8). This is best detected by serial horizontal sectioning of biopsies of fresh unexcoriated papules or pustules. Perifollicular and perivascular infiltration by eosinophils is also seen. In immunosuppression-associated eosinophilic pustular folliculitis, the inflammation may be more diffuse [3].

Mild to moderate peripheral blood eosinophilia is seen in up to 35% of patients [1,2,8] with classical type and in up to 50% with HIV-associated eosinophilic pustular folliculitis, which usually occurs when the CD4 count is less than 200 cells/mL [9].

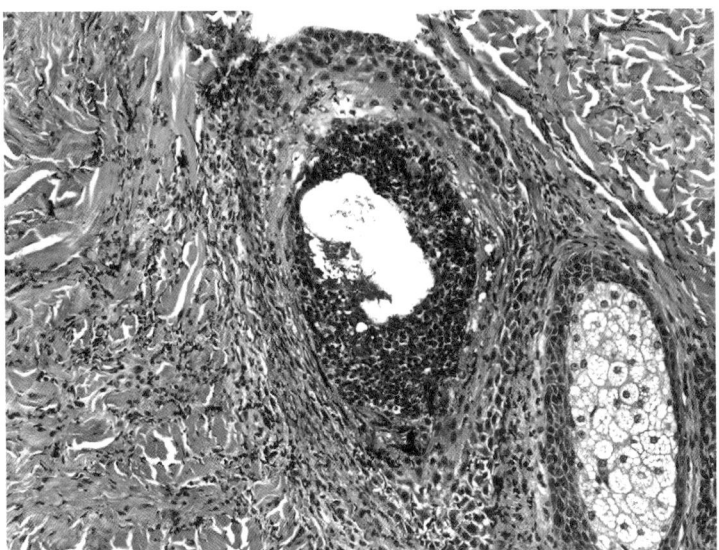

Figure 93.8 Histopathology of eosinophilic pustular folliculitis showing dense accumulation of eosinophils within the follicular canal. (Courtesy of Professor Luis Requena, Universidad Autónoma de Madrid, Spain.)

Genetics

There is no known genetic predisposition.

Clinical features

Classical adult eosinophilic pustular folliculitis

This is a chronic relapsing disease in which crops of sterile follicular papules and pustules coalesce into inflammatory annular plaques with peripheral expansion and central clearing. It takes 7–10 days for the inflammation to subside before the cycle repeats itself a few weeks later [3]. The face is the commonest site of involvement (Figure 93.9a,b): in a review of 91 Japanese cases, the face, trunk and extremities were involved in 88%, 40% and 26%, respectively [8]. Pustular inflammation of the palms and soles may be seen in up to a fifth of cases, even though follicles are not present in palmoplantar skin. This may cause diagnostic confusion with palmoplantar pustulosis [10]. The trunk and the upper outer arms are also frequently involved, legs and scalp occasionally. Widespread involvement has occurred [11].

The inflammatory plaques may reach 3–5 cm in diameter before subsiding to leave slight pigmentation. Lakes of pus and erosions are sometimes seen. Itch is frequent and may be severe but is not invariable. Patients are systemically well. The overall course is chronic with new crops of lesions repeatedly reappearing in affected areas, although a few cases have entered spontaneous remission.

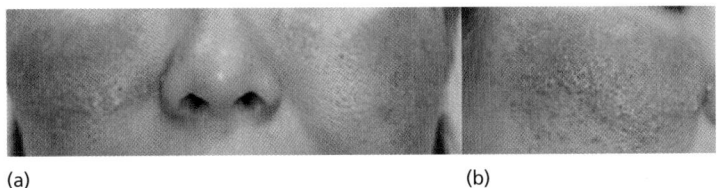

(a)   (b)

Figure 93.9 (a,b) Classical eosinophilic pustular folliculitis: well-defined, dark erythematous plaques with numerous pustules and crusts involving the cheeks. (Reproduced from Ramdial *et al.* 1999 [5].)

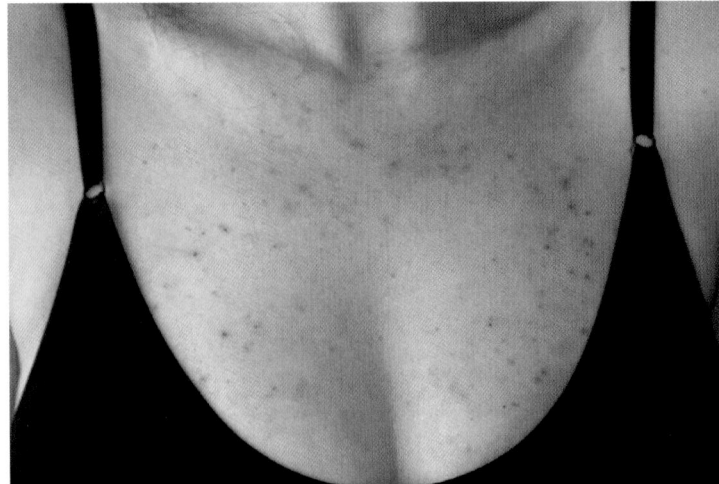

Figure 93.10 Immunodeficiency-associated eosinophilic pustular folliculitis in 32-year-old woman with HIV infection: view of anterior chest. (Courtesy of Professor Luis Requena, Universidad Autónoma de Madrid, Spain.)

Immunosuppression-associated eosinophilic pustular folliculitis

This has been reported predominantly in association with HIV and AIDS [1,9,12,13] (see Chapter 31). It differs in a number of respects from the classical form. It is not restricted to the Japanese and pruritus is typically much more intense. The pustular element is often not as prominent and clustering into plaques is not a characteristic feature [1]. Facial skin is less commonly involved. The clinical signs may be subtle, sometimes with just scattered follicular papules or excoriations (Figure 93.10), and multiple biopsies may be required to confirm the diagnosis.

Paradoxically, eosinophilic pustular folliculitis may first develop after the CD4 count starts to rise with the introduction of highly active antiretroviral therapy (HAART), in which case it may be accompanied by the immune reconstitution inflammatory syndrome (IRIS).

Management

A comprehensive review of the various treatments showed that no treatment is consistently effective, and treatment has to be tailored to the individual patient [12]. Systemic corticosteroids are usually but not always helpful; potent topical corticosteroids are sometimes of some value. Topical pimecrolimus and tacrolimus have also been advocated [14].

Dapsone is effective in some cases and may be the drug of first choice [15,16].

Oral non-steroidal anti-inflammatory drugs (NSAIDs) are widely used in Japan for the classical form: in a review of published Japanese cases nearly 80% were reported to have responded to indometacin [8]. A proposed mechanism of action of oral indometacin is that it interferes with prostaglandin D2 induced chemotaxis by down-regulating expression of CRTH2 (chemoattractant receptor homologous molecule) on the surface of eosinophils [17].

Other reported therapeutic options include minocycline, isotretinoin, itraconazole, cetirizine, metronidazole and colchicine [8]. UVB therapy was helpful in six HIV-associated cases [18], although maintenance treatment was required.

Treatment ladder

First line
• Potent topical corticosteroids, topical pimecrolimus/
  tacrolimus, indometacin, narrow-band UVB phototherapy

Second line
• Oral corticosteroids, oral antimicrobials (minocycline,
  itraconazole), cetirizine or oral isotretinoin

Infantile eosinophilic pustular folliculitis

Definition and nomenclature
Infantile eosinophilic pustular folliculitis is an inflammatory pustular disorder of infants associated with cutaneous and peripheral blood eosinophilia.

Synonyms and inclusions
• Infancy-associated eosinophilic pustular folliculitis
• Infantile eosinophilic pustulosis

Introduction and general description
Infantile eosinophilic pustular folliculitis is an inflammatory pustular disorder of infants associated with cutaneous and peripheral blood eosinophilia. It was first reported in 1984 by Lucky *et al.* [1]. It is characterized by recurrent outbreaks of non-infective pustules containing eosinophils on the scalp of infants. In the majority of cases, the condition commences before the age of 6 months and remits by the age of 3 years. In two thirds of cases, body areas other than the scalp are affected. The cause is unknown. It was originally considered and is still generally termed a folliculitis, but in a substantial number of cases no follicular involvement has been found [2,3].

Epidemiology

Age
Average age at presentation is 6 months [4].

Sex
More common in boys (male to female ratio 4 : 1).

Associated diseases
A case of HIV-associated infantile eosinophilic pustular folliculitis has been described in an infant [5]. It has also been associated with hyper-IgE syndrome and atopic disease [6].

Pathophysiology

Pathology
Tzanck smear shows an abundance of eosinophils. Biopsy shows an intense follicular polymorphonuclear and eosinophilic infil-

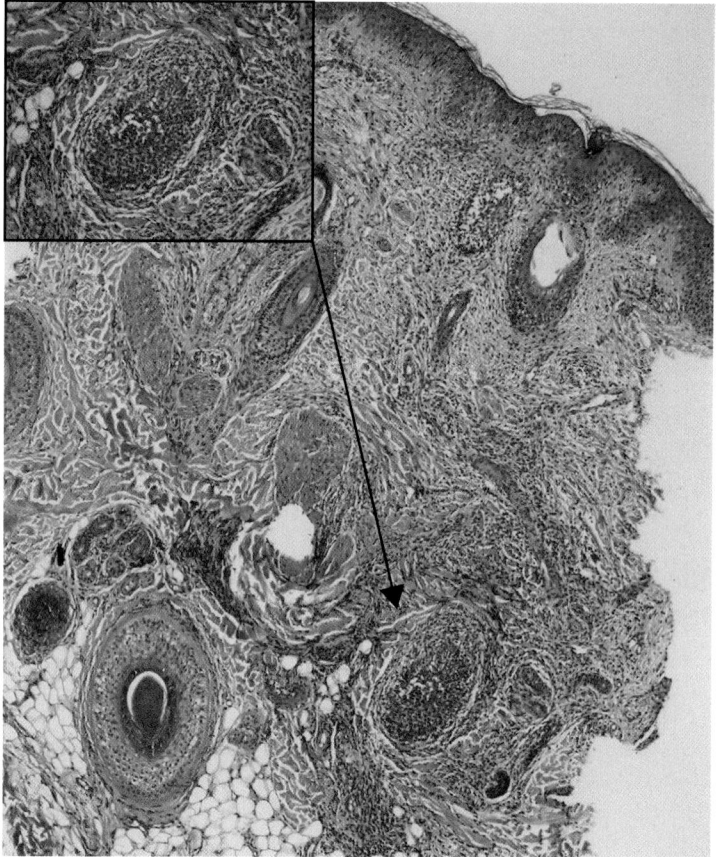

Figure 93.11 Infantile eosinophilic pustular folliculitis with dense infiltrate of eosinophils, spongiosis and microabscess formation within the follicle (inset). (Reproduced from Alonso-Castro *et al.* 2012 [7].)

trate (Figure 93.11). Hair follicles were identified in only 63% of biopsies in a large case series [2].

Causative organisms
Bacteriology is usually negative.

Genetics
It has been reported in brothers [3].

Clinical features

Presentation
It is characterized by recurrent crops of itchy sterile pustules, which recur over several months or years. The sterile pustules develop on the scalp predominantly (Figure 93.12), but lesions may occur at other sites such as the face. Children may develop axillary, inguinal or cervical lymphadenopathy [7]. Pustular lesions resolve spontaneously without scarring [8].

Disease course and prognosis
This is a self-limiting disease in which spontaneous resolution usually occurs from 3 months to 3 years of age.

Differential diagnosis
Other neonatal and infantile pustular eruptions which should be considered in the differential diagnosis are shown in Table 93.1.

PART 8: SPECIFIC CUTANEOUS STRUCTURE

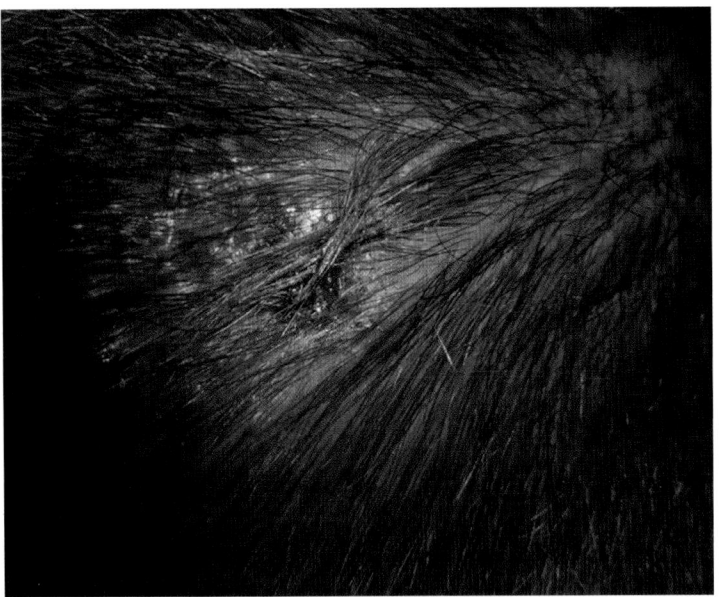

Figure 93.12 Sterile pustules in the scalp of a 23-month-old boy with infantile eosinophilic pustular folliculitis. (Reproduced from Alonso-Castro *et al.* 2012 [7].)

Investigations
Tzanck smear, culture for bacteria and fungi, HIV test and IgE levels.

Management
Because the condition is self-limiting, treatment is not usually indicated; however, with particularly recalcitrant or extensive disease dapsone may be helpful [8].

Treatment ladder

First line
• Expectancy, topical corticosteroids [4]

Second line
• Antihistamines
• Topical tacrolimus [9]

Third line
• Dapsone [8]

Heterotopic sebaceous glands (Fordyce spots)

Definition and nomenclature
Fordyce spots are heterotopic sebaceous glands (i.e. not associated with hair follicles) which are located on mucosal surfaces or glabrous skin of the lips, oral mucosa or genitalia.

Synonyms and inclusions
• Fordyce granules
• Ectopic sebaceous glands

Introduction and general description
These common asymptomatic but readily visible skin and mucosal lesions easily attract the attention of both patients and physicians. Traditionally considered to be ectopic sebaceous glands, they should be considered as within the spectrum of normality.

Table 93.1 Differential diagnosis of infantile eosinophilic pustular folliculitis.

Diagnosis	Incidence	Site	Lesions	Onset	Duration	Peripheral eosinophilia	Tzanck smear	Histology
Infantile eosinophilic pustular folliculitis	Rare	Scalp, trunk (± hands, feet)	Vesicles, pustules, crusts	Birth or later	Cyclical outbreaks for 3 months to 5 years	During outbreaks in some patients	Eosinophils	Eosinophilic spongiosis; subcorneal pustules; eosinophilic folliculitis
Erythema toxicum neonatorum	One-third of neonates	Face, trunk, limbs	Macules, vesicles, pustules	Birth–72 h	Resolves within 1 week	Up to 15%	Eosinophils	Eosinophilic folliculitis; subcorneal eosinophilic pustules
Transient neonatal pustular melanosis	4–5% black infants; 0.1–0.3% of white infants	Neck, trunk, thighs, palms, soles	Vesicles, pustules, pigmented macules	Birth–24 h	Resolves within weeks	May occur	Neutrophils, occasional eosinophils	Neutrophilic intracorneal and subcorneal pustules
Infantile acropustulosis	Rare; mainly in black males	Hands, feet (± scalp, face, trunk)	Pruritic papules, vesicles, pustules	Neonatal period or later	Lesions last 7–10 days, crops recur for 2 months to years	May occur	Neutrophils, occasional eosinophils	Subcorneal pustules containing neutrophils; occasional eosinophils
Langerhans cell histiocytosis	Rare	Scalp, flexures	Papules, pustules, vesicles, crusts	Birth or later	Varies depending on systemic involvement	No	Histiocytes	Infiltrate of Langerhans cells; Birbeck granules on electron microscopy

From Buckley *et al.* 2001 [3] reproduced with permission from Wiley.

Epidemiology

Incidence and prevalence
Fordyce spots on the lips and buccal mucosa are common from an early age and increase in prevalence with age. Fordyce spots were found in 1% of Swedish newborns [1]. The prevalence rises with age: oral or labial lesions were observed in 8% of a large cohort of preschool Brazilian children [2] and in 95% of a large cohort of adult Israeli Jews [3].

Sex
Vulval Fordyce spots are very common in women, with reported rates of 75–95% [4]. Fordyce spots on penile or scrotal skin were incidental findings in 9% of 400 Polish men who sought advice about other genital abnormalities [5].

Pathophysiology

Pathology
Fordyce spots are essentially sebaceous glands in which the duct is connected directly to the overlying epidermal or mucosal surface rather than into a hair follicle. They contain similar lipids to follicle-associated sebaceous glands [6,7].

Clinical features

Presentation
Fordyce spots manifest as multiple smooth, creamy white to yellow well-demarcated papules which may, however, coalesce into irregular plaques. They are usually 1–2 mm in diameter but may be larger and are slightly to moderately elevated above the skin or mucosal surface. They develop most commonly on the vermilion of the upper lip (Figure 93.13a), the buccal mucosa (Figure 93.13b) or the labia minora (Figure 93.13c). Advice is, however, most likely to be sought by adolescents or young men with prominent penile or scrotal involvement (Figure 93.13d).

Clinical variants
Heterotopic sebaceous glands may be located in the coronal sulcus of the penis to either side of the frenulum and in this location have been referred to as the glands of Tyson [8]. They are normal structures and require no treatment.

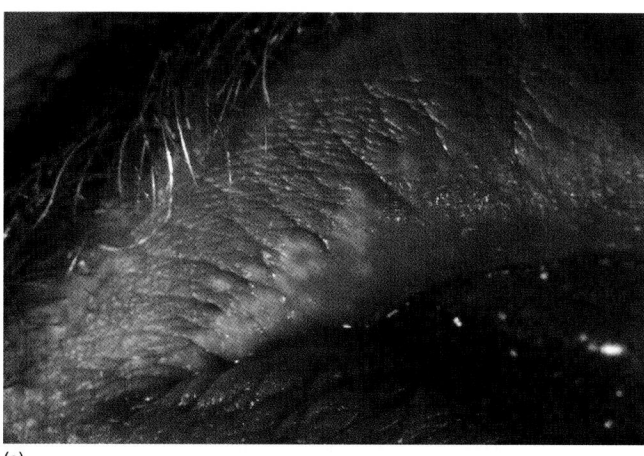

(a)

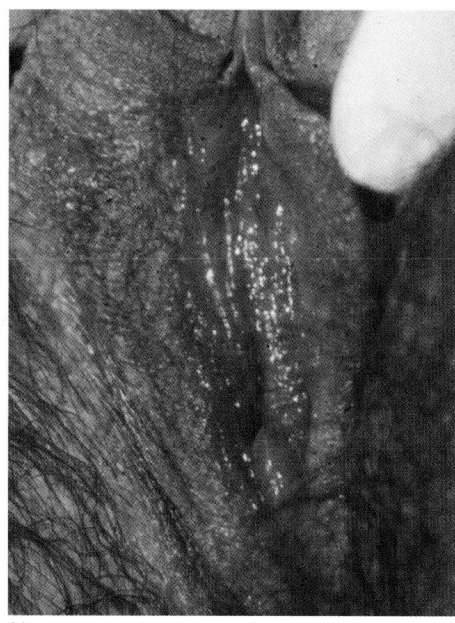

(c)

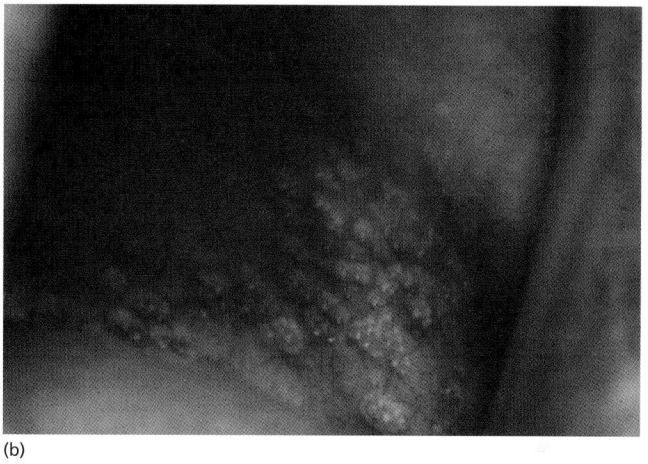

(b)

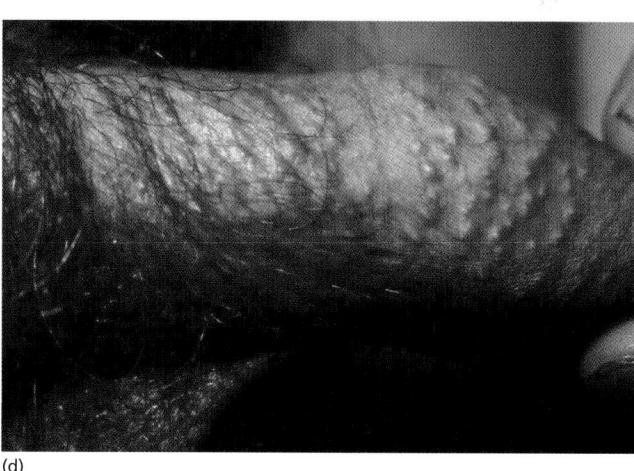

(d)

Figure 93.13 Fordyce spots on the vermilion of the upper lip (a), buccal mucosa (b), labia minora (c, courtesy of Dr Ekaterina Burova, Bedford Hospital, UK) and penis (d).

PART 8: SPECIFIC CUTANEOUS STRUCTURE

Sebaceous glands are found within the tubercles of Montgomery on the areola of the female breast. Typical Fordyce spots on the areolae have, however, been described in a man with coexistent labial and penile lesions [9].

Differential diagnosis
- Leucoplakia.
- Human papillomavirus infection.
- Post-herpetic changes.

Investigations
In cases of doubt, a biopsy will provide the diagnosis.

Treatment ladder

First line
- Reassurance

Second line
- Local destruction with superficial cautery or electrodessication
- Topical trichloracetic acid [10]

Third line
- Systemic isotretinoin [10]
- Carbon dioxide laser evaporation [10]

Resources

Patient resources

http://www.dermnetnz.org/acne/fordyce.html (last accessed August 2015).

Sebaceous gland hyperplasia

Definition
Sebaceous gland hyperplasia presents as scattered clinically obvious flesh-coloured to yellowish papules resulting from hypertrophy of sebaceous glands.

Introduction and general description
Sebaceous gland hyperplasia is characterized by a benign proliferation of sebocytes within normal pilosebaceous units in hair-bearing skin (cf. Fordyce spots). It is most commonly seen in adults but may manifest in the neonatal period due to the passage of maternal androgens across the placenta.

Epidemiology

Incidence and prevalence
Unknown but not uncommon.

Age
Middle-aged or elderly people.

Associated diseases
Immunosuppression in transplant recipients may predispose to sebaceous hyperplasia [1,2].

Pathophysiology

Pathology
The whole pilosebaceous unit is enlarged compared with normal adjacent skin but otherwise appears normal [3].

Genetics
Familial cases presenting at a young age suggest the possibility of a genetic component [4].

Clinical features

Presentation
Insidious in onset, sebaceous gland hyperplasia presents as scattered asymptomatic flesh-coloured to yellowish-pink, often umbilicated papules measuring 1–3 mm in diameter (Figure 93.14). Lesions are occasionally confluent, producing a yellowish hue to the skin. They are seen especially on the forehead, temples and cheeks, but may occur on the upper trunk as well. Their main clinical significance is that they may be mistaken for other disorders presenting with facial papules such as basal cell carcinoma.

Disease course and prognosis
Persistent but asymptomatic.

Investigations
In cases of diagnostic doubt, biopsy will rule out neoplasm or other disorder (see Box 93.1 for differential diagnosis).

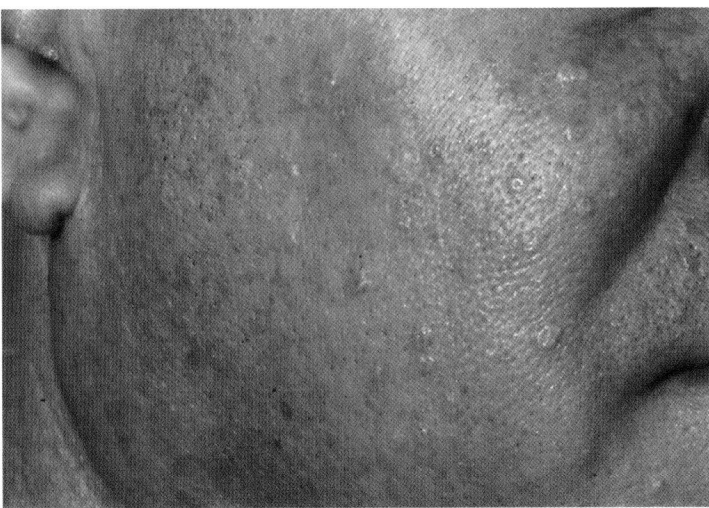

Figure 93.14 Sebaceous gland hyperplasia on the cheek of a 42-year-old man.

Box 93.1 Differential diagnosis of sebaceous gland hyperplasia

- Heterotopic sebaceous glands (Fordyce spots)
- Multiple basal cell carcinomas
- Multiple trichepitheliomas
- Cowden disease (multiple hamartoma syndrome)
- Fibrous papule of the face
- Follicular infundibulum tumour
- Folliculoma
- Granulomatous rosacea
- Lichen nitidus
- Lipoid proteinosis
- Milia
- Molluscum contagiosum
- Muir–Torre syndrome
- Multiple endocrine neoplasia type 1
- Sebaceous adenoma
- Sebaceous carcinoma
- Syringoma
- Trichilemmoma
- Trichoepithelioma
- Trichofolliculoma

Management

First line

Cosmetic camouflage may be used.

Second line

If requested and appropriate, some physical treatments such as gentle cautery, cryotherapy or trichloroacetic acid can be used. Pulsed dye and 1450 nm diode lasers have also been advocated [5,6].

Third line

Oral isotretinoin has been reported to be of considerable benefit in extensive sebaceous gland hyperplasia [7]. A therapeutic trial of oral isotretinoin may help to differentiate between sebaceous hyperplasia and multiple early basal cell carcinomas in transplant recipients, and may avoid multiple biopsies if there are many lesions.

Cyproterone actetate in combination with a combined oral contraceptive preparation has also been used with benefit to induce regression of sebaceous hyperplasia in females [8].

Photodynamic therapy using aminolaevulinic acid has also been shown to be useful for shrinking lesions of sebaceous hyperplasia [9].

Key references

The full list of references can be found in the online version at www.rooksdermatology.com

Pseudofolliculitis

1 Garcia-Zuazaga J. Pseudofolliculitis barbae. Review and update on new treatment modalities. *Military Med* 2003;168:561–4.

Folliculitis keloidalis

3 George AO, Akanji AO, Nduka EU, *et al*. Clinical, biochemical and morphologic features of acne keloidalis in a black population. *Int J Dermatol* 1993;32:714–16.

Necrotizing lymphocytic folliculitis of the scalp margin

1 Kossard S, Collins A, McCrossin I. Necrotizing lymphocytic folliculitis: the early lesion of acne necrotica (varioliformis) *J Am Acad Dermatol* 1987;16:1007–14.

Scalp folliculitis

1 Hersle K, Mobacken H, Möller A. Chronic non-scarring folliculitis of the scalp. Acta Dermatovenereol 1979;59:249–53.

Actinic folliculitis

1 Beukers SM, Van Doorn MBA, van Santen MM, Starink TM. Actinic folliculitis, a rare sunlight-induced dermatosis. *Ned Tijdschr Dermatol Venereol* 2010;20:122–5.

4 Verbov J. Actinic folliculitis. *Br J Dermatol* 1985;113:630–1.

Disseminate and recurrent infundibulofolliculitis

1 Owen WR, Wood C. Disseminate and recurrent infundibulofolliculitis. *Arch Dermatol* 1979;115:174–5.

Eosinophilic pustular folliculitis

1 Nervi SJ, Schwartz RA, Dmochowski M. Eosinophilic pustular folliculitis: a 40 year retrospect. *J Am Acad Dermatol* 2006;55:285–9.

2 Ofuji S. Eosinophilic pustular folliculitis. *Dermatologica* 1987;174:53–6.

12 Ellis E, Scheinfeld N. Eosinophilic pustular folliculitis. *Am J Clin Dermatol* 2004;5:189–97.

13 Soeprono FF, Schinella RA. Eosinophilic pustular folliculitis in patients with acquired immunodeficiency syndrome. *J Am Acad Dermatol* 1986;14:1020–2.

Infantile eosinophilic pustular folliculitis

1 Lucky AW, Esterly NB, Heskel N, *et al*. Eosinophilic pustular folliculitis in infancy. *Pediatr Dermatol* 1984;1:202–6.

Heterotopic sebaceous glands (Fordyce spots)

10 Lee JH, Lee JH, Kwon NH, *et al*. Clinicopathologic manifestations of patients with Fordyce's spots. *Ann Dermatol* 2012;24:103–6.

Sebaceous gland hyperplasia

3 Kumar P, Barton SP, Marks R. Tissue measurements in senile sebaceous gland hyperplasia. *Br J Dermatol* 1988;118:397–402.

CHAPTER 94

Disorders of the Sweat Glands

Ian H. Coulson[1] and Niall J. E. Wilson[2]

[1]Burnley General Hospital, East Lancashire NHS Trust IHC, Burnley, UK
[2]Royal Liverpool and Broadgreen University Hospitals, Liverpool, UK

Introduction

In this chapter the anatomy, physiology and diseases of eccrine and apocrine sweat glands are described. The clinical patterns, causes and associations of excessive sweating on the one hand and of reduced or absent sweating on the other are addressed in detail. Guidance is given on the management of hyperhidrosis and on the choice of appropriate therapy, including topical and systemic agents and surgery. The presentation and management of occlusive and inflammatory disorders of eccrine sweat glands is covered fully, as are the clinical features and management of abnormal sweat odour and colour and of apocrine miliaria. Brief reference is made to conditions associated with sweat gland inclusions; discussion of the latter and of neoplasms derived from sweat gland elements is to be found elsewhere in the book.

ECCRINE GLANDS

Anatomy and physiology of eccrine glands

Human eccrine sweat glands have two distinct functions [1–3,4]. They allow body cooling by evaporation, and have thus contributed in a major way to adaptation to a hot environment by humans; they also moisten the skin on the palms and soles at times of activity, and thus improve their grip.

Eccrine sweat glands are distributed over the whole skin surface including the glans penis and foreskin, but not on the lips, external ear canal, clitoris or labia minora. The number varies greatly with site, from $620/cm^2$ on the soles, about $120/cm^2$ on the thighs to $60/cm^2$ on the back [5]. The total number on the body surface is between 2 and 5 million, and is the similar in different ethnic groups. It has been calculated that the weight of the eccrine glands totals 100 g. The glands vary in size from person to person by a factor of five and this probably accounts for individual as well as regional differences in sweat rate (maximal individual gland secretion rates ranging from 2 to 20 nL/min/gland).

Embryologically, sweat glands are derived from a specialized down-growth of the epidermis at about the third month of intrauterine life on the palms and soles and at about 5 months elsewhere; they resemble adult glands by 8 months. Sweat glands are morphologically normal at birth but may not function fully until about 2 years of age. No new eccrine glands develop after birth. Unlike the apocrine glands they have no developmental relationship with the pilosebaceous follicle, although some glands may eventually come to open into the follicular neck. The gland consists of a secretory coil in the lower dermis (Figure 94.1a) and subcutaneous tissue, and a duct leading through the dermis to the intraepidermal sweat duct unit (Figure 94.1b). Apoeccrine glands have features of

Rook's Textbook of Dermatology, Ninth Edition. Edited by Christopher Griffiths, Jonathan Barker, Tanya Bleiker, Robert Chalmers and Daniel Creamer.
© 2016 John Wiley & Sons, Ltd. Published 2016 by John Wiley & Sons, Ltd.
Companion website: www.rooksdermatology.com

PART 8: SPECIFIC CUTANEOUS STRUCTURE

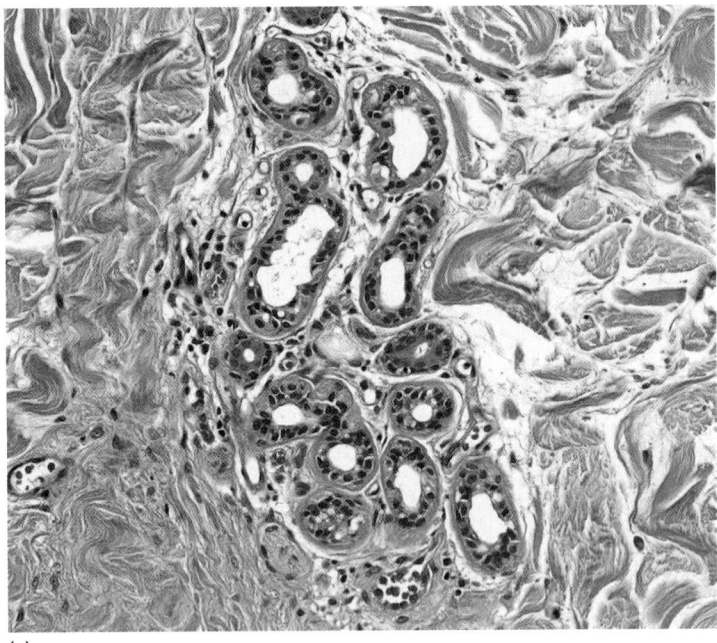

(a)

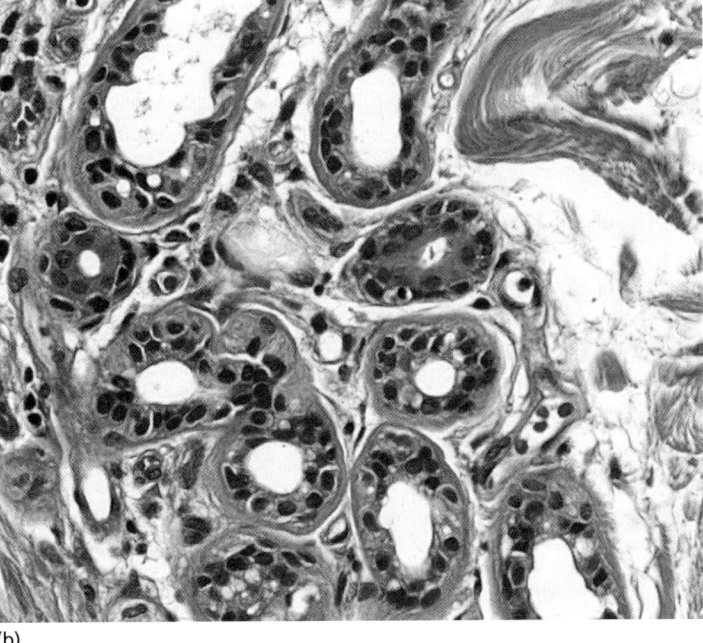

(b)

Figure 94.1 (a) A normal eccrine unit composed of secretory glands and ducts. Magnification 10× (H&E). (b) Closer view of eccrine glands showing the double layer of lining epithelial cells. Magnification 40× (H&E). (Courtesy of Dr Arti Bakshi, Royal Liverpool University Hospital, Liverpool, UK.)

both eccrine and apocrine glands, but seem to be nearer to eccrine in function. They open onto the surface, and produce a copious watery fluid. They may account for 10–45% of adult axillary glands [6].

The *secretory coil* contains three types of cell: large clear cells, which are the main secretory cells, small dark cells, which resemble mucus-secreting cells of other organs but whose function is not known, and myoepithelial cells [7]. The large and small cells of the secretory coil, unlike those of the duct, are attached to the basement membrane, although individual sections may at times suggest a double layer. Outside the basement membrane are the longitudinally arranged myoepithelial cells, whose function is probably to support the gland, but they may also help propel the sweat towards the surface. They respond to cholinergic stimuli. The function of the coil is to produce from plasma a watery isotonic secretion which can subsequently be modified by the duct. Ultrastructurally, the large clear cells are characterized by the presence of many mitochondria and by both intricate basal infoldings and intercellular canaliculi. *Para*-nitrophenyl phosphatase activity, which reflects catalytic activity of Na-K-ATPase is evident in the basal infoldings but not the intercellular canaliculi, suggesting that the basal areas are the sites of active ion transport requisite for sweat secretion. The classic theory suggests that acetylcholine passively increases entry of sodium into the cell, and this is then pumped out by the sodium pump into the intercellular canaliculi rather than directly through the luminal margin. However, there are other theories [4]. Fluid secretion is believed to be mediated osmotically, but the mechanism by which water moves has long been obscure. The discovery of aquaporins (AQPs) may challenge this theory. AQPs are a group of intercellular membrane water channel proteins, which allow movement of large amounts of fluid. In animal models, sweat secretion in AQP5 null mice was markedly decreased [8]. AQP5 has been identified in the dark cells of human eccrine sweat glands but its role in human sweating is still not clear [9,10]. Many different monoclonal antibodies can be shown to react with different portions of the sweat glands, allowing distinction of the gland from other components of the skin [11].

The *duct* consists of two or more layers of relatively uniform cuboidal cells. About one-third of the coil has this histology, as well as the uncoiled part passing up to the epidermis. The basal cells are rich in mitochondria and their entire membranes are rich in Na-K-ATPase activity, suggesting sodium pumping occurs along the entire duct membrane, and performs an active part in modifying the secretion produced by the coil.

It has been suggested that sweat glands do not cool the skin only by evaporation of heat from the surface, but that they also act as heat pipes. According to this theory, evaporation of the fluid at the base of the duct allows water vapour to pass up the duct and condense nearer the surface, and thence return to the deeper parts by capillary action. Such systems are a very effective way of transferring heat quickly [12].

The *intraepidermal sweat unit* is lined by a layer of specialized cells that often may be distinguished only with difficulty from the surrounding epidermis. On the palms and soles, it has a well-developed coil structure that is not so apparent in other sites.

The techniques for studying the function of the eccrine sweat glands [12–14] include the following:
- Collection of sweat in bags or pads at rest, after exposure to heat, or after injection or iontophoresis of pilocarpine or other cholinergic agonists.
- Direct measurement of water loss.
- Microcannulation of the duct or coil [15].

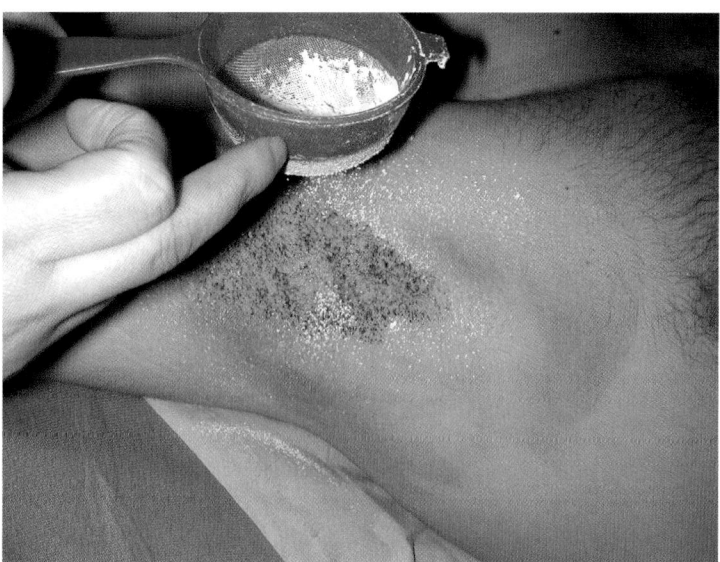

Figure 94.2 Identifying the extent of axillary hyperhidrosis – the skin has been cleaned with povidobe iodine solution and then sprinkled with corn starch powder from a fine culinary sieve. The hyperhidrotic areas are blue-black.

- Measurement of electrical potentials and electrical resistance of the skin, which depends on both the sweat present on the epidermis and the column present within the duct [16,17].
- Visualization of the individual sweat droplets. This may be achieved by direct microscopy, by *in vivo* staining, by forming plastic impressions [18] or by indicators that become coloured on contact with water, such as the starch/iodine technique [19], bromophenol blue [13], quinizarin [20] and the food dye Edicol ponceau. The plastic or silicone impression techniques are probably the most reliable, and can produce a permanent record. A simple modification of the starch/iodine test is to dry the skin, paint it with 2% iodine in alcohol, allow it to dry, and then press the skin against a good-quality paper. The starch in the paper reacts with iodine in the presence of water, so that each sweat droplet shows up as a minute dark spot. Alternatively, the starch may be suspended in castor oil (50 g in 100 mL) and painted onto the iodine-treated skin (Figure 94.2). Special dry starch/iodine powders can be dusted directly onto the skin [21].
- Isolated glands. It is possible to isolate single eccrine glands (and also hair follicles, sebaceous glands and apocrine sweat glands) by the relatively simple technique of shearing tissues with scissors [22,23]. This allows the physiology, biochemistry and tissue culture behaviour to be studied *in vitro*.

Control of eccrine sweating [1–3,4]
Eccrine gland secretion is influenced by a number of stimuli including thermal, osmotic, mental and gustatory factors, mediated by a complex of central and local control mechanisms. As a result, the quantity and composition of sweat is highly variable from minimal basal activity to a maximum of 3 L in 1 h.

Central control
Thermoregulatory sweating is primarily controlled in response to internal body temperature and secondarily influenced by skin temperature [24]. The effect of a rise in core temperature is nine times more efficient than the same rise in skin temperature in stimulating sweating. Central and peripheral changes in temperature influence the thermal receptors in the preoptic area and anterior hypothalamus. An increase in core temperature activates cooling mechanisms including sweating, panting and vasodilatation. Conversely, cooling promotes heat-preservation mechanisms such as vasoconstriction and shivering [25].

Although the precise neural pathway that mediates eccrine sweating in humans is still unclear, evidence from animal studies suggest that the efferent pathway from the hypothalamus includes the medulla, lateral horn of the spinal cord and sympathetic ganglia [**26**].

Osmotic factors also influence the rate of sweat production. Both hyperosmolality and hypovolaemia decrease sweat production, presumably in an attempt to prevent further loss of body fluid [27,28].

Centres and pathways controlling mental sweating are not fully known but areas within the frontal region of the brain have been identified. Functional magnetic resonance studies indicate that neural pathways for thermal and mental sweating are similar [29]. Mental stimuli enhance sweat production particularly from the palms and soles, potentially improving grip at times of stress.

Local control
From the sympathetic ganglia non-myelinated C fibres pass to eccrine sweat glands ending at many cholinergic terminals and a few adrenergic terminals [30]. Although stimulation of adrenergic nerves increases sweating this is much less marked than the response to cholinergic stimulation [31,32,**33**]. The adrenergic nerve supply seems to play little part in the normal modulation of eccrine sweating in humans. In addition, vasoactive intestinal polypeptide, calcitonin gene-related peptide and nitric oxide may play some role in the control of eccrine sweating [24].

Other factors may modify the quantity and quality of sweat in the presence of an intact sympathetic nerve supply including hormones, circulatory changes and axon and spinal reflexes. Sweat coils contain androgen receptors [34], and androgens may be at least partly responsible for the increase in sweating around puberty and for the greater sweat activity in males.

The composition of sweat [**4**,**33**] varies greatly from person to person, time to time and site to site. It has a basic similarity to the plasma from which it is derived. The sweat duct is largely responsible for the modification in sweat constituent concentration that occurs, and this will therefore vary according to how rapidly the sweat is passing through the duct. The most important constituents are sodium, chloride, potassium, urea and lactate. Sweat is hypotonic and this is largely due to reabsorption of sodium in the duct. At increased sweat rates the sodium concentration rises, presumably because there is reduced time for ductal reabsorption. The normal sodium concentration is between 10 and 20 mmol/L at low sweat rates, and up to 100 mmol/L at high rates. Aldosterone can increase ductal sodium reabsorption and in Addison disease high sweat sodium can be demonstrated (70–80 mmol/L). Antidiuretic hormone may reduce sweat rates in humans, but it also induces local vasoconstriction.

An increase in sweat electrolytes occurs in cystic fibrosis and forms the basis of the sweat chloride test [35]. Mutations in the *CFTR* gene in cystic fibrosis result in abnormalities of chloride transport across epithelial cells on mucosal surfaces [36]. A raised level of chloride in sweat (above 60 mmol/L) is considered consistent with a diagnosis of cystic fibrosis although it is recommended that the test is repeated on two occasions [35].

Lactate is found in a concentration of 4–40 mmol/L, which greatly exceeds the concentration found in plasma. It is formed in the gland from glucose from the blood. It is interesting to speculate whether urea and lactate can act to moisturize the stratum corneum.

Glucose is present in small quantities only (usually 0–0.17 mmol/L, although levels up to 0.3 mmol/L may be found). High sweat glucose may be found in uncontrolled diabetes and this may create a favourable environment for skin infections. The pH is 4–6.8.

A variety of other substances may be found in sweat, including pharmacologically active substances and inhibitors, antigens, antibodies and drugs [4]. Some of these seem to be excreted, and have no special function; others may have a definite function, for example a urokinase-type plasminogen activator may play a part in the digestion of glycoprotein plugs in sweat pores [37]. Active excretion or secretion of drugs such as griseofulvin and ketoconazole may contribute to their efficacy.

DISORDERS OF ECCRINE SWEAT GLANDS

Hyperhidrosis

Definition and nomenclature

Hyperhidrosis is defined as excessive production of sweat, that is, more than is required for thermoregulation [1]. It can be defined gravimetrically [2] as greater than 2 standard deviations above mean values of sweat secretion for a normal population in various sites (palmar 50 mg/min/m^2, plantar 50 mg/min/m^2, axillary 150 mg/min/m^2 and facial 50 mg/min/m^2).

Synonyms and inclusions
- Excessive sweating

Introduction and general description

Hyperhidrosis can be a major inconvenience and embarrassment to sufferers. In theory, when there is overproduction of sweat it should be possible to determine whether this is due to abnormal sweat glands, pharmacologically active agents acting on the glands, abnormal stimulation of the sympathetic pathway between the hypothalamus and the nerve ending, or to overactivity of one of the three different 'centres' responsible for thermoregulatory, mental and gustatory sweating. Any difficult case should be approached from first principles in this way.

Most cases of hyperhidrosis can be classified as one of the following:
- Generalized.
- Focal – palmar, plantar, axillary and cranio-facial.
- Localized naevoid.
- Compensatory.
- Hyperhidrosis with extensive anhidrosis (Ross syndrome).

Epidemiology

In a series of Polish medical students, 16% admitted to perceived hyperhidrosis. Less than half of these, however, were determined to have gravimetrically measured sweat secretion rates defined as greater than 2 standard deviations above the reference range for a given site [2]. Generalized and focal naevoid hyperhidrosis are relatively rare. There is no gender or racial preponderance.

Generalized hyperhidrosis

Pathophysiology

There is marked physiological variation in thermoregulatory sweating from person to person in the absence of disease. An increase in the temperature of blood bathing the hypothalamus increases heat loss by sweating and vasodilatation. Some instability of the sweat regulating centre is caused by many febrile conditions, so that sweating may occur at times when there is no fever. This instability may persist for days, or even months, after the fever has subsided, and in some cases is such a prominent feature that the term 'sweating sickness' has been used [3]. Generalized sweating may occur in disorders of unknown aetiology that alter the setting of the thermoregulatory centre and may be associated with episodic hypothermia [1].

For a list of disorders associated with generalized hyperhidrosis see Box 94.1.

Thermoregulatory sweating occurs during or after many infective processes, and may be the presenting manifestation of

---

Box 94.1 Causes of generalized hyperhidrosis

- Febrile infective illnesses: tuberculosis, malaria, brucellosis, endocarditis, etc.
- Metabolic diseases: diabetes, hyperthyroidism, hyperpituitarism, hypoglycaemia, phaeochromocytoma
- Menopause
- Underlying solid malignancy and lymphoma
- Congestive heart failure
- Neurological disorders:
  - Brain disease:
    - Parkinson disease
    - episodic hypothermia with hyperhidrosis
    - generalized hyperhidrosis without hypothermia
  - Peripheral neuropathies:
    - familial dysautonomia (Riley–Day)
    - congenital autonomic dysfunction with universal pain loss
    - cold-induced sweating syndrome
- Drugs: fluoxetine

malaria, tuberculosis, brucellosis, lymphoma, subacute bacterial endocarditis, etc. Night sweats are often part of the clinical picture. A similar mechanism may account for the hyperhidrosis associated with alcohol intoxication or gout, and after vomiting. The mechanism of generalized hyperhidrosis that may be associated with diabetic autonomic neuropathy, hyperthyroidism, hyperpituitarism, hypoglycaemia, obesity, the menopause and malignant disease is unknown. Increased sweating has been documented in some patients with Parkinson disease, but others have noted the combination of patchy anhidrosis and compensatory hyperhidrosis, suggesting autonomic dysfunction. Paroxysmal sweating, tachycardia and headaches strongly suggest a phaeochromocytoma. Hypertension is noted during attacks. Cases have been reported of patients who develop generalized sweating in a thermal pattern, but induced by cold [3].

Hyperhidrosis is seen in association with peripheral neuropathies, as in familial dysautonomia, or Riley–Day syndrome, a recessively inherited disorder of Ashkenazi Jews comprising an absent axon reflex flare after histamine injection, pupillary meiosis, diminished tendon reflexes, diminished pain sensation and absent fungiform papillae of the tongue (see Chapter 85). Excess sweating is thought to be due to sweat centre excitability. Congenital autonomic dysfunction with universal pain loss is similar, but individuals are not Ashkenazi Jews, have a complete absence of pain sensation with accidental self-mutilation, corneal opacities and episodic fever.

Generalized hyperhidrosis may be associated with brain lesions (diencephalic lesions, malformations of the corpus callosum, microgyria) and may be accompanied by episodic hypothermia. Some drugs – for example, fluoxetine – are able to cause generalized hyperhidrosis. In many cases of generalized hyperhidrosis of the thermal type, but with no obvious underlying disease, the aetiology remains unknown, even after extensive investigation.

Focal hyperhidrosis

Pathophysiology

Focal hyperhidrosis includes palmoplantar, axillary and craniofacial ('emotional') hyperhidrosis [4]. Emotional or mental activity increases sweating, especially on the palms, soles, axillae and, to a lesser extent, groin, face and scalp. It should be emphasized that mental activity devoid of any clear emotional content may provoke sweating. Thermal stimuli and physical effort increase this effect in many cases. Most cases of hyperhidrosis presenting to the dermatologist are of this type. Although mental or emotional factors are the usual trigger for this type of sweating, and in some patients deep-seated emotional disturbances may be found, in many there seems to be some facilitation of the nervous pathways causing physiological mental sweating.

Clinical features

Focal hyperhidrosis may be a significant disability and embarrassment, particularly if sweat drips from the hands onto the floor; rusting of metal objects may be an occupational problem, or clothing may be saturated. Patients with axillary hyperhidrosis often

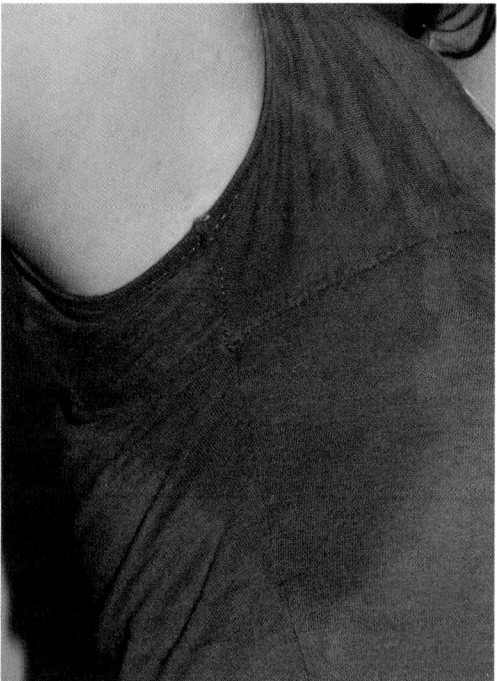

Figure 94.3 Axillary hyperhidrosis: patients often wear white or black garments as the wetness is not as visibly obvious as with coloured clothes.

wear only black or white garments as these show the wetness less obviously than coloured clothes (Figure 94.3).

Hyperhidrosis may be associated with Raynaud phenomenon and reflex sympathetic dystrophy, or may follow cold injury. Frequently there is a family history of excessive sweating.

Palmoplantar hyperhidrosis. Palmoplantar hyperhidrosis (Figure 94.4) occurs in both sexes, and commonly begins in childhood or around puberty. The sweating of the palms and soles may be either continuous or phasic [4]. When continuous, it is worse in the summer, and not so clearly precipitated by mental factors. When phasic, it is usually precipitated by minor emotional or mental activity, and is not markedly different in summer and winter. The hands may be cold and show a tendency to acrocyanosis. Hyperhidrosis may affect the hands, feet and axillae in any combination, but only a minority of patients with axillary hyperhidrosis also have involvement of the palms and soles. Troublesome hyperhidrosis of the feet occurs especially in young adult men. When this is associated with vasomotor changes, so that the sodden skin is also cold and cyanotic, the name 'symmetrical lividity' is sometimes applied. Palmoplantar hyperhidrosis is one component of various syndromes in which palmoplantar keratoderma occurs. It also occurs with the nail–patella syndrome (see Chapter 69).

Axillary hyperhidrosis. This may be continuous, or more commonly phasic, and may or may not be aggravated by heat or mental activity. It is uncommon before puberty. Axillary sweating on undressing is very common. Axillary hyperhidrosis is due to

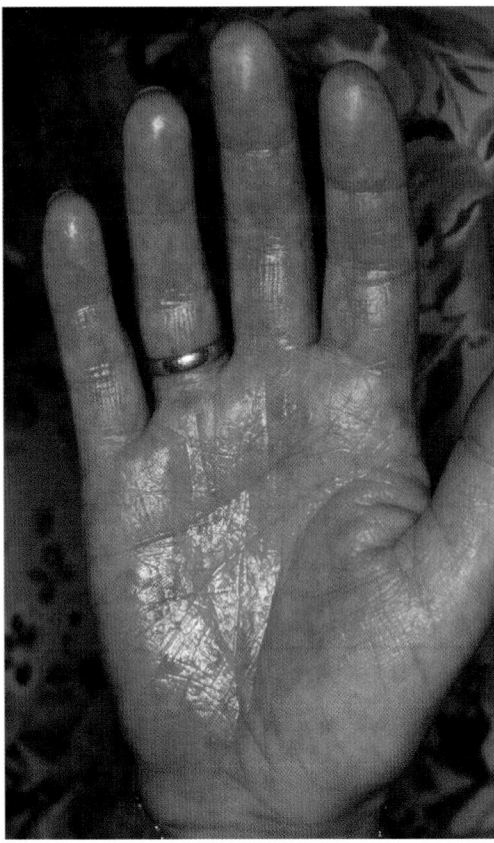

Figure 94.4 Palmar hyperhidrosis.

overactivity of the eccrine glands, unlike axillary odour, which is mainly apocrine in origin.

Cranio-facial hyperhidrosis. Cranio-facial hyperhidrosis (Figure 94.5) is often phasic, occurs in middle age and may be exacerbated by heat, exercise and eating but, unlike true gustatory hyperhidrosis, not exclusively so. It may be more persistent and usually presents

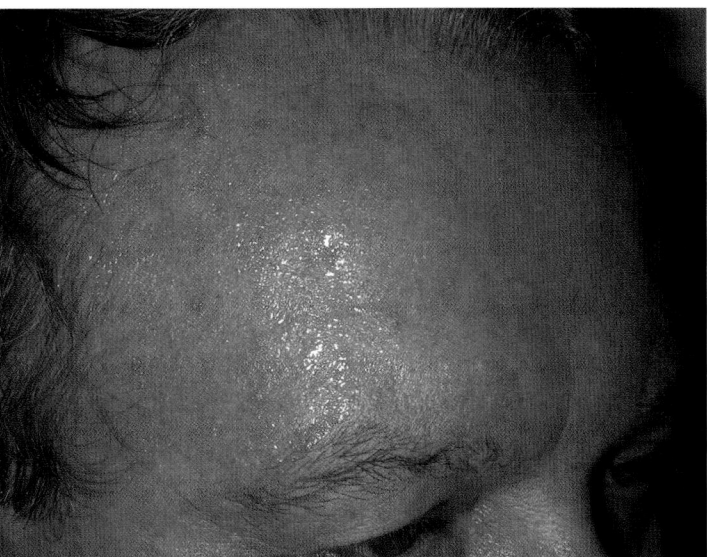

Figure 94.5 Cranio-facial hyperhidrosis. It may be sufficiently profuse to drip off the face and wet the hair.

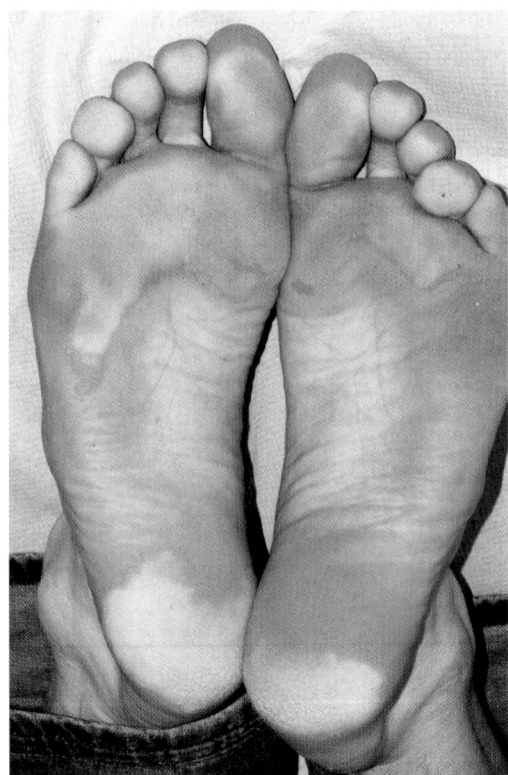

Figure 94.6 Plantar hyperhidrosis showing maceration of the plantar keratin and secondary pitted keratolysis due to infection with *Kytococcus sedentarius*.

at a later age than palmoplantar hyperhidrosis. The entire face and scalp may be affected; sweating sufficient to soak the hair is an additional embarrassment.

Complications and co-morbidities
Palmoplantar hyperhidrosis predisposes to vesicular eczema (pompholyx) and allergic sensitization to footwear constituents; control of sweating may thus reduce the risk of contact dermatitis to footwear materials. Maceration of the skin, particularly in the toe clefts, is common and may predispose to both dermatophyte and bacterial infection (see Chapters 26 and 32). Pitted keratolysis of the feet, due to infection with *Kytococcus sedentarius*, is strongly associated with hyperhidrosis (Figure 94.6).

Disease course and prognosis
Hyperhidrosis may persist for some years, but there is a tendency to spontaneous improvement of axillary and palmar hyperhidrosis after the age of 25 years.

Investigations
Thyroid function and gravimetric determination of sweat rate estimation are seldom contributory.

Localized circumscribed and asymmetrical hyperhidrosis

Pathophysiology
The causes of localized hyperhidrosis are outlined in Box 94.2. Excessive sweating may be due to neurological lesions involving

Box 94.2 Causes of localized hyperhidrosis

- Spinal cord injury:
  - Hyperhidrosis associated with autonomic dysreflexia
  - Hyperhidrosis due to orthostatic hypotension
- Intrathoracic neoplasia
- Gustatory hyperhidrosis
- Frey syndrome
- Granulosis rubra nasi
- Functional and true sweat gland naevi
- Sweating associated with local skin disorders:
  - Glomangioma
  - Blue rubber bleb naevi
  - Pachydermoperiostosis
  - Pretibial myxoedema
  - POEMS syndrome
  - Burning feet syndrome
- Compensatory: after sympathectomy, or with partial anhidrosis
- Idiopathic unilateral circumscribed hyperhidrosis

POEMS, polyneuropathy, organomegaly, endocrinopathy, M protein and skin changes.

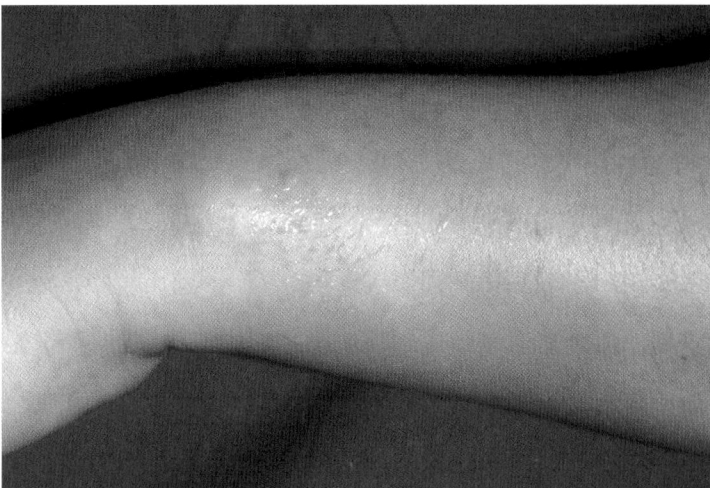

Figure 94.7 Circumscribed (naevoid) hyperhidrosis on the wrist. There is a solitary area of hyperhidrosis with normal sweating elsewhere on the rest of the skin.

any part of the sympathetic pathway from the brain to the nerve ending. It may be the presenting symptom but it is quite exceptional for this to occur as an isolated phenomenon in the absence of other neurological symptoms or signs. Such lesions may be within the central nervous system (cortex, basal ganglia or spinal cord), the sympathetic pathway and ganglia, or in the peripheral nerves [1,5,6,7,8,9,10–14]. It must be remembered that the distribution of the sympathetic nerves does not exactly correspond with sensory dermatomes. One sympathetic grey ramus may supply 10 or more sensory segments, and one white ramus extends over at least five. Asymmetrical sweating may also occur reflexively from visceral disturbances, adjacent to an area of anhidrosis or due to axon reflex stimulation, around a leg ulcer, for example, or around glomus tumours, blue rubber bleb naevi or a sudoriparous angioma.

Compensatory hyperhidrosis occurs in normal sweat glands when those elsewhere are not functioning because of neurological or skin disease, diabetes or after sympathectomy. It is also a component of Ross syndrome (see below).

Functional sweat gland naevi have been reported [13], but must be distinguished from sweat gland hypertrophy associated with local hyperhidrosis of some other aetiology. Areas of skin may be localized (Figure 94.7) [14], termed idiopathic circumscribed hyperhidrosis, or as extensive as one-half of the body [15] and may sweat continuously or, more commonly, with mental activity. They may represent functional naevi, where the eccrine glands show increased sensitivity to cholinergic neurotransmitters. In the absence of other neurological symptoms or signs, they are seldom a manifestation of a progressive neurological lesion.

Cold-induced sweating syndrome

This rare condition presents in infancy with poor feeding and difficulty in suckling, followed in adulthood by paradoxically cold-induced hyperhidrosis and anhidrosis in heat [1]. There is an associated mild neuropathy, kyphoscoliosis, valgus deformity of the elbows, high arched palate and digital syndactyly. Inactivation of a cardiotropin-like cytokine, a second ligand for ciliary neurotrophic factor receptor, has been identified in this syndrome.

Gustatory hyperhidrosis

Pathophysiology

Hyperhidrosis precipitated by eating specific foods can occur physiologically in many people [1]. Hot spicy foods are the most likely cause. The central connections of this reflex are not fully known.

Gustatory hyperhidrosis also occurs in pathological conditions involving the autonomic nervous system. Localized areas of intense hyperhidrosis may occur on the face, and even on the knees [2]. These disorders are very rare, usually start in childhood and are not progressive. Their nature is little understood.

Much the commonest cause, however, is damage to the sympathetic nerves around the head and neck [3–5]. After such an injury, regeneration occurs not only from the proximal ends of the damaged sympathetic nerves, but also from damaged or undamaged parasympathetic nerves. In this way, abnormal connections are made. Thus, the reflex arcs that normally allow chewing or taste stimulation to cause parotid or gastric secretion may cause sweating in a localized zone corresponding to the area of skin in which the sympathetic innervation has been damaged. The commonest site is within the distribution of the auriculotemporal nerve, which may be injured by trauma, abscess or surgery in the parotid region (auriculotemporal or von Frey syndrome). Submental gustatory sweating follows injuries involving the chorda tympani, and sweating in the distribution of the greater auricular nerve commonly follows radical neck surgery [6]. Injury to fibres from the vagus may cause gustatory sweating localized to the upper arm after cervical sympathectomy.

**PART 8: SPECIFIC
CUTANEOUS STRUCTURE**

Box 94.3 Classification of gustatory hyperhidrosis

- Idiopathic
- Central
- Post-herpetic
- Post-peripheral nerve injury:
  - Parotid surgery, injury and abscess
  - Auriculotemporal
  - Chorda tympani
  - Greater auricular
  - Cervical sympathectomy
- Peripheral autonomic neuropathy:
  - Diabetes

Gustatory sweating may occur in diabetes as part of a widespread autonomic neuropathy [7]. It has also followed herpes zoster [8].

Clinical features

Gustatory sweating is by no means uncommon, and occurs in 50–80% of patients subjected to operations on the parotid gland. Usually the symptoms appear 4–7 months after the operation, and either persist indefinitely or wane after 3–5 years. The stimuli required to initiate the reflex vary, as does the severity. Sometimes chewing, without taste sensation, is the most important stimulus. In many cases it is merely a curiosity, but in others it can be a significant disability. As well as sweating there is usually vasodilatation, which in rare instances may occur by itself in the absence of visible sweating. For a classification and list of causes of gustatory hyperhidrosis see Box 94.3. Olfactory hyperhidrosis, in which the trigger stimulus is smell, has also been recorded [9].

Management

Treatment of severe cases may require surgical interruption of the parasympathetic pathway – for example, section of the glossopharyngeal nerve within the skull, or tympanic neurectomy [4]. Excision of the auriculotemporal nerve is usually followed by recurrence. Topical therapy with aluminium chloride [10], topical glycopyrronium bromide [11] or botulinum toxin injections may be helpful [7].

Management of hyperhidrosis

Topical drug treatment

Topical anticholinergics. Atropine-like drugs may be absorbed sufficiently to produce a beneficial local effect without associated systemic side effects, but none of those at present available can be relied upon to do so [1]. Poldine methosulphate, 1–4% in alcohol, suppresses experimentally induced sweating, but unfortunately has not proved to be useful in clinical practice [2]. Topical 0.5% glycopyrronium bromide cream has been successfully used in gustatory hyperhidrosis in diabetics and at

0.5–2.0% for axillary hyperhidrosis [3]. A 2.0% aqueous solution has been used in scalp hyperhidrosis, and may be used to treat axillae.

Eccrine duct-blocking agents. These drugs act by impeding the delivery of sweat to the skin surface. Formalin (40% aqueous solution of formaldehyde) 1% soaks have long been used for treatment of hyperhidrosis of the feet, but are unsuitable for the hands and axillae. Glutaraldehyde 10% in a buffered solution, pH 7.5, swabbed onto the feet three times weekly, has helped some patients [4], but stains the skin so that it is suitable only for the feet. There is a small risk of allergic sensitization both to formaldehyde and to glutaraldehyde.

For axillary hyperhidrosis (as opposed to bromhidrosis), the most commonly used topical applications are aluminium or zirconium salts. Aluminium chloride, the first to be introduced, is in many ways the best, but may be irritant to the skin and damage clothes. Many other salts – for example, the chlorhydrates – are in use in cosmetic preparations [5]. Improved results can be achieved by applying 20% aluminium chloride in absolute ethanol at night after drying the axilla, with or without polythene occlusion. It should initially be applied nightly but may later be required only once every 1–4 weeks [6,7]. Commercial preparations are available. Mild irritation of the skin from such therapy may be helped by a weak topical corticosteroid. The same treatment can also be tried on the hands and feet, or other localized areas of hyperhidrosis, but usually with rather less success. The mode of action of aluminium salts is uncertain, but they can be shown to affect both the duct and the secretory coil [8].

Iontophoresis. One of the more satisfactory methods of controlling hyperhidrosis of the hands and feet is by iontophoresis, using either tap water or anticholinergic drugs such as 0.05% glycopyrronium bromide solution [9–11,12]. The mode of action of tapwater iontophoresis is not known. In very soft water areas, adding sodium bicarbonate to the iontophoresis solution is reported to improve efficacy. Direct current is usually used, with each palm or sole being treated for 30 min with 20 mA, initially three times a week. Once euhidrosis is established, monthly maintenance treatment may be sufficient. Alternating current is less effective, but may usefully be combined with direct current (alternating current offset) to produce a safer, more comfortable treatment [13]. Once control has been achieved, a single treatment may prove effective for some weeks. Minor systemic side effects due to absorption of anticholinergic agents, such as dry mouth and eye symptoms, are not uncommon, and can be avoided if tap water alone is used. The authors' practice is to initiate thrice-weekly treatment on a hospital out-patient basis, and, if this is successful, a small battery-operated home unit can be purchased for maintenance therapy [14]. Less frequent treatment will then be required. When the sweating is controlled, the associated lividity, coolness and oedema improve. Similar treatment has also been used for the axilla, but is less often needed because topical applications or injections of botulinum toxin are more effective in this site. Devices have been designed to deliver iontophoresis to the chest and back affected by post-sympathectomy compensatory hyperhidrosis.

Botulinum toxin A injection. This compound produces prolonged blockade of neuronal acetylcholine release at the neuromuscular junction and in cholinergic autonomic neurons: it has been used to treat dystonic conditions for many years. In recent years, intradermal injection has been used to produce a marked reduction of sweating in hyperhidrotic areas associated with a variety of conditions [15,16–18]. Different preparations of botulinum A toxin have different activities, and dose schedules differ for each product; 0.1 mL of appropriately diluted botulinum toxin administered by high intradermal injection can be given to 1 cm^2 areas of skin appropriately anaesthetized – topical eutectic lignocaine/prilocaine is sufficient for axillary skin, but palms and soles require regional nerve blockade. Each axilla usually requires 12 injections, hands 20 and each foot 24–36. A reduction in sweating is apparent within 48 h and the benefit will normally last for up to 8 months in axillary and 6 months in palmar and cranio-facial hyperhidrosis [19]. Reinjection seems to be effective, and to date resistance has not been seen in hyperhidrosis (although it eventually occurs in 5% of patients treated intramuscularly for dystonia). Botulinum toxin has been used for idiopathic circumscribed and gustatory hyperhidrosis including Frey syndrome, the hyperhidrotic areas in Ross syndrome, and frontal and cranio-facial hyperhidrosis. A sight transient reduction of thenar and hypothenar muscle power is a minor problem after palmar injections [18]. The use of botulinum toxin on the forehead may produce short-lived frown reduction [19].

Systemic drug treatment

Atropine-like drugs have been used to block the effect of acetylcholine on the sweat glands, but their side effects are often more troublesome than the hyperhidrosis itself. These include dryness of the mouth, constipation, urinary retention and disturbances of vision, due to paralysis of accommodation. More serious side effects, for example glaucoma, hyperthermia and convulsions, can occur. Atropine itself is seldom employed. Propantheline may be prescribed in doses of 15 mg three times daily, increasing, if tolerated, to as much as 150 mg daily [20], but overall the results are disappointing. Methantheline at a dose of 50 mg three times a day has recently been advocated [21]. The oral antimuscarinic agent oxybutynin, usually used to treat bladder instability, has been reported to be effective for generalized and focal hyperhidrosis. The dose is escalated from 2.5 mg daily to 5 mg twice a day as tolerated, with an improvement in quality of life in 65% of those treated [22]. Glycopyrollate at a dose of 1–2 mg once to four times a day often gives useful sweat reduction without other marked anticholinergic effects [23]. Clonidine at a dose of 0.1 mg twice daily may be useful, but hypotension may limit its use. Ganglion-blocking drugs can inhibit sweating, but side effects from hypotension are usually too troublesome. Calcium-channel blockers, such as diltiazem [24], have helped some patients. In cases with a pronounced emotional factor, sedative or tranquillizing drugs are often useful, but psychiatric treatment may be necessary. Both clonazepam [25] and amitriptyline have helped isolated cases of unusual localized hyperhidrosis.

Surgical treatment

Sympathectomy. Sympathectomy, whether cervical, transaxillary or endoscopic, causes anhidrosis if complete [26,27]. Sweating may return after a period of some years, due either to regeneration of sympathetic fibres or to fibres that do not pass through the sympathetic ganglia [28]. The former open approach has been largely replaced by an endoscopic procedure, which may be successful in treating palmar, axillary and cranio-facial hyperhidrosis. A pneumothorax is induced, and an operating endoscope inserted into the thorax via a small axillary incision, allowing visualization of the sympathetic trunk. Interruption of the sympathetic fibres between the second and fourth thoracic ganglia can be achieved by surgical transection, radiofrequency ablation, phenol destruction, cautery, clamping or clipping [29]. The latter technique has the potential advantage of partial reversibility. Most surgeons treat both sides at a single session.

With both the open and endoscopic approaches, satisfactory reduction of palmar hyperhidrosis is achieved in over 95% of cases; it is a little less successful for axillary hyperhidrosis. A recent consensus guideline [30] suggested that an international nomenclature should be adopted that refers to the rib levels (R) instead of the vertebral level at which the nerve is interrupted. It states that the highest success rates occur when interruption is performed at the top of R3 or the top of R4 for hyperhidrosis limited to the palms. R4 may offer a lower incidence of compensatory hyperhidrosis but moister hands. For hyperhidrosis involving the upper limbs and/or the axillae, interruptions at R4 and R5 are recommended. The top of R3 is best for cranio-facial hyperhidrosis.

In a series of 1731 patients who underwent endoscopic sympathectomy, the initial failure rate was 9%, and there was recurrence in 2%; overall, 98% of those treated were satisfied with the result. Compensatory hyperhidrosis occurred in 88% of patients, and was severe in 27%. Only 2.5% of patients experienced regret for having the operation [31]. Large case series using endoscopic techniques in children show it to be an acceptable option, with a low recurrence rate [32].

Complications of sympathectomy include haemothorax, pneumothorax, chylothorax, nipple sensitivity and Horner syndrome. There are rare instances of transient or permanent bradycardia complicating the technique. Other disadvantages are that the palms or soles may become excessively dry, and irritant eczema after sympathectomy has been reported. In five patients who had undergone a clipping procedure and subsequently developed compensatory hyperhidrosis, removal of the clips resulted in a return of the palmar sweating and abolition of the compensatory hyperhidrosis [33]. It has been suggested that ablation at the level of the third thoracic ganglion does not produce this side effect. Abolition of severe facial blushing may be a desirable consequence, and resolution of palmar eczema has been reported after endoscopic sympathectomy.

In general, only those patients with severe disability from hyperhidrosis of the hands or axillae warrant surgery, and in these selected cases the results can be very gratifying. Endoscopic sympathectomy has been used successfully in the treatment of severe cranio-facial hyperhidrosis [34]. Pedal sympathetic denervation requires lumbar sympathectomy; if more cranial lumbar ganglia are removed, ejaculatory impotence may occur. A selective retroperitoneal approach has recently been advocated that has no effect on sexual function in either men or women [35]. An endoscopic technique employing clips may also be employed with high patient satisfaction and minimal surgical morbidity.

Excision of the axillary vault. Axillary hyperhidrosis may be greatly helped by local excision of the axillary vault [36,37]. Variations of this technique include subcutaneous curettage of the axillary skin [38], directly trimming the eccrine glands after reflection of the axillary skin using only a short incision [**39**], and tumescent liposuction of the axillae [40]. Microwave devices that ablate eccrine glands in the axillae are under development [41].

Treatment ladder

First line
- Eccrine duct-blocking agents (aluminium chloride hexahydrate)
- Topical anticholinergics (glycopyrrolate)

Second line
- Iontophoresis with tap water or anticholinergics (hands, feet and axillae)
- Intradermal botulinum toxin (axillae, hands and face)
- Oral anticholinergics: propanthelene, methanthelene oxybutynin, glycopyrollate
- Oral clonidine
- Oral β-blockers and anxiolytics

Third line
- Removal or ablation of eccrine glands (axillary)
- Sympathectomy (thoracic or lumbar)

Granulosis rubra nasi

Definition
Granulosis rubra nasi is a rare disorder characterized by hyperhidrosis of the nose and associated skin changes [1].

Epidemiology and pathophysiology
The condition was first described by Jadassohn. The pathogenesis remains obscure but in some cases there is evidence of autosomal dominant transmission [2]. Symptoms develop from as early as 6 months but can occur at any age in childhood and occasionally in adults.

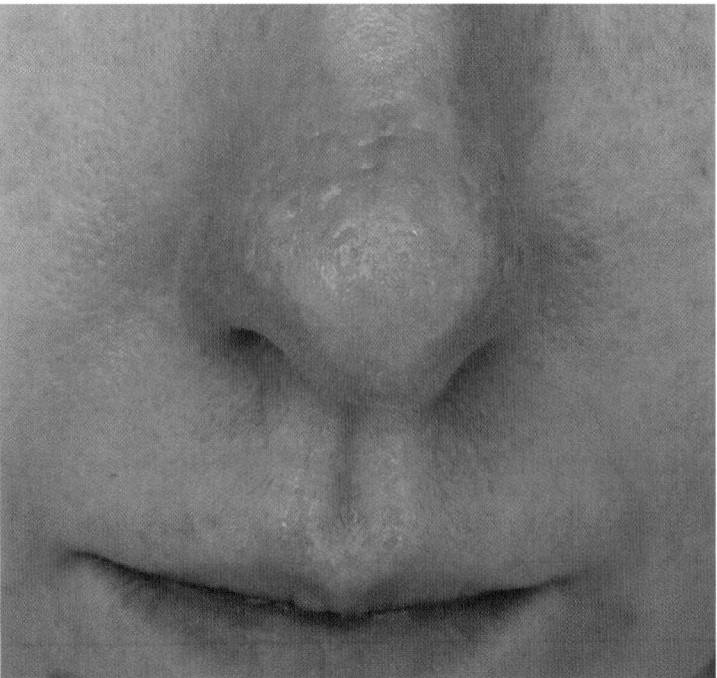

Figure 94.8 Granulosis rubra nasi in young adult female showing localised hyperhidrosis with beads of sweat on nose and philtrum together with multiple vesicles and mild erythema on dorsum of nose. Courtesy of Dr E.P. Burova, Bedford Hospital.

Clinical features
Initial presentation is with excess sweating localized over the tip of the nose. Droplets of sweat are usually visible. With time erythema, papules, vesicles and telangiectasia may develop over the nose, cheeks and upper lips (Figure 94.8) [3]. In the vast majority of cases, resolution occurs around puberty but persistent cases are recognized. Patients may also report peripheral acrocyanosis and palmoplantar hyperhidrosis. A single case has been described in association with phaeochromocytoma [4]. Skin biopsy demonstrates a chronic inflammatory cell infiltrate with dilatation of vascular spaces [3].

Investigations
These are not usually needed.

Management
Reassurance, given the natural history of the condition, is sufficient in most cases. Botulinum toxin has been reported as effective [5].

Anhidrosis and hypohidrosis

Diminished sweat production may be partial (hypohidrosis) or complete (anhidrosis) [1]. Disturbance of any part of the physiological pathway of sweat production may decrease sweating. Causes may be broadly classified as being either of neurological (Box 94.4) or eccrine gland origin (Box 94.5).

Box 94.4 Neurological causes of anhidrosis and hypohidrosis

- Organic brain lesions of hypothalamus, pons and medulla
- Spinal cord lesions:
  - Syringomyelia
  - Sympathectomy
- Congenital insensitivity to pain with anhidrosis
- Degenerative syndromes:
  - Shy–Drager syndrome
  - Ross syndrome
- Peripheral neuropathy:
  - Diabetes
  - Alcohol
  - Leprosy
- Autonomic neuropathy
- Drug-induced blockade of neurotransmission:
  - Ganglion-blocking agents
  - Anticholinergic agents
  - Calcium channel-blocking agents
  - α-adrenergic blockers

Impairment of sweat production interferes with the body's temperature control mechanisms. Symptoms include heat intolerance, fatigue, drowsiness and pyrexia. In severe cases death may result.

Examination of patients with hypo- and anhidrosis is often unremarkable. Autonomic function tests, in particular the quantitative sudomotor axon reflex test and the thermoregulatory

Box 94.5 Eccrine gland disorders producing anhidrosis and hypohidrosis

- Genetic disorders:
  - Bazex syndrome
  - Ectodermal dysplasia
  - Fabry disease
  - Incontinentia pigmenti
- Atrophy or destruction of eccrine glands:
  - Scleroderma
  - Burns
  - Sjögren syndrome
  - Lymphoma
  - Acrodermatitis chronica atrophicans
- Obstruction of sweat ducts:
  - Miliaria
  - Eczema
  - Psoriasis
  - Lichen planus
  - Ichthyosis
  - Porokeratosis
- Drugs affecting eccrine gland function:
  - Topical aluminium salts
  - 5-Fluorouracil
  - Mepacrine
  - Topiramate
- Idiopathic:
  - Acquired idiopathic generalized anhidrosis

sweat test (essentially a heat stress in a warmed room), may help delineate the distribution of anhidrosis and point towards a cause [2]. Skin biopsy is also helpful to identify eccrine sweat gland abnormalities.

Ross syndrome

This rare syndrome is characterized by a triad of segmental anhidrosis, tonic pupils (Figure 94.9a) and absent deep tendon reflexes [3]. It is a progressive degenerative disorder of sensory and autonomic nerves [4,5]. Involvement of the cardiac sympathetic nerve supply has also been reported [6].

The main symptoms are those of heat intolerance and socially disabling compensatory hyperhidrosis (Figure 94.9b), which may

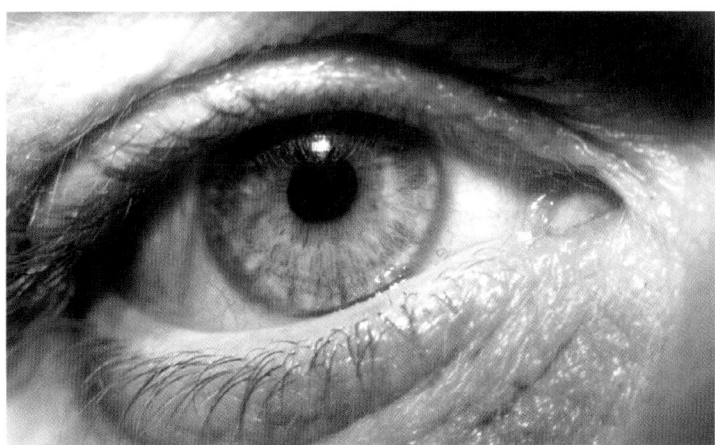

(a)

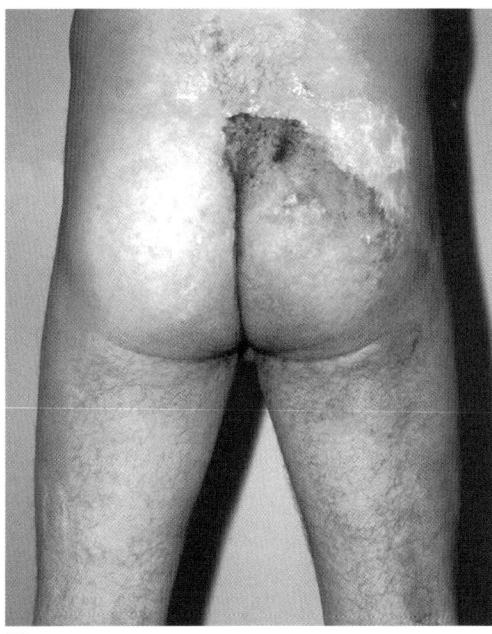

(b)

Figure 94.9 Ross syndrome. (a) The pupils are tonic, asymmetrical and irregular in outline. (b) Most of the skin is anhidrotic but the remaining areas of enervated eccrine glands demonstrate compensatory hyperhidrosis (demonstrated by edicol Ponceau powder, which turns red on hydration).

be asymmetrical, patchy or unilateral. Hyperhidrosis arising in this situation has been successfully treated with iontophoresis and botulinum toxin [4,7].

Acquired idiopathic generalized anhidrosis

This term describes a heterogeneous group of very rare disorders characterized by progressive loss of sweating and heat intolerance [8]. Three subtypes have been proposed: idiopathic pure sudomotor failure, sudomotor neuropathy and sweat gland failure [9]. In a proportion of patients, lymphocytic infiltration of the eccrine glands is seen and the presence of such inflammation may explain the response to oral corticosteroids observed in this condition [10,11].

Miliaria

Definition and nomenclature

This is a common acute or subacute skin condition that arises due to the occlusion or disruption of eccrine sweat ducts in hot humid conditions, resulting in a leakage of sweat into the epidermis (miliaria crystallina and miliaria rubra) or dermis (miliaria profunda) [1–3].

Synonyms and inclusions
- Prickly heat
- Miliaria crystallina
- Miliaria rubra
- Miliaria profunda

Introduction and general description

The three forms of miliaria – miliaria crystallina (sudamina), miliaria rubra (prickly heat) and miliaria profunda – occur as a result of either occlusion or disruption of the eccrine sweat ducts. They differ in clinical form due to the different levels at which occlusion occurs, although some authorities have suggested that disruption of the duct rather than occlusion is responsible [4]. In miliaria crystallina, the obstruction is very superficial, within the stratum corneum, and the vesicle is subcorneal, producing a vesicle containing clear fluid. In miliaria rubra, the later changes include keratinization of the intraepidermal part of the sweat duct, with leakage and then formation of a vesicle around the duct. In miliaria profunda, there is rupture of the duct at the level of or below the dermal–epidermal junction.

Miliaria crystallina can easily be produced experimentally by minimal, non-specific epidermal injury and profuse sweating [5]. It is often seen in febrile illnesses associated with profuse sweating. It occurs commonly in infants due to a delay in patency developing in the sweat ducts.

Miliaria rubra may be produced experimentally in susceptible subjects by epidermal injury [6]. It can be reproduced regularly by occlusion of the skin under polythene for 3–4 days, following which anhidrosis lasts for about 3 weeks. Prolonged exposure of the skin to sweat achieves the same effect. The first event

may be an increase in the skin flora, perhaps with *Staphylococcus epidermidis* being responsible for producing an extracellular polysaccharide substance or slime that blocks the lumen of the sweat duct [1,7]. The parakeratotic plugs, which are a notable feature of the later stages of the disease, are not the primary cause of the obstruction, but arise in the repair process, and may further aggravate the obstruction. Leakage of sweat into the epidermis is responsible for the final production of the lesions, and for their further aggravation.

Miliaria profunda is due to more severe damage to the sweat ducts, and usually follows repeated attacks of miliaria rubra. It may be reproduced by experimental injury.

Rarely, miliaria may be associated with pseudohypoaldosteronism; high sweat sodium levels produce damage of the eccrine ducts, causing lesions similar to those seen in miliaria rubra. It can be precipitated by drugs (bethanechol, isotretinoin and doxorubicin).

Epidemiology

Miliaria crystallina occurs commonly in infants due to a delay in patency developing in the sweat ducts. In a large Japanese study, it was identified in 4.5% of babies, with a peak frequency at 1 week [8]. The incidence of miliaria rubra, and particularly miliaria profunda, is highest in hot, humid conditions, but it may occur in desert regions, affecting up to 30% of people exposed to these climatic conditions. It may begin within a few days of arrival in a tropical climate, but is maximal after 2–5 months. There is a striking variation in individual susceptibility. Infants are especially prone.

Miliaria rubra is common on the trunk in hospitalized patients who have to be nursed on their backs on bedding that has waterproof occlusive membranes below the sheets. It may also commonly be seen after occlusive therapy with polythene. Outbreaks on the legs in miners working in tropical climates have been reported [9].

Clinical features

Clinical features of the three types of miliaria are as follow.

Miliaria crystallina. Clear, thin-walled vesicles, 1–2 mm in diameter without an inflammatory areola, are usually symptomless and develop in crops, mainly on the trunk. In persistent febrile illnesses, recurrent crops may occur. The vesicles soon rupture, and are followed by superficial, branny desquamation.

Miliaria rubra. Typical lesions develop on the body, especially in areas of friction with clothing, and in flexures. The lesions are uniformly minute erythematous papules, which may be present in very large numbers (Figure 94.10). Characteristically, the lesions produce intense discomfort in the form of an unbearable pricking sensation. Relief is often instantaneous when the stimulus to sweating is abolished by a cool shower. In infants, lesions commonly appear on the occluded skin of the neck, groins and axillae, but also occur elsewhere.

Miliaria profunda. This nearly always follows repeated attacks of miliaria rubra, and is uncommon except in the tropics. The

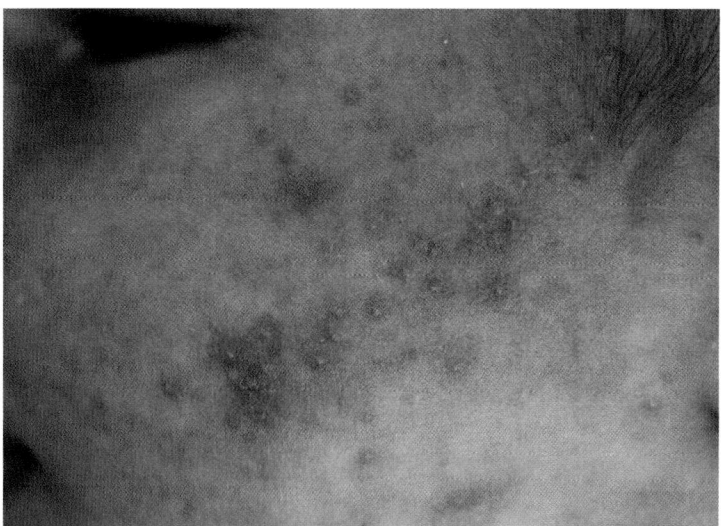

Figure 94.10 Miliaria rubra affecting the cheeks of an infant. (Courtesy of Dr Richard Logan, Bridgend, UK.)

the incidence. The large number of treatments advocated for prickly heat is the best indication of their relative ineffectiveness if sweating is not reduced. In the absence of gross secondary sepsis, the effect of topical or systemic antibiotics or other antibacterial preparations on established miliaria is disappointing, but they may have some role in prophylaxis [1]. Oral ascorbic acid 500 mg twice daily was found to diminish the severity of miliaria, as was the degree of subsequent anhidrosis in experimentally induced disease [12]. Calamine lotion is probably as effective as anything for the relief of discomfort, but because of its drying effect, a bland emollient (e.g. oily cream or menthol in aqueous cream) may subsequently be required to prevent further epidermal damage. Isotretinoin was reported to help a recalcitrant case of miliaria profunda [13].

lesions are easily missed. The affected skin is covered with pale, firm papules 1–3 mm across, especially on the body, but sometimes also on the limbs. There is no itching or discomfort from the lesions.

Patients often wrongly refer to polymorphic light eruption as 'prickly heat'; here the relationship of the rash to light, particularly on newly exposed sites, is usually straightforward.

Disease course and prognosis
This depends mainly on environmental factors. If continued sweating occurs, recurrent episodes lasting a few days are usual, but discomfort may be continuous. However, after a few months some degree of acclimatization occurs, and the disorder becomes less prevalent.

The most important complications of miliaria are secondary infection and disturbance of heat regulation. Secondary bacterial infection is common and sometimes serious. This may present as impetigo. In other cases, the pustules are more clearly related to sweat ducts, although in pustular miliaria factors other than bacterial infection are implicated [10]. Miliaria rubra in young infants may predispose to multiple superimposed staphylococcal abscesses [11]. In most cases of miliaria rubra the changes are reversible if further sweating is avoided, but permanent damage to the sweat duct may occur, especially after miliaria profunda.

Management
The only really effective prevention or treatment for miliaria is avoidance of further sweating. Even if this is achieved only for a few hours a day, as in an air-conditioned office or bedroom, considerable relief is experienced. For the very susceptible person, a move away from tropical climates may be essential. Avoidance of excessive clothing, friction from clothing, excessive use of soap and contact of the skin with irritants will reduce

Treatment ladder

First line
- Control local environment (remove excess bedding, fans, air conditioning)
- Cool the skin (damp compresses, cool showers)
- Avoid tight or excessive clothing

Second line
- Menthol (e.g. 0.5% menthol in aqueous cream)
- Topical antibiotics if there is secondary infection
- Mild topical steroids

Third line
- Removal to cooler climate
- Prophylactic oral vitamin C

Neutrophilic eccrine hidradenitis

Definition and nomenclature
Neutrophilic eccrine hidradenitis refers to a rare clinical condition with non-specific features but characteristic acute inflammation of the eccrine sweat glands, seen on skin biopsy.

Synonyms and inclusions
- Chemotherapy-associated eccrine hidradenitis
- Idiopathic palmoplantar hidradenitis

Introduction and general description
Neutrophilic eccrine hidradenitis (NEH) may arise in a variety of very difficult clinical situations, producing an eruption with very distinct pathological features. It can be classified into the following types:
- Chemotherapy-induced neutrophilic eccrine hidradenitis.
- Infectious neutrophilic eccrine hidradenitis.

PART 8: SPECIFIC CUTANEOUS STRUCTURE

- Palmoplantar neutrophilic eccrine hidradenitis.
- Neutrophilic eccrine hidradenitis with HIV infection.
- Neutrophilic eccrine hidradenitis with Behçet disease.

Epidemiology

This is a rare condition that may be considered a reaction pattern to a variety of stimuli [1,2,3]. Drug-induced NEH is primarily seen in patients receiving cytotoxic chemotherapy, whilst childhood NEH affects otherwise well children [4,5]. Attacks of childhood NEH are reported to be more frequent in the spring and summer. Disease-associated NEH and infectious NEH are both very rare.

Pathophysiology

The key pathological feature of NEH is necrosis of the eccrine epithelium in association with a dense neutrophilic infiltrate. In drug-induced NEH this is most commonly reported with the use of cytotoxic chemotherapeutic agents. Typical histological changes can be induced experimentally by the local injection of bleomycin into human skin, suggesting that the eccrine glands are subject to direct toxicity [6]. Other drugs reported in association with NEH include carbamazepine, tumour necrosis factor α antagonists and cetuximab [7,8,9].

Childhood NEH is not associated with underlying disease. However, it may follow physical exertion and exposure to damp footwear [10].

Infectious NEH is most frequently encountered in immunosuppressed individuals. Causative organisms implicated include *Serratia*, staphylococci, streptococci and *Nocardia* [11–13]. NEH has also been reported in HIV infection, Behçet disease and as a paraneoplastic phenomenon in both haematological and solid organ malignancies [12,13,14,15].

Clinical features

Drug-associated NEH typically occurs 8–10 days after starting chemotherapy. Painful erythematous papules and plaques develop on the limbs, neck and face [2]. Facial erythema and swelling may be severe enough to mimic cellulitis [16]. The condition typically resolves within 2 weeks of treatment ending. Recurrence, however, may occur with subsequent courses of chemotherapy [17].

Childhood NEH has a particular predilection for the soles and less frequently the palms. Typically, tender plaques and nodules are seen. Attacks resolve spontaneously in 3 weeks but the condition may be recurrent [4,5,18].

Investigations

In drug-induced NEH skin biopsy is diagnostic. Associated neutropenia is also common. Further investigations may be necessary to exclude sepsis. Investigation of childhood NEH is not usualsy necessary.

Management

In the majority of cases the condition resolves without any treatment. In adult NEH systemic corticosteroids, dapsone and colchicine have all been recommended [15,19]. Dapsone may also be helpful in preventing recurrent disease [20].

Eccrine syringosquamous metaplasia

Definition

Eccrine syringosquamous metaplasia is used to describe both histological change, seen within eccrine sweat glands, and also a distinct skin eruption associated with the use of chemotherapeutic agents [1].

Pathophysiology

Predisposing factors

Eccrine syringosquamous metaplasia is characterized by the transformation of cuboidal ductal epithelial cells into areas of squamous differentiation [2]. This process has been reported in a wide variety of different settings including pyoderma gangrenosum, panniculitis and infection [3,4]. It is considered a non-specific marker of eccrine duct damage and may be confused histologically with squamous cell carcinoma. Similar histological changes are seen in patients undergoing chemotherapy, presumably forming part of a spectrum of cytotoxic eccrine damage, which includes neutrophilic eccrine hidradenitis [5].

Clinical features

In patients undergoing chemotherapy, eccrine syringosquamous metaplasia has been observed following the use of a range of drugs, most notably cytarabine and protein kinase inhibitors. The eruption develops during or shortly after chemotherapy and slowly resolves spontaneously. Widespread papulovesicular lesions, acral erythema and an intertriginous eruption may all be seen.

Investigations

Skin biopsy is usually diagnostic.

Management

The condition resolves spontaneously but symptom control may be required.

Drugs and eccrine glands

A number of drugs are concentrated and secreted by eccrine glands. This may partially account both for their therapeutic effect and cutaneous toxicity. Drugs known to be secreted include sulfaguanidine, sulfadiazine, amphetamines, arsenicals, iodides, phenytoin, phenobarbitone, carbamazepine, griseofulvin, ketoconazole, fluconazole, ciprofloxacin, diamorphine, cocaine and nicotine [1].

Sweat testing may be used as an alternative to urine testing in the setting of substance abuse [2].

Disorders with sweat gland cellular inclusions

The accumulation of substances within eccrine secretory cells occurs in a number of metabolic conditions summarized in Table 94.1 [1–6].

Table 94.1 Disorders with characteristic eccrine gland inclusion.

Microscopic changes	Disorder
Membrane-bound vacuoles in secretory cells	Mucopolysaccharidoses (Hurler, Hunter and Sanfillipo types)
Intracytoplasmic lipid inclusions	Sphingolipidoses
Secretory cell inclusions	Fabry disease, fucosidosis, Kanzaki disease, adrenoleukodystrophy and maltase deficiency
PAS-positive granules in outer duct cells	Lafora disease

PAS, periodic acid–Schiff stain.

APOCRINE GLANDS

Anatomy and physiology of apocrine glands

Apocrine sweat glands derive their name from the way their secretion appears, on light microscopy, to be derived by pinching off parts of the cytoplasm (from the Greek apo- 'away' and krinein 'to separate'). They are epidermal appendages, and develop as part of the pilosebaceous follicle in the fourth to fifth month of intrauterine life. In the embryo they are present over the entire skin surface, but most glands subsequently disappear, so that in the adult the characteristic distribution in the axillae, perianal region and areolae of the breasts is found [1–3,4]. So-called ectopic glands may be found elsewhere. The mammary glands and ceruminous glands in the external auditory meati are modified apocrine glands. Apocrine glands are poorly developed in childhood, and begin to enlarge with the approach of puberty. The activity of the glands is androgen dependent, and the glands show marked testosterone 5α-reductase activity [5].

The glands are larger than eccrine glands, and in the dissected specimen are visible to the naked eye. They are situated in the subcutaneous tissue. Each consists of a tubule and a duct. The latter is often quite short, and opens into the neck of the hair follicle above the sebaceous gland. Despite their embryological origin from the hair follicle, some apocrine glands eventually come to open on the surface of the skin. The secretory coil is a simple convoluted tube. It is lined by a single layer of columnar or cuboidal cells resting on a basement membrane. The free edge of the cells may show the appearance of apocrine secretion (Figure 94.11). Electron microscopy shows that this may be partly an artefact, but eccrine, apocrine and even holocrine secretion may all be found in places [3,6,7]. The apocrine duct closely resembles the eccrine duct, and consists of a double layer of cuboidal cells. Outside the basement membrane of the gland and duct is a longitudinal layer of myoepithelial cells. Their function is to support the duct and to propel the secretion to the surface, and waves of peristalsis have been seen in them [8]. Where the duct opens into the neck of the hair follicle there is the equivalent of the acrosyringium of the eccrine duct, although it is less obvious [9]. Apocrine sweat glands have an adrenergic sympathetic supply but neural control appears to be unimportant [10].

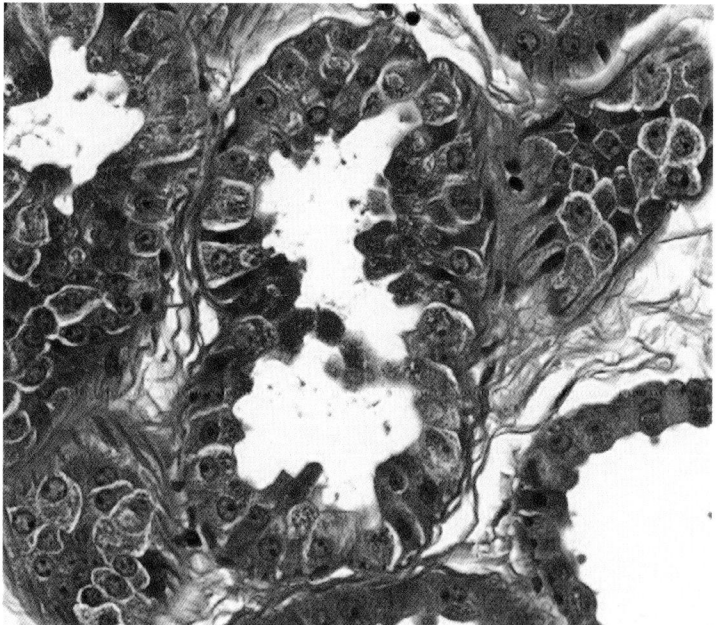

Figure 94.11 Normal apocrine glands lined by cells with abundant eosinophilic cytoplasm and decapitation secretions. Magnification 40× (H&E). (Courtesy of Dr Arti Bakshi, Royal Liverpool University Hospital, Liverpool, UK.)

Apocrine glands secrete small quantities of an oily fluid. This secretion is odourless on reaching the surface of the skin. Bacterial decomposition is responsible for the production of odiferous compounds. In particular, corynebacterial aminoacylase is responsible for the production of 3-methyl-2-hexenoic and 3-hydroxy-3-methylhexenoic acids [11]. Smaller quantities of odiferous sulphanylalkanols and steroids have also been identified [12,13]. The production of these metabolites is under the genetic control of the *ABCC11* gene, which encodes an ATP-driven efflux pump. Individuals homozygotic for a mutation in this gene produce much less odour. Mutation in this gene is predominant in South-East Asians, explaining racial variations in body odour [14].

There is evidence that products of apocrine sweat glands may act as human pheromones but the specific chemicals and pathways involved have not yet been elucidated [15].

DISORDERS OF APOCRINE SWEAT GLANDS

Abnormal sweat odour (bromhidrosis)

Definition and nomenclature

Human skin odour is a matter of concern both to those anxious about emitting it and to those who have to endure it when it emanates from others. It is largely due to the production of volatile chemicals by the actions of bacteria on secreted apocrine sweat.

Synonyms and inclusions
• Osmidrosis

Epidemiology

Human skin odour is largely determined by alteration or degradation of odourless substances secreted by apocrine glands by bacteria, especially *Corynebacterium* species, in the presence of hyperhidrosis [1]. Eccrine secretion is usually odourless but can contain odour-producing substances that are excreted in it, such as drugs, arsenic and garlic. Sebaceous secretion has some odour, as do the decomposition products of keratin, which can cause malodour in some hyperkeratanizing disorders such as keratodermas and Darier disease. On occasion, malodour appreciated only by the patient may be a symptom of monosymptomatic delusion of malodour (olfactory reference disorder) which requires psychiatric intervention [2], or from an organic lesion of the central nervous system.

Incidence

There is marked individual and racial variation in body odour, and what is socially acceptable varies greatly with race and social upbringing.

Age

As apocrine secretion increases under androgen control, malodour usually developes at or after puberty. Cases of generalized bromhidrosis in children have been reported due to chronic retention of nasal foreign bodies, and as a result of precocious puberty.

Sex

Malodour is more evident in men, but men and women seek medical management with equal frequency [3].

Ethnicity

There is anecdotal evidence that axillary malodour is more prevalent in European and African individuals, and less so in East Asians, Chinese and Koreans.

Associated diseases

Recent studies have associated axillary malodour with wet-type ear wax, and this is the result of a single nucleotide polymorphism in the *ABCC11* gene [4]. This gene is responsible for the function of the apical efflux pump and the conjugation of some of the odour-producing thioalcohols. Dry ear wax individuals do not produce these substances.

Pathophysiology

In the axillae, high humidity due to eccrine sweating and sebaceous secretion results in a rich microflora, including bacteria of the genera *Staphylococcus*, *Micrococcus*, *Corynebacterium* and *Propionobacterium*. An increased axillary pH may facilitate the overgrowth of these bacteria. Apocrine secretions are largely odourless, but biotransformation by bacteria, particularly corynebacteria, results in the liberation of short- and medium-chain volatile fatty acids (C2 to C10 branch length), 16-androstene steroids and thioalcohols, each of which may produce its own odour signature [1]. Studies have demonstrated histological differences between normal and bromhidrotic apocrine glands; in the bromhidrotics, the apocrine glands were larger and more numerous [5].

Clinical features

Presentation may be due to the patient being conscious of emitting odour, or as the result of comments from friends and relatives. Sniff testing may result in the appreciation of the character of the malodour, such as 'onion-like and beefy' or a 'lighter fruity' note.

Management

The treatment of axillary bromhidrosis includes the omission of foodstuffs such as garlic from the diet, frequent washing of the axillary regions and local antibacterial substances. There is no evidence that measures used to control axillary eccrine hyperhidrosis – for example, aluminium salts and anticholinergic drugs – have much effect on the apocrine glands, although excessive eccrine excretion may favour the spread of apocrine secretion and facilitate proliferation of the odour-producing microflora.

Deodorants are the mainstay of therapy as the fragrances disguise the undesired odour. A topical glycine-soya sterocomplex agent has shown encouraging improvement on both the intensity and quality of odour in patients with bromhidrosis [6]. A silver-zeolite powder has been shown to have strong antibacterial effects on axillary microflora and to diminish axillary malodour [7]. Botulinum toxin A has been used to treat axillary [8] and genital malodour [9] with good effect: the impact on eccrine sweating and rendering the area anhidrotic may prevent bacterial activity and thus have an effect on odour. Surgical excision of axillary subcutaneous tissue by a variety of surgical techniques (axillary shave and subsection of subcutaneous glands, laser ablation, ultrasound ablation, intradermal alcohol injection and liposuction), which removes both eccrine and apocrine glands, has been performed with good effect in those dissatisfied with conservative measures [10,11,12].

Trimethylaminuria

Definition and nomenclature

This disorder results from excessive amounts of the offensively smelling tertiary amine trimethylamine appearing in eccrine and apocrine sweat, breath and urine, and imparting an unpleasant rotting fish smell to sufferers [1].

Synonyms and inclusions
- Fish odour syndrome

Epidemiology

Incidence

The ability to *N*-oxidize trimethylamine into trimethylamine oxide (which has no odour) is distributed polymorphically, and sufferers are homozygous for an allele that determines this impaired reaction. One per cent of the population are heterozygous carriers of the allele.

Age

Most cases present in their late teens or early twenties.

Sex

The incidence does not vary by gender.

Pathophysiology

Affected individuals are unable to oxidize trimethylamine, which is produced by the intestinal bacterial degradation of choline and carnitine in food, to the odourless trimethylamine N-oxide. This can occur as a primary problem, as a result of a mutation in the flavin-containing mono-oxygenase3 (*FMO3*) gene [2]. Secondary trimethylaminuria can occur when there is an increased burden of trimethylamine, and is seen when there is an increased production of it from its precursors by gut bacteria in conditions such as blind loop syndrome, uraemia and liver disease.

Clinical features

The unpleasant odour, which is often worse after eating seafood, during periods of stress or during menstruation, can be the source of much distress, rejection and resentment. Sufferers are sometimes unaware of their smell, which may be intermittent and may not be detected by physicians when consulted. Trimethylaminuria was found in 7% of a series of individuals who perceived themselves to be malodorous [3].

Investigations

The condition can be diagnosed by direct estimation of trimethylamine in the urine after a marine fish meal. Both affected individuals and heterozygous carriers have abnormally elevated excretion of trimethylamine after such an oral challenge.

Management

A diet low in carnitine and choline may help. Egg yolks, legumes, red meats, fish and beans should be avoided. Short courses of metronidazole or neomycin may temporarily reduce the bacteria that degrade the carnitine and choline in the gut. Charcoal and copper chlorophyllin have been shown to reduce urinary trimethylamine concentrations to normal levels in sufferers [4].

Treatment ladder

First line
- Low carnitine diet

Second line
- Antibiotics (metronidazole and neomycin)
- Oral charcoal
- Oral copper chlorophyllin

Chromhidrosis

Definition

Chromhidrosis is the secretion of vividly coloured apocrine sweat [1,2]. It is most commonly a blue, yellow or green colour and is usually of apocrine origin, and seen in the axilla, areola of the nipple or face.

Clinical features

Apocrine sweat may be tinged with a yellow, green or blue hue in up to 10% of the population. Only rarely does it occur to the striking degree that merits the term chromhidrosis. It results from the secretion of lipofuscins in apocrine sweat, and may be associated with the secretion of coloured breast milk. The more oxidized lipofuscins appear deeper in colour; the lighter-coloured pigments may fluoresce. The diagnosis can be confirmed by finding lipofuscin pigment granules that may fluoresce on fluorescence microscopy in the apocrine secretory cells. Affected individuals' clothes may also fluoresce on Wood's light illumination. The secretion of coloured sweat starts at puberty and persists until there is a gradual regression of apocrine function in old age. Coloured sweat may be discharged from the glands in response to exercise and emotional stimuli, and after manipulation of the skin. The axillae are the most frequently affected sites, although facial [3] and areolar [4] chromhidrosis are recorded.

Management

Treatment ladder

First line
- Topical capsaicin

Second line
- Intralesional botulinum toxin
- Topical capsaicin has satisfactorily reduced facial and nipple chromhidrosis
- Botulinum toxin has been used to successfully suppress facial chromhidrosis [5,6]

Pseudochromohidrosis

Pseudochromohidrosis is the secretion of clear sweat that changes to a coloured secretion after it exits the sweat duct. It may occur due to chromogenic or porphyrin-producing bacteria on the skin [7]. A case of facial red chromhidrosis in a child responded to erythromycin, the antibiotic eradicating a chromogenic bacterium which was felt to be the cause of the abnormal colour [8].

Exogenous chromogens can affect eccrine sweat. Occupational exposure to copper salts has been reported to produce blue eccrine sweat; excessive consumption of a red food dye resulted in red sweat staining of underwear in one reported case [9].

Alkaptonuria (ochronosis) may result in dark perspiration.

Apocrine miliaria

Definition and nomenclature

Apocrine miliaria is a disorder of the apocrine glands comparable to prickly heat of the eccrine glands, and caused by obliteration of the apocrine duct at the infundibulum [1]. It usually presents with an itchy papular eruption in the axillae, ano-genital area or on the areolae of the nipple.

Synonyms and inclusions
- Fox–Fordyce disease

Epidemiology

Incidence and prevalence
It is uncommon.

Sex
It predominates in females. Familial twin and male cases are reported [2].

Pathophysiology
The condition occurs as a result of apocrine sweat duct occlusion by aggregates of epithelial cells of the apocrine or apoeccrine secretory cells [3]. The earliest pathological sign is a small vesicle in the apocrine duct. Later, the apocrine glands are seen to be enlarged, and as a consequence of repeated inflammatory events, perifollicular xanthomatosis with perifollicular foam cells expressing CD68 may develop [4].

Clinical features
The disease occurs mainly in women soon after puberty, but can be postmenopausal [1]. It can occur in males or in children, and has been reported in females with Turner syndrome and in identical twins. In recent years it has been reported after laser axillary hair epilation [5]. Itching, which may be intense, occurs in the axillae, and to a lesser extent in the ano-genital region and around the breasts. Objectively there may be little to see at first, but later skin-coloured or slightly pigmented, dome-shaped, follicular papules develop (Figure 94.12). Hair loss in the axillae usually ensues. The itching is often provoked by those emotional stimuli that normally cause apocrine secretion. The disease runs a very prolonged course, and may persist until the menopause. Some remission may occur in pregnancy.

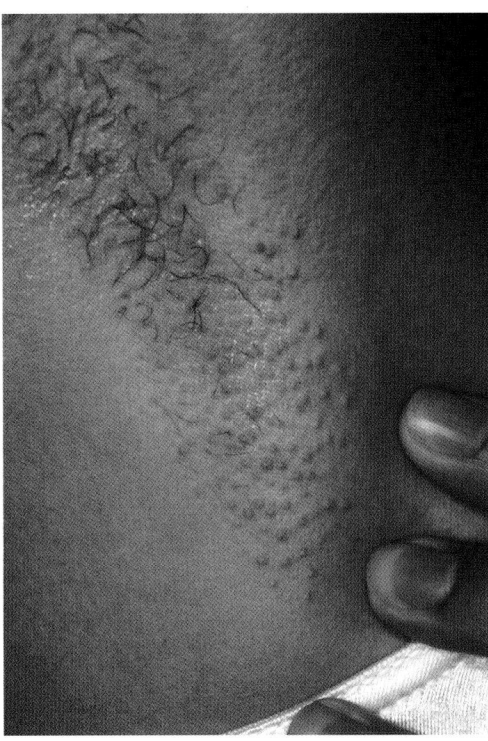

Figure 94.12 Axillary apocrine miliaria (Fox–Fordyce disease).

Differential diagnosis
It is distinctive so is usually easy to diagnose.

Management
Response to treatment is unsatisfactory. Topical and intralesional steroids provide some benefit, but their use is limited by atrophy. Topical clindamycin is reported to have been of help [6]. Treatment with 4–6-weekly doses of ultraviolet radiation, sufficient to cause exfoliation, helps some patients [7]. Topical retinoic acid may also be helpful, as may oral contraceptive agents and oral retinoids [8]. Other cases are sufficiently severe to require electrocautery [9], surgical excision of the affected skin or subcutaneous removal of the apocrine glands [10].

Treatment ladder

First line
- Topical or intralesional steroids
- Topical clindamycin lotion
- Topical retinoids

Second line
- Ultraviolet light
- Oral retinoids

Third line
- Surgery

Key references

The full list of references can be found in the online version at www.rooksdermatology.com.

Eccrine glands

Anatomy and physiology of eccrine glands
4 Sato K, Kang WH, Saga K, *et al*. Biology of sweat glands and their disorders. *J Am Acad Dermatol* 1989;20:537–63, 713–26.
6 Sato K, Leidal R, Sato F. Morphology and development of an apoeccrine sweat gland in human axillae. *Am J Physiol* 1987;252:R166–80, 181–7.
24 Shibasaki M, Crandall CG. Mechanisms and controllers of eccrine sweating in humans. *Front Biosci (Schol Ed)* 2010;2:685–96.
26 Shibasaki M, Wilson TE, Crandall G. Neural control and mechanisms of eccrine sweating during heat stress and exercise. *J Appl Physiol* 2006;100:1692–701.
33 Wolf JE, Maibach HI. Palmar eccrine sweating – the role of adrenergic and cholinergic mediators. *Br J Dermatol* 1974;91:439–46.

Disorders of eccrine sweat glands

Hyperhidrosis
1 Sato K, Kang WH, Saga K, *et al*. Biology of sweat glands and their disorders. *J Am Acad Dermatol* 1989;20:537–63, 713–26.
2 Stefaniak TJ, Proczko M. Gravimetry in sweating assessment in primary hyperhidrosis and healthy individuals. *Clin Auton Res* 2013;23:197–200.
4 Hoorens I, Ongenae K. Primary focal hyperhidrosis: current treatment options and a step-by-step approach. *J Eur Acad Dermatol Venereol* 2012;26:1–8.
6 Chatterjee S, Ghosh K, Banerjee T. An intramedullary tumor presenting with hyperhidrosis. *Neurol India* 2004;52:39.
9 McCoy BP. Apical pulmonary adenocarcinoma with contralateral hyperhidrosis. *Arch Dermatol* 1981;117:659–61.

Gustatory hyperhidrosis

1 Lee TS. Physiological gustation sweating in a warm climate. *J Physiol* 1954;124:528–42.

6 McGibbon BM, Paletta FX. Further concepts in gustatory sweating. *Plast Reconstr Surg* 1972;49:639–42.

Management of hyperhidrosis

1 McMillan FSK, Reller HH, Snyder FH. Antiperspirant action of topically applied anticholinergics. *J Invest Dermatol* 1964;43:363–7.

3 Mackenzie A, Burns C, Kavanagh G. Topical glycopyrrolate for axillary hyperhidrosis. *Br J Dermatol* 2013;169:483–4.

6 Anon. Aluminium chloride for hyperhidrosis. *Drug Ther Bull* 1981;19:101–2.

7 Shelley WB, Hurley HJ. Studies on topical antiperspirant control of axillary hyperhidrosis. *Acta Derm Venereol (Stockh)* 1975;95:241–60.

12 Stolman LP. Treatment of excessive sweating of the palms by iontophoresis. *Arch Dermatol* 1987;123:895–6.

15 Heckmann M, Ceballos-Baumann AO, Plewig G. Hyperhidrosis Study Group. Botulinum toxin A for axillary hyperhidrosis (excessive sweating). *N Engl J Med* 2001;344:488–93.

23 Walling HW. Systemic therapy for primary hyperhidrosis: a retrospective study of 59 patients treated with glycopyrrolate or clonidine. *J Am Acad Dermatol* 2012;66:387–92.

27 Drott C, Gothberg G, Claes G. Endoscopic transthoracic sympathectomy: an efficient and safe method for the treatment of hyperhidrosis. *J Am Acad Dermatol* 1995;33:78–81.

30 Cerfolio RJ, De Campos JR, Bryant AS, et al. The Society of Thoracic Surgeons expert consensus for the surgical treatment of hyperhidrosis. *Ann Thorac Surg* 2011;91:1642–8.

39 Lawrence CM, Lonsdale Eccles AA. Selective sweat gland removal with minimal skin excision in the treatment of axillary hyperhidrosis: a retrospective clinical and histological review of 15 patients. *Br J Dermatol* 2006;155:115–18.

Anhidrosis and hypohidrosis, Ross syndrome, Acquired idiopathic generalized anhidrosis

1 Shelley WB, Horvath PN, Pilsbury DM. Anhidrosis. *Medicine* 1950;29:194–224.

3 Ross AT. Progressive selective sudomotor denervation; a case with coexisting Adie's syndrome. *Neurology* 1958;8:809–17.

9 Chen YC, Wu CS, Chen GS, et al. Identification of subgroups of acquired idiopathic generalized anhidrosis. *Neurologist* 2008;14:318–20.

11 Palm F, Löser C, Gronau W, et al. Successful treatment of acquired idiopathic generalized anhidrosis. *Neurology* 2007;68:532–3.

Miliaria

1 Holzle E, Kligman AM. The pathogenesis of miliaria rubra. *Br J Dermatol* 1978;99:117–37.

2 Leithead CS, Lind AR. *Heat Stress and Heat Disorders*. London: Cassell, 1964.

3 Sargent F, Slutsky HL. The natural history of the eccrine miliarias. *N Engl J Med* 1957;256:401–8, 451.

4 Shuster S. Duct disruption, a new explanation of miliaria. *Acta Derm Venereol (Stockh)* 1997;77:1–3.

7 Mowad CM, McGinley KJ, Foglia A, Leyden JJ. A role of extracellular polysaccharide substance produced by *Staphylococcus epidermidis* in miliaria. *J Am Acad Dermatol* 1995;33:729–33.

Neutrophilic eccrine hidradenitis

2 Harris T, Fine JD, Berman RS, et al. Neutrophilic eccrine hidradenitis. *Arch Dermatol* 1982;118:268.

9 Turan H, Kaya E, Gurlevik Z, et al. Neutrophilic eccrine hidradenitis induced by cetuximab. *Cutan Ocul Toxicol* 2012;31:148–50.

14 Gómez Vázquez M, Peteiro C, Toribio J. Neutrophilic eccrine hidradenitis heralding the onset of chronic myelogenous leukaemia. *J Eur Acad Dermatol Venereol* 2003;17:328–30.

18 Simon M, Jr, Cremer H, von den Driesch P. Idiopathic recurrent palmoplantar hidradenitis in children. Report of 22 cases. *Arch Dermatol* 1998;134:76–9.

Apocrine glands

Anatomy and physiology of apocrine glands

1 Hurley HJ, Shelley WB. *The Human Apocrine Sweat Gland in Health and Disease*. Springfield, IL: Thomas, 1960.

2 Ebling FJG. Apocrine glands in health and disease. *Int J Dermatol* 1989;28:508–11.

3 Montagna W, Parakkal PF. *The Structure and Function of Skin*, 3rd edn. London: Academic Press, 1974.

5 Takayasu S, Wakimoto H, Itami S, et al. Activity of testosterone 5∞-reductase in various tissues of human skin. *J Invest Dermatol* 1980;74:187–91.

7 Schaumburg-Lever G, Lever WF. Secretion from human apocrine glands. *J Invest Dermatol* 1975;64:38–41.

10 Robertshaw D. Neural and humoral control of apocrine glands. *J Invest Dermatol* 1974;63:160–7.

11 Natsch A, Gfeller H, Gygax P, et al. A specific bacterial aminoacylase cleaves odorant precursors secreted in the human axilla. *J Biol Chem* 2003;278:5718–27.

12 Natsch A, Schmid J, Flachsmann F. Identification of odoriferous sulfanylalkanols in human axilla secretions and their formation through cleavage of cysteine precursors by a C-S lysase isolated from axilla bacteria. *Chem Biodiversity* 2004;1:1058–72.

13 Bird S, Gower DB. The validation and use of a radioimmunoassay for 5 alpha-androst-16-en-3-one in human axillary collections. *J Steroid Biochem* 1981;14:213–19.

14 Martin A, Saathoff M, Kuhn F, et al. A functional ABCC11 allele is essential in the biochemical formation of human axillary odor. *J Invest Dermatol* 2010;130:529–40.

Disorders of apocrine sweat glands

Abnormal sweat odour (bromhidrosis)

1 James AG, Austin C, Cox D, Taylor D, Calvert R. Microbiological and biochemical origins of human axillary odour. *FEMS Microbiol Ecol* 2013;83:527–40.

3 Morioka D, Ohkubo F, Amikura Y. Clinical features of axillary osmidrosis: a retrospective chart review of 723 Japanese patients. *J Dermatol* 2013;40:384–8.

4 Nakano M, Miwa N, Hirano A, Yoshiura K, Niikawa N. A strong association of axillary osmidrosis with the wet earwax type determined by genotyping of the ABCC11 gene. *BMC Genet* 2009;4(10):42.

8 He J, Wang T, Dong J. A close positive correlation between malodor and sweating as a marker for the treatment of axillary bromhidrosis with Botulinum toxin A. *J Dermatolog Treat* 2012;23:461–4.

11 Huang YH, Yang CH, Chen YH, Chen CH, Lee SH. Reduction in osmidrosis using a suction-assisted cartilage shaver improves the quality of life. *Dermatol Surg* 2010;36:1573–7.

12 Qian JG, Wang XJ. Effectiveness and complications of subdermal excision of apocrine glands in 206 cases with axillary osmidrosis. *J Plast Reconstr Aesthet Surg* 2010;63:1003–7.

Chromhidrosis

1 Shelley WB, Hurley HJ. Localized chromhidrosis: a survey. *Arch Dermatol Syphilol* 1954;69:449–71.

2 Hurley HJ, Shelley WB. *The Human Apocrine Sweat Gland in Health and Disease*. Springfield, IL: Thomas, 1960.

5 Wu JM, Mamelak AJ, Nussbaum R, McElgunn PS. Botulinum toxin A in the treatment of chromhidrosis. *Dermatol Surg* 2005;31:963–5.

7 Poh-Fitzpatrick MB. 'Red sweat.' *J Am Acad Dermatol* 1981;4:481–26.

Apocrine miliaria

1 Hurley HJ, Shelley WB. *The Human Apocrine Sweat Gland in Health and Disease*. Springfield, IL: Thomas, 1960.

3 Kamada A, Saga K, Jimbow K. Apoeccrine sweat duct obstruction as a cause for Fox-Fordyce disease. *J Am Acad Dermatol* 2003;48:453–5.

4 Bormate AB, Jr, Leboit PE, McCalmont TH. Perifollicular xanthomatosis as the hallmark of axillary Fox–Fordyce disease: an evaluation of histopathologic features of 7 cases. *Arch Dermatol* 2003;144:1020–4.

PART 8: SPECIFIC CUTANEOUS STRUCTURE

CHAPTER 95

Acquired Disorders of the Nails and Nail Unit

David A. R. de Berker[1], *Bertrand Richert*[2] and *Robert Baran*[3]

[1]Bristol Dermatology Centre, Bristol Royal Infirmary, Bristol, UK
[2]Brugmann – St Pierre and Children's University Hospitals, Université Libre de Bruxelles, Brussels, Belgium
[3]University of Franche-Comté, Nail Disease Centre, Cannes, France

PART 8: SPECIFIC CUTANEOUS STRUCTURE

Rook's Textbook of Dermatology, Ninth Edition. Edited by Christopher Griffiths, Jonathan Barker, Tanya Bleiker, Robert Chalmers and Daniel Creamer.
© 2016 John Wiley & Sons, Ltd. Published 2016 by John Wiley & Sons, Ltd.
Companion website: www.rooksdermatology.com

ANATOMY AND BIOLOGY OF THE NAIL UNIT

Structure

Gross anatomy [1,2–5]

The component parts of the nail apparatus are shown in Figure 95.1. The nail is firmly attached to the nail bed; it is less adherent proximally, apart from the posterolateral corners. Approximately one-quarter of the nail is covered by the proximal nail fold, and a narrow margin of the sides of the nail plate is often occluded by the lateral nail folds. Underlying the proximal part of the nail is the white lunula (half-moon lunule); this area represents the most distal region of the matrix [6]. It is most prominent on the thumb and great toe and may be partly or completely concealed by the proximal nail fold in other digits. The reason for the white colour is not known [7–9]. The natural shape of the free margin of the nail is the same as the contour of the distal border of the lunula. The nail plate distal to the lunula usually appears pink, due to

its translucency, which allows the redness of the vascular nail bed to be seen through it. The proximal nail fold has two epithelial surfaces, dorsal and ventral; at the junction of the two, the cuticle projects distally onto the nail surface. The lateral nail folds are in continuity with the skin on the sides of the digit laterally, and medially they are joined by the nail bed. Some authorities term the lateral nail fold and adjacent tissue lateral to the nail fold the nail wall.

The definition of the nail matrix is controversial [10]. There is common acceptance that there is a localized region beneath the proximal nail which produces the major part of the normal nail plate. For those who consider this the sole source of nail it is termed simply the matrix, or germinal matrix. However, there is some evidence that other epithelial parts of the nail unit also contribute to the nail plate, and these are then also attributed matrix status (Figure 95.2). The matrix can be subdivided into dorsal (the ventral aspect of the proximal nail fold), intermediate (germinal matrix or matrix) and ventral (nail bed) sections. The nail bed is also termed the sterile matrix and its role in the production of the nail is unclear. Although it appears that the nail plate may thicken by up to 30% as it passes from the distal margin of the lunula to the end of the nail bed [3], this is not associated with an increase in cell numbers and may represent compaction of the nail from distal tip trauma rather than nail bed or nail plate production [11]. The situation may change in disease, where the nail bed changes its histological appearance to gain a granular layer [12] and may contribute a false nail of cornified epithelium to the undersurface of the nail [5]. The gap beneath the free edge is known as the hyponychium.

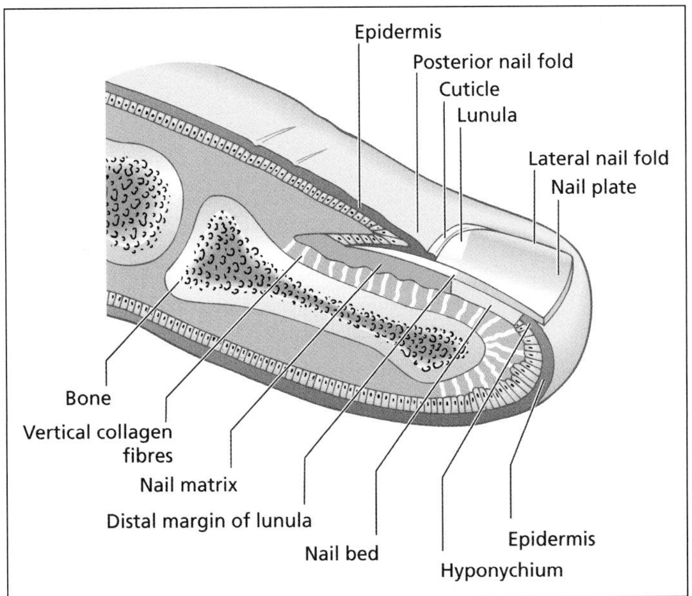

Epidermis
Posterior nail fold
Cuticle
Lunula
Lateral nail fold
Nail plate
Bone
Vertical collagen fibres
Nail matrix
Distal margin of lunula
Nail bed
Epidermis
Hyponychium

Figure 95.1 Longitudinal section of a digit showing the dorsal nail apparatus.

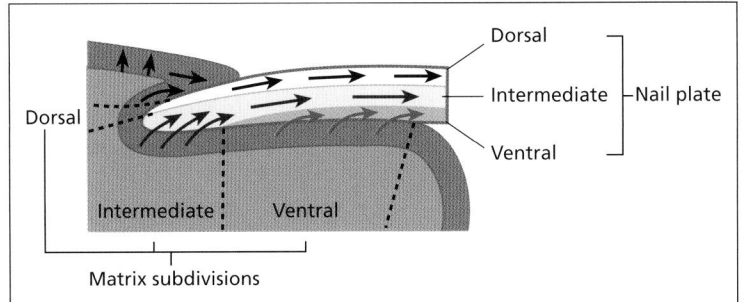

Figure 95.2 Direction of differentiation and cell movement within the nail apparatus.

When the attached nail plate is viewed from above, two distinct areas may be visible: the lunula proximally and the larger distal pink zone. On close examination, two further distal zones can often be identified: the distal yellowish-white margin and immediately proximal to this the onychodermal band [13]. Histologically, it is defined as the most distal attachment of cornified epithelium to the undersurface of the nail and has been termed the nail isthmus [14]. As such, it is structurally significant for the adherence of the nail plate to the nail bed. Once breached, as in conditions such as psoriasis, separation of the nail bed from the nail plate can be progressive.

Microscopic anatomy [15]

Nail folds

The proximal nail folds are similar in structure to the adjacent skin but are normally devoid of dermatoglyphic markings and pilosebaceous glands. There is a normal granular layer. From the distal area of the proximal nail folds, the cuticle adheres to the upper surface of the nail plate; it is composed of modified stratum corneum and serves to protect the structures at the base of the nail, particularly the germinal matrix, from environmental insults such as irritants, allergens and bacterial and fungal pathogens.

Nail matrix (intermediate matrix)

The nail matrix produces the nail plate in the absence of disease (see Figure 95.2). The basal compartment of the matrix is broader than the same region in normal epithelium or in other parts of the nail unit, such as the nail bed [10]. There is no granular layer, and cells differentiate with the expression of trichocyte 'hard' keratin (K31–40 and K81–86) as they become incorporated into the nail plate, alongside normal epithelial keratins [15–17]. During this process, they may retain their nuclei until more distal in the nail plate. These retained nuclei are called *pertinax bodies*. Apart from this, the detailed cytological changes seen in the matrix epithelium under the electron microscope are essentially the same as in the epidermis [18,19].

The nail matrix contains melanocytes in the lowest three cell layers and these donate pigment to the keratinocytes. The presence of 6.5 melanocytes per millimetre of matrix basement membrane can be used as a guide to a normal matrix melanocyte population [20]. The appearance of melanocytes separate from the basement membrane distinguishes them from those found in the nail folds, which are primarily basal [21]. Unlike melanocytes in the proximal nail fold and most other sites, nail matrix melanocytes do not express human leukocyte antigen (HLA)-A/B/C antigens [21]. Matrix melanocytes are further distinguished from those elsewhere by their failure to produce melanin in normal circumstances in white people. This can change, with melanotic streaks presenting in local inflammatory, naevoid or neoplastic disease. In non-white people, brown streaks are common and are almost universal in Afro-Caribbeans by the age of 60 years.

Langerhans cells are detectable in the matrix by CD1a staining, and the matrix appears to contain basement membrane components indistinguishable from normal skin [22].

Nail bed

The nail bed consists of epidermis with underlying connective tissue closely apposed to the periosteum of the distal phalanx. There is no subcutaneous fat in the nail bed, although scattered dermal fat cells may be visible microscopically.

The nail bed epidermis is usually no more than two or three cells thick, although there may be tongues of epithelium that extend obliquely down. The transitional zone from living keratinocyte to dead ventral nail plate cell is abrupt, occurring in the space of one horizontal cell layer; in this regard it closely resembles the Henle layer of the internal root sheath of the epidermis [23]. Nail bed cells do not have any independent movement, and it is yet to be clearly demonstrated whether they are incorporated into an overlying nail plate as it grows distally [24]. The process of nail bed keratinization has been likened to that seen in rat tail epidermis, possibly being affected by pressure changes. The loss of the overlying nail results in the development of a granular layer, which is otherwise present only in disease states [11,25,26].

The nail bed dermal collagen is mainly orientated vertically, being directly attached to the phalangeal periosteum and the epidermal basal lamina. Within the connective tissue network lie blood vessels, lymphatics, a fine network of elastic fibres and scattered fat cells; at the distal margin, eccrine sweat glands have been seen [1].

Nail plate

The nail plate comprises three horizontal layers: a thin dorsal lamina, the thicker intermediate lamina and a ventral layer from the nail bed [4]. This is not always apparent with normal light microscopy using routine stains, where the nail demonstrates a transition between flattened cells dorsally and thicker cells on the ventral aspect. Electron microscopy shows squamous cells with tortuous interlocking plasma membranes [18,19]. At high magnification, the contents of each cell show a uniform fine granularity similar to the hair cuticle [23]. Nail plate thickness can be measured in health and disease using ultrasound or optical coherence tomography [27].

The nail plate contains significant amounts of phospholipid, mainly in the dorsal and intermediate layers, which contribute to its flexibility. The detectable free fats and long-chain fatty acids may be of extrinsic origin. For further details of these and other histochemical changes in the components of the nail apparatus, see these more detailed texts [8].

Nail biology

Genes influencing the presence or absence or malformation of nails have been sought in connection with inherited abnormalities of the nail unit. The role of these genes in normal nail embryogenesis or production are difficult to determine, but it is clear that when there are mutations in the *R-spondin* genes and others influencing the *Wnt* signalling pathway, nail loss or reduction occurs. This first became evident from mutations seen in the *R-spondin4* gene in a family with an autosomal recessive pattern of anonychia [28]. More subtle forms of nail dysplasia can be attributed to defects of *Frizzled6* which in common with *R-spondin4*, enhances the *Wnt* signalling pathway and is found in inherited nail dysplasia [29]. In claw differentiation in knock-out mice, it is associated with expression of keratins K86, K81, K34 and K31; two epithelial keratins, K6a and K6b: all keratins with significance in nail formation and biology. Primary abnormalities in the *Wnt* signalling itself are also associated with inherited nail dysplasias such as Schöpf–Schulz–Passarge syndrome (*Wnt10a*) [30]. Mutations in other genes such as *LMX1B* are associated with multisystem disease such as nail–patella syndrome [31] which may have overlap with elements of *Wnt* signalling.

Keratin represents 80% of nail mass and its distribution and differentiation is pivotal. One classification of keratins is to divide them into 'soft' epithelial keratins or 'hard' trichocyte keratins (K31–40 and K81–86). The latter are characteristic of hair and nail differentiation, where their high sulphur content is responsible for their rugged physical qualities. This is matched by the resistance of trichocyte keratins to dissolution in strong solvent.

Keratin distribution in the nail and associated epithelium has been studied in adult [**14**,15,16], infant [17] and embryonic [32] digits. Immunohistochemistry of the epithelial structures of the normal nail demonstrates that the suprabasal keratin pair K1/K10 is found on both aspects of the proximal nail fold and to a lesser degree in the matrix. However, it is absent from the nail bed. This is reversed when there is nail bed disease, such as onychomycosis or psoriasis, where a granular layer develops and K1/K10 becomes expressed at corresponding sites [23]. The nail bed contains keratin synthesized in normal basal layer epithelium, K5/K14, which is also found in nail matrix. An antibody marking the epitope characteristically associated with keratin expressed in the basal layer is found throughout the thickness of the nail bed, but only basally in the matrix [26].

K6/K16 is identified in the nail bed but not the germinal matrix [16]. This is as proliferation is not a prominent feature. The nail bed has very low rates of proliferation [**10**,33], and it may be that K6/K16 more precisely illustrates a loss of differentiation, often associated with proliferation in skin but representing the resting state of nail bed epithelium.

The location of K6/K16 is reflected in the localization of the features of pachyonychia congenita. In this group of autosomal dominant disorders, there is thickening of the nail plate attributed to disease of the nail bed in variants of the disease attributed to abnormalities in each of these keratins [**34**,35].

Trichocyte keratins 31, 34, 81, 85 and 86 have all been demonstrated immunohistochemically in the nail unit [15,16]. Proximally, these do not extend onto the ventral aspect of the proximal nail fold, sometimes described as the dorsal matrix and distally their expression is limited to a margin taken as corresponding to the lunula. Their distribution appears to define a matrix consistent with the classic description of the germinal matrix.

Blood supply [1]

There is a rich arterial blood supply to the nail bed and matrix derived from paired digital arteries, a large palmar and small dorsal digital artery on either side. The palmar arteries are supplied from the large superficial and deep palmar arcades [2]. The main supply passes into the pulp space of the distal phalanx before reaching the dorsum of the digit (Figure 95.3). Distally, the arteries are extremely tortuous and coiled, which allows them to be distorted without kinking to occlude supply. There are two main arterial arches (proximal and distal) supplying the nail bed and

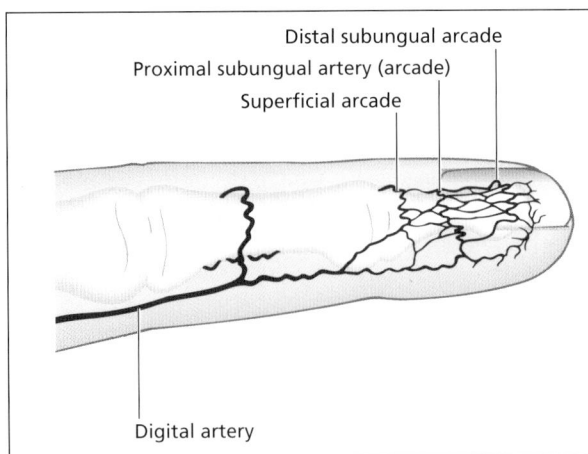

Figure 95.3 Arterial supply of the distal finger.

matrix, formed from anastomoses of the branches of the digital arteries. In the event of damage to the main supply in the pulp space, such as may occur with infection or scleroderma, there may be sufficient blood from the accessory vessels to permit normal growth of the nail. At a microvascular level, there are three patterns. Within the matrix, vessels are longitudinal with helical twisting. The axis becomes more longitudinal in the nail bed without the tortuosity – a pattern that is also seen in the distal proximal nail fold. This orientation is reflected in the appearance of splinter haemorrhages. In the digit pulp, vessels follow the pattern of the dermatoglyphics [**3**]. Nail vessel videomicroscopy can be used as part of a dynamic and anatomical modelling process establishing the parameters of blood flow and vessel anatomy [**4**].

There are many arteriovenous anastomoses beneath the nail – glomus bodies – which are concerned with heat regulation. Glomus bodies are important in maintaining acral circulation under cold conditions: arterioles constrict with cold but glomus bodies dilate [5]. These occupy the subdermal tissues and increase in number in a gradient towards the distal nail bed [6].

Nail growth and morphology

Clinicians experienced in observing the slow rate of growth of diseased or damaged nails are apt to view the nail apparatus as inert, although it is biochemically and kinetically active throughout life. In this respect, it differs from most hair follicles, which undergo periods of quiescence as part of the follicular cycle.

Cell kinetics

The kinetic activity of the matrix has been examined using many techniques. These include immunohistochemistry, autoradiography and direct measurement of matrix product (i.e. nail plate) by ultrasound [1], micrometer or histology.

There is a broad basal compartment of proliferating cells in the matrix, which can be detected immunohistochemically with antibodies to proliferating cell nuclear antigen and Ki-67 (Figure 95.4); both antigens are associated with proliferating cells [2]. The matrix is also the site of maximal inclusion of tritiated thymidine

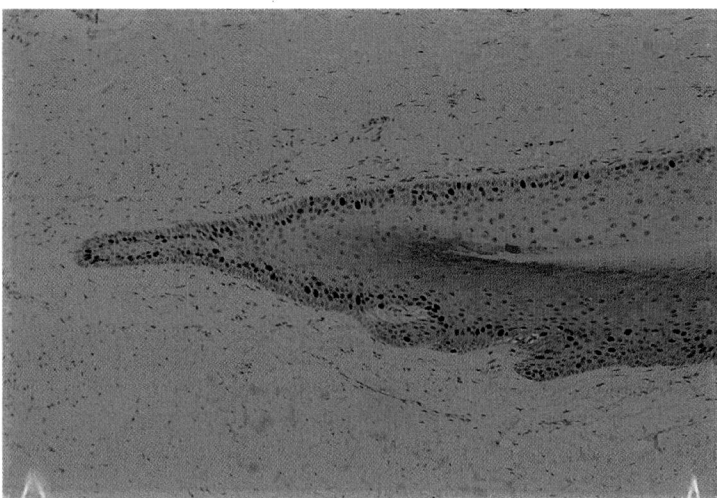

Figure 95.4 Proliferating epithelial cells of the matrix and ventral aspect of the proximal nail fold, staining with the antibody MIB-1.

Table 95.1 Physiological and environmental factors affecting the rate of nail growth.

Faster	Slower
Daytime	Night
Pregnancy [25]	
Right-hand nails	Left-hand nails [27]
Youth, increasing age	Old age [18,27,30]
Fingers	Toes [31]
Summer [18]	Winter or cold environment [32,33]
Middle, ring and index fingers	Thumb and little finger [28,31,34,35]
Male gender	Female gender [27,35]
Minor trauma/nail biting [26,27]	

if injected into the peritoneum of squirrel monkeys and followed subsequently by autoradiography [3]. Although there was some inclusion of thymidine into the nail bed, Zaias and Alvarez [3] interpreted the findings as indicating that the nail bed had no role in the creation of the nail plate. Norton [4] drew a similar conclusion from work with live human subjects where labelled thymidine and glycine were injected locally to act as markers of proliferating and metabolically active keratinocytes, and both primarily labelled the matrix.

However, the earlier work of Lewis [5] suggested on histological grounds that the nail plate is a trilaminar structure originating from three separate matrix zones: the dorsal matrix (ventral aspect of proximal nail fold), intermediate matrix (germinal matrix) and ventral matrix (nail bed). In support of this, Johnson *et al.* [6,7] demonstrated that 21% of the nail thickness is gained as it passes over the nail bed, implying that the nail bed is generating this fraction of the nail plate. De Berker *et al.* [2] noted that the increase in nail thickness did not coincide with corresponding increases of nail plate cells. This challenges the interpretation that nail thickens over the nail bed because of a contribution from underlying structures. An alternative explanation may be appropriate, such as compaction arising from repetitive distal trauma. Others have also debated this issue [8] and, although the nail bed may have a significant contribution to make in disease [9], the evidence for its contribution at other times is conflicting.

Nail morphology

Why the nail grows flat, rather than as a heaped-up keratinous mass, has generated much thought and discussion [10,11–14]. Several factors probably combine to produce a relatively flat nail plate: the orientation of the matrix rete pegs and papillae; adherence to the nail bed; the direction of cell differentiation [15]; and moulding of the direction of nail growth between the proximal nail fold and distal phalanx [16]. Containment laterally within the lateral nail folds assists this orientation, and the adherent nature of the nail bed is likely to be important. In diseases such as psoriasis, the nail bed can lose its adherent properties, exhibiting

onycholysis. In addition, there may be subungual hyperkeratosis. These combined factors make psoriasis the most common pathology in which up-growing nails are seen. Onychogryphosis is characterized by upward growth of thickened nail. In this condition, the nail matrix may become bucket-shaped and the effect of the overlying proximal nail fold is lost.

Linear nail growth [17,18,19]

During the 20th century, many studies were carried out on the linear growth of the nail plate in health and disease; these have been reviewed [20,21] and are listed in Tables 95.1 and 95.2 [22]. Most of these studies have been performed by observing the distal movement of a reference mark etched on the nail plate over a fixed period of time; this may well correlate with matrix germinative cell kinetics but there is no direct proof that it does. However, studies on nail growth in psoriasis, and its inhibition by cytostatic drugs [23,24], suggest that cell kinetics and linear growth rate do have a direct correlation.

Fingernails grow approximately 1 cm every 3 months and toenails at one-third of this rate.

NAIL SIGNS AND THEIR SIGNIFICANCE

It is important for clinicians to understand and accurately describe nail findings if they are to communicate effectively with their colleagues. Signs fall into categories of shape, surface and colour.

Table 95.2 Pathological factors affecting the rate of nail growth.

Faster	Slower
Psoriasis [36]	Finger immobilization [41]
Normal nails [23]	Fever [42]
Pitting	Beau's lines [43]
Onycholysis [37]	Methotrexate [24], azathioprine [24],
Pityriasis rubra pilaris [21,38]	etretinate [39]
Etretinate, rarely [39]	Denervation [44]
Idiopathic onycholysis of women [37]	Poor nutrition
Bullous ichthyosiform erythroderma [13]	Kwashiorkor [45]
Hyperthyroidism [28]	Hypothyroidism [28]
Levodopa [40]	Yellow nail syndrome [13]
Arteriovenous shunts [28]	Relapsing polychondritis [46]

Abnormalities of shape

Clubbing

In clubbing, there is increased transverse and longitudinal nail curvature with hypertrophy of the soft-tissue components of the digit pulp. The nail can be 'rocked' and in causes associated with cardiopulmonary disease there may be local cyanosis.

There are three forms of geometric assessment that can be performed. *Lovibond's angle* is found at the junction between the nail plate and the proximal nail fold, and is normally less than 160°. This is altered to over 180° in clubbing (Figure 95.5). *Curth's angle* at the distal interphalangeal joint is normally about 180°. This is diminished to less than 160° in clubbing (Figure 95.6). *Schamroth's window* is seen when the dorsal aspects of two fingers from opposite hands are apposed, revealing a window of light, bordered laterally by the Lovibond angles (Figure 95.7). As this angle is obliterated in clubbing, the window closes [1]. Assessment of clubbing at the bedside shows poor agreement between examiners [2] in milder cases and there are problems in using firm morphometric analyses that do not lend themselves to routine clinical practice [3]. Ultrasound criteria for diagnosis can also be used [4].

Clubbing appears to be related more to increased blood flow through the vasodilated plexus of nail unit vasculature than to vessel hyperplasia, although MRI studies have also implicated hypervascularity [5]. Altered vagal tone and microvascular infarcts have also been implicated [6,7]. Mutations in the *HPGD* [8] and *SLCO2A1* [9] genes have each been linked to pachydermoperiostosis (primary hypertrophic osteoarthropathy), of which clubbing is a component (see below and Chapter 154): their gene products are involved in prostaglandin metabolism

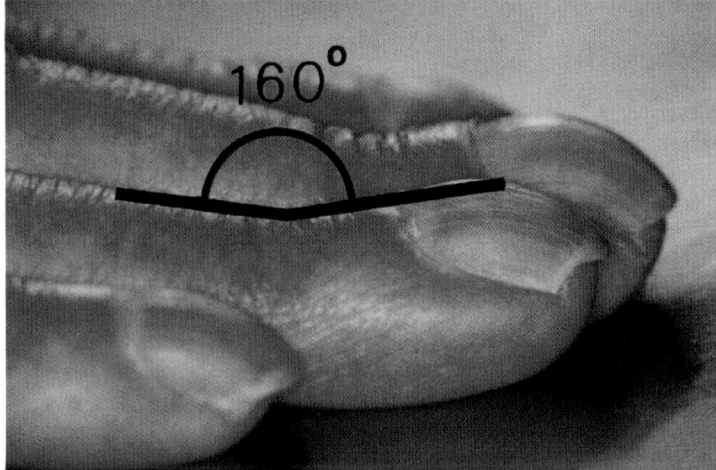

Figure 95.6 Clubbing: Curth's modified profile sign.

and prostaglandin transmembrane transport, respectively, suggesting that prostaglandins may be important. Other factors such as bradykinin and serotonin or reactive factors associated with hypoxia could have relevance.

The list of diseases associated with clubbing has a pattern where chronic inflammation of the bowel and lung are seen with or without precipitating infection. Some of these diseases can be clustered, with tuberculosis associated with underlying fibrotic lung disease or HIV, all of which are found to have independent associations [10]. Vascular causes can be associated with central cyanotic ischaemia, as in heart disease, or local factors such as the unilateral soft-tissue changes of hemiplegia [11]. An isolated subungual tumour located within the mid-proximal zone of the subungual space can displace the nail unit upwards in a form similar to clubbing. However, some of the other features are typically lacking, such as the fluctuant quality of the proximal nail and nail fold [12]. This can be included in the category of pseudoclubbing which arises from local pathology such as osteolysis of the tip of the digit seen in systemic sclerosis.

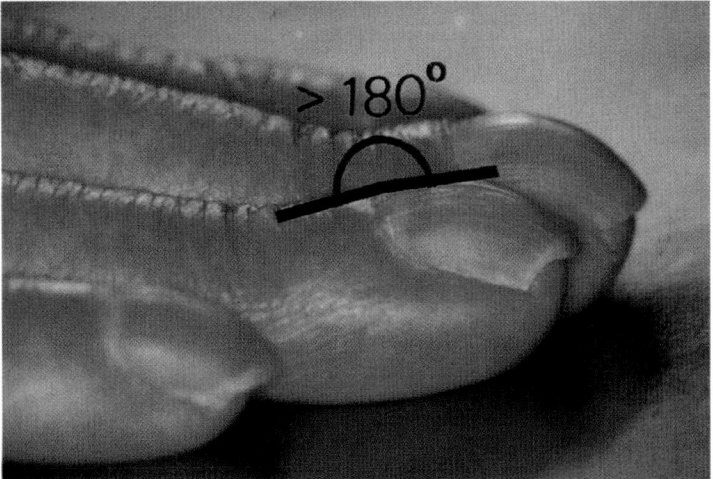

Figure 95.5 Clubbing: Lovibond's profile sign. The angle is normally less than 160° but exceeds 180° in clubbing.

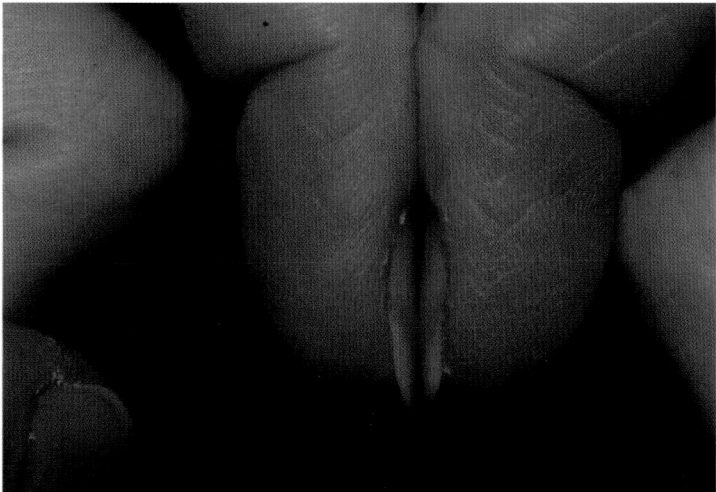

Figure 95.7 Schamroth's window is seen clearly in this image of normal nails.

Table 95.3 Causes of nail clubbing.

Cause	Comment
Asbestosis	Clubbing is found in about 40% of those with asbestosis
Thoracic carcinoma	Includes carcinoma of bronchus, pleura, lymphosarcoma, mediastinal lymphoma and metastatic disease in the lung arising outside the thorax
Cystic fibrosis	This is acquired in adolescence or early adulthood. It can be used as a predictive factor for clinical progression of disease
Cryptogenic fibrosing alveolitis	Clubbing is an indicator of disease morbidity
Mesothelioma	Clubbing is found in about a third of those with mesothelioma and may in some instances be associated with the asbestosis which is a predisposing factor
Nasopharyngeal carcinoma	Clubbing can be an association with nasopharyngeal carcinoma in both children and adults
Pulmonary arteriovenous malformation	Can be found associated with hereditary haemorrhagic telangiectasia
Sarcoidosis	Clubbing can be a local manifestation of sarcoid within the distal digit or a feature of pulmonary involvement
Cyanotic heart disease	Typically a patent ductus arteriosus or septal defect
Infective endocarditis	Clubbing can reverse when the infection is resolved
Hepatopulmonary syndrome	Associated with a shunt that gives rise to breathlessness and cyanosis
Carcinoma of the oesophagus	Usually associated with the pattern seen with hypertrophic osteoarthropathy
Inflammatory bowel disease	May be seen with hypertrophic osteoarthropathy
Laxative abuse	It is not clear whether clubbing resolves if laxative abuse stops
Liver disease	A range of liver diseases is implicated. When treatment is a liver transplant, the clubbing has been seen to reverse
Chronic parasitic infestation	Examples include dysentery caused by *Trichuris trichiuria*
HIV	In one observational study, 37% of HIV patients had clubbing. The mean duration of the HIV was 4 years
Tuberculosis	Pulmonary tuberculosis is often associated with other diseases in turn associated with clubbing, such as HIV or coexisting lung disease
Thyroid disease	The distinction between thyroid acropachy, pachydermoperiostitis and clubbing is not always clear in reports
Lupus erythematosus	A rare association
POEMS syndrome	Found in 70% of patients with this rare syndrome of *polyneuropathy, organomegaly, endocrinopathy, monoclonal gammopathy* and *skin* changes (see Chapter 148)
Hemiplegia	Typically associated with other soft-tissue changes in the hemiplegic hand
Subungual tumour	An isolated subungual tumour can create the shape of a clubbed digit, although the rocking of the proximal nail may be absent

Clubbing is a component of *secondary hypertrophic osteoarthropathy* as well as of pachydermoperiostosis: in both, a subungual lymphocytic infiltrate may be found and, with this, some associated fibrosis which may ultimately create reactive bone changes and osteoarthropathy. In the primary genetic form, pachydermoperiostosis, there is arthritis and subperiosteal new bone formation affecting the long bones. The secondary form has many of the same benign associations as isolated digital clubbing but is much more strongly associated with malignancy, particularly bronchial carcinoma.

A list of conditions associated with nail clubbing is given in Table 95.3.

Koilonychia

In koilonychia (Greek: *koilos*, hollow; *onyx*, nail), there is reverse curvature in the transverse and longitudinal axes giving a concave dorsal aspect to the nail (Figure 95.8) [1]. Fingers and toes may be affected, with signs most prominent in the thumb or great toe.

Koilonychia is common in infancy as a benign feature of the great toenail, although in some infants its persistence may be associated with a deficiency of cysteine-rich keratin [2] in trichothiodystrophy. The most common systemic association is with iron deficiency [3] and haemochromatosis, although the majority of adults with koilonychia demonstrate a familial pattern, which may be autosomal dominant [4]. In dermatoses such as psoriasis and dermatophyte infection, nail bed hyperkeratosis may push the nail up distally to produce a spoon-shaped nail. In mechanics, softening of the nail from contact with oil may be a factor [5], and in hairdressers, permanent wave solutions may be causal [6].

Pincer nail

Synonyms and inclusions
- Involuted nail
- Trumpet nail

Pincer nail describes a dystrophy where nail growth is pitched towards the midline, combined with increased transverse curvature.

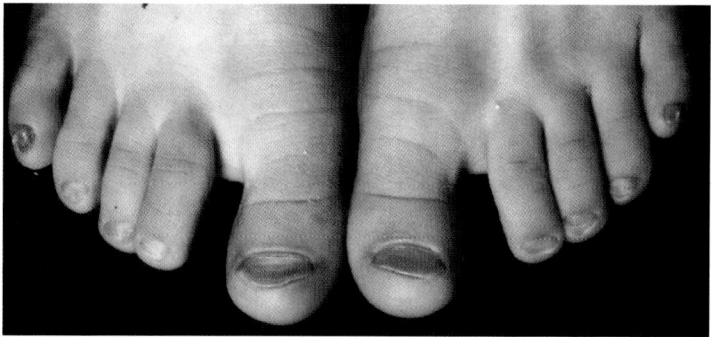

Figure 95.8 Koilonychia. This image is of congenital koilonychia in a young girl.

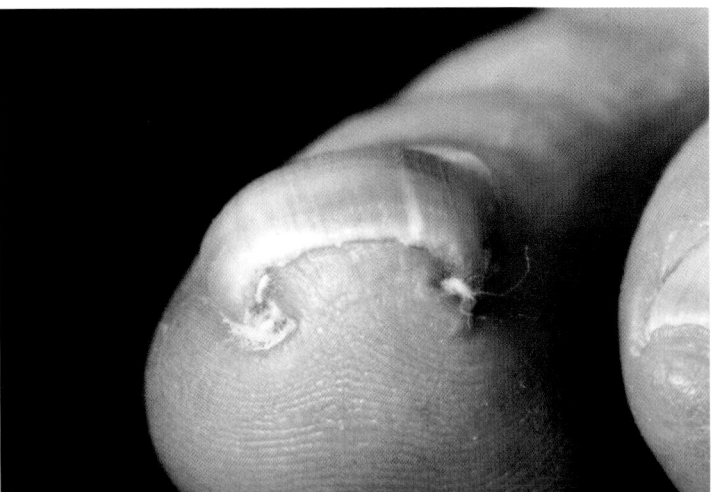

Figure 95.9 Pincer nail.

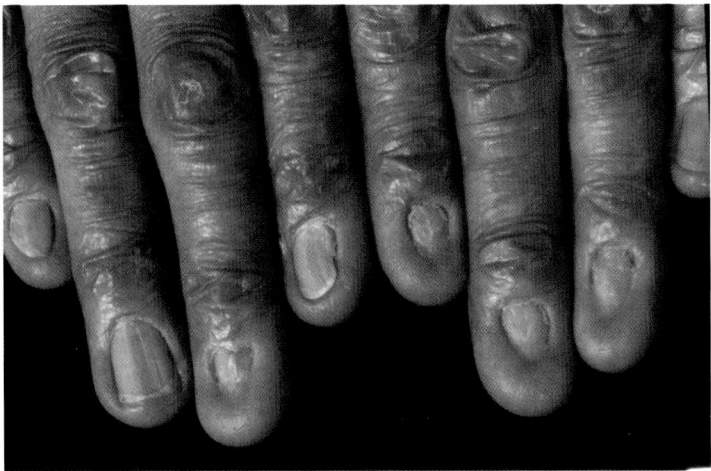

Figure 95.10 Anonychia: nail loss in a 50-year-old man with dominant dystrophic epidermolysis bullosa.

It presents in three patterns [1,2,3]. Probably the most common is in association with psoriasis, where the thumbs and big toes are the most likely to be affected, although the pattern is not as organized and symmetrical as that seen in the inherited version. In the latter, there is often a gradient of involvement, radiating from the thumbs and big toes outwards, which progresses with time (Figure 95.9). The third variant is the individual nail which develops a pincer deformity. In this instance, careful imaging and surgical exploration should be undertaken to exclude an isolated space-occupying lesion beneath the matrix [4,5,6].

Pain may arise due to embedding of the pincer nail in the lateral nail folds and nail bed, which becomes most pronounced distally. Imaging can be helpful. Treatment is usually by surgery to relieve the pain. In the toes, it is usually best to perform a lateral ablation of the most embedded margin. This will sometimes lead to a shift of the nail such that the other side no longer embeds. If both sides require ablation, the dimensions of the toenail may mean that it is better to ablate the entire matrix rather than to leave a central zone of nail. The alternative of corrective surgery in toes has less chance of success, although successful case series are reported. When treating the thumbs or fingers, the chance of success with corrective surgery is higher and the cosmetic and functional handicap of ablation may not be acceptable. Again, a lateral ablation may be adequate, but more complex procedures entail altering the alignment of the matrix [2,7,8], level of the nail bed [9] and addressing any midline hypertrophy of the distal phalanx. Some surgeons advocate a combination of reconstruction and ablation [10]. Nail braces rarely produce long-term benefit, although promising outcomes have been reported [11].

Anonychia

Anonychia is the absence of all or part of one or several nails [1]. It may be congenital, acquired or transient. The underlying genetic abnormality of the congenital form has recently been identified as a mutation in the *R-spondin4*, *Frizzled6* or *Wnt10a* genes (see above: nail biology), which play a part in *Wnt* signalling within the cell [2]. There may be a biological interaction with the underlying phalanx in embryogenesis (see Chapter 69) [3].

Acquired forms are due to scarring of the nail matrix. This can arise through burns, surgery or trauma, or be due to inflammatory dermatoses such as lichen planus where the entire nail matrix is scarred and lost [4]. Similar scarring can occur in variants of epidermolysis bullosa, with irreversible nail loss (Figure 95.10). The transient variant is due to nail shedding. This can occur due to an intense physiological or local inflammatory process, in the absence of scarring.

Abnormalities of nail attachment

Nail shedding

Nails can be lost through different mechanisms as follows:
1 Complete loss of the nail plate due to proximal nail separation extending distally [1] is called *onychomadesis* and is a progression of profound Beau's lines. This may reflect local or systemic disease and in the latter may result in temporary loss of all nails.
2 Local dermatoses such as the bullous disorders and paronychia may cause nail loss. Generalized dermatoses may be manifest, for example toxic epidermal necrolysis (TEN) and severe/rapid onset of pustular psoriasis. Scarring of the nail unit is seen in lichen planus and following TEN, which may both provoke nail loss.
3 Trauma is a common cause of recurrent loss and may reflect the nature of the activity, such as football, or some underlying abnormality of footwear [2] or foot mechanics. It is often associated with subungual haemorrhage [3]. In the long term, athletes often develop thickened dystrophic nails matching a history of recurrent shedding. More severe trauma can result in a degloving event removing all tissue from the end of the phalanx.
4 Temporary loss has also been described due to retinoids [4], and to large doses of cloxacillin and cephaloridine during the treatment of two anephric patients [5].
5 *Onychoptosis defluvium* or alopecia unguium describes atraumatic, familial, non-inflammatory nail loss [6]. It may be periodic and associated with dental amelogenesis imperfecta.
6 Nail shedding can be part of an inherited structural defect, most obviously in epidermolysis bullosa [7], although at times the diagnosis may be occult [8].

Onycholysis

Onycholysis is the distal and/or lateral separation of the nail from the nail bed [1] and can be graded [2]. Psoriatic onycholysis can be considered the reference point for other forms of onycholysis and is typically distal, with variable lateral involvement. Isolated islands of onycholysis present as 'oil spots' or 'salmon patches' in the nail bed: at the border of onycholysis, the nail bed is usually reddish-brown, reflecting the underlying psoriatic inflammatory changes. All the common causes are associated with diminished adherence of the nail to the nail bed as a primary (idiopathic) or secondary event: the latter include trauma, fungal infection, eczema, drug reactions and photo-onycholysis [3].

Idiopathic onycholysis

This is a painless separation of the nail from its bed which occurs without apparent cause. Overzealous manicure, frequent wetting and cosmetic 'solvents' may be the cause but may not be admitted by the patient. There may, however, be a minor traumatic element, as the condition occurs rather more often in persons who keep their nails abnormally long. Maceration with water may also be a factor [3]. It must be distinguished from other causes of onycholysis (see later). The affected nails grow very quickly [4].

The condition usually starts at the tip of one or more nails and extends to involve the distal third of the nail bed (Figure 95.11). Persistent manicure is attempted to remove the debris which accumulates within the onycholytic space, and this can result in a crescentic margin of onycholysis matching the onychocorneal band and appearing similar in all involved digits. Pain occurs only if there is further extension as a result of trauma or if active infection supervenes. More often there is microbial colonization of a mixed nature, including *Candida albicans* and several bacteria, of which *Pseudomonas aeruginosa* is the most common. If the condition persists for several months, the nail bed becomes dark and irregularly thickened. The condition is mostly seen in women and many cases return to normal after a few months. The longer it lasts, the less likely is the nail to become reattached, due to keratinization of the exposed nail bed.

Management [5]

Cut away as much as possible of the loosened nail and apply a topical steroid preparation containing broad spectrum antimicrobials effective against both yeasts and bacteria. Reattachment is slow, and the loosened nail should be recut several times if necessary. Some authorities still recommend 4% thymol in chloroform (not available in the US) as a means of preventing infection and further maceration of the nail bed; however, 2% thymol is often as strong as the patient can tolerate and is usually effective. Where antimicrobial therapy is needed for *Pseudomonas*, gentamicin eye drops can be useful. Drying under the onycholytic nails with a hair-dryer has been advocated in order to desiccate the environment in which *Pseudomonas* would otherwise grow. Soaking the fingertips several nights a week in vinegar or sodium hypochlorite solution (Milton) for 5 min can be useful to prevent recurrence. Domestic vinegar is between 3 and 9% acetic (synonym: ethanoic) acid. At the higher strength it can be irritant, especially if the area being treated is already sore. A dilution of 4 parts water to 1 part vinegar is likely to avoid risk of irritancy. Milton is 1% sodium hypochlorite. A 0.25% solution is suitable for wound care, which means a dilution with 4 parts water to 1 part Milton.

Secondary onycholysis

There are many causes of onycholysis [5–8]. Psoriasis, fungal infection, dermatitis and trauma are amongst the most common. Thirty per cent of psoriatics with nail involvement will have onycholysis, with toenail involvement more common than fingernails [9]. Onycholysis occurs in general medical conditions, including impaired peripheral circulation, hypothyroidism [8], hyperthyroidism [9], hyperhidrosis, yellow nail syndrome and shell nail syndrome. Minor trauma is a common cause, and many occupational cases are due to trauma [10]. Immersion of the hands in soap and water may be considered traumatic, as also may the use of certain nail cosmetics. It has also been described after the application of 5% 5-fluorouracil to the fingertips where it can be used therapeutically for warts [11]. There is a condition of hereditary partial onycholysis associated with hard nails [12]. *Photo-onycholysis* (Figure 95.12) may occur during treatment with psoralens,

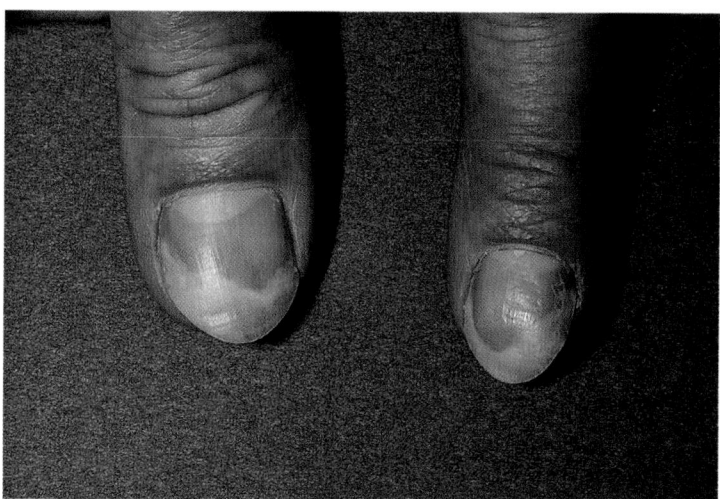

Figure 95.11 Onycholysis: idiopathic type.

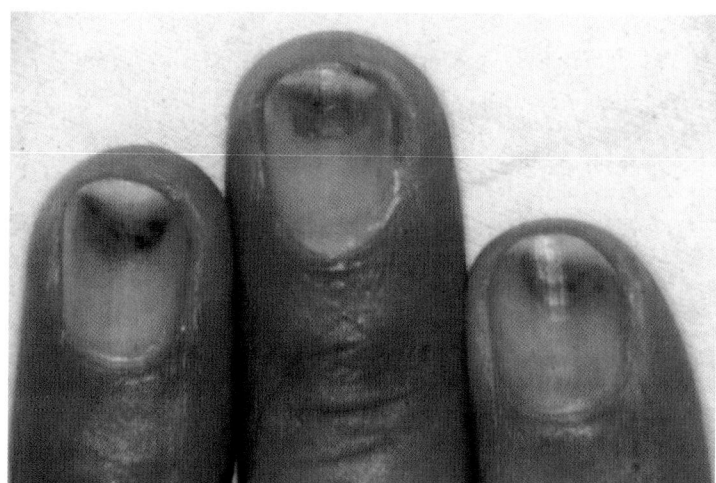

Figure 95.12 Photo-onycholysis with a uniform pattern of discoloured onycholysis in the midline.

PART 8: SPECIFIC CUTANEOUS STRUCTURE

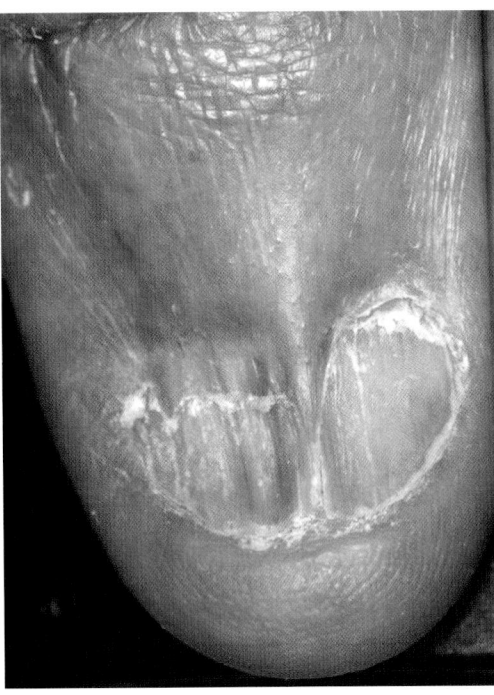

Figure 95.13 Nail pterygium due to lichen planus.

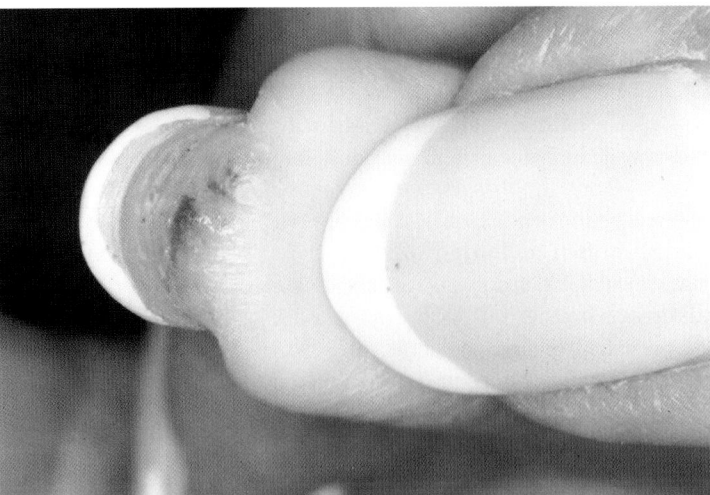

Figure 95.14 Ventral pterygium due to allergy to formaldehyde nail hardener.

PART 8: SPECIFIC CUTANEOUS STRUCTURE

demethylchlortetracycline and doxycycline [13,14], and rarely other antibiotics. This is sometimes associated with cutaneous photosensitivity (see Chapter 24). Drugs such as retinoids [15] and cancer chemotherapy can also be implicated, with taxanes eliciting nail changes in between 19 and 44% of patients, depending on the chemotherapy regimen [16]; cooling the hand with a specialized glove has been demonstrated to help diminish or delay onset of these adverse effects [17,18].

Pterygium [1]
The term pterygium describes the winged appearance achieved when a central fibrotic band divides a nail proximally in two (Figure 95.13). However, the fibrotic tissue may not always grossly alter the nail and can extend from the lateral nail fold as well as the more typical proximal nail fold. A large pterygium may destroy the whole nail.

An inflammatory destructive process precedes pterygium formation. There is fusion between the nail fold and underlying nail bed and matrix. The fibrotic band then obstructs normal nail growth. Superficial abnormal vessels may be seen and there are no skin markings. It most typically develops in trauma or lichen planus and its variants, including idiopathic atrophy of the nail [2] and graft-versus-host disease [3]. It can also occur in leprosy, where it may represent scarring secondary to neuropathic damage and secondary purulent infection [4].

Ventral pterygium
Ventral pterygium (Figure 95.14) or pterygium inversum unguis [1,2] occurs on the distal undersurface of the nail, with forward extension of the nail bed epithelium dislocating the hyponychium and obscuring the distal groove. Causes include trauma, systemic sclerosis [2,3], Raynaud phenomenon, lupus erythematosus,

familial subungual pterygium [4] and infections [5]. The overlying nail may be normal, but adjacent soft tissues can be painful.

Changes in nail surface

Longitudinal grooves
Longitudinal grooves may run all or part of the length of the nail in the longitudinal axis, and need to be distinguished from ridges which are proud of the nail surface [1]. Grooves may be full or partial thickness.

The *median canaliform dystrophy of Heller* [2] is the most distinctive form (Figure 95.15) [3]. The author has seen it in children under

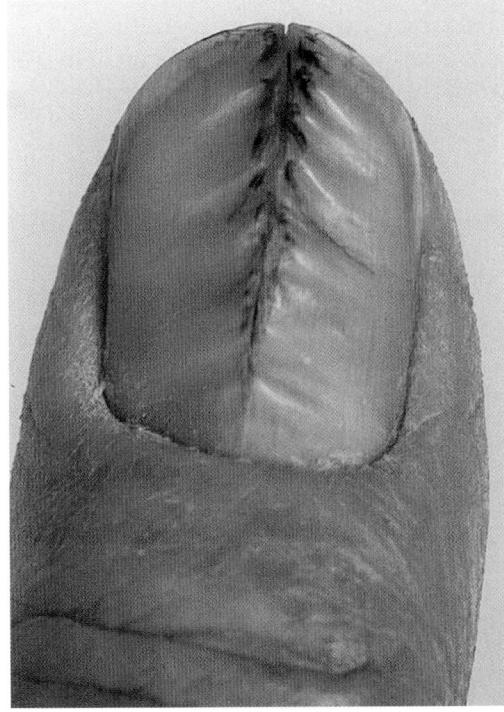

Figure 95.15 Median canaliform dystrophy of Heller.

10, but the literature is potentially misleading due to the confusion between midline transverse ridging of habit tic and true canaliform dystrophy [4]. The nail is split, usually in the midline, with a fir-tree-like appearance of ridges angled backwards. The thumbs are most commonly affected and the involvement may be symmetrical. The cuticle may be normal, as distinct from the cuticle in habit tic deformity ('washboard nails'). After a period of months or years the nails often return to normal, but relapse may occur [5] and a ridge may replace the original defect. Some patients give a definite history of trauma [1] and rarely the disorder can be attributed to oral retinoids [6]. Although familial cases have been recorded, the majority of cases are sporadic and of unknown cause [7].

Tumours (e.g. viral warts, myxoid cysts, periungual fibromas) pressing on the matrix, or a proximal nail fold pterygium, may produce a longitudinal groove.

Transverse grooves and Beau's lines [1,2]

Transverse grooves may be full or partial thickness through the nail. When they are endogenous they have an arcuate margin matching the lunula. If exogenous, such as those due to manicure, the margin may match the proximal nail fold and the grooves may be multiple as in washboard nails associated with a habit tic [3]. When multiple, it may be difficult to distinguish a habit tic from psoriasis. Transverse grooves may occur on isolated diseased digits (trauma, inflammation or neurological events) [4] or may be generalized, reflecting an acute systemic event such as a drug reaction [5], myocardial infarction, measles, mumps or pneumonia. If there is a systemic cause, they are usually referred to as *Beau's lines* [2]. They arise through temporary interference with nail formation and become visible on the nail surface (Figure 95.16) some weeks after the precipitating event. The distance of the groove from the nail fold is related to the time since the onset of growth disturbance. The depth and width of the groove may be related to the severity and duration of disturbance, respectively. In many cases, grooves are seen on all 20 nails but are most prominent on the thumb and great toenail, and are deeper in the midline of the nail. Full-thickness grooves can be associated with distal extension of the plane of separation of the nail plate. This can lead to nail loss, termed *onychomadesis*.

Nail pitting

Nail pitting presents as punctate erosions in the nail surface. Individual pits may be shallow or deep, with a regular or irregular outline. The individual pits of psoriasis are said to be less regular in form and in overall pattern than those of alopecia areata, but this is not always the case. When numerous, they appear randomly distributed upon the nail surface or have a geometric pattern. The latter may cause rippling or create a grid of pits. Mild pitting may also occur in association with different patterns of eczema, but is usually more subtle or localized than psoriatic pitting. Extensive pitting combined with other surface irregularities results in the appearance of *trachyonychia*. An isolated large pit may produce a localized full-thickness defect in the nail plate termed *elkonyxis*, which is found in reactive arthritis, psoriasis and following trauma.

Histologically, pits represent foci of parakeratosis, reflecting isolated nail malformation [1,2] and are present in the fingernails of about half of psoriatics with nail involvement.

Trachyonychia

Trachyonychia presents as a rough surface affecting all of the nail plate and up to 20 nails (20-nail dystrophy) [1,2]. The original French term was 'sand-blasted nails', which evokes the main clinical feature of a grey roughened surface (Figure 95.17). It is mainly associated with alopecia areata [3], psoriasis and lichen planus, although the most common presentation is as an isolated nail abnormality. In the isolated form, histology shows spongiosis and a lymphocytic infiltrate [4] of the nail matrix. It may present at

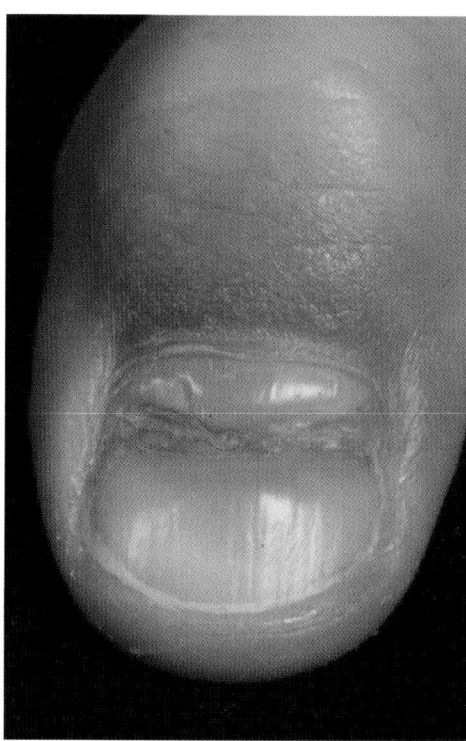

Figure 95.16 Beau's lines present as transverse grooves in the nail matching the proximal margin of the nail matrix and lunula.

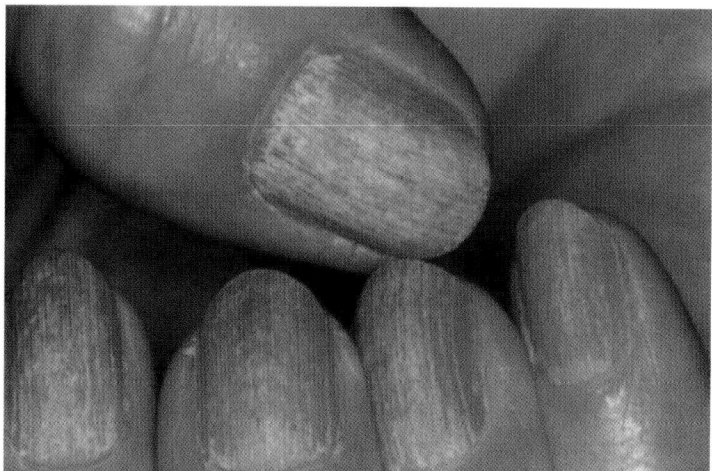

Figure 95.17 Trachyonychia: roughened surface of up to 20 nails.

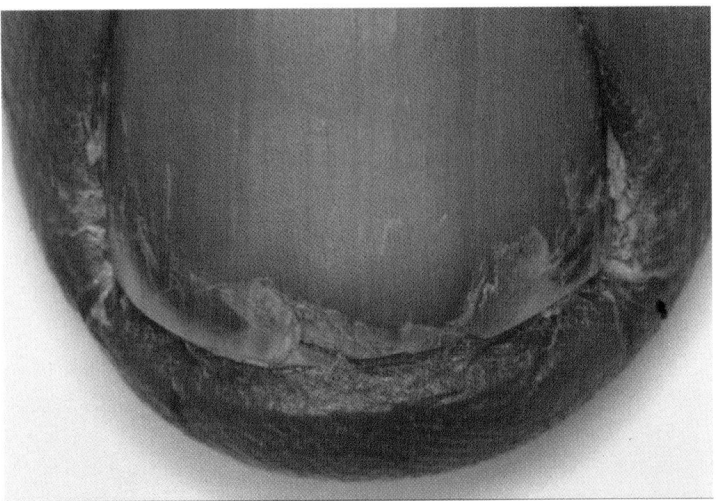

Figure 95.18 Onychoschizia (lamellar splitting).

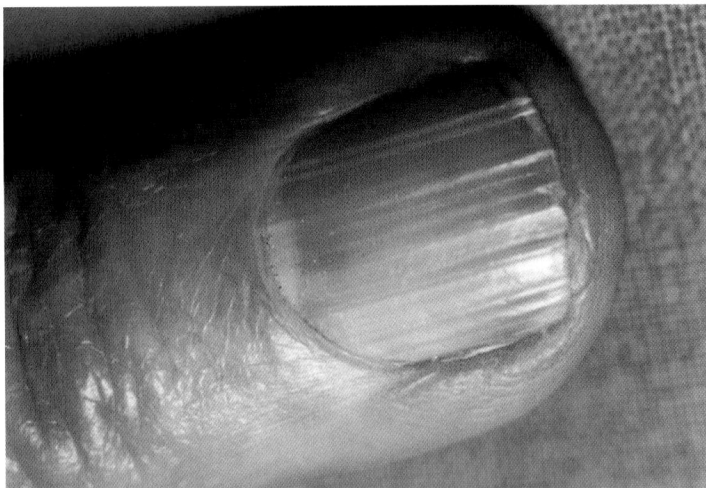

Figure 95.19 Longitudinal ridging of the nail.

birth, as a self-limiting condition in childhood or as a more chronic problem in adulthood. There is some response to potent topical, locally injected and systemic steroids, but this may be temporary.

Onychoschizia (lamellar dystrophy)

Onychoschizia is also known as lamellar nail dystrophy and is characterized by transverse splitting into layers at or near the free edge (Figure 95.18) in fingers and toes, especially in infants [1]. There is a subtle distinction between the static features, such as types of split, and the subjective experience of having brittle nails. Usually these characteristics coincide, although clinicians and patients may prefer to use one term over the other. The different features can be assessed within a scoring system [2]. Variants include splitting at the lateral margins alone and multiple crenellated splits at the free edge. It is seldom associated with any systemic disorder, although it has been reported with polycythaemia [3], HIV infection [4] and glucagonoma [5] and has been referred to as a 'syndrome' [2].

Scanning electron microscopy illustrates the tendency of the lamellar structure of the nail to separate after repeated immersion in water [6], although case–control studies show that occupation is not a major determinant of the condition [7]. However, efforts at retaining hydration (gloves, emollient and base coat with nail varnish) may help reverse clinical changes. Biotin has been used as systemic therapy, but the evidence for its efficacy is weak [8].

Beading and ridging

Beading and longitudinal ridging of the nails are common minor nail surface abnormalities which become more prominent with age (Figure 95.19). They are not an indication of disease.

Changes in nail colour [1–7]

Alteration in nail colour may occur because of changes affecting the dorsal nail surface, the substance of the nail plate, the under-surface of the nail or the nail bed.

Nail plate pigmentation

Exogenous pigment on the upper surface is easy to demonstrate by scraping the nail. If the proximal margin of the pigment is an arc matching the proximal nail fold, this is a further clue confirming an exogenous source. Nicotine is a typical pigment with the 'quitters' nail, which demonstrates the cessation of smoking and nicotine-free fingers for 2 months. Henna and spray tan are other common causes. Where there is onycholysis, the ventral surface of the nail can also become pigmented (Figure 95.20) and the most common instance is the green colour seen from colonization with *Pseudomonas* (Figure 95.21).

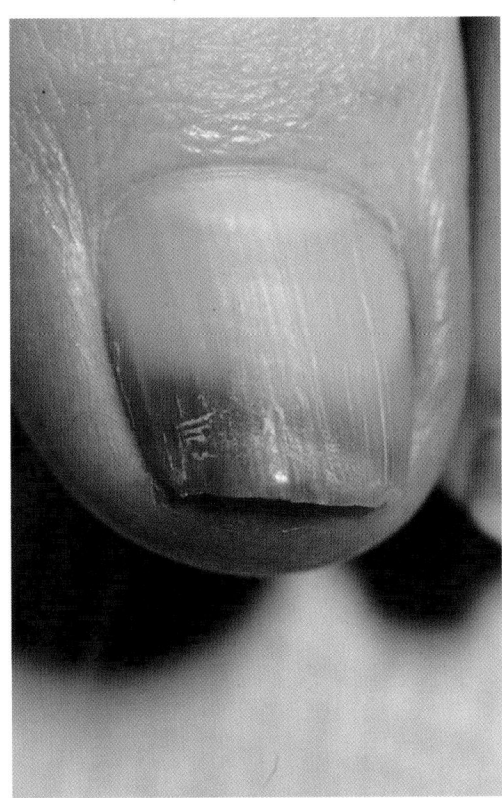

Figure 95.20 Orange pigmentation of onycholytic toenail due to orange dye from work-boots.

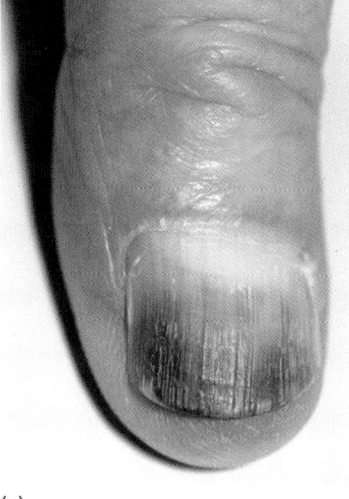

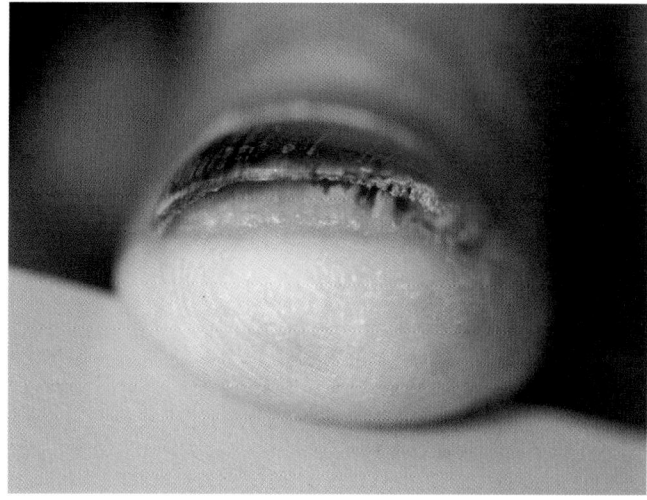

Figure 95.21 Green pigmentation of onycholytic fingernail due to *Pseudomonas*.   (a)

(b)

Nail colour can be changed by the incorporation of pigment into the nail plate, most commonly in the form of melanin produced by matrix melanocytes during nail formation. This produces a brown longitudinal streak the entire length of the nail. In white people this is abnormal and requires thorough assessment and, in some instances, biopsy. In darker-skinned people it is a common normal variant. The incorporation of heavy metals and some drugs into the nail plate via the matrix can also alter nail colour, such as the grey colour associated with silver or the grey-blue discoloration due to antimalarials or phenothiazines.

Loss of nail plate lucency
Nail colour may also be affected by alterations in the normal cellular and intercellular organization, such that there is loss of normal lucency. The disruption of normal nail plate formation by disease, chemotherapy, poisons or trauma can result in waves of parakeratotic nail cells or small splits between cells within the nail. Both make the nail less lucent and produce the white marks of true leukonychia (see later). Transmission electron microscopy suggests that there is a change in keratin fibre organization, which might provide an intracellular basis for altered diffractive properties. This disruption may occur at nail formation or subsequently in the case of fungal nail infection, where discoloration may start distolaterally rather than via the matrix.

Subungual disturbances
Subungual hyperkeratosis as from dermatophyte infection or psoriasis may also change the apparent colour of the nail.

Subungual haemorrhage produces a variety of colour changes ranging from bright red to black. Splinter haemorrhages result from leakage of blood from nail bed capillaries and may be due to local trauma or to microemboli, classically from infective endocarditis.

Nail bed changes
Vascular abnormalities can affect apparent nail colour as in blue nails from cyanosis and bright red nails from carbon monoxide poisoning. In addition to such generalized vascular changes there can be localized changes, as seen with nail bed tumours. The

increased vascularity of a glomus tumour in comparison with the surrounding nail bed may be the sole method of determining its location.

Dermoscopy can be very helpful in the assessment of nail plate pigmentation and underlying nail bed changes [7].

Leukonychia

True leukonychia
This is a white discoloration of the nail attributable to matrix dysfunction; it occurs in a variety of patterns [1,2].

True hereditary leukonychia
In this rare condition, the nails are milky porcelain white. If the whole of the nail plate is affected it is called total leukonychia (Figure 95.22) [3]. In subtotal leukonychia, the proximal two-thirds are white, becoming pink distally. This is attributed to a

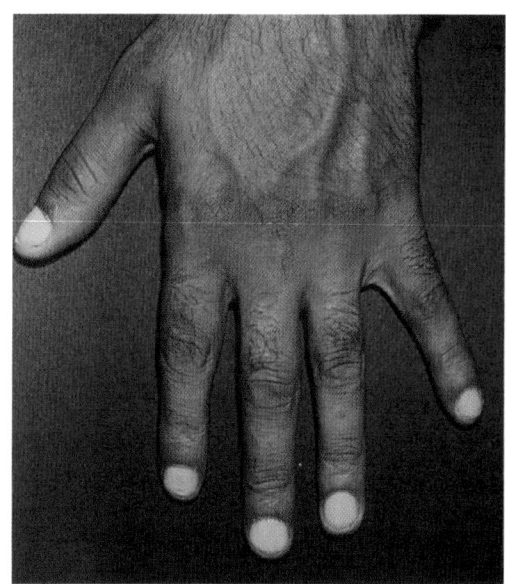

Figure 95.22 Total leukonychia.

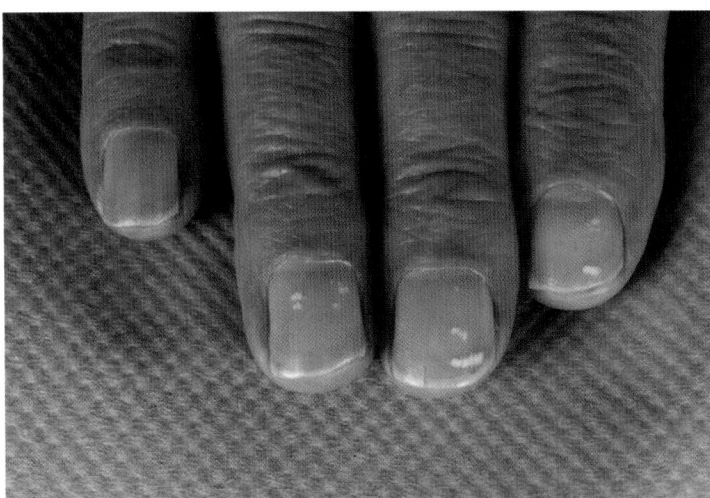

Figure 95.23 Punctate leukonychia.

delay in keratin maturation, and the nail may still appear white at the distal overhang.

Transverse leukonychia (Mees' lines) reflects a systemic disorder, such as chemotherapy or poisoning [4], or systemic infection [5] affecting matrix function. The 1–2 mm wide transverse band is in the arcuate form of the lunula and is analogous to a Beau's line, with which it is occasionally found.

Punctate leukonychia comprises white spots of 1–3 mm diameter attributed to minor matrix trauma (e.g. manicure) (Figure 95.23); it is also seen in alopecia areata. The pattern and number of spots may change as the nail grows. With longitudinal leukonychia, there is a parakeratotic focus in the matrix, sometimes attributable to Darier disease or a small tumour. Striate leukonychia is a term used in different settings. It could be argued to occupy the middle ground between the marks of Mees' lines and punctate leukonychia being reported in both alopecia areata and chemotherapy.

Apparent leukonychia
Here, changes in the nail bed are responsible for the white appearance [1,2]. Nail bed pallor may be a non-specific sign of anaemia, oedema or vascular impairment. It may occur in particular patterns which have become associated with certain conditions.

Terry's nail is a term used to describe nails which are white proximally and normal distally and is attributed to cirrhosis, congestive cardiac failure or diabetes [3]. Nail bed biopsy reveals only mild changes of increased vascularity.

Half-and-half nails describes nails where there is a proximal white zone and distal (20–60%) brownish sharp demarcation, the histology of which suggests an increase of vessel wall thickness and melanin deposition. It is seen in 9–50% of patients with chronic renal failure and after chemotherapy (Figure 153.3).

It is unclear whether the variant Neapolitan nails, where there are bands of white, brown and red, is a version of half-and-half or Terry's nails, or a feature of old age.

Muehrcke's paired white bands are parallel to the lunula in the nail bed, with pink between two white lines. They are commonly associated with hypoalbuminaemia, the correction of which by albumin infusion can reverse the sign. They have also recently been reported following placement of a left ventricular assist device in a patient with congestive heart failure [4].

Colour changes due to drugs and chemicals [1]
There are a number of colour changes which can be caused by drugs. Yellowing of the nail is a rare occurrence in prolonged *tetracycline* therapy, which can also produce a pattern of dark distal photo-onycholysis, Topical *5-fluorouracil* may also cause yellow nails: the whole nail is affected and returns to normal when the drug is discontinued [2,3]. A bluish colour, is seen with *mepacrine* (quinacrine) [4], the nails fluorescing yellow-green or white when viewed under Wood's light. Normal nails show slight fluorescence of violet-blue colour. *Hydroxyurea* has been reported to result in blue lunulae [5]. *Chloroquine* may produce blue-black pigmentation of the nail bed [6]. Other *antimalarials* may produce longitudinal or vertical bands of pigmentation on the nail bed or in the nail [7].

Hyperpigmentation due to increased melanin in the nail and nail bed has been noted in children after 6 weeks of treatment with *doxorubicin* (adriamycin) [9,10]. Other similar cytotoxic drugs may cause a variety of patterns of increased pigmentation [1]. However, in AIDS, longitudinal melanonychia may be seen in untreated cases [11,12] as well as in those receiving zidovudine [9,13].

Argyria may discolour the nails slate blue [8], and inorganic arsenic may produce longitudinal bands of pigment or transverse white (*Mees' lines*).

Yellow nail syndrome

The nails in yellow nail syndrome are yellow due to thickening, sometimes with a tinge of green possibly due to secondary infection with *Candida* or *Pseudomonas*. The lunula is obscured and there is increased transverse and longitudinal curvature of the nail plate with and loss of cuticle (Figure 95.24). Occasionally, there is

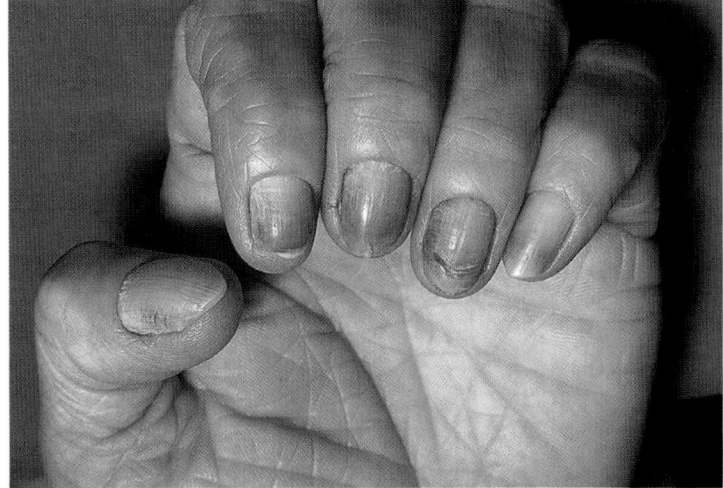

Figure 95.24 Yellow nail syndrome.

chronic paronychia with onycholysis and transverse ridging [1]. The condition usually presents in adults, but may occur as early as the age of 8 years [2]. It does not appear to run in families [3]. Some of the clinical features may overlap with lichen planus [4], although the latter does not have the other systemic features normally seen in this syndrome.

The feature nail changes are usually accompanied by lymphoedema [5] at one or more sites and by respiratory or nasal sinus disease. The nails grow at a greatly reduced rate: 0.1–0.25 mm/week for fingernails compared with the lowest normal rate of 0.5 mm/week. All 20 nails may be involved, although often a few are spared. Histologically, in the nail bed and matrix, dense fibrous tissue is found replacing subungual stroma, with numerous ectatic endothelium-lined vessels [6]. A foreign-body reaction has been noted [7]. It has been suggested that obstruction of lymphatics by this dense stroma leads to the abnormal lymphatic function found in the affected digits in some [8] but not all [9] cases.

The oedema is variable and may affect the legs, face or hands and occasionally it is universal. In some instances, the oedema has been shown to be due to abnormalities of the lymphatics, either atresia or, in some cases, varicosity [10]. Other cases have normal lymphatics, suggesting that a functional rather than an anatomical defect may be present [11], or that perhaps only the smallest lymph vessels are defective. Although the nail changes may draw attention to the underlying lymphatic abnormality, they are found only in a minority of patients with congenital abnormality of the lymphatics. Recurrent pleural effusions have been noted [12,13]. Chronic bronchitis and bronchiectasis may also occur [12]. The condition may be associated with an increased incidence of malignant neoplasms [10,14,15]. Other associations include D-penicillamine therapy [5] and nephrotic syndrome [16].

In hypothyroidism and AIDS [17] there may be yellow nails, but it is debatable whether these represent yellow nail syndrome or simply the discoloration of nail associated with retarded growth [18]. There does not appear to be an inherited element in spite of original reports [19,20].

Nail features can fluctuate enormously over time. Attempted treatments include oral and topical vitamin E, oral zinc, prednisolone and the treatment of chronic infection at other sites [20,21,22–25]. There is debate as to whether itraconazole is of value as treatment. The drug has been demonstrated to increase the rate of longitudinal growth, but an open trial in eight patients demonstrated that half gained no benefit with respect to nail changes [26]. It is reported that results are better when itraconazole or fluconazole are combined with oral vitamin E [27]. Many authorities achieve about a 50% resolution rate, but it is not clear how much of this is part of the natural time disease course [28].

Red lunulae

Erythema of all or part of the lunula may affect all digits, but is usually most prominent in the thumb. Duration of the change will depend on the cause. When associated with cardiac failure, it may follow the course of management of the cardiac disease. When due to a subungual tumour such as a myxoid cyst or glomus tumour, it will remain until the tumour is removed. Inflammatory connective tissue causes may also result in a fluctuating course.

Erythema is less intense in the distal lunula, where it can merge with the nail bed or be demarcated by a pale line, and can be obliterated by pressure on the nail plate. The appearance can fade over a few days. A single report of histological features failed to reveal vascular or epidermal changes [1]. Dotted red lunulae have been reported in psoriasis and alopecia areata, but otherwise the list of associations is so broad that it is unconvincing [2].

The exception to this is a red lunula seen in a single digit. In this setting, it often indicates a local disturbance of vascular flow, which is most likely to be a benign tumour. Glomus tumours and subungual myxoid cysts are the most common [3] and the colour may vary between blue and red.

Longitudinal erythronychia (Figure 95.25)

A longitudinal red streak in the nail can have several causes [1,2]. All will have a corresponding band of thinned nail plate as part of the defect. The effect of this is a strip where blood in the underlying nail bed is seen more easily not only because the nail plate is thinner but also because blood pools in the underlying nail bed capillaries as a result of reduced compression by the overlying nail. Splinter haemorrhages may lie longitudinally within the strip. Such strips of thinned nail arise because of focally reduced proliferation within the matrix. This can be due directly to matrix pathology or may be secondary to focal pressure on the matrix with secondary loss of function.

The matrix pathology includes a spectrum of epidermal disorders. The most common are *lichen planus* and *Darier disease*, where thin longitudinal red streaks may terminate at the free edge with a split. In Darier disease, there may be a small subungual keratosis [3]. Acantholytic dyskeratotic naevus and warty subungual dyskeratoma [4] may both represent localized forms of Darier disease. Longitudinal erythronychia is also a component of acrokeratosis verruciformis of Hopf in which there is both clinical and pathological overlap with Darier disease.

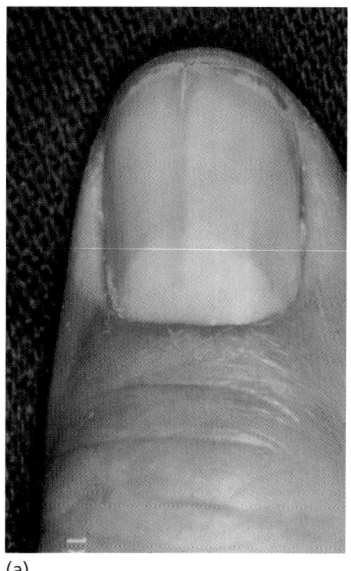 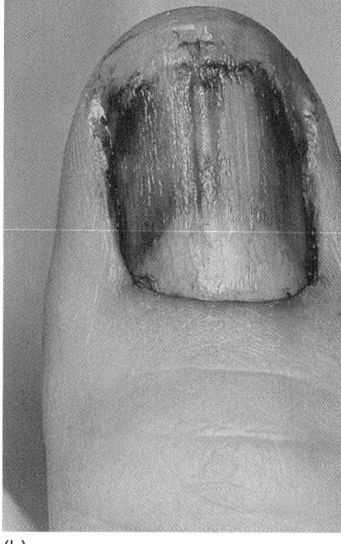

(a)   (b)

Figure 95.25 (a) Longitudinal erythronychia. (b) The longitudinal ridge in the nail bed corresponds to the groove on the undersurface of the nail plate.

Pressure on the matrix may be exerted by any of the full range of dermal tumours as well as tumours of the bone and cartilage that arise from the distal phalanx.

For instances where no primary disease can be identified to explain erythronychia affecting multiple nails the descriptive term 'idiopathic polydactylous erythronychia' has been proposed [5].

Baran and Perrin have coined the term 'onychopapilloma' to describe the isolated benign warty distal nail bed lesions found in association with longitudinal erythronychia for which no underlying cause can be identified [6]. The papilloma is a secondary element, given that it is found distally in the nail bed while the cause lies proximally within the matrix. However, there is a category of this disease where the matrix disease remains unclear and the distal papilloma represents the identifiable entity. Isolated longitudinal erythronychia needs careful assessment, however, as a similar clinical presentation can be due to conditions such as Bowen disease [6] or basal cell carcinoma [7] of the matrix. Biopsy may be warranted if the erythronychia is observed to change.

Not all causes of longitudinal erythronychia conform to these rules. This is particularly the case where there are multiple red streaks associated with a dermatosis and additional nail changes. It can be a feature of lichenoid diseases of the nail unit, discoid lupus erythematosus, psoriasis, Langerhans cell histiocytosis and a number of other diseases where there is patchy nail atrophy. It can be difficult to decide whether histology is needed to ensure a benign diagnosis or one with no systemic implications. A narrow band (approximately 2 mm) that is not changing over 12 months or more with no other elements of the history or examination to cause concern would normally mean that continued monitoring alone would be sufficient management.

Splinter haemorrhages

Splinter haemorrhages represent longitudinal haemorrhages in the nail bed conforming to the pattern of subungual vessels [1–4]. They are most frequently seen in the distal nail bed and on the fingers of the dominant hand, reflecting trauma as the cause. In dermatological practice, they are often found in association with psoriasis, dermatitis and fungal infection of the nails. As they occur under so many conditions, their importance as a sign of disease is often exaggerated. Focal pathology may also represent a cause, as in longitudinal erythronychia and onychomatricoma (see above).

Large numbers of proximal haemorrhages with no obvious traumatic origin may indicate a systemic cause [5], such as bacterial endocarditis, antiphospholipid syndrome [6] or medication [7]. Nail bed psoriasis may dispose to splinter haemorrhages in the most used digits. Unilateral splinter haemorrhages may arise after arterial catheterization on the involved side. Examination under oil with a dermoscope may reveal greater detail.

TRAUMATIC NAIL DISORDERS

Nails may show signs of acute trauma, scars following acute trauma or chronic repetitive trauma.

Acute trauma

Acute trauma is classified with respect to severity, ranging from a small haematoma to digit amputation (Table 95.4) [1].

Subungual haematoma [1,2]

Subungual bleeding is a common sign. It may present as a feature of acute trauma, with pain due to the recent event in combination with pain arising from the pressure exerted by the subungual accumulation of blood. A haematoma arising within the matrix will be incorporated into the nail plate [3]. Where the haematoma is associated with acute trauma, there is usually pain and the diagnosis is obvious. However, with less extreme trauma, a haematoma may not develop immediately and may be painless. This is most common in the toes and may give rise to clinical uncertainty as to whether it represents early subungual melanoma. A history of traumatic sporting hobbies is useful, and signs of symmetrical nail trauma and inappropriate footwear all indicate trauma as the cause of the appearance. Dermoscopy will nearly always resolve the situation [2,4], but if it does not, making a small punch in the surface of the nail may reveal old blood as the source of pigment. Malignancies can bleed and so confirmation of blood does not refute the possibility of a tumour; however, as an isolated finding in the absence of other clues, this test should be sufficient to obviate the need for surgical exploration. An alternative is to score a transverse groove in the nail at the proximal margin of the pigment and observe over a few weeks as the discoloration grows out. If pigment continues to spread proximal to the groove, surgical exploration is warranted.

The only treatment that can be offered is to relieve the pressure, and if dealt with soon after the injury this can be done by puncturing the nail, for instance with a hot pointed implement, cautery, small drill or punch biopsy. This procedure will relieve pain and may save the nail. The possibility of an underlying fracture must be considered for larger haematomas [1].

It is stated that if more than 50% of the visible nail is affected, the nail plate should be removed. However, there is evidence to challenge this rule. A comparison between two groups of children having exploration and repair or trephination alone showed fewer

Table 95.4 Classification of acute nail trauma. (From Van Beek *et al.* [1].)

Type	Effect	Therapy
I	Small haematoma associated with a small break in the nail bed	Fenestration of nail over the haematoma
II	Large haematoma with significant nail bed injury	Remove nail in order to identify site and nature of subungual damage
III	Large haematoma, nail plate displaced	X-ray may reveal fracture of terminal phalanx, usually in association with nail bed laceration which requires resorbable 6/0 suture
IV	Severe crush injury	Avulsion needed to reveal matrix, with multiple lacerations requiring careful reconstruction
V	Amputation of tip of digit, may include parts of matrix	If tip can be retrieved, it should be used as a graft. Otherwise nail bed from other sites may provide autologous grafts

complications in the latter group and considerably less investment in medical time [5]. A literature review failed to find clear evidence for avulsion [6].

Nail bed laceration

The nail bed may be lacerated by incisions, crush and avulsion injuries. In simple injuries there is displacement of the nail plate. Initially, the nail bed damage should be assessed by avulsion, and then the nail can be replaced after any necessary nail bed repair has been performed. The nail plate can be used as a useful splint [1]; a small window for drainage of blood and exudate is made in the nail [2]. More complicated injuries may require flap or graft reconstructions and, in some instances, vascularized composite nail grafts are used with microvascular anastomoses. When the wounds arise from crush injury, fracture is relatively common. If the distal tuft has been fractured to leave fragments of bone dispersed in the soft tissues, long-term morbidity may be prevented if these are removed [3].

Delayed trauma

The most common kind of chronic deformity following an acute injury is a split nail or reduction in the length of the nail bed with consequent overcurvature of the tip of the nail.

Cure of a split nail deformity is difficult, with only a modest chance of success [1]. Sometimes, there is an associated pterygium. Treatment entails excision of the nail bed and matrix scar and, in the case of a pterygium, a split-skin graft or part of the nail plate may be placed on the ventral aspect of the proximal nail fold to help prevent recurrence of the pterygium. It is important to keep the wounded aspects of nail bed or matrix separate from the overlying nail fold after surgery, and this is often best done by returning the nail plate after soaking it in antiseptic during the procedure.

If treatment is required for a shortened distal phalanx with nail bed changes, there are two choices [2]: the entire nail can be phenolized, or a V–Y advancement flap can be performed based on two neurovascular pedicles.

Chronic repetitive trauma

Chronic repetitive trauma may take several forms. Some have been considered in other sections detailing transverse ridges produced by a habit tic (Figure 95.26), the canaliform dystrophy of Heller (Figure 95.27) and chronic paronychia (Figure 95.28).

Nail biting

The nail plate, periunguium and nail bed are all subject to nail biting and picking. Although fingers are most commonly involved, rarely toenails are also bitten [1]. Nail biting produces distinctive features, which are found in 60% of children, 45% of adolescents and 10% of adults [2]. The majority of moderate nail biters have no associated psychiatric disorder [3]. Focal abnormalities, such as viral warts, are often a complication, whether as a cause or as a result of the Koebner effect after biting. Severe damage may be associated with self-mutilating disorders such as Lesch–Nyhan syndrome. Dental problems can arise due to nail embedded in gums or between teeth [4].

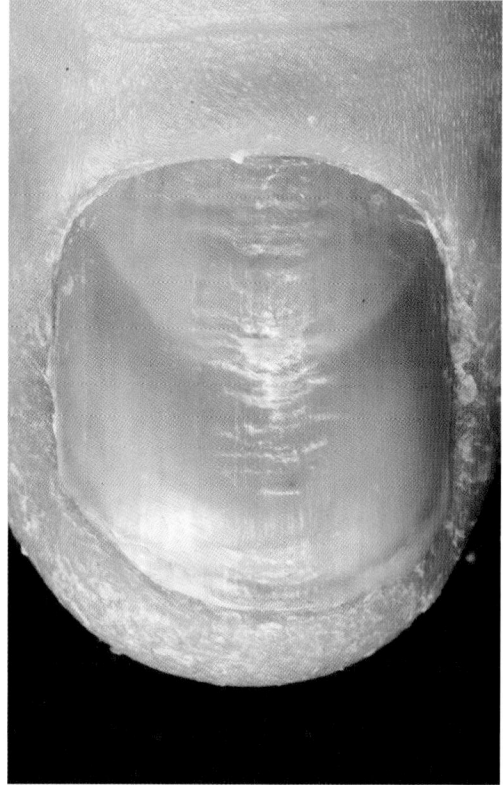

Figure 95.26 Transverse ridges resulting from habit tic.

The nails are typically short, with up to 50% of the nail bed exposed. The free edge may be even or ragged. Surface change may include splitting of the nail into layers or a sand-papered effect, and the nail may acquire a brown longitudinal streak [5]. The most aggressive nail biting (onychotillomania/onychophagia) can produce subungual haemorrhage, strips of nail loss, with residual

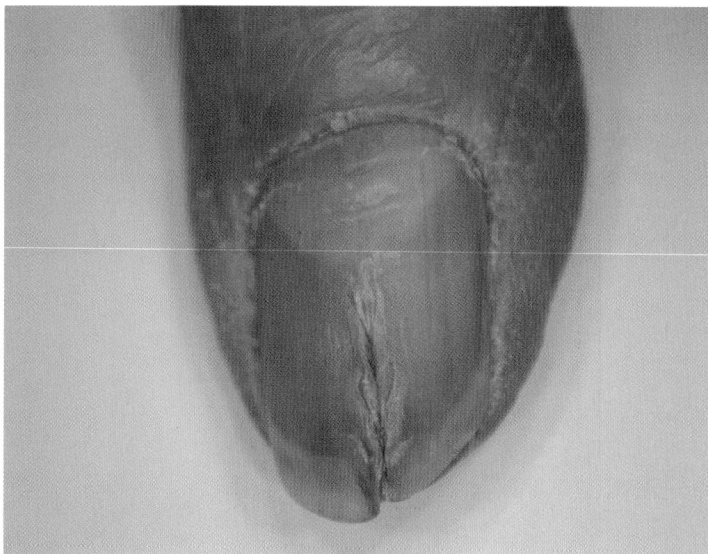

Figure 95.27 Median canaliform dystrophy of Heller affecting distal portion of nail plate; the enlarged lunula and transverse ridging seen proximally reflect chronic trauma.

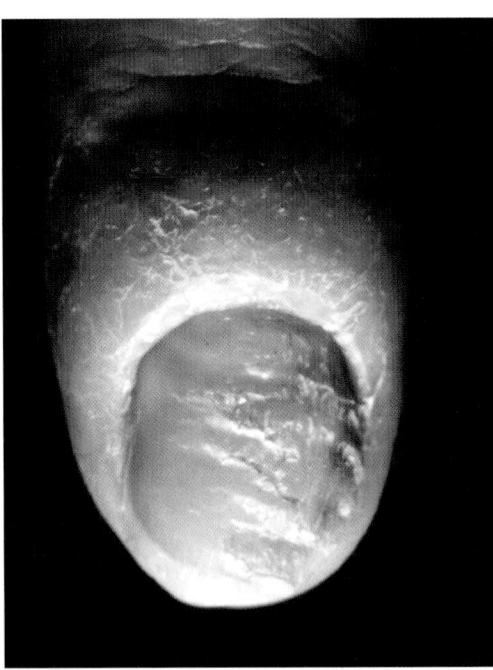

Figure 95.28 Chronic paronychia.

spurs or loss of the entire nail (Figure 95.29). Onychotillomania may be allied to parasitophobia when the patient picks off pieces claiming that they contain parasites [6]. A rough and irregular nail and nail fold may result with haemorrhage in the nail fold also. Many fingernails are involved. Oral pimozide may be beneficial [7].

Trauma followed by secondary infection involving the matrix may make nail loss permanent or result in pterygium formation. The nail folds are sometimes bitten in addition to, or as a substitute

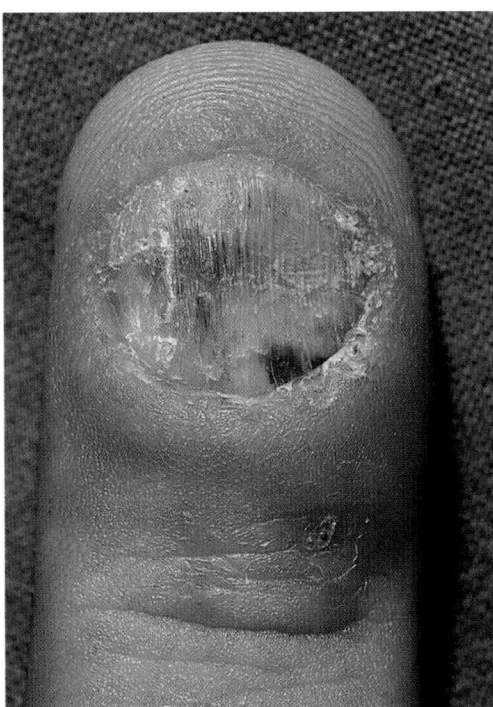

Figure 95.29 Nail biting can be extensive, with damage to the nail folds and nail plate causing subungual haemorrhage.

for, the nail. This can lead to bleeding and chronic paronychia with acute infective exacerbations. This in turn may lead to nail plate damage or ridging and nail fold scarring. In cases associated with infection, osteomyelitis of the terminal phalanx can develop [8,9]. Subjects will sometimes deny nail biting and attribute the appearance to a disease that stops nail growth. Transverse grooves scored proximally in the nail plate will confirm that the nail is growing by moving distally with time. In aggressive nail biting, the groove may be eroded from the surface.

Trauma is sometimes inflicted by other nails, with pushing back of the proximal nail fold as part of a habit tic (see above). This results in serial transverse ridges and depressions running up the midline of the nail, associated with loss of the cuticle (see Figure 95.29). In more conscious forms of self-damage, sharp instruments are used to produce dermatitis artefacta of the nail unit, and the nail fold is commonly preserved [10].

Management
Treatment is often unsuccessful and cure relies largely on the motivation of the patient. Where the patient acknowledges an element of self damage, they may comply with the use of paper surgical tape as a dressing over the tip of the digit 24 h a day for 2–3 months. This needs to be replaced several times a day in some instances. In the first month, it may be helpful to combine the tape with moderate potency topical steroid to suppress any inflammation. Ensure there is no infection prior to this. Local antiseptics and antimicrobial ointments may help settle the infection secondary to nail unit damage. Antiseptics or treatments with the most bitter taste are often prescribed in the belief that this will discourage biting. This is seldom the case. Antidepressants [11] and behavioural therapy [12] have been used with some success in limited studies.

Damage from nail manicure instruments

Metal instruments, such as a nail file or scissors, wooden or plastic orange sticks, or nail whitener pencils may create acute or chronic injuries in the nail area. Onycholysis may result from using the sharp point for cleaning under the nail plate. Nails, however, are best cleaned with a nail brush and soap, because overzealous manicure, pushing back the cuticles, may result in white streaks across several nails. Cleaning around the nail with contaminated instruments may lead to acute or chronic paronychia. According to Brauer and Baran [1], it is not advisable to cut or clip the nail plate, as this produces a shearing action that weakens the natural layered structure and promotes fracturing and splitting. An emery board is preferred for shaping the fingernail by filing from the sides of the nail towards the centre.

Trauma from footwear

Onychogryphosis and nail hypertrophy [1–5]
Onychogryphosis is an acquired dystrophy usually affecting the great toenail, which is thickened, yellow and twisted. It is most commonly seen in the elderly often made worse because of difficulties in self care of the feet [1,2,4]. Trauma and biomechanical foot problems may, however, precipitate similar changes in middle age or earlier.

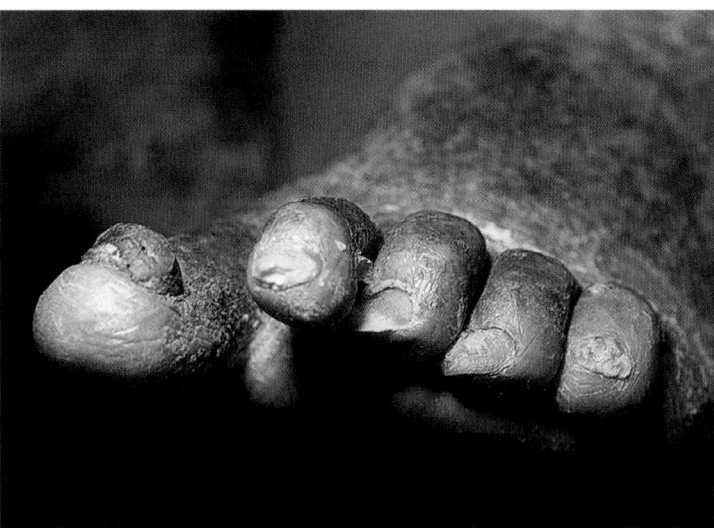

Figure 95.30 Early onychogryphosis of the left great toenail.

At one time, onychogryphosis was known as ostler's nail, because some cases could be traced to injury caused by a horse trampling on the foot of the ostler. Competitive sport is a more contemporary cause. The injury, once sustained, is aggravated by footwear. As the nail becomes longer and thicker, damage from footwear becomes progressively more important. Nail hypertrophy implies thickening and increase in length, whereas onychogryphosis implies curvature also.

Some cases of nail hypertrophy are intrinsic, and this applies especially to toenails other than the nail of the great toe. The nail becomes thick and circular in cross section instead of flat, and thus comes to resemble a claw.

In onychogryphosis, one or more nails become greatly thickened (Figure 95.30) and, with neglect, increase in length, becoming curved like a ram's horn (Figure 95.31). The nails of the great toes are most often involved, but no toenail is exempt. It is possible that the nail plate distortion produced by chronic untreated onychomycosis may be partly responsible for onychogryphosis at a later stage. In extreme cases, the free edge may press on or even re-enter the soft tissues of the foot.

Treatment of onychogryphosis and nail hypertrophy may be either radical or palliative. Radical treatment consists of surgical removal of the nail and matrix and is recommended in those

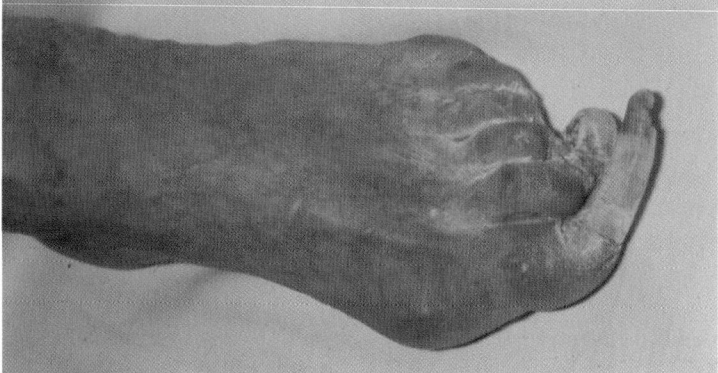

Figure 95.31 Severe onychogryphosis resulting from neglect.

with good circulation (Figure 95.32). Palliative treatment requires regular paring and trimming of the affected nails, usually by a podiatrist using nail clippers and a file or mechanical burr. The thickened nails are extremely hard and trimming is difficult. Other causes of thickened nails include psoriasis, pityriasis rubra pilaris, Darier disease, fungal infections, pachyonychia congenita, congenital ectodermal defects and congenital malalignment of the great toenails [6].

Ingrowing toenail [1,2,3]

Synonyms and inclusions
- Onychocryptosis

The nail can ingrow on any of its four margins, although lateral ingrowing is the most common pattern and is usually found on the big toe. The soft tissue at the side of the nail (lateral nail fold) is penetrated by the edge of the nail plate, resulting in pain, inflammation and, later, the formation of granulation tissue [4]. Infection is not typically associated, although the combination of pain, redness and swelling with ooze will dispose to treatment with antibiotics. Penetration of the nail fold is often caused by spicules of nail at the edge of the nail plate which have been separated from the main portion of the nail. The great toes are those most often affected. The main cause for the deformity is lateral compression of the toe due to ill-fitting footwear, and the main contributory cause is cutting the toenails in a half-circle instead of straight across. Anatomical features, such as an abnormally long great toe and prominent lateral nail folds, are important in some cases. Sport, with the toe impacting on the inside of the shoe through kicking or other movements, can be a contributory factor.

Nail can embed in the proximal nail fold when there is disturbance of nail growth, usually through trauma. This results in dislodging of the nail upwards with a new nail growing beneath. The proximal aspect of the old nail then impacts on the ventral aspect of the proximal nail fold and this creates the same features of inflammation, ooze, swelling, redness and pain as seen when the lateral nail fold is affected. Proximal nail ingrowing is known as retronychia and is self-limiting over a matter of several months as eventually the older nail is shed. During that time, nothing effectively relieves the problem and avulsion is the treatment of choice. The replacement nail usually grows back without any problem [5].

In infancy, ingrowing toenail most commonly occurs before shoes are worn and is associated with crawling, 'pedalling' or wearing undersized 'jumpsuits' [6]; acute paronychia may be associated. Rarely, it is congenital [7] and even familial [2]. In children, ingrowing is commonly distal rather than lateral. Management is conservative in most instances, with topical steroid and antiseptic preparations. Surgery is occasionally required [8].

Clinical features

The first symptoms are pain and redness, shortly followed by swelling and pus formation. Granulation tissue then forms and adds to the swelling and discharge. More severe infection may

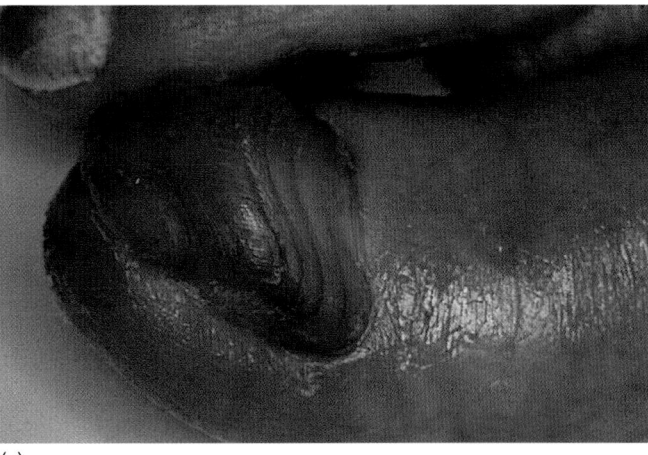

(a)

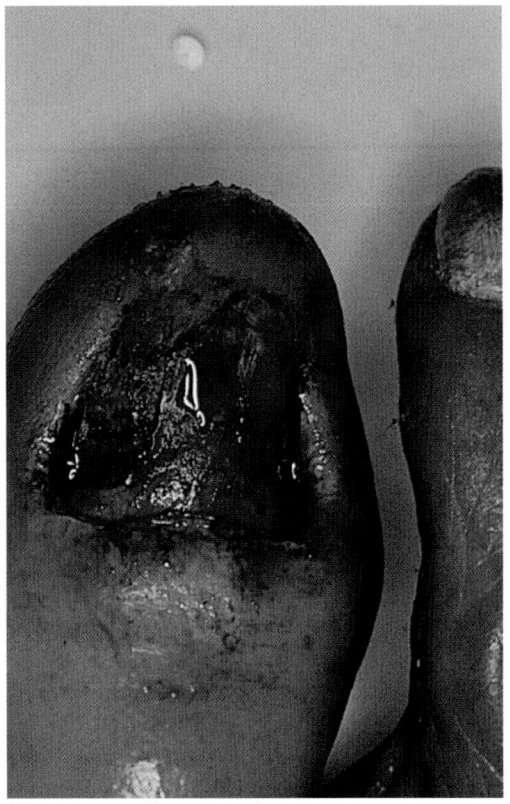

(b)

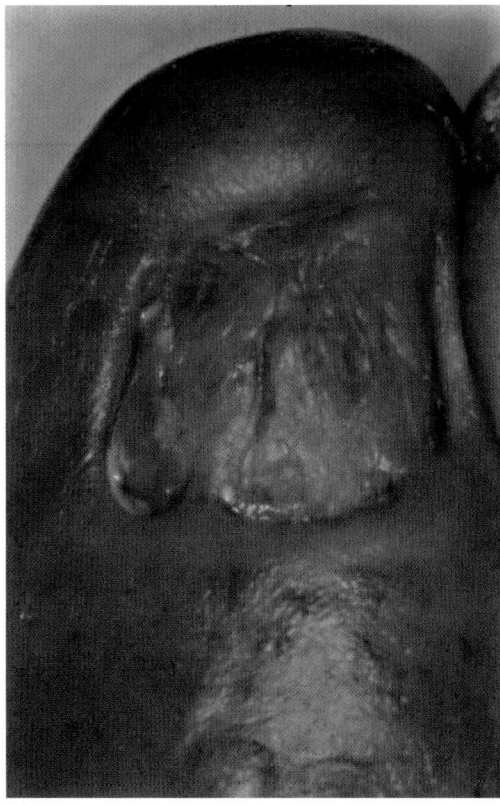

(c)

Figure 95.32 (a–c) Onychogryphosis is often best treated with ablation of the nail matrix.

follow (Figure 95.33a,b). There is seldom any difficulty with diagnosis. Excess nail fold granulation tissue can also be a feature of amelanotic melanoma and reactions to medications such as retinoids, ciclosporin, antiretroviral drugs and chemotherapy [9–15].

Management (see Nail surgery section)

Treatment may be difficult and prolonged. The first essential is to insist that the patient wear shoes sufficiently wide, high and pliable to remove lateral pressure [16]. Any abnormality of foot/toe function should be corrected. The patient must also be instructed to cut the nail straight across instead of in a semicircle. The nail must be allowed to grow until its edges are clear of the end of the toe before it is cut; this prevents the further formation of marginal spicules. In the early stages, the infection may be overcome by the application of antiseptics and by inserting a pledget of cotton-wool under the edge of the nail. Taping the toe or applying plastic gutters between nail edge and nail fold are alternatives [17]. These can be supplemented with acrylic nail to build up a smooth surface able to push the nail fold away and relieve ingrowing [18].

Twice-daily warm water baths followed by careful drying and powdering are helpful. Potent topical corticosteroids can help to diminish inflammation and suppress granulation tissue. They should, however, only be used after infection has been ruled out or is being actively managed. If the infection is more severe with local cellulitis, an appropriate systemic antibiotic should be administered. When granulation tissue forms this should be destroyed by cauterization with a silver nitrate stick. It is important that an

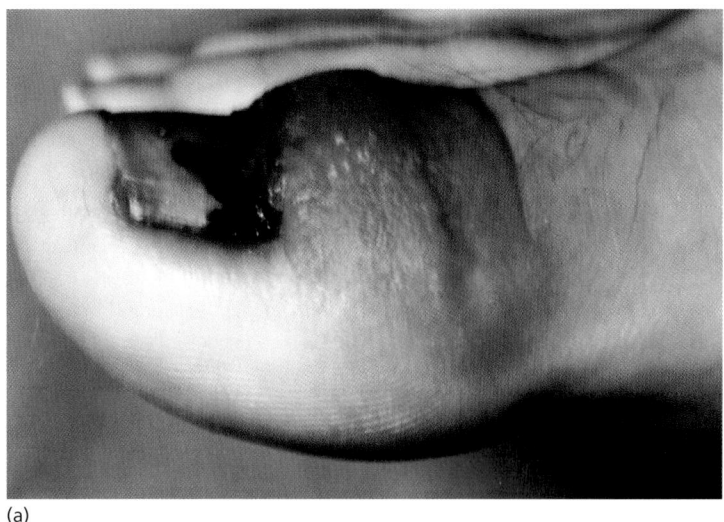
(a)

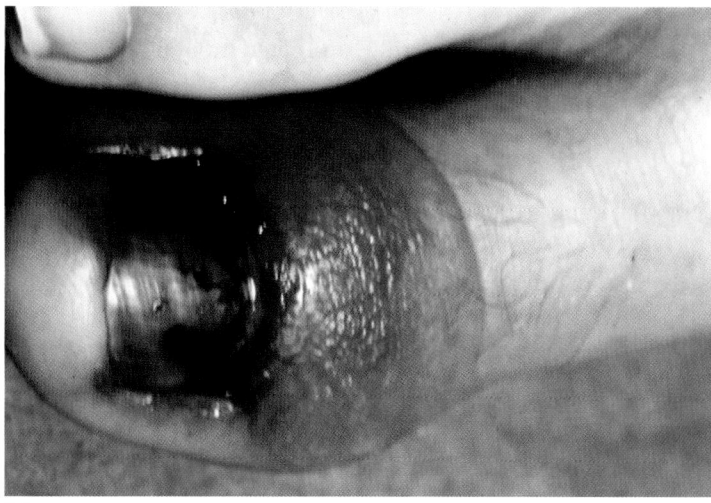
(b)

Figure 95.33 (a,b) Ingrowing great toenail complicated by proximal ingrowing (retronychia).

amelanotic melanoma is not missed [19], and if there are atypical features a biopsy should be performed.

If conservative measures fail, operative intervention will be necessary. Removing the nail alone is likely to result in recurrence of ingrowing when the nail returns [20] and so should be combined with a curative procedure such as phenolization of the relevant part of the matrix [4,21]. Although surgical excision of the matrix can provide an excellent result, it is more dependent than phenolization on the skill of the practitioner. In large studies, phenol treatment results in a greater cure rate and less morbidity (see Nail surgery section) [21].

TUMOURS UNDER OR ADJACENT TO THE NAIL

Benign tumours

Lobular capillary haemangioma (pyogenic granuloma) of nail apparatus

Definition and nomenclature
Pyogenic granuloma (PG) is a common acquired benign vascular tumour frequently encountered at the nail apparatus (nail bed and folds).

Synonyms and inclusions
- Nail pyogenic granuloma

Introduction and general description
Although lobular capillary haemangiomas (PGs) may occur at many different sites (see Chapter 137), they have a particular predilection for the soft tissues around the nail.

Pathophysiology
Nail PGs are due to a range of causes that act through different pathogenetic mechanisms which are as yet not clearly understood.

Predisposing factors
Nail PGs are secondary to four main causes as follows:
1 Trauma: local trauma is the most common cause of PGs involving the nail apparatus. Ingrowing nail, retronychia [1], friction from footwear [2], a range of self-induced disorders (onychotillomania, onychophagia and aggressive manicure) and accidental penetration of a foreign body may also promote the development of PG [3].
2 Drugs: the main characteristic of drug-induced nail PGs is the involvement of multiple digits, both fingers and toes. Several drugs have been implicated including retinoids (systemic and topical) [4,5–8], antiretroviral therapies (indinavir, lamivudine) [4,9–11], mitozanthrones [12], ciclosporin [13] and systemic 5-fluorouracil [14]. A number of new targeted therapies have become an increasingly important cause of PG. The antineoplastic therapies which are very commonly associated with multiple PGs are epidermal growth factor receptor (EGFR) inhibitors (cetuximab, gefitinib) [4], agents of the fluoropyrimidine family (capecitabine) [15–17] and agents of the taxan family (docetaxel, paclitaxel) [4,18,19]. Multiple eruptive PGs have also been reported in association with anti-CD20 antibody treatment for severe rheumatoid arthritis [20].
3 Peripheral nerve injury: different conditions, all having in common injury to the peripheral nerves, have been reported to be associated with nail changes and PGs of the proximal nail fold. Plaster cast immobilization is one such condition, where poor application technique may result in peripheral nerve damage from mechanical compression [21]. Patients will often complain of paraesthesiae and pain. A few days after cast removal, the nail plate detaches proximally from the bed (onychomadesis) and is associated with periungual swelling and PG formation under the proximal nail fold. Similar nail changes have been observed in reflex sympathetic dystrophy [22]. Periungual PGs

have also been reported after Guillain–Barré syndrome [23], in patients with hemiplegia [24] and after multiple episodes of hypoxia [25].

4 PGs due to inflammatory systemic diseases: periungual PGs involving multiple fingernails and toenails have been reported in cutaneous sarcoidosis, psoriasis and seronegative spondyloarthritis [4].

Pathology

Histopathology shows the characteristic features of PG, irrespective of cause and location (see Chapter 137).

Clinical features

History

The patient's history usually identifies the cause of the PG.

Presentation

A PG starts as a minute red papule that rapidly grows to the size of a pea or even a cherry. It bleeds easily, and the surface may become eroded by necrosis of the overlying epidermis.

Clinical variants

PGs are commonly located at the proximal nail fold, but may develop distally in the hyponychium or on the nail bed. In the latter instance, which often results from prolonged frictional trauma, the PG is associated with onycholysis (Figure 95.34).

Differential diagnosis

When a PG is single, especially if it involves the nail bed, histological examination is necessary to rule out melanoma and squamous carcinoma.

Complications and co-morbidities

In some instances PG may promote local infection.

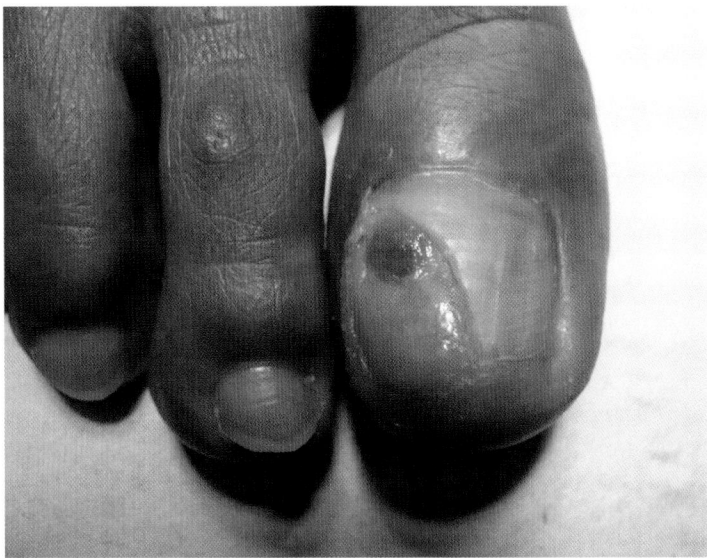

Figure 95.34 Pyogenic granuloma resulting from friction of the overlapping second toe against the lateral aspect of the great toenail.

Disease course and prognosis

If local trauma is suspected, the cause should be addressed (nail spur in ingrowing toenail, surgical removal of foreign body, stopping nail manipulation in onychotillomania, etc.). For drug-induced PGs, conservative treatment is recommended as they are likely to recur until the responsible drug is discontinued or replaced if necessary with a different agent. PG due to cast immobilization usually heals with topical corticosteroids. PGs due to reflex sympathetic dystrophy or to systemic diseases are more difficult to treat and often need several cycles of topical therapy or surgical removal [4].

Investigations

Histological examination should always be undertaken to rule out amelanotic melanoma or squamous cell carcinoma when faced with a single PG without a clear aetiology.

Treatment ladder

First line
• Potent corticosteroid cream (class I) under an occlusive dressing (best for drug-induced PGs) for up to 6 weeks

Second line
• Curettage under local anaesthesia

Third line
• Remove cause (drug, plaster cast, etc.) if feasible

Glomus tumour

Definition and nomenclature

Glomus tumour, a benign tumour of the myoarterial glomus (see Chapter 137), is an important cause of severe pain under the nail [26].

Synonyms and inclusions
• Glomangioma

Epidemiology

Incidence and prevalence

This is an uncommon neoplasm which represents about 1–2% of all hand tumours [26].

Age

Glomus tumour occurs mainly in patients in their forties.

Sex

It affects predominantly women (up to 90% of cases) [27].

Pathophysiology

Glomus tumours arise principally in the pulp or nail bed or matrix of the distal phalanx, where the glomus bodies of Masson are numerous.

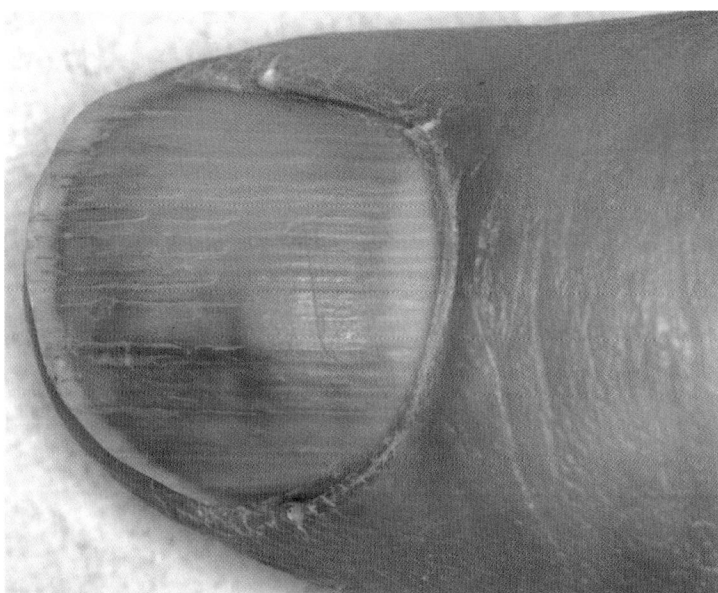

Figure 95.35 Painful glomus tumour of the nail bed. Note the bluish hue.

Pathology

A solid glomus tumour is composed of clusters of glomus cells surrounding capillaries. Glomus cells are uniform and round with pale eosinophilic cytoplasm, and a centrally located round nucleus. A basal lamina, highlighted by periodic acid–Schiff (PAS), surrounds each cell [28].

Presentation

Pain is the predominant symptom of a subungual glomus tumour. The pain may be pulsating, spontaneous or provoked by the slightest trauma. Variations in temperature, especially cold, may trigger pain radiating to the shoulder. Pain is sometimes described as worse at night. One case reports that even polishing the nail was unbearable [29].

Clinical variants

There are two main clinical presentations of subungual glomus tumour as follows:
- A small reddish or bluish spot (<1 cm) seen through the nail plate (Figure 95.35).
- A longitudinal erythronychia with distal notching or overlying longitudinal fissure.

Differential diagnosis

Differential diagnosis includes all causes of nail pain (Box 95.1). Exceptionally, glomus tumour might be totally painless.

Complications and co-morbidities

Pressure of the glomus tumour on the underlying phalanx may induce bone erosion in 50% of cases [**27**,30].

Disease course and prognosis

Patients have been wrongly referred to psychiatrists due to misdiagnosed glomus tumour where no nail alteration was visible and no proper work-up performed.

Box 95.1 Causes of nail pain

Tumours
- Glomus tumour
- Subungual keratoacanthoma
- Subungual exostosis
- Subungual horn
- Osteoid osteoma
- Enchondroma
- Intraosseous implantation cyst
- Metastasis

Inflammatory, infectious
- Bacterial paronychia
- Herpetic whitlow
- Osteomyelitis of terminal phalanx
- Onychomycosis

Inflammatory, non infectious
- Ingrowing toenail
- Nail psoriasis
- Dermatomyositis

Vascular
- Frostbite
- Acrosclerosis

Iatrogenic
- Taxanes
- Epidermal growth factor receptor inhibitors
- Retinoids
- Protease inhibitors

Investigations

Glomus tumour is the main indication for MRI of the nail unit [31]. It offers the highest sensitivity and best assessment of the extent of the tumour. The signal behaviour varies with the histological nature (vascular, cellular, myxoid) of the lesion [32]. MRI accurately determines the spatial location of the tumour, enabling a precise and radical surgical resection to be carried out [33]. Recurrent symptoms can usually be attributed to small synchronous satellite lesions [34].

Management

Treatment consists of surgical removal of the tumour. Two approaches are possible: the direct approach after nail plate avulsion through the nail bed or the matrix followed by meticulous repair [35,36] or the lateral approach on the volar aspect of the lateral nail fold. The latter gives a more restricted view of the tumour with a higher chance of incomplete excision compared with the transungual approach [**27**,37]. It should be recommended only for lesions that are proximal and deep seated [38].

Subungual exostosis

Definition

Subungual exostosis is an isolated slow-growing benign osteochondral outgrowth from the distal phalanx.

Most authors consider it to be a distinct clinicopathological entity [39], but some classify them with osteochondromas [40].

Epidemiology

Incidence and prevalence

Subungual exostosis is probably considerably underreported. The prevalence is unknown.

Age

Patients within their twenties are mostly affected [41,**42**,43].

Sex

The sex ratio varies from series to series but is most probably 1 : 1.

Pathophysiology

Subungual exostosis was previously thought to be a reactive process. It is now considered a true neoplasm harbouring a pathognomonic translocation t(X;6)(q22;q13-14) [44].

Predisposing factors

Trauma seems to be the most important aetiological factor [41].

Pathology

Histopathology shows a bony tumour with a hyaline cartilaginous cap.

Clinical features

History

The association of nail deformity and pain is highly suggestive, but pain is often not present.

Presentation

All large series (*n* = 19–45) have shown that the great toenail is affected in three quarters of cases [41,**42**,45]. Subungual exostosis usually elevates the nail plate as it emerges from the hyponych-ium (Figure 95.36a) or from a lateral sulcus. In its early stages, the tumour may have a porcelain white hue with superficial telangiectases and a collarette surrounding its base. As the tumour enlarges, it develops a thick hyperkeratotic surface.

Clinical variants

Dorsal subungual exostoses may present as a nondescript erythematous patch seen through the nail plate, with or without onycholysis (Figure 95.36b,c).

Differential diagnosis

Differential diagnosis includes verruca vulgaris, fibrokeratoma, PG, ingrowing toenail, squamous cell carcinoma and amelanotic melanoma.

Complications and co-morbidities

Erosion and secondary infection of the nail bed may give rise to a subungual PG-like outgrowth [46] (Figure 95.37).

Investigations

Radiographic examination is the cornerstone in the diagnosis of subungual exostosis. Early lesions, mostly formed from cartilage, may not be visible.

Management

Treatment is resection of the outgrowth under full aseptic conditions.

Digital myxoid pseudocyst

Definition and nomenclature

Digital myxoid pseudocysts are the second most common benign tumours of the digits.

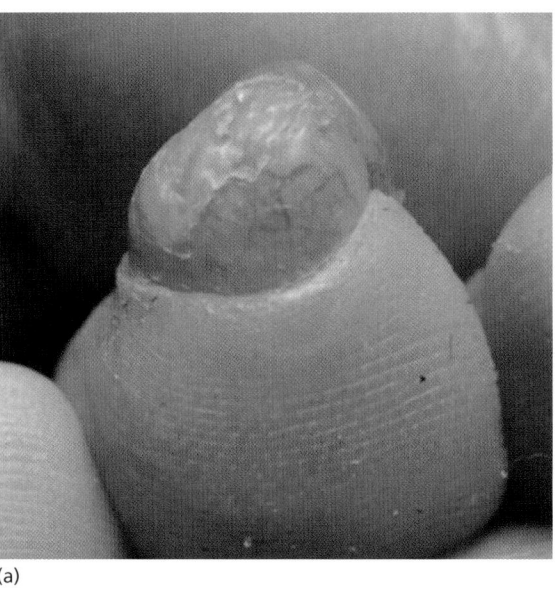
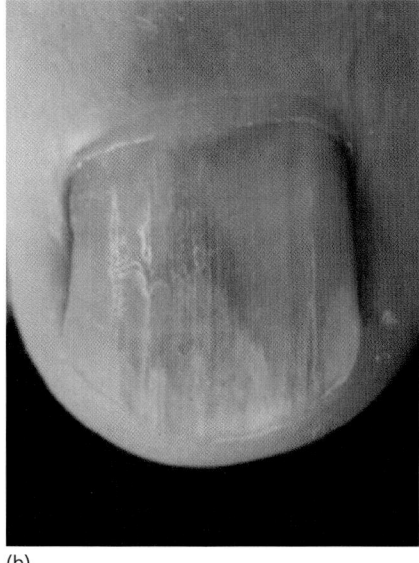
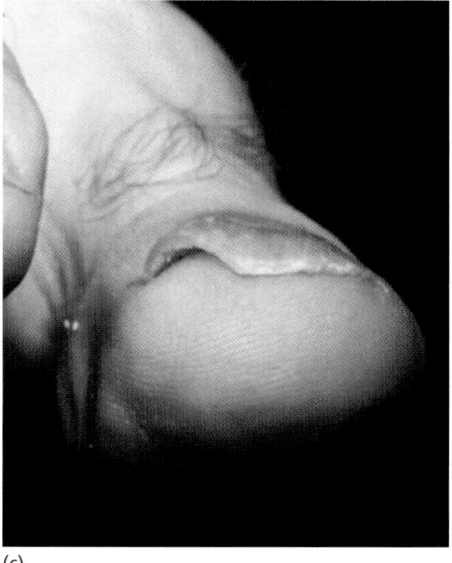

(a)　　　　　　　　　　　　　　　　(b)　　　　　　　　　　　　　　　　(c)

Figure 95.36 Subungual exostosis: exophytic growth of bone emerging from under the nail plate through collarette of skin (note the telangiectases) (a); exostosis from the dorsal surface of the terminal phalanx presenting as painful onycholysis (b,c).

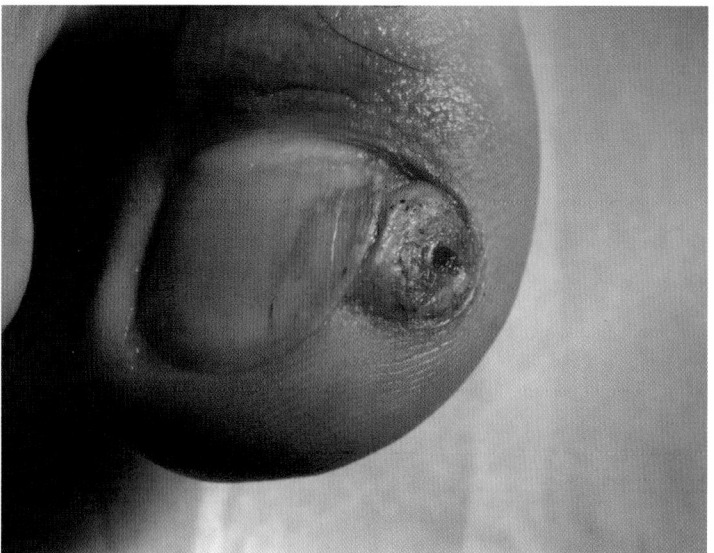

Figure 95.37 This lesion was mistaken for an ingrowing toenail. X-rays confirmed the presence of subungual exostosis.

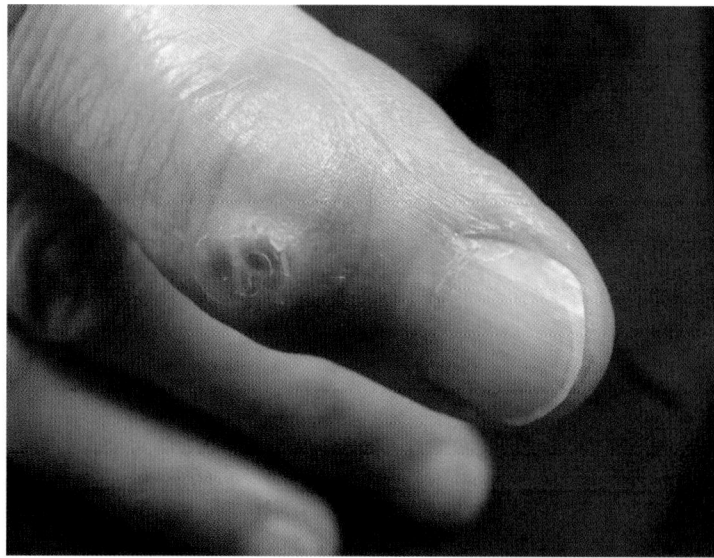

Figure 95.38 Digital myxoid pseudocyst type A.

Synonyms and inclusions
- Digital myxoid cyst
- Ganglion cyst
- Digital synovial cyst

Epidemiology

Incidence and prevalence
The exact incidence and prevalence are not known.

Age
Over 50 years old.

Sex
It is estimated that women are affected more than twice as often as men [47].

Associated diseases
Osteoarthritis.

Pathophysiology
It is now believed that digital myxoid pseudocysts result from leakage of synovial fluid through a breach in the joint capsule of the distal interphalangeal joint [48], as could be demonstrated in more than 85% of cases in a study using MRI [49].

Predisposing factors
The presence of osteophytes and reduction of the joint space from osteoarthritis or repetitive occupational trauma [50] promote leakage of joint fluid.

Pathology
Digital myxoid pseudocysts manifest as well-circumscribed but unencapsulated cyst-like dermal swellings, devoid of any lin-ing. They consist of large mucin-filled spaces containing spindle-shaped and stellate fibroblasts without atypia [28].

Presentation
The clinical features depend upon their location in relation to the nail apparatus. De Berker *et al.* classified them into three subtypes [51,52] as follows:
- Type A: the most common presentation, the digital myxoid pseudocyst presents as a nodule between the distal interphalangeal joint and the proximal nail fold (Figure 95.38).
- Type B: the digital myxoid pseudocysts is in the proximal nail fold and presses on the underlying matrix resulting in a longitudinal groove in the nail plate (Figure 95.39a,b). The groove often varies in depth according to the fluctuating volume of the cyst (Figure 95.39c). A small keratotic tip protruding from under the proximal nail fold may also be observed.
- Type C: the digital myxoid pseudocyst exerts pressure from under the matrix, giving rise to a reddish or bluish lunula (Figure 95.40).

Differential diagnosis
Main differential diagnosis is fibrokeratoma in subtype B.

Disease course and prognosis
In most instances, digital myxoid pseudocysts are asymptomatic but unsightly and therefore may bother the patient. Increased pressure within the joint may be responsible for pain.

Investigations
None are necessary except for type C, for which ultrasound or MRI may be needed.

Management
Numerous treatments have been recommended for this condition. Their aim is to obliterate the leakage from the joint, by inducing fibrosis around the capsule.

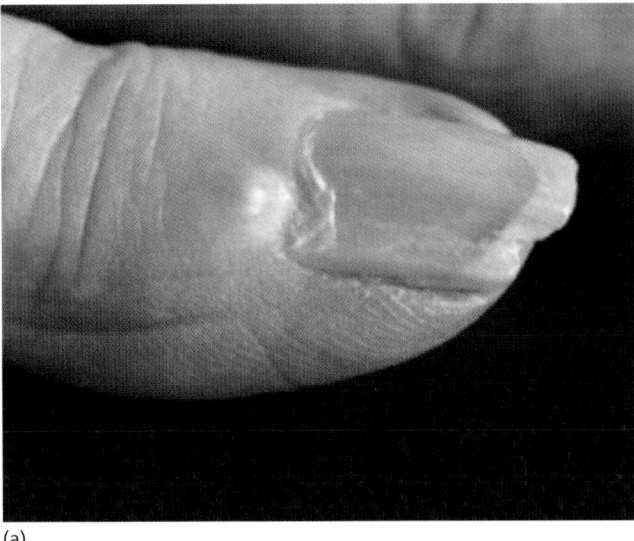
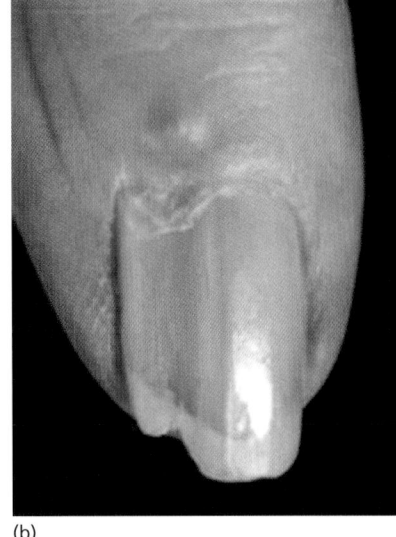
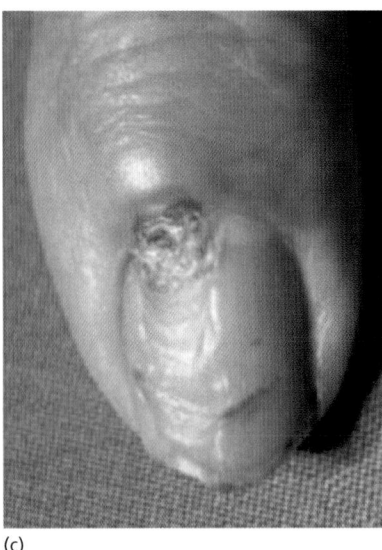

(a)   (b)   (c)

Figure 95.39 Digital myxoid pseudocyst type B. Note the longitudinal groove arising from underneath the proximal nail fold where the matrix is compressed by the overlying pseudocyst and extending to the free edge of the nail (a–c); any tumour compressing the matrix may give rise to a longitudinal gutter as shown in (a) and (b) but only a myxoid pseudocyst, which commonly fluctuates in size and therefore the pressure exerted on the matrix, may give rise to the irregular guttering as seen in (c).

Treatment ladder

First line
- Cryotherapy should be tempted at least twice for type A

Second line
- Methylene-blue guided surgery for ligature of the leak of joint fluid is a quick and effective technique as it provides a very highest success rate on the fingers (94%) [48]

Acquired ungual fibrokeratoma

Definition and nomenclature
Acquired ungual fibrokeratoma is a solitary benign asymptomatic nodule with a hyperkeratotic tip that forms in the periungual area or, rarely, within or under the nail plate.

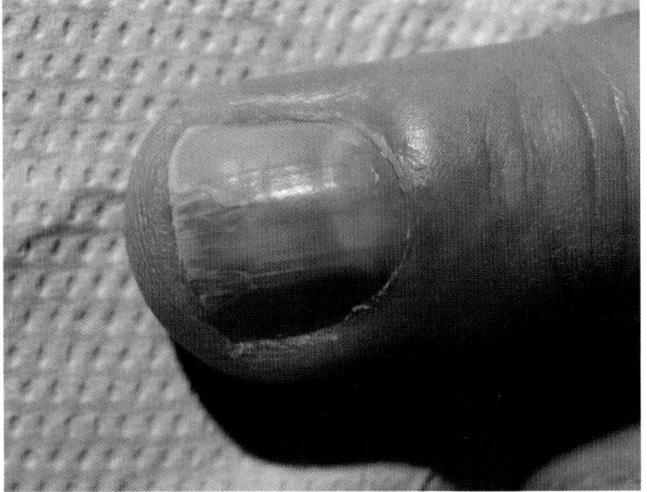

Figure 95.40 Digital myxoid pseudocyst type C. Note the red macule within the lunula.

Synonyms and inclusions
- Garlic clove fibroma
- Acquired periungual fibrokeratoma

Pathophysiology
Trauma is thought to be the major causative factor.

Pathology
Acquired ungual fibrokeratomas are pedunculated fibroepithelial lesions. The epidermis is hyperkeratotic and acanthotic, with thickened, often branching, rete ridges. The core of the lesions is composed of fibroblasts and dense collagen fibres. The vascular component is sometimes prominent [28]. No histogical difference has been found between isolated acquired ungual fibrokeratomas and the Koenen tumours of tuberous sclerosis [53].

Presentation
Most of them emerge from under the proximal nail fold and lie in a longitudinal groove which extends to the free edge of the plate. Their size varies considerably from tiny to prominent (Figure 95.41); they may sometimes be bifid.

Clinical variants
Rarely, an acquired ungual fibrokeratoma may originate from the matrix and grow into the nail plate (intraungual fibrokeratoma) (Figure 95.42) to eventually emerge in the middle of the nail. Subungual fibrokeratomas arising from the nail bed are also rare.

Differential diagnosis
Fibroma, keloid, Koenen tumours, recurring digital fibrous tumour of childhood, cutaneous horn, exostosis.

Investigations
Histology is mandatory as Bowen disease may present as a pseudofibrokeratoma [54,55].

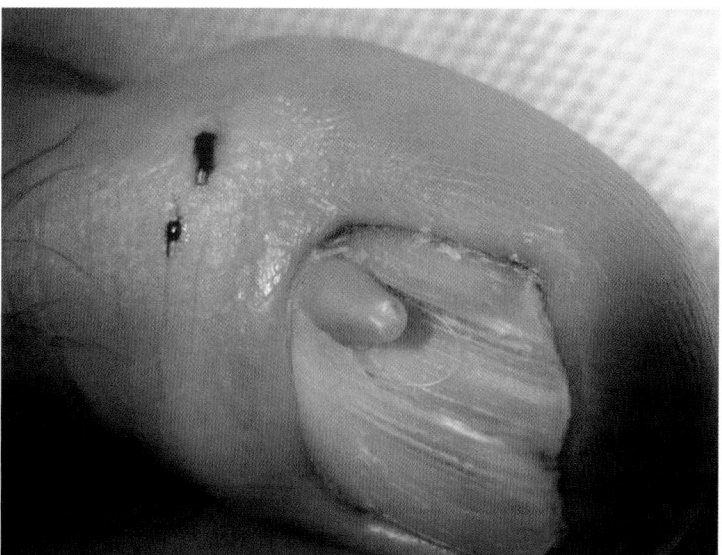

Figure 95.41 Submatricial fibrokeratoma pressing onto the underlying matrix with subsequent longitudinal smooth groove.

When lesions are present on several digits, tuberous sclerosis should be ruled out. The lesions are then called Koenen tumours (Figure 95.43). They develop most commonly on the toes around puberty and their number increases with age.

Management
Surgical removal.

Subungual keratoacanthoma

Definition
Subungual keratoacanthoma is a rare benign but rapidly growing and aggressive tumour that is usually situated in the most distal portion of the nail bed.

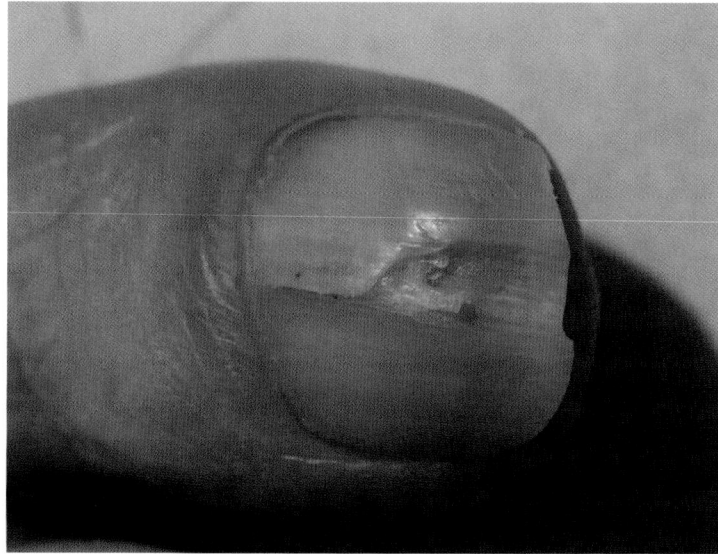

Figure 95.42 Intraungual (dissecting) fibrokeratoma. The lesion grows within the nail plate and emerges at its distal half.

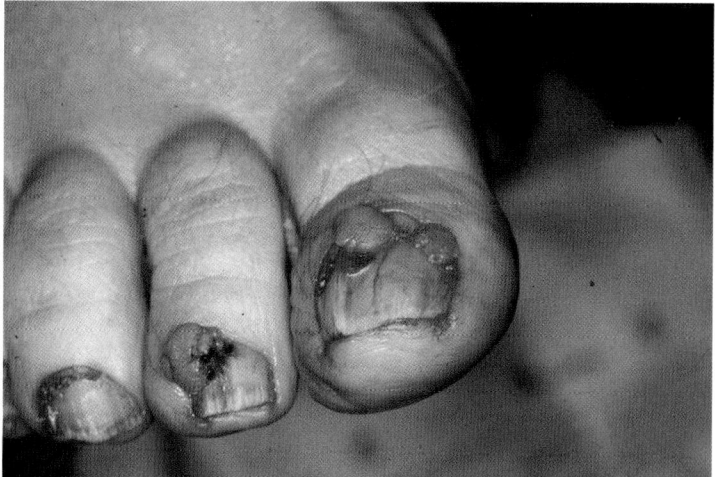

Figure 95.43 Multiple soft fibrokeratomas in tuberous sclerosis.

Epidemiology

Incidence and prevalence
Unknown.

Sex
Subungual keratoacanthoma occurs predominantly in males (75% of cases) [56].

Pathophysiology
The pathogenesis not understood.

Predisposing factors
Trauma [56], oncogenic human papillomavirus [57] and, in one case of steel wool [58], have each been suggested as contributory factors.

Pathology
Microscopic examination shows a squamoproliferative lesion with a focal crateriform pattern and overlying hyperkeratosis with ortho- and parakeratosis. Lobules of squamous epithelium are often well differentiated, composed of large keratinocytes with copious 'glassy' eosinophilic cytoplasm. Dyskeratotic cells are numerous, but atypia and mitotic figures are rare. Tumour protein p53 and proliferation marker Ki-67 can help distinguish subungual keratoacanthomas from subungual squamous cell carcinomas [28].

Genetics
In women, the development of multiple subungual keratoacanthomas may represent a late manifestation of incontinentia pigmenti.

Clinical features

History
Subungual keratoacanthomas are rapidly growing tumours (within weeks) which are always painful and are most often located on the distal part of the nail bed. They are most commonly

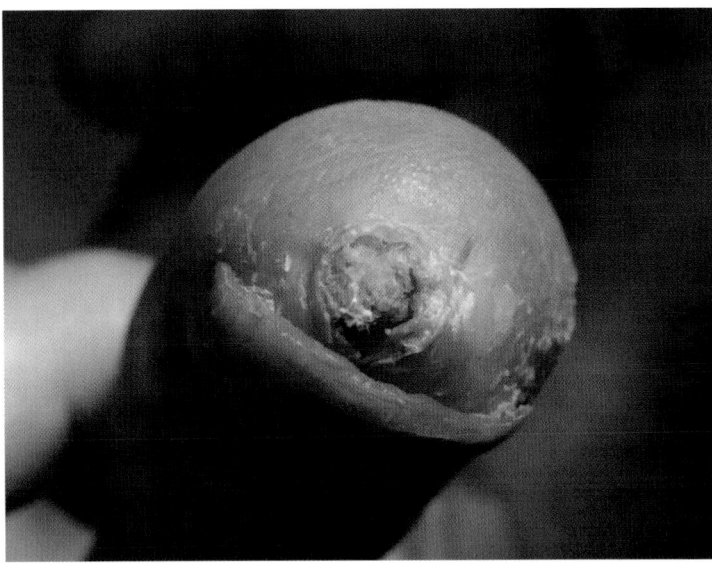

Figure 95.44 Subungual distal keratoacanthoma. Note the keratotic plug on the distal bed.

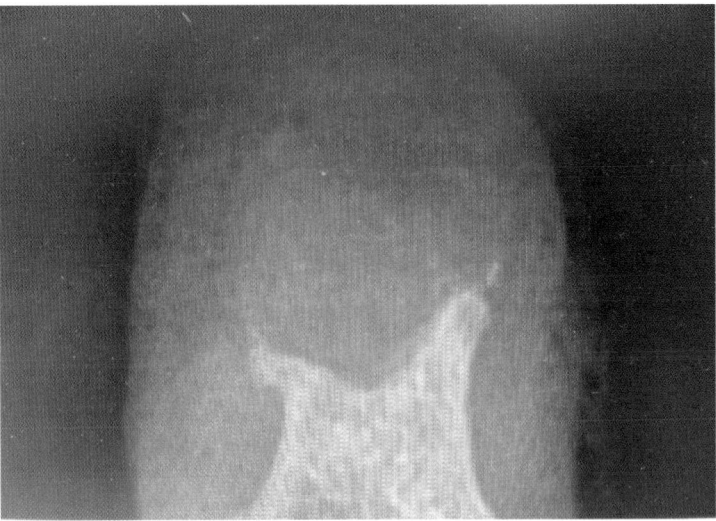

Figure 95.45 X-rays showing massive osteolysis of the distal bony phalanx associated with subungual keratoacanthoma.

located on the thumb but the index and middle fingers are also well-recognized sites [56].

Presentation

The tumour may start as a small and painful keratotic nodule just under the free edge of the nail, rapidly growing to 1–2 cm in diameter within 4–8 weeks. After clipping of the overlying nail plate, the typical gross appearance resembles that of keratoacanthoma at other sites as a dome-shaped nodule with a central crater plugged by keratinous material (Figure 95.44). The tumour may rapidly plunge deeper and erode the underlying bony phalanx.

Clinical variants

If located more proximally under the nail fold, subungual keratoacanthomas may present as a painful chronic paronychia [56,59].

Differential diagnosis

The three main differential diagnoses are: epidermoid implantation cyst, subungual wart and squamous cell carcinoma.

Complications and co-morbidities

Lonlasting lesions may lead to complete destruction of the distal bony phalanx.

Investigations

Standard X-rays consistently demonstrate a well-defined cup-shaped erosion of the underlying bone (Figure 95.45). The margins of the defect show no evidence of sclerosis or any sign of periosteal reaction [60]. This lytic effect is attributed to the very rapid compression from the tumour rather than tumour invasion [61]. Long-term radiological follow-up data following subungual keratoacanthomas are sparse, but failure to reossify [58], partial repair of the bony defect [62] and spontaneous regression with full reossification [63] have all been reported.

Treatment ladder

First line
- Removal of the entire tumour with curettage of the cavity

Second line
- Amputation: only for multiple recurrences or massive bony destruction

Third line
- Acitretin 1 mg/day may be attempted when subungual keratoacanthoma is associated with incontinentia pigmenti

---

Onychomatricoma

Definition and nomenclature

Onychomatricoma is a rare benign tumour of the matrix, with peculiar clinical and pathological features, first described in 1992 by Baran and Kint [64].

Synonyms and inclusions
- 'Onychoblastoma', 'unguioblastoma' and 'unguioblastic fibroma' are similar tumours of the nail matrix [65,66]

Epidemiology

Incidence and prevalence

Unknown.

Age

All published cases were adults except one in a child, in whom the diagnosis was purely clinical and without histopathological verification [67].

Ethnicity

The overwhelming majority of cases are reported in white people, and only exceptionally in non-Europeans [68].

Pathophysiology

The origin of the tumour remains obscure. It most probably stems from a disturbed differentiation of nail matrix cells. The tumour digitations are onychogenic and responsible for the thickening of the nail plate.

Pathology

Histopathology is unique.

Two different zones may be observed as follows:

1 The distal zone is characterized by multiple 'glove finger' papillary projections covered by a matrix-type epithelium devoid of stratum granulosum that keratinizes through an eosinophilic keratogenous zone.

2 The proximal zone is dome shaped in transverse sections and lined by a papillomatous matrix-type epithelium, with vertically oriented deep invaginations into the stroma. These invaginations surround optically empty cavities in a characteristic V-shaped configuration [28].

Clinical features

History

The condition is indolent and patients mostly seek medical advice for cosmetic purposes, when the tumour has been evolving for several years.

Presentation

Single fingers are most commonly affected (75%), mainly the middle finger [69]. Few reports mention involvement of the lesser toes [70] or exceptionally of several digits [71].

Several clinical signs are striking enough to either make the diagnosis or at least to arouse suspicion (Figure 95.46) as follows:

• Thickening of the nail plate, of various width, often sparing a part of normal pinkish nail.
• Transverse and longitudinal overcurvature of the affected portion of the nail.
• Xanthonychia of the affected part of the nail.
• Longitudinal ridging, sometimes quite prominent on the surface of the nail.
• Splinter haemorrhages, mostly proximal but sometimes distal.
• Woodworm cavities at the free edge of the thickened nail plate (Figure 95.47).

Clinical variants

Some unusual clinical variants have been reported: giant form [72], association with dorsal pterygium [73,74] or associated with onychomycosis and longitudinal melanonychia [75]. Only rarely is the length of the digitations such that clipping of the free edge of the nail induces bleeding [76].

Differential diagnosis

Clinical presentation is characteristic but onychomycosis and Bowen disease [77] should be ruled out.

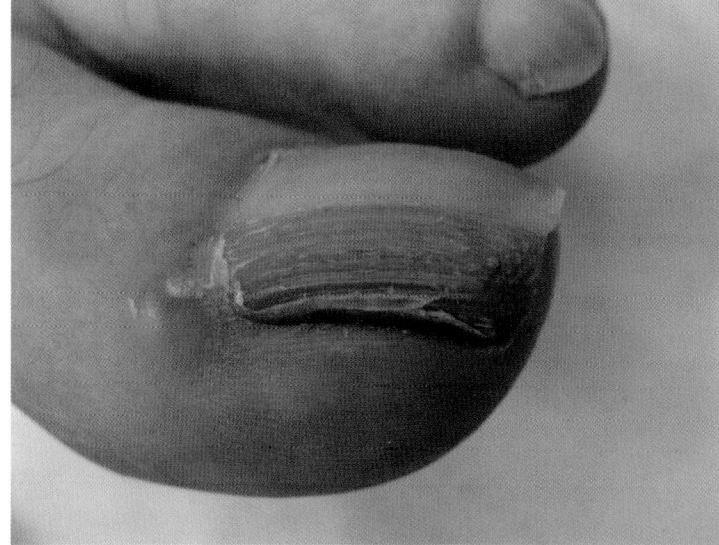

Figure 95.46 Onychomatricoma, pigmented variant: note the very well-delimited longitudinal thickening of the plate.

Disease course and prognosis

Excellent prognosis if skilled surgeons perform the surgery. Longlasting lesions may end in complete destruction of the nail plate.

Investigations

Dermoscopy confirms diagnosis in showing the woodworm perforations at the distal edge of the nail. Recently, nail clipping of the diseased part of the nail has been shown to be a minimally invasive method to achieve the correct diagnosis of onychomatricoma [78]. MRI is typical and reveals a tumour emerging from the nail matrix [79]. Ultrasonic examination seems promising [80]. Nail avulsion is diagnostic as it exposes a villous tumour, reminiscent of a sea anemone, emerging from the matrix while the nail appears as a thickened funnel, storing filamentous

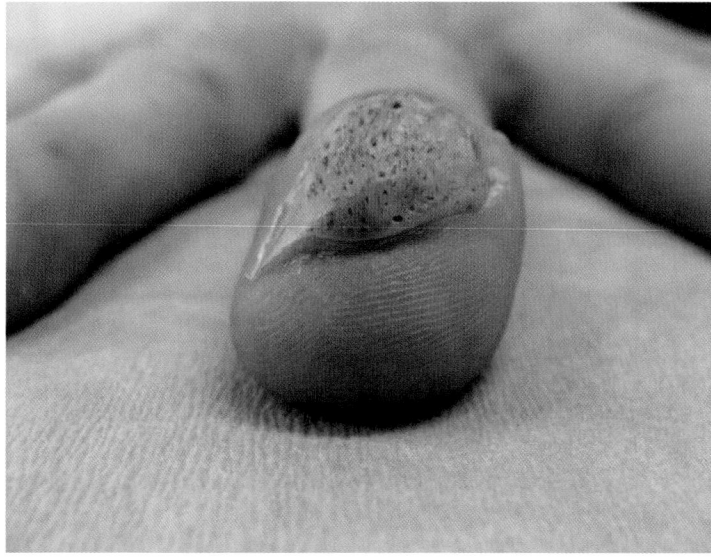

Figure 95.47 Onychomatricoma: 'woodworm' cavities in the nail plate are especially visible in this longstanding case (>40 years).

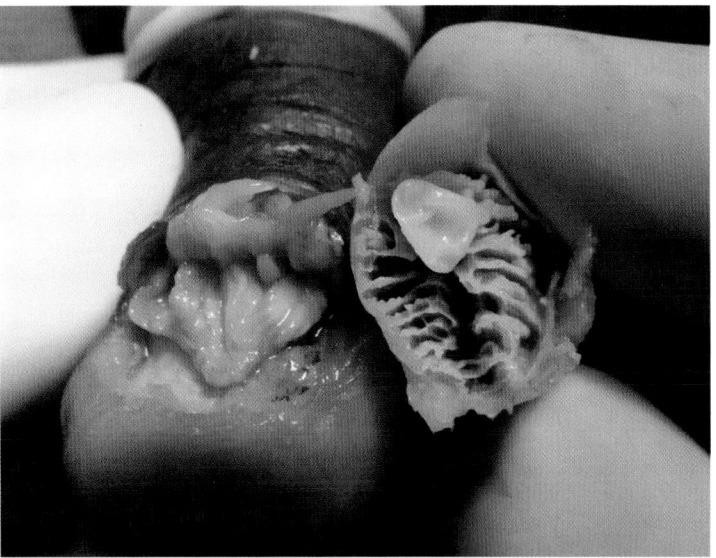

Figure 95.48 Onychomatricoma: showing the sea anemone-like matrix tumour and the cavities in the avulsed nail plate into which digitate projections from the tumour had infiltrated.

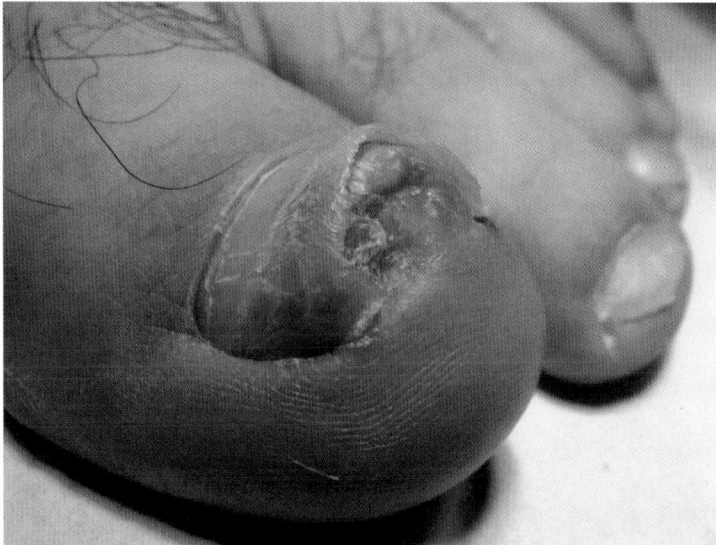

Figure 95.49 Superficial fibromyxoma of the nail bed elevating the distal plate.

digitations of matrix fitting into the holes of the proximal nail extremity (Figure 95.48).

Management
Surgical removal of the tumour is the only option. The tumour should only be shaved from the underlying matrix [35].

Superficial acral fibromyxoma

Definition and nomenclature
Superfical acral fibromyxoma is a rare slow-growing soft-tissue tumour which has a predilection for the subungual and periungual regions of the fingers and toes in adults [81]. It is a distinct clinicopathological entity, recognized by Fetsch *et al.* in 2001 [82].

Synonyms and inclusions
• Digital fibromyxoma

Epidemiology

Incidence and prevalence
Unknown.

Age
Middle-aged adults.

Sex
Males are more commonly affected than women (male to female ratio: 1.6 : 1).

Pathology
It presents as a relatively well-circumscribed but unencapsulated dermal tumour composed of spindle-shaped cells integrated in a fibromyxoid matrix, sometimes invading the subcutis, often with accentuated vasculature and increased numbers of mast cells. Nuclear atypia is slight or absent and mitotic figures are infrequent. Immunohistochemically, more than 90% of cases are positive for CD34. CD99 and epithelial membrane antigen (EMA) are often focally positive [28,83].

Presentation
Superficial acral fibromyxoma is normally diagnosed on histology and its clinical presentation has not been well characterized. The tumour is located in the nail bed or nail folds. Some reports describe a dome-shaped, well-circumscribed, whitish to pink firm tumour, sometimes surrounded by a basal collarette, lifting up the plate (Figure 95.49) and covered with very thin fissured keratin; if located deep in the lateral nail fold, it presents as a swollen fold covered with normal skin. It may or may not be painful [84,85].

Clinical variants
Exceptionally, superficial acral fibromyxoma may be located beneath the matrix [86].

Differential diagnosis
Lipoma, schwannoma and neurofibroma.

Complications and co-morbidities
Bony involvement occurs in one third of cases [86].

Disease course and prognosis
No metastases were observed in a recent series of 124 cases with a mean follow-up of 35 months [**87**].

Investigations
Radiological imaging should be performed to rule out bony involvement.

Management
Complete surgical resection, as it has a propensity for local recurrence if incompletely excised [87].

Onychopapilloma

Definition and nomenclature

Onychopapilloma is a benign longitudinally oriented subungual tumour of unknown aetiology.

Synonyms and inclusions
- Multinucleate distal subungual keratosis [88]
- Nail-producing papilloma [89]

Pathophysiology

Pathology

Onychopapilloma is characterized by: acanthosis and papillomatosis, mostly of the distal part of the nail bed; matrix metaplasia of the nail bed with an onychogenous zone; canaliform deformation of the ventral part of the nail plate; and a keratinous mass under the distal nail plate [28].

Clinical features

History

Patients seek medical advice either because of pain or because they catch the fissured free edge of the nail.

Presentation

Onychopapilloma usually presents as an isolated pink longitudinal nail streak (erythronychia) extending from the distal matrix to the free edge, from under which emerges a fine filiform subungual keratosis. It may be accompanied by distal onycholysis or a fissure. Distal splinter haemorrhages are also common (Figure 95.50).

Clinical variants

Onychopapilloma may, albeit rarely, present as longitudinal melanonychia [90] or leukonychia [91].

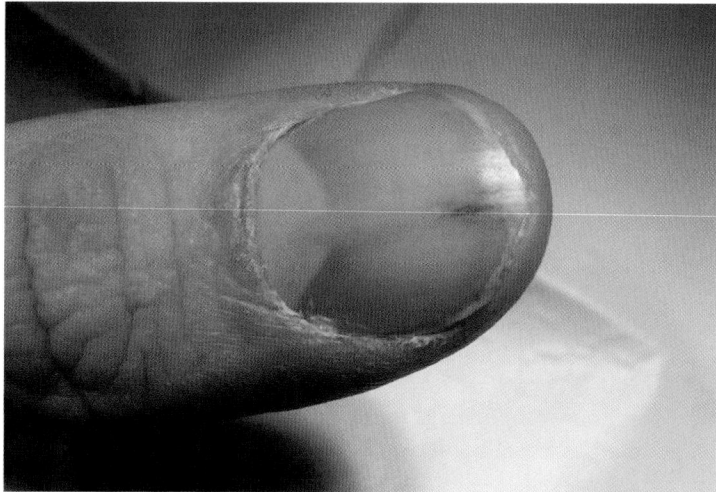

Figure 95.50 Onychopapilloma: note the longitudinal erythronychia starting in the distal matrix, the distal splinter haemorrhages and the onycholysis at its distal end. The nail was longer at that place because the papilloma impaired nail clipping (pain).

Differential diagnosis

Bowen disease [89] and nail lichen planus [92] may present in rare instances as an onychopapilloma.

Management

The onychopapilloma is usually excised only if it bothers the patient or to rule out other tumours.

Malignant tumours

Squamous cell carcinoma

Definition

Squamous cell carcinoma is the most frequent malignant tumour of the nail apparatus, where presentation as *in situ* squamous cell carcinoma (Bowen disease) is more common than invasive squamous cell carcinoma.

Epidemiology

Age
The mean age at presentation is 60 years [93,94–96).

Sex
Three quarters of cases occur in males [93,95,96].

Pathophysiology

Predisposing factors
One third of patients with squamous cell carcinoma of the nail apparatus have a personal history of human papillomavirus-associated genital disease (genital warts, dysplasia or cancer of the cervix) or a similar history in a sexual partner. The average time between the onset of the genital disease and the appearance of the nail tumour is around 12 years [95]. It is estimated that genito-digital transmission of human papillomavirus is responsible for up to 60% of cases of squamous cell carcinoma of the nail apparatus (both *in situ* and invasive forms). Prolonged unprotected contact with chemical mutagens is another possible predisposing factor.

Pathology
The picture is identical to that of Bowen disease in other skin areas [97]. The most important feature to look for is the intact basement membrane defining the *in situ* form.

Causative organisms
Human papillomavirus, especially serotype 16, which is isolated in three quarters of cases [95], but also serotypes 2, 6, 11, 18, 26, 31, 34, 35, 56, 58 and 73 [98–101].

Environmental factors
Ionizing radiation, arsenic and pesticides have been suggested as potential causative factors [95].

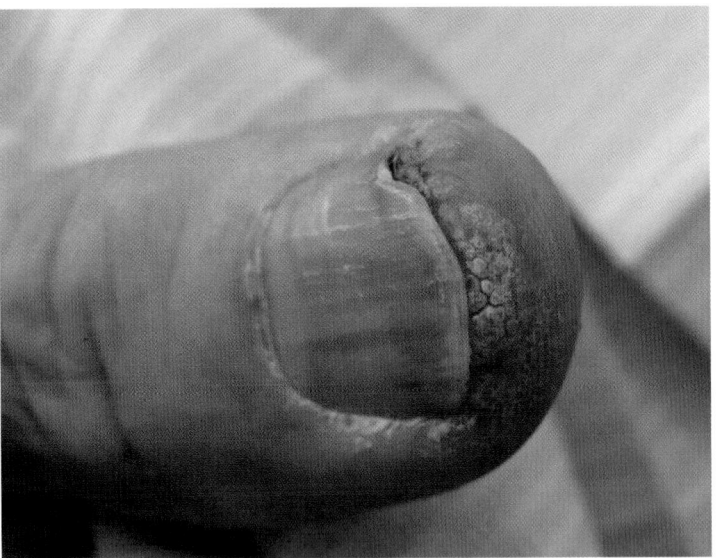

Figure 95.51 Bowen disease: warty lesion of the distal bed and hyponychium. The lesion was treated for several years as a wart.

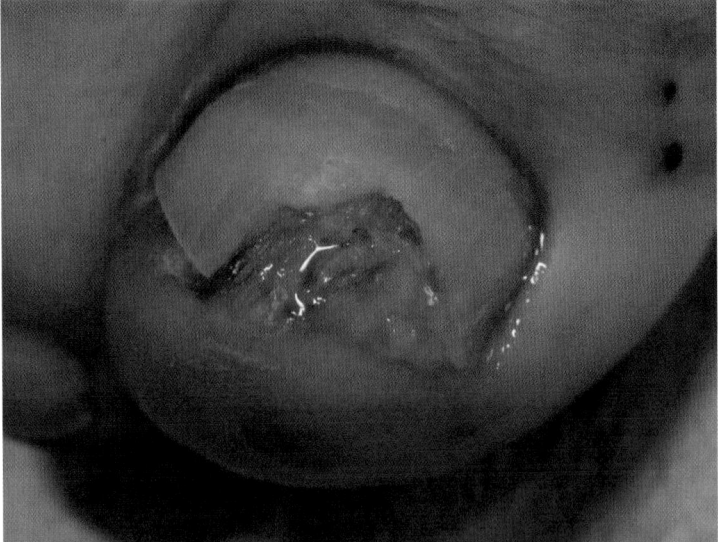

Figure 95.52 Onycholysis and oozing of the great toenail bed due to invasive squamous cell carcinoma.

Clinical features

History
Patients are often not bothered by this indolent and painless condition and therefore tend to seek medical advice very late (mean delay 6 years) [93,102].

Presentation
The clinical presentation is protean, accounting for the delay in diagnosis. The largest published series identifies the right index and middle fingers as the most commonly affected. This finding is in agreement with the postulated genito-digital transmission of human papillomavirus [93]. The condition is usually solitary but, uncommonly, tumours may arise in more than one digit [103–105]. The most common clinical findings are, in decreasing order of frequency, subungual hyperkeratosis (Figure 95.51), onycholysis (Figure 95.52), oozing and nail plate destruction. Oozing is an underrecognized sign and is only occasionally reported in the literature [93,106].

Clinical variants
Squamous cell carcinoma may also present as longitudinal melanonychia [107], an onychopapilloma [89], a fibrokeratoma [54] or may simulate an onychomatricoma [77].

Verrucous carcinoma (carcinoma cuniculatum) of the nail apparatus is a rare low-grade variant of squamous cell carcinoma, characterized by a local aggressiveness but a low potential for metastasis. Only 13 cases have been reported in the literature [108,109]. It presents clinically as a slowly enlarging warty papillomatous plaque and, of reported cases, were most commonly located on the thumb, the hallux or the fifth toe.

Differential diagnosis
The main differential diagnosis is a wart [93].

Disease course and prognosis
Prognosis both of *in situ* and of invasive forms is good: metastases are exceptional [98,110] and only three deaths have been reported [96,111,112].

Investigations
Radiological imaging should be performed to rule out bony involvement, which was however detected in only 2% of cases in the largest reported series of squamous cell carcinoma of the nail unit ($n = 58$) [93].

Management
The goal of treatment is eradication of the tumour. However, even with sophisticated surgical techniques, recurrences are not uncommon, probably because human papillomavirus is difficult to eradicate [93].

Treatment ladder

First line
- Mohs surgery

Second line
- Conventional surgery with micrographic control of the margins on fixed tissue

Third line
- Imiquimod cream [113], 5-fluorouracil cream [114,115] with or without prior curettage, photodynamic therapy [116,117] and intra-arterial infusion with methotrexate [118]. None of these techniques allows histological control of tumour margins and they should therefore be considered as a treatment option only in special cases where surgery is not feasible

Fourth line
- Amputation is mandatory only when bone involvement occurs

Basal cell carcinoma

Definition
Basal cell carcinoma very rarely involves the nail apparatus: 20 cases only have been reported in the literature.

Epidemiology

Age
The average age at diagnosis is 65 years.

Pathology
The pathological features are identical to those observed on the skin (see Chapter 141).

Environmental factors
One basal cell carcinoma of the proximal nail fold was reported in a respiratory specialist using radioscopy for 30 years [119] and another in a worker dealing with azo dyes [120].

Clinical features

History
In the published cases, diagnosis was delayed by an average of about 10 years.

Presentation
The classical clinical features as observed on the skin are very rarely encountered. There is no typical clinical presentation (see Differential diagnosis). Two cases presented as longitudinal melanonychia. Diagnosis was histological in all cases. The thumb is most frequently involved, followed by the hallux [121].

Clinical variants
Longitudinal melanonychia is a rare presentation [121,122].

Differential diagnosis
Chronic paronychia, PG, amelanotic melanoma, squamous cell carcinoma, bacterial or a mycotic infection and habit tic [123].

Investigations
Radiographic imaging to rule out bony involvement.

Management
Surgical removal.

Treatment ladder

First line
• Mohs surgery [124]

Second line
• Conventional excision

Third line
• Amputation if bone involvement

Melanoma (see Chapter 143)

Definition
Melanoma of the nail apparatus is rare but associated with poor prognosis.

Very early recognition and excision provides the best chance of survival.

Epidemiology

Incidence and prevalence
The prevalence ranges from 0.18 to 2.8% of all cutaneous melanomas [125]. The incidence has been estimated at 0.1/100 000/year [126].

Age
Average age of onset is between the sixth and seventh decade. Melanoma of the nail apparatus is exceptional in children, with only 13 reported cases to date [127].

Ethnicity
The proportion of melanomas involving the nail apparatus is much higher in populations of African and East Asian ethnicity than in white people: about 25% of melanomas are located at the nail apparatus in Japanese and African Americans. However, the absolute incidence may well be similar in all racial groups [125].

Pathophysiology
Trauma is often mentioned as a potential causative factor, but no clear link can be established with certainty [128]. UV radiation is not responsible as the nail plate acts as a barrier to penetration of UV [129]; furthermore, the similar frequency of melanoma of the nail apparatus in dark- and fair-skinned peoples suggests that pigmentation is not protective [125].

Pathology
Most cases are acral lentiginous melanoma. In melanoma of the nail apparatus, the histological subtype, the Clark's level, and the Breslow thickness are difficult to assess because of the peculiar nail anatomy [28]. Immunochemistry is particularly helpful for the diagnosis of early disease and for the determination of excision margins: HMB-45 is more sensitive than Mart-1 for detecting intraepithelial melanocytes and the latter is in turn more sensitive than S-100 protein. In invasive melanoma of the nail apparatus, however, S-100 protein is the most sensitive and was the only positive marker in cases of desmoplastic melanoma and in areas with chondroid differentiation [130].

Clinical features

History
Diagnosis is very often delayed and associated with poor prognosis. Patients do not suspect cancer at that site and by the time they consult the melanoma is already advanced with a thick Breslow index [131]. It has been shown that only one third of patients with longitudinal melanonychia seek medical advice [125].

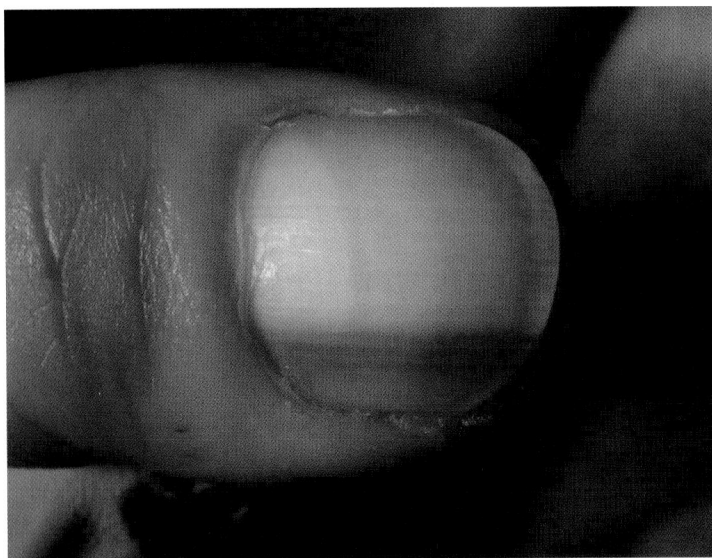

Figure 95.53 Narrow longitudinal melanonychia on a thumb. Dermoscopy showed loss of parallelism that prompted excisional biopsy. Histological examination revealed melanoma *in situ*.

Presentation

In three quarters of cases, melanoma of the nail apparatus starts in the matrix and presents as longitudinal melanonychia [132] (Figure 95.53). In the remainder, it arises from the nail bed and presents as a pigmented or amelanotic nodule, ulceration with bleeding, nail fold pigmentation, unexplained paronychia and/or partial destruction of the nail plate [133] (Figure 95.54).

Clinical variants

As many as 20–30% of melanomas of the nail apparatus are amelanotic [**125**]. Melanoma of the nail apparatus is even more treacherous when it manifests as isolated onychorrhexis [134] or as a fissure in the nail [135].

Hutchinson's sign describes the presence of pigment on the proximal, lateral or distal nail fold. It represents the radial growth

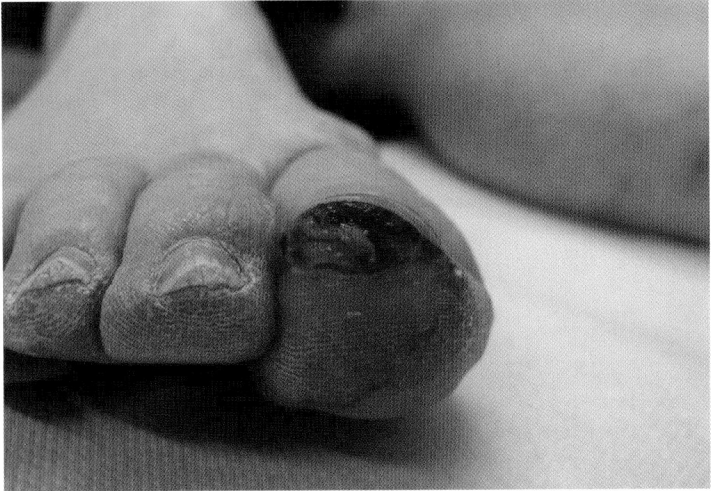

Figure 95.54 Friable granulation tissue under the plate of the great toenail in an old lady wearing sandals all year round. Pyogenic granuloma was suspected but histology revealed an amelanotic melanoma. (Courtesy of M. Caucanas, Toulouse, France.)

phase of subungual melanoma. Although this sign is highly suggestive of melanoma it is not pathognomonic.

Differential diagnosis

All causes of longitudinal melanonychia and tumours of the nail bed (squamous cell carcinoma, PG, etc.).

Complications and co-morbidities

Metastasis.

Disease course and prognosis

Survival rate for *in situ* melanoma is reported as 100%. The 5-year survival rate was 88% for a Breslow thickness of less than 2.5 mm but only 40% for a thickness greater than 2.5 mm [136].

Investigations

The dermoscopic pattern is well established (brown background with brown to black lines which are unevenly pigmented, irregularly spaced, of variable thickness and with or without interruption of parallelism) [137–139]. Some authors have performed matrix dermoscopy after nail avulsion and identified four dermoscopic patterns which showed high sensitivity and specificity [140]. The recent development of intraoperative reflection confocal microscopy examination of the nail matrix has enabled one-step surgical management [141].

Incisional biopsy is not recommended, as it does not allow complete histological examination of the pigmented lesion. Several excisional biopsy techniques are available [142,143]. Sentinel lymph node biopsy for melanomas of the nail apparatus greater than 1 mm in thickness is probably warranted but firm evidence of its benefit in this situation is lacking.

Management

Studies have demonstrated that amputation confers no survival advantage as long as the tumour is fully excised [125,143,144]. Only one study compared local excision to amputation in patients with melanoma of the nail apparatus. In this study of 62 patients with melanoma of the nail apparatus of mean thickness 1.68 mm, no significant differences in recurrence or survival rates were detected. Overall disease-free survival at 5 years was 92% [145].

Excision margins for melanoma of the nail apparatus remain controversial. Surgery poses a challenge because of the lack of surrounding soft tissue [146]. As the matrix is fixed to bone, it is difficult to achieve deep excision margins, without amputation or removal of a layer of bone [147]. Many publications report that treatment of *in situ* melanoma of the nail apparatus by *en bloc* removal of the nail unit with 5–10 mm margins followed by a full-thickness skin graft [146,148–152] results in excellent survival rates with optimal cosmetic and functional results. As there is no evidence that aggressive amputation is associated with higher survival rates, amputation should be aimed at retaining the greatest function possible [153].

Adjuvant systemic chemotherapy and isolated limb perfusion have been used, but no survival benefit has been demonstrated.

Treatment ladder

First line
- *In situ* melanoma of the nail apparatus: *en bloc* removal of the nail unit with 5–10 mm margins
- Invasive melanoma of the nail apparatus: amputation guided by a balance between tumour thickness and conservation of function

PERIONYCHIAL DISORDERS

Nail fold infections

Infections of the nail fold are represented by inflammation, swelling and abscess formation. They can be acute or chronic, isolated or associated with PG.

Synonyms and inclusions
- Onychia

Acute paronychia

Most patients are children and adolescents.

Acute paronychia is a common complaint usually due to staphylococcal infection, but herpes virus, orf virus and some fungi as well as pemphigus can cause acute paronychia. Cytology (Tzanck smear) may be useful in distinguishing non-bacterial from bacterial paronychia [1]. The latter may result from local injuries, a prick from a thorn in a lateral nail groove, a splinter, torn hangnails or nail biting, the two latter being the most common predisposing factors. It also occurs frequently as an episode during the course of chronic paronychia, when other organisms may be involved including streptococci, *Pseudomonas aeruginosa*, coliform organisms and *Proteus vulgaris*. Bacterial paronychia may also present as a subacute infection.

Acute paronychia presents as a painful red swelling of the lateral paronychial area (Figure 95.55). If superficial it may point close to the nail and can easily be drained by incision with a pointed (no. 11) scalpel without anaesthesia. Sometimes a bullous pyoderma brings to light a narrow sinus. This may be a part of a 'collar-stud' abscess that may communicate with a deeper necrotic inoculation zone. This must be laid open and excised. Deeper lesions should be treated with penicillinase-resistant antibiotics initially. If there is no clear sign of response within 2 days, surgical intervention under local anaesthesia is required, particularly in children. We recommend the removal of the proximal third of the nail plate cut transversally with nail-splitting scissors without initial incisional drainage. This gives more rapid relief and more sustained drainage. In associated subungual infection probing will determine the most painful area and provide an indication of where the nail plate should be cut away. Soaking the finger twice a day in an antiseptic solution such as chlorhexidine results in rapid healing.

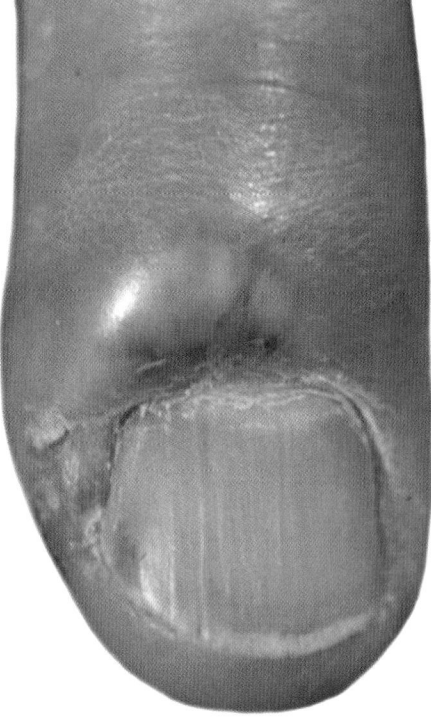

Figure 95.55 Acute bacterial paronychia (whitlow).

Complications of acute paronychia may include osteitis and amputation. Acquired periungual fibrokeratoma after staphylococcal paronychia has been reported [2].

As trauma and terminal phalanx fractures can mimic acute paronychia, radiography is advised when the latter occurs after trauma.

Herpetic paronychia

Synonyms and inclusions
- Herpetic whitlow

This uncommon condition appears mostly in children under 2 years old. It is due to primary inoculation of the herpes simplex virus from herpes stomatitis or herpes labialis and presents as single or grouped blisters close to the nail; it may give a honeycomb appearance. Clear at first, the blisters soon become purulent and may rupture and be replaced by crusts (Figure 95.56). The infection is usually very painful and takes about 3 weeks to resolve, with pain for half that time. Lymphangitis sometimes occurs and may precede vesiculation. Diagnosis may be established by recovering the virus from a recent blister and by cytological examination of the blister floor (Tzanck smear) [3]. Transmission to contacts may occur, explaining the appearance of herpetic whitlow in dental workers or nurses who do not wear gloves and come into contact with herpes labialis.

Treatment probably does little to shorten the course of the disorder, but cleaning with chlorhexidine followed by application of a bland cream is recommended. Relapse may occur as with other primary herpetic infections. Long-term treatment with thymidine analogues, such as oral aciclovir, famciclovir and valaciclovir, may be useful if recurrences are frequent.

PART 8: SPECIFIC CUTANEOUS STRUCTURE

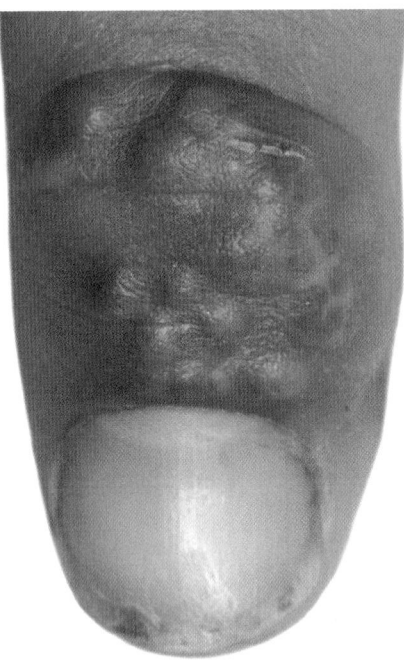

Figure 95.56 Herpetic whitlow.

Numbness of the finger has been reported following infection, as well as persistent lymphoedema. Herpetic paronychia may cause complete destruction of the nail, bacterial superinfection and systemic spread that may cause meningitis [4]. Longstanding cases, particularly in patients with HIV infection, may have an atypical, often verrucous appearance.

Orf paronychia

Orf virus has been reported in subjects who have had a history of contact with animals.

Erythema multiforme secondary to viral infections

In this condition, erythema and oedema of the proximal nail fold often occur. It can be observed in patients with paronychial infection caused by orf or herpes viruses [5].

Paronychia of the great toe of infants

Undersized infant jumpsuits can be responsible for paronychia of the great toe. The undersized garments most probably produce primary trauma with subsequent infection or possible focal ischaemia, increasing the risks of infection after minor trauma [6].

Chronic paronychia

Chronic paronychia is an inflammatory dermatosis of the nail folds which causes retraction of the periungual tissues with resultant secondary effects on the nail matrix, nail growth and soft-tissue attachments (Figure 95.57a–c). It may be associated with infection secondary to an underlying chronic dermatosis, for instance an irritant contact dermatitis from wet work or exposure to caustic materials. Alternatively, it may be secondary to atopic eczema or psoriasis, where minor provocation can result in active disease [7].

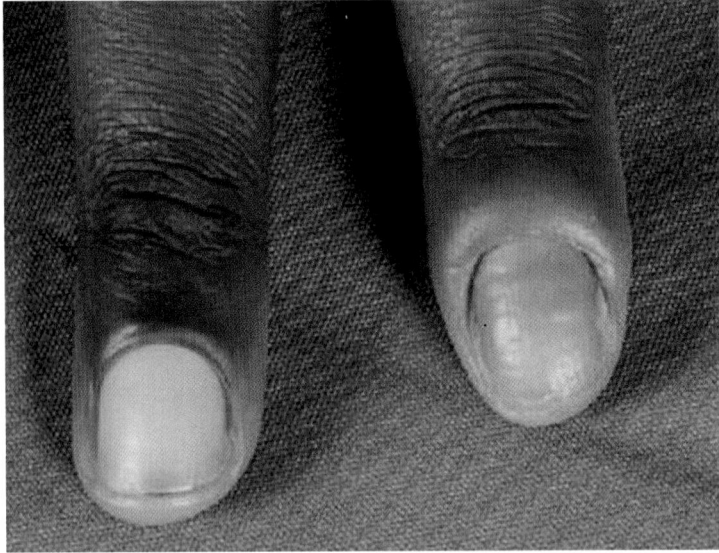

(a)

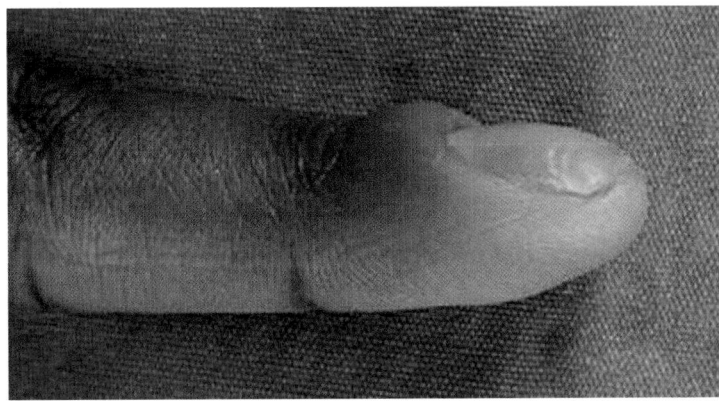

(b)

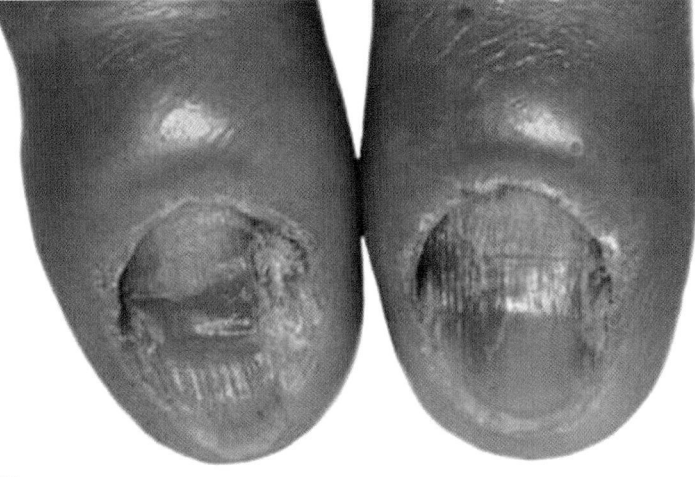

(c)

Figure 95.57 (a–c) Chronic paronychia: paronychial swelling, loss of cuticle and mildly dystrophic nail in early disease (a,b); severe nail dystrophy in more advanced disease (c).

Cold wet hands are predisposed to chronic paronychia. Handling of wet foods represents a particular hazard, as these often combine several predisposing factors including wet working conditions, a cold environment and irritation from the food itself. Chronic paronychia is predominantly a disease of domestic and catering workers, bar staff and fishmongers. The majority of cases are in patients of working age, although it is also seen in children, especially as a result of finger or thumb sucking.

Any finger may be involved, although it is most frequently the index and middle fingers of the right hand and the middle finger of the left. These fingers may be more subject to minor trauma than the others. The condition begins as a slight erythematous swelling of the paronychial tissues. It may be painless but, if tender, is much less so than in acute paronychia, except when pressed. The cuticle is lost and pus may form below the nail fold. Inflammation adjacent to the nail matrix disturbs nail growth, resulting in irregular transverse ridges and other surface irregularities, which may be combined with discoloration.

There is some evidence that the darkening of the lateral edges of the nail plate may be due to the pigment of *Candida* spp. though it is sometimes associated with *Pseudomonas* infection of the nail [8]. The lateral discoloured edges of the nail plate become cross-ridged when the disease mainly affects the lateral nail fold. Repeated acute exacerbations produce numerous irregular transverse ridges or waves on the nail surface, which often becomes rough. Yeast fungi may cause chronic or acute paronychia. *Candida* paronychia can be observed in children who have oral candidosis or a habit of thumb sucking. *Neoscytalidium dimidiatum* may also produce darkening of the lateral edges of the nail plate; by contrast, paronychia due to moulds such as *Fusarium* spp. is often associated with proximal leukonychia. Dermatophytic paronychia is rare.

In longstanding cases, the size of the nail may be reduced, and this reduction is exaggerated by the bolstering of the fold all around the nail. Most of the nail deformity is due to inflammation, which interferes with the formation of the nail, but a true *Candida* infection of the nail plate is occasionally seen, especially in patients with immunodeficiency.

Much of the chronic inflammation seen in this disorder probably arises from an irritant reaction to material sequestered beneath the proximal nail fold. The loss of the cuticle means that detergent and other solvents may gain access to this tight space and act like a prolonged irritant patch test. Acute exacerbations occur from time to time and are due to secondary bacterial infection. Various organisms may be found, including *Staphylococcus aureus* or *Staph. epidermidis*, *Proteus vulgaris*, *Escherichia coli* and *Pseudomonas aeruginosa*.

Besides this most common type of chronic paronychia, a long list of causes of paronychia is provided (see Table 95.5 online at www.rooksdermatology.com).

Management

Treatment is a combination of avoidance of precipitants, hand care and medication. Perhaps the most important part of the treatment, but the one most difficult to achieve, is keeping the hands dry. Patients involved in wet work should be advised to wear cotton gloves under rubber or plastic gloves and avoid manicure of the proximal nail fold. General hand care with emollients and protection from trauma and irritants is helpful. If these precautions are not followed, the condition is unlikely to settle whatever medical treatment is given.

Topical therapy requires a combination of steroid and antimicrobial. A potent steroid may be used for short periods if there is adequate antimicrobial cover. Injected triamcinolone (2.5 mg/mL)

is very useful. Topical imidazoles are usually sufficient to treat *Candida* and may provide modest activity against some bacteria. More potent topical antibacterials may occasionally be needed. Twice a day application of Dakin solution (sodium hypochlorite) is very effective against *Pseudomonas* infection.

When significant nail dystrophy ensues and medical therapy has been unsuccessful, chronic paronychia can be treated surgically with good results and resolution of the dystrophic nail. In patients who experience repeated acute flares associated with chronic paronychia, additional removal of the base of the nail plate is useful.

Primary syphilis on the finger

The finger accounts for 5–14% of extragenital primary syphilitic chancres. It may present as a deep painful horseshoe-shaped whitlow with diffuse induration of paronychial tissues and associated regional lymphadenopathy. Pain and tenderness of the fingertips with swelling and serous discharge may also be observed [9].

Periungual toe infections in neutropenic patients

In neutropenic patients with haematological or solid-organ malignancy, the most common causes of paronychia with cellulitis of the toe are *Fusarium* and, less frequently, *Aspergillus*. The key to successful management is early removal of the infected nail for diagnosis and institution of appropriate therapy [10].

Subungual abscess

In this uncommon form of nail infection, pockets of pus form directly beneath the nail plate without coexisting paronychia (Figure 95.58). There is a yellow discoloration of the nail and onycholysis may affect the distal third of the nail. The severe throbbing pain is similar to that associated with a subungual haematoma and is caused by pressure.

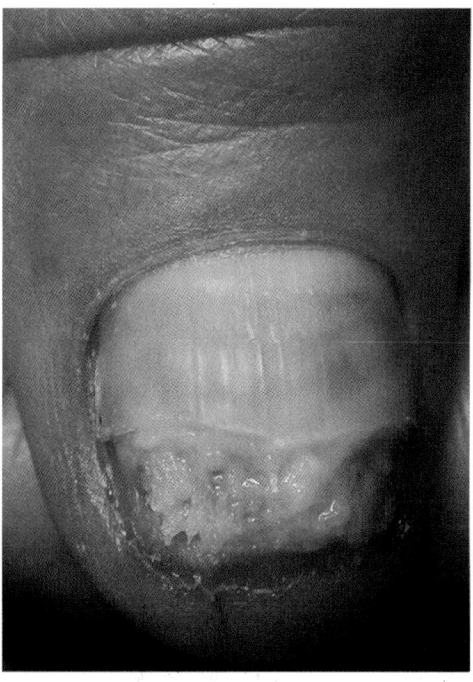

Figure 95.58 Subungual abscess in neutropenic patient receiving cancer chemotherapy. (Courtesy of B. Fouilloux, France.)

The treatment is simple: a red hot wire (e.g. from a heated paper clip) applied to the nail allows release of the pus and bacterial culture. Partial avulsion of the abnormal nail area allows the nail bed to be treated with chlorhexidine, mupirocin or fusidic acid [11].

Other disorders of the perionychium

Drug-induced paronychia

Paronychia may be caused by certain drugs such as isotretinoin and can involve multiple digits [1].

Periungual tissues subject to trauma – onychotillomania

Hangnails are small portions of the horny epidermis that have split away from the lateral nail fold. They are often triangular in shape, with a hard pointed distal end and an adherent base (Figure 95.59). Hangnails are common in people who handle irritants or who work primarily with their hands. Inflammation is usually present causing pain, particularly if the hangnails are interfered with (onychotillomania). Attempts to remove them may be complicated by acute or chronic paronychia. In addition to classical hangnails, scaling of the nail folds with scattered small haemorrhages and focal erosions or necrosis may be observed, typically involving the toes. Hangnails should be snipped off using sharp-pointed scissors. Mupirocin or fusidic acid ointment may prevent or clear low-grade infection.

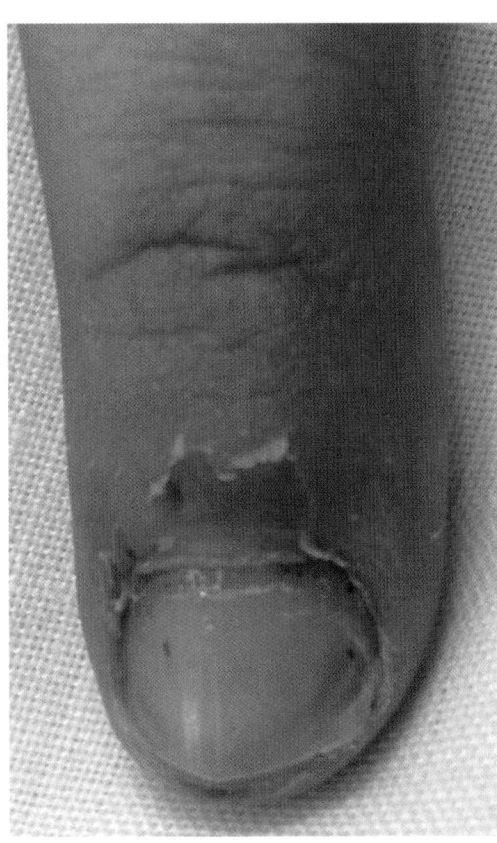

Figure 95.59 Hangnail.

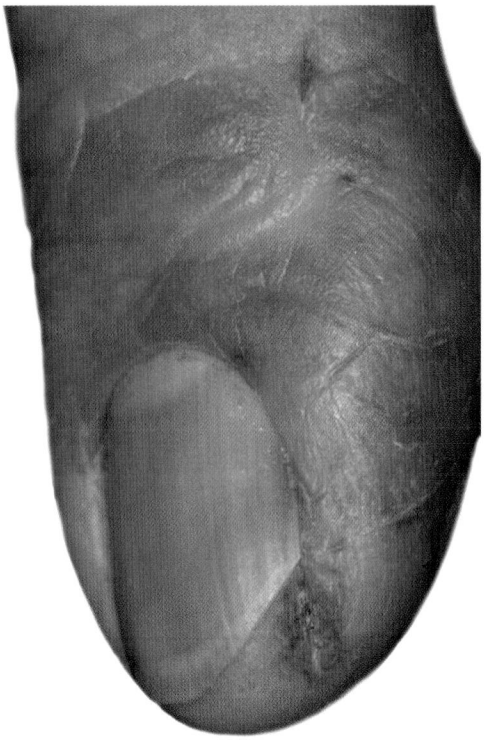

Figure 95.60 Painful dorsolateral fissure of the fingertip.

Painful dorsolateral fissure of the fingertip

This condition is not uncommon and occurs particularly in manual workers involved in wet work or in contact with irritants or solvents; it is also seen in patients receiving chemotherapy or targeted therapies where the fissures, often painful, are associated with xerosis and become infected [12]. Interestingly, the fissures are distal to and in line with the lateral nail groove (Figure 95.60). The discomfort experienced by the subjects may render many subtle tasks difficult and even impossible. There appears to be no anatomical basis for the site of fissure, though it could reflect some structural weakness distal to the lateral nail grooves.

Hypertrophy of the lateral nail fold

This condition is usually the result of longstanding ingrown nails in adults. Inflammation may range from the subclinical to severe. It is also seen as a congenital condition appearing as overgrowths of the lateral nail folds of both halluces shortly after birth. Hypertrophy of the lateral nail fold resolves spontaneously during the first year of life [13].

DERMATOSES AFFECTING THE NAILS

Nail psoriasis (see also Chapter 35)

Psoriasis is probably the most common disorder affecting fingernails, with consequent dystrophy. Between 1.5 and 3% of the population have psoriasis, and up to 50% of psoriatics have nail involvement [1]: over a lifetime, this proportion may cumulatively increase to 80–90% [2]. De Jong *et al*. [3] reported that 93% of people with nail psoriasis considered it a significant cosmetic handicap, 58% found that it interfered with their job and 52% described pain as a symptom.

In children with psoriasis, the reported prevalence of nail involvement ranges from 7% [4] to 39% [5]; pitting has been observed in the first week of life of a neonate whose mother had severe psoriasis [6].

Psoriatic nail changes are prominent in childhood nail disease, parakeratosis pustulosa: approximately one third of affected children will develop manifest psoriasis over time, a smaller fraction will have variants of eczema and half of the total will get better [7].

Pathophysiology

Nail unit psoriasis is a localized form of the process active elsewhere in the body and the features represent a combination of local skin changes and secondary effects on nail plate growth. The occlusion of the nail bed by the nail plate means that scale produced by the latter cannot be shed in the normal way, resulting in subungual hyperkeratosis, loss of nail plate adhesion (onycholysis) and oil spots: the latter are thought to arise from a combination of focal onycholysis and exudation.

High-resolution MRI illustrates the close relationship between the soft-tissue attachments of the distal interphalangeal joint and the proximal element of the nail unit. Consequently, inflammation of the joint seen in psoriatic arthritis has a close association with inflammation of the nail matrix. The extensor tendon of this joint is the main relevant soft-tissue attachment in this area and its inflammation is termed an enthesopathy. There is good evidence of a correlation between the presence of an enthesopathy and changes in the nearby nail [8,9].

Clinical features

In order of reducing frequency, nail signs of psoriasis include pits, onycholysis, subungual hyperkeratosis, nail plate discoloration, uneven nail surface, splinter haemorrhages, acute and chronic paronychia, and transverse midline depressions in the thumbnails [10]. These features can be recorded using the Nail Psoriasis Severity Index (NAPSI), an instrument for precise documentation of nail abnormalities for use in trials and, more generally, for assessing response to interventions [11]. An alternative instrument is Baran's Nail Psoriasis Severity Index, which has been validated by a Polish team [12,13].

Pits

Pits more commonly affect fingers than toes (Figure 95.61). They represent punctate surface depressions arising from proximal matrix disease (Table 95.6). Zaias [1,14] has demonstrated small columns of pathological parakeratotic nail falling off the upper surface of the nail plate to produce a pit. Some authorities advocate nail plate histology as a means of diagnosing nail psoriasis [15]. This can be useful for the exclusion of fungal infection, although the specificity of nail plate changes in psoriasis is yet to be established. The origin of pits means that they can be influenced by disease in the proximal nail fold and it is thought that injection of triamcinolone into the nail fold alone can suppress this clinical

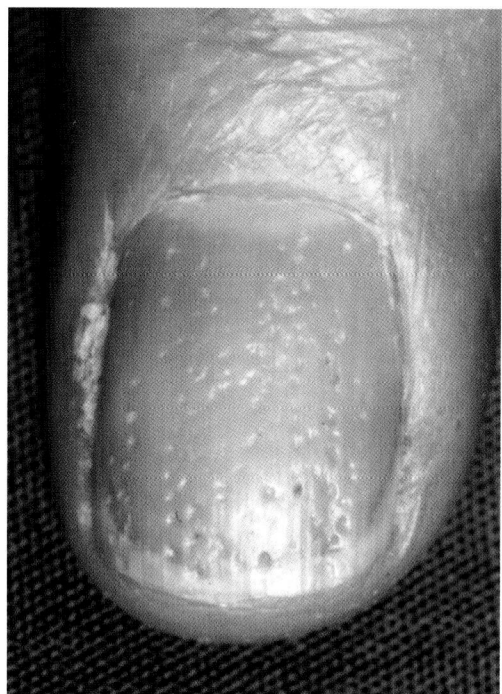

Figure 95.61 Psoriasis: pitting.

feature. The pattern of pitting may be disorganized or occur in transverse/longitudinal rows as seen in alopecia areata [2]. Pits may be shallow or large [14], to the point of leaving a punched-out hole in the nail plate (elkonyxis).

Onycholysis

Focal nail bed parakeratosis produces an 'oil spot' or 'salmon patch'. Extension of this area to the free edge results in onycholysis, which typically has a reddish-brown proximal margin

Table 95.6 Relationship between clinical features and site of disease activity in psoriasis of the nail. (From Zaias [1].)

Clinical feature	Area of disease	Duration of disease
Changes in nail plate	*Matrix*	
Pits	Proximal matrix	Episodic: short
Transverse furrows	Proximal matrix; distal extension depends on depth of furrow	1–2 weeks
Crumbling nail plate	Entire matrix	Prolonged
Leukonychia with rough surface	Proximal matrix; leukonychia may involve distal matrix	Variable
Changes in nail bed and hyponychium	*Nail bed*	
Splinter haemorrhages	Nail bed dermal ridge haemorrhage	Short
Oily spot/onycholysis	Nail bed psoriasis	Prolonged
False nail following onychomadesis	Nail bed psoriasis	Prolonged
Subungual hyperkeratosis	Nail bed psoriasis	Prolonged
Yellow/green discoloration of nail bed	Secondary infection by yeasts or *Pseudomonas*	Prolonged

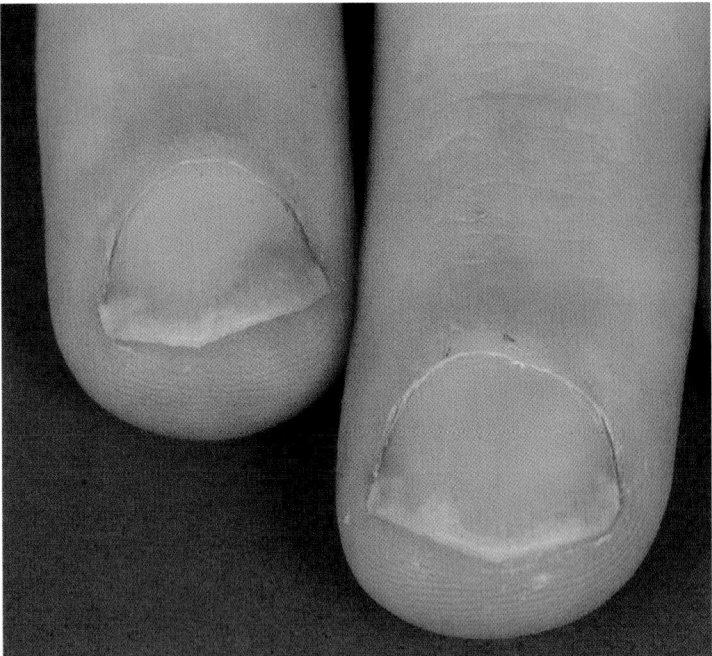

Figure 95.62 Psoriasis: salmon patches progressing to onycholysis.

(Figure 95.62). Alternatively, onycholysis may commence at the distal edge (Figure 95.63), representing disruption of the onychocorneal band [16]. Once this band of firm attachment has been breached, the process is often progressive. Minor manicure, wet work and leverage from long nails exacerbate the problem.

Discoloration

Discoloration in psoriasis is multifactorial. The major factors are nail thickening and subungual hyperkeratosis. Both of these contribute to a yellow appearance, particularly common in the toenails. It is possible that repeated trauma at this site elicits the isomorphic reaction, with local exacerbation of psoriasis. The coincidence of onychomycosis and psoriasis is also commoner in the toenails [17] and can modify the clinical appearances. *Candida* spp. and *Pseudomonas* infection can result in green discoloration.

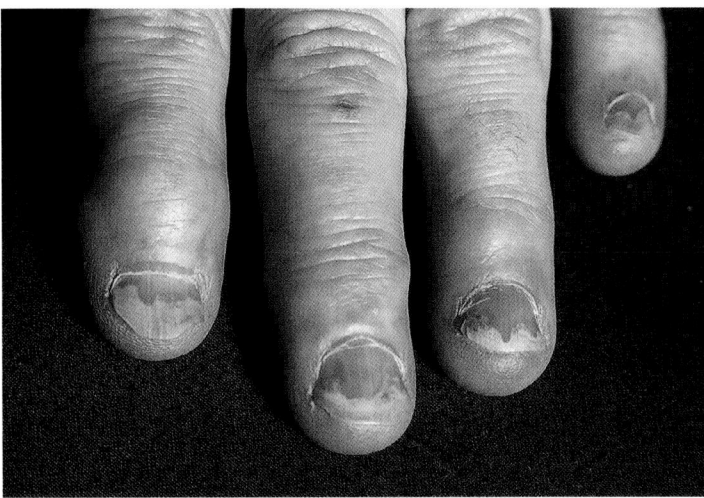

Figure 95.63 Psoriasis: distal onycholysis.

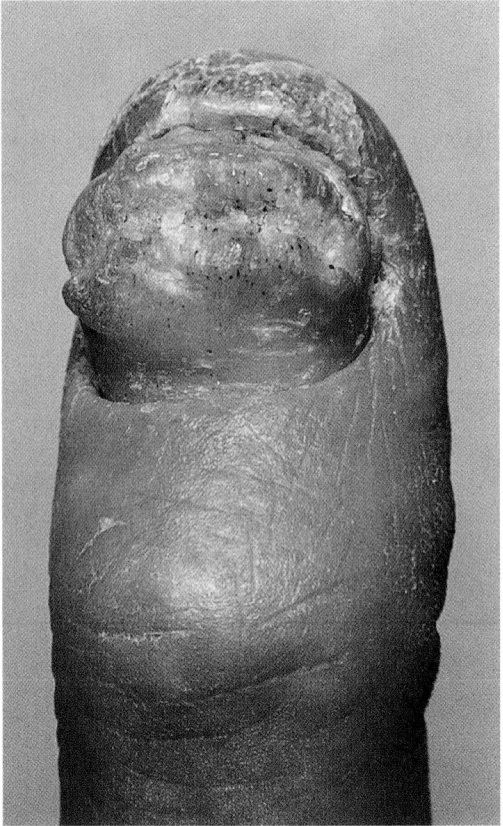

Figure 95.64 Psoriasis: subungual hyperkeratosis.

While non-dermatophytes and bacteria are common, dermatophyte infection is rare [1].

Subungual hyperkeratosis

Subungual hyperkeratosis represents nail bed disease (Figure 95.64). Substantial nail plate thickening may result: it is most marked distally and extends proximally. The fingertip may become very tender where there is gross thickening, as the nail plate attachment is greatly reduced and the nail can easily be caught and tug on the matrix attachment. Subungual hyperkeratosis is a prominent feature of pityriasis rubra pilaris affecting the nails and is often associated with splinter haemorrhages [17,18].

Nail plate abnormalities

Splits, atrophy and fragility may be seen. The nail may also thicken, independently of subungual hyperkeratosis. Transverse midline depressions resembling the nail changes seen in 'washboard nails' [19] are also seen. The latter are normally attributed to the habit tic of disrupting the cuticle (Figure 95.65) and although this may play a part in psoriasis, it appears that there is a lower threshold for their development in the presence of psoriasis.

Splinter haemorrhages

Splinter haemorrhages are seen in the nail bed of 42% of fingernails and 6% of toenails [20]. This may be due to the increased capillary prominence and fragility in nail bed dermis in psoriasis and to the presence of dystrophy. Where transverse overcurvature occurs for reasons other than psoriasis, splinter haemorrhages are also common, suggesting that mechanical factors may be important.

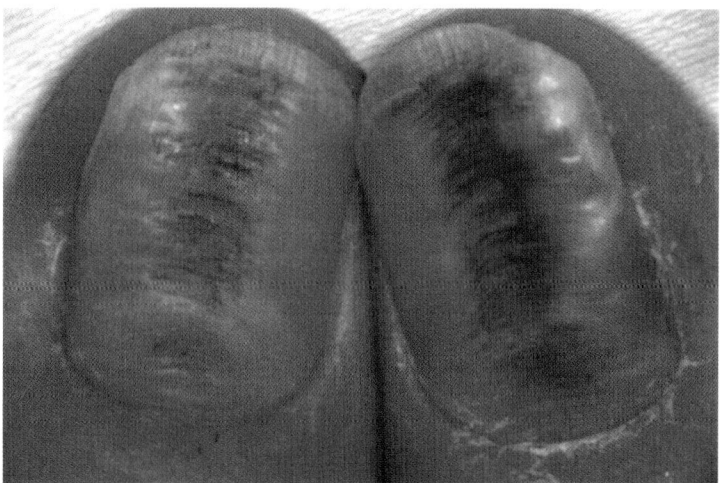

Figure 95.65 Multiple transverse grooves of the thumbnails.

Subacute and chronic paronychia

Periungual involvement may be dramatic and inflammatory, giving rise to gross disruption of the nail matrix. Loss of the nail may follow, with scaling of the nail bed or a deep transverse furrow. Chronic psoriatic paronychia causes loss of the cuticle. The nail plate can become thin [21], although this may be offset by matrix disease, which can result in thickened nail. The nail fold may be scaly, as in psoriasis elsewhere.

Acropustulosis

This form of psoriasis involves destructive pustulation of the nail unit. It may present as a component of pustular psoriasis, palmoplantar pustulosis [22], acrodermatitis continua of Hallopeau or, on isolated digits, as parakeratosis pustulosa [23], which is seen typically in young girls. The nail plate may be lifted off by sterile pustules in the nail bed and matrix (Figure 95.66). There is associated erythema and discomfort of the end of the digit. There may be long-term nail loss, except in parakeratosis pustulosa, which usually resolves spontaneously.

Parakeratosis pustulosa may affect only part of one digit. There is pitting and ridging combined with fine scaling erythema of the periunguium and only very rarely pustules. It is usually interpreted as a form of psoriasis [6], although it shares histological features with eczema [23], and some consider it a variant of eczema [24].

Acrodermatitis continua of Hallopeau (see Chapter 35) can be very aggressive and result in resorptive osteolysis [25] or loss of the toes and distal parts of the fingers [26]. In a study of 20 patients with the condition, seven were male and 13 female, with a mean age of 46 years, and all had involvement of only one digit, with no features of psoriasis elsewhere [27]. Clinical experience suggests that occurrence on multiple digits is also a common pattern.

Differential diagnosis

When the diagnosis of psoriatic nail dystrophy is in doubt, the main differential diagnoses are onychomycosis and lichen planus, and less commonly eczema or reactive arthritis (Reiter syndrome) where pitting may be seen [28]. Onychomycosis more commonly affects the toenails, whereas the fingernails are more commonly involved in psoriasis. Equally, there are often changes on the nail surface

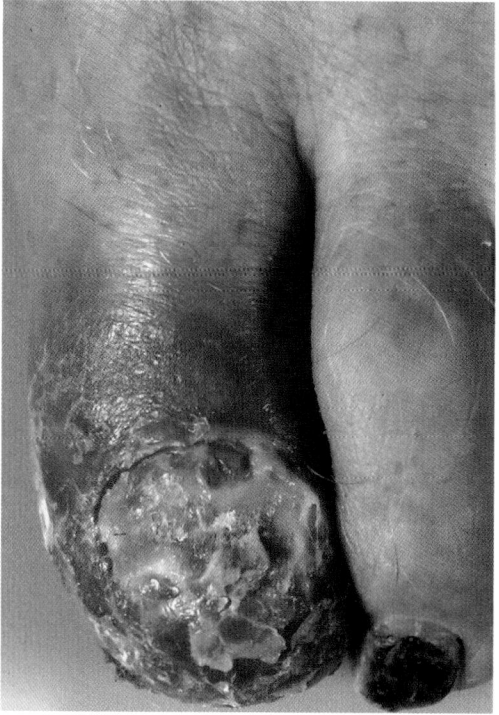

Figure 95.66 Acropustulosis: nail plate has been destroyed by intense pustular inflammation.

alone in psoriasis, whereas in onychomycosis there are usually visible abnormalities within or beneath the nail plate. Onychomycosis of the fingernails tends to involve only one or a minority of digits, in contrast with psoriasis where multiple digits are often affected.

Some forms of fingernail lichen planus are very difficult to distinguish from psoriasis. Both may result in roughened nails (trachyonychia) with subungual hyperkeratosis. If pits are prominent the diagnosis of psoriasis can be made, but if they are subtle and difficult to distinguish from other surface changes, they may be part of lichen planus. The nails in reactive arthritis and pityriasis rubra pilaris can also be difficult to differentiate from psoriasis [29], where distal subungual hyperkeratosis and splinter haemorrhages are common [8]. Aggressive forms of atypical nail psoriasis presenting in later life may represent acrokeratosis paraneoplastica of Bazex (see Chapter 147). The patient is usually male, with subungual hyperkeratosis and scaling of the periunguium, ears and nose associated with malignancies of the upper gastrointestinal or respiratory tract [30–32].

Arthritis of the distal interphalangeal joint suggests a psoriatic cause of any associated dystrophy [33], with the exception of changes due to a myxoid pseudocyst associated with adjacent osteoarthritis. Baker *et al.* [34] found that there was no strict relationship between which joints are arthritic and which nails are dystrophic, although Jones *et al.* [35] noted that in a group of 100 psoriasis patients with arthritis and nail involvement there was a significantly greater chance of joint disease in the adjacent distal interphalangeal joint. There was also a significant correlation between the PASI (Psoriasis Area and Severity Index) score and the NAPSI score, and between the latter and duration of psoriasis. A variant of nail psoriasis presents with pain and soft-tissue swelling of the distal digit associated with psoriatic nail changes and underlying bone erosion and periosteal reaction. This can develop in the absence of joint involvement and has been given the unwieldy term 'psoriatic onychopachy-dermoperiostitis' [36].

Histopathology

Histopathology varies according to the clinical focus of the disease [1,37]. The matrix and nail bed develop a granular layer. Conversely, the hyponychium, where a granular layer is normally present, no longer has one [1]. Where there is subungual hyperkeratosis, there are mounds of parakeratotic keratinocytes beneath the nail plate. Neutrophils may be found throughout these mounds and Munro microabscesses may form. Similar features are seen in acrodermatitis continua of Hallopeau [25]. Amorphous material interpreted as glycoprotein may accumulate within the keratotic mass [1]. Acanthosis and elongation of the rete ridges is present, with increased dilatation and tortuosity of the capillaries of the dermal papillae. Where the nail is lost, the nail bed may form a false nail of compacted hyperkeratosis [38]. The matrix can become quiescent, which can be demonstrated immunohistochemically by the absence of synthesis of the hard keratin 31, which is normally a major constituent of the nail [39].

The nail plate may show faults, clinically manifest as transverse splits and pits, which are lined with parakeratotic cells. These probably originate from the most proximal part of the matrix, or the ventral aspect of the proximal nail fold [1].

Management [40–43]

General hand care is important to avoid provocation of the isomorphic (Koebner) response, whereby minor trauma may elicit psoriasis. These measures include avoiding manicure, keeping the nails short, wearing gloves for wet work and heavy or greasy manual work, avoiding direct exposure to solvents and encouraging emollient usage. Concealment with nail lacquer is a reasonable approach to milder forms of psoriasis, and surface irregularities can be smoothed by the use of nail gel. This is a polymer, applied by a beautician and hardened by exposure to a table-top UVA source. The gel can then be shaped and buffed. Gel or other forms of sculptured or adherent artificial nails have the potential for aggravating onycholysis and are not usually recommended if this is a prominent feature.

Active treatments are mainly directed at the more dystrophic forms of nail involvement and may sometimes help with onycholysis. Often the focus of therapy is the proximal nail fold, where active psoriasis is disturbing the underlying matrix and lack of cuticle is promoting chronic paronychia. Medical treatments include the following.

Local steroids. Clobetasol propionate ointment may be used without occlusion, rubbed into the nail fold. Duration of treatment is limited by local atrophy. It is useful for psoriatic paronychia where there are secondary nail plate changes. Onycholysis may benefit if the nail is clipped back to the point of nail plate attachment and the nail bed treated topically. *Candida* is a frequent colonizer of this space and warrants treatment at the same time. Triamcinolone acetonide may be used by injection into the nail fold or nail bed with regional or digital ring block. Using 0.1 mL injections of 10 mg/mL

triamcinolone acetonide at matrix and nail bed sites on no more than two or three occasions, de Berker and Lawrence reported a good response in subungual hyperkeratosis, nail plate thickening and ridging [44]. However, onycholysis and pitting improved in only 50% of nails. Alternative regimens employ more dilute triamcinolone (2.5–5 mg/mL) and are routinely used more than two or three times per digit, infiltrating the proximal nail fold alone and making a ring block optional. The Dermojet® may also be used to inject corticosteroid directly into the skin of the nail fold under pressure but there are risks of blood splash back and, in one report, of bone damage.

Topical vitamin D analogues. Calcipotriol can be useful where there is subungual hyperkeratosis and nail thickening [45]. It has also been used in combination with topical steroid on an alternating basis (a.m./p.m.) [46] and it is can be used as a combined steroid and calcipotriol ointment or gel. Calcipotriol has the advantage of avoiding the risk of atrophy with long-term use when used without combined steroid, but it is not as effective at treating the nail fold inflammation and consequent changes in proximal matrix function, which manifest as ridging and pitting.

Maintenance treatment with calcipotriol may also be one of the most effective topical therapies for pustular nail psoriasis [47].

Photochemotherapy. Nails may improve in response to general psoralen and UVA (PUVA) therapy or with local PUVA to the nail unit. The latter can be administered using either topical or systemic psoralen. Specially designed high-dose UVA handsets have been advocated. Eighteen of 26 patients showed a greater than 50% improvement in nail changes following whole-body PUVA, although pitting was unresponsive [48]. Four of five patients improved with local therapy: onycholysis was more responsive than pitting, but one patient with severe pitting showed improvement [49].

Retinoids. The nail plate is thinned by acitretin. This reduces subungual hyperkeratosis and good clinical results have been reported [50,51]. Pustulation may be improved. Topical tazarotene 0.1% gel can be helpful for onycholysis and pitting when applied under occlusion [52].

Others. A Cochrane review of therapies for nail psoriasis concluded that quality of data was in general poor and that, although the systemic agents including biological agents appeared to be beneficial, the length of follow-up was insufficient to provide adequate safety data [53]. Systemic methotrexate and ciclosporin may both help the nail unit but would not usually be advocated as therapy for nail disease alone [52,54]. Biological agents can also be effective, although they are usually given in the context of severe disease elsewhere [55–57]. Paradoxically, there are reports of psoriasis precipitated by biological agents given for rheumatological diseases [58]. Acrodermatitis continua of Hallopeau and psoriatic onychopachydermoperiostitis [59] may cause sufficient distress to warrant systemic therapy in the absence of disease elsewhere: they may respond to methotrexate.

There is very anecdotal evidence of benefit from topical ciclosporin [60] and from topical 1% 5-fluorouracil 1% in either 20%

urea [61] or in propylene glycol [62]. Pitting and subungual hyperkeratosis were thought to respond well to the urea formulation. 5-fluorouracil should not be used in the presence of onycholysis. Superficial radiotherapy [63] and electron beam therapy [64] have been shown to be of only temporary benefit and are not usually recommended. Treatment of coincident fungal infection may provide clinical benefit, although it is seldom a dermatophyte and positive cultures may merely represent colonization.

Darier disease of the nails [1,2,3–5]
(see Chapter 66)

Nail involvement is common in Darier disease; 96% of patients are reported to have acral changes of which nail changes are the most common [2]. These include red and/or white longitudinal streaks in the nail, often terminating in a V-shaped nick (Figure 95.67). The streak may represent a zone of fragile or thinned nail, which makes it prone to fragmentation at the tip with the consequent nick. In severe cases, the nails are almost lost by extension of the fragmentation process to involve the entire matrix. Subungual hyperkeratotic papules can be found in the hyponychium. Histologically, matrix and nail bed changes resemble the acantholysis seen in involved skin, with the addition of multinucleate giant cells and epithelial hyperplasia in the nail bed [5]. These histological features make it possible to diagnose Darier disease when it is confined to the nail [1]. Excess ridging and a rough nail surface may also be found, as may total leukonychia. Occasionally, marked thickening of the nail plate occurs. It is probable that the nail is sometimes affected in the absence of disease elsewhere [1].

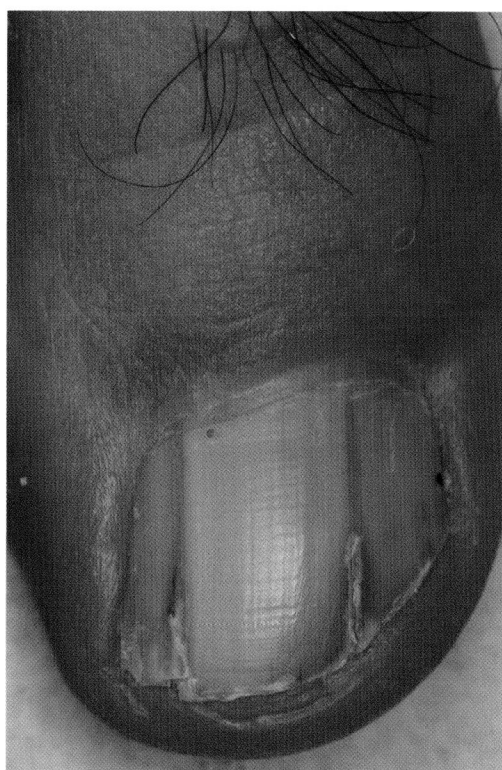

Figure 95.67 Darier disease: white and red longitudinal lines and distal notching.

Hailey–Hailey disease has some histological similarities and may also present with longitudinal white streaks [2]. However, the disease does not have the same destructive effect and is not associated with hyperkeratoses or pain and loss of function associated with the nail splits and disintegration sometimes seen in Darier disease.

A case of squamous cell carcinoma developing in a nail bed with chronic changes of Darier disease has been reported [6]. Pain or conspicuous uncharacteristic features in a nail apparatus affected by Darier disease may therefore be indications for biopsy.

Eczema involving the nails

Nail changes in eczema may be seen in the context of eczema elsewhere, with hand eczema, or as an isolated finding with periungual and subungual features. Endogenous and exogenous factors may contribute. The nail changes may reflect this division, in that they may be in response to a systemic atopic disposition, with pitting in the absence of inflammation, or may demonstrate the effects of local eczema in the nail unit influencing nail formation.

The common allergens such as nickel, fragrance and medicaments rarely have particular bearing on nail abnormalities. However, rubber, chrome and irritant dermatitis are significant factors in hand dermatitis. These materials, and hand dermatitis in general, are associated with particular occupations. Selective exposure to such allergens or strong irritants is as important as chronic low-grade irritation from milder irritants such as water and detergents seen in catering workers. High concentrations of and prolonged exposure to allergens and irritants can result from sequestration beneath the free edge of the nail.

Cyanoacrylates used in prosthetic nails can provoke local and distant allergic reactions. Formaldehyde, occasionally used as a nail hardener, can provoke painful onycholysis if the patient becomes sensitized, or sometimes when acting solely as an irritant. Some allergens may cause nail dystrophy without associated inflammation.

A combination of atopy and an exogenous irritant or allergic contact reaction is common.

Clinical features
Nail matrix disturbance is reflected in thickening, pits, nail loss, transverse ridges, Beau's lines and furrows in a pattern similar to psoriatic nail disease [1] (Table 95.7).

Nail bed disease can manifest as subungual hyperkeratosis, splinter haemorrhages, onycholysis or pain.

Nail changes may betray eczema elsewhere and the nails may be buffed smooth and shiny, indicating their use as a tool for rubbing.

Associated hand dermatitis may show vesicles, scaling, erythema, cracks and swollen fingers, although the presence of vesicles will not always distinguish the condition from psoriasis, which should be sought at other sites. The distribution on the hand or foot may give some clues as to possible local causes, such as gloves, shoes, prosthetic nails or nail varnish. Hands and feet should always be examined together, as the presence of disease in both diminishes the likelihood of a contact dermatitis. Associated disease can present as periorbital eczema in contact allergy to nail

Table 95.7 Differential diagnosis between four common nail disorders: fungal infections, psoriasis, chronic paronychia and dermatitis.

	Fungal infections	Psoriasis	Chronic paronychia	Dermatitis
Colour	Often yellow or brown; part or whole of nail	May be normal or yellow or brown	Edge of nail often discoloured brown or black	May be normal
Onycholysis	Frequent	Frequent	Usually absent	Confined to tip or absent
Pitting	Infrequent	Often present and fine	Uncommon	Coarse pits frequent
Filaments or spores in potash preparations	Filaments, usually abundant	Absent	May be spores in edge of nail; filaments and spores in scrapings from nail fold	Absent
Cross-ridging	Absent	Uncommon	Frequent	Frequent
Other	Associated fungal infections elsewhere	Associated psoriasis elsewhere or family history of psoriasis	Predominantly women; wet work and cold hands cause predisposition	Recent history of dermatitis on hands

cosmetics [2], though often there may be no evidence of inflammation on or around the nails themselves.

Defining the presence of atopy or patch testing can be useful even in the absence of active eczema as subungual hyperkeratosis and discomfort may be disproportionate to the cutaneous features [3].

Management

General hand care is important, with the avoidance of soap, irritants, wet work and any identified cause. Protective gloves should be used, with copious emollient application. Barrier creams are not usually adequate protection once features have developed. Potent topical steroids may be needed, sometimes with additional topical or systemic antimicrobial therapy. These should be rubbed in around the nail folds. In the young, steroids may precipitate premature closure of the phalangeal epiphyses if too potent or used for too long [4]. Osteomyelitis has also been reported in children using potent topical steroids in this area.

Hand or foot PUVA can help.

Lichen planus of the nails and related conditions (see also Chapter 37)

Nails are involved in about 10% of cases of disseminated lichen planus [1]. In a study of 24 adults with nail lichen planus, nail changes were the sole manifestation of the disease in 75% [2,3], and the proportion may be higher in children (Figure 95.68) [4,5], in whom lichen planus of all types is rare. This suggests only a modest degree of overlap between the disease process in the nail unit and at other sites. Although the skin lesions may itch intensely, nail disease may be relatively asymptomatic except when nails are shed.

Clinical features

The disease can involve the proximal nail folds with bluish-red discoloration. Nail plate changes include thinning or thickening, onychorrhexis, brittleness, crumbling or fragmentation, and accentuation of surface longitudinal ridging. All these features are secondary to disease affecting the matrix, which can also produce transient or permanent longitudinal melanonychia [6], longitudinal erythronychia [7] or leukonychia as a post-inflammatory phenomenon (Figure 95.69). When inflammation is intense and

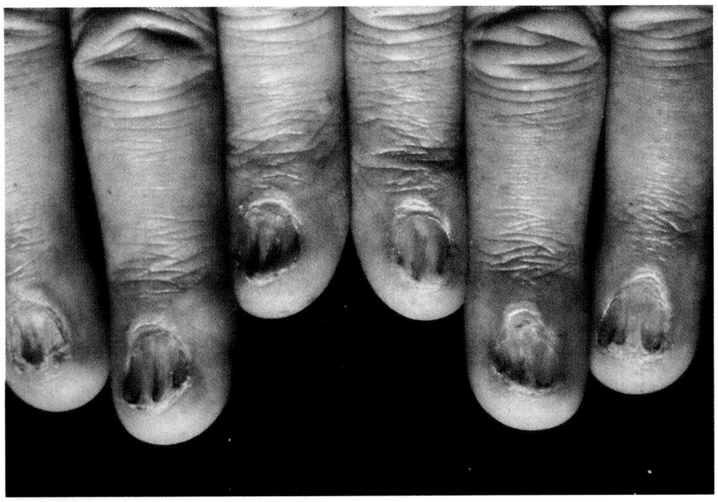

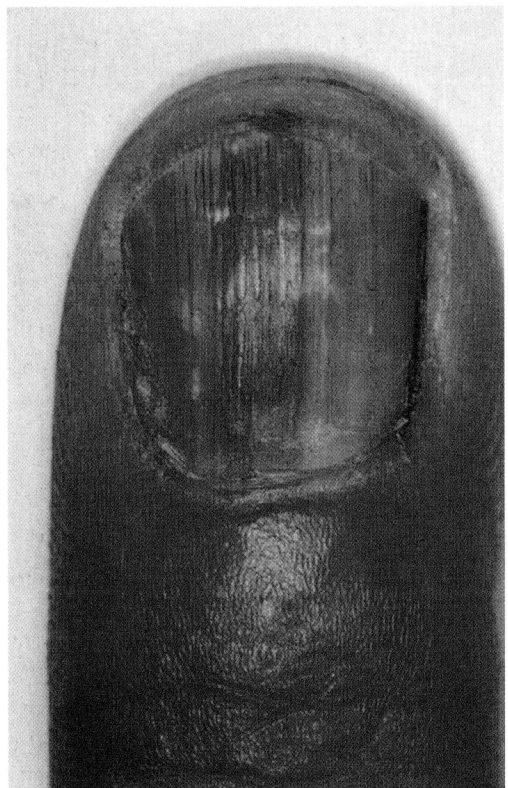

Figure 95.68 Severe onychatrophy from juvenile onset lichen planus of nails.

Figure 95.69 Lichen planus with longitudinal melanonychia.

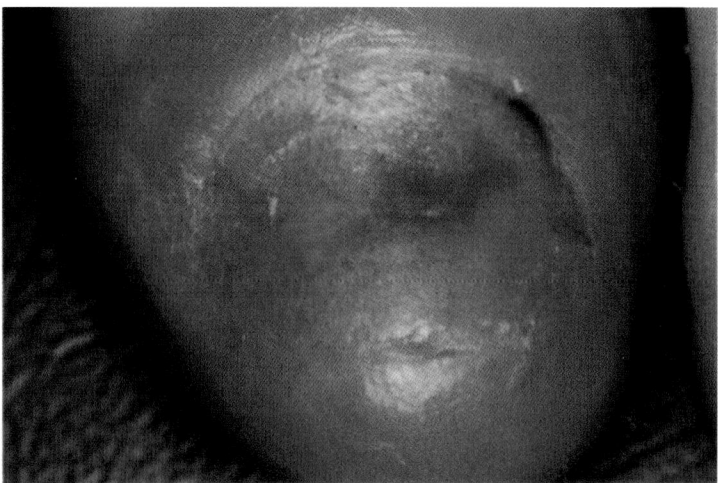

Figure 95.70 Anonychia following lichen planus.

widespread within the nail apparatus, nails may be shed. Single longitudinal depressions in the nail, with a distal notch or entire split, may arise from a pterygium: this is a fibrotic band of tissue fusing the proximal nail fold with the nail bed and matrix following destructive local inflammation. Surviving proximal matrix is unable to push growing nail through the scar tissue, with a consequent split. Thickening, with features resembling yellow nail syndrome, is a less common pattern of presentation [7]. Where this occurs there is usually little difficulty in making the distinction in the fingernails as the prominent surface changes and/or atrophy of lichen planus are seen. However, these changes are less obvious in the toes, where yellow discoloration due to thickening can be marked [8].

Nail bed disease can produce subungual hyperkeratosis and onycholysis. Ulcerative lichen planus may affect the soles of the feet but may also involve the toenails: permanent anonychia may follow [9] (Figure 95.70).

Clinical variants
Twenty-nail dystrophy, in which there is stippling of the nail plate (trachyonychia: see Figure 95.17), may involve all 20 nails but may affect as few as four or five. It is seen in a range of autoimmune diseases [10], especially in *alopecia areata* [3] but also in primary biliary cirrhosis and possibly in pemphigus [11]. In itself, it does not indicate the diagnosis of lichen planus, but is one of the recognized forms of the disease. It is one of the more common childhood patterns of presentation in which the nails feel rough and lose their

lustre [12]. It has a reasonably good prognosis, in contrast with *idiopathic atrophy of the nails*, which may also occur in children. In this form, the surface change is less marked and the change in overall nail morphology greater, with thinning and disintegration of the nail plate. Although nail biopsy is seldom undertaken in children, it may be warranted where the diagnosis of lichen planus needs to be explored. If destructive lichen planus is not treated in childhood, there will be lifelong loss of nails. In the related disorder, *lichen nitidus*, numerous pits giving a fine rippling effect have been reported [13]. Longitudinal ridging, beads and thickening may occur and the nails may become brittle.

In *keratosis lichenoides chronica*, although the skin condition may resemble hyperkeratotic lichen planus, the nail changes may mimic psoriasis; 30% have nail involvement, with hyperkeratotic hypertrophy of periungual tissues. Lichen planus nail changes are seen in *graft-versus-host disease* [14] and in the *disseminated lichenoid papular dermatosis of AIDS*. There can be an overlap between lichen planus and *discoid lupus erythematosus*, both in the skin and nails. Coexistence of skin and nail *lichen sclerosus* has been reported [15]. *Lichen striatus* may extend down a limb to the nails [16].

The differential diagnosis for the range of appearances of lichen planus in the nail unit includes *Stevens–Johnson syndrome*, infection, peripheral vascular disease, trauma and radiodermatitis. Scarring inherited abnormalities such as *dyskeratosis congenita*, *Schöpf–Schulz–Passarge syndrome*, *Darier disease* and variants of *epidermolysis bullosa* can also present with nail atrophy and scarring with overlap with the appearance of lichen planus.

Histology
In twenty-nail dystrophy, there is a granular layer in the nail bed and matrix with marked spongiosis [3]. The hypergranulosis is believed to reflect the disordered keratinization that causes both subungual hyperkeratosis and the poor nail plate formation. In other forms of nail lichen planus, in addition to hypergranulosis, there is occasionally saw-toothing of the rete pattern but colloid bodies are rarely seen [2,17,18].

In twenty-nail dystrophy, it may be useful to perform a screen for organ-specific antibodies because of the association with alopecia areata and the related autoimmune diathesis [3].

Management
Treatment needs to be commenced early and at sufficient potency to ensure that the disease does not progress whilst treated (Table 95.8). Once scarring has progressed sufficiently to cause a pterygium, there will be an irreversible component. In mild forms, where there

Table 95.8 Systemic therapies in common dermatological diseases affecting the nail.

	Ciclosporin	Methotrexate	Prednisolone	Acitretin	Fumaric acid esters	Azathioprine	Biologicals
Psoriasis	++	+	–	+	+	–	++
Lichen planus	+	–	++	+	–	+	–
20-nail dystrophy	+	–	++	–	–	–	–
Eczema	++	+	+	–	–	+	–

Justification for all systemic treatments in nail disease may be based on the combined presentation of skin and nails. It is less common to prescribe on the basis of nail disease alone. Course duration can usually be limited to pulses of 3 months in a 9–12-month period, repeated if needed. Doses are as for the cutaneous disease.
++Good choice, with moderate evidence supporting its use.
+Reasonable choice, with case reports or small series supporting use.
–Little or no published evidence.

is just nail fold redness and subtle nail surface changes, potent topical corticosteroids rubbed into the nail folds for 2–3 months may be adequate. Triamcinolone acetonide may be injected into the proximal nail fold under local anaesthetic. In children, potent systemic steroid therapy puts them at risk of premature closure of the phalangeal epiphyses and prolonged courses should be administered with the collaboration of a paediatrician. Oral steroids at up to 60 mg/day have been used to arrest severe scarring nail lichen planus [2]. Triamcinolone acetonide can be given intramuscularly at a dose of 0.5–1 mg/kg per month for 3–6 months [12]. There are reports of moderate success in the treatment of severe disease in children with systemic agents including oral prednisolone, dapsone and acitretin usually combined with topical therapy [19]. Ciclosporin can also be of benefit and azathioprine has been used to good effect in erosive disease [20]. Methotrexate is mentioned in review articles [21] and alitretinoin [22] in case reports. Ulcerative lichen planus of the nail unit may benefit from grafting the nail bed.

NAILS IN CHILDHOOD AND OLD AGE

Childhood [1]

In early childhood, the nail plate is relatively thin and may show temporary koilonychia. This is particularly prominent on the great toes. Under the age of 5 years, nails are also prone to terminal onychoschizia (lamellar splitting). This can be most prominent on the sucked thumb, but is also seen on the toes. Sucking may also lead to paronychia, which can be a troublesome condition in childhood, with pain and nail dystrophy (Figure 95.71).

Ingrowing can also cause pain and may present in different forms. At birth, there is often a degree of distal ingrowing, particularly in the great toe, as the nail has not surmounted the tip of the digit in its development [2]. In a more gross form, this may present as congenital hypertrophic lip of the hallux, where soft-tissue overgrowth may resemble fibrous tumours of the digit before spontaneously disappearing [3]. Painful distal embedding can lead

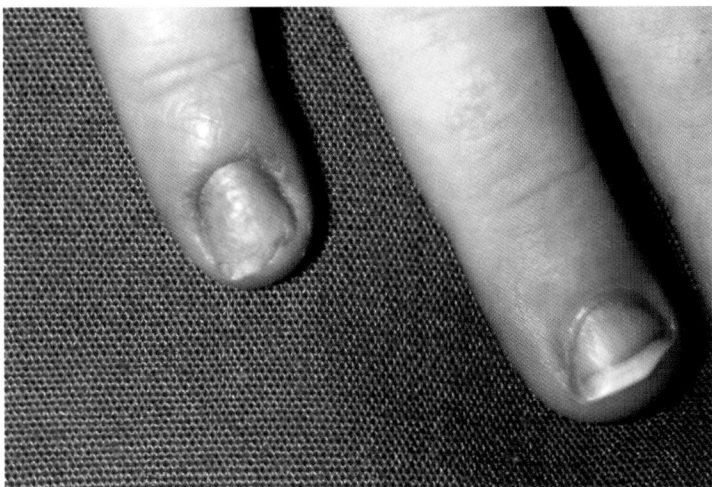

Figure 95.71 Paronychia of the little finger in a 2-year-old child.

to infection, but as long as the toenail is properly orientated with respect to the underlying phalanx, the condition usually subsides. In one series of seven children, two needed surgery due to painful persistence of the problem [4]. The changes associated with congenital malalignment of the great toe may also subside within 5–10 years in about 50% of children. In this condition, there is deviation of the tip of the great toenail laterally, rotating on the distal phalanx. The nail is yellow, triangular, thickened and has transverse ridges [5].

Fungal infection is relatively uncommon in children, with a prevalence of 0.3% [6] to 0.44% [7]. Terbinafine is not licensed for use in children in most countries, although there is evidence of its efficacy and it is sometimes used [7].

Beau's lines can be seen in up to 92% of normal infants between 8 and 9 weeks of age [8]. Normal surface markings of the nail can differ in children from those seen in adults. A herringbone pattern is common and gradually diminishes with time [9], which may reflect a gradual change in the pattern of matrix maturation.

Old age

With age, altered arterial and venous supply and cumulative trauma affect the feet more than most other body sites [10]. Elastic tissue changes diffusely affecting the nail bed epidermis are often seen histologically. The whole subungual area in old age may show thickening of blood vessel walls with vascular elastic tissue fragmentation [11]. Nail growth is inversely proportional to age [12].

The nail plate becomes paler, dull and opaque with advancing years, and white nails similar to those seen in cirrhosis, uraemia and hypoalbuminaemia may be seen in normal subjects. Longitudinal ridging is present to some degree in most people after 50 years of age and this may give a 'sausage links' or beaded appearance.

For details of the common traumatic abnormalities and changes due to inadequate pedicure or neglect, detailed texts should be consulted [1,12]. Nail problems in the elderly are often associated with more widespread mechanical changes of the foot, and it is often more important to direct treatment at maintaining mobility rather than the restoration of normal nails [13,14].

Onychomycosis is one of the most common nail diseases of the elderly, and is often combined with an element of traumatic dystrophy that will predispose to relapse after treatment. There are concerns that drug interactions in this group might make systemic therapy a poor choice [15]. This is not borne out by one large study designed to examine the effects of terbinafine. But the study also revealed that complete cure at the conclusion of the trial occurred in only 28% of cases, a factor which should be considered before instigating therapy [16].

IMAGING OF THE NAIL

X-ray examination

Under normal circumstances, X-ray examination reveals little of the soft structures of the nail unit. It can, however, be useful in identifying a range of pathologies including underlying exostoses, bone

Box 95.2 Causes of acquired acroosteolysis

- Vinyl chloride exposure
- Drugs (phenytoin, ergot)
- Snake or scorpion venom
- Connective tissue diseases
- Thermal injuries
- Biomechanical stress
- Neuropathic diseases
- Hyperparathyroidism

cysts, acroosteolysis, psoriatic arthropathy and reactive changes; it has also been used to measure nail bed thickness in a study of finger clubbing. Pincer nail deformity or trauma, including nail biting, can be associated with radiologically detectable osteomyelitis.

Most isolated nail dystrophies should be X-rayed prior to surgical exploration. Benign space-occupying lesions may compress the underlying bone with corresponding upward convexity in the nail. Osteoid osteoma may be manifest through a characteristic nidus, although X-ray is not sufficient to rule out this pathology and may need to be supplemented with bone scan or MRI. Chondroid tumours may be located externally to the bone, but may be detected by X-ray as a lucency within the bone. Similarly, X-ray may reveal bony invasion by locally invasive or metastatic malignancy: in invasive subungual squamous cell carcinoma, up to 55% of patients will have radiological evidence of involvement of the underlying phalanx.

Acquired acro-osteolysis, acronecrosis and distal phalangeal erosive lesions

Acro-osteolysis in adults is a predominantly bilateral lysis of the distal phalanges of the digits. Radiographs are poor at differentiating longitudinal from transverse acro-osteolysis [1]. Acquired varieties (Box 95.2) are by far the most frequent and usually secondary to a medical condition, trauma or toxins. Investigation of the cause is based more on clinical and laboratory data than on imaging. Idiopathic acro-osteolysis in adulthood may be sporadic or familial.

Occupational acro-osteolysis

Workers involved in the polymerization of vinyl chloride have developed acro-osteolysis. The other features of this occupational condition are Raynaud phenomenon and scleroderma-like skin changes (see Chapter 130). Exposure to vapours of synthetic materials used in the production of other plastic products may occasionally produce similar abnormalities. The acro-osteolysis begins as small cortical erosions which enlarge to produce transverse defects in the terminal phalanges (Figure 95.72a). The isolated phalangeal tuft may then fragment and resorb. If exposure is eliminated, healing may occur with coalescence of phalangeal fragments resulting in a pseudoclubbing, the thumb being more commonly affected than other digits.

Connective tissue diseases

Transverse acro-osteolysis, is rarely associated with Raynaud phenomenon, rheumatoid vasculitis, psoriasis or scleroderma. When present, acro-osteolysis is almost certainly secondary to vascular compromise.

Bony erosions of the phalanges occur in 40–80% of patients with systemic sclerosis. Gradual resorption of the tuft leads to 'pencilling' of the phalanx and in some patients all of the distal phalanx may be destroyed. The presence of sclerodactyly and/or calcinosis cutis helps indicate the correct diagnosis. 'Whittling' or 'pencilling' of the tufts also occurs in psoriasis and can result in a peg-shaped phalanx (Figure 95.72b) [1]. In acronecrosis, the final stage of acro-osteolysis, the soft tissues in the fingertip telescope around the shortened tuft resulting in pseudoclubbing.

Thermal/biomechemical/neuropathic injuries

Thermal injuries (i.e. frostbite [2], electrical and chemical burns) can result in acronecrosis long after the initial insult and may be due to a combination of mechanical and vascular injury. Phalangeal microgeodic syndrome is an uncommon benign condition firstly described by Maroteaux in 1970 [3]. Clinical manifestations include swelling and redness of one or more phalanges of one or both hands. Radiological signs encompass multiple small osteolytic areas and sclerosis compatible with acro-osteolysis. A relation to cold exposure has been suggested since patients often present this during the colder months of the year [4]. Acro-osteolysis has been reported in young guitar players [5] probably related to persistent mechanical injury resulting in vascular compromise and avascular necrosis.

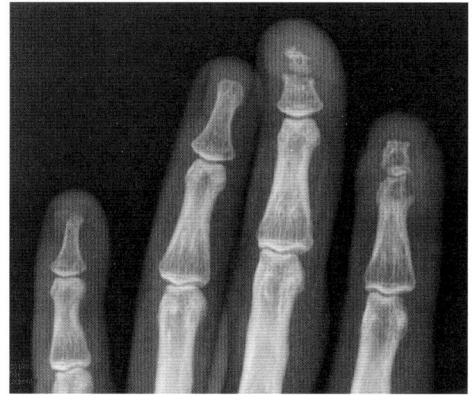
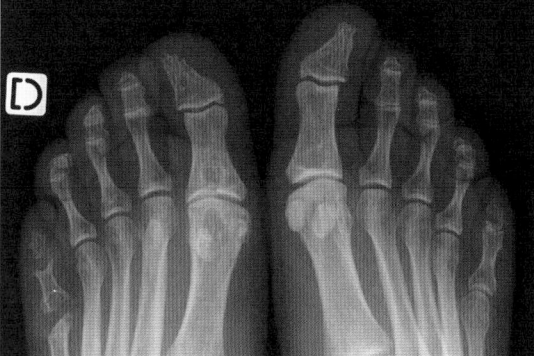

Figure 95.72 Transverse acro-osteolysis of the fingernail (a); acro-osteolysis of the toenail (b). (Courtesy of J. L. Drapé, France.)

(a)   (b)

Hyperparathyroidism

In hyperparathyroidism and renal osteodystrophy, increased levels of parathyroid hormone produce excessive bone resorption and altered bone formation. The earliest radiological sign of this disease is cortical resorption of the phalangeal tuft [6].

Many other diseases can cause distal phalangeal destruction.

Soft-tissue lesions

Epidermoid implantation cyst. This appears after a crush or a penetrating injury. On radiographic examination, it is characterized by a well-defined cystic lucency in the distal phalanx. It occurs more commonly in the phalangeal tuft, rather than at its base.

Glomus tumour. This hamartoma of hypertrophied elements of the normal glomus body is usually a well-encapsulated, soft pink or purple mass, smaller than 1 cm in diameter. When there is osseous involvement, it is characteristically an extrinsic pressure erosion, although occasionally, a more 'punched-out' appearance develops. Glomus tumour may demonstrate particular radiological features. Mathis and Schulz [7] reviewed 15 such tumours on the digit and found that nine had characteristic changes of bony erosion. This was smooth and concave in most cases, but occasionally had a punched-out appearance on the phalangeal tuft. Van Geertruyden *et al.* [8] noted bone erosion or alteration in 36% of 51 cases of subungual glomus tumour. Arteriography may reveal a star-shaped telangiectatic zone but generally, ultrasound or MRI is thought to be more useful in delineating and characterizing the tumour.

Keratoacanthoma. Bony destruction of the distal phalanx is present in virtually all cases of subungual keratoacanthoma and may be seen on radiographs even when examined shortly after clinical presentation. The destruction is characteristically well-defined, smooth, circular and limited to the tip of the phalanx [9].

Osseous neoplasms

Enchondroma is a benign tumour arising from mature hyaline cartilage. It is a small well-defined cystic lucency in the phalanx, sometimes having scalloped margins or a sclerotic rim, and is most commonly located centrally in the bone. In the distal phalanx, the enchondroma is typically located at the base of the phalanx, abutting the articular surface.

Osteoid osteoma is a benign osteoblastic lesion consisting of a small oval or round mass, called a nidus, usually smaller than 1 cm. All those affecting the terminal phalanx have a similar appearance characterized by a sclerotic nidus with a radiolucent halo ('ring sequestrum') [10].

Aneurysmal bone cysts and giant cell tumours rarely occur in the distal phalanges. Both may have similar radiological features characterized by lytic expansive lesions involving the entire phalanx [11].

Haemangiomas may arise in the bone or soft tissue of the distal phalanx. When primary in the bone, they have a characteristic radiographic appearance of linear striations parallel to the shaft of the bone. Soft-tissue haemangiomas are more common and may manifest as local soft-tissue masses, localized bony overgrowth, phleboliths in the soft tissue and pressure erosion of the underlying bone.

Ultrasound imaging

Ideally, a compact linear and variable-frequency probe that works in the range of frequencies from 7 to 22 MHz is used for performing the examination (Figure 95.73a). The machines are capable of detecting the blood flow of the nail bed in real time. Three-dimensinal ultrasound reconstructions may also provide valuable information concerning tumour size, location, shape and internal characteristics (Figure 95.73b). The nail unit is comprised of three main areas: the nail plate, the nail bed and the paronychial tissues. The dorsal and ventral plates present a bilaminar hyperechoic structure (two parallel lines) separated by a very thin hypoechoic layer (interplate space). Low-velocity arterial and venous vessels are usually detectable within the nail bed (colour Doppler with spectral curve analysis) (Figure 95.73c). The distal insertion of the lateral bands of the extensor tendon in the distal phalanx shows a fibrillar hyperechoic pattern, typical of tendinous structures. The bony margin of the distal phalanx shows a continuous hyperechoic line following the contour of the cortex of the bone that is only interrupted by the anechogenicity of the distal interphalangeal joint space, which contains fluid and cartilage (Figure 95.73d) [12].

Optical coherence tomography

Optical coherence tomography (OCT) is an optical analogue of ultrasound, using infrared instead of acoustic waves [13] The reflection of infrared light from the tissue is measured by interferometry, and 2D grey scale images are generated. Images reflecting the different layers may be either horizontal or vertical (similar to ultrasound). Functional aspects such as speckle variation and vascular flow may be included in some equipment. Three-dimensional images can be generated. The axial resolution is <5 and lateral resolution <7 μm; the scanning depth is up to 2 mm, limiting its use to very superficial tissues. It has been widely investigated in dermatology, particularly in non-melanoma skin cancers.

It has been claimed that OCT can differentiate morphological details and nail thickness better than high-resolution ultrasound and thus it has been advocated as an assessment tool for onychomycosis. Furthermore, OCT imaging is consistent with both physical and ultrasound findings in patients with symptomatic psoriatic nail disease. Surprisingly, OCT of diffuse psoriatic nail dystrophy as assessed on clinical examination has shown relative normality of the superficial nail but abnormalities at the nail plate anchorage to the nail bed. Given that OCT can also measure nail plate thickness, OCT has the potential to provide more objective

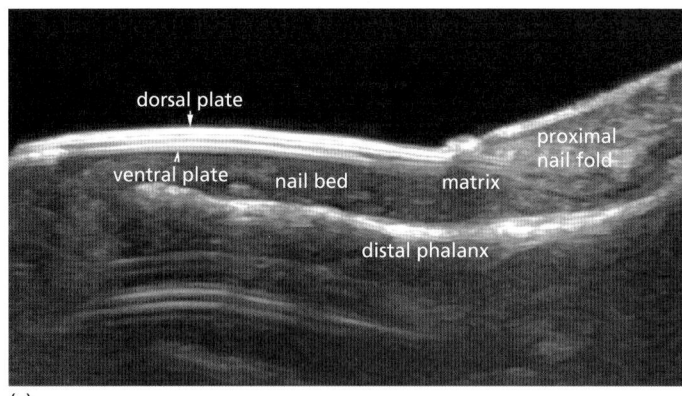

(a)

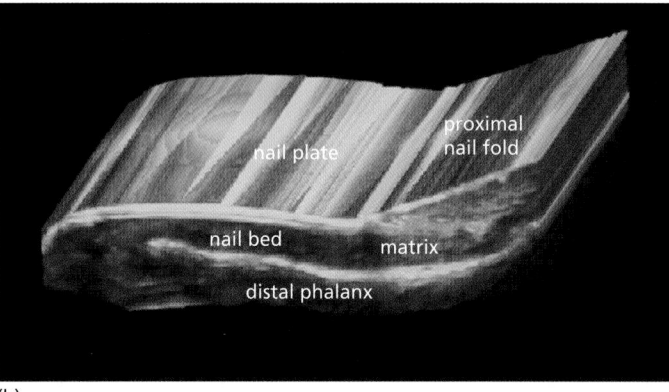

(b)

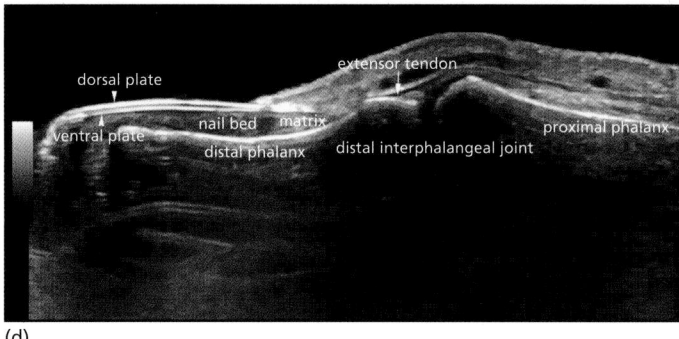

(c)

(d)

Figure 95.73 Ultrasound: grey scale ultrasound (longitudinal view) demonstrates the normal sonographic anatomy of the nail (a); 3D ultrasound reconstruction of the nail (longitudinal view) (b); power Doppler ultrasound (longitudinal view) shows the blood flow within the nail bed (c); extended field of view of the nail and periungual structures (longitudinal view) (d).

and informative quantitative data for use in outcome measures for interventional trials in psoriatic nail disease. In one study, OCT detected subtle abnormalities in 12 clinically normal nails and in 41 nails with normal ultrasound findings [14].

Confocal microscopy

Reflectance confocal microscopy (RCM) focuses infrared light in a specific focal plane, so that structures above and below this plane do not interfere with the image. RCM give horizontal images of the analysed tissue with an axial resolution of <1.25 μm and a lateral resolution of <5 μm, i.e. cellular level, to a depth of 350 μm. No stains are required for RCM imaging. Skin and nails are ideal locations for exploration by RCM, because they are easily accessible sites. The unique properties of RCM make it possible to explore the capillary nail fold at a cellular level.

The nail plate can be scanned from the surface to the lower part adjacent to the underlying nail bed. Three different layers can be differentiated by RCM according to the intensity of the reflection. The superficial layer shows a brighter reflection, followed by a zone with a poorer signal, followed again by a brighter zone in the deepest part.

Two main applications have interested dermatologists so far as follows:

1 Confocal microscopy and onychomycosis. As attempts to document fungal infection by potassium hydroxide (KOH) preparations and fungal culture are sometimes unsatisfactory, Hongcharu *et al.* [15] first reported the possible application of *in vivo* RCM for the diagnosis of onychomycosis. The author correlated RCM findings with the results from routine KOH preparations. RCM was found to be faster and more accurate than the conventional microscopy used with KOH preparations in the diagnosis of onychomycosis [16].

2 Confocal microscopy and melanonychia. Intraoperative dermoscopy and RCM have recently been advocated for better visualization of nail matrix pigmentation during exploratory nail surgery for melanonychia (Figure 95.74) [17]. In most cases, the RCM images obtained either *ex vivo*/*in vivo* were sufficiently reliable to make a diagnosis; the slight loss of quality sometimes observed *in vivo* because of subtle movements, did not adversely affect their diagnostic value. Intraoperative RCM revealed sufficiently atypical cytological and architectural features to accurately indicate the correct final diagnosis of melanoma. A good correlation between RCM and histopathology was found: subungual melanoma was diagnosed intraoperatively and in seven out of eight cases proved to be melanomas by histological examination [18].

In skin and nails, RCM combines the advantages of dermoscopy (non-invasive examination of the whole area of interest without alteration of the epithelial surface) and histopathology (resolution at a cellular level). RCM enables melanocytes to be distinguished readily from adjacent structures and permits the visualization of the architectural and cytological features of the melanocytic proliferation. *Ex vivo* examination can be used as a complementary technique if the data provided by *in vivo* examination are not diagnostically valid.

PART 8: SPECIFIC CUTANEOUS STRUCTURE

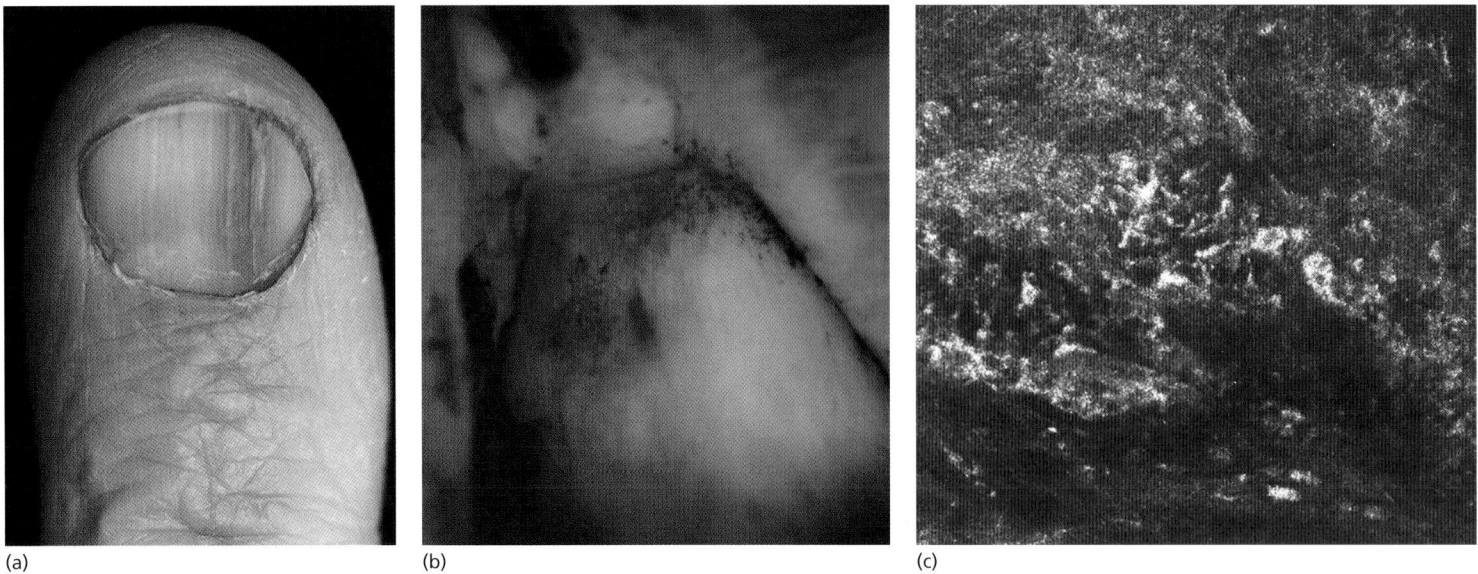

(a)   (b)   (c)

Figure 95.74 Nail melanoma: clinical presentation (a); dermoscopy (b) and *in vivo* reflectance confocal microscopy (c) of the nail matrix in the same patient. (Courtesy of L. Thomas, France.)

Magnetic resonance imaging

MRI is a medical imaging technique used in radiology to investigate the anatomy and physiology of the body. MRI scanners use strong magnetic fields and radio waves to form images of the body. Small surface coils dedicated to digit imaging are now available in all high-field MRI units [19]. MRI can detect tumours as little as 1 mm in diameter; it also defines their location and their tissue characteristics, all of which facilitates surgical management. T1-weighted sequence allows morphological evaluation of lesion contour and anatomical extent; T2-weighted sequence defines tissue characterization from signal intensity emitted by the tumour; gadolinium highlights the vascularization of tumours and may improve definition of lesion contours. The signals obtained in the various sequences are characteristic and can distinguish the most common tumours encountered in the nail region.

MRI can be helpful for investigating a range of periungual neoplasms and cysts. It is the gold standard for assessing glomus tumours of the nail unit and is particularly useful for myxoid (synovial) cysts, where even normal soft tissues can be distinguished and an *in vivo* anatomical assessment made (Figure 95.75a–c and Figure 95.76). MRI can help identify the inflammatory changes of psoriatic arthritis, where it has consequences for the soft-tissue element of the nail unit resulting in abnormal nail growth and appearance.

Proximal nail fold capillaroscopy

Proximal nail fold capillaroscopy is a simple *in vivo* non-invasive and reliable technique used for evaluating superficial microvascular structures. The capillaroscope is composed of an optical microscope with a 50× to 200× magnification. A cold light source

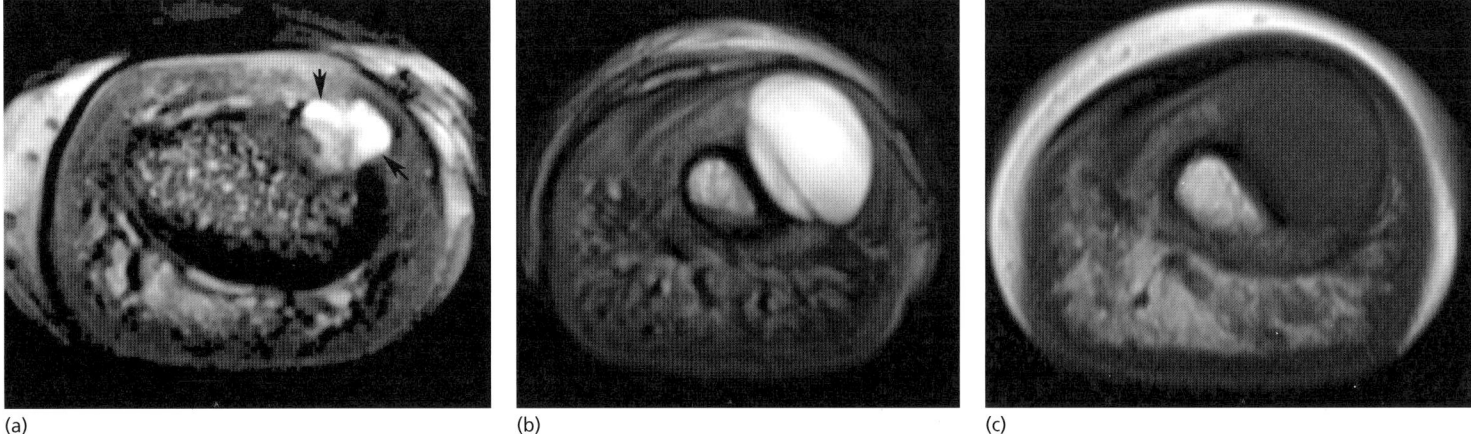

(a)   (b)   (c)

Figure 95.75 Axial T2-weighted image at the level of the distal interphalangeal joint (arrows): pedicle of the myxoid pseudocyst connected with the joint (arrows) (a). Axial T2 (b) and axial T1 (c) at the level of the nail cul-de-sac: lifting of the matrix and the root of the nail plate due to the cyst; bone scalloping of the dorsolateral aspect of the distal phalanx. (Courtesy of J. L. Drapé, France.)

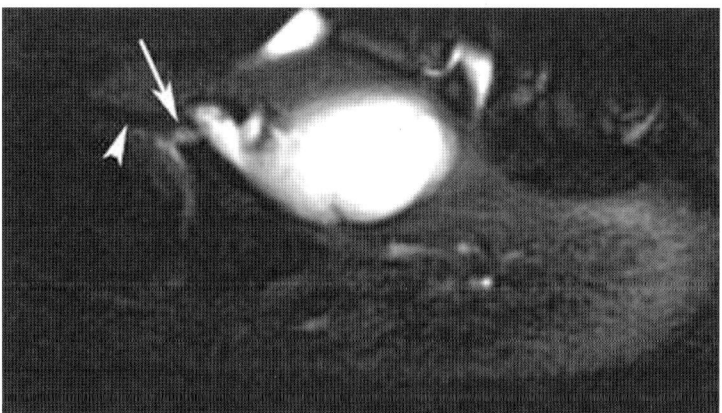

Figure 95.76 Sagittal section T2 fat saturated image: pedicle connecting with the joint (arrow) under the extensor tendon (arrow heads). (Courtesy of the copyright holder J. L. Drapé, France.)

is used in order to avoid vasodilatation. It is of particular value for examining the microvasculature of the proximal nail fold, with its special arrangement of vascular loops parallel to the skin surface, which cannot be well visualized by the naked eye.

Skin is 'prepared' with an ointment of cedar oil or liquid petrolatum in order to improve optical transmission. Second, third, fourth and fifth fingernails of both hands are examined consecutively. Some authors have suggested that a dermoscope (or an ophthalmoscope) can be used for capillaroscopic examination of the proximal nail fold. The lower magnification permits visualization of megacapillaries, but is insufficient to explore other components of the bloodstream in detail.

Useful information can be obtained by an overall examination of the microvascular structure of the proximal nail folds. Capillary loops physiologically have a hairpin shape and are arranged in two parallel longitudinal rows: usually 12–18 loops are found per millimetre (Figure 95.77a). Proximal to and arranged perpendicu-

larly to them, the subpapillary veins can be visualized. It is important to recognize a number of different patterns of no pathological significance: these include a glomerular conformation and elongated and tortuous loops. Pathological changes include ramified vessels, elongated loops, megacapillaries, loss of the normal parallel arrangement of loops and microaneurysms. Under the highest magnification, blood flow can be directly observed: either a normal continuous flow or a pathological intermittent flow with irregular interruptions occurring over time. Vasomotor tone can be evaluated subjectively by detailed observation of a vascular field. It is overactive in idiopathic Raynaud phenomenon and decreased in acrocyanosis. In lupus erythematosus, rapid and marked changes in vasomotor tone can be observed within the same capillary loop. It should be noted that deep epidermal pigmentation may reduce the visibility of the capillary loops.

Examination of the background may also yield useful information. In lightly pigmented skin, the background colour is pinkish, but can be orange if there is venous stasis. A pericapillary halo can be observed in inflammatory conditions and in cases of vascular stasis. A 'hazy' appearance may be seen in systemic sclerosis. Haemorrhages are observed in cases of evolving microangiopathy: a 'pearl necklace' appearance differentiates these from trauma-induced haemorrhages where the appearance is blotchy.

Acrosyndromes

Raynaud phenomenon

Raynaud phenomenon may be either idiopathic, Raynaud disease, or associated with a connective tissue disease (Raynaud sign or symptom). The most important indication for capillaroscopy is in the differential diagnosis between these two situations with very different prognoses. In Raynaud disease capillaroscopy is normal. Rarely, efferent capillaries can be found to be somewhat enlarged and some subtle haemorrhages can be observed. During

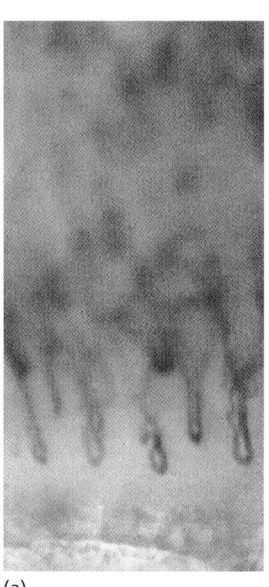
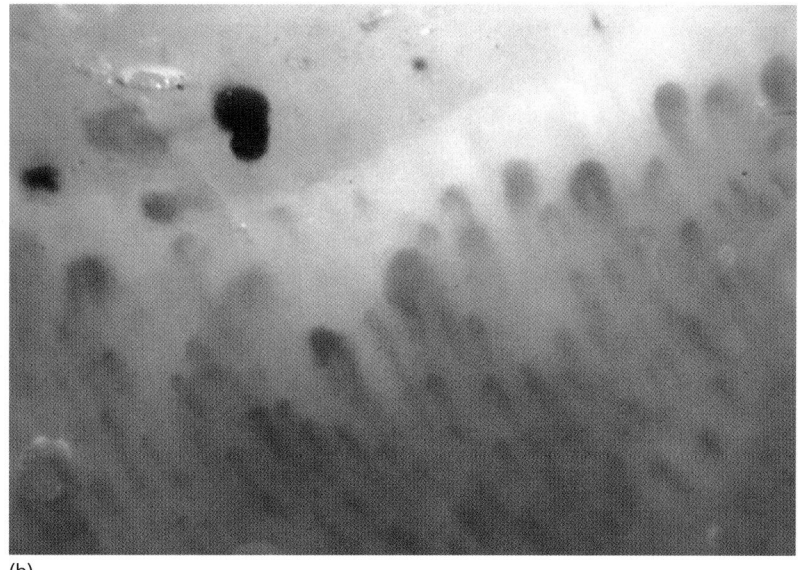
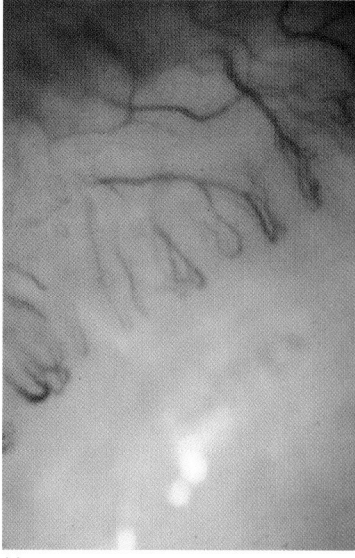

(a)　　　　　　(b)　　　　　　　　　　　　　　　　　　(c)

Figure 95.77 Normal nail fold capillaries (×60) (a); acrocyanosis showing dilatation of the nail fold capillaries, stasis and thrombosis of many vessels (b); rheumatoid arthritis showing rather elongated capillary loops (c).

the vasoconstrictive phase, a whitish background and a reduction in the number of visible capillaries can be observed. The appearances in connective tissue disease are discussed below.

Acrocyanosis

Acrocyanosis is clinically characterized by a painless distal cyanosis often with hyperhidrosis and cold extremities. This disease is worsened by exposure to cold. Capillaroscopy shows a normal or slightly increased number of capillaries of slightly enlarged diameter (especially in the efferent part of the loop). The loops are often tortuous over a cyanotic background. The blood flow is slowed and often has a granular appearance (Figure 95.77b).

Livedo

In livedo reticularis capillaroscopy shows enlarged efferent loops intermixed with normal loops and the blood flow is slowed. In livedo racemosa ('broken livedo') microvasculitis can sometimes be detected.

Chiblains (perniosis)

In chilblains affecting the fingers, homogeneously dilated vascular loops are observed in association with normal loops.

Systemic autoimmune diseases

Rheumatoid arthritis

Signs of dermal vasculitis are observed with tortuous and ramified capillary loops (Figure 95.77c). In some cases, short parallel loops in a 'fish shoal'-like pattern are observed. Background is not hazy and the blood flow is granular and fast.

Dermatomyositis

The clinically visible telangiectases of the cuticle correspond to megacapillaries as seen under the capillaroscope (Figure 95.78).

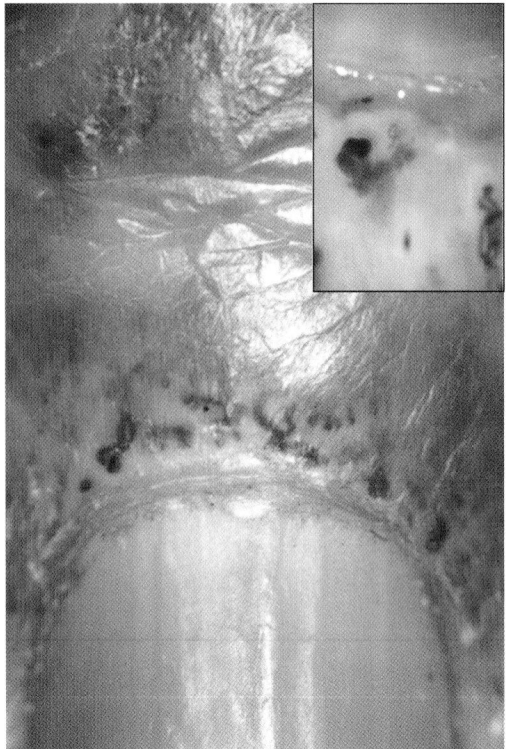

Figure 95.78 Dermatomyositis showing dilated nail folds capillaries and obstructed and thrombosed capillaries (×60) (inset).

However, in contrast with systemic sclerosis, there are no avascular areas.

Lupus erythematosus

In lupus erythematosus, observed abnormalities are morphological and rheological. Elongated loops, irregular enlargement of the afferent and/or efferent vessels, ramified and in some cases tortuous loops, and microaneurysms are the most common morphological changes (Figure 95.79a).

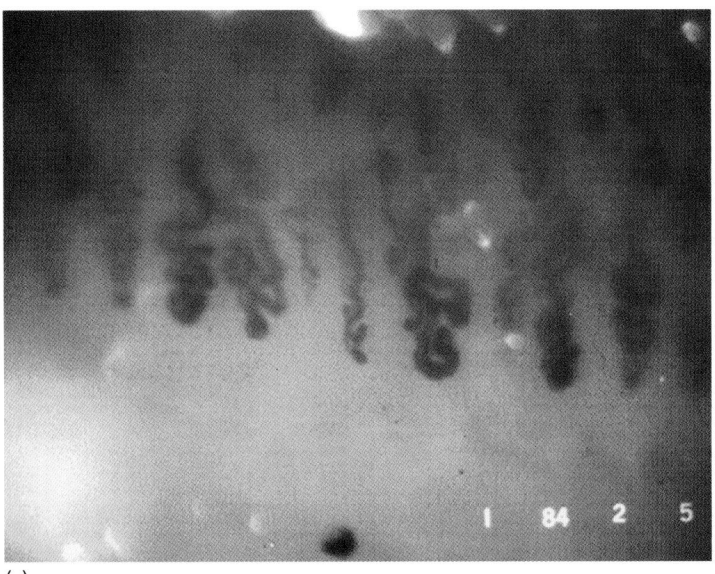

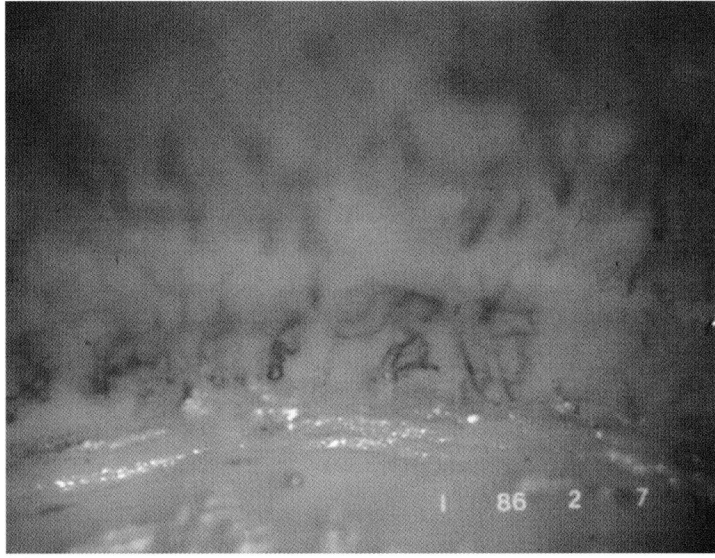

(a)   (b)

Figure 95.79 Lupus erythematosus (a) and systemic sclerosis (b). (Courtesy of the copyright holder C. Mathis, Belgium.)

Systemic sclerosis

Typical changes are observed in systemic sclerosis (Figure 95.79b) and nail fold video-capillaroscopy [20] is at present the most valuable tool for allowing an early diagnosis as follows:

- Rarefaction of the capillary loops with avascular areas.
- Megacapillaries of different size and shape often corresponding to the clinically visible telangiectases of the cuticle.
- Granular blood flow.
- Few haemorrhages.

Four stages are usually recognized as follows:

- Stage I: appearance of a few 'open' loops, 'U-shaped' and a few slightly enlarged capillaries.
- Stage II: slight decrease in the number of capillary loops, a few megacapillaries among many normal loops, hazy background.
- Stage III: marked decrease in the number of capillary loops, many megacapillaries, atrophic capillary loops, very hazy background.
- Stage IV: many avascular areas, reduced number of megacapillaries, very hazy background.

Psoriasis

Cutaneous microcirculation is different in psoriatic patients and normal individuals.

Vascular changes have been reported in nail folds. For this reason, Ribeiro *et al.* [21] studied psoriatic nail fold video-capillaroscopy in 46 patients (mean age 50.5, median disease duration 10 years) and 50 healthy controls and found lower capillary density, increase of avascular areas and morphologically abnormal capillaries in psoriatic subjects. No association between changes in capillary density and duration, extent or severity of the disease was noted. However, the presence of avascular areas was more common in patients whose nails were affected by the disease (pitting or dystrophy).

Toxic diseases

Vinyl chloride poisoning produces sclerodactyly. Capillaroscopy shows megacapillaries without decreased vascular density or avascular areas. The background is not hazy.

NAIL SURGERY

Introduction and general description

Patients often fear nail surgery because of anticipated pain, both during anaesthesia and postoperatively. The potential for causing permanent postoperative nail dystrophy frightens the practitioner.

A good knowledge of anaesthetic techniques, nail anatomy and surgical procedures is a prerequisite for a successful nail surgery with almost no pain and minimal scarring. It is also mandatory to involve a dermatopathologist who is familiar with the histological idiosyncrasies of the nail unit.

Anaesthesia

Premedication

Premedication may be useful in anxious patients. Short action molecules should be preferred: hydroxyzine, diazepines, orally or sublingually, the latter acting more rapidly. The combination of hydroxyzine 25 mg the night before the operation with 0.5 mg lorazepam sublingually 1 h prior to surgery is very effective [1]. Midazolam is favoured by some surgeons as it has short-acting hypnotic, anxiolytic and retrograde amnesic properties [2]. The use of EMLA under occlusive dressing prior to surgery will alleviate only the pain caused by needle insertion but not that due to injection of local anaesthetic and distension of tissues [3].

Equipment

Injections into the nail apparatus encounter high resistance and the use of a Luer lock syringe is mandatory. Using very thin needles (30 G) will decrease pain from puncture and limit the anaesthetic flow and rate of distension of the soft tissues. It is common for the physician to spend more time administering the anaesthesia than performing the surgical procedure.

Anaesthetics

Plain lidocaine 1 or 2% is the reference local anaesthetic. It acts for 60 min. As it is acid, pain during infusion may be reduced by prior alkalinization [4]. Warming the anaesthetic to 37°C also reduces the pain associated with infusion [5].

Lidocaine with epinephrine (adrenaline) is safe in the digits [6,7,8,9] except in patients with vasospastic, thrombotic or severe medical conditions. However, the use of epinephrine is of little interest in nail surgery as, to achieve a bloodless field, a tourniquet must be placed at the base of the digit in almost all procedures. Bupivacaine 0.5% acts after 45 min for up to 480 min [10]. It may be added to lidocaine to lengthen the postoperative analgesia. An alternative is to inject 0.5–1 mL of bupivacaine immediately postoperatively into the lateral aspect of the digit: this will act as a 'volumetric' tourniquet and prevent further bleeding [11]. Ropivacaine has the same quick onset as lidocaine, provides better postoperative pain relief [12–14] and is less cardiotoxic than bupivacaine [15]. Pain at infiltration depends on concentration. For routine use, a 2 mg/mL concentration provides a very comfortable anaesthesia with full sensation restored by 7 h. Ropivacaine produces slight vasoconstriction at low dosages [16].

Procedures

The so-called 'ring block' is still very popular but it should not be recommended any more. Its main drawbacks are the 'late' anaesthetic effect, requiring up to 20 min to develop, and the potential hazard of compression and trauma to neurovascular bundles with subsequent postoperative oedema and prolonged pain [17].

The distal digital block is the technique of choice in nail surgery. The injection site is 1 cm proximal and lateral to the junction of the proximal nail fold and the lateral nail fold. The needle is pushed at a 45° angle directed distally, down to the bone. 0.5 mL of anaesthetic will anaesthetize the branches of the dorsal nerve. The needle is then partially withdrawn and pushed down vertically skimming the lateral aspect of the phalanx towards the pulp where another 0.5 mL are deposited to block the branches of the palmar nerves. For complete anaesthesia, the procedure should be repeated on the opposite side. Anaesthesia takes effect immediately.

Instrumentation

Basic nail surgery requires only very few specific instruments. The classical tray should include an elevator to detach the plate from its attachments (e.g. Freer or Locke elevator, or a dental spatula), a nail splitter, straight haemostat, fine iris or Gradle scissors, no. 15 surgical blade, fine-toothed Adson forceps, a fine-needle holder, 3/0 and 4/0 non-absorbable sutures.

Diagnostic surgery

Proximal nail fold biopsy
Three techniques are available for biopsying this area as follows:
- When the indication is similar to a biopsy elsewhere on the skin, a punch biopsy (not over 3 mm) may be taken on the proximal nail fold, taking care that its distal margin is always preserved.
- The shave biopsy technique is also very useful for this area. Haemostasis can be obtained with aluminium chloride solution.
- When more tissue is required, as in collagen diseases, a crescent-shaped excision, 2–3 mm wide, is carried out from one side to the other. This amount of tissue allows histology, immunohistology and electron microscopy to be performed [18]. The procedure is the same as the surgical treatment of chronic paronychia (see later).

Nail bed biopsy
Indications for nail bed biopsies are diseases of the nail bed presenting as onycholysis, subungual hyperkeratosis or tumour. In the absence of onycholysis, a partial or total nail avulsion (see later) should be performed to expose the area to be biopsied. As for skin, incisional biopsy is performed with a punch and excisional biopsy with a blade. The punch should be pushed down to the bone. No suture is required, as a defect up to 4 mm across will heal by secondary intention without dystrophy.

Elliptical biopsy of the nail bed is indicated to remove larger specimens (e.g. small tumours). The elliptical excision should always be orientated in a longitudinal axis. The nail bed is very fragile and tightly adherent to the bone so that reapproximation of the margins may be difficult. To overcome this, lateral undermining of the edges should be generous. Suturing may leave a gap that will heal by secondary intention.

Nail matrix biopsy
Matrix biopsies are most useful for longitudinal melanonychia. An accurate histological diagnosis requires examination of the entire pigmented lesion and therefore incisional biopsies are not recommended and only excisional biopsies should be performed. Dystrophic sequelae are unlikely if the pigment is confined to the distal matrix, as the latter synthesizes the ventral part of the nail plate. The only consequence will be a nail plate thinned from below. Fortunately, in the majority of cases longitudinal melanonychia originates in the distal matrix [19]. If the pigment is located within or extends to the proximal matrix, a nail plate dystrophy is highly probable, as this part of the matrix generates the upper third of the nail plate.

Several techniques are available according to the width and shape of the band. Each of the following procedures starts identically in order to expose the nail matrix. Using an elevator, the proximal nail fold is detached from the nail plate; two lateral incisions at 45° enable it to be reflected. Then, a lateral avulsion ('sardine tin' avulsion) of the proximal third of the nail plate exposes the whole matrix and the most proximal part of the nail bed.

1 For a well-circumscribed round pigmented lesion of <3 mm in diameter located in the distal matrix, the punch biopsy technique is best [20]. A 3 mm punch encompassing the whole pigmented macule is pushed vertically into the matrix down to the bone (Figure 95.80a–d). The defect is left open and the nail plate is laid back in place and sutured to the lateral nail fold. Punching through the nail plate at the origin of the longitudinal melanonychia before avulsing is very useful when dealing with lightly pigmented bands: the process of avulsion often detaches the superficial layers of the matrix epithelium and the origin of the band may then be difficult to identify. By performing a punch in this manner, the area to biopsy can be clearly seen once the nail plate has been avulsed [21].

2 If the source of pigment is oriented longitudinally, it should be excised using a longitudinal ellipse with minimal margins. The edges of the incision are widely undermined and reapproximated with 5/0 or 6/0 absorbable sutures (Figure 95.81a–d). The nail is laid back in place and sutured to the lateral nail fold. The proximal nail fold is returned to its anatomical position and the lateral incisions are sutured [21].

3 If the source of pigment is oriented horizontally, a crescent-shaped excision should be performed with the convex portion of the incision matching the contour of the lunula. The borders of the defects are generously undermined and the edges are gently reapproximated with 5/0 or 6/0 absorbable sutures. The avulsed nail plate and proximal nail fold are then replaced as described above.

4 For very extensive pigmentation (>6 mm in diameter) the tangential excision is recommended. A shallow incision is carried out around the pigmented zone. The scalpel is then held horizontally and with sawing motions the lesion is removed from the deep dermis. It should not be thicker than 0.5 mm. The specimen is placed on filter paper and properly oriented for the pathologist. The avulsed nail is put back and secured to the lateral fold. This technique has proven sufficient to allow adequate diagnosis in all cases. Its main drawback is a recurrence of the pigmentation in about three quarters of cases [22]. This technique should be restricted to large pigmented bands that were formerly an indication for immediate total ablation of the nail unit (Figure 95.82a–d). This technique avoids mutilating surgery in cases where the pigment derives from a large benign lesion. If histopathology shows that the lesion is malignant, further surgery is required.

Biopsy of whole structures of nail apparatus
The lateral longitudinal biopsy permits study of all components of the nail unit: proximal nail fold, matrix, nail bed, nail plate and hyponychium. This is the most rewarding biopsy technique when dealing with a disease presenting as alterations of the nail plate

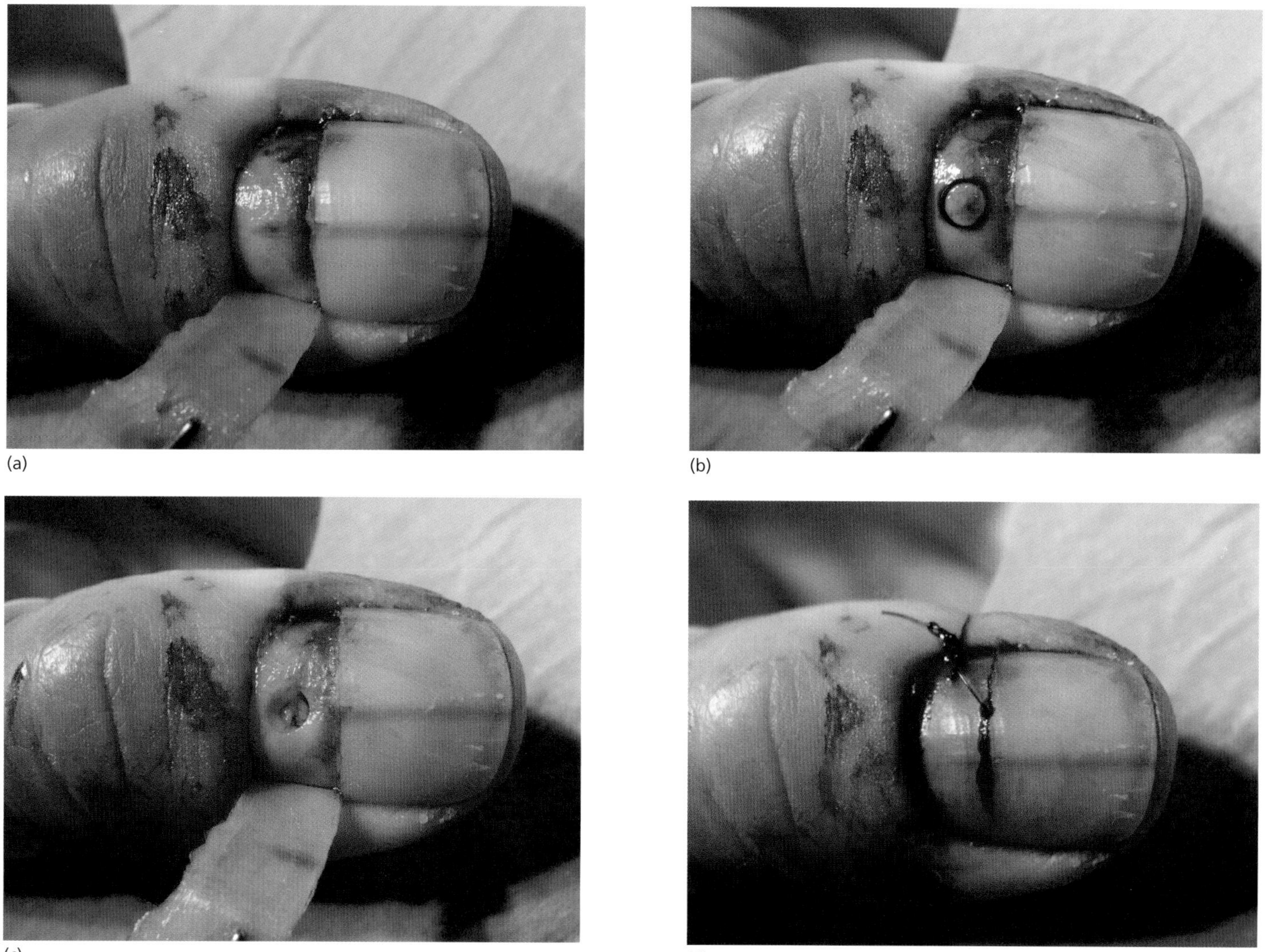

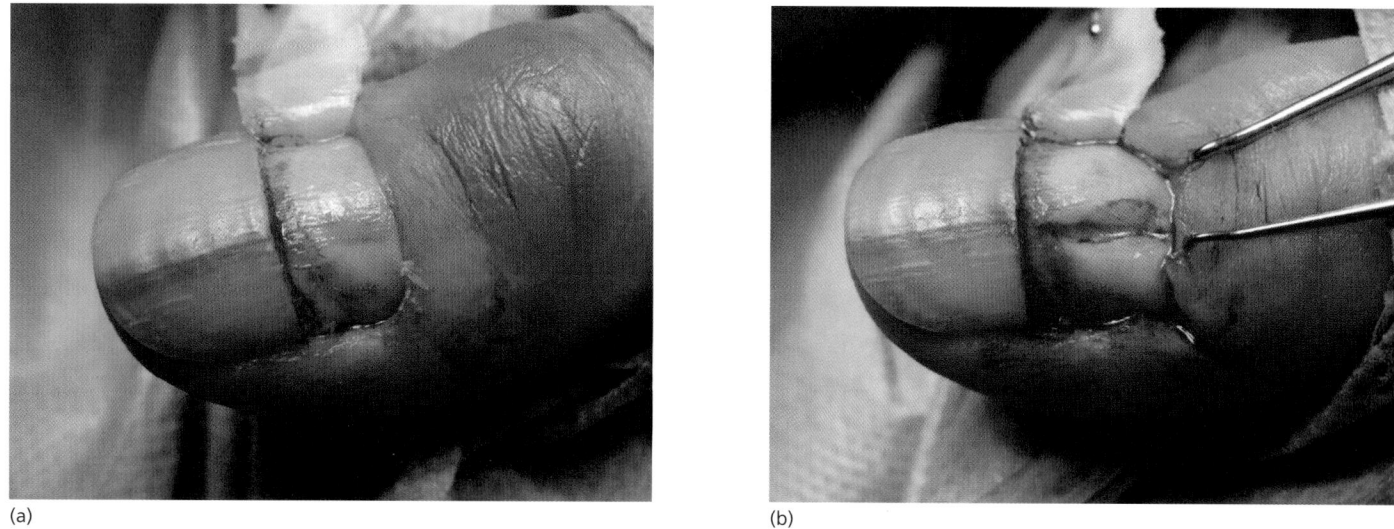

(a)

(b)

(c)

(d)

Figure 95.80 (a) Avulsion of the proximal third of the plate exposes the pigment area responsible for the longitudinal pigmentation. (b) A 3 mm punch is performed around the whole pigmented area. (c) The specimen is removed down to the bone. (d) The plate is put back in place and secured to the lateral fold.

(a)

(b)

Figure 95.81 (a) Avulsion of the proximal third of the plate demonstrates that the pigment area responsible for the pigmentation extends longitudinally on the matrix. (b) The whole pigmented area is removed in a longitudinal elliptical excision. (*Continued*)

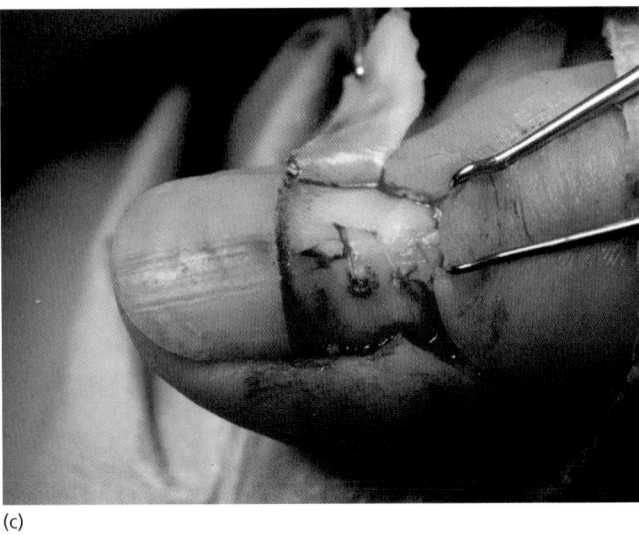
(c)

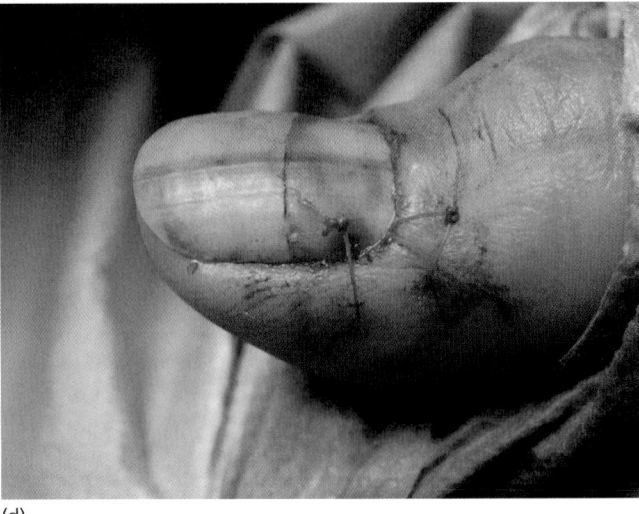
(d)

Figure 98.81 (*Continued*)
(c) After undermining the wedges, the defect is reapproximated with absorbable sutures. (d) The plate is put back in place and secured to the lateral nail fold.

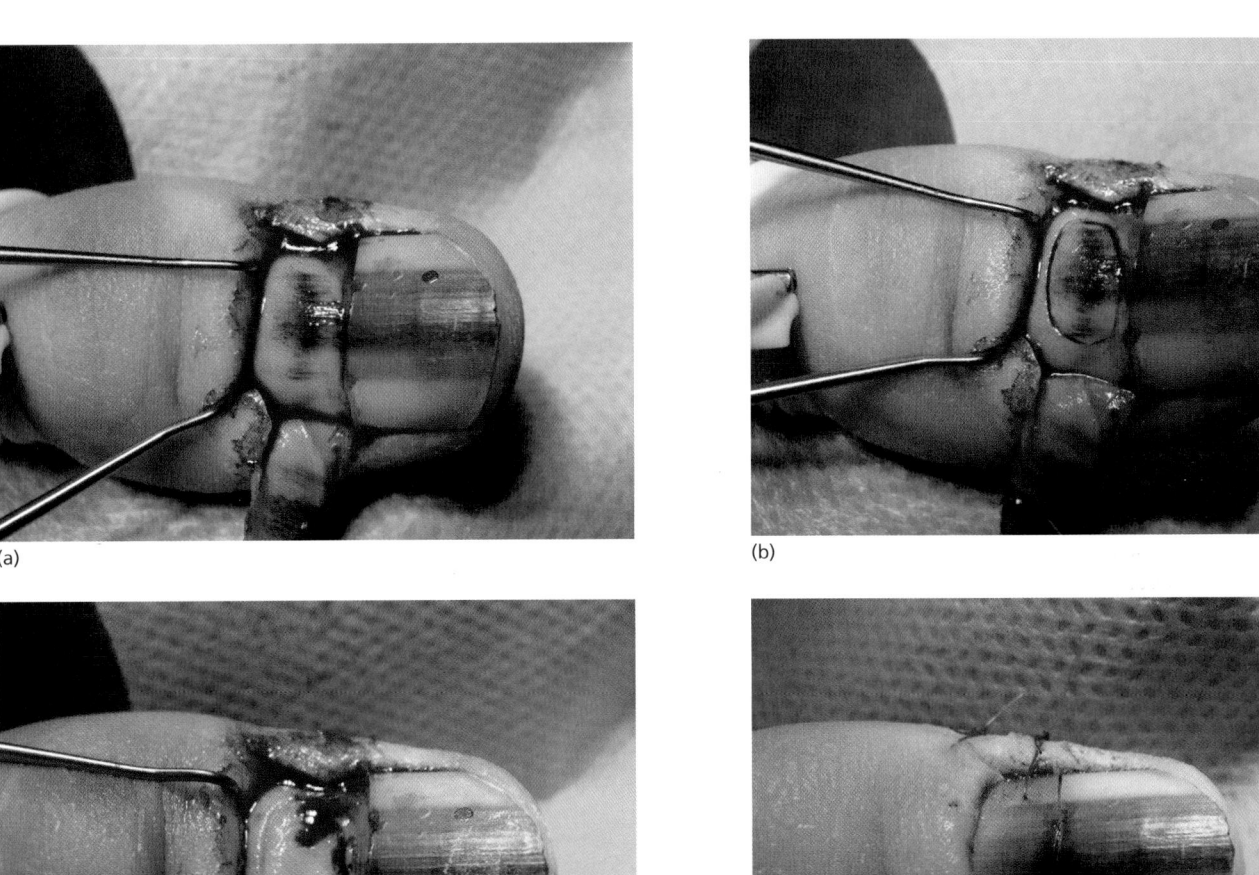
(a)

(b)

(c)

(d)

Figure 95.82 (a) Avulsion of the proximal third of the plate exposes the wide pigment area responsible for the longitudinal pigmentation. (b) An incision is carried out all around the whole pigmented area. (c) The specimen is tangentially removed as a whole. (d) The plate is put back in place and secured to the lateral nail fold.

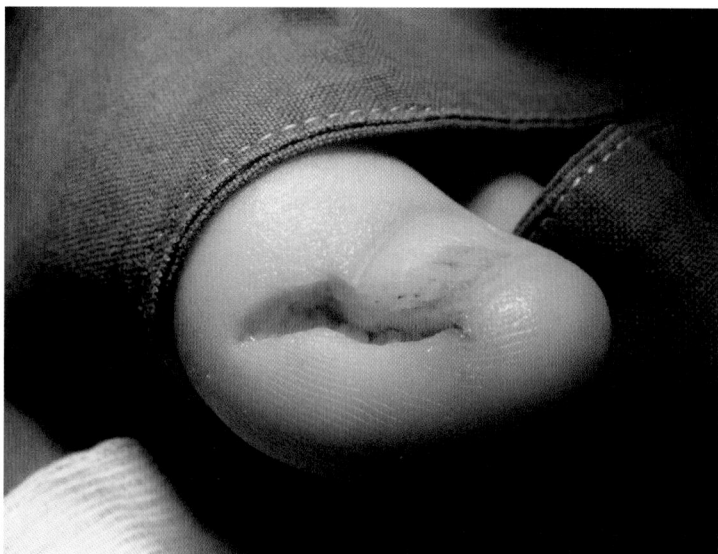

Figure 95.83 Lateral longitudinal biopsy. Note the sigmoid shape of the defect that can be easily closed.

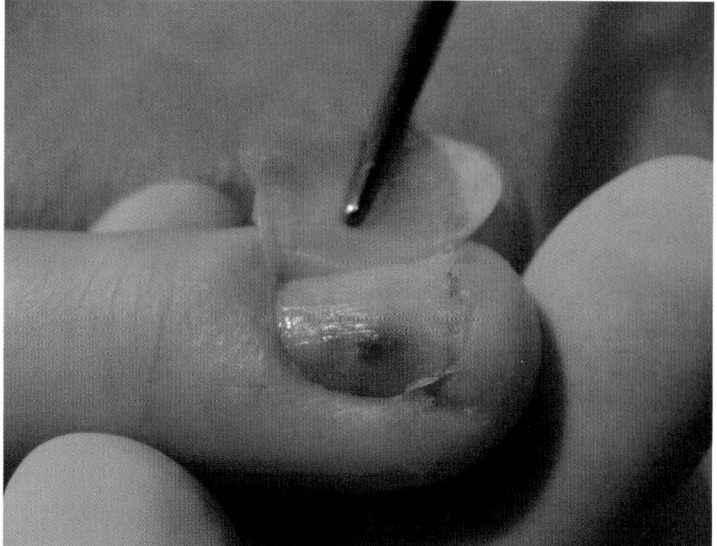

Figure 95.84 Lateral avulsion ('sardine tin' avulsion) allows exposure of the complete nail bed and excisional biopsy of the nail bed tumour.

surface. This will narrow the nail permanently due to the partial amputation of the lateral horn of the matrix. In order to avoid any postoperative lateral deviation, the specimen should not exceed 3 mm in width [23]. The incision starts half way between the cuticle and the crease of the distal interphalangeal joint and runs distally through the proximal nail fold, the nail plate and its bed to the hyponychium. At the junction of the lateral and proximal nail fold, the incision should follow a laterally curved direction extending halfway down the lateral aspect of the finger as far as the distal interphalangeal joint, in order to ensure removal of the lateral horn of the matrix. A second incision, starting from the distal extremity of the previous one, runs from the hyponychium into the lateral sulcus and joins the proximal end of the previous incision. The resulting sigmoid biopsy specimen (Figure 95.83) is then carefully detached from the bone with fine scissors. At the proximal end of the biopsy, care must be taken to include the matrix by avoiding lifting the scissors too soon and thus foreshortening the specimen. The defect is reapproximated with horizontal mattress sutures in order to recreate a lateral nail fold [24].

Excisional surgery

Nail avulsion

Nail avulsion is a core procedure in nail surgery: it allows inspection of and access to a subungual lesion in the nail bed or matrix for biopsy or excision (Figure 95.84); it is an adjuvant treatment in onychomycosis as it reduces the fungal mass; it is part of the treatment of an acute paronychia and of ingrowing toenail. Total surgical removal should be discouraged: the distal nail bed may shrink and become distorted dorsally. In addition, the loss of counterpressure from the nail plate allows dorsal expansion of the distal pulp, promoting distal embedding. Partial nail avulsion should always be favoured. However, in some instances (e.g. prominent dystrophic total onychomycosis) total avulsion is unavoidable.

Total surgical nail avulsion

This may be carried out using either a distal or a proximal approach.

Distal approach

An elevator is gently slid under the proximal nail fold in a back-and-forth motion from side to side, so avoiding injuring the fragile longitudinal nail bed ridges, until the proximal nail fold is freed from the nail plate. The elevator is then pushed under the nail plate from the distal free edge until the elevator gives way (meaning the elevator has reached the matrix area to which the nail plate is loosely attached). Caution must be taken to detach the lateral horns of the nail plate fully. A jaw of a sturdy haemostat is slid under the whole length of a lateral portion of the nail plate and grasped firmly. In an upward rotating motion, the nail plate is avulsed [25].

Proximal approach

The proximal approach is advised when the distal subungual area strongly adheres to the nail plate (e.g. thick hyperkeratosis) and it is then difficult to find a cleavage plane between the plate and the bed. The proximal nail fold is detached as described above. The elevator then reflects the proximal nail fold and is delicately inserted under the base of the nail plate where the adherence to the matrix is weak. The procedure is repeated along the whole width of the nail root. The avulsion progresses distally following the natural cleavage plane up to the hyponychium [25].

Partial surgical nail avulsion

The considerable advantage of this technique is that it leaves a large portion of normal nail plate that still exerts a pressure on the underlying soft tissues, reducing the risk of distal embedding. It is a must in the treatment of some types of onychomycosis (longitudinal streaks, lateral disease, dermatophytoma, onychomycosis due

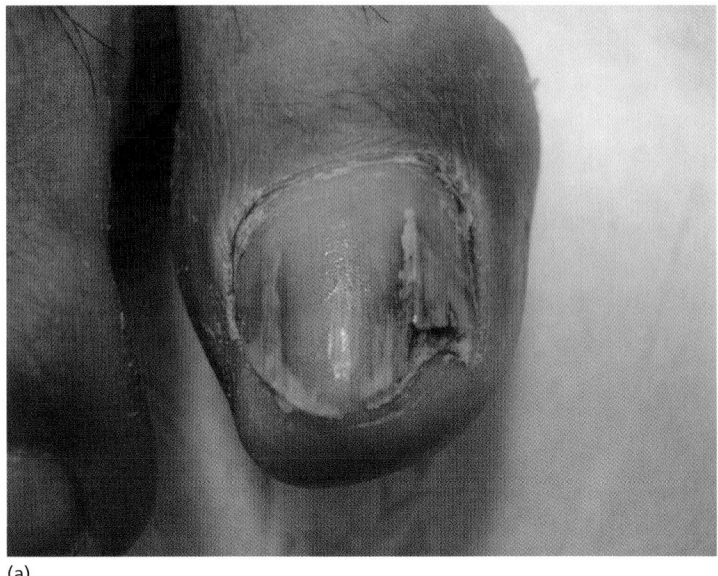

(a)

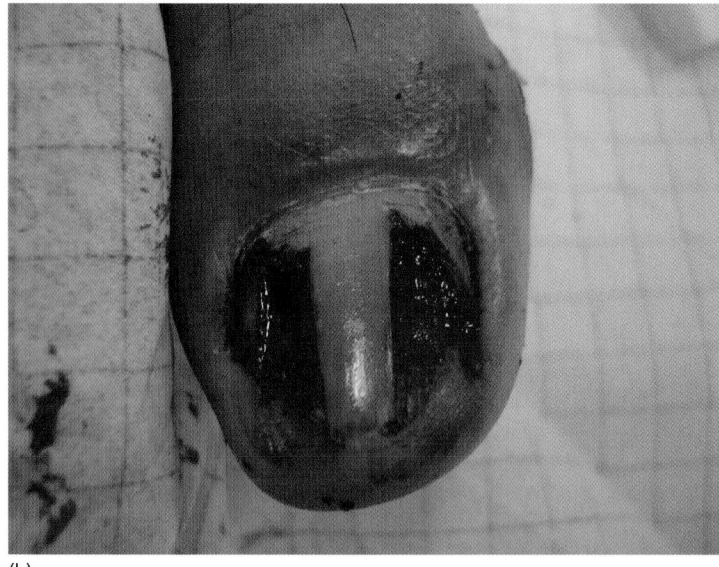

(b)

Figure 95.85 (a) Dermatophyte onychomycosis with longitudinal spikes. (b) After surgical removal of the yellow streaks.

to moulds) [26] (Figure 95.85a,b). Partial nail avulsion is part of many surgical procedures: chemical cautery of a part of the matrix in ingrowing toenails, treatment of acute paronychia, surgical exploration of any nail bed or matrix tumour. It is performed in the same way as the distal approach method of total surgical nail avulsion, but restricted to a limited portion of the nail plate. For exposure of the matrix area, avulsion of the proximal third of the nail plate is best. It starts with two lateral incisions on the proximal nail fold at 45° enabling it to be reflected. A jaw of a nail splitter is inserted under the lateral border of the nail plate, approximately 5 mm distal to the lunula. The plate is cut horizontally to the other side. A haemostat grasps the lateral portion of the plate and lifts it up laterally, as for a sardine tin, exposing the whole matrix area (see Figures 95.80a, 95.81a and 95.82a). After surgery, the plate is laid back in place and sutured to the lateral fold.

Acute paronychia

Acute paronychia generates a lot of pain and prolonged pressure from the swollen paronychial soft tissues onto the matrix may impair the normal regrowth of the nail plate. Incision of the proximal nail fold is discouraged as it may result in a deformed eponychium. If the pus collection is located under the proximal nail fold, the best treatment is avulsion of the proximal third of the nail plate (see Partial nail avulsion earlier) to allow drainage of the pus. If the collection is in the lateral nail fold, avulsion of a lateral strip of nail plate should be carried out. Systemic antibiotics are prescribed empirically and adapted if necessary once culture results are known [27].

Chronic paronychia

Surgical treatment is indicated when medical treatment has failed. An elevator is inserted into the proximal nail groove under the proximal nail fold in order to protect the matrix and the extensor tendon. With a no. 15 surgical blade, a crescent-shaped excision of the proximal nail fold is performed: the incision should run

from one side to the other, reaching its maximum width (5 mm) in the midline of the proximal nail fold. The incision should include the five most proximal millimetres of the lateral nail folds. The blade should be held obliquely at 45° down to the nail plate (Figure 95.86a,b). Complete healing by secondary intention will restore the proximal nail fold with its cuticle in less than 5 weeks (Figure 95.86c). However, the nail plate will appear a bit longer with a larger lunula [28]. This technique is also adequate for small very distal type B myxoid pseudocysts.

Fibrokeratoma resection

For a fibrokeratoma arising from the ventral surface of the proximal nail fold, reflection of the latter with two oblique incisions at 45°, exposes the whole nail pocket (Figure 95.87). In most instances, the fibrokeratoma originates from the most proximal part of the ventral proximal nail fold. The tumour should be delicately dissected up to its base using fine iris scissors and then severed. Injuring the matrix is impossible as the nail plate is still in place. The proximal nail fold is then laid back and secured with 5/0 stitches or adhesive strips [29].

For a fibrokeratoma arising from the nail bed, a nail avulsion is required in order to expose the nail bed (Figure 95.88). The tumour is excised in the same manner as an elliptical biopsy of the bed (see Nail bed biopsy earlier). In both forms, incomplete resection leads to recurrence.

Chemical cautery for ingrowing toenails

The therapeutic aim of this procedure is a selective cautery of the lateral horns of the matrix to obtain a permanently narrowed nail plate that will solve the 'nail plate–lateral nail fold conflict' once and for all. This technique may be performed on both sides of pincer nails and suppresses immediately the 'pincer' effect of the lateral edge of the nail plate on the soft tissues. Chemical cautery with phenol is easy to learn and is very effective (<3% recurrence rate). It is the recommended procedure in several Cochrane reviews as

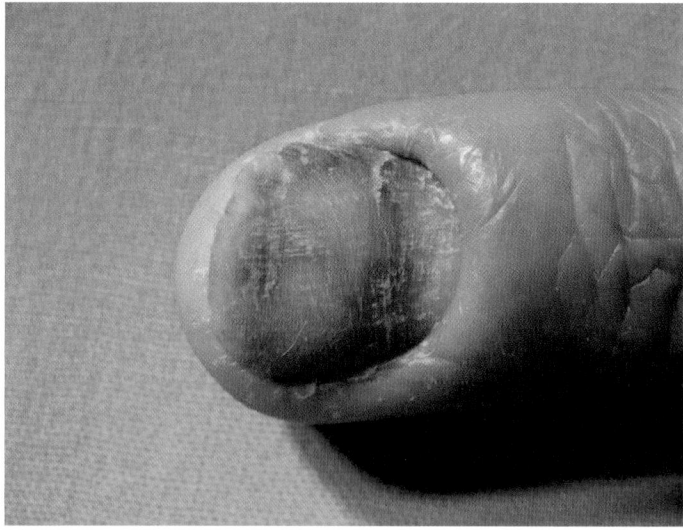

(a)

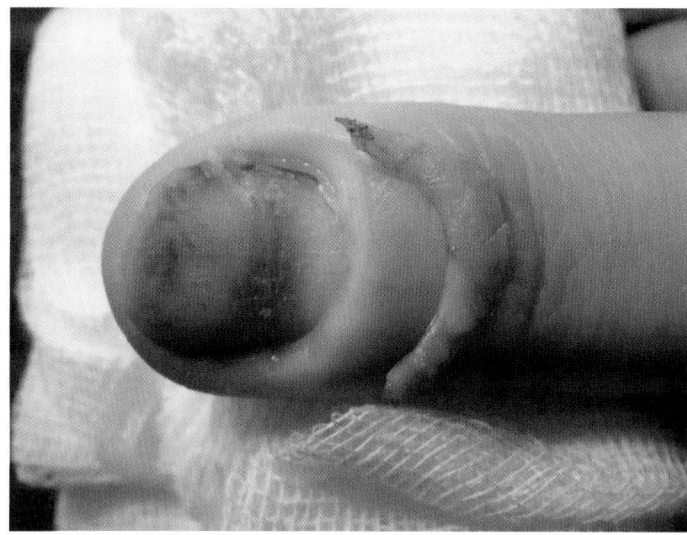

(b)

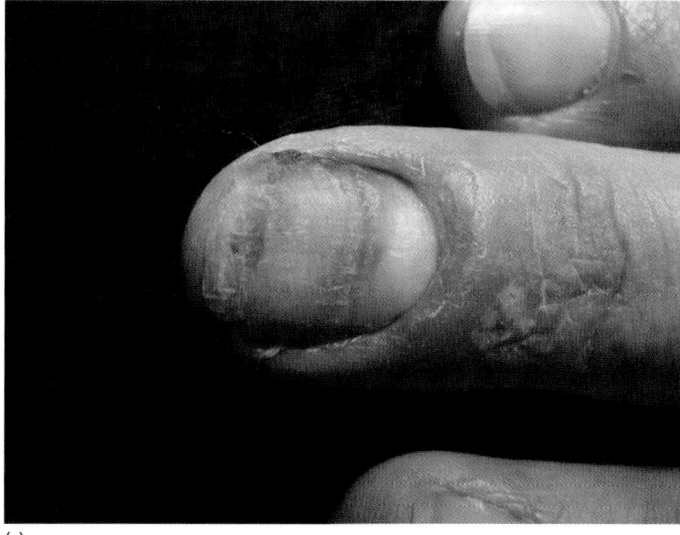

(c)

Figure 95.86 (a) Chronic paronychia resistant to topicals and steroid injections. (b) Crescent-shaped excision of a part of the proximal nail fold. (c) Complete re-epithelialization at day 8. Note that the nail is now apparently longer.

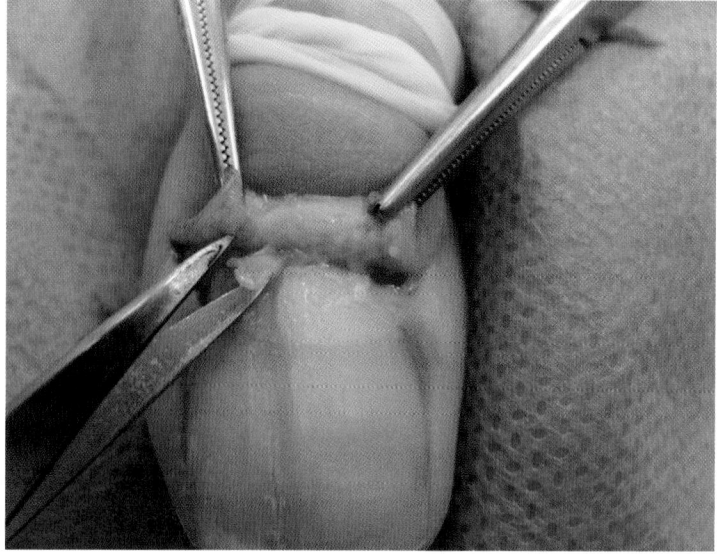

Figure 95.87 Two lateral incisions at 45° allow reflection of the proximal nail fold; visualization of the tumour and its removal.

it has a high success rate with low morbidity [30,31]. After a distal digital block, a 3–5 mm wide lateral strip of nail is avulsed up to its most proximal part. This partial nail avulsion exposes the lateral horns of the matrix at the proximal part of the cavity. Chemical cautery of the lateral horns of the matrix is carried out with a cotton-tipped applicator dipped into 88% phenol and then pushed into the cavity (Figure 95.89a–c). The applicator is left in place for 4 min [32]. To ensure the effect of the phenol, it is essential to work in a bloodless field using a tourniquet. Spillage of phenol onto the periungual tissues should be avoided as this causes unnecessary burns. For beginners, application of a greasy ointment onto the perionychium prior to cauterization may protect the tissues. After the procedure, applying alcohol will not 'neutralize' the phenol but only dilute it [33]. Phenol induces coagulation of proteins from the matrix epithelium. Once coagulated, the epithelium becomes

PART 8: SPECIFIC CUTANEOUS STRUCTURE

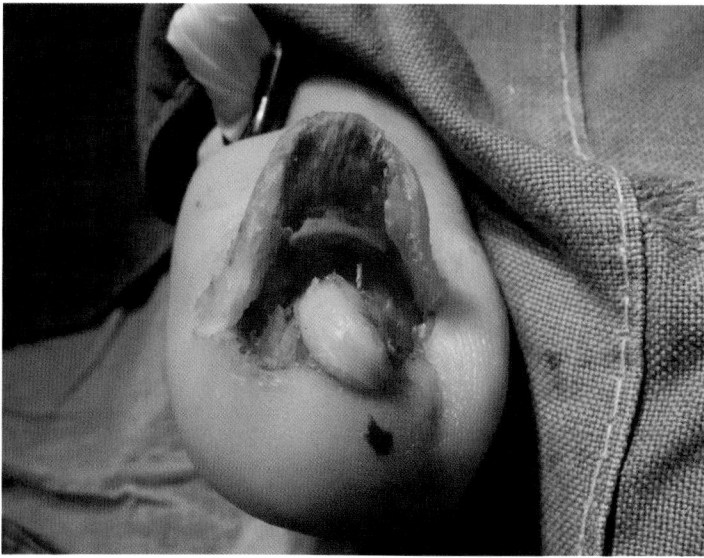

Figure 95.88 Trap door avulsion permits access to the nail bed tumour. The latter will be removed in a longitudinal excision.

PART 8: SPECIFIC CUTANEOUS STRUCTURE

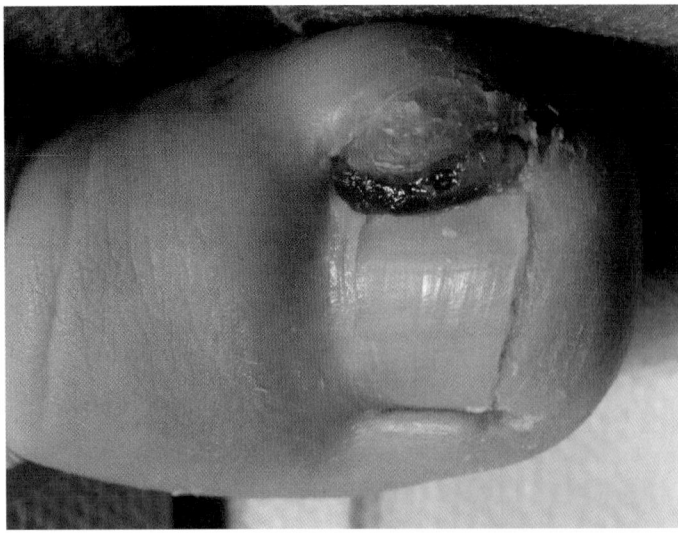

(a)

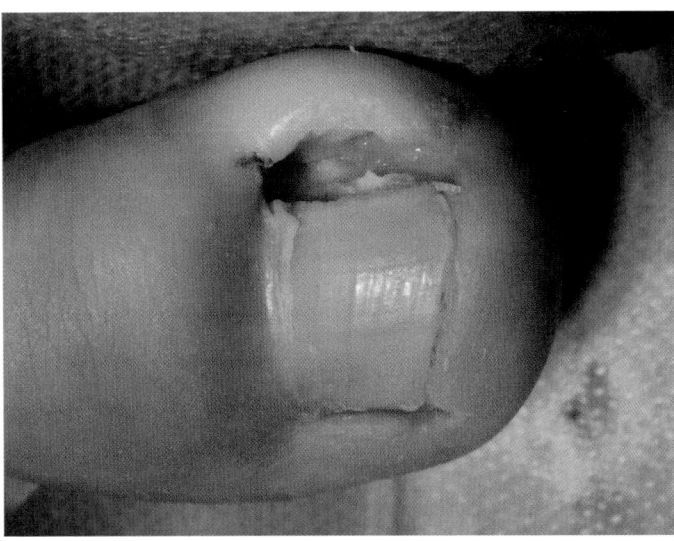

(b)

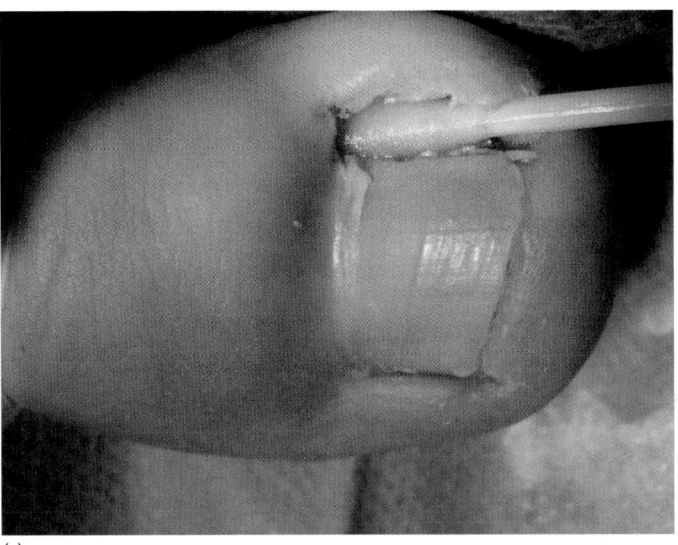

(c)

Figure 95.89 (a) Ingrowing toenail with pyogenic granuloma. (b) After curettage of the pyogenic granuloma, a lateral strip of nail is avulsed. (c) A cotton-tipped applicator, dipped into 88% phenol is pushed into the cavity. Note the bloodless surgical field.

impermeable to any liquid. Release of the tourniquet will allow the blood proteins to inactivate any residual phenol [21]. Patients have little postoperative pain as phenol has, apart from its caustic effect, important antiseptic and anaesthetic properties. The major drawback of this technique is the prolonged oozing from the phenolic burn. This may last up to 5 weeks. Daily home care (soakings and antiseptic ointment) are required until the wounds are completely dry. The ooze should not be mistaken for infection. Very high success rates can be achieved with other caustics including 10% KOH [34] and 100% trichloracetic acid [35].

Longitudinal melanonychia removal
See matrix biopsies.

Postoperative care

Dressings should include generous amounts of antiseptic ointment covered with petrolatum gauze to avoid adhesion to the wound and to facilitate removal of the dressing. Two to three fine-mesh gauze squares and either tubular elastic net or elastic bandage complete it. A narrow bandage (4 cm) is a more flexible form of dressing which enables pressure to be applied more precisely over the wound. The dressing should provide no more than light compression in order not to compromise the blood flow. This bulky dressing will enable postoperative bleeding to be absorbed and will provide some protection against trauma. The limb should be kept elevated for 48 h to ease throbbing and facilitate healing. The patient should wear a sling if the surgery involves a finger, or keep the foot elevated for 2 days for toe surgery. This also means that the patient should not plan to drive home following surgery. Painkillers should be prescribed for 3 days. The dressing should be removed on day 2, if necessary after soaking. Further care includes twice-daily dressings with antiseptic ointment covered by a plaster until complete healing has been achieved.

THE NAIL AND COSMETICS

Nail coatings represent an attractive nail enhancement. They may harden upon evaporation (nail varnish) or polymerize (sculptured nails, gels, preformed artificial nails) [1].

Coatings that harden upon evaporation

Nail varnish
The term 'nail lacquer' is sometimes used to include enamels, top coats and base coats, either as separate entities or combined in one product. Although chemically similar, they contain different ratios of the same constituents to lend different characteristics. The base coat is used to improve the adhesion or bonding of enamel to the nail. A top coat improves the depth and lustre of the enamel and increases its resistance to chipping and abrasion. Nail polishes consist of solids and solvent ingredients, the former representing about 30%, the latter 70% of the product. The ingredients can be divided into six principal groups (Box 95.3).

Box 95.3 Ingredients of nail polish

1 Cellulose film formers (e.g. nitrocellulose): provide gloss, body and gel structure
2 Resins (e.g. tosylamide formaldehyde resin; previously known as toluene sulphonamide formaldehyde resin): improve gloss and adhesion of the film
3 Plasticizers (e.g. camphor): give the film pliability, minimize shrinkage, and soften and plasticize the cellulose
4 Thixotropic suspending agents (e.g. bentonite) for non-settling and flow: keep pigments in suspension by preventing the particles from clogging together, so that they will disperse on shaking
5 Solvents and diluents: keep nitrocellulose, resin and plasticizer in the liquid state and control the application and drying time
6 Colour substances: these are either inorganic (iron oxides) or a variety of certified organic colours (such as D and C yellow aluminium lakes). 'Pearls' or 'frosts' are produced by bismuth oxychloride and titanium dioxide coated with mica and guanine (obtained from fish scales). 'Clears' contain a small tint

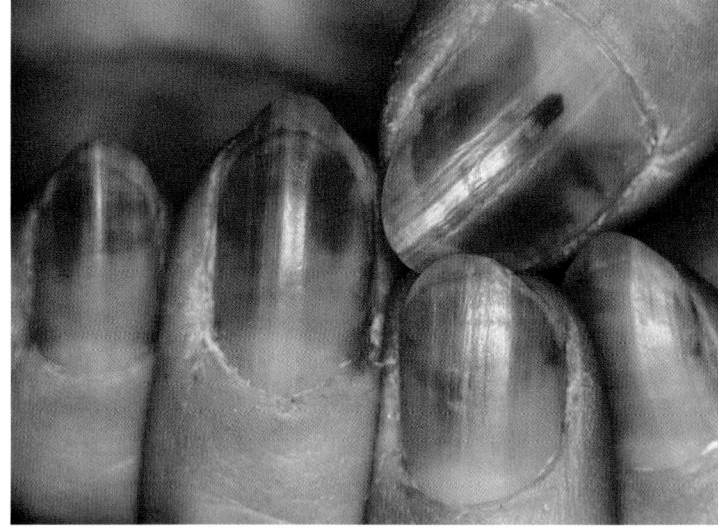

Figure 95.91 Staining of the nail plates from nail varnish.

The base coat is formulated in a manner similar to standard lacquer, but it has a lower non-volatile content (less nitrocellulose) and lower viscosity, because a thinner film is desirable; it may also contain hydrolysed gelatine. In the top coat, the nitrocellulose content is increased and the resin reduced. A slight increase in plasticizer content improves the elasticity of the film. There is no pigment. The top coat often has an added sunscreen.

Reactions such as an allergic contact dermatitis to nail varnish frequently appear on any part of the body accessible to the nails, with paradoxically no signs in or around the nail apparatus [2]. The most commonly involved areas are the eyelids (Figure 95.90), the lower half of the face, the sides of the neck and the upper chest. Sometimes the use of nail polish on stockings to stop 'runs' or on nickel-plated costume jewellery to prevent nickel dermatitis may induce nail polish dermatitis on the legs or at the site of the metal contact. Connubial or transfer nail polish dermatitis may occur in the user's partner or other close contacts. Although any ingredient may account for distant allergic contact dermatitis, tosylamide for-maldehyde resin is the most common culprit. After the nail polish is removed, the dermatitis usually clears rapidly unless secondary infection or lichenification has occurred. Eluate from uncoated metal pellets present in some bottles to keep the varnish in a liquid state may cause nickel reactions and onycholysis.

Nail plate staining from the use of polish is most commonly yellow-orange in colour (Figure 95.91). It typically starts near the cuticle, extends to the nail tip and becomes progressively darker from base to tip. With time, the dyes penetrate the nail too deeply to be removed. Injury to the nail plate from nail lacquers is rare. However, 'granulation' of nail keratin, a superficial friability, can be observed in some instances where individuals leave nail lacquer on for many weeks or where there is poor formulation of the product.

For patch testing, several nail lacquers should be used and tested 'as is' using occlusive chambers (e.g. Finn Chambers® or IQ Ultra Chambers®); the lacquers should be allowed to dry for 15 min before application of the patches, because the solvents and diluents may cause false-positive reactions.

The substances listed in Box 95.4 should be included in the test battery.

Various cosmetic companies now make varnishes that are formulated without the sensitizing resin and are toluene free. The presence of nickel in any product can be detected using the dimethylglyoxime spot test, which is highly specific.

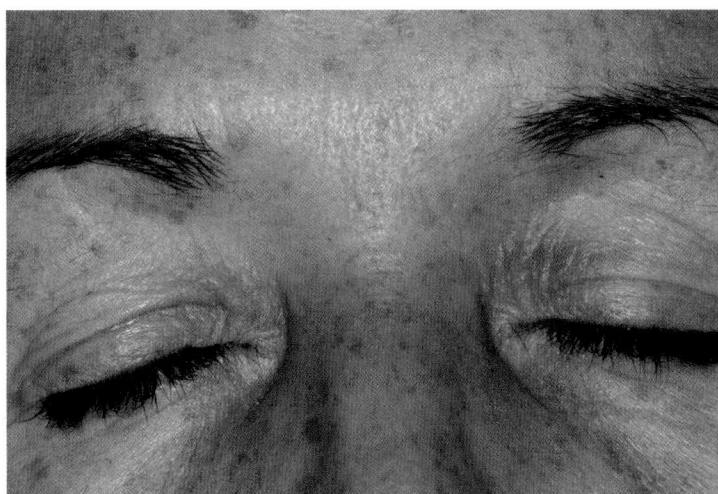

Figure 95.90 Allergy to nail varnish presenting as an eyelid dermatitis.

Box 95.4 Test battery for nail plate staining

- Tosylamide formaldehyde resin (10% in petrolatum)
- Nickel sulphate hexahydrate (2.5% in petrolatum)
- Glyceryl phthalate resin (polymer resin) (10% in petrolatum)
- Pearly material; guanine powder (as is)
- Formaldehyde (1% aqueous)
- Colophony (20% in petrolatum)
- Drometrizole trisiloxane (10% in petrolatum)

Nail polish removers. These are composed of various solvents such as acetone. Occasionally, nail polish removers cause trouble by excessive drying of the nail plate, and may be responsible for some inflammation of the nail folds.

Coatings that polymerize

Sculptured nails

The nail is first thoroughly cleansed and painted with antiseptic and antifungal solutions. The nail is frequently dried with a diethyl ether based nail dehydrating agent and sometimes 'primed' with methacrylic acid/solvent adhesion promoter which works like a double-sided adhesive tape, sticking to both the nail and to the acrylic.

Self-curing acrylic resins are obtained by blending a methyl, ethyl or isobutyl methacrylate monomer which comes in a liquid form and a polymethyl or ethyl methacrylate polymer, which is a powder. The monomer also contains a stabilizer such as hydroquinone and N,n-dimethyl-p-toluidine as an accelerator. The polymer contains benzoyl peroxide as a polymerization initiator. Liquid monomer and powder polymer are mixed and the compound has to be moulded on the natural nail. Self-curing acrylic resins harden at room temperature. When hardened, the compound produces a prosthetic nail that is enlarged and elongated by repeated applications. The prosthesis can be filed and manicured to shape, as the plate grows out, further applications of acrylic can be made to maintain a regular contour.

Allergic reactions

Allergic reactions due to sculptured nails may occur 2–4 months, or even as long as 16 months, after the first application. The first indication is an itch in the nail bed. Paronychia, which is usually present in allergic reactions, is associated with excruciating pain in the nail area, and sometimes with paraesthesia. The nail bed is dry and thickened, and there is usually onycholysis. The natural nail plate becomes thinner, splits and is sometimes discoloured. It takes several months for the nails to return to normal. Permanent nail loss is exceptional, as is intractable prolonged paraesthesia [3].

Irritant reactions

Irritant reactions to monomers occur. These manifest as a thickening of the nail bed's keratin layer, which can sometimes cause the entire nail bed to thicken with or without onycholysis. Nonetheless, the overwhelming majority of cases result from physical trauma or abuse.

Damage to the natural nail is not unusual after 2–4 months of wear of a sculptured nail. If it becomes yellow or crumbly, this means that the product was applied and maintained incorrectly. The patient should find a better-qualified nail technician. The problem may well not be the acrylic nail materials but rather the thinning of the nail due to excessive filing with heavy abrasives.

Primer (methacrylic acid) is a strong irritant, which may produce third-degree burns. It is hazardous if the cuticles are flooded or spills are not washed out immediately. Primer can permeate the plate and soak into the nail bed if the nails are too thin. Soap or baking soda dissolved in water are excellent neutralizers. If primer gets into the eye, it should be rinsed with water for at least 15 min and a Poisons Information Centre should be contacted.

Light-cured gels

Gel system products are a premixed variant of sculptured nails in a semi-liquid form, either acrylic based (14% of the market) or cyanoacrylate based (1% or less of the market). Their virtual lack of odour makes gels popular in full-service beauty salons. UV light-cured gels are the best known of the different gel technologies. These gels contain urethanes and (meth)acrylate compounds, a photoinitiator and cellulose, which necessitates anti-yellowing agents and a UV light unit. The proportion of resins to monomers determines the gel consistency. When the gel is exposed to light of an appropriate wavelength, polymerization occurs, resulting in hardening of the gel. UV gels never involve catalysts and often do not require primers. Depending upon their composition, the gels can be used for different purposes as follows:

- Instead of the sculptured nail technique. However, they do not permit the formation of nails which are as long and resistant as those from the classical liquid–powder technique.
- Over preformed plastic tips: the nail surface is buffed. After disinfection, the preformed plastic tip is simply fixed with cyanoacrylate glue on the distal half of the nail.
- To protect a natural or varnished nail: this procedure is known as 'nail capping'.
- Capping with fabric (silk, linen or fibreglass fixed with cyanoacrylate glue) adds strength and is known as 'nail wrapping'.

The gel nails are useful in patients seeking treatment for cosmetically disfigured nails with the exception of psoriasis, where the risk of the Koebner phenomenon is high [4].

Gel enhancement products shrink by up to 20%, which may result in lifting and tip cracking. As an effect of excessive shrinkage, clients may comment that the enhancement feels tight on the nail bed. Other symptoms include throbbing or warmth below the nail plate. This may lead to tender and sore fingertips. Photobonded acrylate has been observed to cause nail reactions, sometimes with nail loss and paraesthesia. Hemmer *et al.* [4] have patch tested 'hypoallergenic' commercial products in patients wearing photobonded acrylic nails who had perionychial and subungual eczema. Triethyleneglycol dimethacrylate, hydroxyfunctional methacrylates, and (meth)-acrylated urethanes proved to be relevant allergens in photobonded nail preparations. Methacrylated epoxy resin sensitization was not observed. The omission of irritant methacrylic acid in UV-curable gels does not reduce the high sensitizing potential of new acrylates. Contrary to the manufacturers' declarations, all 'hypoallergenic' products continue to include functional acrylate monomers, and therefore retain the potential for allergic sensitization. Gels and acrylics, being chemically distinct entities, will not necessarily cross-react.

Unreacted UV gel in the dusts and filings may produce distant allergic reactions. Although sensitization to butyl-hydroxytoluene is possible, gels usually contain acrylated oligomers and monomers. Acrylates are far more likely to cause sensitization than methacrylates or stabilizers.

Finally, thick and ornately painted gel false nails that may be difficult to remove present a real challenge to pulse oximetry. It appears to be the polish more than the sculpted nail that interferes with the readings.

Gel polish

This is a new manicure system applied in a salon by a nail technician. The application involves a base coat that is cured under a UV lamp, two layers of a proprietary nail varnish, and a top coat. During the curing process with a UV lamp, the manufacturer states that solvents evaporate and leave tiny 'tunnels' in the layer of varnish, connected by acetone-dissolvable polymers.

Preformed plastic nails

Preformed plastic nails are packaged in several shapes and sizes to conform to the normal nail plate configuration. Such nails are trimmed to fit the fingertip and are fixed with cyanoacrylate adhesive supplied with the kit. The usefulness of these prosthetic nails is limited by the need for some normal nail to be present for attachment. Normal physical and chemical insults to the nails cause the preformed plastic nails to loosen. If the preformed nails remain in place for more than 2–3 days, they may cause onycholysis and nail surface damage. Eczematous painful paronychia due to cyanoacrylate nail preparations may be observed after about 3 months. Dystrophy and discoloration of the nails may become apparent and last for several months. In some cases, distant contact dermatitis of the face and eyelids occurs. On patch testing, the patients react far more often to the adhesive than to the prosthetic nails (Figure 96.92). Suggested test substances are *p*-tertiary butylphenol resin (1% petrolatum); tricresyl ethyl phthalate (5% petrolatum); cyanoacrylates and other glues (5% in methylethylketone).

Nail-mending kits

These include paper strips of a basic film-forming product to create a 'splint' for the partially fractured nail plate. The split is first bonded with cyanoacrylate glue, then the nail is painted with fibred clear nail polish. A piece of wrap fabric is cut and shaped to

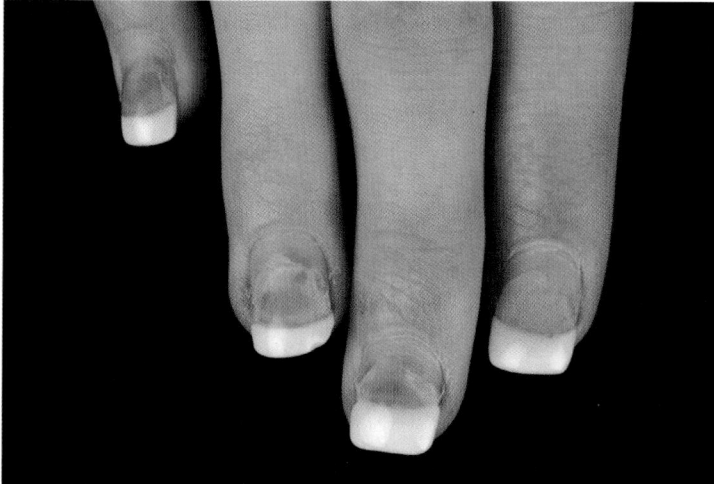

Figure 95.92 Complication of nail extensions: allergy to acrylate adhesive presenting as onycholysis.

fit over the nail surface. This is then embedded in varnish of high solid content, and several coats are applied.

Removal of nail coatings that polymerize

The most commonly used solvent for removal of self-curing acrylic is acetone. Warming the solvent with great care can cut product removal time in half. However, most gels are difficult to remove because they are highly cross-linked and resistant to many solvents. Therefore, if gel enhancements have to be removed, they should be slowly filed (not drilled) with a medium-grit file, leaving a very thin layer of product. They should then be soaked in warm product remover and, once softened, the remaining product may be scraped away with a wooden pusher stick.

Cuticle removers

These are lotions or gels containing approximately 0.4% sodium or KOH. The lotion is left in place for 1–3 min and then washed off. Creams containing 1–5% lactic acid (pH 3–3.7) are also used.

Nail hardeners

There are two main groups of products that make nail-hardening claims.

Products in the first group provide a protective coating, therefore the implied benefits come from the added strength and durability of the coating itself, rather than changes to the physical properties of the nail plate. Some consist of nail polish modified by the addition of extra ingredients including nylon fibres, acrylate resin and hydrolysed proteins: they function either as a base coat for nail polish or as a stand-alone treatment. Others applied as a base coat are essentially a modification of clear nail polish with different solvents and combinations of polyester, acrylic and polyamide resins designed to provide better adhesion of the coloured nail coating.

The second type of hardener chemically alters the structure of the nail. These products may contain up to 5% formaldehyde tissue fixative, but are designed to be applied only to the free edge of the nail while the skin is shielded. Most products never exceed 3% formaldehyde and the more widely sold brands contain less than 1%. Higher concentrations of formaldehyde can adversely affect both the nail plate and the surrounding tissue.

Nail changes due to hardeners may include pain, subungual haemorrhage and bluish discoloration of the nail. Formaldehyde nail hardeners have also been reported as causing onycholysis and both irritant and allergic contact dermatitis. Patch testing should be performed with formaldehyde (1 or 2% aqueous).

Silicone rubber nail prosthesis

For a wide variety of nail problems, ranging from deformed nail to complete loss of the terminal phalanx, a silicone rubber thimble-shaped finger-cover may be indicated. This prosthesis is easily fitted onto the finger stump, encasing the entire distal phalanx; it must be fine and flexible to maintain pulp sensitivity and have the same marking and colouring as the finger. The fixation is excellent and the nail form accepts nail varnish well. The most well known are Pillet Hand Prostheses® (PHPs), which are available in the US and some European countries. When there has been loss of tissue from the distal phalangeal pulp, a 'sub-mini' digital prosthesis is also available.

Nail cream

This is an ordinary water-in-oil moisturising cream, with low water (30%) and high lipid content. It is applied, after cleaning the hands, to prevent or diminish brittleness.

Nail buffing

Weekly buffing may be indicated for removing small particles of nail debris, thus enhancing the lustre and smoothness of the nail plate. Buffing creams, which contain waxes and finely ground pumice, and buffing powders are abrasive and should not be over-used on thin nails.

Nail whitener

This is a pencil-like device with a white clay (kaolin) core used to deposit colour on the undersurface of the free edge of the nail.

Infection risks

Medical staff with artificial nails or nail extensions may put patients at risk through carriage of pathogens. The UK guidelines now require medical staff not to wear such embellishment. Nail varnish is also thought to be associated with bacterial carriage when it becomes chipped, although the evidence for this is less strong. Infection through nail salons and the manicuring process is a further factor that adds to the risks for those with artificial nails.

Conclusion

Nail beauty therapy is a flourishing and innovative industry with low overall risks of serious adverse events. It may certainly produce an attractive enhancement of normal nails and can be very valuable for disguising unsightly nail conditions: it is not recommended for psoriatic nails as it may provoke the Koebner phenomenon. Potential hazards include damage from instrumentation and allergic contact dermatitis.

Key references

The full list of references can be found in the online version at www.rooksdermatology.com.

Structure
1 Zook EG. Anatomy and physiology of the perionychium. *Hand Clin* 2002;18:553–9.
10 de Berker D, Angus B. Markers of epidermal proliferation are limited to nail matrix in normal nail. *Br J Dermatol* 1996;135:555–9.
14 Perrin C. Peculiar zone of the distal nail unit: the nail isthmus. *Am J Dermatopathol* 2007;29:108–9.
28 Blaydon DC, Ishii Y, O'Toole EA, *et al*. The gene encoding R-spondin 4 (RSPO4), a secreted protein implicated in Wnt signaling, is mutated in inherited anonychia. *Nat Genet* 2006;38:1245–7.
29 Cui CY, Klar J, Georgii-Heming P, *et al*. Frizzled6 deficiency disrupts the differentiation process of nail development. *J Invest Dermatol* 2013;133:1990–7.
30 Nagy N, Wedgeworth E, Hamada T, White JM, Hashimoto T, McGrath JA. Schöpf–Schulz–Passarge syndrome resulting from a homozygous nonsense mutation in WNT10A. *J Dermatol Sci* 2010;58:220–2.
34 Spaunhurst KM, Hogendorf AM, Smith FJ, *et al*. Pachyonychia congenita patients with mutations in KRT6A have more extensive disease compared with patients who have mutations in KRT16. *Br J Dermatol* 2012;166:875–8.

Nail growth and morphology
3 Zaias N, Alvarez J. The formation of the primate nail plate. An autoradiographic study in squirrel monkeys. *J Invest Dermatol* 1968;51:120–36.
4 Norton LA. Incorporation of thymidine ³H and glycine-2 ³H in the nail matrix and bed of humans. *J Invest Dermatol* 1971;56:61–8.
10 Baran R. Nail growth direction revisited. Why do nails grow out instead of up? *J Am Acad Dermatol* 1981;4:78–84.
18 Bean WB. Nail growth: 30 years of observations. *Arch Intern Med* 1974;134:497–502.

Clubbing
9 Busch J, Frank V, Bachmann N, *et al*. Mutations in the prostaglandin transporter SLCO2A1 cause primary hypertrophic osteoarthropathy with digital clubbing. *J Invest Dermatol* 2012;132:2473–6.

Pincer nail
1 Baran R, Haneke E, Richert B. Pincer nails: definition and surgical treatment. *Dermatol Surg* 2001;27:261–6.

Onycholysis
2 Daniel CR III, Iorizzo M, Piraccini BM, Tosti A. Grading simple chronic paronychia and onycholysis. *Int J Dermatol* 2006;45:1447–8.

Yellow nail syndrome
20 Maldonado F, Tazelaar HD, Wang CW, Ryu JH. Yellow nail syndrome: analysis of 41 consecutive patients. *Chest* 2008;134:375–81.
21 Baran R, Thomas L. Combination of fluconazole and alpha-tocopherol in the treatment of yellow nail syndrome. *J Drugs Dermatol* 2009;8:276–8.

Longitudinal erythronychia
1 de Berker DA, Perrin C, Baran R. Localized longitudinal erythronychia: diagnostic significance and physical explanation. *Arch Dermatol* 2004;140:1253–7.

Subungual haematoma
1 Dean B, Becker G, Little C. The management of the acute traumatic subungual haematoma: a systematic review. *Hand Surg* 2012;17:151–4.
3 Oztas MO. Clinical and dermoscopic progression of subungual hematomas. *Int Surg* 2010;95:239–41.

Nail bed laceration
2 Tos P, Titolo P, Chirila NL, Catalano F, Artiaco S. Surgical treatment of acute fingernail injuries. *J Orthop Traumatol* 2012;13:57–62.

Nail biting
3 Pacan P, Grzesiak M, Reich A, Kantorska-Janiec M, Szepietowski JC. Onychophagia and onychotillomania: prevalence, clinical picture and comorbidities. *Acta Derm Venereol* 2014;94:67–71.
12 Silber KP, Haynes CE. Treating nailbiting: a comparative analysis of mild aversion and competing response therapies. *Behav Res Ther* 1992;30:15–22.

Ingrowing toenail
1 Baran R, Bureau H. Congenital malalignment of the great toenail as a cause of ingrowing toenail in infancy. *Clin Exp Dermatol* 1983;6:619–23.
4 Baran R, Haneke E, Richert B. Pincer nails: definition and surgical treatment. *Dermatol Surg* 2001;27:261–6.
5 de Berker DA, Richert B, Duhard E, Piraccini BM, André J, Baran R. Retronychia: proximal ingrowing of the nail plate. *J Am Acad Dermatol* 2008;58:978–83.
8 Piraccini BM, Parente GL, Varotti E, Tosti A. Congenital hypertrophy of the lateral nail folds of the hallux: clinical features and follow-up of seven cases. *Pediatr Dermatol* 2000;17:348–51.
16 Wernick J, Gibbs RC. Pedal biomechanics and toenail disease. In: Scher RK, Daniel CR, eds. *Nails: Therapy, Diagnosis, Surgery*. Philadelphia: Saunders, 1990:244–9.
18 Arai H, Arai T, Nakajima H, Haneke E. Formable acrylic treatment for ingrowing nail with gutter splint and sculptured nail. *Int J Dermatol* 2004;43:759–65.

Tumours under or adjacent to the nail

4 Piraccini BM, Bellavista S, Misciali C, Tosti A, de Berker D, Richert B. Periungual and subungual pyogenic granuloma. *Br J Dermatol* 2010;163:941–53.

27 Van Geertruyden J, Lorea P, Goldschmidt D, *et al*. Glomus tumours of the hand. A retrospective study of 51 cases. *J Hand Surg* 1996;21B:257–60.

42 De Berker DA, Langtry J. Treatment of subungual exostoses by elective day case surgery. *Br J Dermatol* 1999;140:915–18.

48 de Berker D, Lawrence C. Ganglion of the distal interphalangeal joint (myxoid cyst): therapy by identification and repair of the leak of joint fluid. *Arch Dermatol* 2001;137:607–10.

56 Baran R, Mikhail G, Costini B, Tosti A, Goettmann-Bonvallot S. Distal digital keratoacanthoma: two cases with a review of the literature. *Dermatol Surg* 2001;27:575–9.

71 Perrin C, Goettmann S, Baran R. Onychomatricoma: clinical and histopathologic findings in 12 cases. *J Am Acad Dermatol* 1998;39:560–4.

87 Hollmann TJ, Bovée JVMG, Fletcher CDM. Digital fibromyxoma (superficial acral fibromyxoma): a detailed characterization of 124 cases. *Am J Surg Pathol* 2012;36:789–98.

89 Baran R, Perrin C. Longitudinal erythronychia with distal subungual keratosis: onychopapilloma of the nail bed and Bowen's disease. *Br J Dermatol* 2000;143:132–5.

93 Lecerf P, Richert B, Theunis A, André J. A retrospective study of squamous cell carcinoma of the nail unit diagnosed in a Belgian general hospital over a 15-year period. *J Am Acad Dermatol* 2013;69:253–61.

125 Thai KE, Young R, Sinclair RD. Nail apparatus melanoma. *Australas J Dermatol* 2001;42:71–81; quiz 82–3.

Perionychial disorders

1 Dardu M, Ruocco V. Clinical cytologic features of antibiotic resistant acute paronychia. *J Am Acad Dermatol* 2014;70:120–6.

2 Sezer E, Bridges AE, Koseoglu D, Yuksek J. Acquired periungual fibrokeratoma developing after acute staphylococcal paronychia. *Eur J Dermatol* 2009;19:636–7.

6 Walker S. Paronychia of the great toenail of infants. *Clin Pediatr* 1979;18:247.

7 Baran R. Nail alterations in hand eczema. In: Alikhan A, Lachapelle JM, Maibach HI, eds. *Textbook of Hand Eczema*. Berlin: Springer-Verlag, 2014:37–47.

8 Hay RJ, Baran R. Onychomycosis: a proposed revision of the clinical classification. *J Am Acad Dermatol* 2011;65:1219–27.

11 Fleming TE, Brodell RT. Subungual abscess: a bacterial infection of the nail bed. *J Am Acad Dermatol* 1997;37:486–7.

12 Dawber RPR, Baran R. Painful dorso-lateral fissure of the fingertip: an extension of the lateral nail groove. *Clin Exp Dermatol* 1984;9:419–20.

Nail psoriasis

1 Zaias N. Psoriasis of the nail. A clinical–pathologic study. *Arch Dermatol* 1969;99:567–79.

8 McGonagle D, Tan AL, Benjamin M. The nail as a musculoskeletal appendage: implications for an improved understanding of the link between psoriasis and arthritis. *Dermatology* 2009;218:97–102.

10 Brazzelli V, Carugno A, Alborghetti A, *et al*. Prevalence, severity and clinical features of psoriasis in fingernails and toenails in adult patients: Italian experience. *J Eur Acad Dermatol Venereol* 2012;26:1354–9.

11 Rich P, Scher RK. Nail Psoriasis Severity Index: a useful tool for evaluation of nail psoriasis. *J Am Acad Dermatol* 2003;49:206–12.

53 de Vries AC, Bogaards NA, Hooft L, *et al*. Interventions for nail psoriasis. *Cochrane Database Syst Rev* 2013;(1):CD007633.

Darier disease of the nails

2 Burge SM, Wilkinson JD. Darier–White disease: a review of the clinical features in 163 patients. *J Am Acad Dermatol* 1992;27:40–50.

Lichen planus of the nails

12 Tosti A, Piraccini BM, Cambiaghi S, Jorizzo M. Nail lichen planus in children: clinical features, response to treatment, and long-term follow-up. *Arch Dermatol* 2001;137:1027–32.

19 Pandhi D, Singal A, Bhattacharya SN. Lichen planus in childhood: a series of 316 patients. *Pediatr Dermatol* 2014;31:59–67.

21 Manousaridis I, Manousaridis K, Peitsch WK, Schneider SW. Individualizing treatment and choice of medication in lichen planus: a step by step approach. *J Dtsch Dermatol Ges* 2013;11:981–91.

Nails in childhood and old age

1 Baran R, Barth J, Dawber RPR, eds. *Nail Disorders*. London: Dunitz, 1991:78–101.

2 de Berker D. Childhood nail diseases. *Dermatol Clin* 2006;24:355–63.

3 Hammerton MD, Shrank AB. Congenital hypertrophy of the lateral nail folds of the hallux. *Pediatr Dermatol* 1988;5:243–5.

4 Piraccini BM, Parente GL, Varotti E, Tosti A. Congenital hypertrophy of the lateral nail folds of the hallux: clinical features and follow-up of seven cases. *Pediatr Dermatol* 2000;17:348–51.

5 Baran R. Congenital malalignment of the toe nail. *Arch Dermatol* 1980;116:1346.

12 Brauer E, Baran R. Cosmetics: the care and adornment of the nail. In: Baran R, Dawber RPR, de Berker DAR, Haneke E, Tosti A, eds. *Diseases of the Nails and Their Management*, 3rd edn. Oxford: Blackwell Science, 2001:366–8.

14 Helfand AE. Assessing onychial disorders in the older patient. *Clin Podiatr Med Surg* 2003;20:431–42.

Imaging of the nail

1 Destouet JM, Murphy WA. Acquired osteolysis and acronecrosis. *Arthritis Rheum* 1983;26:1150–4.

12 Baran R. Nail tumours: Clinical overview. In: Wortsman X, Jemec GBE, eds. *Dermatologic Ultrasound with Clinical and Histologic Correlations*. Heidelberg: Springer, 2013:409–18.

13 Gambichler T, Jaedicke V, Terras S. Optical coherence tomography in dermatology: technical and clinical aspects. *Arch Dermatol Res* 2011;303:457–73.

Nail surgery

1 Richert B. Basic nail surgery. *Dermatol Clin* 2006;24:313–22.

2 Abimelec P, Dumontier C. Basic and advanced nail surgery. In: Scher RK, Daniel CR, eds. *Nails: Diagnosis, Therapy, Surgery*, 3rd edn. Philadelphia: Elsevier Saunders, 2005:265–89.

9 Chowdhry S, Seidenstricker L, Cooney DS, Hazani R, Wilhelmi BJ. Do not use epinephrine in digital blocks: myth or truth? Part II. A retrospective review of 1111 cases. *Plast Reconstr Surg* 2010;126:2031–4.

19 Baran R, Kechijian P. Longitudinal melanonychia (melanonychia striata): diagnosis and management. *J Am Acad Dermatol* 1989;21:1165–75.

22 Richert B, Theunis A, Norrenberg S, André J. Tangential excision of pigmented nail matrix lesions responsible for longitudinal melanonychia: evaluation of the technique on a series of 30 patients. *J Am Acad Dermatol* 2013;69:96–104.

23 De Berker DA, Baran R. Acquired malalignment: a complication of lateral longitudinal nail biopsy. *Acta Derm Venereol* 1998;78:468–70.

24 de Berker DA. Lateral longitudinal nail biopsy. *Australas J Dermatol* 2001;42:142–4.

26 Baran R, Richert B. The management of onychomycosis. *Ann Dermatol Vénéréol* 2003;130:1260–71.

28 Baran R, Bureau H. Surgical treatment of recalcitrant chronic paronychias of the fingers. *J Dermatol Surg Oncol* 1981;7:106–7.

31 Eekhof JAH, Van Wijk B, Knuistingh Neven A, van der Wouden JC. Interventions for ingrowing toenails. *Cochrane Database Syst Rev* 2012;(4):CD001541.

21 Richert B. Surgical management of ingrown toenails: an update overdue. *Dermatol Ther* 2012;25:498–509.

PART 8: SPECIFIC CUTANEOUS STRUCTURE

CHAPTER 96

Acquired Disorders of Dermal Connective Tissue

Christopher R. Lovell

Department of Dermatology, Royal United Hospital and Royal National Hospital for Rheumatic Diseases, Bath, UK

CHANGES IN DERMAL CONNECTIVE TISSUE DUE TO AGEING AND PHOTODAMAGE

Introduction and general description

Both intrinsic ageing and UV exposure result in alterations in dermal connective tissue which affect the appearance of the skin in old age [1,2]. The relative contributions of each vary in the individual from body site to body site and in the population at large according to environmental factors, particularly cumulative photodamage and cigarette smoking. The skin becomes increasingly thin and atrophic in elderly people. Changes in both the epidermis and the dermis result in age-related skin fragility characterized by translucent, lax and wrinkled skin with a tendency to easy bruising and stellate scars. The term 'dermatoporosis' has been coined to describe these changes [3]. The relative contribution of intrinsic ageing and environmental factors to the changes in dermal connective tissue which manifest as skin ageing determine the clinical appearance. Much of what is perceived as aged skin is due to photodamage with the development of actinic elastosis, lax skin and wrinkles. Recent research has helped to elucidate the pathomechanisms underlying these changes. There is reduced collagen biosynthesis and increased production of matrix metalloproteinases, which both inhibit collagen fibril synthesis and promote fragmentation of collagen fibrils, leading to a reduction in healthy collagen but accumulation of damaged collagen. The topic is discussed in detail in Chapter 155. Some specific clinical manifestations associated with aged and photoaged skin are described later.

Wrinkles

Definition and nomenclature

Wrinkles are a characteristic of ageing skin. They may be defined as creases or furrows in the skin surface.

Synonyms and inclusions
- Rhytides

Introduction and general description

Wrinkles are particularly prominent in hypertrophic skin photodamage (see Chapter 155). Cigarette smoking is also a potent independent cause of wrinkling. The so-called 'cigarette face' is characterized by pale grey wrinkled skin with rather gaunt features, so that heavy smokers can often be recognized from their facial appearance alone. Heavy smokers are five times more likely to be wrinkled than non-smokers of the same age, and cigarette smoking probably has at least as much effect on facial wrinkles as sun exposure [1].

Clinical features

They are particularly prominent in hypertrophic skin photodamage (see Chapter 155). Cigarette smoking is also a potent independent cause of wrinkling. The so-called 'cigarette face' is characterized by pale grey wrinkled skin with rather gaunt features, so that heavy smokers can often be recognized from their facial appearance alone. Heavy smokers are five times more likely to be wrinkled than non-smokers of the same age, and cigarette smoking probably has at least as much effect on facial wrinkles as sun exposure [1].

Wrinkles can be classified into three morphological types [2] as follows.

1 Crinkles. This is a very fine wrinkling which occurs in aged skin, even in areas protected from sunlight. These fine wrinkles disappear when the skin is slightly stretched. They are caused by deterioration of elastin, especially the vertical subepidermal fine elastic fibres which keep the epidermis in tight apposition to the dermis [3,4]. Ultrastructural studies have shown that even in normal people the elastic fibres begin to deteriorate from the age of 30 years onwards, regardless of the amount of sun exposure, although sunlight undoubtedly increases the damage [5]. Crinkles are seen in a marked form in mid-dermal elastolysis.

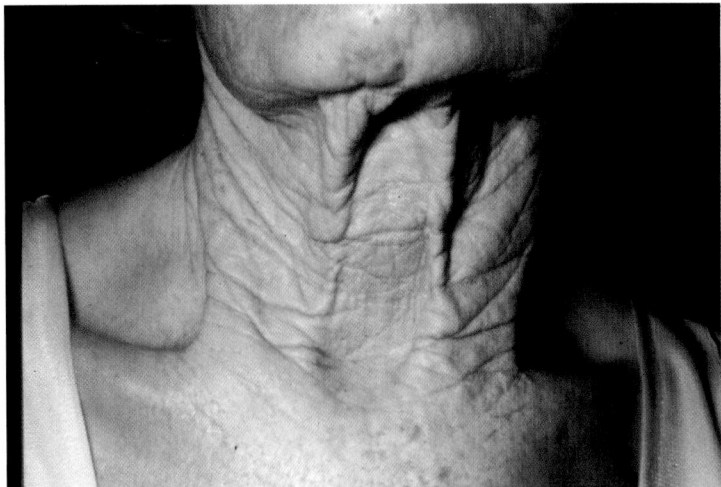

Figure 96.1 Actinic elastosis on the neck of an elderly female patient.

2 Glyphic wrinkles. These creases are an accentuation of the normal skin markings. They occur on skin which has been prematurely aged by elastotic degeneration caused by sunlight, for example on the sides and back of the neck (see Actinic elastosis).
3 Linear furrows. These are long, straight or slightly curved grooves that are usually seen on the faces of elderly people. They include the horizontal frown lines along the forehead, the 'crows' feet' radiating from the lateral canthus of the eye and the creases from the nose to the corners of the mouth.

Actinic elastosis

Definition and nomenclature

Actinic elastosis is another component of hypertrophic skin photodamage. It is characterized clinically by yellowish discoloration and thickening of the skin (Figure 96.1), and histologically by a reduction in collagen and an accumulation of amorphous masses of degenerate elastic fibres in the papillary and upper reticular dermis (Figure 96.2) [1].

Synonyms and inclusions
- Solar elastosis

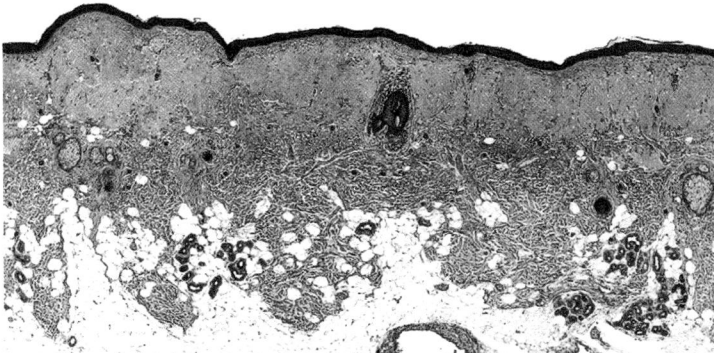

Figure 96.2 Actinic elastosis showing confluent masses of amorphous basophilic material in the papillary and upper reticular dermis with atrophy of the overlying epidermis.

Introduction and general description

Actinic elastosis usually results from prolonged exposure to sunlight [1], but it can also follow infrared (IR) radiation [2].

Epidemiology

Incidence and prevalence

It is related to the cumulative lifetime exposure to UV radiation rather than to episodes of intense UV exposure: it is more common in outdoor workers and in those living in sunny climates. There is, however, considerable variation in susceptibility between individuals.

Age

It does not usually present until the fourth decade or later but cumulative sun exposure is more important than chronological age alone.

Ethnicity

Fair-skinned people are the worst affected, although the condition can occur in black people [3].

Associated diseases

Severe elastosis may occur in photosensitized skin, for example in porphyria cutanea tarda.

Pathophysiology

Pathology

See Chapter 155.

Environmental factors

Cumulative UV exposure is the main exacerbating factor, although other factors, such as IR irradiation, may play a part [2].

Clinical features

History

The characteristic changes develop gradually over the course of years.

Presentation

The light-exposed areas are affected, particularly the forehead, bald scalp and the back of the neck. Mild degrees of elastosis may not be apparent until the skin is pinched up, when it may assume a wrinkled appearance. Elastosis is usually more advanced in the tissue than the clinical appearance would suggest.

The affected skin is diffusely thickened and yellowish (see Figures 96.1 and 155.2b), and on the neck it may be divided by well-defined furrows into an irregular rhomboidal pattern (cutis rhomboidalis nuchae) (see Figure 155.3). There may also be more sharply marginated, thickened plaques on the face or neck. These are usually, but not always, symmetrical. Recent studies suggest that the elastotic skin itself is protected from epithelial neoplasia [4].

Actinic elastosis may also be complicated by actinic granuloma (see later).

Clinical variants

Actinic comedonal plaque (synonyms Favre–Racouchot syndrome, nodular actinic elastosis with cysts and comedones). Actinic elastosis may form into confluent plaques studded with comedones. This is most commonly seen in periorbital skin (see Figure 96.3a,b). It is usually symmetrical, but unilateral and circumscribed forms have been reported [5]. Rarely, a variant has been described with vesicular changes within zones of severe actinic elastosis [6]. Occasionally, similar plaques may form elsewhere than on facial skin, such as the forearm [7].

Elastotic nodules of the ear. In this variant of actinic elastosis, single or multiple firm papules occur on the anterior crus of the antihelix, usually in middle-aged or elderly males. Their significance is that they sometimes have a pearly edge, clinically suggesting basal cell carcinoma (BCC), but histology reveals large aggregates of amorphous elastotic material, sometimes with degradation of underlying cartilage [8–10].

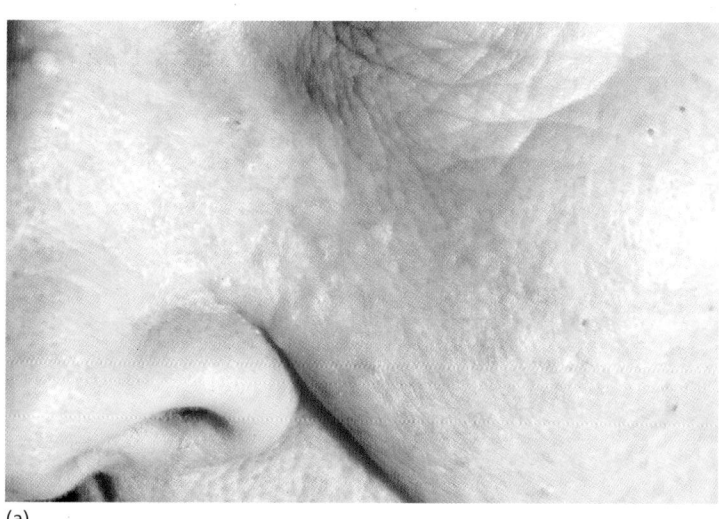
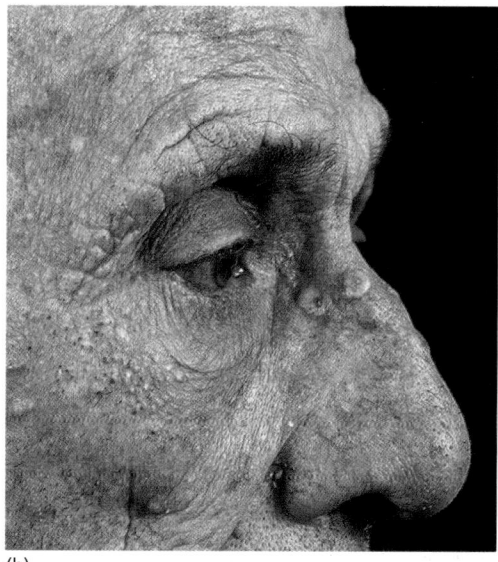

(a)   (b)

Figure 96.3 (a,b) Nodular actinic elastosis with comedones and cysts (Favre–Racouchot syndrome): early stages in a 78-year-old woman (a) and advanced stage in an elderly man (b). (Part b courtesy of Professor R. Marks, St Vincent's Hospital, Melbourne, Australia.)

Differential diagnosis

Plane xanthoma, pseudoxanthoma elasticum (PXE) and colloid milium may sometimes cause confusion, but the combination of the clinical and histological features is distinctive.

Classification of severity

Of cosmetic significance.

Disease course and prognosis

The process may be halted but not reversed by stringent photoprotection. Stopping smoking may be presumed to slow down progression [11].

Investigations

Skin biopsy if there is doubt about diagnosis. Histological changes may be more florid than the clinical appearance.

Management (see also Chapter 155)

Sunscreens protect against the development of photodamage both in humans and animals [12]. In hairless mice exposed to UVB radiation, synthesis of subepidermal collagen has been demonstrated in animals protected with a sunscreen [13]. Topical application of α-hydroxy acids ('fruit acids'), i.e. lactic, glycolic and citric acids, has been shown to lead to a modest improvement in photodamaged skin [14]. More impressive results have been obtained with topically applied tretinoin cream [15]. A double-blind study demonstrated a decrease in papillary dermal collagen type I in photodamaged skin, and subsequent treatment with 0.1% tretinoin cream for 10–12 months resulted in an 80% increase in dermal collagen [16]. Several studies have shown clinical and histological improvement after prolonged use [17]. Tretinoin may also repair skin changes due to intrinsic ageing [18]. Retinoids reduce matrix metalloproteinase 1 (MMP-1) expression *in vitro*, partially restoring levels of fibrillin 1 and collagens I and VII in the papillary dermis [19]. Similar results have been obtained in double-blind trials of topical isotretinoin [20] and tazarotene cream [21]. Antioxidants play a part in the prevention of photoageing [22] and may have a therapeutic role in established photodamage [23]. Non-ablative lasers, including the 1320 nm Nd : YAG and 1540 nm erbium glass lasers, are claimed to wound the upper dermis without epidermal damage [24]. Restoration of fibrillin I in the microfibrillar network of the papillary dermis may prove a useful 'biomarker' for the efficacy of topical products used in actinic elastosis [25,26].

Treatment ladder

First line
• Prevention by photoprotection

Second line
• Topical retinoids

Collagenous and elastotic marginal plaques of the hands

Synonyms and inclusions
• Digital papular calcific elastosis
• Keratoelastoidosis marginalis

Collagenous and elastotic marginal plaques of the hands is an acquired dermatosis affecting dermal connective tissue in which papules and plaques form on the dominant hand along the radial aspect of the index finger, the first web space and the ulnar aspect of the thumb (Figure 96.4a) [1,2]. Histologically, there is

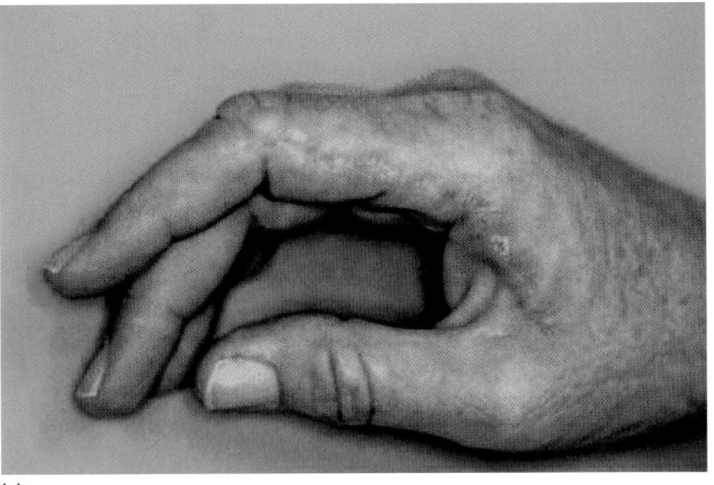
(a)

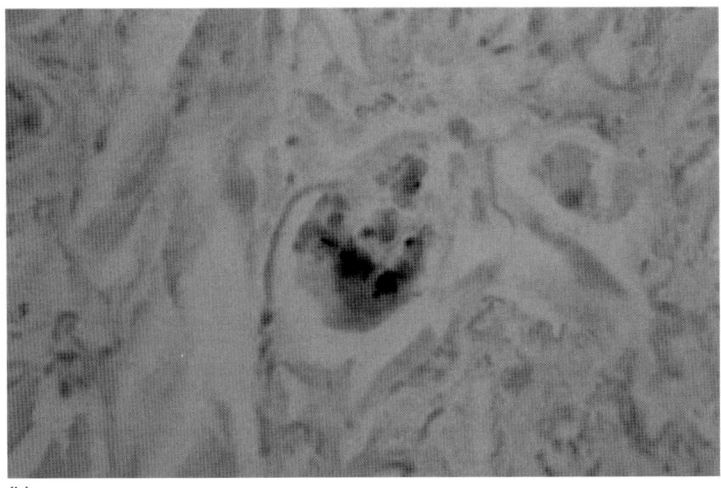
(b)

Figure 96.4 (a,b) Collagenous and elastotic marginal plaques of the hands: linear plaque involving radial aspect of the right index finger of a 49-year-old woman from Queensland, Australia (a); calcium deposits within collagen bundle (b). (From Mortimore and Conrad 2001 [7], with permission from John Wiley.)

hyperkeratosis, with sawtoothing of the rete ridges. The dermal collagen fibres are thickened and arranged haphazardly; there are basophilic elastotic masses, often containing calcium, in the upper reticular dermis (Figure 96.4b) [3]. Cases are sporadic, unlike the clinically similar disorders acrokeratoelastoidosis and focal acral hyperkeratosis (see p. 96.28) [4].

Chronic friction and photodamage have been proposed as aetiological factors; the condition has been reported in manual workers and entirely from geographical areas with high solar irradiation. It is regarded as a variant of actinic elastosis [5] although actinic damage is not always observed clinically [6]; furthermore the papillary dermis is relatively spared by the elastotic process and the basophilic areas containing calcium differ from the changes normally seen in actinic elastosis.

Adult colloid milium and colloid degeneration of the skin

Definition and nomenclature

Colloid degeneration of the skin is defined histologically by the presence of colloid in dermal papillae and presents as yellowish, translucent papules, nodules or plaques on light-exposed skin. There are several clinical variants of which the commonest is adult colloid milium, which manifests as multiple milia-like papules on light-exposed skin, particularly on the face.

Synonyms and inclusions
- Colloid degeneration of the skin
- Colloid pseudomilium
- Nodular colloid degeneration
- Elastosis colloidalis conglomerata

Introduction and general description

Colloid degeneration of the skin is a rare but probably underdiagnosed dermatosis which requires biopsy for definitive diagnosis [1]. It is defined histologically by the presence of colloid in dermal papillae and presents as yellowish translucent papules, nodules or plaques on light-exposed skin. There are several clinical variants of which the commonest is adult colloid milium, which manifests as multiple milia-like papules on light-exposed skin, particularly on the face. The differential diagnosis is presented in Table 96.1.

Epidemiology

Incidence and prevalence
Rare but usually affects fair-skinned, outdoor workers living in sunny climates [1,2].

Pathophysiology
The exact cause of adult colloid milium is uncertain but sunlight exposure is strongly implicated and actinic elastosis is usually evident as well [3]. Occupational exposure to mineral oils has also been implicated [4,5]: an outbreak among refinery workers in the

Table 96.1 Differential diagnosis of colloid milium.

Deposition disorder	Clinical findings	Pathological characteristics	Staining pattern
Adult colloid milium	Multiple symmetrical yellow to flesh-coloured facial papules; associated with sun exposure	Homogeneous eosinophilic colloid masses in papillary dermis from degenerating elastic fibres, often with subepidermal Grenz zone	PAS + Congo red ± Cotton dye − Cytokeratin −
Juvenile colloid milium	Multiple translucent yellowish papules on cheeks, nose, perioral skin; onset before puberty; familial; associated with ligneous conjunctivitis	Secondary to UV-induced degeneration of keratinocytes	PAS + Congo red ± Cotton dye − Cytokeratin +
Nodular colloid degeneration	Flesh-coloured nodule on face, scalp or chest; usually solitary	May be associated with myeloma; lacks plasma cells	PAS + Congo red ± Cotton dye −
Acrokeratoelastoidosis of Costa	Multiple tiny skin-coloured umbilicated papules at sides of hands and feet; familial; commonest in black skin	Fragmentation and degeneration of elastic fibres	Congo red − Cotton dye −
Collagenous and elastotic marginal plaques of the hands	Skin-coloured papules and plaques along radial border of index finger and ulnar border of thumb	Fragmentation and degeneration of elastic fibres	Congo red − Cotton dye −
Nodular amyloid	Single flesh-coloured nodule	Deposition of monoclonal immunoglobulin light-chain fragments from localized plasma cell infiltrate	Congo red + Cotton dye +

Adapted from Mehregan and Hooten 2011 [1].
PAS, periodic acid–Schiff.

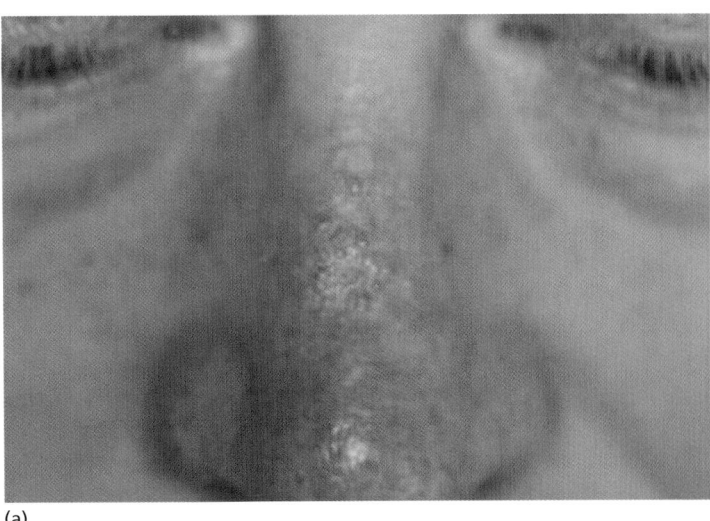
(a)

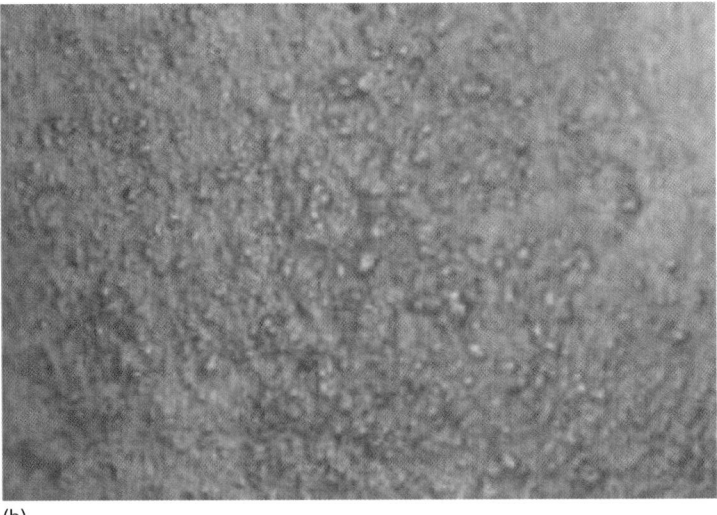
(b)

Figure 96.5 (a,b) Adult colloid milium with multiple tiny yellowish translucent papules on the dorsum of the nose (a) with close-up view of papules on the cheek (b). (From Mehregan and Hooten 2011 [**1**], with permission from John Wiley.)

tropics was attributed to trauma and prolonged contact with photodynamic phenols in oxide fuel (gas oil) [4]. Cases have also been reported in association with ochronosis after the long-term application of strong hydroquinone bleaching creams [6].

Histopathology

The earliest histological change is the appearance of colloid globules at the tips of the dermal papillae. Homogeneous fissured masses of amorphous colloid occupy the upper dermis, each surrounded by bands of collagen. There is characteristically a subepidermal uninvolved Grenz zone. The colloid is usually eosinophilic but may be basophilic. Within it, small blood vessels and the nuclei of fibroblasts are well preserved. In the larger, plaque-like lesions, the colloid change occurs diffusely throughout the dermis. The source of the colloid material is uncertain. It could be a protein synthesized by fibroblasts or it could be derived from degraded elastic fibres [2,7].

Environmental factors
UV exposure.

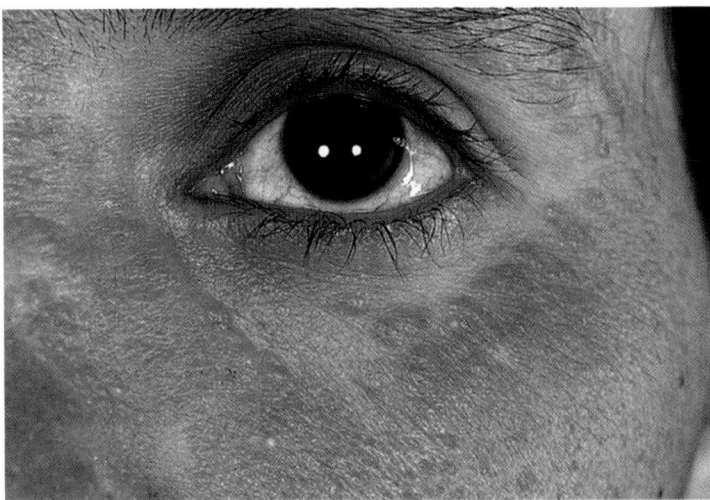

Figure 96.6 More advanced adult colloid milium manifesting as confluent plaques of the infraorbital region but with individual papules discernible at the margins.

Clinical features

Presentation

Small dermal papules 1–5 mm in diameter, yellowish brown and sometimes translucent, develop slowly and more or less symmetrically in irregular groups in areas exposed to sunlight (Figures 96.5 and 96.6) [1]. They feel soft and may release their gelatinous contents when punctured. The most frequently involved sites are the face, especially around the orbits, the dorsa of the hands, the back and sides of the neck and the ears. There are usually other signs of actinic damage. The changes induced by prolonged light exposure are associated to varying degrees. Although colloid milium may become more severe and more extensive over the years, most cases reach their maximum development within 3 years and then remain unchanged.

Differential diagnosis (see Table 96.1)
The rare juvenile form manifests before puberty and is often familial [8,9]. It is thought to derive from degeneration of keratinocytes rather than elastic fibres [10].

Clinical variants
Nodular colloid degeneration presents usually as a single nodule up to 5 cm in diameter though multiple nodules may occur. It may be associated with myeloma [11] (see Table 96.1).

Management
No completely satisfactory intervention has been found for this condition. Good results have been claimed for dermabrasion [12] and for the long-pulsed Er : YAG laser [13].

OTHER CAUSES OF CUTANEOUS ATROPHY

Introduction and general description

Atrophy of the skin is a term which is applied to the clinical changes produced by a decrease in the dermal connective tissue.

Box 96.1 Selected acquired forms of cutaneous atrophy

Generalized cutaneous thinning
- Ageing (see above)
- Rheumatoid disease (see Chapter 154)
- Glucocorticoids (exogenous or endogenous)

Acquired poikiloderma

Striae

Atrophic scars
- Stellate pseudoscars

Spontaneous atrophic scarring of the cheeks

Acrodermatitis chronica atrophicans (Lyme borreliosis)

Atrophodermas
- Follicular atrophoderma
- Linear atrophoderma (Moulin)
- Atrophoderma of Pasini and Pierini

Paroxysmal haematoma of the finger (Achenbach syndrome)

Panatrophy
- Local panatrophy
- Facial hemiatrophy

It is characterized by thinning and loss of elasticity. The skin usually appears smooth and finely wrinkled, and it feels soft and dry. Veins or other subcutaneous structures may be unduly conspicuous. There is often associated loss of hair follicles, and telangiectasia may also be present, due to the loss of connective tissue support of the capillaries. There may or may not be an associated atrophy of the epidermis.

Atrophy of the skin occurs in varying degree in a large number of skin conditions, including naevi, and the underlying histological changes are also variable, because the several components of the connective tissue may be involved to a different degree. Atrophy that includes subcutaneous tissue or even deeper structures is referred to as *panatrophy*. Box 96.1 lists the main acquired disorders in which cutaneous atrophy is prominent.

Atrophy due to corticosteroids

Introduction and general description

Both systemic and topical glucocorticoid therapy can produce cutaneous atrophy by a dose-related pharmacological effect [1]. The effect is more severe with the more potent steroids (as assessed by the vasoconstrictor assay test) but both fluorinated and non-fluorinated topical steroids can cause atrophy. The effect is most marked when potent steroids are applied topically under an occlusive dressing. The skin becomes thin, fragile and transparent, and striae may develop (see later) (Figure 96.7).

Severe dermal atrophy can follow injection of intralesional steroids, such as triamcinolone acetonide (particularly if the higher concentration of 40 mg/mL is used, instead of the more usual 10 mg/mL, which is less likely to cause atrophy) (Figure 96.8). Inhaled corticosteroids also induce dermal thinning in adults and in children [2]. See Chapters 18 and 19, respectively, for more general discussions of topical and systemic glucocorticosteroids.

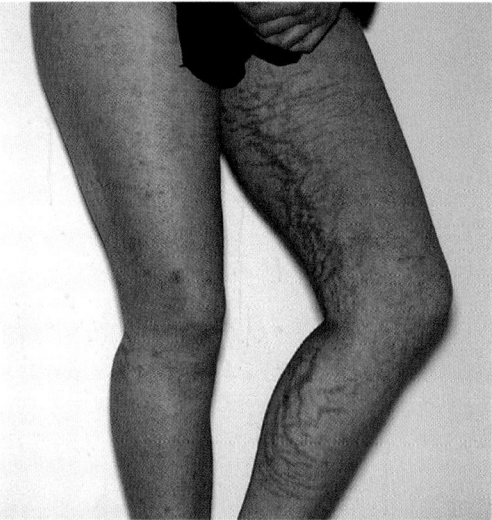

Figure 96.7 Striae of the legs due to long-term application of a potent topical steroid in a young woman with psoriasis.

Pathophysiology

Predisposing factors

Steroids are known to inhibit the formation of glycosaminoglycans. Hyaluronate and the major cell surface hyaluronate receptor CD44 are depleted in atrophic skin [3]. Topical corticosteroids rapidly suppress hyaluran synthase 2 in the dermis; this precedes alteration of dermal collagen [4]. The fibroblasts become shrunken, although their numbers do not decrease, but the number of mast cells is markedly reduced. Topical steroids also inhibit the activity of enzymes involved in collagen biosynthesis [5], and they have been shown to depress synthesis of types I and III collagen *in vivo* [6,7,8]. Type III collagen synthesis is preferentially reduced in fibroblast cultures [7]. They can also

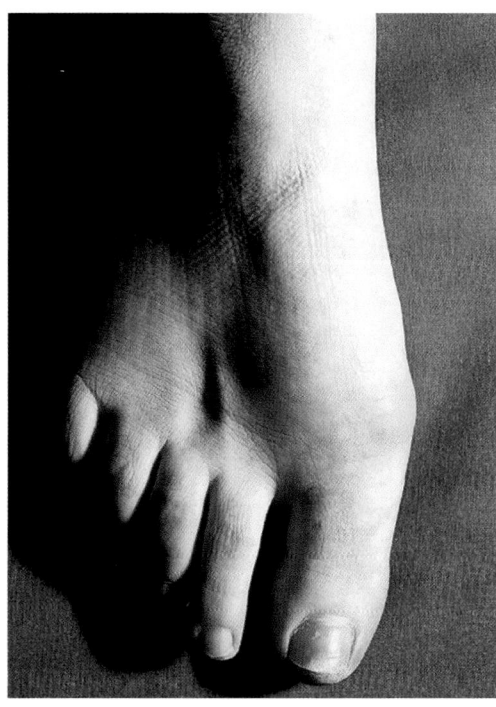

Figure 96.8 Localized atrophy due to injection of a steroid (triamcinolone 40 mg/mL) into the skin between the second and third metatarsals.

PART 8: SPECIFIC CUTANEOUS STRUCTURE

depress collagenase production and collagen breakdown [9], and the rate of collagen turnover is probably decreased. Even a weak steroid, such as hydrocortisone, can suppress the stimulatory effect of cyclic nucleotides on collagenase production. Studies of the effect of topical steroids on collagen and elastic fibres *in vivo* have given conflicting results [10–12]. Capillaroscopic studies have shown that steroid-induced vasoconstriction involves the superficial capillary network, and prolonged superficial ischaemia could also play a role in producing atrophy [5].

Pathology

The earliest histological change is marked thinning of the epidermis, with flattening of the rete ridges and decreased corneocyte size [**13**]. This is followed a few weeks later by thinning of the dermis, which can be measured by skinfold calipers, ultrasonography or a radiographic technique [14–16].

The epidermal thinning probably results from a reduction of mitotic activity in the germinal layer [17], but the mechanism by which dermal thinning is produced is uncertain.

Loss of dermal ground substance leads to a reorganization of the dermal architecture. The spaces between the collagen and elastic fibres become smaller, so that the dermis becomes more compact but thinner [10].

Collagen microfibrils may form globular microfibrillar bodies, although the changes are not specific for steroid atrophy [18]. These ultrastructural changes can develop in the early stages before there is clinical or histological evidence of atrophy. Digestion of collagen fibrils in the endocytic vesicles of fibroblasts may be involved in the production of steroid-induced atrophy [9].

Environmental factors

Systemic, topical, intralesional or inhaled corticosteroids are implicated.

Clinical features

History

A careful history should be taken, including enquiry about the use of corticosteroid inhalers (Figure 96.9).

Presentation

The skin becomes thin and fragile with easy bruising. Changes are generalized in patients on systemic corticosteroids, although the changes are more marked at sites of photodamage and trauma. Thinning due to topical corticosteroids may be localized to the site(s) of application. Severe dermal atrophy can follow injection of intralesional steroids.

Differential diagnosis

Other causes of cutaneous atrophy.

Complications and co-morbidities

Corticosteroid-induced skin thinning leads to delayed wound healing and easy bruising, often after trivial trauma. Measurement of bone density is advisable in at-risk patients, although extensive skin thinning is not necessarily associated with steroid-induced osteopenia [7].

Investigations

Consider measuring blood glucose and bone density, if systemic steroid toxicity is suspected.

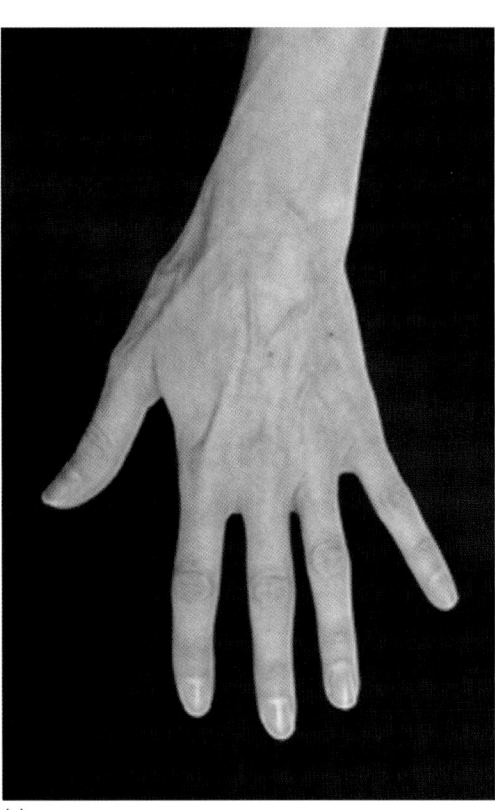

(a)

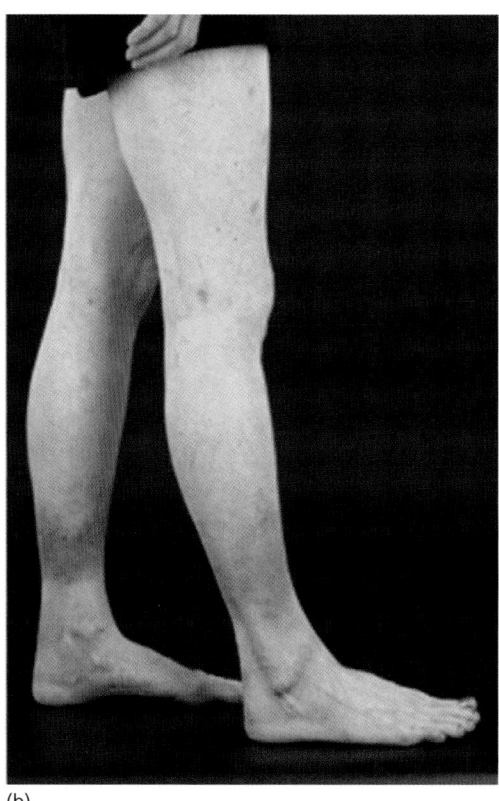

(b)

Figure 96.9 (a,b) Severe generalized cutaneous atrophy in a 29-year-old female as the result of using inhaled corticosteroids for asthma since the age of 7; (b) note haemosiderosis on the lower legs as a result of ready bruising of her atrophic skin.

Management

It has been suggested that local and oral vitamin C therapy might help restore the normal skin thickness [19]. Concurrent application of retinoic acid may partially prevent the epidermal atrophy due to steroids [20]. Intralesional saline injections can restore surface contour [21]. Hyaluronate fragments are reported to induce skin thickening in corticosteroid-induced atrophy [22].

Prevention is clearly the best approach, including the use of steroid-sparing systemic drugs and topical agents such as calcineurin inhibitors to treat skin disease. In the future, more selective corticosteroid receptor agonists, with potentially less atrophogenic effect may be developed [23].

Striae

Definition and nomenclature

Striae are visible linear scars which form in areas of dermal damage produced by stretching of the skin. They are characterized histologically by thinning of the overlying epidermis, with fine dermal collagen bundles arranged in straight lines parallel to the surface.

Synonyms and inclusions
- Striae distensae
- Striae atrophicans
- Stretch marks

Introduction and general description

Aetiology

The factors which govern the development of striae are poorly understood. Many authors have suggested that striae develop as a result of stress rupture of the connective tissue framework [1], but others disagree. It has been suggested that they develop more easily in skin which has a critical proportion of rigid cross-linked collagen, as occurs in early adult life [2]. They are common during adolescence [3], and they seem to be associated with rapid increase in size of a particular region. They are very common over the abdomen and breasts in pregnancy, and they may develop on the shoulders in young male weight lifters when their muscle mass rapidly increases [4]. They are a feature of Cushing disease, and they may be induced by local or systemic corticosteroid therapy [2,5]. The effects of glucocorticoids on the dermal connective tissue are outlined above. Together with other steroid effects, striae have been reported in HIV-positive patients receiving the protease inhibitor, indinavir [6].

Epidemiology

Incidence and prevalence

Striae are very common, and occur in most adult women, as they readily develop at puberty or during pregnancy.

Age

Adolescent striae may first develop soon after the appearance of pubic hair.

Sex

Abdominal striae gravidarum are extremely common in pregnancy.

Striae are often associated with growth spurts in adolescent males (Figure 96.10).

Associated diseases

Most striae occur in otherwise healthy individuals, although they are a feature of Cushing syndrome and Marfan syndrome.

Pathophysiology

Predisposing factors

Striae are associated with growth spurts, e.g. body building or pregnancy, more rarely they may reflect structural abnormalities of connective tissue such as Marfan syndrome or the effect of glucocorticoids.

Pathology

In the early stages, inflammatory changes may be conspicuous; the dermis is oedematous and perivascular lymphocytic cuffing is present. In the later stages, the epidermis is thin with flattening of the dermal papillae [7,8]. The dermal collagen is layered in thin eosinophilic bundles, orientated in straight lines parallel to the surface in the direction of the presumed stress. Scanning electron microscopy shows amorphous sheet-like structures [9]. With Luna stain, the elastic fibres are numerous, close together, fine and straight, and in the same direction as the collagen bundles [10]. On scanning electron microscopy in collagen-free preparations there is an abundance of thin, curled and branched elastic fibres.

Genetics

The importance of genetic factors in determining susceptibility of connective tissue is emphasized by their presence as one of the (minor) diagnostic criteria for Marfan syndrome [11], and congenital arachnodactyly, associated with mutations of the *fibrillin-1*

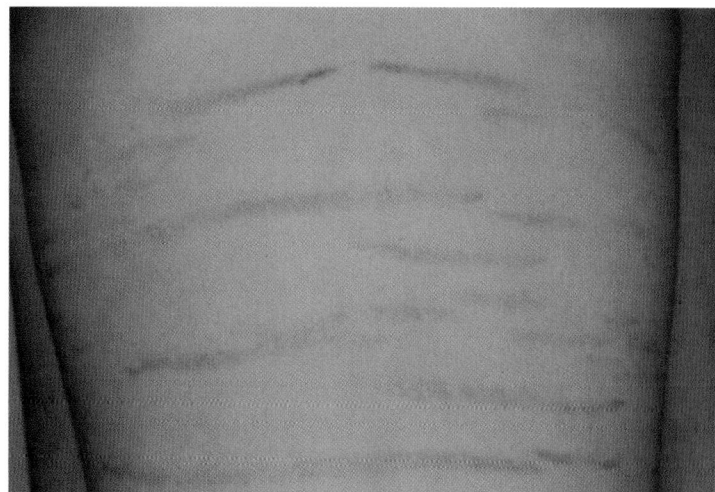

Figure 96.10 Pubertal growth striae across the back of an adolescent boy: note that these are normally all horizontally arranged right across the back (compare with Figure 96.11).

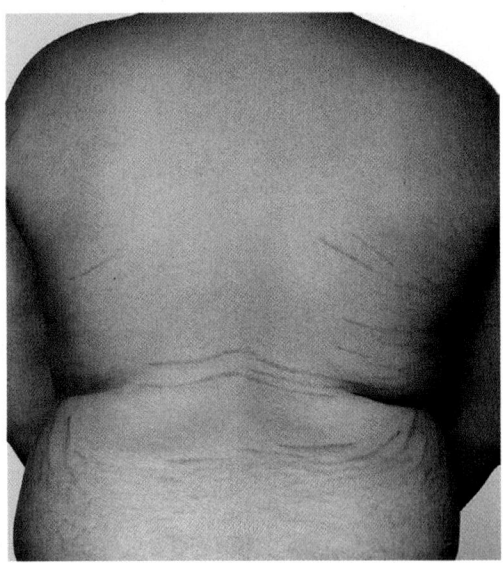

Figure 96.11 Striae due to obesity in a young man.

and *fibrillin-2* genes, respectively. Striae may occur in the absence of other phenotypic features of Marfan syndrome [12], and their presence may be predictors for aortic dissection [13]. They are commonly absent in pregnancy in Ehlers–Danlos syndrome.

Recent genome-wide association analysis of apparently otherwise normal individuals with striae has revealed associations with genes affecting expression of matrix proteins such as collagen, elastin and fibronectin [14].

Clinical features

The commonest sites for obesity-related striae are the outer aspect of the thighs and the lumbosacral region in boys (Figure 96.11), and the thighs, buttocks and breasts in girls, but there is considerable variation, and other sites, including the outer aspect of the upper arm, are sometimes affected. Pubertal growth striae are concentrated symmetrically over and on either side of the spine (see Figure 96.10).

Early lesions may be raised and irritable, but they soon become flat, smooth and livid red or bluish in colour. Their surface may be finely wrinkled. They are commonly irregularly linear, several centimetres long and 1–10 mm wide. After some years, they fade and become inconspicuous. They are then generally paler than the surrounding skin.

The striae in Cushing syndrome or those induced by steroid therapy may be larger and more widely distributed, and involve other regions, including sometimes the face. In pregnancy, the striae appear first and are most conspicuous on the abdominal wall, and later on the breasts, but may involve most or all of the pubertal sites [15]. The striae induced by topical corticosteroid therapy occur particularly in the flexures, but may appear in other sites if occlusive plastic films increase absorption (see Figure 96.7) [16,17].

Differential diagnosis

The diagnosis of striae is usually simple. The possibility of Cushing syndrome must be considered, although this is rarely the cause. Lay people may mistake adolescent growth striae for signs of physical abuse. In linear focal elastosis the lesions are yellow and palpable.

Complications and co-morbidities

Usually striae are no more than a cosmetic problem, but occasionally, if extensive, they may ulcerate or tear easily if traumatized.

Disease course and prognosis

Striae gravidarum generally improve after delivery and adolescent striae have an excellent prognosis. Even corticosteroid-induced striae may disappear or become less conspicuous when treatment is stopped.

Investigations

Exclude Cushing syndrome if suspected.

Management

In the case of common adolescent striae, the patient may be reassured that in time they will become less conspicuous. Numerous unproven remedies are available from cosmetic companies and there is no well substantiated evidence that topical therapies prevent or accelerate healing of striae [18,19].

Some cases appear to respond to treatment with topical tretinoin cream (0.05% daily), although weekly superficial dermabrasion is claimed to be better tolerated [20]. The erythema of 'younger' striae is claimed to respond to the 585 nm pulsed dye and Nd : YAG lasers [21,22]. Fractional photothermolysis has been used in chronic striae [23]. The application of silicone gel may be beneficial [24].

There is no proven treatment.

Acquired poikiloderma

Poikiloderma is a descriptive term, comprising atrophy, macular or reticulate pigmentation and telangiectasia. There may be associated areas of scaling, hypopigmentation and petechiae and signs of inflammation such as lichenoid papules. Congenital poikiloderma is a feature of several inherited disorders, including Kindler syndrome (see Chapter 71), dyskeratosis congenita, Rothmund–Thomson and Weary syndromes (see Chapter 77) and erythrokeratoderma variabilis (see Chapter 65).

Poikiloderma may occur as a pattern of cutaneous response to injury by cold, heat or ionizing radiation [1]. So-called poikiloderma of Civatte (see Chapter 88) is a similar reaction mediated by photosensitizing chemicals in cosmetics. Some inflammatory dermatoses, such as lichen planus, may also give rise to poikilodermatous changes.

Poikiloderma is a feature of some systemic autoimmune diseases, and is a marker of disease severity in dermatomyositis [2]. It is also seen in lupus erythematosus and rarely in systemic sclerosis. Poikiloderma atrophicans vasculare is an early presenting feature of cutaneous T-cell lymphoma (mycosis fungoides), typically stage IA–IIA; it predominantly affects males. It usually responds well to phototherapy and has a good prognosis [3] (Figure 96.12).

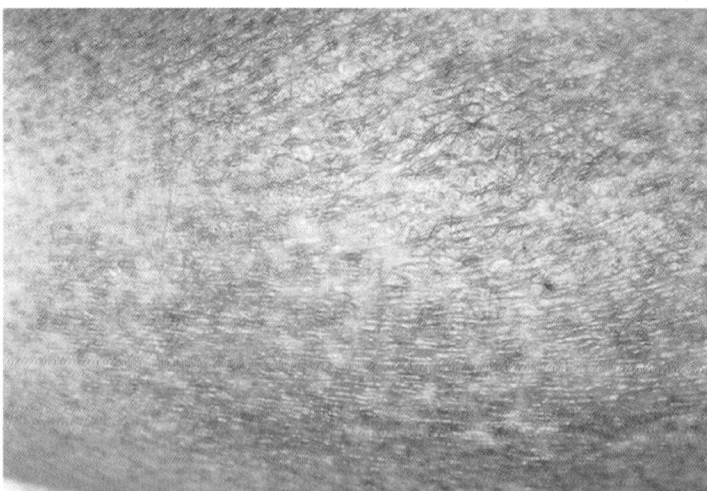

Figure 96.12 Poikilodermatous mycosis fungoides.

Atrophic scars

Definition
Scars resulting from the destruction of connective tissue by trauma or by inflammatory changes.

Introduction and general description
The distribution and character of the atrophic lesions may be so distinctive as to betray their origin, and is sometimes of considerable importance in diagnosis. Viral infections, such as varicella, can leave widespread small circular atrophic scars [1]. The scars left by tertiary syphilis, certain tuberculides and some deep mycoses, especially sporotrichosis, are usually completely atrophic. Onchocerciasis may result in extensive areas of dermal atrophy [2] (Figure 96.13). Areas of cutaneous lupus erythematosus may also leave atrophy without clinical evidence of sclerosis. Lupus vulgaris, the chronic follicular pyodermas and some cases of lupus erythematosus leave a combination of atrophy and sclerosis, in which the latter predominates. Lesions that have been treated by intralesional steroid injections may also leave atrophic scars.

Exposure to ionizing radiation gives rise to a very striking combination of atrophy, pigmentation and telangiectasia (poikiloderma).

The wide atrophic scars which follow injuries in Ehlers–Danlos syndrome (see Chapter 73) emphasize the importance of constitutional factors in determining the pattern of dermal response to a known external injury.

Stellate pseudoscars are white, irregular or 'star-shaped' atrophic scars (Figure 96.14). They are common on light-exposed skin, particularly on the extensor aspects of the forearms, often in association with purpura. These are seen in 20% of patients aged 70–90 years, and a much less common presenile form occasionally occurs before the age of 50 years. These pseudoscars are secondary to mild trauma, and are probably always preceded by haemorrhage into the dermis [3,4].

Stellate scars following trivial trauma can also occur in other conditions which cause fragile skin, for example porphyria cutanea tarda and prolonged use of potent topical steroids.

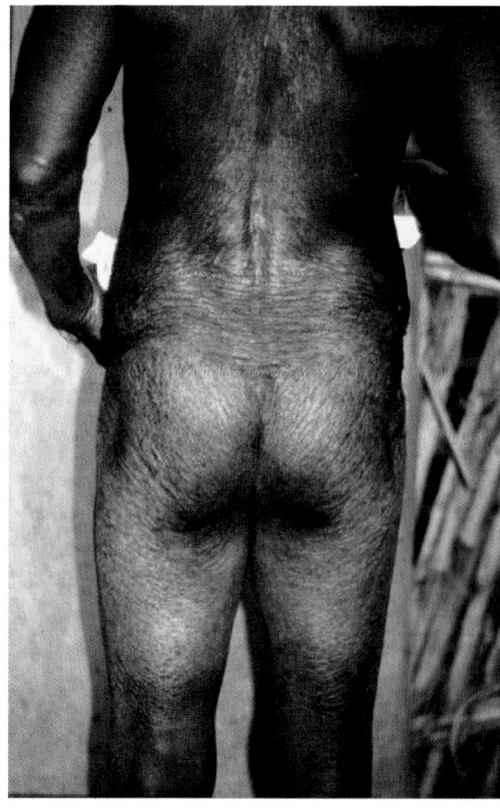

Figure 96.13 Atrophy due to onchocerciasis. (From Murdoch *et al.* 1993 [2], courtesy of Dr M. Murdoch, West Hertfordshire Hospitals NHS Trust, Hertfordshire, UK.)

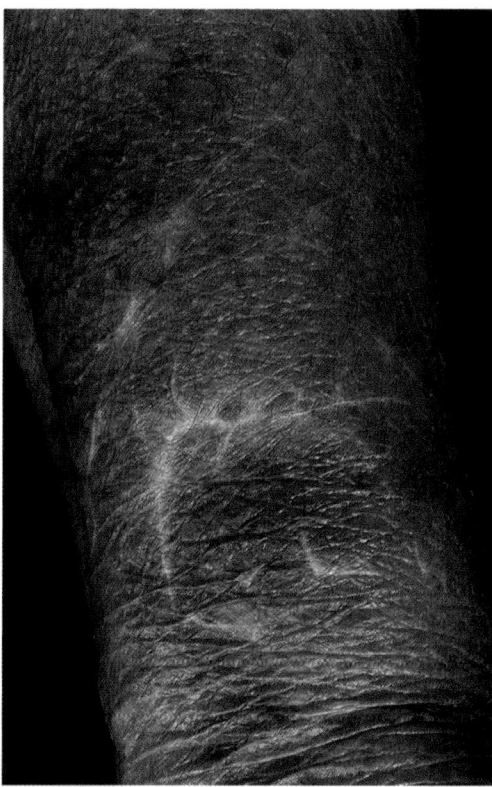

Figure 96.14 Stellate pseudoscars on the forearm of an elderly woman. There was no history of trauma.

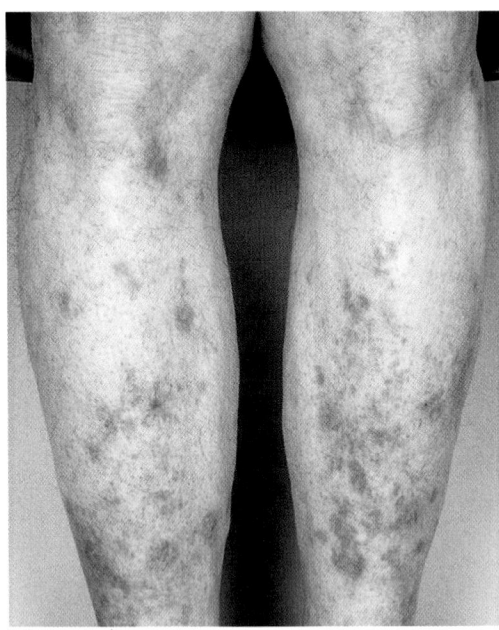

Figure 96.15 Brown pseudoscars of the legs due to diabetic dermopathy. There was no history of trauma.

Brown pseudoscars may also develop over the shins of diabetic patients with no history of trauma (diabetic dermopathy) (Figure 96.15) (see also Chapter 64). Histology reveals that the pigmentation is due to dermal deposition of haemosiderin and melanin [5].

Congenital erosive and vesicular dermatosis with reticulate scarring [6,7,8,9]

This rare congenital condition, which was first described in 1985 [6], presents at birth with signs suggestive of congenital viral infection, including erythema, blistering, erosions and crusting often involving more than 75% of the skin surface. The skin heals over the course of a few months with soft reticulate scarring, which on the limbs tends to follow the long axis of the limbs (Figure 96.16). A recent review of 28 known cases [7] con-

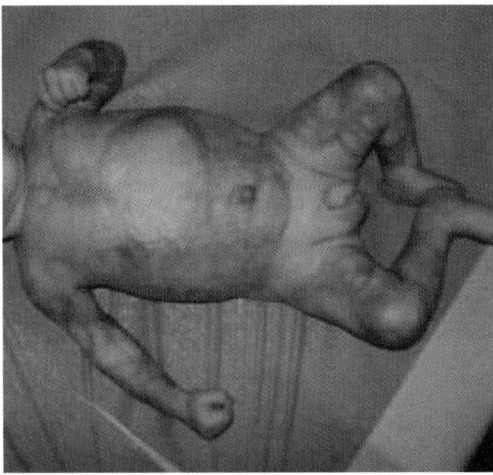

Figure 96.16 Congenital erosive and vesicular dermatosis with reticulate scarring. (From De Lange et al. 2009 [9], with permission from John Wiley.)

firmed that it occurred predominantly in preterm infants (79%) and that there was often a history of maternal chorioamnionitis (43%). Neurodevelopmental problems were common. Histological examination in the early stages shows epidermal necrosis and subepidermal blistering but no evidence of viral infection or vasculitis. This is succeeded by scar formation with loss of appendageal structures, especially eccrine glands. The differential diagnosis includes Goltz syndrome, Rothmund–Thomson syndrome and aplasia cutis [7,8]. An infant was treated successfully using a silicone sheet dressing [9].

Spontaneous atrophic scarring of the cheeks

Synonyms and inclusions
- Varioliform atrophy
- Atrophia maculosa varioliformis cutis

This is a very rarely reported condition in which spontaneous scars develop on the cheeks (Figure 96.17) in young adults [10,11] or children [12]. It may, however, be much commoner than the lack of reports suggests. The shallow atrophic lesions have sharp margins and may be linear, rectangular or varioliform. They may be preceded by slight erythema and scaling. Histology shows mild loss of collagen or elastic fibres; there may be thickening of the stratum corneum [13]. Familial cases are recorded [10,14]; inheritance is probably autosomal dominant [15]. The differential diagnosis includes atrophoderma vermiculatum (see Chapter 87), chickenpox scars and artefact.

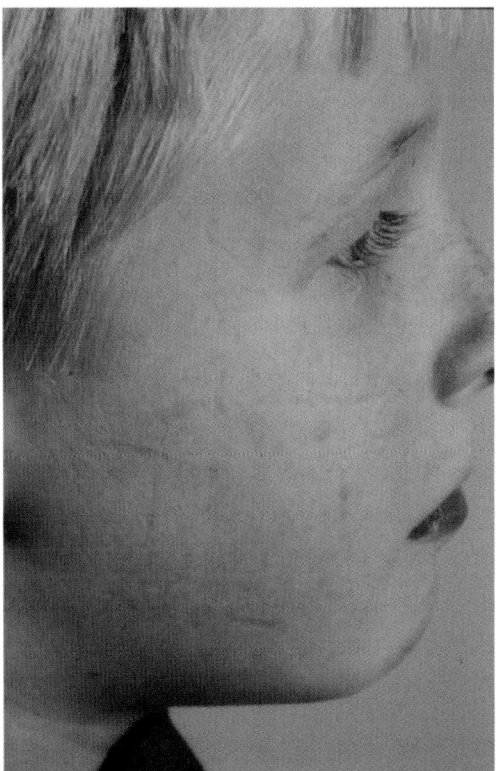

Figure 96.17 Spontaneous atrophic scarring of the cheeks (varioliform atrophy).

Acrodermatitis chronica atrophicans

Definition and nomenclature
This is a late skin manifestation of Lyme borreliosis (see Chapter 27). It is characterized by the insidious onset of painless, dull-red nodules or plaques on the extremities, which slowly extend centrifugally for several months or years, leaving central areas of atrophy.

Synonyms and inclusions
- Chronic atrophic acrodermatitis
- Late-phase Lyme borreliosis

Introduction and general description
The condition is due to infection with a spirochaete, *Borrelia burgdorferi sensu lato*, which is transmitted by ticks [1].

Epidemiology

Incidence and prevalence
The disease occurs mainly in northern or central Europe, Italy and the Iberian Peninsula. Occasional cases occur in other parts of Europe and Africa, but it is very rare in the UK, America, Australia and Asia [2]. These geographical variations are related to different strains of the organism [3–5].

Age
Mostly between the ages of 30 and 60 years.

Pathophysiology

Pathology [6]
During the early stages, there is non-specific dermal oedema with perivascular inflammatory infiltration. Subsequently, the epidermis becomes atrophic and the epidermal appendages are destroyed. Beneath a subepidermal zone of degenerate connective tissue lies a dense, band-like infiltrate, predominantly consisting of lymphocytes, histiocytes and plasma cells. Ultimately, the infiltrate is reduced to narrow bands between collagen fibres. In some patients, scleroderma-like changes may develop [7,8]. More typically, the dermis shows signs of atrophy; the swelling and homogenization of collagen and elastic fibres is followed by their disappearance [9]. *Borrelia afzelii* has been cultured from the atrophic skin [7] but culture is usually negative. *Borrelia afzelii* can be identified by polymerase chain reaction (PCR). The organism may be resistant to attack by the complement system and may lurk in immunologically protected areas such as fibroblasts and endothelial cells. Expression of pro-inflammatory cytokines, such as interferon-γ (IFN-γ), is increased [10].

Causative organisms
Borrelia afzelii is the predominant species associated with acrodermatitis chronica atrophicans [11]. This species is transmitted by ticks in Western Europe, but is rare in the USA, where *Borrelia burgdorferi sensu stricto* predominates [12].

Environmental factors
It is transmitted by bites from ticks, notably *Ixodes* spp., which favour scrubland [12].

Clinical features

History
Most cases occur in country-dwellers. There is usually a history of a tick bite. The onset is usually insidious, and constitutional symptoms are exceptional [13].

Presentation
Dull-red or bluish-red nodules or plaques, more or less infiltrated, develop on the feet or legs, and less often on the forearms and hands. The lesions themselves are typically painless, but there may be associated acral pain or paraesthesiae. Erythema chronicum migrans (see Chapter 27) may have been present at the same site some years earlier. Extension to the trunk and the greater part of the body, including the face, is sometimes seen. Single or multiple lesions may be present. They slowly extend centrifugally, the active inflammatory stage persisting for months, years or even decades. Marginal extension may continue once the central areas have already entered the atrophic phase, in which the skin is smooth, hairless and tissue-paper-like, dull red, pigmented or poikilodermatous (Figure 96.18).

Subcutaneous nodules may develop around the knees or elbows, and fibrous bands along the ulnar margin of the forearms. Gaiter-like

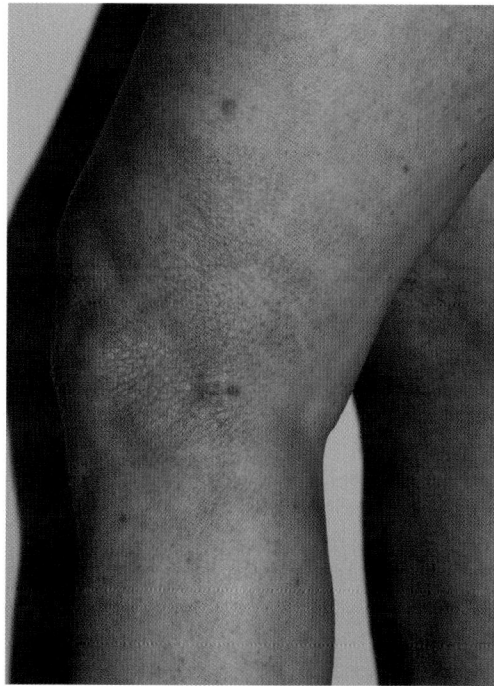

Figure 96.18 Acrodermatitis chronica atrophicans: image captured soon after commencement of antibiotic therapy; note atrophic wrinkled appearance of the skin at the side of the knee. (Courtesy of Dr Ian Coulson, Burnley Hospital, UK.)

sclerosis of the lower third of the legs, often accompanied by ulceration, is a further complication. Morphoea of the trunk and lichen sclerosus (both genital and extragenital) have also been reported in association [2,14]. Conversely, *Borrelia* antibodies have been found in some patients with morphoea [14,15], although this does not appear to be a common finding [16].

In some cases, involvement of the joint capsule or bone results in limitation of movement of the joints of the hands and feet, or of the shoulders.

Clinical variants
Occasional patients develop erythematous plaques, clinically and histologically suggestive of mycosis fungoides [17].

Differential diagnosis
The early cutaneous phase of Lyme borreliosis, erythema chronicum migrans, may be confused with other annular erythemas, although a history is often obtained of a recent tick bite at the site. When it occurs on the lower legs, it may mimic venous insufficiency [18], with thick cyanotic itchy skin.

Complications and co-morbidities
Very rarely, squamous carcinoma has developed in the atrophic skin, and lymphoma has also been reported in non-affected skin [19–21]. Other late manifestations of Lyme borreliosis (lymphocytoma, neurological, etc.) have been fully reviewed by Steere [1].

Disease course and prognosis
The bacteria can be eradicated with systemic antibiotics but some systemic features, such as neuroborreliosis, may persist.

Investigations
In the atrophic stage, diagnosis is usually readily made, and can be confirmed histologically.

Immunoblotting, using *B. afzelii* flagellar antigen (41 kDa) is confirmatory [5]. Serology is used to confirm the diagnosis of Lyme disease, but false-negative and false-positive results are common. In chronic atrophic acrodermatitis, however, the antibody titre is very high. Serology may be positive on enzyme-linked immunosorbent assay (ELISA) but negative on immunoblotting, particularly in patients with neurological disease [22]. A high titre of antibodies may reflect occult central nervous system involvement, when the antibodies can also be demonstrated in colony-stimulating factor [23].

Management
Oral antibiotics should be given for 1 month, for example doxycycline or amoxicillin in standard doses [1]. Improvement occurs gradually and may not become apparent until several weeks after the course of treatment. There may be no improvement if treatment is delayed until atrophy has already developed. If the antibody titre is high or there are clinical features of systemic disease (e.g. neuroborreliosis), intravenous benzylpenicillin, ceftriaxone or cefotaxime should be given for 3 weeks [23]. There may be a case to be made for introducing public health measures such as chemoprophylaxis programmes or eventually a vaccine in endemic areas [24].

Elevated immunoglobulin G (IgG) and IgM antibodies may persist after treatment; this does not reflect treatment failure [25].

Treatment ladder

First line
- Oral antibiotics (e.g. doxyxycline or amoxicillin)

Second line
- Intravenous antibiotics (e.g. benzylpenicillin if significant systemic manifestations)

Atrophodermas

Follicular atrophoderma

Definition
This distinctive abnormality manifests as dimple-like depressions at the follicular orifices and is usually associated with one of a small number of genetic syndromes but may be sporadic. It may be manifest at birth but may not become apparent until late in childhood. It usually involves the backs of the hands (Figure 96.19) and the feet, and sometimes the elbow region. It may be associated with the following conditions [1]:
1 Conradi–Hünermann–Happle syndrome (calcifying chondrodysplasia) (see Chapter 65) [2].
2 Bazex–Dupré–Christol syndrome (see Chapter 68) [3].
3 Hyperkeratosis palmoplantaris, follicular keratosis or palmoplantar hyperhidrosis.

It may also occur as an isolated defect of limited extent.

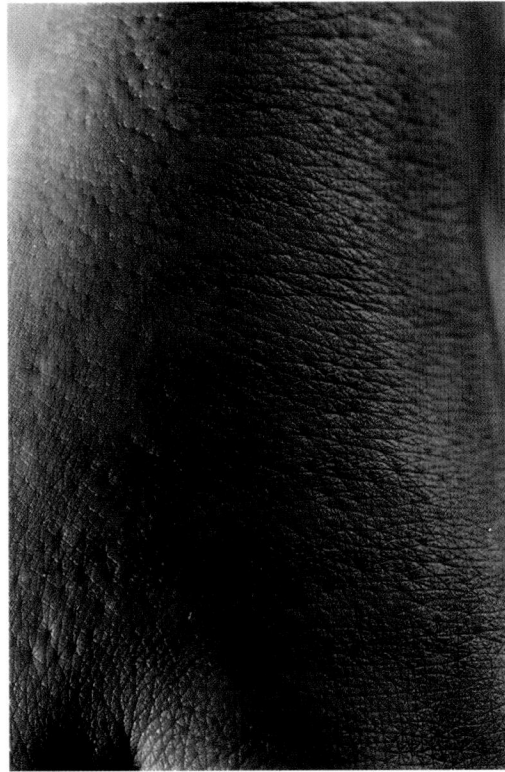

Figure 96.19 Follicular atrophoderma in Conradi syndrome.

Pathophysiology

Pathology
Histology shows widened follicular ostia with thickening of the connective tissue sheath of the follicle.

Genetics
It appears to be associated with a variety of genetic defects.

Clinical features

Presentation
Follicular depressions on the backs of the hands (see Figure 96.19), feet and occasionally elbows.

Management
No proven treatment.

Linear atrophoderma

> **Synonyms and inclusions**
> • Atrophoderma of Moulin

Introduction and general description
It is probable that this and atrophoderma of Pasini and Pierini are atrophic variants of morphoea [4,5].

Epidemiology

Incidence and prevalence
Cases are sporadic and worldwide.

Age
Most cases are described in childhood and adolescence.

Associated diseases
Leuconychia has been associated [6].

Pathophysiology

Pathology
Histologically, the epidermis is normal apart from hyperpigmentation in the basal layer. There is a perivascular lymphocytic infiltrate in the dermis [7]. The collagen bundles are normal or thickened; there is diminished periadnexal and subcutaneous fat [8].

Genetics
The condition may reflect mosaicism following a postzygotic mutational event [7,9].

Clinical features

History
Lesions are usually asymptomatic and insidious in onset.

Presentation
Linear atrophic hyperpigmented plaques in the distribution of Blaschko's lines, sometimes having a zosteriform appearance [8].

Differential diagnosis
Atrophic variants of morphoea strongly resemble this syndrome, and may be identical.

Investigations
Laboratory investigations are normal [8]. Skin biopsy is helpful if there is clinical doubt.

Management
One case of successful treatment with methotrexate is reported [10].

Atrophoderma of Pasini and Pierini

Definition
This condition is probably an atrophic variant of morphoea (see Chapter 57) in which one or more patches of skin become bluish and sharply depressed, with no surrounding erythema [11–13].

Epidemiology

Incidence and prevalence
Cases are mostly sporadic and rare.

Age
Most cases present in childhood or adolescence.

Associated diseases
There is a probable association with morphoea. Familial cases have been reported [14], together with an association with phenylketonuria [15].

Pathophysiology

Predisposing factors
The cause is unknown, although, as in morphoea, *Borrelia burgdorferi* has been implicated [16].

Pathology
The histological changes are often slight [13]. There may be increased pigmentation of the basal layer. During the earlier stages, the collagen in the lower dermis may be oedematous, and elastic tissue clumped and scanty. There may be a dermal perivascular infiltrate consisting of macrophages and T lymphocytes. Immunofluorescence studies may show IgM and C3 staining in the dermal blood vessels [17]. Later, the oedema subsides and there is some reduction in the total thickness of the dermis. Collagen bundles appear homogeneous and clumped in the reticular dermis. Eventually there may also be some epidermal atrophy.

PART 8: SPECIFIC CUTANEOUS STRUCTURE

Causative organisms
In common with morphoea, *Borrelia burgdorferi* has been implicated [16].

Genetics
No genetic factor has been reliably incriminated, although familial cases have been reported [14], and morphoea and atrophoderma of Pasini have occurred in siblings with phenylketonuria [15].

Clinical features

History
The lesions are generally asymptomatic.

Presentation [13,18,19]
The lesions, which may be single or multiple, range in size from 2 cm to many centimetres in diameter, and are round or oval in shape, but may become confluent to form irregular patches (Figure 96.20). They are smooth, slate-coloured or violet-brown, and are slightly depressed below the level of the entirely normal surrounding skin. The back is almost always involved, the chest and abdomen frequently, and the proximal parts of the limbs occasionally.

Differential diagnosis
Atrophic morphoea and linear atrophoderma may represent the same condition. Clinical differentiation from morphoea, possibly an academic exercise, is based on the ivory-white indurated plaque with an oedematous lilac ring so characteristic of the latter. Histologically, sclerosis may be prominent in morphoea and is usually absent in atrophoderma.

Complications and co-morbidities
An overlap with juvenile idiopathic arthritis has been described [20].

Disease course and prognosis
The patches extend very slowly, increase in number for 10 years or more, and then usually persist unchanged. The eventual development of sclerodermatous changes within the patches has been observed, as has the presence in the same patient of lesions typical of atrophoderma and of morphoea.

Investigations
Serological tests for *Borrelia burgdorferi* are typically negative [13] although there are case reports of an association (e.g. see [16]).

Management
No treatment is of proven efficacy, but psoralen and UVA (PUVA) has helped some patients. Hydroxychloroquine has been used [21]. A case apparently associated with *Borrelia burgdorferi* responded to doxycycline [16].

Paroxysmal haematoma of the finger

Definition and nomenclature
This condition presents with the sudden spontaneous onset of one or more painful haematomas in the fingers (Figure 96.21).

Synonyms and inclusions
- Achenbach syndrome
- Acute idiopathic blue finger

Epidemiology

Age
Usually middle age.

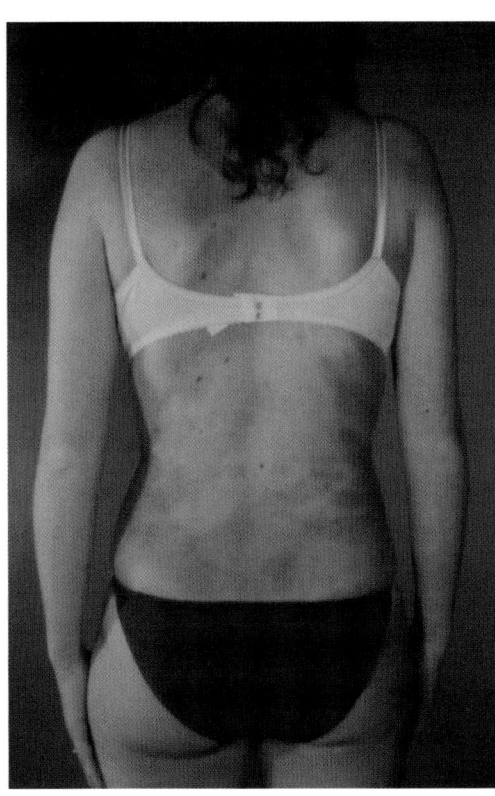

Figure 96.20 Atrophoderma of Pasini and Pierini.

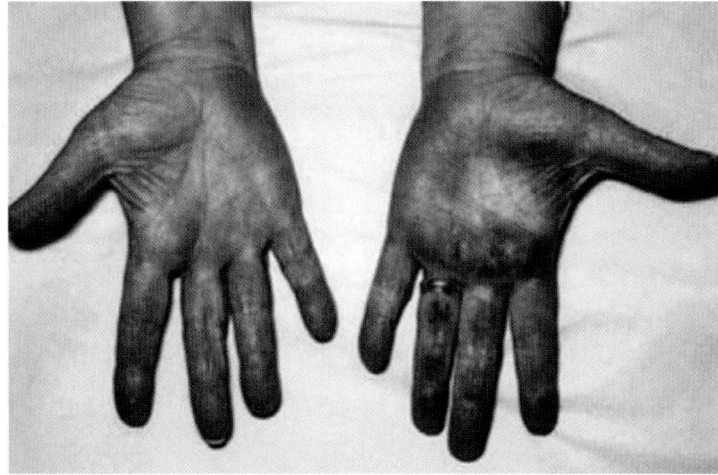

Figure 96.21 Paroxysmal haematoma of the finger. (Courtesy of Dr J. Verbov, Royal Liverpool University Hospitals, Liverpool, UK.)

Sex
Female predominance.

Associated diseases
None.

Pathophysiology

Predisposing factors
The cause is unknown but has been hypothesized to be due to a localized acquired fragility of vascular connective tissue.

Pathology
There is no evidence of vasculitis or amyloid on skin biopsy.

Clinical features

History
Sudden onset of often painful haematoma.

Presentation
Sudden bruising of the volar aspect of a finger may occur spontaneously or after minor trauma; the bruising resolves within days and the patient is asymptomatic between flares [1,2,3,4]. The wrist may sometimes be involved [5]. There is no evidence of ischaemia [6].

Differential diagnosis
It may be mistaken for easy bruising due to steroid atrophy. The absence of ischaemic features and rapid improvement exclude occlusive vascular disease.

Complications and co-morbidities
There are no co-morbidities.

Disease course and prognosis
It may recur at intervals for several years. Although troublesome, it is a benign condition.

Investigations
Although subtle angiographic abnormalities have been described [7], investigation of the patient for significant vascular disease is unnecessary [8].

Panatrophy

Definition
Local panatrophy is a rare disorder involving partial or total loss of subcutaneous fat and atrophy of overlying skin, sometimes associated with atrophy or impaired growth of muscle or bone. A primary neurogenic disturbance has been postulated but not proved. The syndrome may represent the end result of more than one pathological process, but many cases may be due to a variant of morphoea. They are discussed further in Chapter 57.

The atrophic areas exhibit a reduced sympathetic response and aberrant production of non-esterified fatty acids after stimulation with norepinephrine (noradrenaline), and it has been suggested that there may be a primary abnormality of the sympathetic nervous system [1].

Two groups of cases can be differentiated.

1 Panatrophy of Gower: no scleroderma or other sclerotic process accompanies or follows the loss of subcutaneous tissue. Most cases have occurred in women, usually in the second to fourth decades.

2 Sclerotic panatrophy: either typical morphoea or similar sclerotic change in dermal collagen precedes the atrophy [2].

Clinical features
Clinical features of these two groups are as follows.

Panatrophy of Gower [3,4]. Sharply defined areas of atrophy, irregular in size, shape and distribution, develop over a period of a few weeks, without preceding inflammatory stages. In each affected area, the subcutaneous tissue disappears and the overlying skin appears atrophic but is otherwise normal. There may be a single area of atrophy or two or more. In size they range from 2 to 20 cm across, and in shape they are very variable but are sometimes triangular or quadrangular. Most lesions have occurred on the back, buttocks, thighs or upper arms, but some have involved the forearms or lower legs. The atrophy reaches its maximum extent within a few months and then remains unchanged indefinitely.

Sclerotic panatrophy. Atrophy of the subcutis, and sometimes of underlying muscle and bone, may follow clinically and histologically typical morphoea, especially when the process begins in childhood and involves a limb (see Chapter 57).

Sclerotic panatrophy may also occur in the absence of morphoea. The sclerosis involves subcutaneous tissue and muscle, and dense sclerotic scar-like linear bands develop along a limb, or encircle the trunk in a metameric distribution, or encircle a limb. These lesions have also usually occurred in childhood. They cease to progress after a few months and, although new areas may be involved, most lesions have been solitary.

It is probable that Gower's panatrophy and linear morphoea are at the ends of a continuous disease spectrum. The histology of linear morphoea reveals thickened bundles of collagen, which appear to be intact on B-scan ultrasound imaging [5].

In the differential diagnosis of panatrophy, the various forms of *panniculitis* must be excluded. The preceding inflammatory changes are the single most distinctive feature, but they are not always easy to distinguish.

Facial defects can be corrected by autologous fat grafting [6].

Facial hemiatrophy (see also Chapter 57)

Synonyms and inclusions
• Parry–Romberg syndrome

Introduction and general description
Facial hemiatrophy is an atrophic dysplasia of the superficial facial tissues, but the underlying muscles, cartilage and bone may also be affected [1].

Epidemiology

Age
This rare disease usually starts within the first two decades of life.

Sex
The sexes are equally affected.

Associated diseases
Some cases have been associated with syringomyelia, epilepsy or cerebrovascular disease, but in 90% of cases no such association is demonstrable.

Pathophysiology

Predisposing factors
The cause is unknown, but it may be a disorder of the sympathetic nervous system in some cases.

Genetics
There is no evidence that it is usually genetically determined, but it appears to be hereditary in a few pedigrees.

Clinical features

History
Occasionally, there may be premonitory muscle spasms or neuralgia [2] but often it is asymptomatic.

Presentation
The first manifestation is usually increased or decreased pigmentation in irregular patches on the cheeks, forehead or lower jaw. Progressive atrophy gradually develops in the affected sites, involving skin, subcutis, muscle and bone, and may extend in area — and sometimes in depth — for months or years with temporary remissions. The skin becomes dry, thin and atrophic, but may be scar-like and adherent in some areas. When the atrophy is fully developed, the contrast between the sunken, haggard, pigmented affected half of the face and the unaffected half is dramatic. The hair may be lost in the fronto-parietal region on the affected side but is often normal; occasionally, localized canities is an early change. A variety of neurological signs have been reported, of which Horner syndrome is the most frequent. Heterochromia of the iris has developed at the same time as the facial atrophy in about 5% of cases, and retinal changes may also be present [3], including central retinal artery occlusion [4]. There can be ipsilateral cerebral atrophy [5].

The degree of bone atrophy as established radiologically is usually much less than the clinical appearance suggests, and is severe only in some cases of early onset. In such cases, the cerebral cortex may also be affected, and contralateral epilepsy may result.

Differential diagnosis
When the cutaneous involvement is early and conspicuous, the diagnosis presents few difficulties. Hypoplasia following radiotherapy given in infancy, perhaps in treatment of a naevus in the region of the temporo-mandibular joint, could cause confusion. If the skin changes are slight, or of later onset, physiological asymmetry, unilateral mandibular agenesis, hemihypertrophy and atrophy secondary to facial paralysis must be excluded. Hemihypertrophy is always congenital. When the limbs are involved, infantile hemiplegia and lipodystrophy must also be considered.

Lupus panniculitis results in subcutaneous atrophy which can be hemifacial. Atrophic morphoea of the 'coup de sabre' paramedian form may be associated with some degree of facial hemiatrophy, especially if it begins early in life. However, it is generally a more superficial process than progressive facial hemiatrophy. The skin in scleroderma is bound down and adherent, and loss of hair and pigmentary changes are conspicuous. In progressive facial hemiatrophy, the skin may remain mobile and grossly normal. The two processes have been confused frequently in the literature, and may coexist [6].

Complications and co-morbidities
There may be associated segmental vitiligo [7]. Spontaneous fracture of the jaw has also been reported [8].

Disease course and prognosis
The atrophy may remain limited both in extent and depth. It may be confined to the distribution of one division of the trigeminal nerve or involve the whole of the side of the face, sharply demarcated at the midline. Rarely, it may be bilateral, and very rarely may involve half the body, usually on the same side as the face but exceptionally the opposite side — crossed hemiatrophy. The atrophy may, in such cases, begin on the trunk or a limb and only later involve the face.

Management
Plastic surgery using large buried pediculated flaps of dermis and fat, or silicone implants, offers some cosmetic benefit [9–11]. Autologous fat grafts have a variable 'take' although they remain the treatment of choice [12]; supplementation with stromal vascular fraction-supplemented cell therapy may improve the long-term result [13].

DISORDERS OF ELASTIC FIBRE DEGRADATION

Introduction and general description

The capacity of the skin to adapt to local or general changes in body size and contour, and to allow for movement of head and limbs and a wide range of facial expression, depends upon its tension, elasticity and tensile strength. These properties may be congenitally defective or modified by ageing or disease [1–3]. Acquired disorders of elastic tissue have been reviewed in detail by Lewis et al. [4,5].

Elastic fibres are abundant in the skin, arteries, lungs and ligaments. They provide tissues with resilience and elasticity, enabling the skin to resume its original shape after deforming forces have ceased to act. There is wide individual variation, but a tendency for elastic fibres to become less plentiful with age. Cutaneous elasticity is also reduced in a variety of skin disorders including cutis laxa. Additionally, elastic fibres provide adhesion for cells and play a role in regulating growth factors (e.g. transforming growth factor β (TGF-β)) [2].

Tensile strength

The tensile strength of the skin is the degree to which it can be elongated before it tears. It is greatest in infancy and decreases with age, but is also abnormally low in diseases associated with qualitatively or quantitatively abnormal collagen such as Ehlers–Danlos syndrome and Cushing syndrome [3].

Lax skin

Increased laxity of the skin due to ageing (accelerated by dermal photodegradation) is extremely common, but cutaneous laxity can occasionally result from marked weight loss (especially after gross obesity) or can follow recovery from severe oedema. Less commonly, the skin may become lax due to localized or generalized defects in elastic tissue resulting from other causes, and these may be grouped as follows:

1 Generalized elastolysis (cutis laxa):
  (a) congenital (see Chapter 72): it may be a component of inherited disorders including PXE, SCARF syndrome (skeletal abnormalities, cutis laxa, craniostenosis, ambiguous genitalia, retardation and facial abnormalities), de Barsy syndrome, geroderma osteodysplastica;
  (b) acquired: numerous associated disorders, e.g. inflammatory skin disease, multiple myeloma, systemic lupus erythematosus, hypersensitivity reactions, complement deficiency, penicillamine therapy.
2 Localized elastolysis:
  (a) anetoderma;
  (b) blepharochalasis;
  (c) chronic atrophic acrodermatitis (due to Borrelia) (see earlier);
  (d) granulomatous slack skin (due to lymphoma);
  (e) other localized lesions, including mid-dermal elastolysis, post-inflammatory elastolysis and cutis laxa (PECL), elastic tissue naevi, etc.

It is probable that many of the above conditions are variations of the same disease, and there is considerable overlap. They share a similar pathological process, namely elastophagocytosis (the phagocytosis of elastic fibres by histiocytes and/or multinucleate giant cells) [1].

Acquired cutis laxa

Definition and nomenclature

Cutis laxa presents clinically as lax skin which hangs in folds, together with loss of dermal elastic tissue histologically. Congenital forms are discussed in Chapter 72.

Synonyms and inclusions
- Generalized elastolysis
- Generalized elastorrhexis
- Generalized dermatochalasia

Introduction and general description

Cutis laxa may be acquired following inflammatory skin disease [1] or following exposure in utero to drugs such as penicillamine [2]. An immunological pathogenesis has been suggested in many cases.

Epidemiology

Associated diseases

Cutis laxa has been reported in association with urticarial eruptions, nephrotic syndrome [3], complement deficiency, sarcoidosis, syphilis, primary amyloidosis and multiple myeloma [4,5], drug hypersensitivity and the Klippel–Trenaunay syndrome [6]. Focal elastolysis can also occur in association with lupus erythematosus [7], severe rheumatoid arthritis [8] and coeliac disease [9]. D-penicillamine disrupts elastic fibre formation and may cause cutis laxa, elastosis perforans serpiginosa and pseudoxanthoma-like changes [10,11]. Congenital cutis laxa may also occur in offspring of mothers taking penicillamine [2].

Pathophysiology

Predisposing factors

Immunological or chemical disruption of dermal elastic fibres.

Pathology

In acquired cutis laxa, dermal elastic tissue is markedly reduced, although collagen is normal. Fibroblasts express increased elastolytic activity (cathepsin G). Levels of serum α_1-antitrypsin and elastase inhibition are decreased [12].

Genetics

There may be an underlying genetic susceptibility, for example defects in the interaction of elastin and fibulin 5 results in elastic fibres that are more susceptible to degradation by matrix metalloproteinases [13].

Clinical features

History

Cutis laxa may rarely develop at any age following episodes of urticaria or angio-oedema, extensive inflammatory skin disease (such as systemic lupus erythematosus or erythema multiforme) or febrile illness (Figure 96.22). It may also follow hypersensitivity reactions such as penicillin allergy [14].

Presentation

There may be widespread massive folds of lax skin, or the changes may be mild and confined to a limited area, in which case it cannot be distinguished from anetoderma. Purpura may follow slight

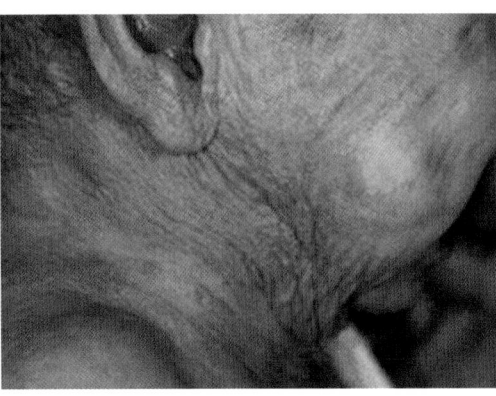

Figure 96.22 Acquired cutis laxa following a generalized inflammatory dermatitis in an 18-month-old child. (From Haider *et al.* [17], with permission from John Wiley.)

trauma and fibrotic nodules may form over bony prominences. Organs other than the skin may also be involved. Emphysema, gastric fibromas and tracheobronchomegaly have been reported [15].

Clinical variants

Post-inflammatory elastolysis and cutis laxa (Marshall syndrome) (Figure 96.23a–c) was originally described as a distinctive syndrome in African children but subsequently reported worldwide, Clinical features are intermediate between anetoderma and cutis laxa [16,17,**18**]. It is preceded by an inflammatory process, often with a neutrophilic component (e.g. Sweet syndrome [19,20]) or an insect bite. The preceding inflammatory lesions may be urticaria-like or multiple red papules, which slowly enlarge to form rings 2–10 cm in diameter [17]. It has been associated with α_1-antitryspin deficiency, which may enable matrix metalloproteinases to destroy dermal elastin, and screening for this enzyme deficiency is recommended [20].

Differential diagnosis

The history should enable the condition to be distinguished from congenital cutis laxa. In Ehlers–Danlos syndrome, the skin is

hyperextensible but not lax, and it recoils quickly. In PXE, the skin may be lax, but it is yellowish and the face is usually spared. It is distinguished histologically by the presence of calcification. There may be circumscribed folds of lax skin in neurofibromatosis, and loose folded skin may also occur in leprechaunism, Patterson syndrome and trisomy 18, but these conditions are distinguished by their associated features.

In severe actinic damage, there may be marked skin laxity due to damage to elastic fibres. There is doubtless considerable overlap with other elastolytic conditions described later.

Investigations

The diagnosis, which is suggested by finding loose skin that recoils only slowly after stretching, may be confirmed by histological confirmation of a reduction in elastic fibres. Investigations for emphysema may be indicated, with referral to a pulmonary physician if necessary. Underlying inflammatory disease may require investigation.

Management

Plastic surgery ('face-lift') may substantially reduce the cosmetic disability [18].

Anetoderma

Definition and nomenclature

The term anetoderma (*anetos:* slack) refers to a circumscribed area of slack skin associated with a loss of dermal substance on palpation and a loss of elastic tissue on histological examination. 'Primary' anetoderma implies that there is no associated localized underlying cutaneous disease, whereas 'secondary' anetoderma can be attributed to some associated condition.

Synonyms and inclusions
- Macular atrophy

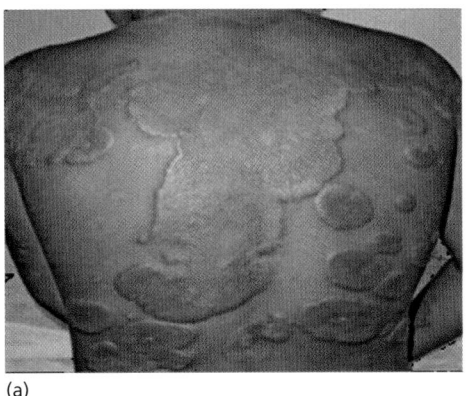
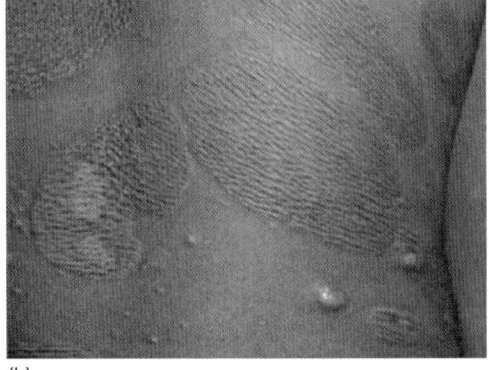
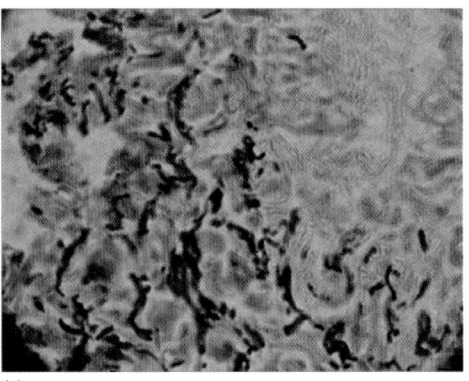

(a)   (b)   (c)

Figure 96.23 Post-inflammatory elastolysis and cutis laxa (Marshall syndrome) in a 6-year-old boy showing acute inflammatory phase (a) progressing to large plaques of lax wrinkled skin (b). Histology shows shortened and fragmented elastic fibres in the reticular dermis (c). (Reproduced from Fontenelle *et al.* 2013 [18] with permission from Sociedade Brasileira de Dermatologia.)

Introduction and general description

Previously, cases of 'primary' anetoderma were divided into the *Jadassohn–Pellizzari* type, in which the lesions are preceded by erythema or urticaria, and the *Schweninger–Buzzi* type, in which there are no preceding inflammatory lesions. This is now of historical interest only, because in the same patient some lesions may be preceded by inflammation and others may not, and the prognosis and histology are identical in the two types [1,2,3].

Epidemiology

Incidence and prevalence
Rare.

Age
Mainly 20–40 years, but is occasionally reported in infants and older patients.

Sex
Mainly in women [2].

Associated diseases
Primary anetoderma is strongly associated with antiphospholipid syndrome [4,5,6] with or without features of systemic lupus. In older reports, this may have led to a misdiagnosis of syphilis in many cases, although there is a definite association with the disease and its treatment [7]. Secondary anetoderma has been reported in association with tuberculosis and leprosy [8], urticaria pigmentosa [9], pityriasis versicolor [10], granuloma annulare [11,12], Stevens–Johnson syndrome [13], B- and T-cell lymphoma [14–16] and other conditions. Some reported associations may be coincidental, but it is probable that many inflammatory diseases may occasionally be complicated by anetoderma.

Localized anetoderma may occur in premature infants, possibly due to the application of transcutaneous oxygen monitoring devices [17,18]. Localized anetoderma-like changes on histology have been reported in association with pilomatricoma [19], dermatofibroma [20], juvenile xanthogranuloma [21] and hamartomatous congenital naevi [22]. Lesions resembling anetoderma occur in post-inflammatory elastolysis and cutis laxa (Marshall syndrome) (Figure 96.23b). Penicillamine-induced anetoderma has also been reported [23].

Pathophysiology

Predisposing factors

Primary anetoderma
Recently, it has become apparent that 'primary' anetoderma is strongly associated with antiphospholipid antibodies, with or without a prothrombotic state (Figure 96.24) [4,5]. It is probable that these antibodies underly the association historically noted with syphilis, and more recently with borreliosis [27] and systemic lupus.

In a few cases, there appears to be an underlying structural defect of connective tissue. Familial cases are reported [24–26] and

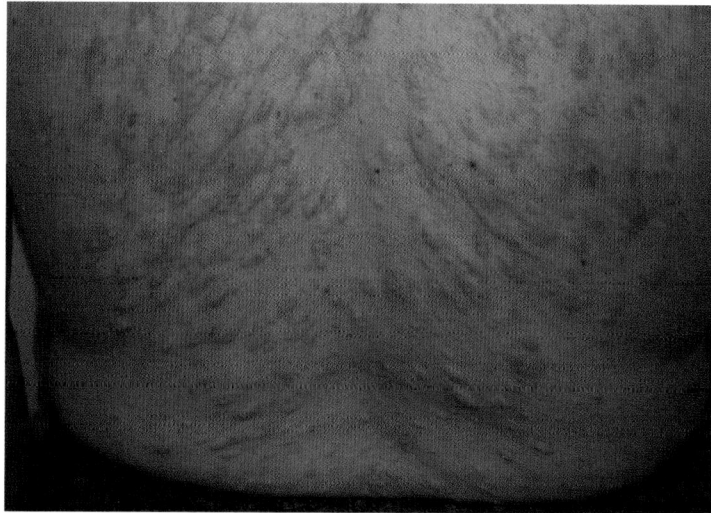

Figure 96.24 Primary anetoderma associated with antiphospholipid antibodies. (From Eungdamrong *et al.* [26], with permission from *Dermatology Online Journal*.)

there is an association with inherited bony or ocular abnormalities. The Blegvad–Haxthausen syndrome comprises anetoderma, blue sclerae and osteogenesis imperfecta (OI).

The histology of anetoderma suggests that the basic abnormality is focal elastolysis [1,28,29]. This may be secondary to the release of elastase from inflammatory cells which are probably always present in the early stages. Metalloproteinases are increased in lesional skin [30].

Complement activation may be involved, as C3 is deposited on the remaining elastic fibres [31]. It has been suggested that decay-accelerating factor (DAF) and vitronectin (an inhibitor of the membrane–attack complex) may protect elastic fibres against this type of damage [32]. Abnormalities in the protective system could play a role in primary anetoderma.

Secondary anetoderma
This is seen in association with another identifiable disease, and has occurred in association with systemic [33] or chronic cutaneous lupus erythematosus [34], not always in relation to the lesions. Anetoderma is also associated with lupus profundus [35,36].

Some cases of primary anetoderma have direct immunofluorescence findings similar to those of either chronic cutaneous or systemic lupus erythematosus, even though there may be no other features of lupus erythematosus [38,39]. Biopsy shows a focal loss of elastic tissue, and a perivascular infiltrate with prominent plasma cells [1,2]. Generalized elastolysis (cutis laxa) has also occurred [37].

Antibodies have not been demonstrated against elastic fibres [39].

Pathology [2,27]
During the early stages, the dermis is oedematous, and a lymphocytic infiltrate (predominantly helper T cells) surrounds the blood vessels and appendages [1,29]. Plasma cells and histiocytes, with some granuloma formation, may also be seen. Later, the oedema

and perivascular infiltrate subside and elastic fibres become scanty. The persistence of fine, irregular or twisted elastic fibres is common. The dermal collagen may also be diminished, but the fragmentation and disappearance of elastic tissue is the essential change, beginning superficially in the subpapillary zone and extending downwards. Electron microscopy shows phagocytosis of elastic fibres by macrophages [40–42].

Causative organisms

Serological evidence of *Borrelia burgdorferi* infection has been observed in some cases [27].

Genetics

Familial cases are reported [24–26].

Environmental factors

It is perhaps more frequent in central Europe than elsewhere, which suggests a possible relationship to chronic atrophic acrodermatitis (due to *Borrelia* spp.) in some cases [27].

Clinical features

History

There may be a history of a previous inflammatory, perhaps urticated, lesion at the site. Often lesions are asymptomatic.

Presentation

In primary anetoderma crops of round or oval pink macules 0.5–1.0 cm in diameter develop on the trunk, thighs and upper arms, less commonly on the neck and face and rarely elsewhere. The scalp, palms and soles are usually spared. Each macule extends for a week or two to reach a size of 2–3 cm. Sometimes, there are larger plaques of erythema, and nodules have also been reported as a primary lesion [43]. Slowly, each lesion fades and flattens from the centre outwards to leave a macule of wrinkled atrophic skin, which yields on pressure, admitting the finger through the surrounding ring of normal skin (Figure 96.25). The colour varies from skin colour to grey, white or blue. The number of lesions varies widely, from less than five to 100 or more.

In some cases, the lesions are initially urticarial weals which, after a succession of exacerbations and remissions, perhaps continuing for many weeks, are succeeded by atrophy. They may become confluent, to cover large areas, especially at the roots of the limbs and on the neck.

The atrophic areas in secondary anetoderma do not always develop at the sites of the known inflammatory lesions. They are soft, round or oval areas which occur mainly on the trunk.

Clinical variants

'Confetti-like macular atrophy' [44] may be a variant of anetoderma, although the lesions are not depressed or herniated. Hypopigmented shiny atrophic patches occur on the upper limbs and trunk. Histology shows an atrophic epidermis with disorganized, hyalinized coarse collagen bundles in mid-dermis, with elastic fibre loss and fragmentation in the upper dermis.

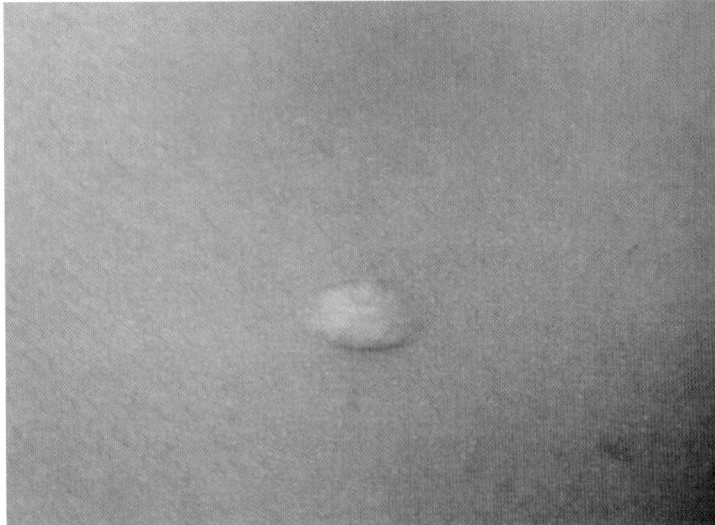

Figure 96.25 Secondary anetoderma in chickenpox scar. (From Veraldi A, Schianchi R, Chickenpox, impetigo, and anetoderma *Pediatric Dermatology* 2006;23:305–6. With permission from John Wiley.)

Differential diagnosis

Extragenital lichen sclerosus (see Chapter 57) presenting as white spots around the base of the neck and shoulders should not be confused with anetoderma. Histological examination establishes the diagnosis if there is doubt.

Focal dermal hypoplasia and atrophic scars must also be considered.

Aquired cutis laxa (see earlier) and anetoderma are closely related, and may represent different forms of the same condition.

The diagnosis of 'primary' anetoderma can be established only by excluding the presence of any of the diseases known to be associated with 'secondary' atrophy, e.g. perifollicular elastolysis (see later).

Disease course and prognosis

The lesions remain unchanged throughout life, and new lesions often continue to develop for many years. If the lesions coalesce they form large atrophic areas, which are indistinguishable from acquired cutis laxa [2].

Investigations

In patients with primary anetoderma it is important to test for antiphospholipid syndrome and treat appropriately, e.g. with aspirin or warfarin.

Management

No specific treatment exists. In the case of secondary anetoderma, treatment should be directed against underlying disease or infections.

Penicillin and the antifibrinolytic drug ε-aminocaproic acid have been advocated [45], but Venencie *et al.* [2] studied 16 patients and found no treatment was beneficial once the atrophy had developed. Colchicine may prevent some atrophic changes [46]. Ablative (e.g. carbon dioxide) lasers may reduce scarring [13].

Mid-dermal elastolysis

Definition and nomenclature

Idiopathic loss of the elastic fibres in the mid-dermis leads to widespread wrinkling of the crinkle type in otherwise healthy young or middle-aged women (Figure 96.26) [1,2]. The exact relationship between this condition and other elastolytic disorders such as acquired cutis laxa and anetoderma is uncertain. Localized areas may clinically resemble PXE, although they are histologically distinct [3,4].

Synonyms and inclusions
- Elastolysis mediodermalis
- Perifollicular elastolysis

Epidemiology

Incidence and prevalence
Sporadic cases.

Age
Young to middle age.

Sex
Mostly female.

Ethnicity
Fair-skinned.

Associated diseases
Cases have been associated with a prothrombotic state [5], suggesting a similarity to anetoderma.

Pathophysiology

Predisposing factors
It has been reported to follow granuloma annulare [6] and other inflammatory conditions.

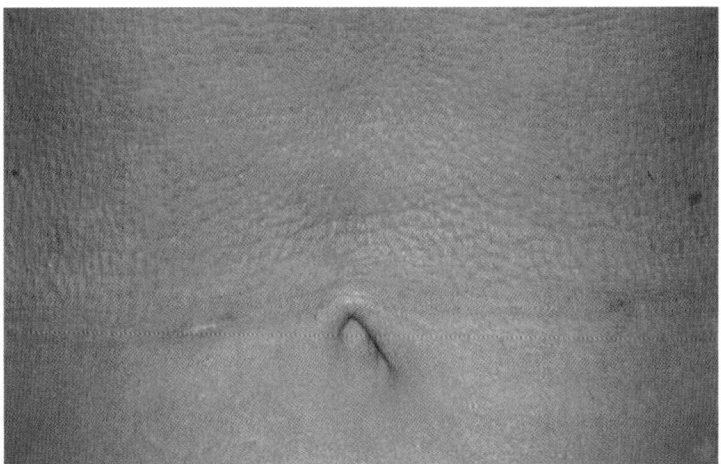

Figure 96.26 Idiopathic mid-dermal elastolysis. (Courtesy of Dr L. Ostlere, St George's Hospital, London, UK.)

Pathology

Ultrastructural studies of mid-dermal elastolysis demonstrate elastic fibres engulfed by macrophages [7]. In the perifollicular variant histology shows a non-inflammatory perifollicular loss of elastin fibres [8]. Immunological studies of affected skin show a non-specific profile of immune activation [9]. Cultured fibroblasts from lesional dermis exhibit increased elastolytic activity and reduced elastin mRNA compared with normal skin [10]. Maghraoui *et al.* [11] have distinguished post-inflammatory elastolysis, with or without features of cutis laxa, from non-inflammatory elastolysis.

The histology of idiopathic mid-dermal elastolysis is similar to that of PECL (see earlier). Those lesions are preceded by inflammatory lesions, but the lesions of idiopathic mid-dermal elastolysis may also occasionally be preceded by erythema, urticaria or a burning sensation, and the two conditions are similar, if not identical.

Causative organisms
Elastase-producing strains *of Staphylococcus epidermidis* have been implicated in the perifollicular variant [**12**].

Environmental factors
UV light may trigger elastophagocytosis [13]. The condition has also been reported in a patient receiving haemodialysis [14] and near the site of insertion of a pacemaker [15].

Inflammatory triggers may include UV radiation, insect bites, varicose veins, borreliosis and acute neutrophilic dermatosis [16,17].

Clinical features

History
The condition is typically asymptomatic.

Presentation
Millimetre to centimetre large, well-circumscribed or net-like areas of crinkly skin (cigarette paper-like fine wrinkling).

Clinical variants
Three variants have been described [18] as follows:
- Type 1: cigarette paper-like fine wrinkling (crinkle) affecting the trunk and upper arms.
- Type 2: perifollicular papules [8,12]. Lesions are small, grey–white, finely wrinkled, round or oval areas, each with a central hair follicle. Some exhibit a balloon-like bulge above the surface. They occur on the upper trunk, neck, earlobes and arms. Similar changes are more commonly seen in acne scars (see Chapter 91).
- Type 3: reticular variant; orange-red inflammatory papules precede net-like areas of atrophy, chiefly on the arms [15,18]. Localized areas may clinically resemble PXE, although they are histologically distinct [3,4]

In addition to these, a linear lumbar variant has also been described [19].

Upper dermal elastolysis

Definition and nomenclature
Selective loss of elastic tissue in the papillary dermis was originally described in an otherwise healthy 86-year-old woman, who presented with numerous yellowish papules on the neck and upper trunk, and associated coarse wrinkles [20]. Since, there have been several other reports, mostly in women aged 60–70 years [21,**22**,23]. This condition may be a unique variant or related to acquired PXE [23].

> **Synonyms and inclusions**
> • Papillary dermal elastosis

Differential diagnosis
The histology of idiopathic mid-dermal elastolysis is similar to that of PECL, which occurs in young African girls (see earlier). Those lesions are preceded by inflammatory lesions, but the lesions of idiopathic mid-dermal elastolysis may also occasionally be preceded by erythema, urticaria or a burning sensation, and the two conditions are similar, if not identical.

Management
No definite treatment exists but topical retinoic acid (0.01% gel) produced some cosmetic improvement in one patient [9]. Reduction of degradation by metalloproteinases would be desirable, as in other elastophagocytic disorders [24].

Blepharochalasis

Definition and nomenclature
Laxity of the eyelid skin due to a defect in the elastic tissue.

> **Synonyms and inclusions**
> • Ascher syndrome

Epidemiology

Incidence and prevalence
Rare, mostly sporadic.

Age
Usually around the time of puberty.

Ethnicity
Most cases are reported in white people.

Associated diseases
Some cases may be a localized form of post-inflammatory elastolysis or follow angio-oedema [1].

Pathophysiology

Predisposing factors
Presumably inflammatory stimulus to elastophagocytosis.

Pathology
In the early stages, there may be a mild dermal lymphocytic infiltrate, and in the later stages the elastic fibres in the lids fragment and decrease [2]. Normal elastin gene expression suggests other factors may be involved in elastic fibre loss [3]. IgA deposition may be detected on fibres, implying an immunopathogenic mechanism may be relevant [**4**]. Disintegration of collagen fibres has also been observed in one case [5].

Causative organisms
None known.

Genetics
Some pedigrees show autosomal dominance, although most cases are sporadic.

Clinical features

History
There may be a history of previous transient episodes of painless eyelid swelling lasting for 2–3 days.

Presentation
Blepharochalasis is an uncommon condition that usually develops insidiously. Attacks of painless swelling of the eyelids are followed by laxity, atrophy, wrinkling and pigmentation, predominantly of the upper eyelids (Figure 96.27). There may be multiple telangiectases. These changes produce an appearance of tiredness, debauchery or premature ageing.

Reduplication of the mucous membrane of the upper eyelid is associated with blepharochalasis in about 10% of cases, and this may make the eyelids appear thick.

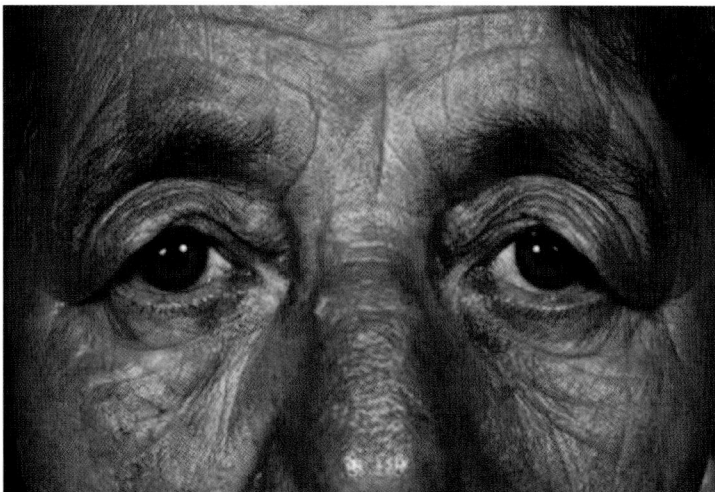

Figure 96.27 Blepharochalasis.

PART 8: SPECIFIC CUTANEOUS STRUCTURE

Clinical variants

Ascher syndrome

Ascher syndrome is the association of blepharochalasis with progressive enlargement of the upper lip due to hypertrophy and inflammation of the labial salivary glands [1–3,6,7,9–11,**12**,13,14]. The lip feels soft and lobulated and there may be excessive salivation. In some cases, the accessory lacrimal glands are also affected, with increased thickness of the eyelids. Goitre (enlargement of the thyroid) has also been reported as part of the syndrome [6].

Differential diagnosis

1 The many other causes of eyelid swelling must be excluded (see Chapter 109). Ptosis is easily distinguished because the skin appears normal. Blepharochalasis is occasionally a manifestation of generalized cutis laxa, and it may form part of Ascher syndrome (see later).
2 Laxity of the eyelid skin is most commonly an age-related phenomenon (dermatochalasis) due to degenerative changes in the connective tissue of the eyelid. Laxity also occurs in Ehlers–Danlos syndrome but other features of this syndrome will also be present. Occasionally laxity, particularly affecting the upper eyelid, occurs in otherwise healthy individuals [8].

Treatment ladder

First line
• Plastic surgery (levator tuck) can be performed, but the condition may recur [2]

Actinic granuloma and annular elastolytic giant cell granuloma

Definition and nomenclature

Actinic granuloma is an uncommon condition affecting actinically damaged skin that results from a low-grade reactive inflammatory process in which degenerate elastic fibres are phagocytosed by multinucleate giant cells and histiocytes. It is the commonest type of annular elastolytic giant cell granuloma, in which abnormal elastic fibres are progressively destroyed by an expanding ring of elastolysis and granulomatous inflammation.

Synonyms and inclusions
• Elastolytic actinic giant cell granuloma
• O'Brien granuloma
• Miescher granuloma of the face
• Atypical annular necrobiosis lipoidica of the face and scalp
• Granuloma multiforme (see later)

Introduction and general description

Annular elastolytic giant cell granuloma (AEGCG) is an uncommon granulomatous cutaneous reaction pattern in which dam-

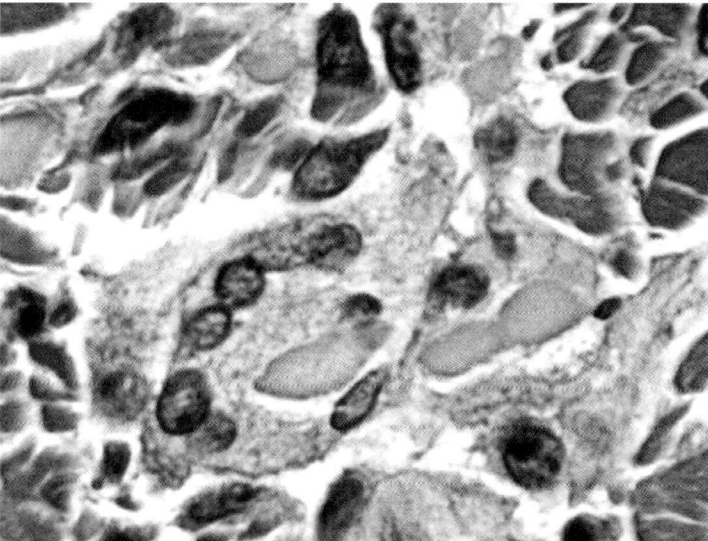

Figure 96.28 Annular elastolytic giant cell granuloma: high-power view showing fragments of degenerate elastic fibres engulfed by multinucleate giant cells. (Courtesy of Professor Luis Requena, Universidad Autónoma de Madrid, Spain.)

aged dermal elastic fibres are slowly eliminated by a process of phagocytosis by multinucleate giant cells and histiocytes (Figure 96.28) [1]. The commonest form, actinic granuloma, occurs in sun-exposed skin and manifests as one or more slowly enlarging annular plaques with an elevated erythematous margin, leaving behind a central area of atrophy devoid of elastic fibres (Figure 96.29) [2]. Actinic granuloma is associated with diabetes in up to 40% of cases: it has been postulated that hyperglycaemia may alter the immunogenicity of elastic fibres

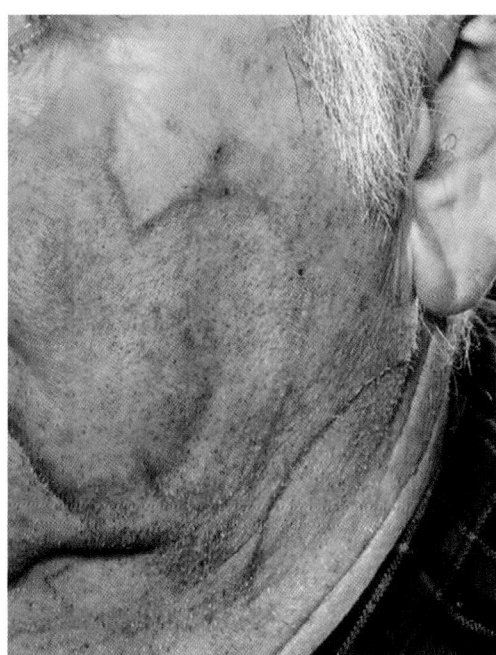

Figure 96.29 Typical actinic granulomas on the face and neck of an elderly man.

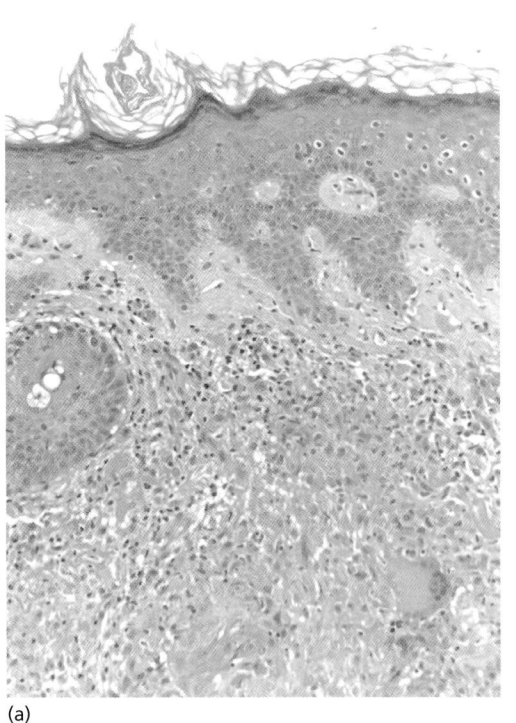

(a)

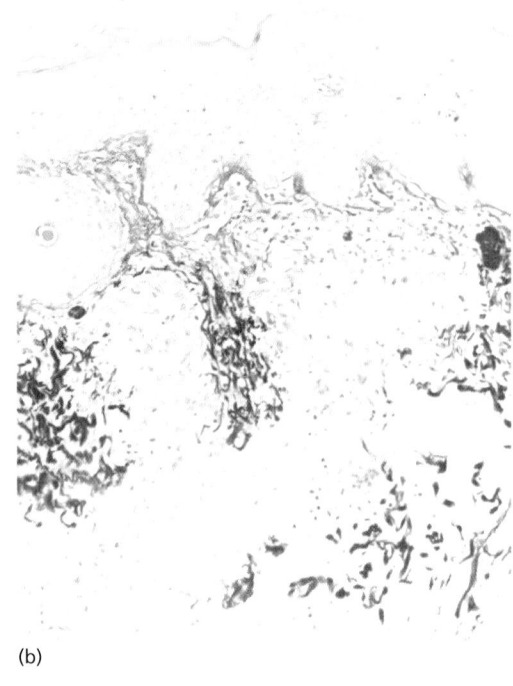

(b)

Figure 96.30 (a,b) Annular elastolytic giant cell granuloma: low-power view showing intense granulomatous inflammation (a) and elastorrhexis with loss of elastic fibres (b). (Courtesy of Dr Leigh Biddlestone, Royal United Hospitals, Bath, UK.)

PART 8: SPECIFIC CUTANEOUS STRUCTURE

[1,3]. There are other less common variants of AEGCG including an annular form of sarcoidosis which typically presents around the temples and forehead and was originally described as atypical necrobiosis lipoidica [4,5]; AEGCG in sun-protected skin [6,7,8]; and AEGCG occurring in burn scars [9,10]. It has also been associated with prolonged doxycycline photosensitivity [11], prolonged sunbed exposure [12] and with the onset and recurrence of acute myeloid leukaemia [13]. The common theme would appear to be damage to elastic fibres provoking a granulomatous inflammatory response.

Epidemiology

Incidence and prevalence
The condition is more common in sunny countries.

Age
Usually over the age of 30.

Ethnicity
Fitzpatrick skin type I are particularly susceptible.

Associated diseases
Diabetes.

Pathophysiology

Pathology
The histological appearances are characteristic [1,2,14,15,16,17,18]. A biopsy taken radially across the thickened edge of the lesion and stained with elastic van Gieson stain shows three distinct zones in the dermis. In the external 'normal' skin, there is actinic elastosis. In the thickened annulus, there is a histiocytic and giant cell inflammatory reaction in relation to elastotic fibres (Figure 96.30a,b), and in the centre, within the annulus, little or no elastic tissue remains. The cellular infiltrate slowly expands outwards, leaving behind a central area from which elastic fibres have been removed by 'elastoclasis'.

The epidermis may be normal or it may show signs of actinic damage.

Environmental factors
Chronic photodamage.

Clinical features

History
Lesions are typically asymptomatic.

Presentation
Lesions may be single or multiple. They normally develop in sun-exposed skin such as the dorsa of the hands and forearms, the vee of the neck or the bald scalp (Figure 96.31). Fair-skinned or freckled subjects are particularly susceptible. The lesions start insidiously as small pink papules, which slowly extend centrifugally to form a ring of firm superficial dermal thickening which is smooth and slightly elevated (see Figure 96.29). The ring initially measures a few millimetres across but gradually expands, often attaining a diameter of several centimetres. The centre may become slightly atrophic and variable depigmentation may

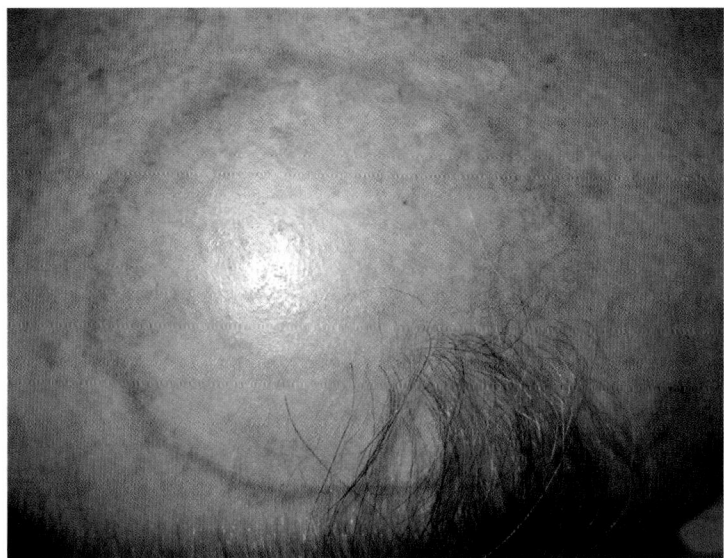

Figure 96.31 Actinic granuloma on a bald scalp. (Courtesy of Professor Luis Requena, Universidad Autónoma de Madrid, Spain.)

occur. The lesions are usually asymptomatic but a sunburn reaction may provoke severe erythema and irritation. Hair growth is not affected (see Figure 96.31).

Clinical variants
See introduction: some cases of AEGCG may represent an annular form of cutaneous sarcoidosis [19].

Granuloma multiforme is a condition which many would regard as a variant of AECGC (see later).

Differential diagnosis
- Granuloma annulare
- Necrobiosis lipoidica
- Elastosis perforans serpiginosa
- Sarcoidosis

Complications and co-morbidities
Diabetes (see earlier).

Disease course and prognosis
The condition can improve with adequate sun protection.

Investigations
Skin biopsy.

Management
No treatment is of proven benefit. Topical steroids are generally unhelpful.

Anecdotal reports of successful treatment include intralesional triamcinolone, and oral hydroxychloroquine, isotretinoin (0.5 mg/kg/day) [20] acitretin 25 mg/day [21], dapsone, methotrexate and ciclosporin and topical tacrolimus [22].

Granuloma multiforme

Introduction and general description
Granuloma multiforme is a dermatosis reported in dark-skinned people mainly from Africa and India [1,2,3–8]. It shares many similarities with AEGCG in that it is characterized by annular plaques with giant cell granuloma formation at the periphery and loss of elastic tissue centrally [1]. As with AEGCG, it presents with papules which enlarge to form annular plaques with raised edges which may attain many centimetres in diameter. Histologically, the condition is difficult to distinguish from AEGCG except that focal necrobiosis and dermal mucin may be seen, which is not the case in AEGCG. Many authorities believe that granuloma multiforme should be regarded as a form of AEGCG [1].

Its importance lies in its superficial resemblance to tuberculoid leprosy, which is an important differential diagnosis. Leiker *et al.* [2,3,4] first described granuloma multiforme and distinguished it from tuberculoid leprosy. Leiker called it Mkar disease, after the town where it was first studied. The condition is endemic in certain villages in eastern Nigeria, where the local inhabitants refer to it in the Ibo tongue as 'Ununo Enyi' (elephant ringworm) [5,8]. The disease appears to occur predominantly in females over the age of 40 years [5,8,9]. Intense sun exposure over many years in people able to withstand acute photodamage appears to be a common feature. The difference in skin type and other unknown factors may explain the rather minor histopathological differences from AEGCG as seen in fair-skinned individuals.

Clinical features

Presentation
The upper, uncovered parts of the body are predominantly affected. The initial lesions are small flesh-coloured papules which become aggregated into plaques or form the elevated rims of annular lesions. In larger annular lesions, the central area is often hypopigmented. Pruritus may be prominent. The condition lasts for many months or years, and may persist indefinitely.

Differential diagnosis
Leprosy is endemic in the same regions where granuloma multiforme is found, and can look very similar. However, there is no loss of sensation or sweating, or other evidence of neural involvement in granuloma multiforme.

Management
No treatment is known to be effective.

Other elastolytic conditions

Granulomatous slack skin is characterized by the slow development of pendulous folds of lax erythematous skin, which on histological examination contain a dense granulomatous dermal infiltrate, with destruction of dermal elastic tissue. It is now considered to be a type of cutaneous T-cell lymphoma (mycosis fungoides) (see Chapter 140) [1,2].

Acquired pseudoxanthoma elasticum-like syndromes

Perforating pseudoxanthoma elasticum

Synonyms and inclusions
- Perforating periumbilical calcific elastosis

Transepithelial elimination (TEE) of altered elastic fibres can occasionally occur in generalized hereditary forms of PXE (see Chapter 72), but it can also occur as a localized acquired defect in patients who do not have the other features of PXE [1]. These localized lesions usually occur in the periumbilical area in obese, multiparous black or Asian women, and it is possible that this represents a response to repeated cutaneous stretching (e.g. ascites or previous abdominal surgery) [2,4]. Similar lesions on the breast have been reported in patients undergoing haemodialysis [2,5].

Clinically, asymptomatic yellow macules and papules coalesce into well-demarcated hyperpigmented plaques which slowly enlarge. The surface may be atrophic, grooved, fissured or verrucous, and compression of the edge of the lesion may produce a liquid discharge.

It seems likely that most cases previously described as elastosis perforans serpiginosa in association with PXE were really examples of perforating PXE [6]. The histology of the two conditions is similar, but in perforating PXE there is transepidermal elimination of altered basophilic, calcified, elastic fibres [7], which are short, fragmented, curled and predominantly in the mid-dermis, whereas in elastosis perforans serpiginosa the fibres are abnormally large, non-calcified, eosinophilic and straight. The condition is similar to, or identical with, papillary dermal elastolysis (see earlier) [8].

Spontaneous resolution has been reported [9].

Acquired pseudoxanthoma elasticum

Synonyms and inclusions
- Pseudo-pseudoxanthoma elasticum

Iatrogenic
Skin changes which are virtually identical to those of PXE can rarely be produced by penicillamine (e.g. in the treatment of Wilson disease), although the systemic features do not occur [1,2]. The skin changes can be explained by the known effect of penicillamine in inhibiting collagen and elastin cross-linking, with the production of vastly increased amounts of abnormal elastin in the dermis [3]. Transepidermal extrusion of elastin has been reported in this condition [4].

Toxic
Lesions clinically resembling PXE are reported in the eosinophilia–myalgia syndrome; dermal calcification is absent on histology [5]. Eosinophilia myalgia syndrome is defined by: (i) incapacitating myalgias; (ii) a blood eosinophil count greater than 1000 cells/µL; and (iii) no evidence of infection (e.g. trichinosis) or neoplastic conditions that could account for these findings, and related to toxic oil syndrome, caused by ingestion of contaminated L-tryptophan or other less well-characterized toxic substances (see Saltpetre disease later).

Depositions
Yellowish papules and plaques resembling PXE are seen in some patients with amyloidosis; amyloid deposits are seen and, again, dermal calcification is absent [6,7].

Haematological disease
PXE–like lesions are described in several haemoglobinopathies, including congenital anaemia, sickle cell disease and thalassaemia [8]. These patients may develop systemic manifestations such as peripheral vascular occlusive disease and retinal neovascularization and haemorrhage [9].

Saltpetre disease [1,2,3]

A condition which resembles the skin changes of PXE clinically, histologically and ultrastructurally has been described in a group of elderly farmers, who decades earlier had spread a fertilizer containing calcium-ammonium nitrate (Norwegian saltpetre). The patients developed cutaneous ulcers at sites of exposure (including antecubital fossae). These quickly healed to leave yellowish-white papules and plaques. None of the patients had a positive family history or other signs of PXE.

Acrokeratoelastoidosis

Synonyms and inclusions
- Acrokeratoelastoidosis
- Focal acral hyperkeratosis
- Hereditary papulotranslucent acrokeratoderma
- Marginal papular acrokeratoderma

Acrokeratoelastoidosis is an uncommon asymptomatic disorder which manifests as multiple tiny crateriform keratotic papules along the margins of the hands and feet, particularly in people of African descent (Figure 96.32a–c). The name derives from the histological appearances which include not only epidermal acanthosis and hyperkeratosis but also fragmentation of underlying dermal elastic fibres [1]. The mechanisms involved are not understood.

It is inherited in an autosomal dominant fashion but does not usually present until after puberty; sporadic cases also occur [2]. As elastorrhexis cannot always be demonstrated, alternative names for clinically indistinguishable cases have been proposed: these include focal acral hyperkeratosis and marginal papular acrokeratoderma [3,4]. There is still controversy as to whether these should be regarded as separate entities.

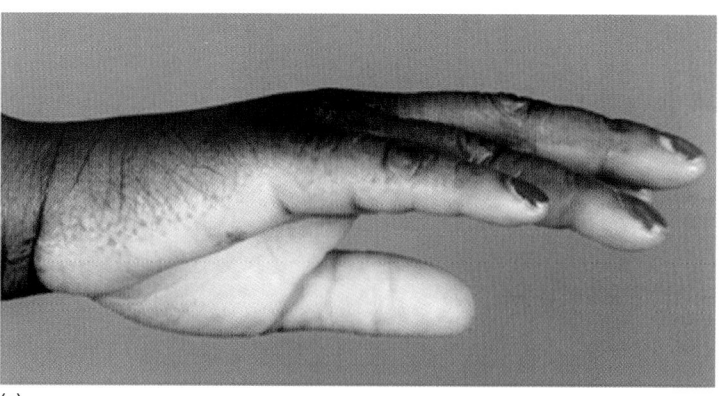

(a)

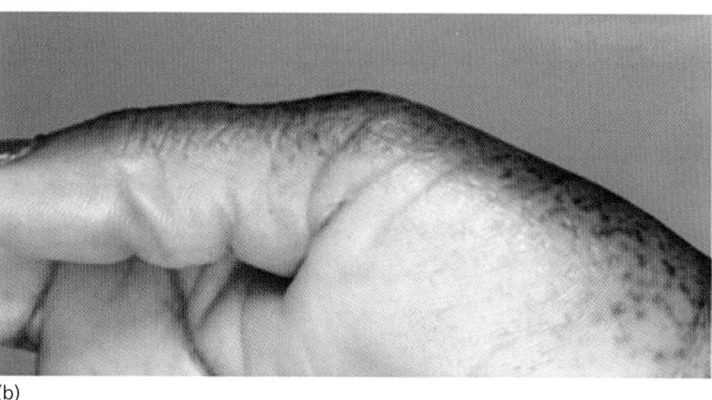

(b)

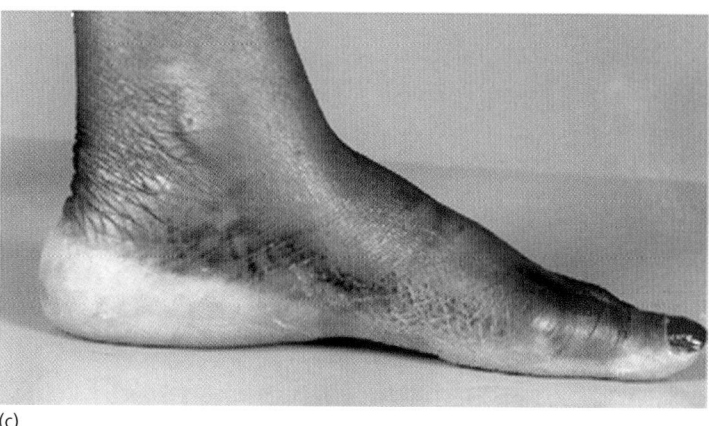

(c)

Figure 96.32 (a–c) Acrokeratoelastoidosis.

ACQUIRED DISORDERS OF ELASTIC TISSUE DEPOSITION

Linear focal elastosis

Definition and nomenclature
This condition is characterized by asymptomatic yellow linear bands arranged horizontally on the lower back [1,2–4]. It less commonly occurs on the legs and shoulders.

> **Synonyms and inclusions**
> • Elastotic striae

Introduction and general description
This condition may represent a keloidal reaction to striae distensae.

Epidemiology

Incidence and prevalence
Case reports are mostly sporadic. It may be commoner than reports suggest.

Age
Initially reported in elderly males [1], although subsequently reported patients are chiefly adolescents [5,6,7].

Sex
Predominantly male.

Ethnicity
White people, Asiatic and Afro-Caribbean [5].

Pathophysiology

Predisposing factors
The lesions may be associated with a growth spurt, similar to adolescent growth striae [6].

Pathology
Ultrastructural studies reveal active elastogenesis. The middle and lower dermal collagen is separated by bluish grey fine fibrillar material, which is composed of thin wavy elastic fibres and fragmented elastic fibre bundles. Early lesions may, in contrast, show elastolysis, with decreased elastin and microfibrillar proteins [8]. The elastic fibres are near to or even in contact with fibroblasts [9]. Elastogenesis may occur in response to local trauma, UV light or perhaps following the development of striae distensae [10]. However, these mechanisms do not adequately explain the increasing number of cases reported, particularly in the young, and it may be that intrinsic defects of elastic fibre metabolism play a role [4].

Causative organisms
None known.

Genetics

There may be an underlying defect of elastic tissue, as yet unidentified [4]. Familial cases are reported [5,11].

Clinical features

History

Insidious onset of asymptomatic lesions chiefly on the lower back.

Presentation

Superficially, the lesions resemble striae distensae, but they are palpable rather than depressed and yellow rather than purplish or white. Linear focal elastosis has been reported adjacent to striae distensae [10,12] and in one case following potent topical corticosteroids [13].

Differential diagnosis

Striae (which often coexist).

Classification of severity

Of cosmetic importance only.

Complications and co-morbidities

Associated with striae in many cases.

Disease course and prognosis

Unknown. Lesions probably regress with time.

Investigations

None needed.

Late-onset focal dermal elastosis

Yellowish papules with a peau d'orange appearance appear on the flexures. Clinically and histologically, the lesions resemble elastomas, but this rare condition has only been reported in elderly Japanese men [1,2].

Elastofibroma dorsi [1,2–8]

Elastofibroma occurs predominantly in elderly women. Most cases are reported from Southern Japan. There may be a history of prolonged manual labour. The painless or slightly tender swelling beneath the lower angle of the scapula, from 2 to 10 cm in diameter, is often discovered fortuitously. It may enlarge slowly, displacing neighbouring structures, and it can be clinically confused with a sarcoma. This is a benign lesion, however, despite the fact that it is poorly circumscribed. The growth is composed of mature fibrous tissue, containing fibres which stain as elastic fibres. The lesions may be solitary or multiple.

Histologically, the lesion contains abundant large elastic fibres, some broken into irregular masses, and large amounts of relatively acellular collagen. The elastic f]ibres are composed of true elastin surrounded by a large amount of hydrophilic material forming an orderly array of tubules [4]. It is generally regarded either as a type of reactive hyperplasia, or as a hamartoma, arising either from dermis, subscapular connective tissue or periosteum [6]. It is

cured by simple excision [7], although there is a high complication rate after surgery; postoperative suction is recommended [8] and there is a risk of recurrence [8,9].

Elastoderma

Elastoderma is a very rare condition which is due to excessive elastogenesis, as distinct from acquired cutis laxa, where there is a loss of elastic tissue. A young woman developed a localized defect of the skin of one arm, which became pendulous and lax, but lost its elastic recoil. Histological and biochemical investigation showed this was due to accumulation of excessive elastin, with derangement of elastin fibrillogenesis [1].

In further cases, also affecting young women, clinically uninvolved skin showed thin elastic fibres on haematoxylin and eosin staining, without calcification [2]. Transmission electron microscopy showed irregular elastic tissue fibres with electron dense extensions; fibroblasts were abundant, possessing widened rough endoplasmic reticulum [3]. Despite the skin laxity, there is no joint hypermobility [3].

Papular elastorrhexis

This is a rare variant of connective tissue naevus. Adolescents or young adults present with multiple non-follicular oval white or yellowish papules on the trunk or limbs; dermal elastic fibres are decreased and fragmented on histology. Most case reports are sporadic, with no family history and no extracutaneous manifestations [1–3]. The differential diagnosis includes acne scars, in which the papules are follicular, with decreased elastin but no elastorrhexis; familial cutaneous collagenoma is histologically similar, but cases of papular elastorrhexis are sporadic [4]. Similar lesions are seen in some patients with Buschke–Ollendorff syndrome (see Chapter 75), in which osteopoikilosis is also a feature. To add to the confusion, abortive forms of Buschke–Ollendorff syndrome have been described, lacking osteopoikilosis [5]. A family has been described with this variant [6]. It is possible that papular elastorrhexis is not a separate entity [7]. Intralesional triamcinolone may be beneficial [8], if treatment is necessary.

FIBROMATOSES AND OTHER CAUSES OF DIFFUSE FIBROSIS

Introduction and general description

Fibrous overgrowth of dermal and subcutaneous connective tissue occurs most readily in certain sites and at certain ages, and some of the resulting syndromes are clinically and histologically distinctive and well defined. There are some cases, however, that defy precise classification, and others in which histological criteria may be a poor guide to prognosis. Invasiveness and a high local recurrence rate may or may not be associated with a tendency to metastasize. The borderline between simple overgrowth and a benign tumour may be equally difficult to define.

Abnormal fibrosis is a feature of many debilitating systemic disorders, such as cirrhosis and pulmonary fibrosis. A closer understanding of the myofibroblast and the regulatory pathways of cytokines and growth factors, such as TGF-β, should enable the development of effective and specific antifibrotic drugs [1].

Fibromatoses

Fibromatosis is a benign fibrous tissue proliferation, which is intermediate between benign fibroma and metastasizing fibrosarcoma. The lesions of fibromatosis tend to infiltrate and recur when removed, but they do not metastasize. The term should not be applied to reactive fibrous proliferation, or to keloid, which is usually secondary to injury. The lesions in fibromatosis may be single or multiple, and the likelihood of recurrence after surgical removal varies with the location of the lesion and the age of the patient. The fibromatoses occur in two major groups:

1 Superficial fibromatoses (fascial fibromatoses):
   (a) palmar (Dupuytren);
   (b) plantar;
   (c) penile (Peyronie);
   (d) knuckle pads.
2 Deep fibromatoses (non-metastasizing fibrosarcoma). These are rapidly growing tumours that usually involve the musculature or aponeuroses. Their tendon-like consistency accounts for their alternative name of desmoid tumours. They are discussed in more detail in Chapter 137.

Palmar fascial fibromatosis

Definition and nomenclature
This is a fibromatous hyperplasia of the palmar aponeurosis, which is characterized by nodular thickening of the fascia with associated flexion contractures of one or more digits (Figure 96.33a,b).

Synonyms and inclusions
• Dupuytren contracture

Introduction and general description
The condition seems to be due to a reactive proliferation of fibroblasts with no inflammatory component; the basic cause is obscure.

Epidemiology

Incidence and prevalence
The prevalence in the general adult population is around 2–6% [1], but it may approach 20% or more in elderly males [2,3,4], in diabetic patients and in patients with AIDS.

Age
Age of onset is generally 30–60 years.

Sex
It is generally commoner in men. Some families are described in which there is a predominantly female expression [5].

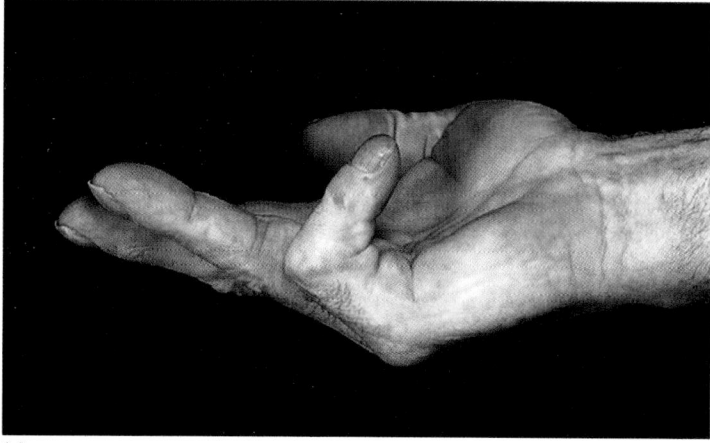

(a)

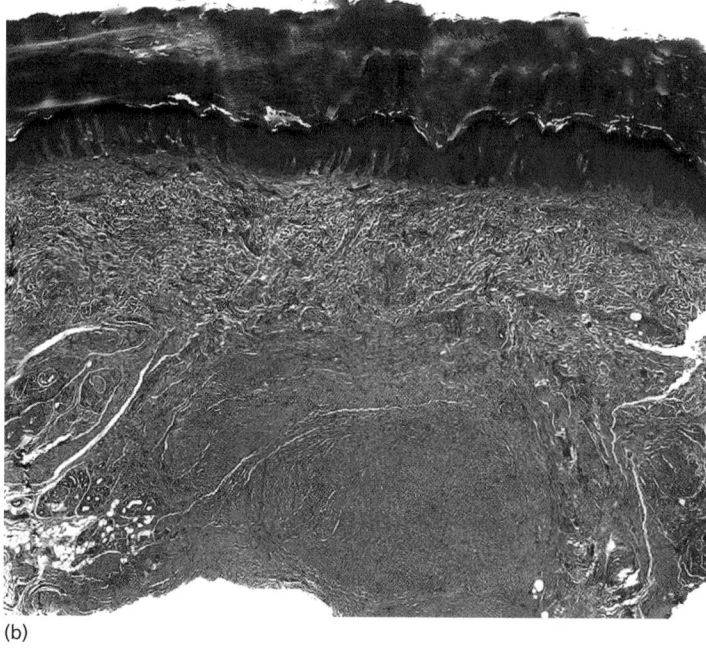

(b)

Figure 96.33 (a,b) Palmar fascial fibromatosis: clinical image illustrating (a) typical fixed contraction of the little finger, and (b) low-power photomicrograph showing grossly thickened deep fascia with nodules of proliferating fibroblasts surrounded by dense collagen. (Part b courtesy of Professor Luis Requena, Universidad Autónoma de Madrid, Spain.)

Ethnicity
Relatively uncommon in people of African or Asian descent.

Associated diseases
In about 5% of patients, the condition is associated with other fibromatoses such as knuckle pads or keloids. This has been termed the polyfibromatosis syndrome.

It occurs more commonly in patients with alcoholic cirrhosis, epilepsy [6] and diabetes [4,7], but the prevalence is decreased in rheumatoid arthritis [8]. Other conditions which have been less convincingly claimed to be associated include periarthritis of the shoulder, chronic lung disease, gout, trauma and ulnar nerve damage [9].

Phenytoin appears to stimulate fibrosis in the polyfibromatosis syndrome [10] and it may also cause gingival hypertrophy by stimulating fibroblasts and increasing collagen production [6,10,11]. There is one case report of a girl aged 14 years who developed Dupuytren contracture while receiving growth hormone therapy for hypopituitarism [12].

High alcohol consumption, smoking and trauma, notably the use of vibrating hand tools, have also been implicated [13].

Pathophysiology

Free radical production secondary to ischaemia may be involved: the concentration of hypoxanthine substrate capable of releasing free radicals is greatly increased in the affected tissue [14]. Localized ischaemia has been thought to play a part, and in animal studies allopurinol (a competitive inhibitor of xanthine oxidase) has been shown to limit the damage associated with acute ischaemia [15]. High concentrations of free radicals are toxic, but in low concentration they stimulate fibroblast proliferation [14]. The contractures, which are a late complication, appear to follow the conversion of the fibroblasts to contractile myofibroblasts [16].

The presence of CD3 lymphocytes and the expression of major histocompatibility complex (MHC) class II proteins in the affected tissue imply that palmar fascial fibromatosis is a T-cell mediated autoimmune disorder [17].

Pathology

Fibroblasts in affected fascia appear to be identical to those in normal palmar fascia but their density is increased and they tend to be clustered around narrowed small vessels [18,19]. In the early stages, there are nodules in the subcutaneous tissue or within the fascia: they are composed of proliferating fibroblasts with irregular hyperchromatic nuclei but there is no excess of collagen. Later stages are characterized by the presence of myofibroblasts, which have a fibrillary cytoplasmic ultrastructure and seem to have some other properties of smooth muscle. The nuclei are deeply indented, possibly due to the contractile properties of the cell. The cells also have altered surface membrane properties which enable attachment to neighbouring cells and stroma. Myofibroblasts have also been identified in the normal aorta and in granulation tissue, hypertrophic scars, keloids, liver fibrosis, dermatofibromata, etc. [16], in which their contractile properties may be important. The advanced stages of palmar fascial fibromatosis are characterized by dense fibrous connective tissue with a few elongated cells. An increased concentration of type III collagen is present in the nodules [20]. This may be due to decreased degradation resulting from increased levels of tissue metalloproteinase inhibitors in the lesions [21]. Structural abnormalities of glycosaminoglycans, notably dermatan sulphate, may predispose to abnormal fibrillogenesis [22].

Genetics

Palmar fascial fibromatosis is often familial, and may be inherited as an autosomal dominant trait [23], in which case the onset tends to occur at an earlier age [24]. Genome-wide studies show increased expression levels of metalloproteinases 1, 3 and 16, fibroblast growth factor and several collagen genes [25].

Environmental factors

Occupational exposure to hand-transmitted vibration may be an exacerbating factor [13].

Clinical features

History

Nodules may be painful initially, although the condition typically develops insidiously over several months or years.

Presentation

The earliest sign is the development of a palmar nodule, usually in the ulnar half of the hand. There are usually no symptoms, but there may be a dull ache or tingling. Insidious progression of the fibrosis over several years causes flexion contractures of the affected fingers. There is often puckering of the overlying skin.

Clinical variants

Plantar and penile fibromatosis are closely related conditions (see later).

Differential diagnosis

In most cases, the diagnosis is straightforward. There may be a histological resemblance to fibrosarcoma, but the latter is more pleomorphic, with larger nuclei and more mitoses. Juvenile aponeurotic fibroma may produce palmar or plantar nodules, but palmar fascial fibromatosis does not occur in young children.

Disease course and prognosis

The condition tends to progress more slowly in women [9]. Eventually, the function of the hand is impaired due to fixed flexion of one or more digits. If left untreated, there may be some improvement after many years.

Investigations

The possibility of one or more of the associated disorders, e.g. diabetes, should be considered and investigated if appropriate.

Management

The advice of an orthopaedic or hand surgeon should be sought. Traditionally complete removal of the palmar aponeurosis has been recommended [26], although minimally invasive subtotal fasciectomy and direct closure is more generally favoured [27,28].

Initial encouraging placebo-contolled trials of collagenase injections [29] have been supported by subsequent experience, and the technique is now more widely practised [30].

Medical treatments are disappointing. Allopurinol may help by decreasing free radical production [31], and it has been suggested that vitamin C might prevent progression of the disease by acting as a free-radical scavenger [2].

Many other non-surgical approaches have been tried, including continuous slow skeletal traction, radiotherapy, dimethyl sulfoxide, vitamin E, steroid injections and interferon, although none has been proven to be clinically useful [32].

High-dose tamoxifen following minimally invasive surgery reduces the risk of recurrent fibrosis in the short term, but the effect is lost on discontinuing the drug [33]. Intriguing results have been reported from the use of relaxin gene therapy on Dupuytren myofibroblasts *in vitro*, with the potential for use *in vivo* [34].

Plantar fascial fibromatosis [1,2]

Definition and nomenclature
This is a rarer condition than palmar fascial fibromatosis, although often associated; a survey from Reykjavik found that 15% of men with the latter had plantar fibromatosis [3]. It most commonly affects the medial half of the mid-foot, presenting as one or more nodules which may become painful and may ulcerate (Figure 96.34). In 25% of cases it is bilateral. The fibromatosis rarely results in contractures but tends to be locally invasive and to recur.

Synonyms and inclusions
• Ledderhose disease

Clinical features

Differential diagnosis
The differential diagnosis includes keloid and fibrosarcoma. Magnetic resonance imaging may confusingly demonstrate the cerebriform pattern typically seen in fibromyxoid sarcoma [4].

In younger patients, aggressive infantile fibromatosis and aponeurotic fibroma must also be considered [5]. Complications are rare, although squamous carcinoma has been reported occurring within a lesion of plantar fibromatosis [6]. Similar nodules have been described symmetrically affecting the anteromedial aspects of the heel pad in children. They are asymptomatic and may resolve spontaneously [7,8]: surgery is contraindicated.

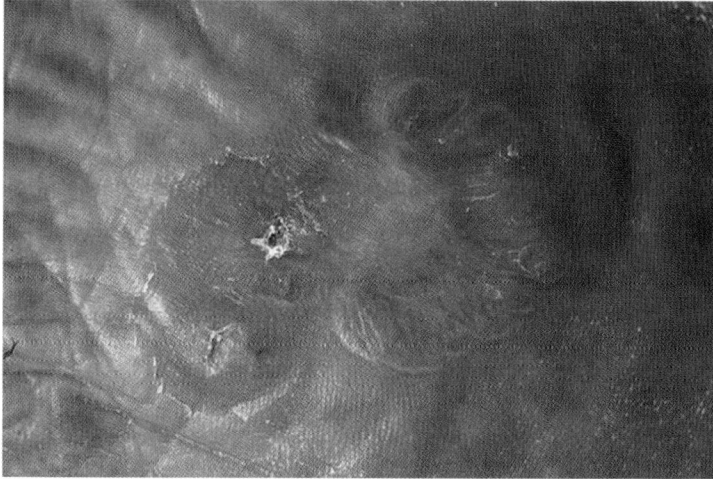

Figure 96.34 Plantar fibromatosis.

Management
Conservative management may be best in the early stages [9]. High-energy shockwave therapy reduces pain [10]. Total excision of the lesion and the entire plantar fascia seems to give the best results, with the lowest incidence of recurrence.

Penile fibromatosis

Definition and nomenclature
Penile fibromatosis is characterized by one or more irregular dense fibrous plaques in the penile shaft. These commonly result in painful erections and curvature of the erect penis.

Synonyms and inclusions
• Peyronie disease
• Plastic induration of the penis
• Fibrous sclerosis of the penis

Pathophysiology
Penile fibromatosis may occur as an isolated abnormality, or as one component of polyfibromatosis in association with palmoplantar fibromatosis, keloids and knuckle pads. Atheroma predisposes to the condition, and it is now thought that the reported association with the use of α-adrenoreceptor blocking drugs was probably attributable to concomitant atheroma [1,2]. There may be a genetic factor, but reliable studies of the mode of inheritance are lacking. The condition is rare below the age of 20 years, and the highest incidence is between 40 and 60 years. It is much less common than palmar or plantar fibromatosis.

Histopathology [3]
The thickened plaque shows cellular fibroblastic proliferation surrounded by dense masses of collagen. Calcification and ossification may occur. The process appears to begin as a vasculitis in the areolar connective tissue beneath the tunica albuginea, whence it extends to adjacent structures.

Presentation
The disease presents with painful erections and curvature of the erect penis due to a thickened subcutaneous plaque, rubbery or hard, usually on the dorsal aspect of the penis in its distal third (Figure 96.35a,b). The erectile deformity may make vaginal penetration impossible, and pain or anxiety about performance may cause secondary impotence. Fibrosis of the underlying cavernous erectile tissue may lead to a constriction or 'waisting' of the penile shaft, leading to flaccidity of the distal portion.

The course is unpredictable [4]. The pain generally subsides within a few months, but the fibrous plaque may resolve, remain unchanged or progress [5].

Investigations
The severity of the disease and the response to treatment can now be evaluated by high-resolution ultrasonography [6], computed tomography [7] or magnetic resonance imaging of the erect penis [8]. If necessary, an erection can be induced by the intracavernosal injection of papaverine [9].

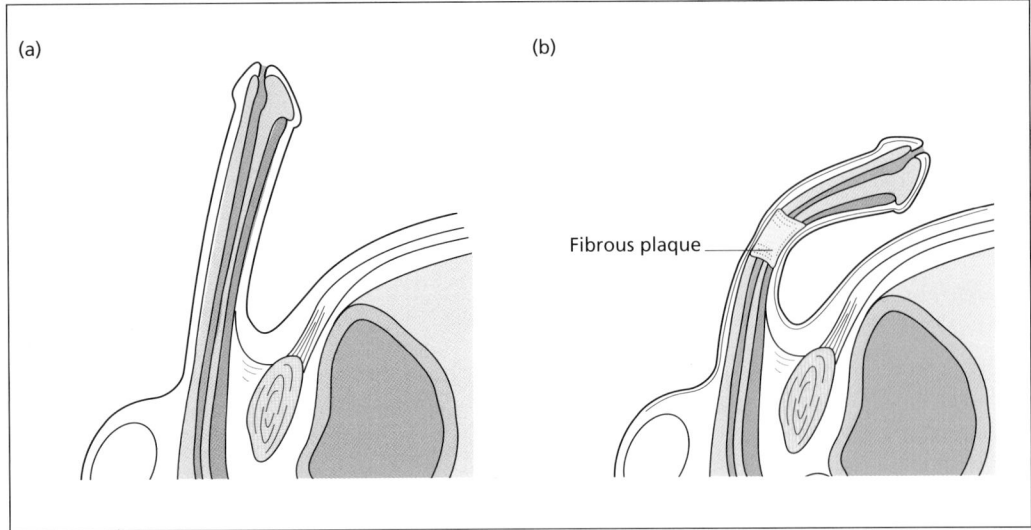

(a)   (b)

Fibrous plaque

Figure 96.35 (a) Normal erect penis. (b) Erect penis with deformation from Peyronie disease showing a fibrous plaque causing 'waisting'.

Management

Many treatments have been tried, but there is little evidence that vitamin E, potassium aminobenzoate, orgotein, radiotherapy, ultrasonic therapy or intralesional steroids affect the long-term outcome, although they may relieve the pain [4,10]. There are case reports of success with more aggressive treatment using pulsed dexamethasone and low-dose cyclophosphamide [10]. Clostridial collagenase injections have given promising results, as in Dupuytren contracture [11–13]. A recent study suggests that iontophoresis with verapamil and dexamethasone ('electromotive drug administration') may reduce the curvature and is well tolerated [14]. Penile traction has its devotees [15].

Surgery is probably the treatment of choice: a bewildering variety of procedures have been employed, including Nesbit's procedure, in which ellipses of normal tunica albuginea are excised from the side of the shaft, opposite the point of maximum curvature. Alternatives include plaque incision and grafting [16] and venous grafting, using the deep dorsal vein [17] A semirigid penile prosthesis may also be inserted.

Knuckle pads

Definition and nomenclature

Knuckle pads are circumscribed thickenings overlying the finger joints. The term is a misnomer as most lesions occur over the proximal interphalangeal rather than the metacarpo-phalangeal joints (knuckles).

Synonyms and inclusions
- Holoderma
- Pulvinus
- Subcutaneous fibroma

Introduction and general description

Knuckle pads were first described in the medical literature by Garrod [1] as an 'unusual form of nodule upon the joints of the fingers'. However, they are probably not so unusual, and they feature in several of Michelangelo's works, including the statues of *David* and the *Sleeping Slave* [1]. They should be distinguished from the 'pseudo-knuckle pads' associated with trauma.

Epidemiology

Incidence and prevalence

The condition is not rare but the true prevalence is uncertain, as most patients ignore the lesions. Mikkelson reported a prevalence of 8.8% in the population of Haugesund, Norway, and of 44.3% in individuals with palmar fibromatosis [2].

Age

Onset is usually between 15 and 30 years of age; however, lesions typically develop slowly and asymmetrically and may not present significant cosmetic problems for several years.

Sex

Probably equal.

Ethnicity

Mostly reported in white people.

Associated diseases

There is a strong association with other fibromatoses such as palmar fibromatosis [2–4]. An association between Dupuytren contracture and other fibromatous lesions has been recorded in some families. In one large family, knuckle pads were associated with sensorineural deafness and with leukonychia (Bart–Pumphrey syndrome) [5]. Knuckle pads have also been associated with epidermolytic palmoplantar keratoderma in a Chinese family due to keratin 9 mutations [6].

Another family has been described with knuckle pads in association with oesophageal cancer, hyperkeratosis and oral leukoplakia [7].

Pathophysiology

Predisposing factors
Although trauma has been implicated, this is more closely linked to 'pseudo knuckle pads'. Familial cases are reported.

Pathology
The epidermis is grossly hyperkeratotic and acanthotic, with elongated rete ridges. The dermal connective tissue is hyperplastic; a proliferative phase is followed by a fibrotic phase. individual collagen fibres may be obviously thickened and arranged in irregular bundles. Spindle-shaped myofibroblasts can be seen on electron microscopy [4,8,9]. Histologically, the changes resemble those of palmar fibromatosis.

Genetics
The condition is usually sporadic but several pedigrees have shown an autosomal dominant inheritance, e.g. the Bart–Pumphrey syndrome [5]. The age of onset and the distribution of the lesions tend to be more or less constant in each family, but show interfamily variation. Similar single nucleotide polymorphisms (SNPs) are found in familial Dupuytren contracture [10]. Knuckle pads are reported in families with palmoplantar keratodermas linked with keratin 9 mutations [6,11]. A family has been reported with familial knuckle pads but no associated conditions [4].

Environmental factors
Trauma is more probably relevant in 'pseudo knuckle pads'.

Clinical features

History
Usually asymptomatic, with insidious onset.

Presentation
Flat or convex, smooth, circumscribed nodules develop slowly and almost imperceptibly over the course of months or years, achieving 0.5–1.5 cm diameter. The lesions may be hypo- or hyperpigmented. In some patients, they become very much raised and obviously indurated, but in others the dermal component is not clinically apparent. They are most commonly seen over the dorsa of the proximal interphalangeal joints (Figure 96.36), but occasionally develop over the knuckles or the distal interphalangeal joints. Any single site or combination of sites may be involved [1,4,8].

Clinical variants
Sites other than the hands are not often affected, but similar lesions on the knees were also present in one family [3].

Differential diagnosis
Knuckle pads should be distinguished from the 'pseudo knuckle pads' associated with occupational trauma, such as in carpet layers, sheep shearers and tailors. Similar lesions are induced by children chewing or biting their fingers or 'knuckle cracking' [12] or playing video games [13]. Unlike true knuckle pads, these lesions

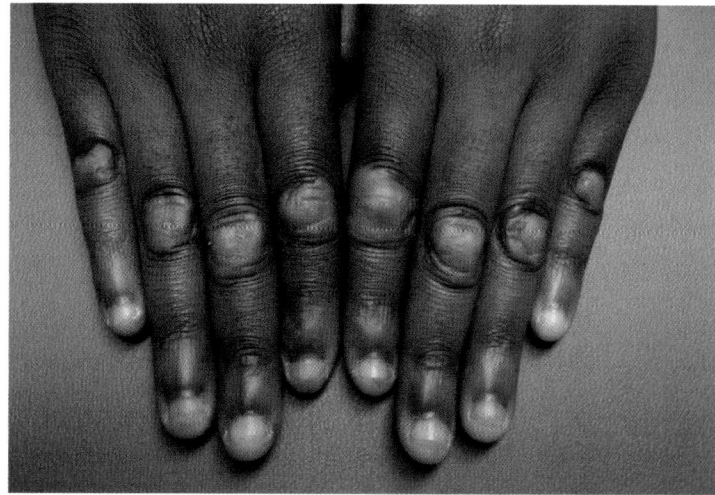

Figure 96.36 Knuckle pads. (From Hyman and Cohen [4], with permission from *Dermatology Online Journal*.)

tend to regress if the traumatic stimulus is removed, and may respond to topical keratolytics.

Heberden nodes of osteoarthritis, pachydermodactyly, granuloma annulare [14], erythema elevatum diutinum and rheumatoid nodules [15] should be excluded.

Classification of severity
A cosmetic embarrassment.

Complications and co-morbidities
Association with other fibromatoses (as noted earlier).

Disease course and prognosis
Lesions gradually enlarge to a maximal size and tend to persist.

Investigations
None usually necessary, unless another inflammatory condition needs to be excluded by skin biopsy.

Management
If the lesions do not bother the patient, conservative management is appropriate. Recurrence and keloidal scarring are common following excision. Intralesional triamcinolone or cryotherapy are ineffective and often painful. Intralesional 5-fluorouracil inhibits fibroblast proliferation and shows promise clinically [16].

Treatment ladder

First line
- Conservative management

Second line
- Consider intralesional 5-fluorouracil

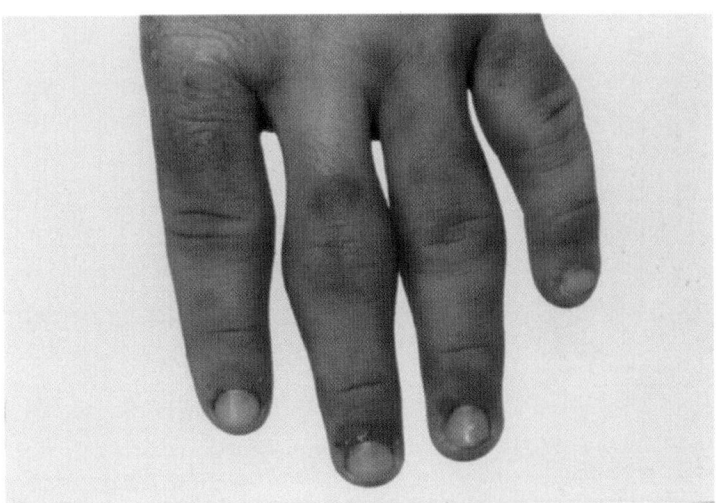

Figure 96.37 Pachydermodactyly. (Courtesy of Dr A. Chamberlain, Churchill Hospital, Oxford, UK.)

Pachydermodactyly

Definition
This is a benign fibromatosis of the fingers (Figure 96.37).

Introduction and general description
This rare condition typically presents in adolescent males, who develop spade-like enlargement of the hands and occasionally the feet [1–9].

Epidemiology

Incidence and prevalence
Rare; incidence uncertain.

Age
Young adults.

Sex
Males are chiefly affected although it has been reported in women [4,5] and two young girls, one of whom had tuberous sclerosis and the other Ehlers–Danlos syndrome [6].

Associated diseases
It may be associated with bilateral carpal tunnel syndrome [2] and varioliform atrophy (p. 96.12) [10].

Pathophysiology

Predisposing factors
It has been suggested that unconscious repeated rubbing and gripping of the fingers, repetitive movements or mechanical injury to the joints may contribute to the condition [3,6,11,12], but pachydermodactyly must be distinguished from occupational callosities and obsessive 'chewing pads'.

Pathology
Histology shows epidermal hyperplasia and marked dermal thickening, with extension of collagenous fibres into the subcutaneous tissue. Types III and V collagen are increased, and electron microscopy shows increased numbers of fine-diameter collagen fibres.

Genetics
Affected families have been reported [13].

Environmental factors
Possible local repetitive trauma.

Clinical features

History
Usually asymptomatic and insidious in onset. A few individuals describe pain of the long bones.

Presentation
It produces a symmetrical diffuse swelling of the skin around the dorsal and lateral aspects of the proximal interphalangeal joints of the index, ring and middle fingers.

Clinical variants
A distal variant has been described in an elderly woman, who also presented with nodules over the extensor aspects of the elbows [14].

Differential diagnosis
Patients may be referred to the rheumatologist with a diagnosis of juvenile idiopathic arthritis [12,15]. It may be confused with knuckle pads [16,17], which may coexist [18].

Classification of severity
The condition is benign.

Complications and co-morbidities
Knuckle pads and pachydermodactyly coexisted in one family [18].

Disease course and prognosis
The condition tends to persist.

Investigations
Patients with the condition can be spared the detailed investigations of a patient with suspected inflammatory arthritis [19].

Management
Most patients do not require treatment. Intralesional triamcinolone has been reported to be beneficial [20], although this is unlikely to be necessary.

White fibrous papulosis of the neck

Asymptomatic small white fibrous papules around the neck have been described in several Japanese [1,2], Iranian and European patients [3,4]. The number of papules ranges from 10 to 100; middle-aged to elderly men are predominantly affected. The papules are round to oval, clearly marginated and non-follicular (Figure 96.38). Histology is unremarkable, showing bundles of thickened collagen fibres in the mid-papillary dermis. Although lesions clinically resemble disorders of elastic tissue, such as anetoderma and Buschke–Ollendorff syndrome, elastic fibres are morphologically

PART 8: SPECIFIC CUTANEOUS STRUCTURE

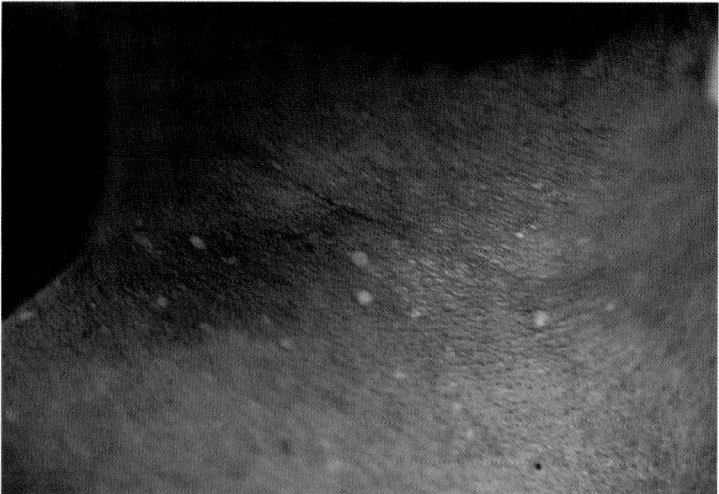

Figure 96.38 White fibrous papulosis of the neck. (Courtesy of Professor H. Shimizu, Sapporo Hospital, Tokyo, Japan.)

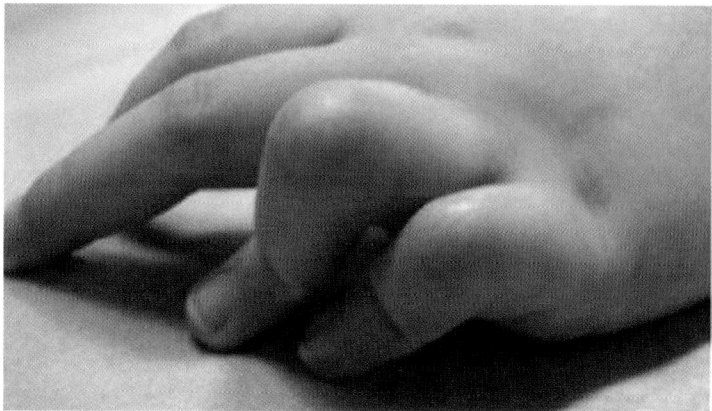

Figure 96.39 Camptodactyly in the ring and little fingers. (From Almeida SF, Monteiro AV, Lanes RCdS. Evaluation of treatment for camptodactyly: retrospective analysis on 40 fingers. *Rev. Bras. Ortop.* 2014;49:134–9, with permission.)

normal on histology. Acquired connective tissue naevi could exhibit similar features, although the late age of onset makes this diagnosis unlikely. The condition appears to have no prognostic significance, and may be underreported. It may reflect intrinsic ageing or photoageing [5].

It has been suggested that there may be a relationship between fibrous papulosis of the neck and acquired elastolysis of the papillary dermis [6,7], indeed lesions of PXE-like papillary dermal elastolysis coexisted in a patient with white fibrous papulosis, suggesting that they are part of the same disease spectrum [8]. These changes are attributed to ageing or photoageing [5,9].

Camptodactyly

Definition
Camptodactyly is a non-traumatic flexion deformity affecting the proximal interphalangeal joint of one or more fingers (Figure 96.39) [1].

Introduction and general description
Camptodactyly should be distinguished from *clinodactyly*, which refers to bending or curvature of the finger in the plane of the hand. Camptodactyly is associated with numerous inherited disorders, the most important of which are described below. It is often depicted in Renaissance art [2].

Epidemiology

Incidence and prevalence
The prevalence of isolated camptodactyly is unclear. The most commonly associated syndrome is microdeletion of 1p36, which affects 1 : 5000 neonates [3].

Age
Most cases are congenital, although some familial cases present in adult life, associated with an erosive arthritis [4].

Sex
Probably equal sex incidence.

Ethnicity
All races may be affected.

Associated diseases
Camptodactyly may be a feature of a variety of syndromes of which several have had molecular defects identified. Clinical features of microdeletion of 1p36 include camptodactyly, facial dysmorphism and low-set ears, cardiac and central nervous system defects; it is responsible for around 1% of idiopathic mental retardation [3].

Congenital camptodactyly is most notably associated with non-inflammatory arthropathy [5]. Additionally, other serous membranes undergo fibrosis leading to constricting pericarditis, coxa vara and pleuritic (camptodactyly, arthropathy, coxa vara and pericarditis =*CAP* or CACP *syndrome*) [6–9]. *Gordon syndrome* encompasses camptodactyly, cleft palate and club foot [10]. The association of camptodactyly, tall stature and hearing loss has been termed the CATSHL syndrome [11]. Familial camptodactyly of later onset has been described in association with an inflammatory arthritis with erosive changes [4]. *Blau syndrome* encompasses familial camptodactyly, granulomatous arthritis, uveitis and an erythematous eruption with phenotypic overlap with early-onset sarcoidosis [12]. In one family, taurinuria was associated [13]. Bilateral camptodactyly is also part of an autosomal recessive disorder (Crisponi syndrome) characterized by muscular contractions of the face, trismus, facial anomalies and death due to fevers. The syndrome is caused by *CRLF1* mutations and is allelic to cold-induced sweating syndrome type I [14].

Sporadic cases of camptodactyly have been linked with accelerated growth and osseous maturation, unusual facial appearance (including large ears, small mouth, broad forehead and hypertelorism), a hoarse, low-pitched cry and hypertonia (*Weaver syndrome*) [15]. Other associated features include pectus excavatum and scoliosis.

Pathophysiology

Predisposing factors
Several genetic disorders (see earlier).

Pathology
Histology of skin lesions may be unremarkable.

Genetics

Many cases are familial. Microdeletion of 1p36 is the most commonly associated abnormality. Mutations in *NOD2/CARD15* have been shown to confer susceptibility to several chronic inflammatory disorders, including Crohn disease, Blau syndrome and early-onset sarcoidosis [16]. CAP (or CACP) syndrome is autosomal recessive, and related to the 1.9 cM interval in the human chromosome 1q25-31; this gene encodes for proteoglycan 4, a surface lubricant for tendons and joints [8]. CATSHL syndrome is associated with mutation in *FGR3* [11], and Crisponi syndrome with a *CRLF1* mutation [14].

Environmental factors

None apparent.

Clinical features

The deformity is asymptomatic.

Presentation

In most cases, the affected child will present with clinical features of a related syndrome.

Clinical variants

Streblodactyly [17,18] (*streblos* = crooked) is inherited as a sex-linked autosomal dominant character. The affected females show from birth a flexion deformity at the metacarpo-phalangeal joints of the thumbs and the proximal interphalangeal joints of the little fingers. Some fingers show swan-neck deformities and hyperextensible metacarpo-phalangeal joints. In one family, there was an abnormal amino aciduria.

Differential diagnosis

Dupuytren disease (palmar fibromatosis) is associated with fibrous scarring affecting the fascia. Juvenile chronic arthritis is typically erosive, whereas the arthritis in CACP syndrome and related disorders is non-erosive [9].

Classification of severity

Morbidity relates to the associated syndrome, if any.

Complications and co-morbidities

Relates to any associated syndrome.

Disease course and prognosis

Lesions are persistent.

Management

Treatment, if required, is surgical [1,19,20]; however, results can be unsatisfactory [21]. Techniques include tendon transfer [21] and a flap with vascular reconstruction [22].

Juvenile fibromatoses

The term juvenile fibromatosis has been applied to a group of disorders occurring in infants and children, and characterized by proliferative activity of the fibroblasts [1–6]. There is a tendency to local recurrence but, unlike fibrosarcomas, they do not metasta-

size. The group includes a number of well-defined clinical entities that affect the skin as follows:

1 Infantile myofibromatosis.
2 Fibrous hamartoma of infancy.
3 Juvenile hyaline fibromatosis.
4 Infantile digital fibromatosis.
5 Calcifying aponeurotic fibroma.
6 Giant cell fibroblastoma.

Infantile myofibromatosis

Definition

Solitary or multiple fibrous nodules developing in infancy in the skin, striated muscle, bone and occasionally viscera [1,2].

Introduction and general description

Although rare, this is the commonest cause of fibrous nodules presenting in infancy. In around 50% of patients, lesions are solitary, predominantly affecting the head and neck. Multiple lesions can occur, with or without visceral involvement.

Epidemiology

Incidence and prevalence

Rare; incidence unknown.

Age

Around 60% of lesions are present at birth, and around 80% by the age of 2 years.

Sex

There is a slight male predominance, around 60% of patients are boys [2].

Ethnicity

May affect all races.

Pathophysiology

Predisposing factors

None known.

Pathology

Histology of a lesion shows characteristic zoning, with peripheral spindle-shaped cells in bundles surrounding a central zone of less poorly differentiated round and polygonal cells. Staining is positive for vimentin and α-smooth muscle elastin, negative for desmin and S-100 [1].

Genetics

Familial cases exhibit autosomal dominant inheritance. Mutations have been described in *PDGFRB* [3,4] and *NOTCH3* [5] genes.

Environmental factors

None known.

Clinical features

History
Lesions are typically asymptomatic.

Presentation
Solitary or multiple nodules, mostly on the head and neck, more rarely the arms. Lesions can occur anywhere on the body. Multiple lesions may be associated with visceral involvement. Lesions may ulcerate.

Clinical variants
Solitary lesions on the upper eyelid may cause amblyopia [6].

Differential diagnosis
The solitary lesions of fibrous hamartoma of infancy usually affect the hand or foot, histology is that of an organoid naevus containing mature adipose cells with a nodular aggregate of fibroblasts and interlacing collagen bands. Juvenile aponeurotic fibromatosis affects the fingers and palms of older children or adults; clinically, it may resemble Dupuytren disease (which is very rare in infants), but histology reveals large dark-staining nuclei in a background of bland fibrosis, with calcification. Bony lesions may be difficult to distinguish from fibrosarcoma.

Classification of severity
A benign process but the presence of systemic involvement considerably worsens the prognosis, with up to 30% mortality [2].

Complications and co-morbidities
Dependent on systemic involvement.

Disease course and prognosis
Many solitary and even multiple cutaneous lesions involute spontaneously [7,8]. Systemic involvement carries a worse prognosis.

Investigations
Histology is essential to differentiate from other tumours and fibromatoses. Full clinical examination, chest and abdominal imaging are advisable in patients with multiple lesions.

Management

First line
Patients without systemic involvement can be managed conservatively. Debulking surgery, without attempting complete removal, may be necessary if the tumour compromises function.

Second line
Systemic disease warrants chemotherapy, e.g. with low-dose vinblastine and methotrexate [9].

Juvenile hyaline fibromatosis

Definition and nomenclature
This is a disorder of glycosaminoglycan synthesis, which is characterized clinically by skin papules or tumours, gingival enlargement, osteolytic lesions and joint contractures, and histologically by deposition of amorphous hyaline material [1–4].

Synonyms and inclusions
- Molluscum fibrosum

Introduction and general description
This, together with systemic hyalinosis, is now regarded as part of the hyaline fibromatosis syndrome (see Chapter 72).

Epidemiology

Incidence and prevalence
The disease is very rare and occurs sporadically, but it has occurred in siblings [6].

Age
Onset in infancy.

Sex
Slight male predominance.

Ethnicity
Most case reports and series originate from the Indian subcontinent.

Pathophysiology

Predisposing factors
The cause is unknown, but increased chondroitin synthesis has been demonstrated in skin fibroblasts cultured from the tumour tissue [1].

Pathology [1–6]
The skin lesions contain 'chondroid' cells embedded in amorphous eosinophilic ground substance in the dermis. In the early lesions, this consists of glycosaminoglycans, but in the later lesions the matrix is mainly composed of chondroitin sulphate [7]. The dermal collagen is decreased and the collagen fibrils are fewer and thinner than in normal skin. The hyaline material may also be present in the muscles and bones. Absence of pro-α_2 chains and type III collagen has been demonstrated in affected skin [8].

Genetics
Inheritance is autosomal recessive. The gene has been mapped to 4q21; there are also mutations in the capillary morphogenesis factor 2 gene [9]. Infantile systemic hyalinosis has been associated with mutations of the *ANTXR2* gene [10,11].

Clinical features

History
The condition presents at birth or early infancy.

Presentation
There may be small pearly papules or nodules, particularly on the face or neck. Large subcutaneous tumours may also occur,

particularly on the scalp. These may be hard or soft, fixed or mobile, and they may ulcerate. Gingival hypertrophy is commonly present, and flexion contractures of the fingers, elbows, hips and knees may develop. Osteolytic lesions can occur in the skull, long bones or phalanges. The musculature is poorly developed [1,9,12–15].

Clinical variants

Infantile systemic hyalinosis is probably an extreme variant, often leading to death in infancy.

Differential diagnosis

Other infiltrative disorders, such as lipoid proteinosis may need to be excluded histologically.

Classification of severity

The condition is a severe disease, with considerable morbidity and reduced life expectancy.

Complications and co-morbidities

Joint contractures are disabling.

Disease course and prognosis

The condition persists into adult life. However, many patients die in infancy and rarely survive beyond the fourth decade [9].

Investigations

Histology is diagnostically helpful.

Management

No treatment is of proven benefit. Surgery may be the treatment of choice [5], although nodules may recur after excision [16]. The tumours do not respond to radiotherapy. Joint contractures may respond to intralesional steroid injections in the early stages and patients may benefit from systemic steroids and physiotherapy.

Other benign fibrous cutaneous nodules

Nodular fasciitis

In this condition, there is fibroblastic proliferation of one or more nodules, usually on the limbs or trunk.

Collagenoma

Collagenoma (collagen naevus) is a form of connective tissue hamartoma (see Chapter 75) which may manifest as a single or localized group of fibrous dermal papules or plaques: the shagreen patch of tuberous sclerosis is an example (see Chapter 80). Multiple fibrous dermal nodules with coarse collagen fibres may develop as sporadic cases (eruptive collagenoma) or as a genetic disorder with a dominant inheritance (familial cutaneous collagenoma).

Albopapuloid form of epidermolysis bullosa

Synonyms and inclusions
• Pasini syndrome

This rare form of epidermolysis bullosa is characterized by the development of ivory-white papules on the trunk, which histologically show connective tissue hyperplasia. Epidermolysis bullosa is discussed in Chapter 71.

Buschke–Ollendorff syndrome

Extensive nodular fibrosis may occur in the Buschke–Ollendorff syndrome (see Chapter 75), in association with juvenile elastoma and osteopoikilosis.

Fibrous digital nodules

In addition to giant cell synovioma and infantile digital fibromatosis, fibrous nodules in the digits may be due to acquired digital fibrokeratoma, fibrous papule of the finger, dermatofibroma (see Chapter 137) or the Koenen tumour (see Chapter 95).

Nephrogenic systemic fibrosis

Definition and nomenclature

A rare fibrosing disorder which occurs in patients with renal impairment exposed to low-stability gadolinium-based contrast agents [1,2].

Synonyms and inclusions
• Nephrogenic fibrosing dermopathy
• Scleromyxoedema of renal disease

Introduction and general description

The condition was first described in 1997 as nephrogenic fibrosing dermopathy [1]. Initially thought to be restricted to the skin, there are several reports of involvement of internal organs including lungs, myocardium and striated muscle, which contribute to a high mortality [3].

Epidemiology

Incidence and prevalence

Rare. With the development of guidelines on the use of gadolinium-based contrast agents [4], it is hoped that the condition will become a matter of historical importance only.

Age

Mostly in elderly adults but several cases have been reported in children [5].

Sex

Equal sex incidence.

Ethnicity

All races may be affected.

Associated diseases
Associated with renal impairment.

Pathophysiology

Predisposing factors
The condition is strongly associated with the prior administration of gadolinium-based magnetic resonance contrast agents, particularly in patients with severe renal disease, typically with a glomerular filtration rate below 30 mL/min/1.73 m² or on dialysis [6]. Gadolinium chelates stimulate an NLRP3 inflammasome-dependent inflammatory response, leading to fibroblast growth, synthesis and differentiation into myofibroblasts [7,8]. Non-ionic linear gadolinium-based contrast agents, particularly gadodiamide, are strongly implicated. Macrocyclic chelating agents, such as gadoterate, are more stable and considerably less likely to induce the syndrome [9]. Additional risk factors include an associated vascular repair (e.g. leaking aortic aneurysm), associated thrombosis or procoagulant state, and concurrent administration of intravenous iron [2]. High-dose erythropoietin is also implicated in some cases; it has a pro-inflammatory action, particularly in the presence of increased iron stores [10].

Pathology
Dermal mucin is detected with Alcian blue staining. Increased collagen and elastic fibres are laid down in haphazard bun-dles in the dermis and subcutis; there are increased numbers of CD68-positive fibroblasts in loose aggregates. Inflammatory changes may predominate, including a septal panniculitis [1,11].

Causative organisms
None proven.

Genetics
None.

Environmental factors
Gadolinium-based contrast agents.

Clinical features

History
A history should be obtained of exposure to gadolinium chelates, although onset may be delayed by several years [7]. Patients may complain of myalgia.

Presentation
Irregular erythematous or brownish indurated plaques, with amoeba-like projections and islands of sparing, occur chiefly on the lower trunk and legs (Figure 96.40). Typically the face is

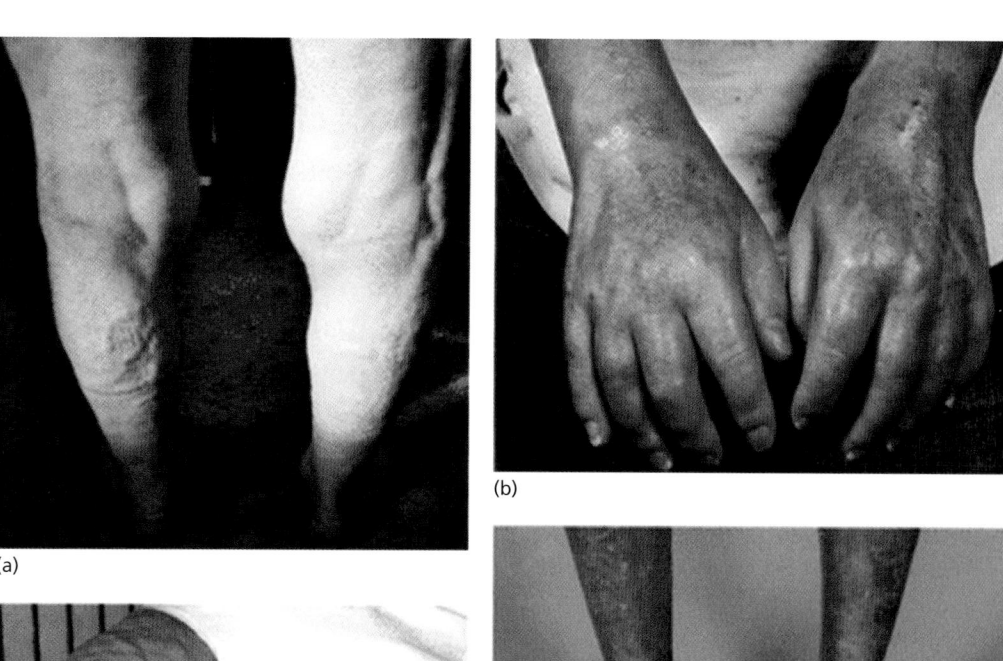

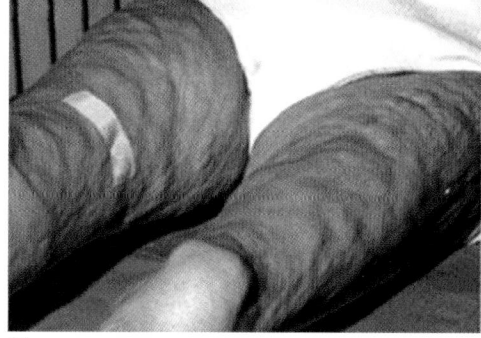

Figure 96.40 Nephrogenic systemic fibrosis: Deep involvement where fibrosis pulls down a linear band of skin on the thighs (a); tightness and hardness of the hands and feet and joint contractures b and d); and firm nodules producing a cobblestone appearance (c). (From Elmholdt TR, Pedersen M, Jørgensen B, *et al.* Nephrogenic systemic fibrosis is found only among gadolinium-exposed patients with renal insufficiency: a case–control study from Denmark. *Br J Dermatol* 2011;165:828–36, with permission from Wiley.)

spared. Sometimes the skin has a 'peau d'orange' texture, which can mimic carcinoma erysipeloides [12].

Clinical variants

The extent of visceral involvement is variable; in some cases the process may involve the testes, myocardium and dura.

Differential diagnosis

Although initially described as 'scleromyxoedema-like', the lesions have a different distribution and morphology, and there is no associated paraproteinaemia [3].

Classification of severity

The condition can be severe, occasionally fatal.

Complications and co-morbidities

Fibrotic obstruction of structures, e.g. superior vena cava obstruction [13] may be a complicating factor. Associated metabolic abnormalities include hypophosphataemia [14].

Disease course and prognosis

Usually, the condition is progressive, although it may remit spontaneously, particularly with the correction of renal abnormalities.

Investigations

A careful history, together with skin or muscle biopsy, can usually confirm the diagnosis. Investigations such as magnetic resonance imaging may be needed to determine the extent of macroscopic visceral involvement.

Management

The most important aspect of management is to maximize renal function. No other treatment is of proven benefit, but thalidomide [15], hydroxychloroquine [16], corticosteroids, immune modulators (e.g. etanercept and rituximab), PUVA, intravenous sodium thiosulphate and extracorporeal photopheresis [17] have been used empirically. Alefacept appears to improve the skin disease [18]. Therapeutic plasma exchange offers pain relief [19]. Renal transplantation is sometimes associated with remission [2].

Prevention should be achieved by adherence to guidelines for the use of gadolinium chelates in radiology [4].

Diabetic thick skin

Some patients with diabetes have thick tight waxy skin and limited joint mobility which is thought to be related to altered collagen. This topic is discussed in Chapter 64.

Environmental and drug-induced scleroderma

A variety of environmental triggers, including drugs and occupational toxins, may stimulate a localized or diffuse scleroderma-like reaction in a genetically susceptible host. Important causes are

---

Box 96.2 Scleroderma-like syndromes due to chemical exposure

Vinyl chloride
Silica dust

Organic solvents
- Aromatic hydrocarbons (e.g. toluene, benzene)
- Aliphatic hydrocarbons
  - Chlorinated (e.g. trichlorethylene, perchlorethylene)
  - Non-chlorinated (e.g. naphtha-n-hexane)

Acrylamide
Epoxy resins
Toxic oil syndrome
Urea formaldehyde foam insulation
Breast augmentation (paraffin, silicone) (unproven)

Drugs
- Reactions to local injection
- Phytomenadione, pentazocine, heparin
- Etanercept
- Reactions to systemic therapy
- Bleomycin
- L-tryptophan (eosinophilia–myalgia syndrome)
- Carbidopa and L-5-hydroxytryptophan
- Penicillamine
- Valproate sodium
- Cocaine
- Appetite suppressants (diethylpropion hydrochloride, amphetamine)
- Diltiazem

---

listed in Box 96.2. Scleroderma-like lesions are seen in a photosensitive distribution in porphyria cutanea tarda. Lesions resembling generalized morphoea are seen in chronic graft-versus-host disease and paraneoplastic scleroderma is associated with neoplasms such as carcinoid. In most cases, the fibrotic process continues after withdrawal of the external stimulus. Sometimes, the ensuing clinical pattern resembles idiopathic forms of morphoea or systemic sclerosis (see Chapters 57 and 56 respectively).

Several occupational disorders resembling systemic sclerosis have been reported. In a Belgian study, men in construction-related occupations (notably electricians) were 10 times more likely to have systemic sclerosis than the general population [1]. Exposure to *vinyl chloride monomer* occurs in workers involved in polyvinyl chloride (PVC) production. One-third of male operatives in a British factory developed a clinical syndrome that included Raynaud phenomenon, dyspnoea, cutaneous sclerosis, pulp atrophy and radiological evidence of acro-osteolysis (Figure 96.41) [2]. Genetic marker studies have demonstrated an increased incidence of human leukocyte antigen (HLA)-DR5 in affected individuals; severe disease is linked with -B8 and -DR3 [3]. A similar syndrome has been reported in gold miners exposed to silica dust [4], which is the most commonly reported occupational association in the literature [5]. Organic solvents, such as trichlorethylene [6] and perchlorethylene [7], which are structurally similar to vinyl chloride, have also been implicated. Exposure to epoxy resin results in an acute syndrome of cutaneous sclerosis, muscle weakness, arthralgia, impotence, lung and oesophageal involvement [8]. The causative agent appears to be a cyclohexylamine. Acrylamide has also been implicated [9].

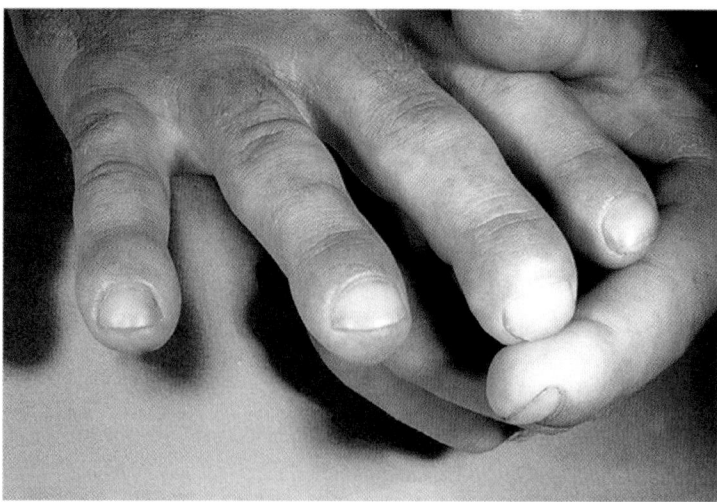

Figure 96.41 Vinyl chloride-induced osteolysis affecting fingertips.

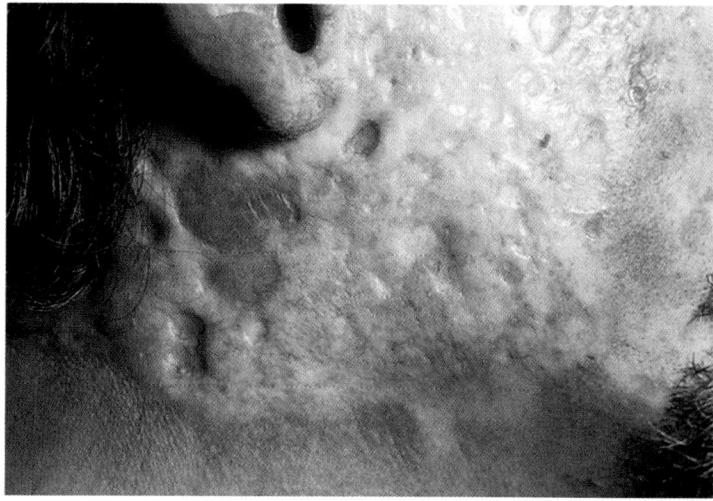

Figure 96.42 Scleroderma and scarring of the face due to porphyria cutanea tarda.

Toxic oil syndrome is a multisystem illness, reported in Spain in 1981. Acute fever, severe but transient pulmonary oedema, myalgia and a pruritic exanthem and eosinophilia were followed after several months by widespread cutaneous sclerosis in 30% of cases [10,11]. The syndrome was probably due to ingestion of imported rapeseed oil mixed with an aniline denaturant, designed to make the oil unfit for human consumption. Toxic oil syndrome bears a striking resemblance to the *eosinophilia–myalgia syndrome* [12–14], linked with consumption of L-tryptophan; this was used as a 'food supplement' to treat insomnia and depression. The offending batches of L-tryptophan contained impurities similar to the contaminants in toxic oil [15,16].

In environmental fibrotic disorders, as in idiopathic scleroderma, subpopulations of fibroblasts appear to be activated to synthesize excess collagen; this property is perpetuated by fibroblasts *in vitro*, indicating that the elevated collagen gene expression is independent of extracellular stimuli [14]. Cytokines appear to stimulate the proliferation of these abnormal clones of fibroblasts; thus, TGF-β and platelet-derived growth factor (PDGF) are elevated in the eosinophilia–myalgia syndrome [17].

Numerous drugs have been reported to induce cutaneous sclerosis. Lesions resembling morphoea may follow injections of pentazocine [18], heparin [19] and vitamin K_1 (phytomenadione) [20–23]; in the case of vitamin K_1, the trigger may be a solvent rather than vitamin K_1 itself [24]. Morphoea-like plaques have also been reported in patients taking penicillamine [25], valproate [26] and etanercept, even in areas remote from the injection site [27]. The case is not proven that silicone breast implants are associated with scleroderma-like disease [28].

Diffuse scleroderma-like changes have been reported following bleomycin therapy [29,30]. A combination of L-5-hydroxytryptophan and carbidopa induced lesions resembling eosinophilia–myalgia syndrome [31]. Phenytoin and diltiazem both induce gingival hypertrophy [32,33]. A patient on phenytoin developed florid hypertrophic retroauricular folds [34]. Thickened skin on the feet has been reported in a patient taking diltiazem [35].

Alcohol can provoke porphyria cutanea tarda, which can produce a sclerodermatous appearance in a photosensitive distribution (Figure 96.42).

Constricting bands of the extremities

Definition and nomenclature
Constricting bands occur around a digit or limb. The bands may be shallow, involving only the skin, or deeper, involving fascia or bone, and in some cases amputation may result. The term *ainhum* (an African word meaning 'to saw' [1]) is applied to a specific type in which a painful constriction of the fifth toe occurs in adults, with eventual spontaneous amputation. *Pseudo-ainhum* is the term applied to other constricting bands which are congenital or secondary to another disease.

Synonyms and inclusions
- Ainhum (dactylolysis spontanea)
- Amniotic bands

Introduction and general description
Constricting bands characteristically present in infants. Patterson [2] has provided a classification of congenital constrictions. Type I describes simple fibrotic rings; the limb distal to the ring is normal. In Type II, there is neurovascular or lymphatic disruption distal to the ring, causing atrophy, lymphoedema and maybe sensory deficit. Type III refers to acrosyndactyly (fenestrated syndactyly), where there is distal fusion of digits which are separated proximally, forming a 'window'. In type IV, there is amputation of the digit or limb (ainhum).

Epidemiology

Incidence and prevalence
Sporadic cases of constricting bands occur rarely worldwide.

Age
Constricting bands typically present in infants and young children (Figure 96.43). Adults in resource-poor countries present with

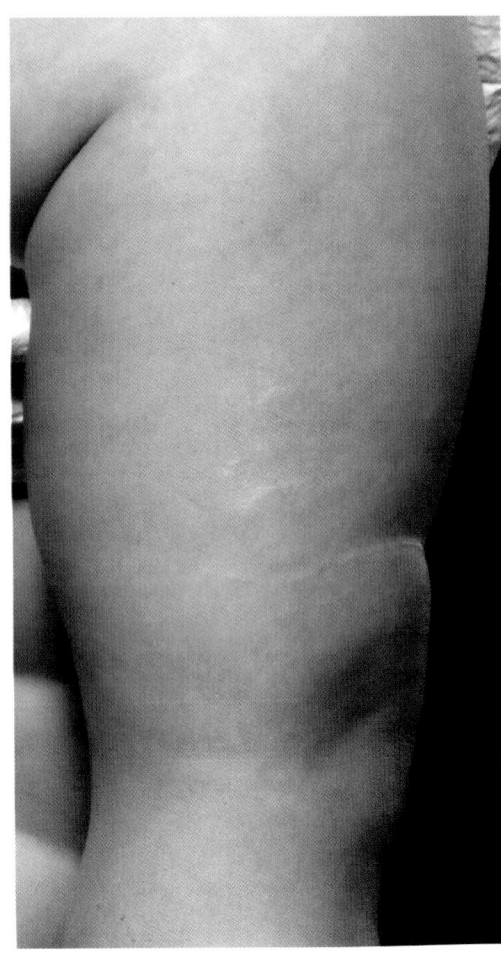

Figure 96.43 Constricting band across the thigh of a 6-month-old infant.

ainhum aged around 30–50 years, although the onset of the condition is probably in childhood [3–5].

Sex
Both sexes are affected.

Ethnicity
Ainhum has been reported chiefly in black Africans and African Americans.

Associated diseases
Constricting bands are often associated with other congenital abnormalities [6].

Pathophysiology
Extrinsic and intrinsic factors are probably equally important. Disruption of the development of the germinal disc in the embryo may predispose to fibrotic bands and associated congenital abnormalities. Rupture of the amnion may result in loss of amniotic fluid and extrusion of all or part of the fetus into the chorionic cavity, with resultant trapping of limbs [6,7]. In adults with ainhum, vascular damage appears to be important, resulting in hypoxia. In some patients, arteriography has shown that the posterior tibial artery is attenuated at the ankle, and the plantar arch and its branches are absent [3].

Predisposing factors
Vascular damage secondary to smoking or diabetes may exacerbate ainhum in adults [3].

Pathology
Fibrosis may be associated with distal degenerative change and osteoporosis, particularly in ainhum.

Causative organisms
Tropical infections have been implicated in ainhum, but are probably coincidental [3,4].

Genetics
Most cases are sporadic, although familial cases of ainhum have been reported.

Environmental factors
Rupture of the amniotic membrane is likely to be an important factor in congenital constrictions. Mechanical factors, including trauma from walking barefoot, may precipitate the development of a groove in the ischaemic toe in ainhum.

Clinical features
Fibrous bands may be solitary or multiple, encasing the limb (usually the leg or foot).

Clinical variants
Ainhum represents the extreme form of the condition, resulting in spontaneous amputation of the digit.

Painful fissuring and hyperkeratosis on the medial aspect of the digit is followed by fibrosis, distal degeneration and osteoporosis. There may be secondary infection and osteomyelitis. The toe becomes dorsiflexed at the metatarso-phalangeal joint, and gradually becomes clawed. Rest pain, coolness and cyanosis of the digit distal to the groove suggest that ischaemia is present. Once the constricting band has encircled the toe, the condition tends to progress rapidly. The toe becomes globular, hangs by a thread of fibrous tissue and is eventually shed (Figure 96.44). Control of secondary infection and protection from trauma may prevent extension of the scarring process. If symptoms are severe, or the dangling digit is a disability, amputation is indicated.

Differential diagnosis

Pseudo-ainhum

Congenital. Congenital pseudo-ainhum may involve a digit, a limb or even the trunk, and it ranges in severity from a superficial groove to amputation *in utero* [6,8,–10]. The cause is unknown, but familial cases have been reported. Some cases of pseudo-ainhum may be due to amniotic bands [11] or adhesions *in utero*, which may arise as a result of tearing of the amnion some time after the 45th day of pregnancy [12]. Cases have occurred in Ehlers–Danlos syndrome and after amniocentesis [12,13]. Several cases are reported where raised limb bands develop in the postnatal period, not always associated with amniotic tears; other possible causes include an early teratogenic insult [1,14].

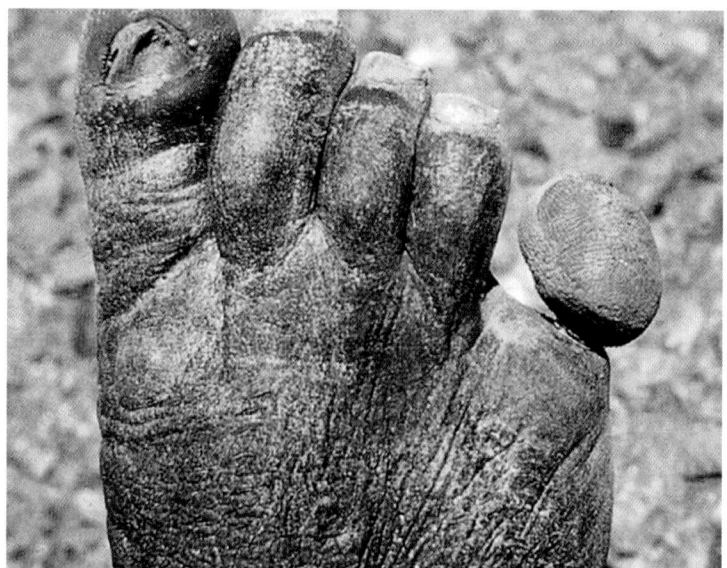

Figure 96.44 Ainhum, just before shedding of the fifth digit. (Courtesy of Dr D. Burley, Princess Margaret Hospital, Swindon, UK.)

Histology of the affected digit or limb reveals broad, finger-like projections of collagen, and coarse elastic bundles that penetrate deep into the subcutaneous fat [10].

Congenital pseudo-ainhum must be distinguished from the following: *aplasia* of the limbs with rudimentary digits; *acromelia* (in which part of the limb does not develop); and *hypoplasia* (in which the parts, although formed, are poorly developed).

Acquired. Pseudo-ainhum may be acquired as a result of infection (particularly leprosy), trauma, cold injury, neuropathy (especially congenital sensory neuropathy), systemic sclerosis, etc. [15], chronic psoriasis [16] and it may occur in association with other hereditary diseases such as palmoplantar keratoderma, particularly Vohwinkel keratoderma (see Figure 65.57b) pachyonychia congenita, erythropoietic protoporphyria [17,18] and Olmsted syndrome (see Chapter 65). Factitial pseudo-ainhum has also been reported due to the self-application of a rubber tourniquet.

Multiple skin creases resembling constrictions may be seen in the Michelin tyre baby syndrome and in 'multiple benign annular creases of the extremity'.

Classification of severity
See Patterson severity grading earlier.

Complications and co-morbidities
Constricting bands may be associated with other congenital defects. In types II–IV, limb mutilation may be caused by fibrotic adhesions [6].

Ainhum results in spontaneous amputation of the digit.

Disease course and prognosis
Some children's constricting bands may involute spontaneously without functional deficit. Most will require surgery to prevent limb deformity or amputation.

Management
Surgical treatments include staged Z-plasty [19]. Good results have been obtained from two-stage sine plasty with removal of the fascial groove and fasciotomy, treating half the limb initially and the other half a week later [20].

ABNORMAL FIBROTIC RESPONSES TO SKIN INJURY

Keloids and hypertrophic scars

Synonyms and inclusions
• Cheloid

Introduction and general description
Keloids and hypertrophic scars represent an excessive connective tissue response to injury, which may be trivial. A keloid is a benign well-demarcated overgrowth of fibrotic tissue which extends beyond the original boundaries of a defect (Figure 96.45a). A hypertrophic scar is similar, but remains confined to the original defect and tends to resolve after several months (Figure 96.45b). Both conditions may represent different stages of the same disorder [1].

Keloids and hypertrophic scars are cosmetically distressing (Figure 96.46), and often painful or pruritic. They appear to be unique to humans, and the lack of an animal model has hampered studies into their pathogenesis. A scar at any site has the potential to become keloidal or hypertrophic, although the earlobes (especially after ear piercing) (Figure 96.47), chin, neck, shoulders, upper trunk and lower legs are especially vulnerable. Burns, scars or tissue infection predispose to hypertrophic scarring. Lesions may follow trivial trauma or inflammatory conditions such as acne. Even chemical trauma, from irritant herbal remedies, can trigger keloid formation. Sometimes keloids appear to develop spontaneously, particularly on the upper chest.

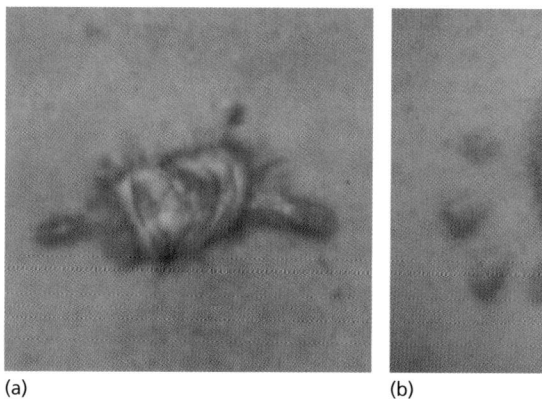

(a)   (b)

Figure 96.45 (a,b) Contrast between two scars from the presternal area: (a) spontaneous keloid, and (b) hypertrophic scar following excision of benign mole; the former shows partial involution after injection of triamcinolone.

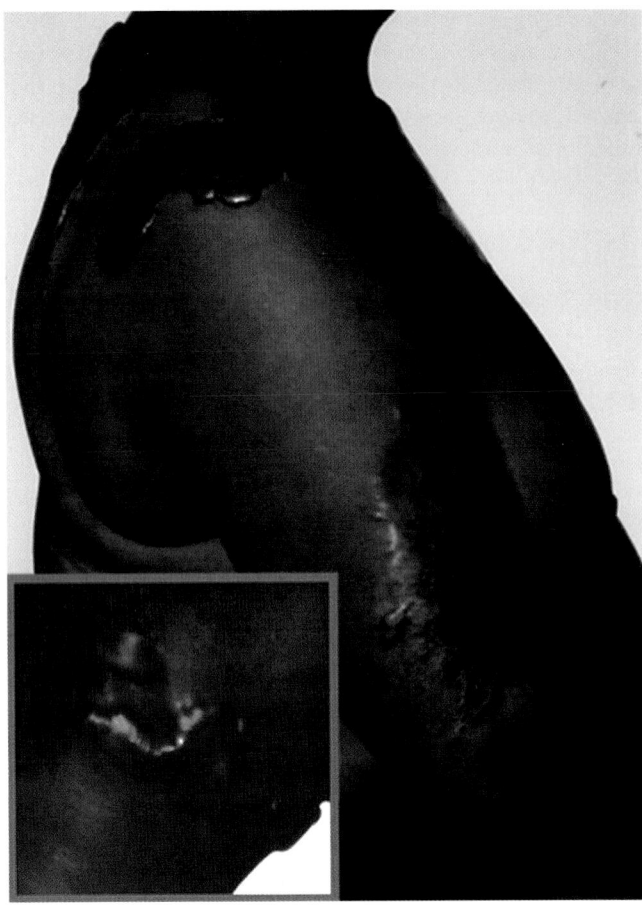

Figure 96.46 Extensive disfiguring keloids affecting an Afro-Caribbean woman.

Introduction of foreign material, either exogenous, such as suture material, or endogenous, such as embedded hairs, is another risk factor. Some African tribes introduce foreign bodies into tribal marks to induce scar hypertrophy. Scarring acne, particularly on the trunk, may become keloid-like (Figure 96.48).

Isotretinoin has been reported to delay wound healing and induce keloids in patients who received argon laser or dermabrasion for acne or rosacea [2], although there is debate as to whether the association is real [3].

Epidemiology

Incidence and prevalence

Keloids or hypertrophic scars occur in 4.5–16.0% of people of African or Hispanic descent [4]. A survey of Taiwanese children reported a prevalence of keloids of 0.3–0.6% [5]. A positive family history is obtained in 5–10% of Europeans with keloids, particularly severe lesions. Family studies suggest an autosomal dominant inheritance with incomplete penetrance [6]. Keloids have been reported in identical twins [7].

Age

Keloids are rare in infancy and old age, occurring chiefly between puberty and age 30 years.

Sex

Women have a greater predisposition in some ethnic groups; keloids may appear or enlarge during pregnancy [8].

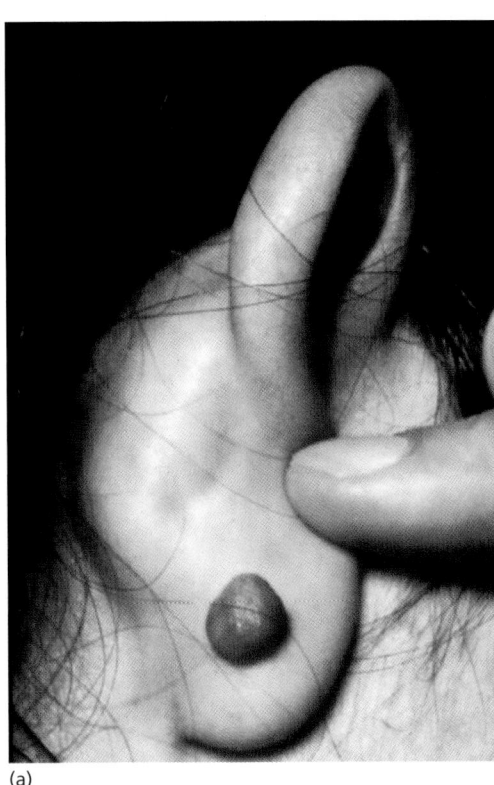

(a)

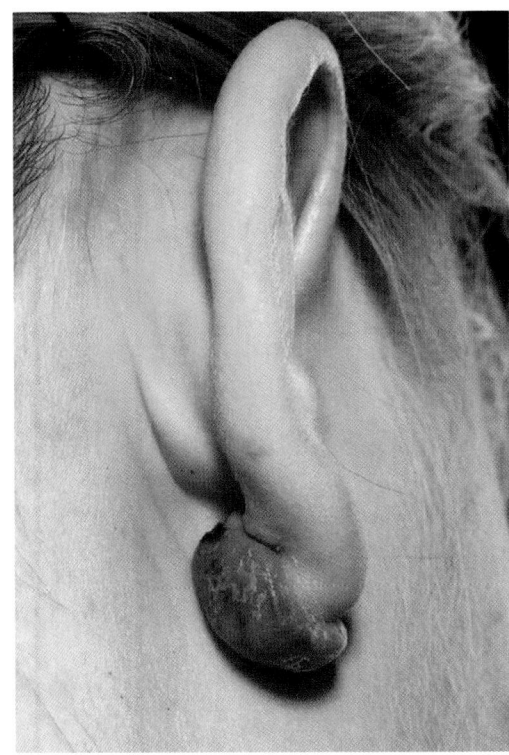

(b)

Figure 96.47 (a,b) Earlobe keloid.

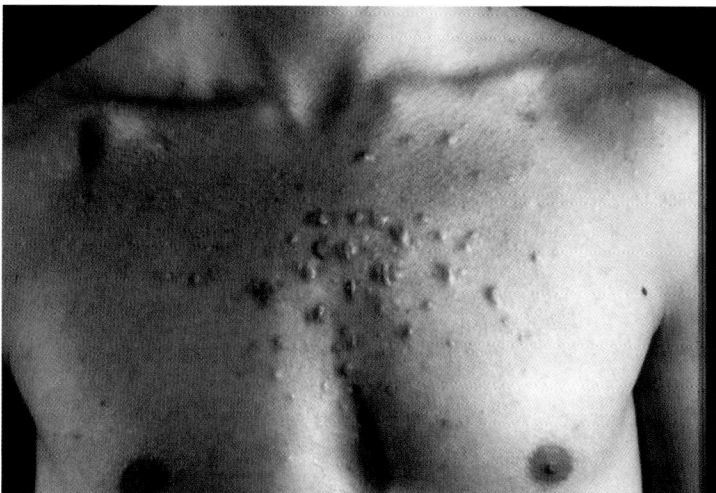

Figure 96.48 Keloid nodules secondary to acne.

Ethnicity

Individuals of African, Hispanic or Asian descent are more prone to keloids (see Figure 96.46) [4].

Associated diseases

Keloids are associated with other fibromatoses such as palmar fibromatosis (Dupuytren contracture) [9], together with genetic disorders such as Ehlers–Danlos syndrome, pachydermoperiostosis [10], Rubinstein–Taybi syndrome [11] and Dubowitz syndrome [12].

Linear keloids occur in athletes abusing anabolic steroids [13]. They form readily in individuals with acromegaly and following thyroidectomy in young patients. Recently, it has been postulated that systemic hypertension may promote the development of keloids [14].

Pathophysiology

Biochemical studies confirm that synthesis of type I and type III collagen is increased in both keloids and hypertrophic scars [15]. Keloids differ from healthy skin in that there is greatly increased dermal cellularity, the ratio of type I to type III collagen is increased and there is greater dermal expression of several extracellular matrix proteins including fibronectin, versican, elastin and tenascin; conversely, there is decreased expression of fibrillin 1 and decorin [16,17]. Hypertrophic scar collagen possesses the reducible keto cross-link, dehydrohydroxylysinonorleucine, normally associated with embryonic skin and granulation tissue [18]. Periostin, in particular, may play an important role in pathogenesis: it is expressed by keloid fibroblasts in hypoxic conditions and, among other actions, stimulates collagen synthesis [19]. Altered expression of proteoglycans may affect the three-dimensional organization of collagen fibres [20]. Keloid fibroblasts, unlike those from hypertrophic scar tissue, are hyperresponsive to TGF-β, which is abundant in healing wounds [21], and to PDGF [22]. They also express increased levels of heat shock protein (HSP) 47, another stimulus to collagen synthesis [23]. Neuropeptide-containing nerves are present [24] and the increased discomfort and itching which may be experienced in hypertrophic scars may be due to up-regulation of opioid receptors [25].

Pathology

Histology may resemble normal wound healing in the early stages, with increased cellularity. In a keloid of recent onset, endothelial proliferation is surrounded by increased numbers of fibroblasts, which form large, irregular nodules or whorls of hyalinized collagen. Later, the lesion matures into an acellular core, made up of thick, poorly vascularized bands of immature collagen [26] (Figure 96.49a,b). There may be focal deposition of mucinous material

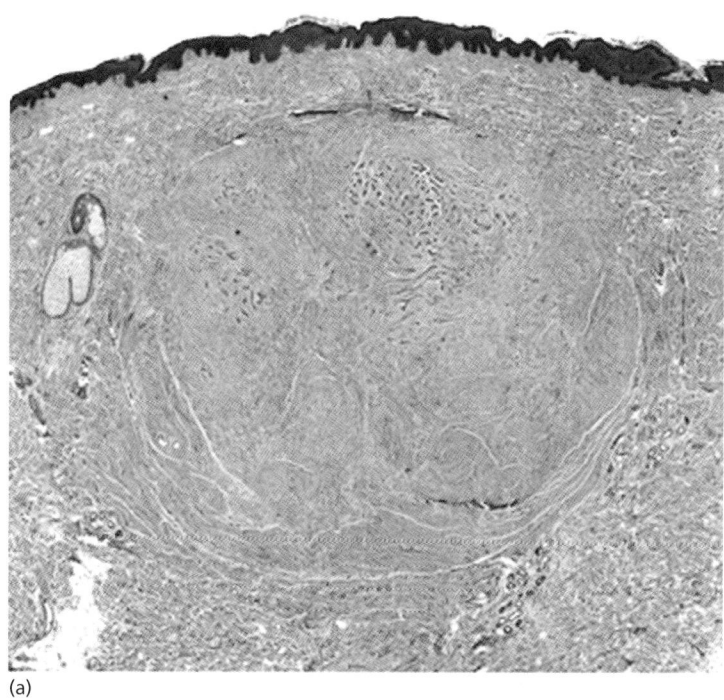

(a)

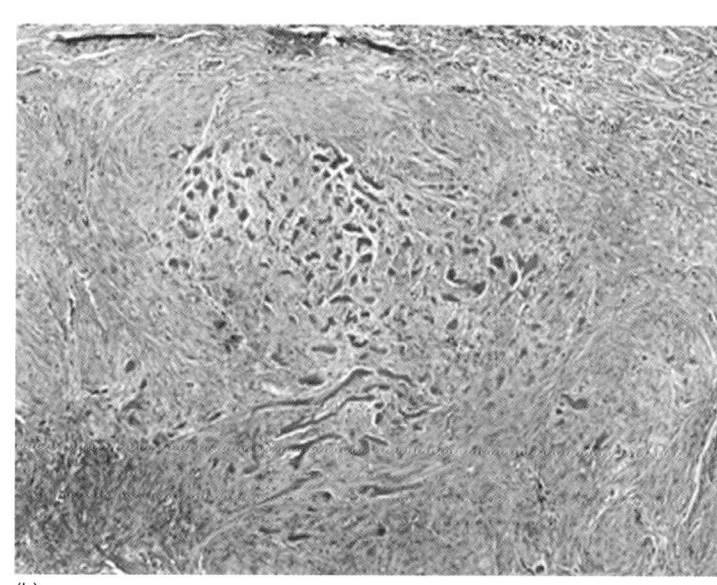

(b)

Figure 96.49 (a,b) Keloid nodule: large well-circumscribed dermal nodule sparing papillary dermis (a); higher-power view with haphazardly arranged thick sclerotic collagen surrounded by whorls of fibroblasts (b). (Courtesy of Professor Luis Requena, Universidad Autónoma de Madrid, Spain.)

in keloids, but not in hypertrophic scars. Mast cell numbers are increased in hypertrophic scars [27]. The epidermis is normal or thinned by the underlying lesion in keloids, but may be thickened in hypertrophic scars [28]. The fibroblasts have a stellate morphology on transmission electron microscopy [28,29]. Scanning electron microscopy reveals a more haphazard organization of collagen bundles than in normal skin or mature scars, with collagen fibrils about half the diameter of those of normal skin.

Genetics
The genetic basis is unknown. Telomere shortening has been described in keloids, and attributed to oxidative stress [30].

Environmental factors
Local trauma, which may be trivial. Hypertrophic scars commonly follow deep burns. Tension on the scar, and the presence of foreign material are aggravating factors in keloids.

Clinical features

History
Hypertrophic scars and keloids typically become raised and thickened within 3–4 weeks of the provocative stimulus, although keloids may develop up to a year later. Lesions are often pruritic and hypersensitive, and sometimes exquisitely tender. They may continue to grow for months or years.

Presentation
Depending on skin colour, lesions may present as firm skin-coloured, pink or red plaques (Figure 96.50); hypertrophic scars remain within the boundaries of the initial wound (see Figure 96.45b), whereas keloids become smoother and rounder and extend outside the wound boundary (Figure 96.45a), often assuming a 'dumb-bell' configuration but sometimes becoming bizarre and irregular (see Figure 96.46).

Clinical variants
Keloids on the beard area sometimes undergo central suppurative necrosis.

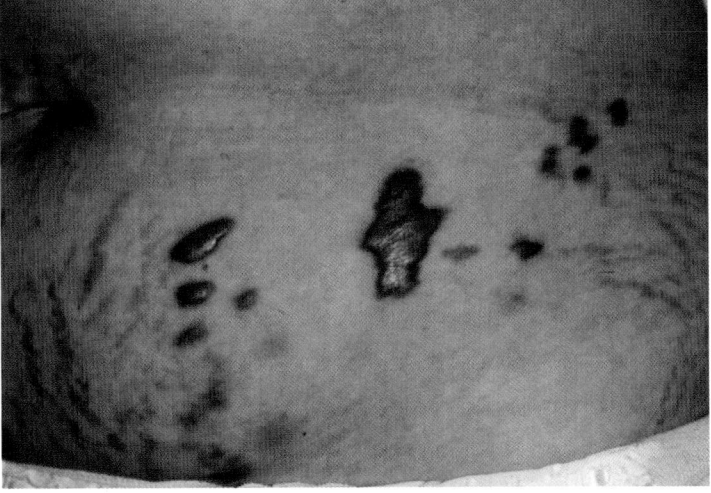

Figure 96.50 Fresh keloids arising in striae gravidarum 3 years after pregnancy.

Differential diagnosis
The diagnosis is usually straightforward if there is a history of trauma or an inflammatory skin lesion. Keloid scarring may follow surgical treatment of BCC, and a sclerotic BCC can mimic a keloid. Other differential diagnoses include fibrosarcoma, dermatofibrosarcoma protuberans, a malignancy developing in a scar or scar sarcoid. In endemic regions, blastomycosis and lobomycosis cause keloidal reactions.

Classification of severity
The Vancouver scar scale (VSS), recording pliability, height, vascularization and pigmentation, is used to quantify disease severity and response to treatment [31].

Complications and co-morbidities
Malignant degeneration is reported [32], although a fibrosarcoma can mimic a keloid clinically.

Disease course and prognosis
Hypertrophic scars typically regress spontaneously, although it may take a few years. Regression of keloids is a much slower process, and keloids can expand gradually over years.

Investigations
A diagnostic skin biopsy is mandatory if the diagnosis is in doubt.

Management
Non-essential surgery should be avoided in sites prone to keloids. Despite numerous small case series advocating a wide range of therapies, there is no level-one evidence for any single treatment [33]. Enthusiastic reports should be assessed critically as there may be racial variation in response to treatment and some studies include both keloids and hypertrophic scars. The follow-up period may be brief, and keloids have a high recurrence rate. Some modalities of treatment may exacerbate the condition. The optimal approach may involve a combination of different modalities of treatment.

First line
Intralesional corticosteroids (most commonly triamcinolone acetonide) inhibit fibroblast proliferation and collagen synthesis [34]. However, there is a risk of telangiectasia, atrophy and pigmentary change. Injections may need to be repeated monthly and recurrence rates can be up to 50% [35].

Second line
Self-adherent silicone gel sheeting may be effective for keloids and hypertrophic scars [36]; they may maintain skin hydration by occlusion but a meta-analysis of 13 trials showed only a weak preventative effect [37]. A cream made of 20% silicone oil applied under occlusion may be beneficial where it is impracticable to use silicone sheeting [38].

Third line
Other treatments include the following:
- Mechanical pressure with custom-made devices or garments can be beneficial, particularly on the earlobe [39] and bras or body corsets for truncal lesions.

- Surgical excision runs the risk of recurrence of an even bigger keloid. Intralesional (core) excision is preferable, and post-surgical intralesional steroids may prevent recurrence [40]. This topic is discussed in greater detail in Chapter 20.
- 5-fluorouracil (5-FU), a pyrimidine analogue, inhibits keloid growth *in vitro* and *in vivo*. Two double-blind studies have demonstrated that intralesional 5-FU is more effective than silicone gel sheeting [41] and intralesional corticosteroids [42] in the treatment of keloids.
- A small case series has demonstrated benefit from bleomycin, using a multiple puncture injection method [43]. A recent Brazilian study reports favourable results from a combination of bleomycin (0.375 IU) and triamcinolone 4 mg injected 3-monthly [44]. Topical mitomycin C may reduce the risk of recurrence after shave biopsy[45]. Similarly, topical imiquimod may reduce the risk of post-surgical recurrence [46].
- Photodynamic therapy has a cytotoxic effect on keloid fibroblasts. A small case series demonstrates reduced blood flow, increased pliability and decreased collagen levels with no recurrence after 9 months [47].
- In a recent randomized study, intralesional verapamil (2.5 mg/mL) gave comparable results to triamcinolone, and was well tolerated [48].
- Laser and light-based treatments have been reviewed recently [49]. Ablative (e.g. carbon dioxide) laser monotherapy carries a high recurrence rate. Pulsed dye and Nd : YAG lasers appear to be more effective, particularly in combination with intralesional corticosteroids or 5-FU. Low-level red and IR light-emitting diodes (LEDs) suppress fibroblast synthesis and achieve cosmetic improvement. Other physical therapies include degenerate wave electrical stimulation [50].
- Inhibitors of pro-inflammatory cytokines such as TGF-β analogues [51] and IFN-α [52] show promise, perhaps in conjunction with intralesional triamcinolone. Recent reviews suggest that a combination of surgery with adjuvant radiotherapy [53] or intralesional 5-FU or corticosteroids [54] is preferable to monotherapy.

PERFORATING DERMATOSES

Definition

Skin disorders in which material is eliminated from the dermis by extrusion through the epidermis to the skin surface by a process of transepidermal (transepithelial) elimination. The primary perforating disorders are particularly associated with diabetes and chronic renal failure in the case of acquired perforating dermatosis and heritable disorders of connective tissue or Down syndrome in the case of elastosis perforans serpiginosum.

Introduction and general description

There has been considerable confusion over the terminology used to describe the perforating disorders, with an array of different terms used to denote what is now thought to represent essentially the same underlying process: biopsies taken at different sites or times from the same patient may show a variety of different patterns depending on whether the lesion involves a follicle and whether it has been modified by excoriation. Perforation is a histopathological construct signifying that material, usually degenerate collagen or elastin, has breached or perforated an epithelium, usually the epidermis, in which case the process is usually referred to as transepidermal elimination (TEE).

The term perforating folliculitis continues to be used in the published literature as a disease entity, though several authorities have recommended that it should be abandoned [1,2]. The term acquired reactive perforating collagenosis fell out of favour some years ago to be replaced by acquired perforating dermatosis when it was demonstrated that both collagen and elastin were commonly involved [2]. Similarly, the distinction between acquired perforating dermatosis and Kyrle disease is not clear-cut [3] and separation of the two is no longer felt to be valid.

Many dermatoses occasionally exhibit the phenomenon of TEE, in which material from the dermis is extruded through the epidermis to the exterior with little or no disruption of the surrounding structures [4]. The extruded material may include inflammatory cells, red cells, microorganisms and extracellular substances, such as mucin or degenerate collagen and elastin [4–7]. In most of these conditions, the TEE is secondary to some underlying disease, such as granuloma annulare or PXE. There is also a rare hereditary disorder, familial reactive perforating collagenosis, which is characterized by TEE of collagen from an early age (see Chapter 72). The primary acquired perforating skin disorders which will be discussed here are therefore limited to acquired perforating dermatosis, which is strongly linked in the majority but not all cases to either diabetes, renal failure or both, and elastosis perforans serpiginosa, which is linked to heritable disorders of connective tissue and Down syndrome.

Acquired perforating dermatosis

Definition and nomenclature
An acquired disorder of transepidermal elimination of degenerate collagen, elastin and other connective tissue components. It is strongly associated with diabetes and chronic kidney disease.

Synonyms and inclusions
- Acquired reactive perforating dermatosis
- Acquired perforating collagenosis

Introduction and general description
Acquired perforating dermatosis is strongly linked with long-standing diabetes (Figure 96.51) and chronic kidney disease, often in association with haemodialysis [1,2,3,4,5,6,7,8]. It is characterized by TEE of both collagen and elastin and presents as a chronic pruritic dermatosis with multiple keratotic crusted papules and nodules.

PART 8: SPECIFIC
CUTANEOUS STRUCTURE

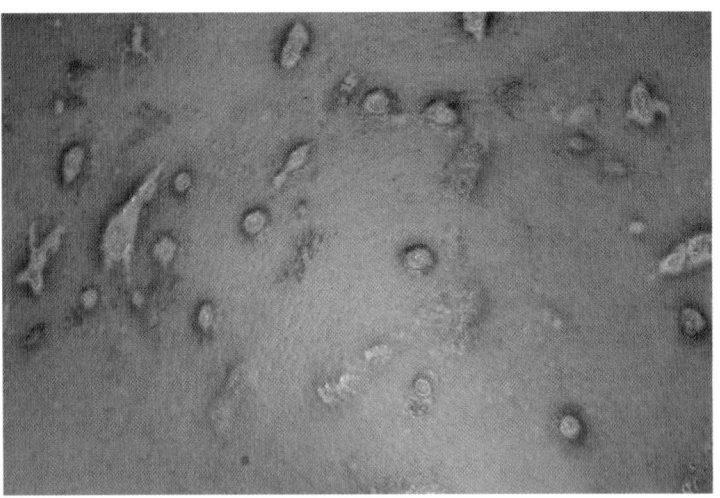

Figure 96.51 Acquired perforating dermatosis: close-up view of the back of a 65-year-old woman with longstanding diabetes.

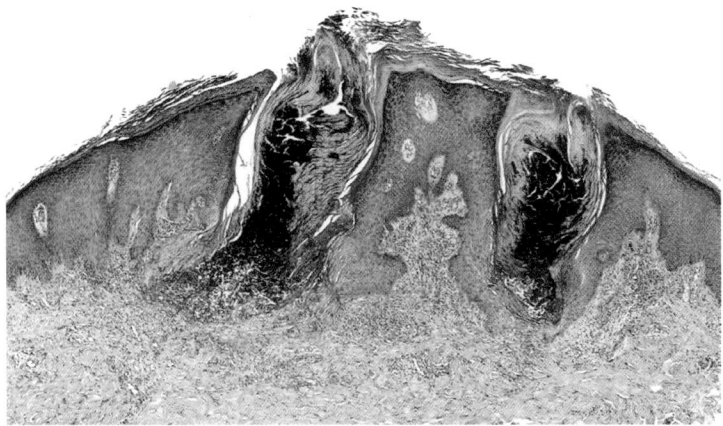

Figure 96.52 Acquired perforating dermatosis: invaginations of the epidermis enable columns of necrotic inflammatory debris to be extruded from the dermis. (Courtesy of Professor Luis Requena, Universidad Autónoma de Madrid, Spain.)

Epidemiology

Incidence and prevalence
Relatively frequent in the commonly affected population with reported rates of 4–11% of patients on haemodialysis [7,8].

Age
Generally occurs in the fifth to sixth decades of life.

Sex
Female to male ratio is 3 : 1 [9,10].

Ethnicity
All races affected.

Associated diseases
Strong association with chronic kidney disease and diabetes. Case reports of association with dermatomyositis [11] and drugs such as natalizumab [12].

Pathophysiology
The bulk of the coarse granular basophilic material which is extruded by TEE appears to derive from the nuclei of polymorphonuclear leukocytes [13]. It has been suggested that lysosomal enzymes derived from leukocytes might be responsible for the altered staining of collagen fibres, the degradation of elastic fibres and the impairment of keratinocyte adhesion, which allows TEE of dermal components [3].

Most patients have chronic renal disease and/or longstanding diabetes.

Pathology
Histology reveals cup-shaped invagination of the epidermis, which is plugged with necrotic inflammatory debris. Collagen bundles are arranged vertically at the base of the lesion and there is transepidermal elimination of collagen fibres (Figure 96.52) [14].

Causative organisms
Generally none, although there is one reported case associated with disseminated histoplasmosis [15].

Genetics
No known genetic factors.

Environmental factors

Clinical features

History
Pruritus, which may be intractable, is a common symptom.

Presentation
Keratotic dome-shaped papules with central crusts develop anywhere on the body but primarily on extensor aspects of the limbs and trunk (Figure 96.53). Dermoscopy with polarized light reveals bright white patches on a featureless grey background, surrounded by reticulate brown lines [1].

Clinical variants

Familial reactive perforating collagenosis [2,9,13,16,**17**,18] is a rare inherited form of TEE in which collagen is extruded through the epidermis. It is usually precipitated by environmental cold or trauma. The basic defect seems to be a type of focal damage to collagen, which is then extruded as a result of necrolysis of the overlying epidermis [19].

The lesion originates in the papillary dermis, where collagen is surrounded and engulfed by focal epidermal proliferation. The collagen appears normal on electron microscopy, but gives an abnormal staining pattern with trichrome and phosphotungstic acid haematoxylin. The central crater which develops contains inflammatory cells and keratinous debris. Elastic tissue is typically absent, and the abnormal collagen is eliminated by transepithelial migration [19,**20**,**21**].

It usually starts in early childhood as small papules on the extensor surface of the hands, the elbows and the knees following

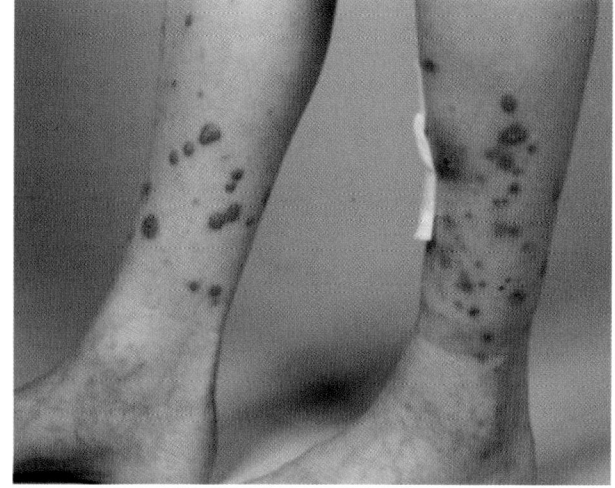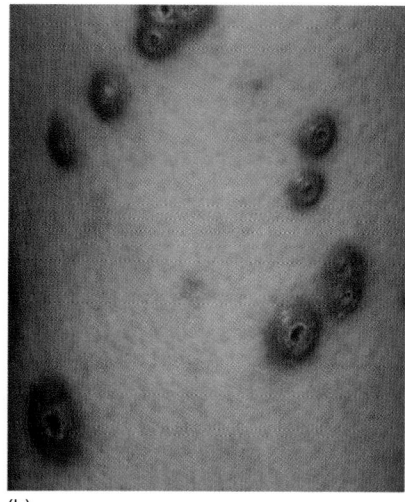

Figure 96.53 (a,b) Acquired perforating dermatosis: a 48-year-old woman with a 25-year history of type 1 diabetes with retinopathy and renal failure; and a 12-year history of skin ulceration with multiple tender crusted sores which were slow to heal.

(a) (b)

superficial trauma. Each skin-coloured papule increases to a size of about 6 mm over 3–5 weeks and then becomes umbilicated, with a keratinous plug [19]. The lesions regress spontaneously in 6–8 weeks to leave a hypopigmented area or slight scar, but new lesions may appear. Lesions can be produced experimentally, and the Koebner phenomenon may result in linear lesions [22]. The papules can also be provoked by inflamed acne lesions, but deep incisions do not produce the lesions. The condition persists into adult life. In some cases, the disease is associated with intolerance to cold and improves in warm weather.

The nosological relationship between familial reactive perforating collagenosis and the acquired reactive perforating dermatosis of chronic kidney disease remains uncertain [23].

Verrucous perforating collagenoma [24,25,26] (synonym collagénome perforant verruciforme). This rarely reported condition appears to be a reaction to the traumatic introduction of foreign materials including fibreglass, vegetable matter, calcium chloride and irritant drugs into the skin. Damaged collagen extruded to the surface by TEE, is manifest as verrucous papules.

Perforating disease due to exogenous agents. Occasionally, a chemical which has been applied to the skin topically or by intradermal injection can be eliminated by the transepidermal route. Eight cases have been reported following occupational exposure to a caustic drilling fluid used in the petrochemical industry [27]. Each patient noted skin irritation following exposure to the fluid and 1 or 2 days later developed tender papules with central umbilication followed by ulceration and crusting. Histological examination demonstrated TEE of altered collagen and debris which stained for calcium.

It is possible that the lesions were due to follicular penetration by the calcium present in the drilling mud. The drilling fluids contain many additives, but calcium carbonate or calcium chloride are often present in high concentrations in the mud. Similar cases have been reported following the use of calcium-containing electroencephalography paste [28].

TEE of altered collagen has also been reported following the use of intradermal steroid injections [29,30].

Differential diagnosis
The condition may be mistaken clinically for molluscum contagiosum, papular urticaria or other perforating disorders, but the histology is characteristic [**14**,18].

Management
Some patients improve spontaneously, particularly if renal function can be improved [7,**10**]. No treatment is of proven benefit, although there are several reports of the use of allopurinol [31,32].

Topical retinoids may reduce the number of lesions. Other treatments which may help include oral isotretinoin, methotrexate, rifampicin, emollient creams, intralesional steroids and topical steroids under occlusion [5,**9**,23]. Narrow-band UVB [33], PUVA [34] and photodynamic therapy [35] have all been used. Associated uraemic pruritus may improve with amitriptyline [36]. Complete remission has been reported after the use of topical tacalcitol [37], however spontaneous resolution can occur.

Elastosis perforans serpiginosa

Definition and nomenclature
A perforating dermatosis in which the material extruded through the epidermis is derived from elastic fibres in the upper dermis [1]. It is closely associated with heritable disorders of connective tissue and Down syndrome.

Synonyms and inclusions
- Perforating elastoma
- Elastoma intrapapillare perforans

Epidemiology

Incidence and prevalence
Rare.

Age
Usually presents between the ages of 5 and 20 years.

Sex
Males are predominantly affected.

Ethnicity
All races affected.

Associated diseases
Some 40% of reported cases have been associated with heritable connective tissue disorders, such as PXE, Ehlers–Danlos syndrome, Marfan syndrome, OI and acrogeria [2,3]. It has also been reported in otherwise healthy individuals and in association with Down syndrome [4–7].

It sometimes occurs in patients receiving penicillamine, which is known to cause the production of abnormal elastin [8–12], and there is an overlap with 'pseudo-PXE' (see earlier).

Pathophysiology

Predisposing factors
The altered elastin resembles that seen in experimental animals subjected to lathyrogens or copper deficiency.

It is probable that the primary abnormality is in the dermal elastin, which provokes a cellular response that ultimately leads to extrusion of the abnormal elastic tissue. It may be significant that the lesions are commonly seen in areas subjected to wear and tear.

Pathology
The earliest detectable change is the focal development of elastotic-staining tissue and basophilic debris in the dermis. This is followed by a reaction of the overlying epidermis, which grows down to engulf the elastotic material. The epidermis surrounding the fully developed lesion is acanthotic and hyperkeratotic (Figure 96.54). The papule consists of a circumscribed area of epidermal hyperplasia traversed by a channel communicating directly with the dermis and containing a mass of tissue, which projects above the surface. This plug consists of horny material in its upper third and of amorphous debris derived from elastin in its lower two-thirds [4,13–16]. In the dermis beneath and around the lesion, there is a foreign-body giant cell reaction. The elastotic material is finally extruded, to leave irregular scarring and warty thickening. Electron microscopy shows an increase in elastic fibres, with fine filaments on the surface similar to those seen in normal embryos. In penicillamine-induced cases the elastic fibres have a characteristic 'bramble bush' or 'lumpy-bumpy' morphology [10,17]. The hydroxylation of dermal collagen is similar to that of newborn skin [14].

Causative organisms
No specific organism identified.

Genetics
The cause is unknown, but a genetically determined defect of elastic tissue may be involved [1]. Often associated with a known heritable disorder of connective tissue.

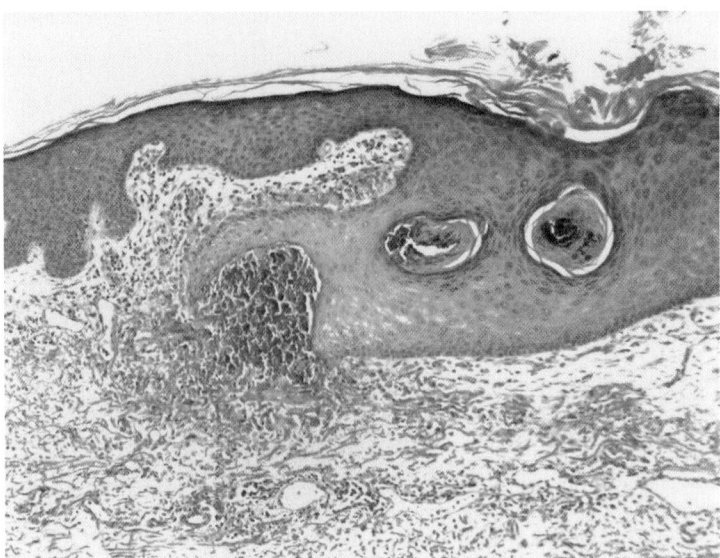

Figure 96.54 Elastosis perforans serpiginosa: note acanthotic epidermis growing downward in order to surround and engulf a focus of basophilic elastotic debris. (Courtesy of Dr Leigh Biddlestone, Royal United Hospitals, Bath UK.)

Environmental factors
The lesions may follow minor trauma such as an abrasion.

Clinical features

History
Lesions are generally asymptomatic.

Presentation
Small, horny or umbilicated papules are characteristically arranged in lines, circles or segments of circles in a serpiginous pattern (Figure 96.55). The individual papules may remain small or may enlarge slightly to assume a crateriform appearance with

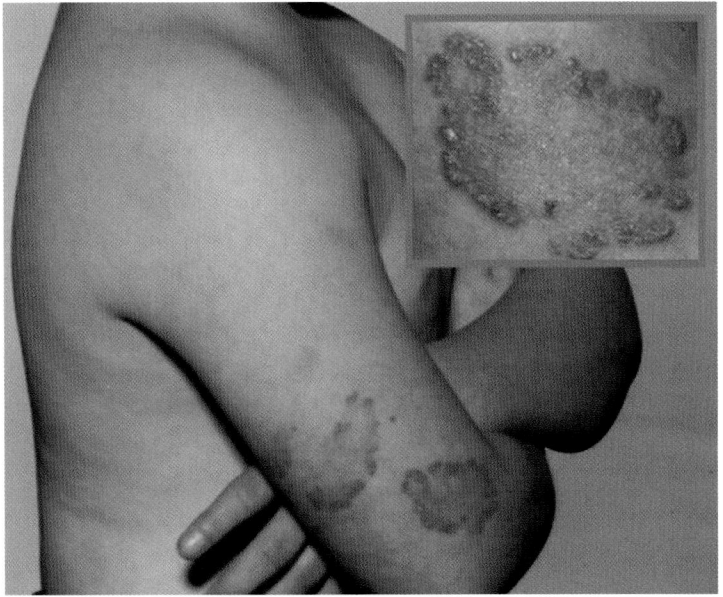

Figure 96.55 Elastosis perforans serpiginosa in a boy with Down syndrome.

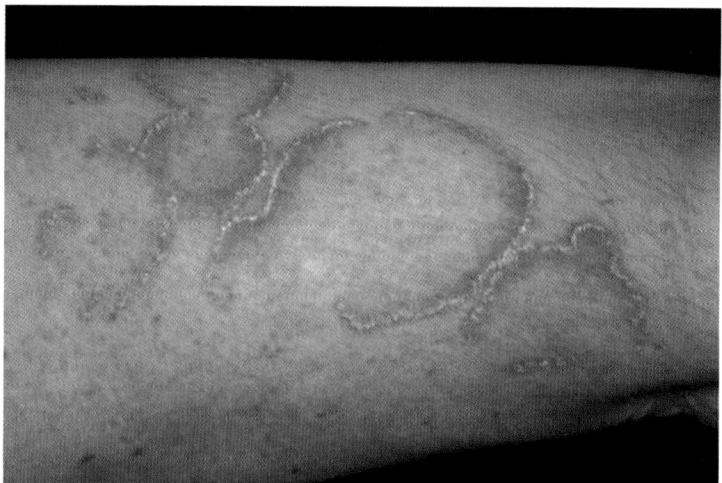

Figure 96.56 Elastosis perforans serpiginosa in a patient with vascular Ehlers–Danlos syndrome.

an elevated edge and a central plug, or further to leave an area of atrophic skin surrounded by smaller papules, each with a horny plug. The rings may reach a diameter of 15–20 cm but are usually smaller (Figure 96.56). The back and sides of the neck are most commonly affected, but the lesions may also occur on the cheeks or on the arms or thighs, and are sometimes bilaterally symmetrical [1,16,**18**,19].

Differential diagnosis
The annular or linear arrangements of the papules and their distribution suggest the diagnosis, which is confirmed by the characteristic histology. Conditions which may cause confusion include porokeratosis of Mibelli, familial reactive perforating collagenosis and perforating granuloma annulare.

A similar histological appearance can occur in acquired perforating dermatosis (see earlier) [20].

Classification of severity
Not of prognostic significance in its own right, but may reflect an underlying heritable disorder of connective tissue.

Complications and co-morbidities
Associated connective tissue disease.

Disease course and prognosis
They may persist for several years, but eventually involute spontaneously to leave reticulate atrophic scars.

Investigations
Skin biopsy is diagnostic, but biopsy scars readily become keloidal.

Management
The condition tends to be self-limiting, and no treatment is of proven benefit [**18**]. However, careful removal of the nodules with a curette under local anaesthesia may give a reasonable cosmetic result. Freezing has been recommended [**18**,21,22]. Excision should be avoided, and dermabrasion may make the condition worse [4]. In a child with Down syndrome and associated vitamin A deficiency, clinical improvement was observed with oral retinoid therapy, even though the treatment produced side effects [6]. Isotretinoin has been used successfully in a patient with penicillamine-induced disease [23]. There are reports of improvement following Sellotape® stripping of the surface keratinous material [24], tazarotene [25], imiquimod [26] and calcipotriol [27]. Treatment with the pulsed dye [28], ultrapulsed carbon dioxide [29,30] and Er : YAG [31] lasers have also been advocated [2].

Treatment ladder

First line
- Conservatism

Second line
- Trial of cryotherapy initially to test site

Third line
- Curettage

Key references

The full list of references can be found in the online version at www.rooksdermatology.com

Changes in dermal connective tissue due to ageing and photodamage

Wrinkles
1 Smith JB, Fenske NA. Cutaneous manifestations and consequences of smoking. *J Am Acad Dermatol* 1996;34:717–32.
2 Kligman AM, Zheng P, Lavker RM. The anatomy and pathogenesis of wrinkles. *Br J Dermatol* 1985;113:37–42.
3 Tsuji T, Yorifuji T, Hamarta T, *et al.* Light and scanning electron microscopic studies on wrinkles in aged person's skin. *Br J Dermatol* 1986;114:329–35.

Actinic elastosis
1 Kligman AM. Early destructive effects of sunlight on human skin. *J Am Acad Dermatol* 1969;210:2377–80.
3 Braverman IM, Fonferko E. Studies in cutaneous aging. II. The microvasculature. *J Invest Dermatol* 1982;78:444–8.

Collagenous and elastotic marginal plaques of the hands
1 Burks JW, Wise LJ, Clark WH. Degenerative collagenous plaques of the hands. *Arch Dermatol* 1960;82:362–6.
2 Jordaan HF, Rossouw DJ. Digital papular calcific elastosis: a histopathological, histochemical and ultrastructural study of 20 patients. *J Cutan Pathol* 1990;17:358–70.
3 Menegesha YM, Kayal JD, Swerlick RA. Keratoelastoidosis marginalis. *J Cutan Med Surg* 2002;6:23–5.

Adult colloid milium and colloid degeneration of the skin
1 Mehregan D, Hooten J. Adult colloid milium: a case report and literature review. *Int J Dermatol* 2011;50:1531–4.
2 Innocenzi D, Barduagni F, Cerio R, Wolter M. UV-induced colloid milium. *Clin Exp Dermatol* 1993;18:347–50.
3 Dummer R, Laetsch B, Stutz S, *et al.* Elastosis colloidalis conglomerata (adult colloid milium, paracolloid of the skin) a maximal manifestation of actinic elastosis. *Eur J Dermatol* 2006;16:163–6.
7 Hashimoto K, Miller F, Bereston ES. Colloid milium: histochemical and electron microscopic studies. *Arch Dermatol* 1972;105:684–94.

12 Netscher DT, Sharma S, Kinner BM, Lyos A, Griego RD. Adult-type colloid milium of hands and face successfully treated with dermabrasion. *South Med J* 1996;89:1004–7.

13 Ammirati CT, Giancola JM, Hruza GJ. Adult-onset facial colloid milium successfully treated with the long-pulsed Er:YAG laser. *Dermatol Surg* 2002;28:215–19.

Other causes of cutaneous atrophy

Atrophy due to corticosteroids

1 Henqqe VR, Ruzicka T, Schwartz RA, *et al.* Adverse effects of topical corticosteroids. *J Am Acad Dermatol* 2006;54:1–15.

2 Turpeinen M, Raitio H, Pelkonen AS, *et al.* Skin thickness in children treated with daily or periodical inhaled budesonide for mild persistent asthma. The Helsinki early intervention childhood asthma study. *Pediatr Res* 2010;67:221–5.

4 Averbeck M, Gebhardt C Anderegg U, *et al.* Suppression of hyaluran synthase 2 expression reflects the atrophogenic potential of glucocorticoids. *Exp Dermatol* 2010;19:757–9.

6 Autio P, Oikarinen A, Melkko J, *et al.* Systemic glucocorticoids decrease the synthesis of type I and type III collagen in human skin in vivo, whereas isotretinoin has little effect. *Br J Dermatol* 1994;131:660–3.

13 Barnes L, Kaya G, Rollason V. Topical corticosteroid-induced skin atrophy: a comprehensive review. *Drug Saf* 2015;38:493–509.

20 McMichael AJ, Griffiths CEM, Talwar HS, *et al.* Concurrent application of tretinoin (retinoic acid) partially protects against corticosteroid-induced epidermal atrophy. *Br J Dermatol* 1996;135:60–4.

Striae

2 Shuster S. The cause of striae distensae. *Acta Derm Venereol Suppl (Stockh)* 1979;59(85):161–9.

4 Carr RD, Hamilton JF. Transverse striae of the back. *Arch Dermatol* 1969;99:26–30.

9 Zheng P, Lavker RM, Kligman AM. Anatomy of striae. *Br J Dermatol* 1985;112:185–93.

14 Tung JY, Kiefer AK, Mullins M, *et al.* Genome-wide association analysis implicates elastin microfibrils in the development of nonsyndromic striae distensae. *J Invest Dermatol* 2013;133:2628–31.

16 Chernovsky ME, Knox JM. Atrophic striae after occlusive corticosteroid therapy. *Arch Dermatol* 1964;90:15–19.

19 Al-Himdani S, Ud-Din S, Gilmore S, *et al.* Striae distensae: a comprehensive revision and evidence-based evaluation of prophylaxis and treatment. *Br J Dermatol* 2014;170:527–47.

Acquired poikiloderma

1 Okazaki M, Kikuchi I. Radiodermatitis. An analysis of 43 cases. *J Dermatol* 1986;13:356–65.

2 Carroll CL, Lang W, Snively B, *et al.* Development and validation of the Dermatomyositis Skin Severity Index. *Br J Dermatol* 2008;158:345–350.

3 Bloom B, Marchbein S, Fischer M, *et al.* Poikilodermatous mycosis fungoides. *Dermatol Online* J 2012;18(12):4.

Atrophic scars

3 Colomb D. Stellate spontaneous pseudoscars. Senile and presenile forms: especially those forms caused by prolonged corticoid therapy. *Arch Dermatol* 1972;105:551–4.

7 Tlougan BE, Paller AS, Schaffer JV, *et al.* Congenital erosive and vesicular dermatosis with reticulated supple scarring: unifying clinical features. *J Am Acad Dermatol* 2013;69(6):909–15.

10 Marks VJ, Miller OF. Atrophia maculosa varioliformis cutis. *Br J Dermatol* 1986;115:105–9.

12 Paradisi M, Angelo C, Conti G, *et al.* Atrophia maculosa varioliformis cutis: a pediatric case. *Pediatr Dermatol* 2001;18:478–80.

Acrodermatitis chronica atrophicans

1 Steere AC. Lyme disease. *N Engl J Med* 1989;321:586–96.

2 Coulson IH. Acrodermatitis chronica atrophicans with coexisting.morphoea. *Br J Dermatol* 1989;121:263–9.

9 Müller KE. Damage of collagen and elastic fibres by *Borrelia burgdorferi*: known and new clinical and histological aspects. *Open Neurol* J 2012;6:179–86.

11 Grygorczuk S, Péter O, Kondrusik M, *et al.* Assessment of the different *Borrelia* burgdorferi sensu lato species in patients with Lyme borreliosis from north-east Poland by studying preferential serologic response and DNA isolates. *Ann Agric Environ Med* 2013;20:21–9.

12 Stinco G, Ruscio M, Bergamo S, *et al.* Clinical features of 705 *Borrelia burgdorferi* seropositive patients in an endemic area of northern Italy. *Sci World J* 2014;2014(1)414505.

13 Burgdorf WHC, Worret W, Schultka O. Acrodermatitis chronica atrophicans. *Int J Dermatol* 1979;18:595–601.

24 Stanek G, Strle F. Lyme borreliosis. *Lancet* 2003;362:1639–47.

Atrophodermas

1 Curth HO. The genetics of follicular atrophoderma. *Arch Dermatol* 1978;114:1479–83.

2 Hartman RD, Molho-Pessach V, Schafer JV. Conradi–Hünermann–Happle syndrome. *Dermatol Online* J 2010;16(11):4.

3 Viksnins P, Berlin A. Follicular atrophoderma and basal cell carcinoma. The Bazex syndrome. *Arch Dermatol* 1977;113:948–51.

4 Moulin G, Hill MP, Guillaud V, *et al.* Bandes pigmentées atrophiques acquises suivant les lignes de Blaschko. *Ann Dermatol Vénéréol* 1992;119:729–36.

5 de Golian E, Echols K, Pearl H, *et al.* Linear atrophoderma of Moulin: a distinct entity? Pediatr Dermatol 2014;31:373–7.

7 Villani AP, Amini-Adlé M, Wagschal D, *et al.* Linear atrophoderma of Moulin: report of 4 cases and 20th anniversary case review. *Dermatology* 2013;227:5–9.

11 Kee CE, Brothers WS, New W. Idiopathic atrophoderma of Pasini and Pierini with co-existent morphea. A case report. *Arch Dermatol* 1960;82:154–7.

12 Miller RF. Idiopathic atrophoderma, report of a case and nosologic study. *Arch Dermatol* 1965;92:653–60.

13 Beuchner SA, Rufli T. Atrophoderma of Pasini and Pierini. *J Am Acad Dermatol* 1994;30:441–6.

17 Berman A, Berman GD, Winkelmann RK. Atrophoderma (Pasini–Pierini) findings on direct immunofluorescent, monoclonal antibody and ultra-structural studies. *Int J Dermatol* 1988;27:487–90.

Paroxysmal haematoma of the finger

1 Achenbach W. Das paroxysmale Handhämatom. *Medizinische* 1958;52:2138–40.

3 Layton AM, Cotterill JA. A case of Achenbach's syndrome. *Clin Exp Dermatol* 1993;18:60–1.

8 Thies K, Beschorner U, Noory E, *et al.* Achenbach's syndrome revisited. *Vasa* 2012;41:366–70.

Panatrophy

3 Barnes S. Gower's case of local panatrophy. *Br J Dermatol* 1939;51:377–80.

4 Sakamoto T, Oku T, Takigawa M. Gowers' local panatrophy. *Eur J Dermatol* 1998;8:116–19.

Facial hemiatrophy

1 El-Kehdy J, Abbas O, Rubeiz N. A review of Parry–Romberg syndrome. *J Am Acad Dermatol* 2012;67:769–84.

Disorders of elastic fibre degradation

4 Lewis KG, Bercovitch L, Dill SW, *et al.* Acquired disorders of elastic tissue: Part 1. Increased elastic tissue and solar elastotic syndromes. *J Am Acad Dermatol* 2004;51:1–21.

5 Lewis KG, Bercovitch L, Dill SW, *et al.* Acquired disorders of elastic tissue: Part II. Decreased elastic tissue. *J Am Acad Dermatol* 2004;51:165–85.

Acquired cutis laxa

1 Nanko H, Jepson LV, Zachariae H, *et al.* Acquired cutis laxa (generalised elastolysis): light and electron microscopic studies. *Acta Derm Venereol Suppl (Stockh)* 1979;59:315–24.

2 Harpey J-P. Cutis laxa and low serum zinc after antenatal exposure to penicillamine. *Lancet* 1983;ii:858–9.

12 Fornieri C, Quaglino D, Lungarella G, *et al.* Elastin production and degradation in cutis laxa acquisita. *J Invest Dermatol* 1994;103:583–8.

18 Fontenelle E, de Almeida APM, de Almeida Souza GMA. Marshall's syndrome. *An Bras Dermatol* 2013;88:279–82.

Anetoderma

1 Venencie PY, Winkelmann RK. Histopathologic findings in anetoderma. *Arch Dermatol* 1984;120:1040–4.

2 Venencie PY, Winkelmann RK, Moore BA. Anetoderma: clinical findings, associations, and long term follow-up evaluations. *Arch Dermatol* 1984;120:1032–9.

5 Hodak E, David M. Primary anetoderma and antiphospholipid antibodies: review of the literature. *Clin Rev Allergy Immunol* 2007;32:162–9.

28 Venencie PY, Winkelmann RK, Moore BA. Ultrastructural findings in the skin lesions of patients with anetoderma. *Acta Derm Venereol Suppl* (Stockh) 1984;64:112–20.

30 Ghomrasseni S, Dridi M, Gogly B, *et al*. Anetoderma: an altered balance between metalloproteinases and tissue inhibitors of metalloproteinases. *Am J Dermatopathol* 2002;24:118–29.

Mid-dermal elastolysis, Upper dermal elastolysis

1 Brenner W, Schmint FG, Konrad K, *et al*. Non-inflammatory dermal elastolysis. *Br J Dermatol* 1978;99:335–8.

12 Dick GF. Elastolytic activity of *P. acnes and Staph. epidermidis* in acne and normal skin. *Acta Derm Venereol Suppl* (Stockh) 1976;56:279–82.

22 Rongioletti F, Izakovic J, Romanelli P, *et al*. Pseudoxanthoma elasticum-like papillary dermal, elastolysis: a large case series with clinicopathological correlation. *J Am Acad Dermatol* 2012;67:128–35.

Blepharochalasis, Ascher syndrome

4 Grasseger A, Romani N, Fritsch P, *et al*. Immunoglobulin A (IgA) deposits in lesional skin of a patient with blepharochalasis. *Br J Dermatol* 1996;135:791–5.

7 Harris WA, Dortzbach RK. Levator tuck. A simplified blepharoptosis procedure. *Ann Ophthalmol* 1975;7:873–8.

12 Ali K. Ascher syndrome: a case report and review of the literature. *Oral Surg Oral Med Oral Pathol Oral Radiol Endod* 2007;103:e26–8.

Actinic granuloma and annular elastolytic giant cell granuloma

1 Hanke CW, Bailin PL, Roenigk HH. Annular elastolytic giant cell granuloma: a clinicopathologic study of five cases and a review of similar entities. *J Am Acad Dermatol* 1979;1:413–21.

2 Gutiérrez-González E, Pereiro M, Toribio J. Elastolytic actinic giant cell granuloma. *Dermatol Clin* 2015;33:331–41.

3 Aso Y, Izaki S, Teraki Y. Annular elastolytic giant cell granuloma associated with diabetes mellitus: a case report and review of the Japanese literature. *Clin Exp Dermatol* 2011;36:917–19.

5 Wilson-Jones E. Necrobiosis lipoidica presenting on the face and scalp. *Trans St John's Hosp Dermatol Soc* 1971;57:203–20.

7 Ishibashi A, Yokoyama A, Hirano K. Annular elastolytic giant cell granuloma occurring in covered areas. *Dermatologica* 1987;174:293–7.

9 Pestoni C, Pereiro M, Toribio J. Annular elastolytic giant cell granuloma produced on an old burn scar and spreading after a mechanical trauma. *Acta Derm Venereol* 2003;83:312–13.

16 O'Brien JP. Actinic granuloma: an annular connective tissue disorder affecting sun and heat-damaged (elastotic) skin. *Arch Dermatol* 1975;111:460–70.

Granuloma multiforme

1 Kumari R, Thappa DM, Chougule A, Adityan B. Granuloma multiforme: a report from India. *Indian J Dermatol Venereol* 2009;75:296–9.

2 Leiker DL, Kok SH, Spaas JAJ. Granuloma multiforme: a new skin disease resembling leprosy. *Int J Lepr* 1964;32:368–76.

Acquired pseudoxanthoma elasticum-like syndromes

Perforating pseudoxanthoma elasticum

1 Premathala S, Yesudian P, Thambiah AS. Periumbilical pseudoxanthoma elasticum with transepithelial elimination. *Int J Dermatol* 1982;10:604–5.

2 Kazakis AM, Parish WR. Periumbilical perforating pseudoxanthoma elasticum. *J Am Acad Dermatol* 1988;19:384–8.

Acquired pseudoxanthoma elasticum

2 Na SY, Choi M, Kim MJ, Lee JH, Cho S. Penicillamine-induced elastosis perforans serpiginosa and cutis laxa in a patient with Wilson's disease. *Ann Dermatol* 2010;22:468–71.

3 Light N, Meyrick-Thomas RH, Stephens A, *et al*. Collagen and elastin changes in d-penicillamine-induced pseudoxanthoma elasticum-like skin. *Br J Dermatol* 1986;114:381–8.

Saltpetre disease

2 Neilson AO, Christensen OB, Hentzer B, *et al*. Saltpetre-induced dermal changes electron microscopically indistinguishable from pseudoxanthoma elasticum. *Acta Derm Venereol Suppl* (Stockh) 1978;58:323–7.

Acrokeratoelastoidosis

3 Rongioletti F, Betti R, Crosti C, Rebora A. Marginal papular acrokeratodermas: a unified nosography for focal acral hyperkeratosis, acrokeratoelastoidosis and related disorders. *Dermatology* 1994;188:28–31.

Acquired disorders of elastic tissue deposition

Linear focal elastosis

1 Burket JM, Zelickson AS, Padilla RS. Linear focal elastosis (elastotic striae). *J Am Acad Dermatol* 1989;20:633–6.

7 Jeong JS, Lee JY, Kim MK, *et al*. Linear focal elastosis following striae distensae: further evidence of keloidal repair process in the pathogenesis of linear focal elastosis. *Ann Dermatol* 2011;23(Suppl. 2):S141–3.

Late-onset focal dermal elastosis

1 Tajima S, Shimizu K, Izumi T, *et al*. Late-onset focal dermal elastosis: clinical and histological features. *Br J Dermatol* 1995;133:303–5.

Elastofibroma dorsi

1 Nagamine N, Nohara Y, Ito E. Elastofibroma in Okinawa: a clinicopathologic study of 170 cases. *Cancer* 1982;50:1794–805.

9 Karakurt O, Kaplan T, Gunal N, *et al*. Elastofibroma dorsi management and outcomes: review of 16 cases. *Interact Cardiovasc Thorac Surg* 2014;18:197–201.

Elastoderma

3 de Waal AC, Blocx WA, Seyger MM, *et al*. Elastoderma: an uncommon cause of acquired hyperextensible skin. *Acta Derm Venereol* 2012;92:328–9.

Papular elastorrhexis

7 Ryder HF, Antaya RJ. Nevus anelasticus, papular elastorrhexis and eruptive collagenoma: clinically similar entities with focal absence of elastic fibres in childhood. *Pediatr Dermatol* 2005;22:153–7.

Fibromatoses and other causes of diffuse fibrosis

Fibromatoses

Palmar fascial fibromatosis

3 Evans RA. The aetiology of Dupuytren's disease. *Br J Hosp Med* 1986;35:198–9.

13 Palmer KT, D'Angelo S, Syddall H, *et al*. Dupuytren's contracture and occupational exposure to hand-transmitted vibration. *Occup Environ Med* 2014;71:241–5.

21 Ulrich D, Hrynyschyn K, Pallua N. Matrix metalloproteinases and tissue inhibitors of metalloproteinases in sera and tissue of patients with Dupuytren's disease. *Plast Reconstr Surg* 2003;112:1279–86.

24 Becker K, Tinschert S, Lienert A, *et al*. The importance of genetic susceptibility in Dupuytren's disease. *Clin Genet* 2015;87:483–7.

25 Forrester HB, Temple-Smith B, Ham S, *et al*. Genome-wide analysis using exon arrays demonstrates an important role of expression of extracellular matrix, fibrotic control and tissue remodelling genes in Dupuytren's disease. *PLOS One* 2013;8(3):e59056.

26 Rodrigo JJ, Niebauer JJ, Brown RL, *et al*. Treatment of Dupuytren's contracture. Long-term result after fasciotomy and fascial excision. *J Bone Joint Surg Am* 1976;58:380–7.

28 Gelman S, Schlenker R, Bachoura A, *et al*. Minimally invasive partial fasciectomy for Dupuytren's contracture. *Hand (NY)* 2012;7:364–9.

30 Meals RA, Hentz VR. Technical tips for collagenase injection treatment for Dupuytren's contracture. *J Hand Surg* 2014;39A:1195–200.

32 Hurst LC, Badalamente MA. Nonoperative treatment of Dupuytren's disease. *Hand Clin* 1999;15:97–107.

Plantar fascial fibromatosis

1 Allen RA, Woolner LB, Ghormley RK, *et al*. Soft tissue tumours of the sole with special reference to plantar fibromatosis. *J Bone Joint Surg Am* 1995;37:14–26.

3 Gudmundsson KG, Jónsson T, Arngrimsson R. Association of morbus ledderhose with Dupuytren's contracture. *Foot Ankle Int* 2013;34:841–5.

8 Jacob CI, Kumm RC. Benign anteromedial plantar nodules of childhood: a distinct form of plantar fibromatosis. *Pediatr Dermatol* 2000;17:472–4.

9 Veith NT, Tscherning T, Hirsting T, *et al*. Plantar fibromatosis: topical review. *Foot Ankle Int* 2013;34:1742–6.

PART 8: SPECIFIC CUTANEOUS STRUCTURE

Penile fibromatosis

1 Chilton CP, Castle WM, Westwood CA, *et al.* Factors associated in the aetiology of Peyronie's disease. *Br J Urol* 1982;54:748–50.

5 Williams JL, Thomas GG. The natural history of Peyronie's disease. *J Urol* 1970;103:75–6.

Knuckle pads

4 Hyman CH, Cohen PR. Report of a family with idiopathic knuckle pads and review of idiopathic and disease-associated knuckle pads. *Dermatol Online J* 2013;19(5):18177.

Pachydermodactyly

1 Al Hammadi A, Hakim M. Pachydermodactyly: case report and review of the literature. *J Cutan Med Surg* 2007;11:185–7.

White fibrous papulosis of the neck

1 Shimizu H, Nishikawa T, Kimura S. White fibrous papulosis of the neck: a review of 16 cases. *Jpn J Dermatol B* 1985;95:1077–84.

Camptodactyly

1 Engbar WD, Flatt AF. Camptodactyly. An analysis of sixty-six patients and twenty-four operations. *J Hand Surg* 1977;2A:216–24.

19 Goffin D, Lenoble E, Marin-Braun F, *et al.* Camptodactyly: classification and therapeutic results. *Ann Chir Main* 1994;13:20–5.

Juvenile fibromatoses

Infantile myofibromatosis

2 Mashiah J, Hadj-Rabia S, Dompmartin A, *et al.* Infantile myofibromatosis: a series of 28 cases. J Am Acad Dermatol 2014;71:264–70.

Juvenile hyaline fibromatosis

13 Fayad MN, Yacoub A, Salman S, *et al.* Juvenile hyaline fibromatosis. Two new cases and a review of the literature. *Am J Med Genet* 1987;26:123–31.

Nephrogenic systemic fibrosis

2 Chopra T, Kandukurti K, Shah S, Ahmed R, Panesar M. Understanding nephrogenic systemic fibrosis. *Int J Nephrol* 2012; Article ID 912189.

15 Streams BN, Liu V, Liegois N, *et al.* Clinical and pathologic features of nephrogenic fibrosing dermopathy: a report of two cases. *J Am Acad Dermatol* 2003;48:42–7.

Environmental and drug-induced scleroderma

3 Black CM, Pereira S, McWhirter A, *et al.* Genetic susceptibility to scleroderma-like syndrome in symptomatic and asymptomatic workers exposed to vinyl chloride. *J Rheumatol* 1986;13:1059–62.

11 Iglesias JL, De Moragas JM. The cutaneous lesions of the Spanish toxic oil syndrome. *J Am Acad Dermatol* 1983;9:159–60.

12 Phelps RG, Fleishmajer R. Clinical, pathologic, and immunological manifestations of the toxic oil syndrome. *J Am Acad Dermatol* 1988;18:313–24.

15 Varga J, Jimenez SA. Chemical exposure-induced cutaneous fibrosis. Lessons from 'experiments of nature'. *Arch Dermatol* 1994;130:97–100.

18 Kaufman LD, Gruber BL, Gomez-Reion JJ. Fibrogenic growth factors in the eosinophilia–myalgia syndrome and the toxic oil syndrome. *Arch Dermatol* 1994;130:41–7.

22 Pujol RM, Puig L, Moreno A. Pseudoscleroderma secondary to phytomenadione (vitamin K1) injections. *Cutis* 1989;43:365–8.

Constricting bands of the extremities

2 Patterson T. Congenital ring constrictions. *Br J Plast Surg* 1961;69:532–69.

5 Browne SG. Ainhum. *Int J Dermatol* 1976;15:348–50.

12 Lockwood C, Ghidini A, Romero R, *et al.* Amniotic band syndrome: reevaluation of its pathogenesis. *Am J Obstet Gynecol* 1989;160:1030–3.

14 Latteo SA, Taylor AE, Meggitt SJ. Raised limb bands developing in infancy. *Br J Dermatol* 2006;154:791–2.

Abnormal fibrotic responses to skin injury

Keloids and hypertrophic scars

1 Köse O, Wasseem A. Keloids and hypertrophic scars: are they two different sides of the same coin? *Dermatol Surg* 2008;34:336–46.

4 Oluwasanmi JO. Keloids in the African. *Clin Plast Surg* 1974;1:179–95.

6 Marneros AG, Norris JEC, Olsen BR, *et al.* Clinical genetics of familial keloids. *Arch Dermatol* 2001;137:1429–34.

7 Brown JJ, Bayat A. Genetic susceptibility to raised dermal scarring. *Br J Dermatol* 2006;161:8–18.

16 Jumper N, Paus R, Bayat A. Functional histopathology of keloid disease. *Histol Histopathol* 2015;30:1033–57.

17 Sidgwick GP, Bayat A. Extracellular matrix molecules implicated in hypertrophic and keloid scarring. *J Eur Acad Dermatol Venereol* 2012;26:141–52.

31 Bloemen MC, van der Veer VM, Ulrich MM, *et al.* Prevention and curative management of hypertrophic scar formation. *Burns* 2009;35:463–75.

33 Ud-Din S, Bayat A. Strategic management of keloid disease in ethnic skin: a structured approach supported by the emerging literature. *Br J Dermatol* 2013;169(Suppl. 1):71–81.

34 Jalali M, Bayat A. Current use of steroids in management of abnormal raised skin scars. *Surgeon* 2007;5:175–80.

35 Gauglitz GG, Korting HC, Pavicic T, *et al.* Hypertrophic scarring and keloids: pathomechanisms and current and emerging treatment strategies. *Mol Med* 2011;17:113–25.

37 O'Brien L, Pandit A. Silicone gel sheeting for preventing and treating hypertrophic and keloid scars. *Cochrane Database Syst Rev* 2006;(1):CD003826.

40 Tzitotzios C, Profyris C, Sterling J. Cutaneous scarring: pathophysiology, molecular mechanisms, and scar reduction therapeutics. Part II. Strategies to reduce scar formation after dermatologic procedures. *J Am Acad Dermatol* 2012;66:13–24.

47 Ud-Din S, Thomas G, Morris J, *et al.* Photodynamic therapy: an innovative approach to the treatment of keloid disease evaluated using subjective and objective non-invasive tools. *Arch Dermatol Res* 2013;305:205–14.

49 Mamalis AD, Lev-Tov H, Nguyen D-H, *et al.* Laser and light-based treatment of keloids: a review. *J Eur Acad Dermatol Venereol* 2014;28:689–99.

Perforating dermatoses

Elastosis perforans serpiginosa

3 Mehta RK, Burrows NP, Payne CM *et al.* Elastosis perforans serpiginosa and associated disorders. Clin Exp Dermatol 2001;26:521–4.

11 Light N, Meyrick-Thomas RH, Stephens A *et al.* Collagen and elastin changes in d-penicillamine-induced pseudoxanthoma elasticum-like skin. Br J Dermatol 1986;114:381–8.

18 Mehregan AH. Elastosis perforans serpiginosa. A review of the literature and report of 11 cases. Arch Dermatol 1968;97:381–93.

Acquired perforating dermatosis

1 Ramirez-Fort MK, Khan F, Rosendahl CO, *et al.* Acquired perforating dermatosis: a clinical and dermatoscopic correlation. *Derm Online J* 2013;19(7):18958.

2 Patterson JW. The perforating disorders. *J Am Acad Dermatol* 1984;10:561–81.

5 Rapini RP, Herbert AA, Drucker CR, *et al.* Acquired perforating dermatosis: evidence of combined transepidermal elimination of both collagen and elastic fibres. *Arch Dermatol* 1989;125:1074–8.

8 Gagnon IAL, Desai T. Dermatological diseases in patients with chronic kidney disease. *J Nephropathol* 2013;2:104–9.

9 Patterson JW. Progress in the perforating dermatoses. *Arch Dermatol* 1989;125:1121–3.

10 Akoglu G, Emre S, Sunqu N, *et al.* Clinicopathological features of 25 patients with acquired perforating dermatosis. *Eur J Dermatol* 2013;23:864–71.

14 Kim SW, Kim MS, Lee JH, *et al.* A clinicopathological study of thirty cases of acquired perforating dermatosis in Korea. *Ann Dermatol* 2014;26:162–71.

17 Kanan MW. Familial reactive perforating collagenosis and intolerance to cold. *Br J Dermatol* 1974;91:405–14.

20 Fretzin DF, Beal DW, Jao W. Light and ultrastructural study of reactive perforating collagenosis. *Arch Dermatol* 1980;116:1054–8.

21 Millard PR, Young E, Harrison DE, *et al.* Reactive perforating collagenosis: light, ultrastructural and immunohistological studies. *Histopathology* 1986;10:1047–56.

26 Moulin G, Balme B, Musso M, Thomas L. Le collagénome perforant verruciforme, une dermatose par inclusion exogène? A propos d'un cas induit par le chlorure de calcium. *Ann Dermatol Vénéréol* 1995;122:591–4.

CHAPTER 97

Granulomatous Disorders of the Skin

Johnny Bourke

South Infirmary-Victoria University Hospital, Cork, Ireland

Granuloma annulare, 97.1	Cutaneous Crohn disease, 97.11	Key references, 97.13
Necrobiosis lipoidica, 97.8		

Granuloma annulare

Definition

This is a disease of the skin and subcutaneous tissue characterized by granulomatous annular plaques, nodules or papules containing foci of altered collagen surrounded by histiocytes and lymphocytes.

Introduction and general description

Granuloma annulare (GA) is a distinctive condition affecting all ages [1,2]. The typical presentation is of annular indurated papules and/or plaques on the extremities, which slowly enlarge before eventually flattening and fading over months or years (Figure 97.1). It may occur at any age and is more common in women. Several different clinical types are seen: localized, generalized, subcutaneous and perforating. The aetiology and pathophysiology are uncertain although there are many reports of associated infective and other triggers. The widely reported association with diabetes is probably incorrect, although adequate controlled studies have not been performed to date. Treatment is generally unnecessary. In severe generalized disease many treatments have been reported to be effective although the evidence is largely anecdotal.

Epidemiology

Incidence and prevalence

The population prevalence/incidence is unknown. GA has been estimated to account for approximately 0.1–0.4% of dermatology out-patient consultations in the UK [1,3].

Age

Granuloma annulare is most common in children and young adults but can occur at any age [1]. Generalized GA occurs more commonly in adults with a mean around 50 years in most series [4,5,6,7]. Subcutaneous GA is seen predominantly in children. Perforating GA has been reported in both adults and children.

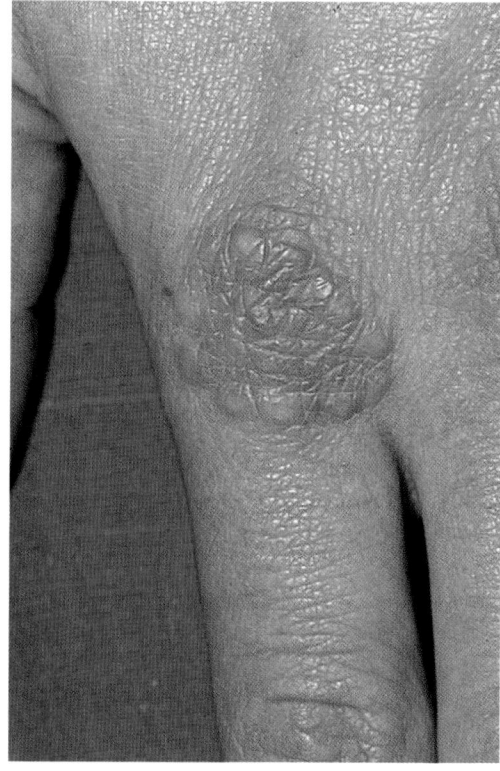

Figure 97.1 Granuloma annulare on the dorsum of the hand – a typical site.

Sex

Granuloma annulare is approximately twice as common in women as in men [8].

Ethnicity

There does not appear to be any racial predilection for GA, with the exception of perforating GA, which is more common amongst ethnic Hawaians [9,10].

Rook's Textbook of Dermatology, Ninth Edition. Edited by Christopher Griffiths, Jonathan Barker, Tanya Bleiker, Robert Chalmers and Daniel Creamer.
© 2016 John Wiley & Sons, Ltd. Published 2016 by John Wiley & Sons, Ltd.
Companion website: www.rooksdermatology.com

Associated diseases

The prevalence of diabetes is probably *not* increased amongst patients with GA [11,12]. However, large-scale studies are needed to address this issue properly. Most publications have reported retrospective surveys, of which some have suggested an association with type 1 diabetes [13–15]. One case–control study [12] showed a lack of association with type 2 diabetes but psoriasis patients were used as controls. The recently recognized association between psoriasis and insulin resistance [16] casts doubt on the findings of this study. Isolated case reports continue, however, to suggest a possible association [17–19].

Both localized and generalized GA has been reported in association with autoimmune thyroiditis in women [6,20–25], including in one case–control study [25]. Generalized GA has also been reported in a patient with a toxic adenoma of the thyroid (Plummer disease) [26]. Two papers suggest the possibility of an association between uveitis and GA [27,28].

The incidence of hyperlipidaemia has recently been reported to be four times higher amongst people with GA than in age-matched controls [29].

Although there are several reports of an association with malignancy, many of the cases were atypical (e.g. painful lesions of the palms and soles). Recent reviews of the literature have concluded that there is no obvious relationship [30,31], although this might not apply to older patients with atypical GA.

There are isolated reports of the coincidence of temporal arteritis [32] and morphoea [33] in patients with GA. Coexistence with necrobiosis lipoidica [19,34–37] and sarcoidosis [38–41] has also been reported.

Pathophysiology

Although the aetiology and pathogenesis of GA are unclear, it appears likely that GA represents a reaction pattern to a variety of triggering factors [8,42]. A miscellany of infections and infestations have been linked; these include scabies [43], hepatitis B [44], *Mycobacterium tuberculosis* [45,46], human papillomavirus [47], varicella/zoster [48–56], Epstein–Barr virus [57,58], parvovirus B19 [59], hepatitis C [60], HIV [61–72] and *Borrelia burgdorferi* [73–75]. The associations reported would appear to be reactive rather than due to any specific mechanism, as evidenced by the heterogeneity of organisms reported and lack of association with persistent viral or bacterial DNA [53,61,75–78].

Traumatic triggers that have been linked to GA have included a variety of immunizations [79–84], tuberculin testing [85], animal and insect bites [86,87], waxing [88] and saphenectomy [89]. Perforating GA has also been reported in the red areas of tattoos [90,91].

Sunlight exposure has been implicated in seasonal GA [92,93] and, more obviously, in cases where there is a clear photo-distribution (Figure 97.2) [94–97]. Generalized GA following psoralen and UVA (PUVA) has also been reported [98]. Whether actinic granuloma is a distinct entity, or represents GA on sun-exposed skin, has been the subject of debate [99–107].

There are several reports of drug-induced GA although some may have been examples of drug-induced interstitial granulomatous reactions [108]. A recent publication from Greece reported that GA was found in almost 4% of rheumatology patients treated with tumour necrosis factor α (TNF-α) blockers [109].

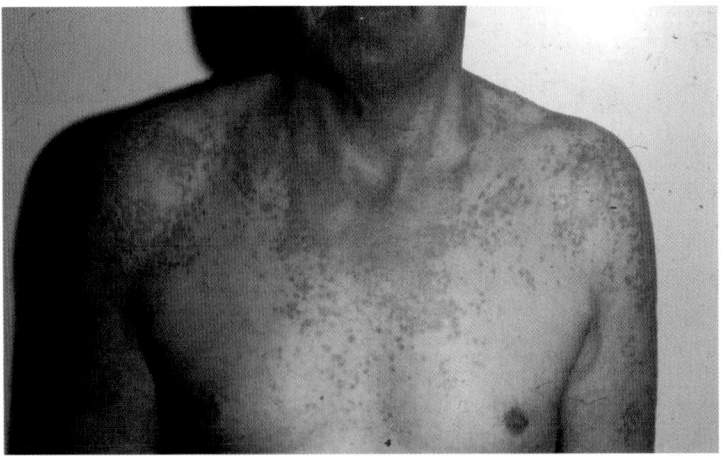

Figure 97.2 Generalized granuloma annulare showing a clear photo-distribution over the 'V' of the neck and shoulders.

There is a report of disseminated GA occurring in the same sites as lesions of erythema multiforme [110].

It has been suggested that an immunoglobulin-mediated vasculitis is the cause of the necrobiotic granulomas in GA [111,**112**], but evidence from immunofluorescence studies is conflicting: some authors have demonstrated immunoreactants in vessel walls [111], whereas others have not [113–114]. An alternative view is that the pathogenetic mechanism is a delayed-type hypersensitivity response [**112**,114–118].

Pathology

The most characteristic histological lesion in GA is the necrobiotic granuloma, but there are three histological patterns that may occur: (i) necrobiotic palisading granulomas; (ii) an interstitial form; and (iii) granulomas of sarcoidal or tuberculoid type [119]. There is some variation in the literature in relation to the prevalence of each of these types in the different clinical patterns of disease [5,121,122]. Observer variation and the existence of more than one pattern in the same section may have contributed to differences in the findings in these series.

Necrobiotic palisading granulomas (Figure 97.3) are situated in the superficial and mid-dermis separated by relatively normal tissue, in contrast to necrobiosis lipoidica. They are characterized by foci of necrobiosis surrounded by histiocytes and lymphocytes, with the histiocytes commonly forming a palisaded pattern. There are varying numbers of multinucleate giant cells in this peripheral zone. T cells in the lymphocytic infiltrate are of the helper/inducer phenotype (CD4+) [123–125], but in two cases associated with HIV infection a predominantly T-suppressor (CD8+) infiltrate was demonstrated [126,127]. A small number of skin-specific clones have been demonstrated together with many non-specific T cells [125], possibly attracted by a high local production of interleukin 2. Mucin, demonstrated by Alcian blue or colloidal iron stains, is present within the foci of the necrobiosis. Small deposits of lipid material may also be present. Collagen alteration, most commonly fragmentation of collagen bundles, was observed in 79% of cases of localized and 53% of cases of generalized GA [5]. There is a marked reduction in or absence of elastic fibres [128,129]. Metalloproteinases are probably involved in the damage to collagen and the elastic fibres [130,131].

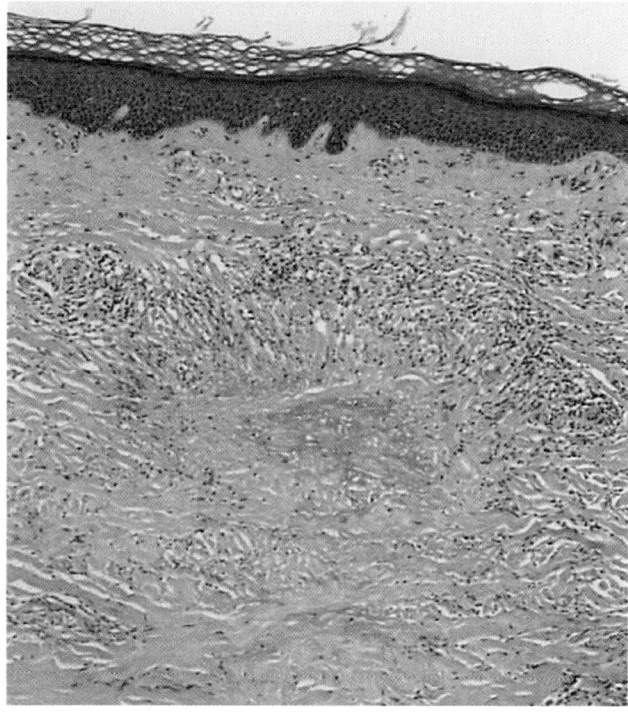

(a)

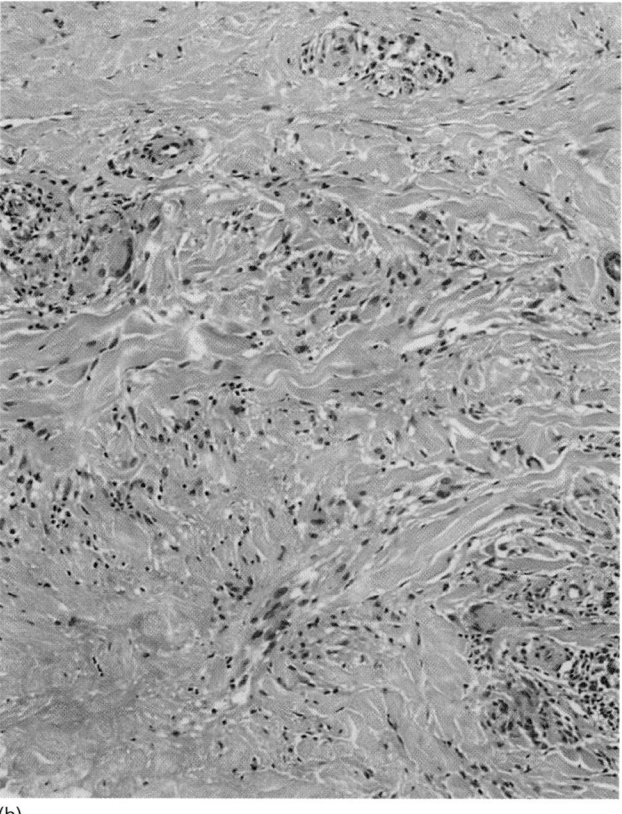

(b)

Figure 97.3 (a) Necrobiotic palisading granuloma showing well circumscribed central necrobiosis surrounded by a palisade of histiocytes. (b) Close-up view showing necrobiotic collagen and multinucleated giant cells.

In the *interstitial* pattern there are no formed areas of necrobiosis. Histiocytes and lymphocytes are present around blood vessels and between collagen bundles, and collagen fibres are separated by mucin.

The *sarcoidal or tuberculoid pattern* is uncommon, and may cause problems in diagnosis. The presence of mucin and eosinophils can help to distinguish GA from sarcoidosis.

Distinguishing features of GA include a perivascular infiltrate of lymphocytes and histiocytes within the lesion and in the adjacent tissue, eosinophils [132,133] and a relative absence of plasma cells. Vasculitic features have been described [134] but not found by others [135]. Histiocytes express the marker PG-M1 [136]. They may show an increased mitotic rate, and recognition of this is important, in particular in differentiating GA from epithelioid sarcoma [136–139].

In perforating GA there is a superficial area of necrobiosis surrounded by palisading histiocytes situated beneath a perforation with varying degrees of epidermal hyperplasia at the margins [119,120,140]. The necrobiotic material is extruded via the perforation.

Subcutaneous GA is clinically and histologically similar to a rheumatoid nodule with large areas of necrobiosis. Alcian blue-stained mucin is the most useful distinguishing feature [141].

Other disorders with similar histological features include mycosis fungoides variants [142–145], interstitial granulomatous dermatitis (interstitial granulomatous dermatitis with arthritis; interstitial granulomatous dermatitis with plaques; palisaded neutrophilic granulomatous dermatitis) [146–152] and interstitial granulomatous drug reaction [153,154].

Causative organisms
There are no confirmed pathogenic organisms.

Genetics
There is an increased prevalence of HLA-Bw35 amongst individuals with generalized GA compared with controls or those with localized GA [155]. There are a few reports of familial cases [156–162].

Clinical features

History
Patients with subcutaneous GA may complain of tenderness and generalized GA may be itchy, but most patients are asymptomatic. Acute, painful, acral lesions have been described [163]. Commonly, the annular lesions will have been treated with antifungal agents before the correct diagnosis is reached.

Presentation and clinical variants
There are four commonly recognized clinical variants, which typically appear independently, although some patients may exhibit more than one variant [164,165].

Localized GA. This accounts for about three-quarters of cases and typically presents as a ring of small, smooth, flesh-coloured or erythematous papules (Figure 97.4a). Stretching the skin enables the papules to be seen more readily (Figure 97.4b). The surface of the skin over the papules is intact and there is usually no scaling. Annular lesions tend to enlarge centrifugally before eventually clearing. They may be solitary or multiple, and may occur anywhere on the skin, although the dorsa of the hands (Figure 97.5a), knuckles (see Figures 97.1 and 97.4), fingers (Figure 97.5b) and feet (Figure 97.5c) are the commonest sites. Some, typically acral, lesions enlarge as nodules rather than as annular plaques.

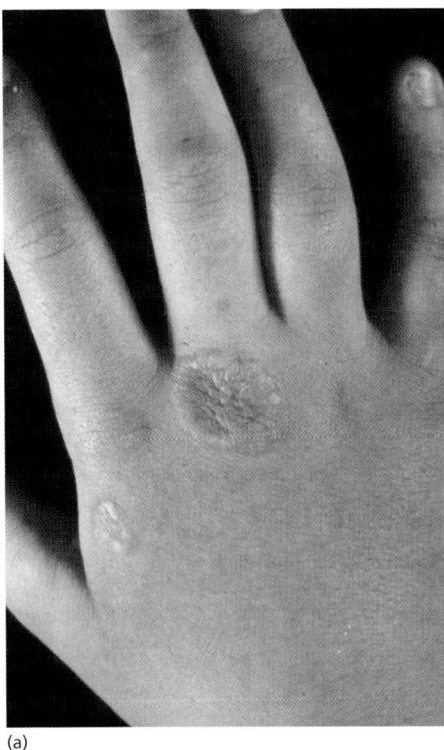

(a)

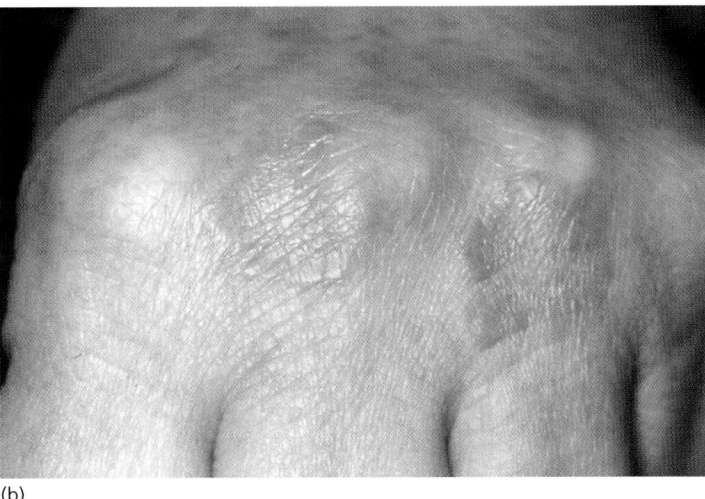

(b)

Figure 97.4 (a) Typical appearance of localized granuloma annulare over the knuckles. (b) Appearance of granuloma annulare over the knuckles on clenching the fist.

Generalized or disseminated GA. Generalized or disseminated GA makes up 10–15% of cases [6,8], is seen predominantly in adults and is twice as common in females. Pruritus may be the presenting feature. Interestingly, it is the commonest form seen in HIV patients [166–170]. The lesions are often ill-defined with skin-coloured or erythematous macules, papules and/or plaques in an annular pattern surrounding a faintly violaceous central area on the trunk and limbs (Figure 97.6) [6,170–173]. The sparing of vaccination sites in a case of generalized GA is an interesting phenomenon [174].

Perforating GA. This is uncommon [175] but has been described in all ages including infancy [176] and in HIV [167]. Localized or generalized papules develop yellowish centres and discharge a little

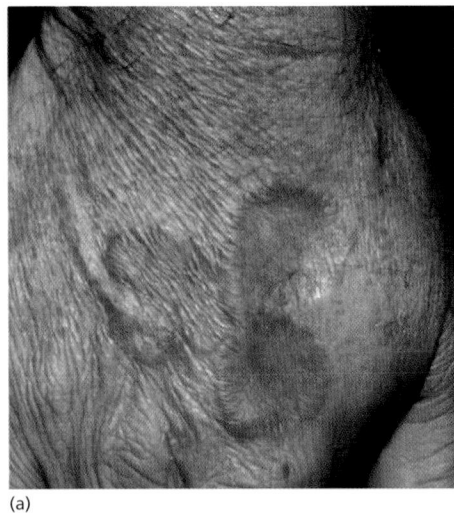

(a)

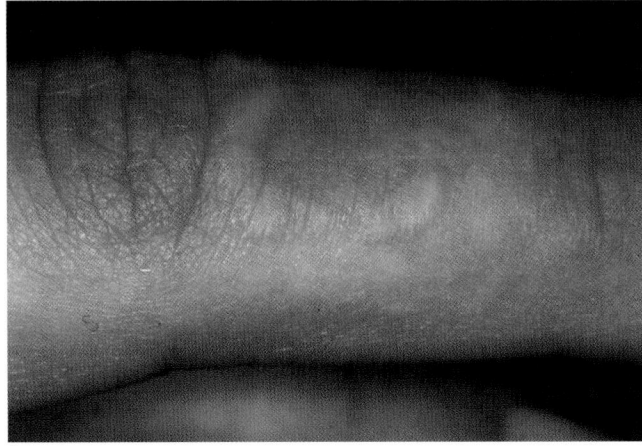

(b)

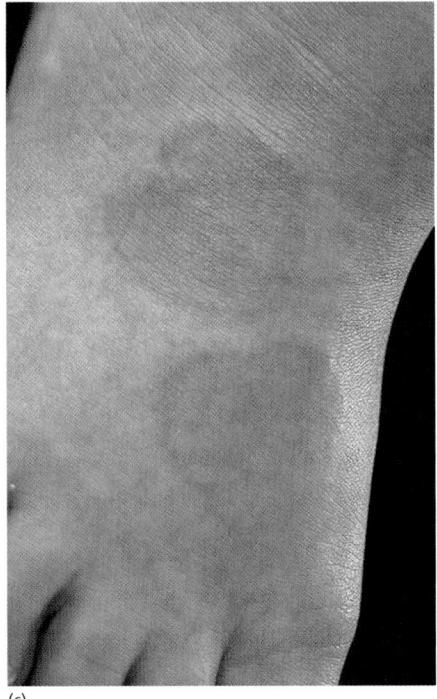

(c)

Figure 97.5 Common sites of localized granuloma annulare. (a) On the dorsum of the hand; note the atrophy in the centre of the lesions. (b) On the dorsum of a finger. (c) On the dorsum of a child's foot; this is often mistaken for tinea, but there is no scale and tinea in this site would be unlikely in a child.

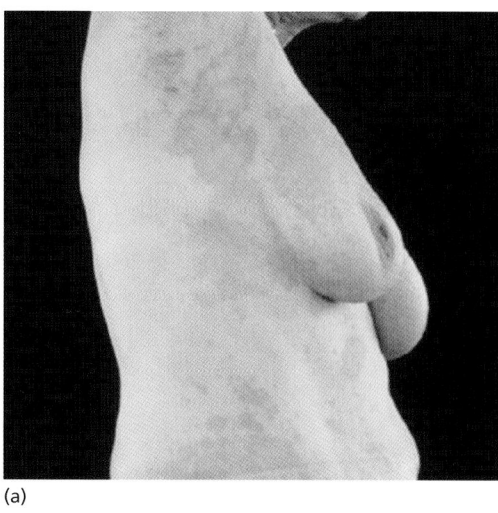

(a)

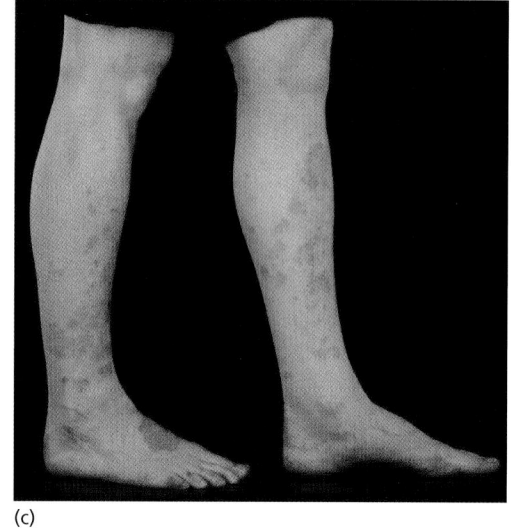

(c)

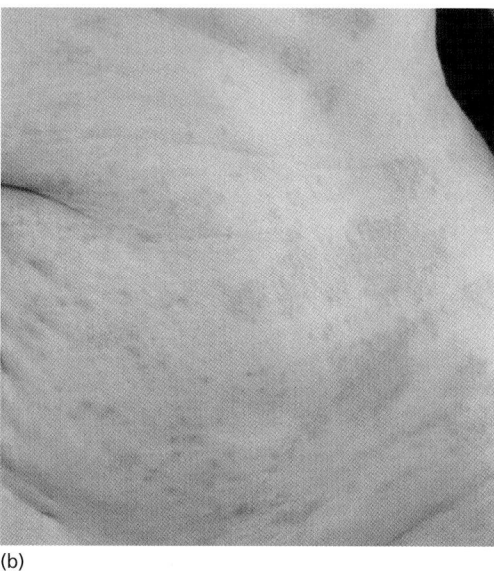

(b)

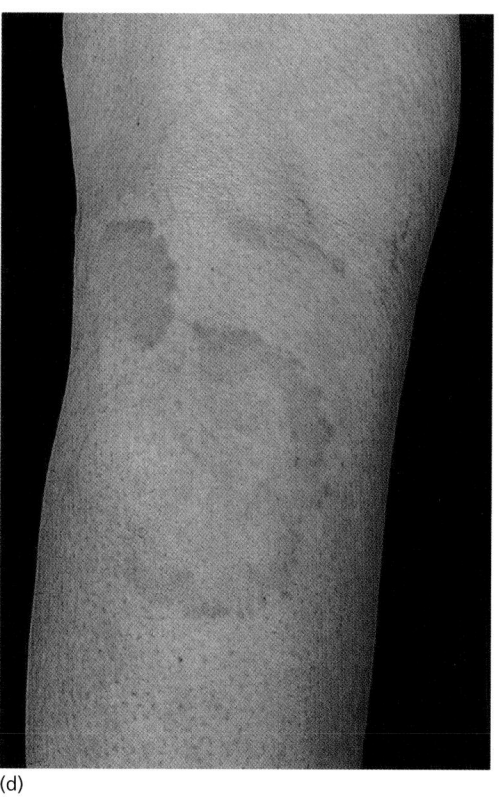

(d)

Figure 97.6 Common sites of generalized granuloma annulare. (a) Right flank. (b) Abdomen. (c, d) Involvement of the lower extremities.

clear, viscous fluid that dries to form a crust, eventually separating to leave a hypo- or hyperpigmented scar (Figure 97.7) [177–178].

Subcutaneous GA. This is also uncommon. It occurs predominantly in children (Figure 97.8) and has been given a variety of names, including benign rheumatoid nodules [179], pseudorheumatoid nodules [180,181], deep granuloma annulare [182,183], subcutaneous palisading granuloma [184], isolated subcutaneous granuloma and subcutaneous necrobiotic granuloma [185]. Lesions are nodular and occur predominantly on the scalp and legs, particularly in the pretibial region [157,186,187], but unusual locations include the periorbital area, palm [188,189] and penis [190]. Rarely, there may be subperiosteal lesions [191]. A congenital case has been recorded [192]. Magnetic resonance imaging features are diagnostically helpful [193–195].

Other reported variants of GA include a papular umbilicated form on the dorsa of the hands in children [196], a case of 'follicular pustulous' GA, in which palisading necrobiotic granulomas occurred in a perifollicular distribution [197], pustular generalized perforating GA, in which a dense infiltrate of neutrophils was present in areas of necrobiosis [198], linear GA [199,200], and 'patch' GA, in which erythematous patches occurred on the trunk and limbs [201]. It has been suggested that cases with 'linear' lesions may be examples of interstitial granulomatous dermatitis, and those with 'patch' lesions may represent examples of the interstitial granulomatous form of drug reaction [202].

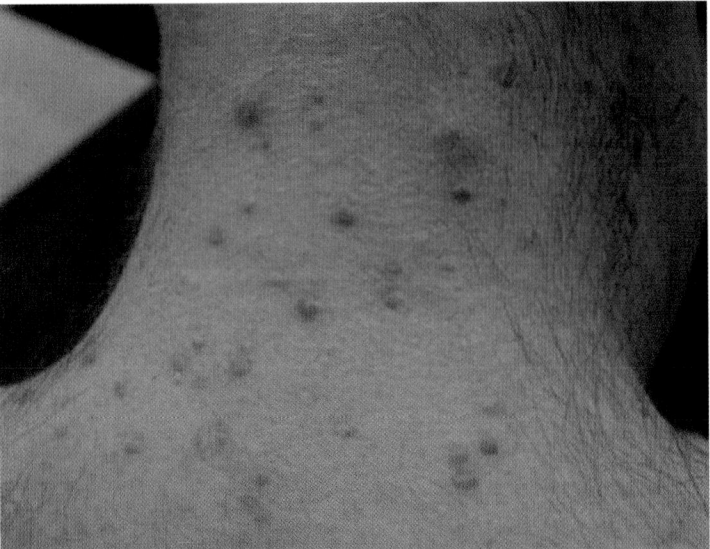

(a)

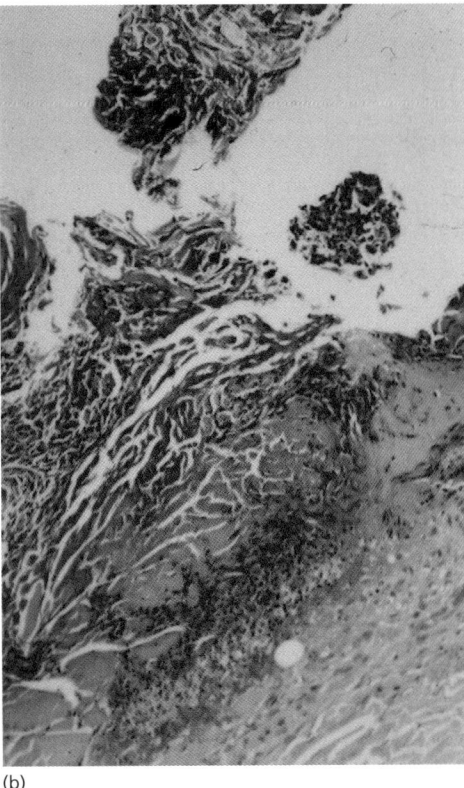

(b)

Figure 97.7 (a) Perforating granuloma annulare on the neck and (b) histology showing transepidermal elimination of necrobiotic collagen.

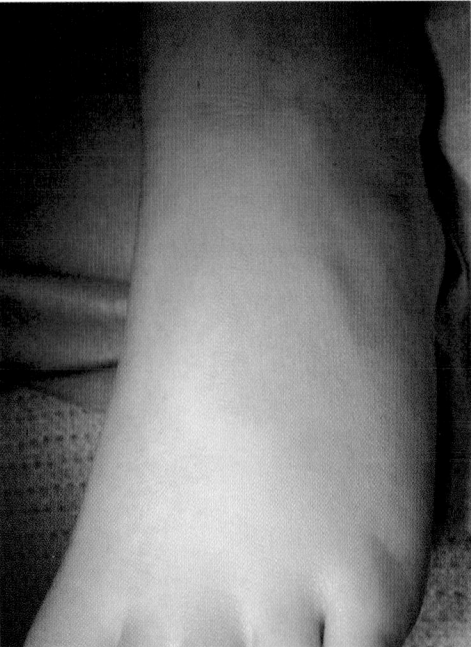

Figure 97.8 Subcutaneous granuloma annulare with nodules visible on the dorsolateral aspect of a child's foot.

may cause diagnostic confusion, including annular lichen planus, erythema annulare centrifugum, erythema migrans of Lyme disease, tuberculides [219] and tertiary syphilis [220]. The morphology and distribution of lesions may simulate mycosis fungoides [221].

Uncommon sites for lesions of GA are the ears (Figure 97.9), where the perforating variety is particularly unusual [203], penis [204–209], palms [210] and periocular regions [211–216]. Mucous membranes are spared, although there is a report of involvement of the oral mucosa in a patient with HIV infection [168]. A destructive form has been described causing damage to soft tissues, tendons, bones and joints [217,218].

Differential diagnosis
Non-dermatologists may mistake GA for tinea or erythema multiforme. Other annular lesions and granulomatous conditions

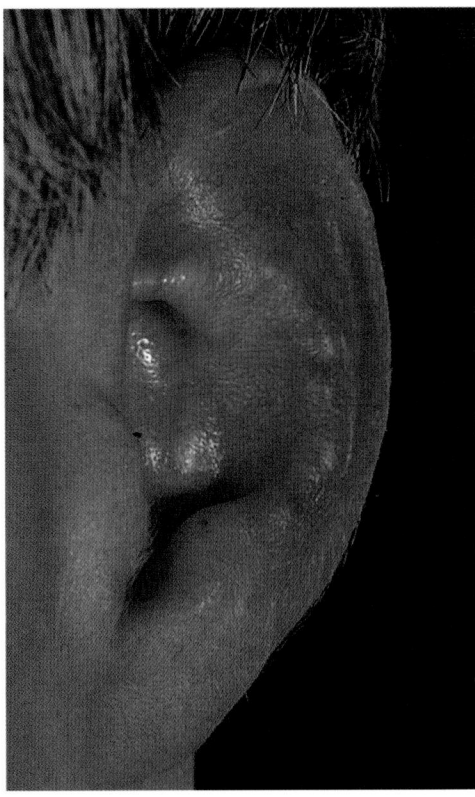

Figure 97.9 Granuloma annulare on the ear. Note the nodules overlying the auricular cartilage of the antihelix.

The differential diagnosis of subcutaneous GA is extensive, including trauma, infection, tumours, sarcoidosis and rheumatoid nodules. A diagnostic biopsy will usually be necessary.

The differential diagnosis of perforating GA includes molluscum contagiosum [222], other perforating disorders (see Chapter 96), sarcoidosis and papulonecrotic tuberculide [223,224]. Epithelioid sarcoma may also masquerade as perforating GA [136–139].

Mycobacterium marinum infection has histologically simulated interstitial GA [225]. Other histological differential diagnoses include granulomatous mycosis fungoides [226], interstitial granulomatous dermatitis and interstitial granulomatous drug reaction.

Complications and co-morbidities

There are reports of anetoderma secondary to generalized GA [227], and mid-dermal elastolysis occurring with GA [228] and subsequent to lesions resembling GA [229]. In another case, loss of elastic fibres was presumed to be responsible for the development of open comedones on the rim of GA lesions occurring on light-exposed areas [230].

Disease course and prognosis

The postal questionnaire survey carried out by Wells and Smith [1] revealed that in about 50% of patients the lesions resolved within 2 years. However, about 40% of those whose lesions cleared had a recurrence, in the majority of cases at the same sites as the original lesions. In this study, there did not appear to be any difference in prognosis between individuals with single lesions and those with multiple lesions, and although there is an impression that spontaneous resolution is less likely to occur with generalized GA there does not appear to be any documented confirmation of this.

Levin *et al.* [231] have discussed the resolution of lesions following biopsy and have noted the paucity of information relating to this phenomenon in the literature. There appears to be anecdotal evidence of its occurrence, but little documentation. However, it is of interest, in this context, that scarification is one form of physical treatment that has been advocated in the past [232–234].

Investigations

Biopsy may be necessary in nodular, subcutaneous, perforating, generalized and atypical forms. Investigation for diabetes, thyroid disease, malignancy and/or hyperlipidaemia are probably necessary only in exceptional cases.

Management

In most cases, particularly in children, reassurance of eventual resolution is all that is needed. As with other conditions that spontaneously resolve, assessment of the efficacy of reported treatments is difficult. There is no high-quality evidence of the efficacy of any intervention for any form of GA and most recommendations rely on anecdotal case reports or small uncontrolled case series.

In persistent localized GA, a trial of topical steroid or tacrolimus/pimecrolimus is reasonable although often ineffective [235,236] even under occlusion. Cryotherapy and intralesional steroid injection [237] may be appropriate for symptomatic localized lesions although the risk of permanent scarring or atrophy is significant. Nitrous oxide has been reported in one study to give a better cosmetic result [238].

For generalized disease, PUVA appears to give the best results [239–247], with one retrospective study of 33 patients showing 50% clearance and a further 31% good to moderated improvement [**248**]. UVA1 has also been reported to be effective in two case series [249,250]. Of the systemic therapies, dapsone [251–253], retinoids [254–262], antimalarials [263–265], fumaric acid esters [266–268] and methotrexate [269,270] have been most extensively reported. None of these has been shown to be reliably beneficial. The potential toxicity of these agents [271] must be weighed against the benign nature of the disease.

Other agents that have been claimed to be effective in localized GA include imiquimod [272,273], isotretinoin [274], local injections of low-dose recombinant interferon γ [275], photodynamic therapy [276], and pulsed dye [277], neodymium:yttrium-aluminium-garnet (Nd:YAG) [278], carbon dioxide [279] and excimer [280] lasers.

For generalized disease, potassium iodide has been shown to be ineffective [281]. There are anecdotal reports claiming efficacy for topical tacrolimus [282] and pimecrolimus [283], ciclosporin [284–287], low-dose chlorambucil [**5**,289–290,291], nicotinamide (niacinamide) [292], pentoxifylline [293], tranilast [294], clofazimine [295], topical vitamin E [296], a combination of vitamin E and a 5-lipoxygenase inhibitor [297], defibrotide [298] and oral calcitriol [299]. Infliximab [300,301], adalimumab [302–305], etanercept [306] and efalizumab [307] have also been reported to be effective; however, in a small series of patients reported by Kreuter *et al.* [3.5] there was either no change or deterioration during therapy with etanercept. The development of GA in patients on TNF-α blockers would also argue against the use of these agents.

Most of the treatments mentioned above have been employed in patients with perforating lesions, with varying degrees of success [309,310]. Lesions of subcutaneous GA should be left to resolve spontaneously once the diagnosis has been confirmed [311].

Treatment ladder

First line
- No treatment/expectant
- Cryotherapy
- Intralesional corticosteroid
- Potent topical corticosteroid

Second line
- Topical tacrolimus
- Pimecrolimus
- Imiquimod
- Narrow-band UVB phototherapy[a]
- PUVA[a]
- Dapsone[a]
- Ciclosporin[a]
- Fumaric acid esters[a]
- Methotrexate[a]

Third line
- Photodynamic therapy
- Laser

[a]Principally for generalized disease.

**PART 8: SPECIFIC
CUTANEOUS STRUCTURE**

Resources

Patient resources
British Association of Dermatologists, patient information leaflet: http://www
.bad.org.uk/for-the-public/patient-information-leaflets/granuloma-annulare/
DermNet NZ, granuloma annulare: http://dermnetnz.org/dermal-infiltrative/
granuloma-annulare.html.
(Both last accessed May 2015.)

Necrobiosis lipoidica

Definition and nomenclature

Necrobiosis lipoidica is a distinctive skin disorder characterized clinically by well-demarcated waxy red-brown plaques with an atrophic centre, most commonly located on the shins, and histologically by full-thickness dermal lymphohistiocytic perivascular infiltration with extensive areas of necrobiosis.

Synonyms and inclusions
• Necrobiosis lipoidica diabeticorum

Introduction and general description

Necrobiosis lipoidica is a distinctive skin condition characterized by well-defined red-brown indurated plaques with an atrophic yellow centre (Figure 97.10). It is most commonly seen on the legs and may ulcerate, causing considerable pain. Histologically, there is a full-thickness lymphohistiocytic infiltrate with extensive necrobiosis of collagen. It is associated with diabetes (both type 1 and type 2) and glucose intolerance. Treatment is generally unsatisfactory.

Epidemiology

Incidence and prevalence

Necrobiosis lipoidica is relatively uncommon. In patients with diabetes, reported prevalences range from 0.3% [1] to 1.2% [2]; it appears to be rare (0.06%) in childhood diabetes [3]. Its prevalence amongst non-diabetics is not well established.

Age

Necrobiosis lipoidica may occur at any age. It is uncommon in childhood and is most commonly seen in young adults and in early middle age. When associated with type 1 diabetes, it is seen at a younger age (third decade) than in type 2 or those without diabetes (fourth decade).

Sex

The female to male ratio is 3 : 1.

Associated diseases

There is no doubt that necrobiosis lipoidica is associated with diabetes, although only about 1% of diabetics develop it [1,2,3,4]. In a much quoted study from a large, specialist, tertiary referral centre, two-thirds of 171 patients with necrobiosis lipoidica had known diabetes at presentation [1]. This is unlikely, however, to be a true reflection of the overall incidence of diabetes in patients with necrobiosis lipoidica. In another study, however, 55 of 65

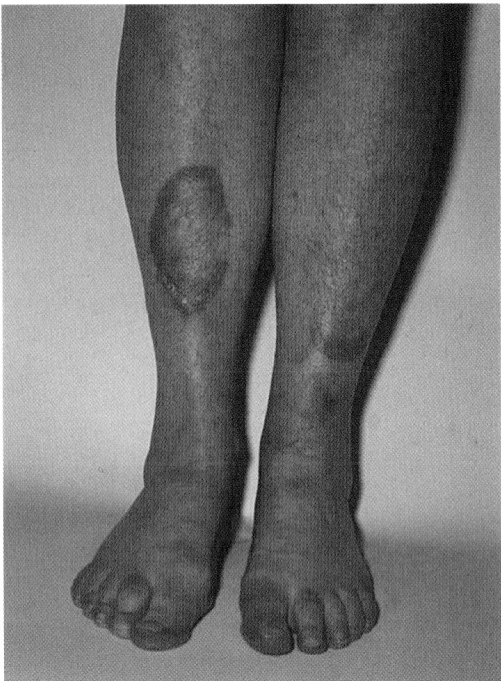

(a)

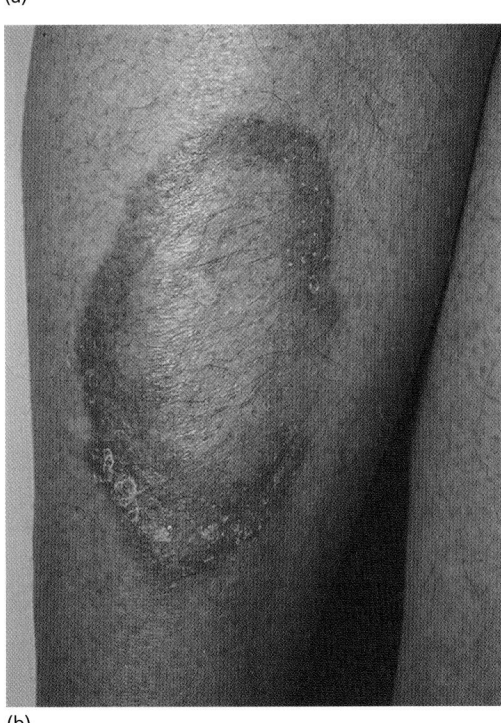

(b)

Figure 97.10 (a) Necrobiosis lipoidica of the shins in a 50-year-old woman. (b) Close-up view of the shin.

patients with necrobiosis lipoidica (85%) had no evidence of diabetes or impaired glucose tolerance at presentation. Only three of 42 patients re-evaluated between 5 and 15 years after initial presentation were found to have abnormal glucose handling [5].

There is some evidence that diabetic patients who have necrobiosis lipoidica are at higher risk of retinopathy and nephropathy than diabetics who do not [6,7,8]. Necrobiosis lipoidica has also been described in association with a number of other conditions including ulcerative colitis [9], Crohn disease [10] and after jejunal bypass surgery [11]. Reports of its occurrence with granuloma annulare have been mentioned previously (see the section on GA). It has also been reported in association with sarcoidosis [12,13].

Pathophysiology

The precise pathogenesis of necrobiosis lipoidica remains unknown [14]. Some authors have considered vascular changes to be important: these might explain the association with diabetes. An altered plasma protein profile [15], elevated factor VIII-related antigen [16] and fibronectin [17] have been proposed as contributory factors. However, in Muller and Winkelmann's histopathological study, vascular involvement was very mild in about a third of the cases [18]. Furthermore, studies investigating blood flow in plaques of necrobiosis have yielded conflicting results. Boateng *et al.* [19] reported reduced blood flow compared with healthy controls and Brungger [20] demonstrated reduced transcutaneous oxygen. However, Ngo *et al.* reported increased blood flow [21].

The possible role of an antibody-mediated vasculitis as an initiating event in necrobiosis lipoidica has also provoked debate as the results of immunofluorescence studies differ. Laukkanen *et al.* [22] did not demonstrate immunoreactants in lesional skin, but others have shown immunoreactants, principally IgM, C3 and fibrin, in vessel walls in the involved skin, and IgM, C3 and fibrinogen at the dermal–epidermal junction [23,24]. Dahl [25] has discussed immunofluorescence findings in necrobiosis lipoidica.

Predisposing factors

The link with diabetes is discussed in Associated diseases.

Pathology [26–28]

The histological appearances are similar to those of granuloma annulare, but some features differ. The epidermis is normal or atrophic, and absent if there is ulceration. There are changes involving the full thickness of the dermis and these often extend into the subcutaneous fat (Figure 97.11). Early lesions show a perivascular and interstitial mixed inflammatory cell infiltrate. Areas of necrobiosis are usually more extensive and less well defined than in granuloma annulare. There is degeneration of collagen and elastin within the lesions [29]. Histiocytes border the areas of necrobiosis. There are variable numbers of Langhans or foreign-body giant cells. A perivascular inflammatory infiltrate includes occasional eosinophils and, in contrast with granuloma annulare, plasma cells. Lymphoid nodules containing germinal centres may be present in the deep dermis or subcutaneous fat [30]. Lipid can be demonstrated in the necrobiotic areas, and cholesterol clefts may be present [31]. Mucin may be present in the dermis, but it is not as prominent as in granuloma annulare.

Small superficial blood vessels are increased in number and are telangiectatic. Deeper dermal blood vessels often show thickening of their walls and proliferation of endothelial cells. The walls are often infiltrated with periodic acid–Schiff-positive, diastase-negative material. Histologically, comedo-like plugs at the periphery of lesions represent the elimination of necrotic material through hair follicles [32,33]. Anaesthesia in the lesions appears to be related to a decreased number of nerves within them [34]. In old atrophic lesions there is considerable fibrosis in the dermis and subcutis.

Genetics

Familial cases are rare [35,36].

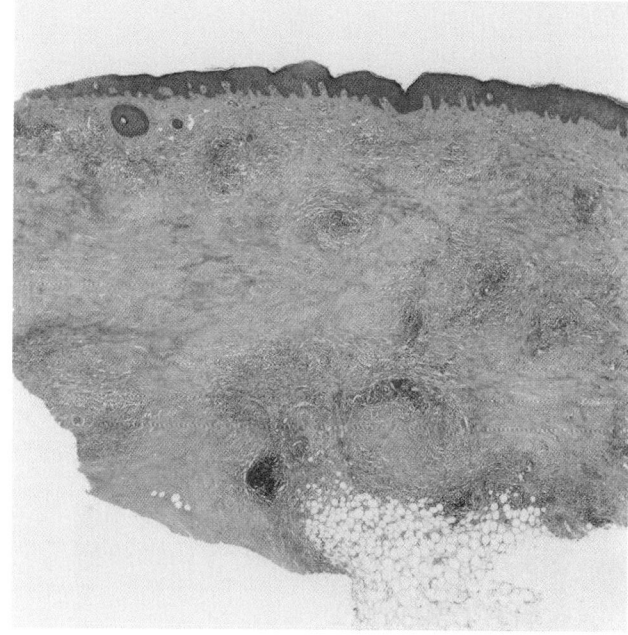

Figure 97.11 Necrobiosis lipoidica showing extensive necrobiosis in the dermis.

Clinical features

History

The lesions are normally asymptomatic unless ulcerated, which is generally a late feature of the condition.

Presentation [37–39]

Necrobiosis lipoidica may occur at any age, but usually develops in young adults and in early middle age. In insulin-dependent diabetics the age of onset is earlier than in non-insulin-dependent and non-diabetic individuals [40]. It is rare in childhood [41,42].

Typical lesions occur on the pretibial skin, and begin as a firm, dull red papule or plaque that enlarges radially to become a yellowish atrophic plaque with an erythematous edge (Figures 97.10 and 97.12). The surface is often glazed in appearance and telangiectatic vessels may be prominent (Figure 97.13). Hypohidrosis and hypoaesthesia or anaesthesia may develop [38,43,44]. Comedo-like plugs may occur at the periphery of lesions [45]. In most cases lesions are bilateral, and they are similar in appearance whether occurring in diabetic or non-diabetic individuals [37]. They tend to be persistent and may ulcerate [46]: in one study [40], ulceration correlated with sensory impairment. Squamous cell carcinoma may develop in longstanding lesions [47–54].

Lesions can occur on other parts of the body, including the trunk [55] and penis [56,57], and rarely may be diffuse [58]. Koebnerization at sites of trauma may also occur (Figure 97.14) [59–62]. The number of lesions and their rate of progress are very variable.

Differential diagnosis

A distinctive condition typically affecting the skin of the head and neck of middle-aged women previously described as 'atypical necrobiosis of the face and scalp margins' [63] or Miescher granuloma [64] has now been accepted by most as being more closely related to O'Brien actinic granuloma [65]. In both conditions there is granulomatous inflammation affecting sun-exposed skin with

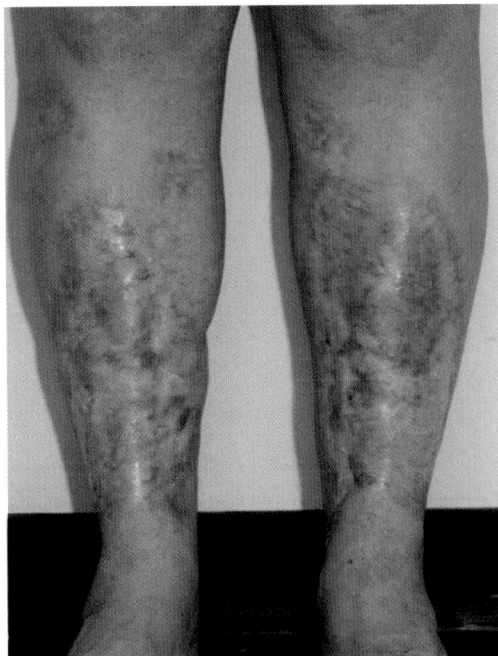

Figure 97.12 Chronic necrobiosis lipoidica (over a 20-year period) in a 41-year-old patient with insulin-dependent diabetes. Note the marked atrophy and telangiectasia.

prominent elastophagocytosis and complete loss of elastic tissue. A unifying term of 'annular elastolytic giant cell granuloma' was proposed in 1979 by Hanke *et al*. [66] and has been widely adopted [67] (see Chapter 96).

Lesions with marked fatty infiltration, particularly when not on the legs, may be mistaken for xanthomas. Necrobiotic xanthogranuloma is a rare, destructive, non-Langerhans cell histiocytosis, in which red-orange or yellowish indurated plaques most frequently involve the periorbital regions and trunk [68,69]. It is associated with systemic lesions and a monoclonal gammopathy (see Chapter 136).

Complications and co-morbidities
Ulceration is the principal complication, affecting up to 35% of patients (Figure 97.15) [1]. Squamous cell carcinoma has also been reported but is rare [47–54].

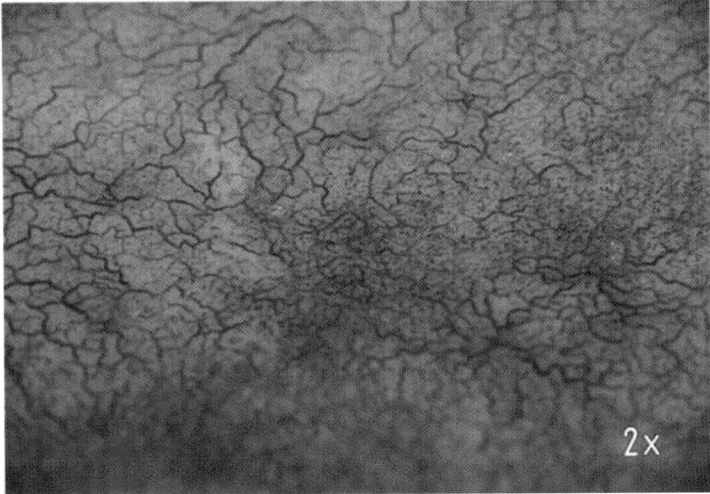

Figure 97.13 Prominent telangiectasia in an area of necrobiosis.

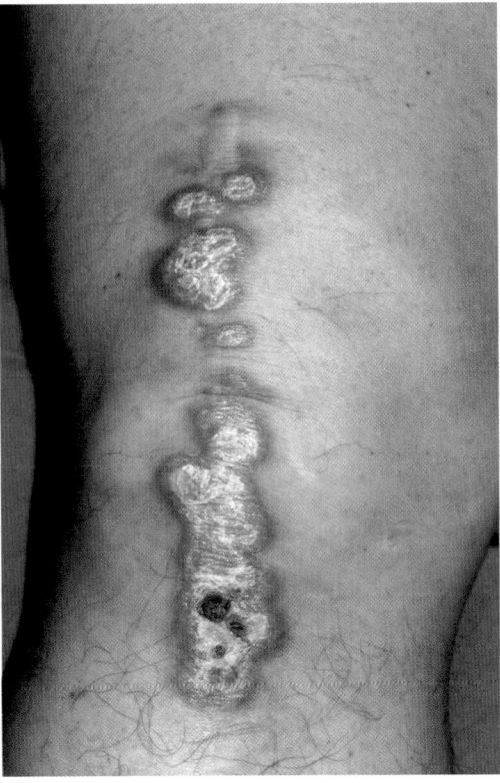

Figure 97.14 Necrobiosis lipoidica Koebnerizing in a scar from previous knee surgery.

Disease course and prognosis
Slow extension over many years is usual, but long periods of quiescence, or resolution with variable atrophy and scarring may occur (Figure 97.16).

Investigations
Skin biopsy is not usually necessary except in atypical cases. Annual screening for diabetes is recommended.

Management
The response of necrobiosis lipoidica to therapeutic intervention is generally disappointing. Many treatments have been reported to be effective but there are virtually no controlled trials and no

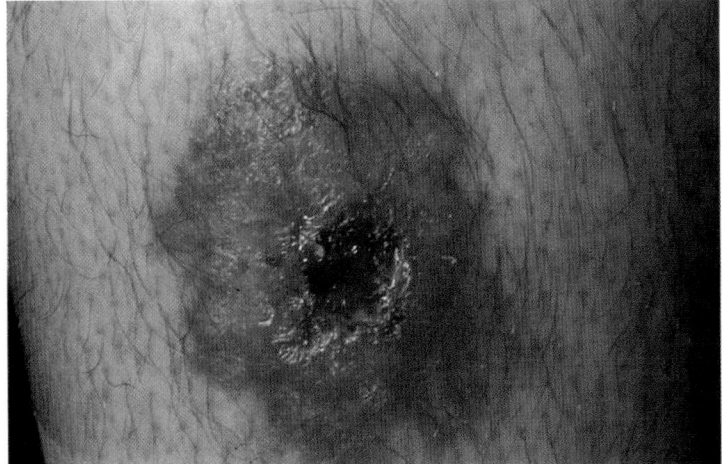

Figure 97.15 Ulcerated necrobiosis lipoidica in a 34-year-old woman with diabetes.

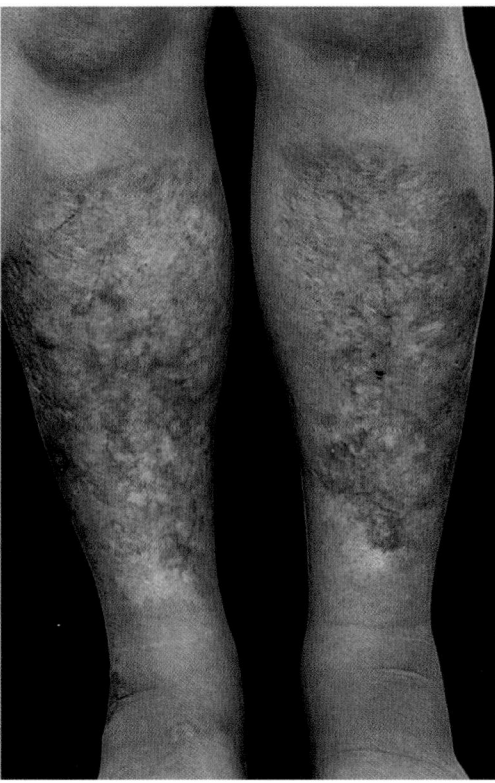

Figure 97.16 'Burnt out' necrobiosis lipoidica – marked atrophy is evident.

convincing evidence that any intervention significantly alters the course of the disease.

Potent topical corticosteroids, particularly if applied beneath an occlusive dressing and changed weekly may help [70]. Locally injected triamcinolone delivered by needle or jet injector [71] can improve the appearance, but atrophy usually remains. As there is evidence of extension of the inflammatory infiltrate into apparently normal skin surrounding active lesions, the injection of steroids into perilesional areas has been advocated to help limit progression [72]. The use of oral steroids may be of benefit [73,74]. Petzelbauer *et al.* [74] employed short-course steroid therapy that resulted in cessation of disease activity in all six patients treated and no recurrence in a mean follow-up period of 7 months.

There are reports of benefit from PUVA [75–81], topical tacrolimus [82], fumaric acid esters [83], thalidomide [84], chloroquine [85], photodynamic therapy [86], a combination of split-thickness autografting and immunomodulatory therapy [87] and etanercept [88]. The response to UVA1 phototherapy has been mixed [89].

Other treatments that have been advocated in the past include fibrinolytic agents [90], high-dose nicotinamide [91], clofazimine [92], pentoxifylline [93–96], tretinoin (0.05%) [97], prostaglandin E1 [98,99] and aspirin or an aspirin/dipyridamole combination [100–102]. Aspirin alone was subsequently shown to be ineffective [103,104] and, in a randomized double-blind comparison with placebo, patients treated with an aspirin/dipyridamole combination did not show any significant improvement [105].

Pulsed dye laser has been employed and may improve the telangiectatic and erythematous components [106] but skin breakdown can occur [107].

Ulcerated necrobiosis lipoidica has been treated by excision and grafting [108–110], although recurrence tends to occur unless the excision is deep [110]. Other treatments that have been advocated for this problem include oral steroids [111], ciclosporin [112–114], mycophenolate mofetil [115], topical granulocyte–macrophage colony-stimulating factor [116,117], infliximab [118], intravenous immunoglobulin [119], hyperbaric oxygen [120,121], topically applied bovine collagen [122] and grafting with bioengineered dermal tissue [5,124].

Treatment ladder

First line
- No treatment
- Topical steroids
- Intralesional steroids
- Topical tacrolimus

Second line
- PUVA
- UVA1

Third line
- Multiple therapies of uncertain value

Resources

Patient resources

British Association of Dermatologists, patient information leaflet: http://www.bad.org.uk/for-the-public/patient-information-leaflets/necrobiosis-lipoidica/.

Changing Faces: The Squire Centre, 33–37 University Street, London WC1E 6JN; www.changingfaces.org.uk.

DermNet NZ, necrobiosis lipoidica: http://dermnetnz.org/dermal-infiltrative/necrobiosis-lipoidica.html.

(All last accessed May 2015.)

Cutaneous Crohn disease

Definition and nomenclature

This is a granulomatous inflammation of the skin in patients with underlying Crohn disease.

Synonyms and inclusions
- Granulomatous cheilitis
- Oro-facial granulomatosis
- Metastatic Crohn disease

Introduction and general description

Cutaneous disease is common in patients with Crohn disease but manifests most commonly as reactive disorders such as erythema nodosum and pyoderma gangrenosum (see Chapter 49) or from the effects on the skin of nutritional deficiency (see Chapter 63).

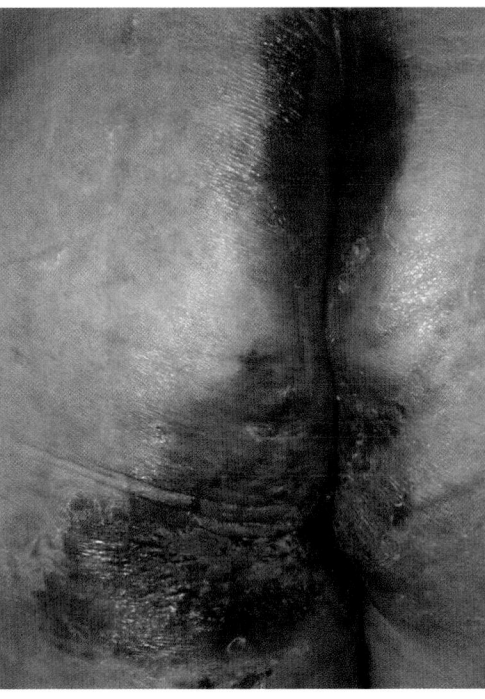

Figure 97.17 Severe perianal Crohn disease.

Granulomatous involvement of the skin may occur by extension of Crohn disease particularly in the lips, perineum, umbilicus and at the sites of surgery or around a stoma. It is characterized by sinuses, abscesses and induration (Figure 97.17) (see Chapter 152). It is usually seen in the presence of active underlying Crohn disease but may predate its diagnosis, particularly in children [1].

Oro-facial granulomatosis (Figure 97.18) may be associated with sarcoidosis or food allergy or be part of the Melkersson–Rosenthal syndrome (see Chapter 110). When isolated, it is regarded by many as a localized form of Crohn disease. It may predate intestinal Crohn disease by many years.

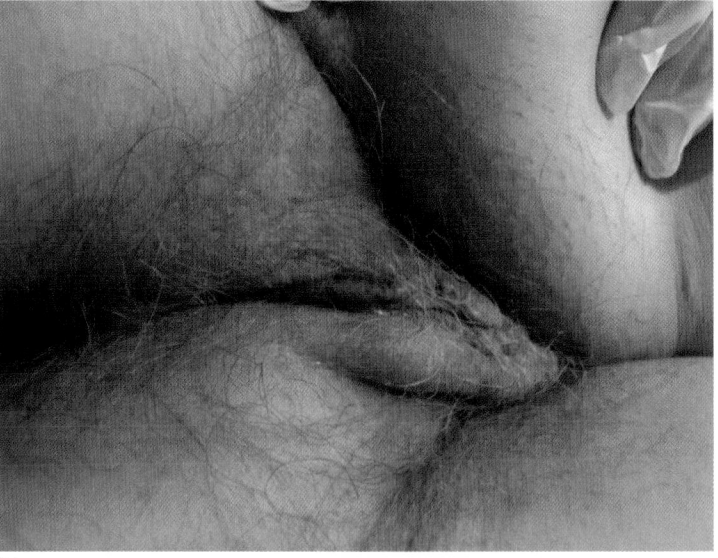

(a)

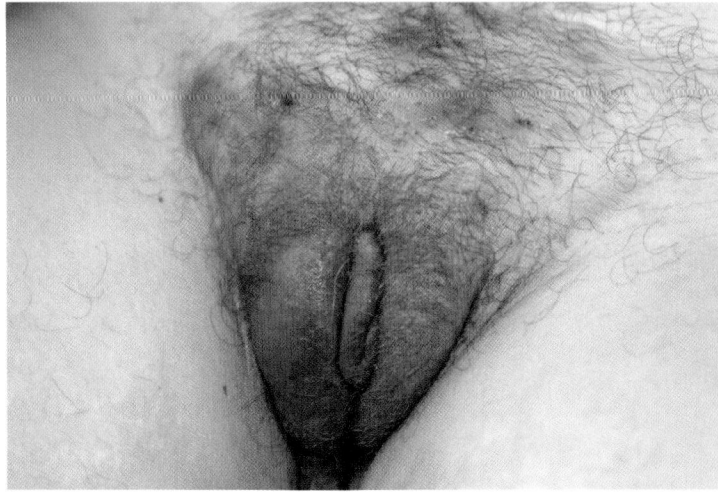

(b)

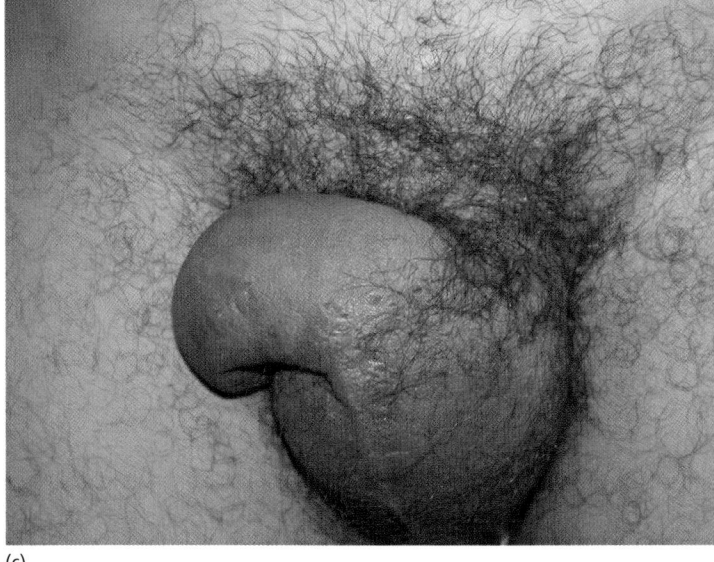

(c)

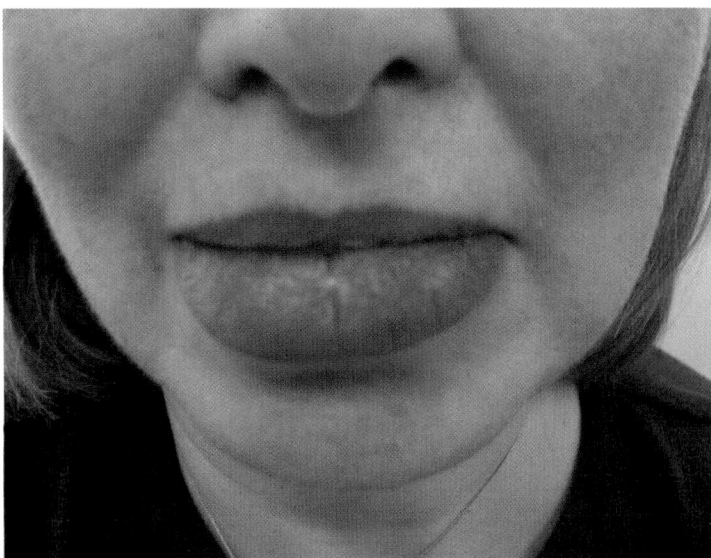

Figure 97.18 Lip swelling due to oro-facial granulomatosis developed in this patient some 5 years before she presented with severe intestinal Crohn disease. (Courtesy of Dr E. P. Burova, Bedford Hospital, UK.)

Figure 97.19 (a) Vulval swelling due to Crohn disease presented in the same patient as shown in Figure 97.18 about 1 year after she developed intestinal Crohn disease. (b) More advanced Crohn disease affecting the mons pubis and vulva; this developed 2 years after presentation with intestinal Crohn disease. (c) Peno-scrotal lymphoedema that presented together with perianal fistulae 5 years after the onset of intestinal Crohn disease. (Part a, courtesy of Dr E. P. Burova, Bedford Hospital, UK; c and d, courtesy of Professor L. Requena, Universidad Autónoma de Madrid, Spain.)

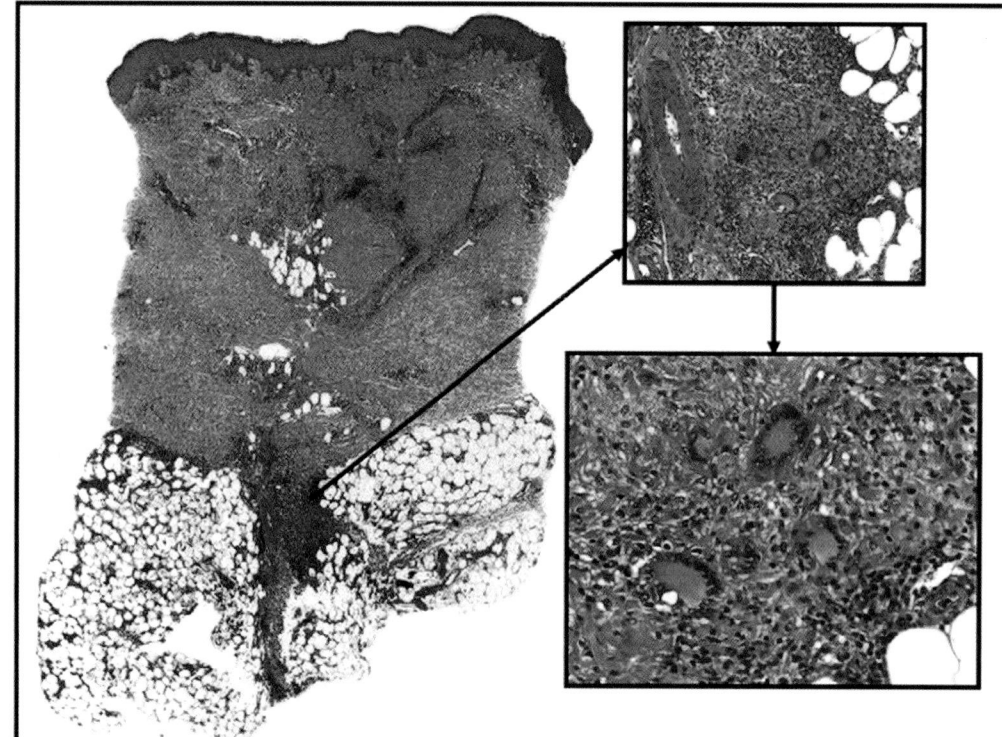

Figure 97.20 Cutaneous Crohn disease showing superficial and deep perivascular dermal infiltrates and a predominantly septal panniculitis. At higher magnification the granulomatous nature of the infiltrate involving the connective tissue septa of the subcutis is clearly evident, with granulomas composed of epithelioid histiocytes and multinucleated giant cells arranged in a perivascular fashion. (Courtesy of Professor L. Requena, Universidad Autónoma de Madrid, Spain.)

The skin may also rarely be involved at distant sites, sometimes called metastatic Crohn disease. The presentation is variable with ulcers, nodules, plaques, papules, pustules or abscesses. It has been reported at many body sites including the face, ears, nipples, palms, soles, lower limbs and abdomen [2]. Involvement of the perineum and genitalia without direct extension is sometimes considered in this category. This may present with oedema and swelling of the perineum and/or genitalia (Figure 97.19). Several deep biopsies may be needed to confirm the diagnosis (Figure 97.20).

Treatment of cutaneous Crohn disease is usually dictated by the severity of the intestinal involvement. For localized disease, topical tacrolimus has been reported to be of benefit [3] although systemic treatment along similar lines to that used in intestinal disease is likely to be necessary for satisfactory resolution. There is no consistent relationship between the appearance of skin lesions and the severity of the intestinal disease, and treatment of the intestinal disease does not necessarily affect the cutaneous features of Crohn disease [4,5].

Key references

The full list of references can be found in the online version at www.rooksdermatology.com.

Granuloma annulare

1 Wells RS, Smith MA: The natural history of granuloma annulare. *Br J Dermatol* 1963;75:199–205.

2 Thornsberry LA, English JC, 3rd. Etiology, diagnosis, and therapeutic management of granuloma annulare: an update. *Am J Clin Dermatol* 2013;14(4): 279–90.
5 Dabski K, Winkelmann RK. Generalized granuloma annulare: histopathology and immunopathology. Systematic review of 100 cases and comparison with localized granuloma annulare. *J Am Acad Dermatol* 1989;20:28–39.
6 Dabski K, Winkelmann RK. Generalized granuloma annulare: clinical and laboratory findings in 100 patients. *J Am Acad Dermatol* 1989;20:39–47.
8 Muhlbauer JE. Granuloma annulare. *J Am Acad Dermatol* 1980;3:217–30.
11 Cox NH. Diabetes and the skin: an update for dermatologists. *Expert Rev Dermatol* 2007;2:305–16.
31 Hawryluk EB, Izikson L, English JC, 3rd. Non-infectious granulomatous diseases of the skin and their associated systemic diseases: an evidence-based update to important clinical questions. *Am J Clin Dermatol* 2010;11(3):171–81.
112 Dahl MV. Speculations on the pathogenesis of granuloma annulare. *Australas J Dermatol* 1985;26:49–57.
248 Browne F, Turner D, Goulden V. Psoralen and ultraviolet A in the treatment of granuloma annulare. *Photodermatol Photoimmunol Photomed* 2011;27:81–4.

Necrobiosis lipoidica

1 Muller SA, Winkelmann RK. Necrobiosis lipoidica diabeticorum. A clinical and pathological investigation of 171 cases. *Arch Dermatol* 1966;93:272–81.
4 Reid SD, Ladzinski B, Lee K, Baibergenova A, Alavi A. Update on necrobiosis lipoidica: a review of etiology, diagnosis, and treatment options. *J Am Acad Dermatol* 2013;69:783–91.
5 O'Toole EA, Kennedy U, Nolan JJ, *et al.* Necrobiosis lipoidica: only a minority of patients have diabetes mellitus. *Br J Dermatol* 1999;140:283–6.
6 Boulton AJM, Cutfield RG, Abouganem D, *et al.* Necrobiosis lipoidica diabeticorum: a clinicopathologic study. *J Am Acad Dermatol* 1988;18:530–7.

Cutaneous Crohn disease

1 Keiler S, Tyson P, Tamburro J. Metastatic cutaneous Crohn's disease in children: case report and review of the literature *Pediatr Dermatol* 2009;26(5):604–9.

CHAPTER 98

Sarcoidosis

Joaquim Marcoval[1] *and Juan Mañá*[2]

[1]Department of Dermatology, Bellvitge University Hospital, Barcelona University, Barcelona, Spain
[2]Department of Internal Medicine, Bellvitge University Hospital, Barcelona University, Barcelona, Spain

Definition

Sarcoidosis is an antigen-mediated disease of unknown aetiology characterized by the presence of non-caseating epithelioid cell granulomas in multiple organs. It involves mainly the lungs, mediastinal and peripheral lymph nodes, eyes and skin. Less frequent but usually severe manifestations can occur in the liver, spleen, central nervous system, heart, upper respiratory tract and bones. Cutaneous lesions of sarcoidosis may be specific, showing histopathologically sarcoid granulomas, or non-specific, mainly erythema nodosum (EN). Cutaneous lesions are frequently the presentation of the disease and skin biopsy enables early diagnosis. Moreover, some types of lesions have prognostic significance and may help to predict the outcome of the systemic disease.

Introduction and general description

Sarcoidosis is a multisystem granulomatous disease of unknown aetiology that mainly involves the lungs, mediastinal and peripheral lymph nodes, eyes and skin. Cutaneous involvement in sarcoidosis is important for several reasons. Skin involvement may be the presenting sign of systemic sarcoidosis. Skin biopsy is easy to perform, enabling early diagnosis with a minor invasive procedure. Some types of cutaneous sarcoidosis have prognostic significance and may help to predict the outcome of the systemic disease. Although cutaneous sarcoidosis almost never causes significant morbidity or mortality, it may be grossly disfiguring and have a strong psychosocial impact.

Epidemiology

Incidence and prevalence
The incidence of sarcoidosis varies widely throughout the world [1,2]. Sarcoidosis seems to be most prevalent in developed countries, ranging from 10 to 40 per 100 000 in the US and Europe [3].

Age
Sarcoidosis occurs more frequently between 20 and 40 years. There is a second peak of incidence around the age of 60. It is less common in the elderly and rare in children [4].

Rook's Textbook of Dermatology, Ninth Edition. Edited by Christopher Griffiths, Jonathan Barker, Tanya Bleiker, Robert Chalmers and Daniel Creamer.
© 2016 John Wiley & Sons, Ltd. Published 2016 by John Wiley & Sons, Ltd.
Companion website: www.rooksdermatology.com

Sex

Sarcoidosis is slightly more common in women than men. In the subpopulation with Löfgren syndrome there is a clear predominance in women [3,5,6].

Ethnicity

In the US, sarcoidosis has been shown to be particularly common in African Americans, with reported incidence rates between 3 and 17 times higher in that population than in white people. Some studies have detected a high prevalence in Scandinavians, in Puerto Ricans in New York and in Irish immigrants in England [2,3]. There is also a significant heterogeneity in disease presentation and course. African Americans and Indians have been shown to have more severe and chronic disease than their white counterparts [7,8], while asymptomatic disease and Löfgren syndrome are more common in white people [9].

Associated diseases

An increased risk of developing lymphoproliferative diseases [10], mainly Hodgkin lymphoma, has been reported in sarcoidosis [11]. The relationship between sarcoidosis and solid tumours is less clear-cut [12,13], although it has been suggested that immunological abnormalities mediated by sarcoidosis or the effects of treatment may increase the risk [14,15]. Several case reports have described the concomitant association of sarcoidosis with a number of autoimmune diseases, including Sjögren syndrome, systemic sclerosis, rheumatoid arthritis, vasculitis, psoriasis, autoimmune chronic hepatitis and primary biliary cirrhosis [16–19]. Autoimmune thyroid disease, particularly Graves disease and Hashimoto thyroiditis, has been associated with sarcoidosis as well [20–22].

Pathophysiology

Pathology

The histopathological changes are similar in all organs affected by sarcoidosis [23]. The cardinal feature is the sarcoid granuloma, defined as aggregates of epithelioid cells with a sparse lymphocytic component [23,24], the so-called 'naked granuloma' (Figure 98.1a,b) [23,25,26]. In the skin, sarcoid granulomas are usually observed in the dermis but can also extend to subcutaneous tissue. There is no particular relation to skin appendages, although in some cases linear granulomas may follow dermal nerves [27]. Granulomas usually contain few or no giant cells, generally of Langhans type, that tend to be more abundant in old lesions (Figure 98.1c) [25]. In some cases, tuberculoid granulomas (non-caseating granulomas with lymphoid cuff >25% of the granuloma diameter) are also observed [27,28]. Although caseous necrosis is typically absent [23,29], discrete foci of fibrinoid or coagulation necrosis can be detected [27,30,31]. Palisading necrobiotic granulomas are rarely observed [27,32].

Although it is considered that the epidermis is usually normal, 49 of 62 cases in a series displayed epidermal abnormalities [33].

Lichenoid changes [27] and transepidermal elimination have also been reported [27,32,34]. In subcutaneous sarcoidosis, the granulomatous infiltrate is limited to subcutaneous tissue (Figure 98.1d) [35,36]. It is predominantly lobular with minimal or no septal involvement, appearing as a lobular panniculitis [36], sometimes with intense fibrosis [37,38].

Giant cells can contain inclusion bodies. Schaumann bodies are basophilic, round or oval concentric, lamellar structures composed of lipomucoglycoproteins impregnated with calcium and iron [25,39]. Asteroid bodies are considered to be formed from trapped collagen bundles and have an eosinophilic central body surrounded by radiating spicules giving the impression of an open umbrella (Figure 98.2a) [40]. None of these bodies is specific to sarcoidosis; they have been observed in other granulomatous processes such as tuberculosis, leprosy, Crohn disease and berylliosis [23,24,41]. Polarizable foreign bodies (Figure 98.2a,b) are observed in 22–50% of cutaneous sarcoidosis [27,31,42,43], suggesting that foreign bodies may be an inciting stimulus for granuloma formation in sarcoidosis [42,44].

CD4 helper/inducer T lymphocytes are present at the centre of the granuloma and a smaller population of CD8 suppressor/cytotoxic T lymphocytes at the periphery [45]. Immunofluorescence studies have shown, in some cases, immunoglobulin M (IgM) within blood vessel walls and at the dermal–epidermal junction, and IgG within and around the granuloma [46].

Histological differential diagnosis

Lupus vulgaris may be difficult to differentiate but usually shows a marked lymphocytic infiltrate around granulomas and significant central necrosis [25]. Tuberculous leprosy granulomas follow nerves and therefore appear elongated and show small areas of central necrosis more often than sarcoidosis [25]. In sarcoidosis the nerves are intact and stains for acid–fast bacilli are negative [27]. Rosacea granulomas are usually perifollicular [25]. Lupoid leishmaniasis, granulomatous cheilitis, Crohn disease and orofacial granulomatosis (see Chapter 110) may also pose difficulties. Plasma cells and coagulative necrosis are features of syphilis [39]. Foreign-body granulomas can also resemble sarcoidosis. The presence of polarizable foreign bodies does not exclude sarcoidosis. Moreover, an exaggerated response to foreign bodies, coexistence with other types of skin lesions of sarcoidosis and the involvement of other organs favours sarcoidosis.

EN associated with sarcoidosis shows the same histological appearance as idiopathic EN [25].

Immunopathogenesis

Bronchoalveolar lavage fluid from patients with pulmonary sarcoidosis shows an increase in CD4+ T cells [47–50]. These activated CD4+ T cells secrete interleukin 2, interferon γ (IFN-γ), interleukin 12 and tumour necrosis factor (TNF)-α, characteristic of the Th1 phenotype [51–53]. IFN-γ activates macrophages and induces transformation into giant cells while TNF-α induces its differentiation into epithelioid cells [54]. Macrophages also release IFN-γ, TNF-α, and chemokines such as CXCL10, attracting additional T cells of CD4/TH1 phenotype [55,56]. It is

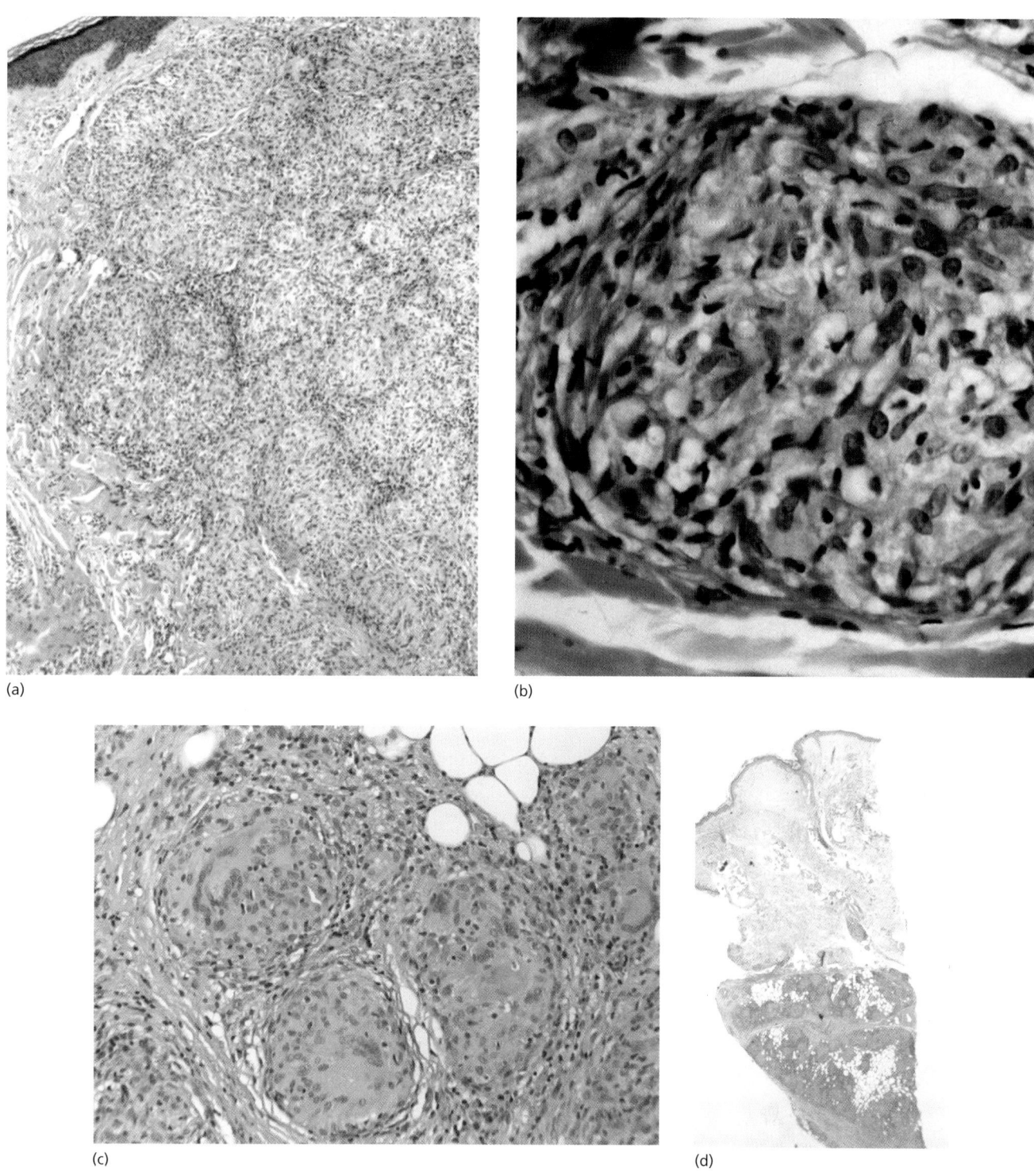

Figure 98.1 (a) Sarcoid granulomas in the dermis in a specific cutaneous lesion of sarcoidosis. (b) Sarcoid granulomas are mainly composed of epithelioid cells with sparse lymphocytic component, without necrosis. (c) Sarcoid granulomas with prominent giant cells. (d) Low-power view of subcutaneous sarcoidosis. The granulomatous infiltrate is limited to the subcutis and is mainly lobular with the appearance of a granulomatous lobular panniculitis.

postulated that IFN-γ inhibits apoptosis in macrophages through the expression of high levels of P21, which leads to granuloma perpetuation [57]. TNF-α is considered the main cytokine in the development and maintenance of the granuloma [58,59], and it is considered the cause of pulmonary fibrosis by stimulating fibroblast proliferation and collagen synthesis [60]. For these reasons, it was considered that anti-TNF-α agents might be beneficial in sarcoidosis. However, the results of clinical trials are conflicting [61] and cases of sarcoidosis induced by TNF-α inhibitors are being reported [62].

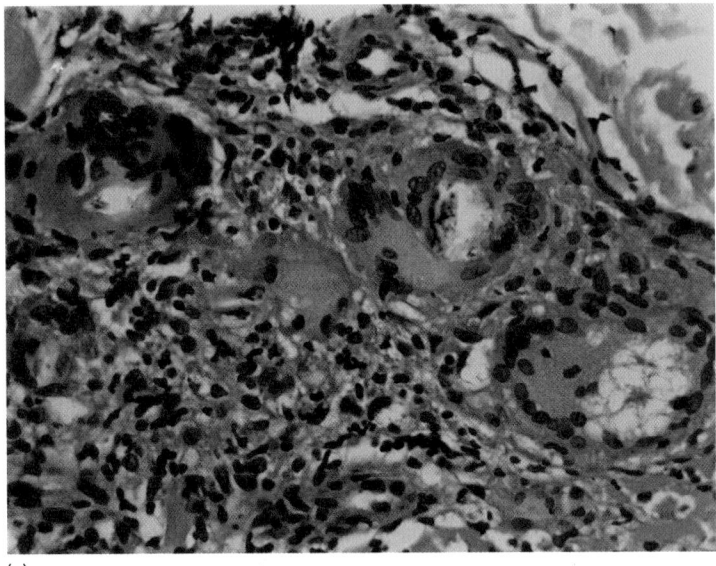

(a)

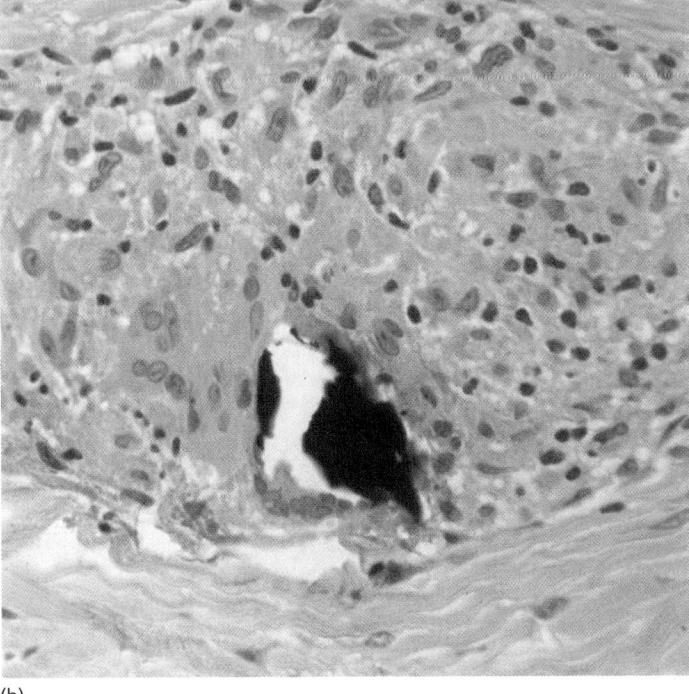

(b)

Figure 98.2 (a) An incipient asteroid body and two foreign bodies in a sarcoid granuloma. (b) A foreign body is observed in a sarcoid granuloma.

Multiple cases of sarcoidosis have been reported in association with IFN-α for hepatitis C but also for melanoma [13,63–69]. It has been suggested that IFN-α increases IFN-γ and interleukin 2, promoting granuloma formation [64,66,70]. IFN-α-induced sarcoidosis develops at a mean interval of 5.4 months after starting the drug [71] and frequently shows cutaneous involvement (60%) [66]. More than 85% of cases follow a benign course and therapy does not need to be stopped [66,72].

Causative organisms

Histopathological similarities with tuberculosis led to extensive evaluation of *Mycobacterium tuberculosis* as a possible aetiologi-

cal factor. Mycobaterial mycolic acid and fatty acids and antibodies against mycobacteria have been detected in sarcoidosis patients, although more recent work has not confirmed such findings [73–76]. Similarly, the isolation of acid–fast L forms from the blood of patients with sarcoidosis has been reported but later studies failed to observe differences with control subjects [77,78]. The presence of mycobacterial DNA/RNA has been reported in 0–80% of patients with sarcoidosis [79–100]. Recently, *M. tuberculosis* catalase–peroxidase was detected in tissue samples of sarcoidosis [101,102]. However, the absence of caseation necrosis, the negativity of purified protein derivative (PPD), and the lack of response to antituberculous treatment are arguments against mycobacterial involvement in sarcoidosis [100].

Propionibacterium acnes has been isolated from bronchial lavage in pulmonary sarcoidosis and DNA of *Propionibacterium* has also been detected [94,98,103]. However, it is known that *P. acnes* is a commensal in peripheral lung tissues and its presence does not appear to be specific for sarcoidosis [94,98,104]. Other infectious agents proposed by some studies but denied by others include *Rickettsia helvetica* [105,106], *Chlamydia pneumoniae* [107,108], *Borrelia burgdorferi* [109–112] , herpesvirus 8 [113–116] and Epstein–Barr virus [100]. Histoplasmosis and other fungi, which can produce sarcoid granulomas, have also been suspected as possible causes, but geographical limitations rule them out [39].

Genetics

A positive family history of sarcoidosis ranges from 2.7 to 17% [55] and having a first-degree relative with sarcoidosis increases the risk of disease fivefold [117]. The risk of developing sarcoidosis in the co-twin of an affected monozygotic brother was increased 80-fold while in dizygotic twins the risk was only sevenfold higher [118]. However, sarcoidosis is not a disease of a single gene.

The first reported association with specific gene products was the association between class I human leucocyte antigen (HLA)-B8 antigens and acute sarcoidosis [119]. Later, HLA class II antigens were also related to sarcoidosis. The HLA-DR allele DRB1*1101 was significantly associated with sarcoidosis development in both African Americans and white people [120]. Other HLA genotypes predispose to the disease phenotype rather than to susceptibility. For example, HLA-DQB1*0201 and HLA-DRB1*0301 are strongly associated with acute disease and good prognosis [121–123]. Genome-wide scanning for sarcoidosis susceptibility genes has identified several genes associated with increased susceptibility to the disease such as the butyrophilin-like 2 gene and annexin A11 [124–127]. In recent years, other genes have also been implicated [56]. However, the known genetic associations are not yet sufficient to calculate genetic risk profiles in sarcoidosis [55].

Environmental factors

Several environmental agents (e.g. beryllium) may induce sarcoid granulomas [128]. For this reason and the tendency for sarcoidosis to involve organs exposed to the environment such as the lung, eyes and skin, an environmental cause for sarcoidosis has been suspected. Seasonal outbreaks of sarcoidosis also support this possibility [129–133]. Multiple environmental agents have been reported to confer increased risk of sarcoidosis, including exposure to tree pollen [134], inorganic particles [135], insecticides [136] and moulds [136,137]. Occupational studies have shown associations with US Navy personnel [138], metalworking [137], fire-fighters [139] and the handling of building supplies [140]. Also of interest is the fact that following the World Trade Center disaster, New York City fire-fighters developed 'sarcoid-like' granulomatous pulmonary disease at significantly higher than normal rates [141]. However, no single infectious or environmental agent, nor any genetic locus, has been clearly implicated in the pathogenesis of the disease [136].

Clinical features

Systemic manifestations of sarcoidosis

Not infrequently, sarcoidosis is discovered by chance on a chest radiograph. The clinical onset of sarcoidosis may be acute or insidious. Acute or subacute sarcoidosis develops over a period of weeks or a few months and it usually heralds a good prognosis [129]. It is characterized by mild constitutional symptoms such as fatigue, malaise, anorexia, weight loss, low-grade fever, arthralgia and respiratory symptoms. An insidious onset for several months is usually associated with respiratory complaints without constitutional symptoms, or with symptoms referable to organs other than the lung. It correlates with a chronic course and permanent organ damage [7,142,143].

Pulmonary sarcoidosis

Intrathoracic involvement occurs in 90% of cases. Patients may be asymptomatic or may present with dry cough and dyspnoea on exercise. Haemoptysis is rare. Pulmonary sarcoidosis is classically divided into four stages on the basis of the chest radiograph (Table 98.1). Figure 98.3 shows a stage II chest radiograph.

Table 98.1 Chest radiograph stages in pulmonary sarcoidosis.[a]

Chest radiograph stages	% at onset	% with resolution
Stage 0: normal chest radiograph	<10	–
Stage I: bilateral hilar lymphadenopathy without pulmonary involvement	50	60–90 (<10% progress to pulmonary involvement)
Stage II: bilateral hilar lymphadenopathy with pulmonary involvement	30	40–70
Stage III[b]: pulmonary involvement without bilateral hilar lymphadenopathy	10–15	<10–20

From Hunninghake et al. 1999 [3] © American Thoracic Society.
[a]Classification based on chest radiograph. Although high-resolution CT may suggest a different stage, it is not necessary to change the criteria since this test is indicated only in a limited number of patients.
[b]Stage III may be subclassified into stage IV, which includes cases with advanced pulmonary fibrosis (hilar retraction, coarse linear opacities, honeycombing, bullae, emphysematous changes, architectural distortion and pulmonary hypertension).

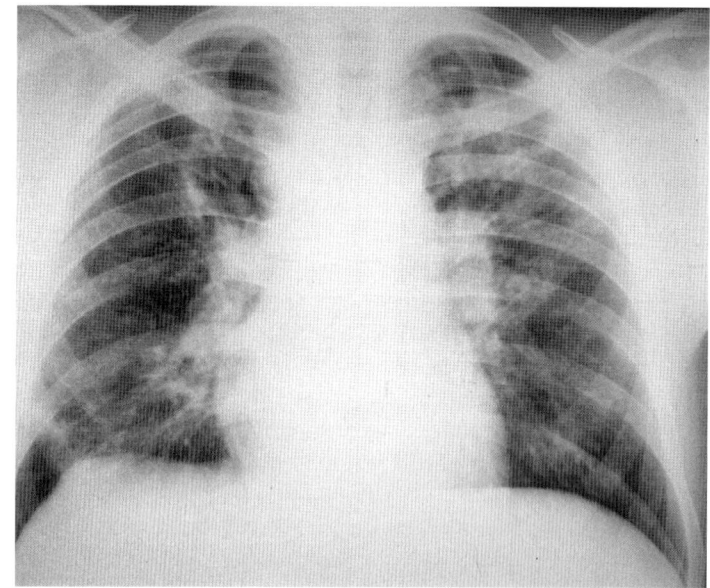

Figure 98.3 Chest radiograph showing stage II pulmonary sarcoidosis (bilateral and right paratracheal lympadenopathy and pulmonary infiltrates with upper and middle lobe predominance).

Atypical radiological findings include large nodules, alveolar infiltrates, hilar calcification, pleural effusion and pneumothorax [144,145]. Sarcoidosis-associated pulmonary hypertension is typically seen in advanced cases, with pulmonary fibrosis, destruction and obliteration of the pulmonary vasculature, and chronic hypoxaemia [146–148].

Extrapulmonary sarcoidosis

Eye. Ocular involvement occurs in 15–20% of patients. Since it may be asymptomatic, slit-lamp and ophthalmoscopic examinations should be performed on every patient with sarcoidosis [149]. The most frequent findings are anterior or posterior uveitis, chorioretinitis, periphlebitis, papilloedema and retinal haemorrhage. Conjunctival follicles, lacrimal gland involvement and keratoconjunctivitis sicca may be present as well [150–154]. Secondary glaucoma, cataract formation and blindness are late complications in untreated cases [155].

Reticuloendothelial system. Peripheral lymphadenopathy involving the cervical, supraclavicular, epitrochlear, axillary and inguinal nodes may be present. In addition to intrathoracic nodes, mesenteric chain and retroperitoneal lymph nodes may be involved. Splenic involvement is frequent, although splenomegaly occurs in only 5–10% of cases, and may result in hypersplenism and pancytopaenia [156]. Bone marrow involvement is rare [2,3].

Liver. Mild hepatomegaly with slight cholestasis occurs in 20–30% of patients. Non-caseating granulomas are present in up to 75% of liver biopsies. Hepatic sarcoidosis affects the periportal areas. Severe chronic cholestasis syndrome, portal hypertension and Budd–Chiari syndrome are rare. Multiple low-attenuation nodules in the liver on CT may be observed [157–159].

Neurosarcoidosis. Five to 10% of patients with sarcoidosis have clinically recognizable neurological involvement [2,3]. The disease has a predilection for the basal meninges, so cranial nerve involvement, particularly facial paralysis, is common. Other manifestations include aseptic meningitis, seizures, pyramidal tract signs, optic nerve dysfunction, papilloedema, hypothalamic and pituitary lesions with diabetes insipidus or hypopituitarism, and cognitive impairment [160–164]. Gadolinium-enhanced MRI may reveal non-enhancing multifocal periventricular and subcortical white matter lesions mimicking those of multiple sclerosis, meningeal enhancement, space-occupying lesions and hydrocephalus [165,166].

Musculoskeletal system. Transient or chronic polyarthralgias are common but frank arthritis is uncommon. Asymptomatic muscle involvement is also common but symptomatic diffuse or nodular myopathy is rare. Bone lesions, usually osteolytic, are not frequent and when present are located predominantly on the hands and feet [2,3].

Heart. Clinical cardiac involvement occurs in 5% of patients. Supraventricular and ventricular arrhythmias and aberrations of atrioventricular or intraventricular conduction may result in complete heart block or sudden death; papillary muscle dysfunction and congestive heart failure may be present. Cor pulmonale is usually secondary to chronic pulmonary fibrosis [167,168]. Cardiac MRI and cardiac PET scans are currently the most useful tests for the diagnosis of cardiac sarcoidosis. Endomyocardial biopsy may reveal granulomas although the diagnostic yield may be low [169,170].

Other manifestations. Parotid involvement is frequent and may produce parotid enlargement, usually bilateral, and xerostomia. Transient or persistent hypercalcaemia, and hypercalciuria, rarely with nephrocalcinosis and nephrolithiasis, may be present. This is due to an increased production of 1.25-dihydroxyvitamin D by granulomas [171]. Interstitial lymphocytic and granulomatous nephritis and renal failure have been reported [172,173]. Sarcoidosis may involve any structure of the upper respiratory tract, most frequently causing nasal stuffiness [174]. Gastrointestinal, genital, endocrine and mammary involvement are rare [2,3].

Course and prognosis. In most patients, particularly those with an acute presentation, the disease resolves spontaneously without sequelae within 2–5 years. Löfgren syndrome has an excellent prognosis. Ten to 30% of patients follow a chronic progressive course, sometimes with irreversible fibrotic changes in spite of therapy [3,129,142]. Occasionally, recurrence of sarcoidosis many years after spontaneous remission occurs, particularly in patients with Löfgren syndrome [175]. Pregnancy is not contraindicated except in severe chronic disease. However, there may be relapses after parturition. Mortality is less than 5%.

Cutaneous manifestations of sarcoidosis
Cutaneous manifestations of sarcoidosis are extremely variable and sarcoidosis is considered one of the 'great imitators' in dermatology. Cutaneous lesions of sarcoidosis are classified as specific and non-specific [176]. Specific lesions are those that histopathologically display sarcoid granulomas [176,177]. The most frequent specific lesions are maculopapules, plaques, lupus pernio, scar-sarcoidosis and subcutaneous sarcoidosis [176,177–181]. The most important non-specific lesion is EN. Cutaneous lesions of sarcoidosis are more frequent in women than in men (2 : 1) and in black people than in other ethnic groups [176].

SPECIFIC FORMS OF CUTANEOUS SARCOIDOSIS

Specific cutaneous lesions develop in 9–37% of patients with systemic sarcoidosis [7,179,182–188]. Although they can appear at any time, they are usually present at the onset of sarcoidosis and the diagnosis is frequently made by dermatologists [31,189,190]. In the initial evaluation of patients with suspected sarcoidosis the entire skin surface must be examined [177]. Because cutaneous biopsy is innocuous, it is a very useful diagnostic procedure that avoids aggressive diagnostic techniques [177] and can provide a rapid diagnosis of sarcoidosis [191].

The presence or absence of specific cutaneous lesions as a whole lacks prognostic significance in the progression of sarcoidosis [177,189,192,193]. However, some types of cutaneous lesions are associated with acute forms of sarcoidosis and others with chronic forms with a less favourable prognosis.

The clinical appearance is due to the presence of epithelioid cell granulomas in the dermis [39]. Specific lesions are red-brown or red-violaceous in colour, generally multiple, and do not cause symptoms. Diascopy reveals the subtle brown-yellow or 'apple jelly' colour characteristic of granulomatous diseases (Figure 98.4a,b) but usually more opaque than in lupus vulgaris [176]. The epidermis rarely appears clinically involved [39]. Diverse types of lesion may coexist in the same patient.

Maculopapular sarcoidosis

Macules and papules are the most common specific lesions [176,177,180,194]. This form includes patients with slightly infiltrated patches as well as those with multiple infiltrated lesions of <10 mm diameter. The lesions are yellow-brown or red-brown in colour without clinically evident epidermal changes (Figure 98.5a–c). They are usually located on the face, mainly around the eyes and in the naso-labial folds, although the occipital area of the neck, trunk, extremities and even mucous membranes may be involved [176,178,179]. They may simulate xanthelasmata, rosacea, secondary syphilis, lupus erythematosus, trichoepitheliomata, sebaceous adenoma, granuloma annulare, lichen nitidus or syringomata [195–197]. They are usually transient and appear to herald the onset of the disease [178]. In some cases papules can enlarge or coalesce to form plaques [176,198].

Maculopapular lesions often resolve either spontaneously or with treatment in less than 2 years without significant scarring. They are commonly associated with acute forms of systemic sarcoidosis such

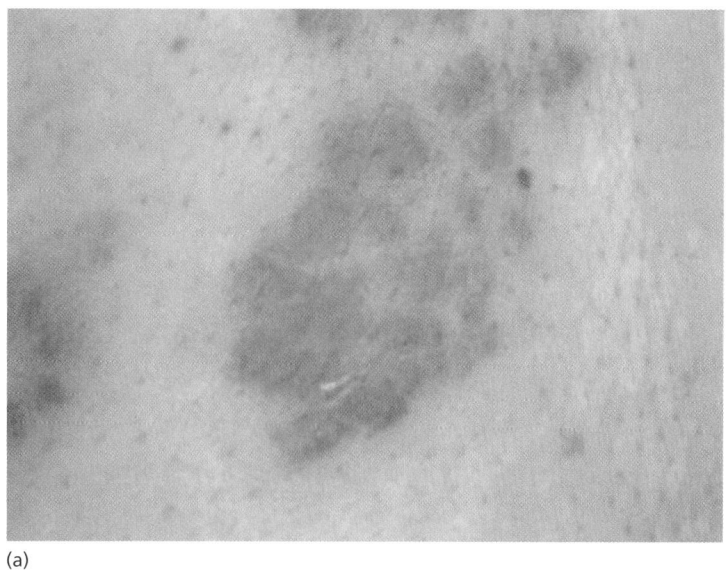

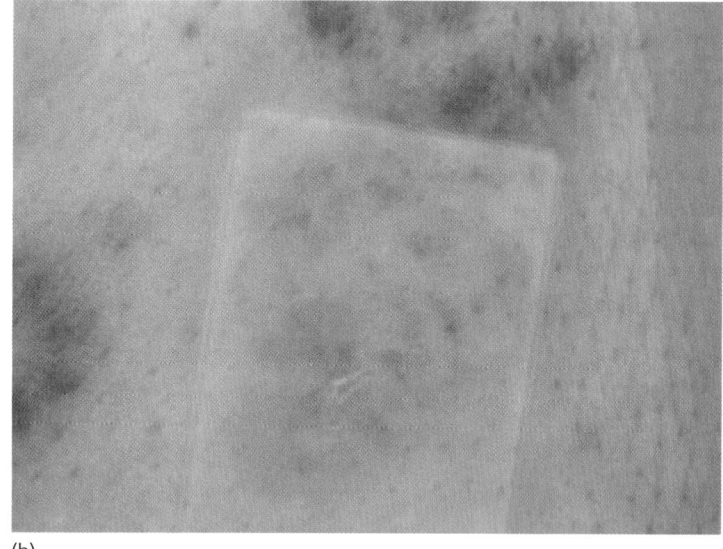

(a)   (b)

Figure 98.4 Sarcoid granulomas (a) revealed under diascopy as 'apple-jelly nodules' (b).

as hilar lymphadenopathy, EN, acute uveitis, peripheral lymph nodes and parotid enlargement [179,**193**,199]. Consequently, maculopapular sarcoidosis is associated with a more favourable prognosis than other forms of cutaneous sarcoidosis [177,**190**].

A particular type of papular lesion involving the extensor surface of the knees has been reported. The papules are grouped over the knees, frequently with a linear arrangement that confers a lichenoid appearance (Figure 98.6a,b) [200]. Polarizable foreign bodies are present in a high proportion of biopsies. These lesions are usually transient and may easily be overlooked. For this reason, the knees should always be examined when sarcoidosis is suspected [200].

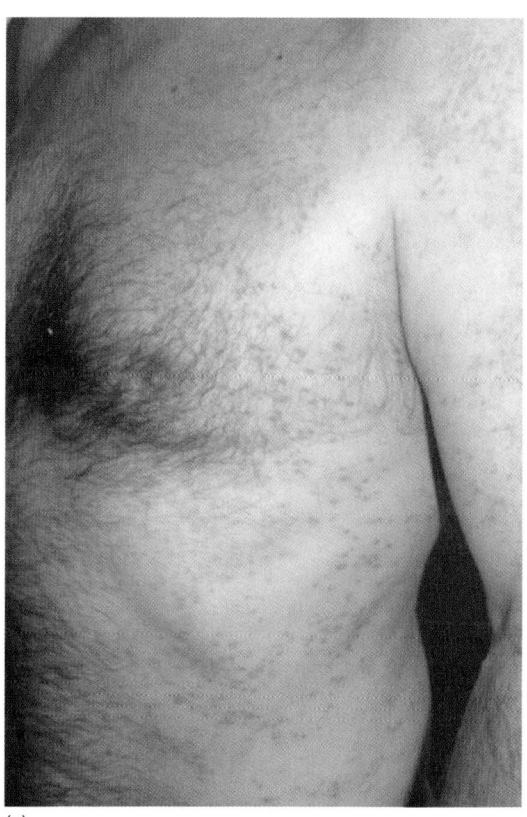

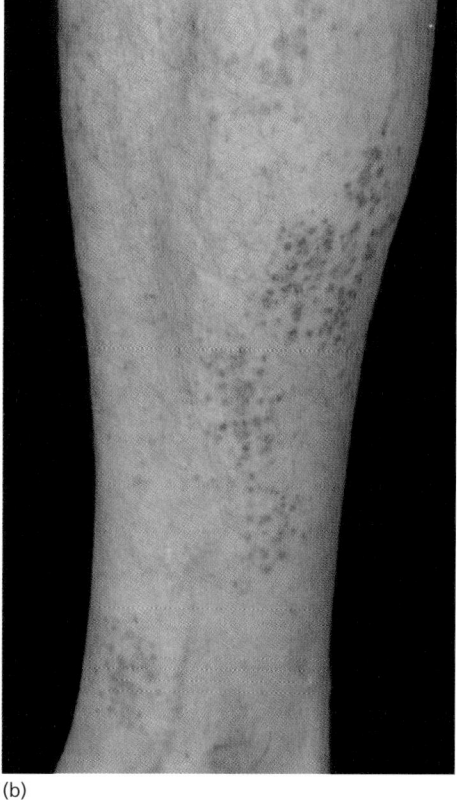

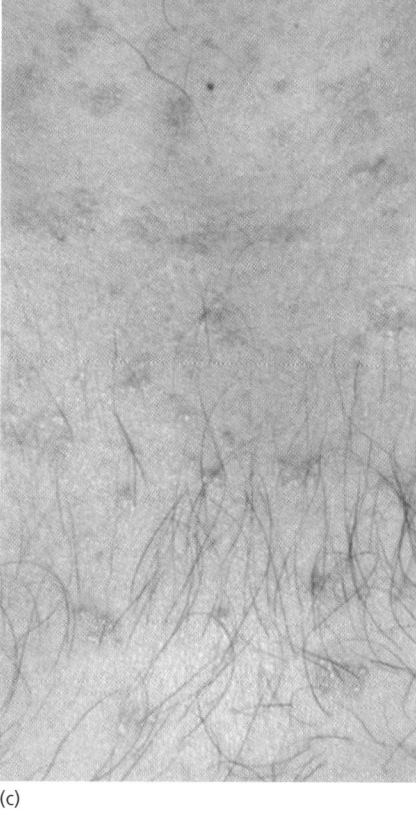

(a)   (b)   (c)

Figure 98.5 (a) Maculopapular sarcoidosis on the chest and arm. (b) Maculopapular sarcoidosis on the leg. (c) Maculopapular sarcoidosis on the pre-sternal area.

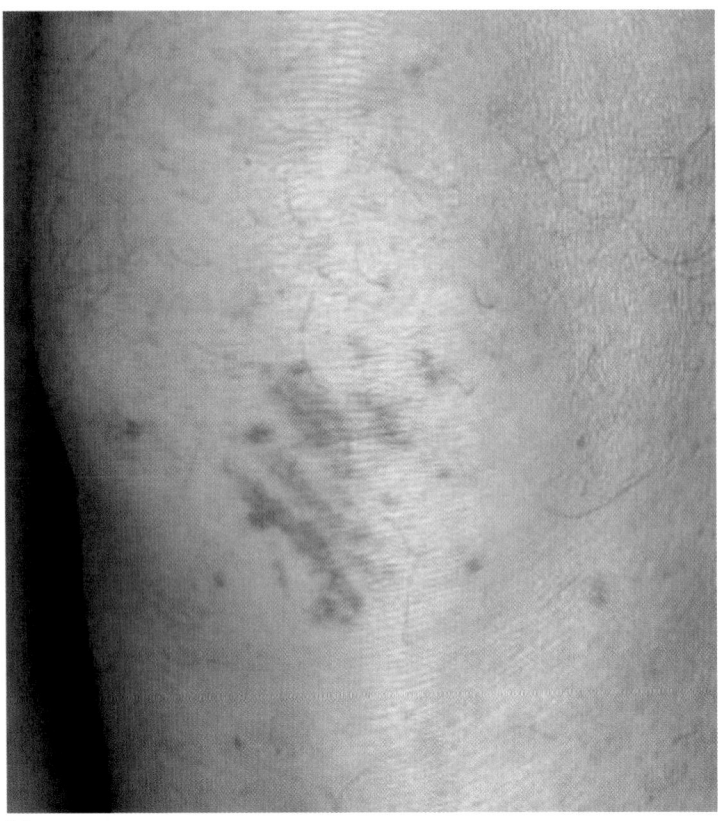

(a)   (b)

Figure 98.6 (a,b) Papular sarcoidosis of the knees.

Nodular and plaque sarcoidosis

This is almost as common as maculopapular sarcoidosis in some studies and more frequent in others [177,201]. It usually presents as multiple round or oval, infiltrated reddish-brown plaques (Figure 98.7) [176,177]. They are larger than 10 mm in diameter, tend to be thicker and more indurated and persistent than papules and are sometimes mammillated (Figure 98.8a,b). Plaques can be associated with nodular dermal lesions (Figure 98.9a,b). They can be located on the face, scalp, back, buttocks and extremities (Figure 98.10a–c) [177]. Plaques can adopt an annular appearance by means of peripheral extension and central clearing, especially on the forehead and neck [179,**193**] (Figure 98.11a,b). Plaques can simulate lupus vulgaris, necrobiosis lipoidica, morphoea, leprosy, leishmaniasis, discoid lupus erythematosus and granuloma annulare [195,202].

After treatment plaques tend to recur; when they do resolve they can leave permanent scarring [**176**,178,179,192,203]. They are associated with chronic forms of sarcoidosis including pulmonary fibrosis, peripheral lymphadenopathy, splenomegaly and chronic uveitis [177,192,193,**194**,199,204]. In patients with plaque-type lesions, the activity of the systemic disease usually persists for more than 2 years [177,**190**,**193**]. However, unlike lupus pernio, plaques are not associated with bony cysts nor with sarcoidosis of the upper respiratory tract [178].

Lupus pernio

Lupus pernio is the most distinctive manifestation of cutaneous sarcoidosis [177]. It tends to appear in older people than other forms of cutaneous sarcoidosis, and is especially frequent in black women [**3**,180,205]. In white people, incidence varies according to

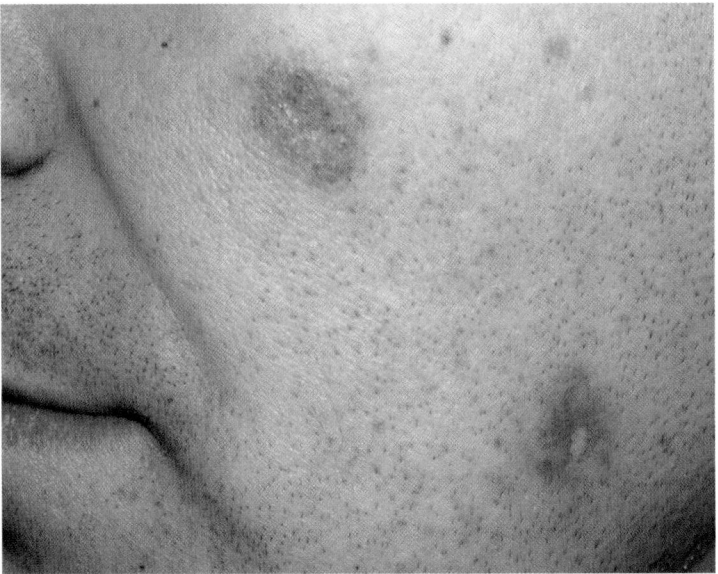

Figure 98.7 Sarcoid plaques on the cheek.

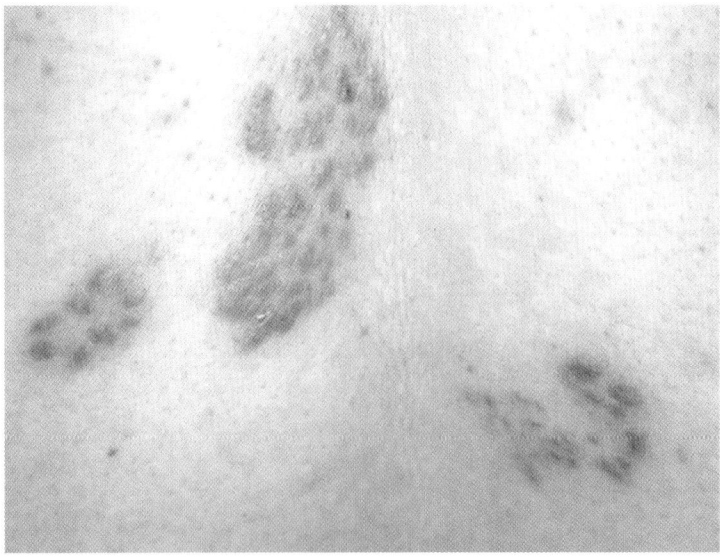

(a)

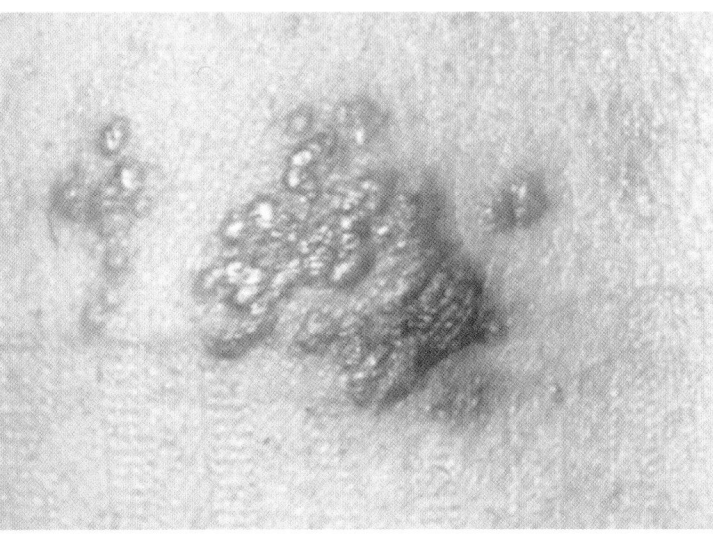

(b)

Figure 98.8 (a,b) Plaque sarcoidosis on the back.

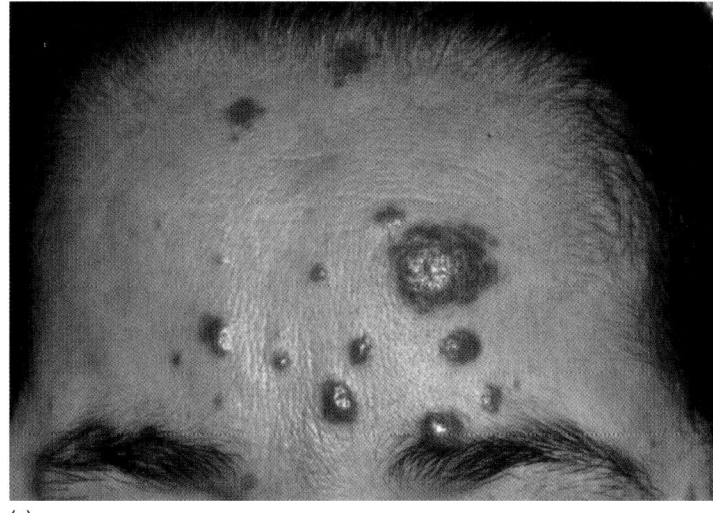

(a)

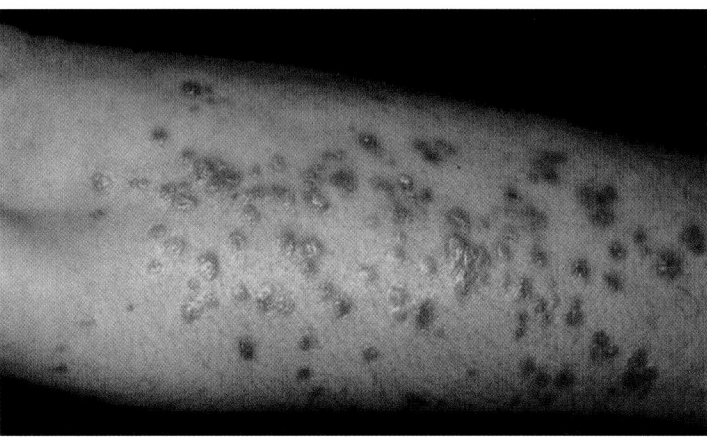

(b)

Figure 98.9 Dermal plaque and nodules on the forehead (a) and nodules on the forearm (b).

the series [**190,193**,206]. Infiltrated erythematoviolaceous plaques involve the nose, cheeks, ears, lips, forehead and fingers [39,**176**] (Figure 98.12a–c). On the cheeks, a prominent telangiectatic component is characteristic. Lupus pernio is usually painless and, as it does not tend to ulcerate [**3**], is not as mutilating as lupus vulgaris [39]. However, unlike other forms of sarcoidosis, lupus pernio can be very disfiguring [207]. It may simulate rosacea, lupus vulgaris or discoid lupus erythematosus [202].

In more than half of cases, lupus pernio is associated with sarcoidosis of the upper respiratory tract [**193**,205,208,209], especially in patients with involvement of the nasal rims [210]. It is also frequently associated with pulmonary fibrosis, chronic uveitis, and bony cysts, particularly affecting the terminal phalanges [**176**,178,205]. When the latter occur the nails are usually dystrophic [211]. Lupus pernio usually follows an extremely chronic course, ranging from 2 to 25 years in published series [178,199]. All patients with lupus pernio in a series presented active chronic disease at 2 years of follow-up [**193**].

Scar sarcoidosis

Scar sarcoidosis can involve scars resulting from surgery, trauma, acne, venepuncture, vaccination, herpes zoster or Mantoux test [39,212–214]. Tattoo sarcoidosis may be considered a variant of scar sarcoidosis [179,215–220] that may occur decades after tattooing and must be differentiated from foreign-body reactions to tattoo pigment [220]. In scar sarcoidosis, the old scars become infiltrated and erythematous and contain sarcoid granulomas histopathologically (Figure 98.13) [55]. Scar sarcoidosis has been observed in 9% of patients with cutaneous sarcoidosis [201] and is frequently located on the knees [39]. The scar infiltration tends to follow the activity of the disease [**176**,179,192,199]. Scar sarcoidosis can appear at the onset of the disease and must be looked for whenever a diagnosis of sarcoidosis is considered [39]. However, more commonly it is associated with longlasting pulmonary and mediastinal involvement, uveitis, peripheral lymphadenopathy, bony cysts and parotid infiltration [178,179,201]. It has been hypothesized that foreign material frequently present in scars can act as an antigenic stimulus for the induction of granulomas [**42**,43,212,221].

PART 8: SPECIFIC CUTANEOUS STRUCTURE

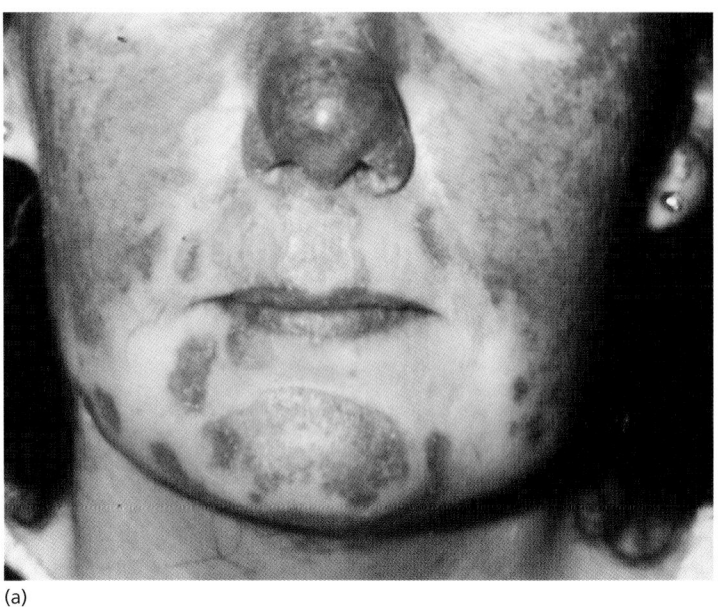

(a)

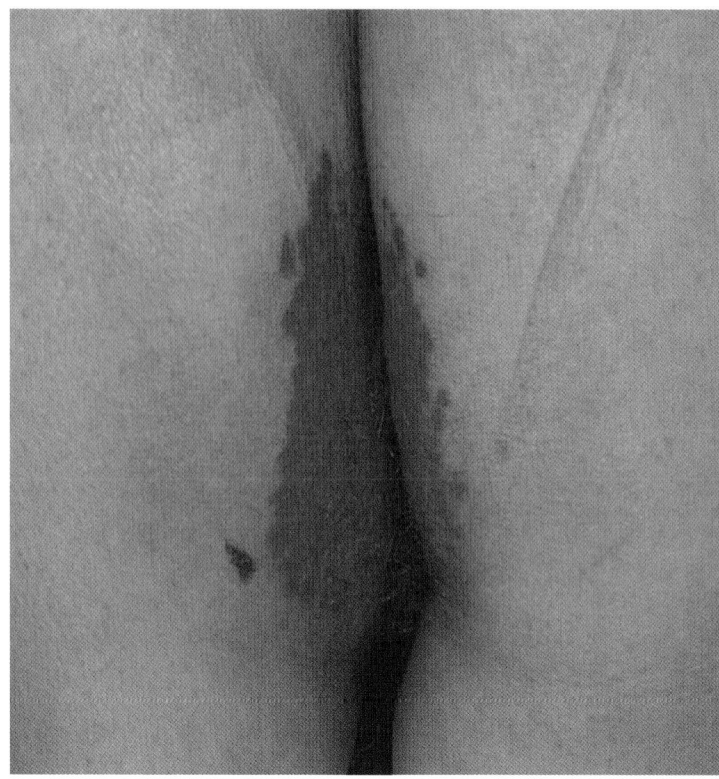

(b)

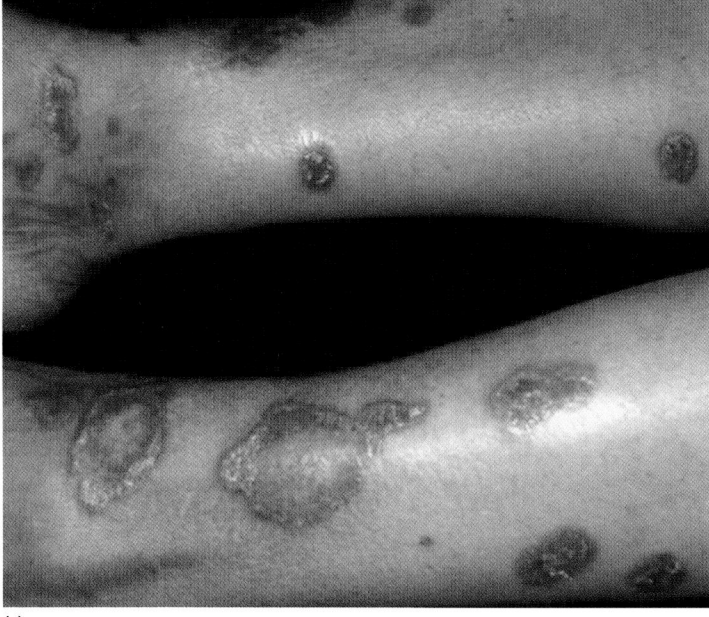

(c)

Figure 98.10 (a) Extensive coalescing plaques of sarcoidosis on the face. (b) Plaque sarcoidosis extending from perianal skin to the buttocks. (c) Plaque sarcoidosis of the lower extremities resembling necrobiosis lipoidica. (Courtesy of the copyright holder Dr J. E. Bothwell, Barnsley District General Hospital, Barnsley, UK.)

Subcutaneous sarcoidosis

In subcutaneous sarcoidosis, sarcoid granulomas are limited to subcutaneous tissue. Although minimal dermal involvement is acceptable for diagnosis [222] it must be differentiated from nodular dermal lesions with extension into subcutaneous fat [35]. It

has been observed in 1.4–6% of patients with systemic sarcoidosis [36,184,223] and represents 12% of specific cutaneous lesions [36]. Most cases occur in white women, mainly in the fifth and sixth decades of life [224]. Multiple indurated subcutaneous nodules are located principally in the extremities. The lesions are painless and covered by normal-appearing skin [**176**,177,225]. Some studies highlight that in most patients the lesions involve the

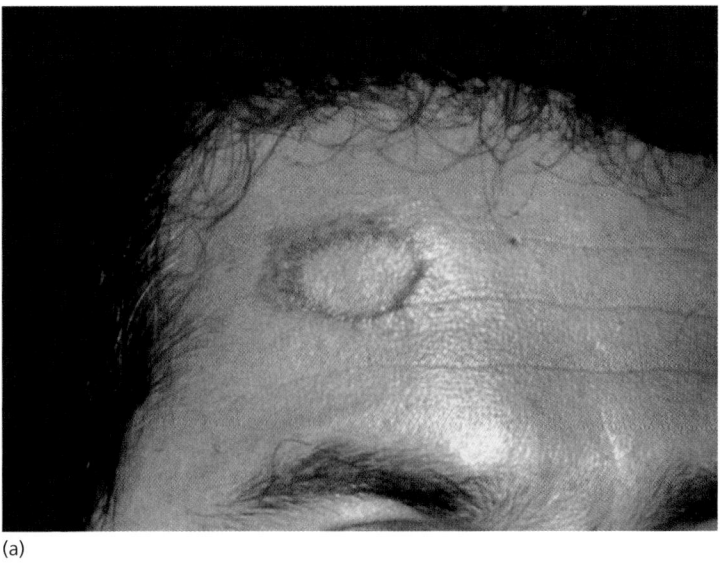

(a)

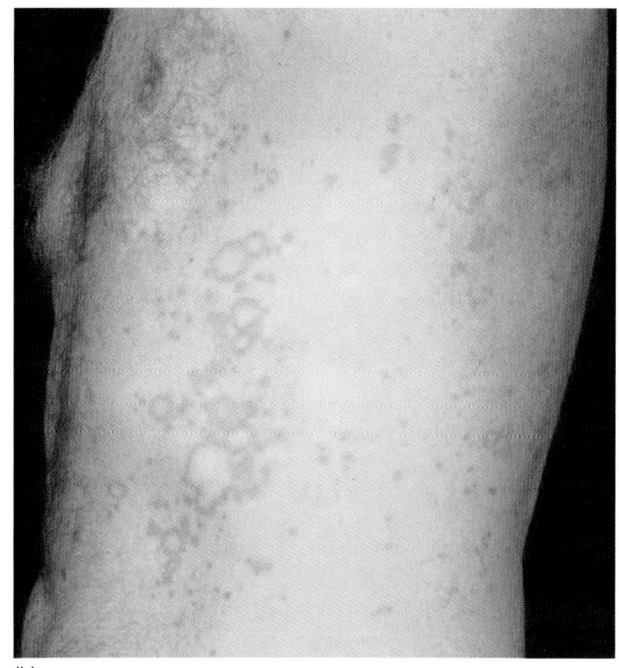

(b)

Figure 98.11 (a) Annular sarcoidosis on the forehead. (b) Extensive truncal annular sarcoidosis.

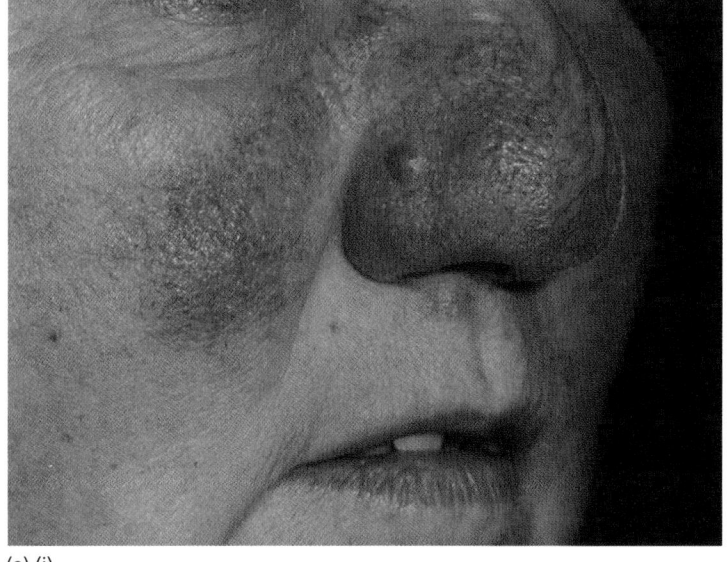

(a) (i)

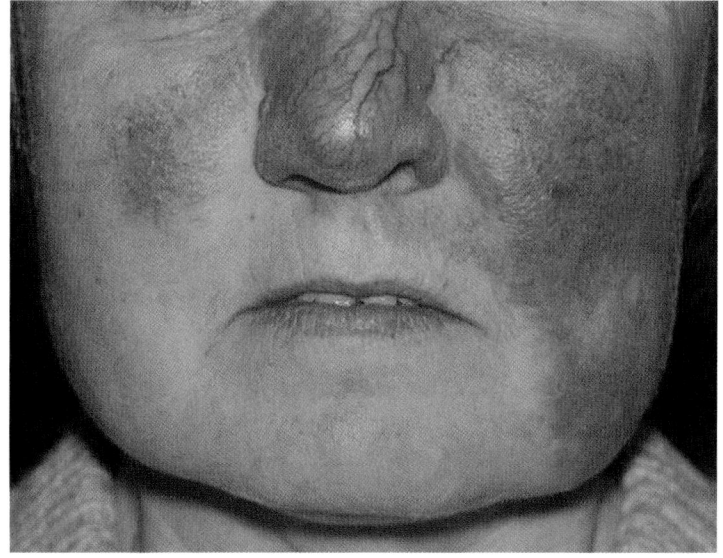

(a) (ii)

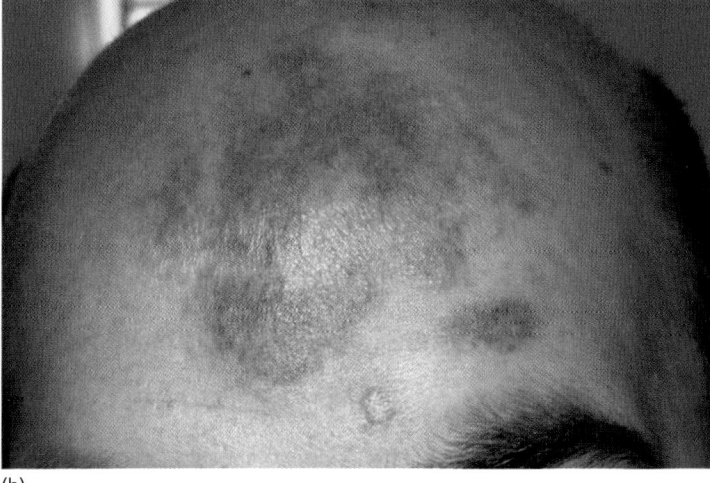

(b)

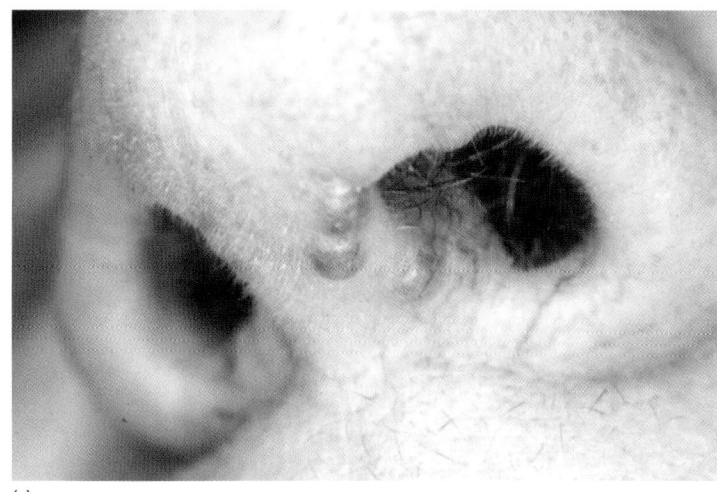

(c)

Figure 98.12 (a) Classical lupus pernio affecting the nose and cheeks. (b) Lupus pernio involving forehead. (c) Sarcoid nodules on columella.

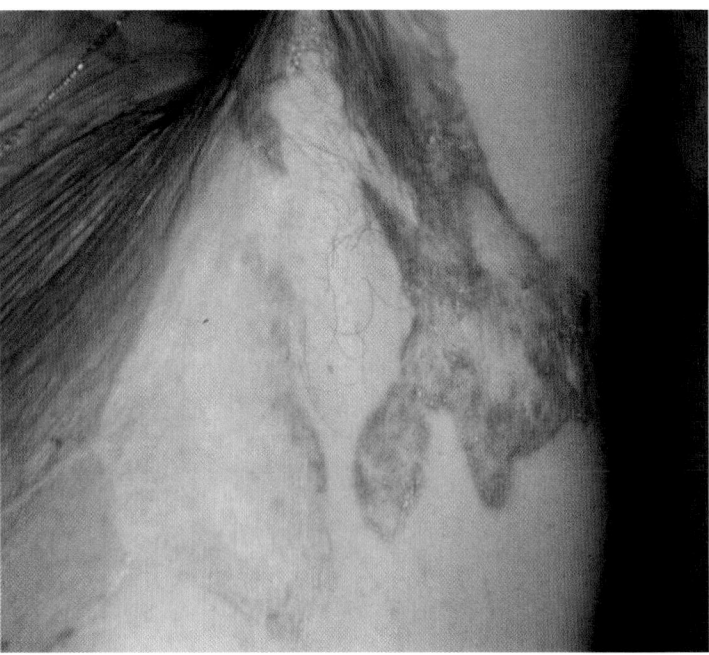

Figure 98.13 Scar sarcoidosis in a burn in the axilla.

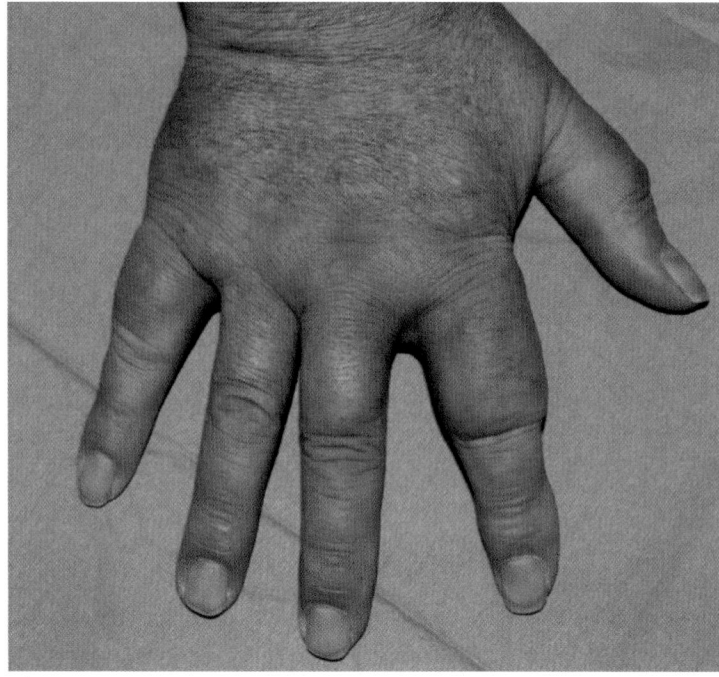

(a)

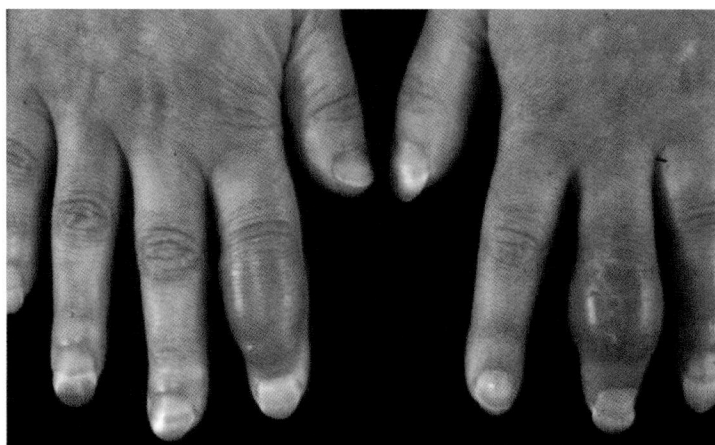

(b)

Figure 98.15 (a,b) Sarcoid dactylitis.

forearms and tend to be fusiform (Figure 98.14) [36,226–229]. The subcutaneous lesions may form indurated linear bands from the elbow to the hand [36,229]. In some cases, the dorsa of the hands are infiltrated and the fingers develop asymptomatic firm fusiform swelling (sarcoid dactylitis) (Figure 98.15a,b) [36,230,231]. Differential diagnoses include epidermal cysts, multiple lipomata, calcinosis, rheumatoid nodules, morphoea, cutaneous metastases and less common conditions such as tuberculosis and deep mycoses [225,232]. Cases of subcutaneous sarcoidosis simulating breast carcinoma have also been reported [233]. It is not unusual for subcutaneous sarcoidosis to coexist with or appear shortly after EN [36]. However, subcutaneous sarcoidosis is not tender, is flesh coloured and is more persistent [223,229].

Subcutaneous sarcoidosis usually appears at the onset of sarcoidosis [36,222,224,225] and is frequently the main complaint at diagnosis [36]. It is associated with stage I changes on chest

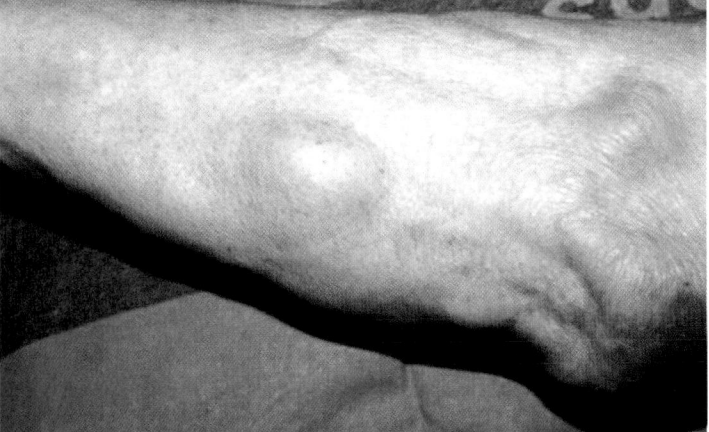

Figure 98.14 Subcutaneous sarcoidosis in the arm with indurated linear bands from the elbow to the hand. (Courtesy of Mañá and Marcoval 2012 [457] © Elsevier.)

radiograph and with less than 2 years' activity of systemic sarcoidosis [**190**].

Less common forms of cutaneous sarcoidosis

Angiolupoid sarcoidosis

This is considered by some authors to be a discrete variant of lupus pernio with prominent large telangiectatic venules. It typically presents in women as a single raised plaque on the bridge of the nose, central face, ears or scalp [202,234]. It has been observed in 8% of patients with cutaneous sarcoidosis in an Indian series [235] and is especially frequent in Taiwan, where it is often associated with eye involvement [236].

Hypopigmented sarcoidosis

Hypopigmented, well-demarcated, round to oval patches are observed mainly on the limbs [176,237]. Erythematous papules can be found in the centre of some lesions, leading to a 'fried egg' appearance [202]. In a series of 145 patients with sarcoidosis, the hypopigmented variant was observed in only eight individuals, most of whom were of Afro-Caribbean ethnicity (Figure 98.16) [184]. It must be differentiated from leprosy, post-inflammatory hypopigmentation, idiopathic guttate hypomelanosis and pityriasis lichenoides chronica [39]. The presence of an interface dermatitis associated with sarcoidal granulomas may explain the hypomelanosis [238].

Lichenoid sarcoidosis

This is more frequent in children [239–245] and is estimated to account for 1–2% of cases of cutaneous sarcoidosis [246]. Multiple 1–3 mm, flat-topped or dome-shaped erythematous or skin-coloured papules may involve extensive areas of the trunk, limbs and face [243,244]. The differential diagnosis includes lichen planus, lichen nitidus, lichenoid drug eruptions, lupus eryhtematosus and papular mucinosis (lichen myxoedematosus) [243]. Wickham striae are absent [244].

Ulcerative sarcoidosis

This usually develops in papulonodular or atrophic lesions on the lower legs and heals with scarring [247,248]. It has been reported in 1.1–4.8% of patients with cutaneous sarcoidosis [193,248] and is more frequent in black and Japanese people [247,249]. Subjacent granulomatous vasculitis has recently been reported [249,250].

Psoriasiform sarcoidosis

Well-demarcated erythematous scaly plaques that may be clinically indistinguishable from psoriasis [202,251,252] are found in 0.9% of patients with sarcoidosis [201]. However, psoriasis plaques have a redder colour and larger scales, and heal without scarring [203].

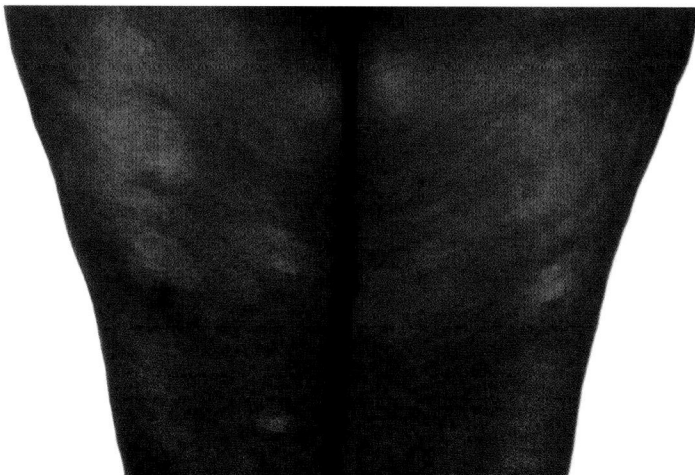

Figure 98.16 Hypopigmented sarcoidosis. (Courtesy of the copyright holder Dr S. Walsh, King's College Hospital, London, UK.)

Verrucous sarcoidosis

This presents as well-demarcated hyperkeratotic papillomatous lesions usually located on the lower extremities [253,254]. Most reported patients have been of African descent with longstanding systemic disease [255,256]. It may resemble warts, nodular prurigo, hypertrophic lichen planus, keratoacanthoma, squamous cell carcinoma or deep fungal infections [254,256].

Necrobiosis-lipoidica-like lesions

Pink to violaceous plaques with depressed centres located on the shins may resemble necrobiosis lipoidica (see Figure 98.12c) [202,257,258]. The granulomatous nature of both diseases may explain this resemblance.

Ichthyosiform sarcoidosis

This is characterized by adherent, polygonal, grey or brown 0.1–1 cm scales most commonly located on the lower extremities of patients of African descent [259–261]. Biopsy reveals both sarcoid granulomas and compact orthokeratosis with a diminished granular layer, mimicking ichthyosis vulgaris [260,261,262].

Erythrodermic sarcoidosis

Slightly infiltrated, erythematous plaques coalesce over large areas. In contrast to classical erythroderma, some areas of skin are spared [202,263]. Some patients with prominent scaling have been reported as acquired ichthyosiform erythroderma. As in other atypical forms of sarcoidosis, histopathological evaluation may be necessary to exclude other more common causes of erythroderma [264].

Morphoea-like lesions

Indurated and atrophic plaques, usually located on the thighs of black women, have been described in sarcoidosis [265,266]. Some cases show a linear distribution resembling linear morphoea [266,267]. In addition to epithelioid granulomas, dermal sclerosis is observed histopathologically [265,267,268].

Livedo

Sarcoidosis may rarely present with livedo. Most reported cases are Japanese women [269,270]. In five cases, biopsy specimens revealed epithelioid cell granulomas around blood vessels conditioning luminal narrowing [269]. Sarcoidosis with livedo is characterized by a high frequency of ophthalmological and central nervous system involvement [269,270].

Other

Less common specific lesions which have been described in cutaneous sarcoidosis may resemble discoid lupus erythematosus [271,272], lichen sclerosus [273], lipodermatosclerosis [274], cellulitis [275] or breast carcinoma en cuirasse [276,277]. Other reported variants include pseudotumoral sarcoidosis [278,279], follicular sarcoidosis [280], photo-induced sarcoidosis [281,282] and variants presenting as palmar erythema [283] or as lower limb oedema, which is generally unilateral [284,285].

SPECIAL LOCATIONS OF SPECIFIC CUTANEOUS LESIONS

Alopecia

Scarring alopecia secondary to sarcoidosis is rare and appears to affect predominantly women of African descent [271,286–290]. Scale is usually absent, although follicular plugging may be present [271]. In extensive cases, the alopecia may be indistinguishable from pseudopelade of Brocq [202], although other cutaneous signs of sarcoidosis are often present [286].

Nails

Splinter haemorrhages, thinning, pitting, thickening, longitudinal ridging, onycholysis, subungual hyperkeratosis, paronychia, pterygium, trachyonychia, and red or brown discoloration of the nail bed all have been reported in sarcoidosis [291–295]. In advanced cases, granulomatous infiltration of the nail matrix can result in total loss of the nail [294]. Nail sarcoidosis is associated in most reported cases with with bony cysts in the underlying terminal phalanx [294,296] and a chronic disease course [39,294].

Oral

Oral involvement is infrequent in sarcoidosis (Figure 98.17) [297,298]. It usually presents as a diffuse submucous thickening or firm nodule in the buccal mucosa [297–299]. Papules, superficial ulcers [297,300] and strawberry gums [301] have also been reported. Differential diagnosis includes oro-facial granulomatosis and Crohn disease [302].

Genital

In the male genitalia sarcoidosis usually presents with testicular or epididymal masses without cutaneous lesions [303,304]. However, several patients with indurated papules, painful

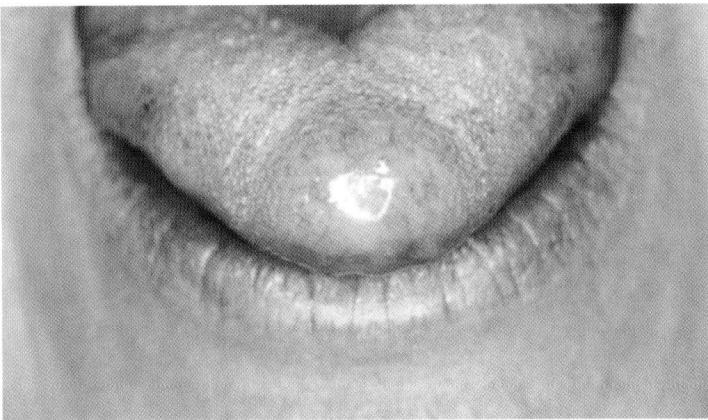

Figure 98.17 Sarcoidosis involving the tongue. (From Marcoval J and Mañá J. Specific (granulomatous) oral lesions of sarcoidosis: report of two cases. *Med Oral Patol Oral Cir Bucal* 2010;15:e456–8 [299]. Reproduced with permission of the copyright holder Medicina Oral S.L.)

nodules or swelling involving the scrotum or penis have been reported [303,305–307]. Vulval sarcoidosis is rare [308,309]. It presents with semi-translucent reddish brown papules and nodules that must be distinguished from tuberculosis, Crohn disease, syphilis, foreign-body reactions and lymphogranuloma venereum [309].

NON-SPECIFIC LESIONS

EN is the most common non-specific lesion of sarcoidosis and is frequently the initial manifestation of the disease (Figure 98.18a–d). It is the marker of acute and benign sarcoidosis and tends to affect younger people than infiltrative cutaneous lesions [**193**]. In recent studies, 10–22% of EN cases were considered to have been caused by sarcoidosis [310]; by way of corollary, about 20% of cases of sarcoidosis are associated with EN [186,201].

The association of EN with bilateral hilar and right paratracheal adenopathies, with or without pulmonary infiltrates, is known as Löfgren syndrome [311–314]. It is more frequent in young women from northern Europe [185,313,315–317] and is the most frequent form of sarcoidosis in Spain [5,188,318]. In Löfgren syndrome, EN can be accompanied by fever, polyarthralgia and uveitis. The prognosis is very good and it usually resolves spontaneously within 1 year [5,314,316,319–321].

When sarcoidosis is associated with EN, it usually runs a benign and self-limited course [317,320,322–324]. In multivariate analysis, the presence of EN proved to be the strongest predictive factor for a favourable prognosis [322]. However, the good prognosis of sarcoidosis presenting with EN seems to be limited to white patients [325].

Less frequent non-specific lesions are erythema multiforme [**176**,326], prurigo [327–330], cutaneous calcinosis [331–334] and digital clubbing [335–339], which is considered a poor prognostic sign [340,341]. Pseudo-clubbing secondary to granulomatous infiltration of the terminal phalanx must be differentiated from true digital clubbing [342,343].

The association of Sweet syndrome with sarcoidosis has been reported in several patients [344–353]. It is typically associated with the onset of acute sarcoidosis [353], which it may precede [352]. Pyoderma gangrenosum has been associated with sarcoidosis [354–358] and, although any association may be fortuitous, one case showed a clear-cut relation between skin biopsy of EN and the development of pyoderma gangrenosum [358].

Investigations

At diagnosis, at least 60% of patients have an increased serum angiotensin-converting enzyme level. Pulmonary function tests reveal decreased forced vital capacity and diffusing capacity for carbon monoxide. Advanced pulmonary fibrosis may cause airway distortion and decreased forced expiratory in 1 s (FEV$_1$) [2,**3**]. Thoracic high-resolution CT is not indicated when the chest radiograph is typical, but it is useful in patients with atypical radiological findings. In addition to the bilateral hilar lymphadenopathy, the most common findings are widespread

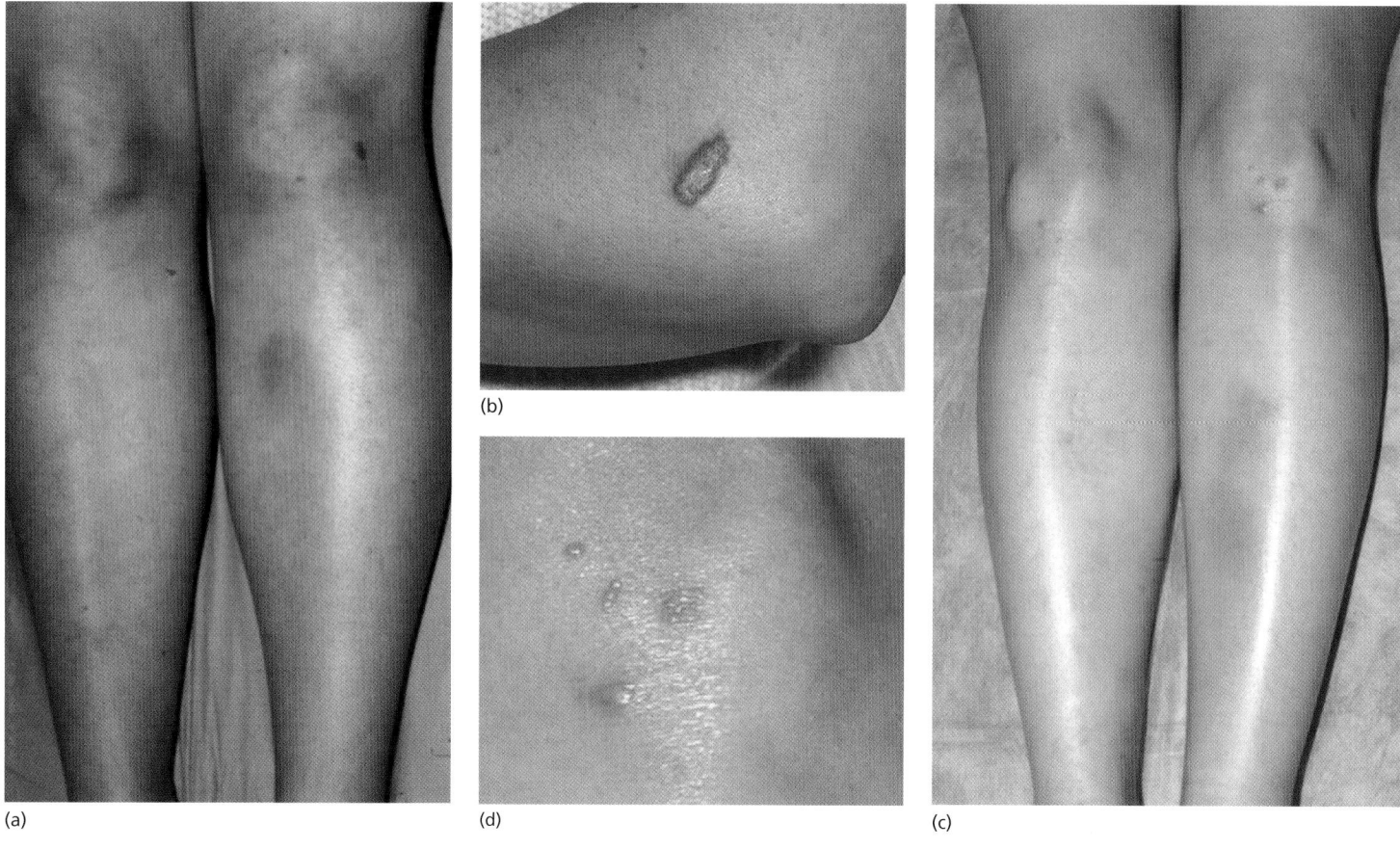

Figure 98.18 (a,c) Erythema nodosum in two patients with Löfgren syndrome with associated papular sarcoidosis in scars on the elbow (b) and knee (c,d).

small nodules with a bronchovascular and subpleural distribution, thickened interlobular septa, ground-glass areas, and confluent nodular opacities with air bronchograms with a predilection for the middle and upper lung areas [359]. The demonstration on bronchoalveolar lavage of a lymphocytic alveolitis with CD4/CD8 >3.5 has a sensitivity of 53% and a specificity of 94%. However, it is not routinely performed unless a transbronchial lung biopsy is indicated. Tuberculin skin test is negative in more than 80% of patients [129]. PET with ^{18}F-fluorodeoxyglucose (^{18}F-FDG PET) is more sensitive than 67-gallium scan for assessing the activity and extension of sarcoidosis (Figure 98.19). ^{18}F-FDG PET/CT is mainly useful in the detection of occult granuloma sites for biopsy and in the detection of residual activity in patients with fibrotic pulmonary sarcoidosis [360].

Diagnostic criteria

The diagnosis of sarcoidosis is based on a compatible clinical and radiological picture, demonstration of non-caseating granulomas with negative cultures for mycobacteria and fungus, and exclusion of other granulomatous diseases [3]. Box 98.1 shows the basic study protocol. The most common biopsies are transbronchial, skin, and peripheral lymph node biopsies. When the clinical and radiological findings are not typical, particularly with stage 0 chest radiograph, it is advisable to obtain at least two positive biopsies. Löfgren syndrome is so recognizable that histological confirmation may not be necessary [3].

Management

Oral corticosteroids are the treatment of choice for systemic sarcoidosis [3]. The recommended dose in pulmonary sarcoidosis is prednisolone 30–40 mg/24 h, with gradual reduction to 5–10 mg/24 h or 10–20 mg/48 h for at least 1 year [3,177]. In patients with severe uveitis, neurosarcoidosis, or symptomatic cardiac involvement, a dose of 1 mg/kg/24 h can be required [3]. When corticosteroids can not be withdrawn, other drugs such as chloroquine or cytotoxic drugs can be considered [3].

Cutaneous lesions usually respond to the treatment administered for the systemic disease but frequently recur when tapering corticosteroids [195,361]. When there is not significant visceral involvement to justify oral corticosteroid treatment, the options for cutaneous lesion treatment are not completely effective and therapeutic recommendations are usually supported by isolated case reports or short series [195,362,363]. For patients with cosmetically insignificant and asymptomatic cutaneous lesions treatment may be unnecessary.

First line

Mild to moderate disease

Cutaneous lesions may respond to potent topical corticosteroids with few adverse effects [364,365]. Intralesional injections of triamcinolone acetonide at concentrations of 5–20 mg/mL repeated every 3–4 weeks may be more effective [366–369].

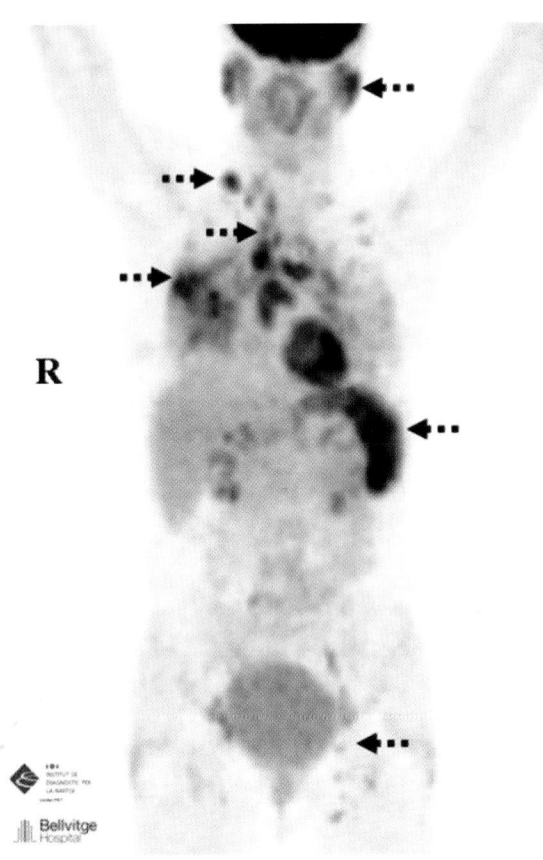

Figure 98.19 Whole body ^{18}F-fluorodeoxyglucose (^{18}F-FDG) PET scan in a 51-year-old women diagnosed with systemic sarcoidosis showing hypermetabolic lymph nodes in the supraclavicular, mediastinal and iliac areas, bilateral pulmonary involvement and increased uptake in both parotid glands and spleen. (Courtesy of the copyright holder PET Unit-IDI, Bellvitge University Hospital, Barcelona, Spain.)

Severe disfigurement or lupus pernio

Prednisolone 20–60 mg/24 h is administered until clinical response (usually 1–3 months) and then tapered by 5–10 mg/week to the lowest dose that prevents relapse [361,367,369]: corticosteroid-sparing agents are indicated when a dose of at least 10 mg of prednisolone daily is required for this [370]. The mechanism of osteoporosis is multifactorial in sarcoidosis and all patients on chronic corticosteroids should have a baseline bone density study. For

---

Box 98.1 Recommended basic assessment of patients with sarcoidosis

- History (including occupational and environmental exposure)
- Physical examination
- Ophthalmological examination (slit-lamp and ophthalmoscopic examination)
- Chest radiograph
- Standard haematological and biochemistry profiles (including urine and serum calcium level, hepatic enzymes and renal function tests), and serum angiotensin-converting enzyme level
- ECG
- Pulmonary function tests (including spirometry and DL_{co})
- Tuberculin skin test
- Biopsies (including culture for mycobacteria and fungus)

---

patients without hypercalcaemia or nephrolithiasis, oral calcium supplements may be used. The addition of vitamin D is less clear-cut. Calcium levels should be checked in the summer months to detect hypercalcaemia. Bisphosphonates have been shown to be useful in treating corticosteroid-induced osteoporosis [371].

Second line

Antimalarials, methotrexate or tetracycline can be used as second line therapy for mild to moderate disease and as corticosteroid-sparing agents in patients with severe disfigurement or lupus pernio. They may be the first option when systemic corticosteroids are contraindicated [363].

Antimalarials

Hydroxychloroquine (200–400 mg daily) and chloroquine (250–500 mg daily) are among the most commonly prescribed drugs [372–374]. They are particularly useful in chronic cutaneous lesions and can be used as corticosteroid-sparing agents in severe cases (Figure 98.20) [177]. In a recent review, 57 of 78 reported patients improved with hydroxychloroquine or chloroquine alone [375]. Hydroxychloroquine has a lower risk of retinopathy but chloroquine seems to be more effective [371,374,376]. Eye evaluation every 6–12 months is usually recommended although there is limited evidence concerning the frequency of ocular toxicity of hydroxychloroquine and the need for routine screening [371].

Methotrexate

Methotrexate has been the most widely studied non-steroidal therapy for systemic sarcoidosis [371]. The overall response rate appears to be greater than 80% for skin lesions [371,377,378]. It is used either for recalcitrant skin disease or as a corticosteroid-sparing agent [379] that can be effective for both pulmonary and cutaneous disease [361,378,380,381]. Patients need to be monitored for neutropenia, renal function, and liver and pulmonary toxicity. Nausea can be reduced with folic acid supplementation [371] (see Chapter 19). The response to methotrexate may take at least 6 months to achieve [379].

Tetracycline

Several non-randomized studies suggest the utility of tetracyclines in cutaneous sarcoidosis [369,382–384]. Minocycline 100 mg twice daily achieved complete resolution of chronic cutaneous lesions in eight of 12 patients and partial response in two [382]. However, poor response to tetracycline has been reported in lupus pernio [385]. Although the mechanism of action is unclear, an anti-inflammatory action of minocycline has been suggested [371]. Because of the relatively benign safety profile of tetracycline, proposed therapeutic strategies include initiating treatment with minocycline for 3 months; if the response is unsatisfactory, hydroxychloroquine can be added, and if the desired improvement is not achieved, methotrexate may then be added to the regimen [363].

Third line

TNF-α antagonists

Several case reports and small series report the utility of infliximab in unresponsive cutaneous sarcoidosis including lupus pernio [385,386–392]. Although in a randomized placebo-controlled

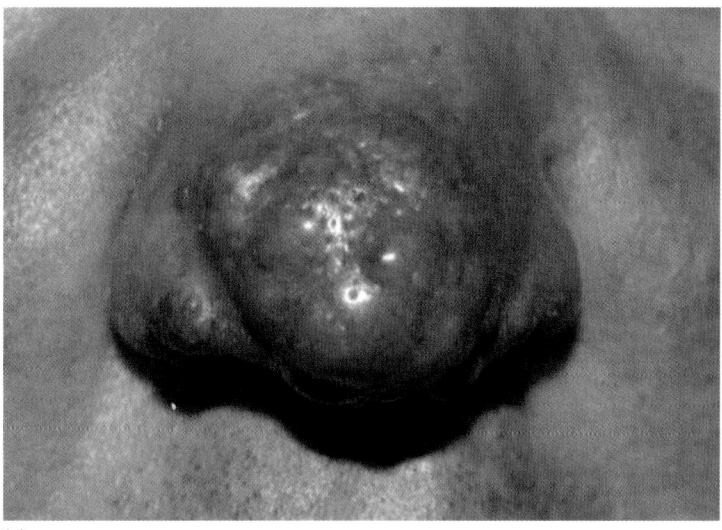

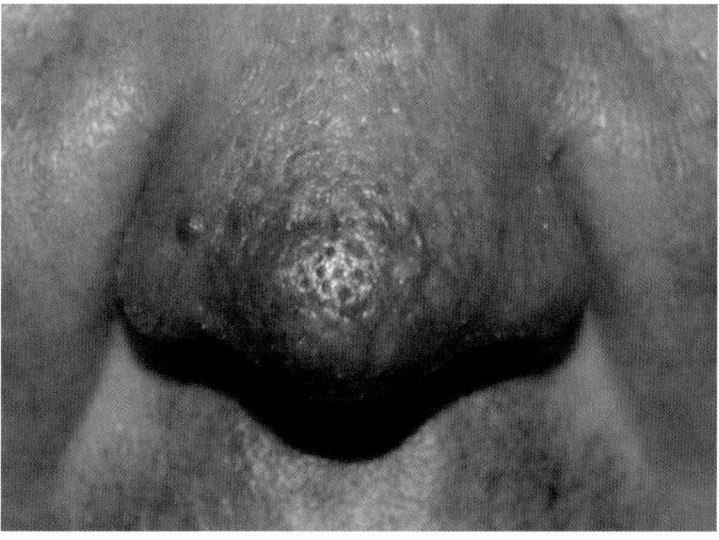

Figure 98.20 (a,b) Lupus pernio before and after treatment with hydroxychloroquine.

trial no significant differences in the appearance of facial lesions were observed [393] and multiple cases of sarcoidosis induced by anti-TNF therapy have been reported [394–404], infliximab is considered a good candidate as a third line therapy for refractory cutaneous sarcoidosis [363,390,392]. Several studies have also reported successful use of adalimumab [391,404–408]. Etanercept is generally not recommended [408–411].

Other reported treatments

Non-systemic

Non-systemic treatments claimed to be useful in isolated cases include topical tacrolimus [412–415], topical psoralen gel and ultraviolet A [416], carbon dioxide laser and pulsed dye laser [417–421], surgical treatment [207,422–425], and topical photodynamic therapy [426–428]. Radiotherapy has rarely been used [429].

Systemic treatments

Isotretinoin [430–432], mycophenolate [433], allopurinol [434–438], pentoxiphylline [439], tacrolimus [440], fumaric acid esters [441,442], psoralens and ultraviolet A (PUVA) [361,443,444], tranilast [445], apremilast [446], chlorambucil [369,447], leflunomide [369,447] and melatonin [448,449] have occasionally been used with apparent benefit. The use of ciclosporin is controversial [369,447]. Thalidomide has multiple effects including the blockage of TNF and has been reported to be effective in patients unresponsive to other treatments [450–455]. However, its use is limited because of its teratogenicity and high risk of neuropathy [455,456].

CUTANEOUS SARCOID REACTION

The histopathological differential diagnosis between cutaneous lesions of systemic sarcoidosis and cutaneous sarcoid granulomas of other aetiology may be very difficult. For this reason, the detection of non-caseating granulomas in the skin is not sufficient to confirm the diagnosis of sarcoidosis in the absence of other organ involvement [3]. Those cases with cutaneous sarcoid granulomas of unknown aetiology are better considered as idiopathic sarcoid reactions. These patients should be followed up because some of them will develop involvement of other organs and thus fulfil the diagnostic criteria for sarcoidosis.

Key references

The full list of references can be found in the online version at www.rooksdermatology.com.

3 Hunninghake GW, Costabel U, Ando M, *et al.* ATS/ERS/WASOG Statement on sarcoidosis. Sarcoidosis Vasc Diff Lung Dis 1999;16:149–73/*Am J Respir Crit Care Med* 1999;160:736–55.

27 Ball NJ, Kho GT, Martinka M. The histopathologic spectrum of cutaneous sarcoidosis: a study of twenty-eight cases. *J Cutan Pathol* 2004;31:160–8.

42 Marcoval J, Mañá J, Moreno A, *et al.* Foreign bodies in granulomatous cutaneous lesions of patients with systemic sarcoidosis. *Arch Dermatol* 2001;137:427–30.

176 Elgart ML. Cutaneous sarcoidosis: definitions and types of lesions. *Clin Dermatol* 1986;4:35–45.

190 Marcoval J, Mañá J, Rubio M. Specific cutaneous lesions in patients with systemic sarcoidosis: relationship to severity and chronicity of disease. *Clin Exp Dermatol* 2011;36:739–44.

193 Veien NK, Stahl D, Brodthagen H. Cutaneous sarcoidosis in caucasians. *J Am Acad Dermatol* 1987;16:534–40.

194 Olive KE, Kataria YP. Cutaneous manifestations of sarcoidosis: relationship to other organ system involvement, abnormal laboratory measurements, and disease course. *Arch Intern Med* 1985;145:1811–14.

360 Teirstein AS, Machac J, Almeida O, *et al.* Results of 188 whole-body fluorodeoxyglucose positron emission tomography scans in 137 patients with sarcoidosis. *Chest* 2007;132:1949–53.

385 Stagaki E, Mountford WK, Lackland DT, Judson MA. The treatment of lupus pernio: results of 116 treatment courses in 54 patients. *Chest* 2009;135:468–76.

393 Baughman RP, Drent M, Kavuru M, *et al.* Infliximab therapy in patients with chronic sarcoidosis and pulmonary involvement. *Am J Respir Crit Care Med* 2006;174:795–802.

PART 8: SPECIFIC CUTANEOUS STRUCTURE

CHAPTER 99

Panniculitis

Luis Requena

Department of Dermatology, Fundación Jiménez Díaz, Madrid, Spain

PART 8: SPECIFIC CUTANEOUS STRUCTURE

ANATOMY AND PHYSIOLOGY OF SUBCUTANEOUS FAT

Introduction

In order to appreciate how subcutaneous fat responds to inflammation, it is important to understand its structure and function. Subcutaneous tissue (subcutis) is composed predominantly of fat cells supported in a connective tissue framework (Figure 99.1). Subcutaneous fat is present almost universally over the body surface between the skin and the deep fascia and, in the normal state, constitutes about 10% of body weight (Figure 99.2). It forms a specialized closely regulated metabolic reserve capable of storing or rapidly releasing energy, typically providing sufficient for about 40 days' requirements [1]. Subcutaneous fat also acts as an insulating layer against heat loss and a protective cushion against external injury. Subcutaneous fat also provides structural support to the overlying skin and has a cosmetic function, for example in the contours of the face.

Subcutaneous fat is absent from the eyelids and the male genitalia. There are obvious sexual differences in the distribution of fat around the body surface, with an increase in thickness resulting in the rounded contours of the female trunk, breasts, hips, pubis and thighs. Subcutaneous fat also varies in thickness with the race, age and endocrine and nutritional status of the individual. Fat also has great social importance as a major contributor to the sexual attractiveness of women on the one hand but, on the other hand, as a cause of misery when present in excess: fat children may be bullied or ostracised at school [2] and fat adults may find it more difficult to get certain jobs.

Brown fat in particular (see later) has a very important thermoregulatory role and acts by increasing the basal metabolic rate [3]. This is particularly important in infancy, and heat production in response to cold exposure is maximal in neonates, who have large quantities of brown fat.

In addition to the above functions, the obesity epidemic in westernized countries and the metabolic consequences of abnormal fat distribution have underlined the fact that the subcutaneous fat, comprising as it does innumerable adipocytes secreting a large

Rook's Textbook of Dermatology, Ninth Edition. Edited by Christopher Griffiths, Jonathan Barker, Tanya Bleiker, Robert Chalmers and Daniel Creamer.
© 2016 John Wiley & Sons, Ltd. Published 2016 by John Wiley & Sons, Ltd.
Companion website: www.rooksdermatology.com

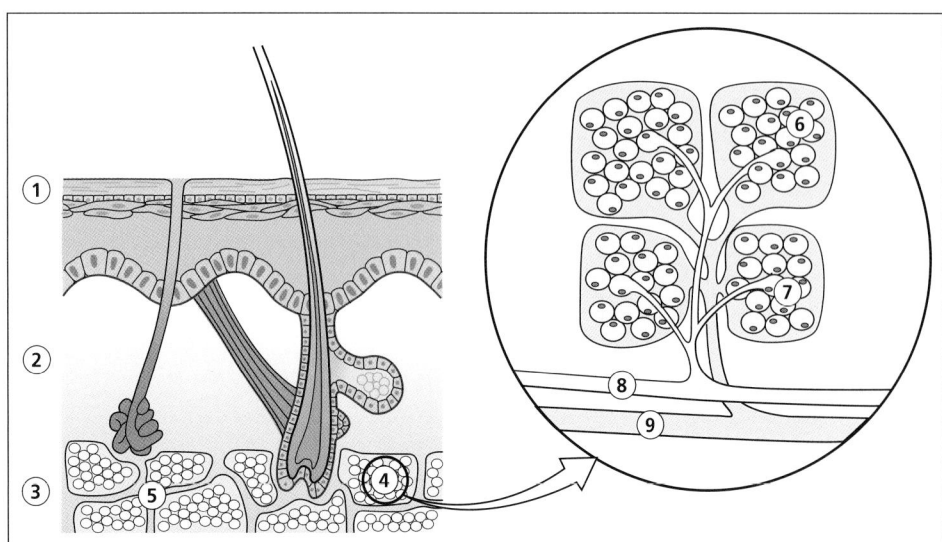

Figure 99.1 Schematic representation of the anatomy of subcutaneous fat with detailed view showing the vascular supply to the fat lobule and its constituent microlobules. (1) Epidermis. (2) Dermis. (3) Subcutis. (4) Fat lobule. (5) Connective tissue septum. (6) Adipocyte. (7) Arteriole. (8) Artery. (9) Vein.

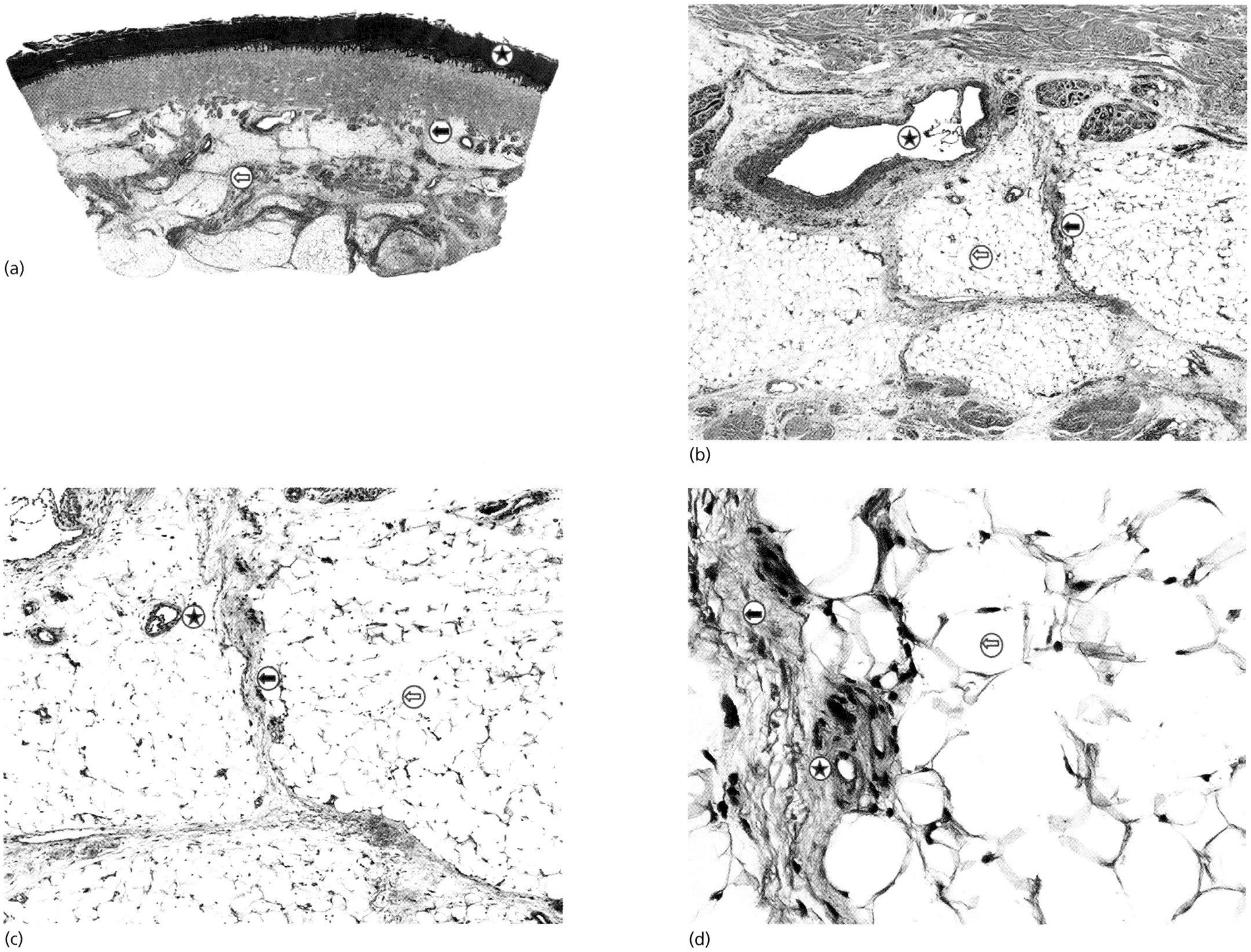

(a)

(b)

(c)

(d)

Figure 99.2 (a) Scanning power view of the normal skin of the sole. The epidermis is covered by a thick compact orthokeratotic horny layer (star). Numerous eccrine units are seen along the interface between the deep reticular dermis and subcutis (black arrow). The subcutis is organized into lobules of adipocytes and connective tissue septa (white arrow) surrounding and demarcating each fat lobule, and associated vessels and nerves. (b) At higher magnification, a large vein (star) may be identified in the deeper dermis because of the presence of valves within its lumen. The subcutis is composed of thin connective tissue septa (black arrow), which delimit lobules of adipocytes (white arrow). (c) At higher magnification, a small venule is seen within the fat lobule (star), as well as the thin septa of connective septa (black arrow) and mature adipocytes of the fat lobule (white arrow). (d) Still higher magnification shows that the connective tissue septa are mostly composed of thin collagen bundles (black arrow). A capillary is seen at the periphery of the fat lobule (star). With H&E stain, adipocytes appear as empty cells with signet-ring morphology. This is due to the fact that the lipid content dissolves in routinely processed specimens and the flat spindle nucleus is displaced to the periphery of the cell by a single large intracytoplasmic vacuole, which contains fat (white arrow).

variety of enzymes, hormones and cytokines, is also a major endocrine organ [4].

Cellular composition of subcutaneous tissue [5,6]

The first fat-containing cell, the pre-adipocyte, appears in the mesenchyme around the 14th week of fetal life. The primitive mesenchymal cell that forms the determined pre-adipocyte is also capable of maturing to form a fibrocyte, myocyte, chondrocyte or osteoblast. Pre-adipocytes can terminally differentiate into either brown adipocytes or white adipocytes.

Brown fat is a special type of granular fat that differs from white fat in its distribution, histology and function. It is multi-locular and is metabolically very active with many mitochondria, so that it is capable of transferring energy from food to produce heat. As it has a much greater capillary network surrounding it compared to white fat (which is partly responsible for the brown colour), heat can be rapidly transferred into the circulation. It is most prominent in the neck and upper thorax of the fetus, and it may be homologous to the hibernating gland fat found in some animals [7]. Brown fat is now known to persist into adult life [8], and it may have a role in preventing obesity [8]. Warm patches develop in the skin 1 h after taking ephedrine orally, and these warm patches may indicate the site of thermogenic brown fat.

Brown fat adipocyte mitochondria uniquely express uncoupling protein 1 (UCP-1), allowing confirmation that brown fat is present in adult white fat depots in variable amounts, and that transdifferentiation from white to brown adipocytes can occur. Development of brown fat begins at the 20th week of gestation, reaches its maximum at birth and then diminishes so that there are no large collections of brown fat in the adult, though fluorodeoxyglucose positron emission tomography (FDG PET) suggests that some adults have supraclavicular areas of brown fat [9]. Evidence for cold induction of brown fat as an adaptive response in humans is at present equivocal [9].

White fat adipocytes are the largest connective tissue cells in the body, with a diameter of up to 100 μm. Much of their differentiation occurs soon after birth. The mature adipocyte has a characteristic signet-ring appearance, because the flat oval nucleus is displaced to the side by a single, large, intracellular, fat-containing vacuole, which is surrounded by perilipin. Originally thought of as an inert store for emergency supplies of energy when necessary, it is now realized that the white adipocyte has a huge array of functions, secreting factors (adipokines) that affect lipid and glucose metabolism, endocrine functions, blood pressure control, coagulation, fibrinolysis, angiogenesis and inflammation. For a full review the reader is referred to Frühbeck [6].

Anatomy of subcutaneous tissue

Subcutaneous tissue is widely distributed throughout the body, forming a true organ as regards both structure and function [4]. Groups of adipocytes are arranged in lobules, each measuring approximately 1 cm in diameter; they are separated from each other by interlobular septa composed of collagen and reticulin fibres. Each lobule may be subdivided into 1 mm diameter micro-

lobules, which represent the functional unit of the subcutaneous fat. Each microlobule is composed of a group of adipocytes arrayed around a central arteriole and surrounded by capillaries and postcapillary venules. Arteries and veins of the subcutis run along the septa. Each individual fat lobule is supplied by a small muscular artery (250–500 μm diameter) branching from the septa to form arterioles (up to 100 μm diameter) that supply every individual microlobule. Each arteriole branches to form a network of capillaries that surrounds each individual adipocyte. In addition to an abundant blood supply, subcutaneous fat also contains a rich lymphatic plexus, which receives vessels from the dermis. These lymph vessels traverse the subcutaneous layer parallel to the skin surface for some distance, before eventually penetrating the deep fascia and draining into the regional lymph nodes. The nature of the adipocyte and its relationship to blood vessels and lymphatics has been reviewed in detail by Ryan and Curri [10]. Both white fat and brown fat are innervated by noradrenergic fibres of the sympathetic nervous system and parasympathetic fibres.

The adipocytes may comprise only 25% of the total cell population of a lobule; the remainder, the stroma-vascular fraction, being macrophages, fibroblasts, mast cells, pericytes, endothelial cells and pre-adipocytes, enabling considerable cross-talk between cells by means of locally secreted cytokines including leptin and adiponectin (see later).

All fat tissue is composed of lobules of fat cells with their supporting connective and stroma-vascular tissue. In addition to the subcutaneous fat, approximately 20% of fat tissue occurs internally, in the mediastinal and retroperitoneal tissues, the mesentery and the bone marrow and in and around individual organs, including blood vessels. This tissue, although it is widely scattered throughout the body, forms a true organ as regards both structure and function [1] but in which depot-specific differences occur [11]. For example, increases in subcutaneous upper body and visceral fat are associated with an increased cardiovascular and metabolic risk but increases in gluteofemoral subcutaneous fat are not [12]. In addition, perivascular adipose tissue shows increased angiogenesis compared to subcutaneous fat [13]. The fact that some genetic lipodystrophy patients lose peripheral fat but fat padding for absorption of mechanical pressure is maintained, is further evidence for depot-specific differences.

The combination of the obesity epidemic and the advent of liposuction has rekindled interest in the structure of subcutaneous fat with MRI scanning as the investigative tool [14]. Subcutaneous fat is divided by the superficial fascia into two compartments, superficial and deep. The fat mass in the superficial (areolar) layer is compartmentalized into lobules by vertical and oblique fibrous septal planes and bands, whilst that of the deeper (lamellar) layer has its septae more horizontally positioned. The superficial layer is fairly constant, but the deeper is more variable, with an increase in fat mass accumulating between split horizontal septae. In females, subcutaneous fat is most abundant in the gluteofemoral region and breasts, resulting in the so-called gynaecoid distribution, whereas in males the android distribution of shoulders and upper arms, neck and lumbosacral area predominates.

Physiology of adipose tissue [5,6,15,16,17,18]

Traditionally, adipose tissue was regarded as an inert energy store with insulating and padding properties. Whilst storage is still a major function, there is now an appreciation that adipocytes and their stroma-vascular tissue have many other highly complex and dynamic actions, including energy homeostasis, adipogenesis, insulin sensitivity and influences on immune and inflammatory responses (see also Chapter 149).

Energy homeostasis

A major function of white adipose tissue is to store energy at times of calorie excess and release it when needed, such as during exercise or starvation. The synthesis (anabolism) and catabolism of fat in the subcutaneous depot depends on many factors, including nourishment and endocrine and neural activity. The role of the autonomic nervous system in regulating fat metabolism is now well established [19], being particularly important for rapid energy need compared to the slower control exerted by neuroendocrine factors [20]. A decrease in parasympathetic activity results in increased lipolysis, as does an increase in sympathetic activity, with the opposites stimulating lipogenesis [21]. Hormones that may affect the energy metabolism of fat cells include insulin, cortisol, norepinephrine (noradrenaline) and several pituitary hormones, including somatotrophin, adrenocorticotrophic hormone (ACTH), thyrotrophin, lipotrophin and natruietic peptide [22].

The fats contained within adipocytes are predominantly triglycerides (triacylglycerols), especially those of palmitic and stearic acids and the unsaturated oleic acid. All the fatty acids have an even number of carbon atoms, predominantly C16 and C18, with a few C14 and C12. Adipose tissue contains 10–30% of water with a small proportion of lipochromes, and less than 2% cholesterol. Fat-soluble substances are also present in varying amounts. These include fat-soluble vitamins and traces of chlorinated hydrocarbons (e.g. aldrin, dieldrin) ingested with the diet, as well as drugs such as acitretin. Adipose tissue *in vitro* has a metabolic rate similar to that of kidney tissue, and approximately half that of liver. Approximately half the triglyceride in the adipose tissue of rats and mice is catabolized and reconstituted in the course of a week or so.

The fat for storage enters the adipocyte as fatty acids, having been converted from lipoproteins by the extracellular enzyme lipoprotein lipase (Figure 99.3). The fatty acids combine with coenzyme A, using the energy of adenosine triphosphate (ATP), to form the corresponding acyl coenzyme A compounds. Some of these are then oxidized to provide energy for the regeneration of ATP, but most are converted to triglyceride by combination with glycerol-3-phosphate derived from glucose.

The adipocyte is one of the few cells to express the insulin-dependent glucose transporter receptor 4 (GLUT-4), which mediates the passage of glucose into the cell and thus facilitates triglyceride formation within the adipocyte via *de novo* lipogenesis, the latter providing only a small contribution to the pool. At the same time, insulin inhibits hydrolysis and breakdown of triglyceride, conserving the energy store.

When the body requires energy, lipolysis occurs. Triglyceride is hydrolysed in the adipocyte, converted to non-esterified fatty acids (NEFA) and glycerol, the rate-limiting enzyme being hormone-sensitive lipase (HSL). The NEFAs are conveyed in the blood to tissues such as liver and muscle, in which fatty acid oxidation readily takes place. In both tissues, the essential part of the process consists of the oxidation in the mitochondria of the long-chain fatty acids. The glycerol of the triglyceride molecule reacts with ATP to form glycerol phosphate, which is oxidized

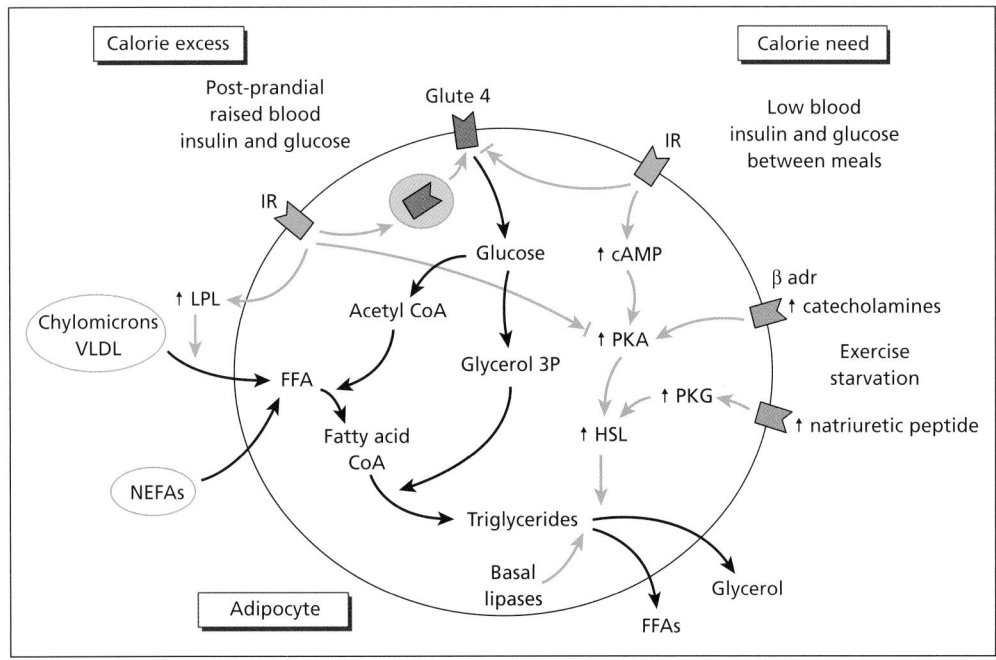

Figure 99.3 Simplified outline of lipogenesis in an adipocyte during energy excess and lipolysis during calorie need. Effects of hormones and enzymes are in blue. FFA, free fatty acid.

to glyceraldehyde-3-phosphate. This in turn may either be converted to glycogen by reversal of glycolysis, or it may be converted to pyruvate. Skeletal muscle readily oxidizes fatty acids but glucose, if available, is preferentially used. In cardiac muscle, fatty acids are a major source of energy. Lipolysis is regulated predominantly through insulin and catecholamines. The latter, elevated during a sudden energy demand, bind to β-adrenergic receptors on the adipocyte and activate HSL through the classic adenosine monophosphate-protein kinase A (AMP-PKA) pathway.

Role of leptin [23]

Leptin is an adipokine involved in energy homeostasis which may have evolved to help adaption from the starved to the adequately nourished state rather than to prevent obesity. Leptin, a product of the *ob* gene, is a 16-kDa polypeptide comprising 167 amino acids with a structural homology similar to other cytokine proteins such as tumour necrosis factor (TNF)-α and interleukin (IL)-6. It is secreted by adipocytes predominantly, but also by the stomach, aiding immediate appetite control. Leptin receptors are present in the hypothalamus, on adipocytes, skeletal muscle, liver, pancreatic β cells, ovary and endometrium. The main effect of leptin is via the satiety centres in the hypothalamus. If excess energy is being stored, rising leptin levels stimulate satiety centres to reduce appetite. Conversely, during starvation low leptin levels stimulate appetite. Circulating levels of leptin correlate with increasing body mass index (BMI), but have little effect on satiety centres, indicating an apparent leptin resistance. Leptin also influences several other functions, including neuroendocrine and reproductive functions, insulin secretion and blood pressure. Patients with congenital leptin deficiency (see Chapter 74) have gross obesity, hyperphagia, delayed pubertal development, abnormal T-cell number and function, and altered thyroid and growth hormone function [24]. In addition, leptin has a role in immune function and inflammation [25]. There is increased expression in chondrocytes and leptin may have a part to play in articular degenerative disease.

Adipogenesis

Adipogenesis refers to the recruitment from multipotent stem cells in the mesenchyme and stroma-vascular tissue, and proliferation of pre-adipocytes followed by their differentiation into mature fat cells. Culture of cell lines has led to the elucidation of many of the transcriptional factors involved in adipogenesis, the major ones being peroxisome proliferator-activated receptor-γ (PPARγ) and the CCAAT enhancer binding proteins (C/EBPs). The precise contribution of adipogenesis towards enlargement of the fat organ at different stages of human development and life changes is uncertain, but it seems maximal before and around birth before diminishing, then possibly continuing at a low rate throughout adult life. Glucocorticoids, growth hormone and insulin stimulate cells to terminal differentiation, but when mature fat cells reach a certain size, recruitment occurs so that the fat organ enlarges through hyperplasia (increased numbers of cells) rather than hypertrophy (increase in size of cells). Control of this hyperplastic response may come from the local adipocyte through paracrine effects involving local growth factors. During adipogenesis the local extracellular matrix also changes, the effects of which might play their own role in differentiation. This is supported by the fact that fat tissue repair is improved if elements of this matrix are included with the donor adipocytes.

Insulin sensitivity

Insulin secretion, stimulated by raised blood glucose levels after meals to reverse hyperglycaemia, has two major effects. It facilitates glucose uptake into most of the body's cells (liver, skeletal muscle and adipocytes) and it suppresses glucose output by the liver. Insulin resistance occurs when a target organ fails to respond normally to insulin, resulting in hyperinsulinaemia. The effect may be incomplete suppression of hepatic glucose output in the liver and/or impaired insulin-mediated glucose uptake in peripheral tissues, including adipocytes. If increased insulin secretion cannot prevent hyperglycaemia, type 2 diabetes results. Adipocytes secrete many factors, some of which have direct and indirect effects on insulin sensitivity.

Adiponectin [26–28]

Adiponectin is a 30-kDa protein composed of 244 amino acids with some structural similarity to both collagen and complement C1q and is currently thought to be secreted exclusively by adipocytes. It has autocrine/paracrine effects locally within adipose tissue as well as endocrine effects distantly. Locally, it can promote pre-adipocytes to become mature fat cells, which with increasing cell size down-regulate their adiponectin secretion to exert some feedback control. Adiponectin receptors are present in many tissues as well as adipocytes. It is likely that adiponectin receptor-activated AMPK (AMP-activated protein kinase) leads to enhanced insulin signalling and therefore insulin sensitivity. If BMI is elevated, the expression of adiponectin is reduced in visceral adipose tissue (VAT) adipocytes in comparison with that in subcutaneous adipose tissue (SAT). Serum adiponectin levels fall with weight gain and rise with weight loss.

Additionally, adiponectin exerts protective anti-inflammatory effects both locally and distantly. Local effects are mediated by inhibiting secretion of IL-6, IL-8, macrophage inflammatory protein 1 and monocyte chemotactic protein 1. It also has distant effects by its direct action on a range of cells including monocytes/macrophages, endothelial cells, hepatocytes and muscle cells, and indirectly by inhibition of TNF-α production.

There is an as yet unexplained paradox concerning adiponectin and its anti-inflammatory effects. Obesity is associated with macrophages in VAT which generate factors, particularly TNF-α, that suppress adiponectin secretion. However, low levels of adiponectin promote inflammation, generating a self-sustaining loop: thus in obesity adiponectin levels are inversely correlated with levels of inflammatory markers. In autoimmune states such as rheumatoid arthritis and systemic lupus erythematosus, adiponectin levels are raised, the level positively correlating with inflammatory markers. To explain this, it has been suggested that the adiponectin system has evolved as a mechanism for adaptation to starvation, a catabolic state [29]. It is therefore raised in other catabolic states such as autoimmune disease and

PART 8: SPECIFIC CUTANEOUS STRUCTURE

inflammatory bowel disease, and did not evolve as a protective device against insulin resistance.

Other adipokines

Many other adipokines have been described [6,18] and most are still being evaluated for their relevance to human biology. The stroma-vascular tissue itself is also responsible for a variety of cytokines. Macrophages secrete TNF-α, IL-1, IL-6, IL-8, IL-10, monocyte chemoattractant protein 1 (MCP-1), macrophage migration inhibitory factor (MIF), angiotensinogen, and endothelial and vascular growth factors. Therefore, as well as affecting energy homeostasis, insulin sensitivity and adipocyte differentiation, the fat organ has influences on inflammation, immune function, vascular inflammation and neoangiogenesis. All of this lends credence to the concept of the fat organ being an endocrine organ in its own right. Whilst these discoveries are of the utmost importance for worldwide obesity-associated morbidity and mortality, their relevance in disorders of subcutaneous fat other than lipodystrophies is unclear.

PANNICULITIS

Introduction and general description

Inflammatory diseases involving the subcutaneous fat comprise a heterogeneous group of disorders named generically panniculitis. These diseases have been classically considered diagnostically challenging both for clinicians and dermatopathologists; the reasons for this difficulty are varied. Firstly, dermatologists usually evaluate different morphological aspects of the skin anomalies to reach a specific diagnosis, but subcutaneous tissue is too deep to be visible to the examining eye. Moreover, cutaneous lesions of panniculitis usually show a disappointing monotony with completely different diseases involving the subcutaneous tissue showing the same clinical morphology, namely erythematous nodules located preferentially on the lower extremities. Secondly, because the lesions are situated deep in subcutaneous tissue, large incisional biopsies are necessary for diagnosis, which is usually based on the correct evaluation of the pattern of the inflammatory infiltrate and the involvement of blood vessels. This requires at the very least that the biopsy specimen should include a fat lobule and its surrounding connective tissue septa. Thirdly, many panniculitides are also histopathologically unsatisfactory, because subcutaneous fat has a limited range of responses and a variety of insults and panniculitic processes of entirely different aetiologies may produce very similar histopathological changes. Moreover, before an accurate histopathological diagnosis may be established, it must be remembered that panniculitides, like other inflammatory cutaneous disorders, are dynamic processes in which both the distribution and composition of the inflammatory cells of the infiltrate may change rapidly over the course of a few days: when biopsies are taken from late or resolving lesions, especially in predominantly lobular panniculitis, they may show completely non-specific findings. For the aforementioned reasons, some authorities have considered that 'the histological septal-lobular dichotomy is sometimes diagnostically useful, but more often there is a mixed picture that adds to interpretative difficulties' [1].

Despite these potential pitfalls, serial sections of an adequate biopsy enable the dermatopathologist in most cases to classify the panniculitic process as either a predominantly septal or a predominantly lobular panniculitis. This first classification step into one of the two general categories of panniculitis is very helpful for diagnostic purposes. However, classification of a panniculitis into a predominantly septal or predominantly lobular panniculitis is no more than an initial descriptive working classification and it should be followed by a search for additional histopathological clues to help reach a more specific clinically relevant final diagnosis. Thus, the next diagnostic step requires assessment of whether vasculitis is or is not present and, when it is present, of the size and nature of the involved blood vessels. The final diagnostic step requires the microscopic identification of the composition of the inflammatory infiltrate involving the septa and/or the fat lobule, the type of adipocyte necrosis and a search for additional histopathological features to enable a specific diagnosis to be reached. Table 99.1 provides a working classification of the panniculitides using this approach for diagnosis [2,3].

There is probably no individual cell of the human body with a better vascular supply than the adipocyte. Postcapillary venules drain into veins which also run along the septa. In each microlobule, the arteriole occupies a central position, whereas the venule runs along the periphery [4]. As a consequence, interference with the arterial supply results in dramatic necrotic changes within the fat lobule (predominantly lobular panniculitis), while venous disorders manifest by alterations in the septal and paraseptal areas (predominantly septal panniculitis) [5]. This peculiar distribution of the vascularization in subcutaneous tissue explains why large vessel vasculitis involving the septal vessels is usually accompanied by little inflammation of the fat lobules, whereas vasculitis involving small blood vessels of the lobule usually causes extensive necrosis of the centrilobular adipocytes and a dense inflammatory response. In contrast with the dermal vascular network, the blood supply of each subcutaneous microlobule is terminal, implying there are no vascular connections between adjacent microlobules or between the dermis and subcutaneous fat. The septa of the subcutaneous fat also contain a prominent lymphatic plexus, which comes from the dermis and traverses the subcutis, first, parallel to the surface of the skin and then vertically penetrating the underlying fascia and draining into regional lymph nodes. The connective tissue septa, which are contiguous with the overlying reticular traverses and with the underlying fascia, provide stability to the subcutaneous tissue by compartmentalizing it. The normal septa are thin, from 200 to 300 µm, and are composed mostly of collagen bundles and thin elastic and reticulin fibres.

Mature normal individual adipocytes are relatively large cells with a diameter up to 100 mm and, in formalin-fixed and H&E-stained sections, appear as empty cells with signet-ring morphology. This is due to the fact that the lipid and triglyceride

Table 99.1 Classification of the panniculitides.

Predominantly septal panniculitides	
With vasculitis	
Veins	Superficial migratory thrombophlebitis
Arteries	Cutaneous polyarteritis nodosa
No vasculitis	
Lymphocytes and plasma cells predominantly	
With granulomatous infiltrate in septa	Necrobiosis lipoidica
No granulomatous infiltrate in septa	Deep morphoea
Histiocytes predominantly (granulomatous)	
With mucin in centre of palisaded granulomas	Subcutaneous granuloma annulare
With fibrin in centre of palisaded granulomas	Rheumatoid nodule
With large areas of degenerate collagen, foamy histiocytes and cholesterol clefts	Necrobiotic xanthogranuloma
Without mucin, fibrin or degeneration of collagen, but with radial granulomas in septa	Erythema nodosum
Predominantly lobular panniculitides	
With vasculitis	
Small vessels	
Venules	Erythema nodosum leprosum
	Erythema induratum of Bazin
Large vessels	
Arteries	Erythema induratum of Bazin
No vasculitis	
Few or no inflammatory cells	
Necrosis at the centre of the lobule	Sclerosing panniculitis
With vascular calcification	Calcific uraemic arteriolopathy (calciphylaxis)
Lymphocytes predominant	
With superficial and deep perivascular dermal infiltrate	Cold panniculitis
With lymphoid follicles, plasma cells and nuclear dust of lymphocytes	Lupus panniculitis
	Panniculitis associated with dermatomyositis
Neutrophils predominant	
Extensive fat necrosis with saponification of adipocytes	Pancreatic panniculitis
With neutrophils between collagen bundles of deep reticular dermis	α_1-antitrypsin deficiency panniculitis
With bacteria, fungi or protozoa	Infective panniculitis
With foreign bodies	Factitious panniculitis
Neutrophilic lobular panniculitis (subcutaneous Sweet syndrome)	
Histiocytes predominant (granulomatous)	
No crystals in adipocytes	Subcutaneous sarcoidosis
	Traumatic panniculitis
With crystals in histiocytes or adipocytes	Subcutaneous fat necrosis of the newborn
	Poststeroid panniculitis
	Sclerema neonatorum
	Gouty panniculitis
	Fungal panniculitis due to zygomycosis, mucormycosis and aspergillosis
With cytophagic histiocytes	Cytophagic histiocytic panniculitis and subcutaneous panniculitis-like T-cell lymphoma[a]
With sclerosis of the septa	Sclerosing post-irradiation panniculitis

[a]Although these disorders are characterized by a neoplastic proliferation of cytotoxic T lymphocytes rather than an authentic panniculitic process, they are included in the classification of the panniculitides because they may mimic panniculitis both clinically and histopathologically.

content dissolves in routinely processed specimens and the single large intracytoplasmic vacuole displaces the flat spindle nucleus without discernible nuclear features to the periphery of the cell. Frozen sections and special stains such as oil red O or Sudan B are required to demonstrate the lipid contents within the cytoplasm of mature adipocytes.

Perivascular adipocytes have been also demonstrated to be powerful endocrine cells capable of responding to metabolic changes and transducing signals to adjacent blood vessels. Cross-talk between perivascular adipose tissue and blood vessels is now being intensely investigated. There is evidence suggesting that perivascular adipose tissue regulates vascular function through a variety of mechanisms and plays an important role in inflammation and vasoreactivity in subcutaneous tissue [6]. Adipocytes also interact with the immune system. Normal subcutaneous fat contains T lymphocytes located between adipocytes of the fat lobule. They differ from those of other tissues and vary between different regions of the body [7]. It has recently been demonstrated that cytotoxic T lymphocytes precede the accumulation of macrophages during the process of inflammation of the fat lobule. *In vitro* co-cultures have shown a vicious cycle of interaction between cytotoxic T lymphocytes, macrophages and adipocytes, suggesting that adipocytes activate cytotoxic T lymphocytes with subsequent recruitment and activation of macrophages [8]. That there is an interaction between adipocytes and lymphocytes is also supported by the demonstration on human adipocytes of the inflammatory receptor CD40, which contributes to intercellular cross-talk between adipocyte and lymphocyte [9]. Co-cultures of adipocytes and lymphocytes have also shown up-regulation of pro-inflammatory cytokines, including IL-6, MCP-1 and plasminogen activator inhibitor 1 (PAI-1), but down-regulation of leptin and adiponectin [9].

Immunohistochemically, adipocytes express S-100 protein, with staining around the periphery of the cell, and vimentin [10]. In contrast with the multivacuolated cytoplasm of sebocytes and foamy histiocytes, which express adipophilin, the single large cytoplasmic vacuole of the adipocyte is adipophilin negative [11,12].

Pattern-based histopathological classification of panniculitis with large vessel vasculitis also requires ascertainment of whether the involved vessel is an artery or a vein. A peculiarity of the veins in the subcutaneous fat of the lower limbs is that they have a thick muscular layer, conferring upon them an 'arterial' appearance [13]. However, it is usually possible to establish this distinction with confidence from H&E preparations, because the middle layer of subcutaneous veins is composed of several muscular fascicles separated by tiny unstained elastic fibres, whereas arteries show a more compact muscular layer. Nevertheless, many authors continue to promote the misleading notion that arteries of the subcutaneous fat of the lower legs have a thicker muscular layer than veins, when in fact veins often have a thicker muscular layer than arteries [13]. In difficult cases, elastic tissue staining allows definite discrimination between artery and vein, because arteries have a well-demarcated, thick and sharp internal elastic membrane, whereas veins have an ill-defined, thin and multilayered internal elastic lamina and tiny elastic fibres interspersed between muscular fascicles of the

PART 8: SPECIFIC CUTANEOUS STRUCTURE

middle layer of the vessel wall. Some authors, however, believe that when inflammation is present within and around the wall of the vessel, all of the studied histological features become less reliable, and that the interobserver reliability of distinguishing arteritis from thrombophlebitis is low [14].

Types of necrosis of the adipocytes

The appearance of necrotic adipocytes is polymorphous and different from other necrotic cells [15–17]. In classical histopathology, nuclear abnormalities such as pyknosis, karyorrhesis and karyolysis are signs of cellular necrosis. In contrast, necrotic adipocytes, regardless of the aetiology of the cell death, show great variability and may appear as either anucleate cells or with complete disintegration of the cellular structure. Unfortunately, these distinctive forms of adipocyte necrosis have little value for diagnostic specificity.

Often, the only sign of necrosis of the adipocytes is the lack of nuclei in the involved cells, and dead fat cells appear as round empty bags with no inflammatory infiltrate among them. The most frequent type of adipocyte necrosis is *lipophagic necrosis*, which consists of the replacement of necrotic adipocytes by foamy macrophages formed by the engulfing of lipid products released from dead adipocytes by macrophages. These lipophages appear quite different from normal adipocytes, with large pale microvacuolated or granular-like cytoplasm and round central vesicular nuclei. Lipophagic granulomatous inflammation, however, is entirely non-specific and many lobular panniculitides show this pattern of fat necrosis at their late or resolving stages. It is usually seen in lipodermatosclerosis and traumatic panniculitis, but may also be present in erythema nodosum and erythema induratum of Bazin.

In contrast, *liquefactive fat necrosis* is a more specific pattern of adipocyte necrosis and it is more often seen in α_1-antitrypsin deficiency panniculitis and in pancreatic panniculitis. Necrotic adipocytes injured by this mechanism appear as granular wisps of amphophilic detritus and their cellular structures are no longer evident. Enzymatic fat necrosis is a specific type of liquefactive fat necrosis characteristically observed in pancreatic panniculitis. It is due to saponification of the adipocyte lipid contents by pancreatic lipase, with secondary deposition of calcium salts, resulting in so-called ghost adipocytes, which consist of adipocytes with no nuclei and granular basophilic cytoplasm.

Hyalinizing fat necrosis is characteristically observed in lupus panniculitis and panniculitis associated with dermatomyositis. In this pattern, necrotic adipocytes appear as mummified anucleated cells, which are surrounded by glassy homogeneous proteinaceous material, effacing the architecture of the fat lobule.

Membranous fat necrosis is also a late-stage and non-specific type of necrosis of adipocytes, in which a leathery eosinophilic or amphophilic rim of collapsed cellular organelles with a crenulated or arabesque appearance is seen: periodic acid–Schiff (PAS) and Sudan III is positive. When membranous fat necrosis is extensive, formation of cystic structures devoid of cellular components and lined by hyaline-crenulated membrane can be observed. Membranous and membranocystic fat necrosis are almost always seen in lipodermatosclerosis, but like other types

of fat necrosis, they may also be seen in late-stage lesions of several types of panniculitis.

Ischaemic fat necrosis is more frequently seen at the centre of fat lobules and is characterized by pallor of adipocytes, which are smaller than normal due to severe impairment of blood supply. Later stages of ischaemic necrosis also show lipophagic granulomata. Ischaemic fat necrosis is frequently seen in erythema induratum of Bazin, but may also be observed in other panniculitides, including calcific uraemic arteriolopathy (calciphylaxis), infectious panniculitis and cutaneous polyarteritis nodosa.

Finally, *basophilic fat necrosis* results from necrosis of adipocytes intermingled with nuclear dust of neutrophils and granular basophilic material, which represent aggregations of bacteria and is characteristically seen in cases of infectious panniculitis.

There are some disorders that should no longer be considered as specific variants of panniculitis. *Weber–Christian disease* is the term that has been classically used to refer to cases of predominantly lobular panniculitis without vasculitis in association with systemic manifestations including fever and involvement of visceral fat tissue. Additional terms such as idiopathic nodular panniculitis, nodular panniculitis and relapsing febrile nonsuppurative nodular panniculitis have been used as synonyms for Weber–Christian disease. However, many cases originally considered as examples of Weber–Christian disease were later reclassified when other variants of lobular panniculitis, including erythema induratum of Bazin (nodular vasculitis), pancreatic panniculitis and α_1-antitrypsin deficiency panniculitis were separated as specific diseases. White and Winkelmann [18] reviewed the clinical and histopathological features of 30 cases of panniculitis previously diagnosed as Weber–Christian disease at the Mayo Clinic and most of the cases could be reclassified: 12 cases as erythema nodosum, six cases as superficial thrombophlebitis (STP), five cases as factitious panniculitis, three cases as traumatic panniculitis, and individual cases as cytophagic histiocytic panniculitis, subcutaneous 'pannicultic' lymphoma and subcutaneous involvement by leukaemia. The authors concluded that the term Weber–Christian disease should be abandoned as a diagnosis for cases of lobular panniculitis because now a more specific diagnosis may be reached in the majority of cases. The same is true for *Rothmann–Makai disease*, a term that was used previously to describe cases of relapsing nodular panniculitis similar to that of Weber–Christian disease but with no fever or other systemic manifestations. These are now considered obsolete terms that should be no longer used.

Superficial migratory thrombophlebitis

Introduction and general description

STP is an inflammation and thrombosis of the superficial veins which presents as painful induration with erythema, often in a linear or branching configuration forming cords (Figure 99.4) [1,2]. The clinical features are fully described in Chapter 103.

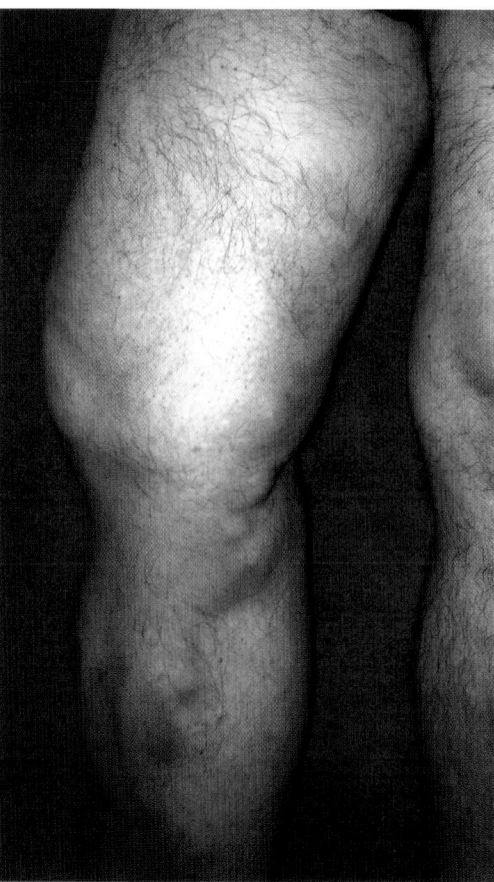

Figure 99.4 Superficial thrombophlebitis. Varicosities and erythematous nodules with linear arrangement involving the right lower extremity.

Pathophysiology

Predisposing factors

STP results from a hypercoagulable state, either primary [3] or secondary [4] (Box 99.1). The causes of secondary hypercoagulable states are varied, but in the majority of cases venous insufficiency of the lower extremities is the only precipitating factor.

Pathology

Histopathologically, cutaneous lesions of STP involve large veins of the septa in the upper subcutaneous tissue. The affected vein exhibits luminal thrombosis and an inflammatory infiltrate within its wall (Figure 99.5). In early lesions, the inflammatory cell infiltrate is composed mostly of neutrophils, whereas in later stages there are lymphocytes, histiocytes and occasional multinucleated giant cells. Granulomatous infiltration participates in the recanalization of the thrombus. A striking feature is that, in spite of the intense damage of the involved vein with dense inflammatory infiltrate in its wall and with marked septal thickening, there is little or no involvement of the adjacent fat lobule, and the process is more vasculitic than panniculitic. Intramural microabscesses in the wall of the involved vein have been described as characteristic of STP associated with Buerger disease [15].

Box 99.1 Primary and secondary hypercoagulable states that cause superficial thrombophlebitis

Primary hypercoagulable states
- Antiphospholipid syndrome
- Deficiencies of
  - Protein C
  - Protein S
  - Heparin co-factor II
  - Antithrombin III
  - Factor XII
  - Tissue plasminogen activator
  - Factor V Leiden [3]

Secondary hypercoagulable states
- Paraneoplastic superficial migratory thrombophlebitis (Trousseau syndrome) [1,5]
- Behçet syndrome [6]
- Buerger disease [7]
- Pregnancy [8]
- HIV-associated immune reconstitution syndrome (IRIS) [9]
- Secondary syphilis [10,11]
- Infectious suppurative thrombophlebitis in children due to *Staphylococcus aureus*, *Escherichia coli*, *Pseudomonas aeruginosa* or fungi [12–14]
- Oral contraceptive pills
- Sepsis, intravenous injections or catheterizations
- Complications of venous sclerotherapy [4]

Clinical features

Patients with STP should be appropriately investigated to rule out hypercoagulable states, paraneoplastic processes (Trousseau sign) and Behçet disease, although by far the most common cause of STP is chronic venous insufficiency of the lower limbs.

Differential diagnosis

The main histopathological differential diagnosis for STP is cutaneous polyarteritis nodosa. In contrast to STP, cutaneous polyarteritis nodosa is characterized by involvement of the small arteries and arterioles of the subcutaneous septa. The process is more inflammatory than thrombotic, with prominent fibrinoid necrosis of the tunica intima, resulting in the so-called target-like arteritis, in which an eosinophilic ring of fibrinoid necrosis replaces the intima of the affected arteriole. In doubtful cases, elastic tissue stain usually resolves any uncertainty, because in cutaneous polyarteritis nodosa the involved artery shows sharp and prominent internal elastic lamina, whereas in STP the damaged vessel is a vein with little or no discernible internal elastic membrane [16]. Some authors, however, believe that when inflammation is present within and around the wall of the vessel, the identification of the internal elastic lamina of the involved vessel is less reliable even with elastic tissue stains, and the smooth muscle pattern has the highest sensitivity and specificity for distinguishing arteries from veins [17]. The recently described type of tuberculid, nodular granulomatous phlebitis, may clinically resemble STP, but this tuberculid is histopathologically characterized by tuberculoid granulomas and multinucleate giant cells involving the walls of the veins of subcutaneous tissue [18,19].

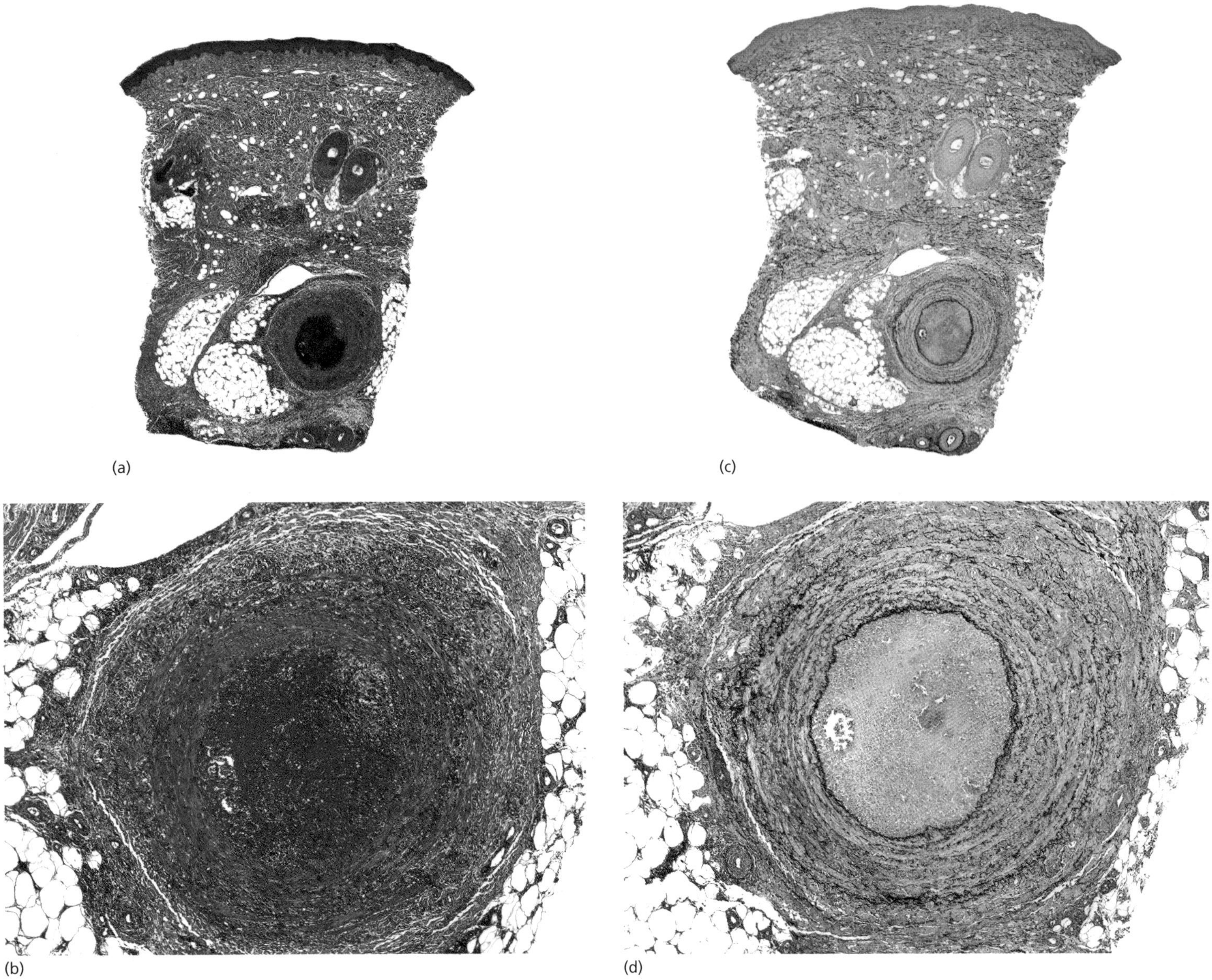

(a)

(c)

(b)

(d)

Figure 99.5 Histopathological features of superficial thrombophlebitis. (a) Scanning view showing involvement of a large vein in the septa of subcutaneous tissue. (b) The involved vein shows thrombosis of its lumen. (c) The same specimen stained for elastic tissue. (d) Several layers of internal elastic lamina are seen around the luminal thrombus.

Cutaneous polyarteritis nodosa

Definition

A cutaneous vasculitis of poorly understood aetiology affecting subcutaneous arteries and arterioles (Figure 99.6). It is strongly associated with circulating antineutrophil cytoplasmic antibodies with peripheral staining (p-ANCA). In contrast to systemic polyarteritis nodosa, there is little or no evidence of systemic disease. It is fully described in Chapter 102.

Pathophysiology

The serum of patients with cutaneous polyarteritis nodosa is usually negative for p-ANCA by enzyme-linked immunosorbent assay (ELISA), but 84% of the patients reveal p-ANCA positivity by

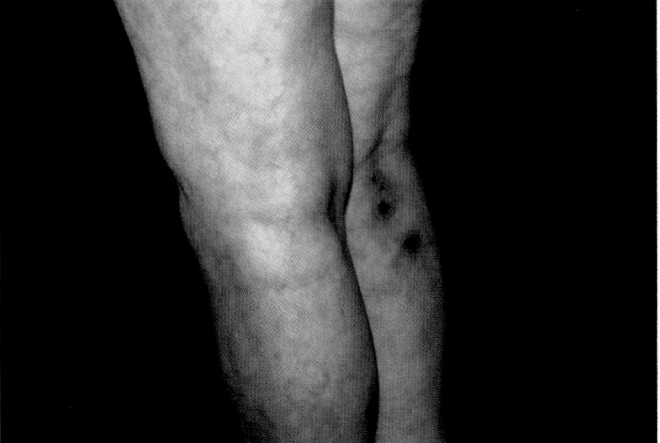

Figure 99.6 Clinical appearance of cutaneous polyarteritis nodosa showing livedo reticularis of the lower extremities with ulcerated nodules on the right calf of a middle-aged woman.

indirect immunofluorescence. Serum lysosomal-associated membrane protein 2 antibody (anti-LAMP-2) levels in cutaneous polyarteritis nodosa patients with p-ANCA are significantly elevated compared with those with negative p-ANCA, which suggests that anti-LAMP-2 antibodies might play an important role in the pathogenesis of the condition [1]. Immunoglobulin G (IgG) antiphosphatidylserine–prothrombin complex (anti-PS/PT) antibodies and/or IgG anticardiolipin antibodies have also been detected in the serum of some patients with cutaneous polyarteritis nodosa [2].

Pathology

Cutaneous lesions exhibit vasculitis involving medium-sized arteries and arterioles at the septa of the upper subcutis (Figure 99.7). Direct immunofluorescence studies of lesions of cutaneous pol-

yarteritis nodosa have demonstrated IgM and complement deposition in the involved vessel walls and consistent absence of IgG [3]. The involved vessel appears with a thickened wall, within which an inflammatory infiltrate is seen. Its composition varies with the stage of evolution of the process. In early lesions, a neutrophilic infiltrate and leukocytoclasis are often seen and, in some cases, eosinophils may be prominent [4]. Characteristically, the intima of the involved artery exhibits an eosinophilic ring of fibrinoid necrosis, giving a target-like appearance to the damaged vessel. In older lesions, lymphocytes are predominant and in a still later stage there is fibrosis of the entire thickness of the vessel wall, leading to the obliteration of its lumen. A rare complication is the formation of periosteal new bone beneath the cutaneous lesions [5]. Although luminal thrombi may be present, they are less frequent than in lesions of superficial thrombophlebitis. Often, arterial involvement is segmental and serial sections throughout the entire specimen are required to demonstrate the pathology. As is the case in superficial thrombophlebitis, lesions of cutaneous polyarteritis nodosa show little or no involvement of the adjacent fat lobule, and the process is exclusively a septal arteritis.

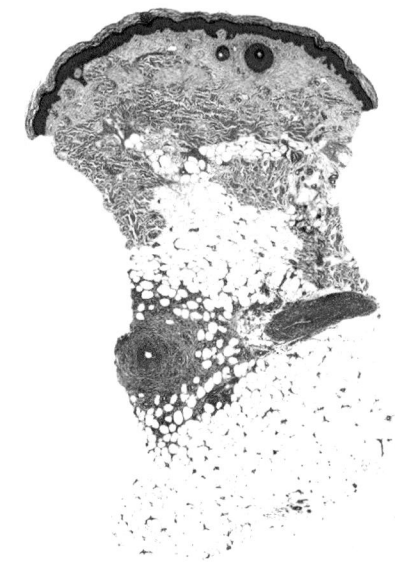

(a)

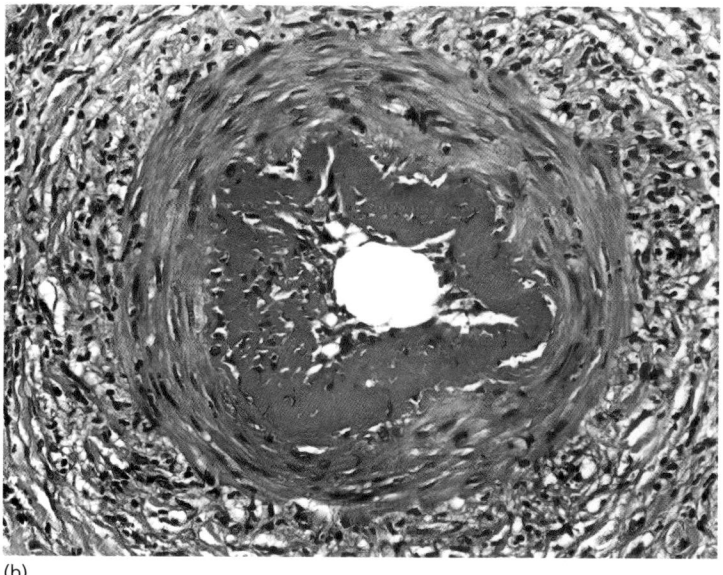

(b)

Figure 99.7 Histopathological features of cutaneous polyarteritis nodosa. (a) Scanning view of a punch biopsy showing involvement of a vessel of the septa of subcutaneous fat. (b) Higher magnification showing fibrinoid necrosis of the intima, giving a target-like appearance to the involved arteriole.

Necrobiosis lipoidica

Definition

Necrobiosis lipoidica is an uncommon skin condition in which degenerated dermal collagen is surrounded by a granulomatous inflammatory response to produce shiny, red-brown or yellowish plaques in the skin, particularly on the shins (Figure 99.8). In severe cases, the affected skin may ulcerate. It is associated in the majority of but not all cases with underlying diabetes, the onset of which it may precede. It is fully described in Chapter 97. It may involve the subcutis but does not cause a true panniculitis, because the palisading granulomatous process involving the subcutis is always a deep extension of the dermal process and, to our knowledge,

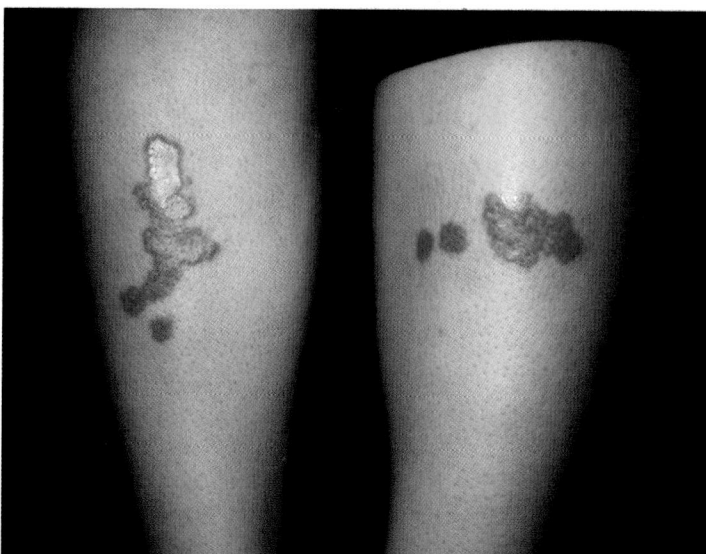

Figure 99.8 Necrobiosis lipoidica showing yellowish indurated plaques on the anterior aspect of the legs in a diabetic woman.

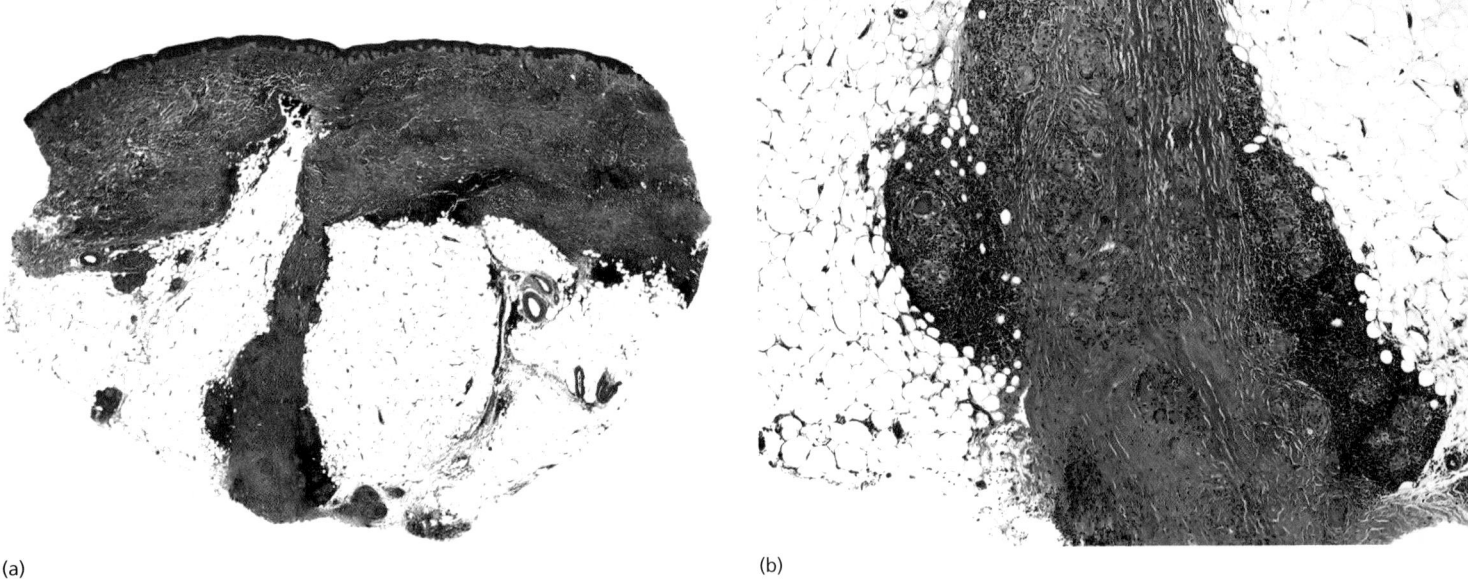

(a)   (b)

Figure 99.9 Histopathological features of necrobiosis lipoidica extending to subcutaneous tissue. (a) Scanning power showing involvement of the full thickness of the dermis and extension to the subcutaneous tissue throughout the septa. (b) Granulomas involving the thickened fibrous septa of the subcutaneous tissue.

there are no descriptions of necrobiosis lipoidica involving only subcutaneous fat.

Pathology

Histopathologically, lesions of necrobiosis lipoidica involve the full thickness of the dermis, and often extend to the superficial subcutaneous tissue causing septal panniculitis [1] (Figure 99.9). There are palisading granulomas with histiocytes surrounding areas of degenerate collagen within widened septa. The most characteristic feature supporting a diagnosis of necrobiosis lipoidica as the cause of an inflammatory process involving the subcutis is the coexistence of similar lesions in the dermis, with alternating horizontal bands of inflammatory cells and fibrosis involving the entire dermis [2].

Early lesions show an inflammatory infiltrate composed predominantly of neutrophils scattered within the septa, whereas in later lesions, histiocytes, lymphocytes and plasma cells, sometimes with lymphoid follicle formation [3], are predominant. Multinucleated giant cells involving the septa are sometimes prominent and in those cases histopathological findings resemble erythema nodosum. Differential diagnosis is, however, straightforward because in the latter condition there are no significant dermal changes other than a perivascular lymphocytic infiltrate.

In chronic longstanding lesions, the dermis and the superficial subcutaneous tissue are replaced by horizontal fibrosis with sclerotic collagen bundles arranged parallel to the epidermis and scattered by plasma cells, closely resembling the findings seen in morphoea. In these late-stage lesions, features of necrobiosis are no longer evident and elastic tissue stains demonstrate dramatic loss of elastic fibres. Some authors have postulated that the finding of vasculitis and leukocytoclasis in lesions of necrobiosis lipoidica is indicative of an underlying systemic disease [4]. Membranous fat necrosis has also been described in late-stage lesions of necrobiosis lipoidica extending to the subcutaneous tissue [5].

Direct immunofluorescence studies have demonstrated IgM and complement in the blood vessels of some lesions of necrobiosis

lipoidica, suggesting that this process is an immune complex vasculitis [6], but extensive histopathological studies identified vascular involvement only in 30% of the cases [7]. The finding of GLUT-1 immunohistochemical expression in areas of sclerotic collagen of necrobiosis lipoidica raises the possibility that a disturbance in glucose transport by fibroblasts may contribute to the histogenesis of necrobiosis lipoidica [8].

Deep morphoea

Definition

A group of related diseases of poorly understood aetiology affecting principally skin and subcutaneous tissue and characterized by variable fibrosis, sclerosis and cutaneous atrophy (Figure 99.10). Within the

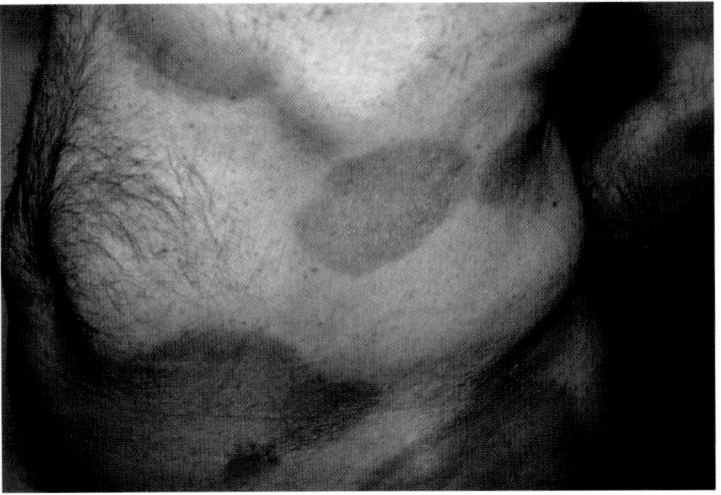

Figure 99.10 Morphoea profunda. The lesions consisted of indurated, hyperpigmented and slightly depressed plaques.

deep morphoea group, three closely related processes are included, namely morphoea profunda, eosinophilic fasciitis and disabling pansclerotic morphoea of children [1]. Although classical morphoea often extends from the deep dermis to the subcutaneous tissue, morphoea is sometimes an entirely panniculitic process with no involvement of the epidermis, cutaneous adnexa or dermis. The process is known variously as morphoea profunda, nodular scleroderma or keloidal scleroderma. These conditions are fully described in Chapter 57.

Investigations

Histopathologically, the lesions show a marked fibrous thickening of the septa of subcutaneous fat (Figure 99.11). As a consequence of

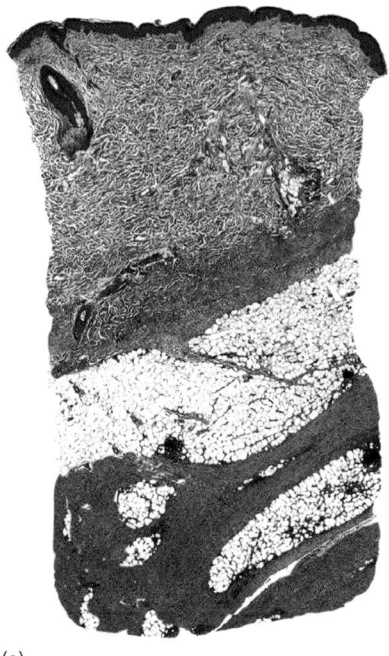

(a)

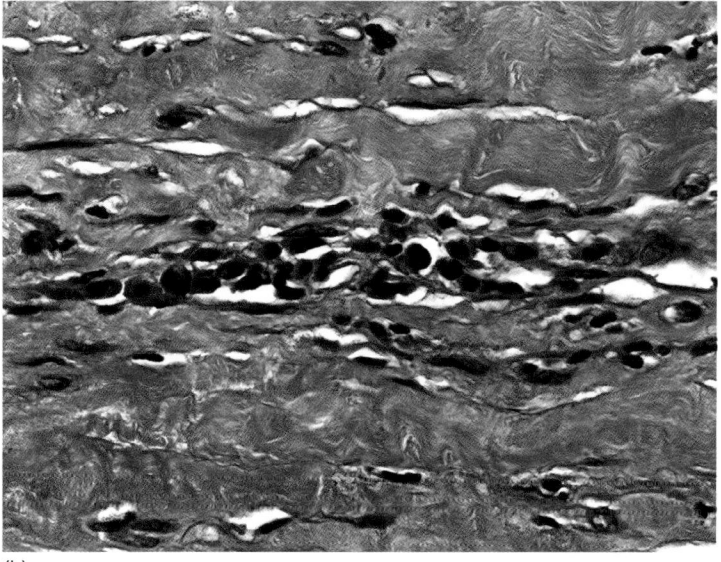

(b)

Figure 99.11 Histopathology of deep morphoea. (a) Scanning power showing sclerosis of the deeper reticular dermis and the septa of subcutaneous tissue. Note that the superficial and mid dermis were spared. (b) Thickened sclerotic collagen bundles with interstitial lymphocytes and plasma cells.

thickening, collagen also replaces the fat normally present around and below the eccrine coils, giving the misleading impression that sweat glands have ascended into the dermis. When the sclerotic process involves both dermis and subcutis, the full thickness of the specimen appears homogeneously eosinophilic. Inflammatory infiltrate is present only in active lesions, consisting of aggregates of lymphocytes surrounded by plasma cells at the interface between the thickened septa and the fat lobules. Plasma cells may be also present arranged interstitially between the sclerotic collagen bundles [2–4]. Active lesions of deep morphoea usually show denser infiltrate than dermal morphoea [4–6].

Eosinophilic fasciitis (Shulman syndrome) is regarded as a variant of deep morphoea in which the thick and sclerotic septa and the fascia show inflammatory infiltrate of lymphocytes, histiocytes, plasma cells and abundant numbers of eosinophils [7–14]. Histopathological study of early stages of eosinophilic fasciitis shows oedema and infiltration by eosinophils, lymphocytes and plasma cells between the collagen bundles of the connective tissue septa of the subcutis and subcutaneous fascia. Lymphoid aggregates may be also present. In the later stages, there is fibrosis and hyalinization of the involved tissues [11].

Disabling pansclerotic morphoea in children is an aggressive clinical variant of morphoea which appears before 14 years of age [15], although adult onset has been also described [16]. The process involves not only the full thickness of the skin, but also the subcutaneous tissues, muscle and bone. Histopathological findings in cutaneous lesions of disabling pansclerotic morphoea show sclerotic replacement of the full thickness of the dermis and subcutaneous fat and the process extends to underlying fascia. In active lesions, a variable infiltrate of lymphocytes and plasma cells is seen between the sclerotic collagen bundles [15].

Subcutaneous granuloma annulare

Clinical features

Presentation

Subcutaneous granuloma annulare is a rare clinicopathological variant of granuloma annulare, characterized by subcutaneous nodules that may appear alone or in association with the classical dermal papular lesions [1,2] (Figure 99.12). It typically presents in children or young adults [3,4]. It is fully described in Chapter 97.

Pathophysiology

An immunoglobulin-mediated vasculitis has been proposed as the underlying mechanism for necrobiotic areas in granuloma annulare [5], although direct immunofluorescence studies failed to demonstrate immune deposits within vessels walls [6]. Additional postulated pathogenic mechanisms include a cell-mediated immune response with increased helper/inducer T cells and CD1a-positive Langerhans cells [7], a Th1 inflammatory reaction with interferon (IFN)-γ-producing lymphocytes eliciting matrix degradation [8], increased collagen synthesis [9] and elastic tissue degeneration [10]. The inflammatory cells release cytokines, including macrophage inhibitor factor, which cause histiocytes

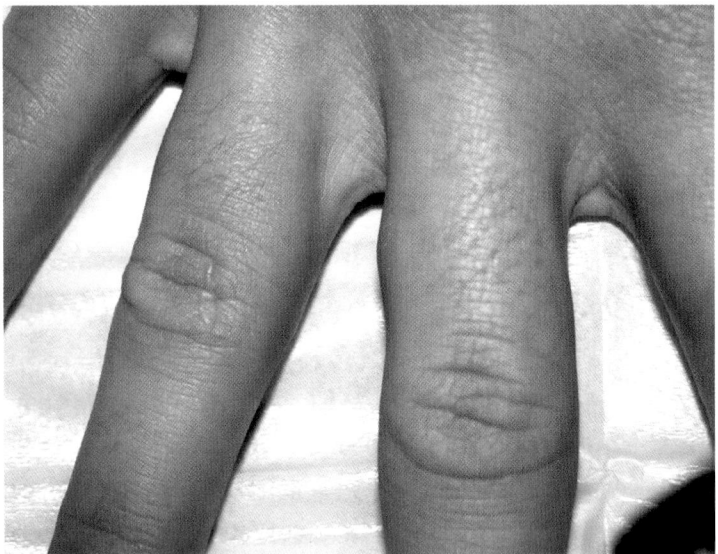

Figure 99.12 Subcutaneous granuloma annulare involving the lateral aspect of the first phalanx of the third right finger in a 14-year-old boy.

to accumulate in the necrobiotic areas and release lysosomal enzymes resulting in degenerate connective tissue [11]. Usually, subcutaneous granuloma annulare is a true panniculitic process with no dermal involvement, although in 25% of patients subcutaneous nodular lesions coexist with the classical presentation of superficial papules [12,13]. In rare instances, subcutaneous granuloma annulare may extend to involve deeper soft tissues and producing a destructive arthritis and limb deformity [14].

Differential diagnosis
Histopathological differential diagnosis of subcutaneous granuloma annulare includes rheumatoid nodule, necrobiosis lipoidica and epithelioid sarcoma.

In contrast with subcutaneous granuloma annulare, which usually exhibits a pale and mucinous centre with a tendency to be basophilic, the central necrobiotic areas of rheumatoid nodules appear homogeneous and eosinophilic with abundant fibrin deposits. Sometimes, however, the differential diagnosis between subcutaneous granuloma annulare and rheumatoid nodule may be impossible on histopathological grounds alone. Old rheumatoid nodules show extensive fibrosis in which necrobiotic areas persist.

Lesions of necrobiosis lipoidica involve the full thickness of the dermis and the subcutaneous involvement is just a deep extension from the dermis into the connective tissue septa of the subcutis. Plasma cells, aggregations of histiocytes and multinucleated giant cells are more common in necrobiosis lipoidica than in subcutaneous granuloma annulare. In the late stages of necrobiosis lipoidica, there is extensive fibrosis and degenerate collagen is no longer seen.

Epithelioid sarcoma (see Chapter 137) is a neoplastic process in which central areas of degenerate collagen are surrounded by epithelioid cells with hyperchromatic and pleomorphic nuclei, some of them showing atypical mitotic figures. Immunohistochemical studies demonstrate that, in contrast with the inflammatory cells in subcutaneous granuloma annulare, the neoplastic cells

in the palisades of epithelioid sarcoma express immunoreactivity for low- and high-molecular-weight cytokeratins, epithelial membrane antigen and CD34; furthermore, their nuclei show no expression of integrase interactor 1 (INI-1) [15–17].

Investigations

Pathology
The histopathological changes seen in subcutaneous granuloma annulare consist of areas of basophilic degeneration of collagen bundles with peripheral palisading granulomas involving the connective tissue septa of the subcutis (Figure 99.13). Usually, the areas of collagen degeneration are larger than in the dermal counterpart of the process. The central necrobiotic areas contain increased amounts of connective tissue mucin and nuclear dust from neutrophils between the degenerated collagen bundles. Elastic tissue is usually absent within the foci of degenerate

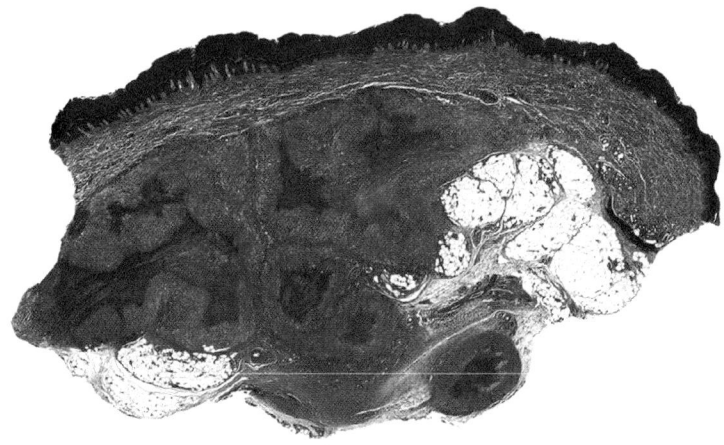

(a)

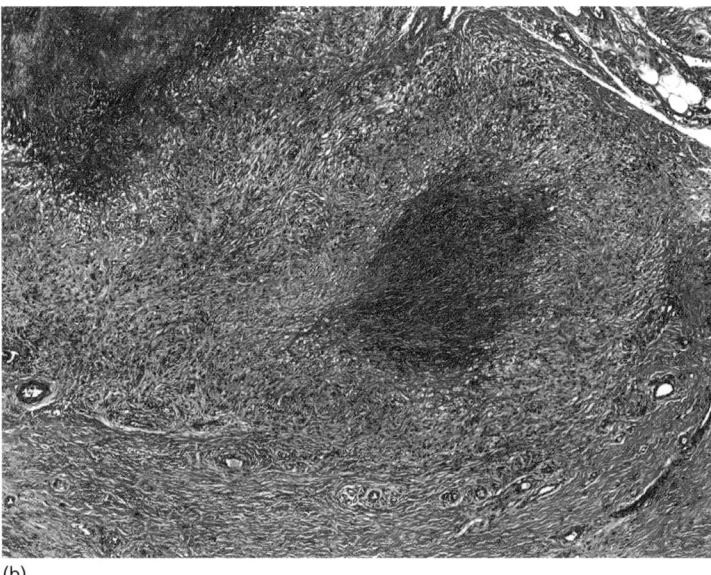

(b)

Figure 99.13 Histopathological findings in subcutaneous granuloma annulare. (a) Scanning power showing the involvement of deeper dermis and subcutaneous tissue. (b) There are several areas of degenerate collagen bundles surrounded by a palisade of histiocytes.

collagen. The peripheral ring is composed of epithelioid histiocytes arranged in a palisade fashion and multinucleated giant cells may also be seen [18,19]. Eosinophils are more common in subcutaneous granuloma annulare than in the dermal superficial lesions [19]. The so-called incomplete or interstitial histopathological variant of granuloma annulare is characterized by histiocytes interstitially arranged between collagen bundles, with mucin deposition but no areas of degenerate collagen. This histopathological pattern, more frequent than the necrobiotic one in dermal lesions, has yet to be described in subcutaneous granuloma annulare and all reported patients with deep forms of the process showed the classical palisading necrobiotic pattern [20]. Immunohistochemical studies showed intense expression of CD68/PGM1 in the histiocytic population and a variable one of lysozyme. T-cell markers (CD3, CD4 and CD8) have been detected mainly in the perivascular lymphocytic infiltrate, with CD4+ T lymphocytes predominating over CD8+ [21].

Rheumatoid nodule

Definition

Rheumatoid nodules are one of the extra-articular manifestations of rheumatoid arthritis. They are usually found in proximity to joints or extensor surfaces (Figure 99.14) and other areas subjected to mechanical pressure. They can also develop elsewhere, including in the pleura and meninges. Nodules vary in size and consistency and are rarely symptomatic. They are described more fully in Chapter 154.

Pathophysiology

The pathogenesis of rheumatoid nodules remains unknown. Because the lesions develop at sites of trauma and pressure, mechanical factors have been postulated as pathogenic factors. Some genetic factor may also be involved, because patients with HLA-DRB1 present with severe rheumatoid arthritis and frequent

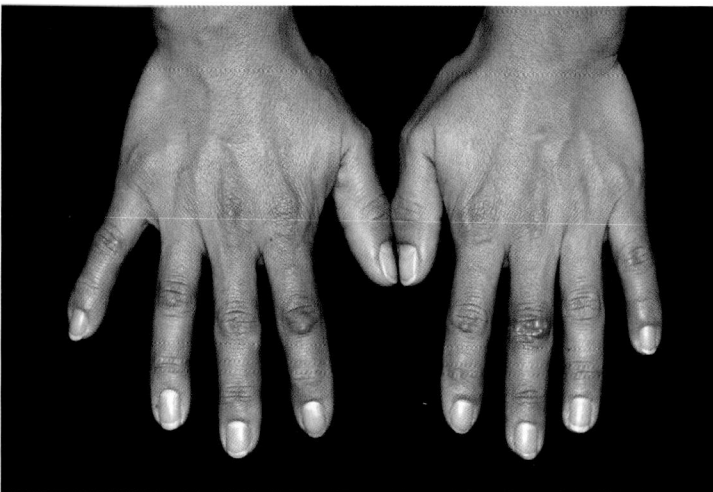

Figure 99.14 Rheumatoid nodules involving the dorsum of the fingers in an adult woman with seropositive rheumatoid arthritis.

rheumatoid nodules, whereas those with HLA-DRw2 have a mild articular disease and infrequent rheumatoid nodules [1–4]. Recently, microchimerism has been demonstrated almost in 50% of the cases of rheumatoid nodules of patients with rheumatoid arthritis. Since microchimerism is genetically disparate, it is possible that microchimerism in rheumatoid nodules serves as an allogeneic stimulus or allogeneic target [5]. Pro-inflammatory cytokines and cell adhesion molecules are very similar in rheumatoid nodules and the synovial lining in rheumatoid joints. The cytokine profile identified within the rheumatoid nodule showed the presence of IFN-γ, but not IL-2, and prominent expression of IL-1β and TNF-α together with IL-12, IL-18, IL-15 and IL-10. These findings support the hypothesis that the formation of rheumatoid nodules is driven by Th1 lymphocytes [6]. An immune complex-mediated mechanism has also been postulated: IgG and IgM have been detected by direct immunofluorescence in the vessel walls of rheumatoid nodules, suggesting that a vasculitic process may be involved [7,8]. The mechanism for the central degeneration of the collagen bundles is also unknown. Although apoptosis has been demonstrated throughout the entire nodule [9], it seems that the proteases, collagenases and other chemotactic factors (e.g. granulocyte–macrophage colony-stimulating factor and fibronectin) secreted by lesional monocytes and macrophages are the main factors inducing degeneration of collagen, mucin deposition and palisading granuloma formation [7,10].

Clinical variants

Accelerated rheumatoid nodulosis (ARN) is the term used to describe the development of new painful rheumatoid nodules in patients with chronic rheumatoid arthritis under treatment with methotrexate. These new nodules develop preferentially on the hands, feet and ears [11–15]. It seems that there is an individual susceptibility to ARN, because it develops more frequently in patients with HLA-DRB1 and seropositive rheumatoid arthritis [1,15]. Genetically predisposed patients appear to be protected against the development of methotrexate-induced ARN by the concomitant administration of hydroxychloroquine [16], D-penicillamine [17], colchicine [18] or sulfasalazine [19]. The pathogenesis of ARN is unknown, although an adenosine A1 receptor promotion of multinucleated giant cell formation by human monocytes has been postulated [20]. ARN is not exclusively related to methotrexate therapy and identical lesions have also been reported in patients with rheumatoid arthritis receiving treatment with azathioprine [21], etanercept [22,23], infliximab [24] and leflunomide [20,25]. Neither is ARN found exclusively in rheumatoid arthritis: similar lesions have been described in patients with psoriatic arthritis [26] and systemic lupus erythematosus [27–30]. ARN has also been described in seropositive, polyarthritic-onset juvenile rheumatoid arthritis after methotrexate treatment [31,32]. In all these patients, the condition causes minimal symptoms and regresses after methotrexate is withdrawn; it does, however, recur when methotrexate is reintroduced.

Differential diagnosis

Histopathological differential diagnosis of rheumatoid nodules includes other palisading granulomas, mainly necrobiosis lipoidica and subcutaneous granuloma annulare. Table 99.2 summarizes the

PART 8: SPECIFIC CUTANEOUS STRUCTURE

Table 99.2 Histopathological differential diagnosis of rheumatoid nodule, subcutaneous granuloma annulare and necrobiosis lipoidica.

	Rheumatoid nodule	Subcutaneous granuloma annulare	Necrobiosis lipoidica
Location	Subcutaneous septa	Subcutaneous septa, often upper and mid reticular dermis involvement	Full thickness of the dermis with extension into subcutaneous septa
Pattern	Massive areas of degenerate collagen with fibrin deposition (eosinophilic necrobiotic granuloma)	Discrete foci of degenerate collagen with mucin deposition (basophilic necrobiotic granuloma)	Fibrosis and ill-defined areas of collagen degeneration (eosinophilic necrobiotic granuloma)
Collagen degeneration	Complete	Complete	Indistinct, elongated areas of degenerate collagen
Fibrosis	Common	Uncommon	Common
Histiocytes	Well-defined palisades of histiocytes	Well-defined palisades of histiocytes	Interstitial histiocytes, no palisading
Inflammatory components	Tuberculoid and sarcoid reaction common	Tuberculoid and sarcoid reaction uncommon	Tuberculoid and sarcoid reaction common
Vascular anomalies	Capillary hyperplasia at the periphery	Perivascular lymphocytes	Capillary wall thickening
Mucin	Variable	Common	Variable
Fibrin	Common	No	Variable

Modified from Hewitt and Cole [38].

main differential diagnostic features among these three necrobiotic disorders. Palisading necrobiotic granulomas have been classified into 'blue' and 'red' granulomas according to the colour of the central area of degenerate collagen stained with H&E [33,34]. Blue granulomas, which show a basophilic centre due to mucin deposition and the presence of neutrophils and nuclear dust, are usually seen in subcutaneous granuloma annulare. Red granulomas exhibit an eosinophilic necrobiotic central area due to fibrin deposition and are seen predominantly in rheumatoid nodules (Figure 99.15). Necrobiosis lipoidica usually shows a more fibrotic pattern and the process always involves the dermis.

Investigations

Histopathological findings in rheumatoid nodules vary according to the age of the lesion. Early lesions show microscopic features of granulation tissue surrounded by mononuclear cells and fibroblasts [35]. In later stages, the lesions show a central area of degenerate collagen admixed with fibrinoid material and surrounded by a palisade of elongated mononuclear histiocytes. The inner central degenerated zone appears as intensely eosinophilic amorphous, granular or fibrillary material containing collagen fibrils, fibrin and cellular debris. Multinucleated giant cells, T lymphocytes, plasma cells, mast cells and eosinophils may also be seen at the periphery. Uncommonly, features of acute vasculitis have been described in the surrounding vessels and sometimes a necrotic blood vessel associated with nuclear debris and sparse neutrophils may be seen at the centre of necrobiotic areas, though these findings probably represent secondary vasculitis. In rare instances, superficial nodules may perforate the epidermis [36]. Longstanding rheumatoid nodules exhibit extensive fibrosis in which clefts and cystic degeneration appear due to liquefactive degeneration of the contents of the nodules [37].

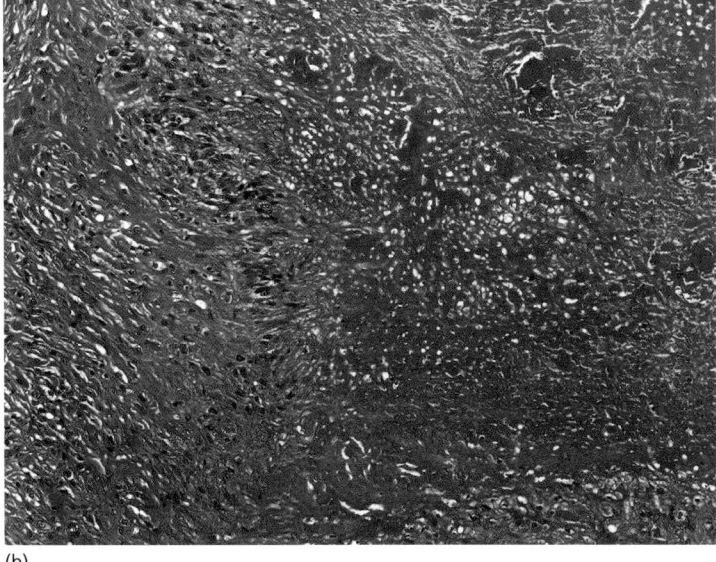

(a)   (b)

Figure 99.15 Histopathological features of rheumatoid nodule. (a) Scanning power showing a diffuse replacement of subcutaneous tissue by a fibrotic process with scattered areas of degenerate collagen. (b) The eosinophilic fibrinoid areas are surrounded by a palisade of histiocytes.

Necrobiotic xanthogranuloma

Clinical features

Necrobiotic xanthogranuloma is a rare histiocytic disorder which causes progressive destruction of the involved cutaneous and extracutaneous tissues. It most commonly presents as multiple indurated yellow-red (Figure 99.16) or violaceous plaques or nodules, preferentially involving periorbital skin. It is described in detail in Chapter 136.

Pathophysiology

The pathogenesis of necrobiotic xanthogranuloma is poorly understood. One proposed mechanism is that the monoclonal paraprotein behaves as a lipoprotein, binding to monocyte lipoprotein receptors to form xanthomata [1]. Intracellular accumulation of lipoprotein-derived lipids in skin macrophages may result from activation of monocytes [2], with both the paraprotein and immune complexes inducing granuloma formation [3]. It has been suggested that the central areas of necrobiosis in lesions of necrobiotic xanthogranuloma may be the consequence of ischaemia [4]. Another proposed pathogenetic mechanism is that an increase in circulating macrophage colony-stimulating factor (M-CSF) levels activates monocytes and favours the accumulation of large amounts of lipid and xanthoma formation [5,6,7]. The finding of *Borrelia* organisms in six of seven cases of necrobiotic xanthogranuloma using focus-floating microscopy has led some authors to propose an infectious aetiology for this process [8].

Differential diagnosis

The histopathological differential diagnosis of necrobiotic xanthogranuloma includes necrobiosis lipoidica, subcutaneous granuloma annulare, juvenile xanthogranuloma and deep xanthomas [5,9]. Subcutaneous granuloma annulare occurs mainly in children

and does not tend to ulcerate. Usually mucin deposits are evident at the centre of degenerate collagen; lymphoid follicles and cholesterol clefts are absent. Necrobiosis lipoidica may extend to subcutaneous tissue and then the differential diagnosis may be challenging. However, xanthomatization, lymphoid follicles and cholesterol clefts are less frequently seen than in necrobotic xanthogranuloma. Juvenile xanthogranuloma and deep xanthomas do not show large areas of degenerate collagen as seen in necrobiotic xanthogranuloma.

Investigations

From the histopathological point of view, necrobiotic xanthogranuloma is not a true panniculitis but a deeper extension of a predominantly dermal process (Figure 99.17). The most characteristic findings consist of a diffuse involvement of the dermis by foamy histiocytes and some Touton-like multinucleated giant cells. From the dermis, the infiltrate extends through the connective tissue septa of the subcutis and underlying soft tissues. Areas of degenerate collagen bundles and cholesterol clefts are often seen within the diffuse infiltrate [10,11]. A palisading granuloma of epithelioid histiocytes is present, at least focally, around the areas

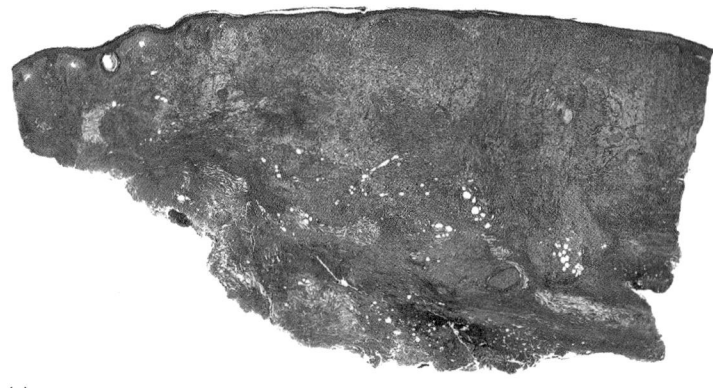

(a)

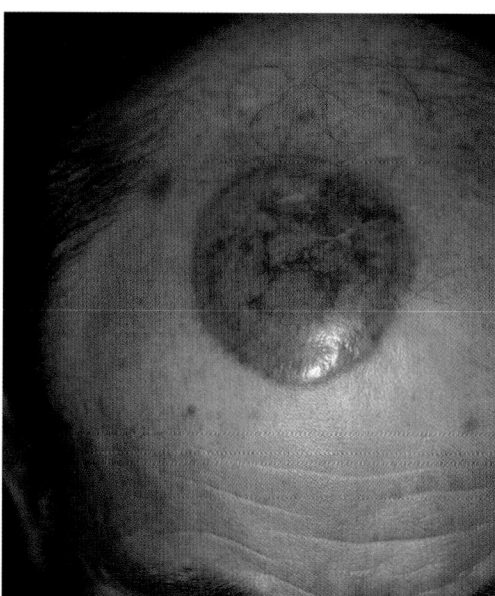

Figure 99.16 Necrobiotic xanthogranuloma. A plaque with yellowish hue involving the scalp.

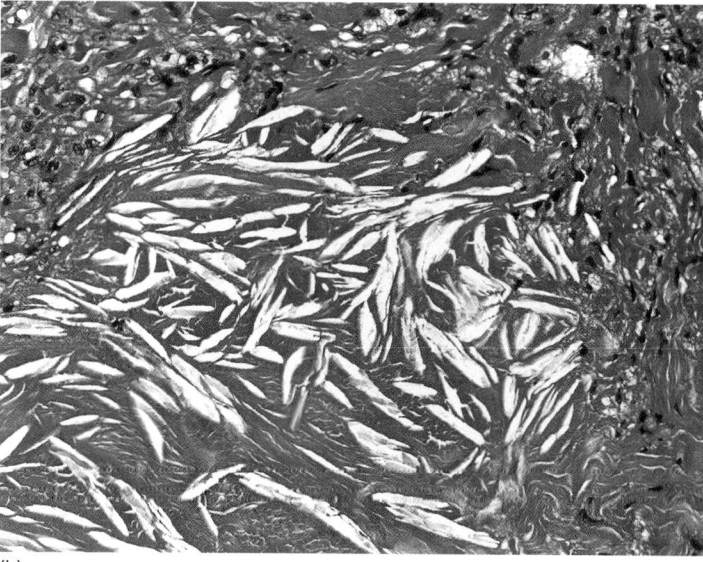

(b)

Figure 99.17 Histopathological features of necrobiotic xanthogranuloma. (a) Scanning power showing diffuse involvement of the entire thickness of the dermis and extension to subcutaneous tissue. (b) Areas of degenerate collagen with abundant cholesterol clefts.

PART 8: SPECIFIC CUTANEOUS STRUCTURE

PART 8: SPECIFIC CUTANEOUS STRUCTURE

of degenerate collagen [9]. Lymphoid aggregates, sometimes with germinal centre formation, and numerous plasma cells at the periphery are often seen around the deeper areas of collagen degeneration [12]. Although there is a diffuse infiltration of the dermis and subcutaneous tissue, some cases exhibit a multinodular pattern [13]. From the immunohistochemical point of view, histiocytes and foamy macrophages express immunoreactivity for lysozyme, CD68, Mac387 and CD11b [14]. In one case, intense histiocytic expression of CD10 was also observed [15].

Immunohistochemistry has demonstrated that, although necrobiotic xanthogranuloma is frequently associated with paraproteinaemia, the skin lesions represent reactive inflammation because the plasma cells present in the cutaneous lesions are polyclonal [16]. Vasculitis is not usually seen, although some lesions may show leukocytoclasis and thrombosis [13,17]. Transepidermal and transfollicular elimination of degenerate collagen and cholesterol clefts have also been reported [18]. Reports of granuloma annulare with subsequent evolution into necrobiosis lipoidica or necrobiotic xanthogranuloma raise the possibility of a general granulomatous process accompanying paraproteinaemia [19,20]. The coexistence of normolipaemic plane xanthoma and necrobiotic xanthogranuloma in the same patient also suggests that these two processes represent part of a spectrum of xanthomatous dermal reactions associated with paraproteinaemia and that they may be more closely related than previously recognized [21].

Erythema nodosum

Introduction and general description

Erythema nodosum is the most common panniculitis. The process usually shows an acute onset and self-limited course. It is clinically characterized by the sudden eruption of several erythematous, tender, non-ulcerating nodules and plaques, typically located on the shins. The condition normally resolves spontaneously without ulceration, scarring or atrophy, but recurrent episodes are common. Erythema nodosum is a cutaneous reactive process that may be triggered by a wide variety of infectious and inflammatory disorders and, less commonly, by malignant neoplasms and medications [1–7,8,9–127] (Table 99.3). The most common triggers are bacterial infections, sarcoidosis and inflammatory bowel disease.

Epidemiology

Incidence and prevalence

The population prevalence of erythema nodosum in a semirural area of England over a 2 year period was 2.4 cases per 1000 population per year [128]. Erythema nodosum accounted for about 0.5% of new cases seen in departments of dermatology in England [95] and about 0.38% of all patients seen in a Department of Internal Medicine in Spain [129]. The average annual incidence of biopsy proven erythema nodosum in persons aged 14 years or more at a hospital in north-western Spain was 52 cases per million population served [8], although this almost certainly underestimated the real incidence of the disease, because only biopsy confirmed cases were included. Most cases of erythema nodosum occur within the

first half of the year [8], probably due to the increased frequency of streptococcal infections in this period; there is no difference in incidence between urban and rural areas [130]. Familial cases are usually attributable to infection; simultaneous occurrence in monozygotic twin sisters has been reported [131].

Age

Erythema nodosum may occur at any age, but most cases appear between the second and fourth decades of life, with the peak between 20 and 30 years of age, probably due to the high incidence of sarcoidosis at this age [132]. Racial and geographical variations in incidence may be explained by differences in the prevalence of aetiological factors.

Sex

Several studies have demonstrated that erythema nodosum occurs three to six times more frequently in women than in men [133], although the incidence before puberty is approximately equal in both genders [134].

Associated diseases

Concomitant presentation of Sweet syndrome and erythema nodosum has been repeatedly reported in the literature [10,135–146]. The simultaneous occurrence of these two reactive processes has been associated with sarcoidosis [136], throat infection [136,137], acute myelogenous leukaemia [138,139] and Crohn disease [139]. The association has been described in up to 15–30% of the patients in some series of biopsy-proven erythema nodosum [140–143], which suggests a common underlying pathogenetic mechanism for both processes [140,146].

Pathophysiology

There are numerous recognized triggers of erythema nodosum [1–7,8,9–127] (see Table 99.3). Aetiological factors show considerable geographical variation related to specific endemic infections. In Europe, streptococcal infections, sarcoidosis and inflammatory bowel disease are important causes. In a significant percentage of cases (ranging between 37% and 60% in reported series), the aetiology of erythema nodosum cannot be determined despite extensive clinical and laboratory investigation [8,38,134,147–150].

A previous episode of upper respiratory infection by group A β-haemolytic Streptococcus is a frequent cause for erythema nodosum in children and young adults. Erythematous subcutaneous nodules usually develop 2–3 weeks after the throat infection and are accompanied by an elevation of the antistreptolysin O (ASO) titre; by the time cutaneous lesions appear, the cultures from throat swabs usually fail to detect microorganisms [8,24]. Tuberculosis is a common cause of erythema nodosum in areas of high endemicity. This used to apply to many parts of Europe but no longer does so [8,147,151]. Erythema nodosum, when triggered by tuberculosis, presents mainly in children at the time of primary pulmonary infection and concomitant with the conversion of the tuberculin test [24].

Many medications have been implicated as the cause of erythema nodosum, although their real pathogenetic role is difficult to establish with confidence. Historically, sulfonamides, bromides and oral contraceptive pills have been the most commonly associated

Table 99.3 Aetiological factors in erythema nodosum [1–127].

Infections

Bacterial infections
Atypical mycobacterial infections [1]
Borrelia burgdorferi infections [2]
Boutonneuse fever [3]
Brucellosis [4]
Campylobacter infections [5]
Cat-scratch disease [6]
Chancroid [1]
***Chlamydia psittaci* infections** [7]
Corynebacterium diphteriae infections [1]
Escherichia coli infections [**8**]
Gonorrhoea [9]
Klebsiella pneumoniae infections [10]
Leprosy [11]
Leptospirosis [12]
Lymphogranuloma venereum [13]
Meningococcaemia [14]
Moraxella catarrhalis infections [15]
***Mycoplasma pneumoniae* infections** [16]
Pasteurella pseudotuberculosis infections [17]
Propionibacterium acnes [18]
Pseudomona aeruginosa infections [19]
Q fever [20]
Rickettsiae [21]
***Salmonella* infections** [22]
***Shigella* infections** [23]
Streptococcal infections [24]
Syphilis [25]
Tuberculosis [26]
Tularaemia [27]
***Yersinia* infections** [28]

Viral infections
Cytomegalovirus [29]
Epstein–Barr virus infection after living-donor liver transplantation [30]
Hepatitis B [31]
Hepatitis C [32]
Herpes simplex [1]
HIV infection [33]
Infectious mononucleosis [34]
Measles [35]
Orf [36]
Parvovirus B19 [37]
Varicella [38]

Fungal infections
Aspergillosis [39]
Blastomycosis [40]
Coccidioidomycosis [41]
Dermatophytes [42]
Histoplasmosis [43]
Sporotrichosis [44]

Protozoal infections
Amoebiasis [45]
Ascariasis [46]
Giardiasis [47]
Hydatidosis [48]
Hookworm infestation [1]

Protozoal infections (cont.)
Sparganum larva [49]
Toxoplasmosis [50]
Trichomoniasis [51]
Visceral larva migrans [52]

Drugs
Acetaminophen [53]
Actinomycin-D [53]
All-*trans*-retinoic acid [54]
Aminopyrine [1]
Amiodarone [53]
Amoxicillin [**8**]
Ampicillin [**8**]
Antimony [1]
Arsphenamine [9]
Azathioprine [53]
Bromides [55]
Busulfan [53]
Cabergoline [56]
Capecitabine [57]
Carbamazepine [53]
Carbenicillin [53]
Carbimazole [58]
Cefdinir [53]
Certolizumab [59]
Chlordiazepoxide [53]
Chlorotrianisene [53]
Chlorpropamide [53]
Ciprofloxacin [53]
Clomiphene [53]
Codeine [53]
Cotrimoxazole [53]
D-penicillamine [60]
Dapsone [53]
Diclofenac [53]
Dicloxacillin [53]
Diethylstilboestrol [53]
Disopyramide [53]
Echinacea herbal therapy [61]
Enoxacin [53]
Erythromycin [8]
Etanercept [62]
Fluoxetine [53]
Furosemide [53]
Glatiramer acetate [63]
Glucagon [53]
Gold salts [64]
Granulocyte colony-stimulating factor [65]
Hepatitis B vaccine [66]
HPV vaccine [67]
Hydralazine [53]
Ibuprofen [53]
Imatinib mesylate [68]
Indometacin [53]
Infliximab [69]
Interleukin 2 [70]
Iodides [53]

(Continued)

Table 99.3 Aetiological factors in erythema nodosum [1–127]. (*Continued*)

Drugs (cont.)	Isotretinoin [71]	***Malignant diseases (cont.)***	Hepatocellular carcinoma [87]
	Leukotriene modifying agents (zileuton and rafirlukast) [72]		Hodgkin disease [88]
	Levofloxacin [53]		Leukaemia [89]
	Lidocaine [73]		Lung cancer [90]
	Meclofenamate [53]		Stomach cancer [**8**]
	Medroxyprogesterone [53]		Myelodysplastic syndrome [91]
	Meprobamate [53]		Non-Hodgkin lymphoma [92]
	Mesalamine [53]		Pancreatic carcinoma [93]
	Meticillin [53]		Parathyroid carcinoma [94]
	Methimazole [53]		Post-radiotherapy for pelvic carcinoma [95]
	Methyldopa [53]		Renal carcinoma [70]
	Mezlozillin [53]		Sarcoma [9]
	Minocycline [74]	***Miscellaneous diseases***	**Acne fulminans** [96]
	Naproxen [53]		Acupuncture therapy and flu-like infection [97]
	Nifedipine [53]		**Adult-onset Still disease** [98]
	Nitrofurantoin [1]		**Ankylosing spondylitis** [99]
	Ofloxacin [53]		Antiphospolipid antibody syndrome [100]
	Omeprazole [75]		**Behçet disease** [101]
	Oestrogens [53]		Breast abscesses [102]
	Oral contraceptives [76]		Chronic active hepatitis [103]
	Oxacillin [53]		**Coeliac disease** [104]
	Paroxetine [53]		Colon diverticulosis [105]
	Penicillin [53]		**Crohn disease** [116]
	Phenylbutazone [53]		Diverticulitis [105]
	Phenytoin [53]		Eosinophilic oesophagitis [107]
	Piperacillin [53]		Granulomatous mastitis [108]
	Progestins [53]		**IgA nephropathy** [109,110]
	Propylthiouracil [77]		**Intestinal bypass syndrome** [111]
	Pyritinol [9]		Jellyfish sting [112]
	Rabies vaccine [78]		**Lupus erythematosus** [113]
	Serotonin reuptake inhibitors [79]		**Pregnancy** [114]
	Sparfloxacin [53]		Primary biliary cirrhosis [115]
	Streptomycin [53]		Radiotherapy [116]
	Sulfamethoxazole [53]		**Relapsing polychondritis** [117]
	Sulfisoxazole [53]		**Reactive arthritis** [118]
	Sulfonamides [80]		Rheumatoid arthritis [119]
	Sulfasalazine [53]		**Sarcoidosis** [120]
	Thalidomide [81]		**Sjögren syndrome** [121]
	Ticarcillin [53]		Smoke inhalation in a house fire [122]
	Trimethoprim [82]		**Sweet syndrome** [123]
	Typhoid vaccination [83]		Systemic lupus erythematosus-like syndrome due to C4 deficiency [124]
	Verapamil [53]		Takayasu arteritis [125]
Malignant diseases	Adenocarcinoma of the colon [84]		**Ulcerative colitis** [126]
	Carcinoid tumour [85]		Vogt–Koyanagi disease [121]
	Carcinoma of the uterine cervix [86]		**Granulomatosis with polyangiitis** [127]

The most well-documented associations are shown in bold.

medications but a large number of drugs have been reported as triggers (see Table 99.3). Oral contraceptive pills have become a rare cause since their oestrogen content was greatly reduced. Where erythema nodosum has arisen in patients receiving antibiotics for infections it is difficult to discern whether the cutaneous reaction is due to the antibiotic or the infectious process.

Sarcoidosis is one of the commonest disorders associated with erythema nodosum in adults [147]. Hilar adenopathy, arthritis around the ankles and erythema nodosum is characteristic of Löfgren syndrome [152]. However, erythema nodosum and bilateral hilar adenopathy do not occur exclusively in sarcoidosis but may also be seen in lymphomas, tuberculosis, streptococcal infections, coccidioidomycosis, histoplasmosis and acute infections by *Chlamydophila pneumoniae* [153,154].

In adults, erythema nodosum is often associated with a flare of inflammatory bowel disease, although the cutaneous eruption may sometimes precede the bowel disease. Crohn disease [106] is more frequently associated than ulcerative colitis [126].

The large list of very disparate processes that may be associated with erythema nodosum indicates that this disorder is a cutaneous reactive process and that the skin has a limited response capacity to very different triggers. Most probably, erythema nodosum results from immune complex deposition in and around veins of the connective tissue septa of the subcutis. In support of this hypothesis is the demonstration of circulating immune complexes [155], complement activation [156,157] and deposits of immunoglobulins in the blood vessels walls of the septa of subcutaneous fat in patients with erythema nodosum [158,159]. Some investigators have, however, failed to demonstrate circulating immune complexes in erythema nodosum patients and a type IV delayed hypersensitivity reaction has been proposed as a possible pathogenetic mechanism [160].

Early lesions of erythema nodosum show a predominantly neutrophilic infiltrate. Recent investigations have demonstrated that patients with erythema nodosum have a fourfold higher percentage of reactive oxygen intermediates (ROI) produced by activated neutrophils in their peripheral blood compared with healthy volunteers. The percentage of ROI-producing cells correlates with the clinical severity of erythema nodosum and ROI may play their pathogenic role by oxidative tissue damage and by promoting tissue inflammation [161].

Patients with sarcoidosis-associated erythema nodosum secrete an uncommon tumour necrosis factor (TNF)-α II due to a nucleotide exchange (G-A) at position -308 in the human TNF-α gene promoter, whereas patients with erythema nodosum without underlying sarcoidosis do not have this genomic anomaly [162]. Conversely, polymorphism of the macrophage *MIF* gene at the position -173 has been associated with a significantly increased risk of developing sarcoidosis in patients with erythema nodosum [163]. These investigations support the hypothesis that sarcoidosis-associated erythema nodosum might be pathogenically linked to altered TNF-α or MIF production due to a genetic promoter polymorphism.

Other investigators have found that the pro-inflammatory cytokine pattern, both in infectious and non-infectious disease related erythema nodosum, is characterized by raised IL-6 serum concentrations [124]. High expression of Th1 cytokines (IL-2 and IFN-γ) has also been demonstrated in most skin lesions and in the peripheral blood of patients with erythema nodosum, whereas this cytokine gene expression pattern was absent or only minimally present in the skin and peripheral blood of control subjects. These results directly demonstrate that a polarized Th1 immune response occurs in the skin lesions of erythema nodosum patients regardless of the wide variety of provoking agents [164].

Recently, it has been demonstrated that adipocytes play an important role in activating inflammatory systems and adaptive immune systems, destroying pathogens throughout the secretion of multiple adipokines and adipocytokines [165]. This immunological role may explain why both coccidioidomycosis [166] and sarcoidosis appear to be less severe and of shorter duration in those patients who develop erythema nodosum, especially if they are carriers of the HLA-DRB1*03-positive leukocyte antigen [167].

Presentation

Clinically, the eruption is quite characteristic and consists of a sudden onset of symmetrical, bilateral, tender, erythematous, warm nodules

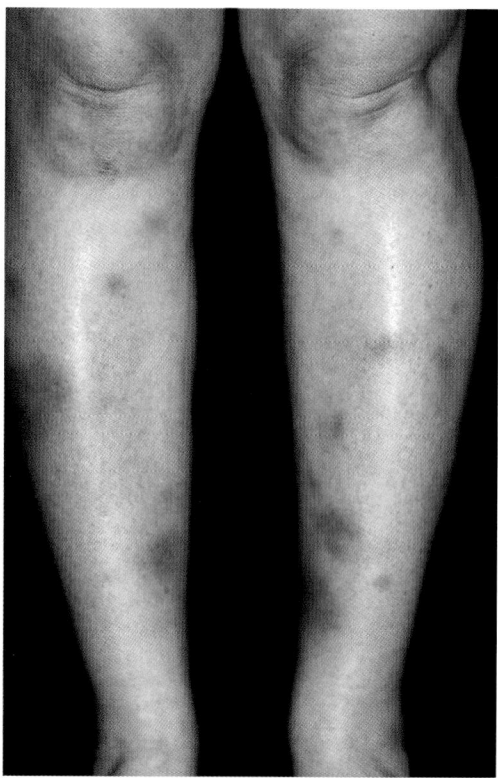

Figure 99.18 Characteristic eruption of erythema nodosum with lesions in different stages of evolution involving the anterior aspect of the legs of an adult woman. Some early lesions consist of bilateral erythematous nodules and plaques, whereas later stage lesions show a bruise-like appearance.

and raised plaques usually involving the shins (Figure 99.18), ankles and knees. The nodules range from 1 to 5 cm or more in diameter and may become confluent resulting in erythematous plaques. Occasionally, lesions of erythema nodosum may appear in other areas, including the thighs, extensor aspects of the arms, neck and even the face. Early lesions show a bright red colour and are raised slightly above the skin. After a few days, they become flat, with a livid red or purplish colour. Finally, they show a yellow or greenish appearance, often taking on the look of a deep bruise, and for that reason the process was classically named 'erythema contusiformis'. Nodules of erythema nodosum never ulcerate and the lesions regress without atrophy or scarring. Often, acute bouts of erythema nodosum are associated with a fever of 38–39°C, fatigue, malaise, arthralgia, headache, abdominal pain, vomiting, cough or diarrhoea. Episcleral lesions and phlyctenular conjunctivitis may also accompany the cutaneous lesions. Rare clinical manifestations associated with erythema nodosum include lymphadenopathy, hepatomegaly, splenomegaly and pleuritis [148]. The eruption persists for 3–6 weeks and regresses leaving no residual marks. Recurrences are common. Duration of erythema nodosum in children is shorter than in adults and arthralgias and fever are less frequent in paediatric cases [168–170].

Clinical variants

The processes described under the names of erythema nodosum migrans [171–174], subacute nodular migratory panniculitis of Vilanova and Piñol [175,176], and chronic erythema nodosum [151] are now all thought to be expressions of different stages of the evolution of erythema nodosum rather than separate entities [177]. In children, there is a rare variant of erythema nodosum characterized by unilateral erythematous nodules involving the palms or soles that appear after physical activity [178–181]. Histopathological study of these palmoplantar lesions shows features of classical erythema nodosum.

Differential diagnosis

Besides authentic erythema nodosum, patients with Behçet disease may present with eruptions that clinically resemble erythema nodosum [101]. However, histopathological study demonstrates that these are not erythema nodosum but show a predominantly lobular panniculitis with leukocytoclastic or lymphocytic vasculitis [182,183]. Furthermore, the frequency of thrombophlebitis is higher in the erythema nodosum-like lesions of patients with Behçet disease compared with individuals with idiopathic erythema nodosum.

Investigations

To identify the responsible aetiological factor in a patient with erythema nodosum, a rational, cost-effective diagnostic approach should be initiated. A complete clinical history should include enquiry about previous diseases, medications, foreign travels, pets and hobbies, and possible familial cases. Initial laboratory investigations should include complete blood count, erythrocyte sedimentation rate, ASO titre, urinalysis, throat culture, intradermal tuberculin test and/or chest X-ray. When the aetiology is unclear, serological tests for those bacterial, viral, fungal or protozoal infections most prevalent in the area should be undertaken. The results of the tuberculin test should be evaluated in the context of the local prevalence of tuberculosis: where tuberculosis is endemic, a significant percentage of healthy adults show positive results for the tuberculin test. A stronger relationship with tuberculosis may be established using an IFN-γ release assay.

When the clinical and laboratory findings are characteristic, a tentative diagnosis of erythema nodosum may be established, but diagnostic confirmation requires biopsy.

Histopathologically, erythema nodosum is the prototype of a predominantly septal panniculitis without vasculitis. The connective tissue septa of the subcutis appear thickened and oedematous and are infiltrated by inflammatory cells that involve mainly the interface between the septa and the fat lobule. Usually, a superficial and deep perivascular inflammatory infiltrate composed predominantly of lymphocytes is also present in the overlying dermis.

As with other panniculitides, erythema nodosum is a dynamic process and the composition of the inflammatory cells involving the septa varies with the stage of the condition. Early lesions of less than 48 h duration show oedema and haemorrhage at the septa, and numerous neutrophils arranged interstitially between collagen bundles [149] (Figure 99.19). Sometimes, if these early lesions show extension of the infiltrate to the periphery of the fat lobule surrounding individual adipocytes in a lace-like fashion, the process may be misinterpreted as a predominantly lobular panniculitis. However, in contrast with a true lobular panniculitis, necrosis of the adipocytes at the centre of the fat lobule is never seen in erythema nodosum. In rare instances, eosinophils may be numerous in early lesions: this finding does not, however, correlate with any specific aetiological factor [184].

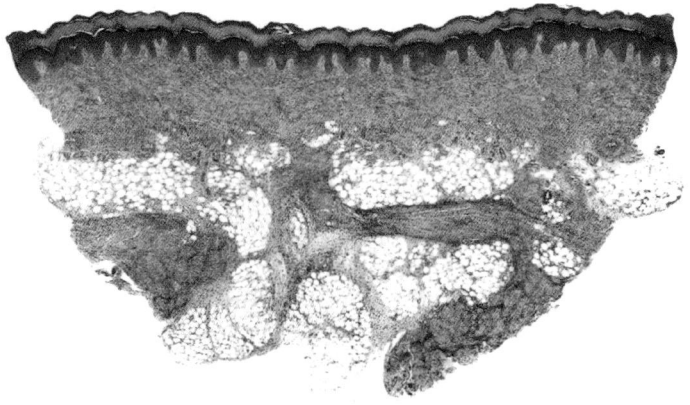

(a)

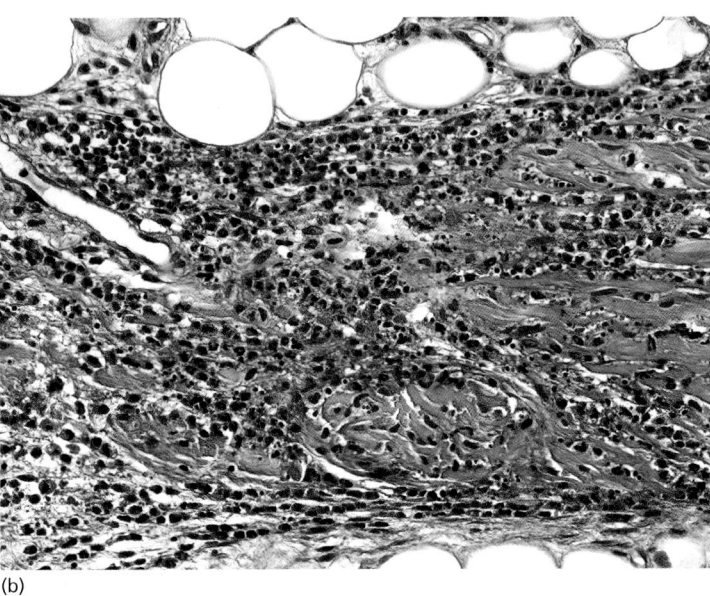

(b)

Figure 99.19 Histopathological features of an early lesion of erythema nodosum. (a) Scanning power showing a mostly septal panniculitis with thickened connective tissue septa of the subcutis. (b) The infiltrate at the septa is mostly composed of neutrophils interstitially arranged between collagen bundles.

A histopathological hallmark of erythema nodosum is the presence of so-called Miescher radial granulomas [185,186,**187**], that consist of small well-defined nodular aggregates of small histiocytic cells around a central stellate or banana-shaped cleft (Figure 99.20). The nature of the central cleft is unknown and, although some authors have considered them to be lymphatic spaces, immunohistochemical and ultrastructural studies have failed to demonstrate any endothelial cell lining. In early lesions, these granulomas are scattered in the septa and are surrounded by neutrophils. In older nodules, histiocytic cells group to form multinucleated giant cells, many of which still retain in their cytoplasm the stellate central cleft as found in Miescher radial granuloma.

Sometimes Miescher radial granulomas are conspicuous in the septa. Occasionally, however, serial sections are required to identify them: if carefully sought, they can be found in almost all stages of erythema nodosum lesions and such a search should always be undertaken to establish a specific diagnosis [**187**]. However, some authors consider that similar granulomas may be found in subcutaneous Sweet syndrome, erythema induratum of Bazin, Behçet

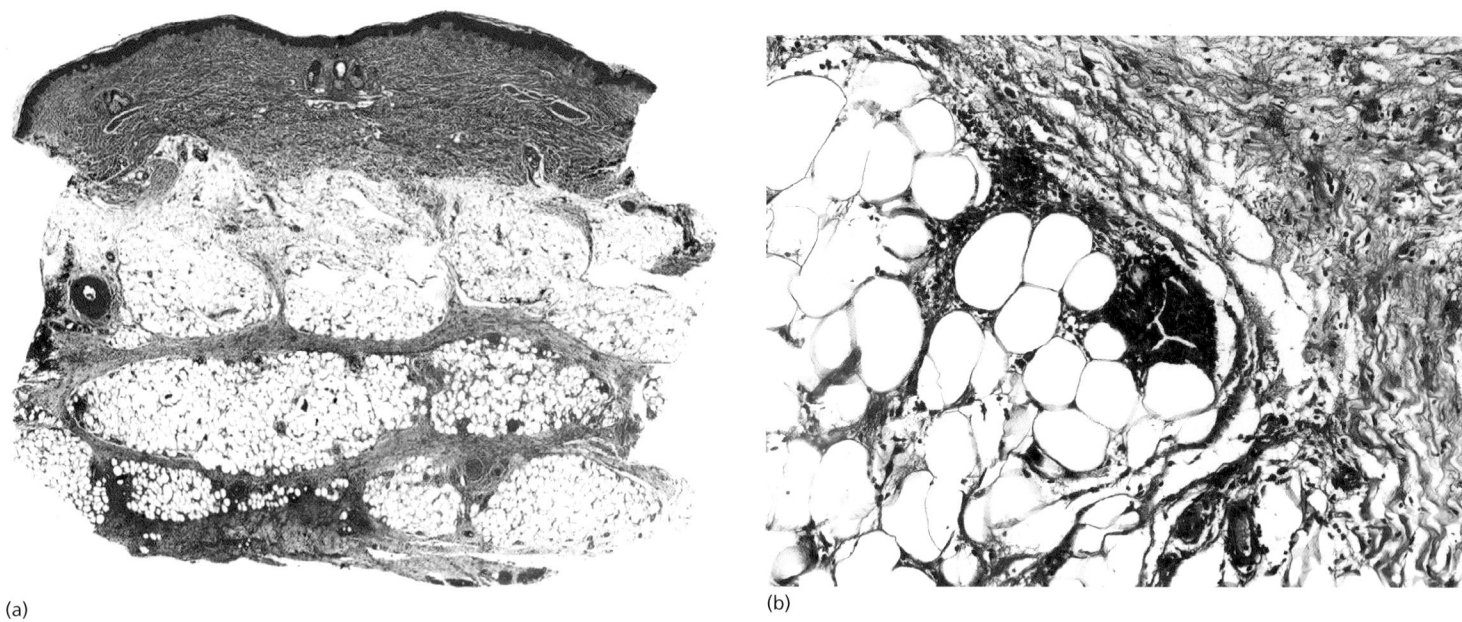

(a)   (b)

Figure 99.20 Histopathological features of a fully developed lesion of erythema nodosum. (a) Scanning power showing thickened septa of the subcutaneous tissue. (b) Higher magnification shows the characteristic features of Miescher radial granuloma: Aggregations of small histiocytes around a central cleft.

disease and necrobiosis lipoidica [177]. Recent immunohistochemical studies have demonstrated that the cells around the central clefts of Miescher radial granulomas express myeloperoxidase [188], in a similar way to those of the small, elongated, twisted-appearing mononuclear cells of the infiltrate in so-called histiocytoid Sweet syndrome [189]. These findings demonstrate that the mononuclear cells that make up Miescher radial granuloma, and those seen in the so-called histiocytoid Sweet syndrome, are actually immature myeloid cells, providing a link between erythema nodosum and Sweet syndrome, two conditions in which neutrophils participate.

Late-stage lesions of erythema nodosum show septal fibrosis and periseptal granulation tissue, partially replacing the fat lobules, with an infiltrate composed of lymphocytes, histiocytes and multinucleated giant cells (Figures 99.21 and 99.22). Despite this fibrotic process involving the septa, it is striking that erythema nodosum resolves completely after some weeks or months.

Vasculitis is not normally seen at any stage in the course of erythema nodosum, although in rare cases a necrotizing small vessel vasculitis with fibrinoid necrosis of the small vessels in the septa has been described [190]. In a detailed histopathological

PART 8: SPECIFIC CUTANEOUS STRUCTURE

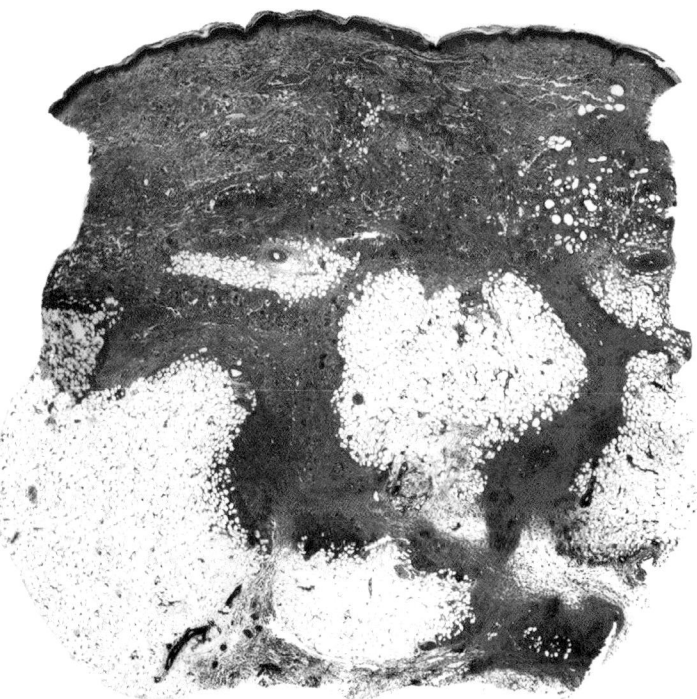

(a)

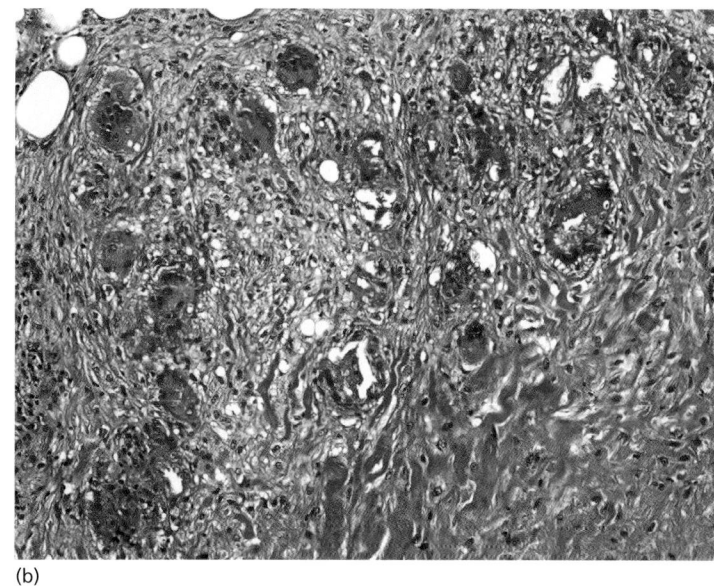

(b)

Figure 99.21 Histopathological features of a late stage lesion of erythema nodosum. (a) Scanning power showing a mostly septal panniculitis. (b) Numerous multinucleated giant cells are present in the infiltrate at the septa.

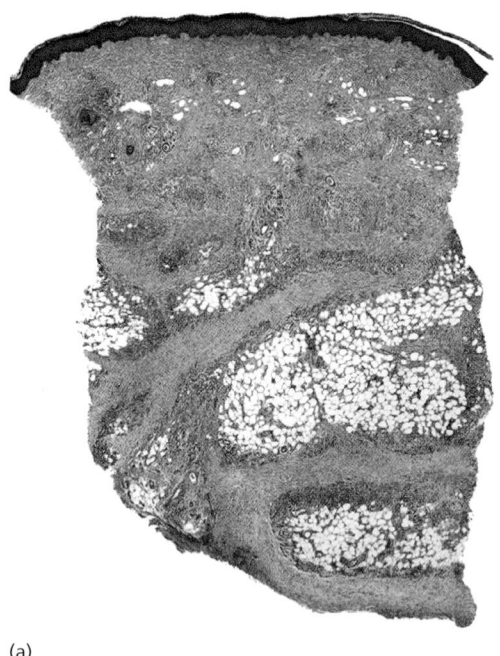

(a)

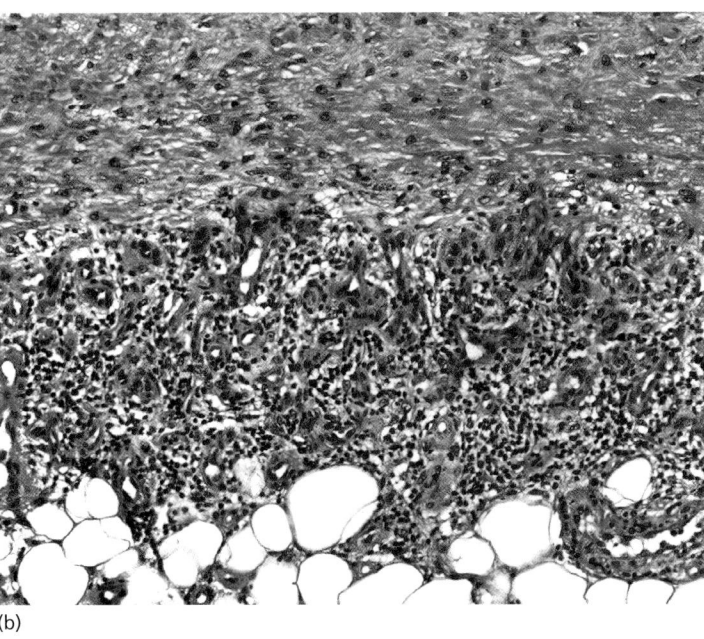

(b)

Figure 99.22 Histopathological findings of a very late stage lesion of erythema nodosum. (a) Scanning power showing very thick connective tissue septa at the subcutis. (b) The infiltrate at the interface shows features of granulation tissue.

study of a series of 79 cases of erythema nodosum, true leukocytoclastic vasculitis was not found [**187**]. The cases described as erythema nodosum with lobular neutrophilic panniculitis and vasculitis involving medium size arteries, are better interpreted as examples of STP, because the involved vessels were medium-sized veins rather than arteries [191]. Ultrastructural studies have also failed to demonstrate true vasculitis in lesions of erythema nodosum [192,193]. Lipomembranous or membranocystic panniculitis [194] and encapsulated fat necrosis ('mobile encapsulated lipoma') [195] may be seen in late-stage lesions of erythema nodosum.

Management

Most cases of erythema nodosum regress spontaneously in 3–4 weeks, but relapses are common. Recurrent episodes of erythema nodosum are more frequent in patients with idiopathic erythema nodosum and erythema nodosum associated with streptococcal upper respiratory tract infections. Complications are uncommon, although cases of retrobulbar optic nerve neuritis during the acute episode of erythema nodosum [196] and erythema nodosum coexisting with erythema multiforme, lichen planus and concomitant reactivation of hepatitis C viral replication [197] have each been described.

Treatment primarily includes identification and management of the underlying cause, especially if infectious. Usually, nodules of erythema nodosum regress spontaneously within a few weeks: limiting physical exercise and bed rest should be recommended. Aspirin, as well as several other nonsteroidal anti-inflammatory drugs, such as indometacin 100–150 mg daily [198] or naproxen 500 mg daily [199] are helpful for pain and for hastening resolution. Non-steroidal anti-inflammatory drugs are contraindicated in patients with inflammatory bowel disease.

In more persistent cases, potassium iodide 400–900 mg daily or a saturated solution of potassium iodide, 2–10 drops in water or orange juice three times per day, may be administered [200–202]. The mechanism of action of potassium iodide in erythema nodosum is unknown, but it probably induces mast cells to release heparin, which suppresses delayed hypersensitivity reactions. The reported response in some patients with erythema nodosum to heparinoid ointment under occlusion also supports this mechanism of action [203]. In addition, potassium iodide inhibits neutrophil chemotaxis [204]. It should be remembered that potassium iodide is contraindicated during pregnancy, because it may induce goitre in the fetus. Severe hypothyroidism secondary to exogenous intake of iodide has also been described in patients with erythema nodosum treated with potassium iodide [205].

Systemic corticosteroids are not usually indicated in erythema nodosum and they should not be commenced unless an infectious aetiology has been excluded. When administered, prednisolone in a dosage of 40 mg/day is followed by resolution of the nodules in few days. Intralesional injection of triamcinolone acetonide at a concentration of 10 mg/mL into the centre of the nodules may also be helpful in solitary persistent lesions.

Some patients have responded to a course of colchicine, 0.6–1.2 mg twice a day [206,207], and to hydroxychloroquine in a dosage of 200 mg twice a day [208].

Recently, cases of erythema nodosum have responded to treatment with anti-TNF biological agents including etanercept [209], adalimumab [210] and infliximab in patients treated with these drugs for inflammatory bowel disease [211]. Paradoxically, however, etanercept [62] and infliximab [69] have been reported to produce erythema nodosum as a cutaneous side effect.

Erythema nodosum leprosum

Definition

Erythema nodosum leprosum is a type II leprosy reaction which is characterized by a necrotizing vasculitis involving small to medium-sized vessels of the deep dermis and subcutis. It is provoked by an immune complex-mediated response to the release of mycobacterial antigens from effete bacilli in patients with multibacillary leprosy (lepromatous and borderline lepromatous), usually after initiation of treatment (Figure 99.23). Leprosy reactions are described in detail in Chapter 28.

Introduction and general description

Type II reactions are due to the formation and deposit of immune complexes in association with excessive humoral reaction: the tissue expression of cytokines is mostly of IL-4 and IL-10. Erythema nodosum leprosum occurs only in patients with lepromatous or borderline lepromatous leprosy and usually occurs during treatment. It represents an immune complex-mediated vasculitis secondary to the deposition of large amounts of mycobacterial antigen, immunoglobulins and complement in the vessel walls [1]. During this type of reaction, patients show an increased CD4/CD8 ratio, due to an increase in T-helper and a decrease in T-suppressor lymphocytes, accompanied by a specific increase in Th2 lymphocytes, which induce plasma cell proliferation and release of immunoglobulins [2,3]. In addition, these patients show a temporary recovery of Langerhans cell antigen-presenting function [4], which is directly proportional to the severity of the leprosy reaction [5,6].

The term 'erythema nodosum leprosum' is inadequate because it may easily be confused with true erythema nodosum, the prototype of septal panniculitis without vasculitis. Erythema nodosum leprosum is a predominantly lobular panniculitis with vasculitis involving the large vessels of the subcutis [7,8].

Histopathological findings in erythema nodosum leprosum vary according to the age of the lesions. Early nodules show oedema of the papillary dermis and a neutrophilic infiltrate with necrotizing

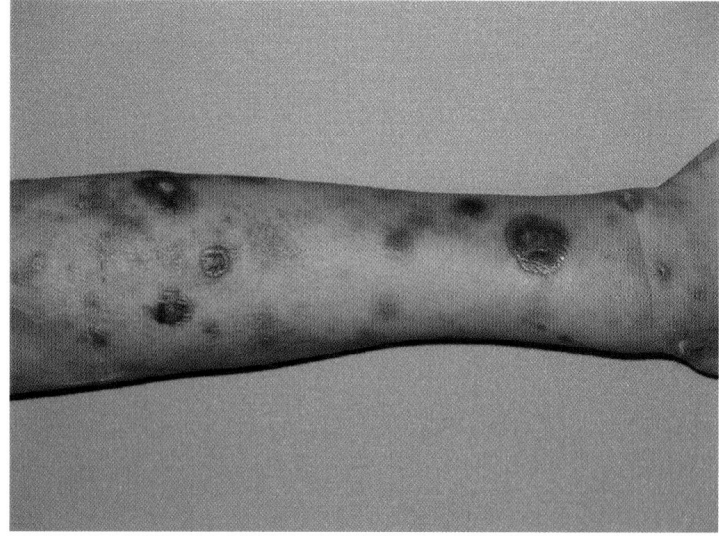

Figure 99.23 Clinical features of erythema nodosum leprosum. Acute onset of erythematous nodules involving the left upper extremity in a patient with lepromatous leprosy.

vasculitis. Although the process is mostly centred in the dermis, it may occasionally extend to subcutaneous tissue, appearing as a predominantly lobular panniculitis with vasculitis involving vessels of the subcutis (Figure 99.24). Later stage lesions exhibit a lymphohistiocytic infiltrate, in which foamy macrophages with numerous mycobacteria are seen within the fat lobule [7–9].

Lucio phenomenon is an uncommon variant of type II leprosy reaction with a unique clinical morphology [8,10–12]. It occurs almost exclusively in Mexican and Central American patients with untreated, diffusely infiltrated, non-nodular lepromatous

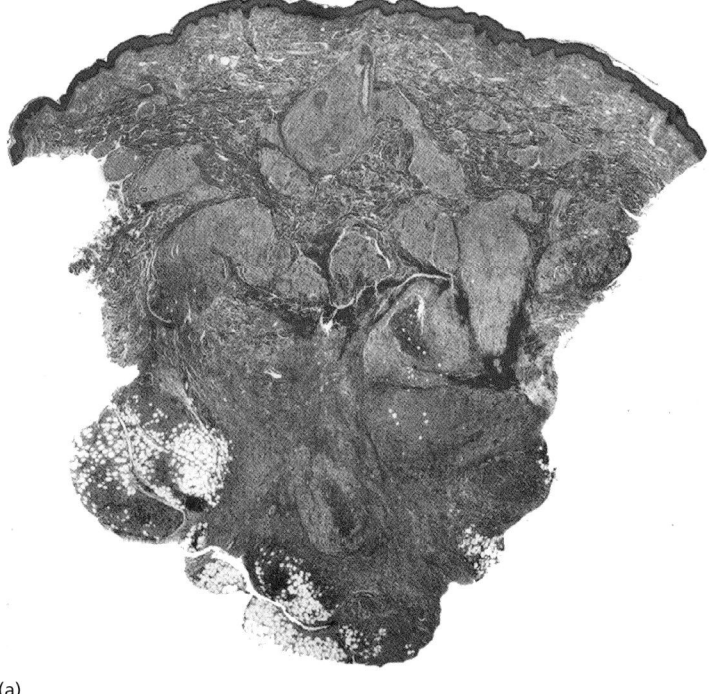

(a)

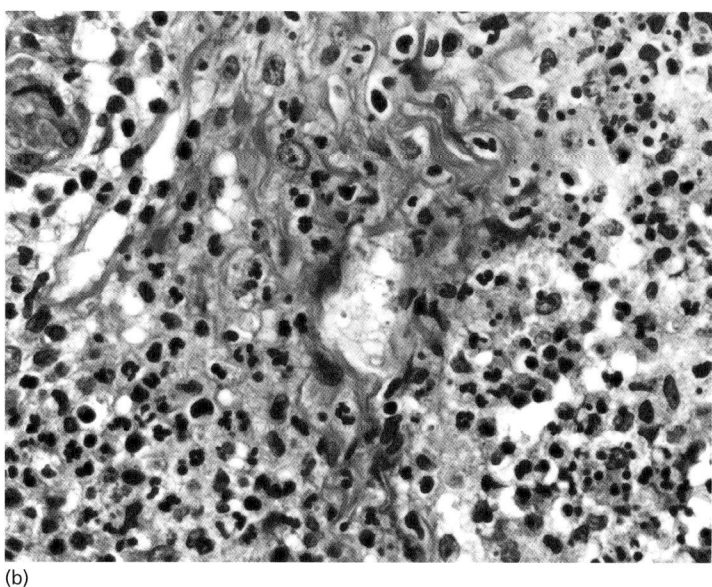

(b)

Figure 99.24 Histopathological features of erythema nodosum leprosum. (a) Scanning power showing dense nodular infiltrates in the dermis and a mostly lobular panniculitis. (b) Some of the small capillaries of the fat lobule show fibrin deposits and neutrophils involving their vessel walls. (*Continued*)

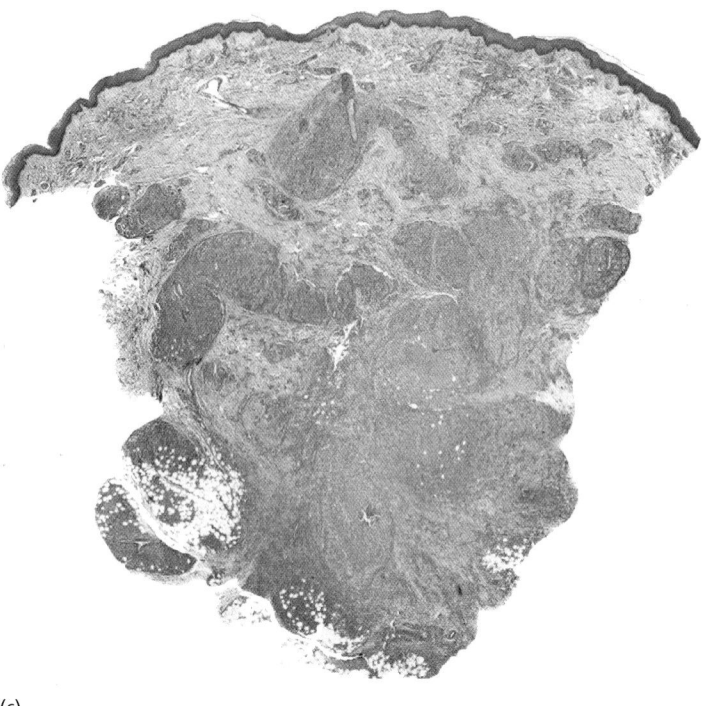

(c)

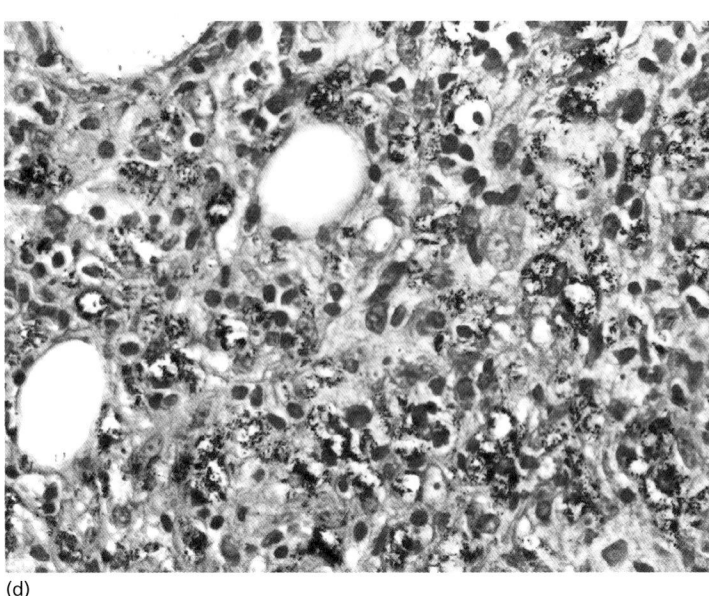

(d)

Figure 99.24 (*Continued*)
(c) A section of the same case stained with Ziehl–Neelsen stain. (d) Higher magnification of numerous microorganisms of *Mycobacterium leprae* within the cytoplasmic vacuoles of the histiocytes.

leprosy and is characterized by multiple haemorrhagic necrotic skin infarcts. It does not result in a panniculitis and subcutaneous tissue is not normally involved. Histologically, there is a necrotizing vasculitis involving the superficial and mid dermis [8,12].

Erythema induratum of Bazin

Synonyms and inclusions
- Nodular vasculitis
- Bazin disease
- Erythema induratum of Bazin

Clinical features

History
Erythema induratum is a chronic recurrent reactive disorder characterized by subcutaneous nodules located preferentially on the posterior aspects of the lower legs of adult women. The nodules commonly develop after exposure to cold and may break down to form irregular ulcers (Figure 99.25). Its clinical features are discussed in greater detail in Chapter 27.

Erythema induratum has historically been regarded as a tuberculid linked to the presence of a distant focus of tuberculosis and, when this is the case, the condition has been referred to as erythema induratum of Bazin. *M. tuberculosis* is not implicated in all cases, however, and the terms erythema induratum of Whitfield and nodular vasculitis have both been used to differentiate such cases from those linked to tuberculosis [1–9]. Whether it makes sense to maintain dif-

ferent terms for what is essentially an identical reactive process is open to question. Although there are still authors who regard erythema induratum of Bazin and nodular vasculitis as separate entities [10,11], no significant clinicopathological differences have been consistently demonstrated between cases related to tuberculosis and those which are not. In recent years, most authors thus consider erythema induratum of Bazin and nodular vasculitis to be a single reactive process that may be provoked by a number of different mechanisms, one of which is active tuberculosis [12]. Box 99.2 shows other suspected aetiological associations which have been reported.

Presentation
From soon after its original description, the relationship between erythema induratum and *M. tuberculosis* has been a controversial issue, because mycobacteria cannot be cultured from the cutaneous lesions. Thus, evidence for the aetiological role of *M. tuberculosis* in erythema induratum has had to be established indirectly from a range of clinical and epidemiological data, including the strong hypersensitivity reaction to tuberculin [25], the presence of concomitant active distant (usually pulmonary) tuberculous infection [26,27], the occasional coexistence in the same patient of erythema induratum and another tuberculid [28,29], the frequent personal or family history of tuberculosis [30,31] and the favourable response to antituberculous chemotherapy [32]. It has been suggested that adipose tissue might constitute a reservoir where the *M. tuberculosis* bacillus could persist for long periods of time and avoid both killing by antimicrobials and recognition by the host immune system [33]. It has, however, never been possible to isolate *M. tuberculosis* from lesions of erythema induratum [34].

Several recent polymerase chain reaction (PCR) studies have demonstrated the presence of *M. tuberculosis* DNA in cutaneous lesions

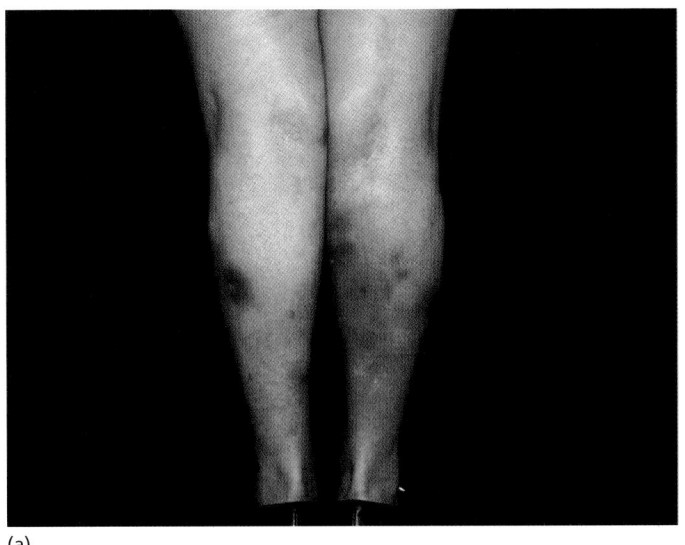

(a)

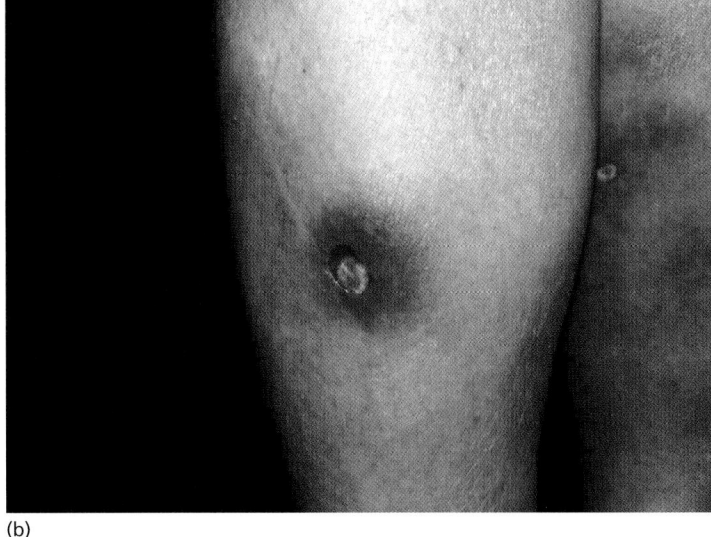

(b)

Figure 99.25 Clinical features of erythema induratum. (a) Erythematous nodules and plaques on the posterior aspect of the legs of an adult woman. (b) Some of the lesions are ulcerated.

of erythema induratum, with frequencies ranging from 25% to 77% of cases, supporting the pathogenic role of *M. tuberculosis* [35–39]. However, in a Spanish study of patients from a region with a high prevalence of tuberculosis, *M. tuberculosis* DNA was detected by PCR in only 14% of cases of erythema induratum [40]. Other investigators have failed to demonstrate the presence of DNA from *M. tuberculosis* or from any other *Mycobacterium* in lesions of erythema induratum [41], supporting the contention that there are likely to be other triggers than tuberculosis.

It has been suggested that erythema induratum results from an immune complex-mediated vasculitis [10], but most authors believe that the disorder results from a type IV, cell-mediated response to an antigenic stimulus [42]. Supporting a delayed hypersensitivity reaction is the presence of abundant number of S-100 positive dendritic cells within the granulomatous infiltrate, which are probably presenting antigens to T cells [43,44]. The pres-

ence in lesional skin of *M. tuberculosis* DNA but not viable tuberculous bacilli suggests that erythema induratum is a hypersensitivity reaction to fragments of tuberculous bacilli.

Investigations

As in other panniculitides, the histopathological findings in lesional skin of erythema induratum vary with the age of the lesions. It is the prototype of a predominantly lobular panniculitis with vasculitis, but the histopathological picture and the composition of the infiltrate in the fat lobule greatly depend on the stage at which the biopsy has been taken [10,26,45,46]. In early stages, the fat lobules are punctuated throughout by discrete collections of inflammatory cells, mostly neutrophils. There may be extensive necrosis of the adipocytes of the fat lobule (Figure 99.26). These necrotic adipocytes elicit a response from histiocytes, which phagocytose lipid and become lipophages. In fully developed lesions, epithelioid and foamy histiocytes, Langhans type or foreign-body multinucleated giant cells and lymphocytes contribute to the granulomatous appearance of the inflammatory infiltrate (Figure 99.27). When intense vascular damage occurs, large areas of caseous necrosis appear and the lesions show all the histopathological attributes of a tuberculoid granuloma. However, stains for acid-fast bacilli, such as Ziehl–Neelsen or Fite, and immunohistochemical stains for mycobacteria are negative. Caseous necrosis may extend to the overlying dermis and secondarily involve the epidermis with ulceration and discharge of liquefied necrotic fat. Previously, the presence of tuberculoid granulomas around the eccrine coils, was regarded as suggestive of a tuberculous aetiology [47], but these findings may also be seen in non-tuberculous cases.

In the literature, considerable controversy persists about whether or not vasculitis is a required histopathological criterion for establishing a diagnosis of erythema induratum. Furthermore, there is no agreement about the nature of the vessels involved in the vasculitis, because some authors have failed to report their nature or size [48], and even when the nature of the involved vessel was specifically stated, there has been disagreement as to whether it is arteries [49,50], veins [51,52] or both [52–57] which are affected. In a recent large study of 101 skin biopsies from 86 patients with

---

Box 99.2 Aetiological associations of erythema induratum

- Chronic hepatitis C [13–15]
- Ulcerative colitis [16]
- Brucellosis [17]
- Paraneoplastic process [18]
- *Nocardia* infections [19]
- Propylthiouracil [20]
- Systemic lupus erythematosus [21]
- Pneumonia due to *Chlamydophila pneumoniae* [22]
- Bacille Calmette–Guérin (BCG) vaccination [23]
- Aortic valve stenosis [24]
- Hepatitis B [25]
- Crohn disease [25]
- Leukaemia [25]
- Rheumatoid arthritis [25]
- Hypothyroidism [25]
- Cold weather [25]
- Chronic venous insufficiency [25]

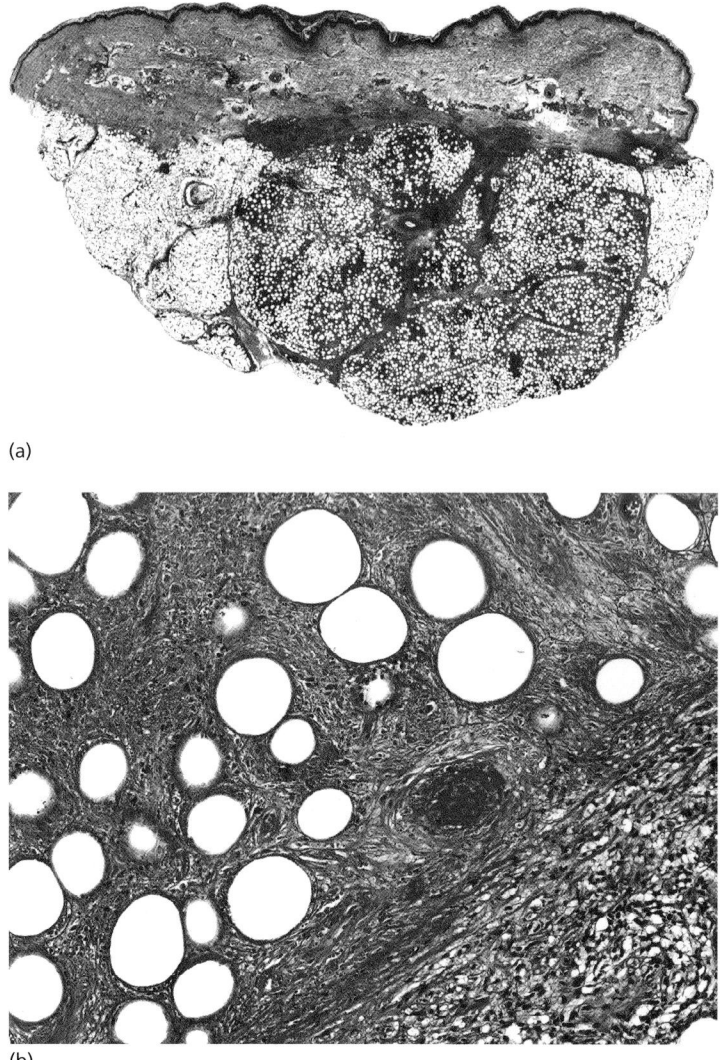

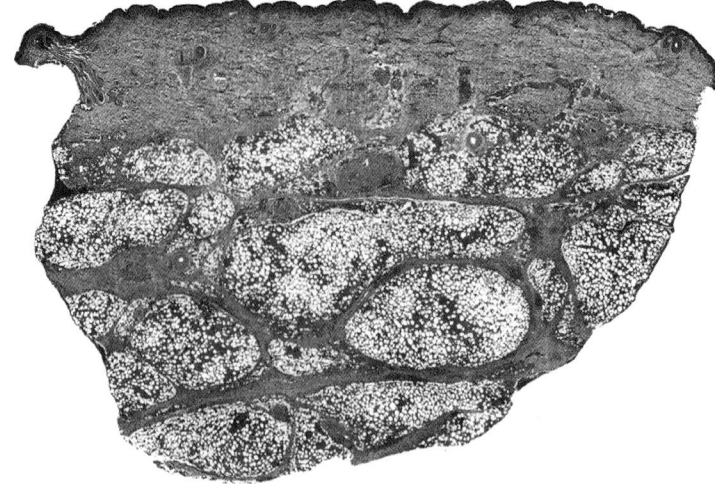

(a)

(b)

Figure 99.26 Histopathological features of an early lesion of erythema induratum. (a) Scanning power showing a mostly lobular panniculitis. (b) Higher magnification showing necrotic adipocytes without nuclei and luminal thrombosis of a small blood vessel.

(a)

(b)

Figure 99.27 Histopathological features of a fully developed lesion of erythema induratum. (a) Scanning power showing a mostly lobular panniculitis. (b) Small granulomas involving the fat lobule.

a clinicopathological diagnosis of erythema induratum, vasculitis was however present in 90% of cases [25] (Box 99.3).

Therefore, although vasculitis can be demonstrated in the majority of cases, there are some cases with all the other clinico-pathological attributes of erythema induratum where vasculitis cannot be demonstrated despite a careful search: its presence should not be considered as an essential criterion for its histo-pathological diagnosis [25].

Box 99.3 Vascular involvement in erythema induratum

- Small venules of the fat lobule (46.5% of cases)
- Both large veins of the connective tissue septa and small venules of the fat lobule (12.8% of cases)
- Only large veins of the connective tissue septa (11.8% of cases)
- Large veins and arteries of the connective tissue septa and small venules of the fat lobule (9.9% of cases)
- Large veins and arteries of the connective tissue septa (8.9% of cases)
- No evidence of vasculitis (9.9% of cases)

From Segura *et al.* 2008 [25]

Sclerosing panniculitis

Definition and nomenclature

Sclerosing panniculitis is a relatively common form of long-term chronic panniculitis associated with chronic venous insufficiency and typically affecting the lower extremities of middle-aged or elderly women. This is manifested as a diffuse sclerosis and pigmentation of the skin and subcutaneous tissue (lipodermatosclerosis) (Figure 99.28). It is discussed in more detail in Chapter 103.

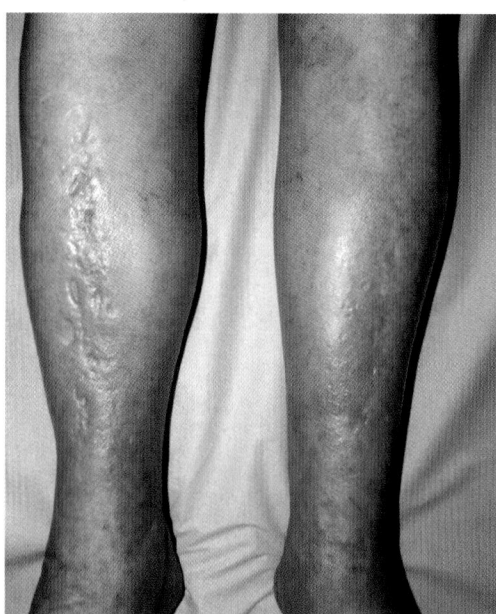

Figure 99.28 Late-stage sclerosing panniculitis showing depressed hard areas with woody induration involving the lower legs.

Synonyms and inclusions
• Lipodermatosclerosis

Clinical features

Presentation

The aetiological role of venous hypertension in the pathogenesis of sclerosing panniculitis is undisputed. Venous hypertension increases capillary permeability, which results in leakage of fibrinogen, its polymerization to form fibrin rings around vessels, with impedance of oxygen exchange and tissue anoxia [1]. Other factors such as trauma and recurrent episodes of cellulitis may also play a role [2,3]. In a study of 128 patients with systemic sclerosis, patients with sclerosing panniculitis had pulmonary hypertension at a significantly higher incidence than those without. The authors suggested that thrombosis caused by venous hypertension of the leg may be the main cause of pulmonary hypertension in patients with systemic sclerosis and sclerosing panniculitis [4].

Reported findings which may be of pathogenetic relevance in sclerosing panniculitis include increased plasminogen activation in affected tissue [5–7], increased expression of vascular endothelial growth factor receptor 1 (VEGFR-1) and angiopoietin 2 (Ang-2) [8], deficiencies of protein C and S [9] and local increased synthesis of collagen [10,11].

Differential diagnosis

Because initial stages of the disease involve only one leg, it may be confused clinically with bacterial cellulitis or erysipelas, although in the latter situation there is accompanying heat on palpation, fever or other systemic symptoms [12]. Early lesions may also mimic erythema nodosum [13]. In longstanding lesions, the differential diagnosis is with other sclerodermiform processes, but the absence of histopathological findings of dermal sclerosis, the

peculiar distribution affecting only the distal part of one or both legs and the presence of features of chronic venous stasis exclude morphoea, scleroderma and acrodermatitis chronica atrophicans. A rare case of sarcoidosis clinically mimicked sclerosing panniculitis [14].

Investigations

Often, clinicians are reluctant to biopsy lesions of sclerosing panniculitis because it is not unusual to induce a chronic ulcer with poor healing at the site of the biopsy [3,15]; most biopsies are thus obtained in the later stages of the disease. However, when a biopsy is performed at the early stages of the process, microscopic study demonstrates a sparse inflammatory infiltrate of lymphocytes in the septa and areas of ischaemic necrosis at the centre of the fat lobules. Necrosis of fat in these early stages is characterized by small pale anucleate adipocytes. The small blood vessels of the fat lobule appear congested, with extravasated erythrocytes, haemosiderin deposits and necrosis of endothelial cells [16]. In fully developed lesions, the septa show marked thickening and fibrosis, whereas lobules appear atrophic, often with lipophagic granulomata at their periphery. In this stage, the inflammatory infiltrate is composed of lymphocytes, histiocytes and foamy macrophages. Blood vessels appear prominent in the septa at all stages.

In late-stage lesions, the inflammatory infiltrate is sparse or absent, septal sclerosis is prominent and fat lobules appear atrophic, with microcysts and focal lipomembranous (membranocystic) changes (Figure 99.29). The latter consist of cystic structures lined by a lipomembrane, which appears as feathery amorphous eosinophilic material, sometimes with a crenellated or arabesque pattern. The thickened undulating membrane is PAS positive, stains for Sudan black and Luxol fast blue and expresses immunoreactivity for CD68 and lysozyme [17–19], suggesting the contribution of these macrophage-derived enzymes in its histogenesis. These changes are not, however, specific for sclerosing panniculitis, because they may be seen in longstanding lesions of various forms of septal and lobular panniculitis. Box 99.4 summarizes the conditions in which lipomembranous fat necrosis has been described in the literature [17–54]. Calcification and elastic tissue degeneration, sometimes with fragmented and calcified elastic fibres resembling those of pseudoxanthoma elasticum (PXE) may be seen in longstanding lesions [55]. These PXE-like fibres are positive for both von Kossa and Verhoeff van Gieson stains and may develop metaplastic ossification [56]. Elastic fibres with PXE-like changes are not specific for sclerosing panniculitis, because they have also been described in uraemic and non-uraemic calcific arteriolopathy (calciphylaxis) [57,58], erythema nodosum, granuloma annulare, morphoea profunda [26,55] and nephrogenic systemic fibrosis [59].

The overlying superficial dermis shows venous stasis changes, with lobules of capillaries and venules of slightly thick-walled vessels in concert with extravasated erythrocytes and haemosiderin deposition. Increased melanin pigment along the basal layer of the epidermis as well as within melanophages in the superficial dermis also contribute to the characteristic hyperpigmentation [60].

Histopathological differential diagnosis of sclerosing panniculitis includes panniculitis of scleroderma and deep morphoea, but these conditions show predominantly septal panniculitis and,

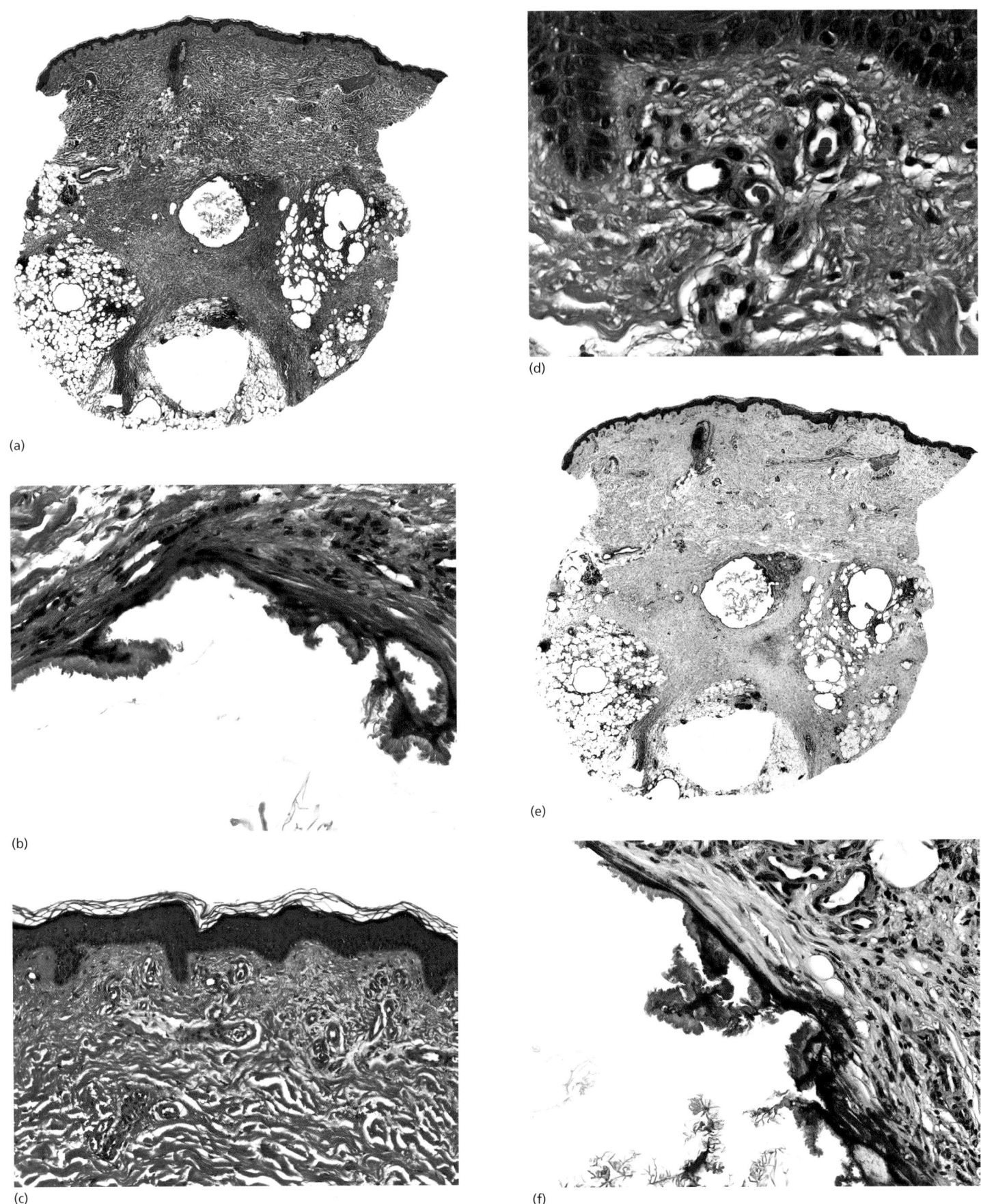

Figure 99.29 Histopathological findings in sclerosing panniculitis. (a) Scanning power showing thickened septa and cystic spaces replacing the fat lobules. (b) A cystic structure lined by a lipomembrane with a crenellated border. (c) Superficial dermis shows stasis changes. (d) Proliferation of thick-walled capillaries and venules in the superficial dermis. (e) A section of the same case stained with periodic acid–Schiff (PAS). (f) PAS positivity of the pseudopapillae with feathery projections into the cystic cavity.

Box 99.4 Panniculitides and other disorders with lipomembranous fat necrosis reported in the literature

Vascular disorders
- Venous insufficiency (lipodermatosclerosis) [16,17,21,26,37]
- Arteriosclerosis [23,24]
- Thromboangiitis obliterans [23]
- Thrombophlebitis [21,25]
- Diabetes [21,25,26,27]

Connective tissue disease/autoimmune disease
- Lupus panniculitis/discoid lupus erythematosus [17,20,21,26,28,29,39–42]
- Morphoea/scleroderma [20,25,30,43,44]
- CREST syndrome [20]
- Dermatomyositis-associated panniculitis [31,37]
- Vasculitis [21,26,33]
- Behçet disease [29,34]

Inflammatory panniculitis
- Erythema nodosum [17,25,26]
- Erythema induratum [17]
- Traumatic panniculitis [17,35]
- Necrobiosis lipoidica [17,26]
- Pancreatic panniculitis [17]
- Factitial panniculitis [28]
- Nodular fat necrosis [45]

Infections
- Atypical mycobacteria [35]
- Erysipelas [17,26]

Neoplastic panniculitis
- Subcutaneous panniculitic-like T-cell lymphoma [36,46]

Miscellaneous conditions
- Splinter granuloma [47]
- Chemotherapy for leukaemia [48]
- Chemotherapy for breast cancer [49]
- Testicular torsion [50]
- Subcutaneous elemental mercury injections [51]
- Mature cystic teratomas of the ovary [52]
- Myospherulosis [53]
- Breast after radiotherapy [54]

Modified from Segura and Pujol 2008 [22].

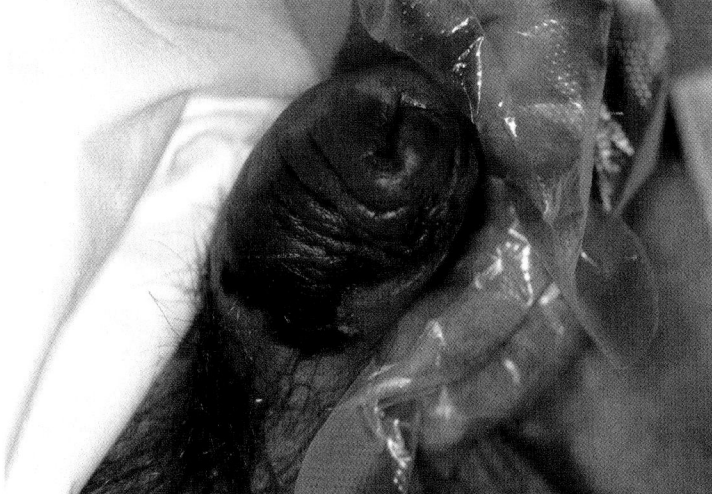

Figure 99.30 Calciphylaxis involving the penis in a patient with end-stage renal disease.

although lipodystrophy and lipophagic changes adjacent to the septa may be seen, they are not prominent.

Calcific uraemic arteriolopathy (calciphylaxis)

Definition

Calcific arteriolopathy (calciphylaxis) is strongly associated with end-stage chronic kidney disease and renal transplantation, particularly in diabetics, though a small proportion of cases arise in the absence of renal disease. It typically presents as irregular exquisitely tender patches of mottled dusky livedoid erythema with pale greyish areas of devitalization before progressing to full-thickness infarction of the skin with consequent necrotic ulceration. These changes commonly extend deeply into subcutaneous fat. Although the most common areas of involvement are the lower extremities and abdomen, the process may also involve other areas including the genitalia (Figure 99.30). The condition is discussed fully in Chapter 61.

Pathophysiology

Three-dimensional studies in calciphylaxis have shown vascular mural calcification as an early feature, which probably precedes endovascular fibrosis [1]. Recent studies in calciphylaxis have revealed the presence of the matrix Gla protein, osteopontin and bone morphogenic protein 2 (BMP-2) in pathologically calcified arteries [2,3]. In involved skin, a significant up-regulation of BMP-2, its target gene *Runx2* and its indirect antagonist sclerostin, as well as increased expression of inactive uncarboxylated matrix Gla protein (Glu-MGP) have been detected. The up-regulation of osteogenesis-associated markers is accompanied by an increased expression of osteopontin, fibronectin, laminin and collagen I indicating an extensive remodelling of the subcutaneous extracellular matrix. Electron dispersive X-ray analysis has revealed calcium/phosphate accumulations in the subcutis of calciphylaxis patients. Widespread medial calcification in cutaneous arterioles is associated with destruction of the endothelial layer and partial exfoliation of the endothelial cells. CD31 immunostaining has revealed aggregates of endothelial cells contributing to intraluminal obstruction and the consequent malperfusion which results in the clinical picture of ulcerative necrosis. These data indicate that vascular calcification in calciphylaxis is an active osteogenic process involving up-regulation of BMP-2 signalling, hydroxyapatite deposition and extensive matrix remodelling of the subcutis [4]. Matrix Gla protein is vitamin K dependent and inhibits vascular calcification. Therefore, oral anticoagulant therapy with warfarin, a vitamin K antagonist, favours vascular calcification in these patients [5]. Other triggering factors that have been recognized as inducers of vascular calcification in calciphylaxis include low levels of albumin, arterial hypertension, obesity, administration of systemic corticosteroids, vitamin D supplementation, blood transfusions, oral phosphate binders, metallic salts, calcitriol, local

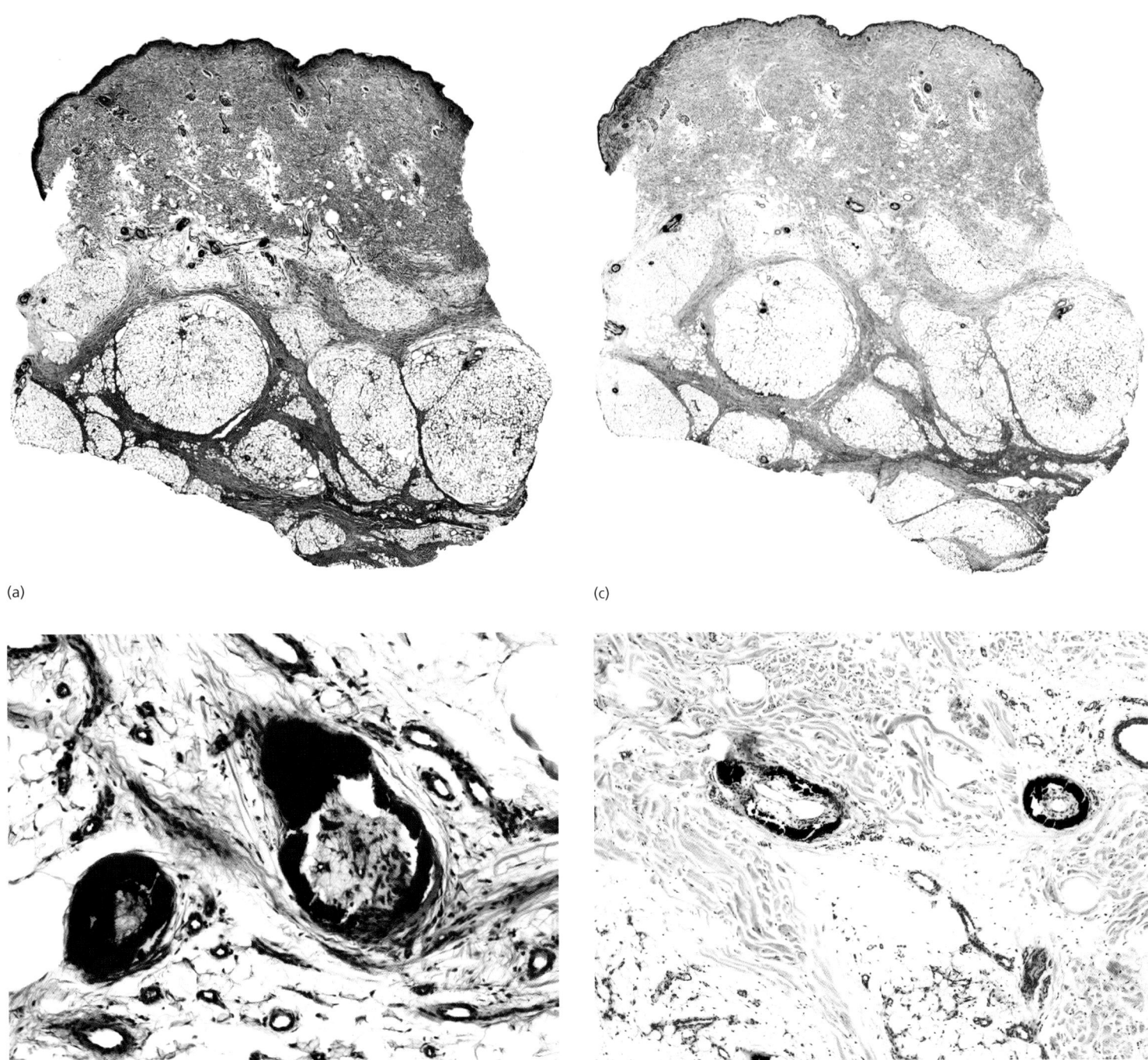

Figure 99.31 Histopathological features of calciphylaxis. (a) Scanning power view showing involvement of the vessels of deeper reticular dermis. (b) Calcification of the vessel walls and occlusion of the vascular lumina. (c) A section of the same case stained with von Kossa stain. (d) Calcification of the vessel walls is positive with von Kossa stain.

trauma, UV light treatment, malnutrition with weight loss and insulin injections [6–12].

Investigations

The most characteristic histopathological finding in calcific arteriolopathy consists in small and medium-sized vessel calcification (Figure 99.31). Small arteries, arterioles and venules may be involved. Vascular calcification is usually extensive within the vessel walls and often exhibits a concentric, circumferential, ring-like pattern. Detailed histopathological studies, however,

have demonstrated that the earliest sites of calcification are the media and/or intima of cutaneous arterioles [13]. Vascular calcification in the arterioles of the deeper reticular dermis or subcutaneous tissue is usually evident with H&E staining but von Kossa stain may help to highlight these deposits. Sometimes the involved vessels also show luminal thrombosis. The affected vessels develop intimal hyperplasia with endovascular endothelial proliferation and intimal fibrosis, resulting in ischaemia of the areas they supply [13,14]. Secondary ischaemic changes include epidermal ulceration and degeneration of dermal collagen.

Box 99.5 Disorders associated with cutaneous vascular calcification

Renal failure and hyperparathyroidism

Other disorders
- Atherosclerosis [23]
- Liver disease (alcoholic cirrhosis) [24–26]
- Crohn disease [27]
- Malignancies: metastatic breast carcinoma [28], cholangiocarcinoma [29], malignant melanoma [30], osteosclerotic myeloma [31], chronic myelomonocytic leukaemia [32]
- Rheumatoid arthritis on long-term steroid and methotrexate treatment [33,34]
- Protein S deficiency [25,33]
- AIDS [35]
- Antiphospholipid antibody syndrome [36]
- POEMS syndrome [37]

Cutaneous vascular calcification as an incidental histopathological finding
- Calcinosis cutis secondary to injections
- Sclerosing panniculitis (lipodermatosclerosis)
- Erythema induratum
- Leukocytoclastic vasculitis
- Traumatic ulcer
- Basal cell and squamous cell cutaneous carcinomas
- Scars

Modified from Dauden *et al*. 2002 and Dauden and Oñate 2008 [15,**22**]

Focal lobular panniculitis is frequently seen [14], although some biopsies show few or no inflammatory infiltrate in the fat lobule adjacent to the calcified vessel. Some authors, however, have described a predominantly septal panniculitis in calciphylaxis [13]. Since vascular calcification may be seen in cutaneous biopsies from other disorders (Box 99.5), additional features may be needed to support a histological diagnosis of calciphylaxis: these include interstitial deposition of calcium in the dermis, fine calcium deposits in and around the adipocytes [15], epidermal and hair follicle calcification [16], perineural calcium deposits [17], and calcified elastic fibres with a PXE-like appearance [18,19]. Perieccrine calcium deposition has been reported as a highly specific histopathological finding in calcific arteriolopathy [20].

Calcific arteriolopathy should be distinguished from metastatic cutaneous calcification, which is a rare phenomenon involving the dermis and subcutis and affecting predominantly uraemic patients with combined hyperphosphataemia and hypercalcaemia, often in the context of hyperparathyroidism (see Chapter 61). It typically presents as firm papules, nodules or plaques in the dermis or subcutis, particularly around large joints or flexural sites. Unlike calciphylaxis, metastatic cutaneous calcification does not lead to tissue necrosis and histopathologically deposits of calcium, appearing blue with H&E and black with von Kossa stains, are seen in the dermis and subcutis with variable surrounding inflammatory infiltrate, but vessel walls are spared [21].

Cold panniculitis

Definition
Cold panniculitis is a form of injury to subcutaneous fat induced by exposure to cold, either environmental [1] or as cold objects applied to the skin (e.g. ice packs) [2–4]. Infants are particularly susceptible. It is not uncommon in children in regions subject to low temperatures [5].

Pathophysiology

Predisposing factors
Cold panniculitis was originally described by Hochsinger in 1902 as submental nodules and plaques in children after cold exposure [6]. Lemez, in 1928, demonstrated infants to be more susceptible to fat necrosis by exposure to cold than adults [7]. Haxthausen in 1941 described similar cases on the cheeks of infants after cold temperatures and named the condition 'adiponecrosis e frigore' [8]. Adams *et al.* in 1954 clarified the pathogenesis of cold panniculitis demonstrating that pigs fed with a diet rich in saturated fatty acids showed higher cold susceptibility due to the higher ratio of saturated to unsaturated fatty acids, resulting in an elevated freezing point of fat [9]. In 1965 Hirsch confirmed than saturated fats solidified at a higher temperature than unsaturated fats [10]. Solomon and Beerman, in 1963, reported the occurrence of panniculitis in a 28-year-old Jamaican woman within hours of cold exposure with lesions which were readily inducible with local applications of ice [11]. Rotman reported similar cases involving the cheeks in two infants of five and eight months of age [12]. A similar process was described under the name 'popsicle panniculitis' on the cheeks of children a few hours after eating ice lollies [2,3,13]. The most extensive histopathological study of cold panniculitis was performed by Duncan *et al.* in 1966, who studied serial skin biopsies after exposing the skin of the child to ice for 2–4 min and performing sequential punch biopsies. Increased duration of ice exposure was required to produce cold panniculitis as the child aged and the reaction no longer occurred at the age of 22 months [4].

Presentation

Neonatal and infantile cold panniculitis
Neonates are particularly susceptible to cold panniculitis. This is thought to be because subcutaneous fat in newborns is rich in saturated fatty acids, particularly palmitic and stearic acids, which have a higher freezing point than unsaturated fatty acids, [10,14] so that a small decrease in an infant's temperature may result in crystallization of subcutaneous fat [1]. The risk in neonates may be increased by cooling for management of birth asphyxia or for infants undergoing cardiac surgery [1,**15**,16]. Cold panniculitis has also been reported in neonates who are administered ice packs to control neonatal supraventricular tachycardia [17,18]. Over the first 2 years of life the subcutaneous fat of children rapidly becomes less saturated, with an increase in the oleic acid content and a consequent lowering of the freezing point and lessening of the risk of cold injury.

In young children, the most commonly involved areas are the cheeks and chin, because they are rich in subcutaneous fat and are normally more exposed to the cold than other body areas. The lesions consist of indolent erythematous or violaceous indurated plaques or nodules with no systemic manifestations. The child is otherwise healthy and the lesions regress without treatment within weeks. Cold panniculitis of the cheeks may also be precipitated by sucking ice lollies (popsicle panniculitis) [2–4].

Cold panniculitis in adults

Adult patients with cold panniculitis are typically obese and predominantly female. The most commonly affected areas are the lateral upper thighs and gluteal region (Figure 99.32). The distribution of the lesions in adults has been postulated to be attributable to the effects of tight-fitting clothing compromising the blood flow in the upper lateral thighs, rendering the ischaemic fat more susceptible to cold injury [19]. These patients often have very cold skin in the affected areas even when they are seen in clinic and perhaps a more plausible explanation is that the skin and immediately subjacent fat is insulated from core body temperature by a thick layer of intervening fat. The tight-fitting clothing offers little protection from low external environmental temperature and the lesions are usually accompanied by some degree of vasodilatation as one would expect with perniosis. It has also been suggested that a diet rich in saturated fatty acids would result in a subcutaneous fat similar to that of a newborn [20]. Some such patients have been found to have cryofibrinogenaemia, which probably predisposed them to cold panniculitis [21].

Cold panniculitis has also been described in healthy adult women with lesions involving the lateral upper thighs after prolonged horse-riding in cold weather. This variant may be regarded as a form of perniosis and has been named 'equestrian cold panniculitis' or horse rider's pernio [19]. Symptoms have been reported to be more pronounced in older women and appear to be aggravated by heavy smoking, by wearing tight riding clothes and by longer riding times [22]. Similar cases have been described in obese women engaged in sporting activities such as cycling and motorcycling in conditions of humidity and wind [23], or riding on open slow-moving vehicles in similar weather conditions [24].

Prolonged application of ice directly to the skin can produce local injury in a manner similar to popsicle panniculitis: 'ice pack dermatosis' has been described on the lower back of adults using ice packs for alleviation of chronic low back pain [25].

Investigations

Histopathologically, cold panniculitis consists of a predominantly lobular panniculitis [26], although a variable septal component is usually present [27]. Inflammation is denser in the lower reticular dermis and dermal–hypodermal interface (Figure 99.33). The

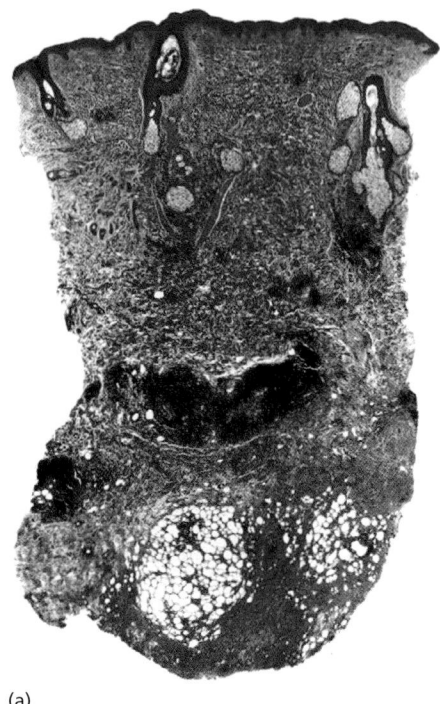

(a)

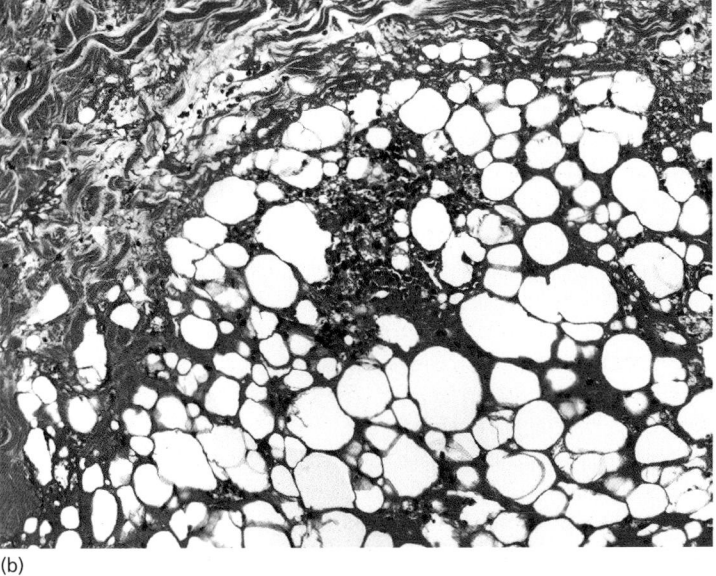

(b)

Figure 99.33 Histopathology of equestrian panniculitis. (a) Scanning power showing dense nodular infiltrates in deeper dermis. (b) Small aggregate of lymphocytes in the fat lobule.

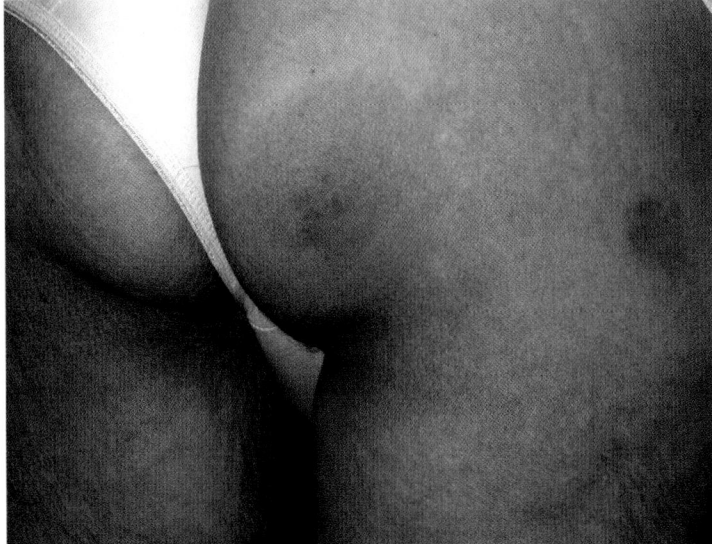

Figure 99.32 Erythematous nodule on gluteal region of a woman with equestrian cold panniculitis.

infiltrate is composed mostly of lymphocytes and some histiocytes involving the fat lobules. The overlying dermis shows a superficial and deep perivascular lymphocytic infiltrate with no vasculitis [26]. Blood vessels of both septa and fat lobules may exhibit endothelial swelling and intramural oedema, but there are no fibrin deposits nor nuclear dust as would be seen in a true vasculitis. Interstitial mucin deposition may also be seen with a histopathological picture closely resembling lupus panniculitis [28].

Duncan *et al.* described the 'lives of lesions' of cold panniculitis in a 6-month-old black male infant by applying an ice cube to his buttocks and taking serial punch biopsies at 30 min, 6 h, 24 h, 48 h, 72 h, 6 days and 2 weeks [4]. Earliest changes were seen in the 24 h specimen, which showed a mild perivascular lymphohistiocytic infiltrate mostly located at the dermal–hypodermal interface, without associated fat necrosis. The changes were more intense in the specimens taken at 48 and 72 h, which showed a denser mixed infiltrate, composed of lymphocytes, scattered neutrophils, histiocytes and foamy macrophages mostly involving the fat lobule. At this time, features of adipocytic necrosis were evident in the form of lipophagic granulomas surrounding small cystic spaces. The inflammatory reaction progressively increased in biopsies taken in the next 2–3 days and then slowly decreased to regress completely by 2 weeks. The subcutaneous nodules regressed leaving no residual lesion.

Differential diagnosis

The clinicopathological differential diagnosis of cold panniculitis includes subcutaneous fat necrosis of the newborn, sclerema neonatorum, lupus panniculitis, poststeroid panniculitis, perniosis and frostbite.

Subcutaneous fat necrosis of the newborn usually appears in the first days of life and has a predilection for the thighs, buttocks, cheeks, back and arms. It may occasionally be associated with symptomatic hypercalcaemia. This panniculitis may be associated with hypothermia, obstetric trauma, maternal diabetes and maternal pre-eclampsia. Histopathology shows a lobular panniculitis with a mostly histiocytic infiltrate including multinucleate giant cells and adipocytes and histiocytes contain needle-shaped clefts that result from lipid crystallization [**15**,16,29,30].

Sclerema neonatorum is an extremely rare disorder which was described in premature or debilitated children who developed a diffuse board-like stiffness due to generalized fat necrosis. The condition appeared in the first days after birth and was usually fatal. Histologically, the adipocytes contain needle-shaped clefts in radial arrays with no inflammatory response [26,31]. There have been no recent reports of sclerema neonatorum and it is likely that the problem has disappeared in places with proper facilities for neonatal care of premature and debilitated newborns.

Lupus panniculitis is rare in children and the few described paediatric cases [32–36] do not differ significantly from lupus panniculitis in adults. Histopathology shows a mostly lobular panniculitis, with an infiltrate composed predominantly of lymphocytes and plasma cells, lymphoid aggregates with germinal centre formation and sclerotic collagen bundles at connective tissue septa. The process is chronic and longstanding lesions show hyaline necrosis of the fat lobule, which is not seen in the more acute and self-resolving process of cold panniculitis.

Poststeroid panniculitis occurs in children receiving high doses of systemic corticosteroids when the dose is rapidly decreased or suddenly withdrawn. The lesions appear as small painful nodules on the cheeks and posterior neck, the areas in which corticosteroid therapy has induced fat deposition. The histopathological picture is identical to that of subcutaneous fat necrosis of the newborn [27,30].

Chilblains appear following cold exposure as bluish macules, papules and plaques involving mostly the acral areas of the skin, but they can also be found on the thighs and buttocks. Histopathologically, the picture may be very similar to cold panniculitis, although chilblains usually show oedema of the papillary dermis, the lymphocytic infiltrate is mostly arranged around eccrine coils and some cases show features of lymphocytic vasculitis in dermal blood vessels. Extension to subcutaneous fat is uncommon in chilblains [36,37].

In early frostbite, there are erythematous and oedematous plaques that may be painful or anaesthetic. In fully developed severe frostbite, there is blistering and necrosis. Histopathology shows subepidermal oedema with blister formation, necrosis of epidermal keratinocytes and a superficial and deep perivascular lymphocytic infiltrate involving the full thickness of the dermis [36].

Management

Treatment of cold panniculitis is not usually required because the condition resolves spontaneously. Prevention of infantile cold panniculitis in children is achieved by avoiding cold exposure and direct contact with ice products [11,16]. For equestrian cold panniculitis in adult women, the use of loose, warm clothing should be recommended when riding, with avoidance of tight-fitting clothes and, where possible, cold exposure [19,38]. Nifedipine has been shown to be ineffective [38]. In one case, a dramatic response to tetracycline was observed, which was also effective prophylactically [39].

Lupus panniculitis

Definition and nomenclature

Lupus panniculitis is characterized by a destructive inflammation of subcutaneous fat. Clinically, lesions consist of indurated plaques which resolve with localized lipoatrophy. Depending on the intensity of inflammation a patient may first present with lipoatrophy rather than induration. The overlying skin may show changes of chronic cutaneous lupus erythematosus. The face, upper arms (Figure 99.34), upper trunk, breasts, buttocks and thighs are most commonly affected. The clinical features are described in detail in Chapter 51.

Synonyms and inclusions
- Lupus erythematosus profundus
- Subcutaneous lupus erythematosus

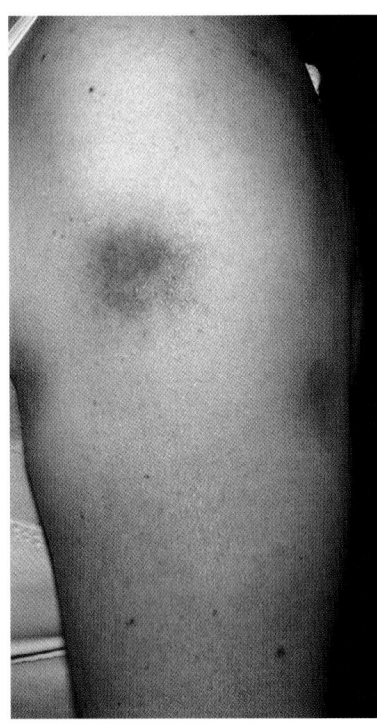

Figure 99.34 Clinical features of lupus panniculitis showing an active erythematous subcutaneous nodule and areas of hyperpigmented lipoatrophy secondary to regressed lesions.

Clinical features

Differential diagnosis

Panniculitis associated with dermatomyositis shares identical histopathological findings with lupus panniculitis [1–13]. Histopathological differential diagnosis of lupus panniculitis also includes cold panniculitis, deep morphoea, persistent nodules after injection of vaccines containing aluminium, panniculitis at the injection sites of glatiramer acetate and subcutaneous panniculitis-like T-cell lymphoma (SPTCL). Differential diagnosis with cold panniculitis is discussed earlier.

Deep morphoea may also display lymphoid nodules at the connective tissue septa of the subcutis, but in contrast with lupus panniculitis the process involves exclusively the septa and the fat lobule is spared.

Persistent nodules at injection sites of a vaccine containing aluminium show similar features to lupus panniculitis, including hyaline necrosis of the fat lobules and lymphoid aggregates, but the correct diagnosis may be suspected by the presence of histiocytes containing fine basophilic granules of aluminium and abundant number of eosinophils [14].

Several patients receiving daily glatiramer acetate injections for the treatment of multiple sclerosis developed localized panniculitis at the injection sites. The lesions consisted of a mostly lobular panniculitis, with lipophagic granulomata, namely histiocytes engulfing the lipids from necrotic adipocytes. In many areas, scattered neutrophils and eosinophils were seen both in the septa and in the fat lobules. Connective tissue septa showed widening and fibrosis in conjunction with many lymphoid follicles, presenting with germinal centre formation. Immunohistochemically, the inflammatory infiltrate of the fat lobule consisted of CD68-positive histiocytes and suppressor/cytotoxic T lymphocytes. In contrast, the lymphoid follicles in the septa and at the interface between septum and fat lobule were mainly composed of B lymphocytes. The clinical history with lesions localized only at the injection sites rules out lupus panniculitis [15,16].

The most difficult histopathological differential diagnosis of lupus panniculitis is SPTCL and overlapping cases of lupus profundus and SPTCL have been described. SPTCL is a peculiar α/β T-cell lymphoma, usually CD8+, which involves subcutaneous fat, without epidermal and/or dermal involvement, and mimics a panniculitic process (see Chapter 140). Magro *et al.* [17] reviewed 32 cases of lymphocytic lobular panniculitis and classified them into three groups: lupus panniculitis, SPTCL and a third group with intermediate features that they named 'indeterminate lymphocytic lobular panniculitis'. Lesions of this third group showed the involvement of subcutaneous fat by atypical lymphocytes with pleomorphic and hyperchromatic nuclei. The same group has recently proposed the term 'atypical lymphocytic lobular panniculitis' for these intermediate cases [18]. The infiltrate showed deletion of one or more pan-T-cell markers (CD3, CD5 and/or CD7) and monoclonal *TCRγ* gene rearrangement by PCR. The authors introduced the concept of subcutaneous lymphoid dyscrasia to encompass the cases with overlapping findings of lupus panniculitis and SPTCL. More recently, Pincus *et al.* [19] reported on five patients and Basisio *et al.* [20] described 11 patients with SPTCL who were unusual in that they also exhibited features of lupus erythematosus. In all cases, attributes indicating SPTCL included an infiltrate of lymphocytes with pleomorphic nuclei involving subcutaneous lobules exhibiting a cytotoxic T-cell (CD3/CD8/βF1) immunophenotype. Additionally, a high proliferation rate and a monoclonal *TCRγ* gene rearrangement were observed in most cases. The manifestations of lupus erythematosus in these patients included a spectrum of clinical and histopathological abnormalities. The clinical manifestations consisted in subcutaneous nodules that healed with lipoatrophy on the face and serological and/or extracutaneous end-organ abnormalities as seen in patients with systemic lupus erythematosus. Histopathological evidences of lupus erythematosus included vacuolar change at the dermal–epidermal interface, interstitial deposition of mucin in the reticular dermis, clusters of CD20+ B cells partially arranged within germinal centres, a few small clusters of CD123+ plasmacytoid dendritic cells within the adipose tissue and positive direct immunofluorescence test on clinically uninvolved and lesional skin. The authors concluded that some patients show overlap between SPTCL and lupus panniculitis and that patients with lupus panniculitis should be monitored for possible evolution into SPTCL. This recommendation is also supported by other reports of T-cell lymphomas with subcutaneous tissue involvement, probably cutaneous γ/δ T-cell lymphomas, with histopathological features similar to those of lupus panniculitis, including vacuolar interface dermatitis and dermal mucinosis [21–23]. In fact, one of these cases was erroneously diagnosed as lupus panniculitis [23]. The most useful criteria now for distinguishing lupus panniculitis from SPTCL are the presence in lupus panniculitis of epidermal involvement, superficial and deep perivascular lymphocytic infiltrate in the dermis, lymphoid follicles with reactive germinal centres, a mixed infiltrate with numerous plasma cells, clusters of

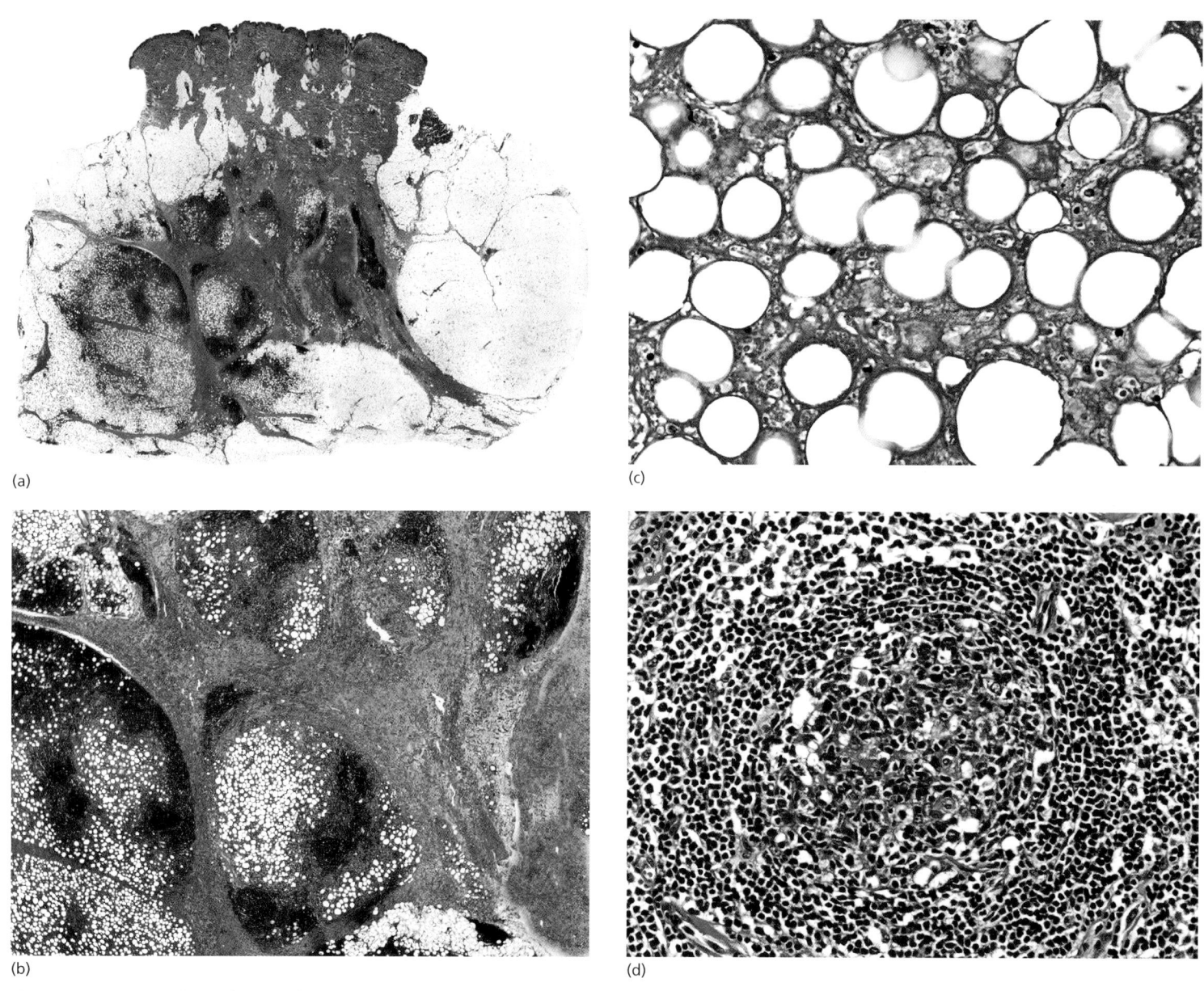

Figure 99.35 Histopathological features of lupus panniculitis. (a) Scanning magnification showing a predominantly lobular panniculitis. (b) Dense lymphoid aggregations at the interphase between the fat lobule and the thickened septa. (c) Hyaline necrosis involving the fat lobule. (d) Reactive germinal centre formation within the lymphoid aggregates.

B lymphocytes, clusters of CD123+ plasmacytoid dendritic cells [24], low proliferative index in lymphocytes and polyclonal *TCRγ* rearrangement [25].

Investigations

Histopathologically, lupus panniculitis is a predominantly lobular panniculitis in which the infiltrate in active lesions involves mainly the fat lobule [26]. Some authors find difficulty in classifying lupus panniculitis as predominantly lobular panniculitis because of the prominent septal component [25,27,28]. The septal component, however, consists of thickening and sclerosis of the collagen bundles in the septa, whereas most of the infiltrate is found in the fat lobule. Active lesions exhibit a picture of a predominantly lymphocytic panniculitis with numerous plasma cells. Longstanding lesions show hyaline necrosis of the fat lobule with little or no infiltrate and replacement by diffuse eosinophilic glassy remnants of adipocytes

[25,29–31]. Lymphoid aggregates, sometimes with germinal centre formation, are also frequently seen in the septa or at the periphery of the fat lobules (Figure 99.35). These lymphoid follicles, although characteristic, are not pathognomonic of lupus panniculitis because they may also be seen in deep morphoea, erythema nodosum, erythema induratum, necrobiosis lipoidica, panniculitis associated with dermatomyositis and necrobiotic xanthogranuloma [32].

Additional histopathological findings consist in calcification, interstitial mucin deposition and features of discoid lupus erythematosus in the overlying epidermis. An uncommon but, when seen, distinctive feature is the presence of nuclear dust within the infiltrate [28,33,34]. Eosinophils are not usually prominent in lesions of lupus panniculitis [25,30] but, in contrast with other forms of cutaneous lupus erythematosus in which eosinophils are characteristically absent, the infiltrate of lupus panniculitis may contain some eosinophils [35].

As with other lobular panniculitides, longstanding and residual lesions of lupus panniculitis may show lipomembranous changes [36]. Lymphocytic vasculitis has been described in lupus panniculitis with variable frequency [37–39]. This vasculitis consists of the presence of lymphocytes in and around the vessel walls, mural fibrin deposition, luminal thrombosis and nuclear dust. Some authors consider that hyaline necrosis of the fat lobule results from the ischaemic process secondary to this lymphocytic vasculitis [40].

Histopathological features of discoid lupus erythematosus at the dermal–epidermal junction in lesions of lupus panniculitis have been described in varying proportions, ranging from 20% to 75% of cases [25,26,29,31,41,42]. These changes include epidermal atrophy with hyperkeratosis, follicular plugging, vacuolar alteration of the basal layer of the epidermis and basement membrane thickening. Additional features of discoid lupus erythematosus are interstitial mucin deposition, telangiectasia, and superficial and deep perivascular dermal lymphocytic infiltrate. Calcification is also a frequent finding in chronic lesions of lupus panniculitis and consists of individual calcification of elastic fibres or large masses of calcium within the lobules and septa [31,43].

Only a few direct immunofluorescence studies have been performed in lesions of lupus panniculitis. The lupus band test at the dermal–epidermal junction is often positive [1,44]. Additional findings consist of IgG deposition at the periphery of adipocytes and around the vessels [42,45].

Immunohistochemical studies have demonstrated that the infiltrate in lupus panniculitis is composed mostly of T lymphocytes, with a slight preponderance of CD4 over CD8 lymphocytes. All of them show α/β immunophenotype. Small aggregates of B lymphocytes are also present at the periphery of the lymphoid aggregates. PCR analyses for *TCRγ* gene rearrangement in the infiltrate has demonstrated its polyclonal nature in most cases [17,28,45–47]. Because of the presence of cytotoxic CXCR3+ lymphocytes in the fat lobules, it has been suggested that lupus panniculitis may be due to a type I interferon Th1 driven immune response [48].

Dermatomyositis-associated panniculitis

Clinical features

Presentation
Panniculitis is less frequent in dermatomyositis than in lupus erythematosus and systemic sclerosis [1,2,3,4–13,14,15]. In a series of 55 adult patients with dermatomyositis and cutaneous lesions studied histopathologically, panniculitis was only found in five cases [1]. Panniculitis has also been described in juvenile dermatomyositis [8,11]. When the inflammation settles it leaves areas of lipoatrophy [4].

In some patients, panniculitis is associated with other characteristic cutaneous lesions of dermatomyositis [8], whereas in others panniculitis is the only cutaneous manifestation of the disease [3,9]. Conversely, there is a report of a patient presenting with panniculitis and vesiculobullous skin lesions but no evidence of muscle involvement [15]. The clinical features of dermatomyositis are discussed in detail in Chapter 53.

Investigations
The histopathological features of dermatomyositis-associated panniculitis are similar to those of lupus panniculitis and consist of a predominantly lobular panniculitis with lymphocytes and plasma cells among the adipocytes. The septal collagen bundles show hyaline sclerosis, and there is progressive replacement of fat with fibrous tissue [2]. Additional histopathological findings include thickening of the blood vessels of the fat lobule, neutrophilic vasculitis with fibrinoid necrosis or lymphocytic vasculitis involving the arterioles of the septa, and calcification. Lymphoid follicles, with or without reactive germinal centre formation, have also been described [5], although this finding is less frequent than in lupus panniculitis or deep morphoea. As in lupus panniculitis, there may be vacuolar change at the dermal–epidermal junction and, in the late stages of the process, membranocystic changes [9,12].

Direct immunofluorescence studies have been reported in only three cases: the results were negative in one case [5]; the second case had deposits of IgM, C3 and fibrinogen in the blood vessels walls of the dermis, but not at the dermal–epidermal junction [9]; and the third case showed deposits of C3 at the basement membrane zone of the dermal–epidermal junction and around the dermal blood vessels, but in the subcutaneous fat only deposits of fibrinogen were detected [5]. As with lupus panniculitis, patients with dermatomyositis-associated panniculitis seem to be a subgroup with a generally good prognosis and no obvious increase in the incidence of malignancy [10]: in fact, malignancy has been reported in only one patient with dermatomyositis-associated panniculitis [3].

More common than pure dermatomyositis-associated panniculitis is panniculitis occurring in association with calcification of muscle and deep tissue. In these cases, the fat lobule shows lipophagic granulomata, calcification and various degrees of acute and chronic inflammation [2].

Pancreatic panniculitis

Synonyms and inclusions
• Enzymatic fat necrosis

Introduction and general description
Pancreatic panniculitis was originally described by Chiari in 1883 [1], but it was not until 1961 when Szymanski and Bluefarb reported the first case in the English literature [2]. There are only a few published series of patients with pancreatic panniculitis [3–7], and most reports include descriptions of no more than one or two cases.

Epidemiology

Incidence and prevalence
Pancreatic panniculitis is uncommon and appears in only about 2–3% of all patients with pancreatic disease [8], although its incidence is higher among males with alcoholism [9,10].

Pathophysiology

The pathogenesis of pancreatic panniculitis remains unclear, but release of pancreatic enzymes, such as lipase, trypsin and amylase, seems to be the most important aetiological factor. It is not completely clear how pancreatic proenzymes become activated in the tissues to produce fat necrosis [11], but trypsin may increase the permeability of the microcirculation within lymphatic vessels [6], allowing lipase and amylase to enter the peripheral circulation. Within the fat lobules these enzymes hydrolyse neutral fat to form glycerol and free fatty acids, which results in adipocyte necrosis and an inflammatory response [12,13]. This theory is supported by the finding of elevated enzyme levels in the blood, urine and skin lesions, even in the absence of detectable pancreatic disease [12], and by the positive intracellular immunostaining of adipocytes with a monoclonal antibody to pancreatic lipase in lesions of pancreatic fat necrosis [14]. However, other factors apart from pancreatic enzymes must also play some pathogenetic role, because there is clear discrepancy between the small number of cases of pancreatic panniculitis compared with the great number of patients with pancreatitis and pancreatic carcinoma who have increased serum levels of pancreatic enzymes but no panniculitis [13,15]. Conversely, some patients with pancreatic panniculitis have had normal serum levels of all pancreatic enzymes [5]. Furthermore, *in vitro* investigations have failed to reproduce pancreatic panniculitis when normal human fat has been incubated with the serum of patients with high levels of pancreatic lipase, trypsin and amylase [5]. Other proposed mechanisms implicate vascular damage [12,16], immune complexes [17], and adipocyte-generated cytokines and adipokines released in response to high levels of free fatty acids. Resistin and leptin have been shown to be potential markers of extrapancreatic fat necrosis [18].

Clinical features

Clinically, cutaneous lesions of pancreatic panniculitis consist of tender, erythematous or red-brown nodules that may spontaneously ulcerate, draining an oily brown, sterile and viscous material that results from liquefactive necrosis of adipocytes (Figure 99.36). These lesions show a predilection for the distal parts of the lower extremities, mostly around the ankles. Venous stasis may promote this process, although lesions in other areas including the knees, thighs, buttocks, arms, abdomen, chest and scalp may also be seen [19]. Ulceration and fistulization of necrotic fat to the skin surface are frequent clinical features in pancreatic panniculitis, but they may also occur in other panniculitides. Although there are no specific clinical findings, it seems that the panniculitis associated with pancreatic carcinoma tends to be more persistent, with more frequent recurrences and a greater tendency to ulceration, fistulization and involvement of cutaneous areas beyond the lower extremities than that related to inflammatory pancreatic disease [10]. Cases of pancreatic panniculitis with a single cutaneous nodule have, however, also been reported [20]. The association of panniculitis with fever, polyarthritis and abdominal pain should raise suspicion of pancreatic disease.

Enzymatic fat necrosis induced by pancreatic enzymes is not confined to subcutaneous fat and often patients have other foci of fat necrosis: when this involves periarticular fat it may cause

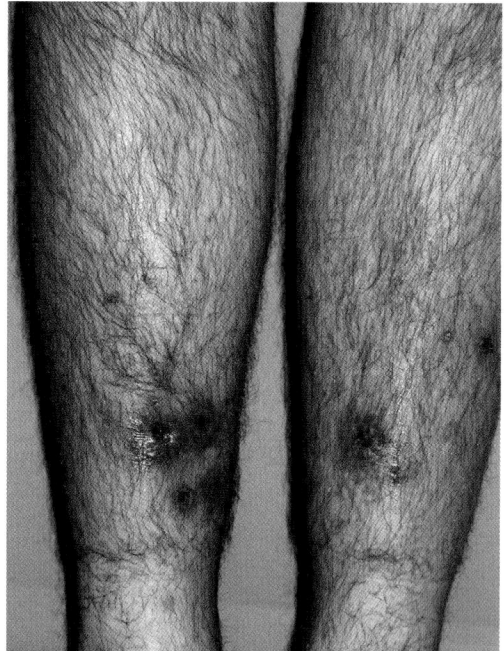

Figure 99.36 Pancreatic panniculitis in an alcoholic male. Nodular lesions, many of them ulcerated around the ankles.

a mono- or oligoarticular arthritis [10,21], which may be symmetrical and can be intermittent, migratory or persistent [16]. This enzymatic arthritis usually involves the small joints of the hands, wrists and feet, but also may affect larger joints such as the elbows, knees and ankles. Aspiration of the involved joint yields a creamy purulent sterile fluid with a few white cells [22]. Joint fluid may also contain lipid crystals with increased levels of amylase, lipase, free fatty acids, triglycerides and cholesterol [22]. In rare instances, this may progress to chondronecrosis and osteonecrosis of the involved joints [23]. Other less common extrapancreatic sites involved by enzymatic fat necrosis rarely cause symptomatology, but autopsies of patients with pancreatic carcinoma and panniculitis have demonstrated fat necrosis in abdominal fat [24] and bone marrow [25]. Radiological images are characteristic, showing osteolytic lesions, moth-eaten bone destruction and periostitis of the involved bone of the extremities due to extensive areas of bone marrow fat necrosis and trabecular bone destruction [26]. The association of panniculitis, polyarthritis and eosinophilia in a patient with pancreatic cancer is known as the Schmid triad and usually carries a poor prognosis [16].

Skin lesions may be the first sign of pancreatic disease and therefore represent an important clue for the diagnosis [1,16,27]. In the literature, there are several reports in which cutaneous nodules of pancreatic panniculitis preceded the detection of pancreatic carcinoma by several months, and the development of panniculitis may also predict progressive or metastatic malignant disease [28]. However, the most frequent underlying associated pancreatic disease is not pancreatic carcinoma, but acute [6] or chronic pancreatitis [29,30] caused by alcohol abuse [6], trauma [31,32], or cholelithiasis [33]. After acute and chronic pancreatitis, pancreatic carcinoma is the next most common cause of pancreatic panniculitis.

Box 99.6 Disorders associated with pancreatic panniculitis

Acute or chronic pancreatitis
- Pancreatitis secondary to alcohol abuse [6]
- Pancreatitis secondary to trauma [31,32]
- Pancreatitis secondary to cholelithiasis [33]
- Pancreatic pseudocyst [34,35]
- Acute fatty liver of pregnancy and pancreatitis [36]

Malignancy
- Acinar cell pancreatic carcinoma [3,13,28,37–42]
- Islet cell pancreatic carcinoma [17,28,43–48]
- Acinar cell pancreatic cystadenocarcinoma [16]
- Liver carcinoma [21]
- Adenocarcinoma of unknown origin [49]
- Cancer-associated fasciitis–panniculitis syndrome [50]

Postprocedural
- Following renal or simultaneous pancreas and kidney transplantation [51–54]
- After endoscopic retrograde cholangiopancreatography [55]

Pancreatic anomalies
- Vascular pancreatic fistulas [56]
- Pancreas divisum [58–60]

Miscellaneous
- Systemic lupus erythematosus [61,62]
- Association with HIV infection and haemophagocytic syndrome [63]
- Hypertriglyceridaemia and nephrotic syndrome [64]
- Sulindac therapy [65]
- Following L-asparginase treatment for acute lymphoblastic leukaemia [66,67]

Rarer disorders that may also cause this panniculitis are listed in Box 99.6.

Differential diagnosis
Clinically, the main differential diagnoses are erythema induratum, α_1-antitrypsin deficiency panniculitis and infectious panniculitis [3,12,17]. Histopathology usually resolves any doubt by finding ghost adipocytes in the saponified fat lobule [12]. Lobular panniculitis at the site of subcutaneous IFN-β injections for the treatment of multiple sclerosis may histologically mimic pancreatic panniculitis [68].

Investigations
Histopathology of pancreatic panniculitis is almost pathognomonic, consisting in a predominantly lobular panniculitis without vasculitis [6,17]. However, some authors have proposed that the earliest feature in pancreatic panniculitis is a predominantly septal panniculitis resulting from enzymatic damage to endothelial cells lining septal blood vessels. These damaged endothelial cells allow pancreatic enzymes to cross from the blood to fat lobules, resulting in necrosis of adipocytes [3,6]. Regardless of this, early states of pancreatic panniculitis show a predominantly neutrophilic infiltrate, with occasional eosinophils and, as the most characteristic finding, ghost adipocytes resulting from coagulative adipocyte necrosis. These ghost adipocytes lose their nuclei and show

a finely granular and basophilic material within their cytoplasm because of calcification. Often ghost adipocytes group in small clusters at the centre of the fat lobule, whereas the neutrophilic infiltrate is present at the periphery [69] (Figure 99.37). Dystrophic calcification in ghost adipocytes results from the hydrolytic action of pancreatic enzymes on fat cells with subsequent calcium deposition, a process known as saponification [5,6]. Often, adjacent lobules show a different stage in the histopathological evolution of the process. In late stages, fat necrosis and ghost adipocytes are less evident and the inflammatory infiltrate is more granulomatous, containing foamy histiocytes, multinucleate giant cells and

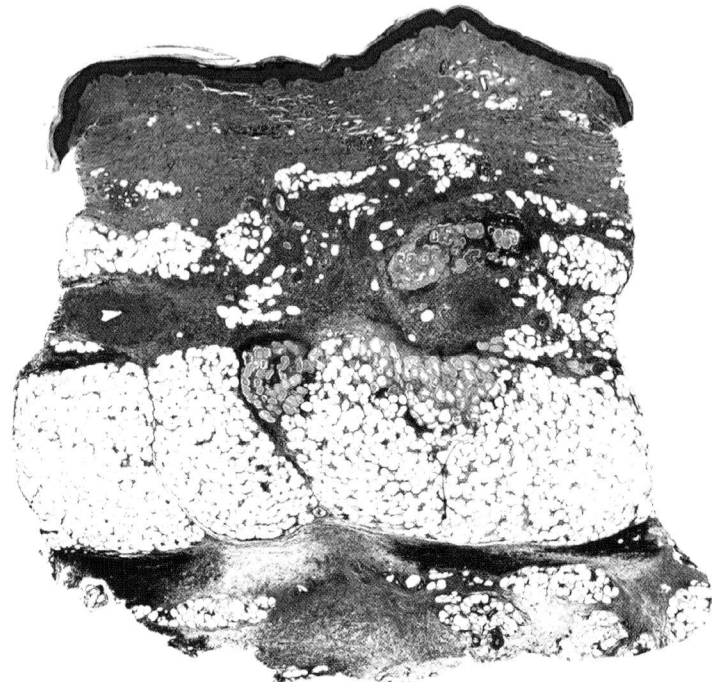
(a)

(b)

Figure 99.37 Histopathological features of pancreatic panniculitis. (a) Scanning power showing a mostly lobular panniculitis. (b) A group of 'ghost' adipocytes surrounded by neutrophils is seen at the periphery of the fat lobule.

haemosiderin deposits [11]. Residual lesions show fibrosis and lipoatrophy. Although ghost adipocytes are very characteristic of pancreatic panniculitis, they are not pathognomonic and similar findings may be seen in mucocutaneous mucormycosis [70] and cutaneous aspergillosis [71]. It has been shown that fungi of the family Mucoraceae produce remarkable amounts of extracellular lipases [72,73] and thus it is likely that the ghost adipocytes result from the local effect of these lipases.

Most patients, although not all, show elevated serum levels of amylase, lipase or trypsin though often one enzyme is within normal levels whilst others are elevated [10]. There is no correlation between the serum levels of pancreatic enzymes and the severity of the cutaneous lesions [74]. In rare instances, patients with pancreatic panniculitis may show high serum levels of pancreatic lipase with no evidence of underlying pancreatic disease [21,75]. A leukaemoid reaction and eosinophilia in peripheral blood are also common haematological abnormalities, particularly in patients with pancreatic carcinoma [75,76]. Other tumour markers such as carcinoembryonic antigen or Ca 19.9 are often elevated in these patients.

Management

Treatment of pancreatic panniculitis should be directed to the underlying pancreatic disease and usually the cutaneous lesions heal once the acute inflammatory pancreatic process has resolved or the pancreatic anomaly has been surgically corrected [3,13,53,77]. Administration of the somatostatin analogue octreotide, a synthetic polypeptide which inhibits pancreatic enzyme production, has been reported to result in a significant improvement in pancreatic panniculitis in some [13,38,78] but not all [17,30,37,48] patients with pancreatic carcinoma. Corticosteroids, non-steroidal anti-inflammatory drugs and immunosuppressive drugs are usually not effective treatments for pancreatic panniculitis [26].

Alpha-1 antitrypsin deficiency panniculitis

Definition

Alpha-1 antitrypsin deficiency is a genetic disorder that manifests as pulmonary emphysema, liver cirrhosis and, rarely, as cutaneous panniculitis. It is characterized by low serum levels of α_1-antitrypsin, the main protease inhibitor in human serum.

Pathophysiology

Genetics

Alpha-1 antitrypsin is the most important serine protease inhibitor produced in the liver. Its principal function is to inhibit trypsin activity, but it also acts as a potent inhibitor of chymotrypsin, plasmin, thrombin, neutrophilic elastase, pancreatic elastase, serine proteases, collagenase, factor VIII, kallikrein, urokinase and cathepsin G. It may also inhibit complement activation, both through a direct effect on complement-related proteases and by inhibiting the neutrophil proteases that activate enzymes of the complement system. Additionally, it is thought to help regulate protease-stimulated activation of lymphocytes and phagocytosis by macrophages and neutrophils. It is an acute phase reactant which is released in stress situations.

Alpha-1 antitrypsin consists of 394 amino acids organized into three β-sheets and nine α-helices. The active site of the protein is a reactive central loop composed of 20 amino acids, which, when in contact with a serine protease, induces conformational changes resulting in inactivation of both α_1-antitrypsin and protease [1]. The gene that encodes this protein, *SERPINA 1* (formerly known as *PI*), is located at 14q32.1. More than 120 allelic variants have been described to date [1]. The most frequent allele, PiM, defined by its protein isoelectrophoretic mobility (M = medium mobility), is associated with homozygous PiMM phenotype and normal serum levels of α_1-antitrypsin (120–200 mg/dL) [2]. Two alleles, PiS (S = slow mobility) and PiZ (Z = very slow mobility), each caused by a single nucleic acid substitution, are considered to be involved in pathological manifestations. In the Z variant, glutamic acid replaces lysine at position 342 [3]. Homozygosity for the Z allele (PiZZ) is associated with very low serum levels of α_1-antitrypsin (20–45 mg/dL), whereas the heterozygous phenotypes PiMZ or PiMS result in a moderate reduction of α_1-antitrypsin serum levels. A null allele variant, without any apparent gene alteration, but with no detectable mRNA produced, has also been described. In individuals who are homozygous for Pi null/null mutations, serum α_1-antitrypsin is not detectable at all [4]. Heterozygosity for pathogenic α_1-antitrypsin mutations (PiMS, MZ, SZ) is estimated to occur in about 10% of the general population [5], with 2% heterozygous for the Z allele [6]. The prevalence of the homozygous PiZZ phenotype is only about 1 in 3500 in northern Europe populations [3]. In heterozygous carriers of the S or Z allele, α_1-antitrypsin production and function are apparently normal but only a small amount of α_1-antitrypsin enters the circulation from its production site in the liver. Both mutations result in a high tendency for the protein to polymerize, especially in the Z variant. In both homozygous and heterozygous phenotypes, polymerized α_1-antitrypsin cannot as a result be released from the liver. Z-type α_1-antitrypsin polymers have been detected in lesional skin, which supports the inflammatory pathogenesis of panniculitis and the potential pro-inflammatory role of polymers [7].

In situations causing tissue injury, such as smoking for emphysema, trauma for panniculitis or hepatotoxins for cirrhosis, the absence or deficiency of α_1-antitrypsin results in uncontrolled activation of lymphocytes and macrophages, lack of inhibition of the complement cascade including C3a–C5a neutrophilic chemotactic factors, and accumulation of neutrophils with release of proteolytic enzymes and secondary tissue damage [8]. The special susceptibility of subcutaneous fat to proteolytic degradation when not protected by α_1-antitrypsin is due to its high fatty acid content. Fatty acids modify elastin conformation and render fat more susceptible to proteolytic degradation [9].

Severe α_1-antitrypsin deficiency is associated with a variety of clinical manifestations including disorders of blood coagulation and fibrinolysis, anomalies in the phagocytic mechanism of the immune response and anomalies in the activation of zymogens and release of hormonal peptides in addition to its effect on the lung, liver and subcutaneous fat.

PART 8: SPECIFIC CUTANEOUS STRUCTURE

Alpha-1 antitrypsin deficiency panniculitis is most severe in homozygous PiZZ individuals. It can, however, also develop in heterozygotes with PiMS [1,9], PiMZ [10], PiSZ [11] genotypes and in homozygotes with PiSS [12] and PiM_1M_1 [13] genotypes. This suggests that other factors than α_1-antitrypsin deficiency may be involved in the pathogenesis. Furthermore, some authors believe that there are patients with the phenotypic features of α_1-antitrypsin deficiency but normal serum levels of α_1-antitrypsin who develop panniculitis because of mutations which do not induce polymerization but which affect the reactive centre loop, resulting in the production of non-functional protein [1,11].

Clinical features

History

Warter *et al.*, in 1972, were the first authors to describe panniculitis in association with α_1-antitrypsin deficiency, although these authors considered the process to be a manifestation of familial Weber–Christian disease [14]. Rubinstein *et al.*, in 1977, described the first two cases of α_1-antitrypsin deficiency-related panniculitis as a specific manifestation of this autosomal recessive inborn error of metabolism [15]. Panniculitis associated with α_1-antitrypsin deficiency is rare, with equal incidence in both genders and the age of presentation ranging from 7 to 73 years, with a mean age of 39.7 years [16], although children may also be affected [17].

Presentation

Dermatologically, panniculitis is the most important clinical manifestation of α_1-antitrypsin deficiency. Inflammation of subcutaneous fat may be the first sign of the disease, although subcutaneous nodules usually appear when other manifestations of the disorder have already developed. The panniculitis presents as erythematous nodules and plaques mainly located on the trunk and around the shoulders and hips [9]. The head and extremities may sometimes also be involved [18]. The earliest lesions resemble cellulitis [6] and show a tendency to ulcerate and exude oily material derived from necrotic adipocytes [18] (Figure 99.38). Healing of lesions leaves atrophic scars. A chronic relapsing course is characteristic. Antecedent trauma at the site of the lesion [9], surgical debridement [18], cryosurgery [19] or injections [20] can precipitate new lesions. Postpartum flares of the process have been attributed to an oestrogen-stimulated increase in proteinase inhibitor levels during pregnancy, followed by a precipitous decline to subnormal levels postpartum [21]. Uncommon cutaneous manifestations associated with α_1-antitrypsin deficiency include vasculitis and acquired angio-oedema [2,22,23]. Visceral extension is uncommon, but involvement of perinephric fat as well as hepatic and splenic sterile abscesses have been reported [12].

Differential diagnosis

Differential diagnosis of α_1-antitrypsin deficiency panniculitis includes other neutrophilic panniculitides with a tendency to ulcerate and fistula formation such as the early stages of erythema induratum, pancreatic panniculitis, factitial panniculitis and infective panniculitis. Most of these panniculitides show specific histopathological findings. When neutrophilic lobular panniculitis is found without indications of other specific diagnoses,

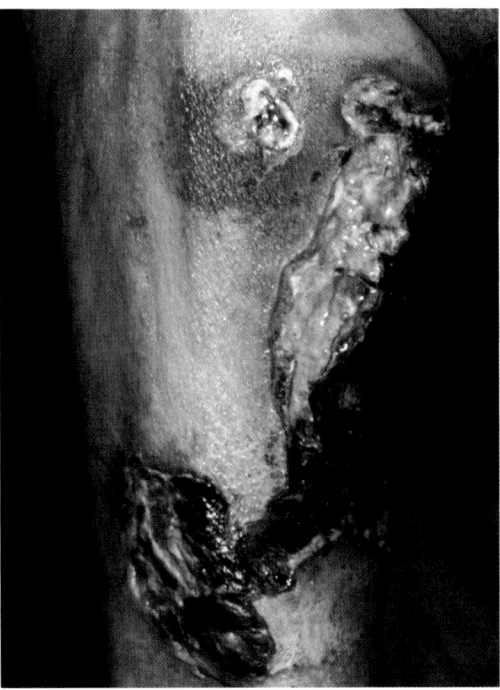

Figure 99.38 Panniculitis associated with α_1-antitrypsin deficiency. Necrotic ulcers exudate oily material that result from necrotic adipocytes.

measurement of serum levels of α_1-antitrypsin and electrophoretic mobility studies should be undertaken.

Complications and co-morbidities

Systemic manifestations of α_1-antitrypsin deficiency include panacinar emphysema, neonatal hepatitis, cirrhosis and liver disease resulting from retention of the abnormal polymerized protein within the liver, pancreatitis, membranoproliferative glomerulonephritis, c-ANCA-positive vasculitis and angio-oedema due to deficiency of protease inhibitor [9,20]. Approximately 50% of ZZ patients will die from emphysema-related complications and 10% will develop liver disease; the MZ phenotype is associated with a slightly higher risk of both lung and liver disease; and no increased likelihood of either lung or liver disease is seen in MS patients [1]. The null/null phenotype is usually accompanied by emphysema, but no liver disease because there is no α_1-antitrypsin synthesis and accumulation in the liver cannot therefore occur [4].

Investigations

Histopathological study of α_1-antitrypsin deficiency panniculitis shows a predominantly lobular panniculitis with no vasculitis. In the early stages, the presence of neutrophils extending into the lower reticular dermis in an interstitial pattern between collagen bundles ('splaying of neutrophils') has been proposed by some authors as a specific clue for the diagnosis [24]. This is, however, a non-specific finding that may be found in any neutrophilic lobular panniculitis. A more specific finding consists in the focal nature of the damage with large clusters of normal adipocytes adjacent to areas of necrosis and dense neutrophilic and histiocytic infiltrates [18, 25] (Figure 99.39). Occasionally, the intense neutrophilic infiltrate may cause collagenolysis and elastic tissue destruction

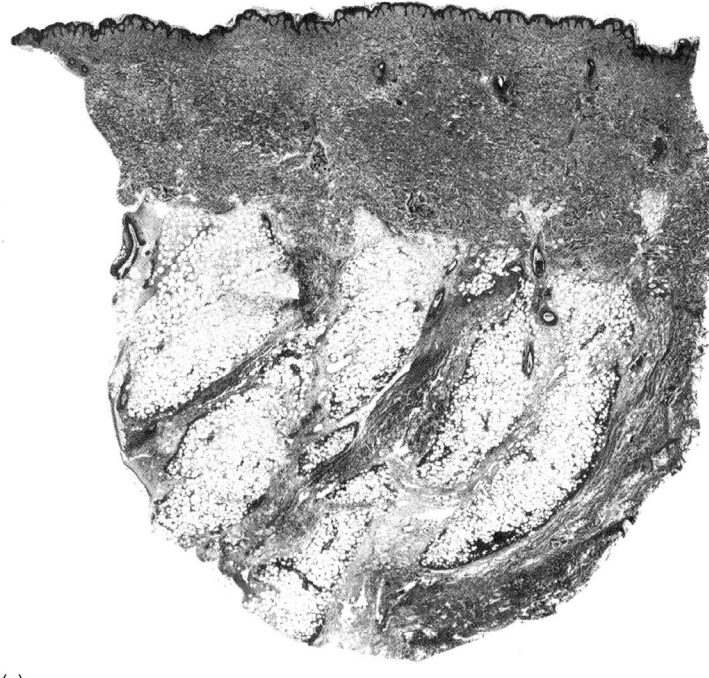

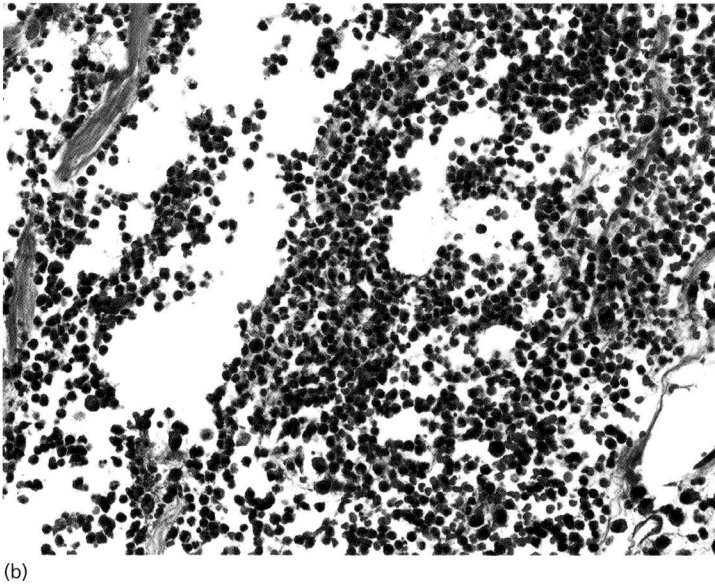

Figure 99.39 Histopathological features of α_1-antitrypsin deficiency panniculitis. (a) Scanning power showing involvement at the septa and the periphery of the fat lobules. (b) Neutrophilic infiltrate and nuclear dust but no evidence of vasculitis.

at the connective tissue septa and then necrotic fat lobules appear to be 'floating' and surrounded by neutrophils [26]. Transepidermal elimination of liquefied dermis may occur as a secondary phenomenon [27]. In late-stage lesions, neutrophils and necrotic adipocytes are less evident and the histopathological picture is dominated by non-specific lipophagic granulomata replacing fat lobules. Some macrophages may engulf nuclear dust of neutrophils and dystrophic calcification may develop [10]. Direct immunofluorescence studies have revealed deposits of complement C3 and IgM around the dermal blood vessels: these are of uncertain significance [9,18].

Laboratory anomalies include absence or significantly reduced levels of α_1 globulin on plasma protein electrophoresis and abnormally reduced levels of α_1-antitrypsin. Sometimes an isoelectrophoretic mobility study for α_1-antitrypsin may demonstrate an abnormal phenotype with normal serum levels. In chronic cases, normocytic normochromic anaemia and hypoalbuminaemia are frequently found [20].

Management

Trauma and surgical debridement should be avoided, as should smoking or exposure to hepatotoxins. Reduction of alcohol intake should be recommended. Several treatments including corticosteroids [9], immunosuppressive drugs, colchicine [19], danazol and antimalarials have shown poor or no response. Doxycycline or minocycline in a dose of 200 mg daily for at least 3 months, may be effective in mild cases, as tetracyclines have anticollagenase activity which may partly re-establish protease-antiprotease homeostasis [5]. Dapsone has also shown to be effective because it inhibits the migration of neutrophils [9,12]. For severe cases with liver and lung involvement, the best option is replacement of α_1-antitrypsin using human pooled plasma from normal donors (Prolastin®). Intravenous infusions in a dosage of 60–100 mg/kg per week, depending on the severity of the deficiency, over a period of 3–7 weeks [3,27–34]. Recurrence after discontinuation of therapy is common, but there is a good response to reinfusion [31]. Other interventions which have been used include plasma exchange [35] and liver transplantation [36]. In one patient α_1-antitrypsin deficiency panniculitis appeared after liver transplant and was successfully treated with retransplant [37]. The role of genetic engineering in producing α_1-antitrypsin is being investigated.

Infective panniculitis

Pathophysiology

Causative organisms

Several bacterial and fungal infections may cause panniculitis as their main clinical manifestation. Full details about cutaneous infections may be found in Chapters 25, 26, 27, 28, 29, 30, 31 and 32.

Bacteria implicated in subcutaneous panniculitis include *Streptococcus pyogenes* [1], *Staphylococcus aureus* [1], *Pseudomonas* spp. [1,2,3], *Klebsiella* [1], *Nocardia* spp. [1,4], *Brucella* [5] and *Borrelia burgdorferi* [6,7]. Most cases of mycobacterial panniculitis reported in the literature have been caused by non-tuberculous mycobacteria [8–19], especially rapidly growing mycobacteria such as *M. chelonae* [14–17] and *M. fortuitum* [18,19], and less frequently by slow-growing mycobacteria such as *M. avium intracellulare complex* [9,11] and *M. marinum* [8,12]. There are exceptional cases due to *Mycobacterium tuberculosis* [12,20] and panniculitis caused by *Mycobacterium leprae* is extremely rare [21]. *M. ulcerans* causes a well-defined clinicopathological entity known as Buruli ulcer, which involves predominantly the subcutaneous fat [22–27].

Fungal infections of the subcutaneous fat may be classified into two main categories: (i) panniculitis in the setting of a disseminated fungal infection; and (ii) classical subcutaneous mycosis.

These two groups differ in their causative microorganisms, their pathogenesis, the setting in which they appear, their prognosis and their treatment. The most common disseminated fungal infections causing panniculitis are *Candida* spp. [1,28,29], *Aspergillus* spp. [30], *Fusarium* spp. [1] and *Histoplasma capsulatum* [31,32], whereas the most common classical subcutaneous mycoses are sporotrichosis due to *Sporothrix schenckii*, eumycetoma caused by *Madurella mycetomatis* [6,33] and chromoblastomycosis caused by pigmented fungi, the most common being *Phialophora verrucosa*, *Fonsecaea pedrosoi*, *Fonsecaea compacta* and *Cladophialophora carrionii* [34,35]. Uncommon subcutaneous fungal infections include phaeohyphomycosis, lobomycosis, rhinosporidiosis and subcutaneous zygomycosis. A case of septal panniculitis caused by cytomegalovirus infection with many cytomegalovirus inclusions in endothelial cells has been described in an immunosuppressed patient [36] and another case of neutrophilic lobular panniculitis due to acanthamoebiasis has been reported in a patient with AIDS [37].

Presentation

With the exception of the classical subcutaneous mycoses, most of these infective panniculitides occur in immunosuppressed patients and are uncommon in immunocompetent hosts. The immunosuppressed population, which has been increasing in recent decades due to HIV infection, organ transplantation and the widespread use of immunosuppressive drugs, is at risk not only of common cutaneous infections but also of opportunistic infections with atypical clinical presentations [38,39].

Bacterial panniculitis may appear in the setting of septicaemia, as the consequence of direct inoculation or by direct spread from an underlying infection. In patients with sepsis, solitary or multiple nodules and abscesses appear as a consequence of the haematogenous dissemination of bacteria. Constitutional symptoms are often absent, but the general condition of the patient is impaired by the underlying disease.

The clinical features of subcutaneous mycobacterial infections vary according to the immune state of the patient. In immunocompromised patients, lesions tend to be widespread due to haematogenous dissemination. Sporotrichoid spread is not uncommon in these patients [40–42] (Figure 99.40) and spread to internal organs may occur [9,40]. In immunocompetent patients, the infection is usually localized and related to trauma, e.g. penetrating injury, surgical procedures, acupuncture, injections or postepilation folliculitis [10,11,15].

Panniculitis in immunosuppressed patients with disseminated fungal infection presents as multiple erythematous subcutaneous nodules, pustules or fluctuant abscesses [28,30,31]. In subcutaneous mycoses, the fungus enters the skin from the soil, plants or wood via a penetrating injury and the lesions are localized mostly to exposed areas of the skin, such as the face, hands, arms or feet [33]. These lesions consist of a solitary painless nodule that spreads slowly; with time, secondary nodules and papules may develop in adjacent skin and may be accompanied by sinuses exuding a serous or oily discharge.

Investigations

The histopathological features of infective panniculitis consist of a predominantly lobular neutrophilic panniculitis without vasculitis

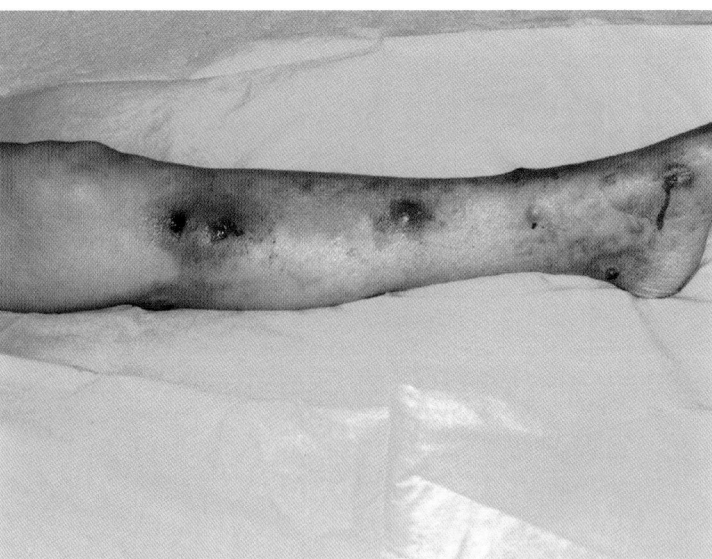

Figure 99.40 Sporotrichoid arrangement of subcutaneous nodules, several of them ulcerated and draining serous or oily discharge in an immunocompromised patient. Cultures isolated *M. chelonae*.

[1,5,41], although in some cases small vessel vasculitis has been described [1]. Apart from the neutrophilic infiltrate in the fat lobule, additional features suggestive of an infective aetiology of a lobular panniculitis are haemorrhage, proliferation of vessels, foci of basophilic necrosis and necrosis of sweat glands [1]. Special stains, including Gram, PAS, Ziehl–Neelsen and methenamine–silver, as well as tissue cultures should be performed.

Rarely, infective panniculitis may resemble SPTCL, as was reported in a case due to *Borrelia burgdorferi* where the lobular infiltrate was composed of atypical lymphocytes with cytotoxic immunophenotye. *Borrelia burgdorferi* aetiology was, however, proven by positive PCR findings, serology and a favourable response to antibiotics [7].

The histopathological findings in panniculitis caused by mycobacterial infections vary according to the organism involved and the immune state of the host. In most cases, the histopathological picture, as in other bacterial panniculitides, is a neutrophilic lobular panniculitis, but mycobacterial panniculitides often contain suppurative granulomata [14,15,18,43] (Figure 99.41) or frank tuberculoid granulomata [12,14,44]. Caseous necrosis is suggestive of tuberculous panniculitis [12].

In Q fever due to *Coxiella burnetii* a 'doughnut-like' lobular granulomatous panniculitis, similar to the changes found in the liver and bone marrow, has been described [45].

Ghost adipocytes reminiscent of pancreatic panniculitis have been documented in cases of mucormycosis [46] and aspergillosis [47] involving subcutaneous fat.

Different histopathological patterns have been described according to the inoculation route of the microorganisms into the skin. Primary cutaneous infections arise either from direct physical inoculation or at the site of an occlusive dressing over an indwelling catheter, whereas secondary cutaneous infections develop either from direct extension to the chest wall in pulmonary infections, or from haematogenous dissemination. In primary cutaneous infections, the epicentre of the inflammation is the superficial dermis,

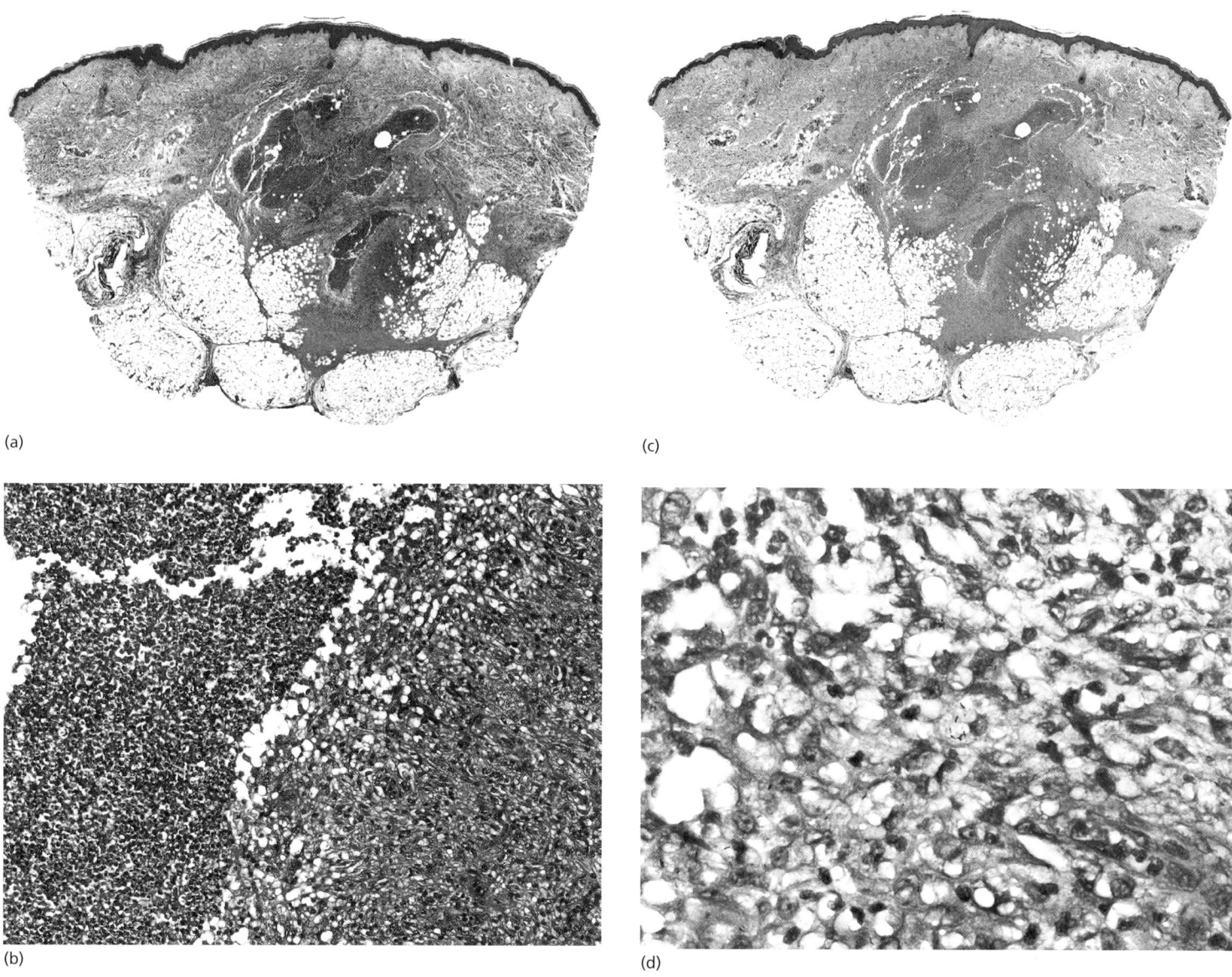

Figure 99.41 Histopathological features in a cutaneous infection by *M. chelonae*. (a) Scanning power showing involvement of the reticular dermis and subcutaneous fat. (b) Suppurative granuloma involving the fat lobule. (c) A section of the same case stained with Ziehl–Neelsen stain. (d) Several acid–alcohol resistant bacillus (BAAR) positive mycobacteria may be seen at the centre of the figure.

and thrombosed vessels do not contain intravascular organisms. In contrast, in secondary cutaneous infections, the epicentre of inflammation is more deeply seated and involves only the deep reticular dermis and subcutaneous fat. The blood vessels are thrombosed and dilated with masses of organisms expanding their lumina [30]. In immunosuppressed patients microorganisms are numerous and they may be easily identified in tissue sections with routine H&E staining or with special stains, but in immunocompetent patients microorganisms are sparse and they may be difficult to detect. In these latter cases, the diagnosis may be established only from culture [1,42]. In cases with few microorganisms, immunohistochemical staining with anti-BCG antibody was proposed as a helpful tool for screening, because this commercially available polyclonal antibody showed cross-reactivity with many bacteria, mycobacteria and fungi, and produced minimal background staining; it might therefore identify microorganisms that could not be seen using conventional stains [48]. However, due to over-purification by the

manufacturer in recent years, anti-BCG antibody no longer has the original wide sensitivity for bacteria and fungi and currently it should be restricted to the search for mycobacteria in formalin-fixed and paraffin-embedded samples. PCR-based methods are also available to test formalin-fixed tissue for specific agents.

Factitious panniculitis

Definition
Factitious or artefactual panniculitides result from external injury to subcutaneous fat. Aetiological factors may be mechanical trauma, chemical substances and thermal injury; the reasons for the injury may be accidental, intentional or iatrogenic. Traumatic and cold panniculitis are covered in other sections of this chapter.

Often factitious panniculitis is a manifestation of underlying psychiatric disorders [1]. In other instances, the process results from iatrogenic injections of drugs or immunization agents.

Pathophysiology

Causative organisms

Recently, the use of injectable filler agents has become widespread in aesthetic dermatology and plastic surgery for the treatment of wrinkles and soft-tissue augmentation. Biodegradable or resorbable agents may induce severe complications but these will usually disappear spontaneously in a few months. Slowly biodegradable or non-resorbable fillers may give rise to severe reactions that show little or no tendency to spontaneous improvement. They may appear several years after the injection, when the patient does not remember which product was injected. Previously, factitious panniculitis frequently resulted from subcutaneous injection of oily materials including mineral oil (paraffin) or vegetable oils (cottonseed and sesame oils) [2]. These products were used over many years to augment the size of breasts or genitalia but often induced subcutaneous foreign-body reactions known as paraffinoma or sclerosing lipogranuloma. Fortunately, most such fillers have now been abandoned by medical professionals, although complications may appear a long time after the injections, even 30 years later, and it still is possible to see cases of paraffinoma or sclerosing granuloma [3]. Although cosmetic fillers currently used for tissue augmentation, such as bovine collagen, silicone, PMMA microspheres (Artecoll®), polymethylsiloxane (Bioplastique®) and hydroxyethylmethacrylate particles in hyaluronic acid (Dermalive®) are better tolerated, they may also sometimes induce factitious panniculitis [4–5,6,7,8]. In recent years, injections with Lipostabil®, a phosphatidylcholine-containing substance, have become a popular therapeutic technique for the treatment of localized fat accumulation and lipomas, causing factitious panniculitis of the injected fat tissue [9]. Mesotherapy injections in an attempt to produce reduction of the thickness of hypertrophic subcutaneous fat produce a granulomatous panniculitis with some cystic fat necrosis [10]. Panniculitis has also been reported at the sites of injection of several therapeutic drugs (Box 99.7)

The extravasation of cytostatic agents during antineoplastic chemotherapy also presents as a severe panniculitis [24,25]. Cupping and acupuncture techniques for the relief of pain may induce factitious panniculitis on the limbs [26,27]. Finally, patients with psychiatric disorders may present with self-inflicted panniculitis due to subcutaneous injections of a wide range of substances including acids, alkalis, farming products, mustard, milk, microbiologically contaminated material, urine and faeces [1,28].

The exact mechanisms involved in factitious panniculitis are uncertain, but vasoconstriction with tissue ischaemia at injection sites, a local inflammatory response elicited by direct contact with drugs or noxious injected substances, immune mechanisms and trauma due to repeated injections may be implicated.

Clinical features

Presentation

The clinical features of factitious panniculitis are variable, depending upon the causative agent. Self-induced factitious panniculitis

Box 99.7 Panniculitis at the sites of injections of medications

- Pethidine [11]
- Pentazocine [12]
- Methadone [13]
- Povidone [14]
- Gold salts (aurothioglucose) [15]
- Phytonadione (vitamin K₁) [16]
- Glatiramer acetate for the treatment of multiple sclerosis [17] (Figure 99.42)
- Tetanus antitoxoid vaccination and antihepatitis vaccines [18]
- Hyposensitization vaccination with vaccines containing aluminium [19]
- Anticancer vaccines such as gangliosides for melanoma and carcinoembryonic antigen and MUC1 for pancreatic cancer [20]
- IFN-β [21]
- Granulocyte colony-stimulating factor [22]
- IL-2 [23]

usually occurs in young adults or middle-aged women with a history of drug addiction or psychiatric disorders (see Chapter 86). Lesions tend to be localized to areas easily accessible to the hands, such as buttocks and thighs, and they are usually solitary or few; when multiple they tend to be grouped. The clinical appearance is bizarre and suspicions should be raised when they do not fit with any well-defined dermatosis. Lesions due to blunt trauma often appear bruised and frequently involve the arm or hand [29]. A particular presentation of self-induced traumatic panniculitis is the so-called Secretan syndrome (l'oedème bleu) [30,31], which consists of a factitious oedema of the hand caused by the frequent application of a tourniquet or repeated trauma. The course is chronic and recurrent, leading to progressive fibrosis of the dorsum of the hand [32].

Self-inflicted injections with contaminated material produce an acute suppurative panniculitis, often with systemic symptoms [33]. Early lesions manifest as inflammatory nodules and plaques secondary to fat necrosis and suppuration. Some cases may show abscess formation and lymphangitic spread. A case of factitious panniculitis masquerading as florid pyoderma gangrenosum was reported in a depressed woman [34]. There is a risk of progression to granulomatous inflammation and fibrosis in longstanding

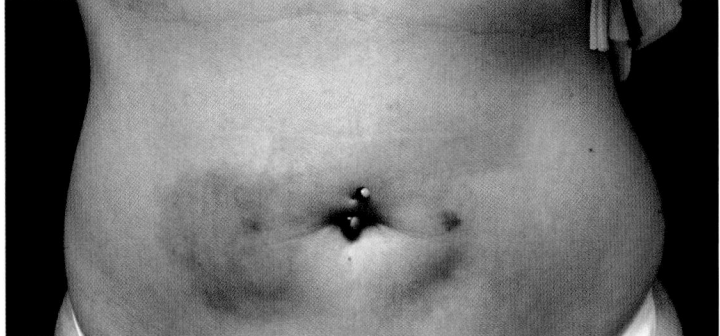

Figure 99.42 Panniculitis on the anterior abdominal wall secondary to subcutaneous glatiramer acetate injections for the treatment of multiple sclerosis.

lesions. Sclerosing lipogranuloma is the term used for factitious lesions of the male genitalia secondary to injections of liquid paraffin intended to augment the size of the penis [35]. Often, these patients deny previous injections, making diagnosis difficult. Lesions similar to sclerosing granuloma may appear in other locations such as the eyelids, lips or gluteal region after injection of liquid silicone [36].

Diagnosis of panniculitis secondary to injection of drugs is usually easy and the location of the lesions provides a clue to their cause. Pentazocine abuse has been described in patients with chronic pain or addiction: repeated injections may induce panniculitis and myositis. Pentazocine panniculitis presents as multiple nodulo-ulcerative lesions of long duration located bilaterally on the buttocks and shoulders [12]. These nodules slowly progress to fibrosis resulting in sclerodermoid plaques that extend to the underlying fascia and muscle [37]. Texier disease is another iatrogenic panniculitis due to vitamin K_1 injections [16]: early lesions have an eczematous appearance, but longstanding reactions mimic morphoea [38]. Procaine povidone was used to treat chronic pain with local infiltrations. Povidone is a synthetic product now widely used in skin care products such as hair sprays and as a dispersing or suspending agent in drugs such as procaine and hormones. Povidone polymers cannot be excreted by the kidney and they are phagocytised and stored permanently in macrophages, resulting in the so-called 'povidone storage disease' [39]. In addition to panniculitis at the sites of injection, povidone may cause pulmonary lesions, lymphadenopathy and visceromegaly [14].

Subcutaneous extravasation of cytotoxic agents causes severe painful necrotic reactions of the subcutis and underlying muscles, which may disable a patient for months. Clinical lesions show red-brown painful oedema which may evolve into necrotic plaques that heal with sclerotic, indurated scars which may become bound to underlying muscle and bone [25].

Investigations

The histopathological findings in factitious panniculitis vary depending upon the causal agent. In most cases, early lesions show features of a predominantly neutrophilic lobular panniculitis, with severe fat necrosis and an intense inflammatory infiltrate. In some instances, eosinophils may be abundant [28], especially in panniculitis arising at the site of cancer vaccines [20], and in sclerosing lipogranulomata of the genitalia [40]. Superimposed infection often complicates self-induced panniculitis. Fully developed lesions show granulomatous infiltrates involving the fat lobule, whereas longstanding lesions are characterized by lipophagic granulomata and surrounding fibrosis. In some cases, polarized light will reveal the birefringent foreign bodies responsible for the panniculitis. In panniculitis due to injected substances, the dermis is also involved by the inflammatory process, which may be a clue to the correct diagnosis.

Sometimes, specific histopathological findings may be helpful in identifying the nature of the foreign material. *Paraffinoma* is characterized by a predominantly lobular panniculitis, in which the subcutaneous fat exhibits a 'Swiss-cheese' appearance, with cystic spaces of variable size and shape, surrounded by foamy histiocytes and multinucleated giant cells; intense fibrosis with sclerotic collagen bundles is seen surrounding the cystic spaces

[41]. Similar findings have been described in the penis following a grease gun injury [42]. Exogenous oils may be highlighted by special stains such as oil red O and osmium tetroxide [2].

Histopathological findings in local reactions to implants of *silicone* are variable depending mainly on the form of the injected silicone. Solid elastomer silicone induces an exuberant foreign-body granulomatous reaction, whereas silicone oil and gel induce a sparser inflammatory response. Silicone particles appear as groups of round empty vacuoles of different sizes between collagen bundles or within macrophages. Silicone particles are not birefringent under polarized light, but sometimes translucent angulated foreign bodies that represent impurities in the silicone are also found [3]. Granulomas from polymethylsiloxane fillers consist of irregularly shaped cystic spaces containing translucent, jagged 'popcorn', non-birefringent particles of varying size dispersed in a sclerotic stroma, surrounded by abundant multinucleated foreign-body giant cells [43].

Granulomas from collagen-based cosmetic fillers containing *polymethylmethacrylate* microspheres show a nodular or diffuse granulomatous infiltrate surrounding rounded vacuoles of similar shape and size, which mimic normal adipocytes and correspond to the implanted microspheres [5].

Injections of lipomas with *phosphatidylcholine*-containing substances induce an early reaction characterized by neutrophilic infiltration with partially destroyed fat cells; late lesions show infiltration of T lymphocytes and macrophages with foamy histiocytes, accompanied by thickened septa and pseudocapsule formation surrounding the inflamed area [9].

Persistent reactions to *aluminium* at the site of injection of hyposensitization vaccines show abundant lymphoid follicles in the subcutaneous tissue with germinal centre formation. They may mimic lupus profundus, pseudolymphoma or deep morphoea, but the abundant eosinophils and the identification of characteristic histiocytes with basophilic granular cytoplasm are the key distinctive features allowing the correct diagnosis [19]. These macrophages contain lysosomes filled with aluminium salts that can be demonstrated with X-ray dispersion microanalysis.

Pentazozine panniculitis is manifested as sclerodermoid plaques that result from thrombosis of small vessels, endarteritis, granulomatous inflammation, lipophagic granulomata and pronounced fibrosis of the dermis and subcutaneous fat [11,44].

Panniculitis secondary to *vitamin K* injections is also characterized by prominent sclerosis of the collagen bundles of the connective tissue septa of the subcutis and an inflammatory infiltrate of lymphocytes, mast cells and plasma cells, which raises the histopathological differential diagnosis with morphoea [16,38]. In contrast with deep morphoea, vitamin K_1 panniculitis usually also involves the fat lobule with lipophagic granulomata.

Povidone panniculitis shows granulomatous infiltration of the fat lobule with focal haemorrhage and necrosis. Many macrophages contain grey-blue foamy material in their cytoplasm, which is positive for Congo red and chlorazol-fast pink [39].

Extravasation of *cytotoxic drugs* shows lobular panniculitis, abundant adipocyte necrosis with little inflammatory infiltrate together with epidermal lesions attributable to direct cytotoxicity. More chronic cases show marked fibrosis and lipomembranous changes [24,45].

Panniculitis secondary to *subcutaneous glatiramer acetate* injections for the treatment of multiple sclerosis consisted of a predominantly lobular panniculitis, with lipophagic granulomata and scattered neutrophils and eosinophils both in the septa and in the fat lobules; the connective tissue septa show widening and fibrosis in conjunction with many lymphoid follicles, some with reactive germinal centres (Figure 99.43). Immunohistochemistry demonstrates that the inflammatory infiltrate of the fat lobule consists of CD68-positive histiocytes and suppressor/cytotoxic T lymphocytes. In contrast, the lymphoid follicles in the septa and at the interface between septum and fat lobule are mainly composed of B lymphocytes [17].

Factitious panniculitis due to repeated *trauma* shows organizing haematomas, focal granulomas and haemosiderin deposition [29].

Management

Early lesions of factitious panniculitis should be treated with systemic antibiotics to cover a wide spectrum of microorganisms. If artefact is suspected, the affected area may be occluded for a week with a bandage: improvement would support a suspicion of self-induced factitious panniculitis, for which appropriate social and psychiatric care should be offered. Regrettably, these offers are usually rejected by patients.

Panniculitis secondary to cosmetic fillers usually require intralesional steroids and, if possible, removal of the implanted material. Panniculitis secondary to injection of drugs usually requires only supportive care and withdrawal of the responsible drug.

Neutrophilic lobular panniculitis

Definition

Neutrophilic lobular panniculitis incorporates a range of different panniculitides in which the fat lobule infiltrate is mostly composed of neutrophils (Box 99.8). According to Cohen, 'neutrophilic lobular panniculitis is not a distinct entity but has a concise pathologic description of specific changes in the subcutaneous fat that have been observed in association with several conditions' [1]. Some of these entities have been covered in other sections of this chapter. Included here is a small group of rare disorders characterized by neutrophilic lobular panniculitis.

Introduction and general description

Subcutaneous Sweet syndrome (see Chapter 49)
Acute febrile neutrophilic dermatosis or Sweet syndrome is a neutrophilic dermatosis characterized by an acute onset of oedematous, erythematous papules and plaques, often accompanied by fever and malaise, which was first described by Sweet in 1964 [2]. Histopathologically, cutaneous lesions show oedema of the papillary dermis and a dense band-like infiltrate of neutrophils involving mostly the superficial dermis, with no vasculitis [3]. Usually,

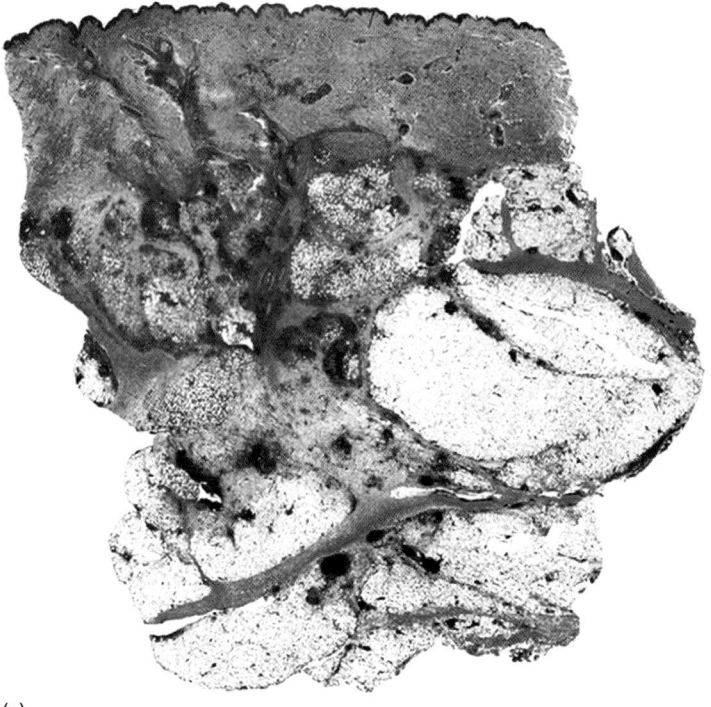

(a)

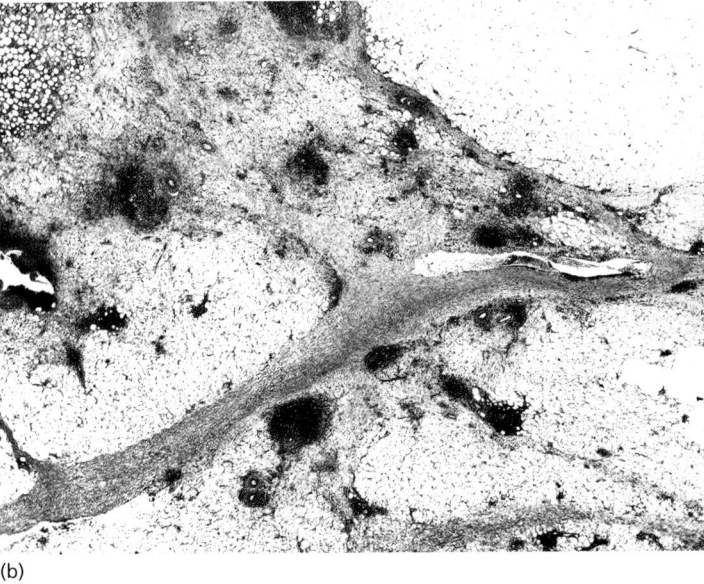

(b)

Figure 99.43 Histopathological features of panniculitis secondary to subcutaneous glatiramer acetate injections for the treatment of multiple sclerosis. (a) Scanning power showing a mostly lobular panniculitis. (b) Numerous lymphoid aggregates are seen at the periphery of the fat lobules.

Box 99.8 Neutrophilic lobular panniculitis

- Alpha-1 antitrypsin deficiency panniculitis
- Pancreatic panniculitis
- Factitious panniculitis
- Neutrophilic lobular panniculitis/subcutaneous Sweet syndrome
- Neutrophilic/pustular panniculitis of rheumatoid arthritis
- Erythema nodosum-like lesions of Behçet disease
- Bowel bypass dermatosis
- Iatrogenic

Adapted from Guhl and García Díez [21].

Sweet syndrome is mainly a dermal process, but even in the original series Sweet reported that the neutrophilic infiltrate may extend into the underlying subcutaneous tissue with an associated neutrophilic panniculitis [2]. Subcutaneous involvement in classic Sweet syndrome is not rare and it has been described in some series with frequencies ranging from 25% to 50% of cases [4–8]. A diagnosis of subcutaneous Sweet syndrome should be made, however, only in those cases in which the neutrophilic infiltrate involves exclusively the subcutaneous tissue with few or no neutrophils in the dermis.

History

Only a few patients have been described with this peculiar variant of Sweet syndrome with exclusively subcutaneous involvement. Cullity *et al.* [9] were the first authors to use the term 'Sweet's panniculitis' or 'acute febrile neutrophilic panniculitis' to describe this entity, although similar cases had been previously reported [4,10]. Most of the cases show a neutrophilic lobular panniculitis, although in rare instances a septal component may be predominant [11]. To date, only 22 well-documented cases of subcutaneous Sweet syndrome have been reported [9–20,**21**,22–26]. Several features support the relationship of neutrophilic lobular panniculitis to Sweet syndrome. In some cases, subcutaneous Sweet syndrome was followed by classical dermal Sweet syndrome [4], whereas another patient presented simultaneously with classical Sweet syndrome and Sweet panniculitis [17]. As in classical Sweet syndrome, many patients with subcutaneous Sweet syndrome had associated myelodysplastic syndromes and haematological neoplasms [9,12–14,18,19,23,24,26–28], and cutaneous lesions showed an excellent response to systemic corticosteroids.

Presentation

Subcutaneous Sweet syndrome, like classical Sweet syndrome, has a median age of onset during the sixth decade of life but appears not to show the female preponderance of the latter [3,8]. Clinically, the lesions consist of erythematous nodules [10–14,16,17] or plaques [9,11] (Figure 99.44). Often the nodules are tender or painful [14]. Frequently, the onset of subcutaneous nodules is preceded or accompanied by systemic symptoms such as fever and malaise [4,9,11,13,15,16]; leukocytosis was found in several patients [11–13,15,16]. The most frequent locations are the lower extremities [10–14,16,17], followed by upper extremities [11,12,14], trunk [9,11,12,14] and head [9]. In one patient, the lesions were associated with all-*trans*-retinoic acid chemotherapy for promyelocytic leukaemia [18]; another patient presented associated dacryoadenitis [19]; and another developed the condition when administered pegylated granulocyte colony-stimulating factor (GCSF) [25].

Investigations

Histopathological study of the lesions demonstrates a dense infiltrate of mature neutrophils involving subcutaneous tissue. The neutrophilic infiltrate may involve septa, lobules or both [1], but in most cases the lobular component predominates [9,11,12,14–17] (Figure 99.45). Vasculitis is usually absent in all cases, but in two patients leukocytoclasia was noted [9,12]. The dermis is, by definition, spared in all patients. Occasionally, some mononuclear cells

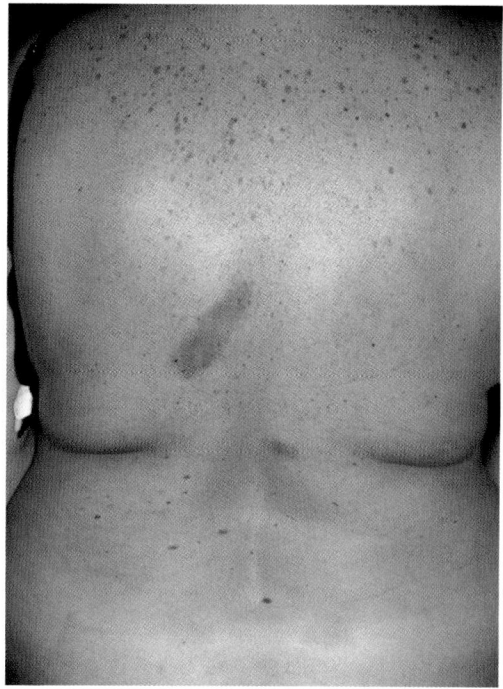

Figure 99.44 Neutrophilic lobular panniculitis showing erythematous plaques and nodules on the back of an adult woman.

may be found in the subcutaneous tissue [9,13]. Rarely, infiltration of myeloperoxidase positive immature granulocytes has been described [20], representing the subcutaneous counterpart of the so-called histiocytoid Sweet syndrome [29]. In summary, Sweet syndrome may involve subcutaneous tissue with two different patterns: (i) with a mostly septal panniculitis and occasionally granulomatous infiltrate, as in classical erythema nodosum associated with Sweet syndrome [30]; and (ii) with a neutrophilic infiltrate mostly involving the fat lobules, as is the case in subcutaneous Sweet syndrome.

Management

Most patients with subcutaneous Sweet syndrome show dramatic response to systemic corticosteroids, such as prednisolone [9,10,13–15]. Dapsone has also been administered successfully in one patient [16].

Behçet disease (see Chapter 48)

In the differential diagnosis of subcutaneous Sweet syndrome are the 'erythema nodosum-like' lesions which occur in approximately 30% of patients with Behçet disease [31,32]. They consist of nodules on the lower extremities [32,33], and sometimes also on the arms [32,33], identical to those of classical erythema nodosum [31]. However, histopathological study demonstrates involvement of both septa and fat lobules [32,33], with necrotizing leukocytoclastic vasculitis involving arterioles and venules [31–34]. In some cases, neutrophilic abscesses are found within the fat lobules [31]. A variable degree of fat necrosis is nearly always present [31]. Therefore, the histopathological findings rule out a diagnosis of erythema nodosum and the vasculitis

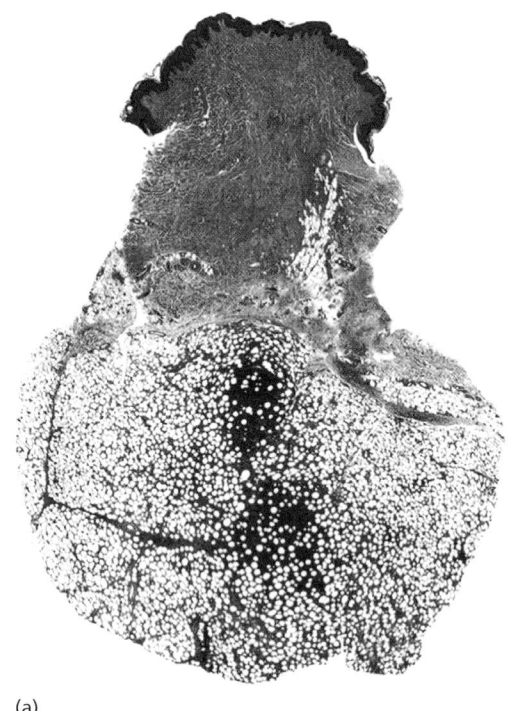

(a)

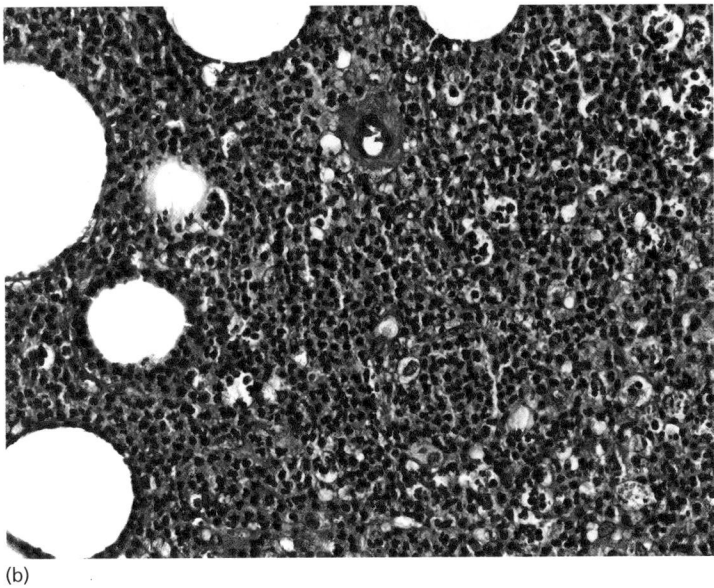

(b)

Figure 99.45 Histopathological features of neutrophilic lobular panniculitis. (a) Scanning power showing a predominantly lobular panniculitis. (b) The lobular infiltrate is composed mainly of neutrophils.

component allows subcutaneous Sweet syndrome to be ruled out [32].

Rheumatoid arthritis (see Chapter 154)

Several cases of neutrophilic (pustular) panniculitis have been described in patients with rheumatoid arthritis [35–41]. In these patients, subcutaneous nodules are mostly located on the lower extremities and they show a tendency to form draining fistulae with a yellowish discharge [36,40–42]. Histopathologically, these lesions are characterized by a lobular infiltrate of neutrophils accompanied by lymphocytes, macrophages and multinucleate

giant cells [36–39,41,42]. Fat necrosis has been found in nearly all cases [36,37,41,42] and leukocytoclastic vasculitis was described in some [36,42].

Bowel-associated dermatosis-arthritis syndrome
(see Chapter 152)

The bowel-associated dermatosis–arthritis syndrome is characterized by recurrent fever, arthralgia and skin lesions after intestinal bypass or bariatric surgery [43,44]. The most frequent skin lesions consist of erythematous papules or vesiculopustules. Lobular neutrophilic panniculitis with tender subcutaneous nodules on the lower extremities has, however, rarely been described in these patients [43–46].

Subcutaneous sarcoidosis

Definition and nomenclature

Minimal dermal involvement is acceptable for a histopathological diagnosis of subcutaneous sarcoidosis [1], but subcutaneous sarcoidosis is considered a specific clinicopathological variant of sarcoidosis involving exclusively the subcutaneous fat and should be differentiated from nodular dermal lesions of sarcoidosis with deep extension into the subcutaneous tissue [2]. Mostly, subcutaneous sarcoidosis is associated with systemic sarcoidosis, although with an indolent and non-aggressive form of the disease [3].

Synonyms and inclusions
• Darier–Roussy sarcoid

Introduction and general description

The most frequent subcutaneous disorder associated with sarcoidosis is not subcutaneous sarcoidosis, but classical erythema nodosum [3]. However, patients with systemic sarcoidosis may also develop sarcoidal granulomas involving the subcutaneous tissue as a specific cutaneous lesion and which is referred to as subcutaneous sarcoidosis. Subcutaneous sarcoidosis is a rare form of cutaneous sarcoidosis [3–6] (see Chapter 98).

Epidemiology

Incidence and prevalence

Subcutaneous sarcoidosis is the least common specific cutaneous manifestation of sarcoidosis. Its frequency varies, ranging in different series between 1.4% and 6% of patients with systemic sarcoidosis [7] and represents 11.76% of specific cutaneous lesions [8]. Its clinical features are described in detail in Chapter 98 (Figure 99.46).

Investigations

Histopathologically, subcutaneous sarcoidosis is characterized by non-caseating granulomas involving fat lobules [3,8] (Figure 99.47). At low-power magnification, the process appears

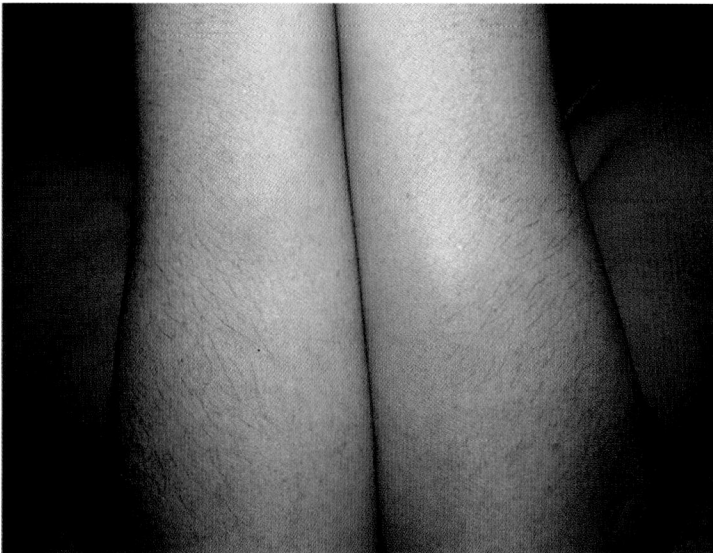

Figure 99.46 Subcutaneous sarcoidosis. Subcutaneous firm nodules on the forearms covered by normal appearing skin.

ous sarcoidosis and this finding should not exclude the diagnosis [12–14].

Traumatic panniculitis

Definition

Traumatic panniculitis refers to damage of subcutaneous tissue induced by physical and chemical agents. The physical injuries may be from trauma, cold, electricity or chemicals. Cold panniculitis and chemical factitious panniculitis have been covered in other sections of this chapter. In general, there is no direct relationship between the severity of the injury and the severity of the resultant panniculitis: even minor trauma often causes nodules of panniculitis on the shins (Figure 99.48).

Presentation

A specific form of traumatic panniculitis is common in women with large pendulous breasts. Large breast masses can form and may be misinterpreted as breast cancer [1].

Another peculiar variant of traumatic panniculitis is the so-called semicircular lipoatrophy that is probably induced by repeated microtrauma (see Chapter 100) [2–7]. These patients, generally adult women, develop horizontal band-like or circular depressions around the anterolateral aspects of the thighs. Lipoatrophy in these areas develops over several weeks without symptoms. Trauma is the most probable cause because the affected areas of the thighs are vulnerable to repetitive trauma from sitting at desks and tables.

Post-traumatic panniculitis may present as a solitary or as multiple subcutaneous nodules caused by traumatic separation and consequent devascularization of pieces of subcutaneous fat from

as a predominantly lobular panniculitis, with minimal or no septal involvement. Sarcoidal granulomas in subcutaneous tissue are usually small, uniform in size, and mainly composed of epithelioid histiocytes, with limited numbers of multinucleate giant cells and a sparse lymphocytic component. Occasionally, small foci of eosinophilic necrosis may appear in the centre of regressing sarcoid granulomas [9], raising the differential diagnosis of tuberculosis [10]. In rare instances, caseating necrosis may be extensive [10]. The development of calcification in these sarcoidal granulomata has also been reported [11]. Foreign refractile particles under polarized light have been detected in some cases of subcutane-

PART 8: SPECIFIC CUTANEOUS STRUCTURE

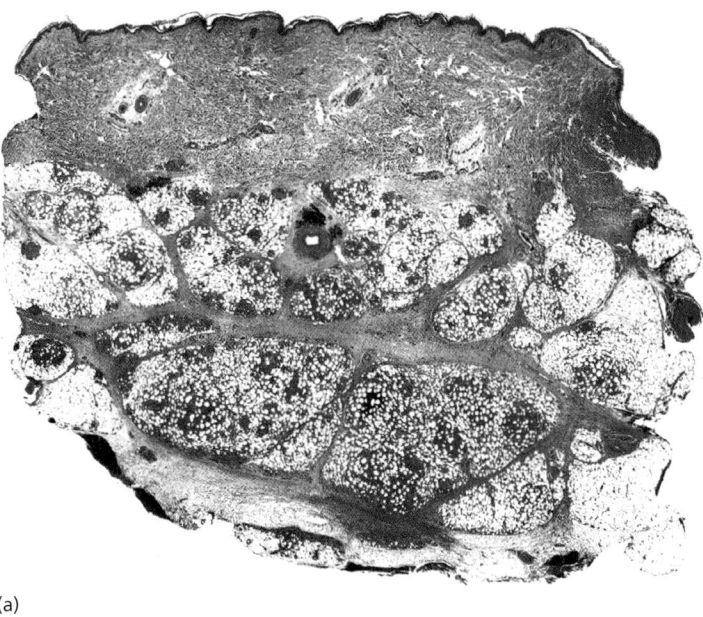

(a)

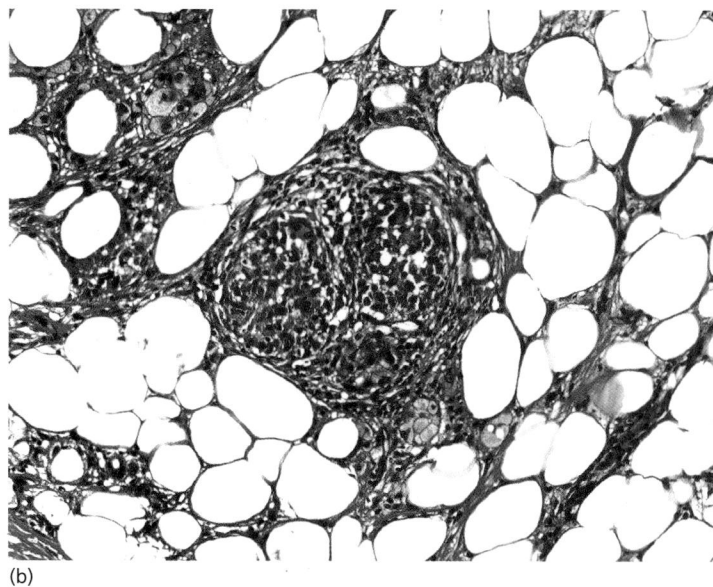

(b)

Figure 99.47 Histopathological features of subcutaneous sarcoidosis. (a) Scanning power showing a predominantly lobular panniculitis. (b) Small non-caseating granulomas involving the fat lobule.

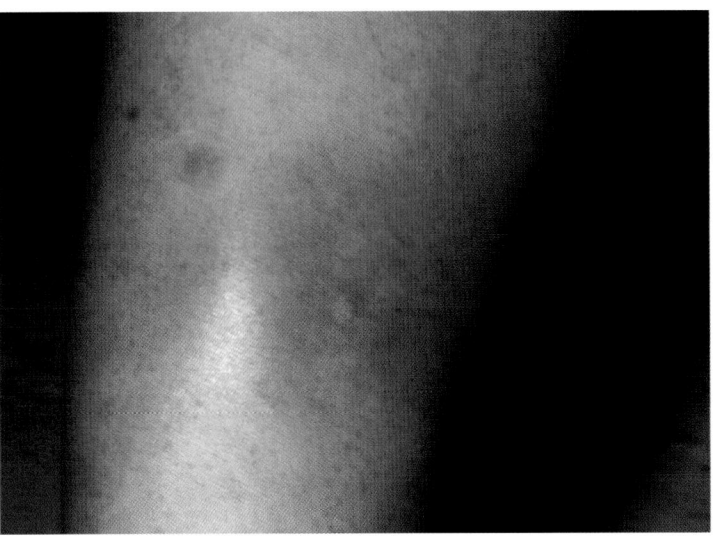

Figure 99.48 Traumatic panniculitis involving the shin.

its blood supply. The resultant walling off of the necrotic fat by fibrous tissue results in so-called encapsulated fat necrosis, otherwise termed nodular cystic fat necrosis or mobile encapsulated lipoma [8–10,**11**,12–17].

Electrical injuries appear at the point of contact of different electrodes causing skin burns with superficial subcutaneous involvement.

Investigations

The histopathological findings in traumatic panniculitis are not specific. Early lesions show intense haemorrhage and an inflammatory infiltrate, mostly composed of lymphocytes and macrophages arranged around septal vessels. Fully developed lesions are associated with cystic areas of fat necrosis surrounded by histiocytes, lipophagic granulomata scattered with haemosiderophages, and some neutrophils and eosinophils. Late lesions

show fibrotic replacement of the fat lobule with residual cystic fat necrosis surrounded by macrophages and foreign-body multinucleate giant cells. Lipomembranous changes are also common in late-stage lesions of traumatic panniculitis [18]. Dystrophic calcification may appear in longstanding nodules.

Biopsy from semicircular atrophy shows inflammatory perivascular changes in early lesions. Nodular-cystic fat necrosis shows extensive necrosis of the fat lobules, with cystic fat necrosis and lipomembranous changes, and, as the most characteristic finding, a thick eosinophilic peripheral fibrotic pseudocapsule with hyaline appearance encircling the nodule and separating it from the surrounding tissues [19] (Figure 99.49).

Management

Traumatic panniculitis is usually a self-limiting disorder and considerable improvement occurs with the time.

Lipoatrophic panniculitis of the ankles in childhood

Clinical features

History

Lipoatrophic panniculitis characteristically involving the ankles was initially reported by Shelley and Izumi in 1970 and they coined the expression 'annular atrophy of the ankles' to name this process [1]. Since then, only a handful of cases have been reported [2–8,**9**,10–19], some of them under the heading of connective tissue panniculitis [3].

Presentation

Many of the reported patients with lipoatrophic panniculitis of the ankles are children with antinuclear antibodies, autoimmune conditions or both, so that this disorder has been included under

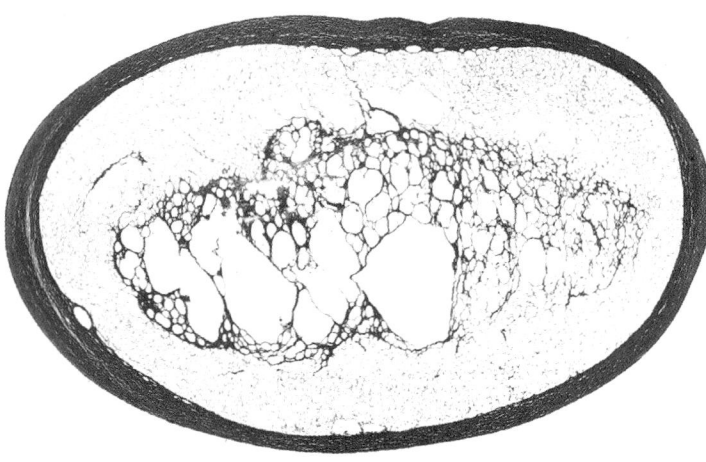

(a)

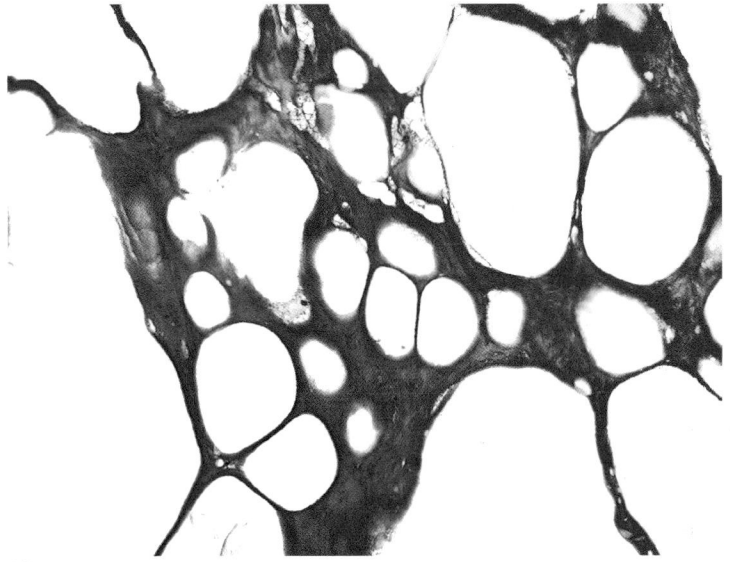

(b)

Figure 99.49 Histopathological features of encapsulated fat necrosis. (a) Scanning power showing an enucleated and very well-circumscribed lesion. (b) Necrotic adipocytes surrounded by hyaline material.

connective tissue panniculitis, together with morphoea, lupus panniculitis and dermatomyositis [4,10].

Clinically, the characteristic annular or semicircular involvement of the ankles makes this a distinctive condition with few if any differential diagnoses. The lesions are tender and the onset of subcutaneous nodules is accompanied by fever, malaise and arthralgia of the ankles. Erythematous nodules and plaques resolve with annular scaling leaving lipoatrophy around the ankles (Figure 99.50).

Investigations

In all except one case in which histopathology has been reported, a mainly lobular inflammation of the subcutaneous tissue has been described, with predominance of histiocytes, lipophagic granulomata and a smaller number of lymphocytes, neutrophils, plasma cells and eosinophils [1–4,9,10–18] (Figure 99.51). One reported case was remarkable for the relative abundance of lymphocytes, some of them mildly atypical [19].

Immunohistochemistry in this case demonstrated that most lymphocytes were positive for CD3 and CD7, with only occasional CD20+ B lymphocytes, and approximately equal numbers of CD4 and CD8 cells. PCR study for B- and T-cell clonality yielded polyclonal results [19]. The authors concluded that their findings of a mostly lymphocytic panniculitis in that case were due to a biopsy performed in an earlier stage of evolution of the lesions of the panniculitic process, compared to previously reported cases [19]. The partial 'rimming' of necrotic adipocytes by lymphocytes, as well as the relatively high proliferative activity disclosed by MIB-1 raised the differential diagnosis of SPTCL, but the other immunohistochemical results and PCR studies ruled out that diagnosis.

Management

Symptomatic treatment with non-steroidal anti-inflammatory drugs provides analgesia and helps resolution. Oral prednisolone usually leads to marked improvement, but some cases have recurred on tapering, and then other drugs such as hydroxychloroquine, methotrexate and azathioprine have been administered with good effect. Residual lipoatrophy of the ankles tends to improve slowly with time.

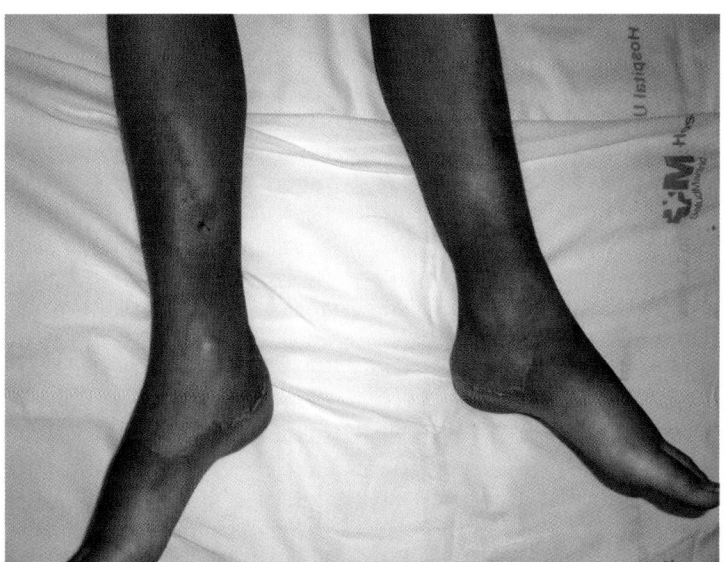

Figure 99.50 Lipoatrophic panniculitis of the ankles in a 12-year-old boy.

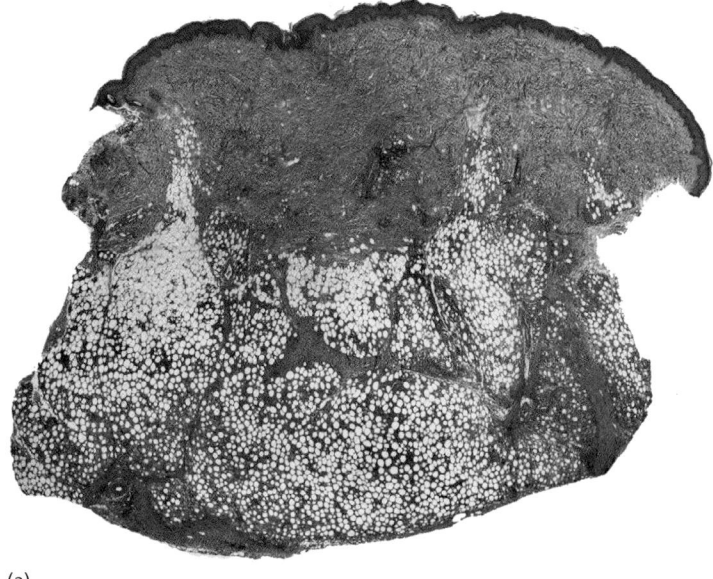

(a)

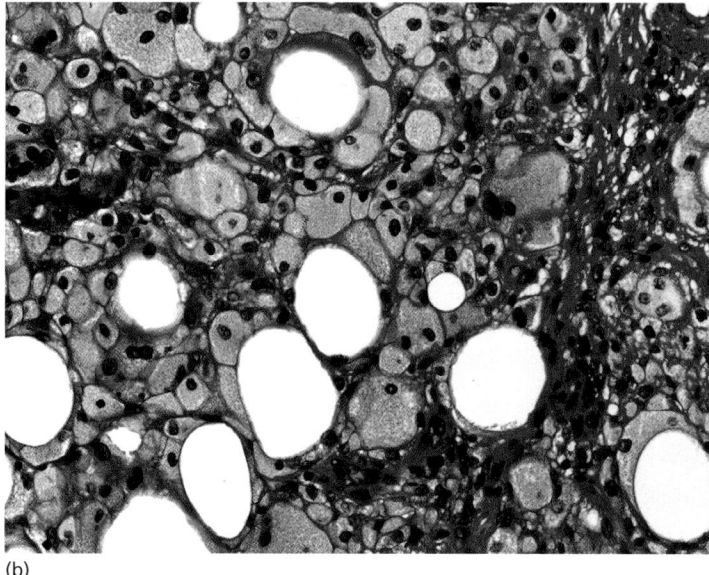

(b)

Figure 99.51 Histopathological findings in lipoatrophic panniculitis of the ankles in children. (a) Scanning power showing a mostly lobular panniculitis. (b) The fat lobule is replaced by a diffuse histiocytic infiltrate. Many histiocytes show a foamy cytoplasm as a consequence of phagocytosis of lipids, resulting in a lipophagic granuloma.

Subcutaneous fat necrosis of the newborn

Pathophysiology

Predisposing factors

The pathogenesis of this disorder is unknown. In many cases, perinatal complications are recorded, such as Rh factor incompatibility, meconium aspiration, umbilical cord prolapse, placenta praevia, birth asphyxia, seizures, congenital heart disease, intestinal perforation, hypothermia, sepsis, anaemia, obstetric trauma, gestational diabetes, pre-eclampsia or maternal abuse of drugs [1–12], but in many instances there is no history or any other associated anomaly. It has been suggested that localized and transient hypoxia may be an aetiological factor [13] and this might explain the predominant location of lesions on the shoulders and buttocks, cutaneous areas where mechanical pressure might compromise the circulation and contribute to hypoxia. Cold may also play a role, because there are several reports of subcutaneous fat necrosis of the newborn in children who have had cardiac surgery and the lesions appeared after cutaneous applications of ice to induce hypothermia [10,14–17]. Cases of subcutaneous fat necrosis of the newborn have been described after whole-body cooling in an infant with polycythaemia and hypocalcaemia [18] and in other newborns after hypothermia treatment of hypoxic ischaemic encephalopathy [19]. Another important predisposing factor may be the particular subcutaneous fat composition in neonates, with a relatively high concentration of saturated fatty acids compared to unsaturated fatty acids, which results in a higher melting point for neonatal fat that confers on it a greater propensity to undergo crystallization under cold temperatures resulting in adipocyte necrosis [20]. It has also been suggested that newborns with subcutaneous fat necrosis might have a transitory protease inhibitor deficiency due to liver immaturity, similar to α_1-antitrypsin deficiency [21]. The histopathological findings of subcutaneous fat necrosis of the newborn are, however, entirely different from those of α_1-antitrypsin deficiency-associated panniculitis, which militates against this theory. Other authors have proposed that subcutaneous fat necrosis of the newborn is a disorder of brown fat, which is present in the most frequently involved areas [12]. Subcutaneous fat necrosis of the newborn has also been described after administration of prostaglandin E_1 for the treatment of congenital heart disease, which supports some pathogenic role of prostaglandin E_1 [22].

Approximately 25% of infants with subcutaneous fat necrosis of the newborn present with hypercalcaemia for unknown reasons: this anomaly is more frequent in infants with extensive lesions and when the trunk is involved [23]. The origin of this hypercalcaemia is not known, but increased calcium absorption due to extrarenal hyperproduction of 1,25-dihydroxyvitamin D_3 (calcitriol) has been detected in several granulomatous processes, including sarcoidosis and subcutaneous fat necrosis of the newborn [23–27]. Elevated parathormone levels have been detected in some cases [28], but autopsy studies failed to reveal any parathyroid hyperplasia. Elevated urinary excretion of prostaglandin E_1 suggests an increased calcium resorption from bone as the explanation for the hypercalcaemia [29,30].

Clinical features

Presentation

Clinically, the lesions consist of multiple symmetrically distributed indurated, smooth, non-pitting mobile subcutaneous erythematous or violaceous nodules or plaques that appear in the first few weeks of life. The most common locations are the shoulders and buttocks (Figure 99.52), but lesions on the face, thighs, back and distal areas of the extremities have been also described [31,32]. These lesions tend to spare the anterior trunk. In rare instances, the nodules may ulcerate, discharge oily contents and heal leav-

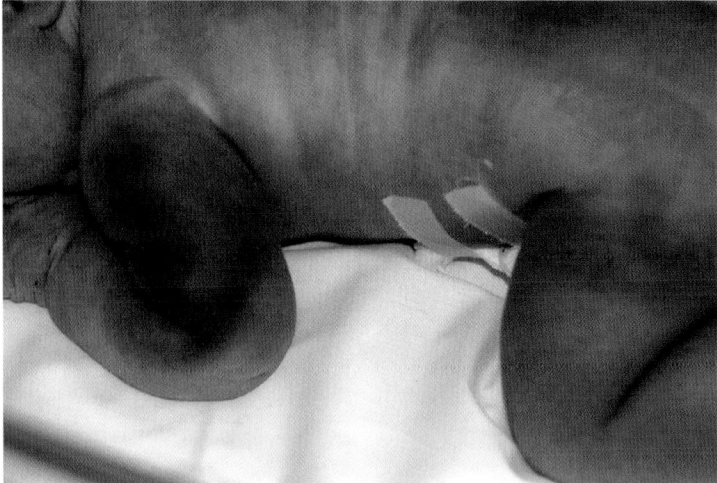

Figure 99.52 Subcutaneous fat necrosis of the newborn. Erythematous and violaceous plaques involving the shoulders, arms and buttocks.

ing atrophic scars. Confluence of the nodules results in extensive erythematous indurated plaques.

Complications and co-morbidities

Most children remain otherwise healthy as the subcutaneous nodules develop, but approximately 25% develop complicating hypercalcaemia [23–30,33,34]. The hypercalcaemia may persist for several weeks after the subcutaneous lesions have regressed, which requires calcium levels to be monitored and associated endocrinological disorders to be ruled out. Other reported laboratory anomalies include transient thrombocytopenia, probably due to platelet sequestration [5,12,13,35], hypoglycaemia due to maternal diabetes and hypertriglyceridaemia [36]. In rare instances, the condition may be fatal, particularly when visceral fat is involved [4]. Nephrocalcinosis persisting several years after resolution of the skin nodules has been reported as a rare complication [37].

Investigations

Histopathologically, subcutaneous fat necrosis of the newborn shows a predominantly lobular panniculitis, with a dense inflammatory infiltrate composed of lymphocytes, histiocytes, lipophages, multinucleate giant cells and sometimes eosinophils interspersed among the adipocytes of the fat lobule. Many adipocytes are replaced by cells with finely eosinophilic granular cytoplasm that contain doubly refractile narrow needle-shaped clefts radially arranged, which represent triglyceride crystallization within adipocytes and stain with oil red O [38] (Figure 99.53). Some of these refractile clefts may also be found within the cytoplasm of multinucleate giant cells. The latter may also contain eosinophilic granules in their cytoplasm [39–41] and their origin from degranulating eosinophils has been postulated [39]. Fibrotic obliteration of small arterioles and calcium deposits in necrotic fat have also been described [42,43,**44**,45]. In late-stage lesions, there is septal fibrosis and areas of calcification and lipoatrophy may appear within the fat lobule [11]. Adipocytes containing needle-shaped clefts radially arranged have been also found during autopsy studies in ventilator-associated tracheobronchitis (VAT) [4,8]. In some cases, the diagnosis was established

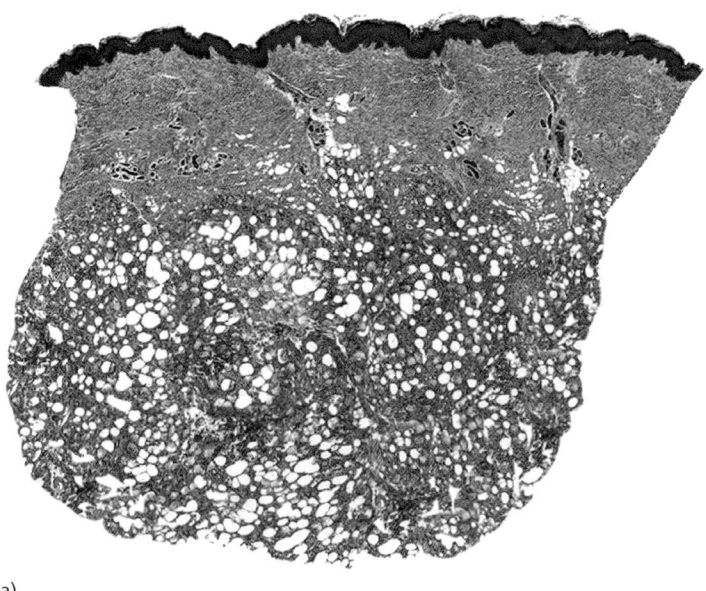

(a)

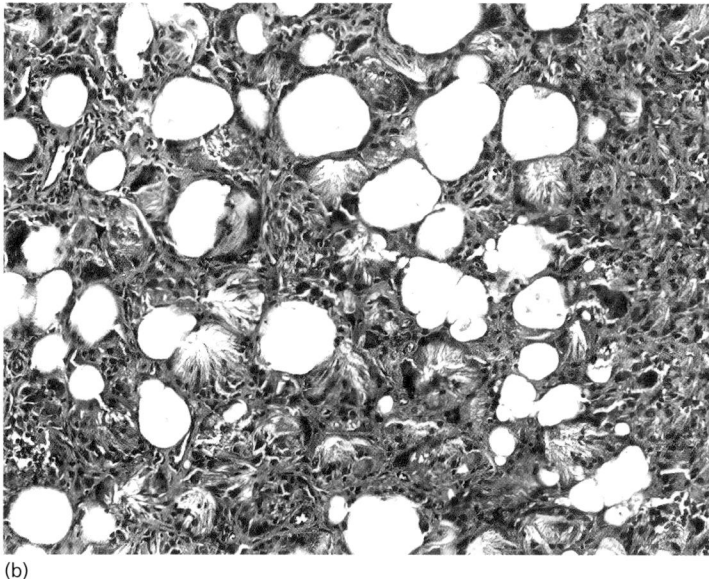

(b)

Figure 99.53 Histopathological features of subcutaneous fat necrosis of the newborn. (a) Scanning power showing a lobular panniculitis. (b) The fat lobule is replaced by a histiocytic infiltrate with some multinucleated giant cells. Many necrotic adipocytes and multinucleated giant cells contain needle-shaped clefts radially arranged.

using touch preparation, which was prepared by pressing a fresh sample biopsy against a glass slide, and fine-needle aspiration techniques [46,47].

Management

In most children with subcutaneous fat necrosis of the newborn, treatment is not required because the problem tends to resolve spontaneously. The main goals are the detection and treatment of hypercalcaemia [23–30,33,34] with avoidance of calcium and vitamin D_3. These measures should be instituted as early as possible with maintenance of adequate hydration with intravenous normal saline. Furosemide has been used to achieve increased calcium excretion by inhibiting calcium reabsorption, but a risk of dehydration and consequent worsening of hypercalcaemia exists. Prednisolone interferes with the metabolism of vitamin D to its active form and also inhibits the production of 1,25-dihydroxy-vitamin D_3 by the macrophages involved in the inflammatory process. Etidronate, a bisphosphonate that decreases bone resorption of calcium, has been helpful in the management of the associated hypercalcaemia [27,28,31–33]. It should be used as a second line drug, because its effects on bone production, growth plates and mineralization in infants are as yet unknown. Pamidronate is also helpful for treatment for hypercalcaemia and may reduce the risk of nephrocalcinosis [48,49]. Calcitonin and citrate may be used as second line therapy for resistant cases.

Poststeroid panniculitis

Clinical features

History

In 1956, Smith and Good [1] reported 11 children with acute rheumatic fever receiving high doses of corticosteroids with rapid taper, of whom five developed erythematous subcutaneous nodules.

Presentation

Poststeroid panniculitis is a rare panniculitis of children and infants on prolonged systemic corticosteroid treatment, and is related to a rapid decrease or a sudden withdrawal of steroid therapy. Only about 20 cases have been described in the literature [2,3,4–15]. It develops in an older age group than sclerema neonatorum and subcutaneous fat necrosis of the newborn, with reported ages ranging from 20 months to 14 years [3]. Although the process is mostly seen in children, there are also a few reported cases in adults [12,13,15]. In one adult patient, the lesions involved the arms and legs and were painless [15].

The lesions vary in size from 0.5 to 4 cm and consist of asymptomatic firm subcutaneous nodules, often with overlying erythema, and tend to be localized in those areas where there is the greatest accumulation of fat from steroid therapy, such as the face, arms and posterior neck [5]. They usually appear 1–10 days after cessation of high doses of systemic corticosteroids.

The disorders for which treatment with high doses of corticosteroids have been administered are varied, including rheumatic fever, leukaemia, nephrotic syndrome, acute exacerbation of chronic obstructive pulmonary disease, erythema nodosum leprosum, autoimmune enteropathy, Sjögren syndrome and brain tumours. Conversely, different oral or intravenous corticosteroid drugs, including prednisolone and dexamethasone, have been associated with this panniculitis. Usually, reinstitution of corticosteroid administration induces improvement of panniculitis, although some authors believe that this is not necessary for its resolution [3].

Investigations

Histopathological findings in poststeroid panniculitis lesions are identical to those of subcutaneous fat necrosis of the newborn.

They consist of a mostly lobular panniculitis with an inflammatory infiltrate of foamy histiocytes and lymphocytes involving the fat lobules [6]. Often, doubly refractile narrow needle-shaped clefts radially arranged are found within the cytoplasm of some histiocytes and necrotic adipocytes, although usually they are not as numerous as in subcutaneous fat necrosis of the newborn.

Management

Lesions of poststeroid panniculitis usually disappear gradually without residual scarring over the course of weeks or months, even without resuming steroid therapy and therefore no treatment is usually necessary. However, readministration of high doses of systemic corticosteroid and a slower and more gradual decrease of the dose is followed by a faster improvement and resolution of the lesions.

Sclerema neonatorum

Definition

Sclerema neonatorum is an uncommon condition which typically affects gravely ill, preterm neonates in the first week of life. It manifests as a diffuse hardening of skin and subcutaneous tissue such that the skin cannot be pitted or picked up and pinched into a fold. Histologically, there is minimal inflammation with extensive fat necrosis. It is associated with a high mortality (see also Chapter 116).

Clinical features

Presentation

Sclerema neonatorum is an extremely uncommon process and almost always appears during the first week of life, although there are also reports of infants born preterm with low birth weight who developed this condition later. In most cases, sclerema neonatorum is a grave illness and it has been associated with a mortality of up to 75% [1,2,3]. However, most case series date from 40 or more years ago, and now the process is very uncommon, probably due to better neonatal care. Prematurity and placental insufficiency have been proposed as pathogenetic factors for its development [3,4]. Affected infants are almost always severely ill from conditions such as septicaemia or other disseminated infections, congenital heart disease, pneumonia, diarrhoea, dehydration, intestinal obstruction or other congenital developmental defects [3]. In a multivariate analysis of risk factors for sclerema neonatorum in preterm neonates in Bangladesh, lower maternal education, signs of jaundice and poor feeding on admission were the main risk factors, although the diagnosis in that study was not histopathologically confirmed [5]. Cold injury has also been proposed as an aetiological factor [6], but it does not appear to be important in most cases.

Lipolytic immaturity in infants born preterm [7] and the different composition of subcutaneous fat in newborns, with a higher proportion of saturated (palmitic and stearic) to unsaturated (oleic) fatty acids, may also be predisposing factors [8,9], because they favour solidification of subcutaneous fat if there is a fall in

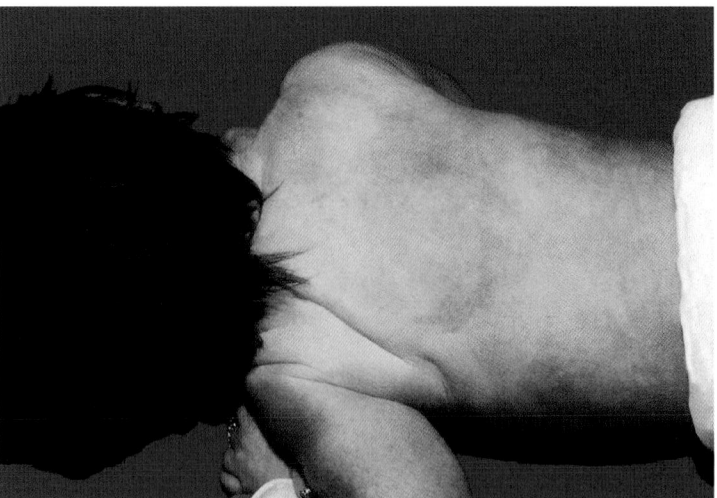

Figure 99.54 Sclerema neonatorum in a newborn with generalized woody induration of the skin.

the temperature of subcutaneous tissue as a result of peripheral circulatory collapse [10]. Sclerema neonatorum is characterized by increased blood lipid peroxidation and diminished superoxide dismutase activity, which raises the possibility that free radicals may also play some role in the pathogenesis of the process [11].

Clinically, infants with sclerema neonatorum typically appear severely ill from birth and during the first days of life they develop generalized woody induration of the skin [10,12] (Figure 99.54). Usually, the process begins on the buttocks and thighs but rapidly extends to involve almost the entire skin surface with the exception of the palms, soles and genitalia. The involved skin has a hard consistency, is non-pitting and is cold to the touch; it is yellowish-white in colour, often with purplish mottling. There is immobility of the extremities and the face shows a mask-like expression. The prognosis is poor and most affected infants die within a few days. However, if the infant survives, the skin recovers its normal appearance and there are no long-term complications such as calcification.

Differential diagnosis

The main differential diagnosis of sclerema neonatorum is subcutaneous fat necrosis of the newborn. This is important because they represent two distinctive clinicopathological processes with very different prognoses [12]. There is a single reported case of coexistence of both disorders in the same infant, but that is a doubtful case because histopathological study was lacking [13]. Usually this differential is straightforward, because subcutaneous fat necrosis of the newborn, which is a localized and self-healing process, does not develop in the first days of life and has characteristic histopathology consisting in a dense histiocytic infiltrate in the fat lobules with radially arranged needle-shaped refractile clefts within adipocytes and histiocytes.

Histopathological changes similar to those of sclerema neonatorum have been described in a patient with gemcitabine-associated livedoid thrombotic microangiopathy. The cutaneous biopsy showed small-vessel occlusion by intravascular fibrin and leukocytes, vessel wall thickening and endothelial cell swelling

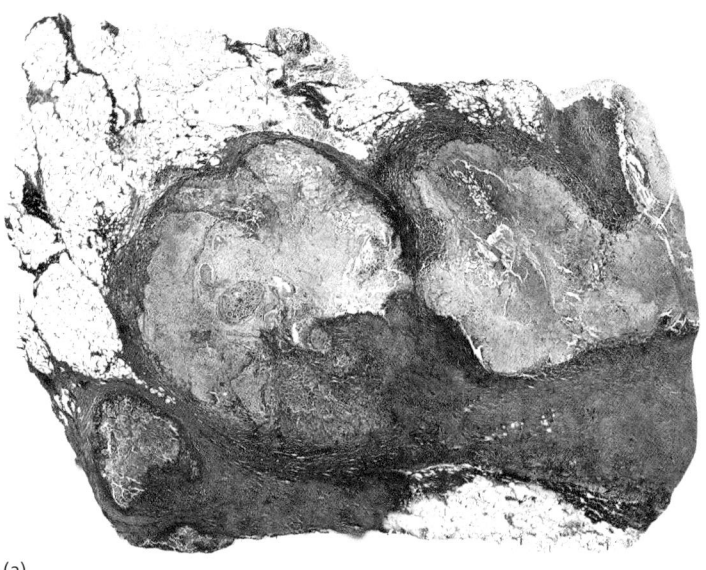

(a)

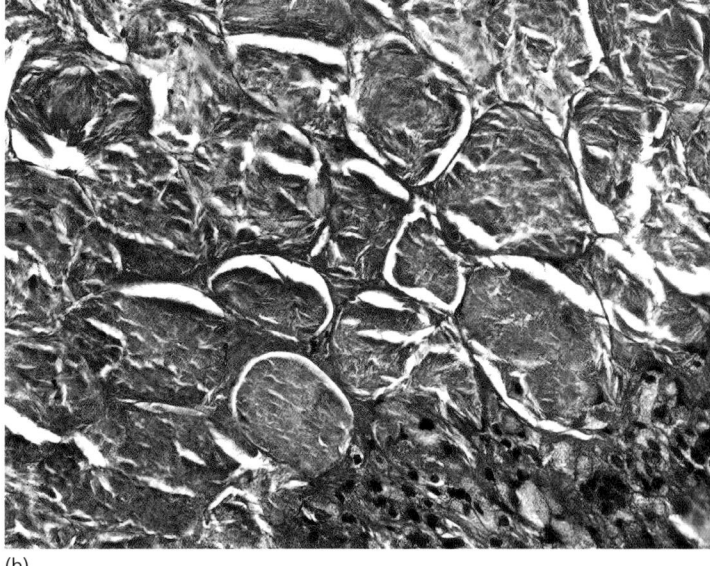

(b)

Figure 99.55 Histopathological features of sclerema neonatorum. (a) Scanning power showing necrosis of the entire fat lobules and thickened connective tissue septa. (b) An entire fat lobule is replaced by granular detritus and the cellular structures of the adipocytes are no longer evident. Many necrotic adipocytes contain needle-shaped clefts.

and some structures arranged radially with needle-shaped clefts resembling those of sclerema neonatorum [14].

Sclerema neonatorum should be not confused with scleredema neonatorum, an entirely different process seen in premature infants with congenital heart disease, which is characterized by distended skin with wax-like appearance that results from dermal oedema with increased amounts of mucin [12].

Investigations

Histopathologically, there is a striking contrast at low-power magnification between the severe damage in the subcutaneous fat and the sparse inflammatory response [9,10,15] (Figure 99.55). Most fat lobules appear to be replaced by amphophilic granular detritus and the cellular structures of the adipocytes are no longer evident. Surprisingly, there is sparse or no inflammatory infiltrate in spite of the intense fat necrosis. The most characteristic histopathological feature consists of the presence of radially arranged needle-shaped refractile clefts in adipocytes and, occasionally, in the few multinucleate giant cells, which result from crystallization of the lipid contents of the adipocytes. X-ray diffraction studies have demonstrated that the clefts in the fat cells are due to crystallization of tryglicerides [16]. In late-stage lesions, thickened connective tissue septa may be the only anomaly [15].

Management

Treatment of sclerema neonatorum is mainly directed to the underlying disease. Systemic corticosteroids have been demonstrated not to be effective [2]. Repeated exchange transfusions may substantially reduce mortality [17,18], but the diagnosis in those cases was not histopathologically confirmed. Intravenous immunoglobulins were used in a newborn with sclerema neonatorum and sepsis, with transitory improvement of the skin induration, but the patient died of respiratory failure [19].

Gouty panniculitis

Definition

Panniculitis is a very uncommon complication of tophaceous gout (see Chapter 154).

Clinical features

Presentation

The usual clinical presentation consists of painful ulcerating nodules on the lower legs [1–5,6,7–9] (Figure 99.56). In most reported

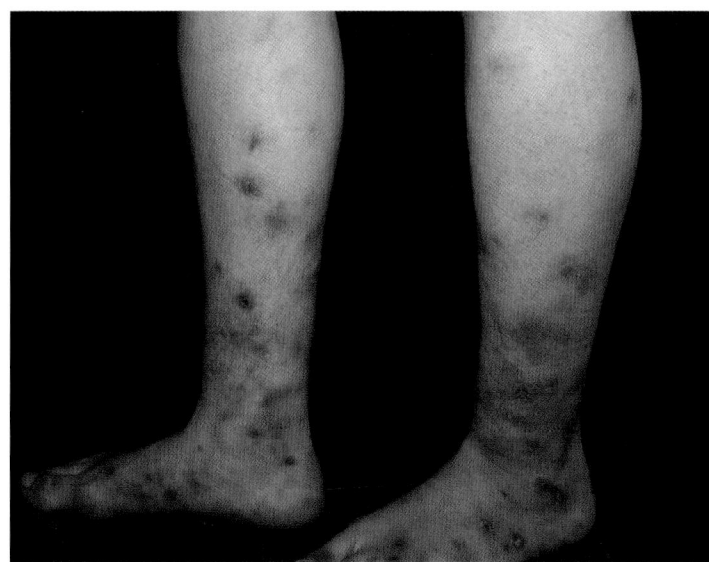

Figure 99.56 Gouty panniculitis. Ulcerated nodules on the lower legs of a patient with hyperuricaemia.

PART 8: SPECIFIC CUTANEOUS STRUCTURE

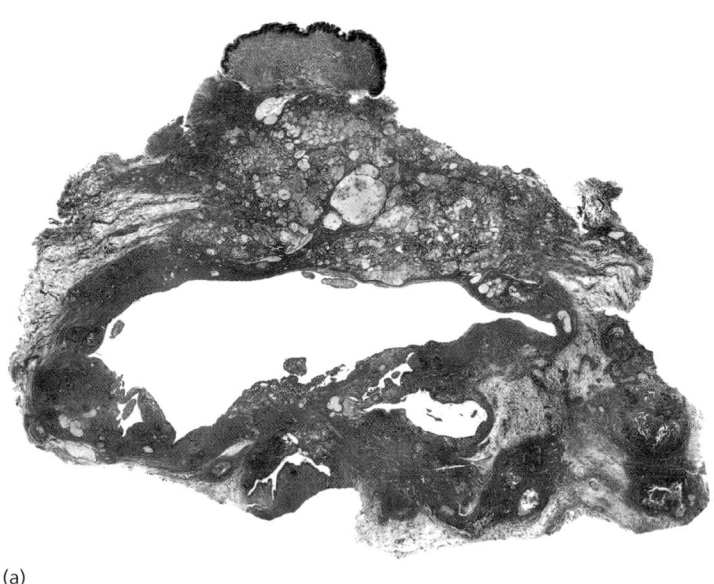

(a)

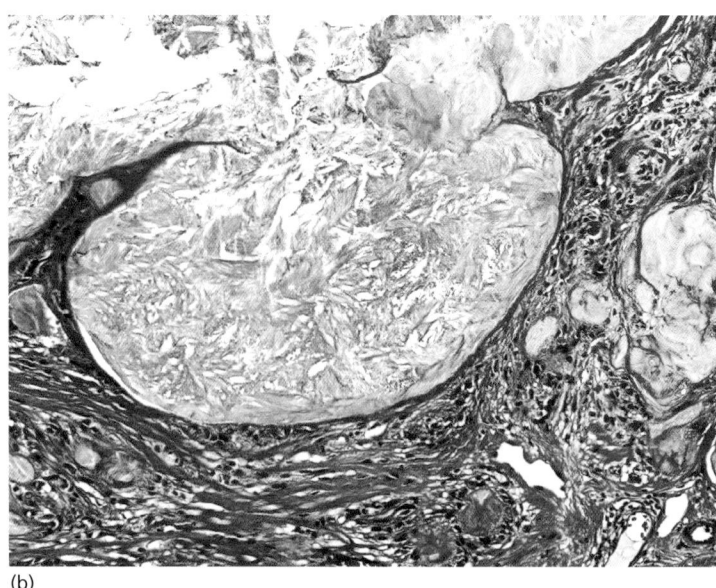

(b)

Figure 99.57 Histopathology of gouty panniculitis. (a) Scanning power showing involvement of the subcutaneous tissue, whereas the dermis is spared. (b) Basophilic amorphous deposits, which are fine needle-like shape urate crystals, appear surrounded by histiocytes.

cases, patients had already sustained severe joint damage by the time panniculitis manifested as subcutaneous nodules, but in some cases panniculitis may be the first manifestation of hyperuricaemia [2]. One of the patients reported also had involvement of bone marrow fat [9].

Investigations

Histopathology shows a lobular, sometimes neutrophilic panniculitis with deposition of needle-shaped refractile crystals within adipocytes (Figure 99.57) [2]. Frequently, histiocytes and multinucleate giant cells form a palisade around the urate crystals.

Fungal panniculitis due to zygomycosis, mucormycosis and aspergillosis

A predominantly lobular panniculitis with fine needle-shaped refractile crystals within adipocytes has been described in subcutaneous fungal infections including zygomycosis [1], mucormycosis [2] and aspergillosis [3] (see Chapter 32). The presumed urate crystals are similar to those found in gouty panniculitis but the mechanism by which they are formed is unknown.

Cytophagic histiocytic panniculitis and subcutaneous panniculitis-like T-cell lymphoma

Introduction and general description

The term cytophagic histiocytic panniculitis was introduced to describe a rare entity characterized by the development of subcutaneous nodules containing lobular infiltrates of macrophages which had phagocytosed lymphocytes, erythrocytes and nuclear debris [1].

With the benefit of modern immunohistochemistry and genetic techniques, it has become evident that most patients who are found to have cytophagic histiocytic panniculitis have one of two types of primary lymphoma affecting subcutaneous tissue [2]: SPTCL or primary cutaneous $\gamma\delta$ T-cell lymphoma. The former is a homogeneous entity with an α/β+ T-cell phenotype, indolent biological behaviour and good prognosis, whereas patients with the latter and a γ/δ+ T-cell phenotype are more heterogeneous and show a very aggressive clinical course with poor prognosis [3–7]. Both entities are discussed in detail in Chapter 140.

However, it seems that there is still a group of patients with cytophagic histiocytic panniculitis in whom a definitive diagnosis of lymphoma cannot be made and in whom molecular studies fail to demonstrate monoclonal rearrangements of infiltrating lymphocytes. Nevertheless the prognosis within this group is often poor, with pancytopenia and fatal outcome from haemophagocytic syndrome involving liver, spleen and bone marrow [8].

Presentation

SPTCL is rare, accounting for less than 1% of all primary cutaneous T-cell lymphomas, with equal incidence in both genders and preferentially involving adult patients, although there are also cases described in children. Clinically, patients present with erythematous subcutaneous nodules that may group into large plaques typically involving the lower extremities (Figure 99.58). A common feature consists of areas of lipoatrophy when the lesions resolve. Less commonly, SPTCL may involve the trunk, head or upper extremities. Approximately, 50% of patients have B symptoms, including fever, fatigue and weight loss; cytopenia and elevation of liver enzymes are frequently found, but a frank haemophagocytic syndrome is rare [9].

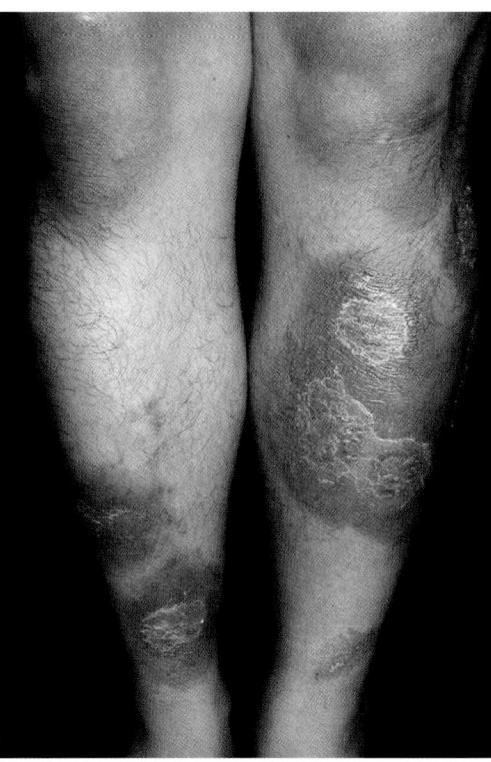

Figure 99.58 Subcutaneous pannicultis-like T-cell lymphoma. Erythematous plaques involving the anterior aspects of the lower extremities.

Investigations

Histopathologically, SPTCL and cytophagic histiocytic panniculitis may be indistinguishable, and only after immunohistochemical and molecular studies can they be differentiated. At low power both disorders mimic a predominantly lobular panniculitis. The fat lobule is involved by small and medium-size atypical lymphocytes with hyperchromatic nuclei. Numerous macrophages are also intermingled with the atypical lymphocytes. A characteristic finding in favour of the diagnosis of SPTCL consists in the sparing of the epidermis and dermis (Figure 99.59). In some areas, atypical lymphocytes are arranged in a circle around necrotic adipocytes, although this rimming is not entirely specific for SPTCL and it may also be seen in other lymphoid processes involving subcutaneous fat [10]. The presence of macrophages with cytophagic activity containing lymphocytes, neutrophils and nuclear debris within their cytoplasm is also a frequent finding in both processes, the so-called 'bean bag' cells. Foamy histiocytes are also frequently found in areas of fat necrosis.

A diagnosis of SPTCL can usually be established with confidence using immunohistochemistry and molecular techniques. Immunohistochemical studies have demonstrated that lymphocytes involving the fat lobules in SPTCL have a TRC-α/β+, CD3+, CD4–, CD8+, TIA-1+, perforin+, granzyme B+, CD30– T-cell immunophenotype. Evidence of Epstein–Barr virus (EBV) infection, either using PCR amplification to detect EBV-encoded RNA and EBV DNA or by immunohistochemical staining for latent membrane protein 1, are characteristically negative. As a consequence of its α/β+ T-cell phenotype, SPTCL expresses βF1 but is negative for CD56, in contrast with primary cutaneous γ/δ+ T-cell lymphoma and other lymphoproliferative processes involv-

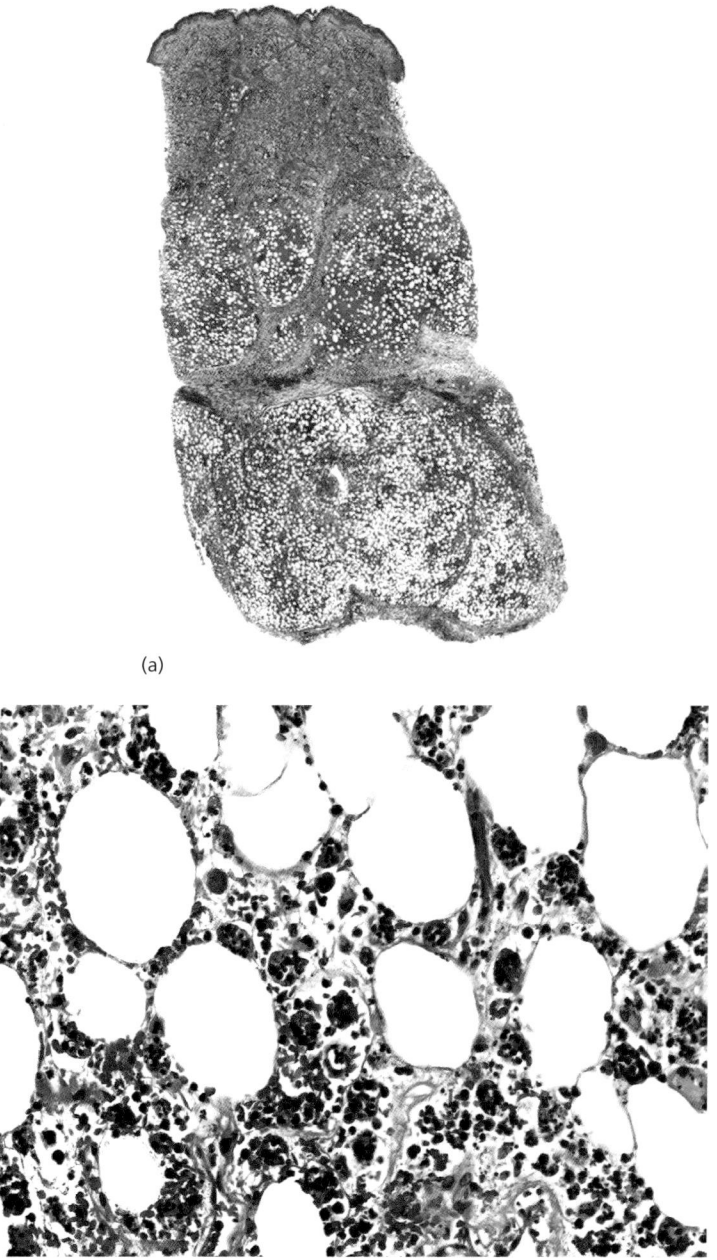

(a)

(b)

Figure 99.59 Histopathological features of subcutaneous panniculitis-like T-cell lymphoma. (a) Scanning power showing features simulating a lobular panniculitis. (b) Numerous macrophages with cytophagic activity containing lymphocytes, neutrophils and nuclear debris within their cytoplasm, the so-called 'bean bag' cells.

ing subcutaneous fat. Monoclonal rearrangement of γ or β genes can usually be detected in lesions of SPTCL using PCR or Southern blot analysis, whereas these rearrangements are not found in patients with cytophagic histiocytic panniculitis.

Sclerosing postirradiation panniculitis

Definition and nomenclature

Sclerosing postirradiation panniculitis is a rare clinicopathological variant of panniculitis that appears months or years after

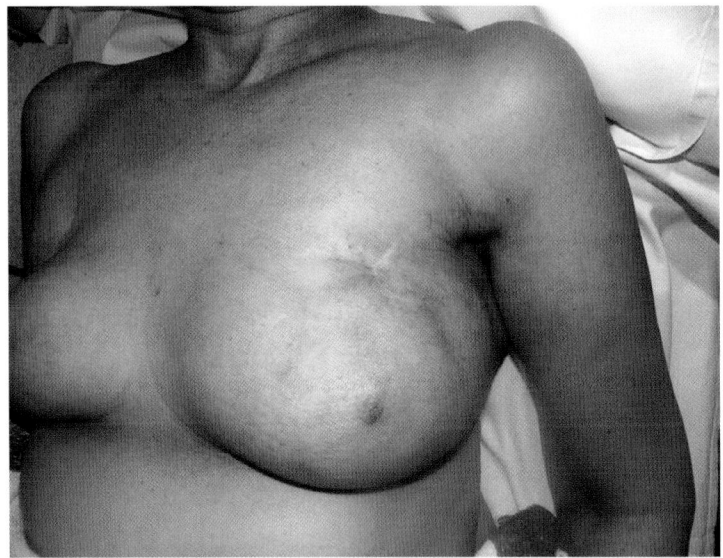

Figure 99.60 Sclerosing postirradiation panniculitis showing a depressed and indurate nodule on the previously irradiated area of the skin.

radiotherapy in the irradiated skin. Clinically, lesions consist of subcutaneous indurated nodules.

Synonyms and inclusions
• Postradiotherapy panniculitis

Clinical features

History
In 1993 Winkelmann *et al.* [1] described the first four cases of pseudosclerodermatous panniculitis after irradiation and, since then, only six additional cases have been published [2–4,5]. This process represents an unusual variant of panniculitis which may rarely occur as a cutaneous complication of radiotherapy.

Presentation
Clinically, sclerosing postirradiation panniculitis presents as an indurated asymptomatic subcutaneous nodule or plaque with little or no change in the epidermis and dermis at the site of previous radiotherapy (Figure 99.60). The most common location is the anterior chest wall following treatment for breast cancer. However, it may appear in any previously irradiated area of the skin [2]. The interval between the radiotherapy and the presentation of the condition varies from months to several years [1–4,5].

Differential diagnosis
The histopathological differential diagnosis includes other diseases showing a septal or lobular panniculitis with sclerosis of the connective tissue septa of the subcutis, such as deep morphoea [6–8] and lupus panniculitis [9]. Deep morphoea consists histopathologically of a septal panniculitis without significant lobular involvement in which there are sclerotic collagen bundles and aggregates of lymphocytes and especially plasma cells at the interface between the connective tissue septa and the fat lobules. In contrast with sclerosing postirradiation panniculitis, deep mor-

phoea does not show lobular involvement and the inflammatory cells within the thickened septa are mainly plasma cells. Lupus panniculitis is a mostly lobular panniculitis with sclerotic septa, but, in contrast with sclerosing postirradiation panniculitis, the inflammatory infiltrate involving the lobules is mostly composed of lymphocytes and plasma cells.

Investigations
The histopathological findings in sclerosing postirradiation panniculitis include a predominantly lobular panniculitis with necrosis of the adipocytes at the centre of the fat lobule and dense inflammatory infiltrates composed mainly of foamy histiocytes. Lipophagic granulomas involving the periphery of the fat lobules and thickening and sclerosis of the connective tissue septa are the most characteristic features in the subcutaneous tissue (Figure 99.61). These histopathological findings may or may not be

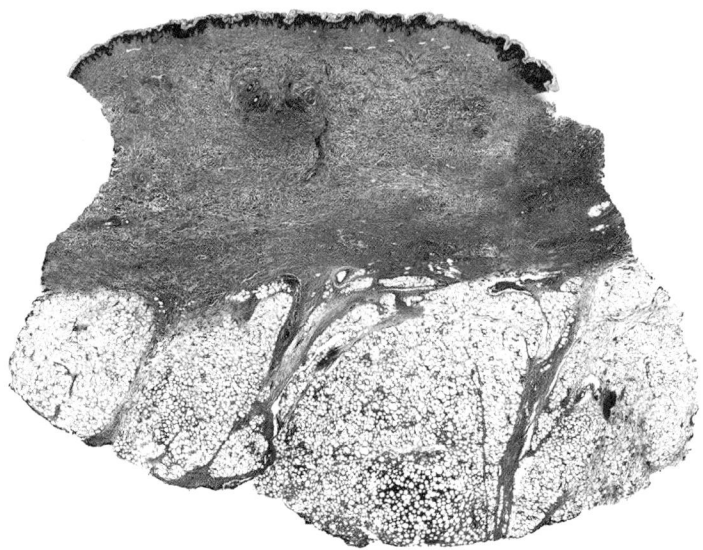

(a)

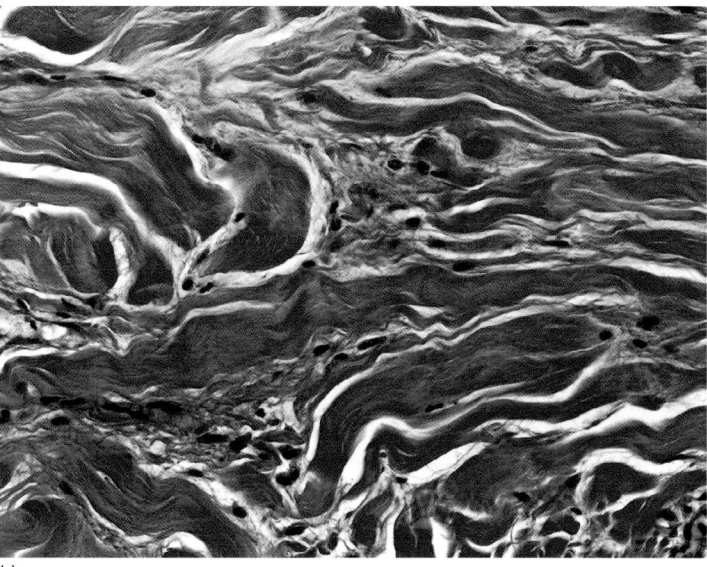

(b)

Figure 99.61 Histopathological features of sclerosing postirradiation panniculitis. (a) Scanning power showing a mostly lobular panniculitis. (b) Sclerotic collagen bundles at the septa of connective tissue of the subcutis.

accompanied by dermal changes secondary to radiotherapy [10–12], namely sclerosis of the papillary dermis, atypical star-shaped fibroblasts scattered amongst dermal collagen bundles and dilated thrombosed blood vessels with endothelial cell swelling and hyaline sclerosis of their walls.

Management

Treatment of sclerosing postirradiation panniculitis is not required and biopsy and subsequent histopathologic study are only performed when the possibility of a subcutaneous metastasis from the previously excised and/or irradiated breast cancer is raised.

Key references

The full list of references can be found in the online version at www.rooksdermatology.com.

Introduction
5 Avram AS, Avram MM, James WD. Subcutaneous fat in normal and diseased states: 2. Anatomy and physiology of white and brown adipose tissue. *J Am Acad Dermatol* 2005;53:671–83.
10 Ryan TJ, Curri SB, eds. *Clinics in Dermatology*, vol. 7. *The Cutaneous Adipose Tissue*. Philadelphia: JB Lippincott, 1989.
17 Avram MM, Avram AS, James WD. Subcutaneous fat in normal and diseased states 3. Adipogenesis: from stem cell to fat cell. *J Am Acad Dermatol* 2007;56:472–92.

Panniculitis
2 Requena L, Sánchez Yus E. Panniculitis. Part I. Mostly septal panniculitis. *J Am Acad Dermatol* 2001;45:163–83.
3 Requena L, Sánchez Yus E. Panniculitis. Part II. Mostly lobular panniculitis. *J Am Acad Dermatol* 2001;45:325–61.

Superficial migratory thrombophlebitis
3 Samlaska CP, James WD. Superficial thrombophlebitis: I. Primary hypercoagulable states. *J Am Acad Dermatol* 1990;22:975–89.
4 Samlaska CP, James WD. Superficial thrombophlebitis. II. Secondary hypercoagulable states. *J Am Acad Dermatol* 1990;23:1–18.

Cutaneous polyarteritis nodosa
4 Díaz Pérez JL, Martínez de Lagrán Z, Díaz-Ramón JL, Winkelmann RK. Cutaneous polyarteritis nodosa. *Semin Cutan Med Surg* 2007;26:77–86.

Necrobiosis lipoidica
1 Peyri J, Moreno A, Marcoval J. Necrobiosis lipoidica. *Semin Cutan Med Surg* 2007;26:87–9.

Deep morphoea
1 Peterson LS, Nelson Am, Su WPD. Classification of morphea (localized scleroderma). *Mayo Clin Proc* 1995;70:1068–76.

Subcutaneous granuloma annulare
1 Requena L, Fernández-Figueras MT. Subcutaneous granuloma annulare. *Semin Cutan Med Surg* 2007;26:96–9.

Rheumatoid nodule
33 Lynch JM, Barrett TL. Collagenolytic (necrobiotic) granulomas: part 1 – the "blue" granulomas. *J Cutan Pathol* 2004;31:353–61.
34 Lynch JM, Barrett TL. Collagenolytic (necrobiotic) granulomas: part II – the 'red' granulomas. *J Cutan Pathol* 2004;31:409–18.

Necrobiotic xanthogranuloma
5 Finan MC, Winkelmann RK. Necrobiotic xanthogranuloma with paraproteinaemia. A review of 22 cases. *Medicine* 1986;65:376–88.

Erythema nodosum
8 García-Porrúa C, González-Gay MA, Vázquez-Caruncho M, *et al*. Erythema nodosum. Etiologic and predictive factors in defined population. *Arthritis Rheum* 2000;43:584–92.
187 Sanchez Yus E, Sanz Vico MD, de Diego V. Miescher's radial granuloma. A characteristic marker of erythema nodosum. *Am J Dermatopathol* 1989;11:434–42.

Erythema nodosum leprosum
3 Murphy GF, Sánchez NP, Flynn TC, *et al*. Erythema nodosum leprosum: Nature and extent of the cutaneous microvascular alterations. *J Am Acad Dermatol* 1986;14:59–69.

Erythema induratum of Bazin
25 Segura S, Pujol RM, Trindade F, Requena L. Vasculitis in erythema induratum of Bazin: A histopathologic study of 101 biopsy specimens from 86 patients. *J Am Acad Dermatol* 2008;59:839–51.

Sclerosing panniculitis
16 Jorizzo JL, White WL, Zanolli MD, Greer KE, Solomon AR, Jetton RL. Sclerosing panniculitis. A clinicopathologic assessment. *Arch Dermatol* 1991;127:554–8.

Calcific uraemic arteriolopathy (calciphylaxis)
22 Dauden E, Oñate MJ. Calciphylaxis. *Dermatol Clin* 2008;26:557–68.

Cold panniculitis
15 Silverman A, Michels E, Rasmussen J. Subcutaneous fat necrosis in an infant, occurring after hypothermic cardiac surgery. *J Am Acad Dermatol* 1986;15:331–6.

Lupus panniculitis
25 Massone C, Kodama K, Salmohofer W, *et al*. Lupus erythematosus panniculitis (lupus profundus): Clinical, histopathological, and molecular analysis of nine cases. *J Cutan Pathol* 2005;32:396–404.

Dermatomyositis-associated panniculitis
2 Winkelmann RK. Panniculitis in connective tissue disease. *Arch Dermatol* 1983;119:336–44.
3 Raimer SS, Soloman AR, Daniels JC. Polymyositis presenting with panniculitis. *J Am Acad Dermatol* 1985;13:366–9.
14 Solans R, Cortés J, Selva A, *et al*. Panniculitis: a cutaneous manifestation of dermatomyositis. *J Am Acad Dermatol* 2002;46(5 Suppl.):S148–50.

Pancreatic panniculitis
3 Dahl PR, Su WP, Cullimore KC, Dicken CH. Pancreatic panniculitis. *J Am Acad Dermatol* 1995;33:413–17.

Alpha-1 antitrypsin deficiency panniculitis
18 Smith KC, Su WPD, Pittelkow MR, *et al*. Clinical and pathologic correlations in 96 patients with panniculitis, including 15 patients with deficient levels of α1-antitrypsin. *J Am Acad Dermatol* 1989;21:1192–6.

Infective panniculitis
1 Patterson JW, Brown PC, Broecker AH. Infection-induced panniculitis. *J Cutan Pathol* 1989;16:183–93.

Factitious panniculitis
6 Sanmartín O, Requena C, Requena L. Factitial panniculitis. *Dermatol Clin* 2008;26:519–27.

Neutrophilic lobular panniculitis
21 Guhl G, García-Díez A. Subcutaneous Sweet syndrome. *Dermatol Clin* 2008;26:541–51.

Subcutaneous sarcoidosis
8 Marcoval J, Maña J, Moreno A, *et al*. Subcutaneous sarcoidosis. Clinicopathological study of 10 cases. *Br J Dermatol* 2005;153:790–4.

PART 8: SPECIFIC CUTANEOUS STRUCTURE

Traumatic panniculitis

11 Hurt MA, Santa Cruz DJ. Nodular-cystic fat necrosis. A reevaluation of the so-called mobile encapsulated lipoma. *J Am Acad Dermatol* 1989;21:493–8.

Lipoatrophic panniculitis of the ankles in childhood

9 Winkelmann RK, McEvoy MT, Peters MS. Lipophagic panniculitis of childhood. *J Am Acad Dermatol* 1989;21:971–8.

Subcutaneous fat necrosis of the newborn

44 Friedman SJ, Winkelmann RK. Subcutaneous fat necrosis of the newborn: light, ultrastructural and histochemical microscopic studies. *J Cutan Pathol* 1989;16:99–105.

Poststeroid panniculitis

3 Roenigk HH Jr, Haserick JR, Arundell FD. Poststeroid panniculitis. *Arch Dermatol* 1964;90:387–91.

Sclerema neonatorum

1 Zeb A, Darmstadt GL. Sclerema neonatorum: a review of nomenclature, clinical presentation, histological features, differential diagnoses and management. *J Perinatol* 2008;28:453-60.

Gouty panniculitis

6 Weberschock T, Gholam P, Hartschuh W, Hartmann M. Gouty panniculitis in a 68-year-old man: case report and review of the literature. *Int J Dermatol* 2010;49:410-3.

Fungal panniculitis due to zygomycosis, mucormycosis and aspergillosis

2 Requena L, Sitthinamsuwan P, Santonja C, *et al*. Cutaneous and mucosal mucormycosis mimicking pancreatic panniculitis and gouty panniculitis. *J Am Acad Dermatol* 2012;66:975–84.

Cytophagic histiocytic panniculitis and subcutaneous panniculitis-like T-cell lymphoma

9 Willemze R, Jansen PM, Cerroni L, *et al*. Subcutaneous panniculitis-like T-cell lymphoma: definition, classification and prognostic factors: an EORTC Cutaneous Lymphoma Group Study of 83 cases. *Blood* 2008;11:838–45.

Sclerosing postirradiation panniculitis

5 Pielasinski U, Machan S, Camacho D, *et al*. Postirradiation pseudosclerodermatous panniculitis: three new cases with additional histopathologic features supporting the radiotherapy etiology. *Am J Dermatopathol* 2013;35:129–34.

CHAPTER 100

Other Acquired Disorders of Subcutaneous Fat

Amy Y.-Y. Chen[1] and Amit Garg[2]

[1]Department of Dermatology, University of Connecticut School of Medicine, Canton, CT, USA
[2]Department of Dermatology, Hofstra NSLIJ School of Medicine, Manhasset, NY, USA

Introduction

This chapter addresses principally non-inflammatory acquired disorders of subcutaneous fat with an emphasis on acquired lipodystrophy, fat hypertrophy, subcutaneous lipomatosis and lipoedema. While some of the entities discussed are very common, such as cellulite and obesity, most are much more rare. Panniculitis and genetic disorders of subcutaneous fat are addressed in Chapters 99 and 74, respectively.

ACQUIRED LIPODYSTROPHY

Acquired lipodystrophy refers to a heterogeneous group of disorders in which there is localized, partial or generalized loss of subcutaneous fat (lipoatrophy), in certain cases accompanied by fat accumulation in other body sites.

Acquired generalized lipodystrophy

Definition and nomenclature

Acquired generalized lipodystrophy (AGL) is a rare disease characterized by a selective loss of adipose tissue from large regions of the body, occurring after birth [1].

Synonyms and inclusions
- Lawrence syndrome
- Lawrence–Seip syndrome

Introduction and general description

After its initial report by Ziegler in 1928 [2], AGL was described in more detail through autopsy findings by Lawrence in 1946 [3]. Although loss of adipose tissue in AGL most often occurs during childhood and adolescence, a few cases report AGL in individuals over the age of 65 years [4,5]. The pattern and extent of fat loss in AGL is variable. Most patients have generalized loss of fat, though fat may be spared in some areas, such as retro-orbital fat. In addition to the loss of adipose tissue, patients often develop severe hepatic steatosis and fibrosis, severe insulin resistance and hyperinsulinaemia, hypertriglyceridaemia and low serum high-density lipoprotein (HDL) levels [6–9].

Epidemiology

Incidence and prevalence

Acquired generalized lipodystrophy is a rare disease and thus its incidence and prevalence are difficult to estimate. Less than 100 cases were identified in a literature review published in 2003 [10]. More recently, in 2012, it was estimated that AGL affects approximately one in 100 000 people in the European Union.

Rook's Textbook of Dermatology, Ninth Edition. Edited by Christopher Griffiths, Jonathan Barker, Tanya Bleiker, Robert Chalmers and Daniel Creamer.
© 2016 John Wiley & Sons, Ltd. Published 2016 by John Wiley & Sons, Ltd.
Companion website: www.rooksdermatology.com

PART 8: SPECIFIC CUTANEOUS STRUCTURE

Age
Most patients with AGL present during childhood or adolescence.

Sex
Women are affected three times more often than men [10].

Ethnicity
The majority of patients have been white, although AGL has also been reported in Hispanic and East Asian patients [10,11].

Associated diseases
Most AGL patients have some degree of metabolic derangement, including fasting and/or postprandial hyperinsulinaemia, hypertriglyceridaemia, low serum levels of HDL, and low leptin and adiponectin [6–9,10]. Diabetes most often occurs subsequent to the onset of AGL, though in some it may present before or at the time of onset [10]. AGL patients usually do not develop diabetic ketoacidosis [12]. Patients may also have increased basal metabolic rate and complain of fatigue and voracious appetite [10].

Hepatomegaly occurs in 70–100% of AGL patients. Hepatic steatosis or non-alcoholic steatohepatitis results in mild to moderate elevation of serum transaminases. Splenomegaly may result from portal hypertension and cirrhosis [10].

Cardiomyopathy may be associated with AGL. In a 2011 study of left ventricular mass in 13 patients with AGL, three had mild and three had moderate ventricular hypertrophy. Abnormalities were seen in five of 11 AGL patients whose electrocardiogram was available for analysis [13].

Muscle and neurological involvement have rarely been reported [5,11].

Reproductive capacity is normal in male patients with AGL. Female AGL patients may have normal reproduction although irregular menses are common [10]. Primary or secondary amenorrhoea rarely occurs [10,14,15]. Single [16] or multiple [17,18] bone lucencies and cysts have been reported in AGL patients, though the clinical significance of these lesions is not clear [18]. Lymphadenopathy has also been reported in some [7,18–20].

Pathophysiology
The mechanism of fat loss in AGL is unknown. Despite reports of a variety of preceding infections, it is not clear that these infections directly cause AGL [21,22]. The classic complement pathway is postulated to be involved in the pathogenesis among AGL patients with autoimmune hepatitis and low serum complement [23,24]. Antibody-mediated destruction or cell-mediated lysis of adipocytes has also been considered [25].

The consequences are that there is an insufficient mass of adipose tissue to store excess energy, which is stored instead as triglyceride in the liver and skeletal muscle, and that there is a perpetual elevation of plasma free fatty acid (FFA), resulting in an impaired β-cell response to glucose and insulin resistance [26–29]. Low serum leptin and adiponectin levels, reflecting the low amount of body fat in these patients, may further contribute to severe insulin resistance and the metabolic complications observed in AGL [30–33].

Pathology
Acquired generalized lipodystrophy is a clinical diagnosis, though histopathology may help confirm the diagnosis. Tissue examination demonstrates a complete or near-complete absence of subcutaneous fat, with the dermis and fascia in direct apposition. If adipocytes are present, they are markedly reduced in number and size and they are arranged in small groups surrounded by abundant connective tissue [34].

Genetics
No known genetic mutation or familial cluster has been identified.

Clinical features

Presentation
In contrast to congenital lipodystrophy, patients with AGL have normal fat density and distribution at birth. The onset of fat loss is typically insidious over months to years (Figure 100.1), although rapid progression over weeks has been observed [10]. Rarely, the process of fat destruction may occur rapidly in one area and stay

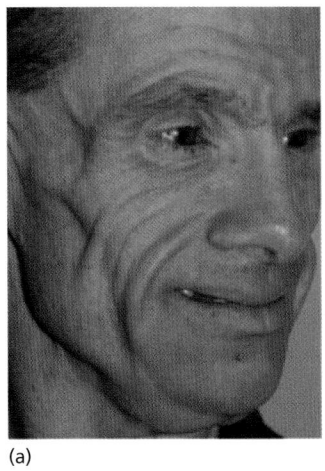
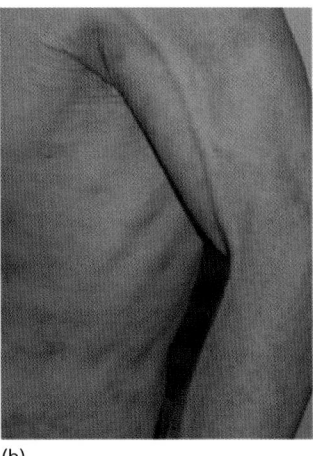
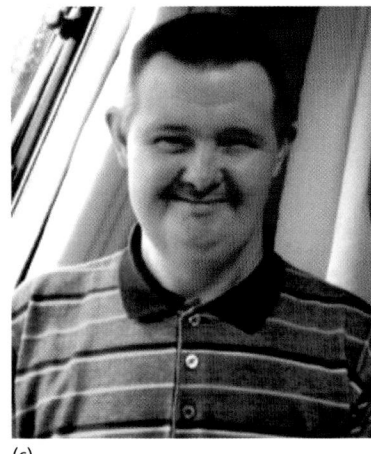

(a)   (b)   (c)

Figure 100.1 Physical examination revealed (a) lipoatrophy of the face and (b) generalized lipoatrophy of the torso with visible subcutaneous veins. (c) A photograph of the patient taken 5 years earlier, in 2008, is shown for comparison. (Reproduced with permission from Aslam A, Savage DB, Coulson IH. Acquired generalized lipodystrophy associated with peripheral T cell lymphoma with cutaneous infiltration. *Int J Dermatol* 2015;54:827–9.)

quiescent over months to years, only to become active again later and result in generalized fat loss [2,10]. The extent and degree of fat loss is variable. Usual sites of involvement include the face (Figure 100.1a), trunk, abdomen and extremities. Underlying veins and musculature become prominent with severe fat loss (Figure 100.1b). In some, loss of fat may also involve the palms, soles and abdominal cavity. Generally, marrow and retro-orbital fat are preserved.

Acanthosis nigricans of the axillae, groin, neck, umbilicus and nipples is noted in 45–64% of AGL patients [10]. Other less common dermatological findings include localized [35,36] or generalized hyperpigmentation [37,38], telangiectasia [19] and hyperkeratosis of the palms and soles [16]. Women with AGL may have mild hirsutism [10,37,39,40]. Rarely, virilization with temporal recession of hair and acne have been reported [14,41]. Alopecia [6] and curly hair [7,10,16,21,37,40,42] have also been observed. Acromegaloid facial features with large hands and feet may rarely be seen [9,10].

In 2003, Misra and Garg proposed new diagnostic criteria applicable to the broad spectrum of AGL patients. Essential criteria include selective loss of body fat affecting large regions of the body, beginning after birth but usually before adolescence. Supportive clinical criteria include loss of subcutaneous fat from the palms and soles, a preceding history of tender subcutaneous nodular swellings, histological confirmation from involved tissue, acanthosis nigricans, hepatosplenomegaly and the presence of other autoimmune diseases.

Supportive laboratory criteria include impaired glucose tolerance, severe fasting and/or postprandial hyperinsulinaemia, hypertriglyceridaemia, low serum HDL, low serum leptin and/or adiponectin, and evidence by magnetic resonance imaging (MRI) of fat loss from large regions of the body with preserved bone marrow fat [10]. The number of these secondary clinical or laboratory criteria needed to support a diagnosis of AGL has not been formally established.

Clinical variants
Acquired generalized lipodystrophy is subdivided into three types. *Type I AGL*, in which initially localized panniculitis precedes generalized fat loss, accounts for approximately 25% of cases [1]. *Type II AGL*, which accounts for another 25% of cases, is associated with autoimmune diseases including haemolytic anaemia, chronic autoimmune hepatitis, Hashimoto thyroiditis, juvenile rheumatoid arthritis, juvenile dermatomyositis and vitiligo [6,23,35,36,43–45]. Juvenile dermatomyositis may have the strongest association with AGL [10]. The remaining patients have the most common subtype, *type III (idiopathic) AGL*, in which no triggers or associated diseases are identified.

Differential diagnosis
Some AGL patients may initially present with localized or partial lipodystrophy and hence may be misclassified as having acquired partial lipodystrophy or localized lipodystrophy.

AGL patients are differentiated from *congenital generalized lipodystrophy* (CGL) patients who have near-complete generalized fat loss at birth (see Chapter 74). Furthermore, CGL patients have advanced bone age and mental retardation. As with AGL, CGL patients may have acromegaloid features, lytic bone lesions and cardiomyopathy [10]. Lytic bone lesions are, however, more common and the

cardiomyopathy more severe in CGL [10,13]. MRI studies of CGL patients show an absence of 'metabolically active' fat in intra-abdominal and intrathoracic regions, and in bone marrow, while marrow fat is preserved in AGL patients [10,46]. Genetic analysis for known mutations may aid in the confirmation of CGL.

While patients with *mandibuloacral dysplasia* may have generalized fat loss, these patient also have skeletal anomalies (see Chapter 72). The identification of associated genetic mutations can help to confirm this diagnosis.

Family histories as well as genotyping will also help differentiate AGL from *autosomal dominant familial partial lipodystrophy* (see Chapter 74) [1].

Complications and co-morbidities
Patients with AGL may suffer complications from metabolic disturbances and other associated co-morbid conditions in association with type II AGL. Retinopathy, nephropathy and neuropathy are common complications because of the patients' longstanding diabetes. Hypertriglyceridaemia may lead to eruptive xanthomas, lipaemia retinalis and acute pancreatitis [10]. These metabolic abnormalities also predispose AGL patients to premature atherosclerosis and coronary heart disease [6,10].

Disease course and prognosis
The loss of subcutaneous fat tissue in AGL patients is permanent. The prognosis of AGL patients largely depends on the course and management of co-morbidities.

Investigations
Laboratory and ancillary testing is pursued to establish the presence and monitor the course of co-morbid diseases. While serum leptin is not useful for establishing the diagnosis, it may predict response to replacement therapy with the synthetic recombinant analogue of human leptin, metreleptin [1].

Management
There is no established management algorithm for AGL. Subcutaneous fat loss is irreversible. To the extent feasible, cosmetic procedures such as filler injections, autologous adipose tissue transfer and muscle tissue transfers may help correct volume losses [1,47,48]. Optimal management of co-morbid conditions requires collaboration between primary care physicians and several specialists.

In one trial, which included three AGL patients among others with various lipodystrophies, 4 months of twice-daily subcutaneous metreleptin injections were shown to be safe and effective. There was a significant decrease in fasting blood glucose level and glycosylated haemoglobin in two patients. In three patients with hypertriglyceridaemia, fasting levels of plasma triglycerides decreased by 83%. In these patients, fasting plasma triglycerides increased soon after discontinuation of the injections and were corrected once again after reinitiation of the therapy [49]. Furthermore, liver volume and serum transaminases decreased significantly during metreleptin therapy, suggesting that it reduced hepatic steatosis [50]. Metreleptin has been approved under the orphan designation for the treatment of AGL in the European Union since July 2012; it remains investigational in the USA.

Acquired partial lipodystrophy

Definition and nomenclature

Acquired partial lipodystrophy (APL) is a rare disease characterized by symmetrical fat loss, usually occurring before the age of 15 years [1,2].

Synonyms and inclusions
- Barraquer–Simons syndrome
- Progressive cephalothoracic lipodystrophy

Introduction and general description

Acquired partial lipodystrophy was first reported by Mitchell [3] and later by Barraquer [4] and by Simons [5]. Although rare, APL is the most common of the non-localized lipodystrophies, other than HIV-associated lipodystrophy. It is characterized by symmetrical and insidious although progressive fat loss starting from the face and scalp and gradually progressing downward to involve the neck, shoulders, upper extremities, thoracic region and upper abdomen. Involvement of the lower extremities is uncommon [1,2].

Epidemiology

Incidence and prevalence

Because it is rare, the incidence and prevalence of APL is difficult to estimate. By 2000, there were approximately 250 cases reported in the English literature [1].

Age

Onset is typically before the age of 15 years, with a median of 8 years [1,2].

Sex

Women are affected approximately three times more commonly than men [1].

Ethnicity

Most reported patients have been white.

Associated diseases

Approximately one-third of patients develop mesangiocapillary glomerulonephiritis (MCGN), usually more than 10 years after the onset of lipodystrophy [1]. Systemic lupus erythematosus has been associated with APL and has occurred 2–28 years after the onset of lipodystrophy [6–9]. Other autoimmune diseases, such as dermatomyositis [10], leukocytoclastic vasculitis [11], dermatitis herpetiformis and coeliac diseases [12], hypothyroidism, pernicious anemia [13], rheumatoid arthritis [8] and temporal arteritis, have also been reported. More recently, APL has been reported in the setting of chronic sclerodermatous graft-versus-host-disease, POEMS (*p*olyneuropathy, *o*rganomegaly, *e*ndocrinopathy, *m*ono-clonal gammopathy and *s*kin changes) syndrome and extrinsic allergic alveolitis, as well as central nervous system (CNS) disorders including epilepsy, sensorineural deafness and mental retardation (see Chapter 148) [14–17].

Pathophysiology

There is evidence to support an autoimmune-mediated destruction of adipocytes in APL. Approximately 80–90% of APL patients have a serum immunoglobulin G named C3 nephritic factor [18,19]. This blocks the degradation of the enzyme C3 convertase, which leads to excessive consumption of C3. As a result, serum C3 levels are low in more than 80% of APL patients [20]. Levels of C1q, C4, C5 and C6 and factors B and P are usually normal, suggesting selective activation of the alternative complement pathway [21]. Lysis of adipocytes may be related to the expression of several complement proteins such as factors D (adipsin), B, H and P [22,23,24]. For example, *in vitro* studies suggest that the C3 nephritic factor causes lysis in adipocytes expressing factor D [22]. Heterogeneity of factor D expression in adipose tissue in different anatomical locations has been postulated to explain the selective loss of upper body fat in APL [23].

In those APL patients without C3 nephritic factor, other immune abnormalities are postulated to be relevant pathogenetic factors. In a paediatric APL patient without C3 nephritic factor, serum tumour necrosis factor α (TNF-α) and interleukin 6 (IL-6) were noted to be elevated [25]. TNF-α has been shown to cause apoptosis in adipocyte cultures, and IL-6 stimulates lipolysis in human adipocytes [26,27]. TNF-α also influences the complement pathway by controlling factor D production in adipocytes [25].

Pathology

Acquired partial lipodystrophy is a clinical diagnosis based on the presentation and progression of disease. Histopathology, in common with AGL, shows complete or near-complete absence of subcutaneous fat, with the dermis and fascia in direct apposition. If adipocytes are present, they are markedly reduced in number and size, and they are arranged in small groups surrounded by abundant connective tissues [28].

Causative organisms

Although fat loss has been preceded by infection in some reported cases of APL, the relationship between APL and infection is unclear [23].

Genetics

LMNB2 mutations have been reported in five patients with APL, although some of these had atypical presentations [29].

Clinical features

Presentation

Fat loss in APL occurs symmetrically, starting on the face and scalp, then gradually spreading to involve the neck, shoulders, upper extremities, thoracic region and upper abdomen (Figure 100.2). Involvement of the inguinal region or thighs is uncommon. Fat in the hips and lower extremities is unaffected. In fact, affected women frequently accumulate excess fat in these regions after puberty. Fat loss typically progresses over a period of about 18 months, although it may continue for several years. Orbital, mediastinal, gluteal, intramuscular, intraperitoneal, perirenal and bone marrow fat is usually unaffected [1,2].

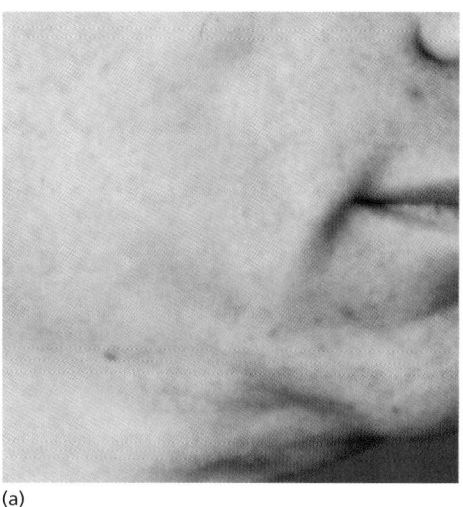

(a)

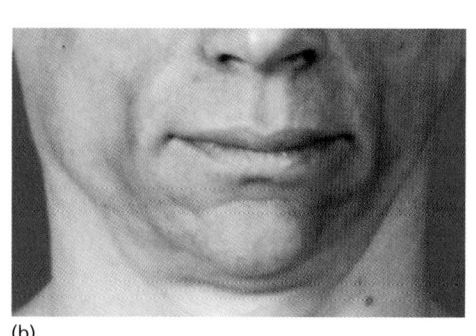

(b)

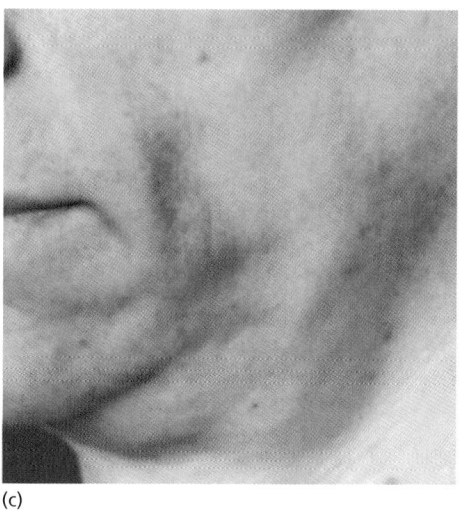

(c)

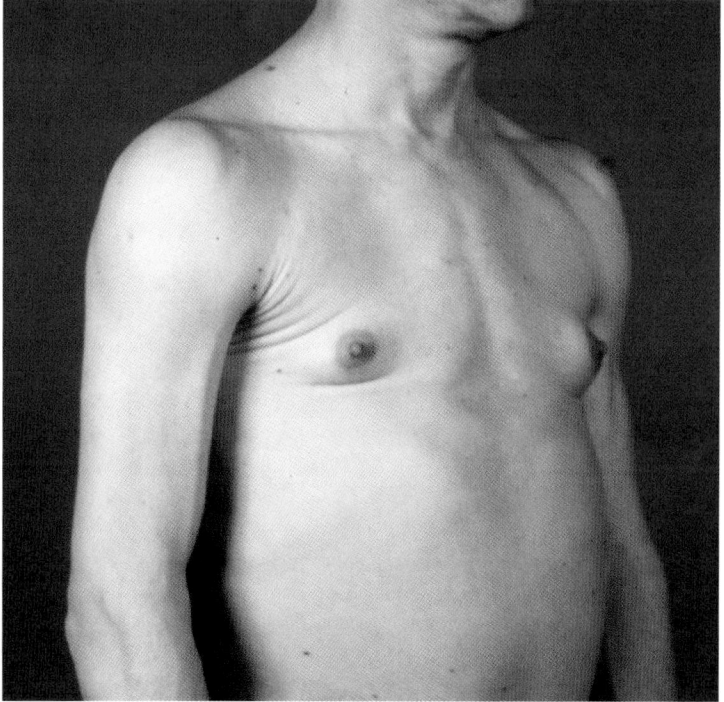

(d)

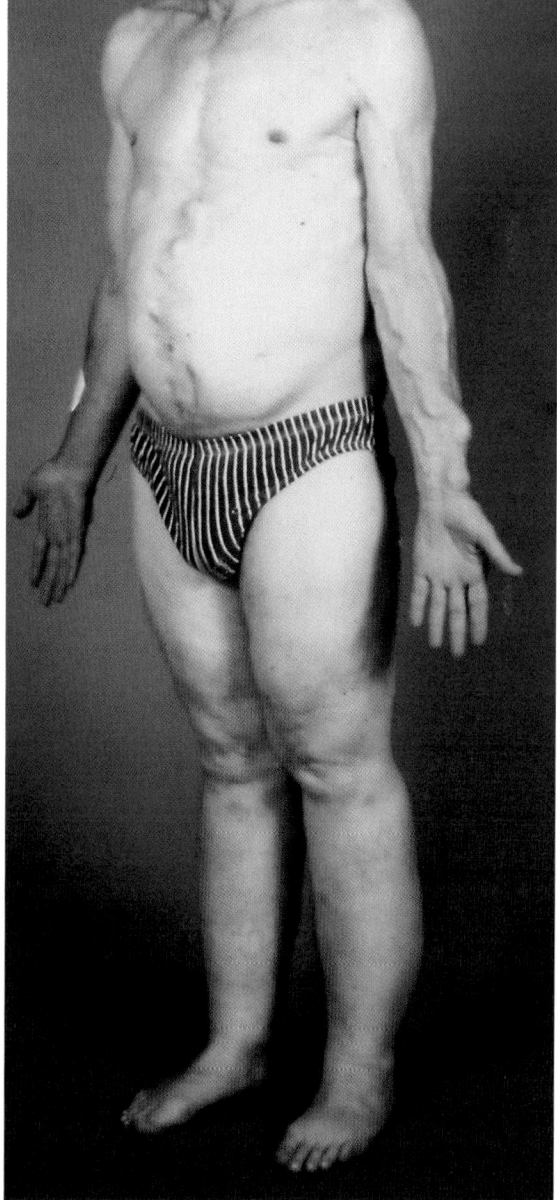

(e)

Figure 100.2 Acquired partial lipodystrophy (APL): (a–c) marked loss of facial fat resulting in a prematurely aged appearance and (d) prominence of arm veins, sternomastoid muscles and breast tissue resulting from subcutaneous fat loss in a 31-year-old man with APL and renal failure; (e) note preservation of subcutaneous fat in the lower half of the body contrasting with dramatic loss of subcutaneous fat in the upper half of the body in a 50-year-old man whose longstanding APL was not recognized until he presented with accelerated hypertension secondary to APL-related glomerulonephritis.

Clinical variants

Three phenotypic subtypes have been recognized: (i) upper body fat loss; (ii) upper body fat loss with hypertrophy of adipose tissue in the lower half of the body; and (iii) hemi-lipodystrophy in which only one side of the face or body is affected.

Differential diagnosis

Acquired partial lipodystrophy is differentiated from familial partial lipodystrophy in which there is a family history of similar lipodystrophy, variations in clinical presentation of fat loss and identified genetic mutations. A history of trauma and medication history can help differentiate other forms of acquired lipodystrophy from APL. APL is differentiated from AGL based on the extent of involvement as well as sparing of the intra-abdominal fat.

Complications and co-morbidities

Unlike in patients with AGL, insulin resistance, diabetes, dyslipidaemia, acanthosis nigricans, hirsutism or menstrual abnormalities are less common in APL patients [1].

Disease course and prognosis

Fat loss is irreversible in APL. Overall prognosis is driven by the presence of co-morbidities.

Investigations

The initial evaluation of APL patients should include serum C3 level and C3 nephritic factor, as well as baseline screening for metabolic derangements with a comprehensive metabolic panel, fasting glucose, lipid panels and insulin level. Evaluation should also include assessment of associated co-morbid conditions. Periodic and continued monitoring for renal disease and autoimmunity is warranted. MRI may demonstrate the extent of fat loss if needed.

Management

There is no established management algorithm for AGL. Subcutaneous fat loss is irreversible. To the extent feasible, cosmetic procedures such as filler injections, autologous adipose tissue transfer and muscle tissue transfers may help correct volume losses. However, the durable efficacy and safety of these approaches have not been extensively investigated. The identification of neutralizing antibodies against C3 nephritic factors in intravenous immunoglobulin (IVIg) has led to treatment of patients who have C3 nephritic factors and type II MCGN with IVIg with encouraging results [30,31]. Optimal management of co-morbid conditions requires collaboration between primary care physicians and several specialists.

HIV-associated lipodystrophy

Definition and nomenclature

Lipodystrophy in patients affected with human immunodeficiency virus (HIV) is associated with highly active antiretroviral therapy (HAART) regimens containing protease inhibitor (PI) or

nucleoside reverse transcriptase inhibitor (NRTI). It is now the most prevalent type of lipodystrophy, in which both lipoatrophy and lipohypertrophy may be observed (see Chapter 31).

Synonyms and inclusions
- Pseudo-Cushing syndrome
- Fat redistribution syndrome
- Maldistribution syndrome
- Protease inhibitor-associated lipodystrophy syndrome

Introduction and general description

The first report of fat redistribution in an HIV-infected individual undergoing antiretroviral therapy including a PI was in 1997 [1]. Lipodystrophy in HIV-infected patients usually appears after patients have been receiving PI- or NRTI-containing HAART regimens for at least 2 years [2]. Currently, there is no consensus on the definition or diagnostic criteria for lipodystrophy in the HIV-infected patient [3]. In 2003, Carr *et al.* established a diagnostic model that included the variables of age, sex, known duration of HIV infection, HIV disease stage, waist to hip ratio, anion gap, serum HDL cholesterol level and trunk to peripheral fat ratio [4]. Although follow-up prospective studies confirmed its high diagnostic sensitivity, the complexity of the model is thought to impede its use in daily clinical practice [5].

Epidemiology

Incidence and prevalence

Lipodystrophy in HIV-infected patients is the most prevalent among lipodystrophies. Due to limitations in the definition, selection of study population and duration of follow-up, there are considerable differences in its reported incidence and prevalence. Prevalence ranges from 8% to 84% with an average of 42% [6]. Average incidence ranges from 7.3 to 11.7 per 100 patient-years [7,8]. Generally, higher prevalence is reported among patients receiving long-term therapy. In pooled analyses, the prevalence is 17% among adults treated with PI-containing therapy for less than 1 year and 43% in those treated for more than 1 year [6]. Each additional 6 months of treatment with HAART is associated with a 1.57 times increased risk of lipodystrophy [7]. It is expected that the prevalence will increase in the future with longer follow-up and continued use of HAART [6].

Age

The risk of developing HIV-associated lipodystrophy increases with age [6,9]. Children receiving PI-containing HAART therapy exhibit a similar redistribution of body fat and metabolic derangements, although children may have a relatively smaller increase in visceral fat in the trunk [10–13].

Sex

Female sex is associated with an increased risk in some studies [3].

Ethnicity

White and East Asian races have been linked to having an increased risk of HIV-associated lipodystrophy [14].

Associated diseases

Patients with HIV-related lipodystrophy may develop hypertriglyceridaemia, although diabetes is less common [2]. There may also be a predisposition to coronary artery disease [15].

Pathophysiology

While the exact cause of HIV-associated lipodystrophy is unknown, both PIs and NRTIs are implicated in the pathogenesis. Because these drug classes are often given together as part of HAART, the individual effects of these drugs on the specific lipodystrophy phenotype remains unclear. It is speculated that while PIs induce peripheral lipodystrophy and metabolic abnormalities, NRTIs may be responsible for the fat accumulation in certain regions such as the buffalo hump [2].

First and second generation PIs have been shown to inhibit adipocyte differentiation and lipogenesis *in vitro* [16]. PIs may also induce insulin resistance by inhibiting glucose transporter-4 expressions [17]. NRTIs, especially zidovudine and stavudine, have been proposed to induce fat loss by inhibiting mitochondrial polymerase γ and causing mitochondrial toxicity [18,19]. This results in production of reactive oxygen species (ROS), which have been linked to lipoatrophy [20]. Excess adipocyte apoptosis was also observed in *ex vivo* fat samples from lipoatrophic areas [21].

The mechanism for the increased amounts of visceral adipose tissue (VAT) observed in HIV-associated lipodystrophy is also unclear. VAT and subcutaneous adipose tissue (SAT) differ in their metabolism, gene expression and inflammatory status [22]. As a result, adipocytes or other cells in VAT and SAT may respond to stimuli (e.g. PIs) in different ways, resulting in hypertrophy in one area and atrophy in another [3].

Predisposing factors

Several factors have been postulated to influence the risk of developing HIV-associated lipodystrophy, including age, gender, ethnicity, duration and status of HIV infection, as well as exposure to both PI- and non-PI-containing HAART [3,6]. Both high and low CD4 counts have been reported in affected patients [23–25].

There is some evidence that first generation unboosted PIs, such as indinavir, are associated with a higher risk of lipodystrophy than are booster PIs [3]. In one study, the incidence of lipoatrophy was lower in patients treated with ritonavir-boosted atazanavir than in those who received unboosted atazanavir [14]. In another study, patients treated with ritonavir-boosted lopinavir developed lipodystrophy by 96 weeks of treatment less frequently than those who received efavirenz, regardless of the type of NRTI used [26].

Genetics

Polymorphisms in genes involved in adipocyte apoptosis and metabolism have also been implicated [3], including ones involved in the pyrimidine pathway or encoding potentially relevant enzymes, cytokines or peptides such as polymerase γ, matrix metalloproteinase 1, TNF-α, IL-1β, IL-6, resistin and mitochondrial haplogroups.

Clinical features

Presentation

Most patients present with a gradual loss of subcutaneous fat from the face, arms and legs. Facial involvement is present in 38–52% of HIV patients with lipodystrophy [3]. Fat loss from the suprazygomatic and temporal regions of the face can be severe enough to impart a stigmatizing emaciated appearance. Patients may also accumulate excess fat over the chin, breasts and waist, as well as over the upper back, producing a so-called 'buffalo hump' (Figure 100.3) [6].

Differential diagnosis

Generalized loss of body fat is commonly seen in HIV-infected patients with AIDS wasting syndrome. Patients with AIDS wasting syndrome have decreased body weight and lean body mass, without accumulation of excess fat over the chin, upper back, breasts or waist. Those with AIDS wasting syndrome also do not develop glucose intolerance or hyperinsulinaemia, although they may have hypertriglyceridaemia [6]. Other differential diagnoses to consider include Cushing syndrome and iatrogenic lipodystrophy related to testosterone therapy.

Classification of severity

Scoring systems have been developed to quantify facial lipoatrophy. In one, the score ranges from 0 (absent) to 4 (severe), depending

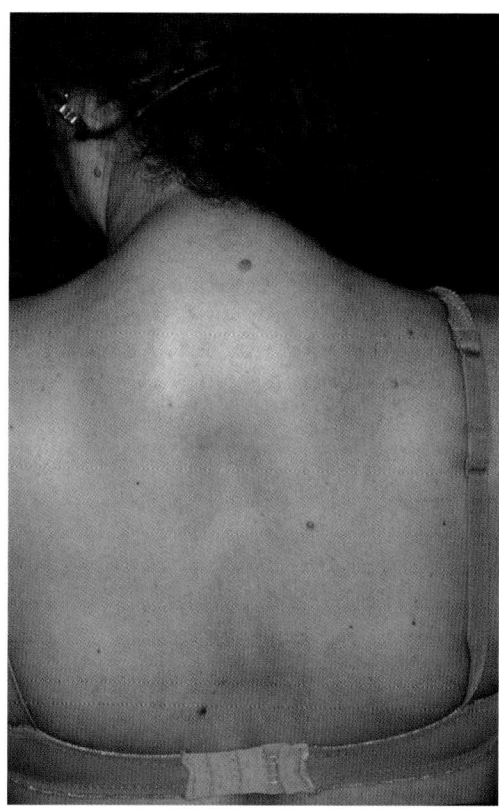

Figure 100.3 Buffalo hump appearance in an HIV patient with lipodystrophy. (Courtesy of Professor L. Requena, Universidad Autónoma de Madrid, Spain.)

on the degree of malar depression, presence or absence of buccal extension and defined melolabial ridge [27]. Other scoring methods involve the use of various imaging modalities which may not be practical in the clinical setting [3].

Complications and co-morbidities

Complications are related to co-morbidities, including dyslipidaemia, impaired glucose intolerance, insulin resistance and coronary artery disease.

Disease course and prognosis

Lipodystrophy is progressive with ongoing HAART therapy [2]. While the possibility of subcutaneous fat recovery exists, it is typically slow and incomplete [3].

Management

There is no established algorithm for the management of HIV-associated lipodystrophy. Management is challenging and requires multidisciplinary input from infectious disease specialists, endocrinologists, nutritionists and primary care physicians. The stigma associated with facial lipodystrophy in particular may have a profound psychosocial impact and psychological support may be required.

Modification of previously successful antiretroviral therapy may increase the risk of treatment failure and must be done in consultation with an infectious disease specialist. Modest improvement in lipoatrophy has been reported with the removal of NRTIs [28]. While metabolic derangements such as dyslipidaemia and insulin resistance seem to be partly reversible if PI therapy is discontinued, lipodystrophy is usually unchanged [3].

Low-calorie or low-fat, high-fibre diets combined with aerobic exercise may improve central fat accumulation [29], although there is little evidence that diet or exercise significantly improves lipoatrophy [29–31]. Thiazolidinediones, which have been shown to induce adipocyte differentiation and increase subcutaneous fat mass, have been tried as pharmacological agents to treat lipoatrophy in HIV-infected patients with inconsistent results [32]. Uridine and pravastatin have been reported to improve lipoatrophy in small randomized trials, but these results need further confirmation [33,34]. Facial fillers such as injectable poly-L-lactic acid as well as autologous fat transfers have both been used to correct severe facial lipoatrophy [35,36].

Switching or discontinuing antiretroviral therapy has not been shown to reduce VAT [37,38]. Since growth hormone deficiency has been associated with visceral adiposity in the general population as well as in HIV patients with lipodystrophy, growth hormone supplementation with doses ranging from 0.33 to 6 mg daily has been tried [39,40]: patients with abdominal lipohypertrophy achieved a 10–20% reduction in VAT and 6–7% reduction in SAT in two studies involving the administration of growth hormone [41,42]. The improvement was lost once therapy was discontinued. Treatment with tesamorelin, a growth hormone-releasing hormone analogue that closely mimics the physiological dose and function of its physiological counterpart, showed a 15.2% reduction in VAT, compared with a 5% increase in VAT in the placebo group ($P <0.001$), at 6 months in a large, randomized, double-blind, placebo-controlled study [43].

Surgical interventions such as liposuction have been used to remove excess fat from the anterior neck, breasts and abdominal compartment [44–46]. However, liposuction cannot remove intra-abdominal visceral fat. Furthermore, approximately 25% of patients will experience recurrence of lipohypertrophy after liposuction.

Localized lipoatrophy and/or lipodystrophy

Localized lipoatrophy and/or lipodystrophy is a heterogeneous group of disorders presenting as one or multiple depressions of various sizes, ranging from a few centimetres to greater than 20 cm in diameter.

Semicircular lipoatrophy

Definition and nomenclature

Semicircular lipoatrophy (SL) is characterized by localized, often bilateral, symmetrical, transverse, semicircular depressions across the anterolateral aspects of the thighs due to atrophy of the underlying subcutaneous fat.

Synonyms and inclusions
- Lipoatrophia semicircularis

Introduction and general description

First described in the German literature in 1974 [1], SL is characterized by localized, symmetrical and often bilateral, transverse, semicircular depressions over the anterolateral thighs [1–3].

Epidemiology

Incidence and prevalence

Semicircular lipoatrophy is probably commoner than the small number of reported cases (about 100) would suggest. [2,4,5].

Age

Most SL cases present in the third or fourth decades of life [6], although it has also been reported among children and the elderly [4].

Sex

The majority of cases occur in women [3].

Pathophysiology

The aetiology of SL is unclear. An older theory related the presence of SL to impaired circulation in the upper leg as a consequence of a congenital abnormality in the lateral femoral circumflex artery [7]. However, patients with arteritis or those whose quadriceps artery has been ligated do not develop SL [8].

An anomaly of fat metabolism in these patients has also been proposed [8,9].

A current and more plausible explanation associates SL with repeated mechanical pressure as a form of microtrauma to the thighs [10,11]. Suggested mechanisms include repeatedly standing or sitting in an unvarying position in which the affected area is constantly compressed by or knocked against various objects [1,12]. Wearing constricting jeans or use of an elastic girdle has also been implicated [3,13–15].

In cases where clusters of co-workers are affected in the same company, repetitive pressure against desk furniture has been identified. In those cases, the height of the depression on the leg measured from the floor plus the height of the shoe heel were constant and the same as the height of the desk [12,16]. In a recent company-wide case–control study, the only statistically significant variables for SL development are female sex and leaning of thighs against the edge of the table [6].

Pathology
The histopathology findings in SL are non-specific. There is partial or complete loss of fat in the affected area with replacement by newly formed collagen [5,17].

Clinical features

Presentation
Semicircular lipoatrophy is characterized by localized, transverse, semicircular depressions, 2–4 cm in width, that are often symmetrical and bilateral. These depressions may also appear band-like, and when more than one is present, they may appear in a parallel arrangement [2,3]. There is no preceding inflammation and the overlying skin is normal. The anterolateral thighs are commonly affected bilaterally. Unilateral cases have been described as well [2,10,11,18]. Multilocular and progressive lesions affecting the trunk and limbs were seen in one patient [19]. Although SL is usually asymptomatic, some patients complained of heavy legs, a burning sensation, cramps or pain after exercising [2,10,18,20].

Differential diagnosis
The differential diagnosis of SL includes other forms of localized lipoatrophy or lipodystrophy as described elsewhere in this chapter.

Disease course and prognosis
Semicircular lipoatrophy has an excellent prognosis as most cases resolve gradually upon withdrawal of repetitive trauma.

Investigations
Semicircular lipoatrophy is a clinical diagnosis and further investigation is rarely required [3,6].

Management
There are no established management guidelines for SL. However, lesions usually regress spontaneously after the removal of microtrauma over months to as long as 8 years [12]. Recurrences are possible, however [7,9].

Localized lipoatrophy due to injected drugs

Localized loss of subcutaneous fat can occur after intradermal, subcutaneous or intramuscular injection of certain drugs. The two most commonly implicated agents are insulin and corticosteroids and these are discussed in detail. Other injected medications or substances that have been implicated as causes of localized lipoatrophy include benzathine penicillin, vasopressin, human growth hormone, methotrexate, iron dextran and diphtheria–pertussis–tetanus (DPT) vaccine [1–4].

Insulin-induced localized lipoatrophy

Definition
Insulin-induced localized lipoatrophy is the loss of subcutaneous fat at the site of insulin injection [1].

Introduction and general description
Insulin-induced localized lipoatrophy was a common complication of insulin therapy prior to the development of purified insulin in the 1970s [2,3]. With the advent of human insulin, the incidence lipoatrophy has decreased dramatically [4].

Epidemiology

Incidence and prevalence
Prior to the introduction of purified human insulin, lipoatrophy occurred in 25–55% of patients using insulin. Since the introduction of highly purified insulin, it is estimated that less than 10% of patients are affected [5,6], although lipoatrophy is still reported with the use of recombinant human insulin, rapid-acting insulin analogues and continuous subcutaneous insulin infusion [4,7–11,12].

Age
Insulin-induced lipoatrophy occurs predominantly in children and young adults [13–15].

Sex
The risk is greater in females than males [16,17].

Pathophysiology
The pathogenesis of insulin-induced lipoatrophy is not completely understood. Lipolytic components or impurities in certain insulin preparations may have resulted in local allergic or immunological reactions. For example, a local immune reaction to insulin crystals with resultant dedifferentiation of adipocytes has been suggested [14,18]. An immune-mediated inflammatory process with release of lysosomal enzymes promoting lipoatrophy has also been proposed [19]. It has also been suggested that mast cells may play a pathogenetic role [12]: in one case series involving five patients with human insulin analogue-induced lipoatrophy, an elevated number of tryptase-positive, chymase-positive degranulated mast cells were seen in the subcutaneous tissue.

Predisposing factors
This form of lipoatrophy is more common among those with prior dermal reactions to insulin [1]. The use of older, less purified forms

PART 8: SPECIFIC CUTANEOUS STRUCTURE

of insulin such as bovine or porcine insulin conveys a higher risk of lipoatrophy [20]. Repeated use of the same injection site also increases the risk.

Pathology
Histopathology shows lobules of small adipocytes and lipomembranous changes [21]. A discrete lymphoid infiltration abutting the blood vessels in the hypodermis may also be observed [22].

Clinical features

Presentation
Insulin-induced lipoatrophy presents as a depressed plaque due to loss of subcutaneous fat at the site of insulin injection. The overlying and surrounding skin appear normal. Lipoatrophy normally presents after 6–24 months of insulin treatment [1]. Interestingly, there is concomitant lipohypertrophy in approximately 25% of patients [23].

Differential diagnosis
Other forms of localized lipoatrophy should be considered.

Complications and co-morbidities
Because insulin absorption from the lipoatrophic area is erratic, continued injection of insulin into affected areas may result in poor glycaemic control [22].

Management
The risk of lipoatrophy may be reduced by regular rotation of insulin injection sites. The importance of this should be explained to all patients who require insulin. Once lipoatrophy develops, continued injection into the lipoatrophic site should be avoided due to erratic absorption of insulin. Spontaneous resolution of established insulin-induced localized lipoatrophy is rare.

There is no generally agreed management algorithm but, if feasible, a change to purified human insulin is recommended. Several authors describe success in restoring fat by co-administration of a corticosteroid such as dexamethasone with the insulin [4,18,24,25]. Other strategies have included using an insulin jet-injection device [26] or a continuous insulin infusion pump [27], although lipoatrophy with the latter has also been reported [7,8]. Twice-daily application of 4% sodium cromoglycate prepared in petrolatum has been claimed to reverse early lipoatrophy and prevent new lesions in one small case series [12].

Localized lipoatrophy due to injected corticosteroid

Definition
Localized lipoatrophy due to injected corticosteroid is the localized loss of subcutaneous fat that occurs after intramuscular or intralesional injection of corticosteroids [1].

Introduction and general description
Injected depot preparations of corticosteroids have been widely used for their sustained systemic antiallergic and anti-inflammatory action for more than half a century. It was recognized at an early stage that they were capable of producing profound lipoatrophy if they were injected into subcutaneous fat.

Epidemiology

Incidence and prevalence
An overall incidence of local reactions following intralesional corticosteroid injection is reported to be 0.5%. These reactions include pain, panniculitis, haemorrhage, secondary infection, pigment alteration, hypersensitivity and atrophy [2]. Of all the persistent local reactions due to corticosteroids, atrophy is the most common [3].

Sex
Women appear to be at significantly greater risk than men [1,4]. In one early study, it was observed that lipoatrophy occurred in six of 14 women but in none of 13 men who received repeated intramuscular or deep subcutaneous injections of triamcinolone diacetate [4].

Pathophysiology
The exact pathogenesis is not clear but several factors are thought to be involved. It is believed that intramuscular injection of triamcinolone has a direct traumatic and a hormonally mediated destructive effect on fat cells [5]. In addition, decreased type I collagen and glycosaminoglycan synthesis has been noted following the injection of corticosteroid [6]. One common finding from histological analyses is the identification of a granular basophilic material in the dermis, thought to represent altered ground substance associated with deposits of corticosteroid crystals [5,7,8]. Cutaneous atrophy has been noted to resolve in parallel with the gradual disappearance of corticosteroid crystals from the tissue [7].

Predisposing factors
Compounds with low solubility, such as triamcinolone acetonide, injected at higher concentrations appear to be associated with greater risks of atrophy. One group of investigators noted that intralesional injections of triamcinolone acetonide at concentrations above 5 mg/cm^3 were associated with increased risks of cutaneous atrophy [9]. However, no lipoatrophy was observed at 6 and 12 weeks after injection in a series of 14 patients with dermatological conditions who had received one or two 30 mg or 60 mg doses of intramuscular triamcinolone acetonide [10].

Pathology
In addition to the presence of granular basophilic material associated with the deposition of corticosteroid, other histological findings include epidermal atrophy, homogenization of collagen, degeneration of sebaceous glands, decreased elastin and involution of subcutaneous fat lobules with small lipocytes separated by hyaline material [1,5,7,8,]. Inflammatory cells are not usually prominent although a sparse mononuclear cell infiltrate can be observed. There is no vascular inflammation [1].

Clinical features

Presentation
Patients present with an oval or circular depressed plaque at the site of prior injection (Figure 100.4). The overlying epidermis is usually normal, although telangiectasia, hypopigmentation or alopecia may occur [3]. There is no associated erythema or tenderness. Atrophy generally begins within weeks to 3 months after injection. The time course and extent of the atrophy depend on several factors, including the solubility and concentration of the corticosteroid used and the depth and anatomical location of the injection [5].

Differential diagnosis
Other forms of localized lipoatrophy should be considered.

Disease course and prognosis
The lipoatrophy may resolve spontaneously over the course of 1–2 years [11–14], although it may persist for longer in some cases [15].

Management
There is no established management guideline. In one small case series, four patients were treated by infiltration of the affected area with normal saline. All four patients demonstrated complete resolution of lipoatrophy and restoration of surface contour after 4–8 weekly injections. The injected volume ranged from 5 to 20 cm^3 per treatment session, depending on the size to be treated. The authors speculated that the efficacy of the treatment may be due to resuspension and redistribution of the poorly soluble corticosteroid crystals by saline solution [3].

Localized lipodystrophy secondary to panniculitis

Localized lipodystrophy may be secondary to inflammation of the subcutaneous fat, of which there are several aetiologies (see Chapter 99).

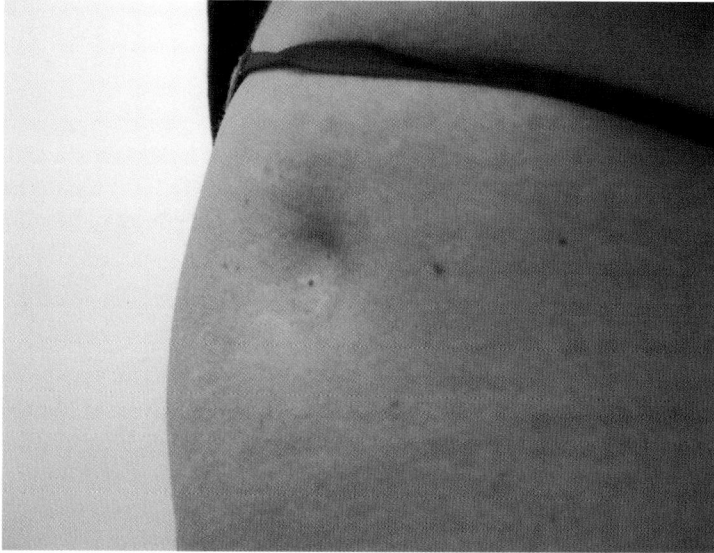

Figure 100.4 Delling of the skin over the right hip due to subcutaneous fat atrophy at the site of depot corticosteroid injection.

Centrifugal lipodystrophy

Definition and nomenclature
Centrifugal lipodystrophy (CLD) is a form of localized lipodystrophy in which atrophic plaques extend centrifugally.

Synonyms and inclusions
• Lipodystrophia centrifugalis abdominalis infantilis

Introduction and general description
Centrifugal lipodystrophy is characterized by localized lipoatrophy that expands centrifugally. Most cases of CLD have been reported from a single region of Japan. The condition predominantly affects children who are otherwise well. Because there have been a few cases of adult onset as well as of involvement of areas other than the abdomen, the term CLD may be more appropriate than lipodystrophia centrifugalis abdominalis infantilis.

Epidemiology

Incidence and prevalence
Centrifugal lipodystrophy is rare: approximately 170 cases have been described [1] since its initial report in 1971 by Imamura *et al.* [2].

Age
The majority (90%) of CLD patients develop the condition in the first 4 years of life with a mean of 2.4 years and a median of 2 years [1]. Very few patients have developed their initial lesions as an adult [1,3].

Sex
Girls outnumber boys by approximately 2 : 1 [1].

Ethnicity
Centrifugal lipodystrophy is reported almost exclusively among children of Asian descent, especially of Japanese origin [1,4,5,6]. There have been a few white patients reported from the USA [7], the UK [8,9], France [10], Italy [11], Germany [12] and Spain [13].

Associated diseases
Most CLD patients exhibit no other signs or symptoms of systemic illness. However, immunological abnormalities that have been reported include positive antinuclear antibodies [1], rheumatoid factor [10], antigliadin antibodies [12] and partial IgA deficiency [10,12].

Pathophysiology
The cause of CLD is unknown. It has been suggested that apoptosis may play a part in the fatty tissue degeneration of CLD but it is unclear if this is a primary event [14]. Fibrous long-spacing collagen has been observed on ultrastructural studies of lesional skin, although the relation of their presence to disease pathogenesis remains to be elucidated [15]. So far, no abnormalities of serum leptin levels have been reported [1].

Pathology

The epidermis and dermis in CLD are unaffected but there is markedly reduced or absent subcutaneous tissue in the affected areas. In the inflamed periphery of the plaque, the loss of subcutaneous fat is accompanied by a moderate mononuclear cell infiltrate. Rarely, multinucleated giant cells, foam cells, swelling of blood vessels, vasculitis and thrombosis have been observed [1].

Genetics

Centrifugal lipodystrophy has occurred in one pair of dizygotic twins and in one pair of affected siblings, which has raised the possibility of a genetic component of the disease [1].

Environmental factors

Although various external factors such as hernia, congenital dislocation of the hip, external pressure, injection or previous skin infection at the sites were reported in about 10% of the cases, no clear relationship has been established between CLD and environmental insults [1].

Clinical features

Presentation

Most cases of CLD begin with a single depressed plaque involving the groin (80%), axillae (20%) or neighbouring regions. Interestingly, in all reported non-Japanese cases, the initial plaque developed exclusively in or near the groin [1]. Less common areas of involvement include the neck, lower chin, retroauricular area or scalp [16,17]. The periphery of the atrophic plaque is typically erythematous while the centre is of normal colour or may have a violaceous or bluish hue. Ulceration of the plaques has been reported to occur rarely [1,18]. Plaques beginning in the groin area may expand to involve the genital region, abdominal wall or even the chest wall. Plaques developing in the axillary region may extend to the chest wall and abdominal wall. During the initial enlargement period, the atrophy may be multifocal. Although most lesions are asymptomatic, some patients report mild discomfort or tenderness [1]. Regional lymph nodes are enlarged in 65% of cases. When the lesion stops expanding, the erythematous rim and lymphadenopathy tend to resolve.

Differential diagnosis

Differential diagnosis of CLD includes other localized lipodystrophies.

Complications and co-morbidities

Patients with CLD usually do not suffer from any complications and co-morbidities, except for rare instances of ulceration involving plaques [1,18]. A case of angioblastoma developing in a non-regressing CLD lesion lasting into adulthood has been reported. The angioblastoma responded to resection followed by radiation therapy [19].

Disease course and prognosis

The atrophic area slowly enlarges centrifugally for 3–8 years, often stopping with the onset of puberty. By 13 years, 82% of cases show no residual inflammation at the periphery and 65% no longer have regional lymphadenopathy.

The atrophic portion may subsequently improve but may remain depressed [1]. Hair regrowth has been observed in cases of scalp involvement [16,17].

Investigations

Results of routine laboratory tests are unremarkable.

Management

There is no established guideline for the management of CLD. Many topical therapies have been tried including topical steroids, pimecrolimus, vitamin A cream and dimethyl sulfoxide. Various systemic therapies have been attempted including corticosteroids, chloroquine, penicillin, vitamin E and ibuprofen. None of these have been effective in preventing enlargement, although topical and systemic steroids occasionally reduced the inflammation at the periphery of the plaque [1]. Psoralen with UVA was reported to be effective in softening the skin and preventing further enlargement in one case [4].

FAT HYPERTROPHY

Fat hypertrophy is a circumscribed expansion of subcutaneous fat and is particularly associated with insulin injection sites. Fat hypertrophy is distinguished from lipomatosis in that the latter involves the formation of multiple foci of proliferating adipocytes.

Insulin-induced localized fat hypertrophy

Definition and nomenclature

Insulin-induced fat hypertrophy is a circumscribed increase in subcutaneous fat at the site or sites of repeated insulin injection by insulin-dependent diabetics.

Synonyms and inclusions
- Insulin-induced lipohypertrophy

Introduction and general description

Insulin-induced fat hypertrophy was, and still is, the most common cutaneous complication of insulin therapy [1]. It is thought to be due to the direct local anabolic and lipogenic effects of insulin on adipocytes.

Epidemiology

Incidence and prevalence

With highly purified human insulin, the prevalence of fat hypertrophy is approximately 30% in patients with type 1 diabetes and less than 5% in patients with type 2 diabetes [2].

Age

No specific age of onset has been identified, although the condition is generally believed to be associated with a young age [2].

Pathophysiology

The fat hypertrophy is thought to be secondary to the anabolic and lipogenic effect of insulin [1,2]. Although insulin antibodies are associated with fat hypertrophy in children and adolescents with type 1 diabetes, it is not known whether they play a role in its pathogenesis [3,4].

Predisposing factors

Several factors have been associated with the development of the fat hypertrophy. These include recent insulin initiation, low body mass index (BMI), use of the abdomen as the injection site and infrequent rotation of the injection site [2].

Pathology

Histological examination shows lobules of large mature adipocytes. Electron microscopy has revealed discrete populations of small adipocytes, suggesting differentiation or proliferation [5].

Clinical features

Presentation

The disorder presents as soft subcutaneous swellings at the sites of insulin injection (Figure 100.5) The overlying epidermis is normal. Because the involved skin tends to be hypoaesthetic relative to uninvolved skin, patients often continue to inject insulin preferentially into affected sites [1].

Differential diagnosis

Localized cutaneous amyloidosis has been associated with insulin injection sites and may be mistaken for insulin-induced fat hypertrophy [6]. Furthermore, insulin *per se* has been identified as one of the proteins that can form amyloid fibrils [7]. Affected skin feels firmer on palpation than that overlying insulin-induced fat hypertrophy and is unlikely to improve after changing the insulin injection site [1].

Complications and co-morbidities

Because the lipohypertrophic nodules have decreased vascularity, impaired insulin absorption at these sites may result in poor glycaemic control [1,8–10].

Disease course and prognosis

Regression of insulin-induced lipohypertrophy is possible once management is instituted.

Management

To prevent the development of fat hypertrophy, patients requiring insulin injections should be advised of the importance of changing injection sites regularly [2]. No universal treatment guideline has been established in the management of this problem. Rotation of injection sites is recommended with the anticipation that existing nodules will regress [1]. Most patients requiring insulin will nowadays be prescribed biosynthetic human insulin analogues, which carry a lower risk of inducing fat hypertrophy. If they are not, changing to human insulin, particularly the short-acting, rapidly absorbed preparations, may help to reverse the condition [11]. Changing the insulin delivery method from injection to continuous subcutaneous infusion using a pump has also been advocated. This method of

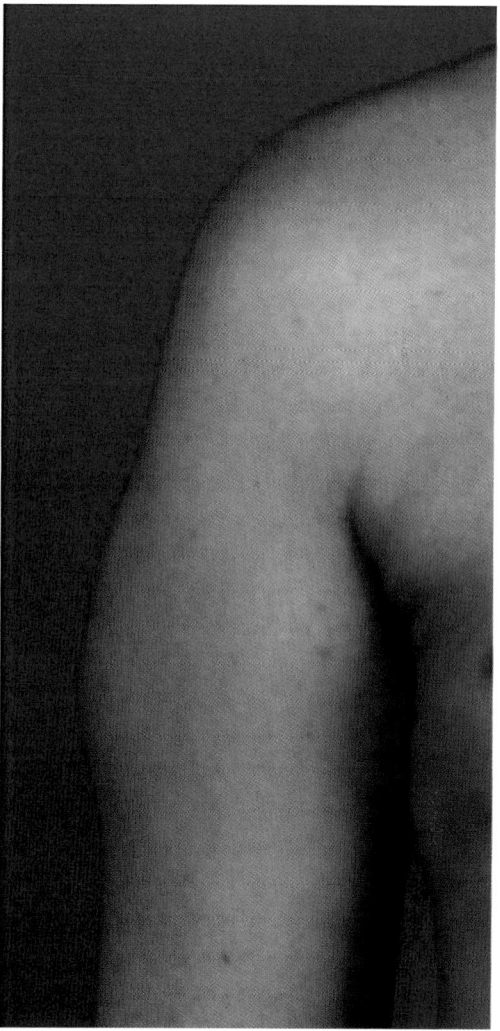

Figure 100.5 Insulin-induced fat hypertrophy of the lateral aspect of the upper arm.

administration reduces overall insulin requirements and is therefore thought to lessen the overall stimulus to lipogenesis [1]. If the above strategies fail, some patients will demand removal of the excess fat. Liposuction has achieved good cosmetic results [12,13].

SUBCUTANEOUS LIPOMATOSIS

Benign symmetrical lipomatosis

Definition and nomenclature

Benign symmetrical lipomatosis (BSL) is an uncommon condition characterized by multiple, symmetrical, unencapsulated fatty tissue deposits throughout the body.

Synonyms and inclusions
- Madelung disease
- Multiple symmetrical lipomatosis
- Launois–Bensaude adenolipomatosis

Introduction and general description

What subsequently came to be known as Madelung disease was first mentioned by Brodie in 1846 [1]. Madelung described a series of patients with the lipomatosis in 1888 [2] and Launois and Bensaude reported it again 10 years later [3]. More recently, the term benign symmetrical lipomatosis has been preferred for this uncommon condition. It is characterized by multiple, symmetrical, unencapsulated fatty tissue deposits involving multiple areas of the body, particularly the neck, shoulder girdle and the proximal upper and lower extremities.

Epidemiology

Incidence and prevalence

The exact incidence and prevalence of BSL is not known. The incidence in Italy has been estimated to be 1 : 25 000 [4]. There are, however, less than 300 cases reported in the literature since its initial description [5].

Age

The age of onset ranges from 30 to 60 years old [6]. However, a few paediatric cases have been reported [7,8].

Sex

Benign symmetrical lipomatosis is a disorder that predominantly affects males, with a reported male : female ratio as high as 31 : 1 [1,6,9–11].

Ethnicity

Historically, BSL has been linked to people of Mediterranean descent [1]. However, cases from non-Mediterranean ethnicities have been described [5,12,13].

Associated diseases

Many conditions are associated with BSL. These include alcohol abuse, chronic hepatic disorders possibly related to the underlying alcohol abuse, lipid abnormalities, arterial hypertension, chronic obstructive pulmonary disease (COPD), gynaecomastia, hypothyroidism, peripheral neuropathy, diabetes, hyperuricaemia and myoclonic epilepsy and ragged red fibres (MERRF) syndrome [1,7,8,10,14–16]. In one study of 22 patients from Spain, 95.5% of the patients had high alcohol intake and 59.1% had some form of hepatic disease. Furthermore, 77% of these patients were reported to be regular smokers. Statistics of reported associations include 41% with dyslipidaemia, 27% with gynaecomastia, 23% with arterial hypertension, 23% with COPD, 14% with hyperuricaemia, 9% with hypothyroidism and 4.5% with type 2 diabetes [1].

Peripheral neuropathy, polyneuropathy and autonomic dysfunction are also common findings among BSL patients [11,17–19,20] and it may be the presenting symptom in some [21]. However, there is controversy as to whether these neurological manifestations are directly related to BSL or are the result of alcoholism.

Compression symptoms affecting the respiratory and digestive tracts are thought to be directly due to fatty masses in the anterior neck and, in one case series, were the symptoms that in all cases occasioned their patients' initial consultation [1].

Pathophysiology

While many theories on the pathogenesis of BSL exist, a role for brown fat in BSL has garnered attention. Although, grossly and histologically, the accumulated adipose tissue in BSL is indistinguishable from mature fat [1], ultrastructural analysis of adipose tissue deposits in BSL suggests that it resembles brown fat [22]. Further support for the role of brown fat in BSL came from another study that demonstrated mRNA expression of brown adipose tissue-specific uncoupling protein-1 (UCP-1) in a lipoma of a patient with BSL, but not in the normal subcutaneous fat from the same patient [23]. Brown fat hypertrophy has been proposed to result from functional sympathetic denervation [22], or from alterations in the synthesis of intracellular cyclic adenosine monophosphate (cAMP) under noradrenergic stimulation [24].

Pathology

Lipomatous tissue in BSL consists of small adipocytes with no atypical features and a slight increase in vascular and fibrous elements. The lipomas are typically not encapsulated and may infiltrate across fasciomuscular and neurovascular planes [25].

Genetics

Genetic alternations in mitochondrial DNA have been demonstrated in BSL patients [18,26]. Most reported BSL cases have been sporadic, although a very small number of familial cases exist for which autosomal recessive inheritance has been proposed [27].

Clinical features

Presentation

Fatty masses develop most commonly on the neck (Figure 100.6), shoulder girdle and proximal upper and lower extremities. Other less common locations include the retroauricular and submandibular areas [28], tongue [21], mammary region [22], abdomen [7] and perineum or scrotum [29]. Although rare, laryngeal involvement resulting in a compromised airway has been described [12,30–33]. The fatty deposits are slow growing and progressive over many years. In contrast to Dercum disease, the fatty growths in BSL are not tender or painful.

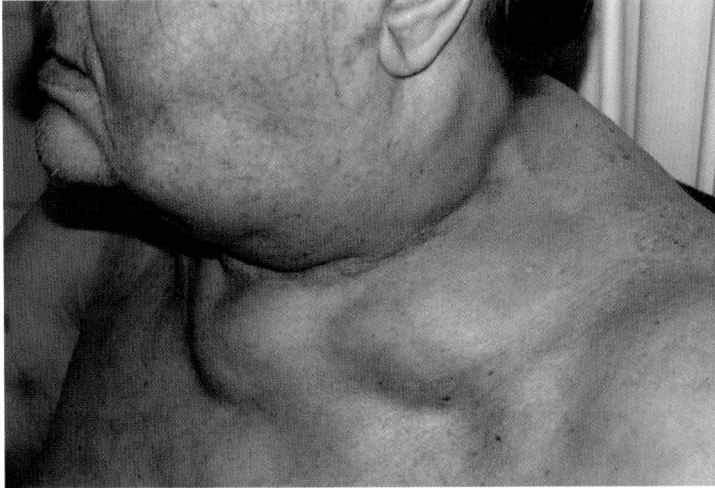

Figure 100.6 Non-tender fatty deposits around the neck in a patient with benign symmetrical lipomatosis. (Courtesy of Professor L. Requena, Universidad Autónoma de Madrid, Spain.)

Clinical variants
Enzi's classification of BSL is the most widely accepted [6]. In type I BSL, fatty deposits are mainly distributed around the neck, shoulders, supraclavicular fossa and proximal regions of the upper extremities. In type II BSL, more caudal regions of the body are involved, while the neck is unaffected. As a consequence, type II BSL patients may appear similar to obese patients.

Differential diagnosis
Differential diagnosis of BSL includes obesity, Dercum disease and familial multiple lipomatosis. Genetic syndromes presenting with multiple lipomas such as Cowden syndrome, Bannayan–Riley–Ruvalcaba syndrome, multiple endocrine neoplasia type 1 (MEN1) and Gardner syndrome can be differentiated from BSL by the presence of other disease-specific clinical features.

Complications and co-morbidities
Respiratory or digestive symptoms may develop if the lipomatosis from the anterior neck is significant enough to compress vital structures. There have been a few cases of head and neck cancer, especially squamous cell carcinoma, reported in patients with BSL [9,34]. However, it is possible that this simply reflects the increased alcohol and tobacco consumption observed among BSL patients. Malignant transformation of lipoma into liposarcomas in BSL has been reported only twice [35,36].

Disease course and prognosis
The lipomatous masses are slow growing and progressive. There are few long-term follow-up data on BSL patients. In one study, however, in which 31 BSL patients were observed for up to 26 years, three of the eight deaths observed were sudden and occurred in patients with autonomic neuropathy in the absence of coronary artery disease or history of cardiac disease [20].

Investigations
The diagnosis of BSL is based on clinical presentation and disease history. Chest radiographs may show abnormal symmetrical mass lesions due to accumulations of adipose tissue. MRI is the best diagnostic tool in evaluation of the spread of adipose tissue, presence of tracheal compression, vascular topography within the fat mass and exclusion of synchronous malignant disease [36,37].

Management
There is no established guideline for the management of BSL. A thorough clinical review, especially for respiratory symptoms, should be carried out at each visit to check for signs of compression or for the rare occurrence of malignant transformation.

Medical treatments have been tried with generally poor results. Oral salbutamol, which induces lipolysis by adrenergic stimulation, has been tested on BSL patients but the results have been disappointing [24]. Fibrate has been claimed to stop the growth or even reduce the volume of fatty masses in BSL patients [38]. Among BSL patients who reported alcohol abuse, abstinence from alcohol has had mixed results in preventing the progression or recurrence of the lesions after surgical treatment [1,39]. General weight loss does not seem to be effective in reducing fatty masses [1].

Open surgery, lipectomy and liposuction, with or without ultrasound assistance, have been tried with varying success rates. Liposuction is less traumatic, has a lower complication rate and produces less scarring than open surgery [40–45]. However, because the fatty deposits are unencapsulated and diffusely infiltrate muscles and vessels without a clear plane for dissection, open surgery with direct observation of important structures is a safer approach in certain anatomical regions where liposuction may be too dangerous [1,45]. Some authors advocate ultrasound-assisted liposuction which can treat multiple areas in a single session and produces limited scarring.

Regardless of the mode of surgical intervention, multiple procedures are often required, especially given the high rates of recurrence [1,46,47]. In one study, BSL patients underwent an average of 3.3 open surgical procedures with a 51% recurrence rate. Isolated lipoaspiration had a 95% recurrence rate in the same study. Recurrence rates vary by anatomical site and are highest following procedures on the arms and pectoral region. The average time taken for fat to reaccumulate after a surgical intervention is approximately 21 months [1].

Emergency intervention is needed when compression symptoms develop. In rare cases where the fatty tissue deposits extend to the mediastinum and compress the trachea, a tracheostomy may be required [20].

Dercum disease

Definition and nomenclature
Dercum disease is a rare disease characterized by generalized overweight status or obesity and pronounced pain in the adipose tissue with or without the presence of lipomas.

Synonyms and inclusions
- Adiposis dolorosa
- Morbus Dercum
- Adiposalgia
- Lipomatosis dolorosa
- Adipose tissue rheumatism
- Neurolipomatosis

Introduction and general description
Dercum disease was first described in 1888 [1]. The disease is characterized by diffuse or localized pain involving adipose tissue, usually affecting those who are overweight or obese. Patients experience a number of other somatoform symptoms, and management of the condition is a challenge.

Epidemiology

Incidence and prevalence
The exact incidence and prevalence of Dercum disease is not known.

Age
Dercum disease most commonly presents between the ages 35 and 50 years [2,3]. While it was initially proposed that Dercum disease

affects postmenopausal women, a recent survey revealed that 86% of patients developed their symptoms prior to the menopause [3].

Sex

Dercum disease is 5–30 times more common in women than in men [3,4].

Ethnicity

No known ethnic predilection has been identified.

Associated diseases

Although various symptoms or diseases have been observed in these patients, none are consistently associated. These include easy bruising, sleep disturbances, impaired memory, depression, difficulty concentrating, anxiety, rapid heart beat, shortness of breath, diabetes, bloating, constipation, fatigue, weakness and joint and muscle aches [3,5].

Pathophysiology

While the exact aetiology of Dercum disease is not known, many theories have been proposed. A local defect in lipid metabolism has been considered. One study showed a difference in the formation of long-chain mono-unsaturated fatty acids between the painful adipose tissue and the unaffected adipose tissue in the same patient [6]. Another study showed that the proportion of monosaturated fatty acids was significantly higher in Dercum disease patients than in healthy controls [7].

Painful adipose tissue from a Dercum disease subject was found to have significantly lower conversion rate of glucose to neutral glycerides than non-painful adipose tissue from the same subject [8]. *In vitro* analysis demonstrated that painful adipose tissue had reduced responsiveness to norepinephrine and lack of response to the antilipolytic effect of insulin compared with non-painful adipose tissue [9].

Roles of various inflammatory factors have also been investigated. Higher levels of IL-13 and significantly lower macrophage inflammatory protein 1β and fractalkine expression were seen in Dercum disease patients. Fractalkine is a unique chemokine that is constitutively expressed by neurons. When fractalkine receptors are occupied, pain and resistance to opioid analgesia are promoted, which is in concordance with symptoms in Dercum disease [10].

Other theories for pain in Dercum disease have included endocrine dysfunction [9,11–16] as well as autonomic nervous system dysfunction [17] and stretching of and pressure on nerves by the growing fatty masses [18,19].

The significance of these observations is, however, unclear and their contribution to disease pathogenesis remains to be elucidated.

Pathology

When lipomas are present, they show the typical histological features of lipomas without inflammation or vascular abnormalities [20].

Genetics

The majority of cases occur sporadically [5]. An autosomal dominant inheritance with variable expression has also been reported [2,21,22,**23**,24,25]. HLA typing has not been revealing [9]. A to G mutation at position A8344 of mitochondrial DNA, which is some-

times associated with familial multiple lipomas, is not detected [24,26].

Clinical features

Presentation

The main symptom in Dercum disease is the either abrupt or indolent onset of pain in adipose tissue [1]. Lipomas may or may not be present in these patients, who are typically obese. Patients have most commonly described the pain as burning or aching of the subcutaneous tissue. Some experience spontaneous paroxysmal attacks of pain [5,27]. The most common locations of painful fat and lipomas are the extremities (Figure 100.7), trunk, pelvic area and buttocks [3]. The head and neck are spared [27]. Interestingly, patients experience more pain in the medial aspects of the involved extremities [5]. Lipomas, when present, vary in size and firmness [3].

While fatigue and psychiatric manifestations were initially included as cardinal symptoms of Dercum disease [28], subsequent literature has not supported this claim. Certainly, not all patients with Dercum disease exhibit psychiatric symptoms [29,30]. More recently, an association between BMI and anxiety and personality disorders has been noted [31]. It has also been proposed that pain and obesity in Dercum disease may contribute to the psychiatric manifestations seen in some patients [5].

Clinical variants

Various classifications have been proposed over the years [5,16,27,28]. In 2012, Hansson and colleagues proposed the following classification [5]:

I Generalized diffuse form: widespread painful adipose tissue without clear lipomas.

II Generalized nodular form: general pain in adipose tissue and intense pain in and around multiple lipomas.

III Localized nodular form: pain in and around multiple lipomas.

IV Juxta-articular form: pain in solitary deposits of excess fat, for example at the medial aspect of the knee.

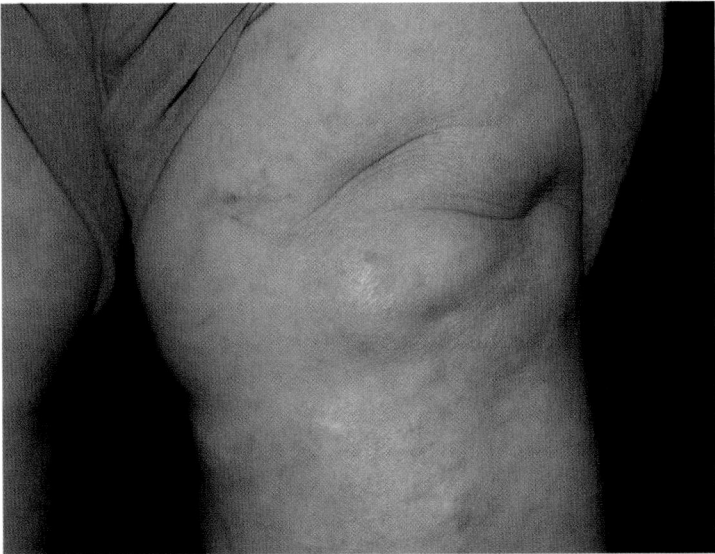

Figure 100.7 Painful lipomas on the lower extremity of a patient with Dercum disease. (Courtesy of Professor L. Requena, Universidad Autónoma de Madrid, Spain.)

Differential diagnosis

Many diseases have similar symptoms to those of Dercum disease. For the generalized diffuse form, fibromyalgia, lipoedema, panniculitis and primary psychiatric disorders may be considered in the differential.

Other types of Dercum disease must be differentiated from conditions that may include solitary or multiple lipomas, as they may also sometimes be painful. These include multiple symmetrical lipomatosis, familial multiple lipomatosis, adipocytic tumours, neurofibromatosis type 1, MEN1 and MERRF syndrome. MERRF syndrome is a disease of mitochondria which is sometimes accompanied by non-painful lipomas.

Complications and co-morbidities

The lipomas in Dercum disease may in rare instances become necrotic [32] or may compress visceral organs [33,34]. Other co-morbidities are mostly related to the associated obesity or the psychiatric morbidity.

Disease course and prognosis

Very little is known about the natural progression of Dercum disease. Several case reports suggest that the pain gets worse over time [25]. However, in one long-term study of patients with the condition, pain seemed to be relatively constant over the 5-year study period [35].

Investigations

Diagnosis is based on clinical criteria after a thorough physical examination and exclusion of the differential diagnoses discussed earlier [5]. There are no laboratory markers for the condition and laboratory tests for inflammatory and autoimmune disease are typically negative [3,36–38].

Management

Overall, there is little evidence on which to base treatment of Dercum disease. Management may be best achieved through a multidisciplinary approach involving multiple specialists including dermatologists, surgeons, pain specialists, psychiatrists and psychologists.

Pain in this setting has been observed to be refractory to traditional analgesics and non-steroidal anti-inflammatory drugs (NSAIDs) [8,20,23,39–46]. However, this experience has been challenged recently after a study found that pain diminished in 89% of patients when treated with NSAIDs and in 97% when treated with narcotics [3].

Topical lidocaine with or without prilocaine [38,47,48], intralesional lidocaine [49] and intravenous lidocaine [8,36,40,42,50–52] have also been tried with varying degrees of success. Pain relief from intravenous lidocaine infusion lasted from 10 h [50] to 12 months [40].

Systemic corticosteroids have been reported to improve pain in some [15,23,53], while worsening it in other patients [54]. Two patients with juxta-articular Dercum disease treated with intralesional corticosteroids experienced dramatic improvement of pain [55]. Methotrexate alone [25] and in combination with infliximab [56], pregabalin or oxacarbazepine [16,37,57,58] has also been used. Two patients with concurrent Dercum disease and hepatitis C were successfully treated with interferon α-2b [59].

A more recent small pilot study involving 10 patients showed that rapid cycling hypobaric pressure may decrease pain [60].

Procedure-based approaches with suction-assisted liposuction [35] and lipectomy [4,18–20,61–63] have also been tried. However, pain often recurs after these procedures.

Infiltrating lipomatosis of the face

Definition

Infiltrating lipomatosis of the face is a disorder where the unilateral overgrowth of unencapsulated benign and mature but invasive adipocytes involves the lower two-thirds of the face.

Introduction and general description

Infiltrating lipomatosis of the face (IL-F) is a disorder characterized by unilateral overgrowth of unencapsulated benign and mature but invasive adipocytes involving the lower two-thirds of the face. Although it usually presents at birth (congenital infiltrating lipomatosis of the face) it may present in adolescence or early adulthood. It is associated with soft tissue and bony hypertrophy [1,2]. IL-F patients have normal psychomotor development [3].

Epidemiology

Incidence and prevalence

Infiltrating lipomatosis of the face is a rare disorder with approximately 50 cases reported in the world literature [1–4,5–12,13,14–26].

Age

Although most cases present at birth, adolescent and early adulthood presentations have also been reported. All reported cases presented during the first three decades of life [23].

Sex

There is no gender predilection [3].

Ethnicity

There is no racial predilection.

Pathophysiology

The pathogenesis of IL-F is unknown. Given the tissue overgrowth, IL-F has been postulated to be part of the spectrum of overgrowth syndromes. *PTEN* and *RET* mutations have been excluded. Though no mutation has been found, IL-F is generally considered to be the result of secondary somatic mutation at some point in early development [13].

A study evaluating the expression of angiogenic and vasculogenic factors refuted a role for neovascularization in the pathogenesis of IL-F [27].

Pathology

In the initial case description, Slavin *et al.* described the histopathological features of IL-F, which include infiltration of mature benign adipocytes into adjacent soft tissue with hypertrophy of the underlying skeleton. They also emphasized the absence of malignant characteristics and lipoblasts but found an increase in fibrous elements with focal fibrosis affecting nerve bundles and vessels with unifocally thickened muscular walls [2].

Causative organisms
Two patients with IL-F have been found to have cytomegalovirus inclusions within the secretory cells of the parotid gland. However, the relationship between cytomegalovirus and IL-F remains unclear [6,8].

Clinical features

Presentation
Patients with IL-F present with unilateral facial swelling that is typically present at birth or in early childhood although it may be delayed until early adult life [23]. The facial swelling is due to the proliferation of unencapsulated benign and mature adipocytes as well as associated soft tissue and bony hypertrophy. There is a wide range of clinical presentations depending on the extent of involvement of the underlying tissue. The lower two-thirds of the face is most commonly involved [1].

Macroglossia and mucosal neuromas on the tongue and buccal mucosa have also been reported [13,19,21], as have dental abnormalities such as abnormal tooth formation[7], root hypoplasia [23] and early eruption of deciduous and permanent teeth on the affected side [13,20,21,23]. A cutaneous capillary blush, usually occurring after resection, has also been reported [13].

Differential diagnosis
Differential diagnosis of IL-F includes other hamartomatous or overgrowth syndromes such as Proteus syndrome, vascular or lymphatic malformations and trauma, as well as benign and malignant neoplasms of the bone and/or soft tissue. MEN2b, Bannayan–Riley–Ruvalcaba syndrome and Cowden syndrome should be considered since they are also associated with mucosal neuromas [13,21]. Congenital hemifacial hyperplasia shares some features with IL-F but this condition does not involve lipocytic infiltration [13,21]. Conditions causing contralateral hypoplasia, such as hemifacial microsomia and progressive hemifacial atrophy (Romberg syndrome) should be excluded [20]. Other disorders of fat tissue infiltration such as liposarcoma or lipoblastomatosis may be ruled out based on histological findings [15,16].

Complications and co-morbidities
Complications and co-morbidities arising from IL-F depend on the extent of involvement of the underlying soft tissue and bone. The lipomatosis itself is benign, although cosmesis may be significantly altered. Resection of IL-F risks injury to vital structures such as the facial nerve.

Investigations
Imaging with MRI provides the best delineation [13].

Management
Management of IL-F involves resection of the tumour followed by reconstruction. The resection is almost always subtotal due to the infiltrative nature of the tumour into vital structures and carries a risk of injury to the facial nerve. On average, IL-F patients undergo at least three surgical procedures [9] with a recurrence rate that is as high as 62.5% with surgical resection alone [14].

The timing of surgery remains controversial. While earlier reports advocated early and wide local excision to prevent extensive lipomatous infiltration [2,9], more recent literature favours delayed resection with temporizing measures such as liposuction, excision of mucosal neuromas and surgery to the upper lip to restore facial symmetry [13]. By delaying the resection until early adulthood it is believed that the chances of facial nerve damage and the total number of debulking procedures required are diminished [5]. It has also been conjectured that growth hormone may play a role in recurrences, implying that mass reduction attempts prior to the end of adolescence may be more likely to fail [13]. Recently, a case of IL-F demonstrating C-KIT and platelet-derived growth factor receptor oncogene expression was treated with imatinib after subtotal surgical resection. At 18 months follow-up, the patient showed no disease progression [1].

Encephalocraniocutaneous lipomatosis

Definition and nomenclature
Encephalocraniocutaneous lipomatosis (ECCL) is a rare, neurocutaneous syndrome characterized by profound mental retardation, early onset of seizures, unilateral temporofrontal lipomatosis, ipsilateral cerebral and leptomeningeal lipomatosis, cerebral malformation and calcification, and lipomas of the skull, eye and heart.

Synonyms and inclusions
- Haberland syndrome
- Fishman syndrome

Introduction and general description
Encephalocraniocutaneous lipomatosis is a rare, sporadic, neurocutaneous syndrome involving tissues of ectodermal and mesodermal origin. It is associated with profound mental retardation, early onset of seizures, unilateral temporofrontal lipomatosis, ipsilateral cerebral and leptomeningeal lipomatosis, cerebral malformation and calcification, and lipomas of the skull, eye and heart [1,2]. The hallmark skin finding is naevus psiloliparus, a fatty hamartomatous malformation, of the scalp [3]. The condition is typically present at birth or shortly after birth.

Epidemiology

Incidence and prevalence
Encephalocraniocutaneous lipomatosis is a rare disorder with about 60 cases reported in the English literature.

Age
Cutaneous and eye findings are usually present at or shortly after birth. Neurological manifestations may present at a later time.

Sex
There is no gender predilection.

Ethnicity
There is no racial or ethnic predilection.

Pathophysiology
The pathogenesis of ECCL is unknown. Most tissues affected in ECCL are of neural crest origin. In addition, because all the CNS anomalies are caused by a mesenchymal defect affecting tissues surrounding the brain or the vessels, and since no primary structural brain malformation is observed, it is postulated that a gene involved in vasculogenesis and the development of multiple mesenchymal tumours may be involved [4,5].

Pathology
The histopathology of naevus psiloliparus shows focal dermal fibrosis with subcutaneous fat in the reticular dermis.

Clinical features

Presentation
Patients with ECCL present with a wide spectrum of clinical manifestations. Naevus psiloliparus of the scalp is the most common skin finding and was present in 44/54 patients studied [6]. Unilateral or bilateral subcutaneous fatty masses are often seen in the frontotemporal or zygomatic region, and they are rarely seen outside the craniofacial region. Patchy or linear alopecia which is typically non-scarring is commonly observed: it may follow the lines of Blaschko or occasionally be scarring. Fibromas, lipomas and fibrolipomas present typically as ipsilateral skin tag-like cutaneous polyps on the eyelid or following a line from the outer canthus to the tragus. Less common cutaneous manifestations include irregular or disrupted eyebrows and café-au-lait macules [6].

Choristomas, with or without other eye anomalies, were observed in 43/54 patients [6] but other ocular abnormalities may also be seen.

Brain anomalies primarily involve the tissue surrounding the brain including blood vessels [4]. Intracranial lipomas are the most prominent feature; other features include meningeal and meningovascular anomalies and spinal cord lipomas, which may be extensive. CNS findings are frequently confined to the same body side as the cutaneous lesions. The spectrum of neurological manifestations of ECCL patients is broad, ranging from normal development to mental impairment of various degrees to intractable seizures. Less commonly, skeletal system involvement with jaw tumours or lytic bone lesions may be present; these may be progressive [5,7–10].

Congenital heart malformation, in particular aortic coarctation, is seen in about 10% of ECCL patients [6].

Differential diagnosis
This includes the Proteus syndrome, oculoectodermal syndrome, oculocerebrocutaneous syndrome and epidermal naevus syndrome [11–15].

Complications and co-morbidities
Complications and co-morbidities depend on the extent of organ system involvement.

Investigations
Investigations for suspected ECCL include a biopsy of suspected naevus psiloliparus lesions or 'skin tags' around the eye. Ophthalmological examination is required to detect associated ocular anomalies. Neuroimaging studies may characterize and assess the extent of CNS involvement [6]. Since fatty masses can involve the spinal cord, it is recommended that MRI of the spine be performed [6]. An electrocardiogram and an echocardiogram may help screen for cardiac problems.

Management
Treatment is symptomatic and requires multidisciplinary care.

LIPOEDEMA

Lipoedema is the term used to describe swelling of tissues due to abnormal accumulation of subcutaneous fat rather than fluid as seen in lymphoedema, with which it may be confused or coexist (lipo-lymphoedema). In the majority of cases it affects the lower extremities but it may also affect the upper extremities and the scalp. Hereafter the term lipoedema, if unqualified, will be used to denote lipoedema of the lower limbs.

Lipoedema of the lower limbs

Definition
Lipoedema is characterized by progressive, symmetrical and bilateral enlargement of involved areas due to subcutaneous deposition of fat.

Introduction and general description
Lipoedema, first described in 1940 [1], is characterized by progressive, symmetrical and bilateral enlargement due to subcutaneous deposition of fat occurring anywhere from the buttocks to the ankles with sparing of the feet [1,2]. Lipoedema occurs independently of lymphatic stasis or venous insufficiency. Imaging studies verify that oedema is minimal and the swelling is in fact due to homogenous enlargement of the subcutaneous compartment [3–8]. Its principal clinical features are summarized in Box 100.1 [2].

Epidemiology

Incidence and prevalence
The exact incidence and prevalence of lipoedema are unknown. It is probably underreported and often misdiagnosed due to unfamiliarity with this disorder [9,10,11,12]. In lymphoedema clinics, up to 15% of referred patients were diagnosed with lipoedema [13,14].

> **Box 100.1 Clinical characteristics of lipoedema** [2]
>
> - Occurrence is almost exclusively in women
> - Bilateral and symmetrical nature with minimal involvement of the feet
> - Minimal pitting oedema
> - Pain, tenderness and easy bruising
> - Persistent enlargement despite elevation of the affected extremities or weight loss

Age
Onset occurs during or soon after puberty [15].

Sex
Lipoedema occurs almost exclusively in women [1,2,9,16]. The condition has been reported only rarely in men [9,17].

Ethnicity
There is no racial or ethnic predilection.

Associated diseases
Most lipoedema patients do not have elevated lipids or other abnormal laboratory values [9,18]. One group of investigators found elevated plasma lipids as well as an abnormal fatty acid composition of tissue triglycerides in lipoedema patients relative to controls. However, the clinical significance of this finding is unclear [19].

Pathophysiology
The aetiology of lipoedema is unknown. Hormones appear to play a role in the development of lipoedema, given that it occurs almost exclusively in women with a typical onset near puberty or during periods of significant hormonal changes [1,2,9,16]. Moreover, male lipoedema cases occurred in those receiving hormonal therapy for prostate carcinoma or with hepatic cirrhosis [12,20].

The anatomy of the lymphatic vessel system in lipoedema patients has been found to be normal or sufficient, as far as the large lymph vessels are concerned [15]. The degree of insufficiency in lipoedema patients, if present, never however reached the level of true chronic venous insufficiency or lymphoedema [10,11,21,22]. The lymphatic transport in lipoedema decreases as the body ages and the fibrosis increases [15]. As a result, in longstanding cases, lipoedema and lymphoedema often coexist [12].

Predisposing factors
Although obese patients may be overrepresented, individuals with normal weight are also affected [1,2,9,16].

Pathology
No histological abnormalities have been identified by haematoxylin and eosin (H&E) stains, fat stains or electron microscopy [9,10,13,14,16–19].

Genetics
A significant portion (16–64%) of affected women have a self-reported positive family history of lipoedema [1,11,14]. *Pit-1* mutation was identified in female members of one family with multiple anterior pituitary hormone deficiency and lipoedema [23]. However, no other genetic mutations have been identified.

Clinical features

Presentation
The onset of symmetrical and bilateral gradual fat deposition starts around puberty in most cases. However, it may also develop during other periods of hormonal changes such as pregnancy or menopause [24].

Enlargement of the lower extremities is disproportionate in relation to the trunk, upper extremities, face and neck [15], even among obese patients [2,13]. Feet are generally spared. Fat deposition of lipoedema begins abruptly above the malleoli, causing a sharp demarcation between the normal and abnormal tissue at the ankles, which is known as the 'cuff sign'. The only sign during early stages of disease may be the disappearance of the retromalleolar sulcus. As the disease progress, this characteristic physical sign becomes more prominent. If the upper extremities are affected, a similar cuff sign that ends sharply above the wrists is seen with sparing of the hands [15]. Although the non to minimal pitting oedema component is mild initially, prominent oedema may eventually develop [15].

Patients often complain of heaviness and discomfort of the involved areas with sensitivity to pressure. The swelling and aching is aggravated by exercise and warm weather [15].

Clinical variants
A classification based on the location of involved areas has been proposed [25]:
- I Mostly buttocks.
- II Buttocks to knees.
- III Buttocks to malleoli.
- IV Mainly arms.
- V Mainly lower legs.

Differential diagnosis
Differential diagnosis of lipoedema includes lymphoedema, obesity, chronic venous insufficiency and lipohypertrophy (Table 100.1) [12,15,26]. In contrast to lipoedema, patients with lymphoedema have a positive Stemmer's sign where there is an inability to pinch a fold of skin at the base of the second toe due to thickening and fibrosis of the subcutaneous tissue. In obesity, the increase in subcutaneous fat is generalized and pain is not usually a feature; furthermore, the typical sparing of the feet is not seen in obese patients. Chronic venous insufficiency is associated with hyperpigmentation and, initially, pitting oedema that can be relieved by leg elevation; with time, however, lymphoedema may supervene. The main difference between lipohypertrophy and lipoedema is the absence of oedema and pain in lipohypertrophy [15]. Other differential diagnoses include Dercum disease and benign symmetrical lipomatosis.

Complications and co-morbidities
Mobility can be significantly impaired.

Table 100.1 Differential diagnosis of lipoedema.

	Lipoedema	Lymphoedema	Obesity	Chronic venous insufficiency
Sex	Female	Both	Both	Both
Family history	Frequent	Rare (except for Milroy disease)	Frequent	In some cases
Effect of leg elevation	Little to none	Initially with moderate improvement[a]	No effect	Marked improvement[b]
History of cellulitis	None	Frequent in secondary lymphoedema	None	Frequent
History of ulcers	None	None	None	Very frequent
Symmetry	Present	Absent	Present	Present or absent
Involvement of feet	No	Yes	Yes	Yes
Tenderness to palpation	Yes	No	No	Yes
Pilling oedema	None or minimal initially[c]	Present with varying severity	Absent	Marked[b]
Tissue consistency	May be soft, fat, or firm	Doughy, similar to gelatin	Soft, like fat	Soft, pitting

[a]Longstanding lymphoedema may not show improvement with leg elevation.

[b]Longstanding venous insufficiency may be complicated by lymphoedema, in which case this may not apply.

[c]Longstanding lipoedema may have pitting oedema.

Disease course and prognosis

Lipoedema is a progressive lifelong disorder.

Investigations

Lipoedema remains a clinical diagnosis. MRI may be used to verify that the swelling is due to homogenous enlargement of the subcutaneous compartment [3–8]. Dynamic lymphoscintigraphy can rule out true lymphoedema. Since venous disease can present concomitantly, duplex ultrasound is advocated by some if patients' complaints cannot be fully explained by lipoedema [15]. No specific abnormalities have been found in phlebograms or arteriograms from lipoedema patients [16,18,19].

Management

Management includes strategies to address the physical as well as psychological impact of the disease, and, as such, a multidisciplinary approach is necessary [15].

Management of diet is important because additional fat laid down in lipoedematous limbs may be abnormally resistant to control by dieting and exercise and will also compound the difficulties of taking adequate exercise, causing further frustration and low self-esteem [15,20,27]. Because BMI and total body weight may not accurately reflect obesity status in lipoedema patients, some authors advocate the use of waist circumference as an indicator for 'healthy weight' [15,28].

Diuretics and leg elevation do not help patients with lipoedema [11,13], although they may benefit patients with concomitant lymphoedema.

Complex physical decongestion therapy, which combines manual lymphatic drainage and compression therapy, is widely accepted as a conservative therapeutic approach [13,20,29,30]. While manual lymphatic drainage reduces the actual volume, compression by stocking or bandage is used to minimize recurrence. Compression therapy may improve, in part, the symptoms of lipoedema and also mitigate the progression of the lymphatic component. Certainly, patients with concomitant chronic venous insufficiency and/or lymphoedema will benefit from compression therapy [15]. In lipoedema patients, however, despite lifelong decongestion therapy, the amount of subcutaneous tissue increases and the disease overall progresses over time.

Tumescent liposuction has become an integral part in the management of lipoedema. Ideally, it should be performed early, and multiple sessions are often required [15]. Patients experience significant improvement in swelling, pain, mobility, appearance and quality of life [24,25,31–33]. Decongestion therapy should remain an integral part of post-liposuction management [24].

Lipo-lymphoedema

Definition

Lipo-lymphoedema is the coexistence of lipoedema and secondary lymphoedema.

Introduction and general description

Secondary lymphoedema may coexist in patients with longstanding lipoedema and the distinction between the two entities can be a challenge. The increased pressure from expansion of fat tissues in lipoedema contributes to the development of lipo-lymphoedema by causing mechanical obstruction of small lymphatic vessels.

Pathophysiology

The lymphatic system in lipoedema is thought to be normal or sufficient, at least as far as the large lymph vessels are concerned. However, the increased pressure from the expansion of fat tissues may cause mechanical obstruction of the small lymphatic vessels in the septa, resulting in mild lymphostasis and oedema of the subcutaneous tissue. Furthermore, lymphatic transport in lipoedema also decreases as fibrosis increases with age, and this can exacerbate the secondary lymphoedema [1].

Pathology

No distinct histological abnormalities have been identified in lipo-lymphoedema by H&E, fat stains or electron microscopy [2–4].

Table 100.2 Imaging characteristics of lipoedema and lymphoedema.

Imaging modality	Lipoedema	Lymphoedema
Lymphangiogram	Normal	Abnormal
Lymphoscintigram	Normal, with mild lymphatic delay in some	Abnormal with delayed lymphatic flow, subdermal collateralization and dermal backflow
Computed tomography	Diffuse and homogenous lipomatous hypertrophy of subcutaneous tissue	Thickening of the calf subcutaneous tissues and perimuscular aponeurosis. Increased fat density. Honeycomb appearance due to fibrous and oedematous stranding of fat
Magnetic resonance imaging	Normal skin thickness, increased fatty tissue	Thickening of the skin and subcutaneous tissue. Honeycomb appearance

Clinical features

Presentation
In addition to the physical examination findings in lipoedema, patients with lipo-lymphoedema may have a positive Stemmer's sign – the inability to pinch a skin fold at the base of the second toe due to oedema or fibrosis of the skin. Stemmer's sign is often present in lymphoedema patients but is usally absent in lipoedema patients [5].

Disease course and prognosis
Lipo-lymphoedema has a chronic and progressive course.

Investigations
Lipo-lymphoedema is a clinical diagnosis. Table 100.2 describes imaging modalities that may assist in identifying lipo-lymphoedema [5].

Management
The lymphatic oedema component of lipo-lymphoedema may improve initially with leg elevation and compression. See also the management section for lipoedema of the lower limbs.

Lipoedema of the scalp and lipoedematous alopecia

Definition and nomenclature
Lipoedema of the scalp (LS) and lipoedematous alopecia (LA) are characterized by the presence of a thick, boggy scalp due to a prominent increase in subcutaneous adipose tissue, which may be associated with varying degrees of hair loss.

Synonyms and inclusions
- Lipoedematous scalp
- Lipoedematous alopecia

Introduction and general description
Lipoedema of the scalp is a rare condition of unknown aetiology where a thick, boggy scalp develops due to a prominent increase in subcutaneous adipose tissue. It can be associated with scarring or non-scarring hair loss, when it is known as lipoedematous alopecia [1]. LS was first described by Cornbleet in 1935 [2] and LA was first described by Coskey *et al.* in 1961 [3]. There is some debate as to whether LS and LA represent clinical variants of the same entity or two different disorders [1]. Since they are both very rare, they will be grouped together for the purposes of this discussion.

Epidemiology

Incidence and prevalence
These are rare conditions with only approximately 45 cases of LS and 30 cases of LA reported in the literature [1,4].

Age
Lipoedema of the scalp and LA are reported most commonly in adults [2,3,5–11,**12**,13–26,**27**,28–31].

Sex
Among reported cases, there is an approximate female to male ratio of 5 : 1 [2,3,**4**,5–11,**12**,13–26,**27**,28,29].

Ethnicity
Both LS and LA have been described in all ethnicities [2,3,4,5–11,**12**,13–26,27,28,29].

Associated diseases
Several conditions have been reported in association with LS or LA but there is no consistent link with any of them [3,5,8,**12**,13,15,16–19,21,23].

Pathophysiology
The exact aetiology is unknown. A failure to maintain the integrity of the dermal–subcutaneous interface with an expansion and invasion of subcutaneous fat into the dermis is likely to be of relevance [27]. Some have speculated that female sex hormones may play a role, since these conditions have a predilection for women [29].

Hair cycle disturbance could occur as a result of lymphangiectasia [1,16,21,24] or oedema [1,9], both of which have been observed histologically in LS and LA. Alternatively, the fat itself might invade and destroy the hair follicle [27].

Pathology
The main pathological feature in both LS and LA is an approximate doubling in scalp thickness resulting from expansion of the subcutaneous fat layer [1]. Dilated lymphatic vessels have been observed in both LA and LS [1,16,21,24]. In LA there is also a loss of hair follicles without any inflammation. Perifollicular fat cells in direct continuity with underlying subcutaneous fat lobules are noted in the dermis, together with fibrous tracks [27] and fragmentation of dermal elastic fibres [1,11].

Genetics
No genetic mutation has been identified in patients with LS and LA. However, an LS mother–LA daughter pair has been reported [23].

Environmental factors

One group of Egyptian investigators observed that all of their patients wore a special tight head scarf called a mandil [19]. The associations between LS, LA and other headwear have not been reported by others.

Clinical features

Presentation

Although LS and LA are usually asymptomatic, some patients may experience pain, pruritus, paraesthesiae or headache [27]. While LA patients may present earlier due to alopecia, most LS patients were not aware of their condition and presented for other reasons [1].

Patients with LS and LA present with boggy thickening of the scalp, predominantly over the vertex, parietal and occipital scalp [12]. The bogginess may gradually extend to the entire scalp. The condition is more easily palpable than visible [1]. The consistency of the scalp has been likened to cotton wadding as used in quilting and upholstering [27]. The involved scalp is easily pressed down to the underlying bone, but returns to its original form immediately pressure is removed [19].

Hair loss in LA is variable and both scarring and non-scarring alopecia have been reported. Hairs do not exceed 2 cm in length and tend to break off easily [3]. Sometimes the hair in the affected area can have a lighter colour than hair from the surrounding unaffected scalp [4].

Of note is the fact that none of the LS and LA patients reported to date have had concurrent lipoedema of the legs.

Differential diagnosis

Differential diagnosis of LS and LA includes naevus lipomatosus superficialis of the scalp, cutis verticis gyrata and encephalocraniocutaneous lipomatosis. Naevus lipomatosus superficialis is usually present at birth and may have solitary or multiple lesions [20]. The scalp in cutis verticis gyrata is furrowed and on biopsy demonstrates closely packed hair follicles and considerable thickening of the collagen bundles of the dermis and subcutaneous tissue [25]. Encephalocraniocutaneous lipomatosis is associated with ophthalmological and neurological abnormalities.

Disease course and prognosis

Both LS and LA are chronic and persistent conditions.

Investigations

Ultrasound or MRI of the involved scalp area can confirm subcutaneous tissue thickening [27]. The average scalp thickness in healthy individuals was 5.8 ± 0.12 mm [32]. In contrast, the scalp thickness in LA and LS patients ranged from 8.5 to 16 mm with an average of 11.4 mm [25]. Biopsy of the affected area may also support the diagnosis.

Management

There is no specific and effective management guideline for LS and LA. Pain, pruritus and paraesthesia are managed symptomatically. Surgical excision of LS has been reported in one patient. At 12-month follow-up, there was no recurrence of LS although residual alopecia remained [27]. Topical minoxidil solutions have not been helpful in regrowing hair [27].

MISCELLANEOUS DISORDERS OF SUBCUTANEOUS FAT

Cellulite

Definition and nomenclature

Cellulite is an architectural disorder of human adipose tissue. It is characterized by the dimpled and nodular appearance of the skin in cellulite-prone areas in postpubertal females [1].

Synonyms and inclusions
- Adiposis oedematosa
- Status protusus cutis
- Dermopanniculosis deformans
- Nodular liposclerosis
- Gynoid lipodystrophy
- Oedematofibrosclerotic panniculopathy

Introduction and general description

The term cellulite was first introduced in the French literature 150 years ago [2]. Cellulite is nowadays among the more common concerns of patients presenting to dermatologists. It is a localized metabolic disorder of subcutaneous tissue that results in a readily visible alteration in the appearance of the female body. Cellulite presents as a change of skin topography evident by skin with dimpling and nodularity that principally involves the pelvic region, lower limbs and abdomen of women. The topographical alteration is caused by herniations of subcutaneous fat through its fibrous connective tissue support matrix.

Epidemiology

Incidence and prevalence

It is estimated that between 85% and 98% of postpubertal females display some degree of cellulite [1].

Age

It first appears after puberty.

Sex

It is almost exclusive to women [1].

Ethnicity

White women are affected more frequently than women of other races [3].

Pathophysiology

The exact pathophysiology of cellulite is not fully understood; many theories seek to explain the structural, architectural, metabolic and biochemical differences between cellulite and non-cellulite fat. In a study performed by Rosenbaum *et al.* [4], biopsies from women with and without cellulite showed an irregular and discontinuous dermal–subcutaneous interface that was characterized by fat protrusion into the dermis. In contrast, the dermal–subcutaneous and connective tissue interface was smooth and continuous in male subjects. These findings suggest that there is a sexual dimorphism in the structural characteristics of subdermal connective tissue that predisposes women to the development of cellulite. Women with cellulite have a higher percentage of thinner, perpendicularly orientated, dermal septa: this appears to facilitate herniation of adipose tissue into the reticular dermis [5,6].

There are also regional differences in both the hormonal responsiveness and metabolic activity of human adipose tissue. For example, adipocytes in the gluteal–femoral region are larger and are influenced by female sex hormones. The gluteal–femoral adipocytes are also metabolically more stable and resistant to lipolysis [1]. Although it has been conjectured that deterioration of the dermal vasculature with oedema and deposition of glycosoaminoglycans in the dermal capillary walls could result in cellulite [3], this observation has not been supported by others [5,6,7]. Similarly, the role of inflammation in the pathogenesis of cellulite remains controversial [2,5,7–10].

Predisposing factors

Excessively high carbohydrate diets provoke hyperinsulinaemia and lipogenesis, leading to an increase in total body fat content, and thereby predispose to cellulite [1,11]. Prolonged periods of sitting or standing may impede normal blood flow and lead to stasis, which alters microcirculation and may increase the risk of cellulite. Finally, fluid retention and the hormonal environment in pregnancy may also be contributory [1].

Pathology

Cellulite is a clinical diagnosis. Tissue sampling is not required for the diagnosis. Histopathological specimens demonstrate indentations of subcutaneous fat into the dermis [5].

Genetics

There seems to be a genetic predisposition to the development of cellulite as most women with cellulite report its occurrence in other family members [12]. However, no specific genetic mutation has been identified.

Clinical features

Presentation

Cellulite presents almost exclusively in postpubertal females and involves the skin of the pelvic region, lower limbs and abdomen. The skin appears dimpled, like the surface of a mattress or of orange peel [1,5]. This surface irregularity is especially apparent when the skin is pinched. Cellulite can affect individuals with both high and low BMI [1].

Differential diagnosis

Obesity is differentiated from cellulite in that obesity is characterized by hypertrophy and hyperplasia of adipose tissue that is not necessarily limited to the pelvis, thighs and abdomen [1]. The skin is not dimpled in obesity.

Classification of severity

Cellulite has been divided into three grades of severity [1]:

Grade I   Skin dimpling is apparent on pinching but not otherwise.

Grade II   Skin dimpling is apparent on standing but not on lying down.

Grade III   Skin dimpling is apparent both on standing and on lying down.

Complications and co-morbidities

There is no associated morbidity or mortality [1].

Disease course and prognosis

Cellulite can be progressive.

Management

Although cellulite is a very common complaint, treatments proposed for it have lacked substantial proof of efficacy. There is no single treatment or treatment combination that has been shown to be reliably effective. The best currently available treatments have resulted in mild to moderate improvement at best. Most of any improvement obtained is not sustained over time and maintenance treatment is often needed.

Weight gain may accentuate the visibility of cellulite. Weight reduction may reduce but, ironically, may also sometimes increase its prominence. One group of investigators has shown, however, that, on average, cellulite severity decreases following weight loss. This is especially true for those with higher BMI and greater cellulite severity grading [13].

Various over-the-counter and prescription topical therapies have been advocated for cellulite. Topical application of 0.3% retinol for 6 months or more has been claimed to improve cellulite [14]. So-called mesotherapy, whereby a variety of substances including phosphatidylcholine, caffeine, theophylline and herbal extracts are injected into subcutaneous tissue in an attempt to dissolve fat, has been widely promoted but, not surprisingly, has not been shown to have any useful place in managing cellulite [14,15,16].

Many non-invasive devices have been promoted for the treatment of cellulite. These include a skin-kneading device, unipolar and bipolar radiofrequency devices, ultrasound devices and selective cryolysis [14].

More invasive procedures such as subcision and liposuction have also been attempted. While subcision may temporarily improve cellulite appearance, long-term efficacy remains to be demonstrated. Liposuction for the treatment of cellulite carries risk. While liposuction reduces fat deposits deeper in the subcutaneous fat, cellulite adipose tissue is deposited more superficially. When liposuction is performed at more superficial levels, there is an increased risk of necrosis and poor cosmetic outcome. Laser-assisted liposuction and/or laser-assisted lipoplasty, which are less invasive than traditional liposuction and offer simultaneous skin tightening, may be the preferred treatment [1].

In the search for a novel approach to managing cellulite, various investigators have looked at peroxisome proliferator-activated receptors (PPARs), which are found on adipocytes and are thought to have an effect on the extracellular matrix, as possible targets for the treatment of cellulite but there is no evidence to date that they are likely to be effective [**14**,17–21].

The ideal management for this condition, which so many women find distressing and for the treatment of which considerable sums have been expended, has yet to be found.

Obesity and the skin

Rates of people being overweight and obese (BMI >25 kg/m^2) have been rising at an alarming rate in many countries of the world in recent years: in England, for instance, 62.1% of adults were overweight or obese in 2013 [1]. The prevalence of obesity (BMI >30 kg/m^2 in adult men and women rose over the 20 years from 1993 to 2013 from 13.2% and 16.4% to 26.0% and 23.8%, respectively [1]. Nearly 10% of all children entering English schools (at age 4–5 years) were classified as obese (weight ≥95th centile for age) [1].

Obesity exposes people not only to well-known metabolic and cardiovascular consequences including type 2 diabetes but also has significant effects on other body systems including the skin [2].

Physiological consequences of obesity on the skin. Subcutaneous fat insulates the body core from the external environment. Whilst this may be of benefit in protecting the body from the effects of exposure to cold it also means that it is harder for the obese to dissipate heat from the core out to the skin surface. This increases the reliance on sweating for thermoregulation in obese people, who tend to sweat more profusely than those who are not overweight [3]. Paradoxically, however, transepidermal water loss is increased in obese people, who are prone to xerosis [4].

Mechanical problems contributing to skin disease in the obese. Friction, sweating and maceration within body folds frequently lead to a painful erosive intertriginous dermatitis with secondary candidosis. Obese women with restricted mobility are more likely to have problems with urinary continence, which can contribute further to inflammation, with an irritant contact dermatitis affecting the genito-crural folds [5]. Stretch marks (striae distensae) are common, particularly if weight gain has been rapid [**2**,5,6]. They tend to be located in the axillary folds, upper thighs, buttocks and abdomen.

The mechanical effects of obesity may impede lymphatic drainage not only in the lower extremities but also elsewhere, for example in abdominal apron folds, resulting in lymphoedema [3]. The chronic high pressure exerted on the skin of the soles of the feet may result in plantar hyperkeratosis and postmenopausal plantar keratoderma (keratoderma climactericum) [**2**,6].

Peripheral vascular and lymphovascular disorders in the obese. Obesity puts strain on the vascular system. Lower limb venous hypertension from whatever cause may be exacerbated in the obese by high intra-abdominal pressures and by immobility. The risks of venous eczema and venous ulceration are increased and they may be more difficult to manage. Chronic lymphoedema frequently supervenes (Figure 100.8) [2].

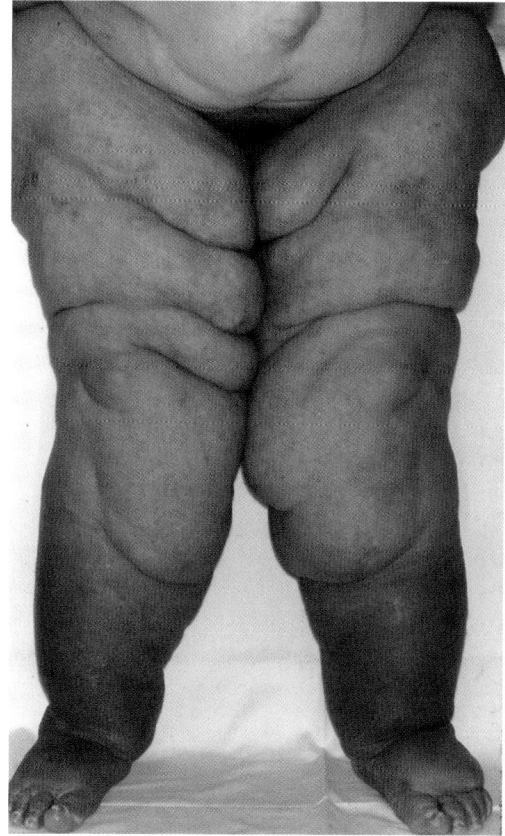
Figure 100.8 Gross obesity with bilateral lymphoedema of lower legs.

Cutaneous infections and obesity. The prevalence of superficial skin infections such as candidosis, dermatophytosis and erythrasma is raised in the obese [2]. Pyogenic infections such as folliculitis and furunculosis are also more frequently seen and may be recurrent. In a large study of patients requiring operative treatment of skin and soft tissue infections by community-acquired meticillin-resistant *Staphylococcus aureus* (MRSA), obese patients were more than three times likely to need further surgical intervention within a year than non-obese patients [7]. Lymphoedema in the obese is commonly complicated by streptococcal cellulitis. Obesity also increases the risk of surgical wound infection and of necrotizing fasciitis [8].

Cutaneous consequences of immunological and endocrine dysregulation in the obese. It is increasingly recognized that adipose tissue has multiple, complex regulatory and hormonal functions in addition to its role as an energy store (see Chapter 99); these functions may be disturbed in the obese. Altered adipocytokine secretion may have an effect on inflammation in the obese [9,10]: for instance, delayed-type hypersensitivity responses are increased in obesity and decline with weight reduction [11]. Adipocytokines may also play a role in the well-recognized link between severe psoriasis and obesity, with evidence that weight reduction, including that achieved by bariatric surgery, can produce significant improvement in psoriasis [**2**,12,13]. There is also some evidence of a link between obesity and atopy including atopic eczema [**2**,13].

The hyperinsulinaemia associated with obesity increases androgen production from adipose tissue and reduces the production

PART 8: SPECIFIC CUTANEOUS STRUCTURE

of sex-hormone-binding globulin, thus increasing circulating free androgen levels. This manifests as increased risks of acne, hirsutism, androgenetic alopecia and polycystic ovary syndrome in the obese [2,15]. Type 2 diabetes is a common complication of obesity and is associated with a variety of specific skin disorders (see Chapter 64).

Genetic disorders associated with obesity. Obesity is a component of a number of genetic disorders of which Prader–Willi syndrome is one of the best known. These are discussed in Chapter 74.

Other skin disorders in the obese. Dercum disease (see earlier in this chapter) is strongly associated with obesity. The presence of obesity may aggravate a variety of other skin disorders including hidradenitis suppurativa and pilonidal sinus. Surgical wound healing is impaired in the obese with an increased risk of incisional hernia [16].

Key references

The full list of references can be found in the online version at www.rooksdermatology.com.

Acquired lipodystrophy

Acquired generalized lipodystrophy
1 Garg A. Clinical review: lipodystrophies: genetic and acquired body fat disorders. *J Clin Endocrinol Metab* 2011;96:3313–25.
10 Misra A, Garg A. Clinical features and metabolic derangements in acquired generalized lipodystrophy: case reports and review of the literature. *Medicine (Baltimore)* 2003;82:129–46.
22 Garg A. Lipodystrophies. *Am J Med.* 2000;108:143–52.
49 Oral EA, Simha V, Ruiz E, *et al.* Leptin-replacement therapy for lipodystrophy. *N Engl J Med* 2002;346:570–8.

Acquired partial lipodystrophy
1 Garg A. Lipodystrophies. *Am J Med* 2000;108:143–52.
2 Garg A. Clinical review: lipodystrophies: genetic and acquired body fat disorders. *J Clin Endocrinol Metab* 2011;96:3313–25.
20 Misra A, Peethambaram A, Garg A. Clinical features and metabolic and autoimmune derangements in acquired partial lipodystrophy: report of 35 cases and review of the literature. *Medicine (Baltimore)* 2004;83:18–34.
21 Sissons JG, West RJ, Fallows J, *et al.* The complement abnormalities of lipodystrophy. *N Engl J Med* 1976 26;294:461–5.
23 Mathieson PW, Peters DK. Lipodystrophy in MCGN type II: the clue to links between the adipocyte and the complement system. *Nephrol Dial Transplant* 1997;12:1804–6.

HIV-associated lipodystrophy
2 Garg A. Clinical review: lipodystrophies: genetic and acquired body fat disorders. *J Clin Endocrinol Metab* 2011;96:3313–25.
3 Domingo P, Estrada V, Lopez-Aldeguer J, Villaroya F, Martinez E. Fat redistribution syndromes associated with HIV-1 infection and combination antiretroviral therapy. *AIDS Rev* 2012;14:112–23.
6 Chen D, Misra A, Garg A. Clinical review 153: lipodystrophy in human immunodeficiency virus-infected patients. *J Clin Endocrinol Metab* 2002;87:4845–56.
14 McComsey G, Rightmire A, Wirtz V, Yang R, Mathew M, McGrath D. Changes in body composition with ritonavir-boosted and unboosted atazanavir treatment in combination with lamivudine and stavudine: a 96-week randomized, controlled study. *Clin Infect Dis* 2009;48:1323–6.
28 Hansen BR, Haugaard SB, Iversen J, Nielsen JO, Andersen O. Impact of switching antiretroviral therapy on lipodystrophy and other metabolic complications: a review. *Scand J Infect Dis* 2004;36:244–53.

Localized lipoatrophy and/or lipodystrophy

Semicircular lipoatrophy
6 Reinoso-Barbero L, Gonzalez-Gomez MF, Belanger-Quintana D, *et al.* Case-control study of semicircular lipoatrophy, a new occupational disease in office workers. *J Occup Health* 2013;55(3):149–57.
12 Senecal S, Victor V, Choudat D, Hornez-Davin S, Conso F. Semicircular lipoatrophy: 18 cases in the same company. *Contact Dermatitis* 2000;42:101–2.

Insulin-induced localized lipoatrophy
1 Richardson T, Kerr D. Skin-related complications of insulin therapy: epidemiology and emerging management strategies. *Am J Clin Dermatol* 2003;4:661–7.
4 Ramos AJ, Farias MA. Human insulin-induced lipoatrophy: a successful treatment with glucocorticoid. *Diabetes Care* 2006;29:926–7.
12 Lopez X, Castells M, Ricker A, Velazquez EF, Mun E, Goldfine AB. Human insulin analog-induced lipoatrophy. *Diabetes Care* 2008;31:442–4.
22 Radermecker RP, Pierard GE, Scheen AJ. Lipodystrophy reactions to insulin: effects of continuous insulin infusion and new insulin analogs. *Am J Clin Dermatol* 2007;8:21–8.

Localized lipoatrophy due to injected corticosteroid
1 Dahl PR, Zalla MJ, Winkelmann RK. Localized involutional lipoatrophy: a clinicopathologic study of 16 patients. *J Am Acad Dermatol* 1996;35:523–8.
3 Shumaker PR, Rao J, Goldman MP. Treatment of local, persistent cutaneous atrophy following corticosteroid injection with normal saline infiltration. *Dermatol Surg* 2005;31:1340–3.
5 Schetman D, Hambrick GW, Jr, Wilson CE. Cutaneous changes following local injection of triamcinolone. *Arch Dermatol* 1963;88:820–8.

Centrifugal lipodystrophy
1 Imamura S. Lipodystrophia centrifugalis abdominalis infantilis: statistical analysis of 168 cases. *Pediatr Dermatol* 2012;29:437–41.
6 Wu MC, Hsu CK, Lee JY. Lipodystrophia centrifugalis abdominalis infantilis: report of four cases. *Pediatr Dermatol* 2012;29:308–10.
12 Muller S, Beissert S, Metze D, Luger TA, Bonsmann G. Lipodystrophia centrifugalis abdominalis infantilis in a 4-year-old Caucasian girl: association with partial IgA deficiency and autoantibodies. *Br J Dermatol* 1999;140:1161–4.
17 Fukumoto D, Kubo Y, Saito M, Arase S. Centrifugal lipodystrophy of the scalp presenting with an arch-form alopecia: a 10-year follow-up observation. *J Dermatol* 2009;36:499–503.

Fat hypertrophy

Insulin-induced localized fat hypertrophy
1 Richardson T, Kerr D. Skin-related complications of insulin therapy: epidemiology and emerging management strategies. *Am J Clin Dermatol* 2003;4:661–7.
2 Hauner H, Stockamp B, Haastert B. Prevalence of lipohypertrophy in insulin-treated diabetic patients and predisposing factors. *Exp Clin Endocrinol Diabetes* 1996;104:106–10.
5 Fujikura J, Fujimoto M, Yasue S, *et al.* Insulin-induced lipohypertrophy: report of a case with histopathology. *Endocr J* 2005;52:623–8.
11 Roper NA, Bilous RW. Resolution of lipohypertrophy following change of short-acting insulin to insulin lispro (Humalog). *Diabet Med* 1998;15:1063–4.

Subcutaneous lipomatosis

Benign symmetrical lipomatosis
1 Brea-Garcia B, Cameselle-Teijeiro J, Couto-Gonzalez I, Taboada-Suarez A, Gonzalez-Alvarez E. Madelung's disease: comorbidities, fatty mass distribution, and response to treatment of 22 patients. *Aesthetic Plast Surg* 2013;37:409–16.
5 Chan HF, Sun Y, Lin CH, Chen RC. Madelung's disease associated with polyneuropathy and symptomatic hypokalemia. *J Formos Med Assoc* 2013;112:283–6.
20 Enzi G, Busetto L, Ceschin E, Coin A, Digito M, Pigozzo S. Multiple symmetric lipomatosis: clinical aspects and outcome in a long-term longitudinal study. *Int J Obes Relat Metab Disord* 2002;26:253–61.
25 Bassetto F, Scarpa C, De Stefano F, Busetto L. Surgical treatment of multiple symmetric lipomatosis with ultrasound-assisted liposuction. *Ann Plast Surg* 2014;73:559–62.

37 Mimica M, Pravdic D, Nakas-Icindic E, *et al.* Multiple symmetric lipomatosis: a diagnostic dilemma. *Case Rep Med* 2013;2013:836903.

Dercum disease

3 Herbst KL, Asare-Bediako S. Adiposis dolorosa is more than painful fat. *Endocrinologist* 2007;17:326–34.
5 Hansson E, Svensson H, Brorson H. Review of Dercum's disease and proposal of diagnostic criteria, diagnostic methods, classification and management. *Orphanet J Rare Dis* 2012;7:23.
23 Brodovsky S, Westreich M, Leibowitz A, Schwartz Y. Adiposis dolorosa (Dercum's disease): 10-year follow-up. *Ann Plast Surg* 1994;33:664–8.
35 Hansson E, Svensson H, Brorson H. Liposuction may reduce pain in Dercum's disease (adiposis dolorosa). *Pain Med* 2011;12:942–52.

Infiltrating lipomatosis of the face

1 Tracy JC, Klement GL, Scott AR. Interdisciplinary management of congenital infiltrating lipomatosis. *Int J Pediatr Otorhinolaryngol* 2013;77(12):2071–4.
2 Slavin SA, Baker DC, McCarthy JG, Mufarrij A. Congenital infiltrating lipomatosis of the face: clinicopathologic evaluation and treatment. *Plast Reconstr Surg* 1983;72:158–64.
3 Urs AB, Augustine J, Kumar P, Arora S, Aggarwal N, Sultana N. Infiltrating lipomatosis of the face: a case series. *J Nat Sci Biol Med* 2013;4:252–7.
4 De Rosa G, Cozzolino A, Guarino M, Giardino C. Congenital infiltrating lipomatosis of the face: report of cases and review of the literature. *J Oral Maxillofac Surg* 1987;45:879–83.
13 Padwa BL, Mulliken JB. Facial infiltrating lipomatosis. *Plast Reconstr Surg* 2001;108:1544–54.

Encephalocraniocutaneous lipomatosis

3 Pardo IA, Nicolas ME. A Filipino male with encephalocraniocutaneous lipomatosis (Haberland's syndrome). *J Dermatol Case Rep* 2013;7:46–8.
4 Moog U, Jones MC, Viskochil DH, Verloes A, Van Allen MI, Dobyns WB. Brain anomalies in encephalocraniocutaneous lipomatosis. *Am J Med Genet A* 2007;143A:2963–72.
5 Moog U, Roelens F, Mortier GR, *et al.* Encephalocraniocutaneous lipomatosis accompanied by the formation of bone cysts: Harboring clues to pathogenesis? *Am J Med Genet A* 2007;143A:2973–80.
6 Moog U. Encephalocraniocutaneous lipomatosis. *J Med Genet* 2009;46:721–9.

Lipoedema

Lipoedema of the lower limbs

11 Harwood CA, Bull RH, Evans J, Mortimer PS. Lymphatic and venous function in lipoedema. *Br J Dermatol* 1996;134:1–6.

15 Langendoen SI, Habbema L, Nijsten TE, Neumann HA. Lipoedema: from clinical presentation to therapy. A review of the literature. *Br J Dermatol* 2009;161:980–6.
16 Rudkin GH, Miller TA. Lipedema: a clinical entity distinct from lymphedema. *Plast Reconstr Surg* 1994;94:841–7; discussion 8–9.
25 Meier-Vollrath I, Schmeller W. [Lipoedema – current status, new perspectives.] *J Dtsch Dermatol Ges* 2004;2:181–6.

Lipo-lymphoedema

1 Langendoen SI, Habbema L, Nijsten TE, Neumann HA. Lipoedema: from clinical presentation to therapy. A review of the literature. *Br J Dermatol* 2009;161:980–6.
5 Warren AG, Janz BA, Borud LJ, Slavin SA. Evaluation and management of the fat leg syndrome. *Plast Reconstr Surg* 2007;119:9e–15e.

Lipoedema of the scalp and lipoedematous alopecia

1 Yasar S, Gunes P, Serdar ZA, Tosun I. Clinical and pathological features of 31 cases of lipedematous scalp and lipedematous alopecia. *Eur J Dermatol* 2011;21:520–8.
4 Zeng YP, Ma DL, Wang BX. Lipedematous scalp with heterochromia of scalp hair in a boy. *Eur J Dermatol* 2011;21:144–5.
12 Scheufler O, Kania NM, Heinrichs CM, Exner K. Hyperplasia of the subcutaneous adipose tissue is the primary histopathologic abnormality in lipedematous scalp. *Am J Dermatopathol* 2003;25:248–52.
27 Yip L, Mason G, Pohl M, Sinclair R. Successful surgical management of lipoedematous alopecia. *Australas J Dermatol* 2008;49:52–4.

Miscellaneous disorders of subcutaneous fat

Cellulite

1 Khan MH, Victor F, Rao B, Sadick NS. Treatment of cellulite. Part I. Pathophysiology. *J Am Acad Dermatol* 2010;62:361–70; quiz 71–2.
6 Querleux B, Cornillon C, Jolivet O, Bittoun J. Anatomy and physiology of subcutaneous adipose tissue by in vivo magnetic resonance imaging and spectroscopy: relationships with sex and presence of cellulite. *Skin Res Technol* 2002;8:118–24.
12 Gold MH. Cellulite – an overview of non-invasive therapy with energy-based systems. *J Dtsch Dermatol Ges* 2012;10:553–8.
14 Khan MH, Victor F, Rao B, Sadick NS. Treatment of cellulite. Part II. Advances and controversies. *J Am Acad Dermatol* 2010;62:373–84; quiz 85–6.

Obesity and the skin

2 Shipman AR, Millington G. Obesity and the skin. *Br J Dermatol* 2011;165:743–50.
6 Scheinfeld NS. Obesity and dermatology. *Clin Dermatol* 2004;22:303–9.

PART 9
Vascular Disorders Involving the Skin

CHAPTER 101

Purpura

Tabi A. Leslie

Royal Free Hospital, London, UK

Introduction

Purpura and bruising, the main terms used to describe bleeding into the skin, may occur as isolated phenomena or as part of a systemic disorder. Purpura is the hallmark of vasculitis affecting smaller vessels of the skin, and may be the dominant feature or a minor part of a systemic vasculitis; otherwise purpura is commonly seen by haematologists due to platelet and coagulation disorders. Vasculitis also causes other cutaneous lesions with a purpuric component, including urticarial lesions, nodules, ulcers, livedo and skin necrosis. Several of these signs also occur in disorders in which vessels are occluded. Morphology and associated features aid the diagnostic approach [1].

The management of purpura may involve a multidisciplinary approach including haematology, general medicine, nephrology, rheumatology and dermatology. Classification of purpura is difficult, as similar clinical patterns may arise from different causes, including vasculitic and non-vasculitic. Aetiology of the purpura or vasculitis may be impossible to determine. Classifications based on morphology or aetiology have limitations. Non-specific capillaritis may be idiopathic, drug-induced or a manifestation of cutaneous T-cell lymphoma. Purpura due to idiopathic thrombocytopenic purpura may be a mixture of diseases [2]. Microvascular occlusion may give rise to palpable lesions and inflammation as a secondary component similar to vasculitis, clinically and histopathologically.

The differential diagnosis of purpura is based on morphology [1], as few patients present with a known aetiology. Haematological causes (thrombocytopenia and clotting factor abnormalities) can be rapidly and easily evaluated by full blood count and laboratory measures of clotting times. More complex haematological disorders (e.g. thrombophilias or abnormal platelet function) [3], vessel wall defects (both structural and others) [4], infections, immunological disorders and thrombotic microvascular occlusion disorders also need to be considered. It is important to differentiate between disorders causing primarily either inflammatory or non-inflammatory lesions [5].

Purpura is discoloration of the skin or mucous membranes due to extravasation of the red blood cells. Petechiae are small, 1–2 mm, purpuric lesions. Ecchymoses (bruises) are larger extravasations of blood. The causes of petechiae and ecchymoses overlap. Thrombocytopenia usually causes petechiae but more extensive bleeding may occur at lower levels of platelet count. Coagulation disorders cause ecchymoses rather than petechiae [6,7]. Haemophilias usually present as bleeding from the umbilical cord or gingivae, or as haematomas or haemarthroses – although dermatologists need to be aware that haemorrhagic subcutaneous nodules may be the first sign of an inherited haemophilia [8]. Gingival bleeding, epistaxis or internal bleeding may occur with platelet or coagulation disorders.

Extravasated blood is broken down to pigments derived from haem, usually within 2 or 3 weeks. Characteristic colour changes

PART 9: VASCULAR

Rook's Textbook of Dermatology, Ninth Edition. Edited by Christopher Griffiths, Jonathan Barker, Tanya Bleiker, Robert Chalmers and Daniel Creamer.
© 2016 John Wiley & Sons, Ltd. Published 2016 by John Wiley & Sons, Ltd.
Companion website: www.rooksdermatology.com

Box 101.1 Causes of purpura and ecchymosis

Platelet disorders
- Thrombocytopenia
- Abnormal platelet function
- Thrombocytosis

Coagulation disorders
- Inherited, e.g. haemophilia or acquired factor deficiency or dysfunction (e.g. antibody inhibitor)
- Drugs, e.g. anticoagulants
- Localized, e.g. heparin injection sites, some insect bites
- Metabolic, e.g. vitamin K deficiency, hepatic failure (decreased synthesis of clotting factors)
- Thrombophilias, e.g. protein C deficiency, protein S deficiency
- Disseminated intravascular coagulopathy and purpura fulminans
- Secondary to systemic disease (often multifactorial, e.g. macrophage activation syndrome)

Other intravascular causes of purpura/microvascular occlusion
- Dysproteinaemias, e.g. hypergammaglobulinaemic purpura (Waldenström), Sjögren syndrome
- Cryoproteinaemias
- Emboli: crystal, fat, myxoma, infective

Mechanical vascular causes of purpura
- Raised intravascular pressure:
  - Coughing, vomiting, Valsalva manoeuvre, tourniquet stasis
- Decreased support:
  - Actinic ('senile') purpura
  - Corticosteroid purpura

- Scurvy
- Amyloidosis
- Inherited disorders of connective tissue (pseudoxanthoma elasticum, Ehlers–Danlos syndrome)
- Abnormal vasculature
- Purpura around vascular lesions, e.g. targetoid haemosiderotic haemangioma, tufted angioma, aneurysmal fibrous histiocytoma

Purpura with inflammation
- Non-thrombocytopenic toxin- and drug-induced purpura
- Contact purpura
- Purpura associated with infections
- Capillaritis (pigmented purpuric dermatoses):
  - Idiopathic
  - Drug-induced
  - Pre-mycotic
- Inflammatory purpura/vasculitis, e.g. Henoch–Schönlein purpura, acute haemorrhagic oedema
- Associated with other inflammatory dermatoses that are not usually purpuric
- Solar purpura

External and other causes of purpura or ecchymosis
- Physical and artefactual causes
- Easy bruising syndrome and purpura simplex
- Paroxysmal finger haematoma (Achenbach syndrome)
- Painful bruising (autoerythrocyte sensitization, Gardner–Diamond syndrome)
- Stigmata

---

include red, blue and purple in the first 5 days, green after 5–7 days and yellow after 7–14 days [9]. Intrinsic factors to the individual and the injury – such as age, sex, skin colour, body site, amount of blood extravasated, depth of bruising and medications that alter bruise dispersion – influence the timescale of colour changes. Smaller, superficial, purpuric lesions may be orange or brown in colour due to residual haemosiderin.

The assessment of traumatic ecchymoses may be important in suspected child abuse.

Unlike purpura, increased intravascular blood in the skin can be blanched by pressure, typically using the technique of diascopy. Not all telangiectatic lesions can be emptied in this way. Small angiomas (e.g. in angioma serpiginosum or the multiple minute variant of Campbell de Morgan spots) and angiokeratomas may cause particular confusion [10]. Observation over several days may be necessary. Capillary microscopy or dermoscopy may also be helpful in determining whether blood is intravascular or extravascular.

Classification of purpura

An aetiological classification of purpura is provided in Box 101.1.

A simple pathogenetic classification of purpura can divide mechanisms of intravascular bleeding into three groups:
1 Simple haemorrhage.
2 Inflammatory haemorrhage.
3 Occlusion/ischaemia.

Simple haemorrhage presents as macules without erythema (Box 101.2), with sufficient haemorrhage into subcutaneous tissue palpable as a haematoma. Inflammatory causes of haemorrhagic lesions usually evolve with increasing erythema in the first 24–36 h, along with increasing purpura. Palpable purpura syndromes may uncommonly produce lesions with retiform or stellate patterning, with accompanying early erythema. By 48 h, erythema and palpability begin to fade in both types of lesions, although the purpura may persist for several days. In contrast, lesions of occlusion/ischaemia usually begin with minimal or no erythema, and may show only modest palpability unless eschar forms. In this situation erythema may develop if sufficient necrosis occurs to induce a wound healing response. Occlusive syndromes tend to manifest retiform or branching patterns of purpura (non-inflammatory retiform purpura), sometimes with accompanying localized livedo reticularis, or as necrotic plaques with minimal erythema.

Box 101.2 Diagnosis of macular non-retiform haemorrhage/petechiae/ecchymosis by size

Lesions <4 mm
- Thrombocytopenia:
  - Immune thrombocytopenic purpura
  - Thrombotic thrombocytopenic purpura
  - Disseminated intravascular coagulation (DIC)
  - Other causes (see Box 101.3)
- Abnormal platelet function:
  - Congenital/hereditary
  - Acquired: drug, systemic disease
  - In myeloproliferative disease
  - Other causes (see Box 101.3)
- With normal platelets:
  - Raised intravascular pressure
  - Trauma
  - Scurvy (perifollicular pattern)

- Hypergammaglobulinaemic purpura (Waldenström)

Intermediate-sized lesions
- Hypergammaglobulinaemic purpura (Waldenström)
- Infection in patients with thrombocytopenia or immune compromise
- Early lesions of vasculitis (sometimes)

Lesions >1 cm (all causes involve a degree of minor trauma)
- Procoagulant defect:
  - Anticoagulation
  - Liver failure
  - Vitamin K deficiency

- DIC (some)
- Poor dermal support:
  - Actinic and corticosteroid purpura
  - Scurvy
  - Hereditary (Ehlers–Danlos syndrome)
  - Amyloidosis
- Platelet deficiency or functional defect
- Other causes:
  - Hypergammaglobulinaemic purpura (Waldenström)
  - Capillaritis
  - Easy bruising syndrome, purpura simplex
  - Physical and artefactual causes
  - Gardner–Diamond syndrome
  - Stigmata

PURPURA DUE TO THROMBOCYTOPENIA OR PLATELET DEFECTS

Thrombocytopenia

Platelets are an essential component of the haemostatic process. Thrombocytopenia or abnormal platelet function from any cause may therefore produce purpura or a bleeding tendency [1,2,3,4,5–8,9].

Platelets exposed to damaged endothelium adhere to one another and to collagen and other subendothelial components. Numerous complex interactions occur, involving von Willebrand factor and its glycoprotein receptor, various integrin adhesion molecules, thrombospondin, fibronectin, laminin, phospholipases and adenosine diphosphate released from damaged cells, as well as collagen and platelets. Platelet activation causes the release of serotonin and thromboxane A_2, both of which cause vasoconstriction, and increase platelet adhesiveness and aggregation leading to the formation of a platelet plug. This process is aided further by the presence of plasma fibrinogen and by thrombin. The production of prostacyclin, a powerful vasodilator and inhibitor of platelet aggregation, is decreased as a result of endothelial damage. Developing platelet plugs are reinforced by fibrin strands formed as a result of activation of the plasma clotting system by platelet factor 3, when this is exposed by alterations in the surface characteristics of the aggregated platelets.

Purpura due to platelet defects can be divided into three groups, the second and third of which are discussed in this chapter:
- Thrombocytopenia, i.e. decreased platelet numbers.
- Abnormalities of platelet function.
- Thrombocytosis, i.e. increased platelet numbers.

Abnormalities of platelet function

Several haemorrhagic syndromes have become recognized in which platelet function is abnormal, although the total count may be normal [1,2–4,5,6]. These may be inherited, idiopathic or secondary to drugs or many other illnesses, including thrombopathia, thrombasthenia, von Willebrand disease, severe anaemia, chronic renal failure and fibrinogen defects. Hermansky–Pudlak syndrome consists of a bleeding diathesis due to storage pool disorder, with oculocutaneous albinism and pigment-containing cells in the bone marrow. Laboratory testing of platelet function is of limited direct relevance to dermatologists [6].

Drugs that may cause abnormal platelet function with clinical bleeding include aspirin, non-steroidal anti-inflammatory drugs (NSAIDs), some penicillin and β-lactam antibiotics (especially high-dose penicillin), alteplase and other fibrinolytic drugs, prostacyclin, thienopyridines (ticlopidine, clopidogrel), glycoprotein IIb/IIIa antagonists, cardiovascular drugs (nitrates, calcium channel blockers, quinidine), antidepressants and phenothiazines, and some chemotherapeutic agents such as mitomycin and daunorubicin [3,4,5]. Volume expanders such as dextran or hydroxyethyl starch, and radiocontrast media, are often forgotten as a cause of platelet dysfunction but can be particularly important in intensive care situations, as can fibrinolytic agents such as streptokinase, and agents that increase platelet cAMP levels such as iloprost or prostacyclin. Natural and herbal remedy agents that can cause platelet dysfunction include fish oil, garlic, cumin, turmeric, *Gingko biloba* and black tree fungus [5].

Thrombocytosis

Abnormally high platelet counts may occur as a result of essential thrombocythaemia or other myeloproliferative disorders, or secondary to a variety of other disease processes

---

Box 101.3 Platelet disorders causing purpura

Thrombocytopenia
- Defective platelet production:
  - Bone marrow abnormality:
    - Aplasia: toxic, immunological, idiopathic
    - Neoplasia: leukaemia, myeloma, carcinomatosis
    - Replacement: myelofibrosis, radiation damage, sarcoidosis
  - Other impaired production: Wiskott–Aldrich syndrome, vitamin B_{12} or folate deficiency
  - Metabolic: uraemia, alcohol, drugs
  - Infections
- Diminished platelet survival:
  - Platelet alloantibodies:
    - Neonatal
    - Post-transfusion
    - Antilymphocyte globulin
  - Platelet autoantibodies:
    - Idiopathic (immune) thrombocytopenic purpura
    - Marrow transplant
    - Antiphospholipid antibodies
    - Systemic lupus erythematosus
- Mechanical: prosthetic heart valves
- Drugs and vaccines
- Infections, sepsis syndrome
- Excessive platelet consumption:
  - Disseminated intravascular coagulation
  - Haemangioma (Kasabach–Merritt)
  - Hereditary haemorrhagic telangiectasia ('mini-Kasabach–Merritt')
  - Thrombotic microangiopathies:
    - Haemolytic–uraemic syndrome
    - Thrombotic thrombocytopenic purpura
- Sequestration:
  - Splenomegaly
  - Hypothermia

Abnormal platelet function
- Inherited and congenital:
  - Von Willebrand disease and defects of the platelet von Willebrand factor receptor

- Hereditary haemorrhagic telangiectasia (often with platelet dysfunction too)
- Bernard–Soulier disease (GpIb/IX/V receptor defect with low platelet count)
- GpIa deficiency
- Glanzmann thrombasthenia (GpIIb/IIIa deficiency)
- MYH9-related disorders (e.g. May–Hegglin abnormality)
- α-granule disorders
- Dense granule (δ-granule) disorders (Hermansky–Pudlak syndrome, Chediak–Higashi syndrome, storage pool disease)
- Abnormalities of signal transduction pathways
- Membrane phospholipids abnormalities (e.g. Scott syndrome)
- Wiskott–Aldrich syndrome (δ-granule abnormality) and X-linked thrombocytopenia (WASP gene mutations)
- Drug-induced
- Uraemia
- Cardiac bypass
- Platelet antibodies:
  - Idiopathic (immune) thrombocytopenic purpura
  - Systemic lupus erythematosus/antiphospholipid syndrome
- Myeloproliferative disorders
- Dysproteinaemias (especially IgA myeloma and macroglobulinaemia)
- Cold-stored (blood bank) platelets

Thrombocytosis
- Essential thrombocythaemia
- Other myeloproliferative syndromes
- Medical diseases and other causes:
  - Blood loss, trauma, burns
  - Post-splenectomy
  - Malignant disease
  - Tuberculosis
  - Sarcoidosis

(Box 101.3). This may lead to a tendency to platelet plugging and thrombosis or, paradoxically, to a bleeding tendency (particularly when the platelet count exceeds $1000 \times 10^9/L$ with a clonal platelet defect such as an acquired form of storage pool disease). Many cases of thrombocytosis do not achieve this high platelet count and are unlikely to cause purpura unless there are additional reasons related to the causative disorder (such as lymphoma or other malignant disease).

Dermatological manifestations and associations of thrombocythaemia include purpura with or without necrosis, livedo reticularis, acrocyanosis, purple (blue) toe syndrome, Raynaud phenomenon, erythromelalgia, other vascular symptoms including gangrene, and associated disorders such as pyoderma gangrenosum [1,2–6,7]. Many of these presentations are also seen in other hyperviscosity and dysproteinaemic conditions.

Platelet hyperreactivity is not usually a dermatological consideration, but it is a factor in peripheral arterial disease and thrombotic

emboli [8]. It is more common in females, linked with higher mean platelet volume and higher fibrinogen levels, and is partly genetically determined.

NON-THROMBOCYTOPENIC VASCULAR CAUSES OF PURPURA AND SYNDROMES OF PRIMARY ECCHYMOTIC HAEMORRHAGE

RAISED INTRAVASCULAR PRESSURE

Gravitational purpura. Gravity and venous stasis are the most important causes of pupura due to raised intravascular pressure, although it may also occur in conjunction with other dermatoses. Many eruptions on the lower leg, especially in the elderly, tend to become purpuric due to a combination of gravitational changes with vascular damage caused by other dermatoses. Rapid development of lower leg oedema may cause an eczematous eruption in which purpura may be prominent [1].

Acroangiodermatitis. Acroangiodermatitis (of Mali, or pseudo-Kaposi sarcoma) may mimic a pigmented purpuric dermatosis, but is discussed here as the purpura is due to abnormal vasculature other than to capillaritis. Occuring more often in men than in women, it is associated with venous insufficiency or with vascular anomalies such as Klippel–Trenaunay syndrome. There are several reports of it occurring as a stump dermatosis in amputees [2], and it has been reported in a patient with a thrombophilic prothrombin mutation [3].

The lesions of acroangiodermatitis occur especially on the lower legs but may extend onto the dorsa of the feet and toes, and up the leg, especially over dilated varicosities. Individual lesions are minute purpuric macules that coalesce to form irregular plaques, which may be several centimetres in diameter. Follicular lesions may occur. The colour of the lesions is not usually the purple colour of fresh purpura but varying shades of yellow (ochre) and brown from haemosiderin and other breakdown products. The epidermis may be normal or show mild eczematous changes. Oedema, sclerosis, ulceration and other signs of venous insufficiency may be associated, but may be entirely absent even in cases of long duration.

Differential diagnosis includes ordinary gravitational dermatitis, Schamberg disease and Kaposi sarcoma. The last mentioned can be distinguished by the staining pattern with CD34 antigen, which stains perivascular spindle cells in Kaposi sarcoma but only the endothelial cells in acroangiodermatitis [4].

Treatment for acroangiodermatitis is unsatisfactory but support hosiery seems logical.

Exercise-induced purpura. Exercise induced pupura is probably an underestimated condition. Histologically, it is a form of leukocytoclastic vasculitis [5]. It is discussed here as it can present as a pigmented purpuric dermatosis related to exercise, where there is no evidence of venous disease. The typical presentation of exercise-induced purpura is with purpuric lesions, which may be urticarial, on the lower legs after prolonged walking (many descriptions are in golfers, marathon runners or long-distance walkers), usually in hot weather. Patients are usually middle aged; however it has also been described in a child with recurrent purpura on the trunk after vigorous exercise [6]. Compression stockings may reduce the occurrence of exercise-induced purpura.

Solar purpura. The term 'solar purpura' is used to describe rapid development of purpuric lesions after exposure to sunlight. This condition is distinct from actinic purpura, which is a manifestation of cumulative sunlight-induced ageing of the skin. The precise nature of solar purpura is uncertain. Some view it as a variant of polymorphic light eruption or arising from solar capillaritis [7,8]. It is distinct from erythropoietic protoporphyria, although purpura clearly occurs in this dermatosis in some patients (Figure 101.1). Some cases may simply be a variation of purpura in dermatoses that are not usually

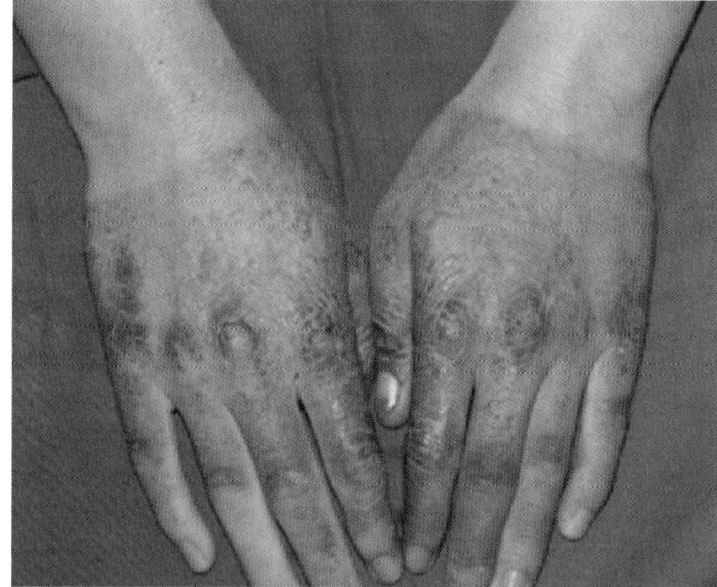

Figure 101.1 Erythropoietic protoporphyria showing marked purpura with sharp cut-off after sunlight exposure.

purpuric, but where profound inflammation has allowed purpura to develop.

ABNORMAL OR DECREASED SUPPORT OF BLOOD VESSELS

Several disorders are associated with abnormal collagen, elastic or other structural proteins, leading to abnormal vessels or poor dermal support or both (Table 101.1). Parent conditions such as Ehlers–Danlos syndrome (collagen), pseudoxanthoma elasticum (elastic) and amyloidosis (abnormal protein) are discussed in more detail elsewhere.

Acnitic purpura. Along with corticosteroid purpura, actinic (also known as Bateman pupura or senile pupura) and corticosteroid purpura are the most common patterns of purpura due to lack of support in blood vessels [1,2]. It occurs most commonly in skin altered by both age and solar radiation, but may occur in premature ageing syndromes. Damage to the connective tissue of the dermis induced by sun exposure presents as purpuric macules on the forearms, hands, face and neck. These resolve after 1–3 weeks, and may leave residual brown pigmentation. Photodamge cannot be reversed, but further damage should be prevented by the use of barriers, such as clothing or sunscreen with UVA and UVB protection [3].

Corticosteroid purpura. Corticosteroid purpura has the same pattern whether due to topical, oral, endogenous (Cushing syndrome) or even inhaled corticosteroids [4]. The purpura occurs mainly in atrophic skin on exposed parts of the hands and forearms, or on the legs. Lesions appear after minor trauma or apparently spontaneously. They are usually asymptomatic and vary in size from a few millimetres to several centimetres across. They are often

Table 101.1 Some dermatologically relevant non-thrombocytopenic causes of purpura, easy bruising or cutaneous bleeding.

Type of disorder	Examples
Inherited defects affecting structural components of the dermis and/or vascular wall	Ehlers–Danlos syndrome[a] Marfan syndrome[a] Osteogenesis imperfecta Pseudoxanthoma elasticum
Acquired defects affecting structural components of the dermis and/or vascular wall	Deposition disorders, e.g. amyloidosis[b] Solar damage (solar/actinic purpura) Scurvy
Haemangiomatous disorders	Cavernous haemangioma[b] Hereditary haemorrhagic telangiectasia[a,b]
Clotting factor and related inherited or acquired deficiencies	Haemophilias Von Willebrand disease Vitamin K deficiency Other nutritional deficiencies (often mixed)
Non-thrombocytopenic platelet abnormalities	See Box 101.3
Biochemical (congenital or acquired)	Homocystinuria Hyperhomocystinaemia[a,b] Diabetes Cushing syndrome
Connective tissue disorders	Systemic sclerosis Dermatomyositis
Paraproteinaemias and hyperviscosity	Waldenström macroglobulinaemia[a] Other paraproteinaemias[a]
Intra- or perivascular inflammation	Capillaropathies Vasculitides Behçet disease Many inflammatory dermatoses
Microvascular occlusion	See section 'Disorders of cutaneous microvascular occlusion'
Infection	Septicaemia, measles, meningococcal infections
Increased pressure within vessels	Valsalva manoeuvre Cough purpura Distal to a sphygmomanometer cuff
Physical	Simple trauma Venous rupture (Achenbach syndrome) Artefactual Chemical and mechanical contact irritants
Drugs	Drugs altering vascular permeability or causing direct endothelial damage Antiangiogenic drugs
Others	Malignant hypertension Autoerythrocyte sensitization

[a] May also have platelet dysfunction.

[b] May also have clotting factor abnormalities.

arranged linearly, and may show a linear or geometric shape. The appearance of the lesions is characteristic, with irregular areas, usually not palpable, that show little inflammatory reaction and that are usually dark purple rather than having the sequential colour changes of a normal bruise. They may persist for several weeks.

Paroxysmal finger haematoma. Also known as Achenbach syndrome, paroxysmal finger haematoma is probably more common than the number of reported cases would suggest [5]. Its importance is that it may be confused with Raynaud phenomenon or acute connective tissue diseases and investigated unnecessarily [6]. In paroxysmal finger haematoma there are recurrent episodes of painful bruising on the palms and palmar aspects of the fingers. It seems likely that the syndrome represents venous rupture, due to frictional trauma.

Scurvy. In scurvy, altered collagenous support for the blood vessels is manifest by either petechiae, especially on the legs, or by small or large bruises on the limbs following mild or inapparent trauma [7]. Large, deep bruises may lead to woody induration, usually of the legs. Perifollicular purpura is typical but is not diagnostic and is frequently absent. Diagnosis is established by the associated symptoms and signs (twisted 'corkscrew' hairs, gingival bleeding), dietary history, laboratory tests and therapeutic response.

Physical and artefactual bleeding

Definition and nomenclature
This is bruising due to trauma.

Synonyms and inclusions
- Black heel and palm
- Talon noir
- Calcaneal petechiae

Introduction and general description
Bruising due to trauma seldom causes diagnostic problems, as there is usually a clear history, except when it occurs as an artefact or in child abuse. Bizarre patterns of purpura may be caused by suction, for example vacuum extractors in the neonate, electrocardiogram leads or around the mouth after sucking out the air from a glass [1]. Cultural remedies such as cupping, coin rubbing (Cao Gio) and spooning (Quat sha) may also produce unusual patterns of purpura that are usually obviously extrinsic in causation. Black heel (talon noire) is a form of purpura due to frictional shearing of vessels. It is pigmentation of the heel (or palm) secondary to extravasation of red blood cells [2].

Epidemiology

Incidence and prevalence
Either sex may be affected by black heel, but the condition is virtually confined to athletic adolescents. Football, basketball, lacrosse and, less often, tennis and squash players are mainly affected. The condition can occur on the hands of weightlifters.

Pathophysiology

Pathology
In black heel, extravasated erythrocytes may be found in the dermal papillae [1], but often the histological changes are limited to

the stratum corneum, where amorphous yellow-brown material may be found in rounded collections having undergone transepidermal elimination. This material is often negative with Perls' stain (which stains haemosiderin) but gives a positive benzidine reaction, showing that it is derived from haemoglobin [3].

Clinical features

History
The condition of black heel results from shear–stress rupture of the papillary capillaries, for example during violent sport, particularly where repeated jumping and sudden stopping or twisting of the heel occurs. Similar circumstances explain occurrences on the palm.

Presentation
In cases of black heel, closely aggregated groups of bluish black specks occur suddenly at the back or side of the heel just above the hyperkeratotic edge of the foot. The metatarsal area has, rarely, been involved. The lesion may resemble a tattoo or even a melanoma [4].

Differential diagnosis
When there is a history of a sudden appearance of the pigmented lesions at a typical site, diagnosis of black heel and palm is rarely in doubt. Viral warts can also produce a black stippled appearance because of extravasation of red cells, but the skin surface is generally abnormal. Occasionally, melanoma or atypical melanocytic hyperplasia [5] will need to be excluded.

Investigations
With black heel, the patient and physician can usually be reassured by carefully paring the affected area, thereby completely removing the abnormality. By epiluminescence microscopy, black heel has highly specific features [6].

Management
The condition is usually asymptomatic, and its importance lies in its resemblance to melanoma. When in doubt as to the diagnosis, carefully paring away the stratum corneum is generally sufficient to remove the pigment.

Dysproteinaemic and Waldenström hypergammaglobulinaemic purpura

Definition and nomenclature
This is a rare skin disease in which the essential features are the presence of purpura with polyclonal hypergammaglobulinaemia.

Synonyms and inclusions
- Benign hypergammaglobulinaemic purpura

Introduction and general description
Walsenström hypergammaglobulinaemic purpura was first described in 1943, with case studies of three women with chronic relapsing purpura, hypergammaglobulinaemia, an elevated erythrocyte sedimentation rate (ESR) and mild anaemia [1]. Purpura may be the presenting and sometimes the only symptom of disturbances in plasma proteins. It may occur at exposed skin sites in cryoproteinaemia and may occur due to monoclonal hypergammaglobulinaemia in myeloma. In such instances there may be platelet dysfunction, but clinical bleeding is usually related to the hyperviscosity syndrome rather than to the altered platelet function.

Epidemiology

Age
In younger patients, Waldenstrom hypergammaglobulinaemic purpura is usually primary. Over time some patients develop the secondary disease.

Pathophysiology

Predisposing factors
This syndrome is associated with severe lung disease and poor prognosis. Other features that have been associated include arthropathy (not uncommon), renal tubular acidosis, chest infections, lymphopenia and immune hypersensitivity pneumonitis.

Pathology
Waldenström hypergammaglobulinaemic purpura is generally taken to imply an idiopathic phenomenon but in fact two of Waldenström's three cases had sicca symptoms, one with sarcoidosis [1]. Hypergammaglobulinaemic purpura is usually a polyclonal disorder with a high presence of specific circulating immune complexes containing IgG or IgA rheumatoid factor. Waldenstrom's is most commonly linked with sarcoidosis, lupus erythematosus, Sjögren syndrome and other autoimmune conditions [2,3,4]. The majority of patients have positive antinuclear antibody and anti-SSA (Ro) or anti-SSB (La) antibodies [5].

Causative organisms
A high antigenic load due to chronic lung infection may be a cause of Waldenström hypergammaglobulinaemic purpura.

Clinical features

Presentation
Waldenström hypergammaglobulinaemic purpura is characterized by recurring crops of petechiae and larger purpuric macules, which commonly burn or sting. It may appear suddenly, mainly affects the lower legs, and is exacerbated by prolonged standing or by tight garments or footwear. Other cutaneous features of paraproteinaemia include various patterns of vasculitis and neutrophilic dermatosis, cryoglobulinaemia, urticaria and systemic capillary leak syndrome, abnormalities of lipid metabolism (notably diffuse plane xanthomatosis), subcorneal pustular dermatosis, and scleromyxoedema, amyloidosis, and features due to hyperviscosity (purpura, mucous membrane bleeding, retinopathy and neurological disturbance) [6,7].

Clinical variants

Some patients with dysproteinaemic purpura present with palpable purpura, rather than the distinctive symptomatic haemorrhagic lesions. Histologically, lesions may be characterized by simple haemorrhage, or by mild perivascular lymphocytic infiltrate or leukocytoclastic vasculitis [8,9].

Differential diagnosis

If there is palpable purpura then a classic cutaneous small vessel vasculitis syndrome may be misdiagnosed.

Complications and co-morbidities

Some patients may develop an autoimmune connective tissue disease, commonly Sjögren syndrome.

Disease course and prognosis

Waldenström hypergammaglobulinaemic purpura can be primary, where lesions usually resolve in about a week, but may become confluent and permanent. In some patients the disease is secondary and will show evidence of an autoimmune connective tissue disease; this is most often Sjögren syndrome, but patients can develop rheumatoid arthritis or lupus erythematosus. Much more rarely, a monoclonal gammopathy or, extremely rarely, a lymphoma or multiple myeloma develops [4].

Investigations

Laboratory evaluation typically reveals polyclonal hypergammaglobulinemia and an elevated ESR. Specific tests for IgG and IgA rheumatoid factor might be performed, since standard assays do not detect these. Where anti-Ro (SS-A) and anti-La (SS-B) antibodies are present, this may indicate a higher likelihood of developing an associated autoimmune connective tissue disease [5].

Management

Treatment is often not required for Waldenström hypergammaglobulinaemic purpura, although prednisolone, NSAIDs, hydroxychloroquine and etamsylate (ethamsylate) have been used. Support stockings have been used, but have also been reported to exacerbate the condition. Avoidance of alcohol, prolonged standing, tight clothing or footwear may be helpful. Where the disease is secondary, treatment should be targeted at the underlying disease.

PIGMENTED PURPURIC DERMATOSES

Five main morphological variants of idiopathic pigmented purpuric dermatosis exist [1,2,3,4,5,6–9]:

1 Schamberg disease (about 50% of cases).
2 Itching purpura (eczematid-like purpura of Doucas and Kapetanakis) (about 10%).
3 Pigmented purpuric lichenoid dermatosis of Gougerot and Blum (about 5%).
4 Lichen aureus (about 10%).
5 Purpura annularis telangiectodes (Majocchi disease) (about 5%).

A further variant, called Favre–Chaix purpura, occurs on the lower leg and comprises purpura and pigmentation associated with oedema, cyanosis and sclerosis; it would appear to be simply a manifestation of venous disease and is not considered further here. However, additional types (such as granulomatous) or subtypes (e.g. segmental variants of the above list) also warrant mention as they may in time prove to be aetiologically distinct. Furthermore, about 20% of cases are unclassifiable [2] and many drugs, systemic diseases or local conditions of the skin may lead to localized, mild purpura with haemosiderin deposition and secondary melanin pigmentation [6].

Pigmented purpurpic dermatosis

Synonyms and inclusions
• Capillaritis
• Purpura progressiva pigmentosa

Introduction and general description

The pigmented purpuric dermatoses are a set of diseases of mostly unknown aetiology, which may be secondary to capillaritis [7]. Distinctive pupuric lesions are characterized by petechial haemorrhage (or extravasation or erythrocytes in the skin with marked hemosiderin deposition). Capillaritis is the generic term for a variety of chronic conditions that share certain histological features. The term 'purpura simplex' has also been applied to this group of disorders, on the basis of the common histological aspects. However, the same term has been applied to other mild and unexplained but morphologically different patterns of purpura such as easy bruising, and it is therefore potentially confusing. The term 'pigmented purpuric dermatoses' may be preferred, at least at present, as it conveys the message of a component beyond simple transient purpura.

Epidemiology

Incidence and prevalence

Schamberg disease is the most common form, occurring in around half of all cases. Other conditions are rare, while granulomatous pigmented purpura is extremely rare.

Age

Adults are mainly affected. There are several cases of Schamberg disease in children, while linear pigmented purpura can occur in children and adolescents, and purpura annularis telangiectodes occurs in adolescents and young adults, especially women [1,8].

Sex

Schamberg disease is seen frequently in middle-aged to older men, as is itching purpura and pigmented purpuric lichenoid dermatitis of Gougerot and Blum.

Pathophysiology

Predisposing factors

The identification of pigmented purpuric dermatoses secondary to a systemic cause is potentially important and is discussed below. Gravity and increased venous pressure are important localizing factors in many cases. Exercise may be a provoking factor.

Pathology

Inflammation and haemorrhage of capillaries and other superficial papillary dermal vessels are the cause of these diseases. There is no association with coagulation abnormality and the reason for the inflammation is unknown.

Pathologically, these disorders are characterized by a narrowing of the lumen and endothelial swelling of superficial small vessels, accompanied by perivascular T-lymphocytic infiltration, extravasation of erythrocytes and haemosiderin deposits in macrophages. An appearance termed 'ectasizing endocapillaritis' has been reported in a study in which the authors divided 22 cases into those that were papular (with an upper dermal band-like infiltrate), macular (with a perivascular infiltrate) or eczematous (with exocytosis and spongiosis) [6], but this has not led to any fundamental advance in understanding these diseases. The cellular infiltrate in all types contains CD4+ T cells in close contact with CD1a+ Langerhans cells [7], suggesting that a cell-mediated immune reaction is operative. A strong expression of the endothelial cell adhesion receptors ICAM-1 (intercellular adhesion molecule 1) and ELAM-1 (endothelial cell leukocyte adhesion molecule-1) may determine the pattern of the infiltrate [7]. Immune complex deposition has also been reported but direct immunofluorescence is often negative. An IgA-associated lymphocytic vasculopathy has been described in eight patients, in six of whom the clinical and histological features were those of a pigmented purpuric dermatosis [7]. The significance of this is unclear but it is notable that many of the subjects had a preceding or associated condition, including viral infection, Henoch–Schönlein purpura, undifferentiated connective tissue disease, lupus erythematosus profundus, Degos disease and Buerger disease.

Clinical features

Presentation

The key characteristics of pigmented purpuric dermatoses are a cluster of petechial haemorrhages. The background is often discoloured yellow-brown because of hemosiderin deposition. Each different subtype of condition displays a particular morphology and location (Table 101.2).

Differential diagnosis

Differential diagnoses include stasis dermatitis, contact dermatitis and purpura secondary to haematological disorders. The petechial haemorrhage of lesions may lead to misdiagnosis of thrombocytopenia or vasculitis.

Complications and co-morbidities

These dermatoses are typically asymptomatic with no systemic findings. Pruritus is prominent in itching purpura.

Disease course and prognosis

Most are chronic but two-thirds may improve or clear eventually [5].

Table 101.2 Presentation of different pigmented purpuric dermatoses.

Syndrome	Clinical features	Location
Schamberg disease	Orange-red flat patches with 'cayenne pepper' spots on the borders Old lesions become yellow-brown patches Oval or irregular outline Pinpoint petechiae inside patches Successive crops	Usually lower legs; also involves trunk, arms, thighs and buttocks Irregularly distributed on both sides with few or many patches
Itching purpura	Pruritic, scaly petechial or pupuric macules, papules and patches Appears similar to Schamberg disease	Usually lower extremities
Pigmented purpuric lichenoid dermatosis of Gougerot and Blum	Combination of Schamberg-like and purpuric red-brown lichenoid thickened papules Chronic, can be pruritic	Usually on lower extremities
Lichen aureus	Isolated, persistent patch Varying colour, purple-brown to golden or rust	Usually lower extremities Commonly overlies a varicose vein
Purpura annularis telangiectodes (Majocchi disease)	Annular brown plaques, 1–3 cm in size. Plaques gradually spread outwards Punctuate telangiectases and petechiae inside border	Trunk, lower extremities (proximal)
Contact allergy		Only affects skin in contact with material responsible (e.g. clothing dye, rubber)
Exercise-induced	Crops of small red spots following prolonged or vigorous exercise Fade to brown and disappear within days Possible burning sensation accompanies new lesions	Commonly on ankles

PART 9: VASCULAR

Investigations

Histology can be helpful. Consider if medication could be causing capillaritis and try discontinuing for several months. Also try avoiding food preservatives and artificial colouring agents for several months. Return to normal if there is no improvement. Usually, no further investigations are necessary.

Management

Lesions may clear spontaneously, but this is usually slow. These disorders may persist for many years and are very resistant to any form of therapy. Explanation without active intervention, or simply support hosiery, is often the most appropriate approach. Topical steroids may be of some help, especially for itch, but prolonged use is best avoided. Emollients can be used as necessary. A rapid response of lichen aureus to topical pimecrolimus has been reported [1]. Psoralen and UVA (PUVA) has proven effective in treating capillaritis of Schamberg, Gougerot–Blum and lichen aureus patterns [10]. Narrow-band UVB (TL01) has been reported as being effective in Schamberg disease [5] and in Gougerot–Blum pigmented purpuric lichenoid dermatitis [1]. Ciclosporin has also been effective in individual reports [8].

DISORDERS OF CUTANEOUS MICROVASCULAR OCCLUSION

Platelet plugging: heparin necrosis

Definition and nomenclature

There are two types of heparin-induced thrombocytopenia (HIT). Type I is a harmless condition that is not due to immune factors, but can cause a reduction in platelet count which is mild and transient. HIT type II is an autoimmune condition leading to low platelet counts and blood clotting. This occurs in 1–5% of patients, usually 5–10 days after starting heparin. In general medical practice, HIT refers to type II heparin-induced necrosis. Ulceration in patients on heparin may be due to other causes of heparin-induced necrosis [1].

> **Synonyms and inclusions**
> - Heparin-induced thrombocytopenia syndrome with heparin-reactive antibodies
> - Heparin-induced thrombocytopenia-associated thrombosis
> - Heparin-associated thrombocytopenia with thrombosis (HATT) syndrome

Introduction and general description

Heparin necrosis may occur with heparin exposure after subcutaneous or intravenous administration. It is an unusual but important iatrogenic syndrome first described in the 1970s. HIT is defined as a clinical event explained by platelet factor 4 (PF4)/ heparin-reactive antibodies (HIT antibodies). In 90% of patients with HIT there is usually an absolute or relative thrombocytopenia with evidence of venous or arterial thrombosis with heparin necrosis in the skin [2].

Epidemiology

Incidence and prevalence

Heparin-induced thrombocytopenia is an uncommon response to heparin and occurs in 1–5% of adults exposed to heparin, with up to 30% developing subsequent thrombosis [3]. This was further confirmed in a study conducted on paediatric patients on intensive care units where the incidence of thrombosis was 2.3%.

Sex

There is some female predominance for HIT [4].

Pathophysiology

Predisposing factors

Unfractionated heparin is three times more likely to be associated with HIT compared with low-molecular heparin, and is more likely to be induced by the bovine-derived unfractionated heparin than the porcine variety [2]. It is caused by an antibody, which binds to PF4 tetramers, a protein which is expressed on the surface of platelets.

The risk of HIT is highest in postsurgical patients requiring heparin and less so in medical and obstetric settings [2].

Pathology

Heparin necrosis is usually mediated by IgG [5], although IgA and IgM class antibodies may play a role. These antibodies can be directed at heparin and other polyanions when bound to PF4, inducing changes in the tetrameric PF4, exposing new epitopes. This may trigger further antibody production so that when anti-heparin/PF4 antibodies bind with heparin/PF4 complexes on the surface of platelets, there is a resulting platelet activation and aggravation. Some antibodies associated with HIT do not bind to heparin/PF4 complexes, but to chemokines or cytokines, including neutrophil-activating peptide-2 (NAP-2) and interleukin 8, leading to the activation of platelets [2,5,6].

Clinical features

History

Patients with HIT often develop an absolute or relative thrombocytopenia (90%) with evidence of venous or arterial thromboses or heparin necrosis in the skin [2]. A better indication of early heparin-induced platelet aggravation can be a proportional drop of over 50% in platelet number from the pre-treatment count rather than an absolute thrombocytopenia of 100–150 × 10^9/L [2]. If heparin has been received within the past 10 days, this may occur immediately on administration. However, two-thirds of patients will have a fall in platelet count between 5 and 10 days after heparin administration, with significant thrombocytopenia taking up to 7–14 days to develop. Occasionally, HIT may develop several days after stopping heparin therapy (delayed-onset HIT). A history of HIT does not necessarily predict that the patient will suffer a second episode, as long as there has been over 100 days between treatments.

Presentation

Cutaneous findings include simple haemorrhage with echymoses and occasionally urticaria or infiltrated plaques [7]. Rarely there

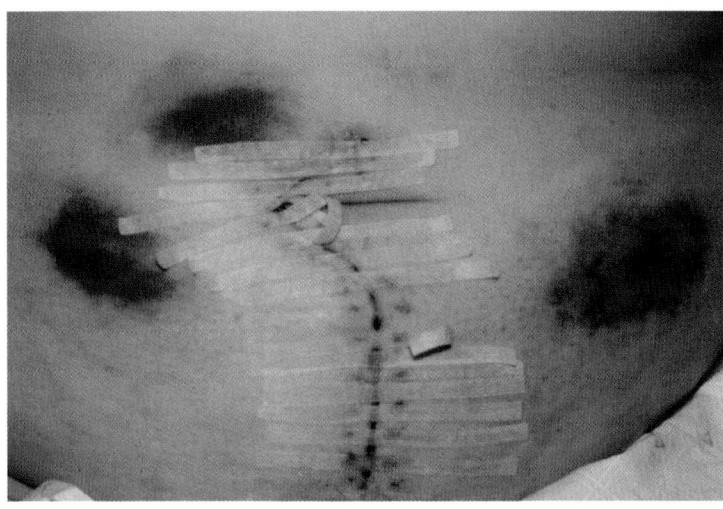

(a)

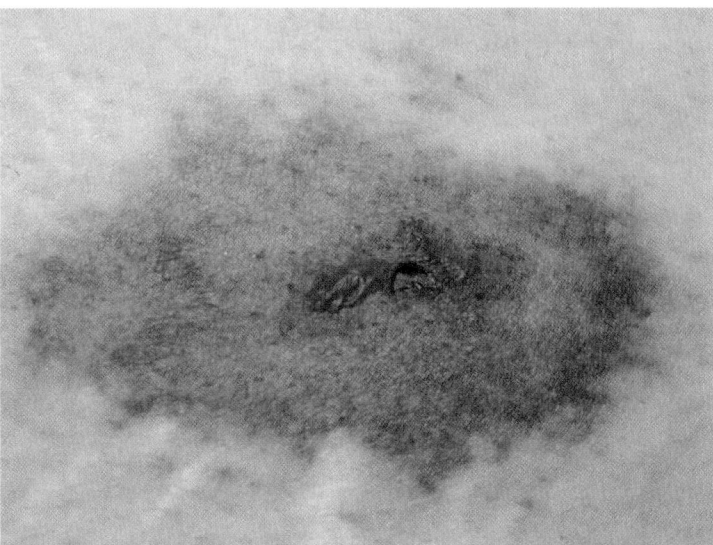

(b)

Figure 101.2 (a) Heparin necrosis at sites of subcutaneous heparin injection. (b) Close-up of a 15 cm lesion on the left abdomen. The lesion is a non-palpable haemorrhage with retiform margins, minimal erythema and central retiform-intense haemorrhage, early necrosis and bullae formation. (From Robson and Piette 1999 [**11**]. Reproduced with permission of Elsevier.)

is cutaneous microvasular occlusion. Some cases present with sharply demarcated, purpuric, tender plaques, with marginal retiform extensions, accompanied by erythema. These lesions are most common at subcutaneous injection sites (Figure 101.2), although they can occur elsewhere, and often develop between day 5 and day 10 of heparin therapy [8]. Patients already sensitized to heparin may develop heparin necrosis much earlier. There is a subset of delayed-onset heparin necrosis, which may take up to 3 weeks to develop after the onset of heparin.

Differential diagnosis

Patients on heparin may develop thrombocytopenia for other reasons, whilst patients without thrombocytopenia may develop arterial or venous thromboses [2]. The history is therefore very important as to whether heparin has been administered in patients

who develop retiform purpura or bland necrosis, with or without thrombocytopenia.

Management

Stopping heparin is important. Previously, substituting heparin with warfarin was thought to be effective but can, in fact, lead to venous limb gangrene. Low-molecular-weight heparin is much less likely to cause HIT, but may be contraindicated in patients with HIT due to other types of heparin.

If patients with a previous history of HIT have not received heparin within 100 days, their antibodies may disappear, allowing them to be treated with heparin, for example during cardiac surgery. The anticoagulants currently used to treat patients with HIT are danaparoid (a heparinoid). Ensure platelet counts return to normal in those who require warfarin monotherapy, as it can decrease protein C activity, leading to a progression of thrombosis and necrosis [9,10].

Platelet plugging: thrombocytosis

Introduction and general description

Thrombocytosis is usually due to essential thrombocythaemia, which is most probably due to a myeloproliferative disorder or polycythemia vera [1]. Thrombocytosis is a common finding with a wide range of primary and secondary causes.

Epidemiology

Incidence and prevalence

Essential thrombocytosis and polycythaemia vera are rare, but are the first and second most common causes of elevated platelet counts, with an increased frequency of thrombotic events and of erythromelalgia [2]. Essential thrombocythaemia has been found to have a 14% risk of thrombosis over 10 years [3].

Age

Thrombocytosis is more common at younger ages.

Sex

Thrombocytosis is more common in women.

Pathophysiology

Reactive or post-splenectomy thrombocytosis at any level is not associated with occlusion, suggesting that thrombosis in the setting of myeloproliferative disease is not a function of thrombocytosis alone. Multiple studies have shown that a specific mutation in the JAK2 tyrosine kinase (JAK2V617F) is found in many patients with essential thrombocytosis, polycythaemia vera and primary myelofibrosis, and a gain-of-function mutation in the thrombopoietin receptor (MPL) is found in a subset of patients with essential thrombocytosis but who are JAK2V617-negative [4]. The mechanisms for ischaemic or occlusive syndromes in myeloproliferative disease must therefore depend on more than platelet number alone.

PART 9: VASCULAR

Predisposing factors

Acquired von Willebrand factors in myeloproliferative disease have been associated with both bleeding and thrombotic complications. Anticardiolipin antibodies, factor V Leiden mutations, abnormal endothelial cell function, and decreased levels of protein C and protein S may be synergistic for thrombosis in chronic myeloproliferative diseases [5,6]. In addition to high platelet counts, abnormal platelet function occurs in myeloproliferative or myelodysplastic disease, although whether this can lead to vascular occlusion at platelet counts of less than $1000 \times 10^9/L$ is controversial. Thrombotic events have been reported at platelet counts of below $600 \times 10^9/L$ in patients with essential thrombocytosis, including some events at normal platelet counts [7].

Pathology

Splenomegaly may be seen in all forms of myeloproliferative syndromes. Ruddy cyanosis is characteristic of polycythaemia vera, as is elevation of haemoglobin, haematocrit and red cell mass. All syndromes may show elevations in white cell count, but this is most characteristic of chronic granulocytic leukaemia, especially in association with elevated eosinophil and basophil counts.

Clinical features

Presentation

Cutaneous lesions are common in thrombocythaemia and other myeloproliferative disorders. Paradoxically, patients with myeloproliferative thrombocytosis may both bleed and clot abnormally. Skin lesions were documented in 22% of 268 patients with essential thrombocythaemia [8], and included urticaria, livedo reticularis, petechiae, ecchymoses, haematomas, erythromelalgia, Raynaud phenomenon, recurrent superficial thrombophlebitis, necrotizing vasculitis, leg ulceration and gangrene. Biopsy findings were variable, but some livedo reticularis and acral infarcts were associated with evidence of microvascular occlusion. Additionally, tender erythematous facial plaques and palmar violet macules and papules were reported as manifestations of platelet plugging in a patient with atypical chronic myeloproliferative disease and a history of Budd–Chiari syndrome, another known thrombotic complication of myeloproliferative disease [9].

Erythromelalgia can occur as a primary or secondary syndrome. This intensely uncomfortable burning associated with paroxysmal erythema of the distal extremities is frequently triggered by skin contact with a warm surface. Although erythromelalgia has been seen in many different settings, the association of purpuric or necrotic areas on the hands and feet with dysaesthetic erythema is exclusively seen with myeloproliferative or myelodysplastic thrombocytosis [10].

Complications and co-morbidities

Patients with essential thrombocythaemia and polycythaemia vera have a higher risk of morbidity from thrombotic complications [1]. Anaemia and altered red cell morphology can occur over time in all patients, and all these diseases have some risk of transition to dyspoiesis and severe anaemia, leukaemia or myelofibrosis.

Disease course and prognosis

Patients with essential thrombocythaemia and polycythaemia vera are likely to present with platelet counts greater than 1 million and to have a good prognosis compared with that of patients with other myeloproliferative disorders [1].

Investigations

The diagnosis of essential thrombocythaemia requires a sustained thrombocytosis with platelet counts of greater than $400 \times 10^9/L$, with the exclusion of reactive causes. The blood film will show thrombocytosis with platelet anisocytosis. There may be an elevated white blood cell count. Bone marrow examination with aspirate and trephine biopsy are usually required, but not always necessary.

Management

Many therapies previously used for myeloproliferative thrombocytosis increase the risk of leukaemic transformation and of complications in fertility and pregnancy. Low-dose aspirin has been widely accepted as effective thrombosis prophylaxis, although definitive proof of its efficacy is lacking. Its dramatic reversal of signs and symptoms in erythromelalgia provides some clinical evidence for its usefulness in thrombocythaemic complications. Because of the platelet origin of occlusion and vascular symptoms in thrombocythaemic erythromelalgia, aspirin administration is notably effective in clearing lesions and alleviating any burning pain, whereas it is much less effective in primary and other secondary forms of erythromelalgia.

In a patient with atypical, chronic myeloproliferative disease and a history of Budd–Chiari syndrome, cutaneous lesions were unresponsive to warfarin, but cleared within 24 h of aspirin administration following the identification of platelet plugs as the cause of previously identified microvascular occlusion.

Hydroxycarbamide is the drug of choice for the prevention of transient ischaemic attacks, but may not be effective in preventing venous thrombosis; anagrelide may reduce the risk of venous thrombosis but appears to increase the risk for arterial thrombosis and haemorrhage. Anagrelide has become an important therapeutic agent, acting to both inhibit platelet activity and decrease the platelet count [11,12]. The JAK2 mutations seem to correlate with leukocyte and platelet proliferation, but the role for the JAK2 and MPL mutations in enhancing thromboses is less clear [13]. Multiple studies suggest that the presence of the JAK2V617F mutation translates into activation of haemostasis, at least in part through increase in platelet-associated tissue factor microparticles and increased platelet–neutrophil aggregates [14].

Cryogelling/cryoagglutination disorders

Introduction and general description

Disorders of cryogelling or cryoagulation, due to type 1 cryoglobulins, cyrofibrinogen or cold agglutinins (uncommon), are occlusive syndromes in the skin triggered by cold exposure.

Cryoglobulins are immunoglobulins that reversibly precipitate or gel in the cold; they were first reported in 1933 and named cryoglobulins in 1947 [1,2,3,4]. In 1974, Brouet *et al.* [1] proposed the now standard subset classification of cryoglobulins into types I, II and III. Type I (single molecule) cryoglobulins are single monoclonal immunoglobulins. Types II and III, termed mixed cryoglobulins, are multiple molecule proteins, typically immune complexes, that gel under laboratory conditions (2–4°C). Cryofibrinogen deposits consist of a complex of fibrinogen, fibrin and fibronectin that forms on cold exposure [5].

Cold agglutinins are immunoglobulins that are able to agglutinate red blood cells below normal body temperatures.

Although the precipitation of cryoglobulins is primarily related to reversible cold-induced denaturation of protein, other factors such as cryoglobulin concentration in the microvascular environment, pH and non-covalent binding factors also influence the likelihood and intensity of precipitation.

Epidemiology

Incidence and prevalence
Type I account for 10–15% of cryoglobulins. Cryofibrinogens and cold agglutinins are rarely the cause of occlusive syndromes triggered by cold exposure, despite being often detected in patients with various illnesses [6].

Age
The median age at diagnosis of cryoglobulinaemia is the early to middle sixth decade.

Sex
Cryoglobulinaemia incidence has a female to male ratio of 2 : 1 [2].

Associated diseases
Type I cryoglobulins are often associated with an underlying lymphoproliferative disorder, especially multiple myeloma or Waldenström macroglobulinaemia [5]. Unless they gel at temperatures close to body temperature, type I and II cryoglobulins are much more likely to cause disease as immune complexes than as cryoproteins, but they can cause disease through either or both mechanisms in any given patient. Rheumatoid factor activity (defined by anti-Fc binding) is detectable in the sera of 87–100% of patients with mixed cryoglobulinaemia [3].

Antibodies to hepatitis C virus (HCV) have been found in more than 50% (42–98%) of patients with type II and III cryoglobulins [2,3,4]. Conversely, 13–54% of patients with HCV have mixed cryoglobulins detected in the laboratory, and the majority of these are type III cryoglobulins (67–91%). Of HCV-infected individuals with cryoglobulins, only 27% had clinical signs consistent with the syndrome of cryoglobulinaemia [2]. The reasons why only a fraction of HCV-infected and cryoglobulin-positive patients develop symptomatic cryoglobulinaemia are unknown.

Although type I cryoglobulinaemia is usually associated with lymphoproliferative disease, it is a much less common type than II and III. The latter two types account for the majority of cryoglobulinaemia-associated lymphoproliferative disease in regions with a high endemic rate of HCV and mixed cryoglobulinaemia [2].

Other syndromes are also associated with cryoglobulins detectable in serum. Patients with connective tissue disease have higher rates of cryoglobulinaemia, including patients with systemic lupus erythematosus (SLE), systemic sclerosis, active rheumatoid arthritis and Sjögren syndrome [2]. In addition to HCV, other chronic infections such as Lyme disease, subacute bacterial endocarditis, Q fever, hepatitis A and B, hantavirus, cytomegalovirus, human T-cell leukaemia virus I and HIV have been reported [2,7]. Chronic inflammatory disease, such as liver cirrhosis from any cause, is also associated with a higher than expected rate of detectable cryoglobulins.

Cryofibrinogenaemia may be idiopathic or can be associated with malignant disorders (especially haematological), thromboembolic disease, IgA nephropathy or various inflammatory, connective tissue or infectious syndromes [8,9].

Monoclonal cold agglutinins are idiopathic or secondary to malignant lymphoproliferative diseases. Polyclonal cold agglutinins are usually associated with infection, especially due to *Mycoplasma pneumoniae*, and less often with HCV, parvovirus B19 or leptospiral infections.

Pathophysiology

Predisposing factors
The presence of cryoglobulins in serum does not invariably predict disease. In fact, despite detectable serum cryoglobulins in the patient groups mentioned, most will not develop symptomatic cryoglobulinaemia [2].

Pathology
Type I cryoglobulins are single monoclonal immunoglobulins, usually IgG or IgM, less commonly IgA, and rarely Bence–Jones protein.

Type II cryoglobulins are composed of monoclonal proteins of IgM, IgG or occasionally IgA class that bind to an antigen present in the blood, most commonly the Fc portion of polyclonal IgG molecules. Those that bind immunoglobulin (usually IgG) by anti-Fc affinity are also, by definition, rheumatoid factors, although only the IgM/anti-IgG rheumatoid factors are recognized by standard rheumatoid factor testing. In up to 95% of type II cryoglobulins with IgM as the antirheumatoid factor immunoglobulin, the IgM contains a κ light chain, which would not be expected by chance alone [3]. Type III mixed cryoglobulins are also most commonly rheumatoid factors, but the IgM, IgG or IgA anti-Fc antibodies in this group are polyclonal rather than monoclonal. In patients with mixed type II and III cryoglobulins, complement levels are usually reduced, especially the C4 component.

Acquired dysfibrinogenaemia may rarely mimic a cryofibrinogen syndrome by acral occlusion, including gangrene. Interestingly, this subset of dysfibrinogenaemia appears to act by greatly increasing red cell aggregation, mimicking occlusion-inducing cold agglutinins. Blood smear preparations show marked rouleaux formation.

In cases of cold agglutinin-related cutaneous occlusion, the agglutination of red blood cells depends on binding of antibody to more than one cell at a time. Pentavalent IgM is almost exclusively responsible for this phenomenon. Just as with cryoglobulins, there are both monoclonal and polyclonal cold agglutinins, usually directed at the I, i or Pr antigens of erythrocytes [**10**].

Clinical features

History
The patient will have undergone exposure to cold temperatures.

Presentation
Occlusion syndromes triggered by cold exposure are suggested by an acral distribution of lesions of necrosis or purpura, often with retiform features, and sometimes associated with acral livedo reticularis. An acral distribution must be distinguished from a dependent distribution of lesions. Both patterns may involve hands and feet, but with a dependent pattern there are typically many more lesions on the feet and legs than on the hands.

Recurrent showers of dependent palpable purpura, sometimes with burning or itching, frequently associated with arthritis or arthralgia, is the classic presentation of mixed (type II and III) cryoglobulinaemia (the combination of purpura, asthenia and arthralgia has been termed Meltzer's triad). Patients with symptomatic cryoglobulinaemia of any type most often present with cutaneous lesions, usually purpura (in 55–100%, especially if HCV associated) [3,11]. Ulceration, haemorrhagic crusts or cutaneous infarction are seen in 10–25% of patients, most often with type I cryoglobulins. Cold-induced acrocyanosis of acral areas, and non-inflammatory retiform purpura are also more typical of type I cryoglobulinaemia. Other reported cutaneous findings include acral cyanosis, Raynaud phenomenon, urticarial lesions, ulceration and livedo reticularis [4,12].

Non-cutaneous clinical findings most frequently include involvement of the joints, peripheral nerves, kidneys and liver [2,3,4].

The most common cutaneous findings in cases of cryofibrinogenaemia are cold intolerance, purpura, necrosis, livedo reticularis, gangrene and ulceration (Figure 101.3) [9,13]. The purpura, or necrosis, typically has a non-inflammatory retiform morphology.

Clinical variants
In addition, the acral distribution of cryo-occlusion syndromes often includes the ears and nose.

Differential diagnosis
A dependent distribution of lesions suggests immune complex-mediated disease, and usually presents as classic palpable purpura or occasionally as inflammatory retiform purpura, not as bland or non-inflammatory purpura or pauci-erythematous necrosis. An acral distribution of lesions is also characteristic of erythema multiforme. However, erythema multiforme presents with target lesions, atypical target lesions or classic palpable purpura, rather than non-inflammatory retiform purpura or necrosis, and it is not associated with livedo reticularis. Chilbains should be considered, although these lesions develop slowly and rarely have acute purpura or necrosis [6].

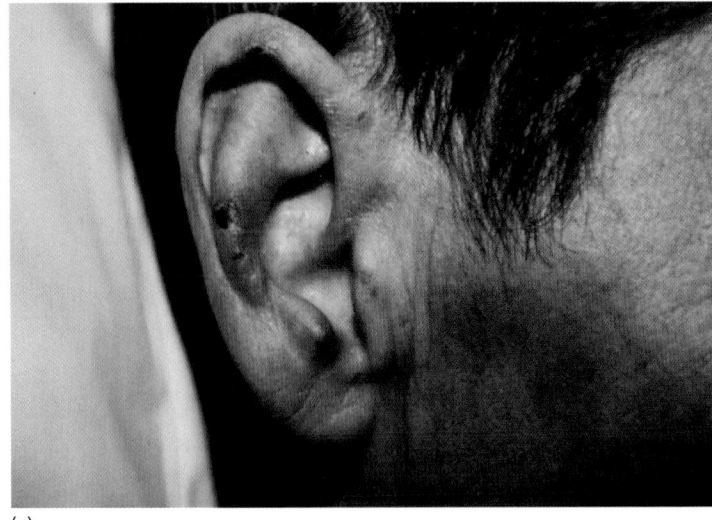

(a)

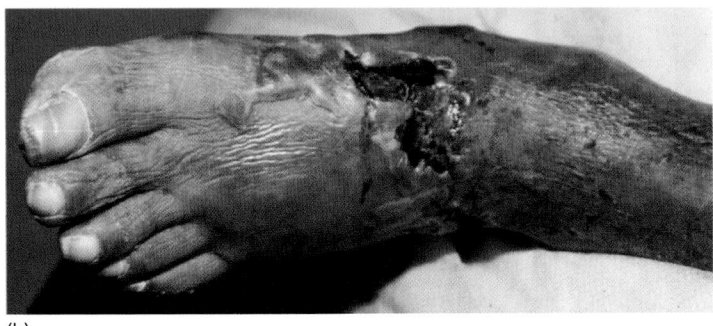

(b)

Figure 101.3 Cold-induced lesions due to cryofibrinogenaemia, (a) on the ear and (b) on the foot. An acral location is typical for cryogelling. The foot lesion shows minimal erythema, retiform bullae and haemorrhage with necrosis.

Although ill patients with immune complex vasculitis may develop dependent lesions on the posterior portions of the ears if supine due to their illness, their other lesions are typically in dependent areas as well, and there is usually no history of cold exposure as the precipitating factor.

Distal occlusion syndromes (cholesterol emboli, acral antiphospholipid antibody syndrome) may also present similarly, but lack a history of cold exposure and the presence of lesions on the nose and ears.

Complications and co-morbidities
There are only two known ways in which cryoglobulins can result in disease. The first is by precipitation within the vascular lumen, typically cold induced, with hyaline plug formation and minor early-phase inflammation. Typical clinical lesions are characterized by minimally inflammatory cutaneous infarction, with or without associated livedo reticularis, or non-inflammatory retiform purpura. Since there is little evidence that cryogelling of monoclonal antibody induces complement activation, cryogelling is the only known mechanism for vascular lesions for type I cryoglobulins [14]. The second mechanism is that of immune complex vasculitis. As nearly all type II and III cryoglobulins are immune complexes, they should all be capable of inducing an immune complex vasculitis, although many do not. If they cryoprecipitate near

Cholesterol embolus   101.15

body temperature, they could also cause vascular injury by simple occlusion, although most appear to gel at temperatures well below 37°C. Cryofibrinogenaemia is common as a laboratory abnormality but is a rare cause of symptomatic clinical disease [15].

Just as with many cryoglobulins and most cryofibrinogens, cold agglutinins are most likely to be asymptomatic. When responsible for disease, reversible acrocyanosis secondary to cold-induced acral agglutination is most common. Livedo reticularis, Raynaud phenomenon, cold urticaria and rarely cutaneous necrosis may occur. In addition to acral lesions on environmental cold exposure, cold intravenous infusions can also trigger localized cutaneous necrosis [16]. Cold agglutinins can induce complement activation after cold-induced binding to red blood cells, followed by lysis and haemolytic anaemia, independent of occlusive syndromes from agglutination.

Investigations

A biopsy of early lesions, before necrosis has had time to trigger a secondary vasculitic histology, should show non-inflammatory occlusion of dermal vessels with cryoprotein or agglutinated red cells.

Careful handling of serum and plasma is necessary to allow the identification of cryogelling proteins, because those most likely to cause disease are those that gel at temperatures very close to normal body temperature. Likewise, the identification of cryoproteins or cryoagglutinins does not prove a cryo-occlusion syndrome, because these may either gel at temperatures that are not relevant to typical cold exposure or may simply represent incidental findings. The latter is especially true of cryofibrinogens and cold agglutinins [2,3].

Despite the presence of monoclonal protein, polyclonal gammopathy is the most frequent finding on serum protein electrophoresis of serum samples (not cryoprecipitate specimens) in patients with type II cryoglobulinaemia [2]. A more sensitive technique, such as immunofixation, is needed to identify the presence of a clonal protein.

Histological demonstration of non-inflammatory hyaline thrombosis is more common in patients with type I cryoglobulinaemia, but some such patients have also been reported to have cutaneous vasculitis [11].

Since cryofibrinogens can be cleaved to form fibrin, plasma rather than serum must be tested to detect these cryogelling proteins. Cryoglobulins should be present in both plasma and sera [5,13]. Biopsy specimens from skin lesions typically show thrombi in small vessels with dermal necrosis [8]. Leukocytoclastic vasculitis has been reported, but is probably due to ischaemic necrosis rather than being a cause [9]. Fibronectin may be a major component of vascular plugs in patients with cryofibrinogenaemia alone, whereas vascular occlusion in patients with both cryofibrinogens and cryoglobulins shows a predominance of cryoglobulin deposition [9].

Management

Treatment of cryoglobulinaemia is often problematic, and prospective or controlled trials are rare [3,4]. If symptoms are mild, no treatment may be needed. If symptoms of acral lesions are precipitated by cold, then the protection of affected areas may be sufficient. Measures to reduce the concentration of a type I cryoglobulin, such as plasmapheresis, plasma exchange or cytotoxic therapy, are occasionally effective, although unfortunately usually only in the short term. For immune complex-related disease, corticosteroids, cytotoxic agents or plasmapheresis may be effective, but relapse is typical once therapy is stopped. Interferon-α has been used to treat HCV-associated cryoglobulinaemia, with or without ribavarin [3,4]. Treatment with these agents has resulted in partial or complete remissions of vasculitic findings, but relapse often follows cessation of therapy. The therapy itself has occasionally been implicated in triggering the onset of vasculitis. In patients with mixed cryoglobulinaemia troubled primarily by recurrent cutaneous vasculitic lesions, colchicine or dapsone therapy may be of some help in reducing the frequency and severity of episodes.

Treatment of cryofibrinogenaemia should be aimed at the underlying disease, where possible, and at protecting areas from cold exposure [17]. Stanozolol, an androgenic steroid with fibrinolysis-enhancing effects, has also been used for treatment of cryofibrinogenaemia, as have other fibrinolytic androgene steroid agents [18]. Patients with cold-induced agglutination syndromes must avoid cold exposure. Therapies such as corticosteroids, cytotoxic agents, danazol, rituxan or interferon-α have been occasionally beneficial [17].

ORGANISMS IN VESSELS

There are a number of cutaneous infections that can produce purpuric lesions:
- Echthyma gangrenosum, caused by *Pseudomonas aeruginosa* (see Chapter 32).
- *Aspergillus* and *Mucor* fungal infections (see Chapter 26).
- Disseminated strongyloides infection (see Chapter 33).
- Lucio phenomenon (erythema necroticans) (see Chapter 28).

EMBOLI

Cholesterol embolus

Definition and nomenclature
Cholesterol emboli resulting from the ulceration of arteriosclerotic plaques and the subsequent release of cholesterol crystals can cause disease of the skin, particularly in the lower extremities.

Synonyms and inclusions
- Blue toe syndrome

Introduction and general description
The most commonly diagnosed cutaneous embolic syndrome is cholesterol embolus, which occurs secondary to fragmentation of ulcerated arteriosclerotic plaques, with distal cutaneous and visceral vessel obstruction.

PART 9: VASCULAR

Epidemiology

Incidence and prevalence

The incidence of cholesterol embolization syndrome (CES) following vascular procedures has ranged from 0.15% to 30%, with large retrospective studies reporting figures of 0.6–0.9% [1,2]. Autopsy studies have shown cholesterol emboli in 77% of patients who underwent aortic aneurysm resection [2]. A prospective study of 1786 consecutive patients aged over 40 years who underwent left heart catheterization found an incidence of cholesterol embolus of 1.4%, with nearly half having definite CES and the remainder having possible CES with primarily renal abnormalities [1]. Patients with cutaneous findings (livedo reticularis, blue toe syndrome or digital gangrene) were considered to have definite CES and comprised 48% of the total. In-hospital mortality was 16% and was associated with progressive renal dysfunction.

Age

As it occurs secondary to atheromatous plaques, it is no surprise that cholesterol embolus is a syndrome reported primarily in men aged 50 years or older.

Associated diseases

Cholestorol embolus is associated with peripheral vascular disease and the known risk factors for atherosclerosis such as diabetes, hypertension and smoking [3]. Blue toe syndrome associated with warfarin use is a syndrome of cholesterol embolus and not of warfarin-induced skin necrosis.

Pathophysiology

Predisposing factors

Although cholesterol embolus may be spontaneous, known triggers include angiography, angioplasty, vascular surgery, intra-aortic pump placement, cardiopulmonary resuscitation (all inducing traumatic rupture of plaques, usually within hours or days), thrombolytic therapy (acute clot lysis in plaque with release of friable plaque within hours or days) and anticoagulation (slow reduction of clot with release of plaque fragments, usually after at least 2 months of therapy) [3,4].

Pathology

On histological examination, the arteriole involved in the skin is usually at the dermal–subcutaneous junction, with elongated clefts within small-vessel lumina along with thrombi [5]. The clefts result from fixation-related dissolving of cholesterol crystals. In experimentally produced cholesterol embolus, a mixed inflammatory infiltrate may be seen in the arterial walls within 24–48 h, followed by multinucleated histiocytes within 3–6 days, and subsequent occasional intimal fibrosis.

Clinical features

Presentation

There are two 'classic' clinical triads of cholesterol embolus. The first comprises leg or foot pain, livedo reticularis and preservation of good peripheral pulses [4]. The second comprises livedo reticularis, renal insufficiency and eosinophilia [6]. Cutaneous findings are frequent in patients recognized as experiencing episodes of cholesterol embolus, including livedo reticularis, gangrene, cyanosis, ulceration, nodules and purpura. Additional clinical findings include fever, myalgia, altered mental status, sudden-onset arterial hypertension, gastrointestinal ulceration and renal insufficiency that may progress to renal failure [4,6].

Investigations

Eosinophilia is a frequent finding in CES, occurring in up to 80% of patients, and may be related to generation of the C5 component of complement [1,7]. Pre-procedure elevation in serum levels of C-reactive protein has been associated with an increased risk of post-procedure CES [1]. Additional laboratory findings may include leukocytosis, thrombocytopenia, pyuria, eosinophiluria, blood-positive urine or stool, elevated values of ESR, creatinine, urea and amylase, and decreased serum levels of complement [3,7].

Management

Treatment of cholesterol emboli involves trying to minimize the risk of further embolization (removal of remaining plaque or perhaps stenting of an atheromatous segment of a major vessel), minimizing damage to end organs, and preventive therapies aimed at slowing the progression of atheromatous disease. Statins, iloprost (prostacyclin analogue), pentoxifylline (oxpentifylline) and steroids have been reported as having limited success in therapeutic interventions to minimize organ damage [2,8]. As anticoagulant use may precipitate cholesterol emboli, avoidance of these agents in patients with known CES seems prudent [2,9]. However, some types of cardiac surgery that may precipitate CES may also require postoperative anticoagulation, for example valvular prostheses [4,9].

Oxalate embolus, cardiac embolus and other emboli

Introduction and general description

Oxalate crystals are a rare cause of symptomatic emboli, but can mimic the cutaneous findings of cholesterol embolism. Although primary (type I) hyperoxaluria is rare, it is the most common cause of oxalate crystal embolus. Atrial myxomas, marantic endocarditis and septic endocarditis can all be associated with cutaneous embolic phenomena. Fat emboli can produce petechiae, which may be few or very numerous [1].

Clinical features

Presentation

Cutaneous manifestations of primary hyperoxaluria are primarily those of oxalate crystal embolization: livedo reticularis, acrocyanosis, and peripheral gangrene, purpura or ulcerations [2]. Secondary hyperoxaluria, especially when due to long-term dialysis, is more likely to lead to extravascular cutaneous deposits of oxalate, producing calcified cutaneous nodules, or firm miliary papules that tend to form on the palmar aspect of the fingers [3].

Symptoms of atrial myxomas may partly mimic those of infectious endocarditis, connective tissue disease, vasculitis or rheumatic fever, with constitutional symptoms such as fever, malaise, arthralgia or weight loss. The obstruction of intracardiac blood flow mimicking valvular disease or embolic phenomena may also occur. Lentigines may be a cutaneous finding in the hereditary NAME (naevi (meaning birthmarks or moles), atrial myxoma, myxoid neurofibromas and ephelides (freckles)) or LAMB (lentigines, atrial and mucocutaneous myxomas and multiple blue naevi) syndrome, which is associated with cardiac myxomas. Cutaneous findings of myxomatous emboli include livedo reticularis, splinter haemorrhages, Raynaud phenomenon, an acral papular eruption with claudication, serpiginous or annular purpuric lesions of the fingertips, red-violet malar flush, petechiae of hands and feet, or toe necrosis [4].

Marantic endocarditis results in the attachment of fibrin vegetations to heart valve leaflets, similar to those seen in acute rheumatic endocarditis and Libman–Sacks (antiphospholipid syndrome) valve disease, and these vegetations can embolize [5]. Infective endocarditis can also produce emboli from vegetations, but these are usually associated with acute bacterial endocarditis. Cutaneous lesions in subacute bacterial endocarditis may be from either emboli or immune complex-related vasculitis. Idiopathic hypereosinophilic syndrome is associated with intracardiac mural thrombi, which can also produce emboli [6]. Documentation of cutaneous emboli is limited, with clinical lesions described as splinter haemorrhages, non-blanching livedoid discoloration, or necrotic, blistering or purpuric lesions [7].

Crystal globulin vasculopathy is a rare syndrome, usually associated with IgG or light-chain paraproteins, which can produce intravascular occlusion by spontaneous crystallization [8]. This syndrome results in rapidly progressive renal failure, polyarthropathy, peripheral neuropathy and skin lesions. Cutaneous lesions include ulcerations, petechiae and ecchymoses, with intravascular thrombus and crystalline deposits [9].

Investigations
Histology can confirm myxomatous emboli, but finding the emboli may require serial sectioning and multiple biopsies [4,5]. An echocardiogram is useful in evaluating patients with a history or physical examination compatible with emboli.

Systemic coagulopathies: protein C/protein S-related disease

Synonyms and inclusions
- Neonatal purpura fulminans: homozygous protein C or protein S deficiency
- Warfarin-induced skin necrosis: severe acquired protein C dysfunction
- Sepsis-related purpura fulminans with disseminated intravascular coagulation: acquired severe protein C deficiency
- Post-infectious purpura fulminans: acquired severe protein S dysfunction

Introduction and general description
Several systemic coagulopathies have a predilection for the cutaneous microvasculature. Cutaneous lesions may be a minor feature of a multiorgan syndrome, a prominent finding of multiorgan involvement or the sole target of occlusion. Recognizing these syndromes is critical in order to begin early, and sometimes syndrome-specific, therapy. Two natural anticoagulant pathways exist in humans. The antithrombin III–heparin/heparan pathway is important for primarily venous large-vessel thrombosis. The only cutaneous lesions related to antithrombin III disorders are stasis ulcers secondary to recurrent venous thrombosis with venous insufficiency. In contrast, disorders of the thrombomodulin–protein C/S anticoagulant pathway are important causes of severe cutaneous occlusion syndromes.

An understanding of this pathway is important in diagnosing and treating these syndromes. The end point of the coagulation cascade is the conversion of prothrombin to thrombin, which rapidly catalyses the conversion of fibrinogen to fibrin and clot formation. When thrombin fails to bind to procoagulant sites on membranes and binds instead to the membrane protein receptor thrombomodulin, this powerful prothrombotic molecule undergoes a transformation. Bound to thrombomodulin, thrombin becomes ineffective at binding and activating clotting factors, and instead rapidly converts protein C in the plasma to activated protein C. Activated protein C, stabilized by certain phospholipids and by protein S, downregulates clotting by cleaving circulating activated clotting factors, including factor VIIIa and most importantly factor Va. It thus exerts an anticoagulant effect; deficiency of protein C, or of its co-factor protein S, therefore creates a procoagulant tendency.

Epidemiology

Incidence and prevalence
The frequency of homozygous protein C deficiency is estimated at 1 in 250 000–500 000 births [1]. Post-infectious purpura fulminans occurs primarily in children as rapidly progressive purpura a few days to weeks after a febrile illness [2,3].

Age
The peak incidence of warfarin-induced skin necrosis is between the sixth and seventh decades.

Sex
The incidence of warfarin necrosis is four times higher in women.

Ethnicity
About 5% of the UK and white North American population are heterozygous for the factor V Leiden mutation. The reported incidence is highest in Cyprus, Sweden and Turkey at 10–15%, and the lowest incidence is in Asia and Africa, and in populations of those ethnicities.

Associated diseases
Homozygous deficiency of either protein C or protein S is associated with neonatal purpura fulminans as well as with cerebral and ophthalmic vessel thrombosis.

The most common associated infections in cases of postinfectious purpura fulminans are varicella zoster and *Streptococcus*. This syndrome has been associated with lupus anticoagulant activity and with autoantibodies to protein S [2,3].

Pathophysiology

Predisposing factors

Protein C and S deficiencies can be inherited autosomally with variable penetrance. Patients who are heterozygous for the deficiency may develop repeated venous thrombosis or pulmonary embolism early in adult life, or may be asymptomatic [1]. One variable affecting the likelihood of thrombosis in individuals with protein C and S deficiencies is co-inheritance of homozygous or heterozygous factor V Leiden mutations [4,5].

The factor V Leiden mutation renders the factor V Leiden molecule much less sensitive to cleavage by activated protein C (APC resistance). This protection from cleavage means that activated factor V Leiden remains longer in the plasma and continues to enhance coagulation. It would be expected then that the factor V Leiden mutation would be synergistic with deficiencies in the thrombomodulin–protein C pathway. However, in some groups of protein C-deficient families, the presence of the factor V Leiden mutation appears to be an important predictor for who will develop large-vessel thrombosis in individuals with similar levels of protein C deficiency.

The risk of warfarin necrosis is increased if loading doses (10 mg or more) of warfarin are used and if a second form of anticoagulation such as heparin therapy is not used to cover the initial phase of anticoagulant therapy [6].

Pathology

The therapeutic effect of warfarin is due to inhibition of γ-carboxylation of the vitamin K-dependent coagulant factors II, VII, IX and X. Although these factors are still produced and may be antigenically detected within the plasma, without γ-carboxylation they are dysfunctional. Importantly, protein C and protein S are also vitamin K-dependent plasma factors, and their inhibition can lead to a prothrombotic state. Protein C and factor VII, with half-lives of roughly 5 h, are particularly vulnerable to early inhibition, whereas protein S and the remaining procoagulant factors with much longer half-lives remain active for a considerably longer period [6]. There is thus a period, after the early inhibition phase, when the anticoagulant effect of protein C has been inhibited but there is an excess of uninhibited procoagulant clotting factors.

The term 'purpura fulminans' is used by physicians for many different situations. It was originally coined in 1887 to describe a syndrome occurring days to a few weeks after some preceding infection, especially varicella zoster or streptococcal infections (now termed 'postinfectious purpura fulminans') [7]. The term purpura fulminans has subsequently been used for widespread cutaneous haemorrhage in patients with sepsis, including infection with *Neisseria meningitidis*, *Staphylococcus aureus*, groups A and B β-haemolytic streptococci, *Streptococcus pneumoniae*, *Haemophilus influenzae* and *H. aegyptius* [2].

Clinical features

Presentation

Retiform (stellate) purpura and necrosis is the most typical cutaneous finding that results from thrombosis within the cutaneous microvasculature. Skin lesions typically begin within a few hours to 5 days after birth, and are most commonly distributed on the extremities, abdomen, buttocks and scalp; they may localize to sites of pressure or previous trauma [1,8].

Warfarin necrosis usually presents as the sudden onset of pain within affected areas 3–5 days after beginning warfarin therapy, followed by well-demarcated erythema progressing to haemorrhage, necrosis and often haemorrhagic bullae or eschar [9]. Although warfarin necrosis may rarely involve acral areas, acral cutaneous purpura in patients on warfarin is more likely to be due to cholesterol embolus – so-called purple (blue) toe syndrome. Warfarin necrosis is more likely to occur in areas with abundant fatty subcutis, such as the breast, hip, buttocks and thigh [9,10].

Cutaneous microvascular occlusion in sepsis with disseminated intravascular coagulation (DIC) presents clinically as non-inflammatory (bland) haemorrhage, usually with a retiform, stellate or branching configuration, with rapid transition to necrosis and eschar [11,12].

Differential diagnosis

Haemorrhage in patients with DIC may be due to septic vasculitis, simple bleeding or microvascular thrombosis. The patterns of cutaneous haemorrhage for each of these different mechanisms are distinctive, and can be a guide to pathophysiology and therapy [13].

Disease course and prognosis

In the absence of appropriate therapy, lesions invariably progress to full-thickness cutaneous necrosis.

Investigations

Laboratory findings are consistent with DIC, with evidence of the consumption of clotting factors (prolonged partial thromboplastin time, PTT), clot lysis (elevated fibrin split products) and often thrombocytopenia.

In a small study, early biopsy of retiform purpuric lesions showed microvascular occlusion with fibrin, and perivascular haemorrhage with minimal to no inflammation; these findings correlated with severe protein C deficiency [12]. This was not true of other forms of purpura in sepsis with DIC.

Management

Traditional treatment included fresh frozen plasma to try to replace deficient protein C or S, or oral anticoagulants to reduce procoagulant factors. Protein C and activated protein C concentrates have been used for the treatment of both acute disease and as prophylaxis against subsequent episodes [14].

Although up to one-third of patients with warfarin-induced skin necrosis may have partial protein C deficiency, the majority of cases appear unrelated to inherited deficiencies of protein C [10]. As warfarin action mimics that of vitamin K deficiency, it would be expected that a depletion of vitamin K would result in warfarin necrosis-like findings, but this has not been documented. Restoration of protein C activity can be accomplished through protein C concentrates, and presumably also through the use of activated protein C. If these are not available, heparin therapy has been recommended.

The protein C pathway is increasingly recognized as critically important in bacterial sepsis, acting to inhibit both coagulation and inflammation [15]. The use of activated protein C concentrate in sepsis appears to be beneficial, especially in severe cases, although whether all patients with sepsis should receive this is not clear [16]. In patients with sepsis, DIC and retiform (occlusion) purpura, it seems reasonable to assume severe protein C deficiency in the acute setting and to treat appropriately. Protein C concentrates and plasma exchange have also been successfully used to replace protein C in purpura fulminans [17,18].

In cases of postinfectious purpura fulminans, replacement of protein S activity is difficult, presumably because this condition is not due to simple clearing of protein S but rather to inhibition of protein S function by an antibody. Such antibody-mediated dysfunction is difficult to overcome by the replacement of factor, and concentrated sources of protein S are unavailable.

Systemic coagulopathies: antiphospholipid antibody/lupus anticoagulant syndrome

Introduction and general description

Another major cluster of systemic coagulopathies with cutaneous microvascular occlusion are those related to lupus anticoagulant activity and antiphospholipid syndrome (APLS). From the original description as recurrent venous or arterial thrombosis, repeated fetal loss and thrombocytopenia, to consensus statement criteria, APLS continues to be redefined [1], most recently by the addition of β_2-glycoprotein I (β_2-GPI) antibodies to the laboratory criteria for diagnosis (Box 101.4) [2]. Although thrombocytopenia

---

Box 101.4 International consensus statement preliminary criteria for antiphospholipid antibody syndrome (definitive diagnosis requires at least one clinical and one laboratory criterion) [2]

Clinical criteria
- Vascular thrombosis: one or more clinical episodes of arterial, venous or small-vessel thrombosis
- Complications of pregnancy:
  - One or more unexplained deaths of morphologically normal fetuses at or after 10 weeks of pregnancy *or*
  - One or more premature births of morphologically normal neonates at or before 34 weeks of gestation *or*
  - Three or more unexplained consecutive spontaneous abortions before 10 weeks of gestation

Laboratory criteria
- Anticardiolipin antibodies, IgG or IgM, present at moderate or high levels on two or more occasions at least 6 weeks apart
- Lupus anticoagulant antibodies on two or more occasions at least 6 weeks apart
- β_2-glycoprotein I antibodies on two or more occasions at least 6 weeks apart

---

was frequently mentioned in early descriptions of APLS, this is no longer a diagnostic criterion for the syndrome.

The mechanisms for clotting in this group are less well understood. Investigators have shown that β_2-GPI–oxidized low-density lipoprotein complexes can frequently be detected in sera from patients with APLS and/or SLE, but not in healthy individuals [3]. Furthermore, patients with APLS have been shown to have autoreactive CD4+ T cells responsive to β_2-GPI in patients with APLS, and which can promote pathogenic IgG anti-β_2-GPI antibody production by autologous B cells. These T cells do not respond to native β_2-GPI, but will respond to chemically reduced or bacterially expressed recombinant β_2-GPI, further supporting the hypothesis that it is a cryptic epitope that is responsible for pathological β_2-GPI antibodies. This insight leads to the possibility of future therapies targeted at depleting or blocking binding domain I-directed β_2-GPI antibodies, or inhibiting their production through the elimination or inhibition of the pathological autoreactive CD4+ T-cell subset [3].

Epidemiology

Incidence and prevalence
Antiphospholipid syndrome may occur as a primary or secondary disorder. In one large study, primary APLS comprised 53% of cases, lupus-associated APLS 36%, lupus-like APLS 5% and other disease associations with APLS 6%, with catastrophic APLS occurring in 0.8% of cases [4].

Age
In a large study the mean age was 42 ± 14 years at study entry, and the onset of symptoms was most often in young to middle-aged patients (2.8% before age 15 years, 12.7% after age 50) [4].

Sex
There is a strong female predominance (82%) [4].

Associated diseases
Compared with primary syndrome patients, lupus patients with APLS are more likely to have arthritis, livedo reticularis, thrombocytopenia or leukopenia [4].

Pathophysiology

Predisposing factors
Precipitating factors include infections, surgical procedures, drugs and the discontinuation of anticoagulation.

Pathology
The most important autoantigen in APLS appears to be β_2-GPI (apolipoprotein H), which binds anionic phospholipids as part of the physiological disposal of apoptotic cells [5]. β_2-GPI is composed of five complement control modules, domains I to V. Infections may trigger β_2-GPI antibodies (e.g. leprosy, leishmaniasis, leptospirosis), as may childhood atopic eczema. These antibodies may differ from those that trigger thrombosis by binding to domain V of the β_2-GPI molecule, rather than to the domain I region which appears to be characteristic of the thrombogenic

subset [6]. Infection-related antibodies, especially in leprosy, are more often IgM than IgG type. In general, IgM β_2-GPI antibodies are seldom implicated in thrombotic events, except perhaps in cerebral stroke. IgG antibodies to β_2-GPI, especially the IgG$_2$ subset, are the most likely to be thrombogenic [7].

Multiple pathways have been implicated by which antiphospholipid antibodies may promote thrombosis: the promotion of procoagulant reactions (interfering with protective membrane proteins such as β_2-GPI or annexin V), interference with anticoagulant pathways (inhibition of protein C/S and antithrombin III pathways), activation of platelets by membrane binding, interference with prostacyclin production and release by endothelium, or interference with fibrinolytic pathways (inhibition of endothelial plasminogen activator or kallikrein activation) [1,8]. However, current investigation points to β_2-GPI antibodies being the likely prothrombotic pathway in most patients. The mechanism of thrombosis with antibody-bound β_2-GPI is thought to occur predominantly through the disruption of a crystal shield of annexin V which covers the membrane and ordinarily prevents the binding of procoagulant molecules [9]. In addition to potential thrombogenesis, β_2-GPI antibody complexes may also be atherogenic.

Clinical features

Presentation

Clinically, APLS can present with a variety of cutaneous findings (Box 101.5) [10]. Livedo is one of the most common, but is not specific since this and retiform purpura or necrosis occur in other microvascular occlusion disorders [10]. In one large study, the frequency of these findings was livedo reticularis 24%, leg ulcers 5.5%, pseudovasculitis 3.9%, digital gangrene 3.3%, cutaneous necrosis 2.1% and splinter haemorrhages 0.7% [4].

Box 101.5 Cutaneous findings in the antiphospholipid antibody syndrome

- Livedo reticularis, with or without retiform purpura or retiform necrosis
- Sneddon syndrome
- Livedoid vasculopathy/atrophie blanche
- Raynaud phenomenon
- Anetoderma-like lesions with thrombosis
- Behçet-like lesions
- Nailfold ulcers
- Widespread cutaneous necrosis (catastrophic antiphospholipid antibody syndrome)
- Leg ulcers, secondary to recurrent thrombosis with stasis, or from conditions in this list
- Cholesterol embolus-like proximal livedo reticularis, with or without distal retiform purpura
- Acral livedo
- Degos (malignant atrophic papulosis) like lesions
- Pseudo-Kaposi sarcoma
- Vasculitis-like lesions
- Pyoderma gangrenosum-like ulcers
- Splinter haemorrhages
- Superficial thrombophlebitis migrans

Clinical variants

Catastrophic APLS is an uncommon but disastrous variant in which patients typically present with widespread cutaneous necrosis and multiorgan failure, especially renal and pulmonary.

The most common extracutaneous manifestations of non-catastrophic APLS include deep-vein thrombosis, pulmonary embolus and central nervous system abnormalities.

Investigations

A variety of serological markers exist, usually detected as antibody against phospholipids (especially cardiolipin) in combination with antigens from a co-factor molecule (e.g. β_2-GPI, prothrombin, annexin V, plasmin, tissue plasminogen activator, thrombin), or as an inhibitor of an *in vitro* coagulation test. The detection of antiphospholipid antibodies is roughly five times more common than the detection of lupus anticoagulant [11].

Mechanisms of coagulation in APLS are most often detected as β_2-GPI antibodies, lupus anticoagulants or antiphospholipid antibodies. The lupus anticoagulant activity is detected, often incidentally, by prolongation of the activated partial thromboplastin time (aPTT), the dilute Russell viper venom time (dRVVT) or the kaolin clotting time [7]. A test of activation of the intrinsic pathway (either aPTT or kaolin clotting time) and direct activation of factor X (dRVVT) are both recommended. Although prolongation of these tests would seem to predict a tendency towards bleeding, individuals with lupus anticoagulant activity very rarely bleed abnormally, but may be paradoxically predisposed to clot formation.

Antiphospholipid antibody activity is detected by one of several antibody assays, the most common being enzyme-linked immunosorbent assay screens for IgG or IgM antibody affinity for cardiolipin, a negatively charged phospholipid molecule found in mitochondrial membranes. Although anticardiolipin antibodies can be detected in the absence of binding to a co-factor, such as β_2-GPI, antiphospholipid antibodies that bind to phospholipid alone without a co-factor molecule are not usually physiologically relevant in inducing thrombosis.

Management

Specific therapy in APLS awaits an understanding of the mechanism by which thrombosis occurs in individual patients, and thus the capability to use tailored therapies to specifically oppose that pathway in a particular individual [12]. Investigation of the role of autoreactive CD4+ T cells driving B-cell production of pathogenic β_2-GPI antibodies may provide more effective therapies in the future. At present, treatment is empirical. Antiplatelet therapy is of uncertain benefit; most therapy depends on acute and often chronic anticoagulation, either with standard or low-molecular-weight heparin initially followed by warfarin [5]. Antimalarial therapy may be of some benefit for atrophie blanche-like or Degos-like syndromes in lupus patients; evidence suggests a protective effect in lupus patients against arterial or venous thromboses [1]. There is evidence that hydroxychloroquine may interfere with the binding of IgG–β_2-GPI complexes on phospholipid bilayers or to a line of cultured human monocytic leukaemia cells, which may provide some rationale for possible prophylactic benefit in APLS patients [13].

VASCULAR COAGULOPATHIES

Sneddon syndrome

Introduction and general description
This syndrome comprises generalized livedo racemosa or livedo reticularis with cerebrovascular lesions that cause focal neurological symptoms or signs [1,2,3,4,5]. Livedo racemosa is usually the first manifestation of Sneddon syndrome, initially affecting the lower trunk and proximal part of the legs, but becoming more generalized. It typically has a broad network pattern (Figure 101.4). Associated Raynaud phenomenon or acrocyanosis may occur, and may be the presenting feature [1,2].

Epidemiology

Incidence and prevalence
This has been estimated at four cases per million people per year [3], and it is usually sporadic, although familial Sneddon syndrome has been reported.

Age
Sneddon syndrome typically presents in the fourth or fifth decade of life.

Sex
Sneddon syndrome is twice as common in women as in men.

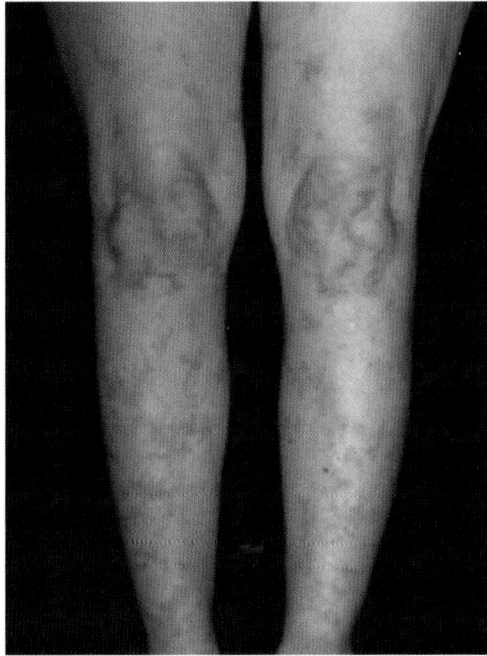

Figure 101.4 Sneddon syndrome showing a typical, broad, racemose livedo patterning.

Pathophysiology
The presence of antinuclear antibodies or of antiphospholipid antibodies/lupus anticoagulant has been reported [4], but some authors only accept the diagnosis of Sneddon syndrome if these antibodies are absent. Differences have been documented between the clinical features of patients with Sneddon syndrome depending on the presence or absence of antiphospholipid antibodies. Those without antiphospholipid antibodies typically have a larger-sized livedo pattern, whereas those with antiphospholipid antibodies have a higher risk of seizures, mitral regurgitation and thrombocytopenia [5]. It is likely that there is a spectrum of disease from APLS to SLE that includes the preferential arteriolar pattern of Sneddon syndrome. Antiprothrombin antibodies were demonstrated in 57% of 46 patients in one series [6], and there are reports of platelet activation in a patient with persistently elevated levels of circulating PF4 [7] and increased levels of antithrombin III [8], factor V Leiden mutation [9] and activated protein C resistance [10].

Pathology
Biopsies may show an endarteritis of dermal arterioles. It has been demonstrated that the most informative biopsies are from the clinically normal centre of any network area rather than from the peripheral 'watershed' area of livedo, and that taking multiple biopsies increases the sensitivity [11]. Initial changes are endothelial swelling with a mixed inflammatory infiltrate, progressing to vascular plugging, subendothelial proliferation and eventual vascular occlusion, fibrosis and disappearance of the inflammatory component [12]. It is possible, if not likely, that the histological findings in patients with antiphospholipid antibodies, especially in association with lupus or lupus-like disease, would be more typical of non-inflammatory occlusion.

Clinical features

Presentation
In addition to the cutaneous livedo, there may be non-specific neurological prodromal symptoms such as headache, migraine, dizziness or vertigo. Transient ischaemic attacks are commoner than completed stroke [13].

Clinical variants
The peripheral nerves may also be affected and hypertension may be present. Hypertension and the neurological aspects are sometimes aggravated by pregnancy or the use of oral contraceptives. There may be renal or cardiac involvement, including valve defects such as mitral regurgitation, although internal organ involvement other than neurological is often asymptomatic [3]. Other features such as shortened digits have rarely been reported.

Differential diagnosis
The differential diagnosis is wide, from both the cutaneous and the neurological perspective. In particular, other causes of livedo and microvascular occlusion syndromes discussed in this chapter need to be considered as well as vasculitic causes (e.g. polyarteritis nodosa). However, it should be noted that other patterns of livedo with anticardiolipin antibodies may be associated with

evidence of cerebral microthrombosis, for example livedo with summer ulceration or livedo with pyoderma gangrenosum-like lesions [14].

Disease course and prognosis

Later neurological features include focal paresis or hemiparesis, focal sensory or hemisensory symptoms, fits and visual defects, and later cognitive changes. Hypertension confers a worse prognosis if untreated.

Investigations

Magnetic resonance imaging (MRI), electroencephalography and arteriography may help to confirm the neurological component; skin biopsy (as above) and exclusion of other causes of livedo are necessary. Patients with positive antiphospholipid antibodies more commonly have infarcts in the distribution of the main cerebral arteries on MRI, whereas those with negative antibodies have small lacunar infarcts [15] and progressive leukoencephalopathy [13].

Management

There is generally no very effective treatment, reflecting the non-inflammatory nature of the disease. Corticosteroids may have some benefit but this is variable and often difficult to assess due to the intermittent nature of the neurological disease; other immunosuppressive agents are often disappointing. The avoidance of smoking and oral contraceptives, and treatment of hypertension and hyperlipidaemia (both of which are commonly present), are important. Thrombolytic agents and vasodilators have been used in the acute situation, and antiplatelet agents appear to be effective in the longer term [5]. In patients with antiphospholipid antibodies or lupus anticoagulants, the maintenance of anticoagulation at an international normalized ratio (INR) of 2–3 seems warranted.

Livedoid vasculopathy/atrophie blanche

Synonyms and inclusions
- Livedo reticularis with summer ulceration
- Segmental hyalinizing vasculitis

Introduction and general description

This syndrome is common as either an idiopathic or secondary syndrome [1].

Epidemiology

Age

This syndrome is most common in young to middle-aged women.

Associated diseases

One of the most commonly noted associations is with chronic venous hypertension and varicosities, although the atrophic scarring in this setting is not usually preceded by small painful ulcerations, nor with surrounding livedo reticularis. It would seem

appropriate to separate venous stasis-related atrophie blanche from more typical forms of the syndrome.

Pathophysiology

The pathogenesis of livedoid vasculopathy is unknown. Clearly, APLS, with or without a lupus association, can produce this clinical syndrome [2]. Multiple pathophysiological abnormalities have been implicated, including platelet activation, factor V Leiden, altered fibrinolysis, antiphospholipid antibodies and hyperhomocystinaemia [1,2,3,4]. In one series of 32 patients, heterozygous factor V Leiden mutation was found in two of nine patients tested (22%), decreased protein C or protein S activity in two of 15 (13%), prothrombin G20210A mutation in one of 12 (8%), lupus anticoagulant in five of 28 (18%), anticardiolipin antibodies in eight of 29 (29%) and elevated homocysteine levels in three of 21 (14%) [5].

Pathology

The most characteristic histological findings in this syndrome are some thickening or hyaline changes in the walls of superficial dermal vessels, and luminal fibrin deposition [1,6]. Red cell extravasation and perivascular lymphocytic infiltrates are expected findings. In a series of 45 skin biopsies from 32 patients, all but one showed intraluminal thrombus and direct immunofluorescence was positive in 86% [5].

Clinical features

Presentation

Persistent, very painful and often punched-out ulcerations of the legs, especially around the malleoli, in women are typical of atrophie blanche [6]. The disease is bilateral in most cases. When accompanied by surrounding livedo reticularis, the term 'livedoid vasculitis' is more likely to be applied. Retiform or stellate purpura or ulcer extension can occur. Healing results in a porcelain-white scar, frequently surrounded by telangiectasia. Besides venous hypertension and antiphospholipid antibody-related syndromes, sickle cell ulcers can show the same porcelain-white scar of atrophie blanche.

Investigations

A skin biopsy may be helpful.

Management

Antiplatelet, anticoagulant and fibrinolytic therapies have been reported to be useful in this syndrome, as well as anabolic steroids such as danazol and stanozolol [2]. PUVA therapy has been reported as effective in some cases [7]. In patients with lupus and atrophie blanche-like lesions, antimalarial therapy may be effective. Rapid relief of pain has been reported with the use of intravenous immunoglobulins [8], postulated to be due to inhibition of the vasoconstrictor chemicals thromboxane A_2 and endothelin which thereby improves perfusion. Lipoprostaglandin E_1 has been used with good response in a patient with livedoid vasculitis and essential cryoglobulinaemia [9], but this may have been mediated by an effect on the cryoprotein levels, which fell dramatically. There are anecdotal reports of response to tetracyclines [10], and dapsone has also been used in patients with underlying myeloproliferative syndromes.

Malignant atrophic papulosis

Definition and nomenclature
Malignant atrophic papulosis is a progressive vasculopathy causing occlusion of small and medium-sized arteries [1].

Synonyms and inclusions
- Degos disease
- Kohlmeier–Degos disease
- Lethal cutaneous and gastrointestinal arteriolar thrombosis

Introduction and general description
Malignant atrophic papulosis is characterized by skin and gastrointestinal lesions, but neurological features are also frequent and postmortem studies show widespread organ involvement. The skin lesions are usually the first feature, and may be the only manifestation over many years. Whether this represents a truly 'benign' variant is uncertain, however it is suggested that the disease should be classified into a malignant systemic form and a benign, cutaneous one [2].

Epidemiology

Incidence and prevalence
It is rare; a review in 1995 suggested that about 120 cases had been reported [3].

Age
It is mainly a disease that presents in young adults, although it can affect any age group [4].

Sex
It has a slight male predominance.

Ethnicity
It is mainly reported in white people.

Associated diseases
Cases have been reported with HIV infection but a causal association is unproven.

Pathophysiology
The pathogenesis probably involves abnormal coagulation, although the precise mechanism is uncertain. Platelet and fibrin thrombi are apparent in dermal, mesenteric and nervous system blood vessels, and both abnormal platelet aggregation and inhibition of fibrinolysis have been reported [4–6]. However, most patients have no clear evidence of a systemic coagulopathy, suggesting that the thrombotic tendency is at the microvascular level. Antiphospholipid antibodies have been documented in a small number of patients, usually in the context of SLE,

although they may also occur even in the benign cutaneous variant [7].

There is also some support for a mechanism involving vascular inflammation. An autoimmune mechanism is suggested by the occurrence of lesions resembling malignant atrophic papulosis in some patients with SLE, rheumatoid arthritis, scleroderma or dermatomyositis [8–11]. Antiendothelial antibodies have also been demonstrated but are probably not the cause of the disease [4]. Circulating immune complexes, or deposition of immune complexes or complement, are not usually demonstrated [2,12]. Although there can be a prominent lymphocytic infiltrate in later lesions, especially around venules, true arteritis and leukocytoclasis are not found [4,13].

Abnormal mucin deposits, which may be thrombogenic, occur even in early lesions although they tend to be more apparent in later lesions [4,13]. It is possible that they may be induced by activated T cells. A viral aetiology was proposed on the basis of electron microscopic demonstration of interwoven tuboreticular structures resembling viral inclusions within endothelial cells, but these are seen in other disorders, including SLE, and can be induced by interferon [4].

Pathology
The histological picture in Degos disease depends upon the duration of the lesion biopsied. Early lesions show a superficial and deep perivascular, perineural and periappendageal chronic inflammatory cell infiltrate [13]. Deep dermal vessels show endovascular inflammation, proliferation and thickening with thrombosis [14]. Mucin deposition is seen at all stages [2,3,13], and fibrin deposition may be demonstrated; fibrinoid necrosis of vessel walls may occur [14]. Immunofluorescence is occasionally positive for IgG or C3. From a histopathological perspective, the presence of lymphocytes, which may be seen within the damaged vessel wall, is viewed as abnormal and has led to the classification of Degos disease as a lymphocytic vasculitis [15] although it is not documented that this is a primary abnormality. Later lesions show a classic 'wedge-shaped' pattern of sclerotic change in the dermis, which is usually only sparsely cellular. Between these stages there is a phase with neutrophilic and eosinophilic infiltrate around adnexae and a dense perivascular lymphocytic infiltrate [13]. The epidermis, initially showing a mild vacuolar reaction, becomes atrophic with slight scaling, resembling that seen in lichen sclerosus and corresponding with the typical porcelain-white colour seen clinically. There may be some associated pigmentary incontinence.

Panniculitis resembling that seen in lupus profundus has recently been reported [16]. Similar changes occur in the intestinal wall, particularly the submucosa. The muscularis mucosae is intact. Blood vessels are thickened and disorganized, with fibrinoid degeneration; platelet–fibrin thrombi are more prominent than in skin biopsy material. Microaneurysms of the bulbar conjunctival vessels have been described. Renal changes include thickening of the afferent glomerular arterioles and of the capillary basement membrane.

Genetics
Familial cases have been reported [17].

PART 9: VASCULAR

Clinical features

Presentation

Cutaneous lesions usually precede systemic manifestations by months to years. They develop as crops over a period of time and are usually asymptomatic, although they may be preceded by slight burning. Skin lesions affect any site, but mainly the trunk and proximal limbs; the face, palms and soles are generally spared. Although they may evolve gradually, and the number of lesions may vary considerably, about 30–40 active lesions are usually present [5]. Oral mucosal lesions are rare but penile lesions may occur [18]; the bulbar conjunctiva is often affected by lesions, which appear as sharply demarcated avascular areas [3]. Peristomal lesions have been reported.

Early skin lesions are pink or red, dome-shaped papules, usually 2–5 mm in size, but sometimes up to about 15 mm. Papules soon become necrotic and umbilicated with a central porcelain-white pallor and scaling, and the pink oedematous border becomes telangiectatic. Most heal rather slowly to leave a small white scar, often surrounded by telangiectases, as in atrophie blanche. Urticaria-like, ulceropustular and gumma-like nodules have been reported. New crops of lesions may continue for several years. Similar lesions occur in many organs. Gastrointestinal lesions are the most important as perforation of the gut is a cause of death [19]. Neurological symptoms are also relatively common.

For features in different systems see Box 101.6.

Differential diagnosis

There is sometimes a resemblance to atrophie blanche or to guttate lichen sclerosus, although the evolution of lesions is different. Identical lesions have been described in cases of various connective tissue diseases [8–11] and in a patient with Crohn disease [20]. The characteristic features are usually hard to confuse with those of other syndromes. A disorder termed 'cutaneous–intestinal syndrome with oropharyngeal ulceration' [21] included a combination of macular, blistering and crusting lesions of the skin, with oro-pharyngeal ulceration and death from perforation of one of many intestinal ulcers. This differed both clinically and histologically from Degos disease. Patients in whom systemic disease precedes skin lesions may cause particular diagnostic problems.

Disease course and prognosis

Although possibly overestimated by reporting bias, and acknowledging that there does appear to be a benign cutaneous ('skin-limited') variant, a mortality of 50% within 2–3 years is reported, and prognosis in males appears to be worse than in females. Systemic manifestations can develop years after the appearance of the skin lesions, including bowel perforation and peritonitis, thrombosis of the cerebral arteries, meningitis, encephalitis and myelitis [22].

Management

There is no consistently effective treatment [2,3]. Steroids do not help, although some benefit in neurological symptoms has been suggested. Aspirin, antiplatelet agents, fibrinolytic agents and pentoxifylline, alone or in combination, may lead to remission and are perhaps most effective in the cutaneous disease [2,3,4,7,23].

Box 101.6 Features of Degos disease in different systems [3]

Gastrointestinal
- Dyspepsia
- Abdominal pain or distension
- Bleeding
- Perforation
- Peritonitis
- Fistulae (enteroenteral or enterocutaneous)
- Obstruction
- Pancreatitis

Neurological
- Cerebral infarction (causing headache, aphasia, dementia, focal epilepsy, hemiparesis, pseudobulbar palsy)
- Cord infarction (paraplegia/quadriplegia, transverse myelopathy)
- Peripheral nerve (cauda equina syndrome, mononeuritis multiplex)
- Various sites (sensory disturbance)

Ocular
- Ptosis
- Diplopia
- Nystagmus
- Ophthalmoplegia
- Optic neuritis
- Papilloedema
- Visual field loss
- Pupillary reaction defects
- Conjunctival avascular lesions
- Posterior subcapsular cataract

Cardiovascular
- Renal artery occlusion
- Pericardial effusion
- Constrictive pericarditis
- Ventricular wall defects

Pulmonary
- Pleuritis

Phenylbutazone has been reported to be effective. Heparin may produce short-term benefits. There is one report of a good response to transdermal nicotine patches [24]. Warfarin, dextrans, chloroquine, immunosuppressive agents and plasma exchange have all been tried. Surgery to treat intestinal perforation may resolve the acute situation but is difficult as there are usually multiple lesions, and there is no long-term benefit from this approach.

Calcific uraemic arteriolopathy

Synonyms and inclusions
- Cutaneous calciphylaxis

Introduction and general description

Calcific uraemic arteriolopathy is a complication of renal failure and dialysis, associated with high mortality rates and characterized by painful skin ulceration [1,2,3]. The original term 'calciphylaxis' referred to an experimental situation of systemic necrosis in rats that were hypercalcaemic due to treatment with vitamin D or with parathyroid hormone, but did not specifically relate to vascular calcification, hence the change in terminology [2].

Epidemiology

Incidence and prevalence
It is rare but appears to be increasing in prevalence [4].

Age
Patients are mainly in the sixth decade of life.

Sex
Women are most at risk, accounting for over 80% of cases.

Associated diseases
It may very rarely occur in other situations, such as alcoholic liver disease, and occasionally after chemotherapy, in patients with normal renal function. Even in non-dialysed subjects about one-third have diabetes [1].

Pathophysiology
Most patients have secondary or tertiary hyperparathyroidism, although the disorder can rarely occur in some with primary hyperparathyroidism. An elevated calcium–phosphorus product is generally expected, but some authors have suggested that this may be present in only a third of cases. Use of vitamin D, or of calcium carbonate (used as a phosphate binder in chronic renal failure), are risk factors [3].

Vascular calcification induces a phenotypic switch of the vascular myofibroblast to one of an osteoprogenitor. Local (paracrine) pro-mineralization chemicals that are involved include osteopontin (stimulated by high glucose levels), bone morphogenetic protein-2 (BMP-2) and Pit-1, as well as matrix metalloproteinases that are stimulated by a catabolic state. Inhibitors of mineralization include parathormone-related peptide (inhibited by vitamin D) and matrix Gla protein (inhibited by warfarin); fetuin A inhibits calcification but is inhibited by vitamin D. Thus vitamin D, a commonly used treatment in chronic renal failure, and warfarin may both provoke this process. It is felt that tensile stress and vascular stasis within calcified areas may also play a part by creating tissue ischaemia.

Predisposing factors
One large institutional study showed that, compared with other patients on dialysis, risk factors included obesity, liver disease, corticosteroid use, elevated calcium–phosphate product and elevated aluminium levels [1]. Hypoalbuminuria (or albumin infusions), recent rapid weight loss, protein C or protein S deficiency, warfarin treatment and hypotension have also been implicated as risk factors.

Pathology
Pathologically, there is calcification in the medial layer of the wall of small subcutaneous vessels, with necrosis of overlying tissue [1,2,3]. Some calcification may occur in dermal vessels, in sep-

tae within the subcutaneous fat, and in adipocytes themselves. Thrombosed vessels are seen occasionally, presumably as a secondary effect as the calcification of small-vessel walls extends more widely than the thrombotic change or the extravascular calcification [3]. Dermal inflammation may occur without ulceration, and bullae sometimes occur.

Clinical features

Presentation
Early lesions tend to present as painful purpuric plaques, often with a retiform or stellate pattern, and may show central necrosis. They may resemble the lesions of hyperoxaluria. Some may become semiconfluent as a 'broken' livedo. The abdomen, thigh and hips are typical sites but the breasts may be involved, and in some patients the disease is mainly acral. Uncommon sites include the penis and the tongue [5] as well as the muscles and internal organs [2]. Woody induration with extending ulcer and eschar formation typically develops.

Disease course and prognosis
The prognosis is generally considered poor, with a mortality of 50–80%, although there are occasional reports of a more benign course [1].

Investigations
A deep skin biopsy for histopathology is usually undertaken to confirm the diagnosis. Blood tests include creatinine and urea, liver function tests, calcium, phosphate and parathyroid hormone. A plain radiograph of the thighs will show extensive vascular calcification.

Management
Parathyroidectomy has been cited as effective, but there is clearly a bias in patient selection for this procedure towards those who can tolerate the procedure and who are therefore a relatively healthy subgroup. Reduction of the calcium–phosphorus product when elevated is recommended (using low-calcium dialysate fluids and non-calcium oral phosphate binders), as is good wound care and attention to possible accompanying infection, which is a common cause of death. Newer treatments that may influence the outcome of this disorder include sodium thiosulphate [6], which increases the solubility of calcium deposits and has an antioxidant function that may improve endothelial cell function, and cinacalcet hydrochloride [7], which is a calcimimetic therapy that suppresses levels of parathyroid hormone. Logically, cinacalcet should be most useful in patients with hyperparathyroidism, and sodium thiosulphate in those patients without (or in whom it is controlled). Hyperbaric oxygen, skin grafting and iloprost infusions can be useful adjuncts in the management of this condition [8].

Key references

The full list of references can be found in the online version at www.rooksdermatology.com.

Introduction
1 Piette WW. The differential diagnosis of purpura from a morphologic perspective. *Adv Dermatol* 1994;9:3–23.

4 Thornsberry LA, LoSicco KI, English JC, 3rd. The skin and hypercoagulable states. *J Am Acad Dermatol* 2013;69(3):450–62.

9 Maguire S, Mann M. Systematic reviews of bruising in relation to child abuse – what have we learnt: an overview of review updates. *Evid Based Child Health* 2013;8(2):255–63.

Purpura due to thrombocytopenia or platelet defects

Thrombocytopenia

1 Shenkman B, Einav Y. Thrombotic thrombocytopenic purpura and other thrombotic microangiopathic hemolytic anemias: diagnosis and classification. *Autoimmun Rev* 2014;13(4–5):584–6.

4 Handin RI. Inherited platelet disorders. *Hematology (Am Soc Hematol Educ Program)* 2005;2005:396–402.

9 Hassan AA, Kroll MH. Acquired disorders of platelet function. *Hematology (Am Soc Hematol Educ Program)* 2005;2005:403–8.

Abnormalities of platelet function

1 Handin RI. Inherited platelet disorders. *Hematology (Am Soc Hematol Educ Program)* 2005;2005:396–402.

5 Shen Y-MP, Frenkel EP. Acquired platelet dysfunction. *Hematol Oncol Clin North Am* 2007;21:647–61.

6 Diz-Küçükkaya R. Inherited platelet disorders including Glanzmann thrombasthenia and Bernard-Soulier syndrome. *Hematology (Am Soc Hematol Educ Program)* 2013;2013:268–75.

Thrombocytosis

1 Champion RH, Rook A. Idiopathic thrombocythemia: cutaneous manifestations. *Arch Dermatol* 1963;87:302–5.

7 Kaszewski S, Czajkowski R, Protas-Drozd, et al. Sweet's syndrome with idiopathic thrombocythemia. *Postepy Dermatol Alergol* 2014;XXXI(1):47–52.

8 Bray PF. Platelet hyperreactivity: predictive and intrinsic properties. *Hematol Oncol Clin North Am* 2007;21:633–45.

Non-thrombocytopenic vascular causes of purpura and syndromes of primary ecchymotic haemorrhage

Raised intravascular pressure

2 Trindade F, Requena L. Pseudo-Kaposi's sarcoma because of suction-socket lower limb prosthesis. *J Cutan Pathol* 2009;36(4):482–5.

5 Ramelet AA. Exercise-induced purpura. *Dermatology (Basel)* 2004;208:293–6.

8 Waters AJ, Sandhu C, Green CM, et al. Solar capillaritis as a cause of solar purpura. *Clin Exp Dermatol* 2009;34:e821–4.

Abnormal or decreased support of blood vessels

1 Bick R. Vascular thrombohemorrhagic disorders: hereditary and acquired. *Clin Appl Thrombosis Hemostasis* 2001;7:178–94.

3 Kaya G, Saurat JH. Dermatoporosis: a chronic cutaneous insufficiency/fragility syndrome. Clinicopathological features, mechanisms, prevention and potential treatments. *Dermatology* 2007;215(4):284–94.

6 Thies K, Beschorner U, Noory E, et al. Achenbach's syndrome revisited. *Vasa* 2012;41(5):366–70.

Physical and artefactual bleeding

1 Metzker A, Merlob P. Suction purpura. *Arch Dermatol* 1992;128:822–4.

2 Lao M, Weisshar A, Siegfried E. Talon noir. *J Pediatr* 2013;163(3):919.

6 Saida T, Oguchi S, Ishihara Y. In vivo observations of magnified features of pigmented lesions on volar skin using video microscope. *Arch Dermatol* 1995;131:248–304.

Dysproteinaemic and Waldenström hypergammaglobulinaemic purpura

1 Waldenström J. Three new cases of purpura hyperglobulinaemica. A study of a long-standing benign increase in serum globulin. *Acta Med Scand* 1952;266(Suppl.):931–46.

2 Miyagawa S, Fukumoto T, Kanauchi M, et al. Hypergammaglobulinaemic purpura of Waldenström and Ro/SSA autoantibodies. *Br J Dermatol* 1996;134:919–23.

9 Lewin JM, Hunt R, Fischer M, et al. Hypergammaglobuulinemic purpura of Waldenstrom. *Dermatol Online J* 2012;18(12):2.

Pigmented purpuric dermatoses

1 Tristani-Firouzi P, Meadows KP, Vanderhooft S. Pigmented purpuric eruptions of childhood: a series of cases and review of literature. *Pediatr Dermatol* 2001;18:299–304.

3 Jensen AL, Vanderhooft SL. Pigmented purpuras. In: Harper J, Oranje AP, Prose N, eds. *Textbook of Pediatric Dermatology*, 3rd edn. Oxford: Blackwell Science, 2011:165.1–165.6.

5 Sardana K, Sarkar R, Seghal VN. Pigmented purpuric dermatoses: an overview. *Int J Dermatol* 2004;43:482–8.

Disorders of cutaneous microvascular occlusion

Platelet plugging: heparin necrosis

9 Mc Kenzie SE, Sachais BS. Advances in the pathophysiology and treatment of heparin-induced thrombocytopenia. *Curr Opin Hematol* 2014;21(5):380–7.

10 Watson H, Davidson S, Keeling D. Guidelines on the diagnosis and management of heparin-induced thrombocytopenia: second edition. *Br J Haematol* 2012;159:528–40.

11 Robson K, Piette W. The presentation and differential diagnosis of cutaneous vascular occlusion syndromes. *Adv Dermatol* 1999;15:153–82.

Platelet plugging: thrombocytosis

1 Harrison CN, Bareford D, Butt N, et al. Guideine for investigation and management of adults and children presenting with a thrombocytosis. *Br J Haematol* 2010;149(3):352–75.

11 Hernandez-Boluda JC, Gomez M. Target hematologic values in the management of essential thrombocythemia and polycythemia vera. *Eur J Haematol* 2014;26(3):428–42.

Cryogelling/cryoagglutination

2 Ramos-Casals M, Stone JH, Cid MC, et al. The cryoglobulinaemias. *Lancet* 2012;379(9813):348–60.

10 Lauchli S, Widmer L, Lautenschlager S. Cold agglutinin disease: the importance of cutaneous signs. *Dermatology* 2001;202:356–8.

15 Michaud M, Pourrat J. Cryofibrinogenemia. *J Clin Rheumatol* 2013;19(3):142–8.

Emboli

Cholesterol embolus

2 Bashore T, Gehrig T. Cholesterol emboli after invasive cardiac procedures. *J Am Coll Cardiol* 2003;42:217–18.

4 Pennington M, Yeager J, Skelton H, Smith K. Cholesterol embolization syndrome: cutaneous histopathological features and the variable onset of symptoms in patients with different risk factors. *Br J Dermatol* 2002;146:511–17.

6 Saric M, Kronzon I. Cholesterol embolization syndrome. *Curr Opin Cardiol* 2011;26(6):472–9.

Oxalate embolus, cardiac embolus and other emboli

1 Akhtar S. Fat embolism. *Anesthesiol Clin* 2009;27(3):533–50.

2 Blackmon JA, Jeffy BG, Malone JC, et al. Oxalosis involving the skin: case report and literature review. *Arch Dermatol* 2011;147(11):1302–5.

4 Greeson D, Wright J, Zanolli M. Cutaneous findings associated with cardiac myxomas. *Cutis* 1998;62:275–80.

Systemic coagulopathies: protein C/protein S-related disease

1 Marlar RA, Montgomery RR, Broekmans AW. Diagnosis and treatment of homozygous protein C deficiency. Report of the Working Party on Homozygous Protein C Deficiency of the Subcommittee on Protein C and Protein S, International Committee on Thrombosis and Haemostasis. *J Pediatr* 1989;114:528–34.

6 Kakagia DD, Papanas N, Karadimas E, et al. Warfarin-induced skin necrosis. *Ann Dermatol* 2014;26(1):96–8.

11 Robson K, Piette W. The presentation and differential diagnosis of cutaneous vascular occlusion syndromes. *Adv Dermatol* 1999;15:153–82.

Systemic coagulopathies: antiphospholipid antibody/lupus anticoagulant syndrome

1 Lim W. Antiphospholipid syndrome. *Hematology (Am Soc Hematol Educ Program)* 2013;2013:675–80.

5 Chaturvedi S, McCrae KR. Recent advances in the antiphospholipid antibody syndrome. *Curr Opin Hematol* 2014;21(5):371–9.

6 Giannakopolulos B, Krills SA. The pathogenesis of the antiphospholipid syndrome. *N Engl J Med* 2013;368:1033–44.

Vascular coagulopathies

1 Sneddon IB. Cerebro-vascular lesions and livedo reticularis. *Br J Dermatol* 1965;77:180–5.

3 Aladdin Y, Hamadeh M, Butcher K. The Sneddon syndrome. *Arch Neurol* 2008;65(6):834–5.

5 Caldas CA, de Carvalho JF. Primary antiphospholipid syndrome with and without Sneddon's syndrome. *Rheumatol Int* 2011;31(2):197–200.

Livedoid vasculopathy/atrophie blanche

1 Chang D, Patel RM. Livedoid vasculopathy. *Cutis* 2012;90(4):179.

2 Acland K, Darvay A, Wakelin S, Russell-Jones R. Livedoid vasculitis: a manifestation of the antiphospholipid syndrome? *Br J Dermatol* 1999;140:131–5.

5 Kerk N, Goerge T. Livedoid vasculopathy – current aspects of diagnosis and treatment of cutaneous infarction. *J Dtsch Dermatol Ges* 2013;11(5):407–10.

Malignant atrophic papulosis

1 Degos R. Malignant atrophic papulosis. *Br J Dermatol* 1979;100:21–36.

2 Theodoridis A, Konstantinidou A, Makrantonaki E, *et al.* Malignant and benign forms of atrophic papulosis (Kohlmeier-Degos disease): systemic involvement determines the prognosis. *Br J Dermatol* 2014;170(1):110–15.

22 Theodoridis A, Makrantonaki E, Zouboulis CC. Malignant atrophic papulosis (Kohlmeier-Degos disease) – a review. *Orphanet J Rare Dis* 2013;8:10.

Calcific uraemic arteriolopathy

1 Weenig RH, Sewell LD, Davis MPD, *et al.* Calciphylaxis: natural history, risk factor analysis, and outcome. *J Am Acad Dermatol* 2007;56:569–79.

2 Hayashi M. Calciphylaxis: diagnosis and clinical features. *Clin Exp Nephrol* 2013;17(4):498–503.

8 Ong S, Coulson IH. Diagnosis and treatment of calciphylaxis. *Skinmed* 2012;10(3):166–70.

PART 9: VASCULAR

CHAPTER 102

Cutaneous Vasculitis

Nick J. Levell and Chetan Mukhtyar

Norwich Medical School, Norfolk and Norwich University Hospital, Norwich, UK

Overview

Definition

Cutaneous vasculitis is inflammation of the blood vessel walls, usually resulting in palpable purpura. Nomenclature of the vasculitides, revised at the 2012 Chapel Hill Consensus conference [1], is based upon the size of blood vessel affected. Some conditions have been renamed, and eponyms have been dropped (Box 102.1).

Introduction and general description

Vasculitis is usually a multisystem disorder that presents in a myriad of ways. Diagnosis is based on a detailed history and careful examination. Patients may present to different specialties and their care should be led by a multidisciplinary team involving physicians with a specialist interest in vasculitis.

Vasculitis can be classified by aetiology or by calibre of the vessel involved. The accepted nomenclature was defined at an international consensus meeting held in 2012 in Chapel Hill, USA. The meeting did not involve dermatologists, and all cutaneous vasculitides could be considered under the umbrella of 'single-organ vasculitis'. It should be recognized that names and classifications will change in the future with greater understanding of the underlying disease mechanisms.

The treatment of primary vasculitis involves immunosuppression. The balance between disease severity and adverse effects of therapy requires expertise and experience in the management of these rare conditions. Secondary vasculitis can be due to infection, drugs, malignancy or inflammatory disease; treatment of the underlying condition may resolve the vasculitis.

Epidemiology

See the specific diseases.

Pathophysiology

The pathophysiology and histopathology varies according to the specific disease.

Clinical features

History

The management of patients presenting with cutaneous vasculitis should begin with a full history. Questions about systemic disease to consider include: (i) complications of vasculitis; (ii) potential malignant and infectious triggers; and (iii) systemic features of systemic vasculitides (Box 102.2). The history should consider diseases that may present with secondary vasculitis including rheumatological diseases (such as systemic lupus erythematosus), thrombo-occlusive disorders and other inflammatory dermatoses.

A full drug history, taken from the patient, the case notes and other relevant clinicians, should focus on medication changes

PART 9: VASCULAR

Rook's Textbook of Dermatology, Ninth Edition. Edited by Christopher Griffiths, Jonathan Barker, Tanya Bleiker, Robert Chalmers and Daniel Creamer.
© 2016 John Wiley & Sons, Ltd. Published 2016 by John Wiley & Sons, Ltd.
Companion website: www.rooksdermatology.com

Box 102.1 Classification of cutaneous vasculitis adapted from the 2012 Chapel Hill Consensus nomenclature [1]

Single-organ (skin) small-vessel vasculitis
- Cutaneous small-vessel vasculitis (see Figure 102.1)
- Urticarial vasculitis (excluding immune complex disease)
- Erythema elevatum diutinum (see Figure 102.9)
- Acute haemorrhagic oedema of infancy
- Recurrent cutaneous necrotizing eosinophilic vasculitis (controversial entity)
- Granuloma faciale (see Figure 102.11)

Cutaneous vasculitis associated with systemic disease or variable vessel size
- Behçet syndrome
- Lupus vasculitis
- Sarcoid vasculitis
- Rheumatoid vasculitis

Small-vessel immune complex-associated vasculitis
- IgA vasculitis (Henoch–Schönlein purpura) (see Figure 102.13)
- Cryoglobulinaemic vasculitis (see Figure 102.14)
- Hypocomplementaemic urticarial vasculitis (HUV)
- Antiglomerular basement membrane vasculitis (anti-GBM/Goodpasture syndrome)

Small-vessel ANCA-associated vasculitis
- Microscopic polyangiitis (MPA)
- Granulomatosis with polyangiitis (GPA/Wegener's granulomatosis) (see Figure 102.20a)
- Eosinophilic granulomatosis with polyangiitis (EGPA/Churg–Strauss syndrome)

Medium-vessel vasculitis
- Polyarteritis nodosa (PAN) (including cutaneous PAN[a]) (see Figure102.3 and Figure 102.25)
- Kawasaki disease

Large-vessel vasculitis
- Giant cell arteritis (GCA)
- Takayasu arteritis

[a]In the paper [1], cutaneous PAN is recognized as cutaneous arteritis (single-organ vasculitis) whereas in this chapter it is considered with PAN.

ANCA, antineutrophil cytoplasmic antibody; IgA, immunoglobulin A.

Box 102.2 Areas in the history of a patient with cutaneous vasculitis that may give clues indicating systemic disease

- Weight loss, fatigue, fever
- Arthralgia, myalgia, arthritis
- Dry eyes, dry mouth
- Red eye, eye pain, vision loss
- Nasal or sinus congestion
- Ear pain
- Oral/nasal ulcers
- Chest pain/dyspnoea
- Abdominal pain, blood in faeces
- Blackouts, weakness, fits

in the days, weeks and months prior to the onset of vasculitis. Occasionally, drugs taken for many years may precipitate reactions. Drugs purchased from pharmacies or borrowed from relatives, herbal treatments, tonics and vitamins should also be considered. Patients may be unwilling to reveal recreational drugs, drugs causing addiction or drugs taken for bodybuilding or sexual purposes. The reason for any drug change should be established.

Vasculitis may be secondary to infection. A history should be taken of infections, both acute and chronic, and their treatments.

Presentation
On general examination, establish if the patient is acutely unwell; patients with systemic vasculitis may have life-threatening internal organ involvement requiring prompt management. All the skin should be examined. Cutaneous vasculitis often results in painful, palpable purpura (Figure 102.1). Leakage of blood from the vasculature into the interstitium causes purpura, which is identified by a failure to blanch on diascopy (pressure with glass). Increased pressure in the venous circulation increases blood vessel leakage and may worsen damage to the vessel walls. Purpura is therefore most apparent on the lower limbs. Prolonged standing exaggerates venous hypertension and thus increases blood leakage and purpura.

The physical signs are determined to some extent by the size of vessel involved (Table 102.1). Severe cutaneous vasculitis will result in painful ischaemia of the skin. Lesional skin will become haemorrhagic (Figure 102.2) and then necrotic and will eventually detach, leaving erosions or ulcers (Figure 102.3), most commonly

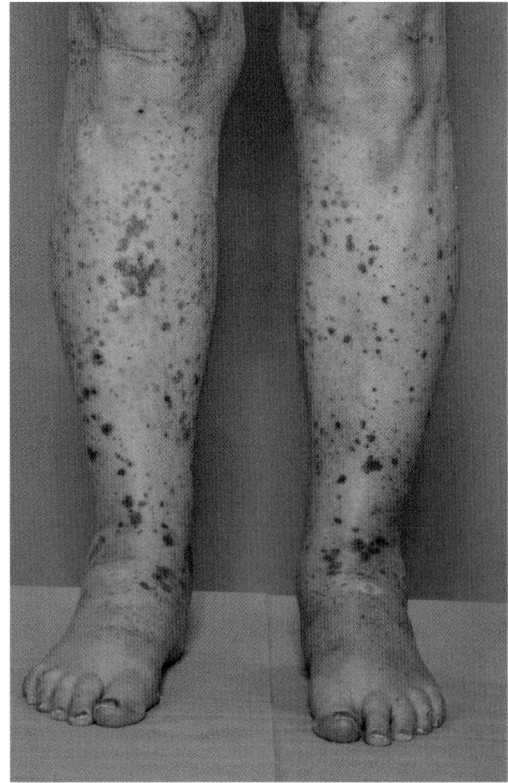

Figure 102.1 Cutaneous small-vessel vasculitis producing palpable purpura. (Courtesy of Andrew Carmichael.)

Table 102.1 Physical signs may give clues as to the predominant vessel size involved in the vasculitis.

Blood vessel size	Physical signs
Small blood vessels	Purpuric macules and papules, haemorrhagic vesicles, urticarial plaques
	Necrosis not usually a major feature
Medium-sized blood vessels	Broken livedo (net/reticulate) pattern, infarction, ulceration, deep nodules

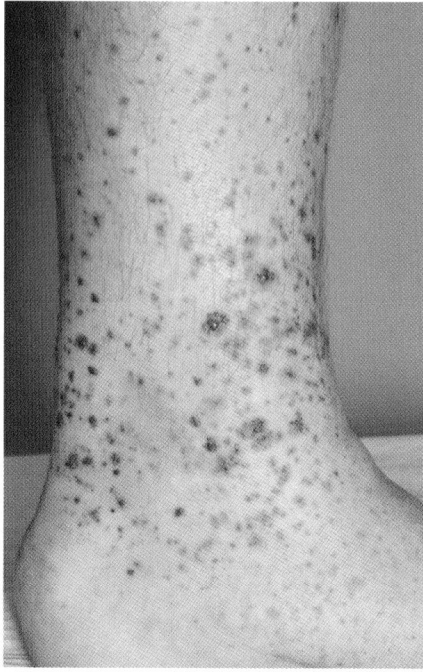

Figure 102.2 Cutaneous small-vessel vasculitis demonstrating a haemorrhagic vesicle. (Courtesy of Andrew Carmichael.)

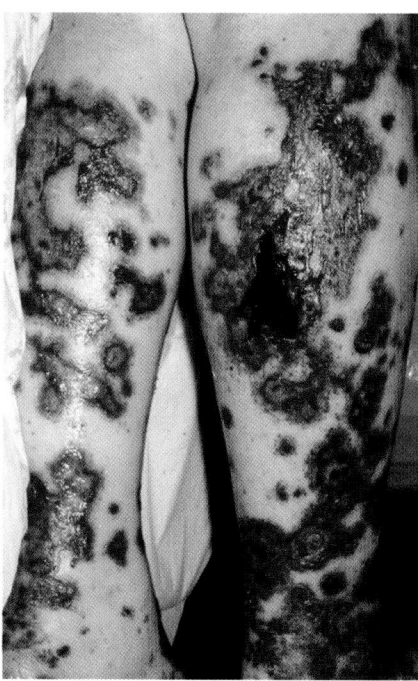

Figure 102.3 Ulcerated necrotic lesions in a livedo distribution suggestive of medium-vessel disease. (Courtesy of Andrew Carmichael.)

Box 102.3 Examination and bedside investigation for systemic vasculitis

- Haematuria, proteinuria (urinalysis), oedema, hypertension
- Congestive cardiac failure, pericardial rub, oedema
- Cough, haemoptysis (examine sputum), wheeze, crepitations
- Abdominal tenderness, melaena, nausea, vomiting, hepatosplenomegaly
- Paraesthesiae, numbness, weakness, abnormal reflexes, psychiatric signs

---

on the lower limbs. These ulcers may then become secondarily infected. The ulcers may be slow to heal, even after resolution of the vasculitis, due to venous stasis, malnutrition, anaemia, lymphoedema, prolonged infection or old age.

The extent of systemic examination will depend on the history and on the overall assessment of the patient. Systemic examination may reveal an underlying infection or malignancy acting as a trigger for the vasculitis. Signs of a systemic primary vasculitis may be found (Box 102.3). Other underlying diseases that may cause secondary vasculitis such as rheumatoid arthritis or lupus erythematosus may be apparent.

Clinical variants

The size of purpuric lesions varies according to the disease. Areas of purpura less than 5 mm in diameter are called petechiae, those larger than 1 cm are ecchymoses. A reticulate (like a net) livedo pattern is seen in some vasculitides and thrombo-occlusive disorders (Table 102.2). A broken livedo (incomplete net) (Figure 102.3) is

Table 102.2 The purpura pattern may give clues as to the disease.

Pattern of purpura	Diseases to consider
Pinpoint, cayenne pepper macular purpura, typically <5 mm	Capillaritis, exercise-induced purpura ('runners' legs'), coughing, ligatures
	Purpura in contact dermatitis (e.g. rubber), venous hypertension, suction induced, fixed drug eruptions, cutaneous T-cell lymphoma
Macular purpura of any size	Purpura due to infections, platelet disorders and thrombocytopenia, other clotting disorders, mild small vessel vasculitis
	Trauma/ artefact
Large macular purpura, typically over 2 cm	Purpura of old age, topical, inhaled or systemic corticosteroid-induced purpura, scurvy
Painful palpable purpura of any size	Cutaneous vasculitis of all types, pityriasis lichenoides, thrombo-occlusive disorders of all types, secondary purpura in tuberculosis or leprosy reactions, neutrophilic disorders, atypical benign or malignant cutaneous growths (e.g. haemangiosarcoma, Kaposi sarcoma, amelanontic melanoma with haemorrhage)
Livedo pattern purpura	Antiphospholipid syndromes, vasculitis in medium-sized blood vessels (e.g. polyarteritis, ANCA vasculitides), thrombo-occlusive disorders of all types including cryoglobulins, chilblains

ANCA, antineutrophil cytoplasmic antibody.

said to be a feature of vasculitis disorders but may also be seen in thrombo-occlusive disease.

Differential diagnosis

Thrombo-occlusive disorders, trauma, inflammatory dermatoses with disordered clotting, purpura due to prolonged running, neutrophilic disorders, cellulitis (particularly in the elderly with oedematous legs), insect and snake bites are often confused with vasculitis.

Disease course and prognosis

See above and specific diseases.

Investigations

The investigation of vasculitis is dependent on the history and examination findings. A thorough assessment may clarify the likely cause and limit the need for extensive investigations. However, investigations are necessary for two main purposes. First, it is important to establish if the vasculitis is primary or secondary. Investigations should be directed to identify underlying rheumatological disease, malignancy, infection or a primary vasculitis. Second, investigations should be carried to demonstrate the presence of vasculitis involving internal organs. Urinalysis to exclude renal disease is useful in most patients.

Skin biopsy in vasculitis, if needed, should be taken from a fresh lesion less than 48 h old. Older vasculitic lesions may develop secondary thrombosis making difficult differentiation from a thrombo-occlusive disorder. Older lesions of thrombo-occlusive disorders may develop secondary vasculitis. A skin biopsy for direct immunofluoresence should be taken if IgA vasculitis is suspected. A 'lupus band' of IgG and complement at the dermal–epidermal junction is of little value as a diagnostic test and is no longer recommended. A vasculitis screen may be used by inexperienced clinicians as a substitute for taking a history and examination and then applying logic. A list of tests is given in Table 102.3 but these should be used in support of clinical findings and intelligent thought.

Management

The management of vasculitis is dependent on the diagnosis and the severity and presence of systemic vasculitis. Triggering drugs should be stopped. Underlying infections should be treated. Malignancy or associated rheumatological diseases should be managed. If systemic vasculitis or vasculitic disease is identified then the treatment is described under the specific diseases in this book. The correction of venous stasis by elevation of the legs, treatment of secondary infection, appropriate dressings in ulcerated areas and pain relief are required.

In systemic vasculitis a multidisciplinary team approach is appropriate. Specialists may be required to deal with disease in almost any organ. In the UK, rheumatologists with an interest in vasculitis often lead or coordinate teams of other specialists to manage complex patients. Early referral is desirable to avoid potentially treatable disease in other organs causing irreversible damage.

Table 102.3 Vasculitis investigations. The 'vasculitis screen' is dependent on the history and examination findings. In acute vasculitis with an obvious infection or drug trigger, investigations may be minimal. The purposes of investigation are threefold: to look for (i) complications of vasculitis; (ii) causes of vasculitis; and (iii) differential diagnoses of vasculitis, such as thrombo-occlusive disorders.

Investigation	Notes
Blood and urine tests	
Urinalysis	Haematuria and proteinuria in renal involvement
Urea and electrolytes	Raised creatinine and urea in renal involvement
Full blood count	Raised white cells in infection/ cryoglobulinaemia Thrombocytopenia may cause purpura
Liver function	Low albumin in renal disease
Erythrocyte sedimentation rate	May be raised in systemic vasculitis, infection and malignancy
C-reactive protein	May be raised in infections
Antineutrophil cytoplasmic antibody (ANCA)	May be present in systemic vasculitides – see text
Antinuclear antibodies	May be present in autoimmune connective tissue disease
Specialist haematological tests for thromboembolic disease such as lupus anticoagulant and anticardiolipin antibodies	If thrombo-occlusive disease is possible from the history, examination or histology
Cryoglobulins	If there is skin, kidney and joint vasculitis. Not necessarily triggered by cold
Tissue tests	
Skin biopsy from early lesion (less than 48 h old) for histopathology	Indicate if vasculitis or thromboembolic disorder Indicate size of blood vessel involvement and predominant cell type Indicate presence of granulomas Indicate certain infections, e.g. mycobacteria
Skin biopsy from early lesion for direct immunofluorescence	Indicate if IgA vasculitis
Skin biopsy for culture	May be useful for chronic infections, e.g. TB
Infection	
Infection screen: cultures, serology and radiology	Depends on age, history of travel and country of residence, history and examination. Screen for acute and/or chronic infections
Malignancy	
Malignancy screen: blood tests and radiology for malignancy	Relevant tests depend on the age of patient, history and examination
Inflammatory disease	
Investigations for other systemic inflammatory disease	If diseases (e.g. inflammatory bowel disease, rheumatoid arthritis) are suspected from history and examination

SINGLE-ORGAN SMALL-VESSEL VASCULITIS

Cutaneous small-vessel vasculitis

Definition and nomenclature

Cutaneous small-vessel vasculitis (CSVV) is a single-organ vasculitis producing leucocytoclastic angiitis of cutaneous vasculature [1,2].

Synonyms and inclusions
- Allergic cutaneous vasculitis
- Allergic cutaneous angiitis
- Hypersensitivity angiitis
- Hypersensitivity vasculitis
- Cutaneous leucocytoclastic angiitis
- Cutaneous leucocytoclastic vasculitis
- Cutaneous allergic vasculitis

Introduction and general description

The American College of Rheumatology (ACR) have produced classification criteria for CSVV. The presence of three of the following five criteria have 84% specificity for CSVV: (i) age greater than 16 years at disease onset; (ii) history of taking a medication at onset that may have been a precipitating factor; (iii) the presence of palpable purpura; (iv) the presence of a maculopapular rash; and (v) a biopsy demonstrating granulocytes around an arteriole or venule [3].

CSVV is a single-organ vasculitis and therefore by definition does not have systemic manifestations. However, the diagnosis should prompt ongoing surveillance because it may be a first manifestation of a more generalized vasculitis. CSVV is a clinical syndrome that encompasses vasculitis due to a variety of causes.

Epidemiology

Incidence and prevalence

The annual incidence of CSVV is reported to be between 15 and 30 per million [4,5].

Age

The mean age at onset is between 36 and 56 years [4,6,7]. However, the age range is wide and extends from the second to the eighth decade of life.

Sex

In a Spanish cohort, men were more commonly affected with a ratio of 1.6 : 1 [4], but in a Singapore cohort, there was a female dominance of 2.1 : 1 [6].

Associated diseases

By definition the condition is localized to the skin, but it may be a precursor for other systemic vasculitides.

Box 102.4 Aetiological triggers for cutaneous small vessel vasculitis (with relevant references)

- Acenocoumarol [12]
- Staphylococcal protein A column immunoadsorption therapy [13–15]
- Anisoylated plasminogen activator complex [16]
- Food allergies [17]
- Propylthiouracil [18]
- Interferon 1B [19]
- Ibuprofen [20]
- Methotrexate [21]
- Warfarin [22]
- Granulocyte colony-stimulating factor [23]
- Ant bite [24]
- Procainamide [25]
- Infliximab [26]
- Maprotiline [27]
- Omeprazole [28]
- Exercise [29]
- Insulin [30]
- Imipenem-cilastatin [31]
- Gabapentin [32]
- Lamotrigine [32]
- Coumarin [33]
- Atenolol [34]
- Solid organ malignancies [35]

Pathophysiology

Predisposing factors

There are many causes of cutaneous vasculitis, but most CSVV is idiopathic [6]. This is a consequence of vasculitis classification systems. For example, if patients with CSVV are found to have viral hepatitis and cryoglobulinemia, they are no longer classifiable as CSVV. There are factors that are thought to contribute to a pure CSVV, which are listed in Box 102.4.

Pathology

Leukocytoclastic vasculitis with segmental inflammation in an angiocentric pattern, swelling of the endothelium, fibrinoid necrosis of vessel walls, extravasation of erythrocytes, and an infiltrate of neutrophils with karyorrhexis of the nuclei (i.e. leukocytoclasia) are major features of CSVV (Figures 102.4 and 102.5). In superficial dermal papillary vessels, IgM or complement C3 perivascular deposits are demonstrated in up to 80% of fresh lesions [8]. Some studies state lower proportions, but this may depend on the timing of the biopsy and also because IgM is relatively poor at fixing complement. IgG is found less often.

Causative organisms

In most patients, CSVV is idiopathic, but a small number of cases (4/138 in [9]) may be related to a bacterial infection.

Genetics

The genetics are not known.

PART 9: VASCULAR

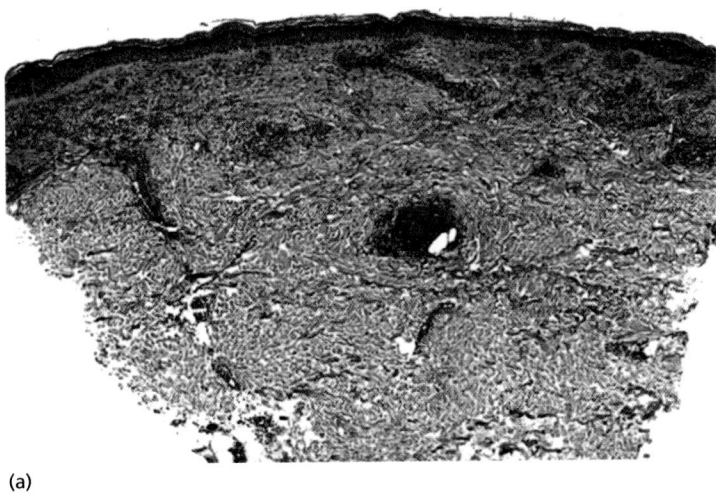

(a)

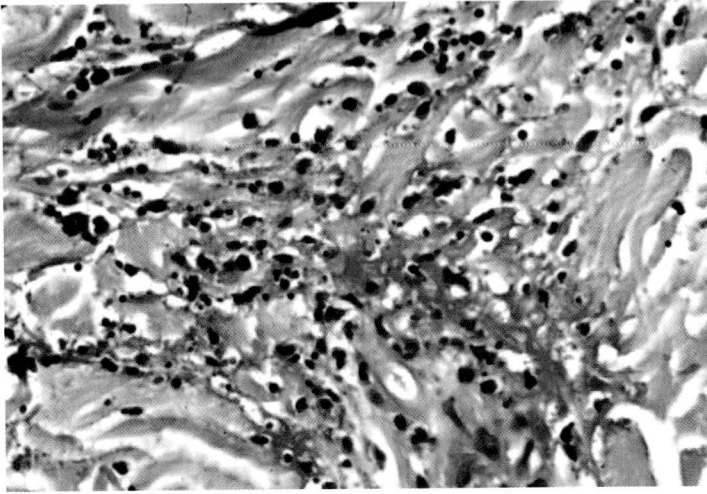

(b)

Figure 102.4 Leukocytoclastic vasculitis. (a) Low-magnification photomicrograph showing perivascular infiltrates and fibrinoid deposits within the vessels of the upper dermis. (b) Higher magnification demonstrating nuclear dust, fibrinoid deposits, vascular alteration and collagen degeneration. (Courtesy of Dr Omar Sangueza, Wake Forest University School of Medicine, Winston-Salem, NC, USA.)

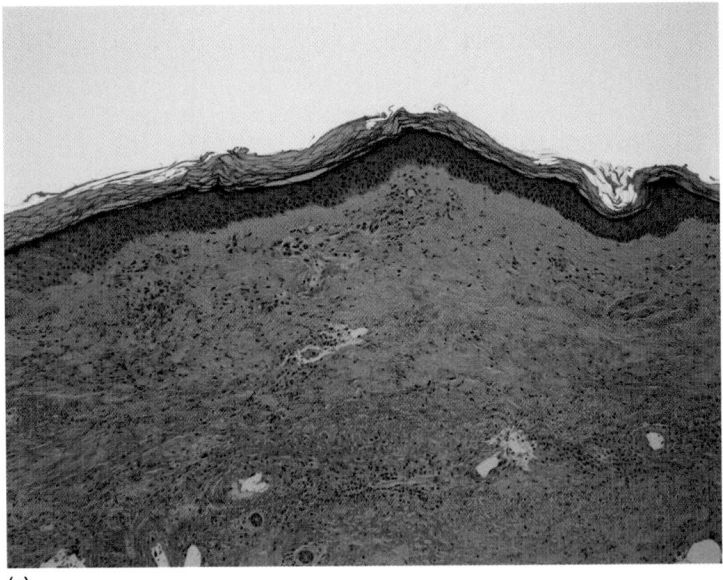

(a)

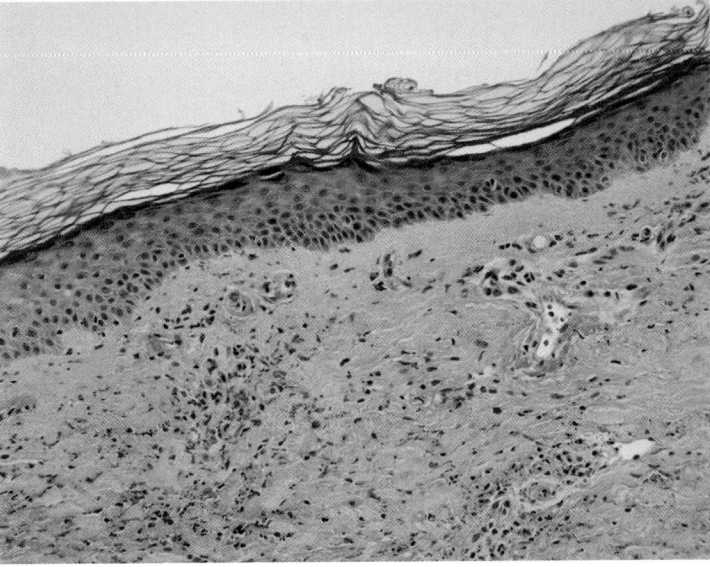

(b)

Figure 102.5 Leukocytoclastic (small vessel) vasculitis at (a) lower and (b) higher magnifications. There is visible vascular wall damage with evidence of red blood cell extravasation, fibrinoid change and extensive leukocytoclasis (nuclear debris from polymorphonuclear leukocytes). (Courtesy of Dr Laszlo Igali, Norfolk and Norwich University Hospital, Norwich, UK.)

Clinical features

History

The skin lesions of CSVV typically arise as a simultaneous 'crop', resulting from exposure to an inciting stimulus. New lesion formation can continue for several weeks. They usually resolve within several weeks or a few months although approximately 10% of patients will have recurrent disease. There are no known risk factors to predict relapses.

Presentation

Lesions typically occur in areas prone to stasis, commonly including the ankles and lower legs (Figures 102.1 and 102.6a), and typically sparing intertriginous regions. CSVV is often asymptomatic, although pruritus, pain or burning may be experienced, as well as systemic symptoms including fever, arthralgia, myalgia and anorexia. The major cutaneous manifestation of CSVV is palpable purpura, ranging in size from 1 mm to several centimetres (Figure 102.6b, c). Sometimes macular in the early stages, such purpura may progress to a wide array of lesions including papules, nodules, vesicles, plaques, bullae or pustules, with secondary findings of ulceration, necrosis and post-inflammatory hyperpigmentation (Figure 102.7).

Clinical variants

Other cutaneous findings include oedema, livedo reticularis and urticaria. The presence of the latter two should prompt consideration of cutaneous polyarteritis nodosa and urticarial vasculitis, respectively.

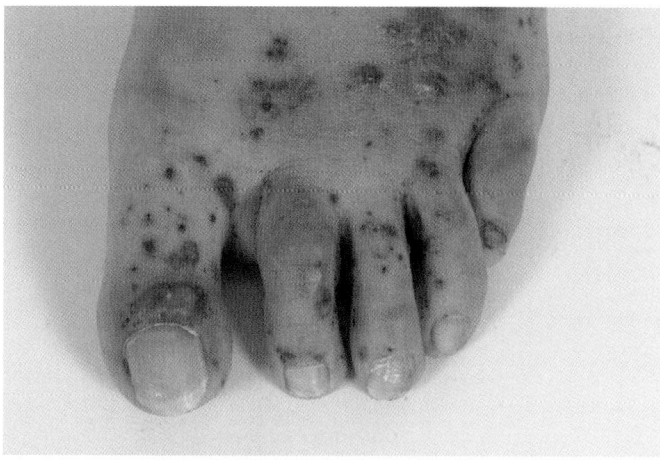

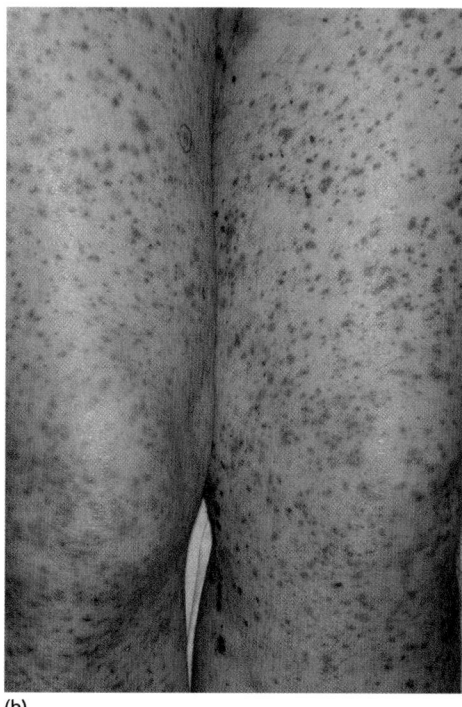

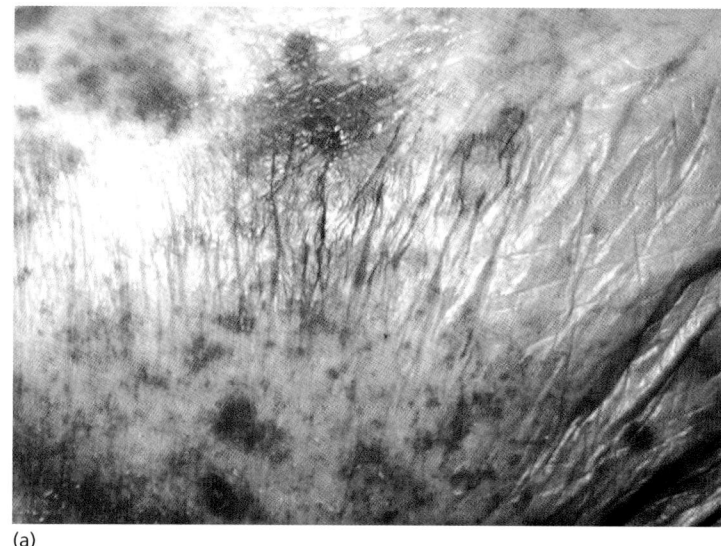

(a)

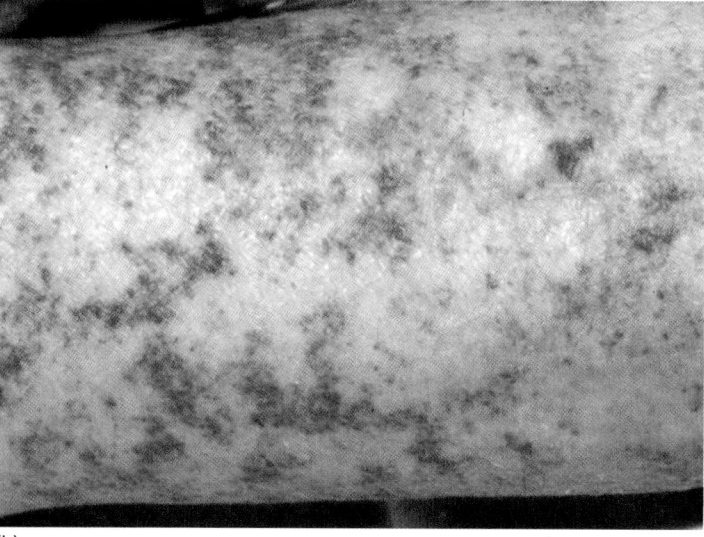

(b)

Figure 102.7 Vasculitis due to sepsis, in a patient with impaired level of consciousness. The necrotic lesion in (a) and the reticulate pattern on the leg in (b) are clues to the involvement of deeper vessels. Histologically, vasculitis due to infection may involve vessels at all levels of the dermis.

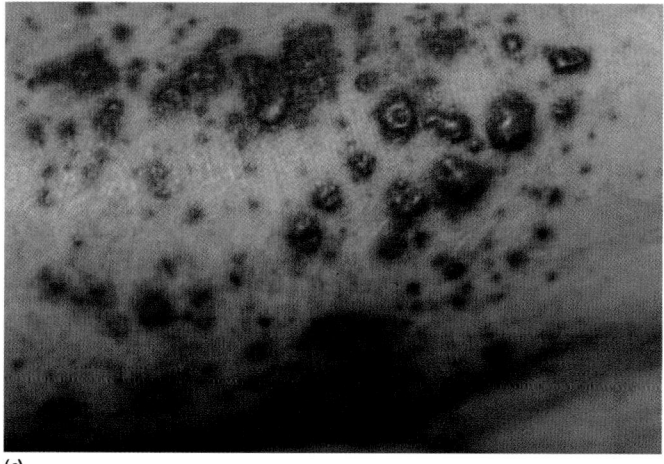

Figure 102.6 Cutaneous small-vessel vasculitis (CSVV). (a) Vesicles in a dependent area on the foot. (b) Purpura on the thighs; there was similar involvement on the lower legs. (c) CSVV progressing to blistering.

Differential diagnosis

The differential diagnosis of CSVV includes many more specifically defined disorders, which are discussed in this chapter and listed in references [2,3,9–11,12,13]. CSVV is a diagnosis of exclusion. Cutaneous vasculitis should prompt a search for a wide array of differential diagnoses, including systemic vasculitides, cancer, infections, allergies, chemical exposures, etc.

Classification of severity

There is no validated biomarker for quantifying disease severity in patients with CSVV. Histopathology is not a good surrogate for severity of disease [10]. The Birmingham Vasculitis Activity Score (BVAS) v3 has been validated to quantify the activity of systemic vasculitis [11]. The validation cohort of BVAS v3 included patients with cutaneous vasculitis and it can be used to create a tangible activity score.

PART 9: VASCULAR

Complications and co-morbidities

Hyperpigmentation and haemosiderosis can take months to resolve. Ulcerated lesions may become infected adding to the morbidity.

Investigations

Investigation of CSVV is guided by the history and examination findings; the range of tests chosen will range from nothing to extensive blood testing, scanning and organ biopsies. The purpose of investigation is twofold: firstly to look for evidence of vasculitis in other organ systems, and secondly to look for evidence of a disease that is predisposing towards CSVV, such as infection or malignancy.

Management

Treatment of CSVV is often unnecessary, as the disease may be self-limiting. The evidence for efficacy of therapy is derived from clinical experience rather than controlled trials. If a triggering agent is identified, such as a drug or infection, it should be removed or treated. Efforts to minimize stasis, such as use of compression hosiery and the elevation of dependent areas, as well as the use of non-steroidal anti-inflammatory drugs (NSAIDs) and antihistamines, may reduce symptoms [10], although not altering the course of the disease.

First line

Oral prednisolone 30–80 mg once daily, tapered over 2–3 weeks, often gives symptom control, although no controlled trials have been carried out to evaluate the treatment of CSVV with oral corticosteroids. Corticosteroid use may be of particular benefit in cases with painful progressive cutaneous lesions. No data support the use of topical corticosteroids or antibiotics in CSVV, although such therapies are commonly used.

Second line

Colchicine 0.6 mg twice daily has been shown to be of benefit by anecdotal evidence and open-label studies [15–17]. Dapsone 50-150 mg daily may be advantageous in the treatment of CSVV [18–21].

Third line

In patients with disease refractory to the above therapies, cytotoxic agents may be considered. Such agents include azathioprine (1–2 mg/kg/day) and methotrexate (15–25 mg/week). The use of ciclosporin (2.5–4 mg/kg/day) and cyclophosphamide is almost never indicated for purely cutaneous disease.

Erythema elevatum diutinum

Definition and nomenclature

Erythema elevatum diutinum (EED) is a rare, chronic, cutaneous eruption. The first descriptions were by Hutchinson and Bury in the 1880s, and the condition was later named in 1894 by Radcliffe-Crocker and Williams. EED is characterized by fibrosing plaques with histological evidence of leukocytoclastic vasculitis.

Synonyms and inclusions

The condition in younger women has been called Bury disease after the early report. Hutchinson's original cases were described in older men. Some early reports make this distinction although the conditions are considered synonymous.

Epidemiology

Incidence and prevalence

Erythema elevatum diutinum is very rare with only a few hundred cases described. There are small case series published but most reports are of single cases only. Few dermatologists have looked after more than a handful of cases.

Age

Erythema elevatum diutinum is most commonly seen in adults in the fourth to seventh decade although occasional childhood cases are reported [1].

Sex

It occurs equally in males and females.

Ethnicity

There has been no description of predilection in any ethnic groups.

Associated diseases

Erythema elevatum diutinum has been associated with autoimmune diseases such as rheumatoid arthritis, coeliac disease, inflammatory bowel disease and type 1 diabetes. Associations with infections, including *Streptococcus*, hepatitis and syphilis, have also been suggested [2–5,6,7,8,9,10,11]. Lesions characteristic of EED have been induced by injection of streptococcal antigen into the dermis [12–15], and have occurred at sites of mosquito bites [10]. EED has been associated with human immunodeficiency virus (HIV) infection. As lesions of EED have responded to antiretroviral and dapsone treatment in HIV-positive patients, it is now recognized as one of the defined reactive dermatoses associated with HIV [16]. EED has been associated with hypergammaglobulinaemia and IgA monoclonal gammopathies, as well as with myelodysplasia, pyoderma gangrenosum and relapsing polychondritis. The association with haematological abnormalities, such as multiple myeloma, is strong; however, EED may precede the haematological disease by several years [17].

Pathophysiology

Although the exact aetiology is unknown, EED is thought to be related to an Arthus-type reaction with immune complex deposition and subsequent inflammation.

Predisposing factors

See the associated diseases.

Pathology

Acute lesions of EED are characterized by leukocytoclastic vasculitis, with little fibrin deposition (Figure 102.8). Eosinophils may also be present in the upper and mid dermis. Depending on the

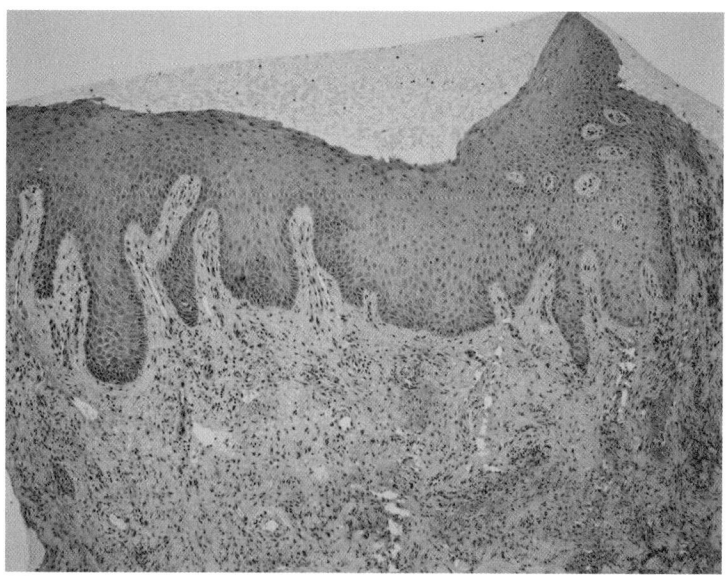

(a)

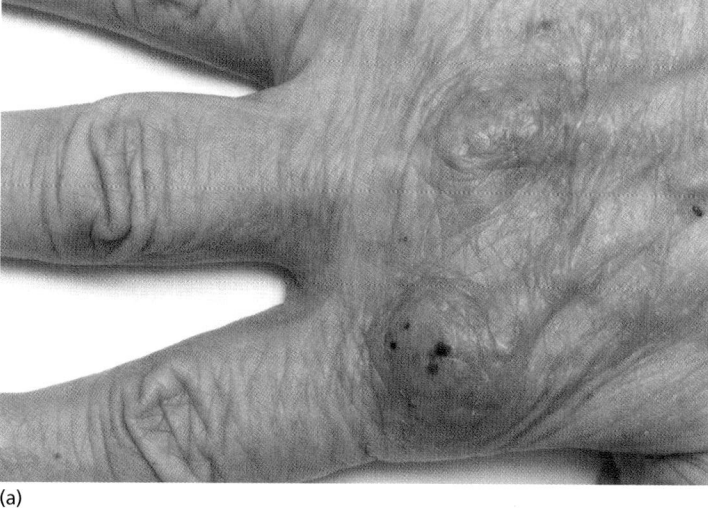

(a)

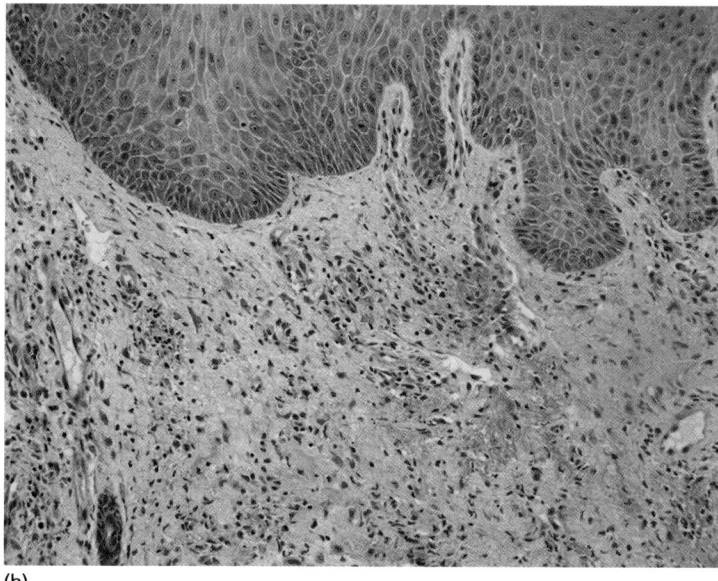

(b)

Figure 102.8 Erythema elevatum diutinum at (a) lower and (b) higher magnifications. There is a perivascular infiltrate containing neutrophils, with leukocytoclasis and some perivascular fibrin deposition. (Courtesy of Dr Laszlo Igali, Norfolk and Norwich University Hospital, Norwich, UK.)

degree of oedema and infiltration into the dermis, unaffected collagen may be present just under the epidermis. Chronic lesions demonstrate angiocentric eosinophilic fibrosis, capillary proliferation and infiltration of macrophages, plasma cells and lymphocytes. Cholesterol deposits in histiocytes and in the extracellular tissue (the latter in a pattern that has been termed 'extracellular cholesterolosis') may be present in older lesions [18]. Dermal nodules of EED contain spindle cells and fibrosis [19].

Clinical features

History
Although they are generally asymptomatic, the lesions of EED may be painful.

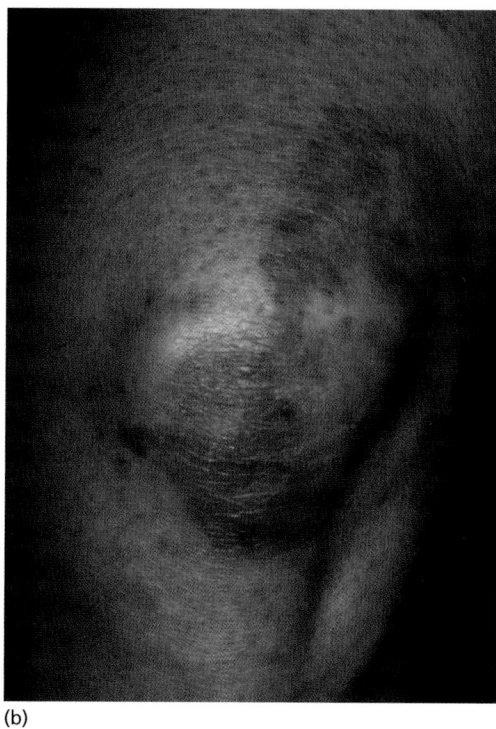

(b)

Figure 102.9 Erythema elevatum diutinum. (a) On the hands. (b) Early non-fibrotic lesions at a typical site on the knee. This patient also had EED on the hands, and pyoderma gangrenosum.

Presentation
Lesions of EED most commonly appear chronically in a symmetrical fashion over the dorsa of the hands, knees, buttocks and Achilles tendons (Figure 102.9). They are red-violaceous, red-brown or yellowish papules, plaques or nodules. Occasionally, the face and ears are also affected by EED. Initially, the lesions are soft, but eventually they fibrose and later leave atrophic scars.

Differential diagnosis
Erythema elevatum diutinum may be difficult to distinguish from CSVV on histology but the clinical presentation enables accurate diagnosis. EED and Sweet syndrome are both described as neutrophilic dermatoses. However, EED differs from Sweet syndrome by

the character of the lesions and their distribution, as well as by histopathological features. The classic assumption that lesions from patients with Sweet syndrome lack histopathological fibrinoid necrosis of the vessel walls has been challenged. In one series, 29% of patients had biopsy specimens showing leukocytoclastic vasculitis [20], although this may have been secondary changes in older lesions. Clinically, the lesions in Sweet syndrome are acute, more often asymmetrical and located on the arms, face and neck [21]. By contrast, EED lesions are chronic, symmetrical and classically located over the dorsum of the hands and knees, buttocks and Achilles tendons. Although leukocytoclastic vasculitis has now been reported as a possible feature of Sweet lesions [2], it is not always present and the fibrosis seen in lesions of EED correlates with the clinical chronicity. Granuloma faciale has been considered in the same group of disorders as EED, but may have features of the IgG4-related sclerosing diseases, such as storiform fibrosis, which is histologically absent in EED [22].

Complications and co-morbidities
Although the lesions can be painful and heal with scarring, complications are rare.

Disease course and prognosis
Erythema elevatum diutinum may last from 5 to 35 years, with crops of new lesions developing every few weeks to months.

Investigations
The demonstration of IgA antineutrophil cytoplasmic antibodies (ANCA) (with various specificities) in six of 10 cases of EED has been suggested to be of some diagnostic value [23]; in this series, seven of the 10 patients had raised IgA levels (monoclonal in three).

Management
Treatment of an associated disorder such as HIV infection or paraproteinaemia may be effective [24].

First line
Dapsone is usually effective in EED [15], although relapse on stopping may occur.

Second line
Niacinamide has also been used with good effect [25]. High potency topical, or intralesional, corticosteroids may minimize the size of lesions in patients with limited disease; 5% topical dapsone gel has been described as effective [26].

Third line
Other therapies used for CSVV may also be effective in treating patients with EED.

Recurrent cutaneous necrotizing eosinophilic vasculitis

Definition and nomenclature
This is a relatively recently described and rare vasculitis consisting of a predominantly centripetal purpuric papular rash, angio-oedema, peripheral blood eosinophilia and an eosinophilic necrotizing vasculitis of small vessels [1,2]. It can be argued that this is a pathological subdivision of CSVV rather than a distinct entity.

Synonyms and inclusions
- Recurrent cutaneous eosinophilic necrotizing vasculitis

Epidemiology

Incidence and prevalence
This is a very rarely described disease with only a few cases in the literature.

Age
The condition has been described in adults aged 17–81 years.

Sex
Either sex may be affected.

Ethnicity
There is no known association.

Associated diseases
Association with connective tissue diseases and with rheumatoid arthritis has been reported [3,4].

Pathophysiology
The cause is unknown. As in other strongly eosinophilic disorders, eosinophil cytokines such as interleukin 5 (IL-5), and toxic eosinophil granule proteins such as the major basic protein, have been demonstrated in serum and tissues, respectively, and presumably play a part in the tissue damage. Neutrophil elastase is prominent around vessels, and mast cell degranulation occurs. Eosinophilic vasculitis has also been reported in a patient with the hypereosinophilic syndrome; in this patient, CD40 (a glycoprotein of the tumour necrosis factor (TNF) receptor family) was considered to be important in pathogenesis [5].

Predisposing factors
There are no known predisposing factors.

Pathology
Histopathology shows fibrinoid deposition and necrosis of small dermal vessels with an infiltrate of eosinophils and absent or minimal leukocytoclasis. Small epidermal vesicles containing eosinophils may be present. Immunoglobulin deposition is not a feature. This eosinophilic small vessel vasculitis may be distinct from other vasculitides such as eosinophilic granulomatosis with polyangiitis (previously known as Churg–Strauss syndrome), in which predominantly medium vessels are affected; and from most drug-induced vasculitis in which eosinophils are generally less prominent.

Causative organisms
There is no known association with causative organisms.

Genetics
The genetics of the condition are unknown.

Environmental factors
There are no reported environmental triggers.

Clinical features

History
Patients may initially present with pruritic papules over the lower limbs. The course is long and recurrent, but fever, arthralgia and visceral involvement are absent.

Presentation
Recurrent pruritic papules and urticarial lesions occur at any site, especially the lower limbs, head and neck, with angio-oedema of the face and extremities. Digital occlusions manifesting as the Raynaud phenomenon or digital gangrene have been reported in patients with cutaneous eosinophilic vasculitis associated with the hypereosinophilic syndrome [5,6], but they can also occur in the hypereosinophilic syndrome in the absence of cutaneous eosinophilic vasculitis [7,8].

Clinical variants
An eosinophilic vasculitis, typically with hypocomplementaemia, also occurs in connective tissue diseases [9].

Differential diagnosis
This condition was recently distinguished from other eosinophilic vasculitides that affect medium-sized vessels (eosinophilic granulomatosis with polyangiitis; see separate section this chapter) and from eosinophilic disorders in which pruritic papules and/or angio-oedema may occur, such as hypereosinophilic syndrome, episodic angio-oedema with eosinophilia, dermatitis herpetiformis, Wells syndrome, polymorphic eruption of pregnancy or drug eruptions.

Complications and co-morbidities
Ulceration and secondary infection of necrotic lesions may occur. By contrast with eosinophilic granulomatosis with polyangiitis, systemic features are not reported.

Disease course and prognosis
A good response to corticosteroids is reported.

Investigations
Investigations are guided by history and clinical examination and will be needed to exclude the differential diagnoses, listed above.

Management

First line
The few cases described have been treated with oral corticosteroids with good effect, intermittently or as prolonged maintenance therapy depending on response [10].

Second line
Secondary infection of ulcerated lesions may require topical or systemic antibiotics according to sensitivities.

Granuloma faciale

Definition and nomenclature
Granuloma faciale is an uncommon condition typified by asymptomatic cutaneous nodules occurring primarily on the face, with occasional extrafacial involvement. Granuloma faciale is limited to the skin, without any systemic manifestations.

Synonyms and inclusions
- Eosinophilic granuloma (not to be confused with Langerhans cell histiocytosis)

Introduction and general description
Granuloma faciale is an uncommon condition of unknown aetiology that is characterized by the presence of benign, purely CSVV. In 1945, Wigley described a 46-year-old woman with recurrent, multiple, raised, discrete, smooth, greyish brown, facial lesions. The histology demonstrated pleomorphic infiltrate with predominant eosinophils, but also polymorphs and plasma cells. In the absence of any bony involvement, this was diagnosed as an eosinophilic granuloma [1]. The term 'granuloma faciale' and 'facial granuloma with eosinophilia' was first used by Boersma in 1951 [2].

Epidemiology

Incidence and prevalence
Granuloma faciale is a rare condition.

Age
It is seen most commonly in 40–60 year olds [3,4].

Sex
Granuloma faciale is commoner in males [3].

Ethnicity
Granuloma faciale has been reported from various parts of the world and does not seem to have any ethnic predilection.

Associated diseases
As noted by Wigley [1], the dermal infiltrate consists of eosinophils and plasma cells. Cesinaro et al. reported a storiform fibrotic pattern and the presence of large amounts of IgG4-staining deposits [5]. This raises the possibility that some patients with granuloma faciale may have IgG4-related disease.

Pathophysiology
Although the aetiology is unclear, this disease is considered to be a histological variant of leukocytoclastic vasculitis with a prominent eosinophilic infiltrate and confined to the skin [4]. The presence of plasma cells and IgG deposition in and around the dermal vasculature has been demonstrated, indicating that granuloma faciale may be immune complex mediated [5]. The reporting of T cells in the tissue is variable. Smoller and Bortz reported large numbers of CD4+ cells that stain strongly for IL-2R antibodies [6],

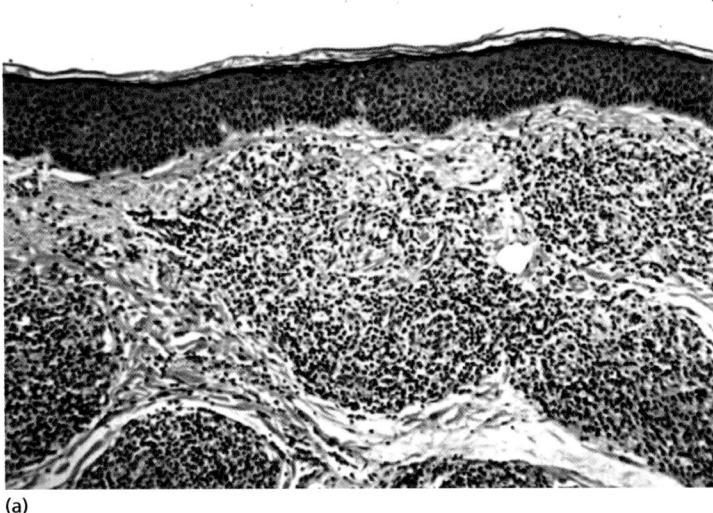

(a)

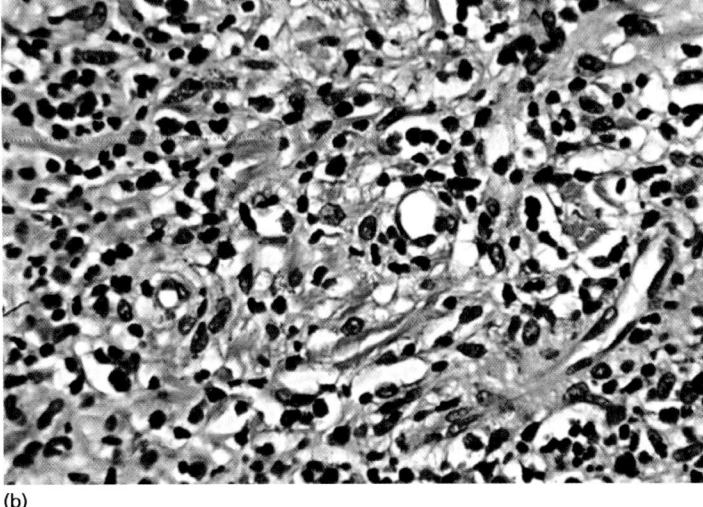

(b)

Figure 102.10 Granuloma faciale. (a) Low-magnification view showing perivascular nodular infiltrates within the dermis. (b) At a higher magnification the infiltrate shows lymphocytes, eosinophils and a few neutrophils. (Courtesy of Dr Omar Sangueza, Wake Forest University School of Medicine, Winston-Salem, NC, USA.)

and Cesinaro *et al.* found T-cell subsets to be variable but with a predominance of GATA-3 lymphocytes [5].

Pathology

Granuloma faciale is a misnomer. The one pathological finding that is almost always absent is a granuloma [7]. It is characterized by a mixed inflammatory infiltrate with a predominance of eosinophils and plasma cells as part of a pleomorphic infiltrate, mainly in the upper half of the dermis but with occasional spread into the lower dermis and subcutaneous tissue (Figure 102.10). A band of normal collagen referred to as a 'Grenz' zone typically separates the inflammatory infiltrate from the epidermis and pilosebaceous appendages. Nuclear dust (fragmented neutrophil nuclei) may be observed near capillaries. The vascular changes may be mild (perivascular distribution of inflammatory cells) to florid (leucocytoclastic vasculitis with fibrinoid necrosis). Perivascular storiform fibrosis and obliterative venulitis have been observed.

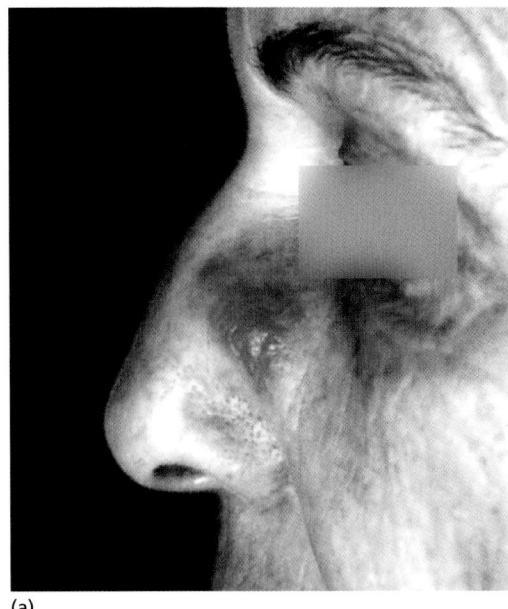

(a)

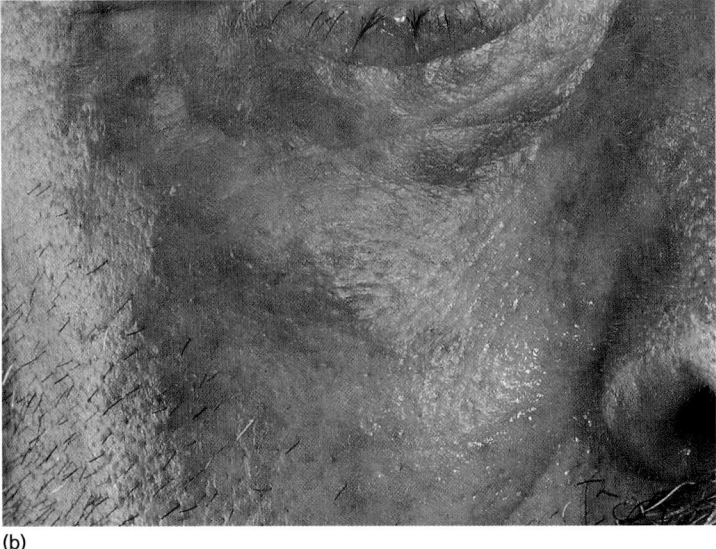

(b)

Figure 102.11 Granuloma faciale. (a) Reddish brown plaque on the nose (courtesy of Dr G. Dawn, Monklands Hospital, UK). (b) Close up of a facial plaque.

Clinical features

History

Lesions of granuloma faciale commonly occur on the face (Figure 102.11); multiple lesions are present in about a third of cases but extrafacial involvement is uncommon, occurring in five of 66 patients in one study [4]. They are almost always asymptomatic, although some patients may describe itching, burning or pain associated with the lesions.

Presentation

The nodules or plaques are soft and red-brown . They are smooth, with prominent follicular orifices and telangiectatic surface changes or scaling. The lesions never ulcerate. Dermoscopy shows parallel, arborizing blood vessels, brown dots and globules and dilated follicular openings [8].

Clinical variants

Extrafacial granuloma faciale is rare, but it has been reported on the scalp, back, shoulders, arms, breast and trunk [9–12]. In a study of 66 patients, only five patients had extrafacial lesions [4]; all these lesions coexisted with facial lesions. Intranasal lesions have been reported.

Eosinophilic angiocentric fibrosis is thought to be a mucosal variant of granuloma faciale that may occur in the nasal passages or upper airways in conjunction with skin lesions of granuloma faciale [13,14]. Eosinophilic angiocentric fibrosis may cause fibrotic stenosis of the affected site with localized extension and damage [15]. For example, epiphora and proptosis have been reported in patients with obstructive sinonasal eosinophilic angiocentric fibrosis [16].

Differential diagnosis

Granulomatous rosacea does not have vasculitis on histology. Sarcoid, TB, cutaneous lupus erythematosus and rarely EED may present with solitary cutaneous lesions.

Disease course and prognosis

Granuloma faciale is a chronic disease with intermittent acute flares that is notoriously resistant to treatment.

Investigations

A definitive diagnosis of granuloma faciale requires clinically consistent lesions and a confirmatory biopsy. Although most laboratory studies are normal, mild peripheral blood eosinophilia may be present [10].

Management

Management of granuloma faciale may be challenging. Topical tacrolimus may be effective but the condition is difficult to treat.

Treatment ladder

First line
- Topical tacrolimus 0.03% or 0.1%

Second line
- Topical or intralesional corticosteroids

Third line
- Dermabrasion [17], laser treatments of various types [17–19], electrosurgery [17], cryosurgery [20], psoralen with ultraviolet A (PUVA) and other systemic treatments including dapsone [21] and tacrolimus [22]
- Some cases have been treated with surgical excision [12]

SMALL-VESSEL IMMUNE COMPLEX-ASSOCIATED VASCULITIS

IgA vasculitis

Definition and nomenclature

IgA vasculitis, previously called Henoch–Schönlein purpura (HSP), is an immune complex vasculitis characterized by IgA1-dominant immune deposits affecting small vessels (predominantly capillaries, venules or arterioles). It often involves the skin and gastrointestinal tract, and frequently causes arthritis. Glomerulonephritis indistinguishable from IgA nephropathy may occur [1].

Synonyms and inclusions
- Henoch–Schönlein purpura
- Anaphylactoid purpura
- Rheumatoid purpura
- Allergic purpura
- Haemorrhagic vasculitis
- Purpura haemorrhagica
- Non-thrombocytopenic purpura

Introduction and general description

William Heberden, in the 1780s, described two children with petechiae, purpura and ecchymosis in conjunction with arthritis. One of the two boys also had abdominal pain, melena and haematuria [2]. In the 19th century, Johann Schönlein and Eduard Henoch independently characterized the condition, which bore their name until the renaming of eponymous vasculitides in 2012 [1].

For the purposes of homogeneity and classification, there are two sets of classification criteria in use. The ACR proposed classification criteria in 1990: if any two of the following four criteria were satisfied, the case could be classified as IgA vasculitis: (i) palpable purpura; (ii) bowel angina; (iii) age <20 years at onset; and (iv) the presence of granulocytes in the vessel wall on biopsy [3]. These criteria were modified in a combined effort by the European League Against Rheumatism and the Paediatric Rheumatology Society for classifying childhood-onset vasculitis. The presence of any one of the following four features in the presence of palpable purpura satisfies a classification of IgA vasculitis: (i) diffuse abdominal pain (ii) any biopsy demonstrating predominant IgA deposition; (iii) any acute arthritis or arthralgia; and (iv) renal involvement in the form of haematuria or proteinuria. [4].

Epidemiology

Incidence and prevalence

The annual incidence of IgA vasculitis is 10–20/100 000 in children [5–7,8], and about 1–1.5/100 000 in adults [9,10]. The incidence of nephritis in conjunction with IgA vasculitis is lower in children at about 3.5/100 000 [11]. A peak incidence

PART 9: VASCULAR

of 70.3/100 000 children between 4 and 6 years of age has been observed [8].

Age

The peak incidence is between the ages of 4 and 6 years [8]. Children developing nephritis are typically slightly older. In one study, children >8 years of age had an odds ratio of 2.7 for developing nephritis [12]. Adult-onset IgA vasculitis can occur at any age.

Sex

There may be a mild male preponderance with reported ratios of 1.8 : 1 [13].

Ethnicity

There is a higher incidence of IgA vasculitis reported from Scotland (20.3-26.7/100 000) [5] than in Taiwan (12.9/100 000) [6] or the Czech Republic (10.2/100 000) [7]. IgA-related nephritis has been more commonly reported in American Indians as compared to Hispanics [14].

Associated diseases

Pathologically, IgA vasculitis in the kidney is indistinguishable from IgA nephropathy. Patients with IgA vasculitis are typically younger and have more extrarenal manifestations [15].

There may be an association of IgA vasculitis with familial Mediterranean fever (FMF). *MEFV* (familial Mediterranean fever) gene mutations have been observed in IgA vasculitis more commonly than the general population [16,17]. The clinical syndrome of IgA vasculitis has been observed more commonly in patients with FMF than in the general population, and some consider it to be a feature of FMF [17–19].

Pathophysiology

Predisposing factors

IgA vasculitis appears to be commoner in the spring, autumn and winter as compared with the summer months [6,20–22]. Respiratory infections may be a precursor in a small number of cases and may be the second hit in patients with a genetic predisposition [21,23]. Streptococcal infections are the most commonly observed predisposing infections [24,25].

Pathology

IgA is thought to be key in the pathogenesis of HSP. Increased levels of IgA in the serum (in 50% with active disease), circulating immune complexes containing IgA, and the deposition of IgA in blood vessel walls and in the renal mesangium are associated with IgA vasculitis (Figure 102.12). In IgA vasculitis, IgA1 rather than IgA2 is the main IgA subclass deposited in skin lesions [26,27]. Diminished glycosylation of the proline-rich hinge region of the IgA1 heavy chain is thought to be an important factor in allowing the IgA to be deposited in the mesangium and in activating the alternative pathway of complement in IgA, as it makes such IgA1 molecules more prone to forming macromolecular complexes [28]. Other IgA antibodies that occur in HSP include IgA ANCA, although this finding is very variable

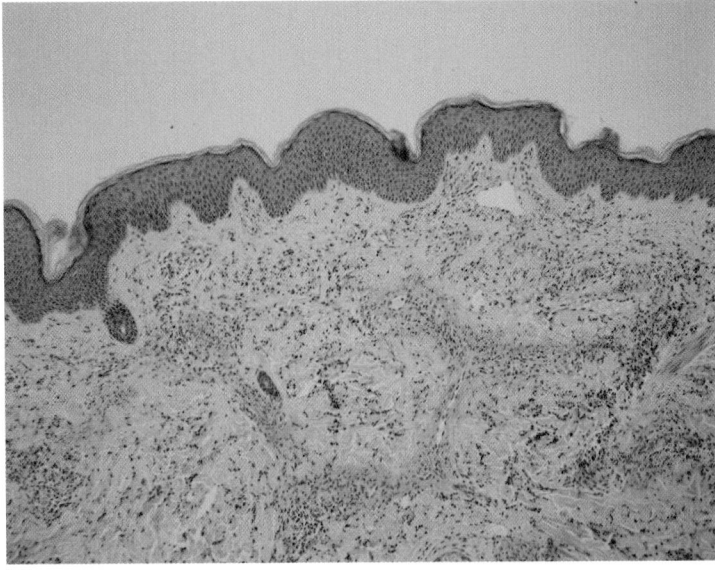
(a)

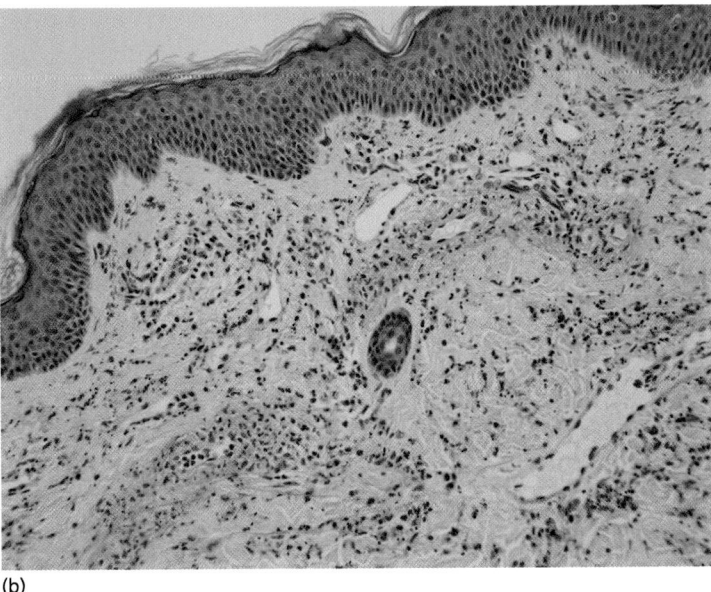
(b)

Figure 102.12 IgA vasculitis at (a) lower and (b) higher magnifications. There is perivascular leukocytoclasis and fibrin deposition, and eosinophils are present. (Courtesy of Dr Laszlo Igali, Norfolk and Norwich University Hospital, Norwich, UK.)

between studies. IgA rheumatoid factor and IgA anticardiolipin antibodies are also sometimes present, as are IgA antiendothelial cell antibodies (AECAs).

The activation of several cytokines is documented, although these are unlikely to be a primary cause. TNF-α levels are increased, and TNF-α can be detected in skin lesions. IL-6, IL-8, transforming growth factor β (TGF-β) and vascular endothelial growth factor (VEGF) levels are all increased in active HSP. TGF-β is of particular interest as blood levels of T cells that produce this cytokine are increased in HSP, and it is known to enhance IgA1 responses. Neutrophil activation, elevated nitric oxide levels, reactive oxygen species and increased urinary leukotriene are all documented.

Causative organisms

There are no definitely causative organisms for IgA vasculitis. Streptococcal infections predispose to IgA vasculitis, and antistreptolysin O titre positivity confers a 10-fold risk of IgA vasculitis [25] but the exact role of the bacteria is unknown. It is likely to be a complex interplay between genetic predisposition, bacterial infection and perhaps other environmental factors. *Bartonella* and *Haemophilus* have been implicated [29,30]; *Helicobacter* antibodies have been reported in adults with IgA vasculitis [31].

Genetics

There is no definite association of any genes with IgA vasculitis. HLA class I genes may be of relevance [32]. *MEFV* gene mutations have been observed to be commoner in patients with IgA vasculitis than in the general population [16,17].

Clinical features

History

Most commonly, IgA vasculitis manifests at the outset with the classic findings of purpura, arthralgia and abdominal pain. Individual lesions usually fade within 5–7 days but crops of lesions can recur for a few weeks to several months.

Presentation

The cutaneous findings are typically erythematous, urticarial papules, which may evolve within 24 h into palpable purpura with haemorrhage. Urticaria, vesicles, bullae (Figure 102.13a) and necrotic ulcers (Figure 102.13b) may develop. A retiform pattern within lesions is characteristic, but not always present. The presentation may be identical to CSVV (see Figure 102.1). Although it typically involves the extensor aspects of the limbs (especially the elbows and knees) and buttocks in a symmetrical fashion, IgA vasculitis may also affect the trunk and face. Renal involvement with IgA vasculitis is common, occurring in approximately 40–50% of patients; 25% have gross haematuria and the remainder microscopic haematuria. Proteinuria occurs in 60% of these, but is uncommon in the absence of haematuria. Gastrointestinal involvement is common (65%), with frank gastrointestinal bleeding in 30% of patients with IgA vasculitis. Painful arthritis is seen in about 75% of patients, most frequently affecting the knees and ankles. Less common manifestations of IgA vasculitis include orchitis (in 10–20% of boys), intussusception, pancreatitis, neurological abnormalities, uveitis, carditis and pulmonary haemorrhage.

Clinical variants

Rarely, gastrointestinal involvement and arthritis can occur in the absence of skin disease.

Differential diagnosis

This includes IgA nephropathy, idiopathic thrombocytopenic purpura, septic shock, acute abdomen and systemic lupus erythematosus (SLE).

Classification of severity

The BVAS (v3) system has been validated to assess the severity of IgA vasculitis alongside several other forms of systemic

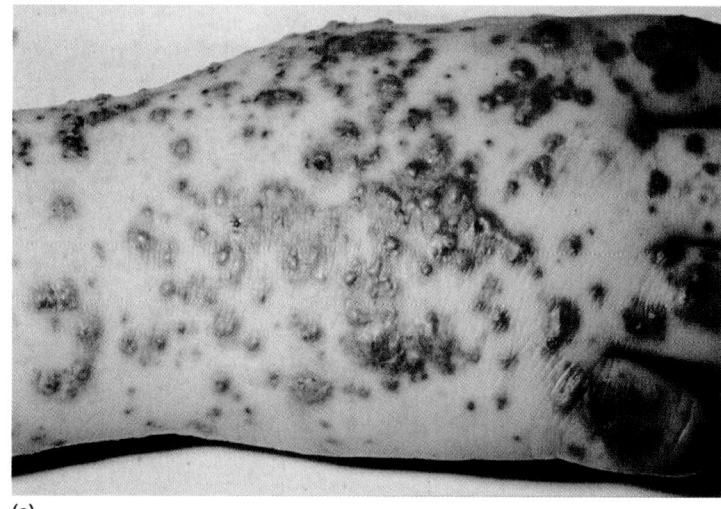

(a)

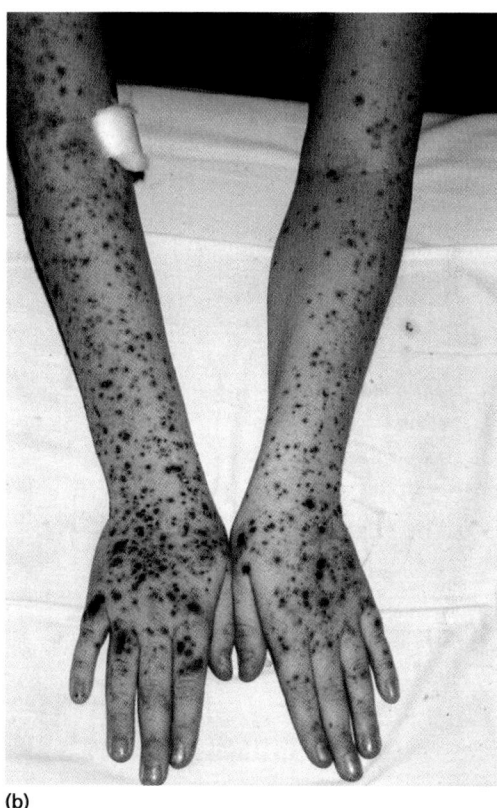

(b)

Figure 102.13 IgA vasculitis. (a) Haemorrhagic vesicles present on the hand. (Courtesy of Andrew Carmichael, South Tees Hospitals NHS Trust, UK.) (b) Vasculitis extending onto the arms.

vasculitides. The tool is able to describe the nature of the clinical involvement, with higher scores suggestive of more severe disease, and is responsive to changes in clinical activity [33].

Complications and co-morbidities

End-stage renal disease is uncommon but, if it occurs, may need renal transplantation. Renal transplant survival is over 80% at 5 years. Uncommonly, IgA vasculitis may recur in the graft and cause graft rejection [34].

Disease course and prognosis

About 25% of patients will relapse, and typically the relapse is mild and easily treated [35]. IgA vasculitis can become chronic in 5–10% of patients, the cutaneous involvement usually lasting between 6 and 16 weeks. Only 1–3% of these patients progress to end-stage renal disease, although one-third to one-half of patients have renal abnormalities on long-term follow-up [13,36].

Investigations

IgA vasculitis is a clinical diagnosis, with confirmation by direct immunofluorescence and routine histology. Perivascular IgA deposits are characteristic of IgA vasculitis and can help to distinguish it from other vasculitides including CSVV, granulomatosis with polyangiitis, eosinophilic granulomatosis with polyangiitis and microscopic polyangiitis. IgA immune complexes are not specific to IgA vasculitis, but can be seen in a variety of patients including those with SLE, endocarditis, dermatitis herpetiformis, alcoholism, IgA nephropathy, inflammatory bowel disease, ankylosing spondylitis, Sjögren syndrome, rheumatoid arthritis, some cancers and in some drug hypersensitivity reactions. No laboratory tests are specific for IgA vasculitis.

Management

The treatment of IgA vasculitis is supportive. The condition is usually self-limiting. There are no controlled studies of any drugs used in IgA vasculitis. Glucocorticoid agents may be of value in children with renal involvement and in most adults. Pulsed intravenous methylprednisolone, ciclosporin A, cyclophosphamide, azathioprine and mycophenolate mofetil have all been tried in open label fashion. There are no convincing data for any of them [37]. Systemic glucocorticoid treatment may be effective in the treatment of abdominal pain, arthritis and nephritis [38]; in this study the dose was prednisolone 1 mg/kg/day for 2 weeks, tapering over a further 2 weeks.

Cryoglobulinaemic vasculitis

Definition and nomenclature

Cryoglobulins are abnormal immunoglobulins that precipitate spontaneously when serum is cooled to a temperature below 37°C. Cryoglobulinaemia is the condition characterized by the presence of circulating cryoglobulins; the accompanying vasculitis that affects the small vessels is due to cryoglobulins deposited as immune complexes. It is mainly the skin glomeruli and peripheral nerves that are affected. Not all cryoglobulinaemia is associated with symptoms. This chapter only deals with the vasculitis manifestations; details of the history, aetiology and pathogenesis of cryoglobulinaemia are provided in Chapter 125.

Synonyms and inclusions
- Type II and type III cryoglobulinaemia
- Mixed essential cryoglobulinaemia
- Cryoglobulinaemia

Introduction and general description

Cryoglobulinaemic vasculitis is a small-vessel vasculitis affecting the skin, joints, peripheral nerves and kidneys. About 80% of cases are secondary to hepatitis C infection [1]. Other causes include B-cell lymphoproliferative disorders, autoimmune diseases like Sjögren syndrome, other viral disorders (hepatitis B, HIV) and essential mixed cryoglobulinaemia.

Cryoglobulins may be divided into three main subtypes:
1. Monoclonal immunoglobulin, usually IgG or IgM, accounts for about 10–25% of cases and is usually associated with lymphoproliferative disease, especially multiple myeloma or Waldenström macroglobulinaemia.
2. Mixed polyclonal (usually IgG) immunoglobulin and monoclonal (usually IgM-κ) immunoglobulin, the latter having rheumatoid factor activity, accounts for about 25% of cases.
3. Polyclonal IgM with rheumatoid factor activity and polyclonal IgG with antigenic activity account for about 50–65% of cases.

Epidemiology

Incidence and prevalence

Cryoglobulinaemic vasculitis is a rare disease and its incidence and prevalence are not known.

Age

The condition is seen usually in adults and is very rare in children.

Associated diseases

Hepatitis C is responsible for about 80% of cryoglobulinaemic vasculitis. The other common associations are Sjögren syndrome and B-cell lymphoproliferative disorders.

Pathophysiology

The mechanism for the production of cryoglobulins by a clonally expanded B-cell population is ill understood. Since most patients with hepatitis C do not develop vasculitis, but have circulating cryoglobulins, there may be a failure of a separate mechanism responsible for the disease manifestations. There are significantly lower circulating T-regulatory cells in patients who develop vasculitis as compared to those with just cryoglobulinaemia [2].

Typically, a polyvalent IgM rheumatoid factor binds to antigen (although other monovalent immunoglobulins can also be responsible) to produce immune complexes that activate complement resulting in endothelial activation and tissue damage.

Predisposing factors

Cold and immobility may precipitate acute episodes.

Pathology

Cryoglobulinaemic vasculitis affects capillaries, arterioles and venules. In the skin, it produces a pandermal leucocytoclastic vasculitis that may extend into the subcutis. Eosinophilic periodic acid–Schiff (PAS) positive globular immune complex deposits and PAS-negative intraluminal fibrin deposits can be visualized. More chronic lesions develop a mononuclear-predominant infiltrate and may become granulomatous. Changes in other organs include

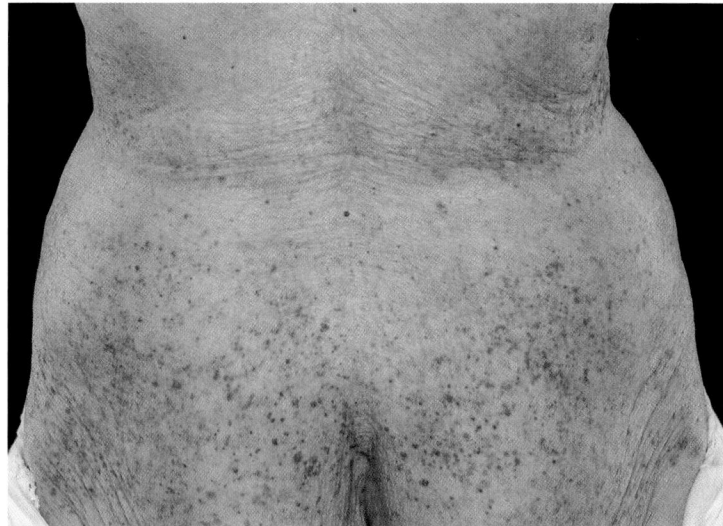

Figure 102.14 Cryoglobulinaemic vasculitis.

membranoproliferative glomerulonephritis, immune complex deposition in the lungs causing bronchiolitis obliterans organizing pneumonia, and vasa nervosa vasculitis causing a peripheral neuropathy.

Causative organisms
The main aetiological factor in mixed cryoglobulinaemia is hepatitis C virus (HCV) infection, which accounts for about 80% of cases. However, although cryoglobulinaemia can be detected in about 50% of subjects with HCV, immune complex vasculitis occurs in less than 5% [3].

Environmental factors
Exposure to cold and immobility can trigger gelling in cryoglobulinaemia, resulting in cutaneous necrosis.

Clinical features

History and presentation
The classic 'Meltzer's triad' of arthralgia, purpura and weakness was described in 1966, but is seen in less than a third of patients [4]. Myalgia, headache, fever and weight loss are common. Palpable purpura, the commonest presenting feature, is nearly universal (Figure 102.14). Sensorimotor neuropathy and mononeuritis multiplex are both commonly documented. Pulmonary involvement is rare. Renal involvement is usually in the form of membranoproliferative glomerulonephritis, and presents with nephrotic range proteinuria [5]. A smaller proportion of patients may present with proliferative mesangial lesions or thrombotic lesions [5]. The Raynaud phenomenon may be seen in patients with associated connective tissue disease.

Differential diagnosis
Cryoglobulinaemic vasculitis should be distinguished from other causes of CSVV because corticosteroid therapy, although sometimes necessary in the short term, may in the longer term worsen the underlying infection that is present in the majority

of cases. Most other causes of leukocytoclastic vasculitis cause a more superficial vasculitis on biopsy specimens, and if cryoglobulin deposits are seen histologically then the diagnosis is usually suspected (although this is much commoner in type I cryoglobulinaemia). Clinically, head and neck involvement, significant livedo, acrocyanosis, Raynaud phenomenon or larger vessel occlusion are all more suggestive of type I cryoglobulinaemia.

Complications and co-morbidities
In patients with hepatitis C-induced disease, the complications are those of liver involvement. Associated glomerulonephritis is common and important and may be more frequent in those with hepatitis C [6]. There is an increased risk of myeloproliferative disorders, particularly a B-cell non-Hodgkin lymphoma [7]. This appears to be fourfold greater in patients without hepatitis C [8]. Sjögren syndrome has been reported in up to 20% of patients [4].

Disease course and prognosis
Cryoglobulinaemic vasculitis per se does not confer a significant mortality risk. In patients with hepatitis C-induced disease, the viral disease will determine the prognosis. In patients without hepatitis C, renal involvement is associated with greater morbidity. There are no large cohort studies to predict outcomes.

Investigations
A pivotal consideration when testing for cryoglobulinaemic vasculitis is transport of the specimen. The greatest care should be taken to ensure that the blood is transported to the laboratory at 37°C to ensure that the tests are not falsely negative. The demonstration of cryocrit in patients with clinical evidence of small-vessel vasculitis is probably the gold standard for the diagnosis (Figure 102.15). A low complement C4 level with a near normal C3 is nearly universal. Rheumatoid factor is positive in high titres. Evidence of viral hepatitis should be looked for. Inflammatory markers will be elevated.

Urine analysis can range from normal to nephrotic range proteinuria. A renal biopsy will often be positive in the presence of significant renal disease, although occasionally the lesions may be due to minimal change disease [5]. A cutaneous biopsy will demonstrate leucocytoclastic vasculitis.

Management
Treatment will depend on the underlying cause. In patients with hepatitis C infection, the treatment should be coordinated with a hepatologist and will need a combination of glucocorticoids, antiviral therapy and immunomodulatory agents [9]. The HCV genotype will dictate the exact choice and duration of the antiviral agent. Interferon a in combination with ribavirin is beneficial, but relapses are common, necessitating long-term treatment [9]. Rituximab may be of benefit in this group of patients [10].

There is little evidence for the management of non-hepatitis C cryoglobulinaemic vasculitis. Consensus from the European League Against Rheumatism recommends a combination of immunomodulatory agents and glucocorticoid treatment based on the model of treating the other small-vessel vasculitides, such as the ANCA-associated vasculitides [9].

PART 9: VASCULAR

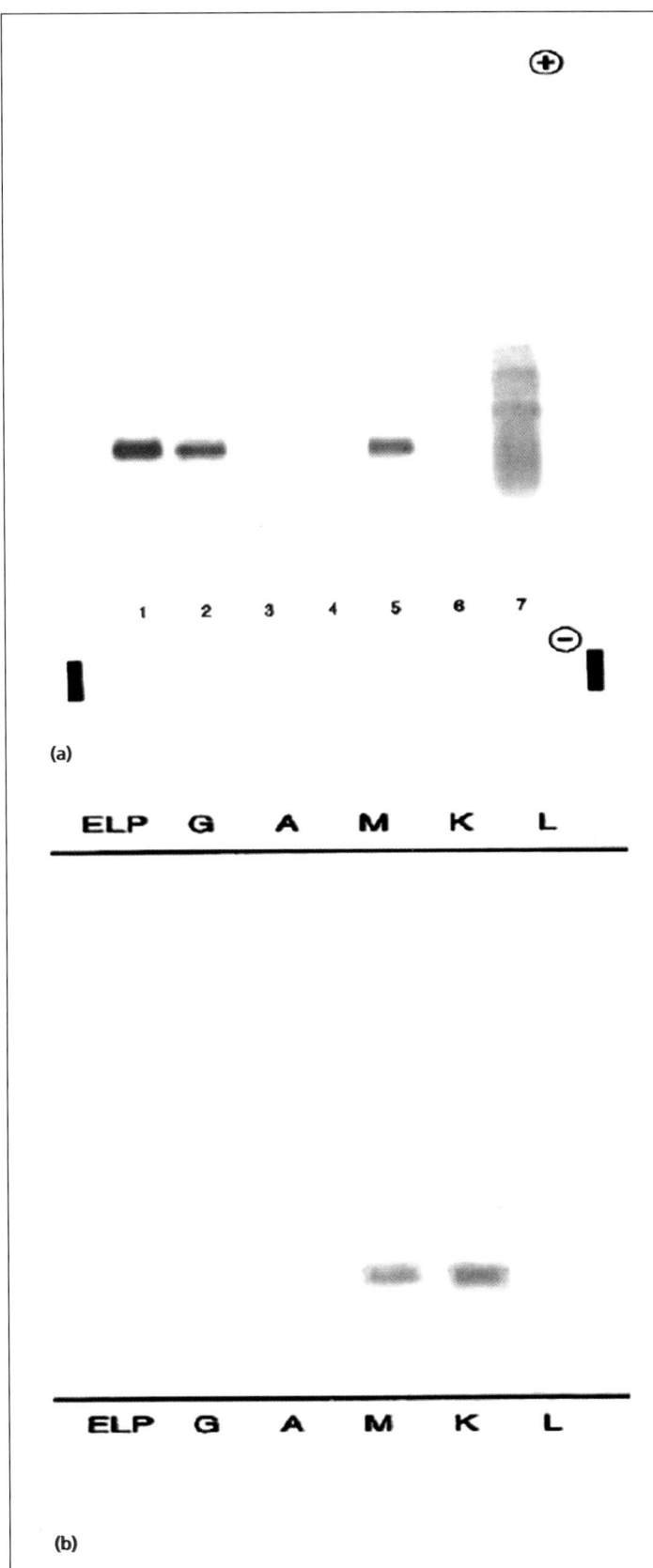

(a)

ELP G A M K L

(b)

Figure 102.15 Serum protein electrophoresis. (a) Demonstrating a clear band in lanes 1, 2 and 5. Lanes 3 and 4 are negative controls and lane 5 is a urine control from a nephrotic specimen. The sample was run on an enhanced urine program and gel for greater demonstration of the migration of low protein concentrations. (b) Demonstrating the same sample as an IgM-κ band. (Courtesy of Ian Thirkettle and Karen Ashurst.)

Hypocomplementaemic urticarial vasculitis

Definition and nomenclature

This section deals with hypocomplementaemic urticarial vasculitis (HUV); other forms of urticarial vasculitis are discussed in Chapter 44. HUV is defined as vasculitis affecting small vessels (i.e. capillaries, venules or arterioles), accompanied by urticaria and hypocomplementaemia and associated with anti-C1q antibodies. Glomerulonephritis, arthritis, obstructive pulmonary disease and ocular inflammation are common [1].

Synonyms and inclusions
- Anti-C1q vasculitis
- MacDuffie hypocomplementaemic urticarial vasculitis
- MacDuffie syndrome

Introduction and general description

The condition is very rare and is characterized by persistant urticarial lesions lasting for longer than 24 h with circulating anti-C1q autoantibodies. Arthritis, glomerulonephritis, pulmonary and ocular disease, leukocytoclastic vasculitis, ocular inflammation and abdominal pain are associated.

Epidemiology

Incidence and prevalence

Hypocomplementaemic urticarial vasculitis is very rare with only a few hundred cases described.

Age

The most common presentation is when a person is in their thirties but childhood cases have been described.

Sex

It is commoner in females [2,3].

Ethnicity

There are no associations.

Associated diseases

It may be associated with SLE [3], and may be linked with increased susceptibility to pyogenic infections.

Pathophysiology

The sera of patients with HUV contains polyclonal IgG with C1q precipitin activity contained within the Fab fragments [4]. These IgG antibodies are directed against the collagen-like region of C1q, resulting in a reduction of C1q in the serum with subsequent activation of the complement pathway [5].

Predisposing factors

These are unknown.

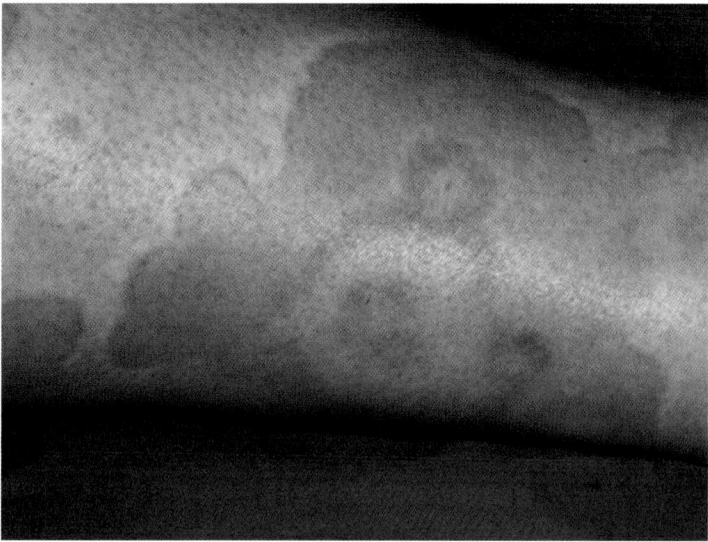

Figure 102.16 Urticarial vasculitis.

Pathology

Lesions of urticarial vasculitis are typically viewed as showing a leukocytoclastic vasculitis. HUV shows a large number of interstitial neutrophils rather than the pleomorphic infiltrate of normocomplementaemic vasculitis [6]. The deposition of immune complexes is present in normal and lesional skin in HUV, as opposed to only lesional skin in normocomplementaemic vasculitis [3,6].

Clinical features

History

Hypocomplementaemic urticarial vasculitis is characterized by weals, which are characteristically painful but can be itchy, and persist for more than 24 h. In HUV, weals resolve with areas of discoloration. Angio-oedema is common and may be a presenting feature.

Presentation

Cutaneous lesions of both the hypocomplementaemic and normocomplementaemic forms of UV are erythematous indurated weals that may contain purpuric foci (Figure 102.16). Angio-oedema and macular erythema may also occur. Livedo reticularis, nodules and bullae may be evident, and may also contain purpuric foci. Patients with the hypocomplementaemic form may have constitutional symptoms.

Differential diagnosis

Hypocomplementaemic urticarial vasculitis has features similar to SLE and may overlap. Signs such as ocular inflammation, angio-oedema and chronic obstructive pulmonary disease may help distinguish the two processes. Pre-bullous pemphigoid, erythema multiforme, Sweet syndrome, other causes of vasculitis and urticaria coexisting with various forms of eczema should be considered, as should mixed cryoglobulinaemia, Muckle–Wells syndrome, Cogan syndrome and Schnitzler syndrome.

Classification of severity

There is no classification.

Complications and co-morbidities

Cough or dyspnoea may indicate pleural and pericardial effusions, emphysema or chronic obstructive pulmonary disease (seen in 20–50%). Proteinuria or haematuria may indicate glomerulonephritis, which may progress to end-stage renal failure, particularly in those with childhood onset. Gastrointestinal symptoms (abdominal discomfort, nausea, vomiting and diarrhoea), arthritis, episcleritis, uveitis, conjunctivitis, aseptic meningitis, nerve palsies and transverse myelitis may occur.

Investigations

If urticarial lesions last for longer than 24 h (which can be determined by drawing around their margin), then they are not ordinary urticaria (except delayed pressure urticaria) and a skin biopsy should be considered. Pain rather than itch, or the presence of purpura, also suggests urticarial vasculitis. History, physical examination and laboratory studies, including C3, C4 and antinuclear antibody, should help to establish the extent of disease and to exclude underlying disease (e.g. hepatitis C) and to evaluate for SLE. Some patients may demonstrate an elevated erythrocyte sedimentation rate (ESR), hypocomplementaemia, a low-titre positive antinuclear antibody and haematuria. A biopsy may help confirm the diagnosis and to exclude other disorders.

Management

The evidence for the treatment of HUV is anecdotal. Systemic corticosteroids are effective. Steroid-sparing agents should be considered, but the evidence for their use is restricted to case reports for cyclophosphamide [7], methotrexate [8], dapsone [9], colchicine [10] and hydroxychloroquine [11]. Some patients require oral antihistamines for the control of angio-oedema and urticaria-like lesions, in addition to therapies directed at the vasculitis.

First line

Although no single treatment is effective for all cases of urticarial vasculitis, the majority of patients respond to systemic corticosteroids.

Second line

Drugs that have been shown to be effective for the treatment of urticarial vasculitis include dapsone (100–200 mg once daily), colchicine (0.6 mg twice to three times daily) and hydroxychloroquine (200 mg once to twice daily).

Third line

For patients with refractory disease, there is limited evidence for the use of cyclophosphamide or mycophenolate mofetil [7,**12**].

Antiglomerular basement membrane vasculitis disease

Definition and nomenclature

Antiglomerular basement membrane (anti-GBM) vasculitis affects glomerular capillaries or pulmonary capillaries, or both, with GBM deposition of anti-GBM autoantibodies. Lung involvement causes pulmonary haemorrhage, and renal involvement causes glomerulonephritis with necrosis and crescents [1].

Synonyms and inclusions
- Anti-GBM syndrome
- Goodpasture syndrome
- Lung purpura with nephritis

Introduction and general description

In 1919, Ernest Goodpasture described two men who he thought had a viral influenza. One of them had the classic changes that came to bear the eponymous diagnosis of Goodpasture syndrome – alveolar haemorrhage and glomerulonephritis with arteriolar vasculitis [2]. The name was formally changed by international consensus to 'anti-GBM disease' in 2012 [1]. The consensus name is flawed because the antibodies bind to pulmonary alveolar capillary basement membranes. Cutaneous involvement is not common, although there are anecdotal reports of non-vasculitic skin changes with immune deposition. [3]. Patients may present to dermatologists with pallor.

Epidemiology

Incidence and prevalence

There are about 0.5 cases/million population per year [4]. The prevalence is unknown.

Age

The disease is known to occur in children [5]; but the peaks seem to occur in the third and seventh decades [6].

Sex

In children the male to female ratio is 1 : 2 [7], whereas this is reversed in those older than 65 years with a M : F ratio of 1.9 : 1 [8].

Ethnicity

The relative ethnic differences are unknown.

Pathophysiology

The condition is due to immune complexes composed of autoantibodies directed against the NC1 domain of the a3 chain of type IV collagen [9]. The distribution of this molecule restricts the condition to the lung and kidney.

Pathology

Perivasculitis and anti-IgM and C3 antibodies at the basement membrane zone in cutaneous lesions have been described in one case [3].

Genetics

Familial instances of the disease have been described including in a pair of identical twins with exposure to hydrocarbon fumes [10].

Environmental factors

It is most common in late spring and early summer.

Clinical features

History and presentation

Haemoptysis, fatigue, dyspnoea and cough may be presenting features. Pallor, oedema, chest signs, heart murmurs and hepatomegaly may be present. Discrete, erythematous, macular lesions on the instep of the foot have been described [3].

Clinical variants

Respiratory features predate renal disease by up to a year in two-thirds of cases, and there may be a gap of up to 12 years.

Differential diagnosis

Granulomatosis with polyangiitis, eosinophilic granulomatosis with polyangiitis, IgA vasculitis and microscopic polyangiitis may all present with renal failure and pulmonary haemorrhage. Identification of anti-GBM antibodies helps diagnosis.

Disease course and prognosis

Untreated outcome is very poor, with near 100% mortality. With treatment, 1-year survival depends on early renal function: there is 100% survival if the serum creatinine is <500 μmol/L, but 65% survival in dialysis-dependent cases [11].

Investigations

Investigations should exclude other systemic vasculitides. ANCA may be positive but antinuclear antibody is usually negative. Specific testing is to anti-GBM antibodies.

Management

First line

Treatment is with corticosteroids, cyclophosphamide and plasma exchange.

Second line

Patients may require renal dialysis if in renal failure or respiratory support if there is severe pulmonary haemorrhage.

SMALL-VESSEL ANCA-ASSOCIATED VASCULITIS

Microscopic polyangiitis

Definition and nomenclature

Microscopic polyangiitis (MPA) is a necrotizing vasculitis, with few or no immune deposits, predominantly affecting small vessels (i.e. capillaries, venules or arterioles). Necrotizing arteritis involving small and medium arteries may be present. Necrotizing glomerulonephritis is very common and pulmonary capillaritis often occurs. Granulomatous inflammation is absent [1]. Historically, MPA was grouped with polyarteritis nodosa, and the two terms were often used interchangeably. It was defined and classified as a separate condition in 1994 at the first Chapel Hill consensus conference [2].

Introduction and general description

Friedrich Wohlwill described two cases with glomerulonephritis and non-granulomatous inflammation of small vessels in 1923 [3]. However, it was not until 1994 that MPA was formally defined by an international consensus [2]. MPA is part of a group of conditions termed ANCA-associated vasculitis (AAV). The other two conditions in this group are granulomatosis with polyangiitis (GPA) and eosinophilic granulomatosis with polyangiitis (EGPA). They are united by their association with antibodies directed against proteinase 3 (PR3) and myeloperoxidase (MPO). PR3 and MPO are proteins that serve as antigens inside the azurophilic granules in the cytoplasm of a neutrophil. Phenotypically, MPA and GPA are very similar in presentation, with the prime difference being the absence of granulomatous inflammation in MPA.

Epidemiology

Incidence and prevalence

The annual incidence of MPA is 2.5–10/million [4,**5**]. However, this rises to 45/million per year in the population over the age of 65 [6]. The point prevalence figures vary from 25 to 100/million population [7–9].

Age

The peak incidence is in populations aged over 65 [6].

Sex

No predilection is known.

Ethnicity

White people are more commonly affected [**10**]. In Japan, the overall incidence of AAV is similar to that in the western European population, but the AAV is exclusively MPA, with almost no GPA [6].

Associated diseases

No associations are known.

Pathophysiology

The exact mechanism of production of vascular inflammation is not known, but ANCA has a prime role in the pathogenesis. Murine models have demonstrated the pathogenicity of MPO ANCA in producing glomerulonephritis and pulmonary haemorrhage [11,12]. ANCA can induce degranulation of neutrophils primed by TNF-α [13]. Primed neutrophils exhibit MPO on their surface. The MPO ANCA can induce a respiratory burst leading to degranulation and the release of toxic oxygen radicals and intracytoplasmic enzymes, which may lead to vascular inflammation [13,14].

Predisposing factors

Farming may predispose to pANCA positivity and MPA [15].

Pathology

Histological specimens from MPA lesions demonstrate segmental vascular necrosis. Neutrophils and monocytes permeate vessel walls, causing leukocytoclasis, the accumulation of fibrin and haemorrhage. Biopsy specimens from lesions of palpable purpura demonstrate leukocytoclastic vasculitis. Focal segmental glomerulonephritis with extracapillary crescents are a characteristic finding in renal biopsies. The presence of glomerulosclerosis is suggestive of the duration of disease and dictates the renal impairment.

Genetics

No culprit genes have been definitely identified, but the geographical distribution of the disease is suggestive of a genetic influence.

Environmental factors

Farming may be associated with MPA [15].

Clinical features

History

Many patients with MPA initially experience constitutional symptoms, including fever, weight loss, myalgia and arthralgia. These may be present for several weeks before the onset of the pulmonary and renal disease that often occurs in patients with MPA.

Presentation

About 40% of patients have palpable purpura on dependent skin sites upon presentation [16]. Mouth ulcers, necrotic lesions on the fingers or toes, splinter haemorrhages and livedo reticularis can all be present. The presence of nodules and livedo reticularis is commoner in polyarteritis nodosa; 80% of patients will have renal involvement. The presentation may be explosive with rapidly progressive glomerulonephritis or pulmonary haemorrhage (Figure 102.17). Peripheral neuropathy is common and is usually

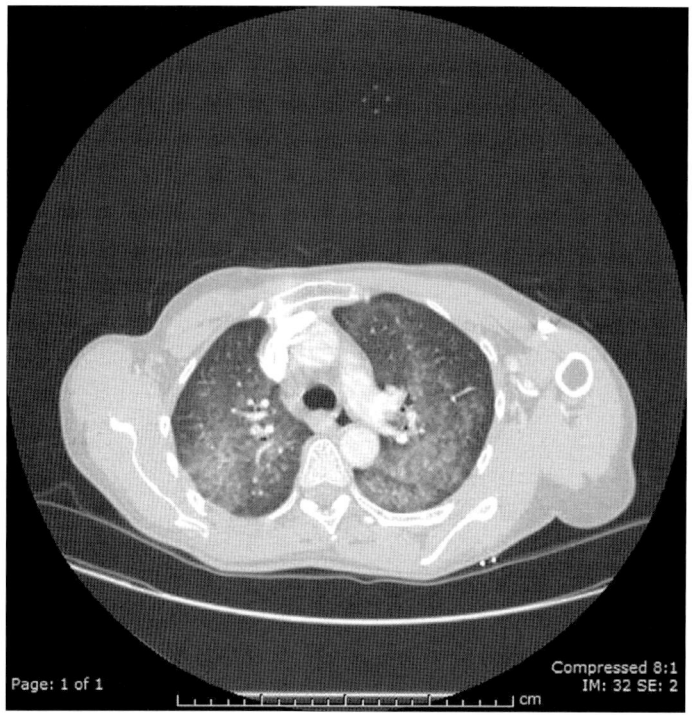

Figure 102.17 Computed tomography of the thorax demonstrating pulmonary haemorrhage affecting both lung fields in microscopic polyangiitis.

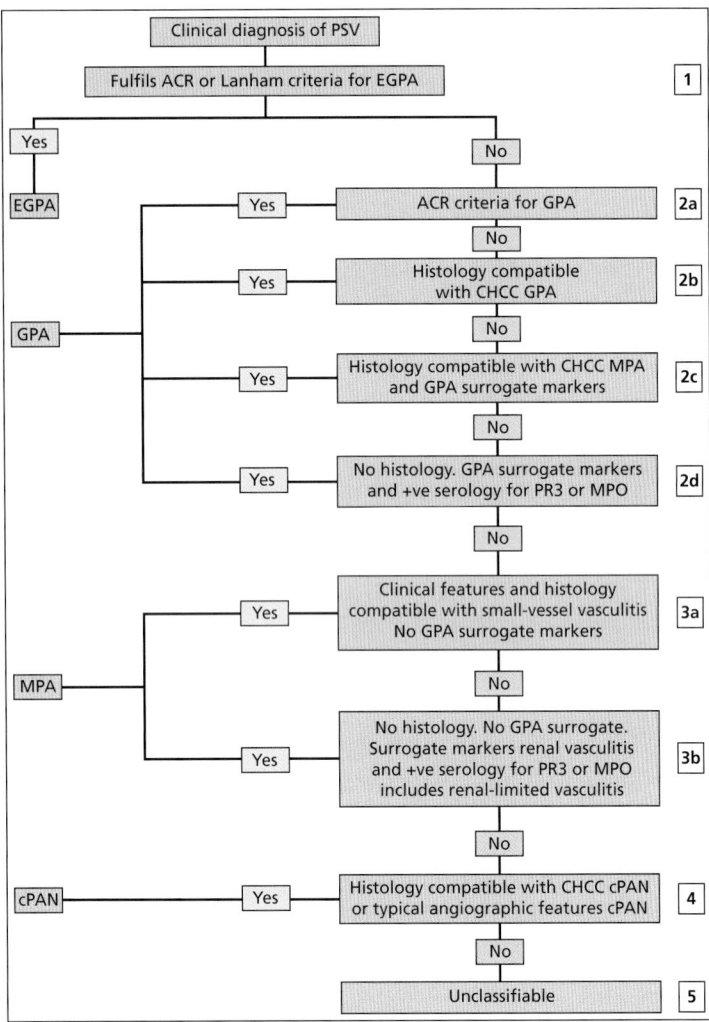

Figure 102.18 Classification of antineutrophil cytoplasmic antibody vasculitides and polyarteritis nodosa (PAN). ACR, American College of Rheumatology; CHCC, Chapel Hill Consensus Conference; cPAN, cutaneous PAN; EGPA, eosinophilic granulomatosis with polyangiitis; GPA, granulomatosis with polyangiitis; MPA, microscopic polyangiitis; MPO, myeloperoxidase; PR3, proteinase 3; PSV, primary systemic vasculitides. (From Watts *et al.* 2007 [17]. Reproduced with permission of BMJ Publishing Group Ltd.)

sensorimotor. Mononeuritis multiplex and even cranial nerve involvement are not unusual.

Differential diagnosis

Microscopic polyangiitis should be distinguished from other ANCA-associated vasculitides and polyarteritis nodosa. The classification of these patients should be set out as suggested by Watts *et al.* (Figure 102.18) [17]. The diagnosis of MPA can be made only in the absence of cardinal features of EGPA and GPA. Significant peripheral eosinophilia, extravascular eosinophils, nasal or paranasal sinus involvement, endobronchial involvement, granulomas on a biopsy, fixed pulmonary infiltrates, cavitating nodules on a chest X-ray, asthma and mastoidal or retro-orbital disease all lead away from a diagnosis of MPA.

Similarly the absence of blood, protein or red cell casts in the urine leads away from the diagnosis of MPA.

Classification of severity

The European Vasculitis Society has classified disease severity in AAV as below [18]:
- *Localized.* Upper and/or lower respiratory tract disease without any other systemic involvement or constitutional symptoms.
- *Early systemic.* Any, without organ-threatening or life-threatening disease.
- *Generalized.* Renal or other organ-threatening disease; serum creatinine <500 µmol/L.
- *Severe.* Renal or other vital organ failure; serum creatinine >500 µmol/L.
- *Refractory.* Progressive disease unresponsive to glucocorticoids and cyclophosphamide.

In practice, there are almost no patients without renal involvement in MPA, and therefore localized and early systemic disease is almost non-existent in this condition.

Complications and co-morbidities

Severe MPA can be associated with renal failure or life-threatening pulmonary haemorrhage. Pulmonary haemorrhage occurs in about 10% of patients and carries a high risk of death [19,20]. In the long term, there is a raised risk of coronary artery disease and hypertension. At 5 years, there is a 16% incidence of cardiovascular events (myocardial infarctions, cerebrovascular accidents or coronary revascularization procedures) [21]. MPO ANCA positivity confers a higher risk of cardiovascular events compared with PR3 ANCA positivity.

Disease course and prognosis

Relapse is common and increases with time. In separate studies it has been documented to be 8% at 18 months [22] and 34% at 70 months [16]. Survival at 12 months is 82–92%, falling to 45–76% at 5 years.

Investigations

Anaemia of chronic disease and laboratory markers of an acute phase response predominate. Urine analysis provides big clues. Most patients will have a blood and protein leak to varying extents. ANCA directed against PR3 or MPO are present in nearly all patients. Imaging helps to establish the extent and severity of disease in patients with lung involvement. Chest X-ray followed by computed tomography (CT) scanning identifies alveolar haemorrhage or pulmonary fibrosis. Histopathology is the gold standard for diagnosis and when possible the kidneys should be biopsied on suspicion of MPA. Other tissues that may provide an answer are the sural nerve, muscle and skin.

Management

Recommendations for the management of MPA have been proposed by the European League Against Rheumatism [18] and the British Society for Rheumatology [23]. Immunosuppressive therapies, including oral or intravenous glucocorticoids, are the mainstay of treatment.

Remission induction

Pulsed intravenous cyclophosphamide (15 mg/kg every 2–3 weeks) or daily oral cyclophosphamide (2 mg/kg/day) form the mainstay of treatment for most patients with MPA. Intravenous cyclophosphamide has the advantage of lower cumulative dose and lower risk of adverse events, but carries a greater risk of relapse [24,25]. Oral prednisolone in a dose of 1 mg/kg/day, to a maximum of 60 mg/day, is commonly used as an adjunct to cyclophosphamide, with the aim of reducing the dose to 15 mg/day at 3 months [18]. At the physician's discretion, intravenous methylprednisolone can be added to speed up the induction of remission at the commencement of cyclophosphamide. Standard practice would be to add 1 g intravenously per day for 3 days. In patients with severe renal disease, plasmapheresis may have a role in saving the kidney [26].

Relapsing and refractory disease
For relapsing disease, rituximab 375 mg/m^2 per week for 4 weeks is superior to pulsed intravenous cyclphosphamide [27,28]. For disease refractory to cyclophosphamide and glucocorticoid, rituximab 375 mg/m^2 per week for 4 weeks has been shown to be of value [29].

Remission maintenance
- *Post-cyclophosphamide.* Due to the cumulative toxicity of cyclophosphamide, azathioprine (2 mg/kg/day) is preferred to maintain remission [22]. The switch over can happen either at the end of six pulses of intravenous cyclophosphamide or after 6 months of oral cyclophosphamide.
- *Post-rituximab.* In patients where rituximab is used to induce remission, current thinking suggests that rituximab should be used at 4–6-monthly intervals over the long term as a remission maintenance agent [30,31].

Granulomatosis with polyangiitis

Definition and nomenclature
Granulomatosis with polyangiitis is a necrotizing granulomatous inflammation usually involving the upper and lower respiratory tract, and necrotizing vasculitis affecting predominantly small to medium vessels (e.g. capillaries, venules, arterioles, arteries and veins). Necrotizing glomerulonephritis is common [1].

Synonyms and inclusions
- Wegener's granulomatosis
- Wegener granulomatosis

Introduction and general description
Friedrich Wegener published three cases in 1937 of patients in their thirties who had a 4–7-month history of spiking temperatures with negative septic screens, raised ESR, predominant upper respiratory tract inflammation with nasal septal involvement and active urinary sediment, resulting in death [2]. Sven Johnsson first used the term Wegener granulomatosis as a distinct diagnosis [3]. The name was changed to 'granulomatosis with polyangiitis' by international consensus in 2013 [1].

The ANCA-associated vasculitides are a group of conditions characterized by their association with the presence of antibodies directed against PR3 and MPO. PR3 and MPO are intracytoplasmic enzymes of neutrophils. GPA is the archetypal ANCA-associated vasculitis, incorporating most of the clinical features of the other two AAVs – MPA and EGPA.

Epidemiology

Incidence and prevalence
The incidence of GPA is 3–10/million per year [4–6,7]. There may be a distinct latitudinal divide, with GPA being commoner in the northern latitudes than in the southern latitudes [6]. The point prevalence of GPA is 24–112/million [8–10].

Age
In children, the median age of onset is 14 years [11,12]. In adulthood, the median age of onset is 50–59 years [10,13,14].

Sex
The condition affects males and females equally.

Ethnicity
The majority of cases occur in white people. GPA is rare in Japan [15], and may be rare in Inuits [16].

Pathophysiology
The exact mechanism of production of vascular inflammation and granulomas is not known, but ANCA has a prime role in the pathogenesis. Murine models have demonstrated the pathogenicity of MPO ANCA in producing glomerulonephritis and pulmonary haemorrhage [17,18]. There is some evidence of *in vitro* pathogenicity of PR3 ANCA [19]. ANCA can induce the degranulation of neutrophils primed by TNF-α [20]. Primed neutrophils exhibit PR3 on their surface. The PR3 ANCA can induce a respiratory burst leading to degranulation and release of toxic oxygen radicals and intracytoplasmic enzymes, which may lead to vascular inflammation [20,21].

There may be a role for a bacterial infection (e.g. *Staphylococcus aureus*), which stimulates autoreactive PR3 producing B cells within granulomas [22,23]. In the autoinflammatory process, granuloma formation occurs prior to vasculitis. The granulomas in GPA have a high proportion of granulocytes, which serve as a source of PR3 [24], which in turn help to continue driving a Th1 cytokine response to further the inflammatory process.

Predisposing factors
Farming and occupational solvent exposure may predispose to GPA [25].

Pathology
Skin histology in GPA may show perivascular lymphocytic infiltrates; however, such non-specific infiltrates may not be related to disease pathogenesis. More specific findings such as leukocytoclastic vasculitis and/or granulomatous inflammation may be

present in up to 50% of skin biopsy specimens (Figure 102.19). Granulomatous inflammation around vessels and palisading necrotizing granulomas are uncommonly demonstrated in skin lesions.

Causative organisms

Clinical observation points to *Staphylococcus aureus* as a potential trigger in some patients. The incidence of chronic nasal carriage of *S. aureus* is significantly higher in patients with GPA compared with healthy individuals and constitutes a risk factor for disease relapse [26,27].

Genetics

There is evidence that GPA has an association with HLA DP, although this may be an association with PR3 ANCA rather than the syndrome of GPA [28,**29**].

Clinical features

History

Features of the classic triad of GPA, including the skin, respiratory tract and kidneys, are not always present early in the course of the disease, making the diagnosis sometimes difficult. In up to 80% of

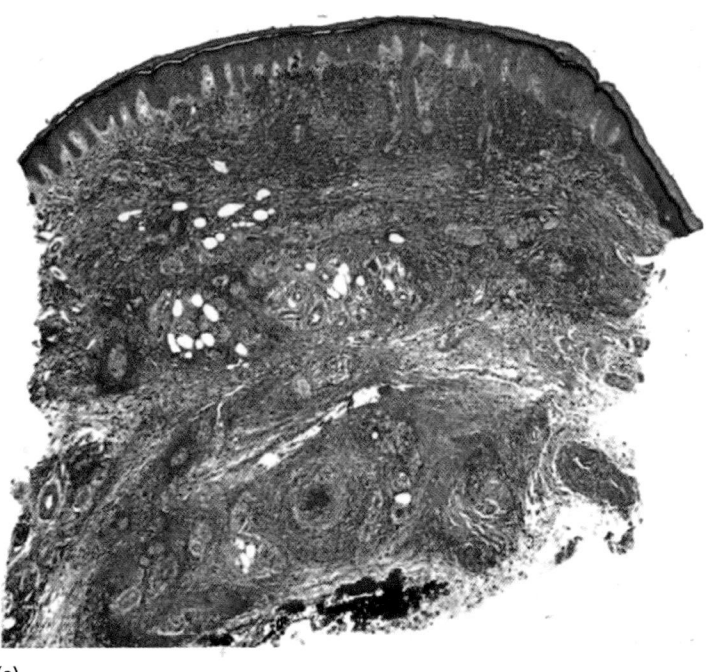

(a)

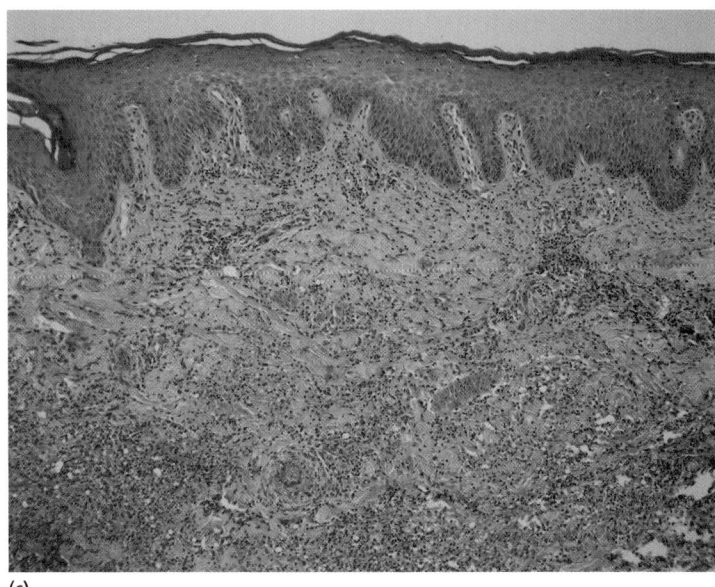

(c)

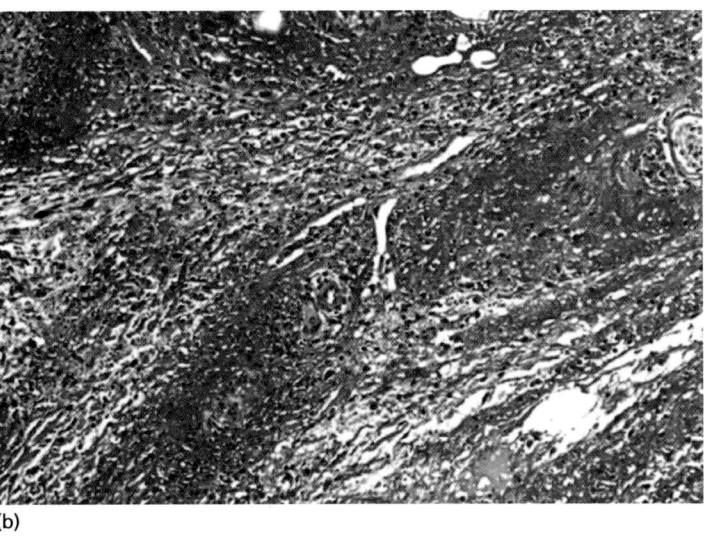

(b)

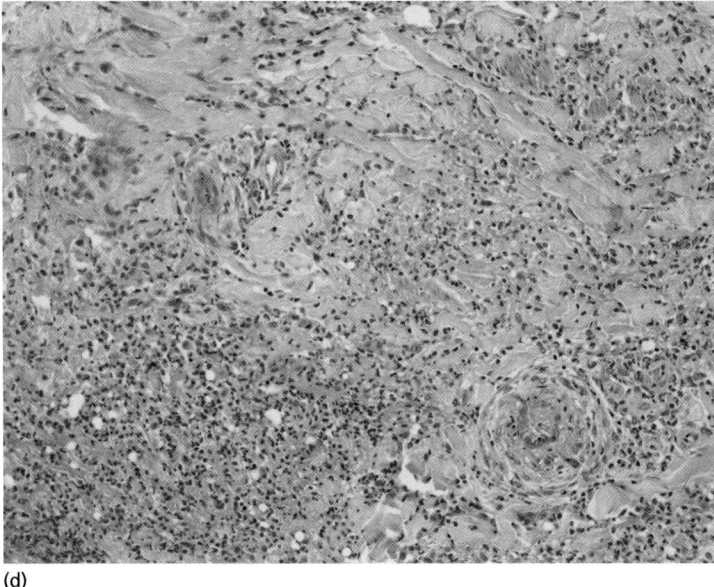

(d)

Figure 102.19 Granulomatosis with polyangiitis. (a) There is extensive leukocytoclastic vasculitis involving the entire dermis. (b) Note the extensive area of collagen degeneration, destruction of vessels and mixed inflammatory infiltrate. (c, d) There is a necrotizing vasculitis with fibrin deposition, red blood cell extravasation and a granulomatous reaction, at lower (c) and higher (d) magnifications. (Parts a and b, courtesy of Dr Omar Sangueza, Wake Forest University School of Medicine, Winston-Salem, NC, USA; c and d, courtesy of Dr Laszlo Igali, Norfolk and Norwich University Hospital, Norwich, UK.)

patients, symptoms involving the upper or lower respiratory tract are present, and at presentation approximately 73% of patients will have nasal, sinus, tracheal or ear involvement.

Less than half present with pulmonary infiltrates or nodules. Renal disease is initially present in only 18%, although approximately 77% will eventually develop glomerulonephritis. Although 40% will eventually manifest skin findings, cutaneous manifestations and oral ulcers are only found in 13% and 6% of patients at initial presentation, respectively.

Presentation

The most common cutaneous manifestation of GPA is palpable purpura on dependent skin sites (Figure 102.20a); digital infarcts (Figure 102.20b), tender subcutaneous nodules, papules, vesicles and petechiae, as well as non-specific ulcers or pyoderma gangrenosum-like lesions may occur. Cases previously diagnosed as having 'malignant pyoderma' may actually have had lesions secondary to GPA. Nodular, or papulonecrotic, lesions occur on the extremities and sometimes on the face and scalp. These may be differentiated from rheumatoid nodules in that they ulcerate, whereas rheumatoid nodules do not.

Oral ulcers are the second most common mucocutaneous sign of GPA. The upper respiratory tract is commonly affected, with otitis, epistaxis, rhinorrhoea and sinusitis as frequent presenting features. A saddle nose deformity may result from necrotizing granulomas of the nasal mucosa. Lower respiratory signs and symptoms include cough, dyspnoea, chest pain and haemoptysis. Nodules, which may be cavitating, may be visible on

imaging (Figure 102.21). Ulcerative lesions in GPA are shown in Figure 102.22.

Differential diagnosis

Granulomatosis with polyangiitis must be differentiated from the other types of AAV. Destructive upper respiratory involvement and severe glomerulonephritis are unusual in EGPA, which typically has asthma and eosinophilia, along with paranasal polypoidal involvement. MPA has predominant renal involvement and is more likely to be associated with MPO ANCA (see Figure 102.18).

Classification of severity

The European Vasculitis Society has classified disease severity in AAV as below [30]:

- *Localized*. Upper and/or lower respiratory tract disease without any other systemic involvement or constitutional symptoms.
- *Early systemic*. Any, without organ-threatening or life-threatening disease.
- *Generalized*. Renal or other organ-threatening disease; serum creatinine <500 µmol/L.
- *Severe*. Renal or other vital organ failure; serum creatinine >500 µmol/L.
- *Refractory*. Progressive disease unresponsive to glucocorticoids and cyclophosphamide.

Complications and co-morbidities

Granulomatosis with polyangiitis or its treatment (especially cyclophosphamide) has a twofold increase in the risk of cancer includ-

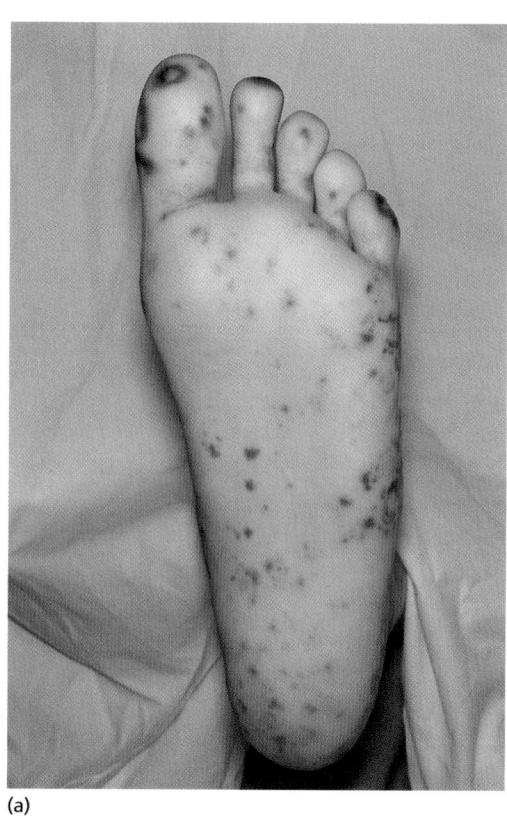

(a)

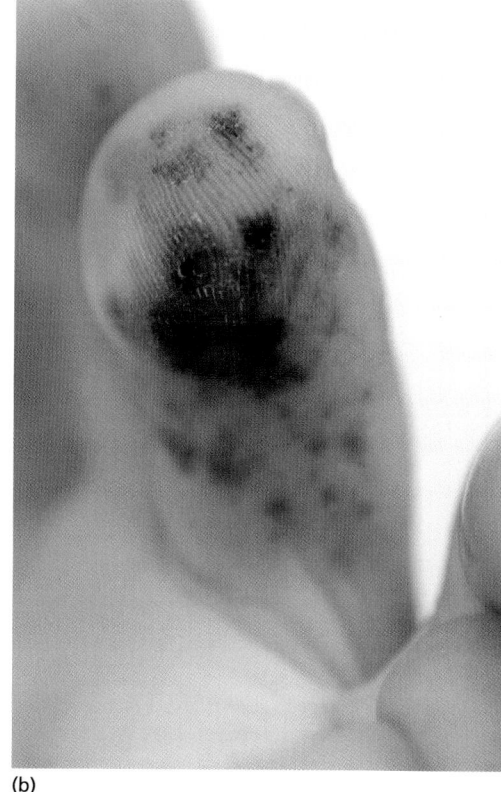

(b)

Figure 102.20 Granulomatosis with polyangiitis. (a) Cutaneous infarction. (b) Digital infarction.

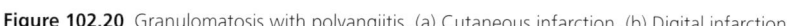

PART 9: VASCULAR

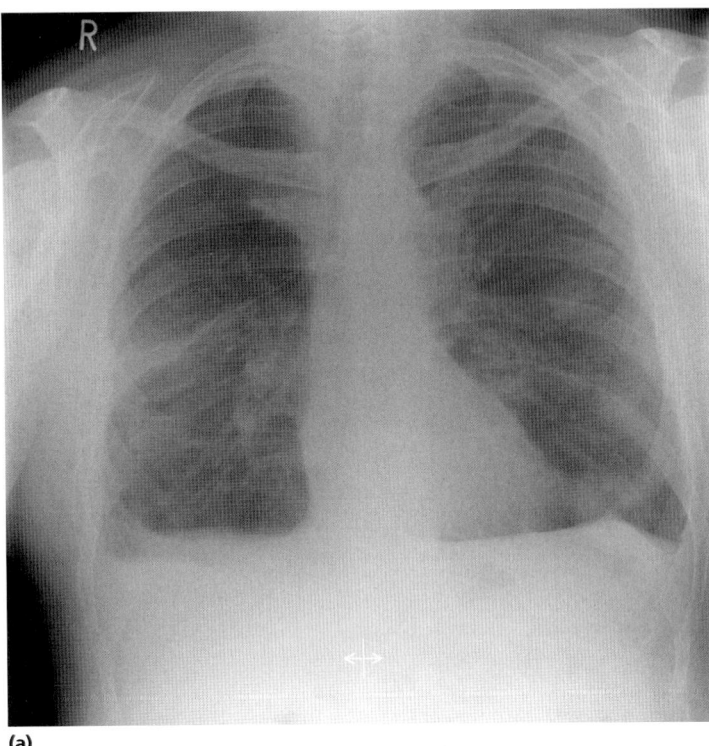

(a)

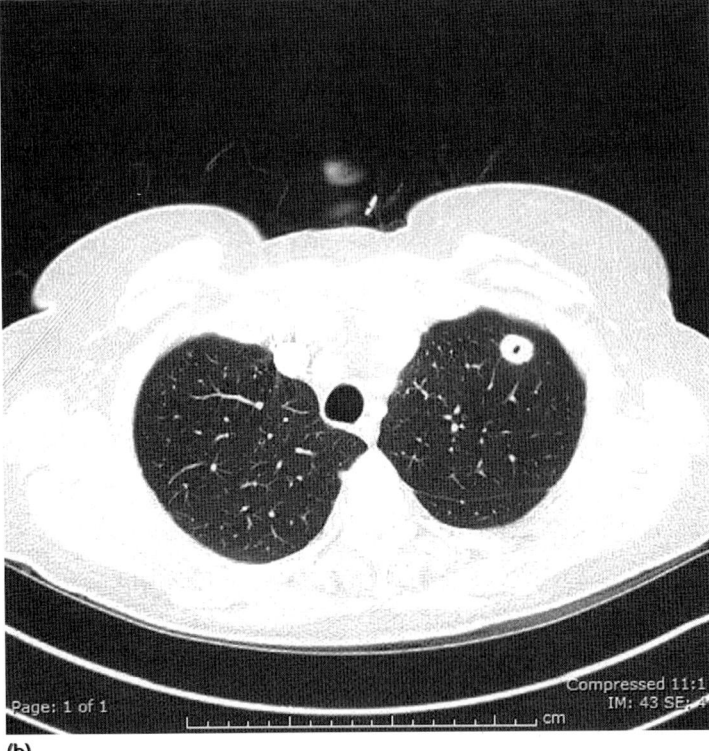

(b)

Figure 102.21 Granulomatosis with polyangiitis. (a) X-ray showing bilateral nodules. (b) Computed tomography of the thorax demonstrating a thick-walled cavity in the right lung field.

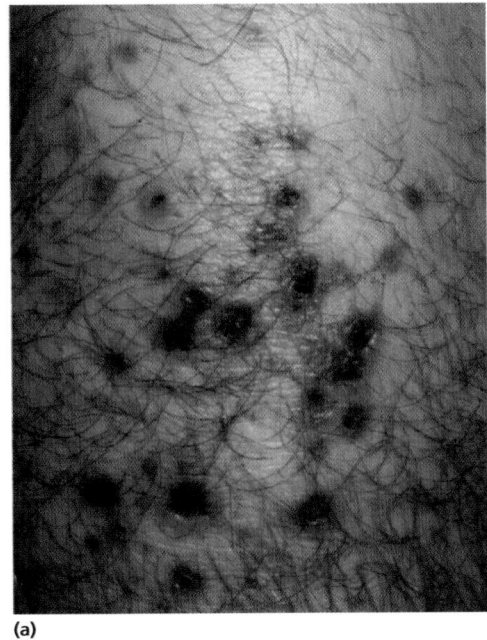

(a)

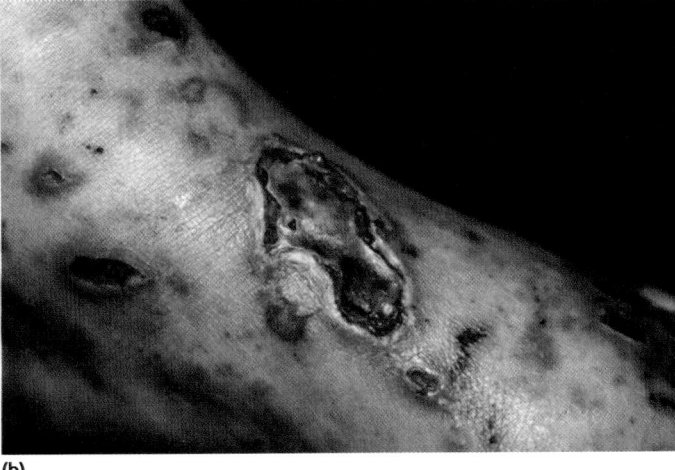

(b)

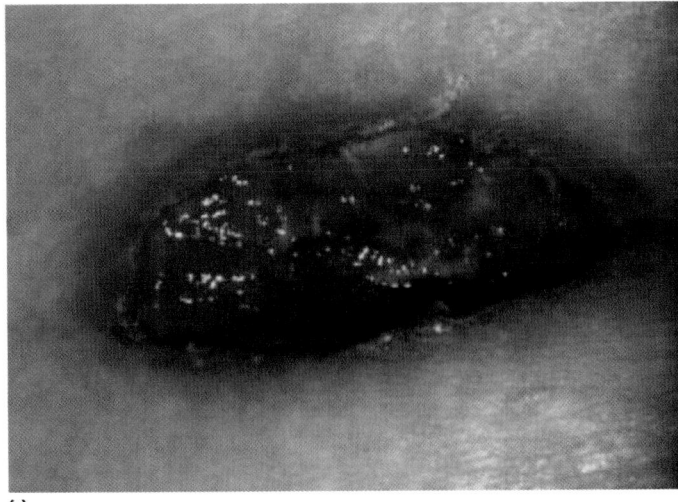

(c)

Figure 102.22 Granulomatosis with polyangiitis. (a) Ulcerated lesions of cutaneous small-vessel vasculitis. (b) Larger ulcerated lesions with background vasculitis. (c) Deep skin ulcer in a person with nasal symptoms.

ing acute myeloid leukaemia, bladder cancer and non-melanoma skin cancers [31,32]. GPA also predisposes to increased cardiovascular morbidity [33].

Disease course and prognosis

Remission can be achieved in up to 90% of patients [34]. At 2 years, the relapse rate is between 18% and 40% [34]. Untreated GPA has a 1-year mortality of 83%; the survival of treated disease at 1 year is >80% [35]. End-stage renal disease occurs in 7% at 12 months, rising to 14% at 5 years and 23% at 10 years [36]. Cancer risk is as discussed above.

Investigations

Investigations are as in MPA.

Management

Recommendations for the management of GPA have been proposed by the European League Against Rheumatism [30] and the British Society for Rheumatology [37]. Immunosuppressive therapy including oral or intravenous glucocorticoid is the mainstay of treatment.

First line

Patients with localized disease can be treated with methotrexate (15–25 mg/week) in conjunction with oral prednisolone 1 mg/kg/day tapering to about 15 mg/day at 3 months [30,38]. The use of methotrexate in preference to cyclophosphamide is associated with a higher risk of relapse [39].

In patients with non-localized disease, cyclophosphamide forms the mainstay of treatment. Cyclophosphamide can be used in a daily oral 2 mg/kg/day dose for 6 months or as pulsed intravenous 15 mg/kg/pulse every 2–3 weeks for six pulses. Intravenous cyclophosphamide has the advantage of a lower cumulative dose and a lower risk of adverse events, but carries a greater risk of relapse [40,41]. Oral prednisolone in a dose of 1 mg/kg/day, to a maximum of 60 mg/day, is commonly used as an adjunct to cyclophosphamide, with the aim of reducing the dose to 15 mg/day at 3 months [30]. At the physician's discretion, intravenous methylprednisolone can be added to speed up the induction of remission at the commencement of cyclophosphamide. Standard practice would be to add 1 g intravenously per day for 3 days.

In patients with severe renal disease, plasmapheresis may have a role in saving the kidney [42].

Second line

Patients with contraindications to cyclophosphamide can be treated with rituximab 375 mg/m^2 per week for 4 weeks instead [43,44].

Third line

Patients with refractory disease to cyclophosphamide and glucocorticoids can be treated with rituximab 375 mg/m^2 per week for 4 weeks [45]. 15-Deoxyspergualin and intravenous immunoglobulin have a role in refractory and persistent disease [46,47].

Remission maintenance

Due to the cumulative toxicity of cyclophosphamide, azathioprine (2 mg/kg/day) is preferred to maintain remission [48]. The switch-over can happen either at the end of six pulses of intravenous cyclophosphamide or after 6 months or oral cyclophosphamide. Methotrexate [49], leflunomide [50] and mycophenolate mofetil [51] are alternative remission maintenance agents. In patients where rituximab is used to induce remission, current thinking suggests that this should used at 4–6-monthly intervals long term as a remission maintenance agent [52,53].

Eosinophilic granulomatosis with polyangiitis

Definition and nomenclature

Eosinophilic granulomatosis with polyangiitis (EGPA) is a very rare systemic disorder characterized by an eosinophil-rich and necrotizing granulomatous inflammation, often involving the respiratory tract, and necrotizing vasculitis predominantly affecting small to medium vessels. There is an association with asthma and eosinophilia. ANCA is more frequent when glomerulonephritis is present [1].

Synonyms and inclusions
- Churg–Strauss syndrome
- Allergic granulomatous angiitis
- Churg–Strauss vasculitis
- Allergic angiitis and granulomatosis
- Allergic granulomatosis
- Allergic granulomatous and angiitis
- Eosinophilic granulomatous vasculitis
- Allergic angiitis
- Granulomatous allergic angiitis

Introduction and general description

This is a rare systemic vasculitis characterized by asthma, peripheral blood and tissue eosinophilia (especially in the respiratory tract) and necrotizing vasculitis with extravascular granulomas. The majority of patients have cutaneous findings in the active phase of the disease. It was originally described by Rackemann and Greene in 1939 as an allergic disease and not classified as periarteritis nodosa; Churg and Strauss later described the syndrome and its histopathological characteristics in 1951 [2]. The condition was renamed EGPA in 2012 by the Chapel Hill Consensus Conference on the Nomenclature of Systemic Vasculitis [1]. EGPA is associated with antibodies directed against MPO and PR3, and, along with GPA and MPA, forms the group of conditions termed 'ANCA-associated vasculitis'.

Epidemiology

Incidence and prevalence

The incidence is 1–2.5 per million [3,4,5] with a prevalence of 10–15 per million [6,7]. The incidence of EGPA in known asthma sufferers may be up to 67/million per year [8].

Age

It is most common in those aged 15–70 years with a peak incidence around the age of 50. It is very rare in children.

Sex
There may be a slight male predilection.

Ethnicity
No connection is recognized.

Associated diseases
It is associated with atopy, particularly asthma and allergic rhinitis.

Pathophysiology
The pathogenesis of EGPA is not precisely known. Allergy probably plays a central role, but the disease is almost certainly multifactorial. As the allergy association might suggest, the inflammatory response is primarily Th2 in nature, although Th1 and Th17 responses are seen [9,10,11]. The Th2 response has been thought to be responsible for eosinophilic activation, and prolonged eosinophil survival. The products of eosinophilic and neutrophilic degradation have been observed in inflamed tissues and are probably responsible for tissue injury [12,13]. The association with ANCA probably suggests a B-cell involvement as well. The role of ANCA in producing vasculitis has been discussed in the GPA and EGPA sections.

Predisposing factors
None are known.

Pathology
EGPA has three key histopathological features: eosinophilic infiltration of tissue, formation of extravascular granulomas in visceral and cutaneous tissues, and vasculitis involving both arteries and veins. The histology of a cutaneous lesion in EGPA may demonstrate any one, if not all, of these features [14]. The granulomas contain necrotic polymorphonuclear leukocytes, eosinophils, severe fibrinoid and fibrillar collagen degeneration, and a proliferation of granulomatous tissue.

Causative organisms
None are known.

Genetics
HLA-DRB4 may be a risk factor for the development of EGPA [15].

Environmental factors
Environmental allergens are associated with more severe asthma.

Clinical features

History
Three phases of EGPA are recognized:
1 The first phase, which may continue for years, consists of asthma with allergic rhinitis and nasal polyps. The asthma typically begins in adulthood in contrast to allergic asthma.
2 The second phase is that of rising peripheral and tissue eosinophilia.
3 The third phase is the predominately vasculitic phase of EGPA, which may affect almost all organ systems, including the cutaneous, cardiac, pulmonary, nervous, gastrointestinal, renal, genito-urinary

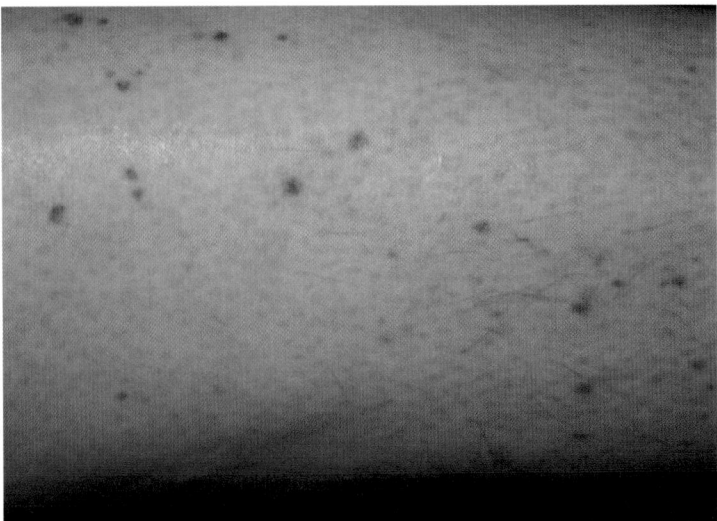

Figure 102.23 Relatively subtle vasculitis on the legs in eosinophilic granulomatosis with polyangiitis. The patient also had eosinophilia and rapidly developed a mononeuritis multiplex.

and musculoskeletal systems. Cardiac involvement is the primary cause of death in patients who do not respond to conventional corticosteroid therapy.

Presentation
In all phases of the disease there may be cutaneous manifestations, with approximately 5% demonstrating cutaneous vasculitis [14]. Palpable purpura and infiltrated nodules (typically located on the scalp or limbs) are the most common skin manifestations, but livedo reticularis, necrotizing livedo (i.e. retiform purpura), migratory erythema, new-onset Raynaud phenomenon, aseptic pustules or vesicles, or infiltrated papules may also be present.

In the vasculitis phase of EGPA, 50–70% of patients have vasculitic skin lesions, most commonly on the lower limbs (Figure 102.23).

Differential diagnosis
The ACR 1990 criteria for the classification of EGPA from other vasculitides needed four of the following six features: (i) asthma; (ii) eosinophilia greater than 10% on a differential white blood cell count; (iii) mononeuropathy (including multiplex) or polyneuropathy; (iv) non-fixed pulmonary infiltrates on chest X-ray; (v) a paranasal sinus abnormality (Figure 102.24); and (vi) a biopsy demonstrating extravascular eosinophils [16].

The Lanham criteria require asthma, peripheral eosinophilia and systemic vasculitis in two or more extrapulmonary organs [17].

The latest in a long line of algorithms to assist classification of the AAV and PAN recommends using either the Lanham criteria or the ACR criteria for classifying EGPA [18] (see Figure 102.18).

Disease course and prognosis
Remission is common in EGPA and achieved in >90% of patients [19]. Relapse rates rise from 10% at 12 months to 20% at 4 years [19]. Survival is better than in the other AAVs. In a pooled analysis, survival at 1 and 5 years was 94% and 60–97%, respectively [20]).

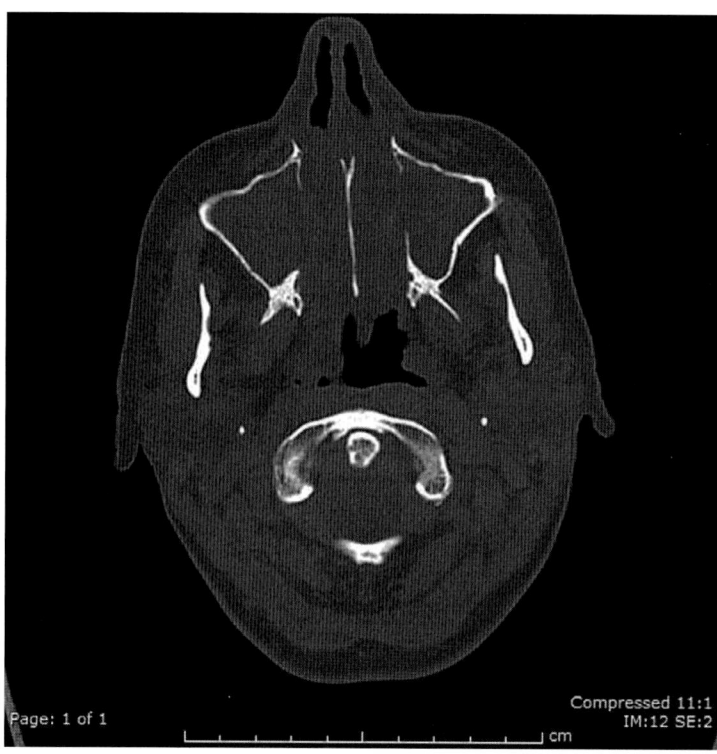

Figure 102.24 Computed tomography scan of paranasal sinuses demonstrating opacification of the maxillary sinuses and bone erosion in eosinophilic granulomatosis with polyangiitis.

Investigations

Peripheral blood eosinophilia is a requisite for the diagnosis of EGPA. Inflammatory markers will be raised and IgE is often elevated. ANCA directed against MPO or PR3 is positive in 30% of patients [21,22]. A urine microscopy demonstrates active urinary sediment in patients with glomerulonephritis. Renal involvement is more likely in ANCA-positive patients [21]. Chest radiographs demonstrate infiltrates. CT scans of the paranasal sinuses are often abnormal and demonstrate mucosal thickening, but rarely bone involvement. The latter is more a feature of GPA. The gold standard remains a biopsy of the affected organ.

Management

There are no randomized controlled trials of any treatment for EGPA. Our knowledge of its treatment comes from open labelled trials and from international consensus-based recommendations [23].

Remission induction

- *Localized disease*. Prednisolone 1 mg/kg/day may be enough to induce remission for most patients with EGPA [24]. However, even in patients without adverse prognostic features, there will be about 10% of patients where this strategy will not result in remission. A further 35% will suffer a relapse. There is currently no way of identifying those who will not do well with steroids alone. International recommendations therefore recommend that in patients without organ- or life-threatening involvement the addition of methotrexate 20–25 mg/week should be considered [23].
- *Systemic disease*. Intravenous pulsed cyclophosphamide 15 mg/kg/pulse at 2–3-weekly intervals (six pulses) with oral

prednisolone 1 mg/kg/day (maximum 60 mg) is the currently preferred regimen for these patients [23].

- *Refractory disease*. Rituximab has been reported to have a beneficial outcome in several case series [9] and the authors have used it beneficially in refractory EGPA.

Remission maintenance

- *Post-cyclophosphamide*. By convention and international consensus, patients are switched to azathioprine 2 mg/kg/day [23].
- *Post-methotrexate*. Remission is maintained by continuing methotrexate long term.
- *Post-rituximab*. There is very little information on post-rituximab maintenance therapy. Current advice would be to use rituximab according to clinical need rather than every 6 months. These patients should be cared for by specialist centres.

MEDIUM-VESSEL VASCULITIS

Polyarteritis nodosa and cutaneous polyarteritis nodosa

Definition and nomenclature

Polyarteritis nodosa (PAN) is a rare necrotizing arteritis of medium or small arteries without glomerulonephritis and without vasculitis in the arterioles, capillaries or venules. It is not associated with ANCAs [1]. Cutaneous PAN (cPAN) is a single-organ vasculitis affecting the skin. It is better termed cutaneous arteritis. It can be considered a limited expression of PAN and does not exhibit systemic involvement [1,2].

Synonyms and inclusions
- Benign cutaneous periarteritis nodosa
- Periarteritis nodosa
- Kussmaul–Maier disease
- Necrotizing arteritis
- Essential polyarteritis

Introduction and general description

A condition described as periarteritis nodosa was described by Adolf Kussmaul and Rudolf Maier in 1866. The first use of the phrase 'polyarteritis nodosa' denoting the pathological extent of the disease involving the arterial wall may have been in 1945 [3]. PAN was used as a term to cover a large variety of vasculitides. In 1994, the label was uniquely applied to a condition that spared small-calibre vessels [4].

This chapter considers cutaneous arteritis as a variant of PAN that is limited to the skin [5]. It may progress to become classic PAN [1], but conversion is exceedingly rare [2]. Although a distinct entity as described by Lindberg in 1931, the diagnosis of cutaneous arteritis should not be made until systemic disease is excluded.

Epidemiology

Incidence and prevalence

The annual incidence of classic PAN is 1–2.5/million [6,7]. The point prevalence has been reported to be 30 per million [8,9]. Cutaneous arteritis is much rarer and there are no formal reports on the incidence and prevalence of this variant.

Age

The peak age is between 40 and 60 years of age. However, it can be observed in all ages, including in children.

Sex

There is no specific predilection.

Ethnicity

No racial predilection has been described.

Associated diseases

Hepatitis B was described as an association in 1970 [10]. PAN can be the first manifestation of hepatitis B and occurs in most cases within 6 months of infection. Successful treatment of hepatitis B results in cure of PAN with disappearance of any aneurysms [11].

Pathophysiology

Predisposing factors

Viral infections have been implicated in provoking classic PAN. Besides hepatitis B virus, as indicated above, Epstein–Barr virus [12], HIV [13], erythrovirus (parvovirus B19) [14] and cytomegalovirus [15] have been reported in new cases of PAN. Other microbial associations reported have been streptococcal infections [16] and coxsackie B4 [17].

Streptococcal infections [18], erythrovirus (parvovirus B19) [19] and *Mycobacterium fortuitum* [20] have been reported in association with cutaneous arteritis. Minocycline has been reported to induce classic PAN-like vasculitis [21] as well as cutaneous arteritis [22].

Pathology

Early in the disease course, there is a predominantly neutrophilic inflammatory infiltrate in the walls of medium-sized arteries and arterioles of septae in the upper portions of the subcutaneous fat. The involved vessels classically demonstrate a target-like appearance resulting from an eosinophilic ring of fibrinoid necrosis. Later in the disease process, the infiltrate becomes less neutrophilic, consisting predominantly of lymphocytes and histiocytes. Complement and IgM deposits in vessel walls of lesions of cutaneous arteritis from some patients may be demonstrated by direct immunofluorescence. Unlike those of systemic PAN, lesions of cutaneous arteritis do not typically involve arterial bifurcations.

Genetics

Recessively inherited missense mutations in *CECR1* (cat eye syndrome chromosome region, candidate 1), encoding adenosine deaminase 2 (ADA2) have been observed in nine unrelated cases from eight families [23]. Similar mutations were found in a separate study of 19 patients of Georgian Jewish descent [24].

Clinical features

History

Although some patients with cutaneous arteritis may report constitutional symptoms, along with mild involvement of the muscles and nerves, cutaneous manifestations are the most striking feature of the disease.

Presentation

Dermal or subcutaneous nodules are most commonly located on the distal lower extremities near the malleoli (Figure 102.25a) and may extend proximally to the thighs, buttock, arms or hands. Patients may report tenderness associated with the nodules, which may ulcerate (Figure 102.25b, c) or more commonly demonstrate necrotizing livedo reticularis, also referred to as retiform purpura (see Figure 102.3). Gangrene of the digits can ultimately occur, most commonly in children with cutaneous arteritis, but this finding should trigger an aggressive search to exclude systemic features of PAN.

Differential diagnosis

Recurrent spiking fevers, polyarthralgia and a macular upper extremity eruption are symptoms shared by both PAN and adult-onset Still disease (AOSD), and can sometimes create a diagnostic challenge. The presence of livedo reticularis (Figure 102.25d) and the finding of a characteristic skin biopsy appearance with PAN help to differentiate it from AOSD.

Those with necrotizing lesions of livedo reticularis must be evaluated for vasculitis or vasculopathy (e.g. antiphospholipid antibody syndrome, cholesterol emboli or other factors that can produce non-vasculitic vessel occlusion; see Chapter 101).

ANCA-associated vasculitis should also be considered as a differential diagnosis (see Figure 102.18) [25].

If nodules are present, they should be biopsied by incisional biopsy methods to assess for a pan-arteritis of muscular arteries which would confirm a diagnosis of PAN.

Cutaneous arteritis is best considered a variant of PAN, so evaluation by history, physical examination, screening laboratory tests and ongoing follow-up for systemic features is required. A multidisciplinary team approach helps accurate diagnosis, and limits the chances of missing or undertreating potentially life-threatening systemic features of PAN.

Classification of severity

Cutaneous arteritis is considered to have a more benign prognosis than PAN with systemic features.

Disease course and prognosis

Gastrointestinal tract, renal, heart and central nervous system involvement are associated with higher mortality [26].

Investigations

Laboratory investigations are usually non-specific, revealing an acute phase response. Screening for potential infective triggers should be undertaken. Diagnosis of PAN requires histological evidence of medium-sized artery vasculitis if possible. Biopsies should be from symptomatic organs. Skin, muscle and nerve

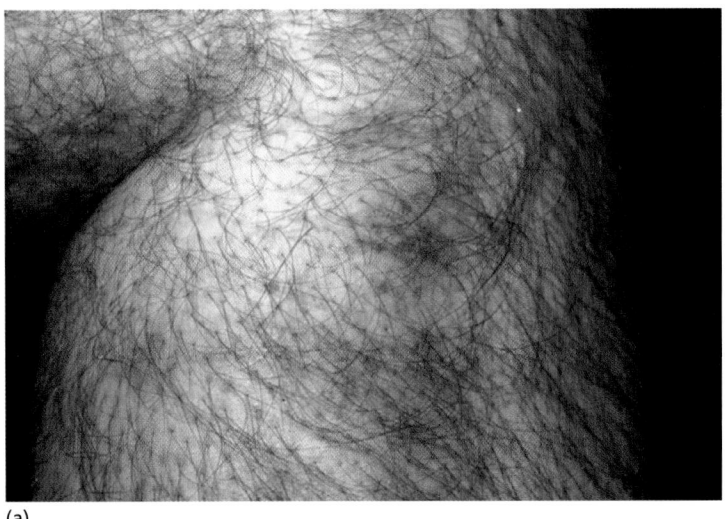

(a)

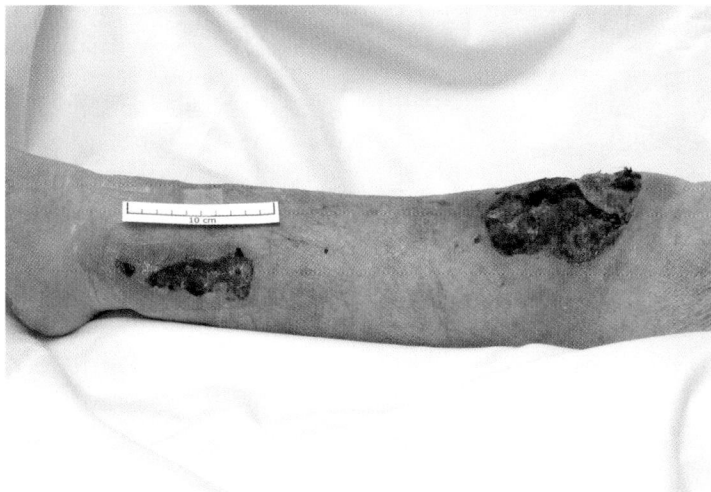

(c)

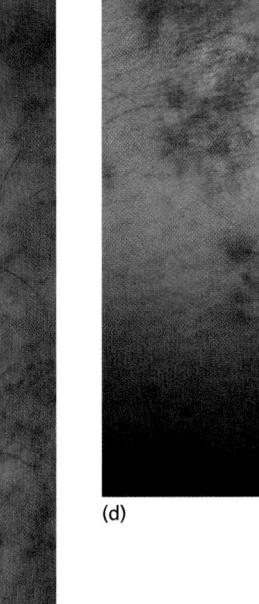

(b)

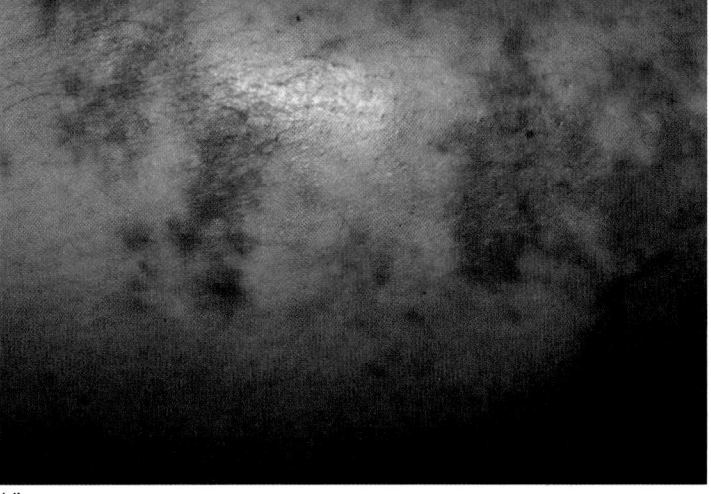

(d)

Figure 102.25 Cutaneous polyarteritis nodosa. (a) Erythematous lesions on the leg. (b) Nodules and ulceration on the leg. (c) Ulcerating lesions on the leg. (d) Livedo of the leg.

histology offer higher diagnostic yield and may be safer. If biopsies are unsupportive, visceral angiography may identify multiple microaneurysms suggesting PAN.

Management

There should be screening for infection (see the section on predisposing factors) and consideration should be given to a trial of discontinuing medication that predates disease. If associated with hepatitis B infection, antiviral therapies form the focus of treatment in combination with immunosuppressive treatment.

First line

Non-steroidal anti-inflammatory drugs and salicylates can be an effective treatment for symptoms of cPAN. High-dose corticosteroids followed by tapering of the dosage over 3–6 months

may occasionally be necessary for some patients. Also without evidence from controlled trials, but based on a strong association with streptococcal infection, penicillin is often used for treatment and prophylaxis in children with cPAN. Screening for recent streptococcal infection with anti-DNAse B or other tests may guide this decision.

Other treatments documented in anecdotal reports include the use of dipyridamole, sulfapyridine, pentoxifylline and dapsone in patients with cPAN. Low-dose weekly methotrexate (7.5–20 mg/week) has been successful in some patients with skin lesions unresponsive to corticosteroids given topically, intralesionally and orally [27]. Chronic leg ulcers resistant to treatment with high-dose corticosteroids have been successfully treated with granulocyte–macrophage colony-stimulating factor (GM-CSF) [28].

Second line

There is an international consensus that PAN requires treatment with a combination of cyclophosphamide and corticosteroids [29]. This combination achieves sustained remission but probably does not alter survival. For patients with hepatitis B-associated PAN, the recommendation is to start with high-dose corticosteroids for 2 weeks, followed by antiviral treatment and plasma exchange [29]. This treatment should be supervised at a specialist centre in conjunction with a hepatologist.

Third line

There are case reports for the use of rituximab in refractory disease [30,31].

Kawasaki disease

Definition and nomenclature

The 2012 Chapel Hill Consensus defined Kawasaki disease as an arteritis associated with the mucocutaneous lymph node syndrome and predominantly affecting medium and small arteries. Coronary arteries are often involved; the aorta and large arteries may be involved. It is usually occurs in infants and young children [1].

Synonyms and inclusions
- Mucocutaneous lymph node syndrome arteritis
- Mucocutaneous lymph node syndrome
- Kawasaki syndrome
- Infantile polyarteritis

Introduction and general description

Kawasaki disease occurs typically in infants and children less than 5 years of age. It was first recognized in 1967 and thought to be a benign, febrile illness associated with mucocutaneous inflammation and lymphadenopathy, until the demonstration of coronary arteritis in 1975 [2]. It is thought to be the commonest cause of acquired heart disease in children. Prompt diagnosis with treatment with aspirin and intravenous immunoglobulins reduces heart complications [3,4].

Epidemiology

Incidence and prevalence

The annual incidence per 100 000 children aged under 5 years is 8.4 in the UK [5]. In a series of epidemiological surveys, Nakamura *et al.* have established that the incidence is rising in Japan every year and had peaked at 240/100 000 in 2010 [6].

Age

The disease almost always occurs in children.

Sex

There is a mild male predilection.

Ethnicity

The disease is much more common in Asia, particularly in Japan.

Associated diseases

Associated diseases include coronary vessel aneurysms and myocardial infarction.

Pathophysiology

Kawasaki disease is thought to be due to an intense inflammatory response to an unidentified infectious agent in genetically susceptible hosts.

Pathology

The angiitis of Kawasaki disease affects nearly all organs, with a very high frequency of cardiac involvement. It is predominantly a vasculitis of medium-sized arteries but can involve any smaller and larger calibre blood vessels. Initially, there is medial oedema associated with neutrophilic infiltration. The inflammatory processes result in the breakdown of internal and external elastic laminae, resulting in aneurysms and thrombosis. The inflammatory processes heal with scarring and resultant stenosis of the affected blood vessel.

Causative organisms

The disease is thought to be triggered by as yet unidentified infectious agents.

Genetics

A functional polymorphism of the *ITPKC* (inositol-1,4,5-trisphosphate 3-kinase C) gene on chromosome 19q13.2 is significantly associated with a susceptibility to Kawasaki disease and coronary artery aneurysms [7]. Single nucleotide polymorhphisms of interest have been found on the *CD40LG* gene [8] and *CASP3* gene [9]. Genome-wide association studies have identified further loci of interest around the FAM167A-BLK region at 8p22-23, the HLA region at 6p21.3 and the CD40 region at 20q13 and the IgG receptor gene *FCGR2A* [10,11].

Clinical features

History

Patients present with at least 5 days of fever, irritability, vomiting, anorexia, cough, diarrhoea, runny nose, weakness and abdominal and joint pain.

The disease typically has an initial acute, febrile stage lasting up to 2 weeks, a second phase lasting 4–6 weeks when the risk of death from coronary aneurysms is greatest, followed by a convalescent phase lasting up to 3 months and characterized by a reduction in the ESR and C-reactive protein (CRP) levels to normal. Larger aneurysms may expand leading to myocardial infarction in the convalescent phase. Those with established heart disease may enter a chronic phase with a risk of late aneurysm rupture even in adult life.

Presentation

The fever is typically spiking and unresponsive to paracetamol. There is acral and perianal erythema and acral oedema, bilateral conjunctivitis with anterior uveitis, fissured lips and a strawberry tongue, and cervical lymphadenopathy, typically a single large cervical node.

Clinical variants

Incomplete Kawasaki disease should be considered in children who do not have all the features of the full disease. Typical echocardiographic features should lead to consideration of treatment as Kawasaki disease in the absence of external clinical features. [12].

Differential diagnosis

Scarlet fever, systemic-onset juvenile idiopathic arthritis and erythema multiforme can mimic Kawasaki disease, as can other localized and systemic infections. The diagnosis should be suspected in a child with prolonged fever.

Classification of severity

The Harada score has been used in some countries as an indication for intravenous immunoglobulin therapy [13]. Four of following seven criteria are needed: (i) white blood count >12 000/mm; (ii) platelet count $<35 \times 10^4$/mm; (iii) CRP >3; (iv) haematocrit <35%; (v) albumin <3.5 g/dL; (vi) age <12 months; and (vii) male sex.

Complications and co-morbidities

There may be hepatic, renal and gastrointestinal dysfunction, myocarditis and pericarditis.

Disease course and prognosis

Deaths may occur due to myocarditis, dysrhythmias, pericarditis, rupture of aneurysms and occlusion of coronary arteries; there is also an increased risk of atherosclerosis due to endothelial cell dysfunction. Coronary aneurysms are demonstrated in around 20% of patients (and in 90% of those who die); some will regress (potentially with stenosis) but giant aneurysms (>80 mm) may require bypass surgery. Clinical factors that predict a higher risk of coronary artery arteritic lesions or aneurysms, or that predict a poor response to treatment, include age below 1 year, low serum albumin, low haemoglobin, high CRP, abnormal liver function and, especially, duration of fever before treatment. Peripheral blood eosinophilia (>4%) after treatment is also associated with treatment resistance. Early intravenous immunoglobulin (IVIg) reduces the coronary aneurysm risk from around 25% to less than 5%. Delaying IVIg beyond day 10 of fever increases the risk of death, particularly in boys under 1 year old.

Investigations

There are no diagnostic tests and Kawasaki disease remains a clinical diagnosis.

Management

Patients should be treated in a specialist paediatric unit. Aspirin and IVIg are the mainstay of treatment.

First line

Intravenous immunoglobulin and aspirin should be given early. Aspirin 100 mg/kg/day is given initially until the fever has settled and is then reduced to 3–5 mg/kg/day for 6–8 weeks in those with no cardiac abnormality, but longer in those with coronary aneurysms. All children should receive IVIg, usually given as a single dose of 2 g/kg over 12 h [4].

Second line

For children who remain febrile 36 h after the first dose of IVIg, a further dose of 2 g/kg can be given. Patients who are unresponsive to IVIg [14] can be treated with high-dose prednisolone 2 mg/kg/day, which should be tapered after normalization of the CRP [15].

LARGE-VESSEL VASCULITIS

Giant cell arteritis

Definition and nomenclature

Giant cell arteritis (GCA) is an arteritis, often granulomatous, usually affecting the aorta and/or its major branches, with a predilection for the branches of the carotid and vertebral arteries. The disease often involves the temporal artery. The onset is usually in patients older than 50 years and is often associated with polymyalgia rheumatica [1].

Synonyms and inclusions
- Horton disease
- Temporal arteritis
- Cranial arteritis
- Giant cell aortitis

Introduction and general description

This is a disease of the elderly, often associated with polymyalgia rheumatica, which presents with headaches and tender palpable arteries, usually the temporal artery. It can rarely cause cutaneous infarction, so presenting to dermatologists [2].

Epidemiology

Incidence and prevalence

The highest mean annual incidence of GCA in people over the age of 50 is recorded at 32.8/100 000 in southern Norway [3]. The age-adjusted (>50 years) annual incidence per 100 000 population is 18.8 in Olmsted county, Minnesota, USA [4] and 22.0 in the UK [5].

Age

This affects people over the age of 50. The age-specific incidence per 100 000 population rises from 2.2 in the sixth decade to 51.9 in the ninth decade [4].

Sex

The disease is 2–3 times more common in women than men [4].

Ethnicity

Giant cell arteritis is considered a disease that particularly targets white people of northern European origin, being less common in African Americans, native Americans and Asians.

Associated diseases

Symptoms of polymyalgia rheumatica are commonly seen in GCA and it is hypothesized that the two conditions may have a similar aetiology, or lie on a disease spectrum.

Pathophysiology

The disease is thought to represent an inflammatory response in predisposed individuals towards an environmental factor. Local dendritic cells recruit and activate CD4 cells in the adventitia. Cytokine cascades involving Th1 and Th17 pathways dominate in the early phase, followed by a chronic smouldering arteritis led by chronic Th1 activation. The end result is a stenosing arteritis.

Predisposing factors

These are unknown.

Pathology

Lesions can be found in all layers of the affected branches of the aorta, particularly the carotid branches. These show segmental and focal pan-arteritis with polymorphic cell infiltrates along with T cells, macrophages and multinucleated giant cells, as well as intimal hyperplasia with a fragmented internal elastic lamina (Figure 102.26).

Causative organisms

None known.

Genetics

There is no known genetic association.

Clinical features

History

Fever and weight loss may occur, and GCA is associated with polymyalgia rheumatica in about 50% of patients. Headache may be localized to the area of the affected artery, that is temporal with temporal arteritis and occipital with vertebrobasilar arteritis. The headache may start abruptly. Facial pain may occur on chewing due to claudication of the jaw muscles. Sudden, permanent visual loss related to ocular or orbital artery involvement may occur. Transient monocular loss of vision (amaurosis fugax) may precede permanent loss. Vertebrobasilar artery involvement may cause ataxia, vertigo or deafness.

Presentation

Patients may present with a new headache on the background of feeling generally unwell or with painless loss of vision. Very rarely, GCA may present with skin infarction. The temporal arteries may be tender, thickened and pulseless. A bruit may be heard over affected arteries (e.g. axillary).

Clinical variants

Isolated aortic inflammation without cranial artery involvement is well recognized.

Differential diagnosis

The temporal artery can be involved in other vasculitides, such as ANCA-associated vasculitides [6,7]. Cancer should always

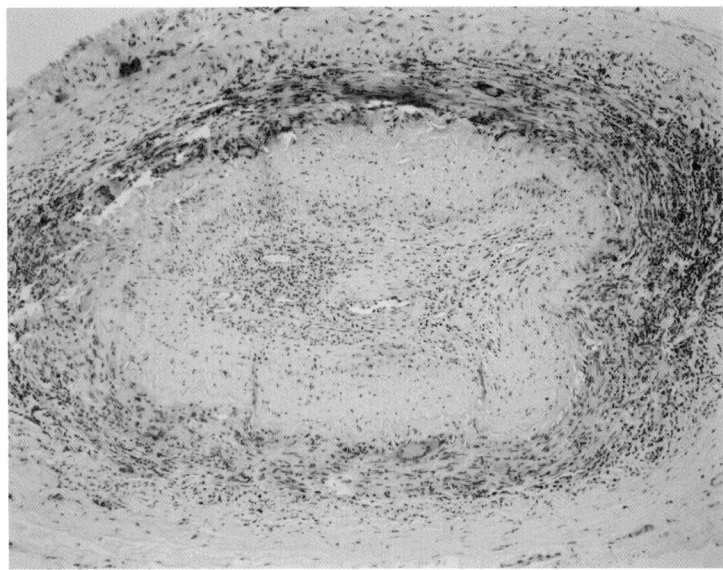

(a)

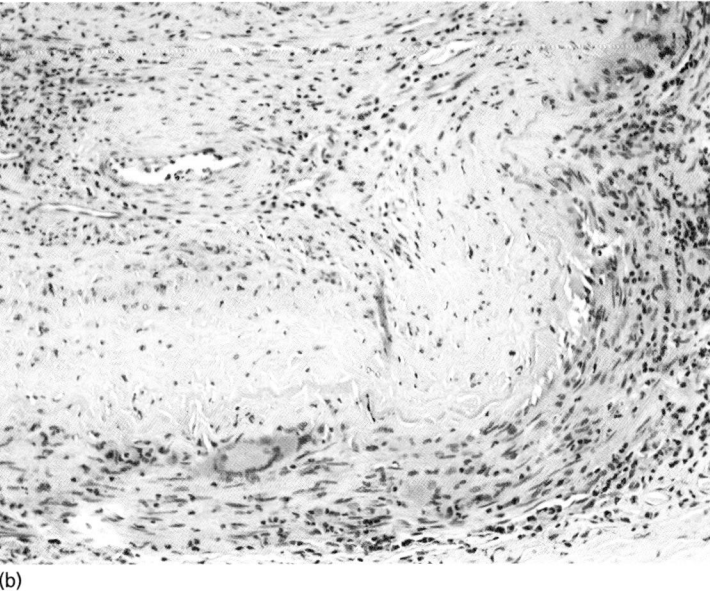

(b)

Figure 102.26 Giant cell arteritis at (a) lower and (b) higher magnifications. There are obliterative vascular changes with a lymphocytic and multinucleated giant cell reaction in the vessel wall. (Courtesy of Dr Laszlo Igali, Norfolk and Norwich University Hospital, Norwich, UK.)

be looked for when the diagnosis of GCA cannot be established beyond doubt [8].

Complications and co-morbidities

Permanent visual loss can be a presenting feature. There is a risk of aortic aneurysms developing as a late complication [9].

Disease course and prognosis

Following a diagnosis of GCA there is a slight excess mortality over 2 years (standard mortality rate 1.52; 95% confidence interval 1.20–1.85)), but not with longer follow-up [10]. The excess mortality was greater in women and in those aged ≤70 years.

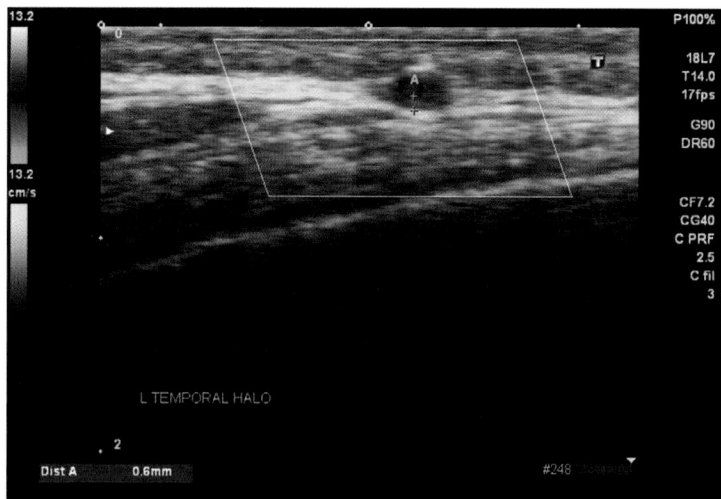

Figure 102.27 Colour Doppler ultrasound of the temporal artery demonstrating vessel wall oedema (the halo sign).

Investigations

Histological diagnosis following biopsy of an affected artery, usually a temporal artery, is the gold standard for diagnosis. The biopsy should ideally comprise a 2 cm length of vessel and, for the greatest chance of obtaining a tissue diagnosis, the biopsy should be performed within 1–2 weeks of commencing corticosteroid therapy. A negative biopsy does not exclude the diagnosis because timing is important and the disease may have skip lesions. The ESR or CRP are almost always elevated. A normochromic, normocytic anaemia, thrombocytosis and raised alkaline phosphatase may all be present. Colour Doppler ultrasound of the temporal and axillary arteries (see Video 102.1 online at www.rookdermatology.com) in steroid-naive patients commonly reveals intramural inflammatory change – the halo sign (Figure 102.27) [11]. Positron emission tomography with 18-fluorodeoxyglucose is of value to demonstrate aortitis [12].

Management

Treatment should be started as soon as the diagnosis is suspected in order to avoid complications; if the diagnosis turns out to be incorrect, the corticosteroids can be withdrawn. Intravenous methylprednisolone 500–1000 mg daily for 3 days, followed by oral prednisolone, is commonly used in those with visual loss, although the visual loss is irreversible. Aspirin is recommended providing there are no contraindications.

First line

Corticosteroids, for example prednisolone 40–60 mg daily, are used for GCA [13]. The dose can usually be reduced slowly in small steps every month, providing that the CRP/ESR levels remain controlled. Treatment is usually for about 2 years [14].

Second line

There is some evidence of the steroid-sparing ability of methotrexate, which can be used in doses of 15–20 mg/week [15].

Takayasu arteritis

Definition and nomenclature

Takayasu arteritis is often granulomatous and predominantly affects the aorta and/or its major branches. The onset is usually in those younger than 50 years [1].

Synonyms and inclusions
- Takayasu disease
- Takayasu syndrome
- Pulseless disease
- Aortic arch syndrome
- Aortitis syndrome
- Occlusive thromboarteriopathy

Introduction and general description

Makito Takayasu, a Japanese ophthalmologist, is credited with the eponym, but the earliest convincing clinical and pathological description in literature of this disease was provided by William Savory's account of a 22-year-old woman's 13-month hospital stay and postmortem examination that demonstrated widespread large arterial inflammation [2].

Epidemiology

Incidence and prevalence

The annual incidence of Takayasu arteritis in Europe and the USA is 0.5–2.5/million [3,4,**5**]. The incidence in Japan is believed to much higher [6].

Age

The disease is seen in younger people, typically below the age of 50, and is found also in children.

Sex

The disease is commoner in females than males.

Ethnicity

It is found in all populations but is commoner in Asians.

Pathophysiology

Pathology

The aorta and its branches are targeted and skip lesions can occur. During the acute phase, a pan-arteritis is present. The inflammatory infiltrate may be predominantly around the vasa vasorum, and fibrosis gradually replaces the inflammatory infiltrates. The vessel lumen may be narrowed secondary to the fibrosing stenotic lesions and/or by intraluminal thrombosis. In older patients there may be superimposed atherosclerosis, and calcification in the wall may occur as a late feature.

Genetics

IL-12B on chromosome 5, MLX on chromosome 17, FCGR2A/FCGR3A on chromosome 1 and HLA-B*52:01 are known associations

[7,8]. Two independent susceptibility loci have been identified in the HLA region (HLA-DQB1/HLA-DRB1 and HLA-B/MICA) [8].

Clinical features

History
Headache, malaise and fever are common presenting symptoms in children. Cutaneous lesions are present in around one-third of patients.

Presentation
Hypertension, pyrexia and pulseless disease are common findings in children. Skin lesions have been reported in up to a third of cases and may comprise erythema nodosum, erythema induratum and pyoderma gangrenosum, as well as ulcerated subacute nodular lesions, papulonecrotic eruptions, papular erythematous lesions of the hands and fingers, facial lupus-like rashes and panniculitis [9]. Cutaneous necrotizing vasculitis has been described resembling nodular vasculitis/erythema induratum. The skin lesions do not appear to relate to the distribution of vascular involvement in any way.

Complications and co-morbidities
Renal artery stenosis, increased arterial stiffness and increased sensitivity of the carotid sinus reflex all contribute to the hypertension. Involvement of the renal arteries can also cause renal dysfunction, and abdominal pain, bleeding or perforation may result from ischaemia or infarction of a viscus. Involvement of the aortic arch and its branches can lead to the 'aortic arch syndrome' with arm claudication, absent radial or brachial pulses (hence 'pulseless disease') or subclavian artery bruits. Aortic regurgitation, coronary artery ischaemia with angina or myocardial infarction, pulmonary hypertension, stroke, syncope and visual disturbances can occur.

Disease course and prognosis
Most patients with Takayasu arteritis will need vascular surgery [10], although restenosis is common [11]. The disease and its treatment both lead to an impairment in quality of life even for patients believed to be in remission [10].

Investigations
Positron emission tomography using 18-fluorodeoxyglucose has replaced conventional angiography as the gold standard for the diagnosis of Takayasu arteritis. However, due to the high radiation dose, magnetic resonance angiography could be used for follow-up monitoring. The ESR and CRP are usually elevated but this may be modest.

Management
There are no proven treatments in Takayasu arteritis.

First line
Prednisolone 1 mg/kg/day is the usual favoured first line treatment [12]. There is some evidence for the addition of azathioprine as an adjunct to corticosteroid therapy [13].

Second line
Cyclophosphamide, infliximab and tocilizumab have been reported to be of anecdotal value.

Key references

The full list of references can be found in the online version at www.rooksdermatology.com.

Single-organ small-vessel vasculitis

Cutaneous small-vessel vasculitis
2 Jennette JC, Falk RJ, Bacon PA, et al. 2012 revised International Chapel Hill Consensus Conference Nomenclature of Vasculitides. Arthritis Rheum 2013;65(1):1–11.
3 Calabrese LH, Michel BA, Bloch DA, et al. The American College of Rheumatology 1990 criteria for the classification of hypersensitivity vasculitis. Arthritis Rheum 1990;33(8):1108–13.
4 Garcia-Porrua C, Gonzalez-Gay MA. Comparative clinical and epidemiological study of hypersensitivity vasculitis versus Henoch-Schonlein purpura in adults. Semin Arthritis Rheum 1999;28(6):404–12.
5 Watts RA, Jolliffe VA, Grattan CE, Elliott J, Lockwood M, Scott DG. Cutaneous vasculitis in a defined population – clinical and epidemiological associations. J Rheumatol 1998;25(5):920–4.
7 Martinez-Taboada VM, Blanco R, Garcia-Fuentes M, Rodriguez-Valverde V. Clinical features and outcome of 95 patients with hypersensitivity vasculitis. Am J Med 1997;102(2):186–91.
8 Boom BW, Mommaas AM, Vermeer BJ. Presence and interpretation of vascular immune deposits in human skin: the value of direct immunofluorescence. J Dermatol Sci 1992;3(1):26–34.
9 Garcia-Porrua C, Gonzalez-Gay MA. Bacterial infection presenting as cutaneous vasculitis in adults. Clin Exp Rheumatol 1999;17(4):471–3.
10 Cribier B, Couilliet D, Meyer P, Grosshans E. The severity of histopathological changes of leukocytoclastic vasculitis is not predictive of extracutaneous involvement. Am J Dermatopathol 1999;21(6):532–6.
11 Mukhtyar C, Lee R, Brown D, et al. Modification and validation of the Birmingham Vasculitis Activity Score (version 3). Ann Rheum Dis 2009;68(12):1827–32.
35 Podjasek JO, Wetter DA, Pittelkow MR, Wada DA. Cutaneous small vessel vasculitis associated with solid organ malignancies: the Mayo Clinic experience, 1996 to 2009. J Am Acad Dermatol 2012;62(2): e55–65.

Erythema elevatum diutinum
6 Planagumá M, Puig L, Alomar A, et al. Pyoderma gangrenosum in association with erythema elevatum diutinum: report of two cases. Cutis 1992;49:201–6.
8 Creus L, Salleras M, Sola MA, et al. Erythema elevatum diutinum associated with pulmonary infiltrate. Br J Dermatol 1997;137:652–3.
10 Sangüeza OP, Pilcher B, Sangüeza JM. Erythema elevatum diutinum: a clinico-pathological study of eight cases. Am J Dermatopathol 1997;19:214–22.
17 Yiannias JA, el-Azhary RA, Gibson LE. Erythema elevatum diutinum: a clinical and histopathologic study of 13 patients. J Am Acad Dermatol 1992;26:38–44.
18 LeBoit PE, Yen TS, Wintroub B. The evolution of lesions in erythema elevatum diutinum. Am J Dermatopathol 1986;8:392–402.
22 Cesinaro AM, Lonardi S, Faccheti F. Granuloma faciale: a cutaneous lesion sharing features with IgG4-associated sclerosing diseases. Am J Surg Pathol 2013;27:66–73.
23 Ayoub N, Charuel J-L, Diemerte M-C, et al. Antineutrophil cytoplasmic antibodies of IgA class in neutrophilic dermatoses with emphasis on erythema elevatum diutinum. Arch Dermatol 2004;140:931–6.
24 Chow RKP, Benny WB, Coupe RL, et al. Erythema elevatum diutinum associated with IgA paraproteinaemia successfully controlled with intermittent plasma exchange. Arch Dermatol 1996;132:1360–4.
25 Kohler IK, Lorincz AL. Erythema elevatum diutinum treated with niacinamide and tetracycline. Arch Dermatol 1980;116:693–5.
26 Frieling GW, Williams NL, Sim SJ. Novel use of topical 5% dapsone gel in erythema elevatum diutinum: safer and effective. J Drugs Dermatol 2013;12:381–4.

Recurrent cutaneous necrotizing eosinophilic vasculitis
2 Chen KR, Pittelkow MR, Su D, et al. Recurrent cutaneous eosinophilic necrotizing vasculitis: a novel eosinophil-mediated syndrome. Arch Dermatol 1994;130:1159–66.
5 Jang KA, Lim YS, Choi JH, et al. Hypereosinophilic syndrome presenting as cutaneous necrotizing eosinophilic vasculitis and Raynaud's phenomenon complicated by digital gangrene. Br J Dermatol 2000;143:641–4.

10 Li W, Cao W, Song H, *et al*. Recurrent cutaneous necrotizing eosinophilc vasculitis: a case report and review of the literature. *Diagn Pathol* 2013;8:135.

Granuloma faciale

1 Wigley JE. Eosinophilic granuloma. Sarcoid of Boeck. *Proc R Soc Med* 1945;38(3):125–6.
3 Marcoval J, Moreno A, Peyr J. Granuloma faciale: a clinicopathological study of 11 cases. *J Am Acad Dermatol* 2004;51(2):269–73.
5 Cesinaro AM, Lonardi S, Facchetti F. Granuloma faciale: a cutaneous lesion sharing features with IgG4-associated sclerosing diseases. *Am J Surg Pathol* 2013;37(1):66–73.
8 Lallas A, Sidiropoulos T, Lefaki I, Tzellos T, Sotiriou E, Apalla Z. Photoletter to the editor: Dermoscopy of granuloma faciale. *J Dermatol Case Rep* 2012;6(2):59–60.
17 Dinehart SM, Gross DJ, Davis CM, Herzberg AJ. Granuloma faciale. Comparison of different treatment modalities. *Arch Otolaryngol Head Neck Surg* 1990;116(7):849–51.
18 Apfelberg DB, Maser MR, Lash H, Flores J. Expanded role of the argon laser in plastic surgery. *J Dermatol Surg Oncol* 1983;9(2):145–51.
19 Ludwig E, Allam JP, Bieber T, Novak N. New treatment modalities for granuloma faciale. *Br J Dermatol* 2003;149(3):634–7.
20 Zacarian SA. Cryosurgery effective for granuloma faciale. *J Dermatol Surg Oncol* 1985;11(1):11–13.
21 Van de Kerkhof PC. On the efficacy of dapsone in granuloma faciale. *Acta Derm Venereol* 1994;74(1):61–2.
22 Caldarola G, Zalaudek I, Argenziano G, Bisceglia M, Pellicano R. Granuloma faciale: a case report on long-term treatment with topical tacrolimus and dermoscopic aspects. *Dermatol Ther* 2011;24(5):508–11.

Small-vessel immune complex-associated vasculitis

IgA vasculitis

1 Jennette JC, Falk RJ, Bacon PA, *et al*. 2012 revised International Chapel Hill Consensus Conference Nomenclature of Vasculitides. *Arthritis Rheum* 2013;65(1):1–11.
3 Mills JA, Michel BA, Bloch DA, *et al*. The American College of Rheumatology 1990 criteria for the classification of Henoch-Schonlein purpura. *Arthritis Rheum* 1990;33(8):1114–21.
8 Gardner-Medwin JM, Dolezalova P, Cummins C, Southwood TR. Incidence of Henoch-Schonlein purpura, Kawasaki disease, and rare vasculitides in children of different ethnic origins. *Lancet* 2002;360(9341):1197–202.
12 Jauhola O, Ronkainen J, Koskimies O, *et al*. Renal manifestations of Henoch-Schonlein purpura in a 6-month prospective study of 223 children. *Arch Dis Child* Nov;95(11):877–82.
13 Trapani S, Micheli A, Grisolia F, *et al*. Henoch Schonlein purpura in childhood: epidemiological and clinical analysis of 150 cases over a 5-year period and review of literature. *Semin Arthritis Rheum* 2005;35(3):143–53.
26 Yang YH, Chuang YH, Wang LC, Huang HY, Gershwin ME, Chiang BL. The immunobiology of Henoch-Schonlein purpura. *Autoimmun Rev* 2008;7(3):179–84.
32 Peru H, Soylemezoglu O, Gonen S, *et al*. HLA class 1 associations in Henoch Schonlein purpura: increased and decreased frequencies. *Clin Rheumatol* 2008;27(1):5–10.
35 Deng F, Lu L, Zhang Q, Hu B, Wang SJ, Huang N. Henoch-Schonlein purpura in childhood: treatment and prognosis. Analysis of 425 cases over a 5-year period. *Clin Rheumatol* 2010;29(4):369–74.
37 Zaffanello M, Brugnara M, Franchini M. Therapy for children with Henoch-Schonlein purpura nephritis: a systematic review. *Sci World J* 2007;7:20–30.
38 Ronkainen J, Koskimies O, Ala-Houhala M, *et al*. Early prednisone therapy in Henoch-Schonlein purpura: a randomized, double-blind, placebo-controlled trial. *J Pediatr* 2006;149(2):241–7.

Cryoglobulinaemic vasculitis

1 Terrier B, Cacoub P. Cryoglobulinemia vasculitis: an update. *Curr Opin Rheumatol* 2013;25(1):10–18.
9 Mukhtyar C, Guillevin L, Cid MC, *et al*. EULAR recommendations for the management of primary small and medium vessel vasculitis. *Ann Rheum Dis* 2009;68(3):310–17.
10 De Vita S, Quartuccio L, Isola M, *et al*. A randomized controlled trial of rituximab for the treatment of severe cryoglobulinemic vasculitis. *Arthritis Rheum* 2012;64(3):843–53.

Hypocomplementaemic urticarial vasculitis

2 Dincy CV, George R, Jacob M, Mathai E, Pulimood S, Eapen EP. Clinicopathologic profile of normocomplementemic and hypocomplementemic urticarial vasculitis: a study from South India. *J Eur Acad Dermatol Venereol* 2008;22(7):789–94.
10 Ashida A, Murata H, Ohashi A, Ogawa E, Uhara H, Okuyama R. A case of hypocomplementaemic urticarial vasculitis with a high serum level of rheumatoid factor. *Australas J Dermatol* 2013;54(3):e62–3.
12 Enriquez R, Sirvent AE, Amoros F, Perez M, Matarredona J, Reyes A. Crescentic membranoproliferative glomerulonephritis and hypocomplementemic urticarial vasculitis. *J Nephrol* 2005;18(3):318–22.

Antiglomerular basement membrane vasculitis disease

2 Goodpasture EW. Landmark publication from the American Journal of the Medical Sciences: the significance of certain pulmonary lesions in relation to the etiology of influenza. *Am J Med Sci* 2009;338(2):148–51.
7 Bayat A, Kamperis K, Herlin T. Characteristics and outcome of Goodpasture's disease in children. *Clin Rheumatol* 2012;31(12):1745–51.
8 Cui Z, Zhao J, Jia XY, Zhu SN, Zhao MH. Clinical features and outcomes of anti-glomerular basement membrane disease in older patients. *Am J Kidney Dis* 2011;57(4):575–82.

Small-vessel ANCA-associated vasculitis

Microscopic polyangiitis

1 Jennette JC, Falk RJ, Bacon PA, *et al*. 2012 revised International Chapel Hill Consensus Conference Nomenclature of Vasculitides. *Arthritis Rheum* 2013;65(1):1–11.
5 Mohammad AJ, Jacobsson LT, Westman KW, Sturfelt G, Segelmark M. Incidence and survival rates in Wegener's granulomatosis, microscopic polyangiitis, Churg-Strauss syndrome and polyarteritis nodosa. *Rheumatology (Oxford)* 2009;48(12):1560–5.
10 Lane SE, Watts R, Scott DG. Epidemiology of systemic vasculitis. *Curr Rheumatol Rep* 2005;7(4):270–5.
18 Mukhtyar C, Guillevin L, Cid MC, *et al*. EULAR recommendations for the management of primary small and medium vessel vasculitis. *Ann Rheum Dis* 2009;68(3):310–17.
22 Jayne D, Rasmussen N, Andrassy K, *et al*. A randomized trial of maintenance therapy for vasculitis associated with antineutrophil cytoplasmic autoantibodies. *N Engl J Med* 2003;349(1):36–44.
23 Ntatsaki E, Carruthers D, Chakravarty K, *et al*. BSR and BHPR guideline for the management of adults with ANCA-associated vasculitis. *Rheumatology (Oxford)* 2014;53(12):2306–9.
27 Stone JH, Merkel PA, Spiera R, *et al*. Rituximab versus cyclophosphamide for ANCA-associated vasculitis. *N Engl J Med* 2010;363(3):221–32.
28 Jones RB, Tervaert JW, Hauser T, *et al*. Rituximab versus cyclophosphamide in ANCA-associated renal vasculitis. *N Engl J Med* 2010;363(3):211–20.
30 Smith RM, Jones RB, Guerry MJ, *et al*. Rituximab for remission maintenance in relapsing antineutrophil cytoplasmic antibody-associated vasculitis. *Arthritis Rheum* 2012;64(11):3760–9.
31 Rhee EP, Laliberte KA, Niles JL. Rituximab as maintenance therapy for antineutrophil cytoplasmic antibody-associated vasculitis. *Clin J Am Soc Nephrol* 2010;5(8):1394–400.

Granulomatosis with polyangiitis

1 Jennette JC, Falk RJ, Bacon PA, *et al*. 2012 revised International Chapel Hill Consensus Conference Nomenclature of Vasculitides. *Arthritis Rheum* 2013;65(1):1–11.
7 Watts RA, Mooney J, Skinner J, Scott DG, Macgregor AJ. The contrasting epidemiology of granulomatosis with polyangiitis (Wegener's) and microscopic polyangiitis. *Rheumatology (Oxford)* 2012;51(5):926–31.
29 Lyons PA, Rayner TF, Trivedi S, *et al*. Genetically distinct subsets within ANCA-associated vasculitis. *N Engl J Med* 2012;367(3):214–23.
30 Mukhtyar C, Guillevin L, Cid MC, *et al*. EULAR recommendations for the management of primary small and medium vessel vasculitis. *Ann Rheum Dis* 2009;68(3):310–17.
31 Faurschou M, Sorensen IJ, Mellemkjaer L, *et al*. Malignancies in Wegener's granulomatosis: incidence and relation to cyclophosphamide therapy in a cohort of 293 patients. *J Rheumatol* 2008;35(1):100–5.

PART 9: VASCULAR

34 Mukhtyar C, Flossmann O, Hellmich B, *et al.* Outcomes from studies of anti-neutrophil cytoplasm antibody associated vasculitis: a systematic review by the European League Against Rheumatism systemic vasculitis task force. *Ann Rheum Dis* 2008;67(7):1004–10.

35 Mukhtyar C, Hellmich B, Jayne D, Flossmann O, Luqmani R. Remission in anti-neutrophil cytoplasmic antibody-associated systemic vasculitis. *Clin Exp Rheumatol* 2006;24(6 Suppl. 43):S93–8.

44 Jones RB, Tervaert JW, Hauser T, *et al.* Rituximab versus cyclophosphamide in ANCA-associated renal vasculitis. *N Engl J Med* 2010;363(3):211–20.

50 Metzler C, Miehle N, Manger K, *et al.* Elevated relapse rate under oral methotrexate versus leflunomide for maintenance of remission in Wegener's granulomatosis. *Rheumatology (Oxford)* 2007;46(7):1087–91.

52 Smith RM, Jones RB, Guerry MJ, *et al.* Rituximab for remission maintenance in relapsing antineutrophil cytoplasmic antibody-associated vasculitis. *Arthritis Rheum* 2012;64(11):3760–9.

Eosinophilic granulomatosis with polyangiitis

1 Jennette JC, Falk RJ, Bacon PA, *et al.* 2012 revised International Chapel Hill Consensus Conference Nomenclature of Vasculitides. *Arthritis Rheum* 2013;65(1):1–11.

2 Daoud MS, Hutton KP, Gibson LE. Cutaneous periarteritis nodosa: a clinicopathological study of 79 cases. *Br J Dermatol* 1997;136(5):706–13.

5 Ishiguro N, Kawashima M. Cutaneous polyarteritis nodosa: a report of 16 cases with clinical and histopathological analysis and a review of the published work. *J Dermatol*;37(1):85–93.

6 Mohammad AJ, Jacobsson LT, Westman KW, Sturfelt G, Segelmark M. Incidence and survival rates in Wegener's granulomatosis, microscopic polyangiitis, Churg-Strauss syndrome and polyarteritis nodosa. *Rheumatology (Oxford)* 2009;48(12):1560–5.

11 Darras-Joly C, Lortholary O, Cohen P, Brauner M, Guillevin L. Regressing microaneurysms in 5 cases of hepatitis B virus related polyarteritis nodosa. *J Rheumatol* 1995;22(5):876–80.

12 Caldeira T, Meireles C, Cunha F, Valbuena C, Aparicio J, Ribeiro A. Systemic polyarteritis nodosa associated with acute Epstein-Barr virus infection. *Clin Rheumatol* 2007;26(10):1733–5.

24 Navon Elkan P, Pierce SB, Segel R, *et al.* Mutant adenosine deaminase 2 in a polyarteritis nodosa vasculopathy. *N Engl J Med* 2014;370(10):921–31.

26 Guillevin L, Lhote F, Gayraud M, *et al.* Prognostic factors in polyarteritis nodosa and Churg-Strauss syndrome. A prospective study in 342 patients. *Medicine (Baltimore)* 1996;75(1):17–28.

29 Mukhtyar C, Guillevin L, Cid MC, *et al.* EULAR recommendations for the management of primary small and medium vessel vasculitis. *Ann Rheum Dis* 2009;68(3):310–17.

30 Krishnan S, Bhakuni DS, Kartik S. Rituximab in refractory cutaneous polyarteritis. *Int J Rheum Dis* 2012;15(5):e127.

Medium-vessel vasculitis

Polyarteritis nodosa and cutaneous polyarteritis nodosa

1 Jennette JC, Falk RJ, Bacon PA, *et al.* 2012 revised International Chapel Hill Consensus Conference Nomenclature of Vasculitides. *Arthritis Rheum* 2013;65(1):1–11.

2 Daoud MS, Hutton KP, Gibson LE. Cutaneous periarteritis nodosa: a clinicopathological study of 79 cases. *Br J Dermatol* 1997;136(5):706–13.

5 Ishiguro N, Kawashima M. Cutaneous polyarteritis nodosa: a report of 16 cases with clinical and histopathological analysis and a review of the published work. *J Dermatol*; 37(1):85–93.

6 Mohammad AJ, Jacobsson LT, Westman KW, Sturfelt G, Segelmark M. Incidence and survival rates in Wegener's granulomatosis, microscopic polyangiitis, Churg-Strauss syndrome and polyarteritis nodosa. *Rheumatology (Oxford)* 2009;48(12):1560–5.

11 Darras-Joly C, Lortholary O, Cohen P, Brauner M, Guillevin L. Regressing microaneurysms in 5 cases of hepatitis B virus related polyarteritis nodosa. *J Rheumatol* 1995;22(5):876–80.

12 Caldeira T, Meireles C, Cunha F, Valbuena C, Aparicio J, Ribeiro A. Systemic polyarteritis nodosa associated with acute Epstein-Barr virus infection. *Clin Rheumatol* 2007;26(10):1733–5.

24 Navon Elkan P, Pierce SB, Segel R, *et al.* Mutant adenosine deaminase 2 in a polyarteritis nodosa vasculopathy. *N Engl J Med* 2014;370(10):921–31.

26 Guillevin L, Lhote F, Gayraud M, *et al.* Prognostic factors in polyarteritis nodosa and Churg-Strauss syndrome. A prospective study in 342 patients. *Medicine (Baltimore)* 1996;75(1):17–28.

29 Mukhtyar C, Guillevin L, Cid MC, *et al.* EULAR recommendations for the management of primary small and medium vessel vasculitis. *Ann Rheum Dis* 2009;68(3):310–17.

30 Krishnan S, Bhakuni DS, Kartik S. Rituximab in refractory cutaneous polyarteritis. *Int J Rheum Dis* 2012;15(5):e127.

Kawasaki disease

3 Baumer JH, Love SJ, Gupta A, Haines LC, Maconochie I, Dua JS. Salicylate for the treatment of Kawasaki disease in children. *Cochrane Database Syst Rev* 2006;Issue 4:CD004175.

4 Newburger JW, Takahashi M, Gerber MA, *et al.* Diagnosis, treatment, and long-term management of Kawasaki disease: a statement for health professionals from the Committee on Rheumatic Fever, Endocarditis, and Kawasaki Disease, Council on Cardiovascular Disease in the Young, American Heart Association. *Pediatrics* 2004;114(6):1708–33.

14 Kobayashi T, Inoue Y, Takeuchi K, *et al.* Prediction of intravenous immunoglobulin unresponsiveness in patients with Kawasaki disease. *Circulation* 2006;113(22):2606–12.

15 Kobayashi T, Saji T, Otani T, *et al.* Efficacy of immunoglobulin plus prednisolone for prevention of coronary artery abnormalities in severe Kawasaki disease (RAISE study): a randomised, open-label, blinded-endpoints trial. *Lancet* 2012;379(9826):1613–20.

Large-vessel vasculitis

Giant cell arteritis

2 Baum EW, Sams WM, Jr, Payne RR. Giant cell arteritis: a systemic disease with rare cutaneous manifestations. *J Am Acad Dermatol* 1982;6(6):1081–8.

5 Smeeth L, Cook C, Hall AJ. Incidence of diagnosed polymyalgia rheumatica and temporal arteritis in the United Kingdom, 1990–2001. *Ann Rheum Dis* 2006;65(8):1093–8.

13 Mukhtyar C, Guillevin L, Cid MC, *et al.* EULAR recommendations for the management of large vessel vasculitis. *Ann Rheum Dis* 2009;68(3):318–23.

15 Mahr AD, Jover JA, Spiera RF, *et al.* Adjunctive methotrexate for treatment of giant cell arteritis: an individual patient data meta-analysis. *Arthritis Rheum* 2007;56(8):2789–97.

Takayasu arteritis

5 Watts R, Al-Taiar A, Mooney J, Scott D, Macgregor A. The epidemiology of Takayasu arteritis in the UK. *Rheumatology (Oxford)* 2009;48(8):1008–11.

9 Frances C, Boisnic S, Bletry O, *et al.* Cutaneous manifestations of Takayasu arteritis. A retrospective study of 80 cases. *Dermatologica* 1990;181(4):266–72.

11 Maksimowicz-McKinnon K, Clark TM, Hoffman GS. Limitations of therapy and a guarded prognosis in an American cohort of Takayasu arteritis patients. *Arthritis Rheum* 2007;56(3):1000–9.

CHAPTER 103

Dermatoses Resulting from Disorders of the Veins and Arteries

Portia C. Goldsmith

Barts Health and Homerton University Hospital, London, UK

ARTERIAL AND ARTERIOLAR DISORDERS

Vasculogenesis, angiogenesis and arteriogenesis

Vasculogenesis is the first step in the development of blood vessels and is the process by which endothelial cells differentiate from their mesodermal precursors. Vasculogenesis leads to the formation of a primary capillary plexus and occurs mainly in embryonal development [1]. Angiogenesis is the process by which new capillaries are formed from existing vessels by sprouting, expanding and remodelling [2]. It is a normal process essential to growth and development. It is pivotal in wound healing but it is also a key element in the pathogenesis of disease [3]. The establishment and remodelling of blood vessels requires a complex orchestration of molecular regulators. In order for angiogenesis to occur, there exists an imbalance in angiogenic growth factors compared to angiogenesis inhibitors. Initially, there is an upregulation of angiogenic growth factors which are released to nearby tissues. The growth factors bind to specific receptors on adjacent vascular endothelial cells leading to cellular activation. The endothelial cells proliferate and secrete matrix metalloproteinases (MMPs) which degrade the extracellular matrix. This permits migration of budding endothelial cells under the influence of angiogenic stimuli, particularly the family of vascular endothelial growth factors (VEGF) A, B, C, D and E, plus placental growth factor and their tyrosine kinase receptors, VEGFR-1, VEGFR-2 and VEGFR-3. Stabilization and maintenance of newly formed vessels occur mainly as a consequence of the angiopoietins [4], Ang1 (expressed by pericytes, smooth muscle cells and fibroblasts) and Ang2 (from endothelial cells) through their Tie receptors. There are many other angiogenic growth factors which are variously important in health and disease such as basic fibroblast growth factor, interleukin-8, platelet-derived growth factor, transforming growth factor β and tumour necrosis factor α [3].

Differentiation into arteries, veins and capillaries is the responsibility of angiogenesis. Neoangiogenesis is an important cause of recurrent varicose veins after stripping [5]. Arteriogenesis produces rapid circumferential growth in the pre-existing collateral vessels, which are less perfused under normal flow conditions. While local tissue ischaemia or hypoxia stimulates angiogenesis, arteriogenesis is mainly induced by inflammation and shear stress [6].

PART 9: VASCULAR

Rook's Textbook of Dermatology, Ninth Edition. Edited by Christopher Griffiths, Jonathan Barker, Tanya Bleiker, Robert Chalmers and Daniel Creamer.
© 2016 John Wiley & Sons, Ltd. Published 2016 by John Wiley & Sons, Ltd.
Companion website: www.rooksdermatology.com

Arterial disease and peripheral ischaemic disorders

Definition and nomenclature

Disorders where the arterial blood supply to the limb (usually the leg) is damaged by atherosclerosis, a chronic disorder that can result in intravascular thrombosis that leads to damage and death of the tissues.

Synonyms and inclusions
- Atherosclerosis
- Peripheral ischaemia
- Peripheral vascular disease

Introduction and general description

Atherosclerosis of the lower limb is a condition most frequently managed by vascular surgeons but patients may present to dermatologists when peripheral ischaemia leads to infarction and ulceration of the skin.

Epidemiology

Atherosclerosis is responsible for more than 90% of all arterial disease in the Western world. It affects 5% of men over the age of 50 years, of which 10% may develop critical limb ischaemia; this increases to 20% if diabetic patients are included [1]. Apart from diabetes, tobacco smoking is one of the most important risk factors for arterial disease. A family history of arterial disease and the presence of hyperlidaemia are the two other major factors associated with atherosclerosis.

Pathophysiology

This is a multifactorial disorder but it is thought that the underlying mechanism is immunological [2]. Evidence suggests that cardiovascular risk factors induce endothelial injury and endothelial dysfunction. Monocytes recruited to the inflamed endothelium of blood vessels differentiate into phagocytic macrophages which scavenge modified lipids to produce foam cells. This is the basis for the development of the lipid-rich atheroma core. In time, there is further influx and inflammation leading to unstable atherosclerotic plaques which can eventually ulcerate through the endothelial lining exposing a highly thrombogenic surface. Platelets adhere to the ulcerated plaque and platelet aggregates (platelet thrombi) may embolize distally or may initiate local thrombosis. Inadequate collaterals, or occlusion by thrombosis or embolism, will lead to tissue infarction (e.g. peripheral gangrene).

Clinical features

The clinical features of peripheral vascular disease are described in Table 103.1

Investigations

The most important investigations are summarized in Table 103.2

Table 103.1 Clinical features of peripheral vascular disease.

History	Claudication–cramping pain on walking, usually in the posterior calf, relieved with rest
	Rest pain at night usually in the foot: indication of critical ischaemia
	Skin ulceration
Presentation	Erythematous or dusky mottled hue to legs, elevation of the leg leads to a white foot (Figure 103.1)
	Trophic changes (including dry skin, cracks, loss of hair, thickened nails) (Figure 103.2)
	Platelet emboli can lodge in the vasculature causing areas of discoloration in the toes and sole of the foot and can appear 'vasculitic-like' (Figure 103.3)
	Ulceration of skin at pressure points and the dorsum of the foot (Figure 103.4)
Clinical variants	N/A
Differential diagnosis	Buerger disease
	Embolism leading to acute ischaemia
	External arterial compression (popliteal entrapment or cervical rib)
	Dissecting aneurysms
	Ergot alkaloid poisoning
	Coagulation disorders (polycythaemia, thrombocytosis)
	Vasculitis
Classification of severity	Mild, moderate and severe peripheral vascular disease (see the ankle–brachial Doppler pressure index in Table 103.2)
Co-morbidities	Cigarette smoking, hypertension, hyperlipidaemia, diabetes, poor diet, obesity, lifestyle, family history of cardiovascular disease
	Cardiovascular: atrial fibrillation and other dysrhythmias, murmurs, heart failure, aortic aneurysm and bruits over stenosed vessels
	Fundi (may show hypertensive changes or cholesterol emboli)
	Peripheral neuropathy
Disease course and prognosis	90% have coronary artery disease and the extent of this determines the overall survival of the patient rather than the peripheral vascular disease [3]

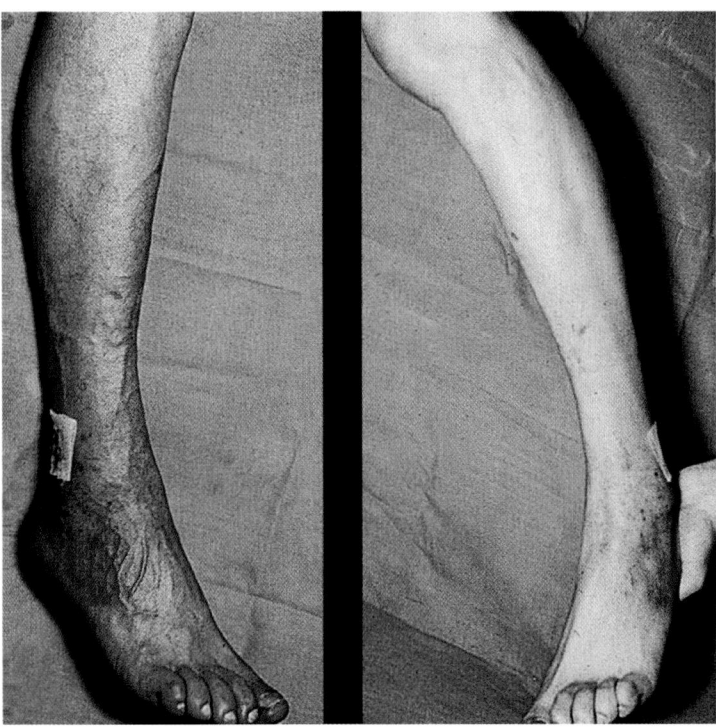

Figure 103.1 Buerger's test showing postural colour change in an ishaemic foot – white when the foot is elevated (right) and red when lowered (left).

Table 103.2 Investigations for patients with suspected peripheral vascular disease.

Doppler ultrasound to measure the ankle–brachial Doppler pressure index
   Normal result = 1
   Ratio 0.71–0.9 = mild peripheral vascular disease
   Ratio 0.41–0.7 = moderate peripheral vascular disease
   Ratio <0.41 = severe peripheral vascular disease
   Ratio <0.2 is usually associated with very severe ischaemia and gangrene
	After the Doppler ultrasound probe has been used to locate the dorsalis pedis or posterior tibial vessel a sphygmomanometer cuff is placed around the limb above the ankle and inflated (Figure 103.5). The red cells flowing past the tip of the ultrasound probe deflect the beam, creating an audible noise. As the cuff is inflated above systolic pressure, flow in the artery ceases and the noise disappears. This ankle–brachial systolic gradient is normally 1.0. A fall in ankle pressure results in a reduction of the pressure index. Falsely high indices may be obtained in some limbs if the vessels are very calcified and fail to compress at systolic pressure. This is especially true for diabetic limbs. In such circumstances a more accurate means of assessment is to measure the Doppler pressures at the toe

Blood tests	Full blood count (to exclude anaemia and polycythaemia), urea and electrolytes (to monitor renal function), glucose, fasting lipids, C-reactive protein (as a marker of inflammation), homocysteine
Cardiovascular and respiratory investigations	Electrocardiogram (to look for ischaemic heart disease and cardiac dysrhythmias), chest X-ray (to look for heart failure, cardiomegaly)
Radiology: to provide a detailed assessment of the anatomy of the arterial tree	
Duplex ultrasound scanning	Duplex ultrasound scanning is often the initial investigation, and is used as a screening test to confirm the major sites of stenosis or occlusion in the vascular tree [**4,5**]. A duplex ultrasound scan provides both a B-mode image of the artery and a measurement of blood velocity; these can be combined to provide a map of stenoses and occlusions within the arterial tree from the aorta to the crural (calf) vessels. The greater the velocity, the tighter the stenosis
Arteriography: choosing the appropriate tests should be made with guidance of the vascular surgeons and interventional radiologists	There are several techniques available. Contrast-enhanced magnetic resonance angiography is favoured but in patients in whom it is contraindicated or not tolerated then use computed tomography angiography

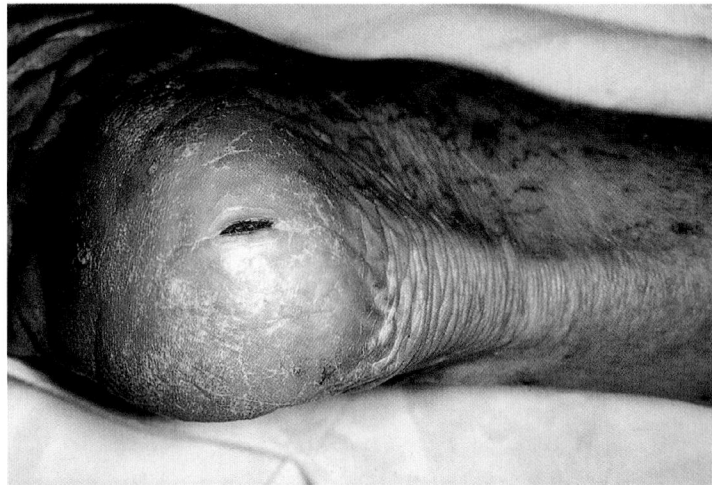

Figure 103.2 Trophic changes including dry skin, cracks, loss of hair and thickened nails (the latter two not shown on figure).

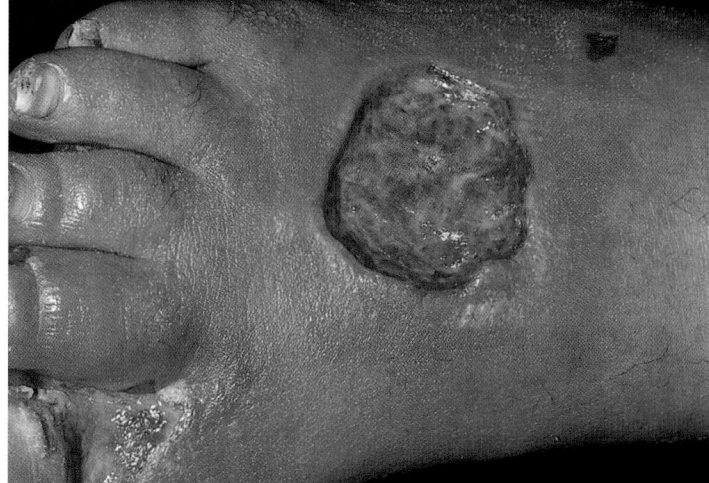

Figure 103.4 Ulceration of the skin at pressure points.

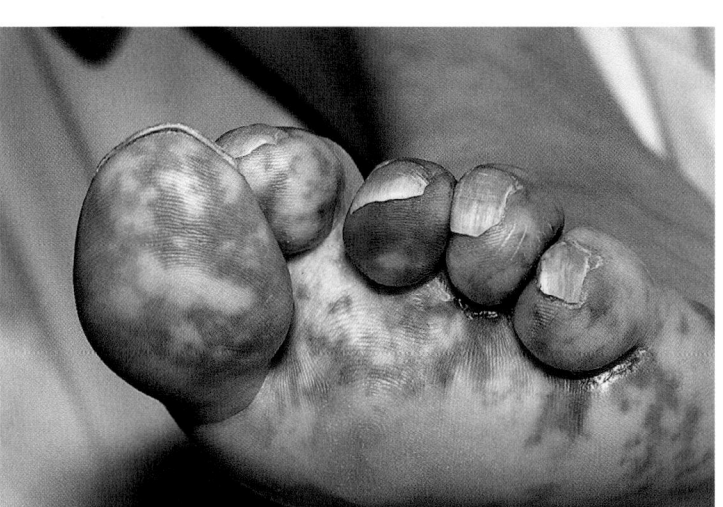

Figure 103.3 Platelet emboli can lodge in the vasculature causing areas of discoloration in the toes and sole of the foot, and can appear 'vasculitic-like'.

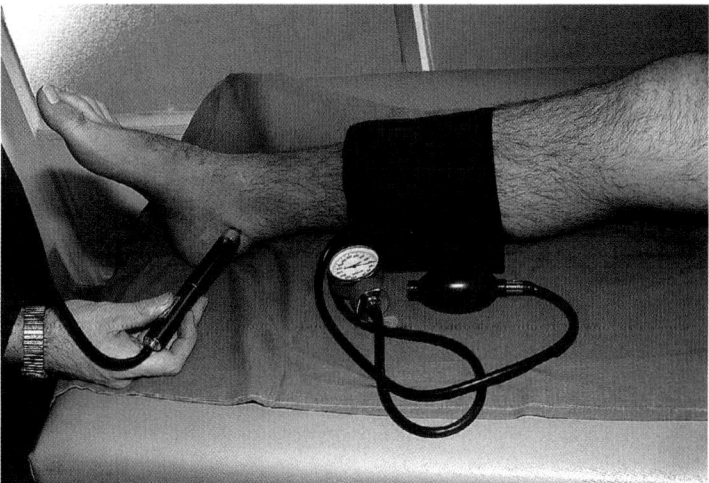

Figure 103.5 Doppler ultrasound to measure the ankle–brachial Doppler pressure index.

Table 103.3 Treatment options for patients with peripheral ischaemia.

Claudication: aim of treatment to relieve symptoms	**First line (conservative)** as only 5% of patients go on to develop rest pain or gangrene Stop smoking, treat hypertension unless lower limb pressures are <80 mmHg and treat diabetes and hyperlipidaemias. Supervised exercise program to try and encourage the development of collateral blood vessels. Antiplatelet agents (clopidogrel and aspirin [**6**]). Aspirin has not been shown to improve claudication itself, but patients with claudication treated with antiplatelet agents have a 25% reduction in subsequent serious cardiovascular events **Second line** Angioplasty and stenting. This technique works best on stenoses in large proximal vessels, and least well on long occlusions of the distal arterial tree. Potential complications include arterial rupture, aneurysm formation, thrombosis and dissection **Third line** Infra-inguinal bypass surgery using an autologous vein whenever possible for people with intermittent claudication Naftidrofuryl oxalate: review progress after 3–6 months and discontinue if there has been no symptomatic benefit
Rest pain and gangrene: aim of treatment to prevent amputation, relieve pain and preserve life	**First line** Manage complicating conditions such as diabetes, dehydration, infection, polycythaemia and anaemia Angioplasty, stenting and bypass surgery where possible to increase the blood flow to the ischaemic areas Control pain with adequate analgesia including opiates **Second line** Amputation
Acute limb ischaemia: aim of treatment to prevent amputation, relieve pain and preserve life	**First line** Urgent angiography to confirm the diagnosis (consider embolism if patient is in atrial fibrillation, has had recent myocardial infarction or if the vascular flow in the other limbs is normal. The cardiac dysrhythmia should be managed) If embolic: balloon angioplasty with or without stenting and sometimes with percutaneous laser atherectomy as an adjunct Peripheral arterial disease: balloon catheter embolectomy with or without stenting and sometimes with percutaneous laser atherectomy and thrombolysis and anticoagulation If stenotic: thrombolysis often via an intra-arterial catheter, followed by anticoagulation. Angioplasty, stenting or surgery may be necessary Platelet emboli should be managed by antiplatelet medication **Second line** Amputation

Management

Once the diagnosis of peripheral vascular disease is made, the patient is best managed by a vascular surgeon who can address the underlying cause. Table 103.3 outlines the basic management strategies. Treatment options differ for patients presenting with claudication, rest pain or gangrene and acute limb ischaemia.

Resources

Further information

Lower limb peripheral arterial disease; diagnosis and management, NICE guideline August 2012, http://guidance.nice.org.uk/CG147

Percutaneous laser atherectomy as an adjunct to balloon angioplasty (with or without stenting) for peripheral arterial disease, NICE guideline November 2012, http://guidance.nice.org.uk/IPG433

Patient resources

Information on peripheral vascular disease (IPG43) http://www.patient.co.uk/health/peripheral-arterial-disease-in-legs

(All last accessed March 2015.)

Thromboangiitis obliterans

Definition and nomenclature

This is a non-atherosclerotic segmental inflammatory disease of the small and medium sized arteries of the distal extremities of predominantly young male smokers [1]. These patients are normally seen by vascular surgeons but may present to dermatologists with erythema and or ulceration of the skin of the fingers and toes.

Synonyms and inclusions
- Buerger disease

Introduction and general description

Thromboangiitis obliterans (Buerger disease) appears to be a distinct condition separate from other forms of vascular occlusion [2,3], with differences in the pathological appearance of the vessel wall, and in the population affected, compared with other arterial diseases [2]. It was first described by Felix von Winiwarter in 1879.

In 1908, Buerger published a pathological description of 11 amputated limbs in young male smokers [4].

Epidemiology

Incidence and prevalence
It is a rare condition. The prevalence is falling in the USA, from 104/100000 in 1947 to 13/100000 in 1986 [5], and in Thailand, the prevalence in one clinic has halved from 1988 to 1995, whilst the prevalence of peripheral vascular disease doubled in the same time period [6].

Age
Most are under 40.

Sex
The number of women with the condition is rising but is about 11% in the USA [5], and less than 3% reported in Thailand [6].

Ethnicity
The prevalence is higher in the Middle East, India and the Far East and less common in Western Europe and North America which is thought to reflect smoking habits more than ethnicity.

Pathophysiology

Predisposing factors
The aetiology of this condition is unknown although tobacco addiction is invariably a major contributing factor, and a failure to overcome this addiction is associated with progressive occlusion of the vessels.

Pathology
Circulating autoantibodies have been identified, in particular antiendothelial cell antibodies are present in high titre in active disease [7]. Antibodies have a pathogenic role and can be used to monitor disease activity [2]. The full thickness of the vessel wall is invaded by lymphocytes, eosinophils, plasma cells and monocytes which disrupt the internal elastic lamina. There is luminal occlusion from thrombosis which is highly cellular. Accompanying nerves and veins may become involved in the inflammatory process. All changes are segmental or focal. At a later stage in the disease, fibrosis occurs, which spreads to involve surrounding structures [2,8].

Causative organisms
Rickettsial infections have been postulated to play a role but evidence is lacking [9].

Genetics
No confirmed genetic basis has been found though studies have been looking at the role of polymorphisms in the T allelle of endothelial nitric oxide synthase [10].

Environmental factors
Ambient temperature may be relevant; two studies have reported that thromboangiitis obliterans is worse in the winter and better in warmer weather [11,12].

Clinical features
The clinical features are summarized in Table 103.4.

Table 103.4 Clinical features of thromboangiitis obliterans.

History	Pain in the upper and lower limbs with cold extremities • intermittent claudication (classically in the arch of the foot) • rest pain • neuropathic pain and increased sensitivity to cold
Presentation	Ulcers: at the sites of trauma and often the sides of the nails or the tips of the digits Gangrene (occurs early) (Figure 103.6) Trophic changes Red or cyanotic peripheries Oedema Venous thrombosis and thrombophlebitis migrans Proximal pulses are present, but dorsalis pedis, posterior tibial and brachial pulses are lost early
Diagnostic criteria [1]	History of smoking Onset of distal extremity ischaemic symptoms before age of 50 Absence of atherosclerotic risk factors other than smoking
Differential diagnosis	Early onset atherosclerosis Multiple emboli Trauma or local lesions (such as entrapment) Collagen vascular disease Diabetic vasculopathy Hypercoagulable states Ergotism, cocaine/amphetamine abuse
Classification of severity	N/A
Complications and co-morbidities	Ulcers and gangrene can lead to sepsis
Disease course and prognosis	If patients continue to smoke, the prognosis is poor as most will require multiple amputations

Investigations
There are no diagnostic tests but angiography shows arterial occlusion and the development of corkscrew collaterals (Figure 103.7). The erythrocyte sedimentation rate (ESR) may be elevated and blood tests should be undertaken to exclude collagen vascular disorders and coagulation abnormalities.

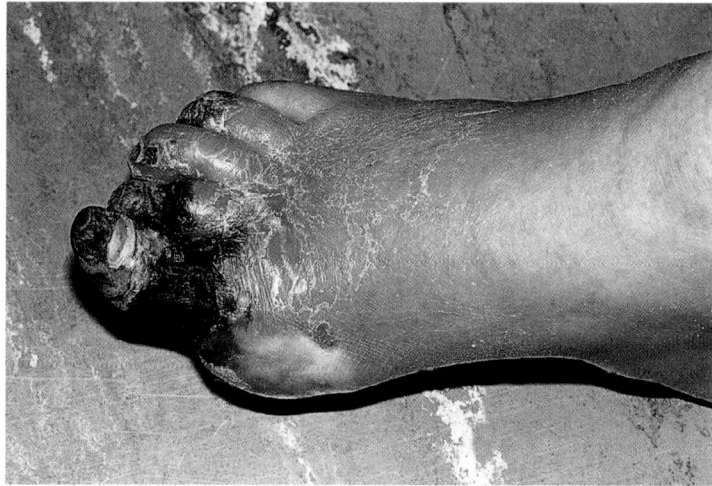

Figure 103.6 Ischaemic toes in Buerger disease.

PART 9: VASCULAR

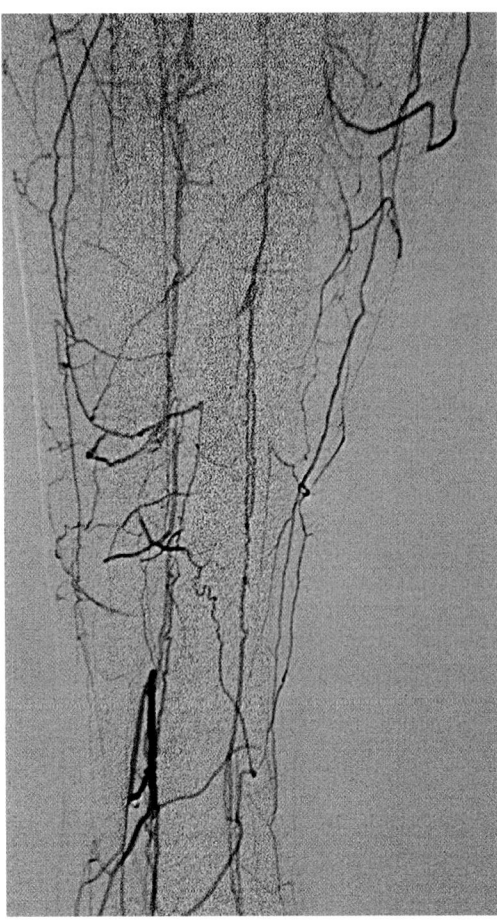

Figure 103.7 Angiography in thromboangiitis obliterans showing vascular occlusion and corkscrew collaterals.

Table 103.5 Management of thromboangiitis obliterans.

First line	Cessation of smoking. This is the only intervention of proven value and is most beneficial if undertaken before the onset of gangrene or tissue loss [1]
Second line	Surgical: • revascularization if possible (most occlusions are not amenable because they are too distal or diffuse and segmental) • amputation for gangrene Medical: prostacyclin analogue infusions, calcium-channel blockers, thrombolytics, anticoagulants Sympathectomy: spinal cord stimulators Stimulating angiogenesis through autologous bone marrow cells rich in endothelial progenitor cells

Management

These patients are best managed by vascular surgeons. Treatment is difficult and many different modalities have been tried (Table 103.5) but evidence for their success is limited [1].

Resources

Patient resources

http://www.patient.co.uk/doctor/buergers-disease-pro (last accessed March 2015).

NEUROVASCULAR DISORDERS

Erythromelalgia

Definition and nomenclature

This is a rare neurovascular disorder in which the extremities are episodically painful and red (see also Chapter 84). A sensation of burning is associated with vasodilatation of the small blood vessels in the affected area.

Synonyms and inclusions
- Mitchell disease (after Silas Weir Mitchell)
- Acromelalgia
- Red neuralgia
- Erythermalgia

Introduction and general description

Erythromelalgia is derived from the Greek *erythros* = red, *melos* = limb and *algos* = pain. The painful burning attacks typically affect the hands and feet but can involve the face and ears. It is a disabling disorder which may be primary idiopathic or hereditary (15% of patients have been shown to have a mutation in the *SCNA9A* gene) or secondary to thrombocythaemia and polycythaemia. It is poorly understood and treatment is often unsuccessful.

Epidemiology

Incidence and prevalence

There is not much data on the incidence of this rare condition. One study from the USA suggested a rate of 1.3/100 000 of the general population with 5% of those having the primary inherited form [1]; another from Norway [2] found the incidence was lower. A study from the Mayo Clinic recorded the incidence as 1 case per 40 000 patients attending the hospital [3]. Dermatologists see this condition rarely even in specialist centres.

Age

Age of onset is variable and though earlier reports from the Mayo Clinic suggested a median onset age in the primary form of 10 years, later studies showed a wide range of onset: 5–91 years, with a median age of 60 overall [1]. In Norway, the range of onset is from 7 to 76 years in the primary group and 18 to 81 years in the secondary group [2].

Sex

There is a small female predominance [1,2].

Ethnicity

There is no current evidence that this is relevant.

Associated diseases

Erythromelalgia may be secondary to myeloproliferative disorders in 9–19% of cases [1,2].

Pathophysiology

Primary erythromelalgia

Erythromelalgia is the first condition in which an ion channel mutation has been associated with chronic pain [4]. Recent advances have identified that 15% of cases are due to genetic mutations. Other cases are thought to have a non-genetic cause or may be mediated by mutations in one or more as yet unidentified genes. Ten mutations in the *SCN9A* gene have been identified in erythromelalgia [5,6,**7**,8,9,**10,11**,12,13,**14**,15]. The *SCN9A* gene codes for the α-subunit of a sodium channel called NaV1.7. Sodium channels transport positively charged sodium ions into cells. They act as threshold sensors and initiate action potentials. The mutations alter the activation profile to produce channels that are open for a longer period of time, leading to more prolonged changes in the membrane potential. NaV1.7 sodium channels are found in nociceptors in the dorsal root ganglion and sympathetic ganglion neurons. The hyperexcitability of the C fibres in the dorsal root ganglion leads to the burning pain that characterizes erythromelalgia. In the sympathetic system, there is hyporeactivity [9] resulting in altered vascular responses to stimuli such as heat and exercise, which causes persistent vasodilatation of the affected skin. It has been shown that the shift in a patient's mutation hyperpolarization activation was less great in milder late-onset primary type erythromelalgia than in a patient with severe early-onset primary erythromelalgia [**16**].

It is unknown why the pain episodes associated with erythromelalgia occur mainly in the hands and feet.

Secondary erythromelalgia

In cases associated with thrombocythaemia, biopsies have revealed arteriolar fibrosis and vascular occlusion due to platelet thrombi [17]. It is thought the abnormally functioning platelets in thrombocythaemia clump in vessels and induce neurovascular damage by triggering inflammation.

Pathology

There are no diagnostic histopathological findings.

Causative organisms

There has been epidemic outbreaks of erythromelalgia reported in students in rural China. The cause is unknown but poxviruses were isolated from throat swabs of several patients in different areas and at different times of the year [18–20].

Genetics

The primary idiopathic form may occur sporadically but when familial it is inherited in an autosomal dominant manner.

Environmental factors

Eating certain fungi, such as *Clitocybe acromelalgia* (Japan) and *Clitocybe amoenolens* (France), has lead to reports of mushroom-induced erythromelalgia which has persisted for up to 5 months following ingestion [21].

In medication-induced erythromelalgia, calcium-channel blockers and bromocriptine can trigger the condition.

Clinical features

Patients may present to general physicians, paediatricians, rheumatologists, vascular surgeons and dermatologists. There may be no abnormal signs at the consultation since the condition is episodic. Consequently, it often takes some time before a diagnosis is made. The clinical features erythromelalgia are shown in Table 103.6.

Table 103.6 Clinical features of erythromelalgia.

History	Intense burning associated with erythema and increased warmth of the extremities (hands, feet, arms, legs, face and/or ears)
	Triggers of attacks may include heat (often wake the patient at night), movement, exercise and emotional distress
	Attacks last from a few minutes to several hours
	During attacks, patients are desperate to cool the affected area
Examination	During attacks, the affected part is very red
	Initially, between attacks, the affected area appears normal. Over time dusky discoloration and acrocyanosis persist and the skin become shiny (Figure 103.8)
Differential diagnosis	Complex regional pain syndrome (reflex sympathetic dystrophy) following trauma
	Thromboangiitis obliterans
	Vasculitis
	Gout
Classification of severity	N/A
Complications and co-morbidities	Skin changes such as irritant dermatitis (Figure 103.9a) and fissuring (Figure 103.9.b) secondary to chronic immersion in cold water to relieve symptoms
	Vascular occlusion in erythromelalgia secondary thrombocythaemia can lead to ulceration, necrosis and gangrene
	Tendency to avoid using the affected limbs leading to oedema and atrophy
	Psychological issues due to chronic pain
Disease course and prognosis	Secondary erythromelalgia due to myeloproliferative disease will respond if the underlying condition is treated successfully
	Primary erythromelalgia is a chronic disorder which is generally unremitting

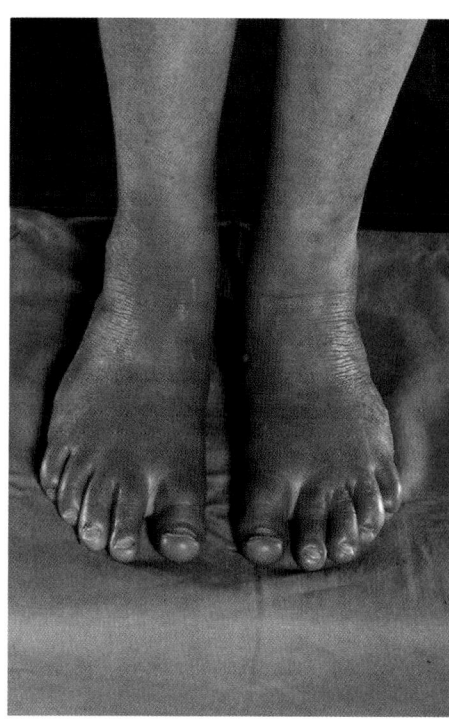

Figure 103.8 Patient during an attack of erythromelalgia.

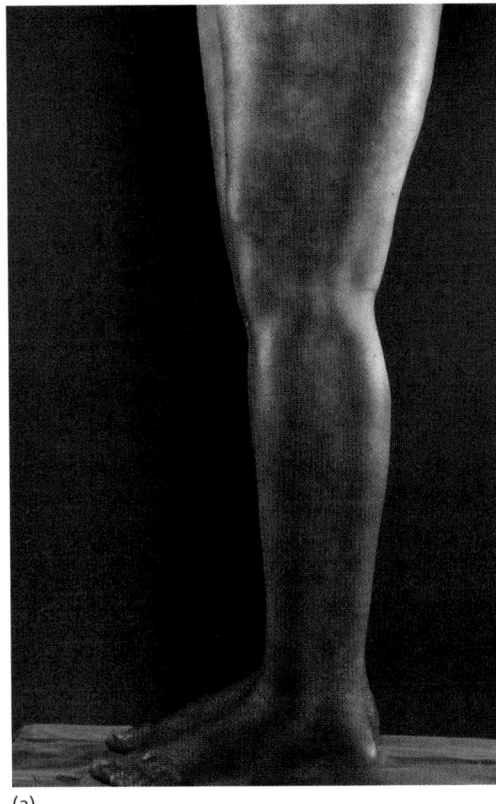

(a)

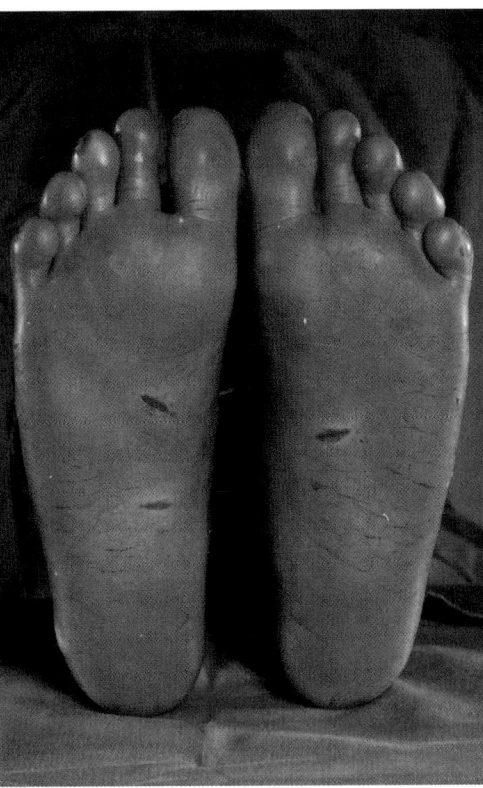

(b)

Figure 103.9 Secondary changes in erythromelalgia due to immersion in water to relieve symptoms (a) irritant contact dermatitis, and (b) fissuring. (Courtesy of Professor Pauline Dowd, University College London Hospital, London, UK.)

Table 103.7 Investigations for a patient with suspected erythromelalgia.

Blood tests	To exclude polycythaemia, thrombocythaemia, collagen vascular disorder, gout, diabetes
Nerve conduction studies	If a peripheral neuropathy is suspected

Table 103.8 Management of erythromelalgia.

Treat underlying cause and supportive measures [22]	If due to myeloproliferative disorder, refer to haematologist. Aspirin for thrombocythaemia
	Advice on avoiding exacerbating factors
	Advise patient against cold water immersion to relieve symptoms
	Neuropathic pain relief: amitriptyline, gabapentin, pregabalin, mexiletine
	Psychological support
	Lidocaine patch [23]
	Referral to pain specialist clinic

Investigations

There are no diagnostic tests for erythromelalgia but investigations should be undertaken to exclude secondary causes and other conditions which can give painful red extremities (Table 103.7).

Management

Treatment is largely symptomatic. There are no large trials comparing supportive measures. The management of erythromelalgia is outlined in Table 103.8.

TELANGIECTASES

Definition and nomenclature

Telangiectases (Latin: *tel* = end + Greek: *angos* = vessel + ectasis from Greek: *ektasis* = expansion) are chronically dilated capillaries or venules.

Synonyms and inclusions
• Telangectasia

Introduction and general description

Telangiectases appear on the skin and mucous membranes as small, dull red, linear, stellate or punctate markings. They represent dilatations (expansion, stretching) of pre-existing vessels without any apparently new vessel growth (angiogenesis) occurring. As such, telangiectases can be bracketed with spider angioma (spider naevi) and capillary aneurysm–venous lakes, whereas vascular malformations represent anomalies of

Table 103.9 Causes of telangiectases.

Primary telangiectases	Secondary telangiectases
Generalized essential telangiectasia	Prolonged vasodilatation (rosacea, venous disease, calcium-channel blocking drugs, smoking)
Hereditary benign telangiectasia	
Hereditary haemorrhagic telangiectasia	
Unilateral naevoid telangiectasia	Chronic UV exposure (ageing skin) and post irradiation
Ataxia-telangiectasia	
Bloom syndrome	Post-traumatic
Vascular naevi (naevus flammeus)	Atrophy (poikiloderma and steroid induced)
Angiomas and angiokeratomas	
Angioma serpiginomum	Collagen vascular disease
Mycosis fungoides and angiotrophic lymphoma	Raynaud phenomenon, CREST syndrome, scleroderma, morphoea lupus erythematosus
Spider naevi	
Naevus anaemicus with telangiectatic vessels	Dermatomyositis
	Mastocytosis: telangiectasia macularis eruptiva perstans
Cutis marmorata telangiectatica	HIV infection
Solitary plaque-like telangiectatic glomangioma	Miscellaneous genodermatoses
	Spider naevi

CREST, calcinosis, Raynaud phenomenon, oesophageal dysmotility, sclerodactyly and telangiectasia.

embryological development (disturbances in vasculogenesis or angiogenesis). Hamartomas include proliferation of other tissue elements, for example melanocytic or eccrine cells, and are not solely vascular [1].

Pathophysiology

The telangiectases are a heterogeneous group of disorders. They can be broadly divided into primary and secondary according to their aetiology though one of the commonest naevi (spider naevi) can be both (Table 103.9). They have varying clinical appearances and are different structurally (Table 103.10).

Table 103.10 Telangiectases with their underlying histology.

Generalized essential telangiectasia (Figure 103.10a,b)	Dilatation of the postcapillary venules of the upper horizontal (subpapillary) plexus
Naevus flammeus (Figure 103.11)	
Angiokeratomas of Fabry and Fordyce (Figure 103.12a,b)	Ultrastructure of the collecting venules shows ectopic development of small valve-containing collecting veins
Hereditary haemorrhagic telangiectasia (Figure 103.13)	Microvascular arteriovenous anastomoses
Cherry angiomas	Spherical and tubular dilatations of capillary loops in the dermal papillae with tortuous cross-connections between individual loops
Telangiectasia macularis eruptiva perstans	Subtle increase in mast cell numbers; mast cells loosely arranged around the dilated vessels of the superficial plexus

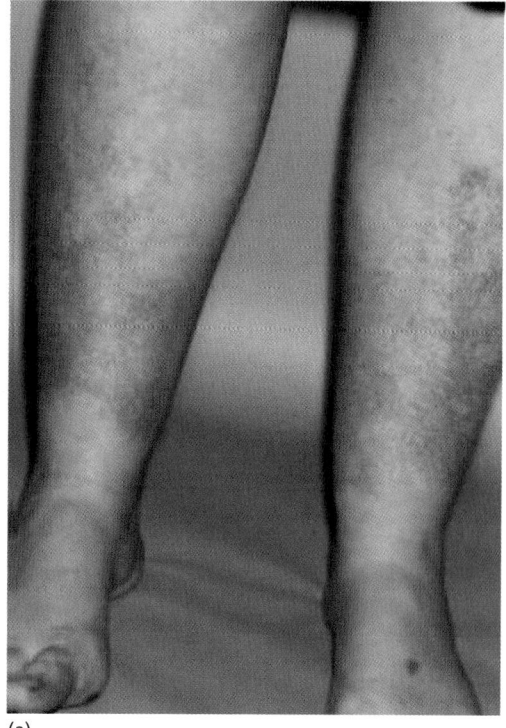

(a)

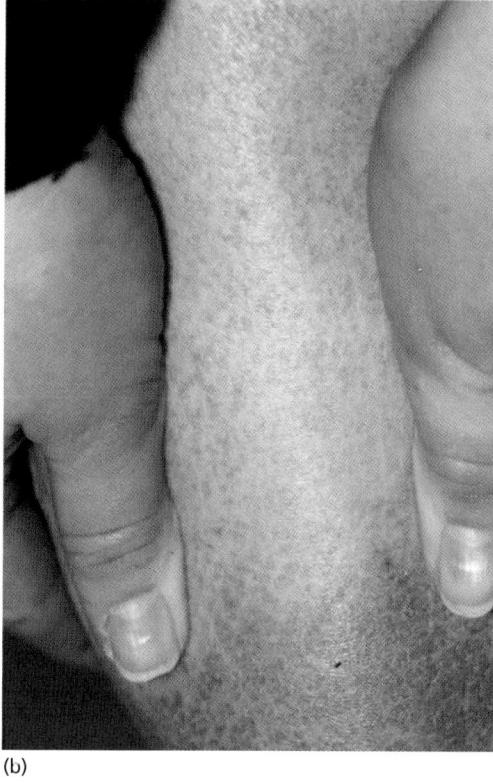

(b)

Figure 103.10 (a) Generalized essential telangiectasia; (b) generalized essential telangiectasia showing blanching with pressure.

PART 9: VASCULAR

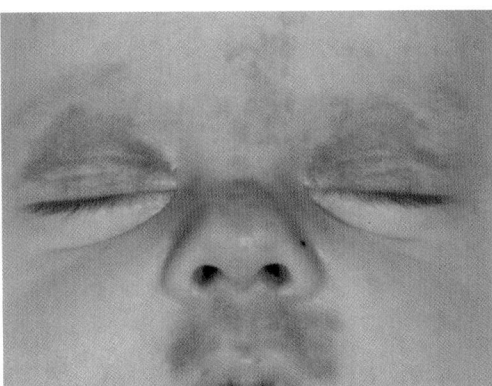

Figure 103.11 Naevus flammeus.

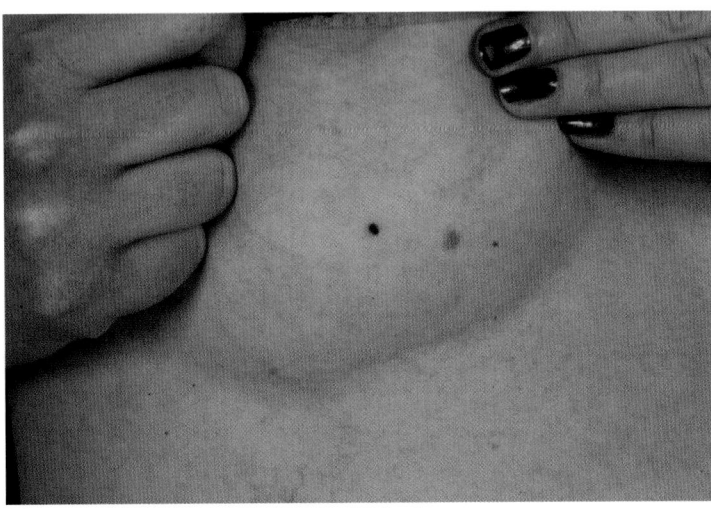

(a)

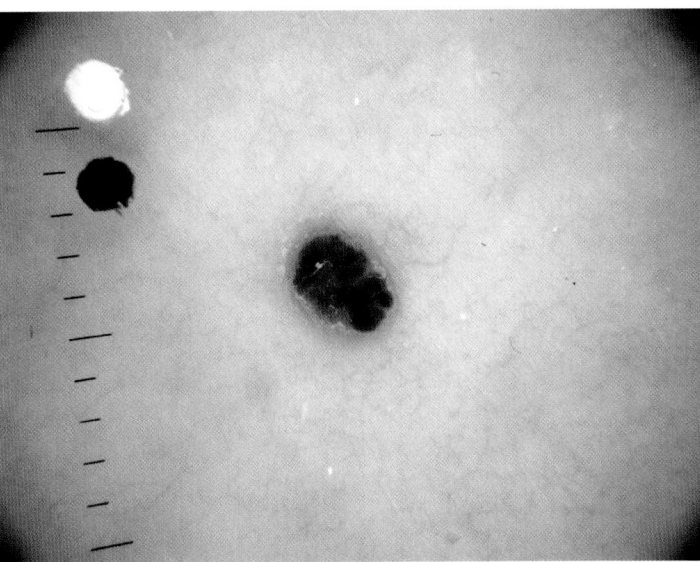

(b)

Figure 103.12 (a) Angiokeratoma; (b) dermoscopic view of angiokeratoma.

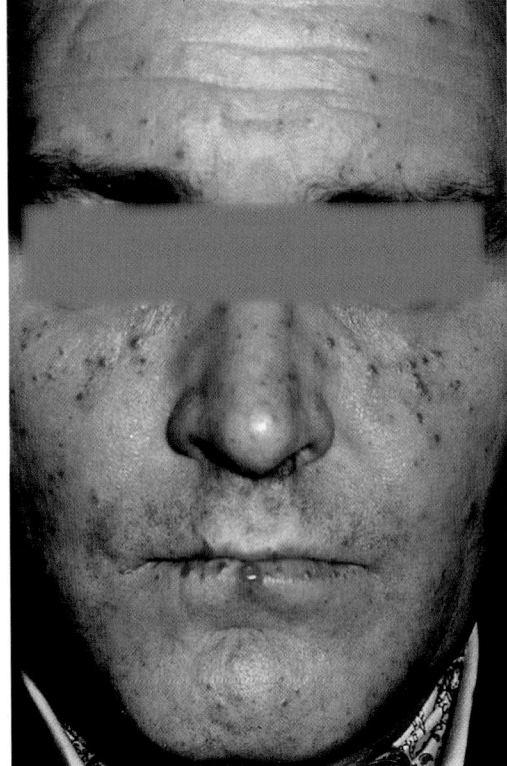

Figure 103.13 Hereditary haemorrhagic telangiectasia.

Spider telangiectases

Definition and nomenclature

These are common small vascular lesions found on the skin of the upper body which are benign. They have a characteristic appearance which can resemble a spider.

> **Synonyms and inclusions**
> - Arterial spider
> - Spider naevus
> - Naevus araneus
> - Spider angioma

Introduction and general description

Spider telangiectases may be solitary or multiple. Their characteristic appearance is due to a central red arteriole (which resembles the body of the spider) surrounded by a circular pattern of thin-walled capillaries (which look like the multiple legs of a spider).

Epidemiology

Incidence and prevalence

Spider telangiectases occur in up to 15% of completely normal persons [1].

Table 103.11 Clinical features of spider telangiectases.

History	Lesions appear suddenly. They are asymptomatic but can be a cosmetic issue
Presentation	Single or multiple
	1–1.5 mm in diameter
	The central body may be raised, and is usually pulsatile on diascopy
	Found on upper body: neck, face, arms and chest , etc. (in the territory of the superior vena cava)
	Often on the hands and fingers in children
	Sometimes at sites of trauma
	May be unilateral [7]
	Classically, when the central arteriole is compressed, the skin blanches and the lesion temporarily vanishes but rapidly returns when the pressure is released (Figure 103.14)
Clinical variants	Can rarely occur on the mucous membranes of the lips and nose
Differential diagnosis	The typical morphology, with a central pulsating vessel, does not occur in other conditions
	In hereditary haemorrhagic telangiectasia, the lesions are macular, punctate or linear; when they are stellate they do not pulsate
Complications and co-morbidities	Trauma may cause bleeding but this stops with simple pressure
	Liver disease
	Number of telangiectases (>20), size (>15 mm) and atypical distribution of lesions (lower body) can predict severity of liver disease and risk of complications such as bleeding varices [8,9,10]
Disease course and prognosis	Lesions can spontaneously resolve in healthy adults and children
	Lesions may disappear at the end of the pregnancy, or with resolution of the liver disorder

Age
They are a frequent finding in healthy children [2].

Sex
Commoner in women (especially when pregnant or on the oral contraceptive pill).

Ethnicity
No difference in racial groups has been reported but the lesions are much more visible in patients with less pigmented skins.

Associated diseases
They occur in large numbers during pregnancy – one or more spider naevi are found in two-thirds of all pregnant women [1]. They may appear in the first few months, but tend to increase in number until term; they usually disappear within 6 weeks of delivery but may persist or recur in the same sites in subsequent pregnancies. They are also characteristically found in patients with liver disease, when they can be a presenting sign [3] and in thyrotoxicosis.

Pathophysiology

Pathology
The main vessel of the spider telangiectasis is an arteriole. The blood flows from this to the periphery, and then passes into a capillary network [4]. The pressure in spider telangiectases rises to 40 mmHg. The lesions consist of a central, ascending, spiral, thick-walled arteriole which ends in a thin-walled ampulla just beneath the epidermis. From the ampulla, thin-walled branching channels radiate peripherally in the papillary dermis. Glomus cells have been described in the wall of the central arteriole [5]. Therefore these lesions actually resemble microarteriovenous malformations. The high oestrogen states that predispose to the lesions (pregnancy and liver disease) are thought to induce vasodilatation of the central arteriole [6].

Clinical features
The clinical features of spider telangiectases are described in Table 103.11.

Investigations
An approach to investigating patients with spider telangiectases in outlined in Table 103.12.

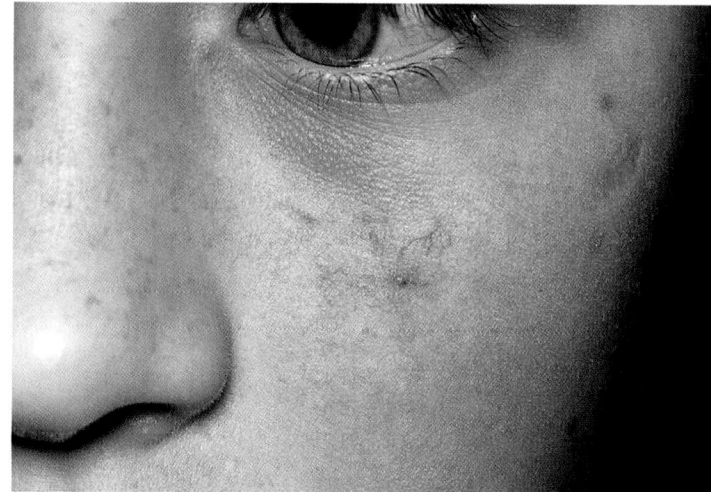

Figure 103.14 Spider telangiectases. Classically, when the central arteriole is compressed, the skin blanches and the lesion temporarily vanishes but rapidly returns when the pressure is released.

Table 103.12 Investigation of patients with spider telangiectases.

Healthy children and adults with single lesions or only a few typical lesions	No investigations needed
Multiple lesions: examine for clinical signs of pregnancy, liver disease or thyrotoxicosis	When concerned about underlying disease: • Blood tests: full blood count, urea and electrolytes, liver function tests, autoantibody screen, hepatitis viral serology, thyroid function tests, α-fetoprotein • Liver: ultrasound if clinical examination and/or blood tests suggests liver disease

Table 103.13 Management of spider telangiectases.

First line	Conservative approach (especially in children and pregnant patients) Many lesions resolve spontaneously Identify and treat underlying disease Cosmetic camouflage
Second line	Electrodessication (small risk of a depressed scar if overtreated and may recur if undertreated) Laser: 585-nm pulsed dye laser produces a high rate of initial clearance [11] but may recur and require a second treatment. Laser is non-scarring but produces purpura KTP 532-nm laser is also highly effective with no post-treatment purpura [12]

Management

Spider telangiectases are asymptomatic and may resolve spontaneously. When on the face, they can be a cosmetic issue. Management is outlined in Table 103.13.

Cherry angiomas

Definition and nomenclature

These are very common, cherry red papules seen in the skin due to abnormal vascular proliferations.

Synonyms and inclusions
• Cherry haemangioma
• Campbell de Morgan spots
• Senile angiomas

Introduction and general description

Cherry angiomas are the commonest angiomas seen in the skin. They are entirely benign and increase in numbers with age.

Epidemiology

Incidence and prevalence

The actual incidence of cherry angiomas is not known. They are very common. One study reported that cherry angiomas were observed in 5% of adolescents and 75% of adults over 75 years of age [1].

Age

They normally spontaneously appear in middle age and increase in number with age though they can first appear in the second decade of life.

Sex

There is no difference between the sexes in the prevalence of cherry angiomas.

Ethnicity

They occur in all ethnic groups, though are more obvious in patients with less pigmented skins.

Associated diseases

There are no significant disease associations although they have been reported to appear in pregnancy [2].

Pathophysiology

Pathology

Cherry angiomas are true capillary haemangiomas, formed by numerous, newly formed capillaries with narrow lumens and prominent endothelial cells arranged in a lobular pattern in the papillary dermis. One study has suggested a possible molecular basis for their pathogenesis. The level of MicroRNA424 is reduced in cherry angiomas when compared to normal skin. This is thought to lead to increased expression of MEK1 and Cyclin E1 which *in vitro* causes endothelial cells to proliferate and could possibly result in the vascular proliferations which make up cherry angiomas [3].

Environmental factors

Exposure to chemicals such as bromides, solvents and mustard gas has been associated with the development of cherry angiomas [4,5,6].

Clinical features

History

They appear as small asymptomatic red dots on the skin usually in the third and fourth decade of life. They often start as pin prick sized lesions which gradually grow. They increase in numbers with increasing age.

Presentation

They may be single or multiple lesions predominantly on the upper trunk and arms [7]. They can arise anywhere on the skin, although rarely on the hands and feet and not on the mucous membranes. Typically, they appear as round to oval, bright red, dome-shaped papules and pinpoint macules varying from less than 1 mm in diameter and up to several millimetres in diameter (Figure 103.15). The larger lesions may be purple in colour.

Differential diagnosis

This includes angiokeratomas, infantile haemangiomas, bacillary angiomatosis and blue rubber bleb naevus syndrome.

Figure 103.15 Cherry angioma.

Complications and co-morbidities
If traumatized cherry angiomas may bleed. They are not associated with underlying disease.

Disease course and prognosis
These lesions are benign and increase in number with age.

Investigations
The diagnosis is usually made clinically, but a biopsy can be confirmatory in doubtful cases.

Management
No treatment is needed in most cases as cherry angiomas are benign and asymptomatic. For lesions that are bleeding, or cosmetically troubling, treatment options include shave excision, hyfrecation, cryotherapy and pulsed dye laser and intense pulsed light [8].

Angiokeratomas

Definition
These are small benign cutaneous vascular lesions which present as red/blue or purple papules.

Introduction and general description
Angiokeratomas are not true angiomas but occur in existing vessels and are characterized by superficial vascular ectasia and overlying acanthosis or hyperkeratosis. They may be solitary or diffuse. There are many different clinical types with similar histology. The main ones are as follows:
- Angiokeratoma of Mibelli – acral skin.
- Angiokeratoma of Fordyce – scrotal skin (see Chapter 111).
- Angiokeratoma corporis diffusum – seen in Fabry disease (see Chapters 81 and 153).

- Angiokeratoma circumscriptum – usually congenital, associated with naevus flammeus, cavernous haemangioma.
- Solitary or multiple angiokeratomas.

Angiokeratoma circumscriptum

These are usually solitary and asymptomatic benign lesions.

Epidemiology

Incidence and prevalence
This is not known, though they are much rarer than other telangiectases such cherry angiomas and spider naevi.

Age
The lesions may be congenital or acquired and therefore can be present at birth. They are more frequently seen in childhood and early adulthood.

Sex
They are commoner in females than males (3 : 1 ratio).

Ethnicity
There is no known ethnic variation in this condition.

Associated diseases
Angiokeratoma circumscriptum may coexist with other types of angiokeratomas and with Klippel–Trenaunay syndrome (KTS), naevus flammeus, cavernous haemangiomas and traumatic arteriovenous fistulas.

Pathophysiology

Pathology
There is a thin layer of hyperkeratosis with papillomatosis and slight acanthosis of the overlying epidermis. There are dilated thin-walled vascular spaces encircled by elongated rete ridges filled with red blood cells. There may be associated telangiectasia in the subcutis.

Genetics
These are not thought to be genetically determined unlike the lesions characteristic of Fabry disease (angiokeratoma corporis diffusum)

Clinical features

History
Generally, these lesions are solitary (though multiple lesions may occur in adulthood) and usually occur on the lower extremities. However, they can occur anywhere on the skin including the tongue and may be multiple and even distributed in band-like formation. They are largely asymptomatic but patients usually present because the lesion has gone very dark or black in colour and there is a concern about it being a malignant melanoma.

PART 9: VASCULAR

Presentation

Angiokeratomas are usually red/blue or purple in colour, sometimes with a slightly rough surface (Figure 103.12). They may appear black if they have thrombosed or if they have been traumatized and bled. Lesions vary from small papules to larger plaques. Dermoscopy can be helpful in revealing blood-filled vascular spaces (Figure 103.12b).

Differential diagnosis

This includes other angiokeratomas, malignant melanoma and cherry angiomas.

Complications and co-morbidities

Trauma may lead to bleeding and/or thrombosis.

Disease course and prognosis

The lesions are benign and generally resolve spontaneously.

Investigations

No investigations are needed for isolated lesions. If there are multiple lesions, Fabry disease should be considered and genetic testing undertaken.

Management

None is needed if the lesions are asymptomatic. If there is diagnostic difficulty, they can be surgically excised. Other treatment modalities that can be adopted are hyfrecation for superficial and small lesions and curettage and cautery and cryotherapy. Different lasers have been used (argon, carbon dioxide, erbium) but the KTP laser or 800-nm diode laser appears to be both effective and the least scarring thus giving the best cosmetic result [1].

Resources

Further information

http://www.pcds.org.uk/clinical-guidance/angiokeratoma

Patient resources

http://dermnetnz.org/vascular/angiokeratoma.html
(All last accessed March 2015.)

Venous lakes

Definition and nomenclature

Venous lakes are composed of dilated venules. They are dark purple/blue papules that appear on the face, lips and ears of elderly patients.

Synonyms and inclusions
• Phlebectases

Introduction and general description

Though venous lakes are entirely benign they can clinically mimic melanoma.

Epidemiology

Incidence and prevalence

The incidence of venous lakes is unknown. A study from a dermatology clinic in Italy identified the prevalence of venous lakes of the lips as 3.7% over a 10-month period [1].

Age

Venous lakes occur in the elderly. The mean age has been reported to be variously 65 [2] and 76.7 years [1].

Sex

They are commoner in men; early studies suggested 95% occurred in men [2] though a more recent report found the male to female ratio to be 1.5 : 1 [1]. Women may present for treatment more readily than men.

Ethnicity

There is no known racial predilection for this condition.

Associated diseases

Menni *et al.* [1] showed a significant increase in solar keratoses in patients with venous lakes.

Pathophysiology

Pathology

Venous lakes are dilated venules. The lesions consist of a single layer of flattened endothelial cells and a thick wall of fibrous tissue. There is often elastosis in the surrounding tissue.

Environmental factors

Sunshine and ageing have been thought to be triggers, and possibly smoking [1,2].

Clinical features

History

The patient usually presents with a painless dark purple/blue papule often on the lip (Figures 103.16 and 103.17) which bleeds if traumatized.

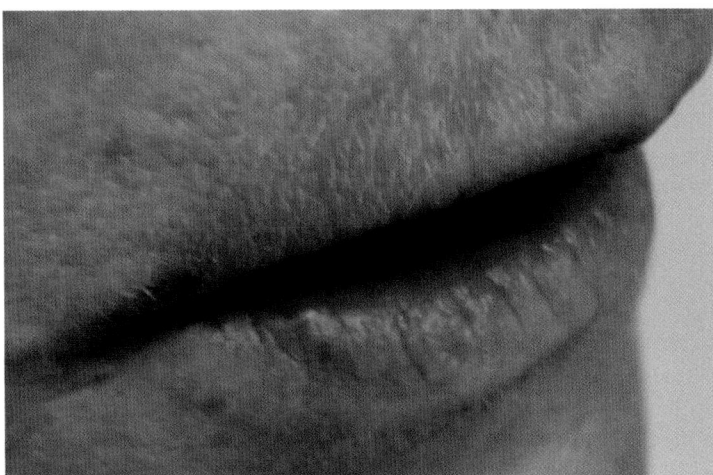

Figure 103.16 Small venous lake.

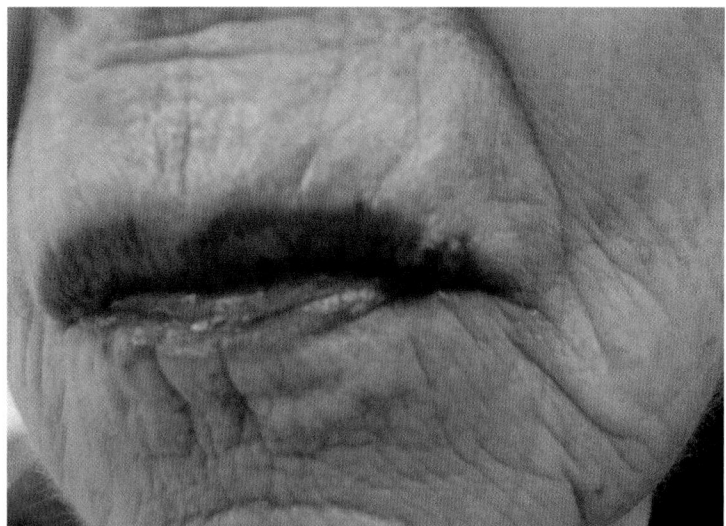

Figure 103.17 Larger venous lakes on upper and lower lips.

Presentation

The papule is soft and compressible. They are usually single but multiple lesions can occur. The commonest sites are the ears, face and lips [2]. If they occur on the lips, the lower lip is the commonest site [1].

Differential diagnosis

The fact that they can be emptied by compression usually excludes malignant melanoma on clinical grounds. Cherry angiomas and angiokeratomas can be similar clinically.

Complications and co-morbidities

Venous lakes are benign and usually asymptomatic but occasionally when traumatized they will bleed and cosmetically they can be an issue for patients.

Disease course and prognosis

Untreated venous lakes persist.

Investigations

None are necessary but biopsy can be confirmatory if the diagnosis is in doubt.

Management

Treatment is only needed if the patient is having problems with bleeding or finds the lesions cosmetically disabling. The lesions can be excised, treated with cryotherapy or laser [3,4,5]. Many different lasers have been used (such as argon, carbon dioxide, pulsed dye and potassium titanyl phosphate lasers). The more destructive the laser treatment, the more likely it is to be effective; however, the risks of scarring are increased.

Resources

Further information

http://www.pcds.org.uk/clinical-guidance/venous-lake (last accessed March 2015).

Primary telangiectasia

Angioma serpiginosum

Definition

Angioma serpiginosum is a rare naevoid disorder affecting the small vessels of the upper dermis.

Introduction and general description

This is a benign vascular condition characterized by small red puncta that cluster together in linear, serpiginous or gyrate patterns, chiefly on the lower limbs in females.

Epidemiology

Incidence and prevalence

This is not known.

Age

The condition may be present at birth and often starts in childhood. Eighty per cent of cases occur before the age of 20 years.

Sex

Ninety per cent of cases occur in females.

Ethnicity

There is no racial predilection for this condition.

Associated diseases

There is one report of a family whose members had oesophageal papillomatosis associated with angioma serpiginosum inherited in an X-linked dominant fashion with the genetic defect linking to Xp11.3-Xq12 [1].

Pathophysiology

Pathology

Generally, it is thought that the condition results from a vascular malformation or neoplasm and is not just a simple telangiectasia. The classical puncta of angioma serpiginosum are caused by either congenital hyperplasia or ectasia of pre-existing superficial dermal capillaries. Histology shows that the affected papillae are distended by a large single ectatic capillary, lined by flattened endothelial cells of normal appearance. Inflammatory changes are not present. Sometimes the vascular spaces disappear due to thrombosis.

Genetics

Most cases are sporadic. However, both autosomal dominant and X-linked dominant inheritance has been recorded and *PORCN* gene mutations or deletions have been reported [2,3].

PART 9: VASCULAR

Table 103.14 Clinical features of angioma serpiginosum.

History	Onset usually in early childhood
	Asymptomatic
	One or more small lesions that grow over a period of months or years
	Growth is irregular with little dots that form satellites that later coalesce
	Predominantly found on the lower limbs and extremities but can be extensive [4]
	Not reported on the hands or mucosae [2]
Examination	Pinpoint violaceous or red macules (may be non-blanching)
	Grouped in areas a few centimetres across, or sometimes form large sheets
	May be annular, serpiginous or linear (Figure 103.18a,b)
	No bleeding, inflammation or pigmentation
	Dermoscopy: well-demarcated red oval or round lagoons can be seen
Clinical variants	Rarely natural resolution leads to atrophic areas [5]
Differential diagnosis	Capillary haemangioma
	Angiokeratomas
Complications and co-morbidities	None
Disease course and prognosis	Lesions often stop growing at puberty and remain unchanged
	Occasionally, they may partially resolve spontaneously

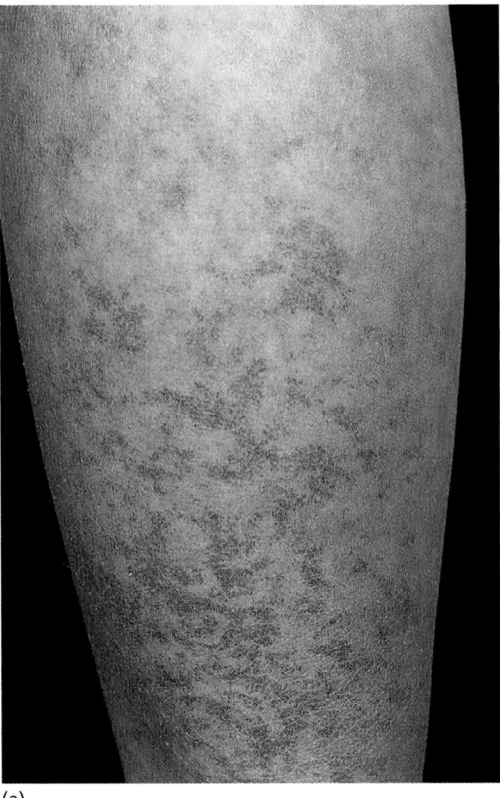

(a)

Clinical features

These are described in Table 103.14.

Investigations

If the diagnosis is in doubt, skin biopsy and imaging can be performed.

Management

Angioma serpiginosum is benign and asymptomatic. Treatment is only indicated for cosmetic reasons. Cosmetic camouflage can be helpful, treatment with pulsed dye laser can be effective [6].

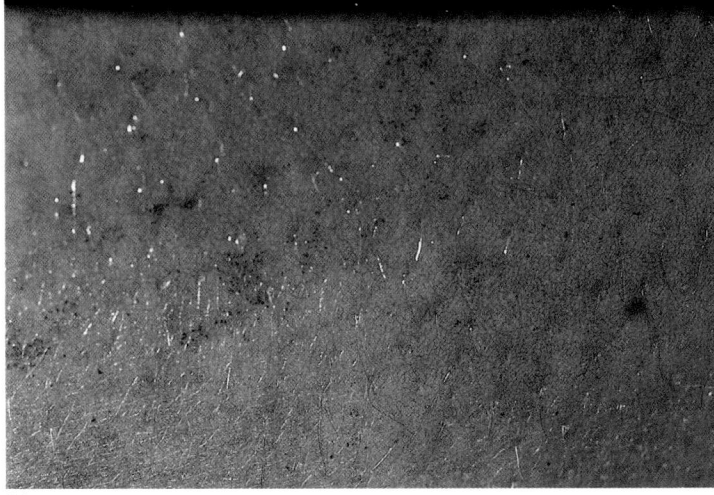

(b)

Figure 103.18 Angioma serpiginosum: (a) grouped lesions, and (b) close up appearance.

Resources

Patient resources

http://dermnetnz.org/vascular/angioma-serpiginosa.html
(last accessed March 2015).

Generalized essential telangiectasia

Definition

This is a syndrome of primary acquired telangiectases with a widespread cutaneous distribution of lesions.

Introduction and general description

This is a benign, non-inherited condition chiefly distinguished from hereditary haemorrhagic telangiectasia by the distribution of the lesions, their arrangement into sheets and the usual lack of bleeding from the lesions.

Epidemiology

Incidence and prevalence

This not known. It is not commonly reported in the literature.

PART 9: VASCULAR

Age
It commonly starts in late childhood or early adult life, although one report of 13 patients found the mean age of onset to be 38 years [1].

Sex
It is much commoner in women (10 out of 13 were females in a study [1]).

Ethnicity
There is no known racial predilection for this condition. Reported cases have largely been in patients with less pigmented skin which may just reflect the fact that the telangiectasia are less noticeable in darkly pigmented skins.

Associated diseases
No known disease associations occur with this condition.

Pathophysiology
The aetiology and pathogenesis of this condition is unknown.

Pathology
There is chiefly dilatation of the capillaries with some dilated post-capillary venules of the upper horizontal (subpapillary) plexus. There are no associated epidermal or dermal changes.

Genetics
There is no known genetic basis for this condition.

Environmental factors
The role of environmental factors in unknown but female hormones, trauma and UVB have been postulated to be of importance [2,3].

Clinical features

History
The eruption frequently starts on the lower limbs as individual lesions but spreads to form red confluent sheets comprised of blanching telangiectasia. It is usually asymptomatic but tingling and numbness has occasionally been reported.

Presentation
The eruption is usually symmetrical. Early lesions are small red or pink linear telangiectases with occasional larger macules arranged in groups. The lesions spread over the skin to become large erythematous sheets and individual telangiectasia can be difficult to distinguish (Figure 103.19). There is a predilection for the lower body but they can occur anywhere and occasionally mucosal and conjunctival lesions have been reported [4]. The sheeted telangiectasiae are usually fixed but will blanch on pressure.

Differential diagnosis
This includes hereditary haemorrhagic telangiectasia, hereditary benign telangiectasia and telangiectasiae triggered by calcium-channel blockers.

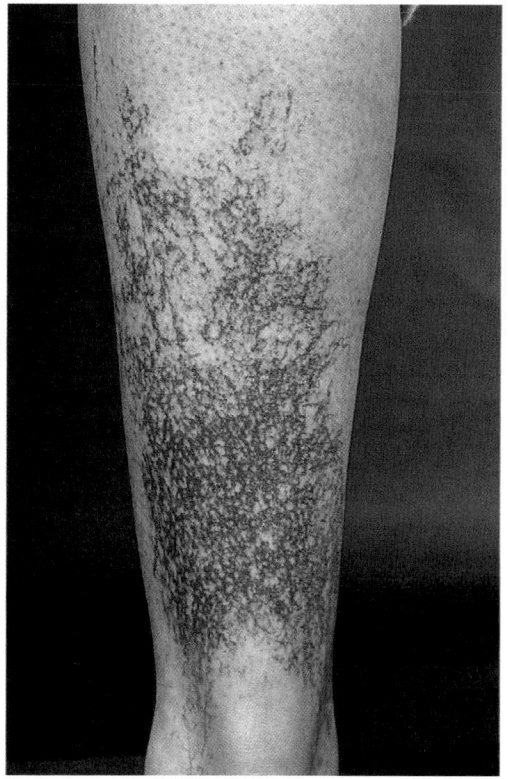
(a)

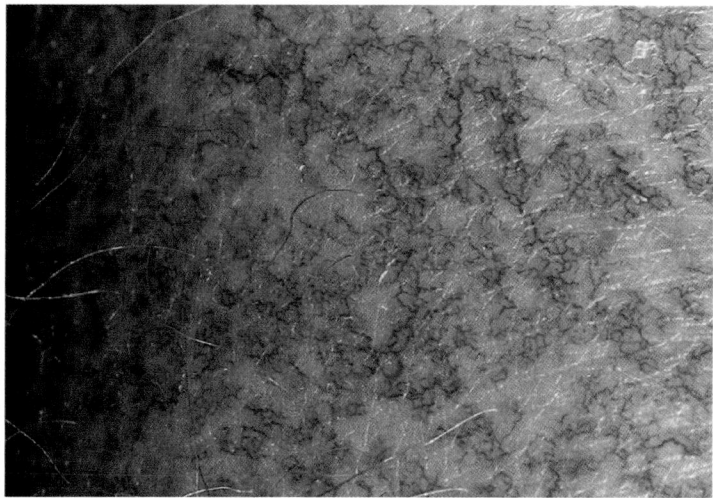
(b)

Figure 103.19 Benign essential telangiectasia: (a) arborizing pattern, and (b) close up appearance.

Disease course and prognosis
This benign condition is progressive and the lesions become fixed with time.

Investigations
None are needed.

Management
Treatment is largely for cosmetic issues. Skin camouflage creams can be helpful but laser (pulsed dye and ND-Yag) treatment is

PART 9: VASCULAR

often attempted. However, the lesions are often so widespread that multiple treatments are needed and those on the lower leg are often very resistant to treatment [5]. Sclerotherapy is not feasible due to the size and number of lesions.

Hereditary benign telangiectasia

This disorder probably has a dominant inheritance [1] and has been mapped to the CMC1 locus for capillary malformation on chromosome 5q14 [2]. It is characterized by the presence of extensive telangiectases, resembling generalized essential telangiectasia, which start in childhood and occur without systemic lesions [3,4]. Less commonly, the telangiectases may be present at birth [5]. They tend to occur more in light-exposed skin. Histology and electron microscopy have been used to distinguish this condition from hereditary haemorrhagic telangiectasia [6]. Distinction from hereditary haemorrhagic telangiectasia is dependent on the lack of bleeding, although lesions do appear related to arteriovenous anastomoses as in hereditary haemorrhagic telangiectasia [7].

Unilateral naevoid telangiectasia syndrome

Definition and nomenclature
A condition of telangiectasiae occurring in a Blaschkoid distribution on the skin.

Synonyms and inclusions
• Unilateral dermatomal superficial telangiectasia

Introduction and general description
This condition was first described by Blaschko in 1899. It may be congenital or acquired and runs a benign course.

Epidemiology

Incidence and prevalence
This is not known. There have been fewer than 100 reported cases [1] but it is not thought to be that uncommon [2].

Age
The congenital form appears during or shortly after the neonatal period. The acquired form often starts at puberty or during pregnancy but can occur at any time.

Sex
The congenital form is commoner in males but the acquired form is much commoner in females.

Ethnicity
There is no racial predilection reported.

Associated diseases
Often there are no associated diseases but in the acquired form it has been seen in patients with liver disease, hyperthyroidism and during pregnancy.

Pathophysiology
The pathogenesis is not understood. The Blaschkoid distribution of the lesions suggests that there is genetic mosaicism that leads to the development of the telangiectasia.

Pathology
Biopsy of lesions shows multiple, dilated, thin-walled vessels lined by pump endothelial cells in the papillary and upper reticular dermis.

Genetics
The congenital form has been reported to be inherited in an autosomal dominant fashion.

Environmental factors
The occurrence of the acquired form of this condition has been reported to be associated with states of oestrogen excess. Increased oestrogen and progesterone receptors have been found by one group in the affected skin [3]. This finding has not been repeated.

Clinical features

History
Patients develop asymptomatic unilateral telangiectases.

Presentation (Figure 103.20)
The telangiectases are often distributed in the third and fourth cervical dermatomes in a Blaschkoid fashion (see Figure 103.23). The lesions are most commonly seen on the upper body especially on the face, neck, shoulder and arm. Sometimes there is a pale ring ('anaemic halo') in the skin surrounding the telangiectases. The lesions blanch on pressure.

Differential diagnosis
Benign essential telangiectasia, angioma serpiginosum.

Complications and co-morbidities
Unilateral naevoid telangiectasia is asymptomatic and benign. There are no complications but it can be associated with high oestrogen states, such as liver disease.

Disease course and prognosis
In most cases of the acquired and congenital form, the lesions are fixed and persist. However, occasionally if the condition is associated with pregnancy or the oral contraceptive pill, the

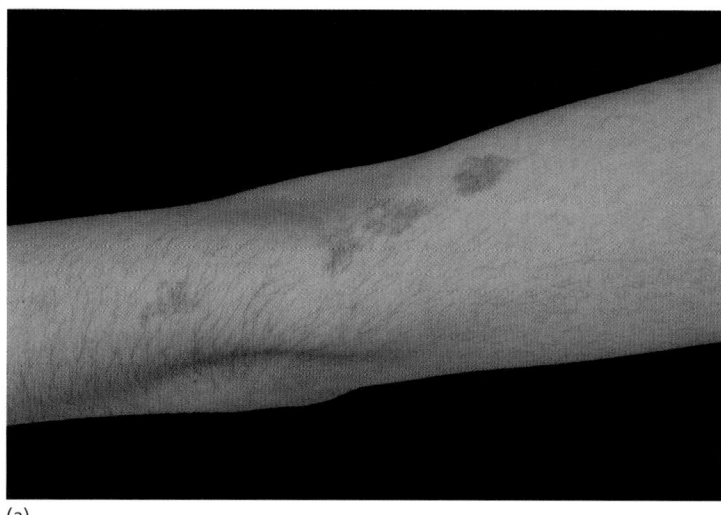

(a)

(b)

Figure 103.20 (a) Unilateral naevoid telangiectasia, and (b) showing grouped lesions in close up.

lesions resolve or improve once the patient's oestrogen levels have fallen.

Investigations
None are necessary but liver function tests and a pregnancy test may be helpful if there are clinical indications of those underlying conditions. A skin biopsy may help if there are diagnostic difficulties.

Management
No treatment is necessary for this benign condition unless the patient finds it cosmetically disabling. Cosmetic camouflage can be helpful. If the patient is pregnant or on the contraceptive pill then waiting to see what happens when the oestrogen levels normalize is advised. Pulsed dye laser can be effective but some authors have reported recurrence [4,5].

MALFORMATIONS

Arteriovenous malformations

Definition and nomenclature
Arteriovenous malformations are fast-flow vascular lesions composed of malformed arterial and venous vessels connected directly to one another without an intervening capillary bed [1,2].

> **Synonyms and inclusions**
> - AV malformations
> - AVMs
> - Arteriovenous anomalies

Introduction and general description
Arteriovenous malformations can occur throughout the body in many different organs and can be fatal in certain instances. For instance, brain arteriovenous malformations account for 1–2% of all strokes. Dermatologists are more likely to encounter arteriovenous malformations when the vasculature affected involves the skin or mucosal surfaces or as an association of hereditary haemorrhagic telangiectasia (see Table 103.15).

Epidemiology

Incidence and prevalence
This is not known for arteriovenous malformations involving the skin but the incidence of brain arteriovenous malformations is ~1/100 000 per year in unselected populations, and the point prevalence in adults is ~18/100 000 [1].

Age
Approximately half are visible in the neonatal period and others become apparent during childhood and adolescence [2].

Sex
There is equal incidence in females and males [2].

Ethnicity
There is no known racial variance in this condition.

Associated diseases
See Table 103.15.

Pathophysiology

Pathology
Arteriovenous malformations consist of arteries connecting directly to veins without the intervening capillary bed. Where

PART 9: VASCULAR

Table 103.15 Conditions associated with arteriovenous malformations.

Condition	Clinical features	Sites of arteriovenous malformations
Familial cases of capillary malformations associated with arteriovenous malformations Autosomal dominant inheritance (inactivating mutation in *RASA1*)	Multiple cutaneous capillary malformations	Subcutaneous, intramuscular, intraosseous and/or cerebral
Parkes Weber syndrome	Soft-tissue and bony hypertrophy associated with the overlying arteriovenous malformation	On an extremity (usually limbs)
Hereditary haemorrhagic telangiectasia (autosomal dominance inheritance)	Epistaxis – spontaneous, recurrent nose bleeds Telangiectases – multiple, at characteristic sites (lips, oral cavity, fingers, nose) Visceral lesions such as gastrointestinal telangiectasia	Lungs, liver, gastrointestinal tract and central nervous system (these may result in massive visceral haemorrhage and death)
Cobb syndrome (cutaneomeningospinal angiomatosis)	Capillary malformation on the skin along the midline of the back	Intraspinal corresponding to the dermatomal distribution of the overlying capillary malformation which may lead to spinal cord damage

they connect is called the nidus. The feeding arteries have a deficient muscularis layer and the draining veins dilate due to the high-velocity blood flow they receive. It is not known how these abnormal connections arise. It is postulated that during early fetal development there of a failure of regression of arteriovenous channels in the primitive plexus that allows these lesions to form which may be due to an aberration in the transforming growth factor β signalling pathway [3].

Genetics
Although most cases of arteriovenous malformations are sporadic, there are a few inherited syndromes whose molecular genetics have been elucidated. A mutation in the gene *RASA1* has been identified on chromosome 5q in families with capillary malformations associated with arteriovenous malformations [4].

Environmental factors
None are known but existing lesions may progress during puberty and pregnancy.

Clinical features
See Table 103.16.

Investigations
1 To confirm the diagnosis and monitor the response to treatment: ultrasound with colour Doppler examination shows low-resistance high-velocity arterial flow, with high diastolic flux, and pulsatile venous flow below the baseline. Arteriovenous shunting is seen within tortuous vessels.
2 To evaluate the extent of the arteriovenous malformation: magnetic resonance imaging (MRI) and magnetic resonance angiography (MRA) demonstrate a collection of vascular flow voids which are the fast-flow vessels that do not enhance with contrast (no tumour aspect); the arteriovenous malformations and its network can be delineated.
If the patient is bleeding, full blood count and clotting studies should be undertaken.

Management
A multidisciplinary approach is essential with specialist vascular surgeons and invasive radiologists and paediatricians where appropriate. Management is challenging. Treatment may be curative but is frequently palliative. Sclerotherapy, embolization and surgery are all options.

Arteriovenous malformations often recur following embolization and surgical resection because incomplete destruction of the lesion leads to rapid recruitment of new vessels from adjacent arteries to supply the nidus, with growth and recurrence of the lesion.

Surgery
The aim of surgery is curative. It may be possible for small and accessible lesions. Sometimes embolization is performed beforehand to reduce intraoperative bleeding.

Embolization
The aim is to temporarily occlude the nidus with either glue or coils. This is usually palliative for bleeding, pain or the control of heart failure or prior to surgery.

Sclerotherapy
Alcohol is injected into the nidus. Sclerotherapy is palliative.

When to treat
For stage I and II arteriovenous malformations in infancy and early childhood, there is no treatment; just monitor (see later for staging system). When the child is older, some clinicians offer surgical resection if the cosmetic result is predicted to be acceptable and the lesion amenable [6]. Follow-up is essential as there is a high rate of recurrence.

For stage II later in childhood, and stage III and IV, surgical treatment (excision and reconstruction) where possible should be considered. However, often the lesions are too deep or extensive for cure and management is only palliative using embolization and partial resection.

Table 103.16 Clinical features of arteriovenous malformations.

History	40–60% are visible at birth
	30% become apparent during childhood
	More common in the head and neck area
	Excessive warmth in the area
	Unusual pain
	Bleeding episodes
Examination	Overlying skin feels warm
	Prominent vessels (Figure 103.21)
	Possible palpable thrill
	Auscultation of the lesion should detect a machinery murmur
Clinical variants	Parkes Weber and Cobb syndrome
Differential diagnosis	Other vascular birthmarks and vascular malformations such as capillary malformations (increased warmth and prominent blood vessels should help make the diagnosis)
	Vascular tumours
	Kaposi sarcoma
Classification of severity (Schobinger staging system)	**Stage I** (quiescent phase)
Patients usually start in stage I in childhood and may remain that way throughout life. Triggers for progression are puberty, pregnancy and trauma	Asymptomatic
	May be clinically not apparent or
	May resemble a port-wine stain or involuting haemangioma
84% may progress to stage II [**5**]	**Stage II** (progressive stage)
	Vascular lesions enlarge and darken
	Lesions deform the integument
	Overlying skin becomes warm
	A pulse or thrill can be palpated
	Stage III (same as stage II plus)
	Deep destruction of tissues occurs with spontaneous necrosis
	Chronic ulceration, pain and haemorrhage
	Stage IV (same as stage III plus)
	Cardiac decompensation due to high-output cardiac failure
Complications	Haemorrhage
	Ischaemia
	Chronic venous insufficiency
	Pain
	Cosmetic deformity
	Limb growth asymmetry
	High output cardiac failure
	Problems related to site of lesion such as impaired vision, difficulty eating or breathing, limb fracture
Disease course and prognosis	Arteriovenous malformations grow with the child
	They do not regress
	It is not known how to predict which patients will go on to stage III and IV
	Morbidity and mortality depends on location, size of lesion (both determine its treatability), presence of severe complications such as heart failure

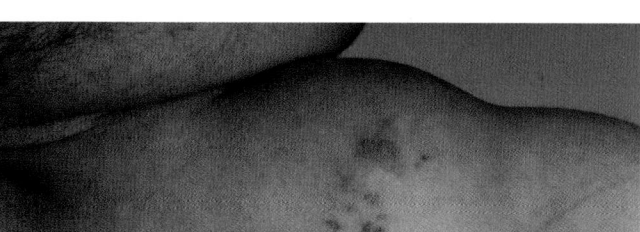

Figure 103.21 Infant with an arteriovenous malformation.

Venous malformations

Solitary venous malformations

Definition and nomenclature
Venous malformations are slow-flow, non-proliferating vascular birthmarks. They are composed of anomalous ectatic venous channels.

Synonyms and inclusions
- Venous angioma
- Cavernous angioma
- Phlebangioma

Introduction and general description

These are the commonest of all vascular anomalies. They are classified as 'slow-flow' lesions. They vary enormously clinically, ranging from single small superficial lesions to deep extensive lesions. They may be single or multiple and can arise in the skin and mucosae and can involve the limbs, the gastrointestinal tract and cranio-facial area. They may be asymptomatic or a major problem for patients with pain, bleeding and disfigurement being the commonest complications.

Epidemiology

Incidence and prevalence

Venous malformations are relatively common and the incidence has been reported to be between 1 and 4% of the population.

Age

The lesions are always present at birth but may not become clinically noticeable until later in childhood as they grow with the child.

Sex

There is no sex difference in venous malformations.

Ethnicity

There is no known racial difference.

Associated diseases

Patients with Turner syndrome may have venous malformations of the intestine and feet. In blue rubber bleb naevus syndrome (Bean syndrome), there are cutaneous and gastrointestinal venous malformations which typically become apparent with age. There may be a risk of severe gastrointestinal haemorrhage. Maffucci syndrome is a rare condition characterized by venous malformations usually on the extremities and dyschondroplasia resulting in enchondromas.

Pathophysiology

The pathogenesis of venous malformations is not understood.

Pathology

The vascular channels of venous malformations are irregular, have narrow lumens lined with flattened endothelial cells and lack smooth muscle cells. The basement membranes are thin and there is no expression of vascular endothelial growth factor or basic fibroblast growth factor.

Genetics

Most cases of venous malformations are sporadic. There have been familial cases of patients with multiple mucosal and cutaneous venous malformations. Genetic analysis has found a mutation in the gene that encodes for the tyrosine kinase domain of the endothelial cell receptor *TIE2* [1]. Others have found somatic mutations in the angiopoietin receptor gene *TEK* associated with solitary sporadic and multiple venous malformations [2].

Environmental factors

Venous malformations do not regress but may expand with trauma, pregnancy and puberty.

Clinical features

The clinical features of venous malformations are outlined in Table 103.17.

Investigations

These are outlined in Table 103.18.

Management

The management of venous malformations depends on the size, depth and complications arising from the lesions [3]. In many cases, the treatment is not curative but supportive. Patients with complex lesions are best managed by multidisciplinary teams in specialist centres. Small localized lesions can be managed with supportive care. Trunk and limb venous malformations are often difficult to manage. Treatment modalities for venous malformations are outlined in Table 103.19. Often treatment modalities may be combined. For instance, for extensive cervico-facial lesions, the lesions may be treated with sclerotherapy, surgical excision and laser.

Table 103.17 Clinical features of venous malformations.

History	Usually visible at birth sometimes just as a blue/purple mark
	May appear more obvious at a later age
	They grow with the child
Presentation	Typically soft blue compressible masses
	More prominent with exercise or
	when the affected area is held in a dependent position
	No palpable thrill
Clinical variants	Glomuvenous malformations (glomangioma)
	Small firmer blue papules or larger pebbly plaques
	Tender to touch
	Pathology: anomalous venous channels lined by cuboidal glomus cells
	Often familial (autosomal dominant) with variable clinical appearance
Differential diagnosis	Haemangiomas (venous malformations do *not* spontaneously regress or go through rapid proliferation phases)
Classification of severity	N/A
Complications and co-morbidities	Pain
	Thrombosis (phleboliths may form even under the age of 2 years)
	Bleeding
	Localized intravascular coagulopathy
	Cervico-facial lesions can cause airway obstruction, speech and dental abnormalities and sinus pericranii
	Limb lesions can be deep and involve muscle, bones and joints with functional difficulty, deformity and pain
Disease course and prognosis	Never regress spontaneously
	Prognosis depends on the lesions' depth and extent and involvement of other organs

Table 103.18 Investigations for venous malformations.

Blood	A full blood count
	Coagulation screen including D-dimers
	Should be undertaken in extensive lesions and if there is bleeding
Plain X-ray	For phleboliths
Direct intralesional injection of contrast	Can outline the vascular anomaly with faint opacification of the draining veins and filling defects at the site of phleboliths
MRI	Most helpful for diagnosis and showing extent of lesion
	Characteristically lobulated margins and round signal voids (due to phleboliths). Contrast enhances lesional tissue and allows differentiation from unenhancing lymphatic malformations
CT scan	Phleboliths seen
	CT with contrast also demonstrates lesion enhancement
Doppler ultrasound	Confirms lesion is 'low flow'
	Assess patency of deep venous system

Table 103.19 Treatment options for venous malformations.

Compression garments (supportive care)	In limb lesions these <ul><li>reduce pain</li><li>protect the overlying skin</li><li>limit swelling</li><li>decrease localized intravascular coagulation</li></ul>
Sclerotherapy (supportive care)	Usually under general anaesthetic by an interventional radiologist
	Multiple sessions are often needed
	Larger lesions usually injected with 95% ethanol
	Smaller lesions injected with 1% sodium tetradecyl sulfate
Laser Nd-YAG and or endovenous laser	This is often used for mucosal lesions
Surgery	Clotting studies and D-dimers should be measured before surgery
	Surgery may be curative in small lesions
	Or to debulk larger lesions

Resources

Patient resources

http://www.gosh.nhs.uk/medical-conditions/search-for-medical-conditions/venous-malformations/venous-malformations-information/ (last accessed March 2015).

Verrucous haemangioma

Definition

This is a congenital vascular anomaly made up of a dermal and subcutaneous capillary vascular component with an overlying warty surface. There has been some debate as to whether it should be classified as a vascular neoplasm [1], though recent evidence supports the original view that it should be regarded as a vascular malformation [2].

Introduction

Verrucous haemangioma was first described in 1967 by Imperial and Hedwig [3], who reported 21 cases and distinguished it from other variants of angiokeratoma and considered it to be a vascular malformation.

Epidemiology [4,5]

Incidence and prevalence

This is a rare condition but the prevalence is unknown.

Age

It is usually noted at birth but can appear during the first 2 years.

Sex

The condition is equal in males and females.

Ethnicity

There is no known racial predilection.

Pathophysiology

The pathogenesis is not understood. The lesions show overlying epidermal hyperkeratosis, papillomatosis and irregular acanthosis with underlying dilated capillary vascular channels in the dermis and also often in the subcutis (Figure 103.22b,c). The vessels are organized in a diffuse or lobular pattern. Most studies show positive staining for GLUT-1 and WT-1, suggesting it is a type of vascular tumour [2]. Recently, however, the largest study to date of 74 patients found most were negative for WT-1 staining, supporting the clinical view that these lesions behave like vascular malformations [5].

Clinical features

History

Over 70% occur on the lower limb but lesions can involve the upper limb and more rarely the trunk; most are solitary.

Presentation

The lesions initially are non-keratotic, soft and bluish-red in colour. They are well-circumscribed linear vascular plaques and vary from a few centimetres to 25 cm in diameter. Over time the surface becomes hyperkeratotic and verrucous (Figure 103.22a). Over 50% are asymptomatic, however the lesions may be painful and itchy.

Differential diagnosis

Angiokeratomas, circumscribed lymphangioma.

Complications and co-morbidities

They may ulcerate and become infected.

Disease course and prognosis

Unlike infantile haemangiomas they do not undergo spontaneous regression and grow in proportion to the child's growth.

Investigations

Skin biopsy and magnetic resonance imaging should be undertaken to confirm the diagnosis and to evaluate the extent of the lesion.

PART 9: VASCULAR

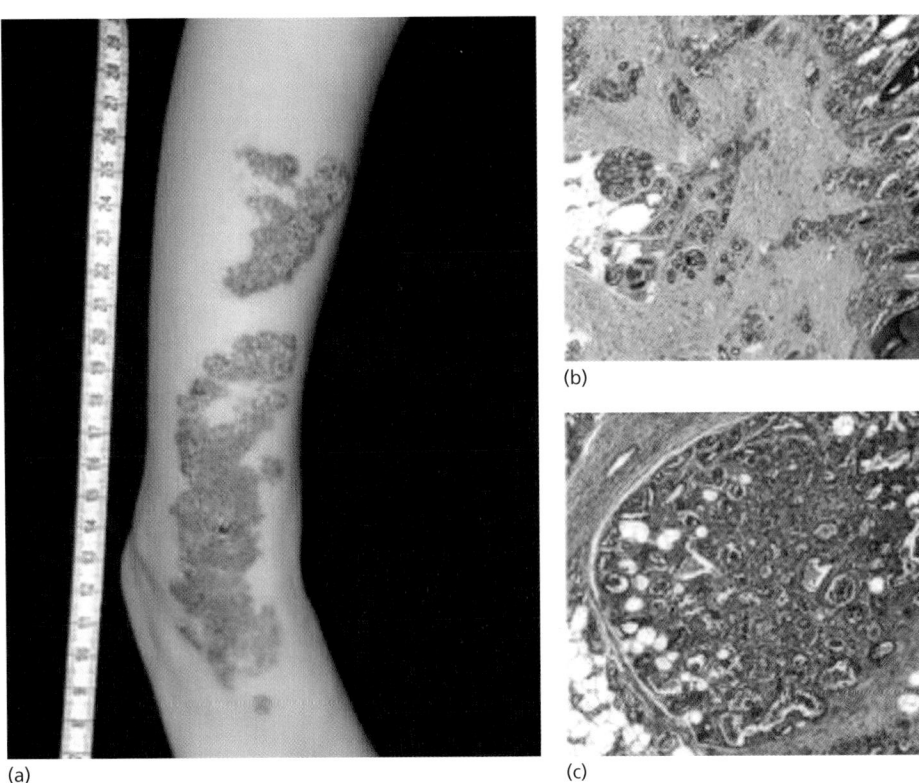

(a)

(b)

(c)

Figure 103.22 Verrucous haemangioma. (a) A linear congenital hyperkeratotic plaque on the lower leg and ankle of a child. (b) Dilated vessels in the superficial dermis and verrucous epidermal hyperplasia. (c) Lobules of capillaries in the subcutaneous tissue. (From Hoeger and Colmenero 2014 [1]. Reproduced with permission from the British Association of Dermatologists.)

Management

Surgery is the treatment of choice. Most can be excised in a single procedure or in stages. However, if lesions are deep and excision is incomplete, recurrence may be a problem. Where excision is not possible, NdYAG laser for plaques and pulsed dye laser for patches can help improve the appearance and relieve symptoms.

Disorders associated with venous malformations

Klippel–Trenaunay syndrome

Definition

Klippel–Trenaunay syndrome is characterized by three features: (i) a capillary malformation (port-wine stain) of the skin associated with (ii) a soft-tissue and bone overgrowth and hypertrophy in combination with (iii) varicose veins, with or without deep venous and lymphatic abnormalities. It can be diagnosed if only two of the three features are present.

Introduction and general description

Klippel–Trenaunay syndrome was first described in 1900, when Maurice Klippel and Paul Trenaunay reported two patients with a capillary malformation, varicosities and hypertrophy of soft tissue and bone in their lower limb [1]. In 1907, Frederick Parkes Weber independently reported several cases similar to those described by Klippel and Trenaunay, though his cases were caused by multiple congenital arteriovenous malformations [2]. KTS most commonly involves the lower limbs, followed by the arms, the trunk and rarely the head and neck. KTS is a congenital condition of unknown aetiology, the management of which is largely supportive [3].

Epidemiology

Incidence and prevalence

It is rare with an incidence <1 : 10 000.

Age

It is a congenital anomaly present at birth but clinically may present later in childhood.

Sex

There is no sex difference in the incidence of KTS.

Ethnicity

There is no known racial predilection.

Pathophysiology

The pathogenesis of KTS is not elucidated. Increased angiogenesis appears to be pivotal.

Pathology

The capillary malformations consist of ectatic capillaries with superficial dilated dermal venules corresponding to nodular lesions within the port-wine stains. When there are lymphatic malformations they appear to be due to lymphatic hypoplasia resulting in lymphatic macrocysts on the pelvis or trunk and microcysts on the abdominal wall, gluteal region and/or limbs. The atypical varicose veins are persistent embryonic veins of the superficial venous system which lack valves and are long and tortuous. The deep venous system is abnormal in 25% of patients with KTS and abnormalities include aneurysmal dilatations, duplications, hypoplasia, aplasia and external compression form anomalous vessels or fibrotic bands. Some patients get perianal and perirectal varicose veins and suprapubic varicose veins can be a sign of atresia of the iliac vein.

Genetics

Most cases of KTS are sporadic. However, there have been reports of a defect in the angiogenic factor VG5Q [4], *RASA1* mutations [5] and a *de novo* supernumerary ring chromosome 18 in KTS patients [6]. A case report of KTS in a monozygotic twin with an unaffected twin suggests the possibility of paradominant inheritance [7].

Clinical features (Figure 103.23)

These are described in Table 103.20.

Investigations

Klippel–Trenaunay syndrome is often diagnosed on the history and examination alone. Physical examination should include auscultation and palpation of the involved area to assess for the presence of an arteriovenous malformation to rule out Parkes Weber syndrome. Duplex ultrasound scanning is the study of choice to evaluate for superficial and deep venous anomalies, and can also be used in differentiating vascular tumours from vascular malformations and arteriovenous fistulae. MRI scans are effective for visualizing the extent of tissue overgrowth of lesions and infiltration of deeper tissues. X-rays may show increased thickness or abnormal density of the affected soft tissue as well as phleboliths. Venograms may be required to delineate the venous abnormality and to exclude deep vein agenesis.

Management

The treatment of KTS is conservative and aimed at relieving the symptoms and preventing the complications of the condition. Patients are often managed best by a multidisciplinary team consisting of the following specialists: paediatricians, dermatologists, vascular surgeons, orthopaedic surgeons, interventional radiologists and pain specialists.

The treatment modalities for KTS are outlined in Table 103.21.

Resources

Patient resources

http://www.gosh.nhs.uk/medical-conditions/search-for-medical-conditions/klippel-trenaunay-syndrome/klippel-trenaunay-syndrome-information/
Patient support group: http://k-t.org/
(All last accessed March 2015.)

Parkes Weber syndrome

Definition

This syndrome was first described by Sir Frederick Parkes Weber in 1907. It is a combined vascular malformation, similar to KTS, characterized by an arteriovenous fistula with varicosities and hypertrophy of the affected extremity. It differs from KTS because of the presence of the arteriovenous fistula and the absence of the

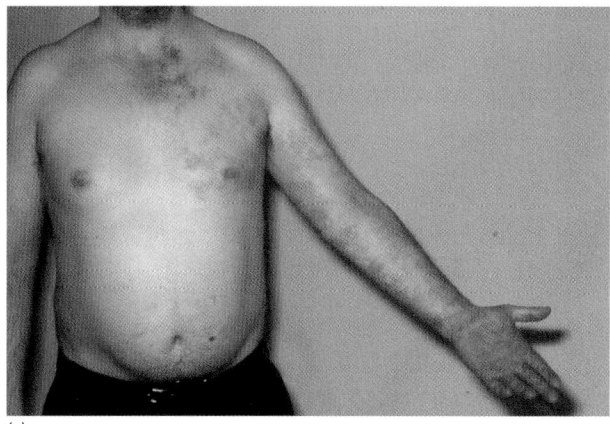
(a)

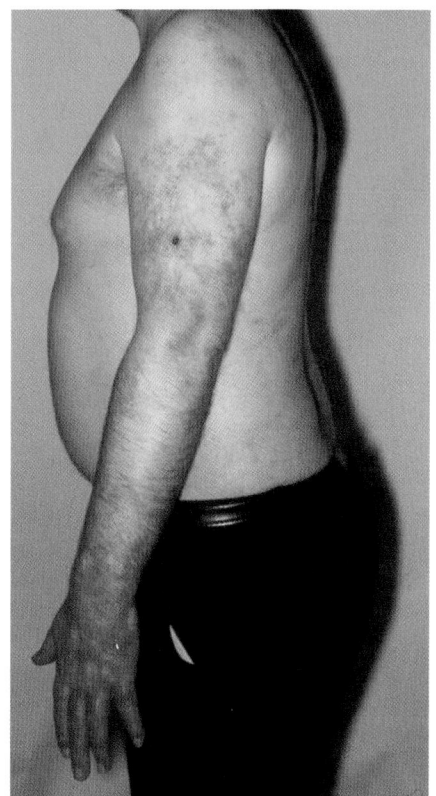
(b)

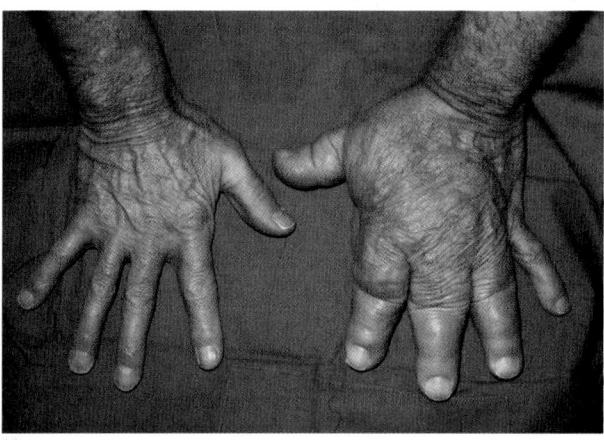
(c)

Figure 103.23 Klippel–Trenaunay syndrome: (a) with capillary/venular malformation; (b,c) abnormal veins and soft-tissue overgrowth.

Table 103.20 Clinical features of Klippel–Trenaunay syndrome (KTS).

History	1 The capillary/venular malformation (port-wine stain); 98% of KTS; usually present at birth; when deep can cause visceral haemorrhage
	2 The abnormal veins; 72%; often not visible until the child is walking; can cause pain, ulceration, thrombosis
	3 Hypertrophy; 67% usually present at birth 63% have all three features and 37% have two out of the three features
Presentation	The capillary/venular malformation (port-wine stain)
	• pink or reddish stain with linear borders, may darken with age to purple
	• 10% are nodular
	• does not cross the midline
	• may be deep and involve underlying organs
	Venous abnormalities
	• dilated tortuous veins
	• if deep venous system involved can lead to skin ulcers and scarring
	Hypertrophy
	• increase in limb girth and/or length
	• bony and soft-tissue enlargement
	• may have hand and feet abnormalities (macrodactyly, syndactyly, ectodactyly, clinodactyly and camptodactyly)
	Lymphoedema
Clinical variants [3]	Simple KTS
	• blotchy or segmental port-wine stain
	• venous malformations and hypertrophy
	Complex KTS
	• geographic port-wine stain
	• venous malformations and hypertrophy
	• higher risk of lymphatic involvement
	• increased risk of complications
Differential diagnosis	Proteus syndrome
	Bannayan–Riley–Ruvalcaba syndrome
	Maffucci syndrome
Classification of severity	N/A
Complications and co-morbidities	Skin
	• stasis dermatitis
	• ulcers
	• secondary infection
	Veins
	• thrombosis
	• thrombophlebitis
	• haemorrhage
	• pulmonary emboli
	Hypertrophy of a limb
	• may lead to subsequent vertebral scoliosis
	• gait problems
	• impaired function
	• premature onset of degenerative joint disease
	Rarer complication depend on the site and depth of the lesions
	Genitourinary haemorrhage
	Gastrointestinal haemorrhage
	Haemothorax
	Pulmonary emboli secondary to venous thrombosis
	Heart failure
	Central nervous system involvement with haemorrhage, infection, hemimegalencephaly, hydrocephalus, atrophy, epilepsy
Disease course and prognosis	Risks of thrombosis and venous complications tend to increase with age

Table 103.21 Management of Klippel–Trenaunay syndrome (KTS).

Compression garments (not helpful in patients with a hypoplastic deep venous system)	To prevent/treat
	• chronic venous insufficiency
	• lymphoedema
	• recurrent cellulitis/ bleeding
Orthotics	To manage asymmetry in the limbs
Orthopaedics	• for small difference in limb length heel inserts can be used
	• larger differences may need osteotomy, epiphysiodesis, epiphyseal stapling
Avoidance of the oral contraceptive pill	To treat and reduce the risk of thrombosis
	• for thrombosis
Anticoagulation	• females with KTS should not use the oral contraceptive pill
	• consider anticoagulation prophylaxis for patients prior to surgical procedures/long haul flights, etc.
Pain management	Pain can be a difficult symptom to relieve and referral to a pain clinic should be considered
Laser	To treat the capillary malformation (port-wine stain) use pulsed dye laser for cosmesis
	• treating ulceration
	To treat the greater saphenous vein to manage varicosities an endovenous laser can be used
Surgery	Treatment of venous malformations and varicosities by venous stripping, ligation, excision and sclerotherapy. This therapy is controversial as there is a high risk of complications and 90% chance of recurrence [8]
	• should only be undertaken if the deep system is normal or shows mild to moderate reflux
	• may help heaviness and recurrent bleeding
	Amputation is a last resort for intractable bleeding, pain or ulceration

following associations: an overlying vascular naevus, a marginal vein malformation and lymphatic malformations. The musculo-skeletal involvement is often less prominent than in KTS [1].

Epidemiology

Incidence and prevalence
This is a rare condition but the prevalence is unknown.

Age
It is present from birth.

Sex
The condition is equal in males and females.

Ethnicity
There is no known racial predilection.

Pathophysiology
The pathogenesis is not fully understood. The pathology of the arteriovenous malformation is described under arteriovenous malformations above.

Genetics

Most cases are sporadic. A mutation in the gene *RASA1* has been identified on chromosome 5q in families with capillary malformations associated with arteriovenous malformations [2].

Clinical features

History

Over 70% occur on the lower limb but Parkes Weber syndrome can involve the upper limb and the head and neck. The tissue overgrowth leads to limb enlargement that continues past puberty and gets progressively worse. There is frequently bone involvement rather than just soft-tissue overgrowth. The arteriovenous malformation may not appear until puberty or after trauma.

Presentation

An obvious pulsatile swelling may be visible with discoloration of the overlying skin and large veins radiating from it. The overlying skin feels warm; there are prominent vessels with a possible palpable thrill. Auscultation of the lesion should detect a machinery murmur. There may be obvious asymmetry of the affected limbs.

Clinical variants

- Capillary malformation – arteriovenous malformation, a new clinical and genetic disorder caused by *RASA1* mutations [2].
- Cloves syndrome (congenital lipomatous overgrowth, vascular malformations, epidermal naevi and scoliosis, seizures and spinal and skeletal abnormalities [3]).

Differential diagnosis

- Klippel–Trenaunay syndrome.
- Proteus syndrome.

Classification of severity

The classification of the severity of arteriovenous malformations is described in Table 103.16.

Complications and co-morbidities

The main risks are complications of the arteriovenous fistula such as tissue ischaemia and high output cardiac failure.

Disease course and prognosis

This is dependent on type, location and severity of the arteriovenous malformation.

Investigations

To confirm the diagnosis and monitor the response to treatment. Ultrasound with colour Doppler examination which shows low-resistance high-velocity arterial flow, with high diastolic flux, and pulsatile venous flow below the baseline and arteriovenous shunting within tortuous vessels.

To evaluate the extent of the arteriovenous malformation. MRI and MRA demonstrate a collection of vascular flow voids which are the fast-flow vessels that do not enhance with contrast (no tumour aspect). The arteriovenous malformation and its network can be delineated.

Management

A multidisciplinary approach is essential with specialist vascular surgeons, invasive radiologists and paediatricians where appropriate. Management is challenging. Treatment is frequently palliative. Sclerotherapy, embolization and surgery are all options. Orthotics and compression garments may help with limb involvement.

VENOUS DISORDERS

Anatomy [1,2,3,4,5,6,7]

Most veins contain semi-lunar valves; these are usually in pairs, but some veins only contain one valve leaflet and sometimes three (tricuspid) valve leaflets are present. These valves are lined by endothelium and are found especially in the smaller veins and at the junction of these veins with larger branches. They prevent the reflux of blood and are particularly important in the leg, where their integrity, and that of the calf muscle pump (the venous heart), counters the gravitational hydrostatic pressure.

There are three venous systems: the deep veins, the superficial veins and the perforating veins (or perforators). The perforating veins are numerous and inconstant, and connect the other two systems. During muscular activity, blood is directed from the superficial to the deep system, up from the foot to the thigh and thence to the abdomen, before venous blood returns towards the heart. Bicuspid valves are found in all three systems. The smallest veins to contain valves lie at the dermal subcutaneous junctions [4] and the valves are extremely variable. Valves may become damaged, thickened or degenerate with age [5]. Thrombosis also causes valvular destruction and a re-canalized post-thrombotic vein is valveless, anatomically distorted and functionally inefficient [5]. The most important perforating veins are considered to be on the medial side of the calf. Incompetence of the valves in these veins has been thought to be important in the causation of venous ulceration [5].

The superficial venous system of the leg begins from the veins on the dorsum of the foot, which join the greater saphenous vein (GSV) (originally called the long saphenous vein) and the short saphenous vein (SSV). They form a dorsal arch, which connects the territory of the SSV with that of the GSV. On the plantar side of the foot, the same venous network joins to a plantar venous arch that also joins both saphenous veins [6,7].

Physiology: the venous macrocirculation [1,2]

Veins act as the capacitance vessels of the circulation. The 'venous return' is the blood returning to the heart via the great veins. Venous return from the lower limbs is achieved by the pumping action of the foot and calf muscles associated with competent valves that prevent backflow [1].

The venous system of the legs contains a volume of 300–350 mL in a healthy standing subject. The venous wall contracts in response to filling, and its function is called 'venous tone'. This acts as counterpressure and automatically changes to attempt to maintain venous pressure at a constant level. The superficial veins drain through the communicating (perforating) veins into the deep system, and only 10% of the venous blood flow from the lower limb passes through the saphenofemoral junction (SFJ).

The deep veins are compressed by each muscle contraction shifting the blood column towards the heart against the pressure of gravity. The venous valves prevent backflow during muscle relaxation. This mechanism is the 'calf muscle pump'. Other muscle groups such as those of the foot also compress veins and aid venous return, but the calf muscle pump is the most important muscle pump of the leg.

Venous thrombosis

Deep-vein thrombosis

Definition
A deep-vein thrombosis (DVT) is a blood clot that forms within the deep veins usually of the leg but can occur in the veins of the arms [1] and in the mesenteric and cerebral veins.

Introduction and general description
Deep-vein thrombosis is a common and important disease. It is part of the venous thromboembolism disorders which represent the third most common cause of death from cardiovascular disease after heart attacks and stroke [2]. Even in patients who do not get pulmonary emboli recurrent thrombosis and 'post-thrombotic syndrome' are a major cause of morbidity.

Epidemiology

Incidence and prevalence
Deep-vein thrombosis and pulmonary emboli are common and often 'silent' and thus go undiagnosed or are only picked up at autopsy. Therefore their incidence and prevalence is often underestimated. It is thought the annual incidence of DVT is 80 cases per 100000 with a prevalence of lower limb DVT of 1 case per 1000 population. Annually in the USA, more than 200000 people develop venous thrombosis; of those, 50000 cases are complicated by pulmonary embolism [3].

Age
Deep-vein thrombosis is rare in children and the risk increases with age, most occurring in the over 40s.

Sex
There is no consensus about whether there is a sexual bias in the incidence of DVT.

Ethnicity
There is evidence from the USA that there is an increased incidence of DVT and an increased risk of complications in African Americans and white people when compared to Hispanics and Asians [4,5].

Table 103.22 Risk factors for deep-vein thrombosis (DVT).

Reduced blood flow	Immobility (bed rest, general anaesthesia, operations, stroke, long haul flights)
Increased venous pressure	Mechanical compression or functional impairment leading to reduced flow in the veins (neoplasm, pregnancy, stenosis, or congenital anomaly which increases outflow resistance)
Mechanical injury to the vein	Trauma, surgery, peripherally inserted venous catheters
	Previous DVT
	Intravenous drug abuse
Increased blood viscosity	Polycythaemia
	Thrombocytosis
	Dehydration
Increased risk of coagulation	
Genetic	Deficiencies in protein C, S or antithrombin III, factor V Leiden
Acquired	Cancer
	Sepsis
	Myocardial infarction
	Heart failure
	Vasculitis, systemic lupus erythematosus and lupus anticoagulant
	Inflammatory bowel disease
	Nephrotic syndrome
	Burns
	Oral oestrogens
	Smoking
	Hypertension
	Diabetes
Constitutional factors	Obesity
	Pregnancy
	Increasing age

Associated diseases
The risk factors for DVT are listed in Table 103.22. In hospital the most commonly associated conditions are malignancy, congestive heart failure, obstructive airways disease and patients undergoing surgery.

Pathophysiology

Pathology
In 1856, Virchow postulated that the main causes of thrombus formation were damage to the vessel wall, alterations in blood flow and hypercoagulability. This is called 'Virchow's triad' and is still valid today.

Maintenance of the fluidity and circulation of the blood and its ability to thrombose are essential for the maintenance of life and are governed by extremely complex homeostatic mechanisms. Thrombosis is a protective mechanism which prevents loss of blood and seals off damaged blood vessels. Fibrinolysis counteracts or stabilizes the thrombosis. The triggers of venous thrombosis are frequently multifactorial, with the different parts of the Virchow triad contributing in varying degrees in each patient, but all resulting in early thrombus interaction with the endothelium. This then stimulates local cytokine production and causes leukocyte adhesion to the endothelium, both of which promote venous thrombosis. Depending on the relative balance between the coagulation and thrombolytic pathways, thrombus propagation occurs.

DVT is commonest in the lower limb below the knee and starts at low-flow sites, such as the soleal sinuses, behind venous valve pockets.

Causes

The risk factors for DVT are shown in Table 103.22.

The most important ones are previous DVT (up to 25% of patients give a previous history of a DVT), active cancer, being postoperative and immobilization. There is now an increasing understanding that the risk factors for DVT often overlap with those of atherothrombosis and that there is a common pathophysiology that includes inflammation, hypercoagulability and endothelial injury [2].

Clinical features (Table 103.23)

Deep-vein thrombosis may be 'silent' in 5% of cases at times making the diagnosis challenging as many patients do not have the classical signs or symptoms; and some of those with 'classical' features do not have DVT when investigated.

Investigations

These are outlined clearly in the National Institute for Health and Care Excellence (NICE) guidelines with a helpful algorithm [7]. Investigations (Table 103.24) that are performed are D-dimers (very sensitive but not very specific) and proximal leg vein ultrasound which when positive indicates that the patient should be treated as having a DVT.

Deciding how to investigate is determined by the 'risk 'of DVT. The first step is to assess the clinical probability of a DVT using the Wells scoring system (Table 103.25). For patients with a score of 0–1 the clinical probability is low but for those with 2 or above the clinical probability is high.

If a patient *scores 2 or above* either a proximal leg vein ultrasound scan should be carried out within 4 h of being requested and, if the result is negative, a D-dimer test should be undertaken. If imaging is not possible within 4 h a D-dimer test should be undertaken and an interim 24-h dose of a parenteral anticoagulant should be given. Then a proximal leg vein ultrasound scan should be carried out within 24 h of being requested.

In the case of a positive D-dimer test and a negative proximal leg vein ultrasound scan, the proximal leg vein ultrasound scan should be repeated 6–8 days later for all patients.

If the patient *does not score 2* on the DVT Wells score but the D-dimer test is positive, the patient should either have a proximal leg vein ultrasound scan carried out within 4 h of being requested. Or again if this is not possible, the patient should receive an interim 24-h dose of a parenteral anticoagulant and a proximal leg vein ultrasound scan should then be be carried out within 24 h of being requested.

In all patients diagnosed with DVT, treat as if there is a positive proximal leg vein ultrasound scan.

Management

The aims of treatment of DVT are to prevent pulmonary embolism, reduce morbidity and prevent or minimize the risk of developing

Table 103.23 Clinical features of deep-vein thrombosis (DVT).

History	Pain (50% of patients)
	Redness
	Swelling (70% of patients)
	Usually of the lower limb but can occur in the arms
Examination	Limb oedema may be unilateral or bilateral if the thrombus is extending to pelvic veins
	Red and hot skin, with dilated veins
	Tenderness
	Pain on dorsiflexion of the foot (the Homans sign)
Clinical variants	In upper limb DVTs
	• 80% have swelling
	• 30% have pain
	• Only 15% have erythema
Differential diagnosis	Cellulitis
	Post-thrombotic syndrome (especially venous eczema and lipodermatosclerosis)
	Ruptured Baker's cyst
	Trauma
	Superficial thrombophlebitis
	Peripheral oedema, heart failure, cirrhosis, nephrotic syndrome
	Venous or lymphatic obstruction
	Arteriovenous fistula and congenital vascular abnormalities
	Vasculitis
Classification of severity	**Provoked**
	Due to acquired states (surgery, oral contraceptives, trauma, immobility, obesity, cancer)
	Unprovoked
	Due to idiopathic or endogenous reasons
	More likely to suffer recurrence if anticoagulation is discontinued
	Proximal (above the knee: affecting the femoral or ileofemoral veins)
	Much more likely to lead to complications such as pulmonary emboli
	Distal (below the knee)
Complications and co-morbidities	Pulmonary emboli (paradoxical emboli if an atrioseptal defect is present)
	Post-thrombotic syndrome
Disease course and prognosis	Many DVTs will resolve with no complications
	Post-thrombotic syndrome [6] occurs in 43% 2 years post-DVT (30% mild, 10% moderate and severe in 3%)
	Risk of recurrence of DVT is high (up to 25%)
	Death occurs in approximately 6% of DVT cases and 12% of pulmonary embolism cases within 1 month of diagnosis
	Early mortality after venous thromboembolism is strongly associated with presentation as pulmonary embolism, advanced age, cancer and underlying cardiovascular disease [6]

the post-thrombotic syndrome. The cornerstone of treatment is anticoagulation. NICE guidelines only recommend treating proximal DVT (*not* distal) and those with pulmonary emboli. In each patient, the risks of anticoagulation need to be weighed against the benefits.

Table 103.24 Investigations for deep-vein thrombosis (DVT).

D-dimers	These are specific cross-linked products of fibrin degradation and are raised in patients with venous thromboembolis
	Sensitivity is high but specificity poor
Compression Duplex ultrasound	Sensitivity 97% for proximal and 73% for distal vein thrombosis compared with phlebography
	Non-invasive, simple, easy to repeat, relatively inexpensive and free of complications
	Two main disadvantages:
	• calf vein thrombosis can be missed, especially when the examination is limited to the popliteal and femoral veins
	• small isolated thrombi in the iliac and superficial femoral veins or within the adductor canal can be difficult to detect and therefore easily overlooked [8]
Radiology	Magnetic resonance venography and CT venography may be useful adjuncts but are expensive and not always available
General investigations	Chest X-ray, routine blood tests (full blood count, liver function tests, urea and electrolytes) urinalysis
If DVT is 'unprovoked' in patients over the age of 40	Mammogram and abdominal pelvic CT scan to look for cancer
	Antiphospholipid antibodies in patients who have had unprovoked DVT if it is planned to stop anticoagulation treatment
	Test for hereditary thrombophilia in patients who have had unprovoked DVT and who have a first-degree relative who has had DVT if it is planned to stop anticoagulation treatment

The greatest area of improved clinical care has been in identifying those at increased risk of thromboembolism in hospital and providing thromboembolism prophylaxis. This takes the form of preventing dehydration, improving mobilization, using antiembolic stockings, using intermittent pneumatic compression in stroke patients and pharmacological prophylaxis with either low-molecular-weight heparin or fondaparinux sodium unfractionated heparin [9].

Treatment of proximal DVT is outlined in Table 103.26.

Table 103.25 Two-level deep-vein thrombosis (DVT) Wells score. DVT is likely with a score of 2 or more.

Clinical feature	Points
Active cancer (treatment ongoing, within 6 months, or palliative)	1
Paralysis, paresis or recent plaster immobilization of the lower extremities	1
Recently bedridden for 3 days or more or major surgery within 12 weeks requiring general or regional anaesthesia	1
Localized tenderness along the distribution of the deep venous system	1
Entire leg swollen	1
Calf swelling at least 3 cm larger than asymptomatic side	1
Pitting oedema confined to the symptomatic leg	1
Collateral superficial veins (non-varicose)	1
Previously documented DVT	1
An alternative diagnosis is at least as likely as DVT	−2

Table 103.26 Treatment of proximal deep-vein thrombosis (DVT).

Anticoagulation	Low-molecular-weight heparin or fondaparinux for 5 days or until INR >2 for 24 h (unfractionated heparin for patients with renal failure and increased risk of bleeding)
	Vitamin K analogues for 3 months
	In patients with cancer consider anticoagulation for 6 months with low-molecular-weight heparin
	In patients with unprovoked DVT consider vitamin K analogues beyond 3 months
	Rivaroxaban is an oral factor Xa inhibitor which has recently been approved by the FDA and NICE and is attractive because there is no need for regular INR monitoring [10]
Thrombolysis	If there is:
	• symptomatic ileofemoral DVT
	• symptoms of less than 14 days duration
	• good functional status
	• a life expectancy of 1 year or more
	• a low risk of bleeding
Compression hosiery	Below-knee graduated compression stockings with an ankle pressure greater than 23 mmHg for 2 years (if there are no contraindications)
Inferior vena cava filters	If anticoagulation is contraindicated
	If emboli are occurring despite adequate anticoagulation

Resources

Further information
http://www.nice.org.uk/guidance/cg144/chapter/guidance
http://www.nice.org.uk/guidance/cg92
(All last accessed April 2015.)

Superficial venous thrombosis

Definition and nomenclature
This is common condition where there is the formation of a thrombus in the veins near the surface of the skin which is usually associated with inflammation of the walls of the vein.

> **Synonyms and inclusions**
> • Superficial thrombophlebitis

Introduction and general description
Superficial venous thrombosis is an uncomfortable but self-limiting condition. It is often seen on the lower leg associated with varicose veins and in hospitals at the sites on intravenous canulae. However, it can be associated with deep thrombosis and the serious consequences of venous thromboembolism.

Epidemiology

Incidence and prevalence
Superficial venous thrombosis is a common condition. The actual prevalence and incidence is unknown. However, up to 25–35% of all hospitalized patients are thought to experience superficial phlebitis at the site of venous cannulae [1].

Age
The mean age of onset is 60 [2].

Sex
It is commoner in females (55–70% occurring in women).

Ethnicity
There is no known racial predilection.

Associated diseases
Migratory thrombophlebitis may be associated with an underlying carcinoma (such as pancreatic cancer) or Behçet disease.

Pathophysiology

Pathology
The pathogenesis of superficial venous thrombosis is similar to that of DVT though trauma to the vein is thought to be the predominant trigger in the Virchow triad (stasis, increased coagulability and vessel wall injury). Several studies have described an association between superficial venous thrombosis and venous thromboembolism. Superficial venous thrombosis located in the main trunk of the saphenous vein has the strongest association with venous thromboembolism [2,3]. Superficial venous thrombosis usually develops in the lower limbs. In 60–80% of cases, the GSV system is involved, and in 10–20% the SSV system [4]. The main cause of superficial venous thrombosis of the lower limbs is varicose veins, which are present in 70% of cases [5]. The main cause of superficial venous thrombosis in the upper limb is iatrogenic, for example intravenous catheters or infusion of drugs such as chemotherapy or heroin. Mondor disease may also be a form of superficial venous thrombosis.

Predisposing factors
These are the same as for DVT [3] and are outlined in Table 103.22.

Clinical features
The clinical features of superficial venous thrombosis are outlined in Table 103.27.

Investigations
The aims of the investigations are to establish the extent of the thrombosis and to exclude involvement of the deep venous system. In patients without obvious risk factors for superficial venous thrombosis, studies to exclude hypercoagulability should be considered. In migratory thrombophlebitis, investigations to exclude an underlying internal malignancy should be considered. These are outlined in Table 103.28.

Management
The treatment of superficial venous thrombosis is outlined in Table 103.29.

Resources

Patient resources
http://www.patient.co.uk/health/Phlebitis.htm
(last accessed March 2015).

Table 103.27 Clinical features of superficial venous thrombosis (Figure 103.24).

History	Gradual onset of localized tenderness
	Redness along the path of a superficial vein
	May have had intravenous catheter at the site
	May have varicose veins
Examination	Overlying skin may be red and hot
	May be swelling
	A tender firm cord extending along the vein on palpation
	If it occurs within varicose veins there may be bleeding
Clinical variants	Migratory thrombophlebitis
	Thrombophlebitis of the superficial veins of the breast and anterior chest wall (Mondor disease)
Differential diagnosis	Cellulitis
	Panniculitis
	Insect bites
	DVT
	Lymphangitis
	Neuritis
	Chronic venous insufficiency
	Baker's cyst
	Haematoma
Complications and co-morbidities	Extension into the deep venous system (DVT and pulmonary embolism)
	If thrombosed veins do not re-canalize patient can develop post-thrombotic syndrome
	Post-inflammatory hyperpigmentation over the affected vein
	Persistent firm subcutaneous nodule at the site
	Secondary infection possibly leading to septic emboli, abscesses and septicaemia
Disease course and prognosis	Prognosis is usually good in uncomplicated disease and symptoms usually resolve within 3–4 weeks
	Recurrence is a risk with superficial venous thrombosis in association with varicose veins

Thrombophlebitis migrans [1,2,3,4]

Definition
This is a form of superficial venous thrombosis which is recurrent and diffuse affecting the large and small veins throughout the body.

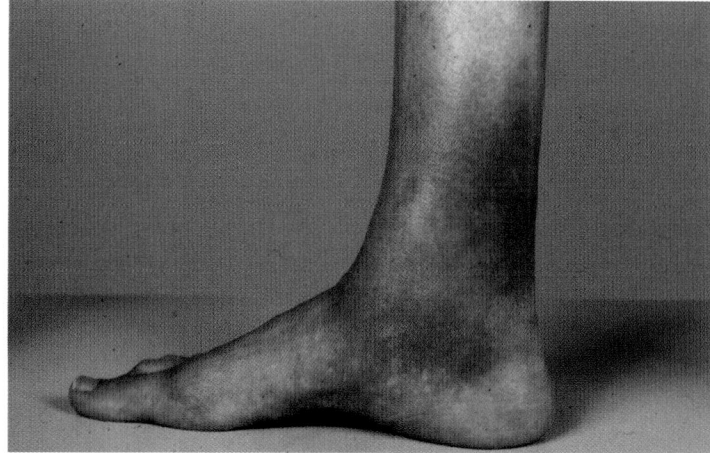

Figure 103.24 Superficial venous thrombosis.

Table 103.28 Investigations for superficial venous thrombosis.

Imaging	Duplex and compression ultrasonography
To detect the location and extent of the superficial venous thrombosis and to exclude DVT	[6] (up to 40% may have proximal DVTs, although the superficial venous thrombosis will be contiguous with the proximal DVT in less than 50% of cases [6])
Consider tests for underlying malignancy	Blood tumour markers, chest X-ray and CT abdomen/pelvis, mammogram in females
If there is migratory thrombophlebitis	
Consider tests for underlying coagulopathy	Factor V Leiden, protein C and S deficiency, antithrombin III deficiency, antiphospholipid antibodies
If there is no obvious trigger	

Table 103.29 Treatment of superficial venous thrombosis of the lower limb.

Medication	**Low-molecular-weight heparin** for 3 months [3]
	Best at reducing local signs and symptoms and reduces the risk of extension to the deep system
	Non-steroidal anti-inflammatory drugs
	Similar in efficacy to low-molecular-weight heparin but easier to administer [3]
	Antibiotics: only of help in suppurative thrombophlebitis
Surgery	**Excision and ligation**
	When a thrombus is found in or near the saphenofemoral junction or saphenopopliteal junction, especially if it extends as free-floating thrombus extending into the common femoral vein or popliteal veins, it should be treated by surgical removal, combined with ligation and stripping and patient started on low-molecular-weight heparin
	Sclerotherapy and stripping of any varicose veins should only be performed some months after the acute superficial venous thrombosis has settled
	Puncture and evacuation
	The thrombus can be squeezed out of the vein through a needle puncture
Compression hosiery or bandages	Used as an adjunct to medical and surgical treatments

Introduction and general description

This is a rare disorder which is important because it is often associated with underlying disease such as internal malignancy (Trousseau syndrome), Behçet disease and Buerger disease.

Epidemiology

Incidence and prevalence

This is not known but it is rare. In one study of 1500 cases of thrombophlebitis, 31 of 77 occurring in association with malignancy were of a migratory type [1]. In this study, carcinomas of the lung and pancreas were the most common sites for the primary tumours, although carcinomas of the breast, colon and stomach were also reported [1]. Other associated diseases are Behçet (between 2 and 20% of all cases; see Chapter 48) and Buerger disease (one study [2] found thrombophlebitis migrans in up to 65.4% of 86 patients). There is no known gender or racial predilection.

Pathophysiology

This is not fully understood. As with superficial venous thrombosis, the mechanism is thought to be within the Virchow triad (stasis, increased coagulability and vessel wall injury). In the thrombophlebitis migrans associated with malignancy, some have suggested that there is a state of chronic disseminated intravascular coagulation [3,4].

Clinical features

History

Patients develop crops of painful red lumps and streaks in the skin. These may resolve and then new ones develop. The lesions appear on the legs, arms, abdominal wall and flanks.

Presentation (Figure 103.25)

The lesions are hot and tender and can be linear or oval subcutaneous lumps or streaks. The overlying skin usually remains intact.

Differential diagnosis

This is wide as there are no pathognomonic features and includes cellulitis, panniculitis, DVT and states with increased coagulability.

Investigations

Ultrasound to confirm the diagnosis, clotting studies and tests to look for an underlying malignancy are all advised. CT scanning, ultrasound, MRI and even positron emission tomographic (PET) scans of the abdomen may be necessary to pick up a pancreatic carcinoma.

Management

Treatment is generally conservative, and patients should be treated with adequate anticoagulation. Lowering triglycerides may be advisable and exercise is good prophylaxis. Medical elastic compression stockings or bandages may alleviate symptoms. In Behçet disease, immunosuppressive medication is given (see Chapter 48)

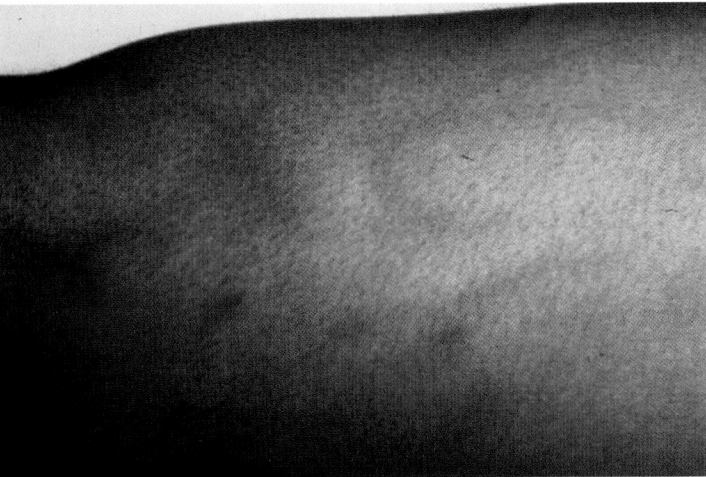

Figure 103.25 Thrombophlebitis migrans.

Mondor disease

Definition

This is a form of superficial venous thrombosis in the chest wall and affects veins that include the lateral thoracic vein, the superior epigastric vein and the thoracoepigastric vein [1,2]. Similar cases have been reported in the antecubital fossa, inguinal area, axilla, penis [3], abdomen and lower limbs.

Introduction and general description

This is a rare, self-limiting and benign condition that was first described in 1939 [1].

Epidemiology

Incidence and prevalence

The incidence and prevalence of this rare condition are unknown. Less than 500 cases have been published in the literature [2].

Penile Mondor disease is rarer still and accounts for less than 10% of cases.

Age

Typically the patients are between 30 and 60 years old.

Sex

The sex ratio is 3 : 1 female : male.

Ethnicity

There is no known racial bias.

Pathophysiology

The pathogenesis of Mondor disease is not understood. As with superficial venous thrombosis the mechanism is thought to be within the Virchow triad (stasis, increased coagulability and vessel wall injury).

In the *chest wall type*, a study [2] of pooled cases of the disease found one-third of cases were idiopathic, most of the rest were related to trauma (injury, muscular strain, poorly fitting bras, surgery, breast prosthesis, etc). Rare causes were underlying breast cancer, hypercoagulable states and connective tissue disorders.

In the *penile type*, surgical trauma, excessive sexual activity, sexual vacuum practices, use of constrictive elements during sexual activity, intravenous drug abuse, prolonged sexual abstinence, local or distant infection, venous obstruction due to bladder distension and pelvic tumours have all been reported [2].

Pathology [3]

It is a two- stage process: initially there is a dense inflammatory cell infiltrate and usually a thrombus occluding the lumen of the affected veins; thereafter, connective tissue proliferation occurs in the vessel leading to a hard cord which resolves when the vessel canalizes.

Clinical features (Figure 103.26)

The features are described according to the latest clinical classification of the disease [2].

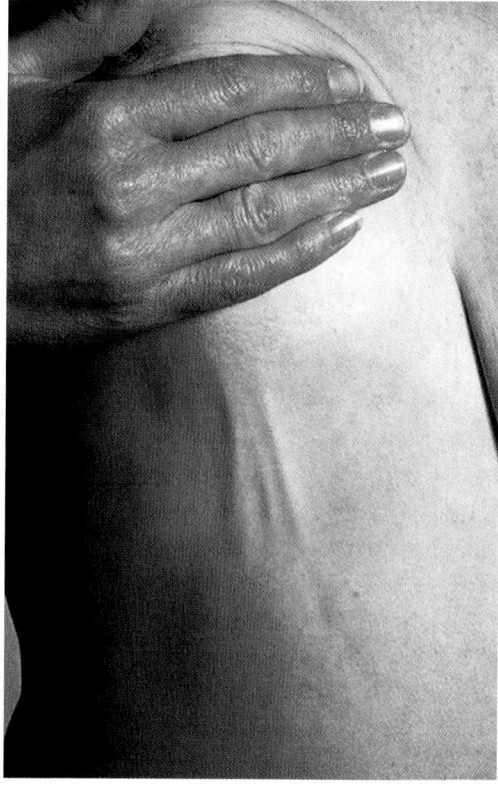

Figure 103.26 Mondor disease.

Mondor disease of the chest wall. The lesions appear and may be painful or asymptomatic. On examination, the lesions may involve any subcutaneous vein on the upper anterolateral chest wall and produce a fibrous painful cord with skin retraction. However, unlike classical superficial venous thrombosis there is *no* overlying cutaneous inflammation.

Mondor disease involving other venous territories. The most usual site of involvement is the penis. A fibrous painful cord with local preputial inflammation but without skin retraction is seen. Other possible sites include the brachial, femoral and calf veins but, unlike chest wall Mondor disease, local inflammation is present.

Mondor disease after breast surgery. This is a subtype described in association with axillary lymph node dissection in breast cancer, and is characterized by retractile scarring of the fascia. Some authors call it axillary web syndrome (AWS). It manifests with palpable cords which 'bowstringing' across the axilla, creating a web of skin. The cords are painful and restrict shoulder movement. They can extend into the ipsilateral arm, and even the forearm, creating linear grooves. There is usually no concomitant superficial venous thrombosis.

Differential diagnosis

The differential diagnosis is wide and includes cellulitis, erythema nodosum, skin metastatic carcinoma, lymphangiectasia and lymphangioma.

Disease course and prognosis

This depends on the site and type of disease.

PART 9: VASCULAR

In *Mondor disease on the chest wall*, this is generally benign and self-limiting with spontaneous resolution usually with 2–8 weeks [2] and only 13% recurrence is reported in one series [4] and none in another [5].

In *Mondor disease involving other venous territories*, the natural history is less well known and, as with other conditions with superficial venous thrombosis, can be associated with deeper thrombosis.

In *Mondor disease after breast surgery*, this usually spontaneously resolves.

Investigations

Diagnosis is largely clinical. Ultrasound examination can diagnose superficial thrombus and exclude a deep thrombus. Mammography can be helpful if there is suspicion of an underlying carcinoma.

Management

This depends on the type of Mondor disease.

In *Mondor disease on the chest wall*, as this is generally benign and self-limiting, no anticoagulation is needed and simple analgesia can be given if the patient is in pain.

In *Mondor disease involving other venous territories*, anticoagulation is recommended and sometimes in penile disease the superficial dorsal vein of the penis is treated with thrombectomy or excision.

In *Mondor disease after breast surgery*, no anticoagulation is needed. If the fascial fibrous bands persist, they can be manually ruptured with immediate return of function and reduction in pain [6].

Varicose veins

Definition and nomenclature

These are visible, dilated and tortuous elongations of the larger superficial venous trunks and their tributaries.

> **Synonyms and inclusions**
> • Venous varicosity

Introduction and general description

Varicose veins are very common and their characteristics and management were described by Hippocrates and Galen [1]. Over the millennia, they have been the subject of controversy and remain so today with much research still being needed to identify their pathogenesis and optimum treatment [2].

Epidemiology

Incidence and prevalence

Varicose veins are common. The incidence of varicose veins is unknown but several studies have reported the prevalence to be high (varying from 10% to 50% of the adult population).

Age and sex

The prevalence increases with age and they are commoner in females. By 20 years of age, the prevalence of varicose veins is 10%; by the age of 40 years, it is 40% in women and 25% in men,

Table 103.30 Pathogenesis of varicose veins.

Primary varicose veins	Pathogenetic features
No known underlying cause	No uniform valvular abnormality found
Associated with valvular incompetence	Intrinsic and structural abnormalities of vein walls are seen
Secondary varicose veins	
Raised endoluminal venous pressure (venous hypertension) due to thrombosis, pregnancy, trauma	Raised venous pressure is thought to cause • Stretching of the endothelium • Expression of cytokines and adhesion molecules • Activation of extracellular signal-related kinases • Free radical production • Dysregulation of transforming growth factor β • Altered fibroblast activity

and varicose veins are present in about 70% of 80-year-old women and 60% of 80-year-old men.

Ethnicity

There is no known ethnic variation in varicose veins.

Associated diseases

Klippel–Trenaunay syndrome where there is a congenital malformation leading to varicose veins.

Pathophysiology [3]

In the healthy venous system, there is venous blood flow through the superficial system into the deep system and back to the heart. One-way valves exist in both systems and in the perforating veins which connect the two. Incompetence in any of the valves can disrupt the normal flow of the blood and cause venous hypertension. The pathogenesis of varicose veins is not fully understood. Valvular incompetence and venous hypertension are thought to be important and interdependent but how they occur remains to be fully elucidated.

Varicose veins can be divided into primary and secondary; however, this is simplistic. The mechanical issues of valve incompetence and raised pressure can occur in both and lead to complex molecular and histopathological alterations in the vessel wall and the extracellular matrix (Table 103.30).

Pathology

The chief findings in varicose veins are intimal hypertrophy, subendothelial fibrosis, luminal dilation and wall thickening.

Genetics

A genetic basis has been thought to be possibly relevant in the pathogenesis of varicose veins, since familial clustering of cases occurs. Genetic studies in twins suggests that *FOXC2* plays a critical role in valve development and function, and that mutations in *FOXC2* may promote varicose veins. Other studies have suggested a link with varicose veins and mutations in the *NOTCH3* gene (thrombomodulin promoter), mutations in the *NDP* gene (which cause Norrie disease) and in the transforming growth factor β receptor 2 gene.

Environmental factors

A population-based cross-sectional survey in Germany of 3072 participants found that the prevalence of varicose veins was twice as high in an urban population as in a rural population [4].

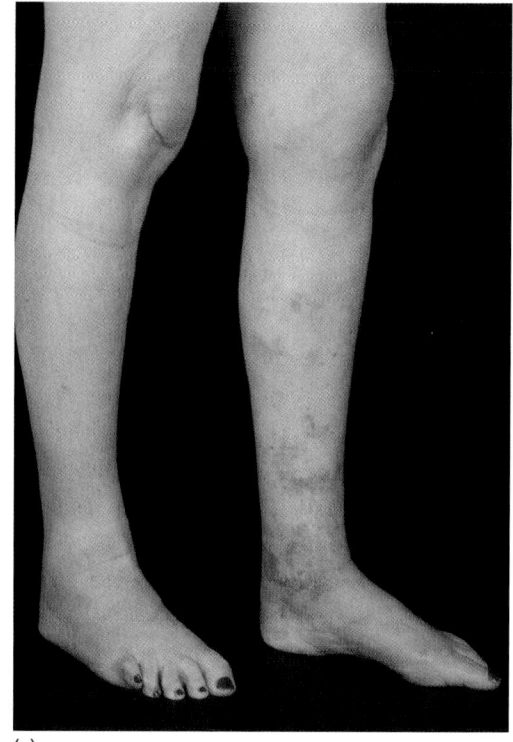
(a)

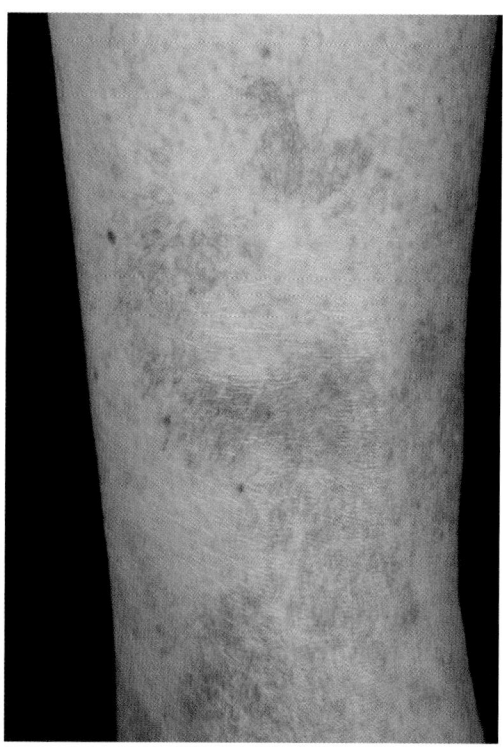
(b)

Figure 103.27 (a) Varicose veins in the left leg, and (b) with superficial telangiectasia.

Clinical features (Figure 103.27)

The severity of symptoms does not necessarily correlate with the size or extent of the visible varices and that in turn does not always correlate with the degree of reflux or severity of venous hypertension.

The clinical features of varicose veins are described in Table 103.31.

Investigations

Colour duplex Doppler ultrasound scanning is used to investigate patients with varicose veins as it provides an anatomical picture of the venous system. It is the investigation of choice for detecting deep-vein reflux. Duplex scanning is also essential to investigate patients with skin changes attributed to venous hypertension. There is some evidence that the incidence of recurrent varicose veins is lower after duplex assessment has been used to plan surgery.

Management

Patients with varicose veins are largely managed by vascular surgeons. The management of varicose veins is outlined in Table 103.32 and is based on the latest NICE guidelines [2].

Resources

Further information
NICE guidelines: http://guidance.nice.org.uk/CG168

Patient resources
http://www.patient.co.uk/health/varicose-veins-leaflet
(All last accessed March 2015.)

Table 103.31 Clinical features of varicose veins.

History	Often asymptomatic but unsightly
	Sometimes there is aching, which is worse on standing
	Ankle swelling
	Symptoms of chronic venous insufficiency: skin discoloration in a gaiter pattern, itching, chronic swelling, pain due to ulceration
Presentation	Visible palpable dilated and tortuous veins in the subcutis
	Reticular veins
	Telangiectases (spider veins)
	Signs of chronic venous insufficiency may accompany varicose veins: pigmentation, eczema, lipodermatosclerosis, ulceration
Differential diagnosis	Thrombophlebitis
	DVT
Classification of severity	**CEAP** classification [5]
	Clinical: C_0–C_6 (from no signs to active venous ulcer) S = symptomatic, A = asymptomatic)
	Etiological: Ec, congenital, Ep, primary; Es, secondary; En, no venous cause found
	Anatomical: As, superficial veins; Ap, perforator veins; Ad, deep veins; An, no venous location identified
	Pathophysiological: Pr, reflux; Po, obstruction; Pn, no venous pathophysiology identifiable
Complications and co-morbidities	Thrombophlebitis
	Bleeding
	DVT and chronic venous insufficiency
Disease course and prognosis	About 4% of patients with varicose veins progress to more severe clinical stages per annum [6]
	3–6% of patients with varicose veins will get venous leg ulcers in their lifetime [2]
	There is a suggestion that obesity, increasing age and genetic factors may be relevant. NICE has recommended that large observational prospective cohort studies are needed to identify the factors that influence progression [2]

PART 9: VASCULAR

Table 103.32 Management of varicose veins [**2**].

Patient advice and information	Discuss the cause and natural history of varicose veins Give advice about weight control Advise light to moderate physical activity
Referral to a vascular unit	If they have any of the following: bleeding varicose veins primary or symptomatic recurrent varicose veins lower limb skin changes, such as pigmentation or eczema, thought to be caused by chronic venous insufficiency superficial vein thrombosis (characterized by the appearance of hard painful veins) and suspected venous incompetence an active or healed venous leg ulcer
Assessment in a vascular unit	Use duplex ultrasound: to confirm the diagnosis of varicose veins to identify the extent of truncal reflux to plan treatment for people with suspected primary or recurrent varicose veins
Interventional treatment: for people with confirmed varicose veins and truncal reflux	Offer *endothermal ablation* and *endovenous laser treatment* of the long saphenous vein If endothermal ablation is unsuitable, offer *ultrasound-guided foam sclerotherapy* If ultrasound-guided foam sclerotherapy is unsuitable, offer *surgery*. If incompetent varicose tributaries are to be treated, consider treating them at the same time If offering compression bandaging or hosiery for use after interventional treatment, do not use for more than 7 days
Non-interventional treatment	Do not offer compression hosiery to treat varicose veins unless interventional treatment is unsuitable
Management during pregnancy	Explain that pregnancy exacerbates varicose veins and that following pregnancy they may improve Do not carry out interventional treatment for varicose veins during pregnancy other than in exceptional circumstances Consider compression hosiery for symptom relief of leg swelling associated with varicose veins during pregnancy

Chronic venous insufficiency

Venous insufficiency

Definition and nomenclature
This is a state which occurs when the blood no longer flows in the correct path from the superficial system into the deep venous system and thence back to the heart. This results in venous congestion and impairment of the venous system. Chronic venous insufficiency may be classified anatomically into three categories (Figure 103.28).

Superficial vein insufficiency. This is indicated by the presence of visible, tortuous, truncal varicose veins. It arises from primary valve failure or when the superficial veins become distended, causing the valves to become secondarily incompetent.

Perforating vein insufficiency. This is a rare condition in isolation, when it is caused by primary valve insufficiency. Secondary perforating vein insufficiency often occurs in combination with deep-vein insufficiency (post-thrombotic limb).

Deep-vein insufficiency. Reflux is the most common type of abnormality, but in about 10% of cases a functional obstruction

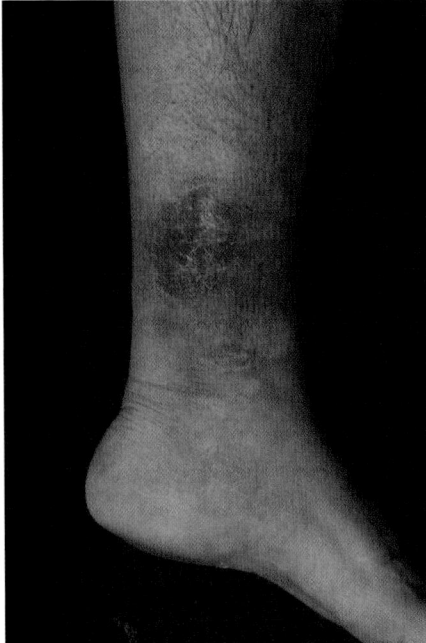

Figure 103.28 Venous eczema.

from thrombosis (non-recanalized thrombosis) will be present, in which case it is likely to be associated with the post-thrombotic syndrome. Avalvulosis is rare unless associated with a mutation of the *FOXC2* gene [1].

If untreated venous insufficiency in either the deep or superficial system causes the progressive syndrome of chronic venous insufficiency.

Synonyms and inclusions
- Post-thrombotic syndrome
- Postphlebetic syndrome

Introduction and general description
Chronic venous insufficiency is common and can be disabling. It is a major aetiological factor globally in the development of leg ulcers.

Epidemiology
Those with superficial venous insufficiency usually present with varicose veins initially. Chronic deep venous insufficiency is most frequently post-thrombotic and occurs in less than half of patients after DVT [2].

Incidence and prevalence
Varicose veins are common. One large study in 30 000 subjects found a prevalence of 7% for varicose veins and 0.86% for 'symptomatic' chronic venous insufficiency [3]. Another screened 1566 subjects and found chronic venous insufficiency in 9.4% of men, and 6.6% of women. Prevalence rose significantly with age: 21.2% in men >50 years and 12.0% in women >50 years [4].

Serious chronic venous insufficiency leading to venous ulcers has an estimated prevalence of approximately 0.3%, although active or healed ulcers are seen in up to 1% of the adult population [5]. In the USA, it is thought that approximately 2.5 million people have chronic venous insufficiency and about 20% of those develop venous ulcers [6].

Age

Chronic venous insufficiency prevalence increases with age.

Sex

Varicose veins are more common in females but studies differ on the sex difference in the prevalence of severe chronic venous deficiency.

Ethnicity

It is not thought that there is any racial difference in the prevalence of chronic venous insufficiency. However, it occurs more commonly in Western society and this probably reflects lifestyle differences such as sedentary or standing occupations, higher rates of obesity and generally reduced levels of physical activity.

Pathophysiology

Changes occurring in the macrocirculation lead to microvascular abnormalities and chronic inflammation which are thought to lead to the physical manifestations of chronic venous insufficiency.

Pathophysiology of venous reflux and chronic venous insufficiency

It is thought that there are two elements to the pathophysiology; the first is abnormal venous blood flow with reflux, and the second occurs at the microvascular level and is a chronic inflammatory process which leads to the skin changes seen in chronic venous insufficiency.

Venous reflux is regarded as the major cause of venous disorders. Reflux is the presence of retrograde flow in a vein in response to a stimulus such as a calf squeeze. It occurs during standing when the valves are incompetent. It can occur in the superficial, deep and perforating veins of the lower extremity.

An elevated and sustained ambulatory venous pressure (venous hypertension) is indicative of chronic venous insufficiency. This may be caused by valvular incompetence or venous outflow obstruction or poor muscle pump function (Table 103.33). Venous outflow obstruction occurs in some patients after a DVT, is more serious than reflux and more difficult to treat. In this situation, when the leg muscles contract, the venous pressure increases, rather than the usual lowering of venous pressure that occurs during ambulation when the vein is not obstructed. Such heightened pressure is transmitted distally as far as the capillary system of the skin, causing capillary hypertension, and eventually leading to destruction of the nutritive capillaries [7]. The current theories on the mechanisms for the pathogenesis of the chronic inflammation in venous disease are outlined by Bergan *et al.* [8] and summarized in Table 103.34.

Table 103.33 Causes of chronic venous insufficiency.

Venous disease	Superficial venous incompetence (varicose veins)
	Deep venous incompetence
	Primary deep venous obstruction (rare)
	Previous deep vein thrombosis
	External compression
Impaired calf muscle pump function	Immobility
	Joint disease
	Paralysis
	Obesity (immobility, femoral vein compression, high abdominal pressures)
Congestive cardiac failure	–

Table 103.34 Pathogenesis of chronic venous disease.

Leukocytes accumulate in leg when there is chronic high venous pressure	Leukocytes are activated by plasminogen activator
	Activated leukocytes shed L-selectin into the plasma and express members of the integrin family (CD11b, which binds to intercellular adhesion molecule 1)
	Integrin binding promotes firm adhesion of leukocytes
	Leukocytes start their migration out of the vasculature and undergo degranulation
	Increased levels of activated leukocytes occur both locally and systemically in patients with chronic venous disease
Degradation of extracellular matrix proteins leads to breakdown of extracellular matrix causing reduced healing and promotes ulceration	Vascular cells and inflammatory cells (e.g. macrophages) produce proteolytic enzymes
	Proteolytic enzymes, including matrix metalloproteinases and serine proteinases, are released as inactive proenzymes and activated by other proteinases, including those produced by mast cells
Capillary proliferation and increased permeability; skin capillaries are elongated; and there is tortuous proliferation of the capillary endothelium	Vascular endothelial growth factor, which is likely to be involved in these changes, has been shown to increase microvascular permeability
Dermal tissue fibrosis: feature of lipodermatosclerosis and ulceration	It is postulated that activated leukocytes migrate out of the vasculature and release transforming growth factor
	Transforming growth factor is a fibrogenic cytokine stimulating collagen production by dermal fibroblasts resulting in dermal fibrosis
Increased capillary permeability and extravasation of red blood cells leads to skin pigmentation: induces the development of a microenvironment that exacerbates tissue damage and delays healing	This leads to elevated levels of ferritin and ferric iron in affected skin
	There is oxidative stress and matrix metalloproteinase activation

Genetics

A genetic basis has been thought to be relevant in the pathogenesis of varicose veins, since familial clustering of cases does occur. Genetic studies in twins suggests that *FOXC2* plays a critical role in valve development and function, and that mutations in *FOXC2* may promote varicose veins. Chronic venous insufficiency may also be a feature of KTS.

Environmental factors

A sedentary lifestyle reduces the efficiency of the muscle pump and thus leads to reduced venous return and occupations with prolonged standing act to increase the risk of higher venous pressures in the legs.

Clinical features

History

The clinical features of chronic venous insufficiency vary from mild oedema to severe incapacitating leg ulceration (outlined in Table 103.35). Patients with superficial venous insufficiency may

PART 9: VASCULAR

Table 103.35 Clinical features of chronic venous insufficiency.

Feature	Description	Pathology
Swelling (oedema)	Pitting oedema (especially around the ankle) Worst at the end of the day Usually disappears at night May complain of a tight feeling Night cramps	The capillary filtration rate increases as a consequence of the increased ambulatory venous (and consequently capillary) pressure and overwhelms lymph drainage. This oedema always has a low protein content
Corona phlebectatica paraplantaris (ankle flare) (see Figure 103.31)	Presence of abnormally visible cutaneous blood vessels at the ankle with several components: 'venous cups', blue and red telangiectases and capillary 'stasis spots'	A direct consequence of increased capillary pressure, which causes these vessels to expand
Hyperpigmentation (see Figure 103.32)	Pigmentation in the 'gaiter skin' Pinpoint or patchy pigmentation may be minimal but may also extend over large indurated skin areas	Haemosiderin accumulates after extravasation of erythrocytes (red cells) Melanin can also be deposited as part of post-inflammatory hyperpigmentation following venous eczema and ulceration
Pressure erythema	Grouped, confluent, very small telangiectasiae develop Often found near incompetent perforating veins. Pressure erythema is often one of the first signs of evolving venous insufficiency	Direct result of increased venous pressure causing vascular dilatation
Venous eczema (see Figure 103.28) Synonyms: stasis dermatitis, hypostatic eczema, dermatitis veineuse	Starts around varicosities at the medial ankle Relatively sharply demarcated Papules and vesicles, which may also extend beyond the main area of eczematous skin Scaling and itching develops Chronic lichenified eczema may develop with time May lead to secondary spread onto adjacent and distant non-contact sites. Itching may develop at any site including the palms and soles Can be complicated by secondary infection Other types of eczema may also occur: • *irritant and allergic contact dermatitis* due to locally applied treatments • *asteatotic dermatitis* (synonym: eczema craquelé). Frequent washing may cause extreme dehydration of the skin. A morphologically similar to eczema with a 'crazy paving' pattern appears	Histopathological features of eczema Aetiology is not completely clear. Homing of activated T lymphocytes appears to be the most reasonable explanation
Lipodermatosclerosis (see Figure 103.29) Pathognomonic of venous and lymphatic hypertension Known to be associated with an increased risk of leg ulcer development	Often found just above the medial malleolus, at the level of the Cockett perforating veins, which are usually incompetent, as is the great saphenous vein When the small saphenous vein is incompetent, the lipodermatosclerosis often affects the lateral side of the calf Early stage lipodermatosclerosis may feel a little indurated and often has an inflamed erythematosus appearance It is also quite often tender and painful. (can be confused with erysipelas, superficial venous thrombosis or even DVT) In longstanding disease, there is a 'woody' hardness to the skin and subcutaneous tissues with pigmentation	Increased matrix turnover is caused by a chronic inflammatory reaction The most characteristic histological findings are dermal and subcutaneous fibrosis, with fat degeneration
Atrophie blanche	Atrophic ivory-white depressed skin lesion often located on the lower legs Usually multiple lesions (diameter 0.5–15 cm) Contains many centrally enlarged capillaries that are visible as red dots Often asymptomatic; however, associated ulceration can be very painful (see Figure 103.30) Not unique to venous insufficiency May also be seen in association with other disorders including lupus erythematosus, scleroderma, vasculitides, cryoglobulinaemia, polycythaemia and leukaemia	The result of decreased capillary density caused by microthrombi and matrix degradation causing hypoxia There is an atrophic epidermis and a thickened, scleroderma-like dermis with proliferative dilated capillaries One or more capillaries are often occluded with fibrinoid material
Varicosities (see section Varicose veins)	Dilated and tortuous veins May be primary varicosities May be secondary, following deep venous thrombosis	
Secondary (high output) lymphoedema	May develop in patients with longlasting chronic venous insufficiency Develops when the previously healthy local lymphatic system fails in the face of an overwhelming filtration load, with eventual structural obliteration of lymphatic routes	
Ulceration (end stage of chronic venous insufficiency) (see Chapter 104)		

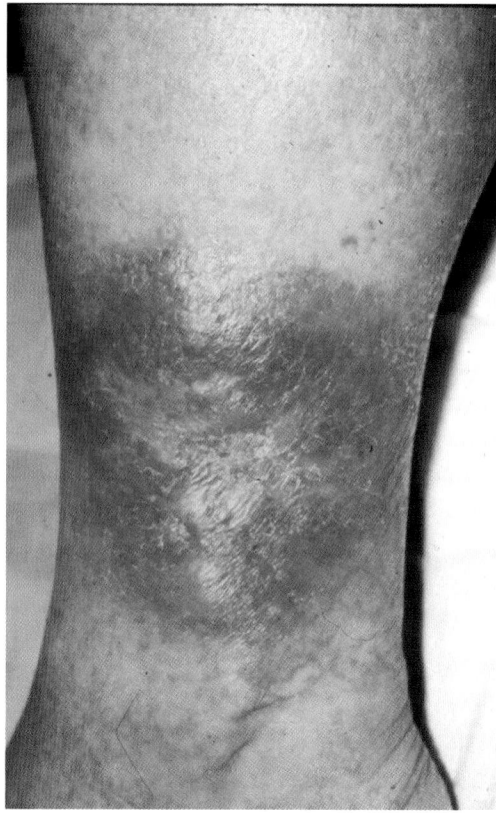

Figure 103.29 Lipodermatosclerosis.

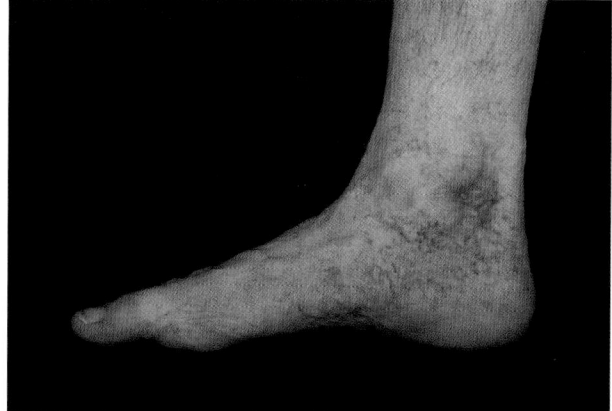

Figure 103.31 Corona phlebectatica paraplantaris.

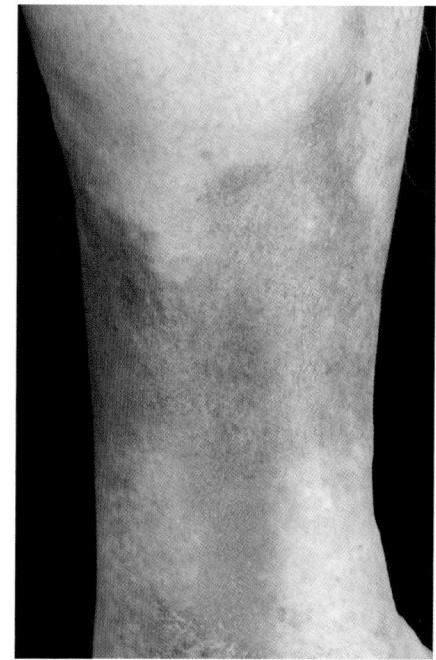

Figure 103.32 Hyperpigmentation secondary to venous insufficiency.

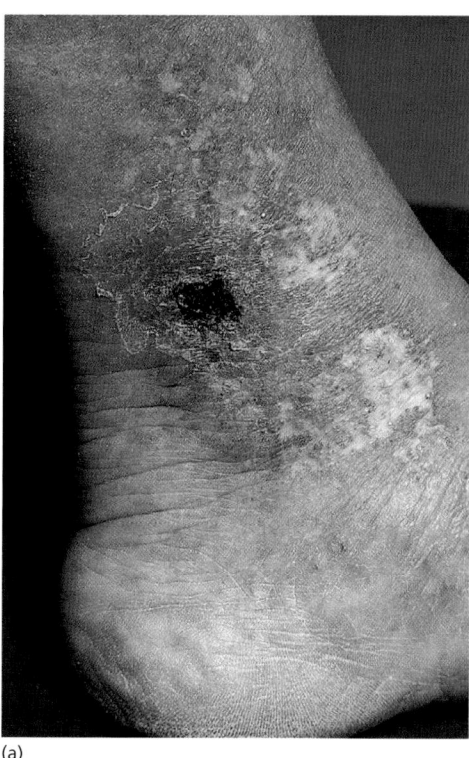

(a)

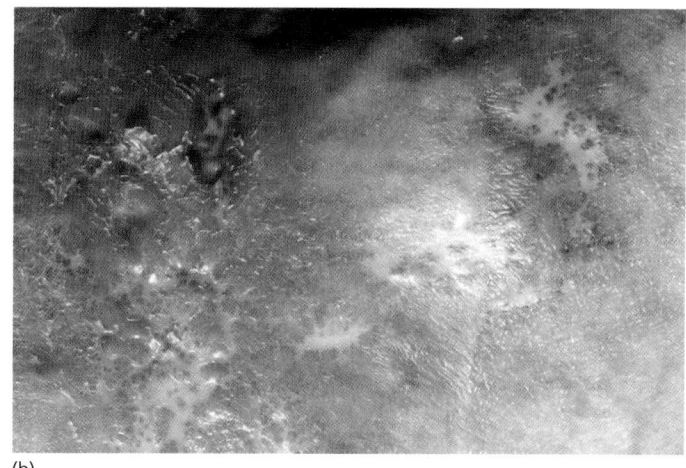

(b)

Figure 103.30 (a) Atrophie blanche: white scars with a central ischaemic ulcer and telangiectasia at the edge of the white areas. (b) Venous ulceration with atrophie blanche.

Table 103.36 Investigations for chronic venous insufficiency.

Duplex ultrasonography	The investigation of choice
Colour flow duplex imaging uses Doppler information to colour code the two-dimensional sonogram	Duplex gives excellent information on venous anatomy and reflux
Accurate but very 'operator dependent'	Allows the communications between deep and superficial veins to be directly assessed
	Indications include: recurrent varicose veins, signs of deep-vein pathology, analysis of the popliteal fossa veins/perforating veins, preoperative marking of varicose veins, assessment of venous malformations, surveillance after treatment, duplex-guided sclerotherapy, evaluation before endovenous interventions, diagnosis of DVT and follow-up after treatment
MRI venography (non-invasive venographic technique)	Most sensitive and specific test for the assessment of deep and superficial venous disease in the lower legs and pelvis
	Also helpful at excluding unsuspected non-vascular causes of leg pain
Phlebography (venography)	Invasive
Contrast injected into a foot vein; is driven into the deep veins by an ankle tourniquet	Largely replaced by MRI venography
Venous pressure measurement	Provides a direct measurement of the severity of chronic venous insufficiency, since it actually measures pressure
A vein in the foot is cannulated	
The patient stands on tiptoe 10 times. The venous pressure drops and the pressure drop is measured. This is defined as the *ambulatory venous pressure*. (should be below 40 mmHg or at least 50% of standing venous pressure)	
The patient stands still until the pressure returns; the time taken for the pressure to return is defined as the *venous refill time* (normally >25 s)	
Venous plethysmography	Bays *et al.* found in chronic venous insufficiency a positive predictive value of venous refill time examined with venous plethysmography of 77% and a negative predictive value of 100% [11]
Photoelectric plethysmographic method of measuring the skin circulation	
The intensity of light reflected from the skin red cells correlates with the blood volume in the skin	
Venous refill time after a standardized exercise is measured	

complain of burning, swelling, throbbing, aching, cramping and heaviness in the legs. Those with deep venous insufficiency almost always have pain. The symptoms are often improved by elevation and rest of the legs.

Classification of severity
The CEAP classification is used for chronic venous insufficiency as it is for varicose veins (see Table 103.31 for explanation).

Complications and co-morbidities
These include thromboembolic disease, venous ulceration and secondary lymphoedema.

Disease course and prognosis
It is not known overall how many patients with chronic venous insufficiency progress to end-stage venous ulceration. About 4% of patients with varicose veins progress to more severe clinical stages per annum. Of patients with varicose veins, 3–6% will get venous leg

ulcers in their lifetime [9]. Patients with lipodermatosclerosis have an increased risk of venous ulceration [10]. About 3% of patients with DVT will go on to develop severe chronic venous insufficiency.

Investigations
The purpose of investigation is to detect venous occlusion, acute or chronic thrombosis, post-thrombotic changes, patterns of obstructive flow and reflux. The most useful and universal investigation is duplex ultrasonography [11]. The chief tools of investigation of chronic venous insufficiency are outlined in Table 103.36.

Management
The aims of treatment are to relieve the symptoms of chronic venous insufficiency and if possible to correct the underlying cause. Patients should be referred to a vascular unit for assessment. Interventional treatments are usually undertaken by vascular surgeons or interventional radiologists. Treatments are outlined in Table 103.37.

Table 103.37 Treatment for chronic venous insufficiency.

Graduated compression	Improve venous dynamics during the day but can be removed when lying down [12,13]
Stockings (class 2, 30–40 mmHg; or class 3, >40 mmHg)	A Cochrane meta-analysis of 22 trials [14] showed that compression stockings were more effective than no compression in healing venous ulcers, and higher compression pressures were more effective than lower ones; multilayer compression bandaging was superior to single-layer bandaging
pressure highest below knee	
available in different lengths	
made from rubber based or synthetic fabrics	In varicose veins and lipodermatosclerosis, compression helps to relieve symptoms. Evidence is lacking for long-term benefit
4-layer bandaging	Compliance may be an issue due to difficulty getting the stockings on
when legs ulcerated and/or very swollen	Patients with severe arterial disease cannot tolerate compression
Interventional treatments [15]	Aim to correct the venous insufficiency by removing the major reflux pathways
Venoablation	Offer *endothermal ablation* and *endovenous laser treatment* of the long saphenous vein
	If endothermal ablation is unsuitable, offer *ultrasound-guided foam sclerotherapy*
	If ultrasound-guided foam sclerotherapy is unsuitable, offer *surgery*
	If incompetent varicose tributaries are to be treated, consider treating them at the same time as surgery

Key references

The full list of references can be found in the online version at rooksdermatology.com.

Arterial and arteriolar disorders

1 Risau W. Mechanisms of angiogenesis. *Nature* 1997;386:671–4.
2 Carmeliet P. Angiogenesis in health and disease. *Nat Med* 2003;9:677–84.
3 Nguyen A, Hoang V, Laquer V, Kelly K. Angiogenesis in cutaneous disease: Part 1. *J Am Acad Dermatol* 2009;61:921–42.
4 Suri C, Jones P, Patan S, *et al.* Requisite role of angiopoietin-1, a ligand for the TIE2 receptor, during embyonic angiogenesis. *Cell* 1996;87:1171–80.
5 De Maeseneer MG, Vandenbroeck CP, Lauwers PR, *et al.* Early and late complications of silicone patch saphenoplasty at the saphenofemoral junction. *J Vasc Surg* 2006;44:1285–90.
6 Simons M. Angiogenesis. *Circulation* 2005;111:1556–66.

Arterial disease and peripheral ischaemic disorders

1 Dormandy JA, Stock G, eds. *Critical Leg Ischaemia: its pathology and management*. Berlin: Springer-Verlag, 1990.
2 Woolard KJ. Immunological aspects of atherosclerosis. *Clin Sci* 2013:125; 221–35.
3 Woolf N, ed. *Pathology of Atherosclerosis*. London: Butterworth, 1982.
4 Koelemay MJW, Den Hartog D, Prins MH, *et al.* Diagnosis of arterial disease of the lower extremities with duplex ultrasonography. *Br J Surg* 1996;83:404–9.
5 Legemate DA, Teeuwen C, Hoeneveld H, *et al.* The potential of duplex scanning to replace aorto-iliac and femoro-popliteal angiography. *Eur J Vasc Surg* 1989;3:49–54.
6 Bendermacher BLW, Willigendael EM, Teijink JAW, Prins MH. Medical management of peripheral arterial disease. *J Thromb Haemost* 2005;3:1628–37.

Thromboangiitis obliterans

1 Dargon PT, Landry GJ. Buerger's disease. *Ann Vasc Surg* 2012:26;871–80.
2 Totemchokchyakarn K. Thromboangiitis obliterans (Buerger's disease). In: Ball GV, Bridges SL, eds. *Vasculitis*. Oxford: Oxford University Press, 2002:460–6.
3 Wessler S. Buerger's disease revisited. *Surg Clin North Am* 1969;49:703–13.
4 Buerger L. Thromboangiitis obliterans: a study of the vascular lesions leading to presenile spontaneous gangrene. *Am J Med Sci* 1908;136:567–80.
5 Lie Jt. The rise and fall and resurgence of thromboangiitis obliterans (Buerger's disease). *Pathol Int* 2008:39;153–8.
7 Adar R, Papa MJ, Halpern Z, *et al.* Cellular sensitivity to collagen in thromboangiitis obliterans. *N Engl J Med* 1983:308:1113–16.
9 Fazeli B, Ravari H, Farzadnia M. Does a species of Rickettsia play a role in the pathophysiology of Buerger's disease? *Vascular* 2012 Dec;20(6):334–6.
10 Adigüzel Y, Yilmaz E, Akar N. Effect of eNOS and ET-1 polymorphisms in thromboangiitis obliterans. *Clin Appl Thromb Hemost* 2010 Feb;16(1):103–6.
11 Tavakoli H, Rezaii J, Esfandiari K, Salimi J, Rashidi A. Buerger's disease: a 10-year experience in Tehran, Iran. *Clin Rheumatol* 2008 Mar;27(3):369–71.
12 Laohapensang K, Rerkasem K, Kattipattanapong V. Seasonal variation of Buerger's disease in Northern part of Thailand. *Eur J Vasc Endovasc Surg* 2004 Oct;28(4):418–20.

Neurovascular disorders

Erythromelalgia

1 Reed KB, Davis MD. Incidence of erythromelalgia :a population-based study in Olmsted County, Minnesota. *J Eur Acad Dermatol Venereol* 2009;231:13–15.
2 Kalgaard OM, Seem E, Kvernebo K. Erythromelalgia: a clinical study of 87 cases. *J Intern Med* 1997;242(3):191–7.
3 Brown GF. Erythromelalgia and other disturbances of the extremities accompanied by vasodilatation and burning. *Am J Med Sci* 1932;183:468–85.
4 Waxman SG, Dib-Hajj SD. Erythromelalgia: a hereditary pain syndrome enters the molecular era. *Ann Neurol* 2005;57:785–8.
5 Yang Y, Wang Y, Li S, *et al.* Mutations in SCN9A, encoding a sodium channel alpha subunit, in patients with primary erythromelalgia. *J Med Genet* 2004;41(3):171–4.

7 Drenth JP, teMorsche RH, Guillet G, *et al.* SCN9A mutations define primary erythromelalgia as a neuropathic disorder of voltage gated sodium channels *J Invest Dermatol* 2005;124(6):1333–8.
10 Harty TP, Dib-Hajj SD, Tyrrell L, *et al.* Na(V)1.7 mutant A863P in erythromelalgia: effects of altered activation and steady state inactivation on excitability of nocioceptive dorsal root ganglion neurons. *J Neurosci* 2006;26(48):12566–75.
11 Han C, Lampert A, Rush AM, *et al.* Temperature dependence of erythromelalgia mutation L858F in sodium channel Nav1.7. *Molecular Pain* 2007;3:3.
14 Sheets PL, Jackson JO, Waxman SG, *et al.* A Nav1.7 channel mutation associated with hereditary erythromelalgia contributes to neuronal hyper excitability and displays reduced lidocaine sensitivity. *J Physiol (Lond)* 2007;581(pt3):1019–31.
16 Han C, Dib-Hajj SD, Lin Z, *et al.* Early and late onset inherited erythromelalgia: genotype–phenotype correlation. *Brain* 2009;132:1711–22.

Telangiectases

Spider telangiectases

1 Bean WB. *Vascular Spiders and Related Lesions of the Skin*. Springfield: Thomas, 1958.
2 Wenzl JE, Burgess EO. The spider nevus in infancy and childhood. *Pediatrics* 1964;33:227–32.
3 Whiting DA, Kallmeyer JC, Simson IW. Widespread arterial spiders in a case of latent hepatitis, with resolution after therapy. *Br J Dermatol* 1970;82:32–6.
4 Martini GA, Staubesand J. Zur Morphologie des Gefässpinnen ('vascular spiders') in der Haut Leberkranker. *Virchows Arch Path Anat Physiol* 1953;324:147–64.
5 Weedon D. Vascular tumors. In: Weedon D, ed. *Skin Pathology*, 2nd edn. London: Churchill Livingstone, 2002.
6 Khasnis A, Gokula RM. Spider nevus. *J Postgrad Med* 2002;48:307.
7 Cunliffe WJ, Dodman B, Butterworth MJ. Unilateral spider naevi. *Br J Dermatol* 1972;87:51–2.
8 Foutch PG, Sulivan JA, Gaines JA, *et al.* Cutaneous vascular spiders and cirrhotic patients; correlation with haemorrhage from oesophageal varices. *Am J Gastroenterol* 1988;83:723–6.
9 Higgins EM, du Vivier AWP. Alcohol and the skin. *Alcohol* 1992;27:595–602.
10 Li CP, Lee FY, Hwang SJ, *et al.* Spider angiomas in patients with liver cirrhosis: role of alcoholism and impaired liver function. *Scand J Gastroenterol* 1999;34:520–3.
11 Sivarajan V, Al Aissami M, Maclaren W, Mackay IR. Recurrence of spider naevi following treatment with 585 nm pulsed dye laser. *J Plast Reconstr Aesthet Surg* 2007;60(6);668–71.
12 Hare McCoppin HH, Goldberg DJ. Laser treatment of facial telangiectases:an update. *Dermatol Surg* 2010;36:1221–30.

Cherry angiomas

1 Murison AR, Sutherland JW, Williamson AM. De Morgan spots. *Br Med J* 1947;1:634–6.
2 Barter RH, Letterman GS, Schurter M. Hemangiomas in pregnancy. *Am J Obstet Gynecol* 1963;87:625.
3 Nakashima T, Jinnin M, Etoh T, *et al.* Down regulation of mir-424 contributes to abnormal angiogenesis via MEK1 and cyclin E1 in senile hemangioma: its implications to therapy. *PLOS One* 2010;5(12):e114334.
4 Cohen AD, Cagnano E, Vardy DA. Cherry angiomas associated with exposure to bromides. *Dermatology* 2001;202:52–3.
5 Raymond LW, Williford LS, Burke WA. Eruptive cherry angiomas and irritant symptoms after one acute exposure to the glycol ether solvent 2-butoxyethanol. *J Occup Environ Med* 1998;40:1059–64.
6 Firooz A, Komeili A, Dowlati Y. Eruptive melanocytic and cherry angiomas secondary to exposure to sulfur mustard gas. *J Am Acad Dermatol* 1999;40: 646–7.
7 Jae-Hong Kim, Hwa-young Park, Sung KA. Cherry angiomas on the scalp. *Dermatology* 2009 Jan–Dec;1(1):82–6.
8 Fodor L, Ramon Y, Fodor A, *et al.* A side-by-side prospective study of intense pulsed light and Nd:YAG laser treatment for vascular lesions. *Ann Plastic Surg* 2006;56 (2):164–70.

Angiokeratoma circumscriptum

1 Gorse SJ, James W, Murison MS. Successful treatment of angiokeratoma with potassium tritanyl phosphate laser. *Br J Dermatol* 2004;150(3):620–2.

Venous lakes

1 Menni S, Marconi M, Boccardi D, Betti R. Venous lakes of the lips: Prevalence and associated factors. *Acta Derm Venereol* 2014;94(1):74–5.
2 Bean WB, Walsh JR. Venous lakes. *Arch Dermatol* 1956;74:459–63.
3 Railan D, Parlette E, Uebelhoer N, Rohrer T. Laser treatment of vascular lesions. *Derm Clin* 2006;24:8–15.
4 Bekhor PS. Long-pulsed Nd:YAG laser treatment of venous lakes: report of a series of 34 cases. *Dermatol Surg* 2006;32(9):1151–4.
5 Wall TL, Grassi AM, Avram MM. Clearance of multiple venous lakes with an 800-nm diode laser: a novel approach. *Dermatol Surg* 2007;33(1):100–3.

Primary telangiectasia

Angioma serpiginosum

1 Blinkenberg EO, Brendehaug A, Sandvik AK, Vatne O, Hennekam RC, Houge G. Angioma serpiginosum with oesophageal papillomatosis is an X-linked dominant condition that maps to Xp11.3-Xq12. *Eur J Hum Genet* 2007;15(5):543–7.
2 Sandhu K, Gupta S. Angioma serpiginosum: report of two unusual cases. *J Eur Acad Dermatol Venereol* 2005;19(1):127–8.
3 Lombardi MP, Bulk S, Celli J, *et al.* Mutation update for the PORCN gene. *Hum Mutat* 2011;32(7):723–8.
4 Katta R, Wagner A. Angioma serpiginosum with extensive cutaneous involvement. *J Am Acad Dermatol* 2000;42:384–5.
5 Gautier-Smith PC, Sanders MD, Sanderson KV. Ocular and nervous system involvement in angioma serpiginosum. *Br J Ophthalmol* 1971;55:433–43.
6 Madan V, August PJ, Ferguson JE. Pulsed dye laser treatment of angioma serpiginosum. *Clin Exp Dermatol* 2009;34(5):e186–8.

Generalized essential telangiectasia

1 McGrae JD, Winkelmann RK. Generalised essential telangiectasia. *JAMA* 1963;185:909–13.
2 Person JR, Longcope C. Estrogen and progesterone receptors are not increased in generalized essential telangiectasia. *Arch Dermatol* 1985;121:836–7.
3 Thieus KP, Haynes HA. Generalised essential telangiectasia with a predilection for surgical scar. *J Am Acad Dermatol* 2009;60:710–11.
4 Ali MM, Teimory M, Sarhan M. Generalised essential telangiectasia with conjunctival involvement. *Clin Exp Dermatol* 2006;31:781–2.
5 Railan D, Parlette E, Uebelhoer N, Rohrer T. Laser treatment of vascular lesions. *Derm Clin* 2006;24:8–15.

Hereditary benign telangiectasia

1 Zahorcsek Z, Schneider I. Hereditary benign telangiectasia. *Dermatology* 1994;189:286–8.
2 Brancati F, Valente EM, Tadini G, *et al.* Autosomal dominant hereditary benign telangiectasia maps to the CMC1 locus for capillary malformation on chromosome 5q14. *J Med Genet* 2003;40:849–53.
3 Gold MH, Eramo L, Prendiville JS. Hereditary benign telangiectasia. *Pediatr Dermatol* 1989;6:194–7.
4 Ryan TJ, Wells RS. Hereditary benign telangiectasia. *Trans St John's Hosp Dermatol Soc* 1971;57:148–56.
5 Watanebe M, Tomita, Y, Tagami H. Hereditary benign telangiectasia – a congenital type. *Dermatologica* 1990;181:152–3.
6 Tsianakas P, Teillac-Hamel D, Fraitag S, *et al.* Etude ultrastructurale des télangiectases héréditaires bénignes. *Ann Dermatol* 1995;122:517–21.
7 Onishi Y, Ohara K, Shikida Y, Satomi H. Hereditary benign telangiectasia: image analysis of hitherto unknown association with arteriovenous malformation. *Br J Dermatol* 2001;145:641–5.

Unilateral naevoid telangiectasia syndrome

1 Dadlani C, Kamino H, Walters RF, *et al.* Unilateral nevoid telangiectasia. *J Dermatol (Online)* 2008;14:3.
2 Guedes R, Leite L. Unilateral nevoid telangiectasia: a rare disease? *Indian J Dermatol* 2012;57:138–40.
3 Uhlin SR, McCarty KS. Unilateral naevoid telangiectatic syndrome. The role of oestrogen and progesterone receptors. *Arch Dermatol* 1983;119:226–8.
4 Cliff S, Harland CC. Recurrence of unilateral naevoid telangiectatic syndrome following treatment with the pulsed dye laser. *J Cutan Laser Ther* 1999;1(2):105–7.

5 Sharma VK, Khandpur S. Unilateral nevoid telangiectasia – response to pulsed dye laser. *Int J Dermatol* 2006;45(8):960–4.

Malformations

Arteriovenous malformations

1 Al-Shahi R, Warlow C. A systematic review of the frequency and prognosis of arteriovenous malformations of the brain in adults. *Brain* 2001;124(10):1900–26.
2 Huang JT, Liang MG. Birthmarks of medical significance vascular malformations. *Ped Clin North Am* 2010;57(5):1091–110.
3 Vikkula M, Boon LM, Mulliken JB, Olsen BR. Molecular basis of vascular anomalies. *Trends Cardiovasc Med* 1998;8:281–92.
4 Eerola I, Boon LM, Mulliken JB, *et al.* Capillary malformation–arteriovenous malformation, a new clinical and genetic disorder caused by RASA1 mutations. *Am J Hum Genet* 2003;73:1240–9.
5 Enjolras O, Logeart I, Gelbert F, *et al.* Arteriovenous malformations: a study of 200 cases. *Ann Dermatol Venereol* 2000;127(1):17–22.
6 Lee BB, Do YS, Yakes W, Kim DI, Mattassi R, Hyon WS. Management of arteriovenous malformations: a multidisciplinary approach. *J Vasc Surg* 2004;39(3):590–600.

Venous malformations

1 Vikkula M, Boon LM, Lii KLC, *et al.* Vascular dysmorphogenesis caused by an activating mutation in the receptor tyrosine kinase TIE2. *Cell* 1996;87:1181–90.
2 Limaye N, Wouters V, Uebelhoer M, *et al.* Somatic mutations in angiopoietin receptor gene TEK cause solitary and multiple sporadic venous malformations. *Nat Genet* 2009;41:118–24.
3 Huang JT, Liang MG. Birthmarks of medical significance vascular malformations. *Ped Clin North Am* 2010;57(5):1091–110.

Verrucous haemangioma

5 Wang L, Gao T, Wang G. Verrucous hemangioma: a clinicopathological and immunochemical analysis of 74 cases. *J Cutan Pathol* 2014;41:823–30.

Disorders associated with venous malformations

Klippel–Trenaunay syndrome

1 Klippel M, Trenaunay P. Du naevus variqueux osteohypoertropiques. *Arch Gen Med* 1900;3:641–72.
2 Parkes Weber F. Angioma formation in connection with hypertrophy of limbs and hemi hypertrophy. *Br J Dermatol* 1907;19:231–5.
3 Redondo P, Aguado L, Martinez-Cuesta A. Diagnosis and management of extensive vascular malformations of the lower limb. *J Am Acad Dermatol* 2011;65:893–906.
4 Tian XL, Kadaba R, You SA, *et al.* Identification of an angiogenic factor that when mutated causes susceptibility to Klippel–Trenaunay syndrome. *Nature* 2004;427:640–5.
5 Eerola I, Boon LM, Mulliken JB, *et al.* Capillary malformation–arteriovenous malformation, a new clinical and genetic disorder caused by RASA1 mutations. *Am J Hum Genet* 2003;73:1240–9.
6 Timur AA, Sadgephour A, Graf M, *et al.* Identification and molecular characterisation of a de novo supernumerary ring chromosome 18 in a patient with Klippel–Trenaunay syndrome. *Ann Hum Genet* 2004;68:353–61.
7 Hofer T, Frank J, Itin PH. Klippel–Trenaunay syndrome in a monozygotic male twin: supportive evidence for the concept of paradominant inheritance. *Eur J Dermatol* 2005;15(5):341–3.
8 Baskerville PA, Ackroyd JS, Browse NL. The etiology of the Klippel–Trenaunay syndrome. *Ann Surg* 1985;202(5):624–7.

Parkes Weber syndrome

1 Redondo P, Aguado L, Martinez-Cuesta A. Diagnosis and management of extensive vascular malformations of the lower limb. *J Am Acad Dermatol* 2011;65:893–906.
2 Eerola I, Boon LM, Mulliken JB, *et al.* Capillary malformation–arteriovenous malformation, a new clinical and genetic disorder caused by RASA1 mutations. *Am J Hum Genet* 2003;73:1240–9.
3 Alomari Al. Characterization of a distinct syndrome that associates complex truncal overgrowth, vascular and acral anomalies: a descriptive study of 18 cases of CLOVES syndrome. *Clin Dysmorphol* 2009;18:1–7.

Venous disorders

1 Browse NL, Burnand KC, Irvine AT, Wilson NM, eds. *Diseases of the Veins*, 2nd edn. London: Arnold, 1999.
2 Tibbs D. *Varicose Veins and Related Disorders*. Oxford: Butterworth–Heinemann, 1992.
3 Gillot C. *Anatomical Atlas of the Lower Limb Superficial Venous Network*. St Gallen: Ganzoni & Cie AG, 2004.
4 Braverman IM, Keh-Yen A. Ultra structure of the human dermal microcirculation. IV. Valve-containing collecting veins at the dermal-subcutaneous junction. *J Invest Dermatol* 1983;81:438–42.
5 Chant ADB, Jones HO, Townsend JCF, et al. Radiological demonstration of the relationship between calf varices and saphenofemoral incompetence. *Clin Radiol* 1972;23:519–23.
6 Caggiati A, Bergan JJ, Glovicki P, et al. Nomenclature of the veins of the lower limb: extensions, refinements and clinical application. *J Vasc Surg* 2005;41:19–24.
7 Weiss MA, Weiss RA, Feied CF, eds. *Vein Diagnosis and Treatment: a comprehensive approach*. New York: McGraw-Hill Professional Publishing, 2001.

Physiology: the venous macrocirculation

1 Browse NL, Burnand KG, Lea Thomas M. Physiology and functional anatomy. In: Browse NL, Burnand KG, Lea Thomas M, eds. *Diseases of the Veins. Pathology, Diagnosis and Treatment*. London: Edward Arnold, 1988;53–69.
2 Summer DS, Zierler RE. Vascular physiology: Essential hemodynamic principles. In: Rutherford RB, ed. *Vascular Surgery*. Philadelphia: Elsevier Saunders, 2005.

Venous thrombosis

Deep-vein thrombosis

1 Kucher N. Clinical practice. Deep vein thrombosis of the upper extremities. *N Engl J Med* 2011;364:861–6.
2 Goldhaber SZ, Bournameaux H. Pulmonary embolism and deep vein thrombosis. *Lancet* 2012;379:1835–46.
3 Silverstein MD, Heit JA, Mohr DN, Petterson TM, O'Fallon WM, Melton LJ 3rd. Trends in the incidence of deep vein thrombosis and pulmonary embolism: a 25-year population-based study. *Arch Intern Med* 1998;158(6):585–93.
4 Pierre-Paul D, Mureebe L, Gahtan V, Kerstein MD. Role of race and sex in diagnosis and one-year follow up of deep venous thrombosis. *Surg Technol Int* 2004;13:215–18.
5 White RH. The epidemiology of venous thromboembolism. *Circulation* 2003;107(23 Suppl. 1):14–18.
6 Kahn SR, Shrier I, Julian JA, et al. Determinants and time course of the post thrombotic syndrome after acute deep vein thrombosis. *Ann Intern Med* 2008;149:698–707.
7 NICE (National Institute for Health and Care Excellence). Venous thromboembolic diseases, NICE Clinical Guideline (June 2012) http://www.nice.org.uk/guidance/cg144 (last accessed April 2015).
8 Michiels JJ, Gadisseur A, van der Planken M, et al. A critical appraisal of non-invasive diagnosis and exclusion of deep vein thrombosis and pulmonary embolism in outpatients with suspected deep vein thrombosis or pulmonary embolism: how many tests do we need? *Int Angiol* 2005;24:27–39.
9 NICE (National Institute for Health and Care Excellence). Venous thromboembolism – reducing the risk, NICE clinical guidelines (2010) https://www.nice.org.uk/guidance/cg92 (last accessed April 2015).
10 NICE (National Institute for Health and Care Excellence). Rivaroxaban for the treatment of deep vein thrombosis and prevention of recurrent deep vein thrombosis and pulmonary embolism, NICE Clinical Guideline (May 2012) https://www.nice.org.uk/guidance/ta261 (last accessed April 2015).

Superficial venous thrombosis

1 Tagalakis V, Kahn SR, Libman M, Blostein M. The epidemiology of peripheral vein infusion thrombophlebitis: a critical review. *Am J Med* 2002;113(2):146–51.
2 Marchiori A, Mosena L, Prandoni P. Superficial vein thrombosis: risk factors, diagnosis, and treatment. *Semin Thromb Hemost* 2006;32:737–43.
3 Di Nisio M, Wichers IM, Middeldoop S. Treatment for superficial thrombophlebitis of the leg. *Cochrane Database Syst Rev* 2007;18:CD004982.
4 Leon L, Giannoukas AD, Dodd D, et al. Clinical significance of superficial vein thrombosis. *Eur J Vasc Endovasc Surg* 2005;29:10–17.

5 Decousus H, Epinat M, Guillot K, et al. Superficial venous thrombosis: risk factors, diagnosis, and treatment. *Curr Opin Pulm Med* 2003;9:393–7.
6 Quéré I, Leizorovicz A, Galanaud JP, et al. Superficial venous thrombosis and compression ultrasound imaging. *J Vasc Surg* 2012;56(4):1032–8.

Thrombophlebitis migrans

1 Lieberman JS, Borrero J, Urdanetta E, et al. Thromboembolism associated with neoplasm: review of 77 cases. *Circulation* 1960;22:780.
2 Fazeli B, Modaghegh H, Ravrai H, Kazemzadeh G. Thrombophlebitis migrans as a footprint of Buerger's disease: a prospective descriptive study in north-east of Iran. *Clin Rheumatol* 2008;27:55–7.
3 Sack C, Levin J, Bell WR. Trousseau's syndrome and other manifestations of chronic disseminated coagulopathy in patients with neoplasms: clinical, pathophysiologic and therapeutic features. *Medicine* 1977;56:1–37.
4 Samlaska CP, Jones WD, Simel DL. Superficial migratory thrombophlebitis and factor XII deficiency. *J Am Acad Dermatol* 1990;22:939–43.

Mondor disease

1 Mondor H. Tronculite sous-cutanee subaigue de la paroi thoracigue antero-laterale. *Mem Acad Chir* 1939;65:1271–8.
2 Laroche JP, Glanaud D, Labau D, et al. Abstracts and Proceedings of the 22nd International Congress on Thrombosis. Nive, France 6–9 October 2012. Mondor's Disease: What's new since 1939? *Thromb Res* 2012;130(S1);S56–9.
3 Alvarez-Garrido H, Garrido-Rios A, Sanz-Muñoz C, et al. Mondor's disease. *Clin Exp Dermatol* 2009;4:753–6.
4 Salemis NS, Merkouris S, Kimpouri K. Mondor's diease of the breast. A retrospective review. *Breast Dis* 2011;33:103–7.
5 Bejanga BI. Mondor's disease, analysis of 30 cases. *J R Coll Surg Edinb* 1992;37:322–4.
6 Salmon RJ, Hamelin JP. Mondor's disease – proposed new pathosociological explanation and treatment. *Oncologie* 2004;6:477–80.

Varicose veins

1 Royle J, Somjen GM. Varicose veins: Hippocrates to Jerry Moore. *ANZ J Surg* 2007;77(12):1120–7.
2 NICE (National Institute for Health and Care Excellence). Varicose veins in the legs (CG168), Nice guidelines (July 2013) https://www.nice.org.uk/guidance/cg168 (last accessed April 2015).
3 Oklu R, Habito R, Mayr M, et al. Pathogenesis of varicose veins. *J Vasc Int Radiol* 2012;23(1):33–9.
4 Rabe E, Pannier-Fischer F, Bromen K, et al. Bonner Venenstudie der Deutschen Gesellschaft für Phlebologie – epidemiologische Untersuchung zur Frage der Häufigkeit und Ausprägung von chronischen Venenkrankheiten in der städtischen und ländlichen Wohnbevölkerung. *Phlebologie* 2003;32:1–14.
5 Eklof B, Rutherford RB, Bergan JJ, et al. Revision of the CEAP classification for chronic venous disorders: consensus statement. *J Vas Surg* 2004;40(6);1248–52.
6 Pannier F, Rabe E. The relevance of the natural history of varicose veins and refunded care. *Phlebology* 2012;27(Suppl. 1):23–6.

Chronic venous insufficiency

1 Mellor RH, Brice G, Stanton AW, et al. Mutations in FOXC2 are strongly associated with primary valve failure in veins of the lower limb. *Circulation* 2007;115:1912–20.
2 Kahn SR, Shrier I, Julian JA, et al. Determinants and time course of the post thrombotic syndrome after acute deep vein thrombosis. *Ann Intern Med* 2008;149:698–707.
4 Ruckley CV, Evans CJ, Allan PL, Lee AJ, Fowkes FG. Chronic venous insufficiency: clinical and duplex correlations. The Edinburgh vein study of venous disorders in the general population. *J Vasc Surg* 2002;36:520–5.
5 Fowkes FG, Evans CJ, Lee AJ. Prevalence and risk factors for chronic venous insufficiency. *Angiology* 2001;52:S5–S15.
8 Bergan JJ, Schmid-Schönbein GW, et al. Chronic venous disease. *N Engl J Med* 2006;355(5):488.
9 Pannier F, Rabe E. The relevance of the natural history of varicose veins and refunded care. *Phlebology* 2012;27(Suppl. 1):23–6.

11 Bays RA, Healy DA, Atnip RG, Neumyer M, Thiele BL. Validation of air plethysmography, photoplethysmography, and duplex ultrasonography in the evaluation of severe venous stasis. *J Vasc Surg* 1994;20:721–7.

13 Erickson CA, Lanza DJ, Karp DL, *et al*. Healing of venous ulcers in an ambulatory care program: the roles of chronic venous insufficiency and patient compliance. *J Vasc Surg* 1995;22:629–36.

14 Cullum N, Nelson EA, Fletcher AW, Sheldon TA. Compression bandages and stockings for venous leg ulcers. *Cochrane Database Syst Rev* 2000;2:CD000265.

15 NICE (National Institute for Health and Care Excellence). Varicose veins in the legs (CG168), Nice guidelines (July 2013) https://www.nice.org.uk/guidance/cg168 (last accessed April 2015).

CHAPTER 104

Ulceration Resulting from Disorders of the Veins and Arteries

Jürg Hafner

Department of Dermatology, University Hospital of Zurich, Zurich, Switzerland

Introduction

Leg and foot ulcers represent a serious burden of disease. Their impact – both physically and psychologically – is underestimated, on both the sufferer and their families and friends. Chronic wounds cause considerable health costs that are estimated to be around 1% of total health care expenses in western countries, and even more (2–3%) when indirect costs are included. Pain is very common, to the detriment of sleep and quality of life.

Nevertheless, surprisingly, many patients suffering from leg and foot ulcers never receive an adequate clinical, vascular and laboratory examination and a rational treatment concept based on a valid diagnostic assessment. The majority of patients with chronic wounds can be effectively treated and healed, and those with refractory lesions can be helped with palliative measures. This, however, requires standardized work-up and treatment planning.

There are four major categories of leg ulcers: venous leg ulcers (VLUs), mixed venous and arterial leg ulcers (MLUs), arterial leg ulcers (ALUs) and hypertensive ischemic leg ulcers (HYTILUs) (Figure 104.1) [1,2]. These groups cover 80% of the underlying causes of leg and foot ulcers.

The CEAP classification system is used to assess venous pathology, pathophysiology and chronic venous insufficiency including venous ulcers. The fundamentals of the CEAP classification include a description of the clinical class (C) based upon objective signs, the aetiology (E), the anatomical (A) distribution of reflux and obstruction in the superficial, deep and perforating veins, and the underlying pathophysiology (P), whether due to reflux or obstruction.

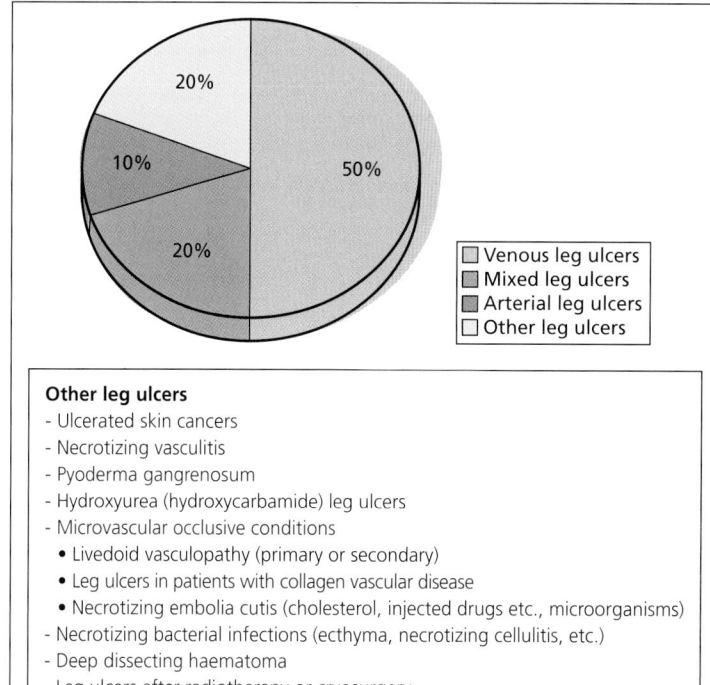

Figure 104.1 Aetiologies of leg ulcers.

Other leg ulcers
- Ulcerated skin cancers
- Necrotizing vasculitis
- Pyoderma gangrenosum
- Hydroxyurea (hydroxycarbamide) leg ulcers
- Microvascular occlusive conditions
  - Livedoid vasculopathy (primary or secondary)
  - Leg ulcers in patients with collagen vascular disease
  - Necrotizing embolia cutis (cholesterol, injected drugs etc., microorganisms)
- Necrotizing bacterial infections (ecthyma, necrotizing cellulitis, etc.)
- Deep dissecting haematoma
- Leg ulcers after radiotherapy or cryosurgery

represent the most advanced grade of chronic venous insufficiency (CVI).

Synonyms and inclusions
- Stasis ulceration
- Venous ulcer
- Gaiter ulcer

Venous leg ulcer

Definition and nomenclature

Venous leg ulcers are chronic skin ulcers at the gaiter area that result from chronic peripheral venous hypertension. They

Introduction and general description

Venous leg ulcers are the most extreme manifestation of chronic venous insufficiency. CVI results from chronic peripheral

Rook's Textbook of Dermatology, Ninth Edition. Edited by Christopher Griffiths, Jonathan Barker, Tanya Bleiker, Robert Chalmers and Daniel Creamer.
© 2016 John Wiley & Sons, Ltd. Published 2016 by John Wiley & Sons, Ltd.
Companion website: www.rooksdermatology.com

PART 9: VASCULAR

venous hypertension caused by venous reflux and/or obstruction, or by neuromusculoskeletal dysfunction of the leg. Venous pathologies involve the deep vein system and/or the superficial vein system and perforator veins. The 'C' grading of the CEAP classification system of venous disease describes the insidious development of chronic venous insufficiency leading from ankle oedema (C3) and reversible morphological skin changes, such as stasis eczema (C4a), over partly reversible morphological changes, such as lipodermatosclerosis (C4b) and atrophie blanche (C4b), to active (C6) or healed (C5) VLUs [1].

Epidemiology

Incidence and prevalence
The lifetime incidence of leg ulcers is around 1%, with a point prevalence of 0.1%. Since approximately half of all leg ulcers are VLUs, the lifetime incidence of VLUs can be calculated at 0.5%, and the point prevalence at 0.05%. The incidence of leg ulcers rises to 4% in the population aged over 80 years.

Age
Venous leg ulcers primarily affect individuals aged over 65 years. Although VLUs can occur in younger adults, the incidence increases with every decade.

Sex
Venous leg ulcers occur equally distributed in women and men. Female patients are overrepresented in wound centres since they have a higher life expectancy.

Ethnicity
Venous leg ulcers occur in any country and population. The incidence and prevalence, however, have been investigated exclusively in western nations. Since VLUs occur more often in people with standing occupations and in obese persons, western lifestyles predisposes to VLUs.

Associated diseases
Box 104.1 lists a number of the associated diseases.

Box 104.1 Disorders associated with venous leg ulcers

- Venous thromboembolism
- Superficial venous thrombophlebitis
- Varicose veins
- Chronic venous insufficiency
- Stasis dermatitis
- Lipodermatosclerosis
- Acroangiodermatitis
- Obesity
- Ankle joint ankylosis
- Rheumatoid arthritis
- Neuromuscular diseases with impact on venous calf pump ejection

---

Pathophysiology [1]
Chronic venous insufficiency and VLU result from peripheral venous hypertension or chronic ambulatory venous hypertension. They exclusively occur in humans. Gravitation, upright walk and dysfunctional venous ejection during leg motion or dysfunctional venous drainage due to obstruction (e.g. chronic occlusion, obesity, pregnancy) are prerequisites to the development CVI and VLUs. Venous reflux can occur at the deep venous system – primarily or secondarily after deep venous thrombosis – or at the superficial venous system (long and/or short saphenous vein). Perforator vein insufficiency rarely occurs in an isolated fashion and contributes less to CVI and VLU than previously suspected. Congenital valvular aplasia is a rare condition leading to severe CVI and VLU early in life. All forms of neuromuscular diseases and/or ankle and knee joint dysfunction can induce CVI and VLUs. Obesity raises the intra-abdominal pressure, which impedes venous drainage. The May–Thurner syndrome describes an endovenous septum at the site where the right common iliac artery crosses the left common iliac vein. It predisposes to CVI and VLU of the left leg, with or without accompanying iliac vein thrombosis.

Venous hypertension induces changes that remain reversible in the early stages of CVI, such as stasis dermatitis and early lipodermatosclerosis (grade C4a in the CEAP classification). In later stages there are irreversible changes, such as severe forms of lipodermatosclerosis (with a leg shape of an inverted champagne bottle) and atrophie blanche (grade C4b). Chronic and recurrent protein-rich oedema and aseptic inflammation induce fibrosis and tissue hypoxia. VLU represents the highest grade of CVI. It can occur spontaneously as a result from dermal and epidermal hypoxia, or after minor trauma to the trophically predamaged gaiter area [1].

Predisposing factors
Predisposing factors include family history, obesity, standing occupation, venous thromboembolism, varicose veins, ankle joint ankyloses and neuromuscular diseases with an impact on venous calf pump ejection.

Pathology
There is sclerosing panniculitis with non-specific skin ulceration. The epidermis is acanthotic, while the dermis is thickened and fibrotic. The subpapillary veins are elongated with wall thickening (pseudo-increased due to more cross-sections of tortuous vessels) (Figure 104.2). There are haemosiderin deposits. The chronically inflamed and fibrotic dermis expands, to the cost of the subcutis. The fascia is thickened and fibrotic; the leg muscles may show fatty degeneration. The ulceration itself is non-specific, exposing fibrin and/or biofilm layers, granulation tissue and a mixed inflammatory infiltrate.

Clinical features

History
There is usually a family history of CVI and VLU and a personal history of venous thromboembolism and/or varicose veins. Other

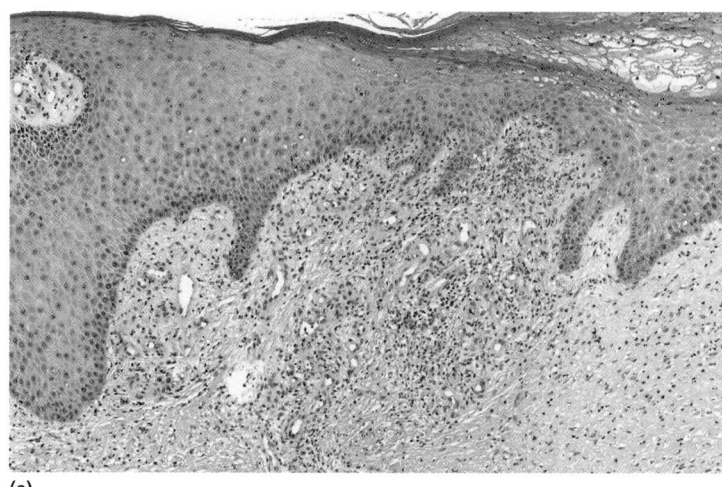

(a)

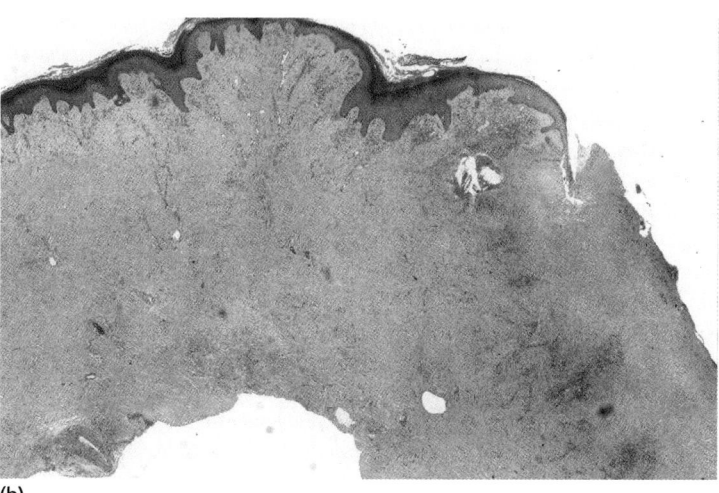

(b)

Figure 104.2 Histology of a venous leg ulcer. (a) Fibrotic dermis and subcutis with an apparent increase of vessels (venules) at the level of the subpapillary plexus. The apparent increase in vessels is caused by multiple cross-sections through tortous subpapillary venules. The vessels have thick walls, changes caused by chronic venous hypertension. (b) Extensive fibrosis extends into the subcutis.

common features are obesity, a standing occupation, neuromuscular disease and joint disease.

Presentation [1]
Chronic skin ulcers are common at the gaiter area, embedded in trophic skin changes attributed to CVI (stasis dermatitis, lipodermatosclerosis, pigmentation, induration, leg shape of an inverted champagne bottle). VLUs are less commonly located in the lateral retromalleolar area (related to deep and short saphenous vein reflux).

Clinical variants
These ulcers may be semicircumferential or circumferential in extensive cases. Patients with an insufficient deep venous system and an insufficient short saphenous vein may develop CVI at the lateral dorsum of the foot and the dorsum of the toes [1,2,3].

Differential diagnosis
This includes MLU, ALU, HYTILU and vasculitic leg ulcer (particularly in patients with chronic hepatitis C with cryoglobulinaemia) and males with Klinefelter syndrome.

Classification of severity
The CEAP system classifies active VLU as C6 and healed VLU as C5. The venous clinical severity score system (VCSS) is also used.

Complications and co-morbidities
These include chronic pain and impairment of quality of life, local wound infection, systemic infection and sepsis, infestation with maggots (fly larvae), secondary squamous cell carcinoma and secondary lymphoedema (periulcer lymphoedema and/or foot and toe lymphoedema).

Disease course and prognosis
Venous leg ulcers are chronic and recurrent unless patients receive an accurate diagnostic assessment on which to base treatment and secondary prevention.

Investigations
Recommended investigations are summarized here:
1 *Vascular investigations*:
   - Assessment of peripheral arterial disease: assessment of *systolic ankle blood pressure* and calculation of *ankle brachial pressure index (ABPI)*.
   - Assessment of venous pathologies: *superficial venous reflux* can be detected with simple continuous wave Doppler ultrasound (if the operator is sufficiently experienced). *Deep venous reflux/obstruction and/or post-thrombotic findings* can only be examined with duplex ultrasound. Venography gives good morphological information.
2 *Wound documentation* [3]. The wound size and its morphological qualities should be documented at every visit. Electronic photographic documentation systems along with their software allow for photometric wound surface area measurement to objectify the healing process.
3 *Microbiology*. In the presence of clinical signs of critical colonization and/or bacterial cellulitis and/or sepsis, wound microbiology must be analysed. A swab from the wound base (after the removal of fibrin layers and biofilms) or a small tissue biopsy from the wound base – if feasible – yield more representative microbiology results than superficial swabs from necrotic material.
4 *Wound histology*. If there is a suspicion of vasculitis, pyoderma gangrenosum, hypertensive ischaemic leg ulcer, ulcerating malignant skin tumour or in any refractory chronic leg ulcer showing no trend to heal after 3 months treatment, a biopsy should be performed. A deep and narrow (3–4 mm wide) ellipse biopsy, usually 3–5 cm long and including the vital wound border and ulcer base, should be taken and sent for routine histology (H&E), direct immunofluorescence and cryoconservation for eventual further examinations. The body of the ellipse biopsy that is sent in for H&E histology should be left intact and

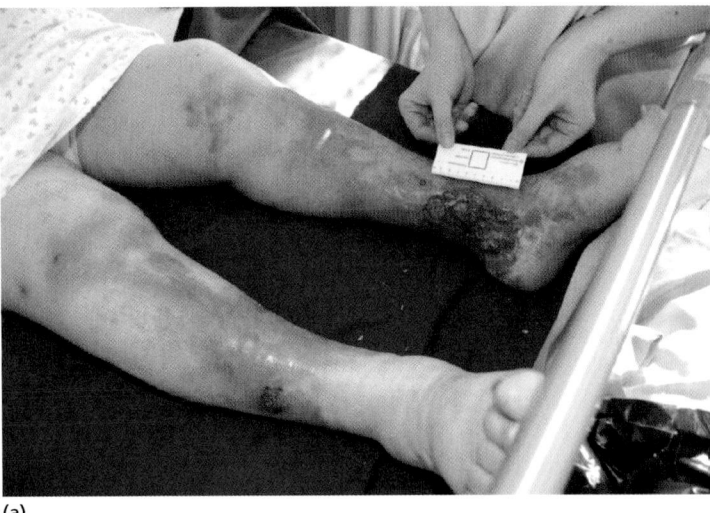

(a)

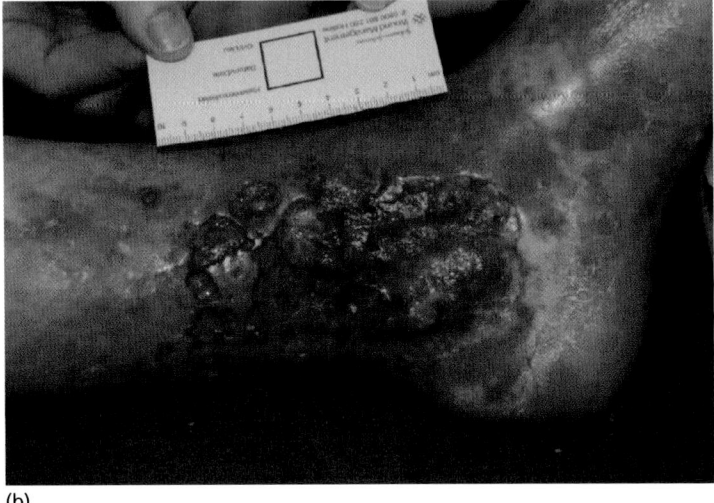

(b)

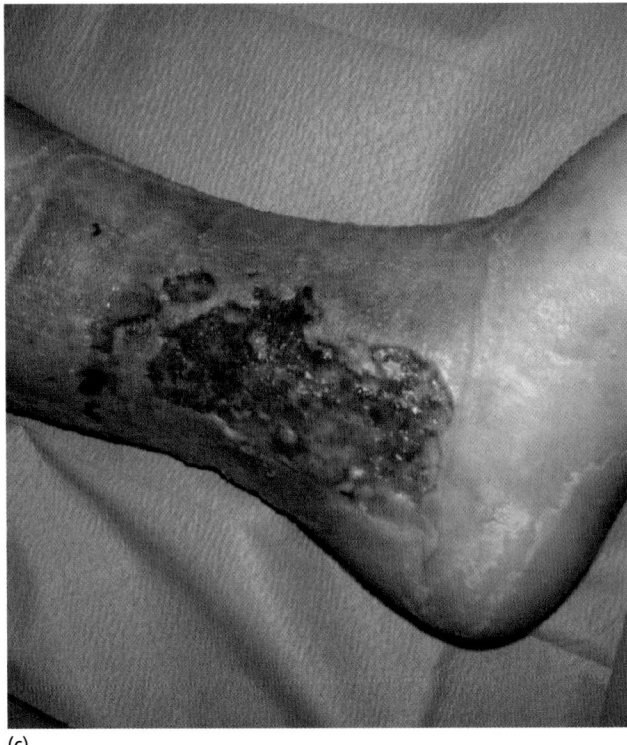

(c)

Figure 104.3 Venous leg ulcer. (a) A 77-year-old patient with chronic venous insufficiency following recurrent venous thromboembolism. There was uncontrolled oedema and non-infectious erythema; vascular assessment showed complete deep reflux and reflux of the long saphenous vein. There was no peripheral arterial disease. (b) Close up view of ulcer. (c) The same patient after 7 days of compression therapy with multilayer bandaging. The oedema and erythema has improved and there is early re-epithelialization.

sectioned lengthwise, in order to get a histological profile from vital skin to the ulceration, extending from the epidermis to the deep subcutis.

5 *Assessment of malnutrition*. Total protein, albumin and lymphocyte count are sufficient to indicate malnutrition in the vast majority of cases. More costly vitamin and/or zinc measurements should be restricted to specific questions.

6 *Pain assessment*. Pain should be assessed at regular (e.g. 4 weeks) intervals, with reproducible methods such as the visual analogue scale (VAS).

7 *Assessment of quality of life*. The use of a standardized QoL questionnaire (e.g. the SF36) is recommended [4].

Management

Compression therapy, either using bandages or stockings, are the mainstay in the treatment of VLUs (Figure 104.3) [5,6]. Manual or mechanical lymph drainage (intermittent pneumatic compression)

can be used as an adjunct [7]. Wound bed preparation considers *tissue* quality, *infection*/inflammation, *moisture* balance and *edge* advancement, according to the TIME concept. There is a large array of synthetic dressings and none are noticeably superior. Dressings have to be selected according to the stage of wound healing and the TIME policy [8,9]. Approximately half of patients with VLU suffer from superficial venous reflux which can be abolished by a variety of methods (flush ligation and stripping, endovenous thermoablation, foam sclerotherapy) [10], whereas patients with predominantly deep venous reflux have less or no benefit from superficial vein surgery [11]. Topical negative pressure (vacuum) significantly enhances healing of superinfected chronic leg ulcers with a substantial tissue loss [12]. Refractory VLUs can be treated with skin equivalents or tangential fibrosectomy with split-skin grafts (shave operation of VLU) (Figure 104.4). VLU recurrence is common (30% in 12 months) [7,13]. Consistent compression therapy and the elimination of superficial venous reflux are key to VLU prevention [5,7,11].

An algorithm of management is summarized in Figure 104.5.

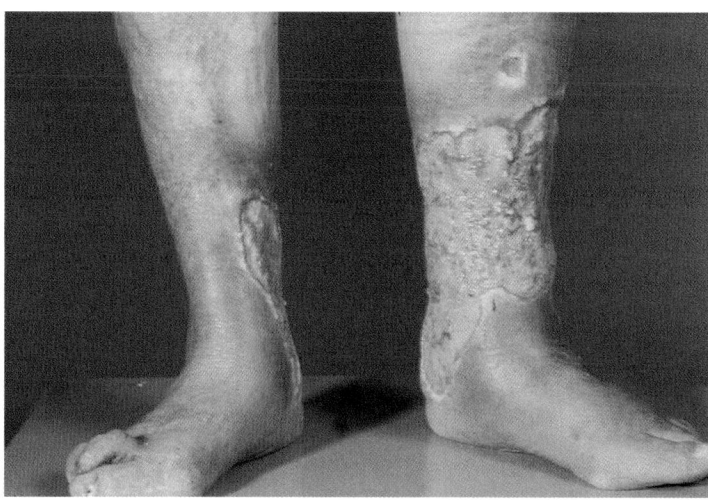

(a)

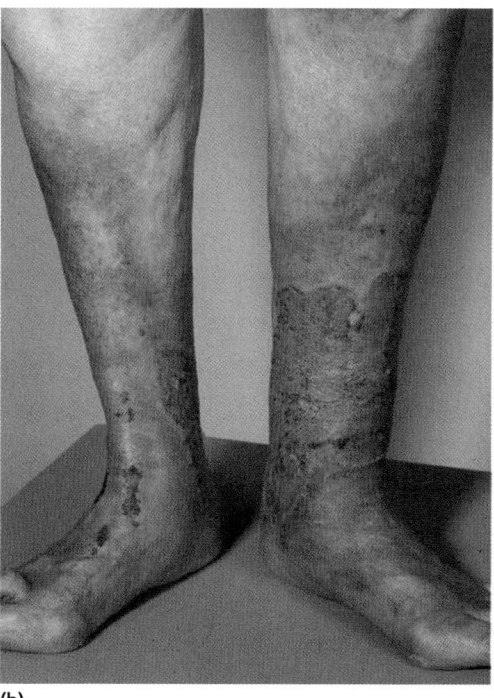

(b)

Figure 104.4 Post-thrombotic syndrome. (a) An 80-year-old patient with recurrent venous thromboembolism. The right leg shows a large chronic venous leg ulcer (VLU) at the medial ankle, the typical location. The left leg has a longstanding (approximately 30 years) circumferential VLU. (b) The same patient after shave operation split-skin grafting.

Resources

Further information

Deutsche Gesellschaft für Phlebologie. *Diagnostik und Therapie des Ulcus cruris venosum.* AWMF-Leitlinien-Register Nr. 037/009 Entwicklungsstufe 3. https://www .phlebology.de/leitlinien-der-dgp-mainmenu/171-diagnostik-und-therapie-des-ulcus-cruris-venosum (last accessed June 2015).

Neumann HAM, Jünger M, Munte K, *et al. S3-Guideline for Diagnostics and Treatment of Venous Leg Ulcers. Developed by the Guideline Subcommittee of the European Dermatology Forum.* http://www.euroderm.org/index.php/edf-guidelines (last accessed May 2015).

Maessen-Visch MB, de Roos KP. Dutch venous ulcer guideline update. *Phlebology* 2014;19(Suppl. 1):153–6.

O'Donnell TF, Passmann MA, Marston WA, *et al.* Management of venous leg ulcers: clinical practice guidelines of the Society for Vascular Surgery® and the American Venous Forum. *J Vasc Surg* 2014;60(Suppl. 2), S3–59.

Mixed leg ulcer

Definition and nomenclature

Mixed leg ulcers are VLUs in a leg with peripheral arterial disease (PAD) [1]. They are harder to heal than VLUs [2]. They cannot be distinguished from VLUs by clinical appearance alone. Diagnosis can only be made after vascular assessment. Bimalleolar (both medial and lateral) ulcer location is more common in MLUs than in VLUs. Clinical grading of CVI follows the CEAP classification, and PAD is graded after the Fontaine classification. Most patients with MLU have Fontaine grade 2 PAD, and do not meet the criteria of chronic critical limb ischaemia.

Synonyms and inclusions
- Mixed venous and arterial leg ulcer

Introduction and general description

Mixed leg ulcers are VLUs occurring in a leg compromised by PAD. Approximately 20% of all leg ulcers are MLUs. They are harder to heal than VLUs and diagnosis can only be made after vascular assessment as they are clinically identical to VLUs. This underscores the need for vascular assessment (arterial and venous examination) in all patients with leg ulcers. Since MLU patients with more advanced PAD do not tolerate compression therapy well, management primarily focuses on improving arterial inflow, mostly by the use of balloon catheter angioplasty (percutaneous transluminal angioplasty (PTA)), thereby transforming the MLU into a VLU. As soon as the arterial inflow is restored, management follows again the algorithm for VLU (see Figure 104.5) [1,3,4,5].

Epidemiology

Incidence and prevalence

The lifetime incidence of leg ulcers is around 1%, with a point prevalence of 0.1%. Since approximately 20% of all leg ulcers are MLUs, the lifetime incidence of MLUs can be calculated at 0.2%, and the point prevalence at 0.02%. Leg ulcer incidence rises to 4% in the population aged over 80 years.

Age

Mixed leg ulcers at a young age is exceptional since PAD mainly affects the population of 50 years and older. MLUs primarily occur in the over 65-year-old population.

Sex

Mixed leg ulcers occur equally distributed in women and men. Female patients are overrepresented in wound centres as they have a higher life expectancy.

PART 9: VASCULAR

PART 9: VASCULAR

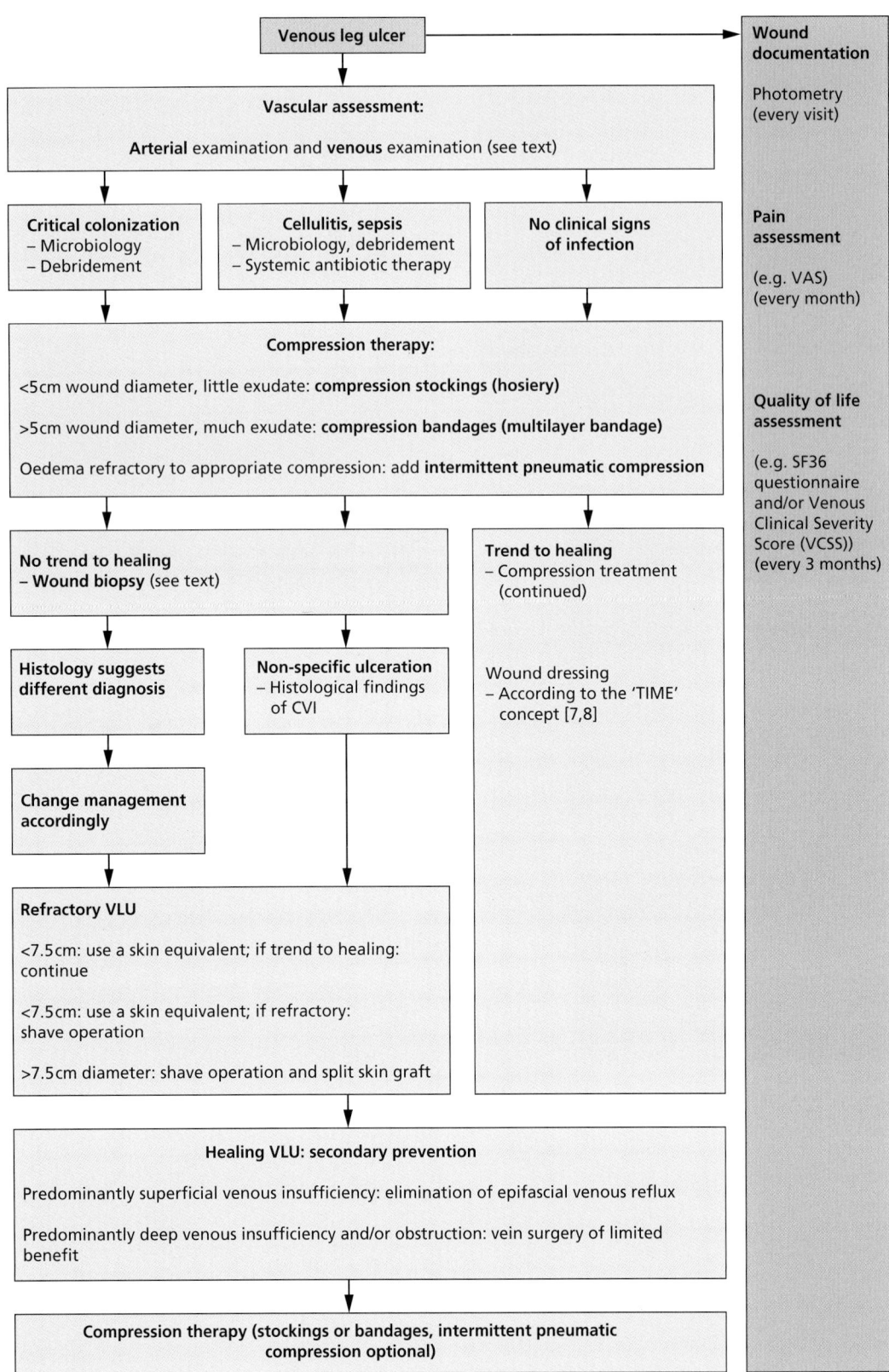

Figure 104.5 Algorithm of the management of venous leg ulcers. CVI, chronic venous insufficiency; VAS, visual analogue scale.

Box 104.2 Disorders associated with mixed leg ulcers

- Venous thromboembolism
- Superficial venous thrombophlebitis
- Varicose veins
- Chronic venous insufficiency
- Stasis dermatitis
- Lipodermatosclerosis
- Acroangiodermatitis
- Obesity
- Smoking
- Diabetes
- Hyperlipidaemia
- Hypertension
- Coronary heart disease
- Stroke

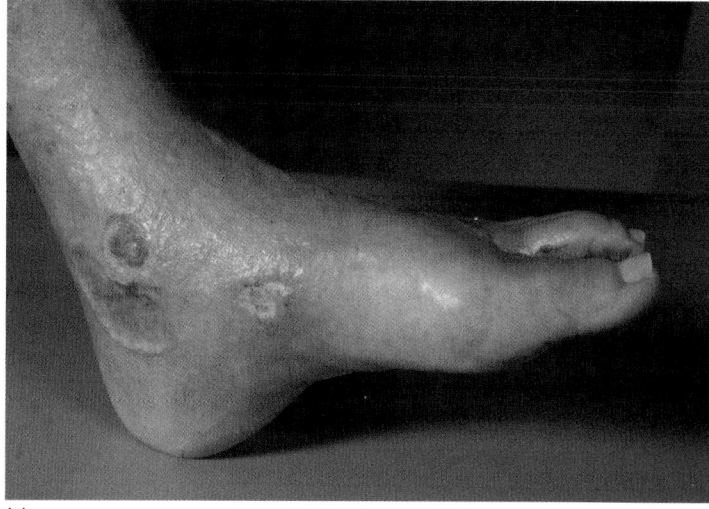

(a)

Ethnicity

These ulcers occur in any country and population. The incidence and prevalence, however, have exclusively been investigated in western nations. Western lifestyle increases the risk for both CVI and PAD.

Associated diseases

Box 104.2 lists a number of the associated diseases.

Pathophysiology

Pathophysiology combines the pathophysiology of VLU and PAD.

Predisposing factors

Predisposing factors include family history, obesity, standing occupation, venous thromboembolism, varicose veins, smoking, diabetes, hyperlipidaemia, hypertension, coronary heart disease and stroke.

Pathology

This is identical to that for VLU.

Clinical features

History

There is usually a family history of CVI and VLU and a personal history of venous thromboembolism and/or varicose veins. Other common features are obesity, a standing occupation, neuromuscular disease and joint disease. There are also cardiovascular risk factors: coronary heart disease, stroke and peripheral arterial disease.

Presentation

Mixed leg ulcers cannot be clinically distinguished from VLUs although a bimalleolar location (both medial and lateral skin ulcers on the same leg) occurs more frequently in MLUs (Figure 104.6).

Clinical variants

These ulcers may be semicircumferential or circumferential in extensive cases, with CVI at the dorsum of the foot in such cases.

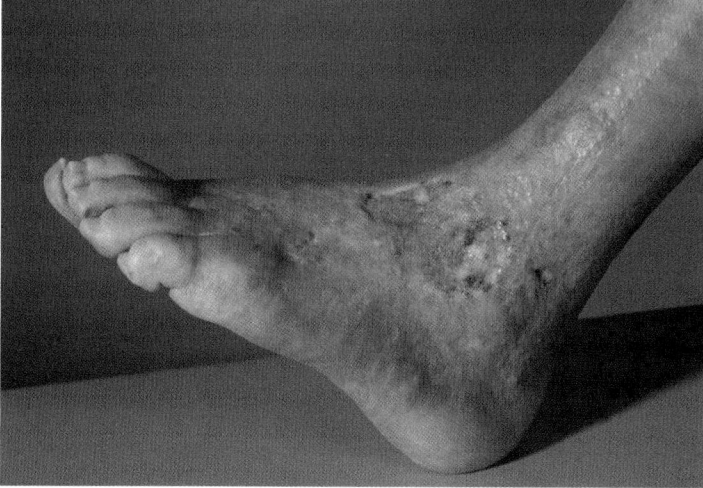

(b)

Figure 104.6 Mixed leg ulcer. (a) An 80-year-old patient with chronic venous insufficiency with lipodermatosclerosis and chronic leg ulceration at the medial ankle region. Vascular assessment demonstrated insufficiency of the superficial femoral, popliteal and posterior tibial veins, as well as peripheral arterial disease (ankle pressure 104 mmHg, ABPI 0.7). (b) The same patient with a chronic leg ulcer at the lateral ankle region (i.e. bimalleolar leg ulcers).

Differential diagnosis

This includes VLU, ALU, HYTILU and vasculitic leg ulcer (particularly in patients with chronic hepatitis C with cryoglobulinaemia) and males with Klinefelter syndrome.

Classification of severity

The CEAP system classifies active VLU as C6 and healed VLU as C5. The Fontaine classification of peripheral arterial disease is also used (see the section on arterial leg ulcers in this chapter).

Complications and co-morbidities

These include chronic pain and impairment of quality of life, local wound infection, systemic infection and sepsis, infestation with maggots (fly larvae), secondary squamous cell carcinoma,

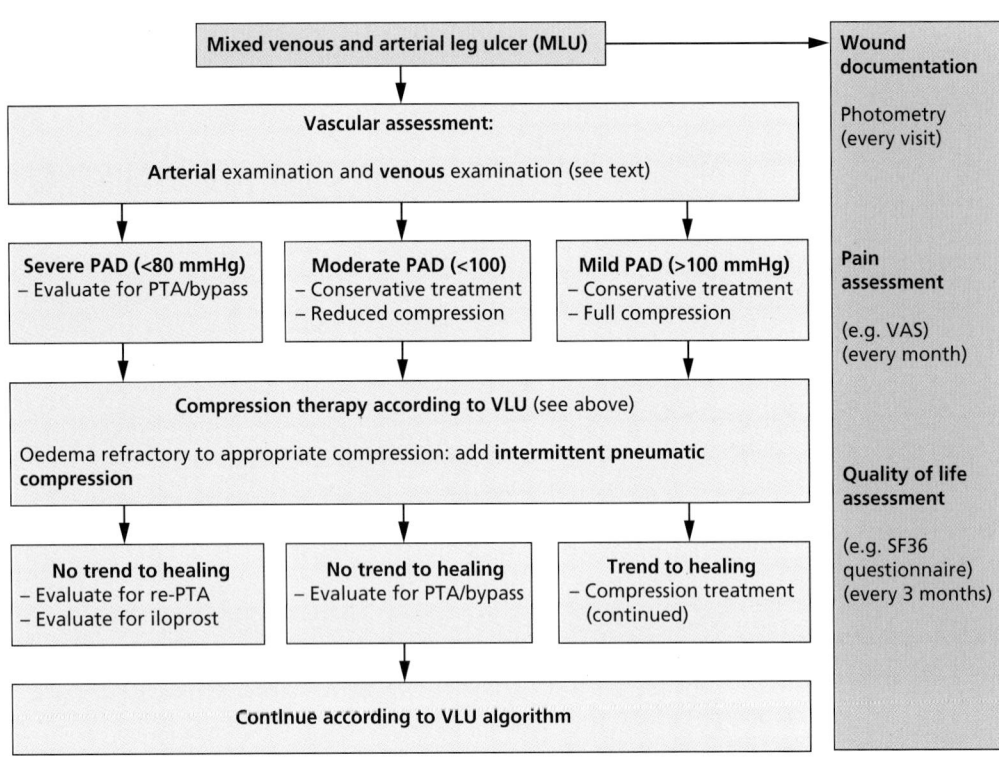

Figure 104.7 Algorithm of the management of mixed leg ulcers. PAD, peripheral arterial disease; PTA, percutaneous transluminal angioplasty; VAS, visual analogue scale.

secondary lymphoedema (periulcer lymphoedema and/or foot and toe lymphoedema) and extensive tissue necrosis requiring major surgery or amputation.

Disease course and prognosis

Mixed leg ulcers have a high risk of recurrence (50% in 12 months). Consistent compression therapy and angiological follow-up to quickly detect and re-treat PAD are key to reducing the frequency of MLU recurrence. Intermittent pneumatic compression (IPC) effectively treats both CVI and PAD. Therefore, IPC can be particularly beneficial to patients with MLU.

Investigations

Recommended investigations correspond to those in VLUs (see earlier section in this chapter).

Management

An algorithm of management is summarized in Figure 104.7.

Arterial leg ulcer

Definition and nomenclature

Arterial leg ulcers are chronic skin ulceration primarily caused by skin ischaemia due to advanced PAD.

Synonyms and inclusions
- Ischaemic leg ulcer
- Leg ulcer in peripheral arterial disease

Introduction and general description

Arterial leg ulcers originate from local skin ischaemia in advanced PAD. They may occur spontaneously or after minor trauma to an area of ischaemic skin that is at risk of ulceration. Initially they present as a black eschar or poorly granulating skin ulceration with a necrotic, black wound border. Delineation is sharp, and the wound border is generally steep [1,2]. The surrounding skin does not exhibit signs of CVI, but looks unchanged and normal. Approximately half of patients with HYTILU exhibit PAD in the same leg (see the next section in this chapter). The distinction between ALU and HYTILU with PAD on the same leg is based on skin and wound biopsy.

The measurement of systolic ankle pressure (AP) and the calculation of the ankle brachial pressure index (ABPI) typically exhibit values of 70–100 mmHg AP, which corresponds to an ABPI of 0.4–0.7, depending on the systolic blood pressure at the arm [1,2]. The criteria for critical limb ischaemia are rarely met: systolic AP <50 mmHg (or <70 mmHg in the presence of trophic skin lesions), systolic toe pressure <30 mmHg (or <50 mmHg in the presence of trophic skin lesions) and transcutaneous oxygen pressure (tcPO$_2$) <30 mmHg [1,2–4,5].

Epidemiology

Incidence and prevalence

The lifetime incidence of leg ulcers is around 1%, with a point prevalence of 0.1%. Since ALUs and HYTILUs together account for approximately 10% of all leg ulcers, the lifetime incidence of HYTILUs and ALUs can be calculated at 0.1%, and the point prevalence at 0.01%.

Age

Arterial leg ulcers generally affect the elderly, that is patients aged 60 years and above. Since PAD mainly occurs in individuals older than 50 years, ALU is very rare in young adulthood.

Sex

Arterial leg ulcers occur equally distributed in women and men. Female patients are overrepresented in wound centres since they have a higher life expectancy.

Ethnicity

These ulcers occur in any country and population. The incidence and prevalence, however, have exclusively been investigated in western nations. Western lifestyle increases the risk for ALUs.

Associated diseases

These include obesity, smoking, diabetes, hyperlipidaemia, hypertension, coronary heart disease and stroke.

Pathophysiology

Peripheral arterial disease leads to tissue ischaemia. The angiosome concept describes how each of the three calf arteries supplies arterial blood to well-delineated segments of the leg [6]. Occlusion of one or several branches of an atherosclerotic calf artery may directly and irreversibly shut down the skin circulation of a well-circumscribed area. The affected skin becomes cyanotic and then necrotic, a process accompanied by severe ischaemic pain. It remains to be shown if the lateral and pretibial skin circulation is less abundant and collateralized than at the medial and dorsal aspect of the leg, which would explain the proneness of these locations.

Predisposing factors

Predisposing factors include smoking, diabetes, hyperlipidaemia, hypertension, coronary heart disease and stroke.

Pathology

The histology of ALU is non-specific. It shows tissue necrosis and – in case of critical colonization – dense inflammatory infiltrates with polymorphonuclear leukocytes.

Clinical features

History

There is a history of cardiovascular risk factors and often symptoms of atherosclerosis of other vascular territories (coronary heart disease, stroke, renal artery stenosis).

Presentation

Arterial leg ulcers arise spontaneously as areas of painful skin necrosis (eschar), generally at the lateral or pretibial aspect of the leg (Figure 104.8). Typically, an ALU develops within normal-looking skin. Wound pain is strong, very strong or excruciating.

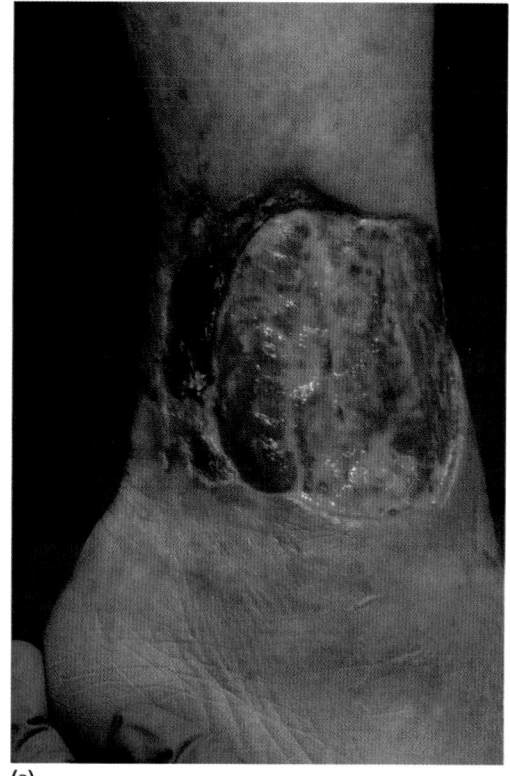

(a)

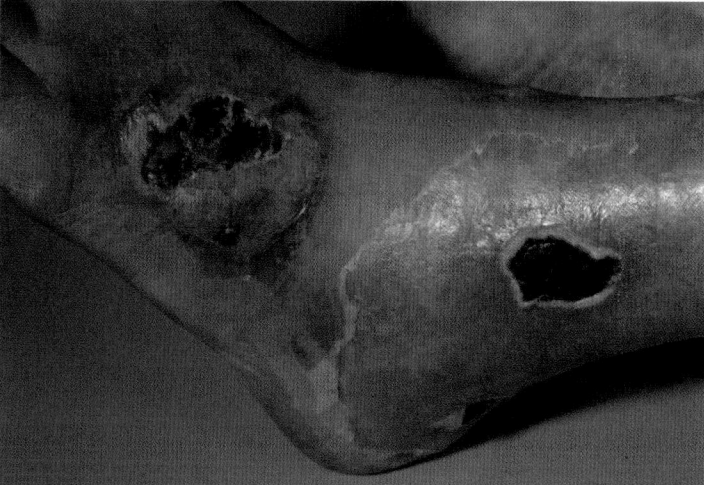

(b)

Figure 104.8 Arterial leg ulcer. (a) An 80-year-old patient with spontaneous and rapidly progressive, painful skin ulceration at the right lateral ankle region. Vascular assessment showed advanced peripheral arterial disease (ankle pressure 72 mmHg, ABPI 0.5). (b) A 51-year-old diabetic patient with skin necrosis with an eschar at the left lateral ankle and dorsum of the foot. Vascular assessment showed critical leg ischaemia (ankle pressure 64 mmHg, ABPI 0.4, tcPo$_2$ 21 mmHg).

The ulcer surface area tends to grow progressively. Clinically, there is a well-delineated zone of skin necrosis covered with eschar or remnants of necrotic wound border. Steep ulcer margins are usual, with a white or black wound base, exhibiting virtually no granulation tissue. Smaller ALUs are round in shape and have a 'punched-out' appearance. Larger ALUs are polycyclic and figurated.

PART 9: VASCULAR

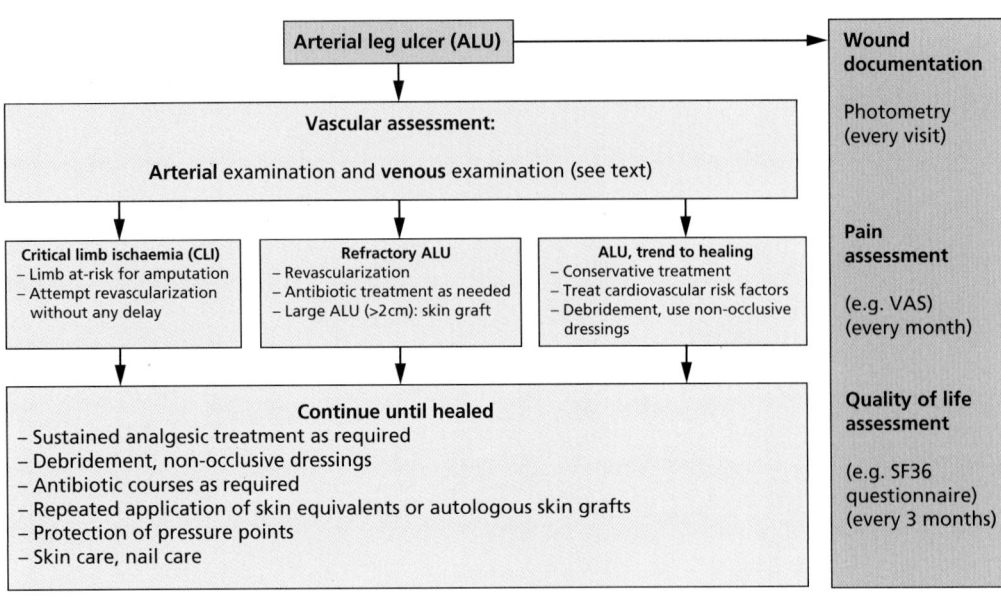

Figure 104.9 Algorithm of the management of arterial leg ulcers (ALUs). VAS, visual analogue scale.

Clinical variants

Arterial ulcers at the dorsum of the foot usually occur in very advanced PAD, in a leg that typically meets the criteria of CLI. ALUs can occur at a medial or dorsal location, however, this is unusual.

Differential diagnosis

This includes HYTILU (in some situations discriminating between ALU and HYTILU is difficult). Necrotizing vasculitis, necrotizing cutaneous embolism, pyoderma gangrenosum, necrotizing cutaneous infections and deep dissecting haematoma.

Classification of severity

Peripheral arterial disease can cause intermittent claudication (Fontaine grade 2), rest pain (Fontaine grade 3) and toe and/or forefoot necrosis (gangrene) (Fontaine grade 4). The higher grades 3 and 4 of PAD commonly fulfil the criteria of chronic CLI, which are defined by systolic ankle (<50 mmHg) and toe (<30 mmHg) pressure, and transcutaneous oxygen pressure (tcPo_2) (<30 mmHg). ALUs do not fit well into the Fontaine classification, but approximately 90% correspond to Fontaine grade 2, even if they do not exhibit intermittent claudication, due to impaired mobility.

Complications and co-morbidities

These include chronic pain and impairment of quality of life, local wound infection, systemic infection and sepsis, infestation with maggots (fly larvae) and extensive tissue necrosis requiring major surgery or amputation.

Disease course and prognosis

If PAD is amenable to PTA (balloon catheter angioplasty), prognosis is favourable. Successful PAD treatment alleviates pain almost immediately. Not all ALUs, however, heal spontaneously after revascularization. The majority benefit from an early skin graft to speed up wound healing and to terminate wound pain. The recurrence of ALUs is exceptional (unlike VLUs and MLUs). In patients who are not amenable to revascularization, iloprost perfusions can add some benefit, and IPC helps improve microcirculation in PAD. Wounds should be kept debrided, and occlusive wound dressings are contraindicated. Courses of antibiotic treatment may be required to treat critical colonization, to reduce peri-wound oedema and to improve the chances of healing. Split-skin grafts should be tried even under suboptimal local conditions (e.g. little granulation tissue).

Investigations

Recommended investigations correspond to those in VLUs (see earlier section in this chapter).

Management

Percutaneous transluminal angioplasty (balloon angioplasty) restores sufficient arterial inflow in the majority of cases. As a result, wound pain improves dramatically, although the wounds do not necessarily start to heal. Most patients still require a skin equivalent or autologous split-skin graft to speed up wound healing. Recurrences of ALUs are exceptional [2].

An algorithm of management is summarized in Figure 104.9.

Hypertensive ischaemic leg ulcer

Definition and nomenclature

Hypertensive ischaemic leg ulcers represent a skin infarction due to ischaemic, subcutaneous arteriolosclerosis occurring in a patient with hypertension.

Synonyms and inclusions
- Martorell hypertensive ischaemic leg ulcer
- Ulcus hypertonicum Martorell
- Angiodermite nécrotique
- Martorell hypertensive ischaemic leg ulcer

Introduction and general description

Hypertensive ischaemic leg ulcers were defined by Martorell in 1945 [1], and by Farber and Hines in 1946–47 [2]. They observed four hypertensive women who developed painful leg ulcers with histologically pathological subcutaneous arterioles. HYTILUs represent a form of skin infarction due to occlusive subcutaneous arteriolosclerosis [3,4,5,6,7]. On approximately 70% of histology slides, the thickened arterioles display striking medial calcinosis [6]. Wound location is highly characteristic. In more than 90% of patients the eschar or wound is located at the laterodorsal aspect of the leg and/or over the Achilles tendon [3,6]. All patients have hypertension, and 60% have type 2 diabetes. Clinically, HYTILU can be confused with pyoderma gangrenosum or vasculitic skin necrosis [6].

Epidemiology

Incidence and prevalence

The lifetime incidence of leg ulcers is around 1%, with a point prevalence of 0.1%. Since ALUs and HYTILUs together account for approximately 10% of all leg ulcers, the lifetime incidence of HYTILUs and ALUs can be calculated at 0.1%, and the point prevalence at 0.01%.

Age

It is exceptional to see HIYTILUs at a young age, since longstanding hypertension and diabetes mainly affect individuals aged 50 years and older. Therefore, HYTLU typically occurs in patients aged over 60 years.

Sex

These ulcers occur equally distributed in women and men. Female patients are overrepresented in wound centres since they have a higher life expectancy.

Ethnicity

These ulcers occur in any country and population. The incidence and prevalence, however, have exclusively been investigated in western nations. Western lifestyle increases the risk for HIYTILUs.

Associated diseases

Associated diseases include obesity, smoking, diabetes, hyperlipidaemia, hypertension, coronary heart disease and stroke.

Pathophysiology

An HYTILU is an ischaemic skin infarction caused by subcutaneous arteriolosclerosis (Figure 104.10). The arterioles regulate blood pressure, and hypertensive arteriolosclerosis is an expression of longstanding hypertension. Most patients with HYTILU have been treated for hypertension for many years and have normal blood

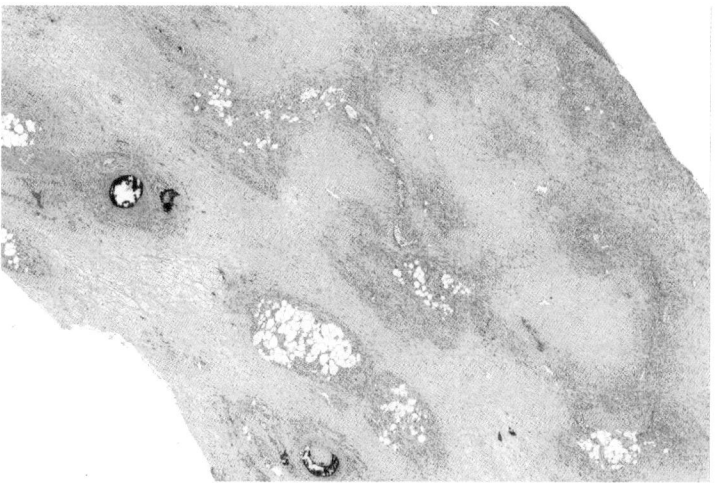

(a)

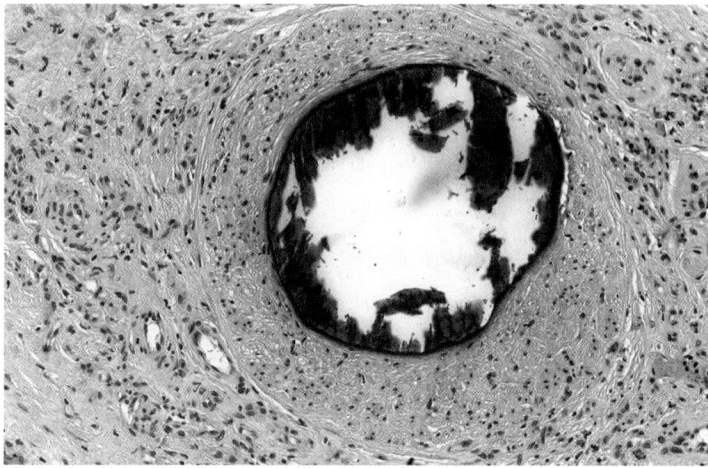

(b)

(c)

Figure 104.10 Subcutaneous arteriolosclerosis. (a, b) Skin biopsy showing subcutaneous arteriolosclerosis with medial calcification. (c) Skin biopsy showing stenotic subcutaneous arteriolosclerosis without medial calcification.

pressure values. Antihypertensive treatment spares large numbers of strokes and myocardial infarctions, leaving an increasingly large elderly population without any macrovascular complications of longstanding hypertension. This increases the likelihood that some well-treated hypertensive persons will develop HYTILUs, usually a non-life threatening, but highly symptomatic, late complication of hypertension.

Both clinically and histologically, Martorell HYTILUs cannot be distinguished from distal calciphylaxis (uraemic calcific arteriolopathy, distal pattern), proximal calciphylaxis (uraemic calcific arteriolopathy, proximal pattern), and 'eutrophication' (calciphylaxis in normal renal and parathyroid gland function). This suggests a common pathophysiology based on shared risk factors: hypertension, diabetes, an elevated $Ca \times PO_4$ product in case of end-stage kidney disease, and/or a dysfunction of the α_2-HS (Heremans–Schmid) glycoprotein (fetuin A), a vitamin K-dependent protein that protects tissues from calcification [8].

The sensitivity and specificity of the histological finding of subcutaneous arteriolosclerosis has yet to be investigated. Sometimes arterioles with an increased wall : lumen ratio can be found in the wound biopsies of venous ulcers. The prevalence of subcutaneous arteriolosclerosis at the laterodorsal aspect of the leg in the elderly or in the elderly hypertensive population is unknown.

Predisposing factors

Predisposing factors include hypertension, diabetes, hyperlipidaemia, smoking, coronary heart disease and stroke.

Pathology

The histology of HYTILUs is highly characteristic. The muscularis of the subcutaneous arterioles is greatly thickened at the expense of a narrow lumen. Approximately two-thirds of arterioles show striking medial calcinosis, comparable to the Monckeberg medial calcinosis of calf arteries (Figure 104.10a, b). The intima can be hyperplastic, adding to the arteriolar stenosis. The skin necrosis in itself is non-specific. It often exhibits biofilm layers that are loaded with bacteria.

Clinical features

History

A history of hypertension, diabetes and atherosclerosis of other vascular territories (coronary heart disease, stroke, renal artery stenosis) is common.

Presentation

The patient usually presents with single or multiple eschars and skin ulcers at the laterodorsal aspect of the leg and/or over the Achilles tendon (Figure 104.11). The wound border is livid or violaceus to black. The ulcer usually occurs within an area of livedo.

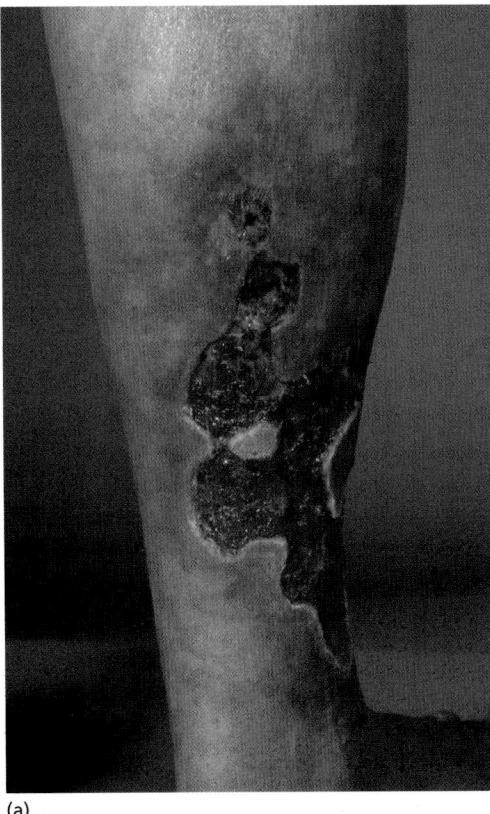

(a)

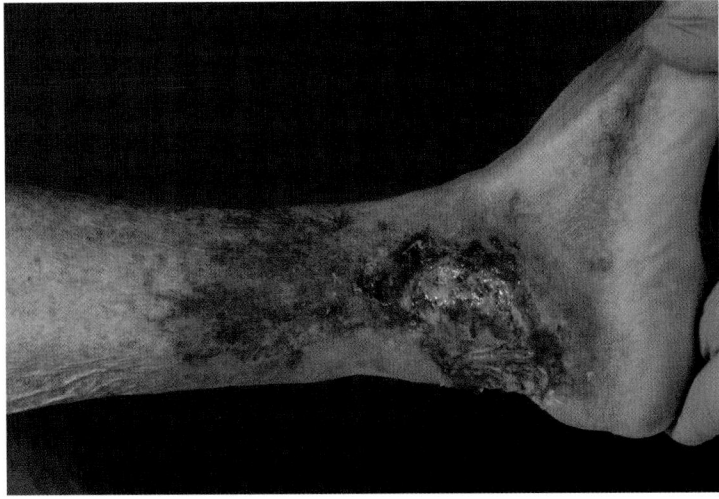

(b)

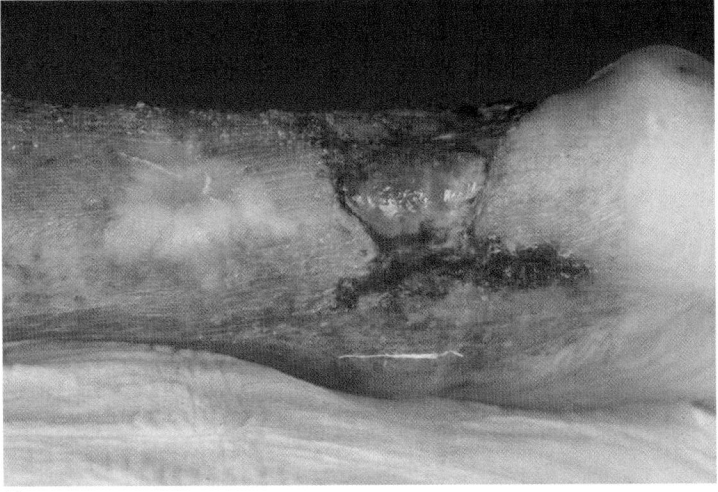

(c)

Figure 104.11 (a) A 65-year-old patient with hypertension (well controlled), diabetes (well controlled) and a polycyclic, figurated, painful ulcer at the laterodorsal aspect of the right leg. Vascular assessment showed no peripheral arterial disease (ankle pressure 132 mmHg, ABPI 1.0). (b) A 73-year-old patient with hypertension, no diabetes and skin necrosis at the right lateral ankle region, extending to the Achilles tendon. Vascular assessment showed no peripheral arterial disease (ankle pressure 146 mmHg, ABPI 0.9). (c) The same patient as Figure 104.3as showing skin ulceration at the left Achilles tendon.

Initially, there is rapid progression accompanied by excruciating pain. The necrosis comprises all skin levels and extends down to the fascia. Arteriolosclerotic skin ulcers can occur in a distal pattern (Martorell HYTILU) or in a proximal pattern involving the medial thighs, groins, abdomen, upper arms and breasts (referred to as 'calciphylaxis in normal kidney and parathyroid gland function' or 'eutrophication').

Clinical variants

A medial or pretibial location is exceptional, but can occur. Isolated skin necrosis over the Achilles tendon as sole manifestation occurs in 10–20% of cases.

Differential diagnosis

This includes pyoderma gangrenosum and vasculitic leg ulcer.

Classification of severity

Different grades of severity exist, but up to now they have not been standardized.

Complications and comorbidities

These include chronic pain and impairment of quality of life, local wound infection, systemic infection and sepsis. Extensive tissue necrosis may require major surgery or, exceptionally, amputation.

Disease course and prognosis

Prognosis is good even though HYTILU represents a severe disease in aged people. Half of patients require not only one, but several, skin grafts to completely heal all their wounds. Even if skin grafts do not 'take', pain is almost immediately alleviated.

Investigations

Recommended investigations correspond to those in ALUs (see earlier section in this chapter).

Management

Treatment consists of necrosectomy, local negative pressure wound treatment and, eventually, skin grafting. An algorithm of management is summarized in Figure 104.12.

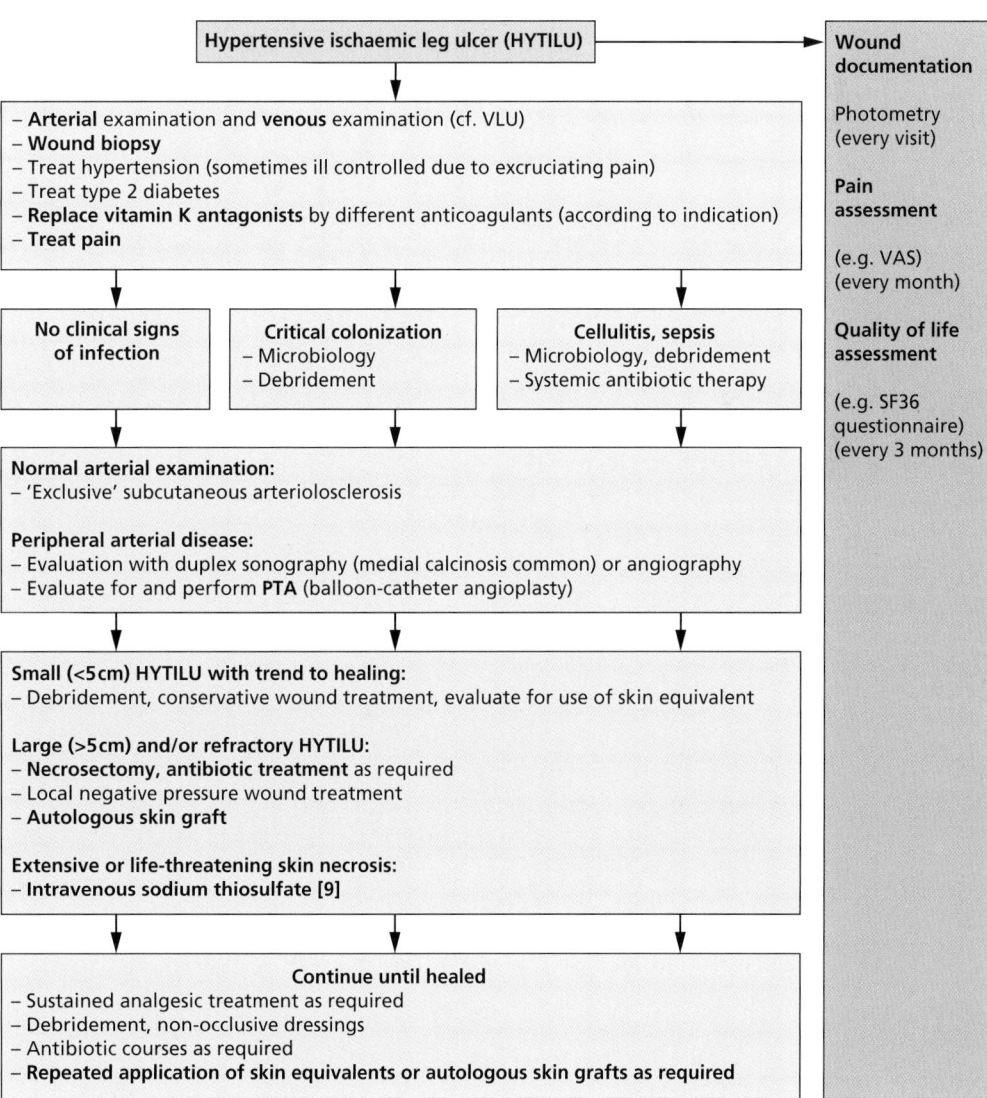

Figure 104.12 Algorithm of management of hypertensive ischaemic leg ulcers. PTA, percutaneous transluminal angioplasty; VAS, visual analogue scale; VLU, venous leg ulcer.

PART 9: VASCULAR

Key references

The full list of references can be found in the online version at www.rooksdermatology.com.

Introduction

1 Läuchli S, Bayard I, Hafner J, *et al.* Healing times and the need for hospitalization for leg ulcers of different etiologies [in German]. *Hautarzt* 2013;64:917–22.
2 Jockenhöfer F, Gollnick H, Herberger K, *et al.* Aetiology, comorbidities and cofactors of chronic leg ulcers: retrospective evaluation of 1000 patients from 10 specialised dermatological wound care centers in Germany. *Int Wound J* 2014, epub ahead of print.

Venous leg ulcer

1 Eklöf B, Rutherford RB, Bergan JJ, *et al.* Revision of the CEAP classification for chronic venous disorders: consensus statement. *J Vasc Surg* 2004;40:1248–52.
5 Mauck KF, Asi N, Elraiyah TA, *et al.* Comparative systematic review and meta-analysis of compression modalities for the promotion of venous ulcer healing and reducing ulcer recurrence. *J Vasc Surg* 2014;60(Suppl. 2):S71–90.
9 Schultz GS, Barillo DJ, Mozingo DW, *et al.* Wound bed preparation and a brief history of TIME. *Int Wound J* 2004;1:19–32.
11 Barwell JR, Davies CE, Deacon J, *et al.* Comparison of surgery and compression with compression alone in chronic venous ulceration (ESCHAR study): randomized controlled trial. *Lancet* 2004;363:1854–9.

Mixed leg ulcer

1 Ghauri AS, Nyamekye I, Grabs AJ, *et al.* The diagnosis and management of mixed arterial/venous leg ulcers in community-based clinics. *Eur J Vasc Endovasc Surg* 1998;16:350–5.

4 Humphreys ML, Stewart AH, Gohel MS, *et al.* Management of mixed arterial and venous leg ulcers. *Br J Surg* 2007;94:1104–7.
5 Obermayer A, Göstl K, Partsch H, *et al.* Venous reflux surgery promotes venous leg ulcer healing despite reduced ankle brachial pressure index. *Int J Angiol* 2008;27:239–46.

Arterial leg ulcer

2 Hafner J, Schaad I, Schneider E, *et al.* Leg ulcers in peripheral arterial disease (arterial leg ulcers): impaired wound healing above the threshold of chronic critical limb ischemia. *J Am Acad Dermatol* 2000;43:1001–8.
3 Norgren L, Hiatt WR, Dormandy JA, *et al.* Inter-society consensus for the management of peripheral arterial disease (TASC II). *Eur J Vasc Endovasc Surg* 2007;33(Suppl. 1):S1–75.
4 Rutherford RB, Baker JD Ernst C, *et al.* Recommended standards for reports dealing with lower extremity ischemia. Revised version. *J Vasc Surg* 1997;26:517–38.

Hypertensive ischaemic leg ulcer

1 Martorell F. Las ulceras supramaleolares por arteriololitis de las grandes hipertensas. *Actas (Reun Cientif Cuerpo Facul) Inst Policlinico Barcelona* 1945;1:6.9.
3 Schnier BR, Sheps SG, Juergens JL. Hypertensive ischemic ulcer: a review of 40 cases. *Am J Cardiol* 1966;17:560–5.
5 Vuerstaek JD, Reeder SW, Henquet CJ, Neumann HAM. Arteriolosclerotic ulcer of Martorell. *J Eur Acad Dermatol Venereol* 2010;24:867–74.
6 Hafner J, Nobbe S, Partsch H, *et al.* Martorell hypertensive ischemic leg ulcer: a model of ischemic subcutaneous arteriolosclerosis. *Arch Dermatol* 2010;146:961–8.

CHAPTER 105
Disorders of the Lymphatic Vessels

Peter S. Mortimer and Kristiana Gordon

St George's Hospital, London, UK

PART 9: VASCULAR

Introduction

Lymphatic dysfunction interferes with fluid homeostasis, tissue immunity and peripheral fat mobilization. Any chronic oedema represents lymphatic failure. If impaired lymph drainage is solely responsible, then lymphoedema results. This produces characteristic skin changes known as elephantiasis as well as increased fat deposition in the subcutaneous tissues. Impaired immune cell trafficking results in an increased risk of infection, particularly cellulitis (erysipelas), which often becomes recurrent. This chapter describes the clinical consequences of lymphatic dysfunction and in particular the impact on the skin and subcutaneous tissues. The sections are divided according to common clinical presentations.

CLINICAL PRESENTATIONS OF LYMPHATIC DYSFUNCTION

Chronic, venous and drug-induced oedema

Definition and nomenclature

Oedema is an excess of interstitial fluid. Any oedema, whatever the cause, is due to capillary filtration overwhelming the lymph drainage for a sufficient period of time [1]. Interstitial fluid is reabsorbed almost entirely by the lymphatic vessels. Contrary to

Rook's Textbook of Dermatology, Ninth Edition. Edited by Christopher Griffiths, Jonathan Barker, Tanya Bleiker, Robert Chalmers and Daniel Creamer.
© 2016 John Wiley & Sons, Ltd. Published 2016 by John Wiley & Sons, Ltd.
Companion website: www.rooksdermatology.com

popular belief, venous reabsorption of interstitial fluid cannot be maintained for any length of time in peripheral tissues. Therefore all peripheral oedema represents lymphatic failure. Most chronic oedemas arise from increased microvascular filtration overwhelming the lymph drainage (relative lymphatic failure). Examples are heart failure, venous disease and nephrotic syndrome. Oedema arising principally from a failure in lymph drainage is lymphoedema (absolute lymphatic failure).

Synonyms and inclusions
- Oedema
- Lymphoedema
- Dependency oedema

Introduction and general description
It is important to determine if oedema (Greek oídēma, a swelling) is due to fluid or another tissue component. Overgrowth syndromes, such as Klippel–Trenaunay syndrome, may have excessive growth of bone, fat or muscle (with or without additional fluid). A plexiform neurofibroma (neurofibromatosis) may cause tissue swelling from both the neural tumour and lymphoedema.

If swelling is fluid it is best not to approach a lower limb chronic oedema clinically by trying to pigeonhole the diagnosis into 'heart failure', 'venous oedema', 'lymphoedema', etc. A far better approach is to consider if the oedema represents pure lymphatic failure, or, as is most common, lymphatic failure due to the lymph drainage being overwhelmed by increased capillary filtration. Most cases of chronic oedema have more than one factor contributing to the impaired lymph drainage and increased capillary filtration (Table 105.1). Consequently, treatment of chronic oedema should be to enhance the lymph drainage and address any factors causing increased filtration.

If lower limb oedema is unilateral or asymmetrical then local factors need to be considered such as pelvic lymph or venous obstruction, post-thrombotic syndrome or inflammation from der-

matitis or infection. Bilateral lower limb oedema suggests systemic factors such as hypoproteinaemia or high central venous pressure (e.g. heart failure). In the obese person, several factors contribute. The weight of a huge abdominal apron causes obstruction of lymph and venous drainage in the thigh or groin when sitting [2]. Poor mobility results in no enhancement of lymph drainage. Sitting with legs dependent causes periods of high venous pressure and consequently high microvascular fluid filtration (falling asleep in a chair without leg elevation is particularly bad). Sleep apnoea syndrome leads to periods of arterial and pulmonary hypertension and fluid retention [3].

Epidemiology
Lymphoedema per se is perceived as uncommon, yet lymphatic insufficiency is a major contributing cause of chronic ankle oedema, which is considered common (particularly in the elderly). Lymphoedema can be a difficult diagnosis, particularly if mild or in the early stages, therefore it is frequently underdiagnosed. One survey, which determined the problem of chronic oedema (as a surrogate for lymphoedema) in the community, ascertained 823 patients in a catchment area of 619 000 in southwest London. This estimated the overall prevalence of chronic oedema as 1.33/1000 population; the prevalence increased with age and was 5.4/1000 in subjects aged over 65 years (i.e 1 in 200). In only a quarter did the oedema arise from cancer treatment [4].

Pathophysiology
Oedema develops when the microvascular (capillary and venular) filtration rate exceeds lymph drainage. Simply put, the blood vessel supplies tissue fluid and the lymphatic drains it away. For oedema to develop either the microvascular filtration rate is high, the lymph flow is low, or there is a combination of the two.

The filtration rate is governed by the Starling principle of fluid exchange. Microvascular filtration of fluid from capillary into interstitium is driven by the hydraulic (water) pressure gradient across the blood vessel wall ($P_c - P_i$) in which P_c indicates capillary

Table 105.1 Causes of chronic oedema.

Increased capillary filtration			Reduced lymph drainage	
↑Capillary pressure	↓Plasma proteins	↑Capillary permeability	Primary lymphatic insufficiency	Secondary lymphatic insufficiency
↑Venous pressure:	↑Loss:	Inflammation:	Germline mutation:	Iatrogenic
Right heart failure	Nephrotic syndrome	Varicose eczema	Genes known (Milroy	Surgery
DVT	Protein-losing enteropathy	Psoriasis	disease, lymphoedema,	Radiotherapy
Venous obstruction	↓Synthesis:	Chronic infection	distichiasis)	Cancer
Calcium channel	Cirrhosis	Urticaria and angio-oedema	Genes unknown (Meige	Infection
antagonists	Advanced cancer	Drugs	disease)	Filanasis
Dependency	Malabsorption		Mosaic mutation:	Cellulitis
Overtransfusion:	Malnutrition		Lymphatic malformation	Accidental trauma
Salt and water overload			Overgrowth spectrum	Obesity
Advanced renal failure				Immobility
↑Blood flow:				Sustained lymph load:
Inflammation				Venous disease
Arteriovenous fistula				Heart failure
				Venous obstruction
				DVT

DVT, deep-vein thrombosis.

pressure and P_i indicates interstitial pressure) and is opposed by the osmotic pressure gradient ($\pi_p - \pi_i$) in which π_p indicates plasma osmotic pressure and π_i indicates interstitial osmotic pressure from tissue proteins), which is the suction force retaining fluid within the vessel. This is the suction force retaining fluid within the vessel. The colloid osmotic pressures influencing filtration across both fenestrated and continuous capillaries are exerted across the endothelial glycocalyx; the osmotic pressure of the interstitial fluid does not directly determine transendothelial fluid exchange. There is substantial evidence that with important exceptions such as the renal cortex and medulla, downstream microvessels are not in a state of sustained fluid absorption as traditionally depicted. Although doggedly persistent in textbooks and teaching, the traditional view of a filtration–reabsorption balance has little justification in the microcirculation of most tissues. Tissue fluid balance thus depends critically on lymphatic function in most tissues [5].

Clinical features

History
Lymphoedema does not usually respond to elevation or diuretics, except in the early stages or when it is compounded by increased capillary filtration. Chronic oedema that does not reduce significantly after overnight elevation is likely to be lymphatic in origin. Chronic oedema associated with bacterial cellulitis indicates lymphatic insufficiency because of the important role the lymphatic plays in tissue immunosuveillance.

A drug history is important because a number of drugs can cause chronic oedema. Calcium channel antagonists are a common cause of peripheral oedema, with amlodipine one of the worst offenders. Other drugs described to cause oedema are corticosteroids, taxanes, non-steroidal anti-inflammatories, clonidine, morphine, gabapentin, olanzapine, pramipexole and thiazolidinediones.

Presentation
Interstitial fluid volume must increase by over 100% before oedema is clinically detectable through pitting or indentation of the skin from pressure. Dermal oedema manifests as 'peau d'orange' due to expansion of the interfollicular dermis, whereas subcutaneous oedema gives rise to pitting.

Lymphoedema differs from all other oedemas (in which increased capillary filtration is the major factor) in that cells, proteins and fat accumulate in addition to water. This results in a 'solid' as well as a 'fluid' component to the swelling, so giving rise to the brawny nature of the oedema, which does not readily pit except in the early stages. The lack of pitting is an unreliable sign in lymphoedema. Easy displacement of tissue fluid on pressure can often be demonstrated, particularly in the early stages. With time, the skin thickens in lymphoedema and becomes more warty. A positive Kaposi–Stemmer sign represents a failure to pinch a fold of skin at the base of the second toe and is pathognomonic of lymphoedema (Figure 105.1).

In circumstances where the cause of the chronic oedema is not obvious a search for reasons for high microvascular fluid filtration should be pursued, for example raised jugular venous pressure in heart failure, local inflammation from dermatitis or infection, and low plasma proteins. In the lower limbs, signs of venous disease causing venous hypertension – for example varicose veins,

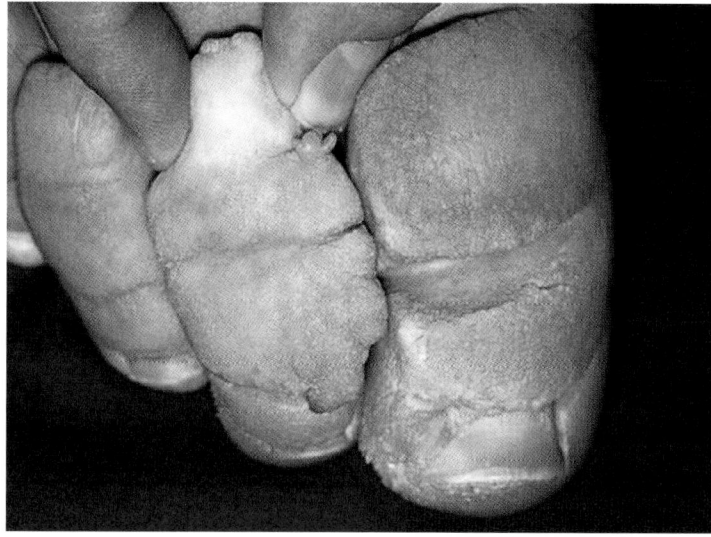

Figure 105.1 The Kaposi–Stemmer sign: an inability to pinch or pick up a fold of skin at the base of the second toe indicates lymphoedema.

haemosiderin deposition (particularly submalleolar), varicose eczema and atrophie blanche – should be carefully assessed. The reason severe venous disease may not exhibit oedema is because lymph drainage is maintained but in most cases it is the associated lymphatic insufficiency that causes the 'venous oedema'.

Investigations
Management of chronic lower limb oedema requires treatment of the underlying cause. If increased microvascular filtration is suspected then the following should be considered and investigated.
1 Causes of high central venous pressure (e.g. heart failure) should be pursued. B-type natriuretic peptide (BNP) estimation is a useful screen. The main clinical utility of either BNP or NT-proBNP (N-terminal pro-BNP) is that a normal level rules out acute heart failure.
2 Plasma albumin should be measured and if low a search for loss (e.g. nephrotic syndrome) or failure (e.g. liver disease, malabsorption or malnutrition) of synthesis should be considered.
3 Local inflammation should be looked for; this will increase microvascular filtration (e.g. infection, dermatitis or underlying arthritis).

There are limited methods available that permit reliable investigation of the lymphatics. Lymphoscintigraphy (isotope lymphography) involves the interstitial (dermis or subcutis) injection of a radiolabelled protein or colloid. Radioactivity, measured using a wide field-of-view gamma camera, is determined over the injection site depot and at regions of interest over vessels or nodes. Measurement of transit times and time activity curves permits a quantitative analysis of lymph drainage [6]. Measurement of tracer uptake within axillary or ilioinguinal lymph nodes at a specified time will discriminate lymphoedema from oedema of non-lymphatic origin (Figure 105.2).

Computed tomography (CT) of lymphoedematous limbs has demonstrated a characteristic 'honeycomb' pattern in the subcutaneous compartment which other oedemas do not show. CT not only provides information through cross-sectional area of volume change in a limb, but will also identify the compartment in which that change takes place. Thickening of the skin is also a characteristic feature of

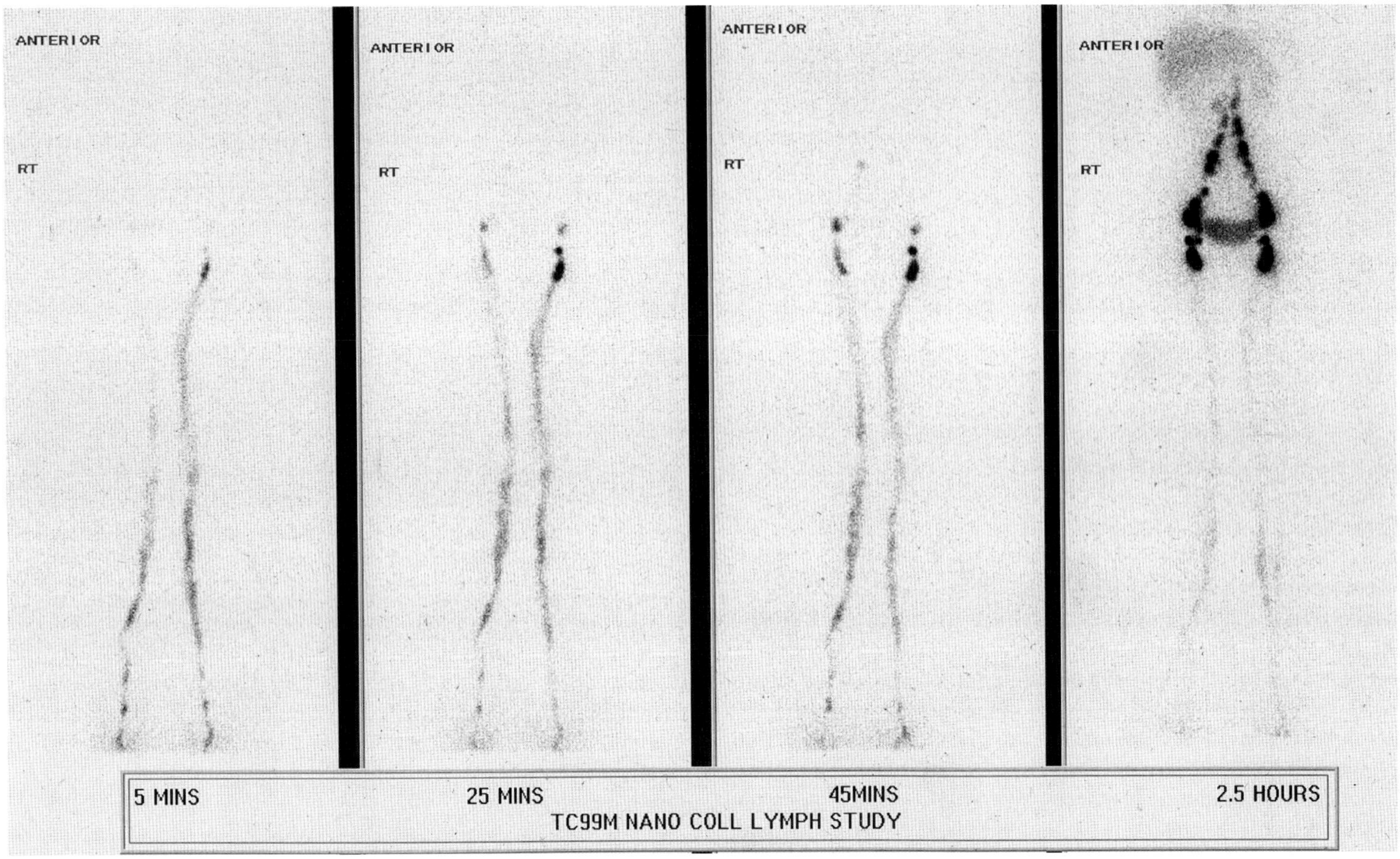

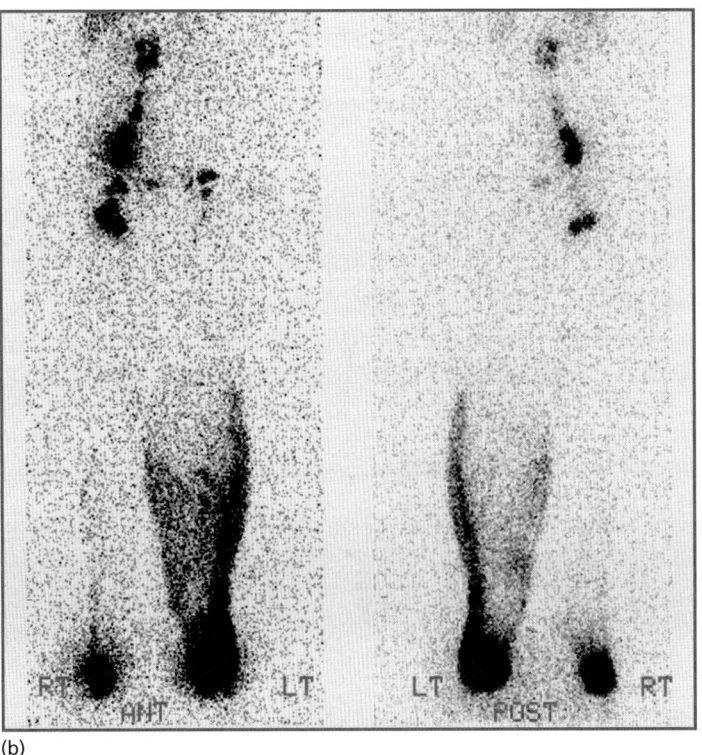

Figure 105.2 (a) Normal lymphoscintigraphy. Images show patent lymph routes draining tracer from the feet to the ilio-inguinal nodes. (Courtesy of Professor A. M. Peters.)
(b) Obstruction of lymph drainage at the groin leads to re-routing of tracer through the skin collaterals (dermal backflow).

lymphoedema, although not specific. Magnetic resonance imaging (MRI) is potentially better than CT for distinguishing types of oedema. Magnetic resonance lymphangiography has recently been introduced to overcome the invasive nature of X-ray lymphography.

Management

Venous oedema results from venous hypertension causing excessive microvascular filtration. Varicose veins or post-thrombotic syndrome are the commonest causes. However, it must be remembered that it is the lymphatics and not the veins that are responsible for the drainage of tissue fluid. If the lymph drainage is compensating, no matter how severe the venous disease, there will be no oedema. By implication, oedema in the presence of venous disease indicates lymphatic failure and treatment needs to address improvements in lymph drainage as well as control of the venous disease. Surgical treatment of varicose veins will often not resolve the 'venous' oedema because lymph drainage is compromised and surgery will not improve it, indeed it may reduce it further. Therefore compression is the treatment of choice for venous oedema because compression garments (hosiery) have the advantage of reducing microvascular filtration (from venous hypertension) while at the same time improving lymph drainage.

In cases of drug-induced oedema (e.g. due to amlodipine), the drug should be replaced or measures introduced to control swelling. The empirical use of diuretics is to be discouraged as they are often ineffective over time.

Swelling of one leg points to a local cause such as venous obstruction from vein compression or a deep-vein thrombosis (DVT). Lymphatic obstruction usually produces whole-limb swelling that is worse proximally. Imaging is required in case of cancer.

Genital oedema occurring in isolation is usually a result of local inflammation, for instance due to infection, ano-genital granulomatosis (cutaneous Crohn disease), hidradenitis suppurativa or sarcoidosis. Genital oedema can be part of more widespread oedema from heart failure or nephrotic syndrome. Primary lymphoedema can affect the genitalia but not usually without lower limb involvement. Lymph or chylous reflux can produce genital oedema often with lymphangiectasia (weeping lymph blisters).

The same physiological principles apply to upper limb oedema as they do to lower limb oedema – that is, microvascular fluid filtration exceeding lymph drainage capacity for a sustained period. Upper limb oedema is much less common than lower limb oedema and usually results from either proximal venous obstruction (e.g. thoracic outlet syndrome) or an inflammatory disorder (e.g. due to infection, arthritis or eosinophilic fasciitis) or lymphoedema.

Chronically swollen leg

Definition and nomenclature

Swelling of the lower limb, due to oedema, is caused by increased microvascular fluid filtration overwhelming lymph drainage. Causes of increased filtration such as increased venous pressure, low plasma proteins and inflammatory states need to be considered as well as reasons for impaired lymph drainage.

Synonyms and inclusions
- Oedema
- Lymphoedema
- Puffiness

Introduction and general description

Swelling of a leg may be caused by oedema, in which case pitting should be evident to some degree, or it may be caused by an increase in volume of other tissue elements, for example bone, muscle or fat. The cause of swollen legs is often multifactorial (Table 105.2); therefore, the patient's individual history and an appropriate physical examination are important. Other differentials

Table 105.2 Causes of a swollen leg.

Genetic			Acquired				
Vascular	**Lymphatic**	**Other**	**Vascular**	**Lymphatic**	**Inflammatory**	**Musculoskeletal**	**Tumours**
Vascular malformation	Lymphoedema	Overgrowth spectrum:	DVT	Lymphoedema:	Cellulitis	Rheumatoid arthritis	Lymphoma
Diffuse phlebectasia	Lymphatic malformation	Fat hypertrophy	Post-thrombotic syndrome	Cancer surgery	Pretibial myxoedema	Ruptured Baker's cyst	Sarcoma
Klippel–Trenaunay syndrome	Lymphangiomatosis	Lipomatosis	Chronic venous reflux	DXT	Varicose eczema	Joint effusion	Metastases
Parkes–Weber syndrome		Lipoedema	Venous outflow obstruction	Filanosis	Psoriasis	Haematoma	
Maffucci syndrome		Proteus syndrome	Dependency syndrome	Podoconiosis	Pompholyx	Torn muscle	
		Muscle hamartoma/ overgrowth	Thrombophlebitis	Trauma	Sarcoidosis	Pathological fracture	
		Gigantism/ hemihypertrophy	Venous injury, e.g. IV drug abuse	Reconstructive surgery	Herpes simplex	Achilles tendonitis	
			Acute arterial ischaemia	Vein harvesting/vein stripping		Myositis ossificans	
			Idiopathic/cyclical oedema of women	Immobility/armchair legs			
			Drugs, e.g. calcium channel antagonists	Factitial			
				Chronic regional pain syndrome			
				Obesity			

DVT, deep-vein thrombosis; DXT, radiotherapy; IV, intravenous.

to consider are a ruptured Baker's cyst, infection, trauma and malignancy. Inflammation of a joint or periarticular structure may cause oedema that is not primarily vascular. MRI is useful in circumstances where the nature of the swelling is uncertain. A patient may perceive one leg to be swollen when in fact the other leg has become smaller, for example through atrophy of muscle or fat. This section addresses fluid-related swelling that is vascular in origin.

Epidemiology

Chronic leg swelling is common but data are few. A recent report from Denmark indicated that of 595 hospitalizations of patients aged 75 years or above in the emergency department, 6.3% were due to suspected DVT or red swollen legs [1].

Pathophysiology

All oedema is caused by microvascular fluid filtration exceeding lymph drainage for a sufficient period of time. As lymph flow is responsible for the drainage of all tissue fluid, except for transient periods of venous reabsorption, a chronically swollen leg due to fluid indicates lymph drainage failure. This failure will be either due solely to lymphatic dysfunction (lymphoedema) or due to excessive microvascular fluid filtration overwhelming lymph drainage capacity [2]. Causes of increased microvascular fluid filtration are: (i) increased venous pressure due to chronic venous insufficiency, post-thrombotic syndrome, venous obstruction or heart failure; (ii) hypoproteinaemia from protein loss (e.g. nephrotic syndrome), malnutrition or a failure of protein synthesis (e.g. cirrhosis); (iii) increased vascular permeability (e.g. inflammatory states such as infection or dermatitis).

In cases of obesity and infirmity, lymph drainage routes in the leg may be patent but non-functional due to lack of mobility, for example in arthritis. In addition sitting for long periods without moving will cause sustained venous hypertension and increased fluid filtration into the legs, while the lack of movement will result in poor lymph drainage. Furthermore, a large obese abdominal apron pressing on the thighs when sitting will obstruct venous outflow. Sleep apnoea syndrome will result in systemic 'fluid retention' due to high heart chamber pressures.

Clinical features

History

Clinical features will depend upon the cause. Features that indicate primarily a lymphatic cause are: (i) persistent swelling, which can be intermittent at first; (ii) oedema that does not resolve with overnight elevation; (iii) a poor response to diuretics; and (iv) recurrent cellulitis.

Presentation

Chronic, non-inflammatory, asymmetrical lower limb oedema should always suggest a cause within the hindquarter (e.g. chronic venous hypertension or lymphoedema). Systemic causes of oedema including cardiac disease, renal disease or hypoproteinaemia should cause bilateral leg swelling. Calcium channel antagonists cause peripheral oedema in up to 30% of cases.

Lymphoedema characteristically produces a thickened skin. With increasing chronicity and severity, so skin changes of hyperkeratosis and papillomatosis (elephantiasis) supervene. A failure to pinch a fold of skin at the base of the second toe (Kaposi–Stemmer sign; see Figure 105.1) is pathognomonic of lymphoedema. In more advanced cases fat deposition and fibrosis lead to a more indurated or 'brawny' swelling that results in bulging folds of skin and subcutaneous tissue.

The chronically swollen red leg usually indicates lipodermatosclerosis. While usually attributed to chronic venous disease, oedema is always a feature and cases do occur with lymphoedema in the absence of venous reflux.

Investigations

Blood tests are important to exclude hypoproteinaemia and heart failure, where measurement of plasma albumin and BNP (or NT-proBNP) should be performed respectively. In cases of suspected venous and/or lymphatic obstruction, imaging such as ultrasound, CT or MRI of the root of the limb (e.g. the ilioinguinal region) should be undertaken. Lymphoscintigraphy is the investigation of choice to confirm a lymphatic aetiology. Venous duplex ultrasound will identify whether venous reflux is contributory to the fluid swelling. A skin biopsy may be necessary if pathologies such as Kaposi sarcoma, pretibial myxoedema or malignancy are considered.

Management

Treatment of a swollen leg is dependent on the cause. In circumstances where systemic causes for peripheral oedema (e.g. heart failure) have lead to, or coexist with, the lymphoedema, then treatment of the internal medical condition must be undertaken before embarking on specific lymphoedema therapy. The general principle for treating a swollen limb is to control for increased microvascular filtration and to enhance lymph drainage. Lymph drainage responds to exercise and movement while wearing compression [3]. This principle will also control venous hypertension.

Phleboedema and mixed lymphovenous disease

Definition and nomenclature

Phlebolymphoedema or mixed lymphovenous disease is a mixed aetiology swelling of the lower limb due to chronic venous insufficiency and lymphatic insufficiency. Phlebolymphoedema refers to chronic oedema arising from chronic venous hypertension causing increased microvascular fluid filtration overwhelming lymph drainage. Over time established lymphoedema results from the compromised lymphatics.

Synonyms and inclusions
- Venous oedema
- Lipodermatosclerosis
- Venous stasis
- Post-thrombotic syndrome
- Venous obstruction
- Chronic oedema
- Elephantiasis

Introduction and general description

Veins and lymphatics are inextricably linked. Their endothelial parentage is identical as lymphatics and veins have a common embryological origin [1]. They have synergistic functions – the venous capillaries and venules filter fluid from circulation to tissue spaces and the lymphatics drain that fluid back (eventually) to the circulation.

Oedema is a common complication of venous insufficiency. It is assumed that venous oedema is the sole consequence of increased capillary filtration from venous hypertension. As lymph drainage is the main buffer against oedema, it is in fact the failure of local lymphatics to compensate for the increased lymph load from filtration that leads to oedema [2]. Lymphoedema associated with venous disease can give rise to the most gross swelling and skin changes owing to the combined effect of impaired lymph drainage in the face of increased lymph load (capillary filtration) (Figure 105.3).

Phlebolymphoedema most commonly occurs in the lower limb but can occur elsewhere in the body in circumstances of venous hypertension – for example a pendulous abdomen (hanging abdominal apron), large pendulous breast and upper limb venous outflow obstruction.

Epidemiology

Oedema is a common finding in chronic venous disease. The Bonn vein study identified up to 20% prevalence depending on age and severity of the venous disease [3].

Pathophysiology

Predisposing factors

Phlebolymphoedema requires raised venous pressure to increase fluid movement from the blood vessels (capillaries and venules)

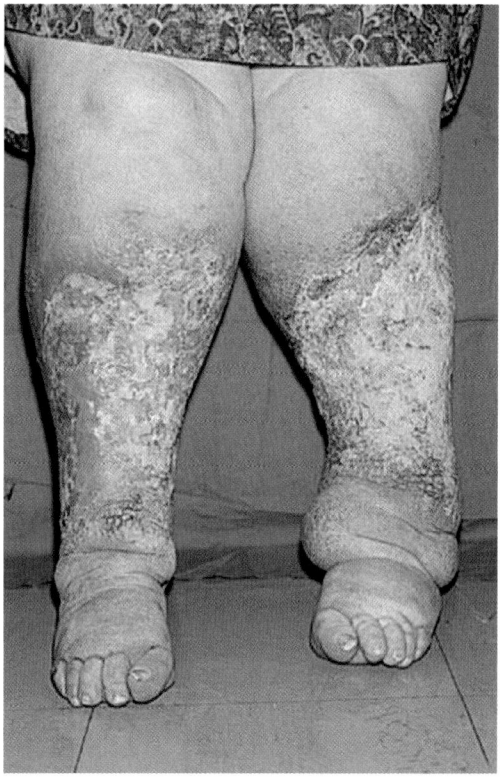

Figure 105.3 Lymphoedema associated with chronic venous disease.

into the tissue spaces. In the lower limbs this may occur from varicose veins, DVT or venous obstruction (Figure 105.4). Because the calf muscle pump is important for venous drainage, long periods spent with the legs dependent and therefore subject to gravitational forces causes sustained periods of venous hypertension.

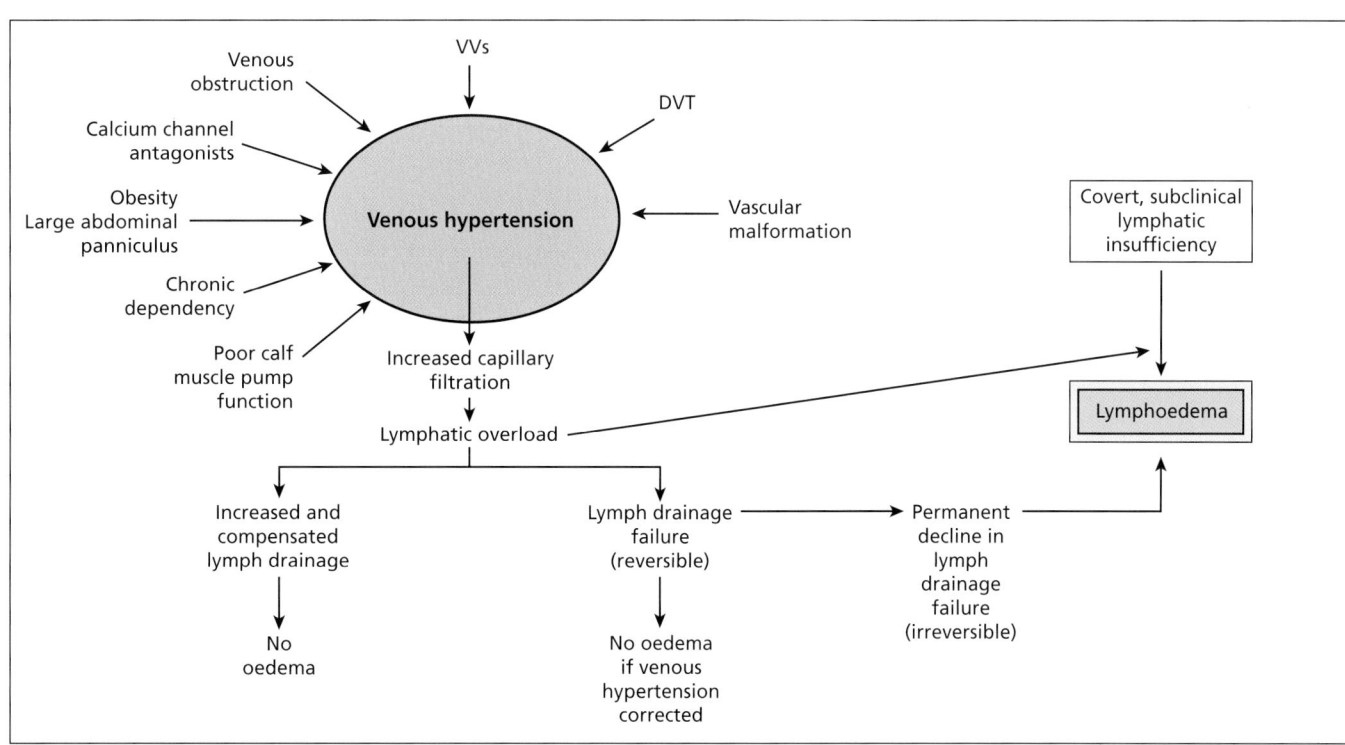

Figure 105.4 Causes of mixed lymphovenous disease and phlebolymphoedema.

Immobility tends to encourage swelling, particularly if gravitational forces (dependency syndrome) encourage ongoing fluid filtration. A common scenario is 'armchair legs', where patients sit in a chair day and night with their legs dependent (otherwise known as elephantiasis nostras verrucosis because of the severe lymphoedema skin changes that ensue). Patients at risk are those with neurological deficit in the legs preventing movement; those with chronic respiratory or cardiac disease, which requires them to sit upright in a chair day and night; and those with sleep apnoea syndrome who cannot lie flat. Obesity can also result in venous obstruction when a large abdomen compresses the thigh veins when sitting upright in a chair.

Treatment with calcium channel antagonists causes lower limb oedema in up to 30% of users [4]. Discontinuing the drug will often resolve the oedema.

Traditional surgical stripping of varicose veins or harvesting of the great saphenous vein for coronary artery bypass grafting could also damage leg lymphatics and lead to phlebolymphoedema. Fortunately, both procedures are rarely performed since the introduction of endovenous therapy and stenting.

Intravenous drug abuse can damage both the veins and lymphatics from both thrombosis and sepsis leading to phlebolymphoedema in the upper and lower limbs.

Pathology

Oedema is an excess of interstitial fluid. Any oedema, whatever the cause, is due to capillary filtration overwhelming the lymph drainage for a sufficient period of time [5]. Contrary to popular belief, venous reabsorption of interstitial fluid cannot be maintained for any length of time in peripheral tissues. Interstitial fluid is reabsorbed almost entirely by the lymphatic vessels. Venous hypertension causes an increase in microvascular fluid filtration that requires greater lymph drainage if oedema is to be avoided. In chronic venous disease the fluid load frequently overwhelms lymph drainage to produce oedema. Over time the high lymph load results in deteriorating lymph drainage and a permanent lymphoedema. Furthermore, high tissue fluid and venous pressure result in lipodermatosclerosis, an inflammatory condition of the most affected skin and subcutaneous tissues.

Genetics

Many primary lymphoedemas for which gene mutations are known also possess venous reflux because of a genetically determined venous valve failure. The best documented is lymphoedema distichiasis syndrome where the mutation is in the *FOXC2* gene [6].

Clinical features

History

Phlebolymphoedema in the lower limb will start as a pitting oedema indistinguishable from any other chronic oedema. There may be a history of varicose veins including past venous surgery (stripping or endovenous therapy), DVT, heart failure, sleep apnoea syndrome, obesity or infirmity with long periods spent with the legs dependent.

Chronic venous disease may result in symptoms such as heaviness, aching, itching (from varicose dermatitis), skin pigmentation (from purpura or haemosiderin). Symptoms worsen towards the end of the day and are relieved by overnight elevation and are usually exacerbated by heat and alcohol. Lipodermatosclerosis will often produce severe pain and tenderness. Poor wound healing can result in a chronic ulcer.

When lymphoedema dominates, the skin becomes harder and swelling does not resolve as much with overnight elevation. Recurrent cellulitis always indicates lymphatic insufficiency.

Presentation

When chronic oedema is associated with symptoms and signs of chronic venous disease then phlebolymphoedema is likely. Oedema is usually confined to below the knee but severe cases can extend into the thigh. When signs of lymphoedema dominate then tissues will be indurated and pitting more difficult to elicite. The Kaposi–Stemmer sign will probably be positive (pathognomonic of lymphoedema) (see Figure 105.1).

Advanced cases develop elephantiasis skin changes with hyperkeratosis and papillomatosis [7]. Recurrent cellulitis can occur due to underlying lymphatic insufficiency and the effect lymphatic dysfunction has on local immune cell trafficking. Such infections will usually cause local signs of inflammation (i.e. pain, redness, heat and swelling), signs that can easily be confused with acute (on chronic) lipodermatosclerosis. Lipodermatosclerosis, however, does not cause systemic upset, an increased white cell count or C-reactive protein (CRP) or respond to antibiotics.

Chronic regional pain syndrome (reflex sympathetic dystrophy) can present like a phlebolymphoedema, but pain (particularly allodynia) and loss of function are distinctive features.

Differential diagnosis

When venous hypertension exists with lymphatic insufficiency then phlebolymphoedema is likely. However, there may be many causes for venous hypertension and more than one cause may coexist – for example, heart failure, obesity, chronic venous disease, dependency, etc.

Complications

Phlebolymphoedema may be complicated by lipodermatosclerosis, dermatitis, ulceration, lymphorrhoea and infection, especially cellulitis. Rarely, malignancy (e.g. lymphangiosarcoma) can complicate the phlebolymphoedema.

Prognosis

Prognosis is poor regarding long-term morbidity unless underlying causes are addressed. Compression therapy with exercise is the only satisfactory treatment.

Investigations

Venous duplex ultrasound is the investigation for chronic venous disease. It can detect venous reflux, thrombosis and some venous obstruction. In cases of mixed vascular malformations and iliac vein obstruction, more specialist imaging with venography may be necessary.

Lymphoscintigraphy is the investigation of choice for detecting lymphatic insufficiency. It is very sensitive but not that specific and can miss lymphoedema, particularly in the presence of venous disease.

Management

First line

Compression and exercise treat both venous disease and lymphoedema. Compression may be achieved through bandaging or compression garments. Bandaging is helpful initially to produce a reduction in swelling and improve limb shape so compression garments fit better. Standard 'venous ulcer' compression bandaging will adequately treat most cases but if there is marked forefoot involvement (swollen or papillomatous toes) or if swelling extends above the knee, then lymphoedema-style treatment in the form of decongestive lymphatic therapy (DLT) is preferred [8]. DLT involving toe and thigh bandaging can only be provided by trained therapists and is generally not available in the community.

Wounds, dermatitis and infection need to be treated before, or at the same time, as compression is applied.

Exercise is to be encouraged in preference to rest but when the patient is resting, the leg should be elevated to heart level. Patients should be discouraged from spending too long in a chair unless it is a reclining chair. In infirm patients pneumatic compression therapy may be helpful [9].

Second line

Superficial venous reflux may be amenable to endovenous therapy. Hopefully this will reduce the lymph load and so reduce oedema but it is often still necessary to wear compression garments afterwards [10].

Lipodermatosclerosis (chronic cellulitis)

Definition and nomenclature

The chronically swollen red leg is a common sight in medical practice. Often wrongly mistaken for bacterial cellulitis, it is frequently mismanaged. Lipodermatosclerosis (LDS) is an inflammatory condition of the skin and subcutaneous tissues affecting the lower third of the leg, and is commonly, although incorrectly, called chronic cellulitis. It is due to sustained 'congestion' – that is, high interstitial fluid and venous pressures. It is most usually described with chronic venous disease but the common denominator is chronic oedema and it can frequently be seen in lymphoedema without any venous reflux. While it resembles bacterial cellulitis there are no systemic symptoms or signs of infection. Bacterial infection (true cellulitis) can, however, frequently complicate LDS but antibiotics alone do not resolve it and the only proven treatment is compression therapy to 'decongest' the tissues.

Synonyms and inclusions
- Chronic cellulitis
- Sclerosing panniculitis

Introduction and general description

Many patients diagnosed with bacterial cellulitis do not have infection and therefore antibiotic treatment is inappropriate. Distinguishing true cellulitis or erysipelas from its many mimics is challenging but critical if unnecessary use of antibiotics, unnecessary in-patient admissions and delays in treatment are to be avoided.

True bacterial cellulitis presents with local redness, heat, pain and swelling at one site (e.g. one leg), combined with systemic upset such as fever or flu-like symptoms. Inflammatory markers including white cell count and CRP are usually raised and there is a good response to antibiotic treatment.

LDS is usually bilateral with no systemic symptoms and no raised inflammatory markers. Its response to antibiotics is poor.

Epidemiology

Of 595 hospitalizations of patients aged 75 years or above in an emergency department in Denmark, 6.3% were due to suspected DVT or red swollen legs [1].

Pathophysiology

Predisposing factors

It is assumed to be chronic venous disease but chronic oedema is the only invariable predisposing factor. It is caused by lymphoedema, chronic venous disease, dependency and immobility and cellulitis.

Pathology

The pathology of LDS is not well understood but has always been considered secondary to chronic venous hypertension. mRNA and protein expression of matrix metalloproteinase 1 (MMP-1), MMP-2 and tissue inhibitors of metalloproteinase 1 (TIMP-1) have been shown to be significantly increased, indicating that LDS is characterized by elevated matrix turnover [2]. LDS is always accompanied by tissue iron overload. It has been suggested that patients with LDS are unable to counteract venous-induced skin iron overload [3].

Clinical features

History

Lipodermatosclerosis is usually bilateral. While redness and oedema are always present, warmth is usually, but not always, present. Induration indicates that the underlying subcutaneous tissues are involved with the inflammatory process (sclerosing panniculitis). Pain and tenderness are ever present but not itch; if itch occurs, varicose/stasis eczema probably coexists. Systemic symptoms and signs are absent as are raised inflammatory markers. Antibiotics have no effect, but because the patient is often admitted and confined to bed, or told to rest with legs elevated, there is an improvement in the inflammation because of a lessening of the congestion [4].

Presentation

There are two forms of LDS: acute and chronic (Figure 105.5). Acute LDS simulates acute cellulitis with a flare of local redness, heat and pain. With time the chronic form supervenes. The skin becomes 'bound down' and retracted as the subcutaneous tissues become more fibrotic and contracted. Eventually redness gives rise

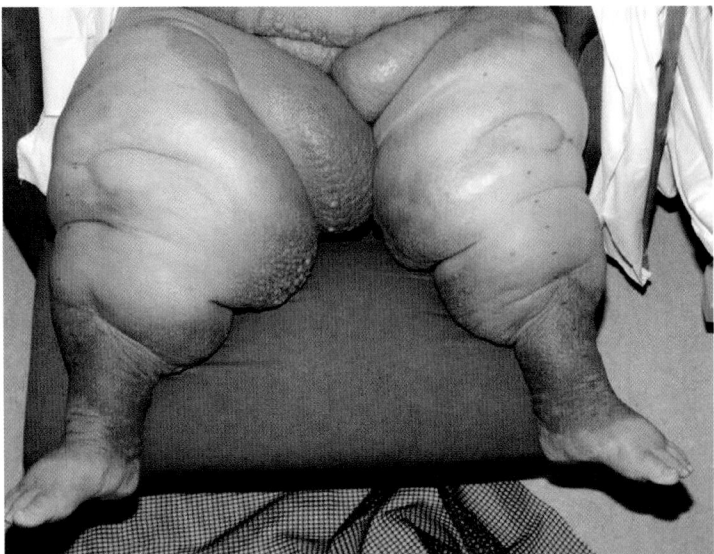

Figure 105.5 Acute and chronic lipodermatosclerosis; the bright red skin (acute) could be mistaken for bacterial cellulitis but it is an inflammatory response to the skin fluid congestion. The treatment is decongestive lymphatic therapy with or without antibiotic cover.

to brown pigmentation and the leg contour takes on an 'inverted champagne bottle' shape. Pitting oedema will continue to exist both above and below the area of LDS and is a common feature (and common denominator) throughout.

Differential diagnosis
The differential diagnosis is acute cellulitis.

Complications
Complications may include lymphorrhoea, infection and ulceration.

Investigations
Lipodermatosclerosis is a clinical diagnosis. Biopsy will reveal 'stasis dermatitis' changes together with a fibrotic panniculitis but there are no specific or diagnostic features. Furthermore, biopsy may induce ulceration if healing is poor.

Management

First line
Compression therapy is the only proven therapy. Compression bandaging will achieve quicker results than compression hosiery but may not be tolerated if the affected tissues are very inflamed and tender. In such circumstances it may be necessary to start with bed rest or even topical steroids before introducing gentle compression. In more chronic cases, where shape change exists, multilayer lymphoedema compression bandaging works better [5]. Bandaging may have to be continued until a more normal contour shape is obtained. Only then will compression hosiery fit and work satisfactorily.

Second line
If superficial venous reflux is proven on duplex ultrasound then endovenous therapy (e.g. radiofrequency vein ablation, laser vein ablation or foam sclerotherapy) could be administered. If endovenous therapy is considered unsuitable then traditional ligation and stripping of superficial veins could be undertaken [6].

Recurrent cellulitis (erysipelas)

Definition and nomenclature
Cellulitis (or erysipelas as it is more usually known in Europe) is one of the most common reasons for emergency admissions to hospital and up to half of patients have repeat attacks. Lymphoedema and leg ulcers provide the greatest risk for cellulitis, particularly recurrent cellulitis. Penicillin is effective in preventing subsequent attacks of cellulitis during prophylaxis, but the protective effect diminishes progressively once drug therapy is stopped [1]. Risk factors such as lymphoedema need to be addressed if recurrence is to be averted.

Synonyms and inclusions
- Erysipelas
- Lymphangitis
- Pseudo-erysipelas
- Pseudo-cellulitis
- Dermatolymphangioadenitis

Introduction and general description
Cellulitis of the leg is a common infection of the skin and subcutaneous tissues. Most infections that affect intact skin are thought to be due to streptococci although other organisms may be responsible if the integrity of the skin is compromised [2]. Cellulitis is a common consequence of lymphoedema irrespective of the cause of the lymphoedema. In recurrent cellulitis, the damage to the lymphatics may make the lymphoedema worse and so predispose to yet further episodes of infection. There is evidence that covert lymphatic insufficiency may predispose to first time attacks of cellulitis [3].

In filarial lymphoedema, episodes of infection – referred to as acute dermatolymphangioadenitis, but to all intents and purposes the same as cellulitis – cause acute morbidity and increasingly severe lymphoedema [4].

In developed countries most patients with cellulitis are treated for the acute episode and discharged, yet the rate of recurrence is high, suggesting that underlying predisposing factors (e.g. lymphoedema) may not be sufficiently managed following the first attack.

Epidemiology
Recurrent cellulitis is common. In a recent study 53% of subjects with a history of cellulitis had at least one recurrence during the 3-year trial [1].

Pathophysiology

Predisposing factors
Several studies have determined risk factors for lower limb cellulitis. Dupuy *et al.*, in a multivariate analysis, calculated an odds ratio of 71.2 for lymphoedema, 23.8 for breaks in the skin barrier (leg ulcer, toe-web intertrigo, dermatitis), 2.9 for venous insufficiency

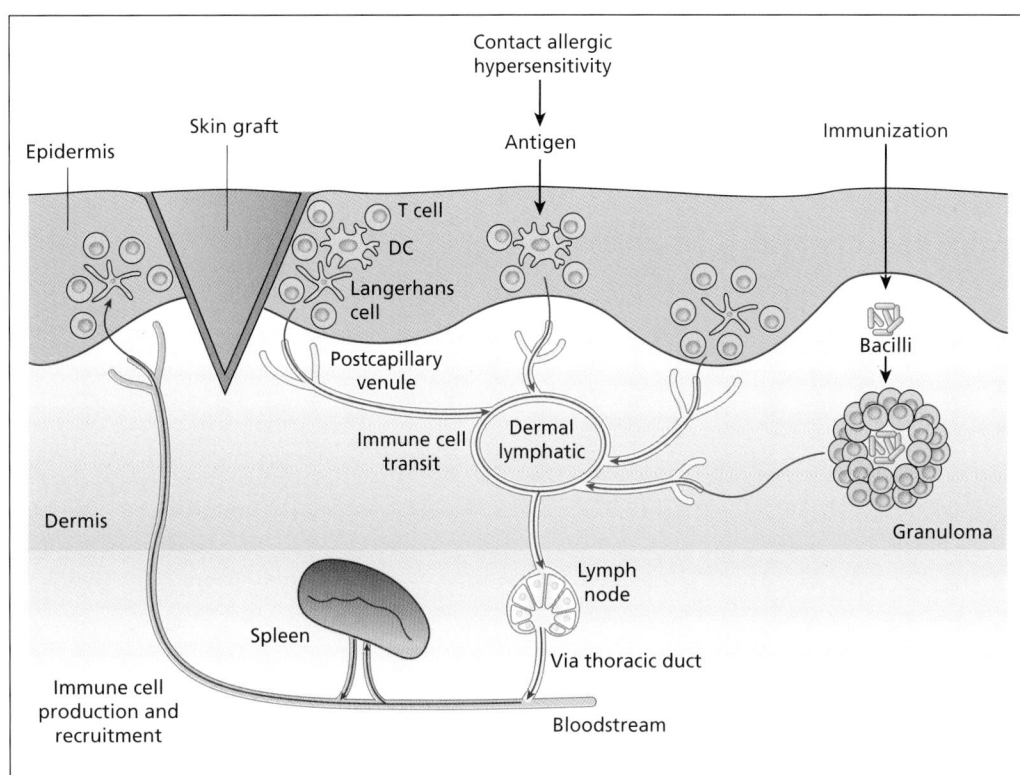

Figure 105.6 The lymphatic vessel sits centre stage for immune cell trafficking within the skin. DC, dendritic cell. (From Mortimer *et al.* 2014 [8].)

and 2.0 for obesity as independent risk factors associated with cellulitis [5]. In another series of 171 patients, 81 (47%) had recurrent episodes and 79 (46%) had chronic oedema. The concurrence of these two factors was strongly correlated (P <0.0002) [6].

Impaired lymph drainage leads to high rates of infection, particularly cellulitis, within the lymphatic basin. In a community-based survey, 29% of those with lymphoedema (64/218) had suffered cellulitis within the previous 12 months, of which 27% (16/64) required admission for intravenous antibiotics with a mean length of stay of 12 days at an estimated cost of £2300 per patient [7].

The afferent lymphatic vasculature provides the major exit route from the skin for soluble antigens and for immunologically active cells (e.g. lymphocytes, dendritic cells and macrophages) (Figure 105.6). It is likely that disturbances in immune cell trafficking compromise tissue immunosurveillance to predispose to infection, but the exact mechanism is not known [8].

Causative organisms

Most episodes of cellulitis are believed to be caused by group A streptococci. However, microbiologists consider *Staphylococcus aureus* to be the cause in most patients [9,10].

Clinical features

History

Cellulitis can vary from patient to patient and episodes can vary in presentation. Some episodes are accompanied by severe systemic upset, with high fever or rigors; others are milder, with minimal or no fever. Increased swelling of the affected area may occur. Inflammatory markers (CRP, erythrocyte sedimentation rate) are usually raised.

Presentation

When associated with established lymphoedema, clinical features may differ from classic cellulitis. Onset may be in minutes (as opposed to hours as in classic cellulitis). Toxicity may be severe with flu-like symptoms, nausea and vomiting, headache and high fever. Systemic symptoms may occur before local signs. The rash may be polymorphic with no defined border. In milder cases, inflammatory markers are not always raised. Episodes may be slow to resolve with oral antibiotics. Recurrence of infection is not unusual after only a week's course of antibiotics (Figure 105.7).

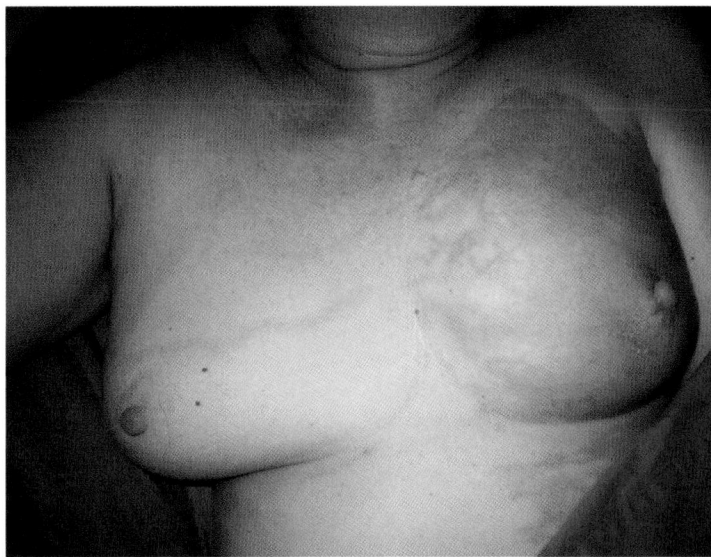

Figure 105.7 Recurrent cellulitis in lymphoedema following breast cancer treatment. Note lymphangitis crossing the watershed to the contralateral lymph node territory.

In some cases, symptoms and signs may grumble over a period of weeks. This is particularly so when associated with breast cancer-related lymphoedema (BCRL) of the breast. The patient may complain only of tiredness and of not feeling very well. Local signs may be redness and swelling with 'flare-ups' of redness from time to time. Inflammatory markers are usually negative and only a prompt response to a prolonged course of antibiotics confirms the diagnosis.

Differential diagnosis

The main differential diagnoses are DVT, necrotizing fasciitis and LDS. Other possibilities include gout, vasculitis, a ruptured Baker's cyst and pannicultis.

Investigations

Cellulitis is a clinical diagnosis supported by a blood neutrophilia and raised CRP. Blood cultures should be performed but may be positive in only 10% of cases [11]. Microbiology of any cuts or breaks in the skin or aspiration of blister fluid should be considered before antibiotics are started.

Management

First line

Cellulitis is best managed by dermatologists because up to a third of patients can be misdiagnosed and over a quarter of cases have associated skin disease, treatment of which is likely to reduce the chances of cellulitis recurrence [12].

Low-dose prophylactic penicillin, phenoxymethylpenicillin 250 mg twice daily, given for a period of 12 months almost halves the risk of recurrence during the intervention period compared with placebo [1]. However, although some level of protection appears to be sustained for several months after the end of prophylactic therapy, this effect is lost by 36 months, a finding that suggests that longer term prophylaxis may be required. Patients with a body mass index (BMI) of 33 or higher, multiple previous episodes of cellulitis or lymphoedema of the leg had a reduced likelihood of a response to prophylaxis. A high BMI, multiple attacks and lymphoedema would all be associated with lymphatic

dysfunction, supporting the view that lymphoedema is a very strong risk factor for cellulitis.

In patients allergic to penicillin, or in whom penicillin prophylaxis fails, alternative antibiotics such as erythromycin should be considered although there are no data on safety or efficacy [13].

In all cases of recurrent cellulitis, risk factors such as lymphoedema, wounds, breaks in skin integrity (particularly interdigital), dermatitis and fungal infections should be treated.

Swollen arm

Definition and nomenclature

Swelling of the upper limb or extremity is invariably due to oedema but overgrowth of tissue can occur. Oedema is likely to be caused either from lymphatic insufficiency (e.g. breast cancer treatment) or from venous obstruction.

Synonyms and inclusions
• Lymphoedema
• Breast cancer-related lymphoedema
• Postmastectomy lymphoedema
• Oedema

Introduction and general description

Swelling of an arm may be caused by oedema, in which case pitting should be evident to some degree, or it may be caused by an increase in the volume of other tissue elements, for example bone, muscle, fat or a tumour (Table 105.3). A swollen arm may be normal but perceived to be bigger if the contralateral limb has shrunk. The commonest reason for upper limb swelling is lymphoedema following breast cancer treatment. Arm swelling can be a presentation of cancer with metastatic disease in the axilla.

Upper limb swelling may due to primary lymphoedema (usually associated with lymphatic abnormalities elsewhere) or with a lymphatic malformation. Secondary lymphoedema can be caused

Table 105.3 Causes of a swollen arm.

Congenital/genetic			Acquired			
Vascular	**Lymphatic**	**Other**	**Vascular**	**Lymphatic**	**Musculoskeletal**	**Tumours**
Vascular malformation	Lymphoedema	Overgrowth spectrum:	Subclavian vein thrombosis:	Lymphoedema:	Rheumatoid	Lymphoma
Diffuse phlebectasia	Lymphatic malformation	Proteus syndrome	Effort thrombosis	Axillary surgery	arthritis	Sarcoma
Klippel–Trenaunay	Lymphangiomatosis	Fat hypertrophy	Venous catheterization	DXT	Haematoma	Metastases
syndrome		Muscle hamartoma	Chemotherapy ports	Cancer	Torn muscle	
Arteriovenous		Gigantism/	Chest radiotherapy	Neurological deficit	Pathological	
malformation		hemihypertrophy	Thoracic outlet syndrome	Chronic regional pain	fracture	
		Lipoedema	Superior vena cava	syndrome	Myositis	
		Dercum disease	obstruction	Lymphangitis (bacterial	ossificans	
		Madelung disease (benign	IV drug abuse	infection, herpes	osteomyelitis	
		symmetrical lipomatosis)		simplex, psoriasis,	Septic arthritis	
				rheumatoid arthritis)		
				Yellow-nail syndrome		

DXT, radiotherapy; IV, intravenous.

by rheumatoid arthritis, psoriatic arthropathy, hand dermatitis, yellow-nail syndrome, chronic regional pain syndrome (reflex sympathetic dystrophy), pretibial myxoedema, sirolimus treatment and following repeated infections such cellulitis and lymphangitis from herpes simplex.

Epidemiology
More than one in five women who survive breast cancer will develop arm lymphoedema [1].

Pathophysiology

Predisposing factors
Upper limb lymphoedema is most commonly caused by cancer treatment (i.e. axillary lymphadenectomy or radiation), but less commonly can be a presenting sign for advanced malignancy.

Venous outflow obstruction may be due to axillary/subclavian vein compression or stenosis (usually due to malignancy or radiation damage) or occlusion from thrombosis. Subclavian vein thrombosis is a rare condition that most often occurs in the context of central venous catheters, pacemakers, trauma, surgery immobilization, oral contraceptive pill use, pregnancy or malignancy. It occurs particularly in cancer patients receiving chemotherapy through central lines. It can also have primary causes such as anatomical anomalies, including thoracic outlet syndrome and Paget–Schröetter syndrome (so-called 'effort thrombosis'). Arteriovenous fistulae for haemodialysis will increase arm size from an increased blood flow but arm oedema will only occur with thrombosis or if lymph drainage is compromised.

Pathology
Upper extremity swelling of vascular origin will be due to oedema or increased vascular volume (e.g. vascular malformation). All oedema is caused by microvascular fluid filtration exceeding lymph drainage for a sufficient period of time. As lymph flow is responsible for the drainage of all tissue fluid, except for transient periods of venous reabsorption, a chronically swollen arm due to fluid indicates lymph drainage failure. This failure will be either due solely to lymphatic dysfunction (lymphoedema) or due to excessive microvascular fluid filtration overwhelming lymph drainage capacity [2]. Increased filtration can be caused by high venous pressures or from enhanced vasular permeability from inflammation (e.g.dermatitis or infection).

Causative factors
Recurrent infections from herpes simplex can lead to upper limb lymphoedema [3]. Non-infective forms of inflammation due to chronic hand dermatitis [4], rheumatoid arthritis [5] or psoriatic arthropathy [6] can lead to lymphoedema.

Genetics
Gene mutations causing tissue overgrowth have recently been identified [7]. *PIK3CA* mutations are frequently associated with a lymphatic anomaly and are usually mosaic/somatic in nature. Primary lymphoedema of the upper limb can be caused by a *CCBE1*, *FAT4* or *GJC2* mutation.

History
In its mildest form BCRL may go unnoticed, even by the patient. Swelling of the hand or wrist may be observed. Alternatively, the patient may notice that their clothes are tight. Aching is frequently experienced.

Presentation
Upper limb BCRL should exhibit pitting oedema but in more advanced cases fat and fibrosis contribute more to the swelling, so the consistency of the swelling may be fatty or firm. The distribution of swelling along the arm varies between patients, and swelling may be confined to a specific region of the upper limb. In some patients the hand may be swollen, whilst in others the hand may be spared despite more proximal swelling of the forearm or upper arm. In cases of incipient or mild BCRL, when the arm is not obviously increased in size, inspection may reveal decreased visibility of subcutaneous veins on the ventral forearm and dorsal hand ipsilaterally (the skin is thickened in lymphoedema and therefore more opaque) with smoothing or fullness of the medial elbow and distal upper arm contours. By pinching up the skin and subcutis of each arm between finger and thumb, the thickened ipsilateral tissues can be palpated [8]. Skin colour is normal except in the presence of venous outflow obstruction when it is red to blue; or with infection when it is pink to red; or with LDS when it is deep to cherry red.

Differential diagnosis
Venous outflow obstruction due to axillary/subclavian vein compression or stenosis, or occlusion from thrombosis, will produce a discoloured (red/blue) painful swollen arm often with parasthesia.

A swollen arm due to overgrowth may be associated with lymphoedema or lymphatic malformation in which case there may be signs of a vascular birthmark often at the root of the limb. There may be overgrowth with fat either from lipohypertrophy, such as in lipoedema, or with lipomatosis, such as Madelung disease (Figure 105.8).

Other differentials to consider are musculoskeletal disorders (e.g. ruptured muscle, arthritis, myofascitis or polymyositis), infection, trauma, a neoplasm (including sarcoma and carcinoma), allergic reaction and factitious causes. Rarely, systemic causes such as heart failure, superior vena caval obstruction and hypoproteinaemia can produce arm swelling.

Complications
The main complication of lymphoedema anywhere is infection and, in particular, cellulitis. Tense lymphoedema can produce lymphangiectasia, that is, surface 'lymph blisters' that can weep lymph (lymphorrhoea). Rarely lymphangiosarcoma can complicate any form of lymphoedema.

Prognosis
Cellulitis complicating upper limb lymphoedema can on occasion be severe and life threatening.

PART 9: VASCULAR

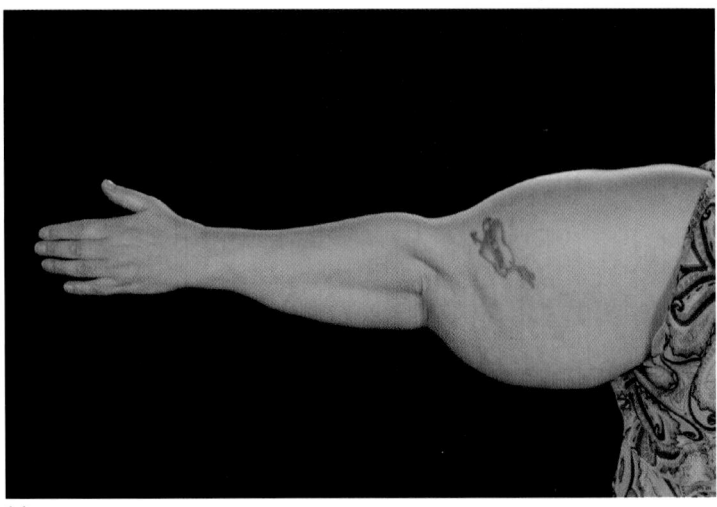

(a)

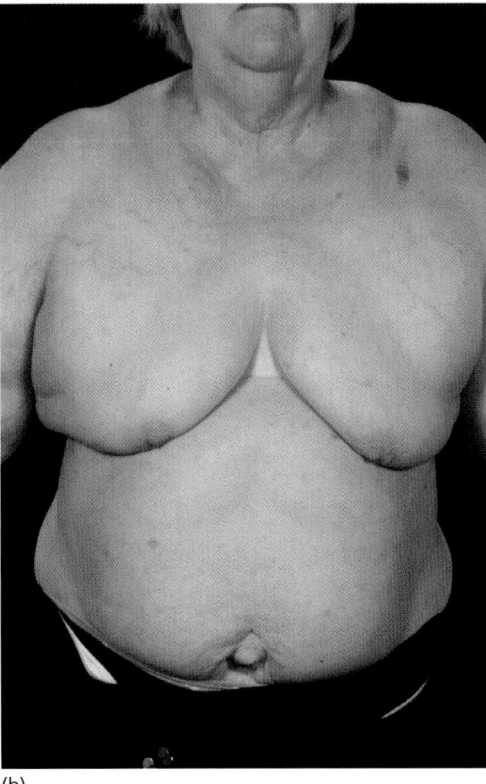

(b)

Figure 105.8 Madelung disorder. (a) Benign symmetrical lipomatosis (also known as benign symmetrical lipomatosis of Launois–Bensaude, Madelung disease, multiple symmetrical lipomatosis and cephalothoracic lipodystrophy) is a cutaneous condition characterized by extensive symmetrical fat deposits in the head, neck and shoulder girdle area. (b) Increased fat (lipomatosis) around the neck and shoulder girdle.

Investigations

Lymphoedema is usually a clinical diagnosis in the context of past cancer treatment. However imaging of the axilla is necessary to exclude a relapse of cancer (e.g. breast cancer or melanoma).

In cases of suspected non-cancer lymphoedema, lymphoscintigraphy is the investigation of choice to confirm impaired lymph drainage. A venous duplex ultrasound examination is the first investigation of choice in suspected venous outflow obstruction, but CT or MRI venography may be necessary in neutral and stress postions to confirm a thoracic outlet obstruction. A thrombophilia screen is indicated in cases of thrombosis.

Where overgrowth is suspected, MRI comparing both upper limbs should identify enlarged muscle or fat. MRI can also help distinguish fat from fluid.

Management

Treatment of a swollen arm is dependent on the cause. In circumstances where systemic causes, for example cancer recurrence or heart failure, have lead to, or coexist with, the lymphoedema, then treatment of the medical condition must be undertaken before embarking on specific lymphoedema therapy. The general principle for treating a swollen limb is to limit increased microvascular filtration and enhance lymph drainage. Lymph drainage responds to exercise and movement done while wearing compression [9].

Where cellulitis, in particular recurrent cellulitis, occurs then prophylactic antibiotics may be indicated [10].

Although surgical decompression and venous angioplasty may be considered for thoracic outlet obstruction, the typical treatment for primary subclavian vein thrombosis is oral anticoagulation only [11]. Venous compression or stenosis may benefit from stenting.

Swollen face, head and neck

Definition and nomenclature

Facial swelling may be generalized or localized, for example to the eyelid(s), lips or one cheek. It may extend beyond the face to involve the head and neck. To be chronic it should persist for more than 3 months.

Synonyms and inclusions
- Puffy face
- Facial lymphoedema
- Rosaceous lymphoedema
- Morbihan disease
- Solid facial oedema
- Oro-facial granulomatosis
- Granulomatous cheilitis
- Melkersson–Rosenthal syndrome

Introduction and general description

Chronic swelling of the face is most often due to fluid oedema but can arise due to an increase in other tissue components, such as blood vessels in a port wine stain (capillary malformation), acromegaly, overgrowth spectrum (hemihypertrophy) or tumours (Table 105.4).

Oedema may extend beyond the face to involve the head and neck, which occurs after surgery and/or radiotherapy for head and neck cancer or with recurrent cancer. Lymphoedema is a frequent late effect of head and neck cancer. Head and neck lymphoedema may be categorized as involving external structures (e.g. the skin and soft tissue of the face and neck) and internal structures, such as the mucosa and underlying soft tissue of the upper aerodigestive tract

Table 105.4 Causes of head and neck swelling.

Congenital/genetic			Acquired		
Vascular	**Lymphatic**	**Overgrowth**	**Tumours**	**Inflammatory**	**Miscellaneous**

Vascular malformation	Syndrome (neck webbing):
	  Turner
	  Noonan
	Generalized lymphatic dysplasia
	Mosaic with segmental
	  lymphoedema
	Lymphangioma/lymphatic
	  malformation
		Macrocephaly, e.g.
		  macrocephaly capillary
		  malformation syndrome
			Metastatic head and neck
			  cancer
			Angiosarcoma
			Radical neck lymphadenectomy
			Radiotherapy
				Rosacea/acne
				Cellulitis/erysipelas
				Oro-facial granulomatosis
				Tuberculosis
				Sarcoidosis
				Dental abscess
				Sinusitis
				Dermatomyositis
				Dermatitis/eczema, psoriasis,
				  contact allergy
				Blepharochalasis
				Pediculosis
				Angio-oedema
					Acromegaly
					Accidental trauma
					  (cauliflower ear)
					Cushing syndrome
					Graves disease

(e.g. the pharynx and larynx). In one study, the most common sites of external lymphoedema were the neck and submental area [1].

Oedema of the upper or lower lip (or both) may be from a vascular anomaly or result from recurrent angio-oedema, oro-facial granulomatosis (OFG), sarcoidosis and infective cheilitis or from the administration of lip fillers for cosmetic purposes.

Chronic oedema of the eyelids is common. Conditions that need to be considered include dermatomyositis, Graves disease and particularly rosacea/acne. Eyelid swelling may be quite simply due to acquired lax skin from photoageing and other processes that have undermined tissue compliance, such as blepharochalasis [2]. Contact allergy or angio-oedema, if persistent or recurrent, may slowly compromise lymphatic function. Equally, one severe attack of facial cellulitis may damage the lymphatics sufficiently to cause lymphoedema.

Chronic inflammatory disorders (e.g. rosacea, psoriasis, eczema), bacterial cellulitis, pediculosis, trauma and primary (congenital) lymphoedema can all lead to localized, lymphoedematous enlargement of the ear. Rosaceous enlargement is called otophyma [3].

Angiosarcoma or Kaposi sarcoma may infiltrate local lymph drainage, and manifest with eyelid oedema. Facial swelling can coexist with obvious primary lymphoedema of one or more limbs, suggesting that there is widespread congenitally determined lymphatic insufficiency.

Epidemiology
There are no data for facial lymphoedema from inflammatory disorder. The European literature reports that 46% of patients developed secondary lymphedema as a late effect of head and neck cancer treatment [4].

Pathophysiology
Oedema is an excess of interstitial fluid. Any oedema, whatever the cause, is due to microvascular (capillary) filtration overwhelming the lymph drainage for a sufficient period of time [5]. Interstitial fluid is reabsorbed almost entirely by the lymphatic vessels. Gravitational factors contributing to increased microvascular filtration do not play a part except overnight when the patient is lying down, hence facial swelling is often at its worst in the morn-

ing. However sustained increased venous pressures (e.g. superior vena caval obstruction) can produce facial oedema.

If primary facial lymphoedema occurs it is invariably present at birth. It is usually asymmetrical and associated with lymphoedema elsewhere. Head and neck oedema occurring *in utero* may regress by birth but can leave signs such as prominent medial epicanthic folds or neck webbing postnatally, as seen in Turner and Noonan syndromes. Congenital eyelid lymphoedema may be associated with conjunctival oedema.

A lymphatic malformation (lymphangioma) of the head and neck is more common than lymphoedema and gives rise to swelling from lymph fluid present within abnormally formed lymphatics (whereas lymphoedema is lymph fluid within the interstitial space). The mouth and particularly the tongue are common sites.

Facial lymphoedema may be secondary to other inflammatory pathologies of the skin such as rosacea or acne vulgaris [6]. The skin or subcutaneous initial lymphatics fail rather than the main regional collecting trunks, but in addition telangiectasia and inflammation contribute to oedema through increased fluid filtration. To what extent granulomatous rosacea, Morbihan disease and solid facial oedema (Figure 105.9) represent advanced versions of

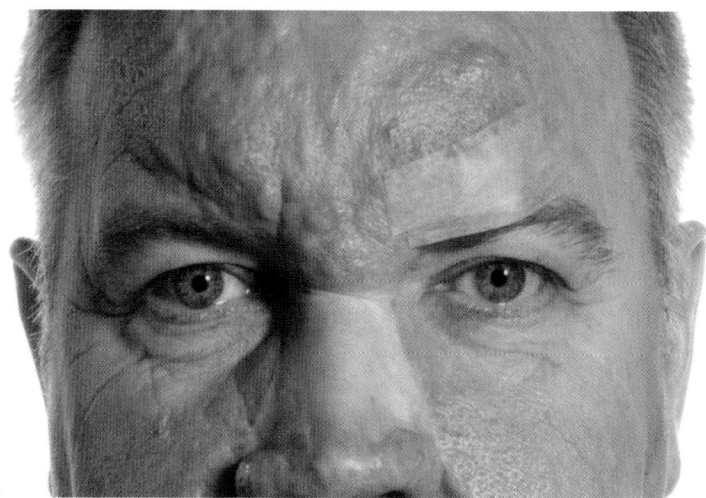

Figure 105.9 Solid facial oedema.

rosaceous lymphoedema remains unclear [7]. Other inflammatory disorders considered to cause facial oedema include eczema, psoriasis, infection, pediculosis [8] and trauma (cauliflower ears). Contact allergy or angio-oedema, if persistent or recurrent, may slowly compromise lymphatic function [9]. One severe attack of facial erysipelas or cellulitis may damage the lymphatics sufficiently to cause lymphoedema.

Chronic oedema of the eyelids is common and may just be due to acquired lax skin from photoageing and other processes that have undermined tissue compliance [2].

Medical conditions to be considered with periocular oedema are dermatomyositis, Cushing syndrome (moon face) and thyroid disease particularly Graves disease. Renal disease, contrary to expectations, does not cause oedema unless associated with hypoproteinaemia (i.e. nephrotic syndrome) or when advanced. Inflammation within underlying structures may manifest with facial oedema (e.g. dental root infection, chronic sinusitis and salivary duct obstruction).

Angiosarcoma or Kaposi sarcoma may infiltrate local lymph drainage routes and manifest with facial lymphoedema.

Oedema of the upper or lower lip (or both) may be congenital or result from chronic dermatitis, recurrent angio-oedema or OFG (Figure 105.10). In OFG it might prove difficult to identify granulomas on biopsy so their absence does not exclude the diagnosis. If present, a diagnosis of OFG (also called granulomatous cheilitis and Melkersson–Rosenthal syndrome) is made, but it remains unclear if the granulomas are cause or effect [10]. Granulomatous inflammation may exist only locally but a thorough search for gastrointestinal Crohn disease or systemic sarcoidosis should be made. Crohn disease of the bowel can become apparent some time after presentation of OFG. Granulomatous inflammation from administration of lip fillers for cosmetic purposes can also cause chronic swelling [11].

Head and neck lymphoedema is becoming increasingly more common as more head and neck cancer is treated by lymph node neck dissection and radiotherapy (Figure 105.11). Fibrosis and secondary infection are frequent complications.

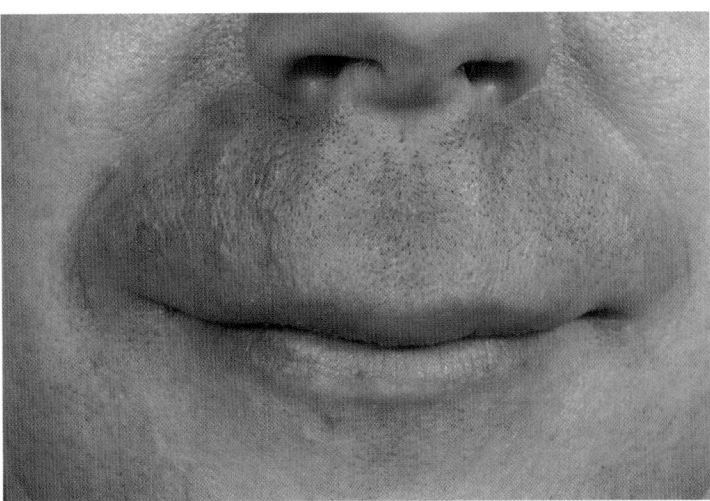

Figure 105.10 Oro-facial granulomatosis exhibiting redness and indurated swelling of the right upper lip.

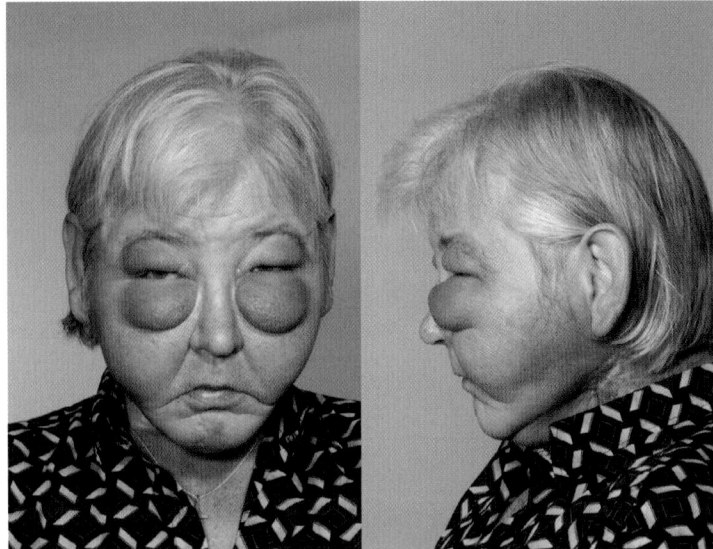

Figure 105.11 Severe facial lymphoedema following treatment for carcinoma of the tongue.

Clinical features

The clinical features of facial lymphoedema depend on the underlying aetiology. Swelling usually affects the central forehead, periocular skin and cheeks where it may be surprisingly asymmetrical. Erythema is always present in rosacea but inflammatory pustules and papules may be conspicuous by their absence. OFG starts with intermittent bouts of swelling resembling angio-oedema affecting the lips or cheeks, but with time the condition may become persistent. An extension of the oedema within the mouth is common and is the reason for the rugose changes on the buccal mucosal and tongue (scrotal tongue).

Lymphoedema may cause facial disfiguration and distress in patients with head and neck cancer [1].

Investigations

Skin biopsy may be helpful if granulomatous disease, rosacea, dermatomyositis, angiosarcoma or Kaposi sarcoma is suspected. Lymphoscintigraphy can be performed on the head and neck but is difficult to interpret. MRI or CT imaging may be useful if an underlying pathology such as cancer, sinusitis or dental root infection is suspected. Such imaging may also help distinguish between swelling from fluids and other tissue components such as fat.

Management

Treatment of facial lymphoedema will depend on the cause. Any inflammation will need to be treated to reduce the higher lymphatic load arising from increased vascular permeability and blood flow. Raising the head of the bed during overnight sleep helps to reduce venous pressure and therefore microvascular filtration. Otherwise the standard principles of enhancing lymph flow through massage techniques and facial exercises apply [12].

In rosaceous lymphoedema, antibiotic therapy appears disappointing in reducing swelling; low-dose isotretinoin has been advocated, but may need to be sustained for 1–2 years [13]. Laser ablation of the telangiectasia may reduce the fluid load on the lymphatics.

There are no data from clinical trials for the treatment of OFG. In one review of 45 patients who required treatment, 24 (53.3%) were treated with topical corticosteroids/immunosuppressants only, whereas 21 (46.7%) received a combined therapy (topical plus systemic corticosteroids/immunosuppressants and/or intralesional corticosteroids). The long-term outcome analysis showed complete or partial resolution of tissue swelling and oral ulceration in 78.8% and 70% of patients, respectively [14]. There are reports of therapeutic success with azathioprine, thalidomide, infliximab and mycophenylate mofetil.

Modified decongestive lymphoedema therapy can be successful in treating head and neck lymphoedema following cancer treatment [15].

Swollen genitalia and mons pubis

Definition and nomenclature
Genital lymphoedema may affect the shaft of penis and/or scrotum plus the mons pubis.

Synonyms and inclusions
- Genital lymphoedema
- Peno-scotal lymphoedema
- Vulval lymphoedema
- Elephantiasis
- Genital oedema
- Massive localized lymphoedema
- Acquired genital lymphangioma

Introduction and general description
Genital lymphoedema may be primary or secondary (Table 105.5). The genitalia have the option of bilateral lymph node drainage. For swelling to occur, drainage pathways to both inguinal regions must fail or local genital lymphatics must become occluded.

In primary genital lymphoedema gene mutations have been identified, including in *GATA2* and *FOXC2*.

Table 105.5 Causes of lymphoedema of the genitalia and mons pubis.

Primary (congenital/genetic)	Secondary
Noonan syndrome	Cancer (advanced primary, inflammatory cancer,
Hennekam syndrome (*CCBE1*,	pelvic relapse, skin infiltration)
FAT4)	Lymphadenectomy (pelvic, bilateral, ilio-inguinal)
Generalized lymphatic dysplasia	Radiotherapy
Chylous reflux	Accidental trauma
Emberger syndrome (*GATA2*)	Obesity
Lymphoedema distichiasis	Crohn disease/ano-genital granulomatosis
(*FOXC2*)	Hidradenitis suppurativa
Yellow-nail syndrome	Infections:
	Filanasis
	Cellulitis
	Lymphogranuloma venereum
	Donovanosis
	Systemic causes (heart failure, nephrotic syndrome)

Secondary lymphoedema may be caused by advanced or local infiltration of cancer, extensive scarring from accidental or surgical trauma, obesity, granulomatous disease such as Crohn disease or ano-genital granulomatosis (Figure 105.12a), hidradenitis suppurativa (Figure 105.12b) and infections such as filariasis, lymphogranuloma venereum and donovanosis.

Mons pubis swelling can develop in isolation but more often is associated with genital or lower limb lymphoedema.

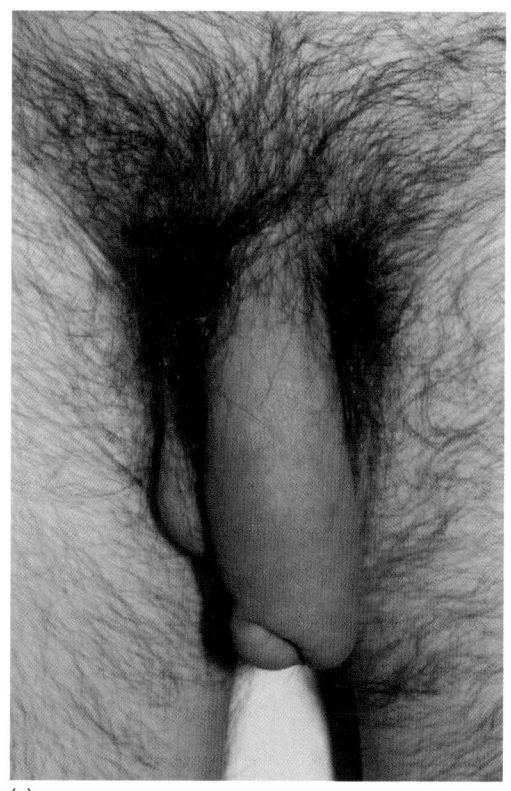

(a)

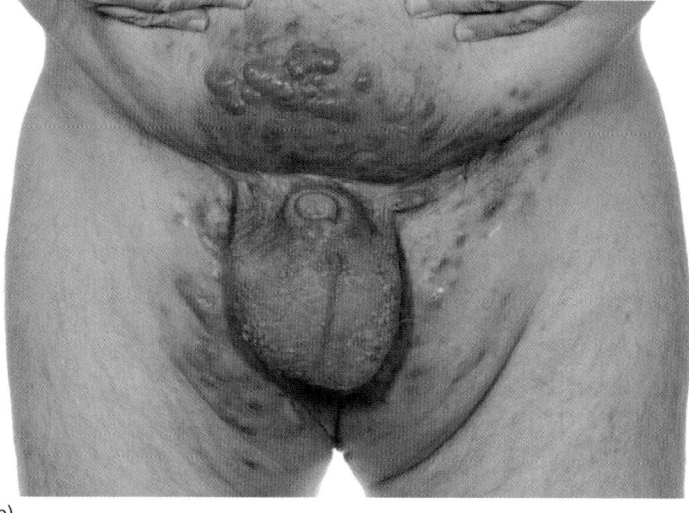

(b)

Figure 105.12 (a) Lymphoedema of the penis secondary to ano-genital granulomatosis. There may be no sign of inflammation. (b) Genital lymphoedema secondary to hidradenitis suppurativa. Note the cutaneous lymphangiectasia that predisposes to lymphorrhoea. (From Thomas *et al.* 2014 [13].)

PART 9: VASCULAR

Pathophysiology

Predisposing factors

For primary cases a genetic predisposition is likely. In both primary and secondary cases an infection or other forms of local inflammation (e.g dermatitis) may cause swelling. Compression of leg lymphoedema, through bandages or pneumatic compression pumps, can push fluid up to the trunk. This can result in genital oedema, especially if care is not taken to redirect the lymph through collateral drainage routes.

Pathology

In all forms of pure lymphoedema the pathology is the same, namely increased dermal and subcutaneous thickness through fluid, increased fat and fibrosis. A non-specific inflammatory infiltrate is invariably present [1]. Lymphatic vessels may be increased in number and expanded due to increased lymphatic pressure but they may also be reduced in number through genetically determined underdevelopment or if obliterated by fibrosis.

Causative factors

In primary lymphoedema a genetic cause is probable. To date there are at least four phenotypes for which mutations are known and which cause genital lymphoedema: Emberger syndrome, lymphoedema distichiasis syndrome, Hennekam syndrome and Noonan syndrome. Genital swelling may be a feature of congenital lymphoedema, particularly if part of a generalized lymphatic dysplasia. Chylous reflux into the scrotum may result from congenitally malformed retroperitoneal aortic and iliac lymphatics giving rise to megalymphatics or from intestinal lymphangiectasia.

Most cases (60%) of genital lymphoedema will be caused by obliteration of the upper thigh, inguinal and iliac lymph vessels for reasons not always apparent. One-quarter of cases will be caused by obliteration of outflow lymphatics from the scrotum and 15% caused by reflux [2].

The commonest cause of genital lymphoedema and hydrocele worldwide is filariasis [3]. Other secondary causes of genital lymphoedema include active cancer and its treatment (e.g. bilateral inguinal lymphadenectomy or radiotherapy), granulomatous disease (e.g. Crohn disease and ano-genital granulomatosis) and extensive local inflammation and scarring (e.g. hidradenitis suppurativa). Genital swelling may occur as part of extensive oedema below the waist in heart failure, hypoalbuminaemia and inferior vena cava obstruction. Less common causes include tuberculous lymphadenitis, lymphogranuloma venereum and dovovanosis [4].

Mon pubis lymphoedema is caused by local radiotherapy, obesity and by local inflammatory disorders such as Crohn disease and hidradenitis suppurativa.

Genetics

Mutations in *GATA2* cause Emberger syndrome in which genital lymphoedema is one phenotypic feature [5]. Mutations in *FOXC2* cause lymphoedema distichiasis syndrome; uncommonly genital lymphoedema and lymphangiectasia can also feature [6]. Mutations in *CCBE1* and *FAT4* cause Hennekam syndrome (lymphoedema–lymphangiectasia syndrome), a form of generalized lymphatic dysplasia; genital lymphoedema is variable as a feature [7]. In Noonan syndrome molecular genetic testing identifies a mutation in *PTPN11* in 50% of affected individuals, in *SOS1* in approximately 13%, in *RAF1* in 3–17% and in *KRAS* in fewer than 5% [8].

Clinical features

History

The development of swelling will be dependent on the underlying cause. The onset may be insidious or sudden with no obvious trigger. Infection (e.g. cellulitis) may be a provoking factor. A history of exposure to filariasis with travel to endemic areas must always be considered. Primary cases invariably have one or both lower limbs swollen at the time of onset of genital lymphoedema.

Presentation

In primary lymphoedema swelling may be present at birth or develop later in life. Genital lymphoedema is much more common in men, probably because of anatomy and the dependent nature of male external genitalia. The various parts of the genitalia – the penis, scrotum and labia – are not always equally swollen.

Longstanding lymphoedema causes thickening and hyperkeratosis of the overlying skin with the production of papillomas. These probably arise from lymph congestion within the dermal lymphatics, which, in the early stages, can appear as 'lymph blisters' on the skin surface before the tissues become organized and fibrotic. This expansion of congested dermal lymphatics due to backpressure (dermal backflow) is called lymphangiectasia (and not lymphangioma, which strictly implies a lymphatic endothelial proliferation). When the 'lymph blisters' are filled with lymph they are translucent but when filled with chyle they are opaque and white. The 'lymph blisters' will rupture on occasion, resulting in a copious release of lymph (lymphorrhoea), mimicking incontinence or excessive sweating. Lymphorrhoea can seriously undermine quality of life and risk a contact dermatitis and cellulitis.

Cellulitis attacks are common with genital lymphoedema. Each attack further undermines lymph drainage routes, leading to worse swelling and a higher risk of infections, so establishing a vicious cycle. Offending organisms may be many and difficult to identify. Gram-negative infections should always be considered [9]. The inguinal lymph glands are often enlarged as a result of infection (filarial or bacterial).

Mons pubis lymphoedema presents as a dome-shaped swelling with peau d'orange skin changes. In the obese it can grow to epic proportions whereupon it resembles a pseudosarcoma and is called massive localized lymphoedema [10].

Differential diagnosis

The characteristic skin changes make a diagnosis of lymphoedema relatively straightforward. However, systemic causes of oedema such as heart failure and nephrotic syndrome should be considered when accompanied by more widespread oedema. Hydrocele and an inguinal hernia can be mistaken for oedema.

Complications

Genital lymphoedema can be complicated by infection (e.g. cellulitis) or the leakage of lymph or chyle with resulting contact dermatitis. Penile swelling may interefere with micturition and sexual function. Impotence may develop. A secondary balanoposthitis may occur.

Prognosis

Prognosis is dependent on the underlying aetiology but established lymphoedema is incurable. The risk of severe attacks of cellulitis is ever present.

Investigations

Filariasis must be excluded by a complement fixation test, or nighttime blood smears if active filarial infection is likely. A skin biopsy is essential to diagnose granulomatous disease or cancer infiltrating dermal lymphatics.

Imaging with a CT or MRI scan is necessary to exclude lymphatic obstruction within the pelvis or ilioinguinal glands from cancer or other pathologies (e.g. retroperitoneal fibrosis). Lymphoscintigraphy may be helpful to identify lower limb lymphatic abnormalities. It may demonstrate tracer within the scrotal lymphatics in cases of reflux.

Management

First line

Decongestive lymphatic therapy aims to reduce swelling through a combination of massage and compression [11]. This should only be undertaken if the underlying causes have been treated, such as cancer, granulomatous disease or infection.

Skin care should be scrupulous. Prophylactic antibiotics may be necessary to counter recurrent cellulitis [9]. Compression is easier on the female genitalia than the male. Custom-made tights or shorts are recommended. Foam inserts can increase local pressure comfortably. A scrotal sling or harness may provide support and compression in the male.

Second line

Surgical reduction may be straightforward and effective [12]. Circumcision may resolve preputial swelling and any redundant foreskin. Hyfrecation or diathermy is best for lymphangiectasia. Antibiotic cover is recommended in all cases.

Obesity-related lymphoedema

Definition

Obesity leads to, and exacerbates, lymphoedema at all sites but particularly in the lower limbs.

Introduction and general description

Obesity is a significant risk factor for lymphoedema of the arms, legs and abdomen. Obesity is the strongest risk factor for BCRL [1]. Furthermore, dieting improves arm lymphoedema beyond that possible through loss of subcutaneous fat alone (from weight loss irrespective of the diet used) [2]. The pathophysiology of lower limb lymphoedema can be complex, with increased fluid filtration from venous hypertension combined with impaired lymph

---

> **Box 105.1 Contributing factors to obesity-related lower limb lymphoedema**
>
> - Poor mobility (to stimulate lymph drainage)
> - Venous hypertension:
>   - Dependency (armchair legs)
>   - Abdominal girth/pendulous abdomen obstructing venous drainage in thighs
> - Sleep apnoea syndrome
> - Drug therapy, e.g. calcium-channel antagonists
> - Co-morbidities, e.g. heart failure or post-thrombotic syndrome

drainage from an indirect effect of reduced mobility being the most important contributors (Box 105.1). The addition of obstructive sleep apnoea/sleep apnoea hypoventilation syndrome results in salt and water retention and heart failure.

Epidemiology

A crude estimate of approximately 15 000 patients attending a US clinic showed almost 75% of morbidly obese patients have chronic oedema of the legs [3].

Pathophysiology

Fat and lymphatics appear to have a close relationship. High-density lipoproteins require transport through the lymphatics to return to the bloodstream during reverse cholesterol transport [4]. In a model of hypercholesterolaemia, lymphatic function was severely compromised, including impaired dendritic cell migration. Removal of cholesterol from the peripheral tissues via reverse cholesterol transport requires lymph drainage [5]. Mice with a heterozygous *Prox1*-inactivating mutation have leaky lymphatic vessels and develop obesity and inflammation [6].

Fat deposition is a striking feature of lymphoedema swelling and the justification for liposuction as a treatment for lymphoedema. Obesity impairs lymphatic transport capacity and impaired lymphatic function promotes adipose deposition. How obesity predisposes to lymphoedema is not clear. Lymph drainage requires movement and exercise to promote flow. In a cross-sectional study, 33% of severely obese participants had lymphoedema and those participants had worse physical function than those without lymphoedema. This association was independent of BMI [7].

It is the lower limb that is most closely linked with lymphoedema. In one study all 10 patients with a BMI between 30 and 53 had normal lower extremity lymphatic function, whereas the five patients with a BMI greater than 59 had abnormal lymphatic drainage consistent with lymphoedema [8]. Using an isotope clearance technique, lymph drainage was found to be significantly lower in obese human subjects when compared with lean controls [9].

A large abdominal apron resting on the thighs during sitting obstructs venous drainage and probably interferes with lymph drainage as well. The pressure in the iliofemoral vein in morbidly obese patients is significantly higher than in non-obese subjects [10]. Abdominal adipose tissue potentially leads to elevated risk for both venous thromboembolism and chronic venous insufficiency. Excess body weight is also related to alterations in the coagulation system, including impaired fibrinolytic activity and elevated plasma concentrations of clotting factors [11].

Clinical features

History
Swelling is usually insidious in onset and progressive. Acute cellulitis may alert patient and carers to the swelling. More often a chronic redness with local pain and tenderness indicative of LDS may develop. Trivial trauma may result in the weeping of fluid from the skin (lymphorrhoea). Persistent weeping will irritate the surrounding skin to promote dermatitis, extensive erosion and even ulceration. Odour may result from bacterial colonization. The constant weeping can discourage the patient from going to bed (to avoid soiling the bed). Consequently, the patient sleeps in a chair, which further increases fluid filtration into the legs. The patient may choose to sleep in a chair anyway for reasons of comfort or sleep apnoea syndrome. As the legs swell more the extra weight further impairs mobility so reducing lymph drainage yet more.

Presentation
Skin changes of LDS and venous hypertension are invariable. Distinction from bacterial cellulitis can be difficult with acute flares of pain and redness. Elephantiasis skin changes are common.

Differential diagnosis
Systemic causes of oedema (including cardiac disease, hypoproteinaemia and abdominal–pelvic malignancy) should always be considered, particularly if bilateral leg swelling is present. Calcium-channel blocking antagonists can exacerbate peripheral oedema.

Complications and co-morbidities
Leg ulceration, heart failure and overwhelming sepsis are common complications. Co-morbidities such as diabetes, sleep apnoea syndrome and right-sided heart failure often coexist.

Prognosis
The prognosis is poor unless the patient loses weight and becomes more ambulant.

Investigations
Standard investigations such as venous duplex ultrasound and lymphoscintigraphy are probably unnecessary as they are unlikely to change management. More important are BNP to exclude heart failure, plasma protein estimation and D-dimers if thrombosis is considered likely.

Management

First line
There are a number of management options to pursue.
1 Systemic conditions such as heart failure and sleep apnoea syndrome should be treated.
2 Compression therapy in the form of multilayer lymphoedema bandaging is the treatment of choice [12]. Standard venous ulcer bandaging will not address toe swelling with skin changes or oedema extending into the lower thighs. Pneumatic compression devices or Velcro wraps can be useful adjunctive therapy. Compression garments should not be used until swelling is controlled and the skin is in good condtion.
3 Exercise if logistically possible. This can be done through walking or static cycling, if safe. Active movements should always be encouraged but passive exercises are better than nothing.
4 Elevation of legs when resting. Encourage sleeping in a bed and not in a chair unless it is a reclining chair.
5 Treat active infection (e.g. cellulitis) [13]
6 Wound care should be undertaken where necessary.
7 Emollients such as 50/50 white soft and liquid paraffin should always be used. For the hyperkeratosis of elephantiasis, 10% salicylic acid is recommended.

Second line
Consider bariatric assessment and intervention.

Abdominal wall lymphoedema

Definition and nomenclature
Abdominal wall lymphoedema is skin and subcutaneous oedema of the lower abdominal wall generated when ilioinguinal lymph drainage is compromised bilaterally, or within a pendulous obese abdomen.

Synonyms and inclusions
- Pendulous abdomen
- Swollen abdominal panniculus
- Elephantiasis nostras verrucosa
- Secondary cancer-related lymphoedema
- Truncal lymphoedema

Introduction and general description
The abdominal wall is not considered a likely place for lymphoedema but is probably more common than generally realized. Diagnosis may be difficult because the soft tissues of the abdominal wall make pitting difficult to elicit. Furthermore, abdominal wall lymphoedema may manifest with more fat than fluid, making distinction from obesity demanding. Peau d'orange skin changes can be a helpful sign and palpation of fluid gives a more solid feel than fat.

Abdominal wall lymphoedema can develop following cancer treatment when ilioinguinal lymph drainage is compromised. In such circumstances lower limb lymphoedema would likely coexist. Cancer relapse must be considered if swelling develops some time after curative cancer treatment. Cancer relapse may be in the pelvis or with infiltration of the abdominal wall skin (e.g. carcinoma erysipeloides).

Non-cancer-related lymphoedema of the abdominal wall is invariably related to obese abdominal panniculus, or in circumstances of extensive oedema such as heart failure, nephrotic syndrome or yellow-nail syndrome. Pretibial myxedema has been described to cause abdominal wall oedema.

Pathophysiology

Compromised ilioinguinal lymph nodes affect all lymph drainage routes below the waist. This usually causes lower limb lymphoedema first, but in more severe cases the lower abdominal wall and genitalia are affected as well. External beam pelvic radiotherapy not only affects the lymph nodes but can also affect smaller collateral lymphatics within the skin and subcutaneous tissue of the mons pubis to cause lymphoedema within the radiation field.

Relapse of cancer with infiltration of the dermal and subcutaneous lymphatics of the lower abdomen can also produce lymphoedema. Advanced cancer can produce profound lymphoedema from the waist downwards, particularly if accompanied by iliac vein or inferior vena cava obstruction.

Obesity is known to cause lymphatic dysfunction and exacerbate lymphoedema. This is particularly so in abdominal panniculus when the abdomen becomes pendulous. This creates venous congestion so increasing fluid filtration into the abdominal wall. Intense oedema complicated by infection often leads to elephantiasis changes (elephantiasis nostras verrucosa). Obese patients often suffer sleep apnoea syndrome, which only further increases systemic salt and water retention.

Causative factors

Causative factors include cancer treatment (e.g. bilateral inguinal or pelvic lymphadenectomy) or radiation therapy for gynaecological, penile, bladder or prostate cancer, as well as relapsed cancer and cellulitis. Obesity where the abdominal panniculus is pendulous is also a major risk factor.

Clinical features

History

The patient may not perceive mild abdominal wall oedema. With progression there may be a sensation of getting fatter, or tightness and discomfort within the affected area. There may be a history of past cancer treatment, obesity or cellulitis.

Presentation

Pitting can usually be demonstrated only over the anterior superior iliac spine. Pinching a fold of lower abdominal skin will reveal thickening with a heavier, more solid feel than just fat. Peau d'orange skin changes may be observed. With time, and progressive accumulation of fat and fibrosis within the swollen area, the tissues will feel more indurated, particularly following an episode of cellulitis. More severe cases can develop marked hyperkeratosis, skin thickening and papillomatosis. These changes produce a warty, cobblestone appearance, referred to as elephantiasis nostras verrucosa (Figure 105.13) [1].

Cellulitis is a frequent occurrence because of the compromised local tissue immunity. Recurrent attacks exacerbate the lymphoedema, leading to a vicious cycle. LDS may develop within the pendulous abdomen from venous congestion and past cellulitis [2].

Differential diagnosis

Abdominal wall oedema may develop in heart failure, hypoalbuminaemia (nephrotic syndrome, liver disease and malnutrition) and inferior vena cava obstruction.

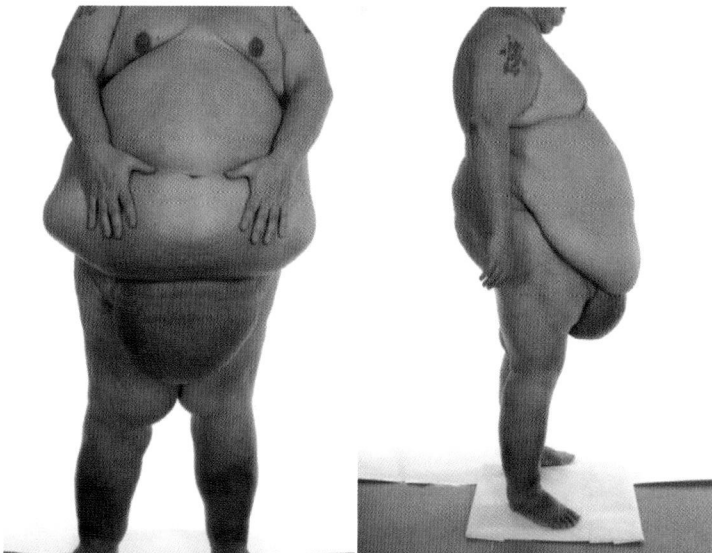

Figure 105.13 Lymphoedema of the pendulous abdomen and mons pubis from obesity.

Complications

Progression of abdominal wall lymphoedema can result in huge swelling, which may hang down as far as the patient's knees, so compromising mobility and risking overwhelming sepsis.

Prognosis

There is a high morbidity and life-threatening sepsis in the very obese.

Investigations

In cancer patients, restaging using abdominal ultrasound or a CT scan is recommended. Skin biopsy may be helpful if infiltrative cancer is considered to be possible. In the severely obese check for the following: (i) heart failure, through BNP estimation; (ii) low plasma albumin; and (iii) sleep apnoea syndrome, through sleep studies.

Management

First line

Correction of any underlying causes is the first priority wherever possible. Diuretics are usually of little help in lymphoedema but may be tried for short periods where physiology involves increased microvascular filtration.

In severe morbid obesity (BMI >50) bariatric intervention should be considered.

Antibiotics should be given if infection is present. Prophylactic antibiotics may be given if there is recurrent infection [3].

Decongestive lymphatic therapy (manual lymphatic drainage and abdominal compression using binding or compression garments) should be administered [4].

Second line

A melon slice surgical apronectomy may be considered but the risk of infection and wound dehiscence is high in obese patients [5].

PART 9: VASCULAR

PART 9: VASCULAR

Cancer-related lymphoedema

Definition and nomenclature
Lymphoedema is rarely a presenting feature of cancer unless the cancer is already advanced but it is a common consequence of cancer treatment and relapsed cancer.

Synonyms and inclusions
- Breast cancer-related lymphoedema
- Postmastectomy lymphoedema
- Radiation-induced lymphoedema
- Malignant lymphoedema
- Carcinoma erysipeloides
- Carcinoma en cuirasse

Introduction and general description
Lymph flow is remarkably well maintained through malignant nodes, therefore cancer does not usually present with swelling. The few exceptions to this general rule are lymphophilic tumours, such as malignant eccrine poroma, Kaposi sarcoma, lymphangiosarcoma and inflammatory breast cancer (Table 105.6). Cancer-related lymphoedema usually results from cancer therapy. Surgical lymphadenectomy, radiation therapy and chemotherapy can all contribute.

Advanced or relapsed cancer can present with lymphoedema. Extensive lymph node involvement can compromise lymph flow but other factors such as venous obstruction and hypoproteinaemia may also contribute to oedema formation. Recurrent cancer should always be considered as a cause of limb swelling, particularly if associated with pain. Full staging investigations should be undertaken in any cancer patient who develops new limb swelling.

Carcinoma erysipeloides (also called lymphangitis carcinomatosa, carcinoma telangiectatica or carcinoma en cuirasse) occurs when cancer cells infiltrate the dermal lymphatics (Figure 105.14). It represents metastatic disease. Bulk disease may be absent and therefore imaging may be normal. By obstructing collateral lymph drainage routes, dermal lymphatic infiltration by cancer is frequently associated with localized, or extensive limb, lymphoedema.

Table 105.6 Causes of cancer-related lymphoedema.

Cancers where lymphoedema is a presenting sign	Cancer treatment
Inflammatory carcinoma	Lymphadenectomy
Lymphangiosarcoma	Radiotherapy
Kaposi sarcoma	Chemotherapy (taxanes)
Malignant eccrine poroma	Breast reconstruction
Advanced primary cancer, e.g. axillary or pelvic lymph node metastases	
Relapsed cancer:	
Lymph node metastases	
Carcinoma erysipeloides	
Lymphangitis carcinomatosa	
Carcinoma en cuirasse	

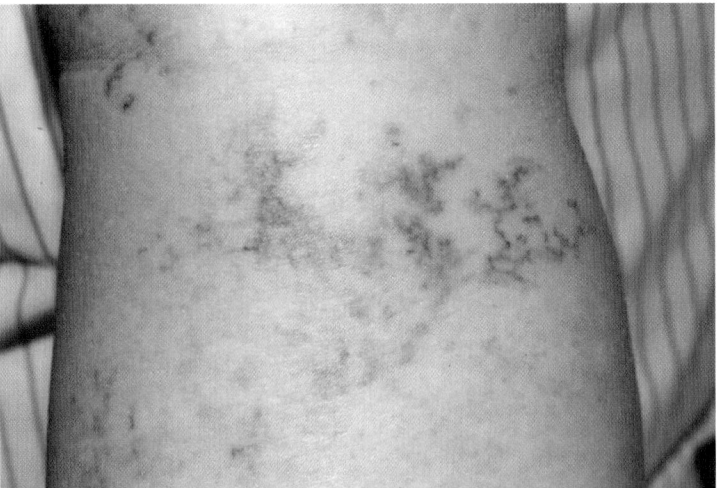

Figure 105.14 Carcinoma erysipeloides (carcinoma telangiectatica): the red vessels are dermal lymphatic vessels infiltrated with adenocarcinoma of the breast.

Epidemiology

Breast cancer-related lymphoedema. More than one in five women who survive breast cancer will develop arm lymphoedema [1]. Taxane chemotherapy significantly contributes to BCRL [2].

Lymphoedema related to cancers of the male and female urogenital tract. The incidence of lower limb lymphoedema following radical hysterectomy alone was estimated at 5–10% [3] but can be as high as 49% by 10 years of follow-up in patients who have also received adjuvant radiation treatment [4]. The incidence after vulval cancer was reported at 28% [5]. For prostate cancer the rate was found to be 0–10% after extended pelvic lymphadenectomy [6]. With extended-field irradiation for carcinoma of the prostate an incidence of about 5% for genital and/or leg oedema has been noted and the oedema remained chronic in the majority of patients [7]. After penile cancer treatment the incidence of lymphoedema may be as high as 33% [8].

Melanoma-related lymphoedema. In a prospective study of lymphoedema after melanoma treatment, moderate lymphoedema (i.e. an increase in limb volume of >10%) occurred in 14.8% after sentinel lymph node biopsy but in 30.4% after therapeutic lymph node dissection [9].

Extremity soft-tissue sarcoma. The incidence of lymphoedema was 28.8% following limb salvage for extremity soft-tissue sarcomas. Nine percent of the cohort of 289 patients developed significant (grade ≥2) lymphoedema [10].

Pathophysiology

Predisposing factors
Extensive surgery (e.g. axillary lymph node dissection, greater number of lymph nodes dissected, mastectomy) and being overweight carried the highest risk for BCRL. Recent evidence suggests

axillary radiation may convey less risk than axillary clearance [11]. Cellulitis may be a trigger as may an insult to the limb such as sterile or non-sterile skin puncture. Extreme resistance exercise such as carrying a heavy suitcase or shopping may trigger the swelling, as may a long haul flight.

Pathology

Breast cancer-related lymphoedema has been the most widely studied form of lymphoedema. The pathology consists of fat as well as fluid, hence the justification for liposuction treatment.

Carcinoma erysipeloides is a form of metastatic spread and occurs most commonly with breast cancer but can occur with melanoma, thyroid, lung, gastric, pancreatic, ovarian, prostate and colo-rectal cancer [12].

Clinical features

History

Lymphoedema following cancer treatment may occur immediately after lymphadenectomy, particularly if complicated by wound infection or 'seroma', or be delayed in onset for many years. Lymphoedema can cause aching but is predominantly painless unless associated with infection, thrombosis or active cancer.

Presentation

Carcinoma erysipeloides manifests clinically with a fixed erythematous patch or plaque resembling cellulitis, but without fever [13]. A network or lattice pattern of telangiectatatic vessels represents the infiltrated dermal lymphatics (Figure 105.14). Inflammatory breast cancer is a rare and very aggressive disease in which cancer cells block the lymph vessels in the skin of the breast. This type of breast cancer is called 'inflammatory' because the breast often looks swollen and red, or 'inflamed'.

Investigations

If relapsed cancer is suspected, restaging investigations such as positron emission tomography (PET)/CT are indicated. Skin biopsy is the investigation of choice for skin metastases. MRI can determine if swelling is fluid and therefore likely to be lymphoedema.

Management

If active cancer is diagnosed then oncology treatment is the priority. If cancer is in remission or stable then lymphoedema treatment (decongestive lymphatic therapy) can be implemented.

Swollen breast and breast lymphoedema

Definition and nomenclature

Unilateral breast oedema is most often caused by breast cancer treatment but can be also caused by infection (e.g. cellulitis), malignancy (e.g. inflammatory breast cancer or angiosarcoma) and inflammatory mastitis. Rarely, it can occur with congestive cardiac failure, nephrotic syndrome and from treatment with mTor (mammalian target of rapamycin) inhibitors.

Synonyms and inclusions
- Breast oedema
- Swollen breast

Introduction and general description

As changes to breast cancer treatment have led to more breast-conserving surgery and increased use of therapeutic radiation to the breast, so the incidence of lymphoedema localized to the breast has risen. The risk is higher in the obese and in women with larger breasts.

Epidemiology

Of 144 women enrolled into one study before cancer treatment, 38 developed breast lymphoedema (26%) [1].

Pathophysiology

Oedema is an excess of interstitial fluid. Any oedema, whatever the cause, is due to capillary filtration overwhelming the lymph drainage for a sufficient period of time [2]. Interstitial fluid is reabsorbed almost entirely by the lymphatic vessels. Inflammation will increase blood flow and vascular permeability, both of which amplify microvascular fluid filtration. Inflammation can be caused by radiation and infection. Lymph drainage may be unable to respond to higher filtration because of effects from axillary surgery in compromising lymph flow. Disturbances in the Starling principle of fluid exchange will be greatest in the most dependent regions of the breast.

Predisposing factors

Carcinoma erysipeloides refers to a red, swollen breast resulting from breast cancer infiltrating the dermal lymphatics overlying the breast. Removal of one or more axillary lymph nodes risks lymphoedema within the drainage basin, that is the ipsilateral upper limb and adjoining quadrant of the chest including the breast. Therapeutic radiation to the breast can also induce/exacerbate breast swelling. Obesity and size of breast increases risk, as may adjuvant taxane chemotherapy [3]. In multivariate analysis from one study, factors associated with the development of breast lymphoedema in the axillary surgery subgroup included baseline BMI ($P = 0.004$), surgical incision location ($P = 0.009$) and prior surgical biopsy ($P = 0.01$) [4].

Other systemic causes for breast lymphoedema include heart failure, low plasma proteins resulting from nephrotic syndrome or liver failure, axillary lymphadenopathy and central vein occlusion. There have been several reports of breast oedema associated with mTor inhibitors [5].

Genetics

Breast lymphoedema is a secondary lymphoedema for which no genetic factors have been yet identified.

Environmental factors

These include surgery, radiation and drugs.

Clinical features

History
Breast swelling can be observed immediately following axillary lymphadenectomy, particularly if a 'seroma' or wound infection has occurred (a seroma is a misnomer as it represents a collection of lymph not serum). The onset of swelling can be delayed for months or years, particularly when arising from radiation effects. Swelling may be triggered by an attack of cellulitis.

Symptoms are breast heaviness, swelling, indentations from a bra and sometimes pain and tenderness. Breast redness may feature, indicating inflammation usually secondary to cellulitis, radiation effects or malignancy.

Presentation
Pitting and peau d'orange skin changes are most noticeable on the undersurface of the breast. Inflammation can be present. Cellulitis can coexist and is difficult to distinguish from post-radiation changes (Figure 105.15).

Differential diagnosis
Oedema can be determined clinically from indentation due to pressure (pitting). Other differential diagnoses include swelling from hormonal effects and fat hypertrophy.

Complications
Infection is a common complication of breast lymphoedema and further exacerbates oedema. Unexplained breast oedema should always be investigated in case of relapsed breast cancer or the development of (lymph)angiosarcoma.

Prognosis
Uncomplicated breast lymphoedema usually settles with treatment and resolves over time.

Investigations
Breast ultrasound is usually sufficient to confirm oedema and exclude malignancy. MRI is an alternative. A skin or breast biopsy may be necessary if malignancy is suspected.

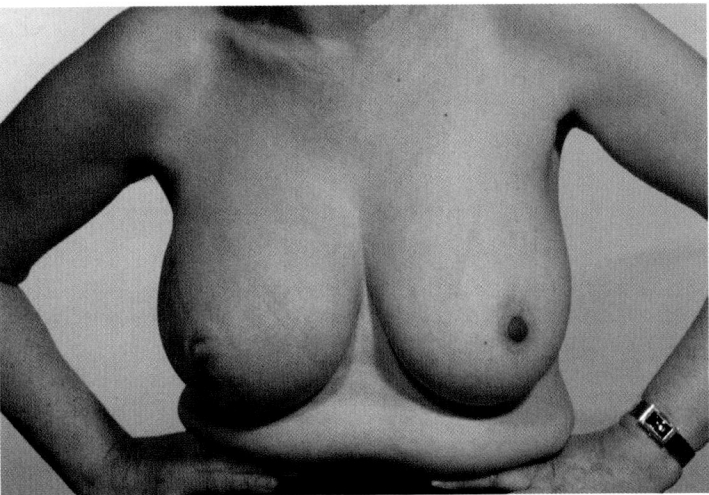

Figure 105.15 Breast lymphoedema following cancer treatment. Note pitting from bra indentations in the skin of the right breast.

Management

First line
An infection, if present, needs to be treated. Malignancy needs to be excluded. Obesity should be addressed and weight reduced to as near normal as possible.

Lymphoedema treatment should involve a supportive bra (a sports bra is often the best). It is recommended that the bra be worn both day and night in order to keep the breast uplifted, which overcomes gravitational factors. Massaging techniques are recommended, such as manual lymphatic drainage therapy, kinesiotaping and water immersion exercises (swimming aerobics), although the evidence base for their use is limited [6].

Second line
Mastectomy is a last resort.

Massive localized lymphoedema

Definition and nomenclature
Massive localized lymphoedema is a benign lymphoproliferative soft-tissue overgrowth in the morbidly obese patient. It represents gross lymphoedema usually confined to one area such as a thigh and appearing like a tumour.

Synonyms and inclusions
- Pseudosarcoma
- Elephantiasis nostras verrucosa

Introduction and general description
Lymphoedema typically affects a limb but uncommonly it can present as a localized mass resembling a tumour. It is not unusual for an area of lymphoedema on the lower inner thigh, leg, inguinal region or abdominal apron to hypertrophy into an enlarged fold and then, under the influence of gravity, progress into a pendulous swelling (Figure 105.16a). Obesity and repeat attacks of infection locally increase risk [1].

Pathophysiology

Predisposing factors
These include obesity, filariasis and recurrent infection.

Pathology
Solid or papillomatous plaques can mimic tumours but biopsy will reveal typical features of lymphoedema, namely oedema, dilated lymphatics, fibrosis, fat, epidermal acanthosis and hyperkeratosis, and inflammatory dermal infiltrate. In one series all 22 cases showed striking dermal fibrosis, expansion of the fibrous septa between fat lobules with increased numbers of stromal fibroblasts, lymphatic proliferation and lymphangiectasia. Multinucleated fibroblastic cells, marked vascular proliferation, moderate stromal cellularity and fascicular growth raised concern among referring pathologists for such conditions as atypical

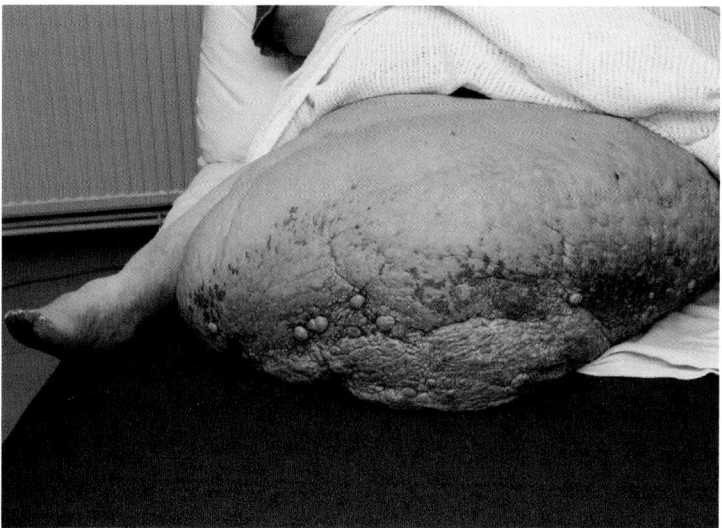

Figure 105.16 Massive localized lymphedema of the right thigh showing marked 'cobblestone' skin changes.

lipomatous tumour/well-differentiated liposarcoma, angiosarcoma and a fibroblastic neoplasm such as fibromatosis [2].

Clinical features

Presentation
An area of lymphoedema becomes raised like a tumour, then under the effects of gravity may become more polypoid-like and feels very heavy. Lesions most resemble a benign tumour such as a pedunculated lipoma although a soft-tissue sarcoma could also be suspected. The overlying skin is markedly thickened skin with a 'cobblestone' appearance with elephantiasis skin changes (Figure 105.16). The structure often appears lobulated and can grow to a considerable size [2].

Differential diagnosis
Differential diagnoses include lipoma, lymphatic malformation, lymphocele and sarcoma.

Complications
Weeping of lymph fluid and ulceration are common. Infection with septicaemia frequently occurs. When very large the 'tumour' can interfere with movement and mobility. A total of 65 cases of massive localized lymphoedema have been described in the literature, nine of which resulted in angiosarcoma (10.3% of all cases) [3].

Prognosis
The likelihood is that the lesion will continue to enlarge and suffer chronic sepsis unless treated.

Investigations
Magnetic resonance imaging typically demonstrates a sharply demarcated, pedunculated mass consisting of fat partitioned by fibrous septae surrounded by a thickened dermis. There is oedema both within the mass and tracking along the subcutaneous septae in a lace-like fashion outwards from the pedicle, outlining large lobules of fat [4].

Management
The only satisfactory treatment is surgical resection with reconstruction. However, this is not without hazard as wound dehiscence and overwhelming infection can present serious life-threatening risks. Intensive multilayer lymphoedema compression bandaging and IV antibiotics given first might reduce the surgical complications and improve prognosis.

Primary lymphoedema

Definition and nomenclature
Primary lymphoedema arises due to an intrinsic abnormality involving a genetically determined aplasia, hypoplasia, malformation or dysfunction of the lymphatic vessels, whereas secondary lymphoedema results from lymphatic damage due to extrinsic factors such as surgical lymphadenectomy, radiotherapy or chronic venous disease. Primary lymphoedema may occur as a non-syndromic Mendelian condition, or less commonly as part of a complex syndromic disorder [1].

Synonyms and inclusions
- Primary lymphoedema
- Lymphatic dysplasia
- Milroy disease
- Meige disease
- Lymphoedema congenita
- Lymphoedema praecox
- Lymphoedema tarda

Introduction and general description
Primary lymphoedema, or lymphoedema due to an underlying genetic abnormality, should always be suspected in a patient presenting with swelling and no obvious underlying medical cause. Suspicion of primary lymphoedema should be raised in those presenting during childhood or early adult years.

Historically, primary lymphoedema was classified into three categories depending on the age of onset of swelling: congenita (lymphoedema present at birth), praecox (lymphoedema developing after birth but before the age of 35 years) and tarda (lymphoedema developing after the age of 35 years). It became apparent that this classification system, based purely on age of onset, was oversimplified and redundant in clinical practice as it failed to facilitate categorization based on more specific phenotypes.

Mutations in several genes are known to cause primary lymphoedema. Some, but not all, of these factors have been shown to play a role in the regulating of lymphangiogenesis. The first two genes to be identified as causative for human lymphoedema were *VEGFR3* (also known as *FLT4*) in Milroy disease [2,3,4,5] and *FOXC2* in lymphoedema distichiasis syndrome [6,7,8]. Since then several new genes for human lymphatic disease have been discovered. Mendola *et al.* recently screened 78 patients for mutations in known primary lymphoedema genes and detected mutations in just 36% of cases [9]. This suggests that other causal genes for primary lymphoedema have yet to be identified.

Developments in clinical phenotyping and identification of the genetic cause of a number of subtypes of primary lymphoedema demonstrate that primary lymphoedema is highly heterogeneous. A new classification system and diagnostic pathway has been developed in order to delineate specific primary lymphoedema phenotypes, and facilitate the discovery of new causative genes [1,**10**]. Phenotyping and genotyping of patients with primary lymphoedema leads to a better understanding of the natural history and management of specific conditions and more accurate recurrence risks for future generations.

Epidemiology

Incidence and prevalence
Limited data exist on the prevalence of lymphoedema. The prevalence of primary lymphoedema was estimated as one in 6000 based on one UK clinic [11]. More recently, chronic lymphoedema (of primary and secondary causes) was estimated to affect as many as 1.33/1000 population in the UK [12]. A similar survey in Derby estimated 4/1000. Further epidemiological studies are needed to establish the true prevalence of primary lymphoedema. Estimates of prevalence have been difficult to calculate as it is presumed that many affected individuals do not come to medical attention.

Clinical features

Presentation
Primary lymphoedema may be present at birth or develop later in life. One or more limbs may be affected, or indeed there may be generalized/whole body swelling, depending on the subtype of lymphoedema.

The clinical signs of lymphoedema can range from mild swelling to that of grotesque enlargement in chronic, poorly managed patients. Protein-rich materials, lipids and debris accumulate in addition to water. This results in 'solid' and 'fluid' components to the swelling, giving rise to the 'brawny' nature of chronic oedema that resists pitting [13]. Skin changes may be present, including brawny fibrotic skin and the presence of the Kaposi–Stemmer sign (the failure to pinch/pick up a fold of skin at the base of the second toe, as a result of its thickness; see Figure 105.1). The Kaposi–Stemmer sign is pathognomonic of lymphoedema [14]. Papillomatosis (small flesh-coloured papules) occurs as a result of dilatation within the upper dermal lymphatics and subsequent fibrosis of the dermis. Lymphangiectasia appears as small blisters on the skin surface as a result of engorgement of lymphatic vessels. Lymph fluid frequently leaks as a result of minimal trauma and is termed lymphorrhoea.

Clinical variants
A number of subtypes of primary lymphoedema exist. They each present with differing age of swelling onset, distribution of lymphoedema and possible associated health problems. Connell *et al*.'s diagnostic pathway provides the simplest approach to classification of the various subtypes. However, the pathway remains a work in progress as new subtypes and causal genes are discovered [**10**]. The primary lymphoedema classification pathway is presented in the form of a colour-coded algorithm to illustrate the five main categories of primary lymphoedema, and the individual subtypes (including genotypes) within these categories (Figure 105.17 and Table 105.7). The main categories are:

1 Syndromic associated with lymphoedema, but where lymphoedema is not the predominant feature) (blue).
2 Localized or generalized lymphoedema associated with systemic/visceral lymphatic abnormalities (pink).
3 Lymphoedema in association with disturbed growth and/or cutaneous/vascular anomalies (yellow).
4 Congenital-onset primary lymphoedema, that is, lymphoedema that is present at birth or develops within the first year of life (green).
5 Late-onset primary lymphoedema, that is, lymphoedema that develops after the first year of life (purple).

These five categories are discussed in turn below, including the clinical phenotypes and causal gene mutations.

Syndromic
Lymphoedema is a recognized feature of many syndromes. Lymphoedema is not the primary problem in these conditions but is an associated feature. These include Turner and Noonan syndromes. Turner syndrome should always be suspected as the cause of congenital hand and/or foot swelling in female infants.

The genetic causes of many of these syndromes are known and testing is available. Table 105.8 provides a list of syndromes that include lymphoedema as part of the phenotype.

Lymphoedema with systemic/visceral involvement
A widespread developmental abnormality of the lymphatic system leads to systemic/visceral involvement and swelling that may not be confined to the limbs.

Lymphatic dysfunction may present prenatally with hydrothoraces or hydrops fetalis. The development of *in utero* oedema may cause dysmorphic facial features such as epicanthic folds, a broad nasal bridge and neck webbing with low-set ears [15].

Systemic lymphatic abnormalities may present with pericardial and pleural effusions, chylous ascites and pulmonary and intestinal lymphangiectasia in the postnatal period. An individual with intestinal lymphangiectasia will complain of abdominal pain and diarrhoea following the ingestion of foods with a high fat content (as the intestinal lymphatics are responsible for fat absorption). Management of systemic lymphatic impairment is not straightforward and a multidisciplinary approach is key. Management includes the drainage of effusions and implementation of a medium-chain triglyceride diet to manage intestinal lymphangiectasia and chylous disorders [16].

Patients with systemic lymphatic abnormalities can be classified into one of two categories depending upon the clinical presentation: a multisegmental lymphatic dysplasia with systemic involvement (MLDSI) or a generalized lymphatic dysplasia (GLD).

Multisegmental lymphatic dysplasia with systemic involvement. Patients with MLDSI have a segmental pattern of lymphoedema. The swelling affects different body parts in association with a systemic lymphatic abnormality. For example, they may have lymphoedema of one or more limbs or body sites (including the

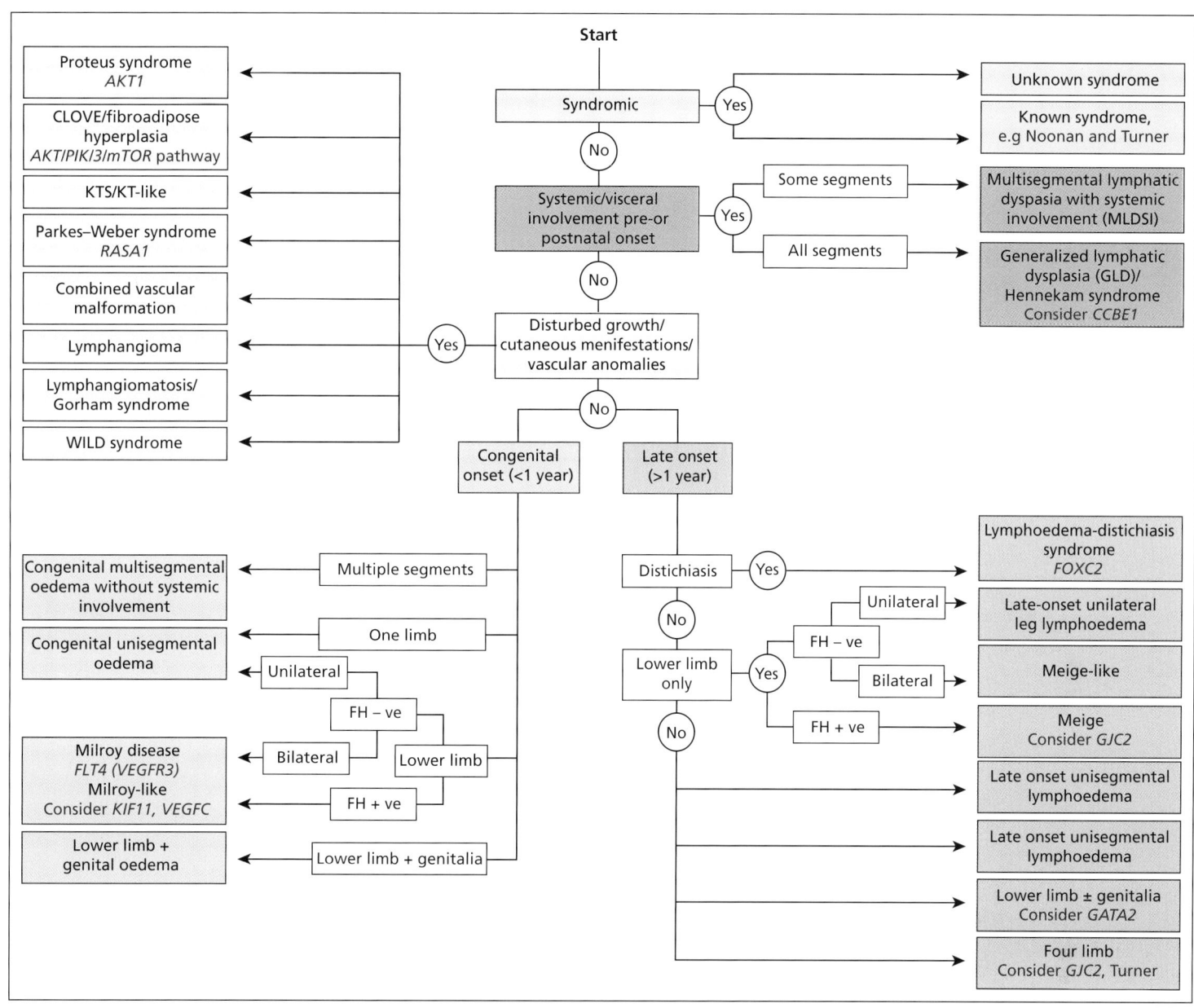

Figure 105.17 Classification pathway for primary lymphoedema. Text in red indicates the suggested genetic test for the subgroup. Please refer to Table105.7 for the definition of other terminology used in the figure [**10**]. FH, family history: +ve, positive; -ve, negative; KT, Klippel–Trenaunay; KTS, Klippel–Trenaunay syndrome. (From Connell *et al.* 2013 [**10**] and Mortimer and Rockson 2014 [**54**].)

Table 105.7 Definition of terminology used in the classification pathway.

Term	Definition
Congenital onset	Onset of lymphoedema before the age of 1 year
Cutaneous manifestations	Naevi/pigmentation variations (e.g. epidermal naevi/vascular malformations)
Distichiasis	Presence of aberrant eyelashes arising from the meibomian glands
Disturbed growth	Hypertrophy (overgrowth) and hypotrophy of bone or soft tissue resulting in altered length of a limb or body part
KT/KT-like	Klippel–Trenaunay/Klippel–Trenaunay-like syndrome
Late onset	Swelling presenting after 1 year of age
Prenatal onset	Detection of lymphatic abnormality in the prenatal period. Isolated pedal oedema is excluded from this definition as this may be a presentation of Milroy disease
Segment	A region of the body affected by lymphoedema (i.e. face, conjunctiva, genitalia, upper limbs, lower limbs – each constitute one body part). Multisegmental refers to more than one segment affected by lymphoedema. Bilateral lower limb swelling is not considered to be multisegmental lymphoedema
Syndromic	A constellation of abnormalities, one of which is lymphoedema
Systemic involvement	Systemic lymphatic problems persisting beyond the newborn period or manifesting at any age thereafter. This includes hydrops fetalis, chylous ascites, intestinal lymphangiectasia, pleural and pericardial effusions and pulmonary lymphangiectasia
Vascular anomalies	Includes congenital vascular abnormalities

Table 105.8 List of known syndromes associated with lymphoedema and the causative gene (or chromosomal abnormality) if known.

Known syndrome	Chromosome/gene
Aagenaes syndrome	Not known
Carbohydrate-deficient glycoprotein types 1a, 1b, 1h	PMM2, PM1, ALG8
Cardio-facio-cutaneous syndrome	RAS-MAP kinase pathway including KRAS, BRAF, MAP2K1, MAP2K2
CHARGE syndrome	CDH7
Choanal atresia-lymphoedema	PTPN14
Ectodermal dysplasia, anhidrotic, immunodeficiency, osteopetrosis and lymphoedema (OLEDAID syndrome)	IKBKG (NEMO)
Fabry disease	GLA
Hennekam syndrome	CCBE1, FAT4
Hypotrichosis-lymphoedema-telangiectasia	SOX18
Irons–Bianchi syndrome	Not known
Lymphoedema-myelodysplasia (Emberger syndrome)	GATA2
Macrocephaly-capillary malformation (MCM)	PIK3CA
Microcephaly with or without chorioretinopathy, lymphoedema and mental retardation (MCLMR)	KIF11
Mucke syndrome	Not known
Noonan syndrome	RAS-MAP kinase pathway PTPN11, KRAS, SOS1 and others
Oculo-dento-digital syndrome (ODD)	GJA1
Progressive encephalopathy, hypsarrhythmia and optic atrophy (PEHO)	Not known
Phelan–McDermid syndrome	22q terminal deletion or ring chromosome 22
Prader–Willi syndrome	15q11 microdeletion or maternal uniparental disomy 15
Thrombocytopenia with absent radius	1q21.1 microdeletion and RBM8A
Turner syndrome	45, X0
Velo-cardio-facial syndrome	22q11 microdeletion
Yellow-nail syndrome	Not known

Adapted from Connell *et al.* 2013 [**10**].

face), in association with previous or current systemic lymphatic abnormalities (e.g. intestinal lymphangiectasia, recurrent chylous pleural effusions). The patient has no syndromic features and is of normal intelligence. The underlying mechanism is thought to be of somatic mosaicism, and no known causal genes have been identified to date. There is a low sibling and offspring recurrence risk.

Generalized lymphatic dysplasia. Patients with GLD have a more global pattern of lymphoedema. Swelling typically affects all body parts and often presents *in utero* with hydrops fetalis. A number of patients with GLD will have a family history of lymphoedema suggestive of autosomal recessive inheritance, inferring a higher recurrence risk than MLDSI. Hennekam syndrome is one type of autosomal recessive GLD and presents with lymphoedema of all

four limbs, intestinal and/or pulmonary lymphatic dysplasia, a variable degree of learning difficulties and characteristic facies (a flat face, flat and broad nasal bridge and hypertelorism) [17]. Associated problems include hypothyroidism, glaucoma, seizures, hearing loss and renal abnormalities [18,19]. Lymphoscintigraphy has rarely been undertaken in this condition but Bellini *et al.* demonstrated abnormal drainage in the upper and lower limbs and the thoracic duct in one patient [18].

Patients with suspected Hennekam syndrome may be screened for mutations in *CCBE1* (collagen and calcium binding EGF domain 1) on chromosome 18q21 [20,21]. However, *CCBE1* mutations only appear to account for 25% of cases, suggesting genetic heterogeneity [**20**]. This is supported by the recent identification of homozygous or compound heterozygous mutations of the *FAT4* gene (a member of the protocadherin family, and not a recognized component of the lymphangiogenesis pathway) in four of 24 *CCBE1* mutation-negative Hennekam syndrome patients [22].

The function of *CCBE1* in humans has yet to be elucidated, but animal studies confirm that *ccbe1* enhances the process of lymphangiogenesis induced by vascular endothelial growth factor C (VEGFC), and is also necessary for the budding and sprouting of lymphangioblasts [23,24].

Lymphoedema associated with disturbed growth and/or cutaneous/vascular anomalies
Lymphoedema may develop in association with vascular abnormalities, disorders of growth and cutaneous abnormalities. Identifying the type of malformation and thereby the vessels involved is important for diagnosis and management.

These patients are challenging as there is considerable overlap in clinical findings and a clear-cut diagnosis based upon phenotype alone is not always possible. The recent identification of *de novo* somatic mutations as the underlying mechanism for some of these conditions may further understanding and improve management. For example, gene abnormalities within the AKT/PIK3/mTOR pathway have been found to cause Proteus and CLOVES syndromes [**25,26**]. This has allowed separation of these conditions within the diagnostic pathway, and has identified gene pathways that could be targeted by pharmacological therapy [**27**]. Conditions with gene abnormalities within the AKT/PIK3/mTOR pathway that are associated with lymphoedema include the following.

CLOVES syndrome.   The spectrum of clinical signs include congenital *l*ipomatous *o*vergrowth, *v*ascular malformations, *e*pidermal naevi and *s*keletal abnormalities (CLOVES). Somatic mosaicism of activating mutations within *PIK3CA* have been reported [26]. The same gene and same mechanism have also been implicated in a few patients with Klippel–Trenaunay syndrome and with fibroadipose hyperplasia [26,**27**]. Lymphatic malformations can arise as part of these conditions. Further molecular studies, together with careful phenotyping, will facilitate the understanding of this spectrum of disease. It is likely that combined vascular malformations may also arise as a result of somatic mosaicism.

Klippel–Trenaunay syndrome. Patients present with a combination of several or all of the following within a single limb: limb length hypertrophy of muscle, fat or bone (e.g. presenting as increased limb length or girth), varicose veins, vascular malformation (e.g. capillary malformations) and lymphoedema. Activating mutations within *PIK3CA* have also been reported [26].

Proteus syndrome. Proteus syndrome is a disease characterized by progressive, segmental overgrowth of the bones, skin and connective tissue. Lymphatic and capillary malformations are the most common vascular changes seen in this syndrome. Clinical signs of Proteus syndrome may not be present at birth but develop during infancy and progress throughout the individual's life. The diagnosis may be established using diagnostic clinical criteria and/or molecular analysis [28]. The majority of individuals with typical Proteus syndrome will have an activating mutation in *AKT1*, arising as a result of somatic mosaicism [25]. AKT acts within the molecular pathway that includes the *mTOR* and *PIK3CA* genes. This pathway is critical as a progrowth and antiapoptosis facilitator. The identification of the PIK3/AKT/mTOR signalling pathway underpinning disease processes gives rise to the potential for therapeutic targets through inhibition of this pathway [**27**].

Congenital multisegmental lymphoedema. Patients with congenital multisegmental lymphoedema without systemic lymphatic impairment have been included within the yellow section of the classification pathway in order to avoid confusion with multisegmental lymphoedema occurring in association with systemic lymphatic abnormalities (in the pink section of the pathway). These patients have an asymmetrical pattern of lymphatic failure with some limb sparing (i.e. some limbs are unaffected) but without overgrowth or cutaneous or vascular abnormalities. It is possible that somatic mosaicism in gene(s) involved in lymphangiogenesis could explain this subtype of congenital primary lymphoedema.

WILD syndrome. This syndrome is a condition comprising clinical signs of *w*arts, *i*mmunodeficiency, *l*ymphoedema and ano-genital *d*ysplasia (WILD) [29]. These patients have extensive, asymmetrical, multisegmental lymphoedema comprising facial and conjunctival oedema, genital lymphoedema, and epidermal naevi and/or capillary malformations typically of the torso and upper limbs. These patients have a sporadic condition, suggesting probable somatic mosaicism [**10**]. The underlying genetic cause has yet to be identified.

Congenital-onset primary lymphoedema
Historically, all cases of congenital lymphoedema were classified as Milroy disease. However, several different types of congenital lower limb primary lymphoedema have been recognized.

Milroy disease. Milroy disease presents with congenital lymphoedema of the lower legs (usually symmetrical). The onset of swelling may occasionally be delayed but will occur within the first year of life. Lymphoedema is typically confined to the feet and ankles, but may progress up to the knees. Up-slanting 'ski-jump' toenails are present as a result of disturbance of the nail bed by oedema. Prominent large-calibre veins are frequently present on the feet and pretibial regions. Varicose veins, typically the long saphenous veins, are a common finding in adults with Milroy disease, but do not appear to affect the paediatric population. A third of affected males have hydroceles [30]. Milroy disease rarely presents in the antenatal

period with hydrops fetalis but the outcome may be favourable (i.e. the swelling may regress and remain confined to the feet), or the hydrops may progress and result in intrauterine death [31,32].

Lymphoscintigraphy in Milroy disease confirms failure of the initial lymphatic vessels to absorb fluid. The term 'functional aplasia of lymphatic vessels' has been used to describe the characteristic lymphoscintigraphy results [**10**]. The initial lymphatic vessels are present (confirmed on histological examination) but unable to absorb interstitial fluid [33].

Abnormalities within the gene that encodes vascular endothelial growth factor receptor type 3 (VEGFR-3) on chromosome 5q35 are causal of Milroy disease [2,31]. Mutations in the tyrosine kinase domain of *VEGFR3* are found in 70% of patients with congenital-onset primary lymphoedema affecting both lower limbs [34]. Inheritance is autosomal dominant but *de novo* cases may occur [2,3].

Milroy-like lymphoedema. Individuals with congenital lower limb lymphoedema who do not have an underlying *VEGFR3* mutation are classified as having Milroy-like lymphoedema. Mutations within the *VEGFC* gene have been identified as causal in several families within this category [**35**,36]. VEGFC is the ligand for VEGFR-3 and controls lymphatic sprouting during embryonic development [23,37]. Affected individuals typically have all the clinical signs of Milroy disease (congenital lower limb lymphoedema, prominent large-calibre veins and hydroceles, inherited in an autosomal dominant pattern) yet their lymph scans are atypical.

MCLID syndrome. *M*icrocephaly with or without *c*horioretinopathy, *l*ymphoedema or *i*ntellectual *d*isability (MCLID) syndrome is an autosomal dominant syndrome comprising congenital lower limb lymphoedema (mimicking Milroy disease) as well as microcephaly and variable degrees of learning difficulties that occur as a result of mutations in the *KIF11* gene on chromosome 10q24 [38]. The presence of chorioretinopathy is variable but should always be excluded by an expert ophthalmology opinion. Lymphoscintigraphy demonstrates the same pattern of lymphatic functional aplasia as that seen in Milroy disease. The KIF11 protein product is involved in spindle formation during mitosis but is not clear how *KIF11* relates to the lymphangiogenesis pathway [39]. MCLID should be considered in all patients with congenital bilateral lower limb lymphoedema and microcephaly.

Late-onset primary lymphoedema
The term late-onset lymphoedema is used to describe a primary lymphoedema that develops after the first year of life (i.e. non-congenital lymphoedema). This section contains a number of assorted conditions, some with life-threatening associated diseases (e.g. Emberger syndrome), but they all share the common finding of non-congenital limb swelling.

Lymphoedema distichiasis syndrome. This condition presents with pubertal onset of bilateral lower limb lymphoedema. Distichiasis (aberrant eyelashes arising from the meibomian glands) is present in 95% of affected individuals and is frequently present at birth but rarely causes symptoms until childhood [40]. Other clinical signs include ptosis, cleft palate and congenital heart disease.

PART 9: VASCULAR

The majority of affected individuals have varicose veins [41]. Lymphoedema distichiasis syndrome occurs as a result of mutations in the *FOXC2* gene on chromosome 16q24 and is inherited in an autosomal dominant manner [7]. *FOXC2* encodes a transcription factor necessary for ensuring normal development of the lymphatic collecting vessels and valves [42]. Lymphoscintigraphy of affected individuals demonstrates reflux of lymph within the lower limbs as a result of valve failure within the lymphatic vessels [43]. Similarly, abnormal venous valves lead to early-onset venous reflux in all patients with *FOXC2* mutations [44].

Meige disease. Meige disease is the most prevalent subtype of primary lymphoedema [10]. It typically presents with bilateral lower limb lymphoedema that rarely extends above the knee. The onset of symptoms is in adolescence or adulthood. There are no other associated features of the condition [45]. Lymphoscintigraphy frequently demonstrates abnormal deep rerouting of lower limb lymph drainage as evidenced by an increased uptake of tracer within the popliteal lymph nodes and impaired main superficial lymphatic tract filling [10]. Family history is consistent with an autosomal dominant pattern of inheritance yet the causal gene of classic Meige disease has not yet been identified.

Emberger syndrome. Emberger syndrome comprises late-onset (but in childhood) bilateral or unilateral lower limb with or without genital lymphoedema together with myelodysplastic syndrome and/or acute myeloid leukaemia [46]. It may also be associated with a high-frequency, progressive sensorineural deafness. Severe cutaneous warts occur as a result of the associated immune dysfunction. Myelodysplasia may develop at any stage and will progress to acute myeloid leukaemia with a high mortality [47]. Lymphoscintigraphy has not been routinely performed on patients with this condition.

Mutations in the *GATA2* gene on chromosome 3q21are causal and are inherited in an autosomal dominant manner [48]. *GATA2* is expressed in lymphatic, vascular and endocardial endothelial cells [49]. Mouse studies suggest the lymphoedema occurs as a result of abnormal lymphatic valve development [50]. *GATA2* is also involved in the regulation of haematopoiesis, hence the association of lymphoedema with myelodysplasia in this rare, yet life-threatening, condition [51].

Late-onset four-limb lymphoedema. An autosomal dominant pattern of late-onset lymphoedema affecting either the lower limbs, or all four limbs, occurs as a result of mutations in the *GJC2* gene [52]. Apart from lower limb varicose veins, no other associated conditions have been reported. Lymphoscintigraphy demonstrates lymphatic tracts that appear normal but with significantly reduced quantification uptake of tracer, reflecting reduced absorption from tissues by peripheral lymphatics in all four limbs [52]. The functional role of *GJC2* within the lymphatic system is unclear as it encodes for the connexin 47 protein located on chromosome 1q42, and is not known to be involved in the lymphangiogenesis pathway.

Differential diagnosis

Secondary lymphoedema that has occurred as a result of an underlying medical cause needs to be excluded, for example lower limb

Table 105.9 Stages of lymphoedema adapted from the International Society of Lymphology Consensus Document [53].

Stage	Clinical signs
Stage 0	A latent/subclinical state where swelling is not evident despite impaired lymphatic transport. This stage may exist for many months or years before oedema becomes evident
Stage I	Early onset of lymphoedema where there is accumulation of tissue fluid that reduces with limb elevation; pitting may be present
Stage II	Accumulation of fluid that does not reduce on elevation; at later stages it may be non-pitting
Stage III	Fibrotic tissue and absent pitting; elephantiasis skin changes develop (e.g. acanthosis, fatty and fibrous tissue changes, and warty overgrowths)

lymphoedema as a result of venous insufficiency. A detailed history, examination (and possible investigation with lymphoscintigraphy or venous duplex imaging) should provide the underlying diagnosis.

Classification of severity

The severity of the lymphoedema may be classified according to the clinical features (Table 105.9), and this may be useful in monitoring response to therapy over a prolonged period.

Complications and co-morbidities

See the section called Complications of lymphoedema later in this chapter.

Management

See the section called Lymphoedema management later in this chapter.

Resources

Patient resources

Lymphoedema Support Network: http://www.lymphoedema.org (last accessed August 2015).

Lipoedema

Definition and nomenclature

Lipoedema is a disorder of adipose tissue that occurs almost exclusively in women, usually at a time of hormonal change. Patients have progressive fatty swelling of the lower limbs, with associated easy bruising, skin tenderness and pain of the lower limbs.

Synonyms and inclusions
- Adiposis dolorosa
- Painful fat syndrome
- Adipositas oedematosa
- Stovepipe legs

Introduction and general description

Lipoedema is a condition characterized by abnormal adipose deposition within the lower limbs. It occurs almost exclusively in females, and is thought to be an inherited disorder. The onset of symptoms typically occurs at a time of hormonal change such as puberty or pregnancy. Patients complain of progressive fatty swelling of the lower limbs, with associated easy bruising, skin tenderness and pain of the lower limbs. Contrary to what the name suggests, oedema is not a key feature and the 'swelling' is caused by adipose tissue and not fluid. Lipoedema was first described by Allen and Hines in 1940 as 'bilateral enlargement of the legs thought to be due to abnormal deposition of subcutaneous fat and accumulation of fluid in the lower legs' [1]. The lack of a clear definition of the disorder has led to significant confusion regarding diagnosis and management. In fact, some clinicians consider it a physiological variant rather than a disease [2]. However, lipoedema recently received acceptance as a medical condition and obtained an MIM number in 2011.

Epidemiology

Incidence and prevalence
Limited prevalence data exist for lipoedema. Some clinicians believe it is a rare disorder [3], but many feel that it is more common than expected and is often misdiagnosed as simple obesity or lymphoedema [4,5,6].

Age
Onset is typically at puberty or other times of hormonal change such as pregnancy or commencement of the oral contraceptive pill.

Sex
Lipoedema occurs almost exclusively in females. Only six cases of lipoedema affecting males have been reported in the literature [7,8,9]. Child et al. identified four unrelated isolated adult males with the condition. All were thought to have developed lipoedema secondary to hormonal disturbances, with reduced testosterone levels being a common factor [7].

Ethnicity
No ethnic differences have been reported.

Pathophysiology

Pathology
The aetiology of lipoedema is still unknown. It has not yet been determined whether the cause of the 'fatty swelling' is due to adipocyte hypertrophy or hyperplasia, or a combination of both. Histological examination of tissue biopsies and liposuction aspirates identified oedema of the adipocytes and/or interstitium, but no other abnormalities were detected [9,10]. One study postulates that activated adipogenesis occurs in lipoedema tissue leading to hypoxia and subsequent adipocyte necrosis and recruitment of macrophages, as occurs in obesity [11]. Child et al. proposed that a hormonal influence was likely to underlie the condition as lipoedema appeared to be expressed most commonly at puberty or other times of hormonal change [7].

Genetics
Frequent observations of mother to daughter inheritance led to the hypothesis that lipoedema is a genetic disorder. Patterns of inheritance of the condition within families are consistent with either X-linked dominant inheritance or autosomal dominant inheritance with sex limitation [7].

Clinical features

History
Affected individuals develop bilateral and symmetrical 'fatty' non-pitting swelling, usually confined to the legs and hips [8]. The feet are spared, giving rise to an 'inverse shouldering' or 'bracelet' effect at the ankles (Figure 105.18). Patients frequently complain of tenderness and easy bruising of the affected areas. The onset of lipoedema is usually at or soon after puberty but can appear to develop at other times of hormonal change such as pregnancy or even menopause [7]. Over time, the patient may develop similar clinical signs in their upper arms. Wold et al. [8] have proposed a set of diagnostic criteria for lipoedema:
1 Occurrence is almost exclusively in women.
2 It has a bilateral and symmetrical nature with minimal involvement of the feet, resulting in an 'inverse shouldering' or 'bracelet' effect at the ankle.
3 Minimal pitting oedema is seen.
4 There is pain, tenderness and easy bruising.
5 Persistent enlargement is found despite elevation of the extremities or weight loss.

Presentation
In the teenager or young adult the lipoedema phenotype is characteristic; the classic disproportionate distribution of fat below the waist, the coexisting features of tissue tenderness and easy bruising and the lack of response to weight-reducing diets all argue against a form of obesity. However, later in life, lipoedema can be complicated by obesity and/or lymphoedema, rendering the diagnosis more difficult to make. In this case historical symptoms are key to the diagnosis [7]. Whilst lipoedema is confused with obesity by many clinicians, associated obesity has, nonetheless, been observed in 50% of patients [12].

Differential diagnosis
Lipoedema must be differentiated from lymphoedema, a more common cause of bilateral lower limb enlargement. However, lymphoedema typically results in asymmetrical oedematous swelling due to the accumulation of interstitial fluid within tissue spaces. Typical cutaneous findings of lymphoedema include brawny, hard and warty changes of the skin and subcutis. Pitting (where the skin remains indented for a few minutes after removal of firm finger pressure for 30 s) is often present during the initial stages of lymphoedema. In contrast, cutaneous changes and pitting are almost always absent in lipoedema [7].

Clinicians may be tempted to confuse lipoedema with Dercum disease, another 'painful fat' disorder. However, patients with

PART 9: VASCULAR

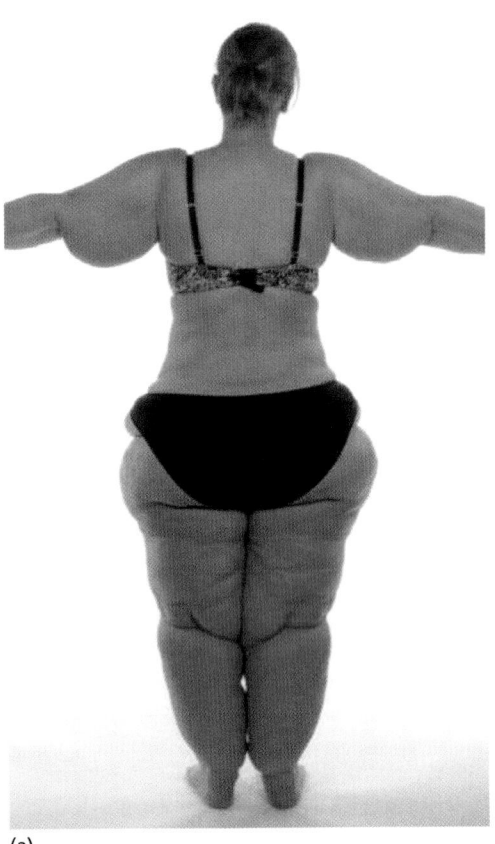

(a)

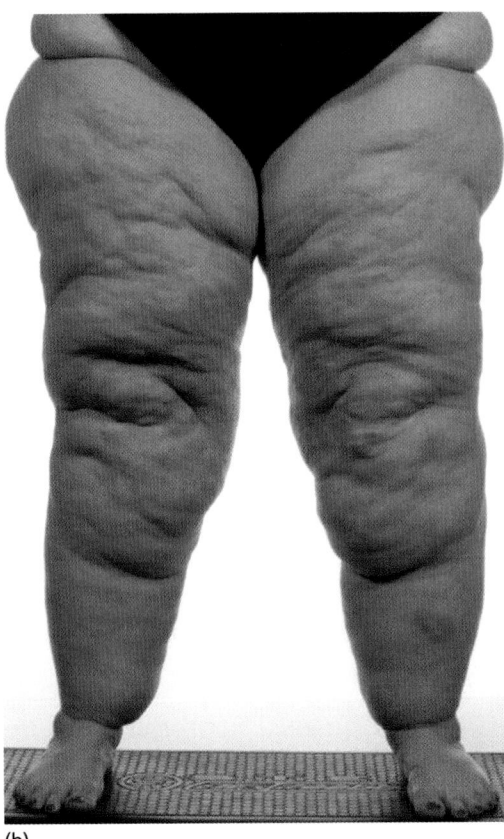

(b)

Figure 105.18 A patient with classic lipoedema. (a) Symmetrical fatty swelling of both lower limbs with sparing of the trunk. Increased adipose deposition of the upper arms is present. (b) Lipoedema features include sparing of the feet with 'inverse shouldering' of the ankles. Fat pads are developing on the medial aspect of both knees.

Dercum disease typically have multiple, painful, diffuse or nodular lipomas (with chronic pain lasting more than 3 months) and a generalized obesity problem. Men may be affected, but there is a female preponderance with a ratio of 5–30 : 1 [13].

Classification of severity
Table105.10 contains the clinical stages of lipoedema as suggested by Schmeller and Meier-Vollrath [3].

Complications and co-morbidities
Lipoedema is frequently complicated by the onset of a secondary lymphoedema, resulting in the clinical picture of lipo-lymphoedema [7]. The clinical features of lipo-lymphoedema range from mild pitting oedema of the feet to severe swelling of the entire lower limbs as a result of impaired lymphatic drainage. Allen and Hines proposed that the progressive oedema formation in lipoedema

was the result of poor resistance of accumulated fat against the hydrostatic passage of fluid from the capillaries into the interstitium [1]. Lymphoscintigraphy performed after the onset of lipo-lymphoedema will confirm the presence of main tracts but lymphatic drainage will be impaired.

Disorder of gait, joint deformities (e.g. genu valgum) and pain may occur as a result of disproportionate adipose tissue of the legs. A number of women complain of knee pain prior to the onset of radiological changes, suggesting that knee pain is part of the lipoedema phenotype (possibly due to an associated disorder of connective tissue) or secondary to the strain put on the knee joint from increased limb volume.

Patients with lipoedema often develop psychological morbidity as a result of their chronic progressive disorder [14].

Disease course and prognosis
Poorly managed lipoedema will undoubtedly progress to lipo-lymphoedema.

Investigations
The diagnosis of lipoedema is currently clinical with no absolute phenotypic features or confirmatory test. Numerous investigations have been undertaken in patients with lipoedema, including lymphoscintigrams, venograms, arteriograms and magnetic resonance lymphangiography, all failing to demonstrate specific abnormalities but suggesting a subclinical reduction in lymphatic function in patients with lipoedema [4,15–17]. None of these investigations demonstrated specific diagnostic signs of lipoedema.

Table 105.10 Stages of lipoedema.

Stage	Clinical signs
Stage I	The skin is smooth and the subcutaneous layer is thickened, soft and with an even structure. This stage can last for several years
Stage II	The skin might be cool in certain areas as a result of functional vascular imbalance. Over time, subcutaneous nodules develop and the skin surface becomes uneven
Stage III	After several decades, patients may develop large amounts of tender subcutaneous tissue and bulging protrusions of fat, mainly at the inner side of the thighs or knees, which lead to an impairment of gait

Adapted from Schmeller and Meier-Vollrath 2006 [3].

High-resolution cutaneous ultrasonography has been proposed as a method for differentiating lipoedema from lymphoedema. Naouri *et al.* reported a significant difference in dermal thickness between the two groups – no dermal thickening detected in lipoedema compared with marked dermal thickness in lymphoedema [18]. However, the experienced clinician will be able to tell the two conditions apart by the soft 'doughy' consistency of excess subcutaneous adipose deposition in lipoedema compared with the pitting, firmer tissue consistency of lymphoedema.

Management

No curative therapies are available for lipoedema. Management goals are aimed at the improvement of subjective symptoms (e.g. pain), prevention of lipoedema progression and prevention of lipo-lymphoedema.

Conservative therapies including manual lymph drainage, intermittent pneumatic compression and multilayered short-stretch bandaging were shown to reduce the perception of pain in patients with lipoedema [19]. However, these treatments have no effect on the reduction of limb volume, unless there is coexistent lymphoedema. Compression therapy has been shown to prevent additional oedema formation [20,21].

The prevention of lipoedema progression is key. Physical activity should be encouraged as it will reduce the risk of obesity and may have a positive impact on the oedema component. Dietary advice and advice on avoiding weight gain is a crucial part of the management plan. Patients should be made aware that obesity is a major exacerbating factor of lipoedema [22].

Liposuction has been accepted as a therapeutic option for lipoedema. Treatment aims to cause a reduction of limb volume/mass, a reduction of pain and improvement in mobility. Reliable criteria for liposuction timing do not exist. It would appear that treatment in the early stages yields a better outcome than when liposuction is used in advanced cases or in lipo-lymphoedema [22,23]. The long-term data on liposuction are still weak but the immediate results appear promising. However, patients must be aware that liposuction does not offer a cure. If the patient does not maintain their weight in the postoperative period then they will return to the original disease state [24].

Resources

Patient resources

Lipoedema UK: www.lipoedema.co.uk.
Lymphoedema Support Network: www.lymphoedema.org.
(Both last accessed August 2015.)

Yellow-nail syndrome

Definition and nomenclature

Yellow-nail syndrome (YNS) comprises overcurved, smooth, translucent, slow-growing nails with a yellow discoloration along with respiratory ailments such as chronic sinusitis, bronchiectasis or pleural effusion, and lymphoedema. Although listed by McKusick

[1] as a genetic condition it more commonly develops late in adulthood as a sporadic condition.

> **Synonyms and inclusions**
> • Lymphoedema and yellow nails

Introduction and general description

The first case series of 13 patients who were given a diagnosis of YNS was described by Samman and White [2]. Typically, the patient has: (i) lymphoedema; (ii) a respiratory disease such as pleural effusion; and (iii) yellow dystrophic nails. Two of these features are required for the diagnosis, since the complete triad is only observed in about one-third of patients.

Epidemiology

A recent systematic review of 150 patients revealed that their median age was 60 years (range: newborn to 88 years). YNS occurred in all age groups but in 78.7% (100/127) patients were aged between 41 and 80 years. The male : female ratio was 1.2 : 1. All cases had lymphoedema and 85.6% had yellow nails. Pleural effusions were bilateral in 68.3%. The appearance of the fluid was serous in 75.3%, milky in 22.3% and purulent in 3.5% [3].

Pathophysiology

The pathogenesis of this condition is unknown. Lymphangiogram abnormalities have been described [4] although a lymphoscintigraphic study demonstrated that a primary lymphatic abnormality is unlikely [5].

Pathology

The pleural effusion in YNS is an exudate in the vast majority of patients. There is a lymphocytic predominance in 96% of cases, with a low count of nucleated cells. In 61 of 66 (92.4%) patients, pleural fluid protein values were >3 g/dL.

Genetics

Wells described a family with eight cases in four sibships of two generations [6]. In the proband, who had yellow nails, lymphoedema began in the legs at the age of 51 years. At times oedema also affected the genitalia, hands, face and vocal cords. Lymphangiograms were interpreted as showing primary hypoplasia of the lymphatics [6].

Govaert *et al.* reported a girl who was born at 33 weeks' gestation with non-immune hydrops and a recurrent left chylothorax to a mother with YNS. The non-immune hydrops in this case was diagnosed on a 29-week ultrasound examination [76]. Slee *et al.* reported a case of a newborn infant who, at 23 weeks' gestation, was found to have hydrops on antenatal ultrasonography; bilateral chylothorax was found at delivery [8]. The mother had YNS with typical nail changes and bronchiectasis. The infant had a recurrent cough, possibly preceding an early onset of bronchiectasis.

Clinical features

History

The average age of onset reported is during the sixth decade. Patients are usually first aware of not needing to cut their nails. The

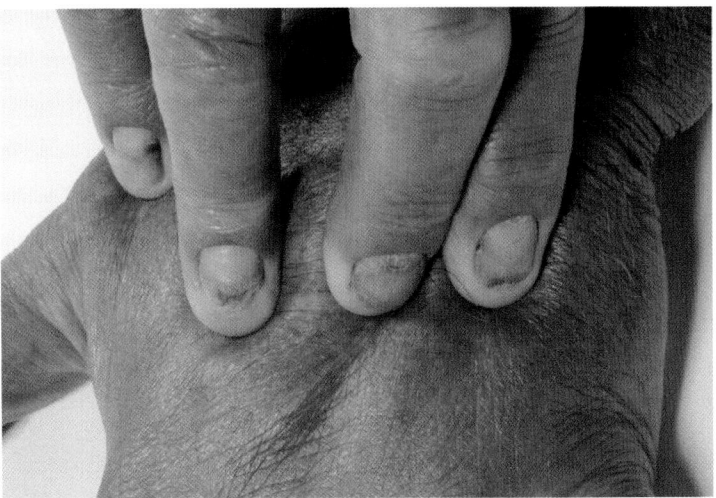

Figure 105.19 Yellow-nail syndrome showing slow-growing, overcurved, thickened nail plates and hand oedema.

nails then become thicker and harder to cut. The nail may discolour yellow but also may lift up and become opaque (due to onycholysis) or go green/black due to secondary haemorrhage or *Pseudomonas* infection. Picking up items may prove difficult due to tactile dysfunction. Nails may fracture or shed. Nail units may become painful, particularly if affected by a paronychia. Cough is the commonest respiratory symptom and may be productive. Shortness of breath may indicate pleural effusion. Peripheral oedema usually starts in the ankles bilaterally but may become very widespread and involve the trunk, genitalia and upper limbs if severe.

Presentation
Nail changes include slow growth, yellow-green discoloration, transverse and longitudinal overcurvature, onycholysis, shedding, cross-ridging and loss of lunulae and cuticles. The nail plate is yellow and overcurved, but remains translucent and smooth (Figure 105.19).

Although lymphoedema is the most consistent association with yellow nails, other associations include bronchiectasis, sinusitis, chronic cough and pleural effusions. Rarely a pericardial effusion can occur.

Differential diagnosis
Nail changes are not unusual with lymphoedema due to secondary fungal infection, although fungus causes a softer and more friable nail plate. A diagnosis of YNS is difficult without the characteristic nail changes. Cor pulmonale can present with respiratory symptoms and peripheral oedema.

Complications
Recurrent chest infections are the commonest complication. Recurrent cellulitis frequently complicates lymphoedema. Acute paronychia can complicate the nail unit changes.

Prognosis
In one study four of the 11 patients had complete recovery of their nails over a mean period of 4–5 years [9]. There are some suggestions that life expectancy is reduced [10].

Investigations
Yellow-nail syndrome is a clinical diagnosis. There is no confirmatory diagnostic test.

Management
The most effective treatments for pleural effusions appear to be pleurodesis and decortication/pleurectomy [3]. The lymphoedema does not respond well to diuretics, which is predictable as diuretics do not improve lymph drainage. Nevertheless diuretics such as spironolactone may be necessary if oedema is widespread and severe. Vitamin E is the most common treatment prescribed for the nail changes but the evidence base for this is weak [11]. Treatment of the chronic paronychia with fluconazole has been claimed to be beneficial in anecdotal reports [12].

Lymphatic malformation and lymphangioma circumscriptum

Definition and nomenclature
Vascular tumours are endothelial neoplasms characterized by increased cellular proliferation. Haemangioma is the most common and is almost exclusive to infants. Vascular malformations, on the other hand, are the result of abnormal development of vascular elements during embryogenesis and fetal life. These may be single-vessel forms (capillary, arterial, lymphatic or venous) or a combination. Vascular malformations do not generally demonstrate increased endothelial turnover [1]. The same principles apply to lymphangioma as to lymphatic malformations.

Synonyms and inclusions
- Lymphangioma circumscriptum
- Cavernous lymphangioma
- Microcystic lymphatic malformation
- Macrocystic lymphatic malformations
- Cystic hygroma
- Lymphangiodysplasia
- Mixed vascular anomaly

Introduction and general description
The term lymphangioma circumscriptum has been in common usage by dermatologists to describe a lymphatic malformation. Strictly, a lymphangioma should be a 'growing lymphatic tumour' involving proliferating lymphatic endothelium. A lymphatic malformation once formed from an abnormal development of lymphatic vessels grows only by expansion/distension, not proliferation, and therefore lymphangioma is an inappropriate term in such circumstances. A lymphatic malformation results from an error in the embryonic development of the lymphatic system.

Lymphangiomatosis is a disorder of proliferative lymphatic vasculature. It is characterized by the progressive involvement of various body tissues and can involve the skeletal system, connective tissues and visceral organs.

Localized congenital lymphatic malformations can be divided into macrocystic (or deep) and microcystic (or superficial) lesions.

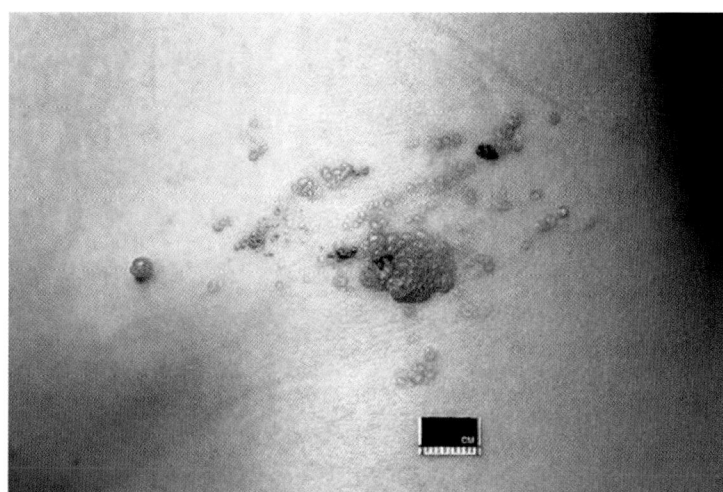

Figure 105.20 Lymphangioma circumscriptum showing fluid-filled vesicles resembling frogspawn. At times the vesicles can contain blood, weep clear fluid (lymphorrhoea) or become warty.

Lymphatic malformations can have both microcystic and macrocystic components. Lymphatic malformations with few but large macrocystic swellings containing clear lymph are called cystic hygromas (hygroma = moist or watery tumour). Most occur in the neck, but they frequently extend into the upper mediastinum. The term tends to be reserved for those congenital lymphatic malformations that present at birth or are diagnosed by prenatal ultrasound. In the neck they presumably arise from an embryonic jugular lymph sac. Individuals with Turner syndrome are particularly prone to both hydrops and cystic hygroma. Exceptionally, a cystic hygroma occurs in the groin, presumably from an embryonic iliac lymph sac. Fetal cystic hygroma can give rise to severe abnormalities, leading to fetal death [2]. Deeper, larger and cavernous lymphatic malformations can be called macrocystic lymphatic malformations. Lymphangioma circumscriptum is a term best reserved for a lymphatic malformation that is localized to an area of skin, subcutaneous tissue and sometimes muscle [3] (Figure 105.20).

Epidemiology

Lymphatic malformations account for 4% of all vascular malformations, but comprise 25% of benign vascular growths in children [4]. Approximately 75% present at birth, while the remainder present by 2 years old. The anatomical location of a lymphatic malformation is most frequently the head and neck (48%). A study has demonstrated that lymphatic malformations involve the left side of the body more frequently (62%) [5].

Pathophysiology

Pathology

A lymphatic malformation is characterized by the size of the malformed channels: microcystic, macrocystic (often known as cystic hygroma if in the neck) or combined (microcystic/macrocystic) [6]. The contraction of thickened muscular linings may increase intramural pressure and cause cystic dilatation [7]. On light microscopy of biopsies, there are marked expanded channels in the dermis, which can extend into the subcutaneous and other deeper tissues. The channels are lined with flattened cells, which express CD31 and D2-40.

Lymphatic malformations can be isolated lesions disconnected from nearby normal lymphatic vessels (atruncular) or they can be connected (truncular) in which case lymphoedema will feature. In such a malformation, lymph fluid is trapped within the ectatic malformed lymph vessels, whereas in lymphoedema the lymph fluid is within the interstitial space of the tissues.

These malformations can be part of a syndrome such as Turner syndrome (due to monosomy X) or overgrowth syndromes, such as Proteus syndrome, Klippel–Trenaunay–Weber syndrome (capillary lymphaticovenous malformation) and CLOVES syndrome due to mutations in the AKT/PIK3 pathway [8].

Causative factors

Following regional lymph node excision or radiotherapy, cutaneous lymphangiectasia may occur [9]. In such circumstances, which commonly affect the external genitalia, the scrotum or vulva is studded with multiple clusters of tiny, translucent vesicles (see Figure 105.26). Previous surgery and/or radiation disrupt the deep collecting channels in the tissue, leading to lymph stasis, lymph backflow and, subsequently, distention of the upper dermal lymphatics. The mechanism for the skin 'lymph blisters' or vesicles is therefore the same as for congenital 'lymphangioma circumscriptum' but the cause is quite different.

Genetics

The lack of familial forms and the unifocality of the lesions suggest that the cause could be a somatic mutation restricted to cells of the lesion. Such a mutation would be too damaging (i.e. lethal) if it occurred germline [8].

Somatic mutations that activate PIK3CA have been identified in patients with CLOVES syndrome and in some with Klippel–Trenaunay–Weber syndrome [10]. All of these proteins are core elements of the AKT/PIK3/mTOR pathway, suggesting that sporadic lymphatic malformations as well as overgrowth syndromes may be caused by somatic changes in the components of this pathway. A recurrent somatic activating mutation has been discovered in the AKT1 pathway in patients with Proteus syndrome [11].

Clinical features

History

Lymphatic malformations manifest at birth or during infancy either as a localized subcutaneous swelling or as 'frogspawn' (groups of watery or haemorrhagic vesicles or lymph blisters) on the skin (see Figure 105.20). They grow proportionally with the affected child. Some show marked progression especially during puberty and may not be noticeable until this time. If the malformation is disconnected from normally draining lymphatic pathways/trunks there will be no lymphoedema (atruncular) (Figure 105.21). If connections exist then limb lymph drainage will be adversely affected and lymphoedema will be observed and may be the presenting feature (truncular) (Figure 105.22) [12].

Lymphatic malformations may occur at any site, although they often appear in the mouth, on the neck or jaw or around the axilla

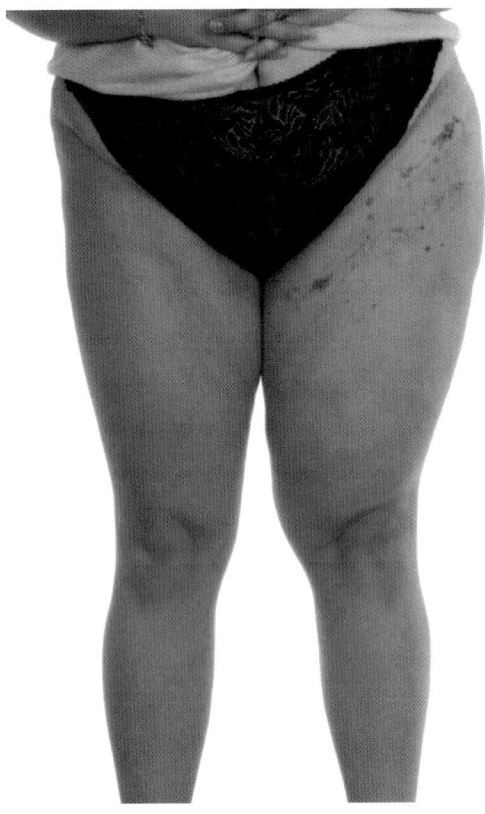

Figure 105.21 Atruncular lymphatic malformation without lymphoedema.

or groin. The most common symptom is recurrent oozing, usually of clear fluid (lymph), known as lymphorrhoea. Infection (e.g. cellulitis) can be a presenting feature because of the dysfunctional immune cell trafficking associated with a lymphatic malformation.

Extensive lymphatic malformations can have a blood vascular component. Consumption coagulopathy and in particular low platelets can complicate them. This may be because the correct separation of the lymphatic and blood vasculatures during embryonic development is dependent on CLEC-2-mediated platelet activation [13].

Presentation

Lymphangioma circumscriptum may present at any age but is usually noted at birth or appears during childhood. The commonest sites are the axillary folds, shoulders, flanks, proximal parts of the limbs and perineum. Clinically, the condition manifests with fluid-filled vesicles ('lymph blisters'), which bulge on the skin surface (see Figure 105.20). They may be translucent when the overlying epidermis is very thin, or they may vary in colour from red to blue-black when they contain blood, which is a frequent occurrence. The surface of the lymphangiomas may appear extremely warty and the lesions may be mistaken for viral warts. Weeping of lymph or blood-stained lymph (lymphorrhoea), or local cellulitis, may be other presentations.

Vascular birthmarks in the skin that look like blood capillary malformations may be mistaken for lymphatic capillary dermal malformations as seen in Proteus syndrome. Biopsy and staining with D2-40 may be necessary to make the distinction although the dermal vessels may be sufficiently undifferentiated to express both blood capillary and lymphatic phenotypes.

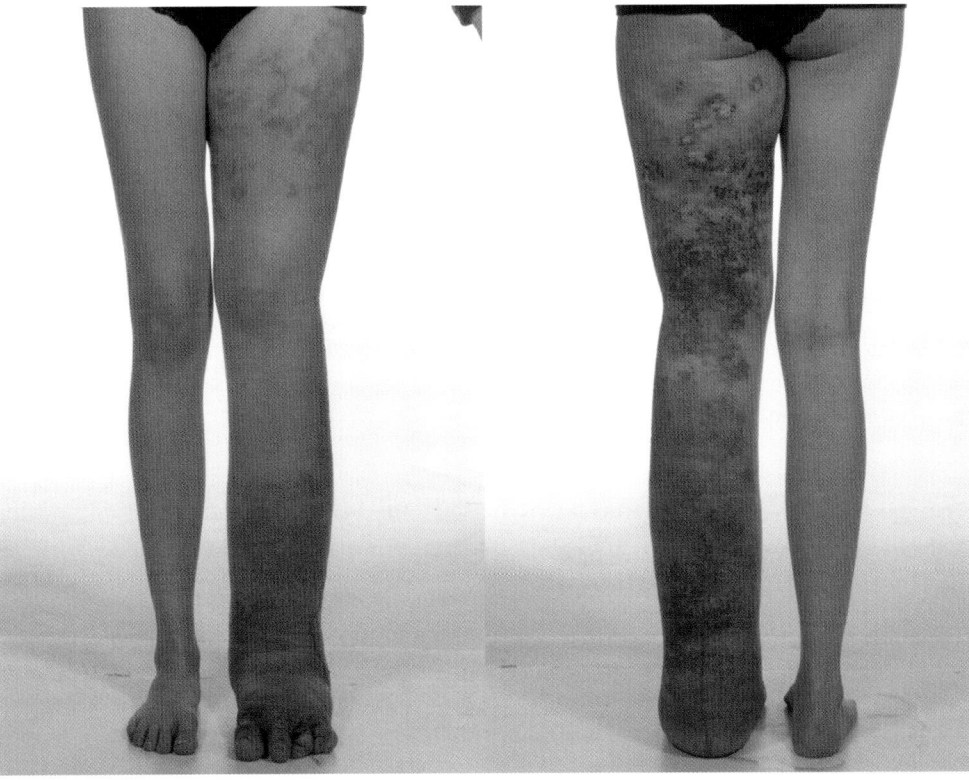

Figure 105.22 Truncular lymphatic malformation with blood-filled cutaneous lymphangiectasia and lymphoedema.

Differential diagnosis

A lymphatic malformation can be mistaken for other vascular malformations, hamartomas or tumours. The surface lymph vesicles can be confused with human papillomavirus warts.

Complications

Lymphatic malformations of the neck region often lead to obstruction of the upper airways. The volume of the malformation increases with infection or trauma. Intracystic haemorrhage is also common. Frequent discharge of lymph fluid (lymphorrhoea), ulceration and infection are the most frequent complications. Pain can be a problem but it is difficult to know if the cause is infection, lymph thrombosis or lymphatic vessel distension from intralymphatic pressure. Squamous cell carcinoma is described arising within lymphangioma circumscriptum [14].

Prognosis

Prognosis is usually excellent, providing there is no lymphangiomatosis. Infection can rarely be severe and life threatening.

Investigations

Biopsy will reveal angulated channels, which stain for CD31 and D2-40. Ultrasound should demonstrate fluid-filled channels, which on duplex will be slow flow. Distinction from a slow-flow venous malformation is difficult. MRI can demonstrate the extent of the lymphatic malformation – that is, extension into muscle or bone. Overgrowth of tissue elements (fat, muscle or bone) may also be seen, as may be any lymphoedema component. Lymphoscintigraphy should be normal in an atruncular lymphatic malformation but abnormal in a truncular lymphatic malformation.

Management

First line

The majority of lymphatic malformations are best managed conservatively. Sclerotherapy is the mainstay of treatment of macrocystic lymphatic malformations, but the response using traditional sclerosants is much less beneficial in microcystic lesions. Sclerotherapy of microcystic lymphatic malformations using bleomycin is effective and safe, giving a complete response in 38% and a partial response in 58% ($n = 31$) in one series [15].

It is generally not possible to excise a lymphatic malformation because of its extent and ill-defined infiltration of surrounding tissues. Indeed, attempted excision may result in further growth of the remaining malformation. Debulking procedures may be necessary for very large malformations causing complications such as the obstruction of vital organs and their functions.

Surface vesicles that weep or bleed should be destroyed by diathermy or laser. Since the vesicles have a tendency to reform, such procedures can be repeated as often as necessary.

Infection should be treated promptly with antibiotics, as in lymphoedema. If recurrent attacks of infection occur then prophylactic antibiotics should be considered [16].

For truncular lymphatic malformations with lymphoedema, compression garments are recommended. In atruncular lymphatic malformations compression may prove fruitless, as the lymph fluid is trapped within the closed vessel system of the malformation [17].

Second line

Sildenafil can reduce lymphatic malformation volume and symptoms in some children [18].

Third line

For those patients with a proven mutation in the AKT/PIK3/mTOR pathway, mTOR inhibitors such as sirolimus may prove helpful. Clinical trials are underway.

Lymphoedema as a result of amniotic band constriction

Definition and nomenclature

Lymphoedema of a limb may occur as a result of amniotic band constriction. This congenital disorder is caused by the *in utero* circumferential entrapment of fetal parts by fibrous amniotic bands. These bands cause constriction and fibrosis, with subsequent impairment of regional lymphatic drainage, resulting in lymphoedema. Early surgical release may prove beneficial, but affected individuals typically suffer lifelong problems with lymphoedema.

Synonyms and inclusions
- Amniotic band syndrome
- Amniotic band sequence
- Amniotic deformity, adhesion and mutilation complex
- Pseudoainhum

Introduction and general description

Lymphoedema of a digit or limb may occur as a result of constriction by amniotic bands. This congenital disorder, often termed amniotic band syndrome (ABS), is thought to occur as a result of *in utero* circumferential entrapment of fetal parts by fibrous amniotic bands formed during the rupture of the amnion during the first trimester of gestation. The rupture results in the formation of adhesions between the amnion and fetal skin. Small strands of amnion envelop the developing digits or limbs, leading to circumferential band-like constrictions.

Aside from circumferential limb constrictions, pseudosyndactyly, intrauterine amputation and umbilical cord constrictions have been reported. The reduction in amniotic fluid and/or limb tethering by amniotic bands may result in reduced fetal movements, scoliosis, limb deformity, lung hypoplasia and hydrops [1]. Examination of the placenta and membranes confirms the diagnosis when aberrant bands are detected.

Amniotic bands rarely present in the antenatal period on routine ultrasound imaging. Isolated amniotic bands are more likely to be detected at birth. If amniotic bands occur with limb deformities with or without necrosis, all attempts are made to salvage a necrotic limb, but amputation may be necessary.

Longer term sequelae of amniotic bands include the development of lymphoedema. The *in utero* circumferential entrapment of fetal parts by fibrous bands causes constriction and fibrosis, with subsequent impairment of regional lymphatic drainage. Impaired drainage of lymphatic fluid will result in lymphoedema, usually within the first few months of life. Patients with milder forms (e.g. amniotic bands that are not fully circumferential) may not develop lymphoedema until later life, if at all.

Epidemiology

Incidence and prevalence
The incidence is less than one in 1 000 000.

Age
Such lymphoedema is found in the neonatal period.

Sex
There is no gender discrepancy.

Ethnicity
There is no ethnic variation.

Associated diseases
There is a strong association between amniotic bands and club-foot (talipes) [2]. Other associated abnormalities include clubhand, haemangioma, cleft lip and/or cleft palate [3].

Pathophysiology

Predisposing factors
A study conducted by the National Center on Birth Defects and Developmental Disabilities (Atlanta, USA) observed that maternal cigarette smoking and aspirin use increased the risk of limb reduction deficiencies accompanied by amniotic bands [4].

Pathology
The pathogenesis of amniotic bands is not yet fully understood. Two theories have been suggested, and most favour the first.

Amniotic band theory. This theory is that bands occur due to a partial rupture of the amniotic sac. The rupture involves only the amnion whilst the chorion remains intact. Fibrous bands of the ruptured amnion float within the amniotic fluid and encircle and constrict parts of the fetus. Subsequently, the fetus grows but the bands do not enlarge, causing constriction of the affected limb or digit. Constriction compromises the vascular supply, causing congenital abnormalities. One or more digits or limbs may require surgical amputation soon after birth if they are necrotic. A number of infants have undergone complete 'natural' amputation of an affected digit or limb prior to birth [5].

Vascular disruption theory. This suggests there must be an 'intrinsic' defect of the vascular circulation as the constricting mechanism of the amniotic band theory cannot fully explain the high incidence of cleft defects occurring with ABS. An underlying mechanism for this theory has not been reported [6].

Genetics
It is a sporadic condition, with rare exceptions: a few affected families have been described [7].

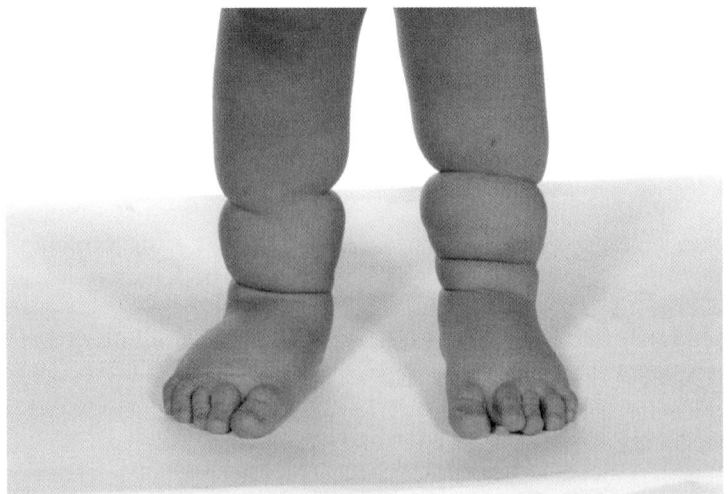

Figure 105.23 Amniotic bands and lymphoedema.

Clinical features

History
Amniotic bands rarely present in the antenatal period on ultrasound. Clinicians may be alerted to their presence if the fetus develops associated problems. Isolated amniotic bands are more likely to be detected at birth.

Presentation
Amniotic bands may affect digits or limbs. There is considerable variation in clinical presentation, depending upon the site of the amniotic band(s). Limb deformity and/or necrosis may be present [2]. Lymphoedema may develop in the antenatal period as a result of circumferential limb constriction by fibrous amniotic bands. The swelling will develop distal to the site of the band, enhancing the appearance of the narrow linear band around the affected limb (Figure 105.23). Milder cases (e.g. amniotic bands that are not fully circumferential) may not develop lymphoedema until later life, if at all.

Differential diagnosis
The differentiation of amniotic bands from Adams–Oliver syndrome should be straightforward. The latter condition is an autosomal dominant disorder characterized by transverse limb reduction defects, cutis marmorata and aplasia cutis congenita over the posterior parietal region with an underlying bone defect [8].

Complications and co-morbidities
Affected individuals have an increased risk of infection (e.g. cellulitis) within the swollen limb due to impaired lymphatic drainage and subsequent reduced immune surveillance within it [9].

Disease course and prognosis
Prolonged constriction of a limb by an amniotic band will result in impaired lymphatic drainage, leading to lymphoedema distal to the band site. If untreated, this will deteriorate over time and cause a deformed, heavy limb with reduced function.

Investigations

Prenatal ultrasound scans may detect swelling of digits or limbs distal to the amniotic band constriction, but the band itself cannot be visualized [5]. Three-dimensional ultrasound and MRI may be used for more detailed imaging when the index of suspicion for ABS is high [10].

Management

First line

Treatment typically occurs after birth, but with the advancement of prenatal radiodiagnosis fetal surgery *in utero* has been attempted [11].

Children with circumferential or near-circumferential amniotic bands may undergo surgical release with a Z-plasty procedure [2]. The aim of surgery is to release the fibrous tissue, thereby relieving constriction of both the vascular supply and draining lymphatic vessels of the limb. Surgery cannot completely reverse the constriction so the child is left with a degree of impaired lymphatic drainage within the affected limb.

Second line

The child will benefit from the input of an experienced lymphoedema therapist to improve limb drainage. Provision of made-to-measure compression hosiery can improve lymphatic drainage if worn on a daily basis.

Lymphangiomatosis, lymphangioleiomyomatosis and non-malignant lymphatic tumours

Definition and nomenclature

Lymphangiomatosis refers to excessive growth of aberrant lymphatic vessels. The process may vary from overgrowth of a lymphatic malformation to a lymphatic tumour. A fundamental requirement is cellular proliferation of lymphatic endothelial cells.

Synonyms and inclusions

- Lymphangioma
- Kaposiform lymphangiomatosis
- Acquired progressive lymphangioma
- Benign lymphangioendothelioma
- Atypical vascular lesions
- Gorham–Stout disease
- Generalized lymphatic anomaly

Introduction and general description

There is no clear distinction between lymphatic malformations, lymphangiomatosis and some non-malignant lymphatic tumours. Lymphangiomatosis implies there is progression through proliferation of aberrant lymph vessels whereas in a lymphatic malformation there should be no progression other than expansion though distension from intralymphatic pressure. Most lymphatic malformations are stable and run a completely benign course.

Conversely, some visceral thoracic and abdominal lymphatic malformations can relentlessly progress, infiltrating vital organs with fatal outcome and making distinction from lymphangiomatosis and frank neoplasia difficult.

Some non-malignant vascular tumours may exhibit a lymphangioma-like appearance with positive staining for lymphatic markers (e.g. tufted angioma, kaposiform haemangioendothelioma, multifocal lymphangioendotheliomatosis with thrombocytopenia, papillary intralymphatic angioendothelioma, retiform haemangioendothelioma and adult-type haemangioendotheliomas). However, it can be difficult to know if these are primarily lymphatic tumours. They can demonstrate locally aggressive behaviour and can be associated with life-threatening systemic complications such as Kasabach–Merritt syndrome.

The central nervous system seems to be spared, presumably because of its lack of lymphatic vessels. Lungs, retroperitoneal tissues and abdominal organs are most commonly affected by lymphatic malformations and lymphangiomatosis.

Chylous reflux may complicate visceral lymphangiomatosis. Disseminated intravascular coagulation can occur and may give rise to thrombosis and haemorrhage [1].

Gorham disease. Gorham disease (Gorham–Stout disease or disappearing/vanishing bone disease) is characterized by proliferation of lymphatic vessels resulting in progressive destruction and resorption of the osseous matrix. Overlying skin changes of lymphangioma may be present. The major distinguishing characteristic is the progressive osteolysis seen in this disease [2].

Generalized lymphatic anomaly. Generalized lymphatic anomaly (GLA) is a rare congenital disease resulting in malformation of the lymphatic vessels involving multiple sites of soft tissues, lungs, abdominal organs or bones but, unlike Gorham disease, is not usually progressive. Findings suggestive of GLA are more extensive involvement, particularly of the appendicular skeleton, the presence of discrete macrocystic lymphatic malformations and visceral organ lesions [3].

Benign lymphangioendothelioma. Acquired progressive lymphangioma (benign lymphangioendothelioma) is a benign tumour that differs from simple 'acquired lymphangioma' or simple cutaneous lymphangiectasia by its clinical behaviour and histopathology [4]. It presents as reddish or bruise-like plaques, which are usually located on the abdominal wall, thigh or calf. Typically, the condition affects young adolescents but may also arise in adults. It is usually localized, flat and grows slowly. Acquired progressive lymphangioma is considered to originate from lymphatic endothelium. The histopathological appearance can mimic a low-grade sarcoma or Kaposi sarcoma [5]. Anastomosing dilated channels, with a tendency to dissect the collagen bundles, are lined by swollen endothelial cells but without cellular atypia. It usually runs a long and benign course. D2-40 and Prox1 immunostains are positive [6].

Maffucci syndrome. Maffucci syndrome consists of diffuse haemolymphangiomatosis accompanied by severe, widespread

PART 9: VASCULAR

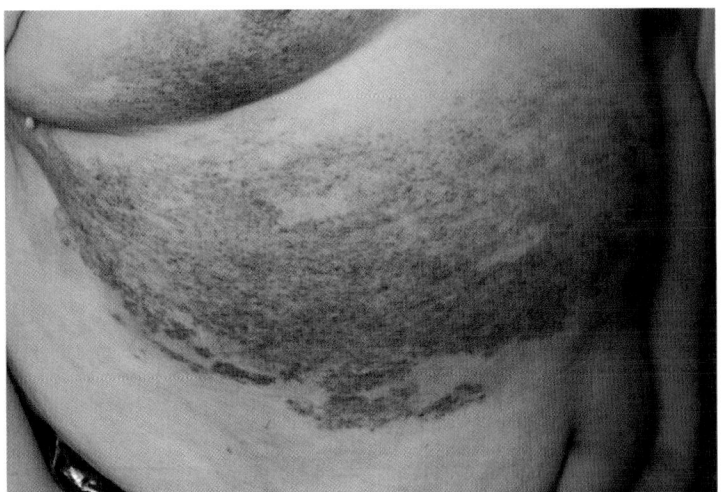

Figure 105.24 Kaposiform lymphangiomatosis showing a Kaposi sarcoma-like rash with localized lymphoedema of the breast and chest wall associated with haemoptysis.

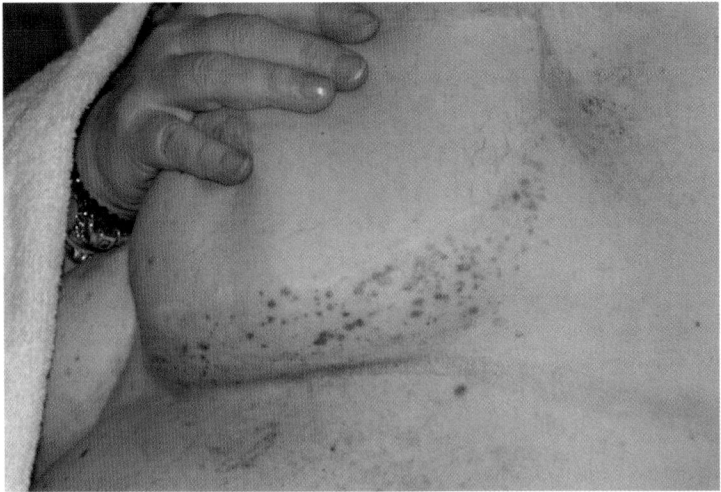

Figure 105.25 Benign lymphangiomatous papules (atypical vascular lesions) post radiotherapy.

deformities of bone and cartilage, notably enchondromas of the digits [7]. The lymphangiomas do not appear, on lymphography, to communicate with the main lymphatic pathways and often possess both blood vascular and lymphatic elements. Bony deformity may be gross; slowly uniting pathological fractures are common. The disease has high malignant potential including the development of lymphangiosarcoma [8].

Kaposiform lymphangiomatosis. Kaposiform lymphangiomatosis is a relatively newly described form of lymphangiomatosis, found mainly in children although adults can be affected. Skin involvement resembles diffuse Kaposi sarcoma and can lead to lymphoedema. It is distinguished from generalized lymphatic anomaly and diffuse pulmonary lymphangiomatosis in part by characteristic haematological abnormalities and haemorrhagic complications, including haemoptysis [9]. Characteristic clusters or sheets of spindled lymphatic endothelial cells (human herpesvirus 8 negative) accompany malformed lymphatic channels histologically (Figure 105.24).

Atypical vascular lesions. Cutaneous vascular proliferations that occur in the field of prior radiotherapy include angiosarcoma and small, cutaneous lesions with a pseudosarcomatous pattern that are reported as atypical vascular lesions or benign lymphangiomatous papules (Figure 105.25) [10]. Microscopically, the lesions are located mostly in the superficial/mid-dermis and are composed of expanded, irregularly jagged, vascular channels lined by a single layer of bland endothelial cells which are invariably D2-40 positive. Lesions can show additional cytological and/or architectural atypia but the prognosis is excellent [11,12].

Lymphangioleiomyomatosis. Lymphangioleiomyomatosis (LAM) is a slowly progressive, low grade, metastasizing neoplasm, associated with cellular invasion and cystic destruction of the pulmonary parenchyma. LAM is almost exclusively seen in women, especially during childbearing age. LAM cells harbour mutations in the tuberous sclerosis genes. Lymphatic manifestations of LAM include thoracic duct wall invasion, lymphangioleiomyoma formation, chylous fluid collections in the peritoneal, pleural and pericardial spaces, chyloptysis, chyle leak from the vagina or umbilicus, chylous pulmonary congestion, and lower extremity lymphoedema. Skin and kidney involvement is frequently found in tuberose sclerosis–LAM. Dermatological manifestations in tuberose sclerosis include angiofibromas, hypomelanotic macules, shagreen patch and ungal fibromas. Serum VEGFD estimation and high-resolution CT can be helpful in diagnosis. mTor inhibitors (e.g.sirolimus) are effective treatment [13].

Lymphangiectasia

Definition and nomenclature
Lymphangiectasia (or lymphangiectasis) means distension, expansion or dilatation of a lymph vessel.

> **Synonyms and inclusions**
> - Lymphangiectasis
> - Acquired lymphangioma
> - Secondary lymphangioma
> - Benign lymphangiomatous papules
> - Cutaneous lymphangiectasia
> - Intestinal lymphangiectasia
> - Chylous reflux

Introduction and general description
Lymphangiectasia can affect any lymph vessel in any tissue (e.g. pulmonary lymphangiectasia, intestinal lymphangiectasia). Intestinal lymphangiectasia can be associated with chylous reflux, which can result in skin manifestations. It can also cause a protein-losing enteropathy and peripheral oedema and so will be included for discussion.

Cutaneous lymphangiectasia represents distended, but otherwise normal, dermal lymphatics engorged with lymph due to a failure of downstream drainage. The surface 'lymph blisters' or

Table 105.11 Causes of cutaneous lymphangiectasia.

Congenital	Acquired (acquired lymphangioma)
Lymphatic malformation (lymphangioma circumscriptum)	Post surgery
	Radiation therapy
Chylous reflux (intestinal lymphangiectasia)	Scarring:
Noonan syndrome	Accidental trauma
Lymphoedema distichiasis	Inflammatory:
	Filariasis
	Crohn/ano-genital granulomatosis
	Hidradenitis suppurativa
	Tuberculosis adenitis/scrofuloderma
	Chylous reflux, e.g. post DXT

DXT, radiotherapy.

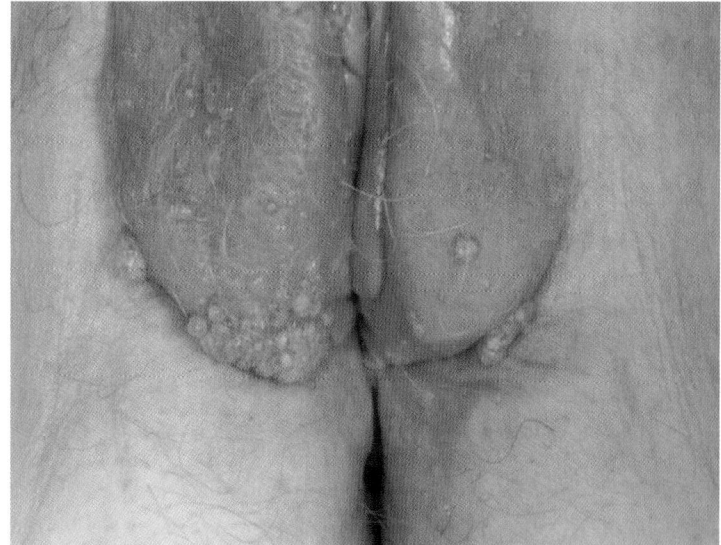

Figure 105.26 Vulval lymphangiectasia showing acquired lymphangiomas (lymphangiectasias) following cervical cancer treatment. The lymphangiomas were mistaken for genital warts.

vesicles seen in cutaneous lymphangiectasia are not necessarily structurally or histologically any different from those seen in a lymphatic malformation or lymphangioma. Acquired or secondary lymphangioma is an alternative term, but confusing as there is no tumour or proliferative component.

Lower limb lesions usually arise in association with lymphoedema following either ilioinguinal block dissection or pelvic surgery and radiotherapy for cancer, or when cancer relapses. Lymphangiectasias/acquired lymphangiomas have been described in association with scarring processes, including recurrent or chronic infections (such as the scrofuloderma variant of tuberculosis), scleroderma, keloid and repeated trauma (Table 105.11). They may also occur as a consequence of defective collagen or elastin, as documented in a report of penicillamine dermopathy [1].

Genital skin is particularly prone to lymphangiectasia. Lymphangiectasia/acquired lymphangioma of the vulva or scrotum is described following cancer treatment, tuberculous inguinal lymphadenitis, hidradenitis suppurativa and genital involvement with Crohn disease or ano-genital granulomatosis [2].

Pathophysiology
Cutaneous lymphangiectasia arises following damage to previously normal, deep lymphatic vessels [3]. The mechanism by which they form is identical to congenitally determined lymphatic malformations [4]. Obstruction to drainage leads to back pressure and dermal backflow, with subsequent congestion and expansion of the upper dermal lymphatics. Lymphangiectases are not true neoplasms or hamartomas, but represent simple expansion and engorgement (lymphangiectasia) of normal dermal initial lymphatic vessels.

Pathology
Histologically the dermis exhibits expanded, angular, lymphatic vessels, which are CD31 and D2-40 positive on staining. Endothelial cell atypia is usually absent.

Clinical features

History
For cutaneous lymphangiectasia, weeping and discharge of lymph or chyle is the commonest symptom. The discharge may be confusingly blood-stained as blood readily enters lymph.

Presentation
The clinical appearance of cutaneous lymphangiectases/acquired lymphangiomas may vary greatly, ranging from clear, fluid-filled blisters to smooth, flesh-coloured papules or nodules. Typically, lymphangiectasia can be seen as translucent, almost flat, papules or vesicles in the skin, which may ooze lymph spontaneously or after trauma. Blood content may make them look black and like angiokeratomas. Genital lesions may become hyperkeratotic on the surface and be mistaken for warts (Figure 105.26). Lesions may be solitary but scattered throughout a lymphoedematous limb, or they may be grouped, as seen in 'lymphangioma circumscriptum'.

Differential diagnosis
Differential diagnoses include human papillomavirus warts and molluscum contagiosum.

Clinical variants
Chylous reflux may manifest as lymphangiectasia. In such circumstances the lymph blisters/vesicles are white or cream coloured due to the milky chyle contained within. Fat is normally absorbed through the gut lacteals and drained through the cisterna chyli to the thoracic duct. Disturbances to this drainage route either within the gut wall (intestinal lymphangiectasia) or mesenteric lymphatics will result in a redistribution of chyle to other sites such as the pleural, pericardial or peritoneal cavities (chylous ascites). An incompetence of valves within the main abdominal lymphatic trunks results in gross reflux of chyle to the lower limbs, perineum and genitalia [5]. The reverse flow to skin or 'dermal backflow' will result in chylous cutaneous lymphangiectasia. Chylous 'blisters' may occur on the toes. Chylous reflux can occur through a fault of lymphatic development such as in Noonan syndrome or be acquired from damage to lymph drainage routes through accidental or surgical trauma, filariasis or malignancy.

Intestinal lymphangiectasia is an uncommon disorder and an important cause of protein-losing enteropathy [6]. The major symptoms are peripheral oedema, and abdominal pain and diarrhoea on dietary fat challenge. Hypoproteinaemia, low serum albumin and immunoglobulin levels are found on investigation. Biopsies of the small intestine showed variable degrees of dilatation of lymph vessels in the mucosa and submucosa. Capsule endoscopy is the investigation of choice [7]. Primary intestinal lymphangiectasia can be associated with the Turner, Noonan and Hennekam syndromes. In secondary intestinal lymphangiectasia, the dilatation of the lymphatics is caused by obstruction of the vessels or an elevated lymph pressure, secondary to elevated venous pressure. Obstruction can be seen in patients with inflammatory bowel disease, sarcoidosis or lymphoma or in patients who have had pelvic radiotherapy. Secondary intestinal lymphangiectasia is observed in children with congenital heart disease who have undergone a Fontan operation [8]. Dietary replacement of fat with medium-chain triglycerides (MCTs) is recommended as MCTs are absorbed and directed to the portal venous system rather than to the intestinal lacteals [9].

Complications
Recognition and appropriate treatment of cutaneous lymphangiectasia is important primarily because the lesions may act as portals of entry for infection. In addition, persistent leakage of lymphatic fluid may be mistaken for urinary incontinence in the case of vulval lymphangiectasia.

Prognosis
Even when treated, cutaneous lymphangiectasia often recurs.

Investigations
Biopsy with D2-40 stain is the definitive investigation.

Management
Treatment of cutaneous lymphangiectasia/acquired lymphangiomas is essentially the reduction of underlying lymphoedema and the control of infection. This may be relatively straightforward on the leg, but is not so easy on the genitalia, where compression is difficult to implement. Destruction of the 'lymph blisters' by laser or diathermy is helpful as palliative treatment [10].

Lymphocele, seroma and lymph fistula

Introduction and general description
Lymphoceles (lymphocysts) occur when afferent lymph vessels are disrupted and lymph fluid accumulates in a potential space without a distinct endothelial lining. When copious lymph fluid drains externally it is referred to as a lymph fistula. A seroma is a pocket of clear serous fluid that also collects in a tissue space usually after surgery. Seromas may be difficult to distinguish from lymphoceles.

Lymphocele
Lymphoceles usually occur following surgery or accidental injury. The wall of lymphoceles is 'false', in that no endothelial lining exists and instead a dense network of fibrin with lymphocytes is

present [1]. Dermatologists might come across groin or axillary lymphoceles as they are superficial and frequently associated with infection and wound complications. In cases of groin lymphoceles, treatment options include observation, serial aspiration and compression, instillation of sclerosing agents, radiation therapy, negative pressure wound therapy, and operative resection of the cavity with or without muscle flap coverage.

Lymphoceles following varicose vein surgery or vein harvesting have become much less common with changes in vascular surgical practice. With increasing levels of plastic surgery, particularly abdominoplasties and thigh lifts, lymphatic complications are likely to become more common.

Seroma
Following lymphadenectomy it is not unusual for a localized swelling containing clear fluid to develop. Often referred to as a seroma, the fluid is not serum but an exudate, equivalent to lymph, that fills the tissue space [2]. Aspirated fluid is indistinguishable from lymph. Repeat aspiration is often necessary until collateral lymph drainage forms. A seroma, particularly if infected, may herald the onset of lymphoedema if alternative drainage routes are not established.

Lymph fistula
A lymph fistula occurs where a lymphatic vessel connects externally to the skin surface and weeps copious amounts of lymph. It usually occurs following trauma or surgery where lymph accesses the skin surface through a wound. It may be a feature of a lymphatic malformation. A chylous fistula drains fat rich lymph externally.

Lymphatic filariasis

Definition and nomenclature
The single largest cause of lymphoedema worldwide is lymphatic filariasis (LF) [1]. It is a parasitic disease caused by microscopic worms that are transmitted by mosquitos. The adult worms live within the human lymphatic system and disrupt drainage, resulting in lymphoedema and hydroceles. Worldwide, 120 million people are infected and 40 million of these have lymphatic problems. Access to health care and lymphoedema treatment is often limited, resulting in a severe burden of disease in endemic countries.

Synonyms and inclusions
- Elephantiasis

Introduction and general description
Infection with one of three parasitic filarial worms causes LF: *Wuchereria bancrofti*, *Brugia malayi* and *B. timori*. *W. bancrofti* infection accounts for 90% of LF worldwide [2] (see also Chapter 33). The adult worms reside within the afferent lymphatic vessels (and/or the lymph nodes) while their larvae, the microfilariae, circulate within the peripheral blood and are able to infect mosquito vectors as they feed, facilitating transmission to other human hosts

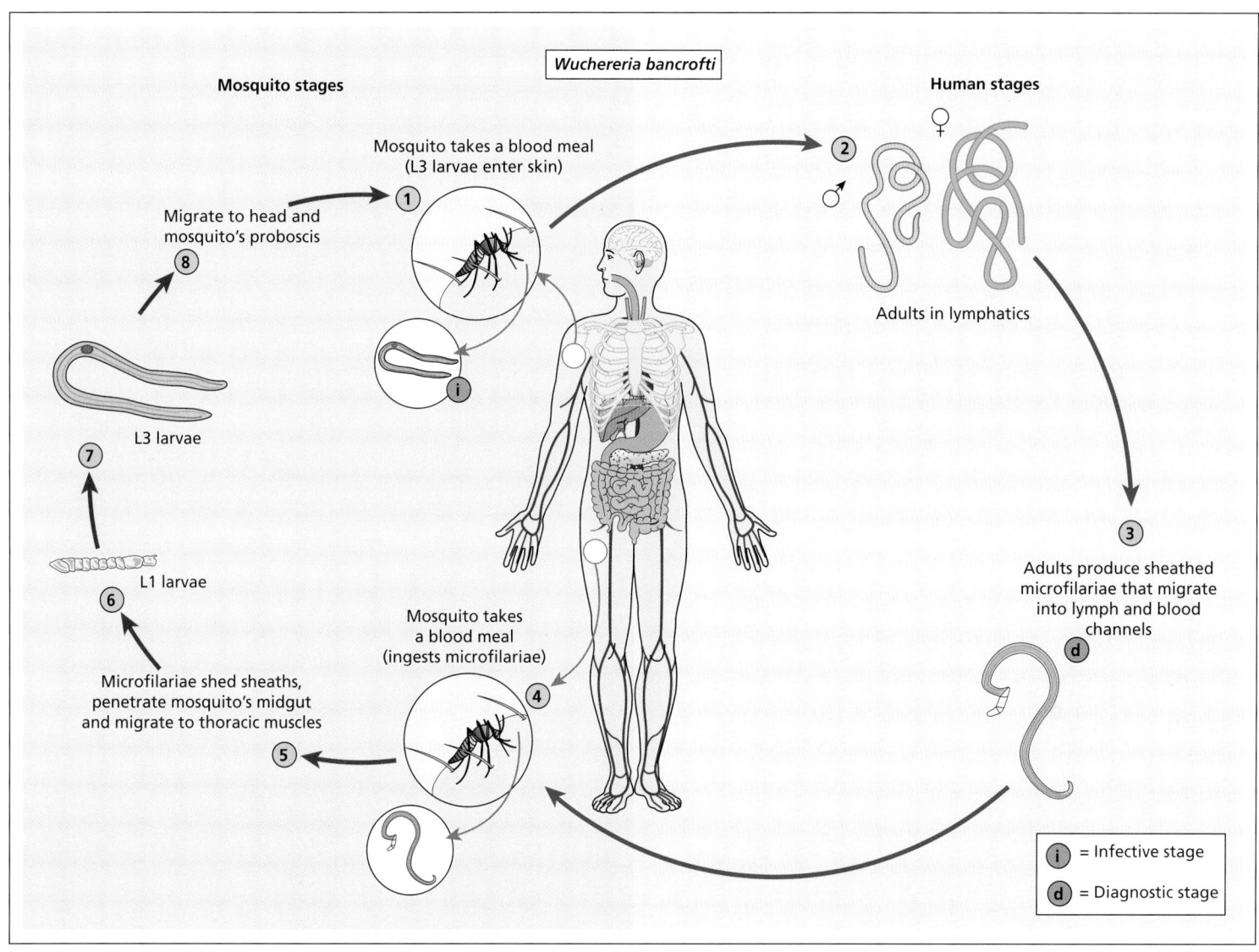

Figure 105.27 The life cycle of filarial nematodes in the human and mosquito hosts. *Wuchereria bancrofti*, *Brugia malayi* and *B. timori* have similar life cycles. The adult worms reside in the lymphatic system of humans and cause filarial disease. The female worm produces offspring (microfilariae), which leave the lymphatic system, enter the blood system of the human host and are taken up by mosquitoes during a blood-meal. The microfilariae undergo development within the mosquito, become infective larvae and subsequently migrate to the mosquito's mouthparts. These larvae may be transmitted to humans when the mosquito takes its next blood-meal. Once transmitted to humans, the larvae take approximately 6–12 months to mature into adult worms. (From Centers for Disease Control and Prevention 2015 [23].)

(Figure 105.27). The adult female worm may survive for more than a decade and is able to release thousands of fully formed microfilariae into the lymphatic circulation of the host every day. Infected patients may be asymptomatic, or demonstrate acute or chronic manifestations. The clinical signs are related to the adult worms residing in the lymph vessels and are not due to the microfilariae. The filarial parasites specifically target the lymphatics and impair lymph flow, which is critical for the maintenance of fluid balance and physiological interstitial fluid transport [3,4].

Epidemiology

Lymphatic filariasis is endemic in 73 countries and 1.2 billion people are at risk of transmission and subsequent infection. An estimated 120 million individuals are currently infected. Approxi-

mately 40 million have chronic lymphatic pathology: 13 million with lymphoedema/elephantiasis and an additional 27 million males have hydroceles as a result of LF [5,6]. Areas where LF is endemic include parts of Africa, South-East Asia, the western Pacific, the Americas and the Middle East. Transmission and morbidity are highest in South-East Asia and sub-Saharan Africa [6].

Age
While infections are contracted throughout life, most individuals remain asymptomatic until symptoms emerge during adolescence and adulthood.

Sex
Males are more likely to be affected than females.

Pathophysiology

Pathogenesis of lymphatic disease

The pathogenesis of filarial disease remains poorly understood and has been a subject of great debate. The clinical consequences of lymphatic filariasis are believed to occur as a result of interaction between the pathogenic parasite, the immune response of the host and secondary bacterial and fungal infections that complicate the situation.

Lymphoedema may occur as a result of live adult worms within lymphatic vessels in the lower limbs and pelvic region. The live worms secrete irritant toxins that cause dilatation of the lymph vessels surrounding the worm [3,7]. This causes a reduction in lymphatic flow. The subsequent oedema promotes fibrosis. Lymphoedema is further aggravated by secondary bacterial and fungal infections that arise as a result of impaired immune surveillance within the lymphoedematous region [8,9].

Lymphatic damage and subsequent lymphoedema may also occur as a direct result of dead adult worms within the lymphatic vessels (worm death due to old age or treatment). The presence of dead worms induces granuloma formation which leads to lymphatic outflow obstruction within the vessel and subsequent lymphoedema [10,11].

Predisposing factors

People residing for prolonged periods in tropical or subtropical areas where lymphatic filariasis is endemic are at the greatest risk for infection. Repeated mosquito bites over several months are required in order to acquire LF. Visiting tourists have a very low risk of acquiring LF [6].

Causative organisms

Numerous parasitic filarial nematodes may infect humans but only *W. bancrofti*, *B. malayi* and *B. timori* species are responsible for LF. *W. bancrofti* is responsible for 90% of cases of LF worldwide [12].

Clinical features

Presentation

Lymphatic filariasis has a range of clinical manifestations, varying from clinically asymptomatic microfilaria-positive individuals to those with disfiguring chronic filarial disease (elephantiasis). Overlap exists between the different symptom groups.

Clinical disease occurs in the minority of those infected with LF. The majority of infected individuals have few manifestations, despite the large number of circulating microfilariae in the peripheral blood. However, most will have some degree of subclinical disease, including microscopic haematuria and/or proteinuria, dilated and tortuous lymphatic vessels seen on lymphoscintigraphy, and scrotal lymphangiectasia in affected males [10,13].

The most common presentation of LF is with acute adenolymphangitis (ADL) in adolescence. ADL is characterized by sudden-onset fever, painful lymph nodes, lymphangitis and transient oedema. Involvement of the genitals appears to occur exclusively with *W. bancrofti* infection [14]. Previously asymptomatic individuals may experience symptoms lasting 4–7 days, with a tendency to develop recurrent episodes [15]. Individuals with established LF and lymphoedema develop more severe and prolonged episodes

of ADL. However, filarial ADL is distinct from acute dermatolymphangioadenitis, a process characterized by plaque-like lesions of cutaneous or subcutaneous inflammation, accompanied by ascending lymphangitis and regional lymphadenitis. These features occur in association with systemic signs of inflammation including fever and chills. Dermatolymphangioadenitis is thought to result from secondary bacterial or fungal skin infections as a consequence of immunodeficiency due to the underlying lymphatic damage [16].

Chronic lymphatic obstruction as a result of filarial worms leads to the development of hydroceles, lymphoedema/elephantiasis skin changes (severe hyperkeratosis, papillomatosis and skin fissuring) and rarely chyluria. Hydroceles are the result of accumulation of clear, straw-coloured lymphatic fluid within the tunica vaginalis as a result of obstruction of lymphatic vessels draining the retroperitoneal and subdiaphragmatic areas. The diameter of the hydroceles may be significant, reaching up to 30 cm.

Lymphoedema occurs as a result of the accumulation of lymphatic fluid within tissues following lymphatic vessel damage. The sites most commonly affected are the lower limbs and scrotum. Other sites can be affected such as the upper limbs and trunk. Initially the lymphoedema is intermittent and pitting in nature, but over time it becomes persistent and fibrotic. It is accompanied by gross skin changes referred to as elephantiasis – profoundly thickened and fibrotic skin with severe papillomatosis and secondary microbial infections [6].

Chyluria is a rare complication of LF and is the result of the presence of chyle (intestinal lymph) within the urinary tract. It occurs as a result of impaired drainage of retroperitoneal lymph below the cisterna chyli with subsequent reflux and flow of the lymph directly into the renal lymphatic vessels, which may rupture and permit flow of chyle into the urinary tract. The urine appears milky white in colour. Serious nutritional deficiencies may occur as a result of the loss of fat and protein within the urine.

Tropical pulmonary eosinophilia syndrome may rarely affect an individual with LF due to *W. bancrofti* or *B. malayi*. They develop respiratory wheeze and a paroxysmal nocturnal cough, similar to asthma. Chest radiographs demonstrate nodular or diffuse pulmonary lesions. Other features of this syndrome include elevated peripheral blood eosinophilia and high levels of serum immunoglobulin E and specific antifilarial antibodies. Unlike other forms of lymphatic filariasis, patients with tropical pulmonary eosinophilia are hyperresponsive to filarial antigens, especially those derived from the microfilarial stage of the parasite. If untreated, the patient may develop restrictive lung disease with interstitial fibrosis. Treatment with diethylcarbamazine is effective [17,18].

Differential diagnosis

The differential diagnosis includes podoconiosis and chronic, poorly managed lymphoedema due to any other cause.

Disease course and prognosis

The clinical course of untreated LF is of progressive skin changes, worsening lymphoedema and increased incidence of secondary infection. A poor quality of life is associated with untreated disease. Elephantiasis and subsequent deformity leads to social stigma, financial hardship from loss of income and increased medical expenses. The socio-economic burdens of isolation and poverty are immense.

Investigations

In endemic areas, adults with lower limb lymphoedema and/or male genital involvement are likely to have LF. A definitive diagnosis can be made by detection of the adult parasitic worm within the lymphatic vessels or accessible lymph nodes. Doppler ultrasound may detect motile adult worms within the scrotum. However, these diagnostic tests are not always suitable for use in developing countries.

Filarial parasites exhibit 'nocturnal periodicity' that restricts their appearance in the blood to the hours of 10 pm to 2 am. The diagnosis of LF has traditionally depended on the nocturnal laboratory examination for microfilaria in peripheral blood smears (stained with Giemsa or haematoxylin and eosin) between these hours to maximize the chances of detection.

In recent years, polymerase chain reaction (PCR) and rapid antigenic assays have been developed. Antigen testing is a simple, sensitive and specific tool for the detection of the *Wuchereria bancrofti* antigen and is being used widely by lymphatic filariasis elimination programmes. The test detects infection within minutes and can be carried out at any time of day, unlike previous tests [19].

Lymphoedema, elephantiasis skin changes and hydroceles may persist in individuals with burned-out infections. Therefore, it is impossible to exclude a diagnosis of filarial-induced disease in the absence of circulating antigens or parasites. This situation may occur in patients who have received multiple courses of treatment or who no longer live in the endemic area.

Management

Drug treatment

The World Health Organization (WHO) launched the Global Programme to Eliminate Lymphatic Filariasis (GPELF) which aims to stop the spread of LF. Pharmaceutical companies have pledged to donate the required drugs. The strategy proposed by WHO to achieve LF elimination comprises two components: (i) the interruption of transmission of filarial infection in all endemic countries by the drastic reduction of microfilariae prevalence levels; and (ii) the prevention and alleviation of disability and suffering in individuals already affected by LF.

The interruption of transmission of infection is only possible if the entire at-risk population is treated by mass drug administration for a prolonged period of time to ensure a reduction in the blood levels of microfilariae to a level where transmission can no longer be sustained. The following drug regimens have been recommended by the WHO to be administered once a year for at least 5 years, with a coverage of at least 65% of the total at-risk population: (i) 6 mg/kg diethylcarbamazine citrate (DEC) in combination with 400 mg albendazole; or (ii) 150 µg/kg ivermectin in combination with 400 mg albendazole (in areas where onchocerciasis is prevalent, in order to avoid adverse drug reactions with DEC) [6].

Lymphoedema, elephantiasis skin changes and acute inflammatory episodes are typically managed with simple measures of improved hygiene, skin care, exercise activities and elevation of affected limbs. The GPELF has pledged to provide access to a minimum package of care for every individual with chronic manifestations of LF in all areas where the disease is present, in a bid to alleviate suffering and improve their quality of life.

Surgical treatment

Males with hydroceles benefit from hydrocelectomy procedures to achieve volume reduction [20].

Lifestyle management

Lifestyle measures can reduce the bacterial and fungal load that contribute to worsening lymphoedema. These include regular washing with soap and water, use of footwear and access to antibiotics and lymphoedema treatment [21]. Prevention of infection can be achieved by avoidance of mosquito bites. Lifestyle measures include sleeping under a mosquito net, using mosquito repellent on exposed skin and wearing long sleeves and trousers.

Resources

Further information

Global Programme to Eliminate Lymphatic Filariasis: http://www.filariasis.org (last accessed August 2015).

Podoconiosis

Definition and nomenclature

Podoconiosis refers to the development of bilateral lower limb lymphoedema, thought to occur as a result of prolonged exposure to irritant mineral-rich soils present at high altitudes (Figure 105.28).

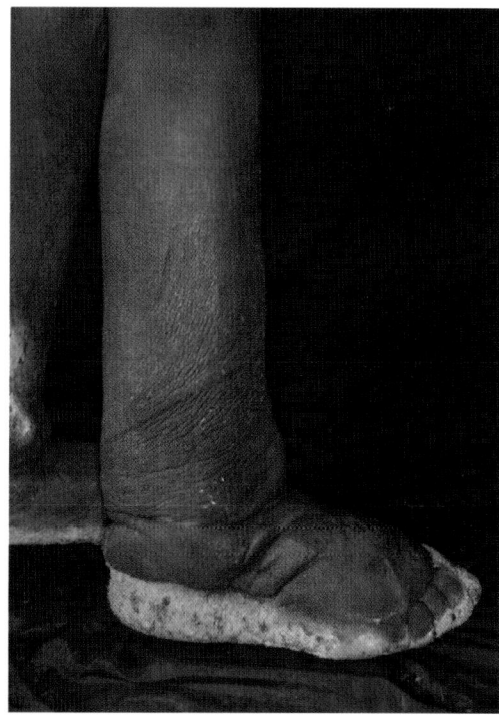

Figure 105.28 Lower limb lymphoedema due to podoconiosis. Note the presence of toe maceration and typical 'mossy' appearance of the foot. (Reproduced with permission from D. Markos.)

PART 9: VASCULAR

These minerals appear to trigger an inflammatory response resulting in impaired lymphatic drainage and subsequent lymphoedema. Development of the condition is closely associated with barefoot living and working. A genetic susceptibility has also been postulated.

Synonyms and inclusions
- Mossy foot
- Verrucosis lymphatica
- Endemic non-filarial elephantiasis

Introduction and general description

Podoconiosis is a leading cause of lower limb lymphoedema of young people in Africa, Central America and north India, yet it remains a neglected condition. It has been prevalent for centuries but was previously encompassed by the umbrella term 'elephantiasis' until the pathogenesis of filariasis was realized in the 19th century. All cases of elephantiasis were then assumed to be filarial in origin until the discrepancy between the widespread distribution of 'elephantiasis' cases and more focal distribution of filaria in North Africa, Central America and Europe prompted a review of this theory.

The term podoconiosis was proposed in the 1980s to describe non-filarial cases of elephantiasis skin changes, and has since gained widespread acceptance. It is derived from the Greek for foot, *podos*, and dust, *konos* [1].

Epidemiology

Incidence and prevalence

It is estimated that 4 million people are affected by podoconiosis, mainly in tropical Africa, Central and South America and South-East Asia. Ethiopia is the country with the highest reported prevalence, with an estimated 1 million people living with the disease [2,3]. Prevalence estimates are limited but have been made in Ethiopia, Cameroon and Uganda. Estimated prevalence is 4% in Ethiopia, 8% in Cameroon and 4.5% in Uganda [4,5,6]. The variation in reported prevalence figures may be attributable to survey size and sampling methods.

Age

Onset is typically in the first or second decade of life, but may occur later.

Sex

Gender ratio results may be unreliable, especially in remote areas affected by podoconiosis. A recent Ethiopian survey reported that females are more likely to be affected than males [4].

Pathophysiology

Predisposing factors

Podoconiosis occurs in the highland areas of tropical Africa, Central and South America and South-East Asia. It has been suggested that podoconiosis was previously prevalent in North Africa (Algeria, Tunisia, Morocco and the Canary Islands) and Europe [7].

However, it has not affected these areas since the use of footwear became customary.

Certain occupations (i.e. those with prolonged contact with soil) are at higher risk of developing podoconiosis, especially farmers.

Podoconiosis is associated with lower levels of income, poor education, being unmarried and the delayed introduction of foot wear [8].

Pathology

The pathogenesis of podoconiosis is not yet fully understood. Current evidence suggests a pivotal role of mineral particles within the soil, in a genetically susceptible individual [9]. One possible theory is that irritant particles cause an inflammatory immune response with subsequent impaired lymphatic drainage of the lower limbs, perhaps as a result of intraluminal lymphatic vessel obstruction by inflammatory cells. Supportive evidence for this theory includes the detection of elemental particles present in irritant clays (e.g. aluminium, silicon, magnesium or iron) within lower limb lymph node macrophages of affected individuals who lived barefoot [10].

Genetics

An association has been reported between podoconiosis and variants in HLA class II loci. Podoconiosis may be a T-cell-mediated inflammatory disease and could be a model for gene–environment interactions, and further research in this area is underway [11].

Environmental factors

The association between podoconiosis and exposure to irritant soil was established when maps of disease occurrence were superimposed onto geological survey maps, confirming a connection with clays derived from volcanic activity [12,13]. A recent study indicated that soil particles including smectite, mica and quartz were associated with podoconiosis prevalence and underpin the process [9].

The climatic factors thought to be necessary for producing irritant clays are high altitude (greater than 1200 m above sea level) and high seasonal rainfall (over 1000 mm annually) [4]. These conditions contribute to the steady disintegration of volcanic ash and the reconstitution of the mineral components into irritant silicate clays.

Clinical features

History

The affected individual typically resides in a high-risk area and will have lived and worked barefoot. Podoconiosis presents with a prodromal phase of pruritus of the forefoot skin and a burning sensation of the feet and lower limbs prior to the onset of elephantiasis skin changes [14–16].

Presentation

Early changes of podoconiosis are similar to that of any other cause of lower limb lymphoedema. The affected individual develops bilateral lymphoedema of the foot and ankle regions. Lymphorrhoea (leakage of lymph), hyperkeratosis, papillomatosis, fibrosis and gross disfigurement of the below-knee regions develop if the condition is untreated. The toes develop a characteristic macerated and 'mossy' appearance, hence the pseudonym 'mossy foot'. Recurrent lower limb cellulitis frequently complicates the clinical picture.

Clinical features of podoconiosis that differentiate it from filarial elephantiasis include the feet and ankles being the initial site of symptoms in podoconiosis, rather than the groin or proximal lower limbs. Podoconiosis affects both lower limbs, whereas filariasis typically presents with unilateral lower limb swelling that extends above the knee. Groin involvement in podoconiosis is extremely rare, unlike in filariasis.

Podoconiosis may be distinguished from leprotic lower limb lymphoedema by the preservation of sensation within the lower limbs, and the absence of trophic ulceration, thickened palpable nerves or involvement of other body sites.

Differential diagnosis
Differential diagnoses include filariasis, endemic Kaposi sarcoma and leprotic lymphoedema.

Complications and co-morbidities
Significant social stigma is attached to podoconiosis. Affected individuals are excluded from school, churches and mosques, and barred from marriage with unaffected individuals because of local beliefs that the condition is contagious [17]. An affected individual is less likely to work and this impacts the patient's financial status.

Disease course and prognosis
Without access to footwear and conventional lymphoedema treatment (skin care and compression), the condition is progressive and complicated by recurrent cellulitis.

Investigations
Typically, affected individuals do not have access to lymphoscintigraphy or other investigative techniques. Filariasis, leprosy and endemic Kaposi sarcoma should be excluded if suspected by the clinician.

Management

Primary prevention
Primary prevention of podoconiosis consists of avoiding prolonged contact between the skin of the feet and irritant soils by using good footwear.

Prevention of disease progression
Prevention of disease progression and recurrent infections may be possible if affected individuals are instructed in the use of foot hygiene (e.g. daily washing of feet with soap and water and the use of antiseptics), and the use of shoes and socks for life. Simple compression bandaging is effective in reducing limb volumes, assuming that elephantiasis changes have not yet developed. A change in occupation or relocation may be beneficial, but may not be feasible for the affected individual.

Advanced disease
Advanced cases of podoconiosis are managed with daily skin care, leg elevation and multilayer compression bandaging, assuming that the affected individual has access to health care providers. Debulking surgery was previously employed, but has since been abandoned

because of disappointing results. The local belief that there is no effective medical treatment acts as a barrier to accessing local health care. Disappointingly, few organizations offer treatment for podoconiosis because of the lack of evidence-based treatment options compounded by patchy acknowledgement that the disease even exists.

Resources

Further information
Footwork (The International Podoconiosis Initiative): www.podo.org (last accessed August 2015).

Pretibial myxoedema

Definition and nomenclature
Pretibial myxoedema (PTM) is a form of cutaneous mucinosis that typically occurs in association with Graves disease, hence the synonym thyroid dermopathy. Deposition of hyaluronic acid within the dermis and subcutis causes the development of asymptomatic 'swelling', nodules and plaques, typically of the pretibal region of both lower limbs. The precise cause of this phenomenon remains uncertain.

Synonyms and inclusions
- Localized myxoedema
- Thyroid dermopathy
- Infiltrative dermopathy

Introduction and general description
Pretibial myxoedema is a form of cutaneous mucinosis that occurs in association with Graves disease (see also Chapter 149). Patients typically present with asymptomatic, pretibial nodules and plaques that may have a yellow-brown hue. Lower limb lymphoedema may develop in severe cases. PTM results from the dermal accumulation of hyaluronic acid and other glycosaminoglycans, secreted by fibroblasts.

Epidemiology

Incidence and prevalence
Pretibial myxoedema affects up to 5% of patients with Graves disease; it affects up to 13% of patients with severe eye disease [1,2].

Sex
It more commonly affects females, with a female:male ratio of 4 : 1 [3].

Associated diseases
Pretibial myxoedema occurs almost exclusively in Graves disease. The classic triad of Graves disease is: (i) pretibial myxoedema;, (ii) ophthalmopathy (e.g. exophthalmos and orbital myopathy); and (iii) thyroid acropachy (swelling of the digits and clubbing). PTM has rarely been reported in association with Hashimoto thyroiditis, primary hypothyroidism and in euthyroid patients [4,5].

Pathophysiology

The hyperthyroidism of Graves disease occurs as a result of stimulation of the thyroid-stimulating hormone receptor (TSHR) on thyroid follicular cells by autoantibodies directed against the receptor. However, the pathogenesis of Graves ophthalmopathy and PTM is less clear. PTM occurs as a result of glycosaminoglycan (GAG) deposition within the dermis. The underlying mechanism of GAG deposition is not clearly understood, but is likely to occur as a result of several processes, including autoimmune, cellular and mechanical factors. For example, TSHR antibodies may bind to and stimulate dermal fibroblasts to increase the production of GAGs [6]. Dermal GAG accumulation (i.e. mucin deposition) results in the separation of collagen fibres, expansion of connective tissues and oedema formation [7]. The obstruction of dermal lymphatic vessels by mucin results in lymphoedema [8]. The involvement of mechanical factors in the development of PTM may explain the lower limb predilection: dependency and trauma have been proposed [9].

Pathology

Characteristic histopathological features of PTM consist of mucin deposition (i.e. GAGs including hyaluronic acid) within the reticular dermis. Alcian blue and periodic acid–Schiff stains demonstrate mucinous material between collagen fibres. With extensive deposition of mucin, the collagen fibres become frayed and fragmented. Stellate fibroblasts may be observed, but the actual number of fibroblasts is not increased. There may be hyperkeratosis of the overlying epidermis.

Mucin deposition restricted to an expanded papillary dermis, with nodular angioplasia, and haemosiderin deposition are more suggestive of stasis dermatitis rather than PTM [10].

Clinical features

History

Pretibial myxoedema occurs almost exclusively with Graves disease. The patient is likely to have a history of thyrotoxicosis (e.g. weight loss, palpitations and hyperhidrosis) and possible ophthalmopathy and acropachy. PTM may develop prior to, during or after the thyrotoxic state as it is not related to thyroid function. It usually occurs 12–24 months after the onset of Graves disease, but may occur up to 12 years after its development [11].

Presentation

Pretibial myxoedema is typically confined to the lower limbs. The shins are the classic site, but the toes may be the only affected site. PTM may occur within surgical scars or sites of trauma [12]. PTM may rarely affect other body sites, such as the head and neck region, torso and upper limbs, presumably triggered by trauma [13–15].

Patients typically present with firm, non-pitting indurated nodules and plaques on the pretibial regions and feet. The lesions may be flesh-coloured or have a yellowish brown hue. A peau d'orange appearance may develop as a result of expansion of the interfollicular dermis. Cutaneous lesions may be asymptomatic, occasionally pruritic, or cause discomfort. Mild cases are usually asymptomatic and only of cosmetic concern. In severe cases of PTM, lesions may coalesce to give the entire extremity an enlarged, verruciform appearance (Figure 105.29). Functional impairment (inability to wear shoes as a result of toe disfiguration) and/or the development of secondary lymphoedema may occur.

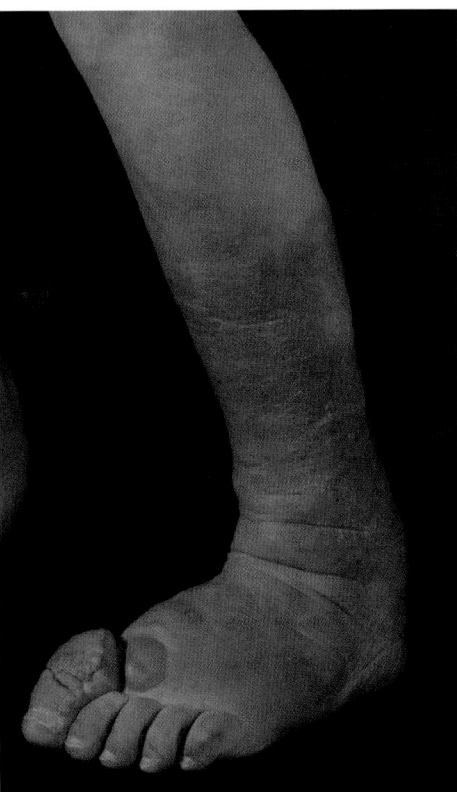
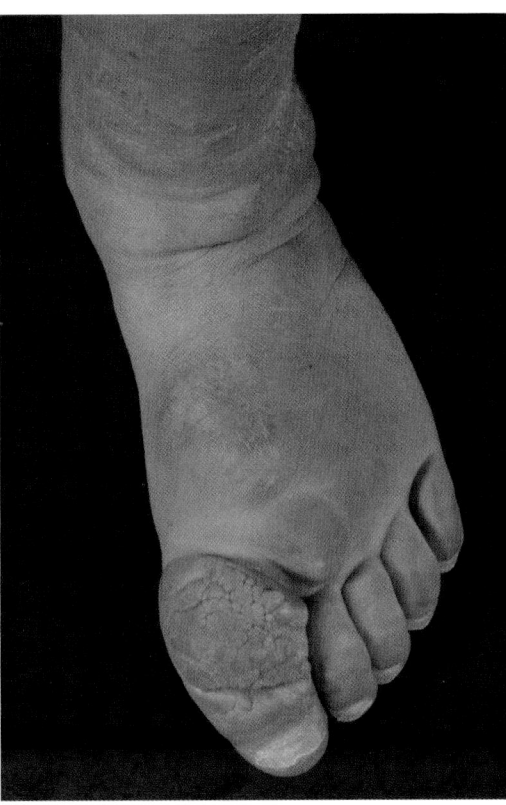

Figure 105.29 Pretibial myxoedema.

Differential diagnosis

Differential diagnoses include lymphoedema, stasis dermatitis, obesity-associated lymphoedematous mucinosis and lichen amyloidosis.

Complications and co-morbidities

Pretibial myxoedema rarely causes significant morbidity. Local discomfort and difficulty in finding footwear may be experienced. Severe forms of the disease may cause lower limb lymphoedema and subsequent complications of increased incidence of infection.

Disease course and prognosis

Few studies exist on the evaluation of PTM outcomes. However, the prognosis for mild cases appears to be favourable. In mild cases, 50% of patients achieve complete remission after several years [16]. The largest series reports after 25 years of follow-up that 70% of mild untreated and 58% of treated severe cases achieved complete or partial remission. Very severe forms appear to be persistent [3].

Investigations

The diagnosis of PTM is possible from the patient's history and characteristic clinical findings. It is rarely necessary to perform a skin biopsy, especially if there is a history of hyperthyroidism or Graves ophthalmopathy. If a biopsy is undertaken, the histopathological findings are characteristic.

The investigation of lymphatic function with lymphoscintigraphy is not routinely performed. However, lymphoscintigraphy and fluorescence microlymphography may confirm structural and functional alterations to the lymphatic drainage. Mucin deposition within the dermis may compress or occlude the initial lymphatic vessels, resulting in lymphoedema [8].

Management

Mild and asymptomatic cases of PTM may not require treatment. If symptomatic, treatment options include the use of potent topical corticosteroids under occlusion at night for several months. Prompt diagnosis and initiation of treatment appear to correlate with better outcomes [17]. The use of compression hosiery or multilayer bandages may be used to manage the associated lymphatic impairment/secondary lymphoedema seen in more extensive and chronic cases.

A small number of case reports suggest surgical excision may be of benefit in select cases [18]. However, surgery should be considered with caution as PTM may develop within areas of trauma.

Several therapeutic agents have been trialed in the treatment of PTM. Evidence of their efficacy is limited. These include intralesional steroids, systemic immunomodulators (e.g. prednisolone, plasmapheresis, intravenous immunoglobulin and rituximab) and octreotide [19,20,21–23,24].

Trauma-induced lymphoedema

Introduction and general description

Lymphoedema and other lymphatic complications, such as lymphocele or lymph fistula, can develop after therapeutic interventions or accidental damage to lymph drainage pathways. The failure of lymphatics to regenerate and re-anastomose satisfactorily through scarred or irradiated tissue is probably responsible for lymphoedema development.

Epidemiology

The incidence of lymphoedema following varicose vein surgery was estimated to be 0.5% [1]. In another series the incidence of lymphatic complications from 5407 surgical procedures for varicose veins was 118 cases (2.2%); a lymphocele on the limb occurred in 1.3%, an inguinal fistula or lymphocele in 0.7% and lymphoedema in 0.2% [2].

Pathophysiology

Trauma to lymphatics, either from elective surgery or by accident, usually needs to be extensive to induce lymphoedema. Indeed, the experimental production of lymphoedema is extremely difficult to achieve owing to the excellent regenerative powers of lymphatics.

It remains a puzzle as to why most women who have a full axillary lymph node clearance following breast cancer surgery do not develop lymphoedema, yet 6% of women who have a single sentinel lymph node biopsy do develop arm swelling [3]. Furthermore, it is not known why breast cancer-related lymphoedema (BCRL) can manifest immediately postsurgery or be delayed for many years. A genetic predisposition may be relevant: mice with a heterozygous mutation in the adrenomedullin gene developed lymphoedema when subjected to surgery but wild-type mice did not [4].

Radiotherapy to lymph nodes can be as much a risk factor towards lymphoedema as surgery [5].

Genetic factors are likely to be important. Obesity increases the incidence of postsurgical lymphoedema, as has been demonstrated following breast cancer treatment [3]. Wound infections increase the incidence of postsurgical and accidental lymphoedema.

Clinical features

Lymphoedema can develop after varicose vein treatment. Varicose vein surgery may be undertaken for reasons of 'venous oedema'. However, the chronic oedema may already reflect a compromised lymph drainage, in which case surgery may further undermine lymph drainage and make swelling worse. With the greater use of endovenous therapy using laser, radiofrequency or foam vein ablation (rather than traditional stripping and surgical ligation) the incidence of lymphoedema is likely to be reduced.

Lymphatics can be damaged and produce lymphoedema during saphenous vein harvesting for coronary artery bypass grafts. However, the increasing use of coronary stents has considerably reduced this risk. Similarly, great saphenous vein harvesting for critical limb ischaemia can result in lymphatic complications such as lymphocele [6].

Lymphoedema can develop at the donor site after reconstructive surgery such as a transverse upper gracilis free flap for breast reconstruction [7].

Resection of excess skin and soft tissue of the thighs after massive weight loss can also cause lymphoedema. The lymphatic collectors of the thigh sit superficial to the veins. Therefore, in a vertical medial thigh lift, choosing a dissection plane superficial to the great saphenous vein is unlikely to preserve the collectors of the ventromedial bundle [8]. Lymphoedema and other lymphatic complications (e.g. cellulitis, lymphocele) are a significant risk. An interruption of lymphatic pathways presumably results in a failure of adequate lymphangiogenesis and repair, resulting in lymphoedema.

Accidental trauma, such as a degloving injury to a limb, will produce lymphoedema distal to the injury if widespread circumferential scarring has occurred.

Self-inflicted injury, such as the repeated application of a tourniquet, will eventually cause permanent lymphatic damage and chronic swelling (Secrétan syndrome) [9]. The abrupt termination of the swelling often coincides with a skin contour change due to subcutaneous atrophy caused by a tight constricting band. Skin pigmentation may also coexist at the site. Factitious lymphoedema can be caused by tourniquets, blows to the arm or repeated skin irritation, usually in patients with known psychiatric conditions. Factitious lymphoedema results in symptoms and signs suggestive of chronic regional pain syndrome [10].

Intravenous drug abuse may cause lymphoedema due to a combination of infection and injected agents causing lymphangitis plus associated venous damage. Puffy hand syndrome is a long-term complication of intravenous drug abuse [11]. It can affect from 7% to 16% of intravenous drug users [12].

Investigations
Lymphoscintigraphy is the investigation of choice to determine lymphatic insufficiency.

Management
Decongestive lymphatic therapy is first line treatment [13]. Infection needs to be treated and prevented [14]. The use of additional therapies such as pneumatic compression therapy and Velcro wraps can be considered.

Lymphoedema due to immobility

Introduction and general description
Lymph drainage, unlike blood flow, requires intermittent changes in local tissue pressure generated by movement and exercise in order to produce initial lymphatic transport. Main limb collector lymphatic vessels pump the lymph supplied from the initial lymphatics. Lymphatic collector vessels rely on innervation and effective smooth muscle contraction for pumping. Consequently, immobility, by reducing initial lymphatic absorption and transport, reduces lymph flow to the collectors. Less pumping promotes swelling, particularly if gravitational forces (dependency syndrome) encourage ongoing fluid filtration into the tissues but without sufficient compensatory lymph drainage.

Lymphoedema is well recognized with certain neurological conditions that restrict movement. Cerebrovascular accident (CVA), spina bifida and multiple sclerosis (MS) are those that are best described.

Post-radiation brachial plexopathy following breast cancer treatment leads to severe lymphoedema with paralysis being the major contributing factor.

Epidemiology
In a review of 240 electronic medical records from an adult spina bifida clinic, 22 patients (9.2%) had lymphoedema [1]. Lower limb oedema is common in MS patients, especially in those with reduced mobility. In one study, 93 patients (45%) of a total of 205 patients with definite MS showed oedema with abnormal findings on lymphoscintigraphy [2].

Pathophysiology
Exercise and movement are essential for stimulating lymph drainage. Any reduction in movement lowers lymph drainage accordingly. Immobilizing any body part in the face of sustained microvascular filtration will result in (lymph)oedema despite patent, and otherwise normal, lymphatic vessels. The lower limb is most commonly affected because of the contribution from dependency/gravitational forces. Paralysis and neurological deficit cause lymphoedema for similar reasons.

Hand oedema after a stroke is not considered to be lymphoedema owing to normal lymphoscintigraphy. However, one would expect lymph drainage pathways to be patent but not functional owing to the lack of movement. Combine that fact with increased microvascular filtration (and high lymph load) due to dependency of the paralysed or spastic limb, and lymphoscintigraphy might be expected to be falsely normal. After all, if the lymphatics are working oedema should be avoided irrespective of cause [3].

It is likely, but unproven, that with neurological deficit a failure of lymphatic pumping due to denervation contributes most to oedema formation, but a lack of isotonic exercise (from muscle weakness or spasticity) will reduce initial lymph flow so making less lymph available for collector pumping.

With time, pathological changes within the failing, but hitherto normal, lymphatics occur. Lymphangiothrombosis or luminal fibrosis leads to an irreversible lymphoedema even if full mobility is restored.

Clinical features
Oedema associated with immobility will usually develop insidiously unless the immobility is sudden in onset (e.g. CVA). Hand or foot swelling is the usual story because of the effect of gravity being maximal in the distal part of the limb. Peripheral oedema can cause pain and tissue tenderness. Extreme oedema may result in the weeping of fluid from the skin (lymphorrhoea).

A common scenario is 'armchair legs', a term coined by Sneddon and Church [4] where patients sit in a chair day and night with their legs dependent (otherwise known as elephantiasis nostras verrucosis because of the severe lymphoedema skin changes that ensue). No premorbid abnormalities of the lymphatics exist, but the immobility results in minimal lymph drainage and a functional lymphoedema due to a lack of movement or exercise to stimulate normal lymph drainage. Dependency of the limb compounds the problem by increasing capillary filtration. The syndrome is not confined to the legs, but can affect any chronically dependent and immobile part, as demonstrated in the pendulous abdomen [5].

Physical examination reveals swelling in which pitting is marked, due to a mixed aetiology of reduced lymph drainage and increased microvascular fluid filtration. Neuropathic limbs take on a particular appearance with a bluish hue and background livedo.

Differential diagnosis
Deep-vein thrombosis should be considered if onset is acute.

Complications
As with all forms of lymphoedema, there is an increased risk of infection and lymphorrhoea.

Investigations
In cases of possible DVT, D-dimers and compression ultrasonography should be considered. In breast cancer patients PET/CT of the axilla should be undertaken to exclude axillary recurrence.

Management
Compression bandaging is the mainstay of treatment but needs to be undertaken with care if sensation is reduced. Oedema should reduce easily but refill occurs rapidly. Therefore, well-fitting compression garments are applied as soon as swelling is reduced. Pressure areas need to be carefully monitored. Skin care is of the utmost importance. The tendency of paralysed limbs to reswell means that bandaging may need to be continued or replaced with Velcro wraps (e.g. Farrow wraps). When resting, elevation of the lower extremities is desirable, either while sitting in a wheelchair or lying in the bed, with the back of the knees and calves supported by pillows. The oedematous limb or limbs should be positioned higher than the hips if possible.

Systems that encourage passive movements can prove helpful [6]. Pneumatic compression pumps may be helpful as they simulate the calf muscle pump.

Lymphangitis

Definition
Lymphangitis is an inflammation of lymphatic vessels. It is most often caused by infection from bacteria, virus or fungus or infiltration by cancer cells.

Introduction and general description
Lymphangitis represents inflammation of the lymphatic collectors and is clinically seen as tender red streaks up the limb corresponding to the inflamed vessels. In the lower limb, oedema is so often an accompanying feature that red streaks, such as are seen with lymphangitis of the arm, are rarely seen. A more diffuse erythema is seen extending up the medial side of the leg and thigh. Distinction from an ascending cellulitis becomes difficult. In some circumstances the inflammatory response may be profound and painful inflammation of the regional lymph glands (lymphadenitis) may arise.

Pathophysiology
Lymphangitis may occur without any demonstrable inflammation or may be recurrent, for example following relapsing herpes simplex infection [1]. Permanent obliteration of lymphatic collectors may follow severe or recurrent lymphangitis. In such cases, if reserve lymphatic capacity is limited, permanent swelling (lymphoedema) can result.

Lymphangitis occurs in filariasis [2]. Sporotrichoid spread (also known as nodular lymphangitis) describes a characteristic pattern of superficial cutaneous lesions that progress along the path of lymphatic drainage. Fungi, and classically sporotrichosis, exhibit this tendency but also nocardiosis, chromoblastomycosis and aspergillosis. Sporotrichoid spread through lymphangitis has been described with leishmaniasis and atypical mycobacterium (e.g. *Mycobacterium marinum*). Cutaneous squamous cell carcinoma can rarely demonstrate sporotrichoid spread as can a hypersensitivity lymphangitis to an arthropod bite [3].

Snake toxin molecules are generally large and cannot directly enter the circulation, but are readily taken up by the lymphatics [4]. Snake bite venom will often cause lymphangitis [5]. Pressure bandaging with immobilization is the recommended first aid treatment with the intention of preventing lymph drainage [6].

Mondor disease is considered to be a form of superficial thrombophlebitis but it commonly complicates lymph node removal, so a form of lymphangitis or lymphatic thrombosis may be more likely [7[. Lymphatic cording or axillary web syndrome following axillary lymph node intervention may be similar. It is also described following a jellyfish sting [8,9]. Lymph can clot and lymphangiothrombosis may occur more often than realized [10].

Sclerosing lymphangitis of the penis is a condition related to vigorous sexual activity, manifesting as an asymptomatic, firm, cord-like swelling around the coronal sulcus of the penis [11].

Carcinoma erysipeloides (lymphangitis carcinomatosa, carcinoma telangiectatica, carcinoma en cuirasse) occurs when cancer cells infiltrate the dermal lymphatics. It is a form of metastatic spread and occurs most commonly with breast cancer but can occur with melanoma and thyroid, lung, gastric, pancreatic, ovarian, prostate and colo-rectal cancer [12]. Carcinoma erysipeloides manifests clinically with a fixed erythematous patch or plaque resembling cellulitis, but without fever [13]. The inflamed area may show a distinct raised periphery and oedema secondary to lymphatic obstruction. A network or lattice pattern of telangiectatic vessels represents the infiltrated dermal lymphatics (Figure 105.14). Inflammatory breast cancer is a rare and very aggressive disease in which cancer cells block lymph vessels in the skin of the breast. This type of breast cancer is called 'inflammatory' because the breast often looks swollen and red, or 'inflamed'.

COMPLICATIONS OF LYMPHOEDEMA

The major complications of lymphoedema are swelling and infection.

Swelling

Limb swelling leads to discomfort, limb heaviness, reduced mobility and, on occasion, impaired function. The size and weight of affected limbs can result in secondary musculoskeletal complications such as back pain and joint problems, particularly in the case

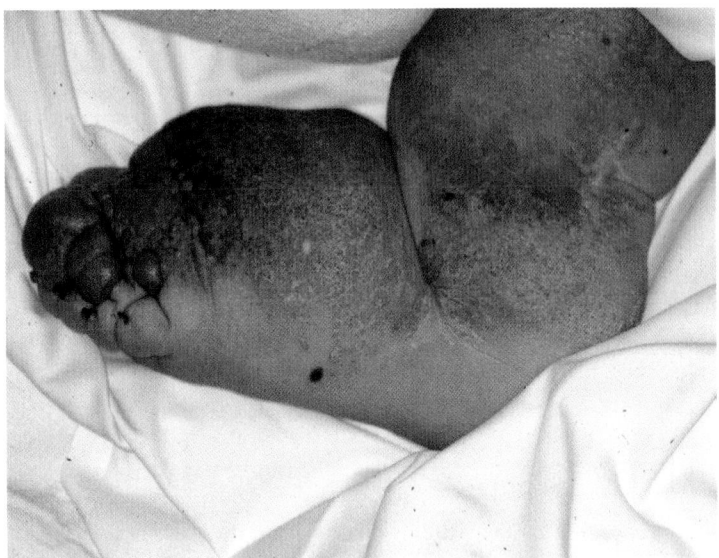

Figure 105.30 Elephantiasis verrucosis nostras showing marked hyperkeratosis and papillomatosis.

of asymmetrical lower limb swelling. Balance can be an issue with asymmetrical limb swelling affecting either the upper or lower limbs [1].

Skin changes

Elephantiasis refers to skin resembling elephant skin. The epidermis becomes hyperkeratotic and warty and the dermis markedly thickened and fibrotic. Distended dermal lymphatics can bulge on the skin surface and, with tissue organization, produce a cobblestone appearance. Elephantiasis skin changes occur in established chronic lymphoedema, particularly in the lower limb or in circumstances of profound lymphatic obstruction (Figure 105.30) [2]. Thickening of the skin impairs joint mobility. Leakage of lymph through the skin (lymphorrhoea) may occur from engorged dermal lymphatics (lymphangiectasia) (Figure 105.31).

Infection

Episodes of secondary infection, particularly cellulitis, are a characteristic feature of lymphoedema. Patients with lymphoedema irrespective of cause are liable to these attacks. It is likely that disturbances in immune cell trafficking compromise tissue immunosurveillance, but the exact mechanism is not known [3].

Constitutional symptoms such as fever, rigors, headache or vomiting can be profound and sudden in onset. Within 24 h, redness appears within the lymphoedematous area but without an advancing border. Pain and heat also feature. Recurrent episodes may be frequent and further impair lymph drainage, so exacerbating the lymphoedema. Thus, a vicious cycle is established. Haemolytic streptococci of group A, B and particularly G have been demonstrated. Toxicity from infection can be extreme and even fatal [4]. It is not unusual for patients to comment that attacks of cellulitis can be induced by strenuous exercise or long car journeys. This suggests a mechanism not dissimilar to herpes simplex where the microorganism is always present but becomes reactivated.

Fungal infections, particularly tinea pedis, are difficult to avoid because of web-space skin maceration from swollen toes (Figure 105.32).

Opportunistic infections are also described in lymphoedema, lending further support to the localized immunodeficiency theory [5].

Psychosocial issues

In one study over 80% of patients (188/217) had taken time off work due to their lymphoedema, with an estimated mean time off work of 10.5 days per year for medical appointments. Overall, 9% stated that the lymphoedema affected their employment status, with 4/209 (2%) respondents having to change jobs and 17/209 (8%) having to give up work because of it [6]. Relationships can also suffer.

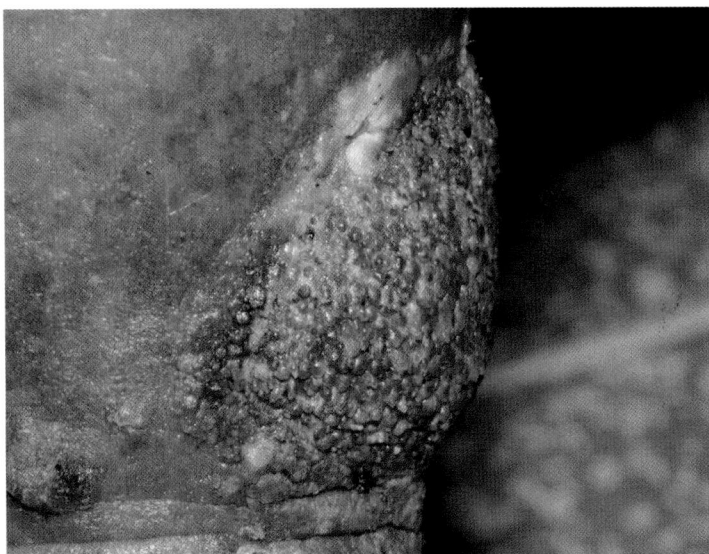

Figure 105.31 Acquired cutaneous lymphangiectasia leading to ulceration of the lower leg.

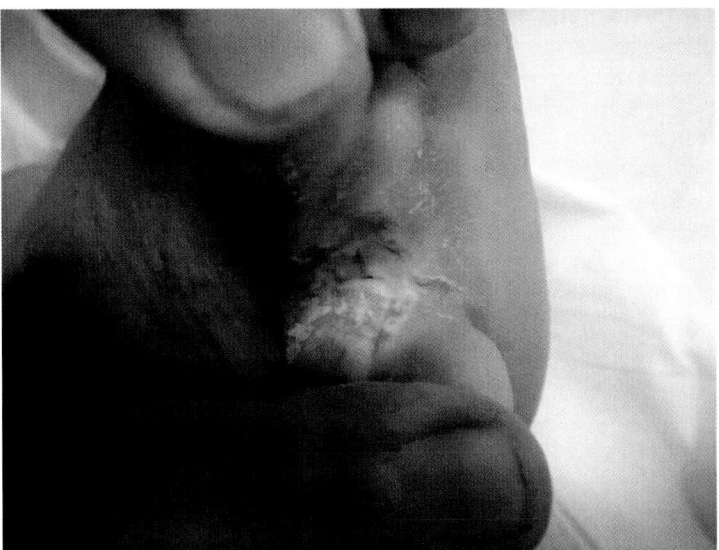

Figure 105.32 Macerated web-space skin leads to bacterial entry points and fungal infection.

The difficulty in finding clothes or shoes to fit creates social problems. Poor footwear will further compound the swelling by discouraging a normal gait or enough exercise.

Patients with arm swelling in relation to breast cancer experienced functional impairment, psychosocial maladjustment and increased psychological morbidity [7].

Malignancy

Chronic lymphoedema has a permissive effect with certain types of malignancies, particularly angiosarcomas, in what is known as Stewart–Treves syndrome [8]. The presumed mechanism is through immunodeficiency of the compromised drainage basin, in a similar way to malignancy complicating systemic immuno-defiency, such as in renal transplant recipients [9]. The Stewart–Treves syndrome describes lymphangiosarcoma developing from well-established postmastectomy oedema. However, lymphangio-sarcoma is now described as occurring with lymphoedema of any cause (Figure 105.33).

Other tumours that have been recorded to develop with lymphoedema include basal cell carcinoma [10], squamous cell carcinoma [11], lymphoma [12–14], melanoma [15,16], malignant fibrous histiocytoma [17], Merkel cell tumour [18] and Kaposi sarcoma [19]. Certain uncommon benign tumours are reported associated with lymphoedema [20].

Miscellaneous conditions

A range of cutaneous conditions has been reported as occurring preferentially at sites of lymphoedematous involvement. These include xanthomatous deposits [21,22], bullous pemphigoid [23],

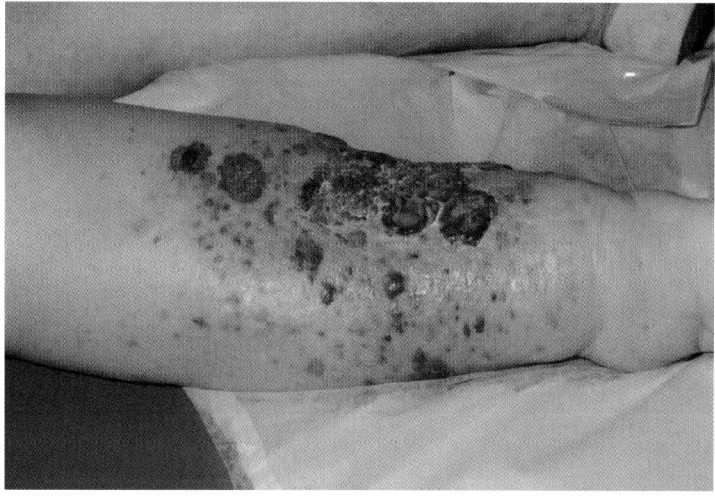

Figure 105.33 Lymphangiosarcoma arising in primary lymphoedema.

toxic epidermal necrolysis [24], atypical neutrophilic dermatosis [25] and severe necrotizing fasciitis [26].

IMAGING OF THE LYMPHATIC SYSTEM

Most patients with lymphoedema are diagnosed from the history and clinical findings. The use and value of imaging techniques is highly dependent on availability and expertise. Table 105.12 compares the different techniques available for imaging the lymphatic system. The techniques used to investigate the lymphatic system are discussed below, but some patients will benefit from additional imaging in order to understand the cause of their swelling. For example, MRI

Table 105.12 Lymphatic imaging techniques and their properties.

Imaging technique	Contrast agent	Depth of imaging	Invasiveness	Availability
Lymphography/ lymphangiography	Intralymphatic injection of a radio-opaque oil (e.g. Lipiodol)	Anatomical imaging of lymphatic collectors and lymph nodes	Very invasive; requires the identification of a lymphatic collecting vessel by exploratory surgery	Rarely performed
Lymphoscintigraphy	Simple intradermal/subcutaneous injection of a radiolabelled tracer protein (e.g. technetium-99-labelled colloid)	Lymphatic collectors and lymph nodes Poor resolution compared with lymphography technique Limited functional data acquired Not anatomical	Minimal	Readily available in hospitals
Fluorescence microlymphangiography	Simple intradermal injection of fluorescent contrast agent (FITC-dextran)	Superficial dermal lymphatic vessels	Minimal	Research tool
Near infrared lymphangiography	Simple intradermal/subcutaneous injection of indocyanine green	Superficial dermal lymphatic vessels and superficial lymph nodes Contractility can be visualized but not quantified	Minimal	Increasing availability in departments offering lymphatic microsurgery
Magnetic resonance lymphangiography	Simple intradermal/subcutaneous injection of a gadolinium-based contrast agent	Lymphatic collectors and lymph nodes Subcutaneous fat and oedema also visualized	Minimal	Research tool

FITC, fluorescein isothiocanate.

PART 9: VASCULAR

and CT scanning may be indicated to assess the presence of intra-abdominal or pelvic pathology or masses obstructing lymphatic drainage. MRI may also be requested to assess tissue hypertrophy or signs of overgrowth (e.g. in Klippel–Trenaunay syndrome). Venous duplex imaging may be requested to investigate the possibility that a patient's lymphoedema is associated with venous incompetence.

Lymphography and lymphoscintigraphy

X-ray contrast lymphography (lymphangiography) remains the gold standard mode of demonstrating lymphatic collectors and lymph nodes. However, it is rarely used as the technique requires the invasive procedure of direct cannulation of the lymphatics [1].

Lymphoscintigraphy (isotope lymphography) is currently the investigation of choice for determining if chronic oedema may be due to lymphatic failure. It involves a simple intradermal/subcutaneous injection of a radiolabelled tracer protein, exclusively cleared by lymphatics. Measurement of tracer uptake and transit through the lymphatics permits qualitative and quantitative analyses of lymph drainage and may discriminate lymphoedema from lipoedema [2,3]. Lymphoscintigraphy has the potential to distinguish between different types of primary lymphoedema and their mechanisms of lymphatic failure, for example initial lymphatic dysfunction in Milroy disease, versus lymph collector reflux in lymphoedema distichiasis syndrome (Figure 105.34). However lymphoscintigraphy suffers from poor spatial resolution and cannot provide functional measurements of flow [4].

Fluorescence microlymphangiography

Fluorescence microlymphangiography (FML) is a research tool that uses a fluorescent contrast agent (fluorescein isothiocanate (FITC) dextran) to provide information on superficial dermal lymphatic

vessels. It has been used to improve understanding of lymphatic disease, including primary lymphoedema. For example, FML in conjunction with immunohistochemistry demonstrated that lymphatic dysfunction, not aplasia, underlies Milroy disease [5].

Near infrared lymphangiography

Near infrared lymphangiography (NIR) using indocyanine green (ICG) is a recently introduced and potentially useful technique used to demonstrate superficial lymphatic vessels [6]. NIR imaging techniques use tracers that fluoresce under the excitation of near infrared waves (750–1000 nm) and external fluorescent detectors. ICG is a dye with properties of NIR absorption and fluorescence emission. ICG-solution is injected intradermally or subcutaneously and enables real-time detection of the lymphatic vessels.

NIR has been used to assess lymphatic vessel structure and function. ICG is administered intradermally in order to map the lymphatic architecture [7]. Fluorescent images have been collated to describe patterns of abnormal lymphatic structure in lymphoedema (e.g. dilated vessels with proximal obliteration) and diffuse constellation-like patches of dye accumulation (termed the 'Milky Way' features). This method has also been used to quantify lymphatic function in the lower limb [7]. NIR is now widely used to assess lymphatic vessel patency prior to lymphatico-venous or lymphatico-lymphatic anastomosis surgery [8].

Magnetic resonance lymphangiography

The use of contrast-enhanced magnetic resonance lymphangiography (MRL) has been reported in the investigation of patients with lymphoedema. MRL has been used to demonstrate the presence of enlarged and tortuous lymphatic vessels in patients with unspecified lymphoedema [9]. It is still a research tool but could prove

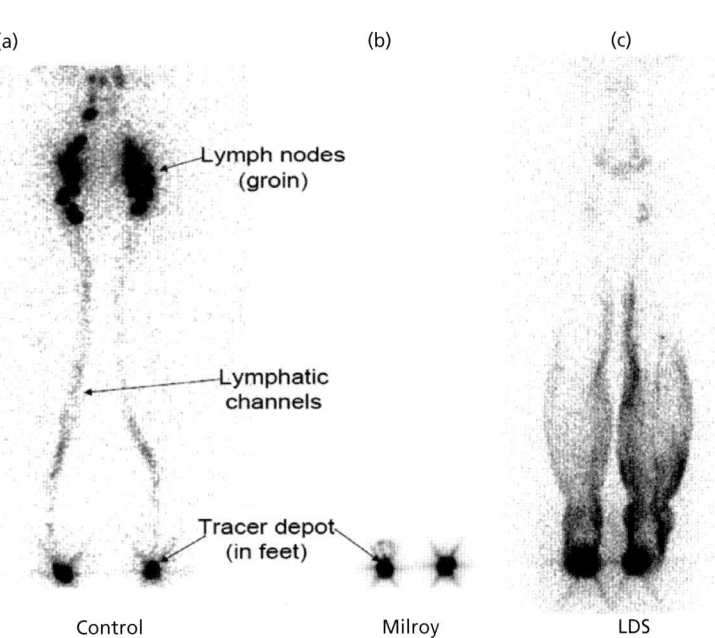

Figure 105.34 Lymphoscintigraphs showing the uptake of technetium-99 in the inguinal lymph nodes (ILNs) at 2 h after injection in the normal lymphatic system and in patients with differing types of lower limb primary lymphoedema. (a) Healthy control. (b) Milroy disease, demonstrating functional aplasia of the lymphatics (i.e. no uptake into the ILNs). (c) Lymphoedema distichiasis syndrome with reasonable uptake to the ILNs but evidence of marked reflux due to lymphatic valve incompetence. (d) Meige disease with poor uptake and evidence of rerouting via the deep lymphatic channels resulting in uptake within the popliteal lymph nodes. (Adapted from Connell *et al.* 2013 [11].)

PART 9: VASCULAR

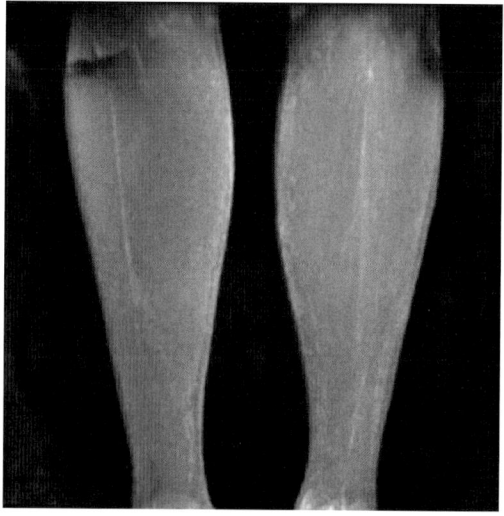
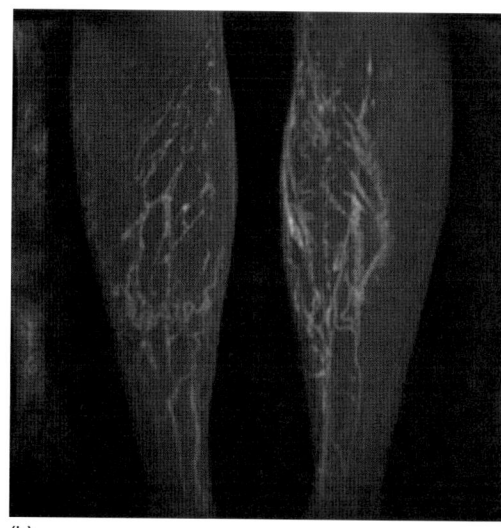

Figure 105.35 (a) Baseline magnetic resonance lymphangiography (MRL) images taken from a patient prior to contrast injection. His phenotype is of lymphoedema distichiasis syndrome (*FOXC2* positive). Two main vessels can be seen within the lower limbs. These could be venous or lymphatic in origin. (b) Post-contrast MRL images demonstrating multiple, dilated, tortuous lymphatic vessels seen in the below-knee regions.

(a)   (b)

useful as it has the potential to provide high-quality images of anatomical abnormalities (Figure 105.35), and may be able to provide quantification of lymphatic function in the future.

Histopathological investigation of the lymphatic system

Skin biopsies may be useful when investigating a suspected lymphatic malformation. The distinction between lymphatic and blood vessels in skin biopsy sections has been made more straightforward by specific lymphatic markers. D2-40 (podoplanin) is considered the most robust as it stains initial lymphatics, pre-collectors and collecting vessels but not blood vessels. LYVE-1 stains initial lymphatics but also macrophages and is down-regulated by inflammation. Prox-1 and VEGFR-3 are also lymphatic-specific and stain larger vessels. A panel of markers is recommended, particularly in vascular malformations where differentiation between venous and lymphatic phenotypes may not be clear-cut [10]. CD31 and CD34 stain both lymphatic and blood vascular endothelium.

LYMPHOEDEMA MANAGEMENT

Lymphatic failure results in the accumulation of protein as well as water within the swollen tissues. Treatment is difficult because of the presence of the 'solid' component in the swelling. The management of lymphoedema varies greatly around the world. In developed countries, the emphasis is more on physical forms of therapy involving massage, exercise and compression designed to stimulate lymph drainage. In poorer, hotter countries where hosiery and appropriate bandages are too costly and uncomfortable, surgery may be the mainstay of treatment. Two particular problems need to be overcome with lymphoedema: the swelling and the predisposition to infections, particularly recurrent cellulitis.

There is limited research to inform evidence-based guidelines on the treatment of lymphoedema. Nevertheless, robust guidelines developed through consensus by experts do exist [1].

Unfortunately there is no proven curative treatment for lymphoedema. Management is aimed at improving swelling through physical treatments designed to stimulate flow through existing or collateral drainage routes. Several surgical techniques have been implemented in recent years in a bid to improve lymphatic drainage, or achieve limb volume reduction via liposuction. However, in the absence of robust data to support most surgical techniques, so-called 'conservative' physical therapies are relied on for the majority of patients.

Medical assessment

Medical assessment aims to identify and exclude other causes of peripheral oedema. In circumstances where systemic causes for peripheral oedema, for example heart failure, have lead to or coexist with the lymphoedema, then treatment of the medical condition must be undertaken before embarking on specific lymphoedema therapy. Where necessary, appropriate investigations should be performed to confirm lymphoedema and to identify treatable underlying causes (e.g. active cancer) or co-morbidities (e.g. superficial venous incompetence).

Physical therapies

All patients with a diagnosis of lymphoedema should be referred to a local trained lymphoedema therapist. Management will focus on the needs of each individual patient. This may include: (i) risk reduction, for example in breast cancer patients; (ii) swelling reduction and improvement of shape; (iii) treatment and prevention of infection; (iv) treating skin problems such as elephantiasis, lymphorrhoea and wounds, as well as discouraging tissue fibrosis; (v) restoring functional independence and correcting posture imbalance; and (vi) pain and psychosocial management. Therapy assessment will include setting the benchmarks against which improvement can be judged, for example limb volume measurement, mobility and functional assessments. A treatment plan will depend on the site and severity of the lymphoedema and the need to engage other services, for example leg ulcer services, oncology or vascular surgeons.

Physical methods of treating lymphoedema have been practised in Europe for many years [2]. Therapy essentially aims to control lymph formation (capillary filtration), including treatment of inflammatory causes and/or venous hypertension; and to improve lymph drainage through existing lymphatics and collateral routes by applying normal physiological procedures that stimulate lymph flow. Physical treatment can, in the majority of cases, improve quality of life considerably. Central to management is getting patients to understand their condition and know what they can do for themselves. Only then can a high level of motivation and adherence to treatment be generated [3]. It is important to explain to patients that, unlike blood which is propelled by the heart, lymph drainage relies on local changes in tissue pressure generated by exercise and movement. Physical treatment exploits these principles, enhancing lymph flow as much as possible within the limits of a compromised drainage system. It should be appreciated that lymph flow still exists in lymphoedema, otherwise swelling would be a relentlessly progressive process.

The essential components of physical therapy include the following.

Care of the skin and prevention of infection

Elephantiasis skin changes are not only unsightly but lead to problems including infection, odour, lymphorrhoea, restricted movement from fibrosis (pseudoscleroderma) and poor wound healing. Regular application of an emollient is important for hydrating the hardened skin, so making it more supple and discouraging hyperkeratosis. Tinea pedis is almost invariable because of the closely apposed swollen toes – circumstances not improved by elastic hosiery. Modern antifungal creams unfortunately macerate skin further and therefore it is suggested that terbinafine cream is applied for 2 weeks followed by an alcohol wipe (assuming the skin is not broken). For deep cracks and crevices that bacteria may readily colonize, regular toilet is necessary followed by an antiseptic soak, for example potassium permanganate. Hyperkeratosis can often be improved through the regular application of 5% salicylic acid ointment, but the best treatment to reverse elephantiasis skin changes is long-term compression. Areas that constantly seep lymph should also respond to sustained compression.

Prevention of infection, particularly lymphangitis/cellulitis, is crucial to the control of lymphoedema. Care of the skin, good hygiene, control of tinea pedis and good antisepsis following abrasions and minor wounds are important in reducing the risk of cellulitis, as maintenance of skin integrity and an effective barrier will reduce the entry of microorganisms.

Exercise

Exercise and movement are crucial to lymph drainage [4]. Dynamic muscle contractions (isotonic exercises) encourage both passive (movement of lymph along tissue planes or through non-contractile lymphatics) and active (increased contractility and therefore propulsion of lymph within contractile lymphatics) phases of lymph drainage. Overexertion and excessive static (isometric, e.g. gripping) exercise increase blood flow, which tends to increase oedema.

External compression

External compression (hosiery, bandage or pneumatic compression) complements the exercise programme. Such compression is not intended to 'squeeze' oedema but to act as a counterforce to striated muscle activity and so generate higher tissue pressures during contractions. This provides the most powerful stimulus to lymph drainage. Compression also limits capillary filtration by opposing capillary pressure. Compression is much less effective without exercise. Multilayer bandaging can be used for limb reduction, but also has the advantage of restoring limb shape so that subsequent use of compression garments (hosiery) is more effective at controlling swelling [5].

Bandaging may be the only method suitable for huge misshapen limbs and for controlling lymphorrhoea. Layers of strong, non-elastic (short-stretch) bandages are applied to generate a high pressure during muscular contractions but low pressure at rest. The use of foam or soft padding helps to distribute pressure more evenly and to protect the skin. The digits are bandaged to control the swelling of fingers and toes. The strategic positioning of rubber pads 'irons out' pockets of swelling and deep skin folds (Figure 105.36). Multilayer bandaging is a skill that takes time to learn and should not be undertaken by any professional without appropriate training. The compression administered may have to be modified in circumstances such as cancer requiring palliative treatment, moderate limb ischaemia or if there is any neurological deficit. Hosiery (below-knee or full-length stockings, half or full tights and sleeves) usually requires high compression and double layers may occasionally be required. Most garments last no more than 6 months. Two garments (or pairs) should be provided, one to wear and one for the wash. Washing is necessary to maintain the compression properties of the garment. The patient's technique for the application, removal and care of garments is crucial for a successful outcome.

Pneumatic compression therapy (intermittent/sequential pneumatic compression) should not be used in preference to exercise and compression but can be useful in mixed lymphovenous oedema and in infirm patients [6]. An inflatable boot, legging or sleeve is connected to a motor-driven pump and lymph is displaced proximally towards the root of the limb. If hosiery is not fitted immediately following compression therapy, the swelling readily recurs. Pneumatic compression softens the tissues and reduces limb volume during treatment, but it is doubtful that any long-term benefit is gained over hosiery and exercise alone.

Massage (manual lymphatic drainage therapy)

Massage is an important component of treatment, particularly for midline lymphoedema where there are few alternatives [2]. Manual lymphatic drainage (MLD) is a massage technique performed by lymphoedema therapists with the aim of re-routing the accumulation of lymph from the swollen region via collateral lymphatic pathways to lymphatic basins that are able to drain normally. The initial step in MLD is to decongest central/proximal areas before massaging the oedematous region. This facilitates the drainage of lymph via lymphatic vessels/pathways that have been stimulated by the massage technique. Tissue movement must be gentle if it is to stimulate lymph flow without increasing blood flow [7].

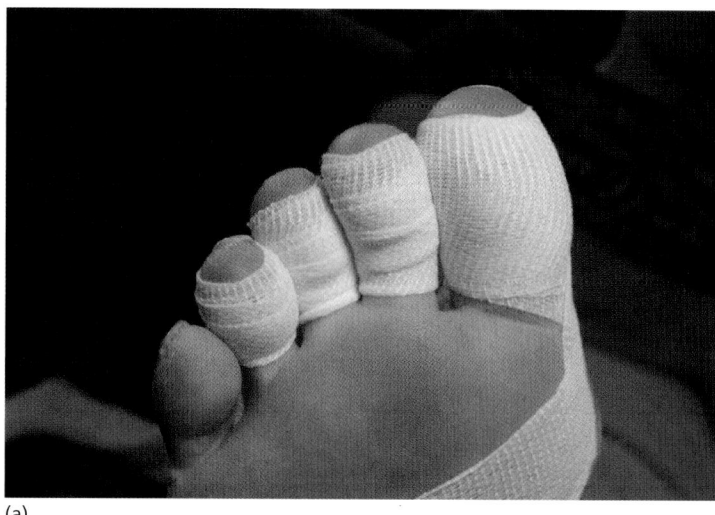

(a)

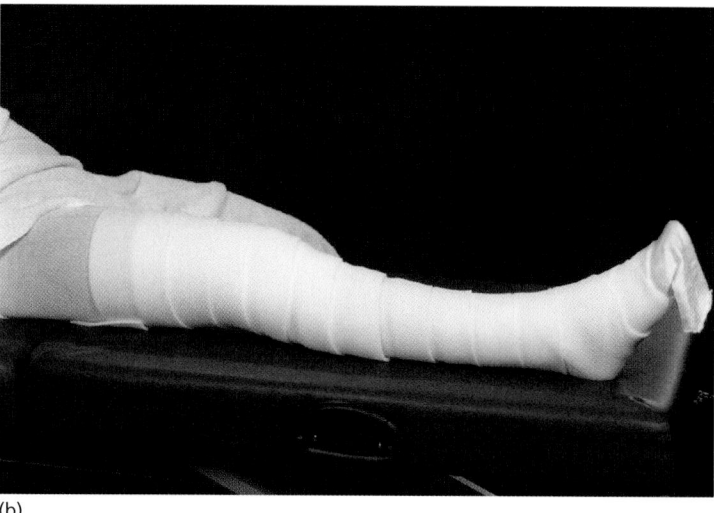

(b)

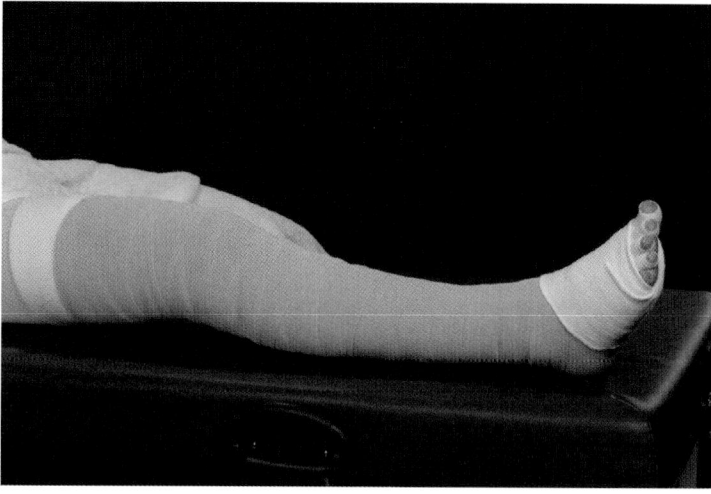

(c)

Figure 105.36 (a) Toe (or finger) bandaging with cotton crepe bandages. (b) Sub-bandage wadding over a tubular cotton bandage. (c) Short-stretch compression cotton bandages applied in layers in a figure of eight and/or spiral style.

A number of MLD techniques are available but no single method appears to be superior. MLD is widely practised and many patients, therapists and physicians advocate the benefits. Continuous MLD delivered by a therapist is expensive and few health care providers will fund this long term. Simple lymphatic drainage is a good alternative to MLD, and can be delivered by a partner or carer trained in the technique.

Breathing, postural exercise, elevation and rest

Breathing and postural exercises are important, particularly for clearance of lymph from the thorax and abdomen. Without the dispersal of truncal lymph, more peripheral limb oedema will not drain. Elevation per se does nothing to improve lymph drainage, but lowering venous pressure (and therefore filtration) can help to reduce swelling. Rest and elevation alone, however, are not the correct treatment for lymphoedema!

Additional therapies that may of benefit include:

1 *Weight loss.* Many patients with lymphoedema are overweight because of morbid obesity as well as fluid retention. Excessive weight gain is likely to impair lymph drainage in the same way as it impairs venous drainage, and obesity reduces mobility (and therefore exercise). Control of weight in combination with physical treatment may be sufficient to resolve oedema completely in some patients. Weight loss irrespective of type of diet has been shown to reduce arm volume over and above what would be expected from fat loss alone in BCRL [8,9].

2 *Hyperbaric oxygen (HBO), low-level laser therapy (LLLT) and kinesiotaping.* There are data recommending the use of HBO and LLLT independently in BCRL [10,11,**12**] although a recent randomized controlled trial failed to demonstrate significant benefits from HBO treatment [13]. However, LLLT may reduce limb volumes and pain in patients with BCRL [14]. Kinesiotaping has been shown to increase lymph flow [**15**].

Intensive and maintenance treatment

Patients with mild limb lymphoedema, no fibrosis and no shape distortion can be started on maintenance treatment with compression hosiery. Intensive therapy, comprising a 2–4-week course of daily skin care, MLD, multilayer bandaging and exercises, is indicated for patients with moderate to severe limb swelling, poor limb shape or tissue changes such as fibrosis, elephantiasis or lymphorrhoea. Once intensive treatment is complete, maintenance treatment with hosiery is commenced immediately. While decongestive lymphatic therapy has become accepted first line therapy, evidence for best treatment is weak [16].

Pharmacological therapies

There is little use for drug therapy in the management of lymphoedema. Diuretics alone demonstrate minimal improvement in lymphoedema, as their mode of action is to reduce capillary filtration by a reduction in circulating blood volume.

Paroven (an oxerutin) and coumarin (a benzopyrone) have been trialled in lymphoedema and may create a small reduction in limb volume by reducing vascular permeability and thus the amount of fluid forming in the subcutaneous tissues. However, this has been shown to be of little clinical benefit to the patient [17].

PART 9: VASCULAR

Animal studies involving vascular endothelial growth factors has stimulated excitement and hope amongst the lymphatic community that successful forms of drug therapy may be possible in the future. Introduction of VEGFC into animal models of postsurgical lymphoedema (using mouse skin and rabbit ears) induced lymphatic vessel growth and a subsequent reduction in lymphoedema [18,19]. A similar study demonstrated regeneration of functional cutaneous lymphatics in skin of *Chy* mice with primary lymphoedema by viral-mediated *VEGFC* gene transfer that caused overexpression of VEGFC [20]. More recent animal studies have incorporated growth factors with lymph node transfer surgical methods. Studies using transplanted lymph nodes that were transfected with VEGFC demonstrated that the lymphatic network in the defective area could be restored, with transplanted nodes and existing vessels becoming incorporated [21,22]. Research is currently being undertaken to optimize growth factor delivery and human trials in patients with secondary lymphoedema should commence in the near future [23].

Surgical options

Surgery has a specific role in the management of lymphoedema [24]. It is of value in limb lymphoedema in a few patients in whom, even after conservative treatment, the size and weight of a limb inhibit its use or interferes with mobility. Surgery involves either removing excessive tissue or bypassing local lymphatic defects. Lifelong non-surgical measures such as hosiery must be continued postoperatively.

Excisional methods

Excisional surgical procedures for the management of lymphoedema, regardless of the underlying cause, have been employed for more than a century [25]. They are now rarely utilized as the postoperative complications can be disastrous. Reduction (excisional) operations remove a longitudinal ellipse of skin and the underlying abnormal subcutaneous tissue down to the deep fascia in a 'melon slice' that permits primary closure of the skin edges (Sistrunk procedure). Undercutting of the skin allows the removal of additional tissue (Homans procedure). This procedure is preferred to circumferential excision and skin grafting (Charles procedure) or to the addition of in-rolling of a skin flap (Thompson buried dermis flap operation). Postoperative complications include skin transplant necrosis, poor cosmetic results and worsening lymphoedema distal to the surgical site. None of the excisional procedures have curative potential as all chances of restoring effective lymphatic transport have been surgically removed. Volume reduction may be achieved through tissue reduction, but not through lymphatic drainage improvement. The indications for this type of surgery should be restricted to rare cases lacking alternative conservative or surgical treatment options. The exceptions to this rule are cases of genital or eyelid lymphoedema, where reduction/debulking surgery is used sooner rather than later [26].

Lymphatico-venous anastomosis surgery

Recently there has been much interest in lymphatico-venous anastomosis (LVA) surgery. LVA is a type of lymphovenous bypass, utilizing a supermicrosurgical technique to anastomose distal subdermal lymphatic vessels with adjacent venules less than 0.8 mm in diameter in an attempt to improve regional lymph drainage and potentially remove the need for use of hosiery (a scenario that many patients are desperate to achieve). It is popular amongst surgeons as it is performed under local anaesthetic and the surgical incisions are small. Postoperative complications include lymphatic vessel occlusion, possibly due to thrombus formation within the lumen [27]. Prior to LVA surgery patients undergo ICG fluorescent imaging to locate functional patent lymphatic vessels within the affected limb.

A review of the literature suggests that the efficacy of LVA surgery is questionable. Postoperative results (within 1 year of surgery) vary greatly between centres, with limb volume reductions of 4–67% [28,29]. There is a lack of long-term data as the technique is relatively new. However, surgeons favour its use because of the low risk of complications. There is currently no method of determining its effect on lymphatic function. The development of imaging techniques could provide a tool to answer the question of its place in lymphatic treatment strategies.

Lymphatico-lymphatic anastomosis surgery

The rationale behind lymphatic grafting surgery is to avoid the problems inherent to LVA surgery caused by coagulation of blood within the lymphatics, by connecting the lymphatic system to itself. Again, there is a lack of robust long-term data regarding efficacy.

Lymph node transfer surgery

Autologous transplantation of normal lymphatic tissue within a local or free flap to a site deficient of lymph nodes and vessels has been performed. The rationale is that the transplant of normal lymph nodes could encourage and improve lymphatic drainage in a previously oedematous region. Few surgeons seem to be performing this type of surgery but reported results appear encouraging, with one case series suggesting 40% of patients were cured of their lymphoedema [30]. However, no long-term data are available on its use. One important concern to raise with this type of surgery is that it relies on the transfer of normal lymph nodes in order to improve lymphatic drainage. This may be possible in a patient with secondary lymphoedema, but may cause complications in patients with primary lymphoedema who may not have 'normal' lymph nodes, or 'normal' lymphatic vasculature, even at unaffected sites. This concern is supported by reports of donor site lymphatic vessel dysfunction in patients undergoing microvascular lymph node transfer surgery for cancer-related lymphoedema [31].

Liposuction

Chronic lymphoedema may be associated with fatty tissue deposition in some patients, although the mechanisms of this are not fully understood. Excess adipose tissue will not respond to decongestive lymphoedema treatments, anastomosis surgery or lymph node transfer procedures. Liposuction creates significant volume reduction in therapy-resistant lymphoedema of the extremities, when combined with lifelong compression therapy [32]. This adjunctive therapy is used in compliant patients willing to wear lifelong compression garments. If patients disregard regular use of their garments, a relapse or worsening of lymphoedema is observed as liposuction may cause injury to remaining subcutaneous lymphatics within the lymphoedematous extremities [32]. However, liposuction has been shown to create a long-term volume reduction of 100% in compliant patients followed for up to 17 years [33]. Liposuction techniques, although not curative, offer an effective symptomatic treatment.

Resources

Further information

Clinical Resource Efficiency Support Team. *Guidelines on the Diagnosis Assessment and Management of Lymphoedema*, 2008. http://www.gain-ni.org/images/Uploads/Guidelines/CrestGuidelines.pdf.

A list of trained therapists can usually be accessed through national professional bodies for lymphoedema, for example:

Australasian Lymphology Association: http://www.lymphoedema.org.au.
Lympoedema Support Network (UK): http://www.lymphoedema.org.
National Lymphedema Network (USA): http://www.lymphnet.org.
(All last accessed August 2015.)

Key references

The full list of references can be found in the online version at www.rooksdermatology.com.

Clinical presentations of lymphatic dysfunction

Chronic, venous and drug-induced oedema

1 Levick JR. *An Introduction to Cardiovascular Physiology*, 5th edn. London: Arnold, 2010.
2 Willenberg T, Schumacher A, Amann-Vesti B, *et al.* Impact of obesity on venous hemodynamics of the lower limbs. *J Vasc Surg* 2010;52(3):664–8.
3 Dreifuss SE, Manders EK. Massive scrotal edema: an unusual manifestation of obstructive sleep apnea and obesity-hypoventilation syndrome. *Case Rep Med* 2013;2013:685–716.
4 Moffatt CJ, Franks PJ, Doherty DC, *et al.* Lymphoedema: an underestimated health problem. *Q J Med* 2003;96(10):731–8.
5 Levick JR, Michel CC. Microvascular fluid exchange and the revised Starling principle. *Cardiovasc Res* 2010;87(2):198–210.
6 Proby CM, Gane JN, Joseph AE, *et al.* Investigation of the swollen limb with isotope lymphography. *Br J Dermatol* 1990;123:29–38.

Chronically swollen leg

1 Strømgaard S, Rasmussen SW, Schmidt TA. Brief hospitalizations of elderly patients: a retrospective, observational study. *Scand J Trauma Resusc Emerg Med* 2014;22:17.
2 Levick JR. *An Introduction to Cardiovascular Physiology*, 5th edn. London: Arnold, 2010.
3 Lymphoedema Framework. *Best Practice for the Management of Lymphoedema*. International Consensus. London: Medical Education, 2006. http://www.lympho.org/mod_turbolead/upload/file/Lympho/Best_practice_20_July.pdf (last accessed August 2015).

Phleboedema and mixed lymphovenous disease

1 Kaipainen A, Korhonen J, Mustonen T, *et al.* Expression of the fms-like tyrosine kinase FLT4 gene becomes restricted to lymphatic endothelium during development. *Proc Natl Acad Sci USA* 1995;92:3566–70.
2 Levick JR, Michel CC. Microvascular fluid exchange and the revised Starling principle. *Cardiovasc Res* 2010;87(2):198–210.
3 Rabe E, Guex JJ, Puskas A, Scuderi A, Fernandez Quesada F; VCP Coordinators. Epidemiology of chronic venous disorders in geographically diverse populations: results from the Vein Consult Program. *Int Angiol* 2012;31(2):105–15.

4 Telinius N, Mohanakumar S, Majgaard J, *et al.* Human lymphatic vessel contractile activity is inhibited in vitro but not in vivo by the calcium channel blocker nifedipine. *J Physiol* 2014;592(2):4697–714.
5 Levick JR. *An Introduction to Cardiovascular Physiology*, 5th edn. London: Arnold, 2010.
6 Mellor RH, Brice G, Stanton AW, et al; Lymphoedema Research Consortium. Mutations in FOXC2 are strongly associated with primary valve failure in veins of the lower limb. *Circulation* 2007;115(14):1912–20.
7 Dean SM, Zirwas MJ, Horst AV. Elephantiasis nostras verrucosa: an institutional analysis of 21 cases. *J Am Acad Dermatol* 2011; 64(6):1104–10.
8 Lymphoedema Framework. *Best Practice for the Management of Lymphoedema*. International Consensus. London: Medical Education, 2006. http://www.lympho.org/mod_turbolead/upload/file/Lympho/Best_practice_20_July.pdf (last accessed August 2015).
9 Zaleska M, Olszewski WL, Durlik M. The effectiveness of intermittent pneumatic compression in long-term therapy of lymphedema of lower limbs. *Lymphat Res Biol* 2014;12(2):103–9.
10 Brittenden J, Cotton SC, Elders A, *et al.* A randomized trial comparing treatments for varicose veins. *N Engl J Med* 2014;371(13):1218–27.

Lipodermatosclerosis (chronic cellulitis)

1 Strømgaard S, Rasmussen SW, Schmidt TA. Brief hospitalizations of elderly patients: a retrospective, observational study. *Scand J Trauma Resusc Emerg Med* 2014;22:17.
2 Herouy Y, May AE, Pornschlegel G, *et al.* Lipodermatosclerosis is characterized by elevated expression and activation of matrix metalloproteinases: implications for venous ulcer formation. *J Invest Dermatol* 1998;111(5):822–7.
3 Caggiati A, Rosi C, Casini A, *et al.* Skin iron deposition characterises lipodermatosclerosis and leg ulcer. *Eur J Vasc Endovasc Surg* 2010;40(6):777–82.
4 Hirschmann JV, Raugi GJ. Lower limb cellulitis and its mimics: part II. Conditions that simulate lower limb cellulitis. *J Am Acad Dermatol* 2012;67(2):177.
5 Lymphoedema Framework. *Best Practice for the Management of Lymphoedema*. International Consensus. London: Medical Education, 2006. http://www.lympho.org/mod_turbolead/upload/file/Lympho/Best_practice_20_July.pdf (last accessed August 2015).
6 National Institute for Health and Care Excellence (NICE). *Varicose Veins in the Legs: the Diagnosis and Management of Varicose Veins*. NICE Guidelines No. CG168. NICE, 2013. http://www.nice.org.uk/guidance/CG168 (last accessed August 2015).

Recurrent cellulitis (erysipelas)

1 Thomas KS, Crook AM, Nunn AJ, et al; UK Dermatology Clinical Trials Network's PATCH I Trial Team. Penicillin to prevent recurrent leg cellulitis. *N Engl J Med* 2013;368(18):1695–703.
3 Damstra RJ, van Steensel MA, Boomsma JH, *et al.* Erysipelas as a sign of subclinical primary lymphoedema: a prospective quantitative scintigraphic study of 40 patients with unilateral erysipelas of the leg. *Br J Dermatol* 2008;158:1210–15.
4 McPherson T, Persaud S, Singh S, *et al.* Interdigital lesions and frequency of acute dermatolymphangioadenitis in lymphoedema in a filariasis-endemic area. *Br J Dermatol* 2006;154(5):933–41.
5 Dupuy A, Benchikhi H, Roujeau JC, *et al.* Risk factors for erysipelas of the leg (cellulitis): case control study. *BMJ* 1999;318:591–4.
6 Cox NH. Oedema as a risk factor for multiple episodes of cellulitis/erysipelas of the lower leg: a series with community follow-up. *Br J Dermatol* 2006;155:947–50.
7 Moffatt CJ, Franks PJ, Doherty DC, *et al.* Lymphoedema: an underestimated health problem. *Q J Med* 2003;96:731–8.
12 Levell NJ, Wingfield CG, Garioch JJ. Severe lower limb cellulitis is best diagnosed by dermatologists and managed with shared care between primary and secondary care. *Br J Dermatol* 2011;164(6):1326–8.
13 British Lymphology Society (BLS). *Consensus Document on the Management of Cellulitis in Lymphoedema*. BLS, 2013. http://www.thebls.com/docs/Cellulitis_Consensus_2013.pdf (last accessed August 2015).

Swollen arm

1 DiSipio T, Rye S, Newman B, Hayes S. Incidence of unilateral arm lymphoedema after breast cancer: a systematic review and meta-analysis. *Lancet Oncol* 2013;14(6):500–15.

2 Levick JR. *An Introduction to Cardiovascular Physiology*, 5th edn. London: Arnold, 2010.

3 Fletcher PG, Sterling JC. Recurrent herpes simplex virus type 2 infection of the hand complicated by persistent lymphoedema. *Australas J Dermatol* 2005;46(2):110–13.

4 Pearce VJ, Mortimer PS. Hand dermatitis and lymphoedema. *Br J Dermatol* 2009;161(1):177–80.

5 Kiely PD, Bland JM, Joseph AE, *et al.* Upper limb lymphatic function in inflammatory arthritis. *J Rheumatol* 1995;22:214–17.

6 Mulherin DM, Fitzgerald O, Bresnihan B. Lymphoedema of the upper limb in patients with psoriatic arthritis. *Semin Arthritis Rheum* 1993;22:350–6.

7 Keppler-Noreuil KM, Sapp JC, Lindhurst MJ, *et al.* Clinical delineation and natural history of the PIK3CA-related overgrowth spectrum. *Am J Med Genet A* 2014;164(7):1713–33.

8 Stanton A, Modi S, Mellor R, Levick R, Mortimer P. Diagnosing cancer-related lymphoedema in the arm. *J Lymphoedema* 2006;1:12–15.

9 Lymphoedema Framework. *Best Practice for the Management of Lymphoedema.* International Consensus. London: Medical Education, 2006. http://www.lympho.org/mod_turbolead/upload/file/Lympho/Best_practice_20_July.pdf (last accessed August 2015).

10 British Lymphology Society (BLS). *What is Lymphoedema?* www.thebls.com/cellulitis (last accessed August 2015).

Swollen face, head and neck

2 Dozsa A, Karoli ZS, Degrell P. Bilateral blepharochalasis. *J Eur Acad Dermatol Venereol* 2005;19:725–8.

5 Levick JR. *An Introduction to Cardiovascular Physiology*, 5th edn. London: Arnold, 2010.

10 Nozicka Z. Endovasal granulomatous lymphangitis as a pathogenetic factor in cheilitis granulomatosa. *J Oral Pathol* 1985;14:363–5.

11 Salles AG, Lotierzo PH, Gemperli R, *et al.* Complications after polymethylmethacrylate injections: report of 32 cases. *Plast Reconstr Surg* 2008;121:1811–20.

12 Lymphoedema Framework. *Best Practice for the Management of Lymphoedema.* International Consensus. London: Medical Education, 2006. http://www.lympho.org/mod_turbolead/upload/file/Lympho/Best_practice_20_July.pdf (last accessed August 2015).

13 Odom R, Dahl M, Dover J, et al; National Rosacea Society Expert Committee on the Classification and Staging of Rosacea. Standard management options for rosacea, part 2: options according to subtype. *Cutis* 2009;84(2):97–104.

Swollen genitalia and mons pubis

1 Daroczy j. Pathology of lymphoedema. *Clin Dermatol* 1995;13:433–44.

3 Dandapat MC, Mohapatro SK, Patro SK. Elephantiasis of the penis and scrotum. A review of 350 cases. *Am J Surg* 1985;149:686–90.

9 British Lymphology Society (BLS). *What is Lymphoedema?* www.thebls.com/cellulitis (last accessed August 2015).

10 Brewer MB, Singh DP. Massive localized lymphedema: review of an emerging problem and report of a complex case in the mons pubis. *Ann Plast Surg* 2012;68(1):101–4.

11 Lymphoedema Framework. *Best Practice for the Management of Lymphoedema.* International Consensus. London: Medical Education, 2006. http://www.lympho.org/mod_turbolead/upload/file/Lympho/Best_practice_20_July.pdf (last accessed August 2015).

12 Garaffa G, Christopher N, Ralph DJ. The management of genital lymphoedema. *BJU Int* 2008;102(4):480–4.

Obesity-related lymphoedema

1 Disipio T, Rye S, Newman S, Hayes S. Incidence of unilateral arm lymphoedema after breast cancer: a systematic review and meta-analysis. *Lancet Oncol* 2013;14(6):500–15.

2 Shaw C, Mortimer P, Judd PA. A randomized controlled trial of weight reduction as a treatment for breast cancer-related lymphedema. *Cancer* 2007;110:1868–74.

4 Randolph GJ, Miller NE. Lymphatic transport of high-density lipoproteins and chylomicrons. *J Clin Invest* 2014;124(3):929–35.

5 Lim HY, Thiam CH, Yeo KP, *et al.* Lymphatic vessels are essential for the removal of cholesterol from peripheral tissues by SR-BI-mediated transport of HDL. *Cell Metab* 2013;17(5):671–84.

6 Harvey NL, Srinivasan RS, Dillard ME, *et al.* Lymphatic vascular defects promoted by Prox1 haploinsufficiency cause adult-onset obesity. *Nat Genet* 2005;37(10):1072–81.

7 O'Malley E, Ahern T, Dunlevy C, Lehane C, Kirby B, O'Shea D. Obesity related chronic lymphoedema-like swelling and physical function. *Q J Med* 2015;108(3):183–7.

8 Greene AK, Grant FD, Slavin SA. Lower-extremity lymphedema and elevated body-mass index. *N Engl J Med* 2012;366:2136–7.

9 Arngrim N, Simonsen L, Holst JJ, Bulow J. Reduced adipose tissue lymphatic drainage of macromolecules in obese subjects: a possible link between obesity and local tissue inflammation. *Int J Obes (Lond)* 2013;37(5):748–50.

10 Arfvidsson B, Eklof B, Balfour J. Iliofemoral venous pressure correlates with intraabdominal pressure in morbidly obese patients. *Vasc Endovascular Surg* 2005;39:505–9.

11 Willenberg T, Schumacher A, Amann-Vesti B, *et al.* Impact of obesity on venous hemodynamics of the lower limbs. *J Vasc Surg* 2010;52(3):664–8.

Abdominal wall lymphoedema

1 Buyuktas D, Arslan E, Celik O, Tasan E, Demirkesen C, Gundogdu S. Elephantiasis nostras verrucosa on the abdomen of a Turkish female patient caused by morbid obesity [Letter]. *Dermatol Online J* 2010;16(8):14.

2 Bull RH, Mortimer PS. Acute lipodermatosclerosis in a pendulous abdomen. *Clin Exp Dermatol* 1993;18(2):164–6.

3 British Lymphology Society (BLS). *What is Lymphoedema?* www.thebls.com/cellulitis (last accessed August 2015).

4 Lymphoedema Framework. *Best Practice for the Management of Lymphoedema.* International Consensus. London: Medical Education, 2006. http://www.lympho.org/mod_turbolead/upload/file/Lympho/Best_practice_20_July.pdf (last accessed August 2015).

5 Ollapallil J, Koong D, Panchacharavel G, Butcher C, Yapo B. New method of abdominoplasty for morbidly obese patients. *ANZ J Surg* 2004;74(6):504–6

Cancer-related lymphoedema

2 Jung SY, Shin KH, Kim M, *et al.* Treatment factors affecting breast cancer-related lymphedema after systemic chemotherapy and radiotherapy in stage II/III breast cancer patients. *Breast Cancer Res Treat* 2014;148(1):91–8.

9 Hyngstrom JR, Chiang YJ, Cromwell KD, *et al.* Prospective assessment of lymphedema incidence and lymphedema-associated symptoms following lymph node surgery for melanoma. *Melanoma Res* 2013;23(4):290–7.

10 Friedmann D, Wunder JS, Ferguson P, *et al.* Incidence and severity of lymphoedema following limb salvage of extremity soft tissue sarcoma. *Sarcoma* 2011;2011:289673.

11 Donker M, van Tienhoven G, Straver ME, *et al.* Radiotherapy or surgery of the axilla after a positive sentinel node in breast cancer (EORTC 10981-22023 AMAROS): a randomised, multicentre, open-label, phase 3 non-inferiority trial. *Lancet Oncol* 2014;15(12):1303–10.

12 Marneros AG, Blanco F, Husain S, *et al.* Classification of cutaneous intravascular breast cancer metastases based on immunolabeling for blood and lymph vessels. *J Am Acad Dermatol* 2009;60:633–8.

13 Finkel LJ, Griffiths CEM. Inflammatory breast carcinoma (carcinoma erysipeloides), an easily overlooked diagnosis. *Br J Dermatol* 1993;129:324–6.

Swollen breast and breast lymphoedema

1 Boughey JC, Hoskin TL, Cheville AL, *et al.* Risk factors associated with breast lymphedema. *Ann Surg Oncol* 2014;21(4):1202–8.

2 Levick JR. *An Introduction to Cardiovascular Physiology*, 5th edn. London: Arnold, 2010.

3 Jung SY, Shin KH, Kim M, *et al.* Treatment factors affecting breast cancer-related lymphedema after systemic chemotherapy and radiotherapy in stage II/III breast cancer patients. *Breast Cancer Res Treat* 2014;148(1):91–8.

4 Boughey JC, Hoskin TL, Cheville AL, *et al.* Risk factors associated with breast lymphedema. *Ann Surg Oncol* 2014;21(4):1202–8.

5 Hille U, Soergel P, Makowski L, Dörk-Bousset T, Hillemanns P. Lymphedema of the breast as a symptom of internal diseases or side effect of mTor inhibitors. *Lymphat Res Biol* 2012;10(2):63–73.

Massive localized lymphoedema

1 Lu S, Tran Ta, Jones DM, *et al.* Localized lymphedema (elephantiasis): a case series and review of the literature. *J Cutan Pathol* 2008;36:1–20.

2 Manduch M, Oliveira AM, Nascimento AG, Folpe AL. Massive localised lymphoedema: a clinicopathological study of 22 cases and review of the literature. *J Clin Pathol* 2009;62(9):808–11.

3 Chopra K, Tadisina KK, Brewer M, Holton LH, Banda AK, Singh DP. Massive localized lymphedema revisited: a quickly rising complication of the obesity epidemic. *Ann Plast Surg* 2015;74(1):126–32.

4 Khanna M, Naraghi AM, Salonen D, *et al*. Massive localised lymphoedema: clinical presentation and MR imaging characteristics. *Skeletal Radiol* 2011;40(5): 647–52.

Primary lymphoedema

4 Karkkainen MJ, Ferrell RE, Lawrence EC, *et al*. Missense mutations interfere with VEGFR-3 signalling in primary lymphoedema. *Nature Genet* 2000;25(2):153–9.

7 Fang JM, Dagenais SL, Erickson RP, *et al*. Mutations in FOXC2 (MFH-1), a forkhead family transcription factor, are responsible for the hereditary lymphedema-distichiasis syndrome. *Am J Hum Genet* 2000;67(6):1382–8.

10 Connell F, Gordon K, Brice G, *et al*. The classification and diagnostic algorithm for primary lymphatic dysplasia: an update from 2010 to include molecular findings. *Clin Genet* 2013;84(4):303–14.

12 Moffatt CJ, Franks PJ, Doherty DC, *et al*. Lymphoedema: an underestimated health problem. *Q J Med* 2003;96(10):731–8.

20 Alders M, Hogan BM, Gjini E, *et al*. Mutations in CCBE1 cause generalized lymph vessel dysplasia in humans. *Nature Genet* 2009;41(12):1272–4.

25 Lindhurst MJ, Sapp JC, Teer JK, *et al*. A mosaic activating mutation in AKT1 associated with the Proteus syndrome. *N Engl J Med* 2011;365(7):611–19.

27 Lindhurst MJ, Parker VER, Payne F, *et al*. Mosaic overgrowth with fibroadipose hyperplasia is caused by somatic activating mutations in PIK3CA. *Nature Genet* 2012;44(8).

35 Gordon K, Schulte D, Brice G, *et al*. Mutation in vascular endothelial growth factor-C, a ligand for vascular endothelial growth factor receptor-3, is associated with autosomal dominant Milroy-like primary lymphedema. *Circ Res* 2013;112(6):956–60.

39 Ostergaard P, Simpson MA, Mendola A, *et al*. Mutations in KIF11 cause autosomal-dominant microcephaly variably associated with congenital lymphedema and chorioretinopathy. *Am J Hum Genet* 2012;90(2):356–62.

48 Ostergaard P, Simpson MA, Connell FC, *et al*. Mutations in GATA2 cause primary lymphedema associated with a predisposition to acute myeloid leukemia (Emberger syndrome). *Nature Genet* 2011;43(10):929–31.

Lipoedema

1 Allen EV, Hines EA. Lipedema of the legs: a syndrome characterized by fat legs and orthostatic edema. *Staff Meetings Mayo Clin* 1940;15:184–7.

3 Schmeller W, Meier-Vollrath I. Tumescent liposuction: a new and successful therapy for lipedema. *J Cutan Med Surg* 2006;10(1):7–10.

5 Harwood CA, Bull RH, Evans J, Mortimer PS. Lymphatic and venous function in lipoedema. *Br J Dermatol* 1996;134(1):1–6.

6 Fonder MA, Loveless JW, Lazarus GS. Lipedema, a frequently unrecognized problem. *J Am Acad Dermatol* 2007;57(Suppl. 2):S1–3.

7 Child AH, Gordon KD, Sharpe P, *et al*. Lipedema: an inherited condition. *Am J Med Genet A* 2010;152A(4):970–6.

8 Wold LE, Hines EA, Jr, Allen EV. Lipedema of the legs; a syndrome characterized by fat legs and edema. *Ann Intern Med* 1951;34(5):1243–50.

13 Hansson E, Svensson H, Brorson H. Review of Dercum's disease and proposal of diagnostic criteria, diagnostic methods, classification and management. *Orphanet J Rare Dis* 2012;7:23.

19 Szolnoky G, Varga E, Varga M, Tuczai M, Dosa-Racz E, Kemeny L. Lymphedema treatment decreases pain intensity in lipedema. *Lymphology* 2011;44(4):178–82.

23 Peled AW, Slavin SA, Brorson H. Long-term outcome after surgical treatment of lipedema. *Ann Plast Surg* 2012;68(3):303–7.

Yellow-nail syndrome

2 Samman PD, White WF. The yellow nail syndrome. *Br J Dermatol* 1964;76:153–7.

3 Valdés L, Huggins JT, Gude F, *et al*. Characteristics of patients with yellow nail syndrome and pleural effusion. *Respirology* 2014;19(7):985–92.

4 Emerson PA. Yellow nails, lymphoedema and pleural effusions. *Thorax* 1966;21:247–53.

5 Bull RH, Fenton DA, Mortimer PS. Lymphatic function in the yellow nail syndrome. *Br J Dermatol* 1996;134:307–12.

6 Wells, GC. Yellow nail syndrome with familial primary hypoplasia of lymphatics, manifest late in life. *Proc Roy Soc Med* 1966;59:447.

8 Slee J, Nelson J, Dickinson J, Kendall P, Halbert A. Yellow nail syndrome presenting as non-immune hydrops: second case report. *Am J Med Genet* 2000;93:1–4.

9 Hoque SR, Mansour S, Mortimer PS. Yellow nail syndrome: not a genetic disorder? Eleven new cases and a review of the literature. *Br J Dermatol* 2007;156(6):1230–4.

10 Maldonado F, Tazelaar HD, Wang C, Ryu JH. Yellow nail syndrome: analysis of 41 consecutive patients. *Chest* 2008;134:375–81.

11 Lambert EM, Dziura J, Kauls L, Mercurio M, Antaya RJ. Yellow nail syndrome in three siblings: a randomized double-blind trial of topical vitamin E. *Pediatr Dermatol* 2006;23(4):390–5.

12 Baran R, Thomas L. Combination of fluconazole and alpha-tocopherol in the treatment of yellow nail syndrome. *J Drugs Dermatol* 2009;8(3):276–8.

Lymphatic malformation and lymphangioma circumscriptum

1 Marler JJ, Mulliken JB. Current management of hemangiomas and vascular malformations. *Clin Plast Surg* 2005;32(1):99–116.

5 Hogeling M, Adams S, Law J, Wargon O. Lymphatic malformations: clinical course and management in 64 cases. *Australas J Dermatol* 2011;52(3):186–90.

6 Greene AK, Perlyn CA, Alomari AI. Management of lymphatic malformations. *Clin Plast Surg* 2011;38:75–82.

7 Whimster IW. The pathology of lymphangioma circumscriptum. *Br J Dermatol* 1976;94:473–86.

8 Brouillard P, Boon L, Vikkula M. Genetics of lymphatic anomalies. *J Clin Invest* 2014;124(3):898–904.

10 Kurek KC, Howard E, Tennant LB, *et al*. Somatic mosaic activating mutations in PIK3CA cause CLOVES syndrome. *Am J Hum Genet* 2012;90(6):1108–15.

11 Lindhurst MJ, Sapp JC, Teer JK, *et al*. A mosaic activating mutation in AKT1 associated with the Proteus syndrome. *N Engl J Med* 2011;365(7):611–19.

12 Lee BB, Kim YW, Seo JM, *et al*. Current concepts in lymphatic malformation. *Vasc Endovasc Surg* 2005;39(1):67–81.

15 Chaudry G, Guevara CJ, Rialon KL, et al. Safety and efficacy of bleomycin sclerotherapy for microcystic lymphatic malformation. *Cardiovasc Intervent Radiol* 2014;37(6):1476–81.

17 Lee BB, Andrade M, Antignani PL, et al; International Union of Phlebology. Diagnosis and treatment of primary lymphedema. Consensus document of the International Union of Phlebology (IUP)-2013. *Int Angiol* 2013;32(6):541–74.

Lymphoedema as a result of amniotic band constriction

1 Yu VY. Neonatal consequences of placental and membrane dysfunction. *Reprod Fertil Dev* 1991;3(4):431–7.

2 Das SP, Sahoo P, Mohanty R, Das S. One-stage release of congenital constriction band in lower limb from new born to 3 years. *Indian J Orthop* 2010;44(2):198–201.

4 Birth Defects Res A Clin Mol Teratol. 2009 January; 85(1): 52–57.

5 Tadmor OP, Kreisberg GA, Achiron R, Porat S, Yagel S. Limb amputation in amniotic band syndrome: serial ultrasonographic and Doppler observations. *Ultrasound Obstet Gynecol* 1997;10:312–15.

6 Sentilhes L, Verspyck E, Patrier S, Eurin D, Lechevallier J, Marpeau L. Amniotic band syndrome: pathogenesis, prenatal diagnosis and neonatal management. *J Gynecol Obstet Biol Reprod* 2003;32:693–704.

7 Blyth M, Lachlan K. Amniotic bands in paternal half-siblings. *Clin Dysmorphol* 2010;19(2):62–4.

8 Mempel M, Abeck D, Lange I, *et al*. The wide spectrum of clinical expression in Adams-Oliver syndrome: a report of two cases. *Br J Dermatol* 1999;140(6):1157–60.

9 Mortimer PS, Rockson SG. New developments in clinical aspects of lymphatic disease. *J Clin Invest* 2014;124(3):915–21.

10 Paladini D, Foglia S, Sglavo G, Martinelli P. Congenital constriction band of the upper arm: the role of three-dimensional ultrasound in diagnosis, counseling and multidisciplinary consultation. *Ultrasound Obstet Gynecol* 2004;23:520–2.

11 Soldado F, Aguirre M, Peiró JL, *et al*. Fetoscopic release of extremity amniotic bands with risk of amputation. *J Pediatr Orthop* 2009;29:290–3.

Lymphangiomatosis, lymphangioleiomyomatosis and non-malignant lymphatic tumours

1 Mazreeuw-Hautier J, Syed S, Leisner R, Harper J. Extensive venous/lymphatic malformations causing life-threatening haematological complications. *Br J Dermatol* 2007;157:558–63.

2 Dellinger MT, Garg N, Olsen BR. Viewpoints on vessels and vanishing bones in Gorham-Stout disease. *Bone* 2014;63:47–52.

3 Lala S, Mulliken JB, Alomari AI, Fishman SJ, Kozakewich HP, Chaudry G. Gorham-Stout disease and generalized lymphatic anomaly – clinical, radiologic, and histologic differentiation. *Skeletal Radiol* 2013;42(7):917–24.

6 Wang L, Chen L, Yang X, Gao T, Wang G. Benign lymphangioendothelioma: a clinical, histopathologic and immunohistochemical analysis of four cases. *J Cutan Pathol* 2013;40(11):945–9.

8 Jermann M, Eid K, Pfammatter T, *et al.* Maffucci's syndrome. *Circulation* 2001;104:1693.

9 Safi F, Gupta A, Adams D, Anandan V, McCormack FX, Assaly R. Kaposiform lymphangiomatosis, a newly characterized vascular anomaly presenting with hemoptysis in an adult woman. *Ann Am Thorac Soc* 2014;11(1):92–5.

11 Gengler C, Coindre JM, Leroux A, *et al.* Vascular proliferations of the skin after radiation therapy for breast cancer: clinicopathologic analysis of a series in favor of a benign process: a study from the French Sarcoma Group. *Cancer* 2007;109(8):1584–98.

12 Flucke U, Requena L, Mentzel T. Radiation-induced vascular lesions of the skin: an overview. *Adv Anat Pathol* 2013;20(6):407–15.

13 Bissler JJ, Kingswood JC, Radzikowska E, *et al.* Everolimus for angiomyolipoma associated with tuberous sclerosis complex or sporadic lymphangioleiomyomatosis (EXIST-2): a multicentre, randomised, double-blind, placebo-controlled trial. *Lancet* 2013;381(9869):817–24.

Lymphangiectasia

1 Goldstein JB, McNatt NS, Hambrick GW. Penicillamine dermopathy with lymphangiectases. *Arch Dermatol* 1989;125:92–7.

2 Harwood CA, Mortimer PS. Acquired vulval lymphangiomata mimicking genital warts. *Br J Dermatol* 1993;129: 34–6.

3 Mallett RB, Curley RK, Mortimer PS. Acquired lymphangiomata: report of four cases and a discussion of the pathogenesis. *Br J Dermatol* 1992;126:380–2.

4 Whimster IW. The pathology of lymphangioma circumscriptum. *Br J Dermatol* 1976;94(5):473–86.

5 Browse NL. Management of lymph and chyle reflux. In: Browse NL, Burnand KG, Mortimer PS, eds. *Diseases of the Lymphatics*. London: Arnold, 2003:259–92.

6 Waldmann TA, Steinfeld JL, Dutcher TF, *et al.* The role of the gastrointestinal system in "idiopathic hypoproteinemia." *Gastroenterology* 1961;41:197–207.

7 Lee J, Kong MS. Primary intestinal lymphangiectasia diagnosed by endoscopy following the intake of a high-fat meal. *Eur J Pediatr* 2008;167:237–9.

8 Braamskamp MJ, Dolman KM, Tabbers MM. Protein-losing enteropathy in children. *Eur J Pediatr* 2010;169(10):1179–85.

9 Bliss CM, Schroy PC, III. Primary intestinal lymphangiectasia. *Curr Treat Options Gastroenterol* 2004;7:3–6.

10 Makh DS, Mortimer P, Powell B. A review of the surgical treatment of vulval lymphangioma and lymphangiectasia: four case reviews. *J Plast Reconstr Aesthet Surg* 2006;59:1442–5.

Lymphocele, seroma and lymph fistula

1 Ferguson JH, Maclure JG. Lymphocele following lymphadenectomy. *Am J Obstet Gynecol* 1961;82:783–92.

2 Watt-Boolsen S, Nielsen VB, Jensen J, Bak S. Postmastectomy seroma. A study of the nature and origin of seroma after mastectomy. *Dan Med Bull* 1989;36(5):487–9.

Lymphatic filariasis

1 Rockson SG. Lymphedema. *Am J Med* 2001;110:288–95.

2 Lymphatic filariasis: the disease and its control. Fifth report of the WHO Expert Committee on Filariasis. *World Health Organ Tech Rep Ser* 1992;821:1–71.

3 Nutman T. Insights into the pathogenesis of disease in human lymphatic filariasis. *Lymph Res Biol* 2013;11(3):144–8.

4 Chakraborty S, Gurusamy M, Zawieja D, Muthuchamy M. Lymphatic filariasis: perspectives on lymphatic remodelling and contractile dysfunction in filarial disease pathogenesis. *Microcirculation* 2013;20(5):349–64.

6 World Health Organization (WHO). Global programme to eliminate lymphatic filariasis. *Wkly Epidemiol Rec* 2014;89(38):409–18.

12 Bennuru S, Nutman TB. Lymphatics in human lymphatic filariasis: in vitro models of parasite induced lymphatic remodeling. *Lymphat Res Biol* 2009;7:215–19.

19 Weil GJ, Lammie PJ, Weiss N. The ICT filariasis test: a rapid-format antigen test for diagnosis of bancroftian filariasis. *Parasitol Today* 1997;13:401–4.

Podoconiosis

1 Price EW. Non-filarial elephantiasis – confirmed as a geochemical disease and renamed podoconiosis. *Ethiop Med J* 1988;26:151–3.

2 Davey G. Recent advances in podoconiosis. *Ann Trop Med Parasitol* 2009;103:377–82.

3 Davey G. Podoconiosis, non-filarial elephantiasis, and lymphology. *Lymphology* 2010;43:168–77.

4 Deribe K, Brooker SJ, Pullan RL, *et al.* Epidemiology and individual, household and geographical risk factors of podoconiosis in Ethiopia: results from the first nationwide mapping. *Am J Trop Med Hyg* 2015;92(1):148–58.

9 Molla YB, Wardrop NA, Le Blond JS, *et al.* Modelling environmental factors correlated with podoconiosis: a geospatial study of non-filarial elephantiasis. *Int J Health Geogr* 2014;13:24.

17 Yakob B, Deribe K, Davey G. Health professionals' attitudes and misconceptions regarding podoconiosis: potential impact on integration of care in southern Ethiopia. *Trans R Soc Trop Med Hyg* 2009;104:42–7.

Pretibial myxoedema

1 Fatourechi V, Pajouhi M, Fransway AF. Dermopathy of Graves disease (pretibial myxedema). Review of 150 cases. *Medicine (Baltimore)* 1994;73:1.

3 Schwartz KM, Fatourechi V, Ahmed DD, *et al.* Dermopathy of Graves' disease (pretibial myxedema): long-term outcome. *J Clin Endocrinol Metab* 2002;98:438–46.

8 Bull RH, Coburn PR, Mortimer PS. Pretibial myxoedema: a manifestation of lymphoedema? *Lancet* 1993;341:403–4.

11 Fatourechi V. Thyroid dermopathy and acropachy. *Best Pract Res Clin Endocrinol Metab* 2012;26(4):553–65.

16 Fatourechi V. Pretibial myxedema. pathophysiology and treatment options. *Am J Clin Dermatol* 2005;6(5):295–309.

17 Takasu N, Higa H, Kinjou Y. Treatment of pretibial myxedema with topical steroid ointment application with sealing cover (steroid occlusive dressing technique: steroid ODT) in Graves' patients. *Intern Med* 2010;49(7):665–9.

19 Deng A, Song D. Multipoint subcutaneous injection of long-acting glucocorticid as a cure for pretibial myxedema. *Thyroid* 2011;21:83–5.

21 Dandona P, Marshall NJ, Bidey SP, *et al.* Successful treatment of exophthalmos and pretibial myxoedema with plasmapheresis. *BMJ* 1979;1:374–6.

22 Antonelli A, Navarranne A, Palla R, *et al.* Pretibial myxedema and high-dose intravenous immunoglobulin treatment. *Thyroid* 1994;4:399–408.

23 Heyes C, Nolan R, Leahy M, Gebauer K. Treatment-resistant elephantiasic thyroid dermopathy responding to rituximab and plasmapheresis. *Australas J Dermatol* 2012;53(1):e1–4.

Trauma-induced lymphoedema

2 Pittaluga P, Chastanet S. Lymphatic complications after varicose veins surgery: risk factors and how to avoid them. *Phlebology* 2012;27(Suppl. 1):139–42.

4 Nikitenko LL, Shimosawa T, Henderson S, *et al.* Adrenomedullin haploinsufficiency predisposes to secondary lymphedema. *J Invest Dermatol* 2013;133(7):1768–76.

5 Kissin MW, della Rovere GO, Easton D, *et al.* Risk of lymphoedema following the treatment of breast cancer. *Br J Surg* 1986;73:580–4.

6 Unno N, Yamamoto N, Suzuki M, *et al.* Intraoperative lymph mapping with preoperative vein mapping to prevent postoperative lymphorrhea following paramalleolar bypass surgery in patients with critical limb ischemia. *Surg Today* 2014;44(3):436–42.

7 Buchel EW, Dalke KR, Hayakawa TE. The transverse upper gracilis flap: eefficiencies and design tips. *Can J Plast Surg* 2013;21(3):162–6.

8 Tourani SS, Taylor GI, Ashton MW. Understanding the three-dimensional anatomy of the superficial lymphatics of the limbs. *Plast Reconstr Surg* 2014;134(5):1065–74.

9 Reading G. Secrétan's syndrome: hard edema of the dorsum of the hand. *Plast Reconstr Surg* 1980;65:182–7.

10 Nwaejike N, Archbold H, Wilson DS. Factitious lymphoedema as a psychiatric condition mimicking reflex sympathetic dystrophy: a case report. *J Med Case Rep* 2008;2:216.

11 Andresz V, Marcantoni N, Binder F, *et al.* Puffy hand syndrome due to drug addiction: a case–control study of the pathogenesis. *Addiction* 2006;101(9):1347–51.

13 Lymphoedema Framework. *Best Practice for the Management of Lymphoedema.* International Consensus. London: Medical Education, 2006. http://www.lympho.org/mod_turbolead/upload/file/Lympho/Best_practice_20_July.pdf (last accessed August 2015).

Lymphoedema due to immobility

1 Garcia AM, Dicianno BE. The frequency of lymphedema in an adult spina bifida population. *Am J Phys Med Rehabil* 2011;90(2):89–96.

2 Solaro C, Ucelli M, Brichetto G, *et al.* Prevalence of oedema of the lower limbs in multiple sclerosis patients: a vascular and lymphoscintigraphic study. *Mult.Scler* 2006;12:659–61.

3 Geurts AC, Visschers BA, van Limbeek J, Ribbers GM. Systematic review of aetiology and treatment of post-stroke hand oedema and shoulder-hand syndrome. *Scand J Rehabil Med* 2000;32(1):4–10.

4 Sneddon I, Church R. *Practical Dermatology*, 4th edn. London: Arnold, 1983: 166.

5 Bull RH, Mortimer PS. Acute lipodermatosclerosis in a pendulous abdomen. *Clin Exp Dermatol* 1993;18:164–6.

6 Dirette D, Hinojosa J. Effects of continuous passive motion on the edematous hands of two persons with flaccid hemiplegia. *Am J Occup Ther* 1994;48(5):403–9.

Lymphangitis

1 Gill MJ, Arlette J, Tyrrell DL, Buchan KA. Herpes simplex virus infection of the hand. Clinical features and management. *Am J Med* 1988;85(2A):53–6.

3 Kennedy JL, Jeffus SK, Platts-Mills TA, *et al.* Seventeen-year-old girl hospitalized for localized swelling, pruritus, tenderness, and lymphatic streaking with eosinophilia. *J Allergy Clin Immunol Pract* 2013;1(3):299–301.

4 Barnes JM, Trueta J. Absorption of bacteria and snake venoms from the tissues: importance of the lymphatic circulation. *Lancet* 1941;1:623–6.

5 Pozio E. Venomous snakebites in Italy: epidemiological and clinical aspects. *Trop Med Parasitol* 1988;39(1):62–6.

7 Marsch W, Haas N, Stuttgen G. Mondor's phlebitis: a lymphovascular process. *Dermatologica* 1986;172:133–8.

8 Moskovitz AH, Anderson BO, Yeung RS, *et al.* Axillary web syndrome after axillary dissection. *Am J Surg* 2001;181:434–9.

10 Lippi G, Favaloro EJ, Cervellin G. Hemostatic properties of the lymph: relationships with occlusion and thrombosis. *Semin Thromb Hemost* 2012;38(2): 213–21.

11 Babu AK, Krishnan P, Andezuth DD. Sclerosing lymphangitis of penis – literature review and report of 2 cases. *Dermatol Online J* 2014;20(7):ii.

12 Marneros AG, Blanco F, Husain S, *et al.* Classification of cutaneous intravascular breast cancer metastases based on immunolabeling for blood and lymph vessels. *J Am Acad Dermatol* 2009;60:633–8.

13 Finkel LJ, Griffiths CEM. Inflammatory breast carcinoma (carcinoma erysipeloides), an easily overlooked diagnosis. *Br J Dermatol* 1993;129:324–6.

Complications of lymphoedema

2 Daróczy J. Pathology of lymphedema. *Clin Dermatol* 1995;13(5):433–44.

3 Mortimer PS, Rockson SG. New developments in clinical aspects of lymphatic disease. *J Clin Invest* 2014;124(3):915–21.

4 Nei T, Akutsu K, Shima A, *et al.* A case of streptococcal toxic shock syndrome due to group G streptococci identified as *Streptococcus dysgalactiae* subsp. *equisimilis*. *J Infect Chemother* 2012;18(6):919–24.

6 Moffatt CJ, Franks PJ, Doherty DC, *et al.* Lymphoedema: an underestimated health problem. *Q J Med* 2003;96(10):731–8.

9 Lee R, Saardi KM, Schwartz RA. Lymphedema-related angiogenic tumors and other malignancies. *Clin Dermatol* 2014;32(5):616–20.

Imaging of the lymphatic system

1 Kinmonth JB. Lymphangiography in man; a method of outlining lymphatic trunks at operation. *Clin Sci (Lond)* 1952;11(1):13–20.

2 Stewart G, Gaunt JI, Croft DN, Browse NL. Isotope lymphography: a new method of investigating the role of the lymphatics in chronic limb oedema. *Br J Surg* 1985;72(11):906–9.

3 Proby CM, Gane JN, Joseph AE, Mortimer PS. Investigation of the swollen limb with isotope lymphography. *Br J Dermatol* 1990;123(1):29–37.

4 Modi S, Stanton AW, Mortimer PS, Levick JR. Clinical assessment of human lymph flow using removal rate constants of interstitial macromolecules: a critical review of lymphoscintigraphy. *Lymph Res Biol* 2007;5(3):183–202.

5 Mellor RH, Hubert CE, Stanton AW, *et al.* Lymphatic dysfunction, not aplasia, underlies Milroy disease. *Microcirculation* 2010;17(4):281–96.

6 Xiong L, Engel H, Gazyakan E, *et al.* Current techniques for lymphatic imaging: state of the art and future perspectives. *Eur J Surg Oncol* 2014;40(3):270–6.

7 Unno N, Inuzuka K, Suzuki M, *et al.* Preliminary experience with a novel fluorescence lymphography using indocyanine green in patients with secondary lymphedema. *J Vasc Surg* 2007;45(5):1016–21.

8 Yamamoto T, Yamamoto N, Azuma S, *et al.* Near-infrared illumination system-integrated microscope for supermicrosurgical lymphaticovenular anastomosis. *Microsurgery* 2014;34(1):23–7.

10 Costa da Cunha Castro E, Galambos C. Prox-1 and VEGFR3 antibodies are superior to D2-40 in identifying endothelial cells of lymphatic malformations – a proposal of a new immunohistichemical panel to differentiate lymphatic from other vascular malformations. *Pediatr Dev Pathol* 2009;12:187–94.

11 Connell F, Gordon K, Brice G, *et al.* The classification and diagnostic algorithm for primary lymphatic dysplasia: an update from 2010 to include molecular findings. *Clin Genet* 2013;84(4):303–14.

Lymphoedema management

1 Medical Education Partnership (MEP). *Best Practice for the Management of Lymphoedema: International Consensus*. London: MEP Ltd, 2006.

5 Badger CMA, Peacock JL, Mortimer PS. A randomized, controlled, parallel group clinical trial comparing multi-layer bandaging followed by hosiery versus hosiery alone in the treatment of patients with lymphedema of the limb. *Cancer* 2000;88:2832–7.

8 Shaw C, Mortimer P, Judd PA. A randomised controlled trial of weight reduction as a treatment for breast cancer-related lymphedema. *Cancer* 2007;110:1868–74.

12 Kozanoglu E, Basaran S, Paydas S, Sarpel T. Efficacy of pneumatic compression and low-level laser therapy in the treatment of postmastectomy lymphoedema: a randomized controlled trial. *Clin Rehabil* 2009;23:117–24.

15 Tsai HJ, Hung HC, Yang JL, *et al.* Could Kinesio tape replace the bandage in decongestive lymphatic therapy for breast-cancer-related lymphedema? A pilot study. *Support Care Cancer* 2009;17:1353–60.

22 Sommer T, Buettner M, Bruns F, Breves G, Hadamitzky C, Pabst R. Improved regeneration of autologous transplanted lymph node fragments by VEGF-C treatment. *Anat Rec* 2012;295(5):786–91.

24 Browse NL, Burnand KG, Mortimer PS. *Diseases of the Lymphatics*. London, Arnold, 2003.

29 Damstra RJ, Voesten HG, van Schelven WD, van der Lei B. Lymphatic venous anastomosis (LVA) for treatment of secondary arm lymphedema. A prospective study of 11 LVA procedures in 10 patients with breast cancer related lymphedema and a critical review of the literature. *Breast Cancer Res Treat* 2009;113(2):199–206.

30 Becker C, Assoud J, Riquet M, Hidden G. Postmastectomy lymphedema: long-term results following microsurgical lymph node transplantation. *Ann Surg* 2006;243(3):313–15.

33 Brorson H. From lymph to fat: complete reduction of lymphoedema. *Phlebology* 2010;25(Suppl. 1):52–63.

PART 9: VASCULAR

CHAPTER 106

Flushing and Blushing

Síona Ní Raghallaigh and Frank C. Powell

Charles Institute of Dermatology, University College Dublin, Dublin, Ireland

Introduction

Flushing and blushing are the result of transient cutaneous vasodilatation that is usually physiological in nature. Although these terms are often used interchangeably, they are distinct processes. A blush signifies a psychosocial response to an experienced emotion, whereas a flush is a thermoregulatory response to increased body temperature. Patients who develop excessive or socially impeding flushing or blushing may present for medical consultation. Frequent blushing can be associated with anxiety states and, in some cases, social phobia. Excessive flushing may be associated with topical agents, food or alcohol intake, or rarely with underlying systemic disease. Clinical features useful in defining the diagnosis include the environmental setting in which the vascular reaction occurs, the extent and pattern of cutaneous involvement, and whether sweating or other systemic symptoms accompany the vasodilatation. Histological evaluation of skin is unhelpful but other investigations may be necessary in particular clinical circumstances. Understanding of the mechanisms by which these cutaneous reactions occur has increased, but treatment options remain limited.

Epidemiology

In the authors' experience, frequent blushing tends to be most problematic in younger individuals (i.e. early teens to mid-twenties) and diminishes with increasing age. Flushing reactions can occur in all age groups. Young male patients appear to be most likely to present for medical management of excessive blushing reactions, mainly due to the associated psychosocial impact (Figure 106.1a, b). With the exception of menopausal flushing, excessive flushing does not appear to have any gender proclivity. Flushing and blushing affects all ethnic groups and skin colours. Pale skinned individuals are most troubled by the social burden of frequent blushing, presumably because the contrast between erythema and unaffected skin is most marked in this group.

Physiology

Physiological transient vasodilatation plays an integral role in thermoregulation. This sympathetically mediated process is regulated by cutaneous arteriovenous anastomoses – the superficial venous plexus, located at the juncture of the papillary and reticular dermis, and the deep horizontal plexus, located at the juncture of the deep reticular dermis and panniculus [1]. Reflex cutaneous vasodilatation in response to an increase in core body temperature involves an initial abolition of the active vasoconstrictor tone that is dominant in normal circumstances. As body heating continues, active vasodilator neural activity to the cutaneous arterioles is enhanced, causing rapid increases in skin blood flow, which is usually coincident with the onset of sweating. Overall, this active vasodilator system is responsible for 80–95% of the increase in skin blood flow that accompanies heat stress. During normothermic conditions, with the body at rest, total skin blood flow is approximately 200–500 mL/min. With full active vasodilatation, skin blood flow can dramatically increase to 8 L/min [2,3]. Neural control of cutaneous vasodilatation involves cotransmission by sympathetic cholinergic nerves, with the release of acetylcholine and one or more cotransmitters, such as substance P (and/or neurokinin-1 receptors), vasoactive intestinal peptide (VIP) and pituitary adenylate cyclase activating peptide (PACAP) [4,5,6]. This neurally mediated increase in blood flow in turn releases nitric oxide (NO) from endothelial cells, which, along with prostaglandins released from local keratinocytes, sustain these vasodilatory effects [7,8,9].

PART 9: VASCULAR

Rook's Textbook of Dermatology, Ninth Edition. Edited by Christopher Griffiths, Jonathan Barker, Tanya Bleiker, Robert Chalmers and Daniel Creamer.
© 2016 John Wiley & Sons, Ltd. Published 2016 by John Wiley & Sons, Ltd.
Companion website: www.rooksdermatology.com

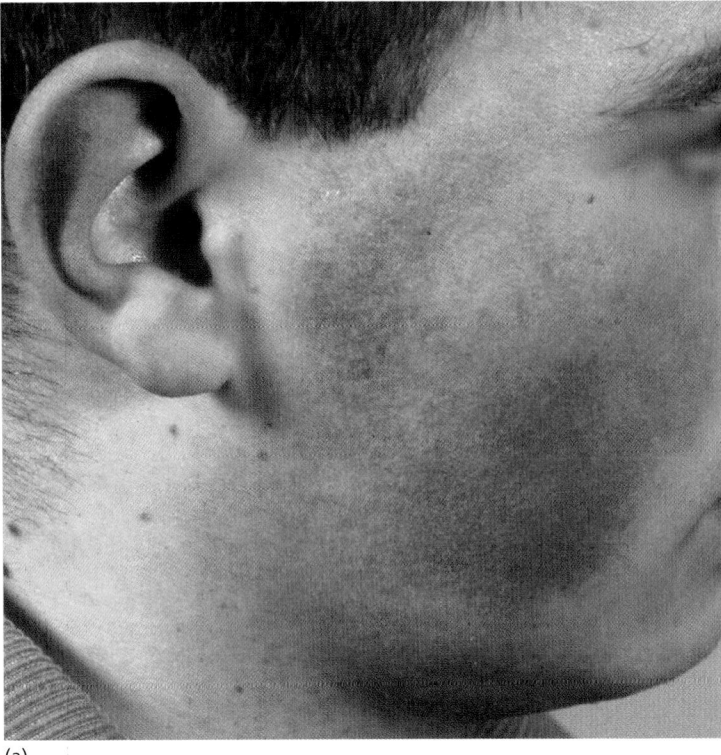

(a)

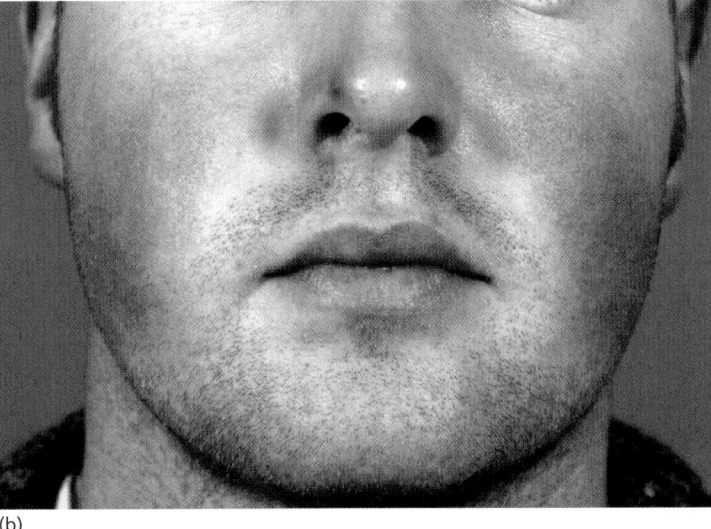

(b)

Figure 106.1 (a, b) These images demonstrate the typical distribution of the blush, as seen in two young men who presented for the management of frequent blushing. Note the 'skip areas' of pallor on the upper lateral cheek in (a). Sparing of the skin around the mouth suggestive of 'circumoral pallor' is evident in both cases. The ears reddened with blushing in both men.

Pathophysiology of flushing

Abnormal, non-thermoregulatory flushing may result from circulating agents that act directly on the vascular smooth muscle, or may be mediated by vasomotor autonomic innervation. Vasoactive mediators can be external or internal. External mediators include

---

Box 106.1 Drugs that cause flushing

- 5-hydroxytryptamine (5-HT) 3 receptor antagonists: ondansetron, ramosetron, tropisetron
- Angiotensin-converting enzyme (ACE) inhibitors: captopril, enalapril, lisinopril, perindopril, ramipril
- β_3 adrenoceptor agonists: fluvoxamine, mirtazapine
- Calcium-channel blockers: nifedipine, verapamil
- Oral or intrasynovial triamcinolone
- Fumaric acid esters
- Hydralazine
- Metronidazole
- Nicotinic acid
- Nitrates: isosorbine mononitrate/dinitrate, glyceryl trinitrate
- Phentolamine
- Pilocarpine
- Prostacyclin
- Prostaglandin E
- Sildenafil, tadalafil, vardenafil, mirodenafil (phosphodiesterase inhibitors)
- Tamsulosin
- Venlafaxine
- High-dose pulsed methylprednisolone
- Morphine and other opiates
- Metrifonate
- Bromocriptine
- Tamoxifen
- Vancomycin
- Rifampicin
- Combination anaesthesia with isoflurane and fentanyl
- Contrast media

With alcohol
- Antimalarials
- Disulfiram
- Chlorpropamide
- Calcium carbonate
- Phentolamine
- Griseofulvin
- Metronidazole
- Ketoconazole
- Tacrolimus ointment

---

those found in food or drugs (Boxes 106.1 and 106.2). Specifically, foods containing tyramine, histamine, higher chain alcohols, monosodium glutamate, aldehyde, nitrites and sulphites, may be associated with flushing [10]. Internal vasoactive mediators include neuropeptides (e.g. substance P, tachykinins, kallikrein,

---

Box 106.2 Food that causes flushing

- Spicy food (especially chilli pepper)
- Caffeine
- Alcohol (especially if alcohol dehydrogenase deficient)
- Fruit (lemons, tomato)
- Vegetables (spinach)
- Cheese (histamine rich – Roquefort)
- Sodium nitrite rich meats (e.g. salami)
- Fish (scombroid poisoning/ciguatoxin)

Box 106.3 Causes of flushing

- Thermoregulatory – heat exposure, exercise, fever
- Food, beverages, medication, alcohol (see Boxes 106.1 and 106.2)
- Menopause
- Rosacea
- Carcinoid
- Phaeochromocytoma
- Mastocytosis
- Anaphylaxis
- Polycythaemia
- Cholinergic urticaria
- Neurological disorders
  - Parkinson disease
  - Migraine
  - Brain tumours
  - Multiple sclerosis
  - Spinal cord lesions
  - Orthostatic hypotension
  - Horner syndrome
  - Trigeminal nerve damage
  - Autonomic epilepsy
  - Autonomic hyperreflexia
  - Frey syndrome
  - Harlequin syndrome
- Renal cell carcinoma
- Medullary carcinoma of the thyroid
- Postsurgery (gastric/prostate/orchidectomy)
- Rovsing syndrome
- Thyrotoxicosis
- Pancreatic cell tumour
- Psychiatric disorders
- Dumping syndrome
- POEMS (polyneuropathy, organomegaly, endocrinopathy, monoclonal gammopathy and skin changes) syndrome
- Basophilic granulocytic leukaemia
- Malignant histiocytoma

kinins, neurotensin, neuropeptide K, VIP, gastrin-related peptide, motilin), catecholamines (e.g. epinephrine, norepinephrine, dopamine), hormones (e.g. oestrogens, adrenocorticotrophic hormone, corticotrophin-releasing hormone, calcitonin), histamine and prostaglandins. As previously described, neurally activated flushing may be associated with sweating ('wet flushing') whereas flushing due to circulating vasoactive mediators does not usually involve sweating, and is referred to as 'dry flushing' [11]. A notable exception to this pattern of associated sweating is the carcinoid syndrome.

Disorders associated with flushing are listed in Box 106.3, with the clinical features of the flush associated with specific disorders described in Table 106.1. Causes of flushing in the paediatric population are listed in Table 106.2.

Psychosocial aspects of blushing

Blushing is a reaction to emotion or social attention, and the blush reaction appears with the development of self-awareness in childhood, usually between the ages of 2 and 3 years [12].

This non-verbal signal of social discomfort has been shown to evoke affiliative, empathic responses in others [13]. While blushing is not exclusive to any particular emotion, it has often been associated with feelings of guilt or shame. Because of this perception (which is often inaccurate), individuals who blush may develop considerable anxiety both during social circumstances and before they venture into them. This can progress to erythrophobia (i.e. an excessive fear of blushing resulting in social phobia and avoidance of social circumstances that might lead to blushing). In addition to blushing, people with social anxiety frequently experience autonomic and motor signs of anxiety during social encounters [14]. Psychologists can assess the degree and impact of blushing using validated questionnaires, such as the 'Blushing Propensity Scale' [15] and the 'Fear of Negative Evaluation Scale' [16]. It is clear that many individuals who blush frequently become very self-conscious of this tendency, and feel that the blush is more severe than in fact it is. The actual intensity of blushing (as measured by laser Doppler fluxemetry or photoplethysmography) has been shown to be unrelated to the perceived intensity of or the susceptibility to blushing [17]. Similar findings have been shown in studies involving patients with rosacea who blush, and who perceive the blush to be more intense than it is [18]. Blushing appears to build up over repeated episodes in people who report that they blush frequently, and frequent blushers have been shown to be more sensitive to vasodilating agents such as niacin [19]. It has been proposed that such individuals may have a physiological predisposition to delayed vascular recovery [20].

Clinical presentation

Patients with excessive blushing complain of an involuntary and prolonged reddening primarily of the facial skin, which is often precipitated by anxiety, emotion or psychological upset. Blushing usually starts on the lateral cheeks and spreads rapidly to involve the entire malar region. Frequently, 'skip' areas of pallor can be observed within the erythematous blush, with sparing of the area around the mouth giving the impression of 'circumoral pallor'. The blush may spread to the forehead and the sides of the neck. The ears characteristically develop an intense erythema, involving primarily the helix and antihelix. Blushing is not usually associated with facial sweating, but there may be accompanying palmar hyperhidrosis and tremor. Because of the tendency to blush in certain social circumstances and their perception that the blush is more marked than it is, individuals may develop a degree of 'anticipatory anxiety' before they venture into these situations [11].

Patients with frequent flushing complain of sudden intense reddening of the face, neck and chest, representing an exaggeration of the normal response to vigorous exercise or temperature change. A flush may evolve in a similar manner to a blush, but often has a more widespread distribution extending to the anterior chest and sometimes the abdomen, particularly the epigastric region. Localized facial sweating may be a feature of flushing. Menopausal women sometimes refer to the sudden onset of flushing and sweating that can occur as a 'drenching flush'. In a minority of

PART 9: VASCULAR

PART 9: VASCULAR

Table **106.1** Disorders associated with flushing.

Disease	Pathogenesis of flush	Characteristics of flush	Associated symptoms and signs	Investigations	Management of flush	Notes
Menopause	The 'hot flush' of menopause is attributed to hypothalamic thermoregulatory dysfunction associated with fluctuations in oestrogen levels. Research suggests that the thermoneutral zone, which is narrowed in women with hot flushes, returns to normal with the administration of oestrogen	Rising feeling of intense heat, profuse sweating and diffuse facial flushing; this may be followed by shivering; typical episodes last from 3 to 5 min and may occur up to 20 times/day	The flush may be associated with considerable discomfort and anxiety, affecting normal daily functioning and sleep patterns. Vasomotor symptoms typically appear in the late menopausal transition period, at which stage an interval of ≥60 days of amenorrhoea is likely to have occurred	FSH AMH Inhibin B	For postmenopausal women with moderate-to-severe vasomotor symptoms (and no history of breast cancer or cardiovascular disease), short-term (2–3 years) oestrogen therapy is the treatment of choice. For women with moderate-to-severe hot flushes in whom oestrogen is contraindicated or not well tolerated, or for women who have stopped oestrogen and are experiencing recurrent symptoms but wish to avoid resuming oestrogen, therapy with gabapentin, SNRI or SSRI may be considered	
Rosacea (see Chapter 91)	Neuroinflammatory mediators have been postulated to play a role in the flushing associated with rosacea. Genes involved in vasoregulation and neurogenic inflammation are upregulated in rosacea patients [37]. Dysregulation of TRPV channels, which are expressed by both neuronal and non-neuronal cells, have been shown to have enhanced gene expression in rosacea [38]. Findings from a study assessing cutaneous vascular responses to acetylcholine in rosacea patients suggest that activation of nociceptive nerve fibres contributes to skin sensitivity in these patients, and that axon reflexes augment flushing in patients with the most severe symptoms [18]	Subgroup – longstanding predisposition to frequent flushing with specific triggers such as spicy food, moving from a cold to warm environment, etc. Not all patients with rosacea flush	May be associated telangiectasia, fixed facial erythema, papules and pustules, phymatous and ocular rosacea, signs of photodamage, and with increased skin sensitivity	Occasionally a skin biopsy may be required to rule out other causes of facial erythema	Avoidance of exacerbants Skin care regime Daily application of sunblock Topical brimonidine	

Carcinoid syndrome					
Carcinoid tumours arise from enterochromaffin cells; they can release many different polypeptides (e.g. kallikrein, bradykinin), biogenic amines (e.g. serotonin, histamine) and prostaglandins CS is typically caused by metastatic tumours of the *midgut* (jejunum, ileum, appendix, ascending colon). Hepatic metastases result in downstream release of tumour products, thereby bypassing the portal circulation and avoiding hepatic metabolism. CS due to *foregut* tumours (bronchial, gastric, duodenum, thymus) is less common. However, as their products are released directly into the systemic circulation, these tumours can result in CS in the absence of metastases. *Hindgut* tumours (distal colon, rectum, genitourinary) are usually hormonally inactive and therefore rarely cause CS The main secretory products of carcinoid tumours are serotonin, histamine, tachykinins, kallikrein and prostaglandins. *Serotonin* does not cause flushing, but results in increased intestinal secretion and motility (diarrhoea), and increased fibroblast growth (cardiac valvular fibrosis) *Histamine* can be produced by primary gastric carcinoids, and causes atypical flushing and pruritus *Bradykinin* (a product of kallikrein cleavage action) is a potent vasodilator and may result in flushing in some carcinoid patients. *Prostaglandins E and F* stimulate intestinal motility and fluid secretion in the normal gastrointestinal tract Some carcinoid tumours secrete *tachykinins (substance P, neurokinin A, neuropeptide K)* which may contribute to flushing and diarrhoea	The flush associated with classic CS (due to midgut carcinoids) begins suddenly and lasts from 30 s up to 30 min. The face, neck and upper chest may flush red to violaceous, with an associated mild burning sensation. Severe flushes are accompanied by hypotension and tachycardia. As the disease progresses, the episodes may last longer and the flushing may be more diffuse and cyanotic The flushes associated with gastric carcinoid tumours are atypical, and tend to be red-brown, patchy, sharply demarcated, with bizarre gyrate or serpiginous patterns that may resolve centrally; usually associated with an intense pruritus In patients with the bronchial carcinoid variant, the flushes can be very severe and prolonged, lasting hours to days. Atypical flushing may be associated with tremor, disorientation, lacrimation, salivation, oedema (including periorbitally) Most flushing episodes occur spontaneously, but they may be provoked by eating, drinking alcohol, defaecation, emotional events, palpation of the liver, and anaesthesia	Flushing is the most common symptom (occurring in 85% of patients with CS). Associated symptoms include secretory diarrhoea, hypotension, tachycardia, abdominal cramping, sweating and bronchospasm. As the disease progresses, valvular heart disease (right-sided fibrosis, tricuspid and pulmonary valves), venous telangiectasia, leonine facies and pellagra (diversion of dietary tryptophan for the increased production of serotonin) may occur	*24-h urinary excretion of 5-HIAA* (5-HIAA is the end product of serotonin metabolism; generally not useful in foregut and hindgut tumours, as these cannot convert 5-HT to serotonin) *Urinary serotonin* (may be of value in the rare patient with a foregut carcinoid in whom CS is suspected; DOPA decarboxylase in the renal parenchyma converts 5-HTP to serotonin) *Chromogranin A* (appropriate tumour marker for patients with an established diagnosis in order to assess disease progression, response to therapy or recurrence after surgical resection) *Imaging studies of* abdomen and pelvis; CT, MRI and SRS (octreoscans) are the primary imaging modalities used to identify carcinoid tumours *Echocardiogram* for patients with clinical evidence of carcinoid heart disease or if major surgery is being planned	*Somatostatin analogues* (e.g. *octreotide*) provide effective symptomatic control. Prophylactic preoperative subcutaneous or intravenous administration of octreotide is recommended for patients with CS undergoing surgery for metastatic disease *Hepatic resection* for patients with liver metastases; can provide long-term symptomatic relief of CS symptoms; useful in resectable disease, benefits need to be weighed in unresectable disease	Carcinoid crisis is a life-threatening form of CS that results from the release of an overwhelming amount of biologically active tumour products; it may be triggered by tumour manipulation (e.g. biopsy, surgery) or by anaesthesia. It is less commonly reported after chemotherapy, hepatic arterial embolization or radionuclide therapy, mostly in patients with markedly elevated serum serotonin or urine 5-HIAA

(Continued)

PART 9: VASCULAR

PART 9: VASCULAR

Table 106.1 Disorders associated with flushing (*Continued*)

Disease	Pathogenesis of flush	Characteristics of flush	Associated symptoms and signs	Investigations	Management of flush	Notes
Mastocytosis (see Chapter 46)	Mast cell accumulation in at least one tissue with both chronic and episodic mast cell mediator release; mediators that may cause increased vasopermeability and vasodilatation include histamine, cysteinyl leukotrienes (LTC4, LTD4, LTE4), prostaglandins (PGD2) and platelet-activating factor	Sudden onset; features may be similar to that of an allergic or anaphylactic reaction; often with identifiable triggers such as narcotics, opioids, non-steroidal anti-inflammatory drugs (NSAIDs), systemic anaesthesia, exercise, massage, alcohol, infection, *Hymenoptera* stings	Skin findings: urticaria pigmentosa, diffuse cutaneous mastocytosis, isolated mastocytoma(s), or telangiectasias (TMEP) Associated pruritus, blister formation, Darier sign Acute release of mediators: pruritus, hypotension, syncope, abdominal pain, nausea, vomiting, diarrhoea, fatigue, headache, collapse Chronic mediator release: cachexia, chronic gastrointestinal symptoms, diffuse musculoskeletal pains, tissue remodelling and organ fibrosis; weight loss, neuropsychiatric symptoms; lymphadenopathy, splenomegaly, anaemia, eosinophilia, osteopaenia, osteoporosis	Skin biopsy (with histopathological staining with Giemsa and/or immunohistochemical staining for tryptase and c-kit) for cutaneous mastocytosis; this will not provide information about systemic involvement but may help to classify cutaneous disease Complete blood count with differential Liver function tests (including serum aminotransferases and alkaline phosphatase) Serum tryptase Metabolites of mast cell activation (24-h urine for N-methyl histamine and 11-β-prostaglandin F2) may be measured Bone marrow biopsy and aspiration	*Avoidance of triggers* *Antihistamines:* H₁ antihistamines (e.g. cetirizine, fexofenadine, hydroxyzine, doxepin) alone may be ineffective; combined blockade of H₁ and H₂ receptors prevents the vasodilatory effects of histamine *Ketotifen* has been reported to have both mast cell stabilizing and H₁ antihistamine properties, but is sedating *Aspirin* (up to 650 mg twice daily) may be used to control flushing, but should be used with extreme caution and only in patients known to tolerate NSAIDs *Cromolyn* *Steroids* (oral and topical) *Psoralen and ultraviolet A* therapy for urticaria pigmentosa *Laser therapy* for TMEP *Epinephrine autoinjector* (e.g. Anapen®) for patients with anaphylaxis	Patients with evidence of systemic mastocytosis, or those with unexplained anaphylaxis or hypotension, should be referred to the appropriate specialties for further investigation and management
Phaeochromocytoma	Catecholamine-secreting tumours that arise from chromaffin cells of the adrenal medulla; release of catecholamines (epinephrine, norepinephrine, dopamine) and other vasomediators (VIP, calcitonin gene-related peptide, adrenomedullin) episodically into the systemic circulation	Flushing of the face, neck, chest and trunk; paroxysmal attacks last 15 min to hours; usually occur spontaneously but may be triggered by deep abdominal palpation, diagnostic procedures (e.g. colonoscopy), induction of anaesthesia, surgery, with certain foods or beverages containing tyramine or with certain drugs (e.g. MAO inhibitors)	Hypertension (60% have sustained hypertension; 40% experience hypertension only during attacks); tachycardia; headaches, hyperhidrosis, piloerection; palpitations, a sense of impending doom,	24-h urine fractionated catecholamines and metanephrines Plasma fractionated metanephrines Radiological tests Biochemical confirmation of the diagnosis should be followed by radiological evaluation to locate the tumour. About 10% are extra-adrenal, but 95% are within the abdomen and pelvis	Avoid precipitants (e.g. glucagon, histamine, metoclopramide) Combined α- and β-adrenergic blockade to control blood pressure and prevent intraoperative hypertensive crises Adrenalectomy	Check for cutaneous stigmata of neurofibromatosis

	Pathophysiology	Clinical presentation	Investigation	Management
		chest pain or abdominal pain associated with nausea and vomiting, pallor, weakness and collapse	*CT/MRI* *MIBG scintigraphy.* If abdominal and pelvic CT or MRI is negative in the presence of clinical and biochemical evidence of phaeochromocytoma, the diagnosis should be reconsidered. If it is still likely, then 123-I-MIBG scintigraphy may be done. *FDG-PET* more sensitive than 123-I-MIBG and CT/MRI for detection of metastatic disease	
Anaphylaxis	Mast cell and basophil vasoactive mediators release	Urticaria, angio-oedema, hypotension, bronchospasm, rhinitis, chest pain, headache, tachycardia, collapse / Typically within minutes of exposure to trigger (if known); rarely presents with flushing alone	Plasma histamine and tryptase C4, C1, C1q levels Test for C1 esterase inhibitor deficiency	During the anaphylactic episode, either IV or IM epinephrine (the latter via EpiPen® (0.3 mg) or 0.3–0.5 mL of 1 : 1000 dilution) should be administered into either the anterolateral thigh muscles or the deltoid muscle every 5 min, as necessary, to control blood pressure and symptoms
Acute alcohol sensitivity	ADH2, ALDH2 and CYP2E1 are important enzymes for the catalysis of the conversion of ethanol to acetaldehyde and to acetate in humans. Genetic polymorphisms have been reported in these enzymes. Between 40 and 80% of several Asian groups have been found to be deficient in ALDH2. The accumulation of acetaldehyde following the ingestion of alcohol triggers catecholamine release from the adrenal medulla and sympathetic nerves	Palpitations, headache, vomiting and sweating / Unpleasant sensation following alcohol ingestion	An ethanol patch test may be a useful initial investigation	Alcohol avoidance / Research suggests that polymorphisms in alcohol dehydrogenase activity may increase an individual's susceptibility to oesophageal and oropharyngeal cancer

PART 9: VASCULAR

5-HT, 5-hydroxytryptamine; 5-HTP, 5-hydroxytryptophan; ADH2, alcohol dehydrogenase; ADH2, alcohol dehydrogenase-2; ALDH2, aldehyde dehydrogenase-2; AMH, anti-Müllerian hormone; CS, carcinoid syndrome; CT, computed tomography; CYP2E1, cytochrome P450 2E1; DOPA, dihydroxyphenylalanine; FDG-PET, 18-fluoro-deoxyglucose positron emission tomography; FSH, follicle-stimulating hormone; HIAA, 5-hydroxyindoleacetic acid; MAO, monoamine oxidase; MIBG, metaiodobenzylguanidine; MRI, magnetic resonance imaging; NSAIDs, non-steroidal anti-inflammatory drugs; SNRI, serotonin–norepinephrine reuptake inhibitor; SRS, somatostatin receptor scintigraphy; SSRI, selective serotonin reuptake inhibitor; TMEP, telangiectasia macularis eruptiva perstans; TRPV, transient receptor potential ion channels of vanilloid type; VIP, vasoactive intestinal polypeptide.

Table 106.2 Paediatric flushing. Many of the systemic diseases outlined in Box 106.3 may also apply to the paediatric population. However, this table outlines disorders which may be of particular relevance in children.

Pyrexia	–
Teething	Parents and professionals frequently attribute symptoms such as irritability, increased salivation and flushed cheeks to the eruption of primary teeth in infants. Little evidence exists to support these observations [31]
Mastocytosis	See Table 106.1
Frey syndrome/ gustatory hyperhidrosis	Also known as auriculotemporal nerve syndrome, gustatory sweating results from a disruption of the auriculotemporal nerve pathways. Damage to the nerve may cause a misdirected regrowth that results in parasympathetic innervation of sympathetic receptors and, therefore, facial sweating and flushing with gustatory stimulation [32]
Raised intracranial pressure	Neurological deterioration associated with flushing involving either upper chest, face or arms in children has been reported. The flush typically lasts 5–15 min, and dissipates quickly. The flushing reaction is postulated to be a centrally mediated response to sudden elevations in intracranial pressure [33]
Nephropathic cystinosis	Children with this lysosomal storage disorder display an inability to produce normal volumes of sweat. This deficiency results in heat intolerance and avoidance, flushing, hyperthermia and vomiting in small children [34]
Oesophageal atresia	Unilateral facial flushing has been reported following surgical repair of oesophageal atresia [35]
Harlequin colour change	A benign phenomenon, presenting as well-demarcated unilateral transient erythema on the dependent side in a neonate. The flush last from 30 s to 20 min. It presents in the first 3 weeks of life, usually on days 2–5. It is believed to be caused by temporary imbalance in the tone of cutaneous blood vessels secondary to hypothalamic immaturity [36]

patients who experience flushing there may be associated systemic complaints, which warrant further investigation. Patients with carcinoid syndrome can experience associated diarrhoea and wheezing. Flushing associated with itch can be seen in patients with mastocytosis. Exertional flushing can sometimes be seen in patients with cholinergic urticaria. Flushing after a warm bath is occasionally reported in patients with polycythaemia. Flushing localized to the nose has been reported as a prodrome to migraine attacks. Men following surgery for prostate cancer may experience postsurgical flushing, particularly if they receive postsurgical oestrogen therapy. The 'dumping syndrome flush' is a combination of flushing, tachycardia and sweating experienced by some patients after gastric surgery.

Investigations

A thorough history, with particular emphasis on precipitating or exacerbating factors, drug usage and food intake, and a detailed

review of systemic symptoms including queries relating to anxiety and stress, is essential in the evaluation of an individual who presents with a complaint of excessive flushing. It may be useful for the patient to keep a record of flushing episodes, detailing possible triggers and associated symptoms such as headache, abdominal pain, wheeze, diarrhoea or chest pain. Patients who flush after alcohol intake can be tested by an ethanol patch test. In individuals deficient of the enzyme alcohol dehydrogenase an area of erythema develops in the tested skin.

If an underlying systemic disorder is suspected, a detailed history and clinical examination should help to direct further workup. Initial investigations should include a full blood count, renal, liver profiles, urinalysis, 24 h urine for 5-hydroxyindoleacetic acid (5-HIAA) (carcinoid syndrome), 24 h urinary fractionated metanephrines (phaeochromocytoma), serum tryptase, 24 h urine histamine and bone marrow examination (mastocytosis). Radiological imaging, when required, should be dictated by the underlying working diagnosis (see Table 106.1 and Figure 106.2).

Management

The management of the *flushing* patient should be tailored to the individual and guided by the underlying cause (see Table 106.1 and Figure 106.3). However, most flushing patients will benefit from general guidance on managing the flush, such as identification of potential triggering factors (e.g. work environment, temperature, foods, alcohol, drugs) and their avoidance; information on histamine-releasing foods and medication; and advice on cooling techniques and temperature regulation (see Figure 106.3).

The management of *blushing* should encompass a comprehensive explanation of the psychosocial nature of the problem and its relationship to anxiety as well as reassurance of the lack of disease association and the possibility of spontaneous improvement in younger patients with time. When blushing is associated with social withdrawal or excessive anxiety, consider referral for psychological counselling and cognitive behavioural therapy. Biofeedback techniques may be useful in these patients.

Topical α-adrenoreceptor agonists, which produce cutaneous vasoconstriction, have shown early promising results in the treatment of flushing associated with rosacea. Brimonidine tartrate is a highly selective α_2-adrenoreceptor agonist used in ophthalmic solution for the treatment of open-angle glaucoma. Topical brimonidine tartrate gel 0.5% has been shown in controlled prospective randomized clinical trials to reduce facial erythema after single and repeated once-daily applications. No major adverse events were noted in this trial, and tolerability was good [21]. Case reports of other α-adrenoreceptor agonists (e.g. oxymetazoline 0.05% solution, and xylometazoline 0.05% solution; applied to the skin in their nasal decongestant formulations) showed a reduction of facial erythema over several hours in patients with erythematotelangiectatic rosacea [22,23].

Low-dose β-blocker therapy may be useful in some patients with either flushing or blushing. Nonselective β-blockers decrease sympathetic activity, thereby resulting in vasoconstriction. In addition, their anxiolytic effects may reduce the anxiety that contributes to

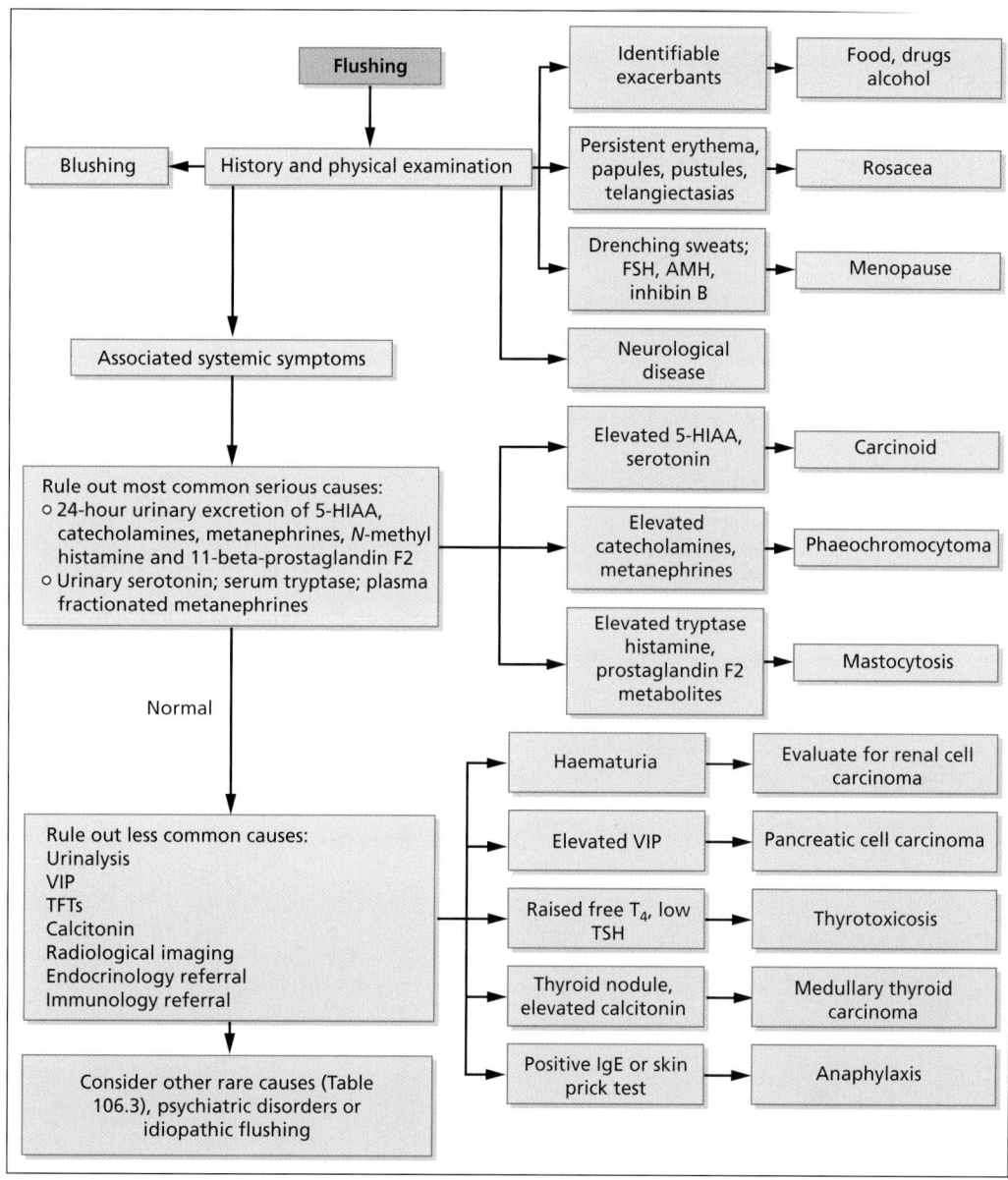

Figure 106.2 Investigations algorithm [**10**].

blushing in some of these patients. Both propranolol (30–120 mg/ day) and carvedilol (titrated from 3.25 mg three times a day to 25 mg/day) have been shown to reduce flushing episodes in patients with rosacea [24,25].

Other drugs reported to be helpful in certain subgroups include aspirin [26], antihistamines [27] and clonidine [28]. The evidence of efficacy of these medications is lacking, and the potential toxicity of these agents should be considered before prescribing.

Laser techniques such as pulsed dye laser, intense pulsed light and potassium-titanyl-phosphate laser may be useful for the treatment of telangiectasia and erythema. Endoscopic transthoracic sympathectomy has been shown to be helpful in some patients with intractable flushing or blushing, but long-term side effects such as compensatory hyperhidrosis are common, and more serious complications may occasionally occur [29]. Botulinum toxin A, which acts presynaptically to abolish the release of all transmitters selectively from cholinergic nerves, has been used with success to treat neck and anterior chest wall flushing [30].

Complications

Patients who are subject to frequent blushing may begin to avoid situations in work or social interactions that they associate with triggering the skin reaction. This may lead to social reclusion and in severe cases clinical depression and suicide risk. Patients who experience severe flushing reactions can experience profound tiredness and lethargy afterwards. Women who experience postmenopausal flushing often complain of sleep disturbance and debilitating fatigue.

Prognosis

Young patients who present with frequent blushing often show a mild degree of social phobia and these patients tend to improve spontaneously with age. If the blushing persists after the midtwenties the likelihood of spontaneous improvement seems to

PART 9: VASCULAR

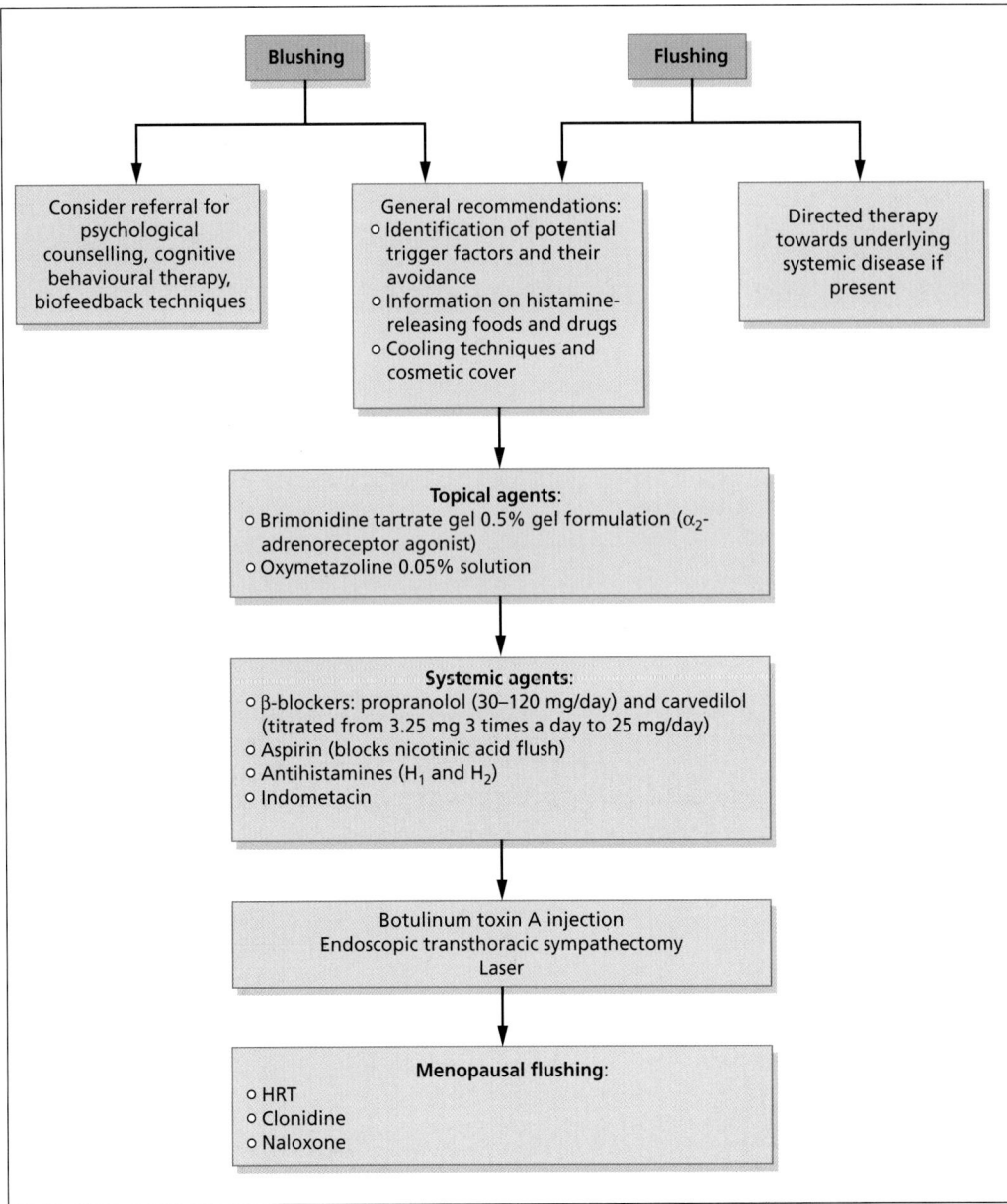

Figure 106.3 Management algorithm.

diminish. Patients with flushing reactions tend to have a chronic course if the cause is undetermined or if treatment is ineffective.

Key references

The full list of references can be found in the online version at www.rooksdermatology.com.

1 Rowell LB. Reflex control of the cutaneous vasculature. *J Invest Dermatol* 1977;69(1):154–66.

2 Johnson JM, Kellogg DL Jr. Thermoregulatory and thermal control in the human cutaneous circulation. *Front Biosci* 2010;S2:825–53.

6 Kellogg DL Jr, Zhao JL, Wu Y, Johnson JM. VIP/PACAP receptor mediation of cutaneous active vasodilation during heat stress in humans. *J Appl Physiol* 2010;109:95–100.

9 Charkoudian N. Mechanisms and modifiers of reflex induced cutaneous vasodilation and vasoconstriction in humans. *J Appl Physiol* 2010;109:1221–8.

10 Izikson L, English JC 3rd, Zirwas MJ. The flushing patient: differential diagnosis, workup, and treatment. *J Am Acad Dermatol* 2006;55(2):193–208.

11 Powell FC. *Rosacea Diagnosis and Management*, 1st edn. New York: Informa Healthcare, 2009.

12 Crozier WR, de Jong PJ. *The Psychological Significance of the Blush*. Cambridge: Cambridge University Press, 2013.

13 Drummond PD, Lazaroo D. The effect of facial blood flow on ratings of blushing and negative affect during an embarrassing task: preliminary findings. *J Anxiety Disord* 2012;26:305–10.

17 Drummond PD, Su D. The relationship between blushing propensity, social anxiety and facial blood flow during embarrassment. *Cogn. Emot.* 2012;26:561–7.

21 Fowler J, Jackson M, Moore A. Efficacy and safety of once-daily topical brimonidine tartrate gel 0.5% for the treatment of moderate to severe facial erythema of rosacea: results of two randomized, double-blind, vehicle-controlled pivotal studies. *J Drugs Dermatol* 2013;12:650–6.

PART 10
Skin Disorders Associated with Specific Sites, Sex and Age

CHAPTER 107

Dermatoses of the Scalp

Paul Farrant[1], Megan Mowbray[2] and Rodney D. Sinclair[3]

[1]Brighton and Sussex University Hospitals, Brighton, UK
[2]Department of Dermatology, Queen Margaret Hospital, NHS Fife, Dunfermline, UK
[3]University of Melbourne, Melbourne; Epworth Healthcare, Richmond, Victoria; and Sinclair Dermatology, Research and Clinical Trials Centre, Melbourne, Australia

SCALING DISORDERS OF THE SCALP

Seborrhoeic dermatitis

Introduction and general description

Seborrhoeic dermatitis is an inflammatory condition of the skin that affects the scalp, face, groin and chest (see Chapter 40). On the scalp there is a range of presentations from fine, dry flakes of skin or dandruff (previously referred to as pityriasis capitis) to thicker, greasy, yellow scales associated with an underlying inflammation of the scalp. The role of infective agents has been debated over the last century with the emerging discoveries of populations of yeast on the scalp and response to anti-yeast treatments providing some evidence of a link.

Epidemiology

Seborrhoeic dermatitis of infancy is probably a distinctive condition and may be a marker of the atopic state (discussed below). For others, the condition becomes more prevalent from puberty, probably driven by an increase in androgens and an increase in sebum production.

At the mild end of the spectrum, seborrheic dermatitis is a very common condition, with around 50% of 20-year-old white males having evidence of dandruff. Inflammatory seborrhoeic dermatitis affects 1–3% of immunocompetent adults [1]. There is a higher prevalence in patients with HIV infection and in this clinical situation the condition is often more severe and harder to treat. There is also an increased prevalence in Parkinson disease, epilepsy and spinal cord injury.

Clinical features

At one end of the spectrum, seborrhoeic dermatitis consists of fine, small, white or grey scales, which may be diffuse or localized in patches (Figure 107.1). Seborrhoea may bind the scale to produce more adherent mounds of yellowish, greasy scales. Under the scale the scalp is often erythematous and moist. There may be associated perifollicular erythema. As well as the scalp, seborrhoeic dermatitis commonly involves the eyebrows, naso-labial folds, chest and groins.

Differential diagnosis

The main differentials of seborrhoeic dermatitis are scalp psoriasis, tinea capitis and lichen simplex chronicus. Psoriasis is often characterized by silvery scales with well-demarcated erythema, often involving the hair line. There may be some overlap of clinical features, which has led to the term 'sebo-psoriasis'. Dermoscopy has been reported as a diagnostic tool to help differentiate these two conditions, with arborizing vessels being a feature of seborrhoeic dermatitis and red dots, globules and twisted red loops being features

PART 10: SITES, SEX, AGE

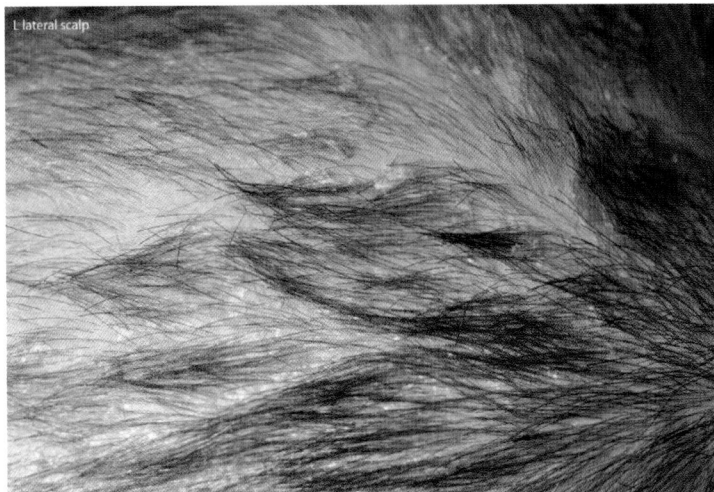

Figure 107.1 Seborrhoeic dermatitis of the scalp.

of scalp psoriasis [2]. Tinea capitis may be confused with seborrhoeic dermatitis, especially tinea due to *Trichophyton* species and one should have a low threshold for taking skin scrapings. Lichen simplex most typically involves the occiput and can be differentiated by itch, which is the characteristic feature of this condition.

Management

All treatments are aimed at control and not cure, and it is important that patients are made aware of this at the outset. Over-the-counter preparations include shampoos that are aimed at dandruff control; the active ingredients in these agents are zinc pyrithione, selenium sulphide, ciclopirox and ketoconazole. Coal tar shampoos can also be helpful in seborrheic dermatitis but are less cosmetically acceptable to patients. Medicated shampoos need to be used at least twice weekly for maintenance therapy to limit relapse.

The more inflammatory end of the seborrhoeic dermatitis spectrum requires the addition of an anti-inflammatory agent, typically a corticosteroid. Topical corticosteroids for scalp use are available in gels, lotions, mousses and shampoos. These should be used for a short period, on an intermittent basis, to avoid side effects.

Systemic oral antifungals agents such as ketoconazole, itraconazole and terbinafine should be reserved for severe unresponsive refractory cases. The evidence for efficacy of systemic antifungals agents is poor [3].

Seborrhoeic dermatitis of infancy

Infantile seborrhoeic dermatitis or 'cradle cap' presents with greasy, yellow scales over the vertex of the newborn. It is often self-limiting and improves within the first year of life for the majority. It is regarded as a manifestation of the atopic state.

Psoriasis

Introduction and general description

Psoriasis is a common inflammatory skin disease that has a particular predilection for the scalp. It is not uncommon for the scalp to be the first site of involvement in psoriasis. The epidemiology, aetiology and pathology are all discussed in Chapter 35. The clinical features and treatment of scalp psoriasis are discussed here.

Epidemiology

Psoriasis affects 2–5% of the population and around 80% of psoriasis sufferers will have scalp involvement at some point.

Pathophysiology

In patients complaining of hair loss associated with psoriasis, scalp biopsies frequently show an increase in catagen and telogen hairs when viewed horizontally. Hair follicles often become miniaturized and there is atrophy of the sebaceous glands.

Clinical features

Psoriasis of the scalp is characterized by well-demarcated plaques, often erythematous in nature, covered in silvery thick scales (Figure 107.2). The scales may become matted together

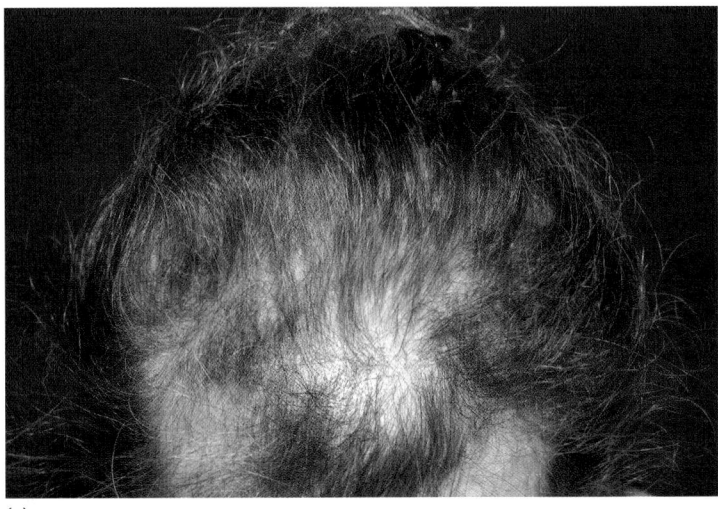

(a)

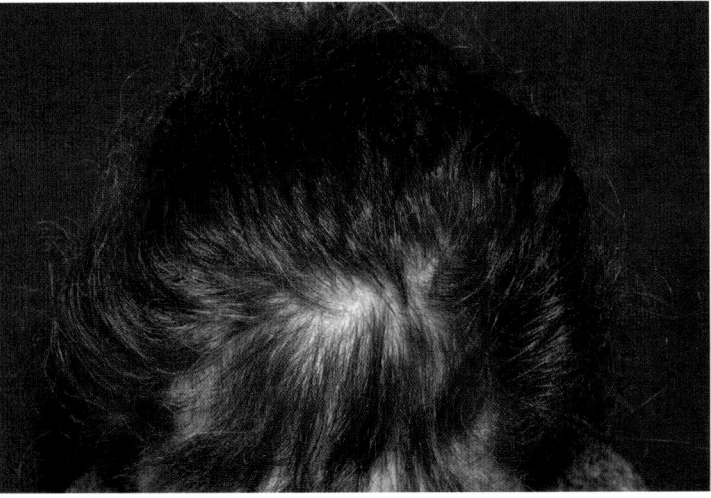

(b)

Figure 107.2 Scalp psoriasis with hair loss. (a) Psoriatic alopecia. (b) Hair regrowth after active management of scalp psoriasis.

to form thickened plaques. Scalp psoriasis can be localized in patches or more diffuse throughout the scalp and occasionally covers the entire scalp. Psoriasis commonly involves the hair line, extending 1–2 cm beyond the hair line onto the forehead or neck. However, the earliest changes may be more subtle with diffuse scaling without specific features, and a diagnosis may only be reached from the involvement of other sites or from a strong family history.

In erythrodermic psoriasis, scalp involvement may lead to marked hair loss. Scalp psoriasis is associated with an increase of hairs in the telogen phase and a degree of hair loss is not uncommon, but often under-recognized. Treatment of the psoriasis often leads to hair regrowth but scarring hair loss associated with psoriasis has been described [1].

Differential diagnosis
The main differential is seborrhoeic dermatitis, as discussed in the previous section. Examination of other body sites often provides clues to the true diagnosis but sometimes the conditions cannot be distinguished. Occasionally, discrete areas of discoid lupus can mimic psoriasis and a solitary scaly plaque on a bald scalp may represent Bowen disease.

Management
There are similarities with the management of scalp psoriasis and body psoriasis but important differences too. The main function of hair in today's society is largely cosmetic and treatments that impact on appearance are rarely tolerated. Creams and ointments that are messy, sticky and greasy need to be replaced with more suitable vehicles for hair-bearing skin such as gels, lotions, mousses or shampoo formulations. Counselling patients about long-term goals and the need for maintenance therapy is important, as the condition is controlled by treatment and not cured. Hair can provide a framework for scales to adhere to so that plaques become thickened and produce a barrier to the absorption of topical treatments. In severe cases of scalp psoriasis, removing these thickened plaques through physical means is an essential first step before the addition of any anti-inflammatory agent.

Medicated shampoos are commonly used in the management of scalp psoriasis and these often contain coal tar, which has mild anti-inflammatory properties and can be soothing for patients with itch. Other active ingredients may include cade oil, arachis oil, salicylic acid, coconut oil and urea. The addition of conditioners to scalp preparations may make them more acceptable to patients. Antidandruff shampoos may also be helpful as part of a regular routine.

In patients that have thickened plaques, efforts should be made to remove the scale. Scale can be softened with the use of oils (e.g. arachis or olive), petroleum-based emollients or pomades containing coal tar, salicylic acid or cade oils. These should be left on for several hours or overnight. Once the scale has been softened, it can be gently combed out, using a blunt tooth plastic comb, avoiding any trauma to the underlying scalp, which may exacerbate psoriasis due to koebnerization. Assistance from a specialist nurse or friend or carer is often needed. If preparations are left on overnight an ordinary shampoo should be applied to the scalp whilst the hair is still dry, rubbed in to produce an emulsion, and then the hair should be wetted and rinsed. For severe cases this procedure may need to be repeated for several days to make sufficient progress before proceeding to anti-inflammatory preparations.

In milder cases of psoriasis or in severe cases that have been de-scaled, treatment is then focused on the underlying psoriasis. Vitamin D analogues, topical corticosteroids and combination products containing both, or topical steroid and additional ingredients such as salicylic acid, are the mainstay of treatment. Very potent or potent topical steroids are superior to vitamin D analogues, while vitamin D and steroid combinations are superior to potent steroid monotherapy [2]. The atrophic potential of corticosteroid treatments for scalp psoriasis remains unclear but has been described in trials investigating clobetasol propionate [3]. Topical corticosteroid or combination products often need to be used frequently at the outset, for example daily for up to a month, and then reduced to twice weekly or so for maintenance. It is important that patients are aware of the different formulations and efforts made to select the most appropriate vehicle. Newer formulations in the form of gels, foams and shampoos are targeted at addressing patient dissatisfaction of older treatments, with the aim of improving compliance [4].

In resistant cases of scalp psoriasis it may be necessary to use systemic agents to control the condition. Ciclosporin used short term can be particularly effective, especially if there is marked hair loss associated with the psoriasis. Ultraviolet therapy is less useful since the hair coverage acts as a barrier to UV light, but excimer laser therapy can be effective for hair line psoriasis in resistant cases [5].

Pityriasis amiantacea

Introduction and general description
Pityriasis amiantacea refers to a scaling pattern on the scalp where the scales overlap like tiles on a roof. The matted scale is attached to the underlying hair shafts. The condition may be localized and confined to a small patch or widespread involving the entire scalp, creating a skull cap-type appearance of scale and crust. Lifting up the scale often results in hairs coming away, revealing a moist erythematous scalp. Hairs usually regrow if the underlying condition is treated. Some consider pityriasis amiantacea to be a form of severe psoriasis whilst others consider this a pattern that can be attributable to a range of causes such as seborrhoeic dermatitis, eczema, lichen simplex and psoriasis.

Pathophysiology
Biopsies from 18 patients were examined by Knight [1]. The most consistent findings were spongiosis, parakeratosis, migration of lymphocytes into the epidermis and a variable degree of acanthosis. The essential features responsible for the scaling are diffuse hyperkeratosis and parakeratosis together with follicular keratosis, which surrounds each hair with a sheath of horn.

PART 10: SITES, SEX, AGE

Management

Scale should be gently removed as described in the treatment of scalp psoriasis. Attention should then turn to treating the underlying condition, which typically involves the use of topical corticosteroids in an appropriate vehicle.

Contact dermatitis

Introduction and general description

Contact dermatitis of the scalp is an inflammatory condition resulting from an external agent and can be separated into irritant (non-immunogenic) or allergic (immunogenic, typically type IV). The scalp is surprisingly resistant to contact dermatitis and this may be due to either a thickened stratum corneum acting as a barrier or impaired antigen presentation from Langerhans cells. Most contact dermatitis from products used on the scalp present in the surrounding skin, such as the hair line, or on the hands of those that apply them, for example hand dermatitis in hair dressers.

Irritant contact dermatitis. The commonest causes of an irritant dermatitis are bleaches, thioglycolates (permanent waving solutions) and heat (blow drying) (see Chapter 129). Shampoos may dry the scalp but the majority of chemicals are washed off after a short contact period. Irritant dermatitis may present on the scalp with burning, soreness or tightness within a short period of time of the contact. There may be associated erythema, oedema and exudation.

Allergic contact dermatitis. Causes include permanent hair dyes, bleaches, permanent waving solutions, hair straighteners and relaxers (see Chapter 128). Contact allergic dermatitis may be iatrogenic and deliberate, such as with the use of diphencyprone in alopecia areata treatment.

Mangement

Contact dermatitis should be managed through identification and elimination of the offending contact irritant/allergen and the use of topical corticosteroids during the acute phase. Hair care practices may need to be altered.

Lichen simplex chronicus

Introduction and general description

Lichen simplex chronicus refers to a localized thickening of skin that results from chronic rubbing and scratching. The dermatoglyphics of the skin are often accentuated. The nape of the neck is frequently affected and can mimic psoriasis.

Epidemiology

Lichen simplex chronicus is rare before puberty and has a peak incidence between 30 and 50 years of age, with women being more commonly affected than men.

Pathophysiology

Typical histological features include hyperkeratosis and acanthosis with localized areas of both parakeratosis and spongiosis.

Clinical features

Lichen simplex chronicus can result from any underlying cause of itch that leads to scratching and rubbing. An underlying cause though may not be identified and it falls within the spectrum of neurodermatitis. The main symptom is itch and the most commonly associated diseases at this site are atopic eczema, seborrhoeic dermatitis and psoriasis.

Management

Management of lichen simplex chronicus requires education of the patient so that they have insight to the cause of the problem; any psychological aspect will need to be addressed. Efforts to break the itch–scratch cycle include treatment to manage the itch, which often involves potent or super-potent topical corticosteroids or intralesional corticosteroids. Occlusion of the affected area after the application of corticosteroid may be beneficial but is difficult to achieve on the scalp. Cognitive behavioural therapy and, in particular, habit reversal can be used in motivated subjects.

Radiodermatitis

Introduction and general description

After the discovery of X-rays in 1895 there were a number of applications for their use in the early 20th century in the management of hair-related problems. X-rays were advocated as a treatment for hirsutism and then subsequently as a treatment for scalp ringworm and this continued until the discovery of griseofulvin in 1958, with an estimated 300 000 children treated in this way. Unfortunately X-rays later were found to induce skin cancers and now their use is limited to the management of malignancy.

Pathophysiology

In chronic radiodermatitis the epidermis becomes atrophic, with a loss of hair follicles and sebaceous glands. Superficial vessels are telangiectactic but deeper vessels may be partially or completed occluded by fibrosis.

Clinical features

Patients may still present many decades after scalp X-ray treatment. Common presentations include the development of a basal cell carcinoma or a localized area of alopecia or finer hairs at the site of treatment. It is not uncommon for patients to refer to previous 'light treatment' for ringworm rather than X-ray therapy. Patients treated with modern radiotherapy for malignancy present with a well-circumscribed patch of cicatricial alopecia. These may be erythematous initially, fading to white in the chronic phase. In chronic radiodermatitis the skin is atrophic. Skin necrosis may occur and skin malignancies can develop years after treatment.

Management

There is no treatment but localized areas of alopecia, malignancy or necrosis may be amenable to surgical excision.

SECONDARY CICATRICIAL ALOPECIA

There are a number of inflammatory conditions that alter the connective tissue of the scalp and lead to secondary cicatricial alopecia. Unlike the primary cicatricial alopecias discussed in Chapters 89 and 93, the hair follicle is not the primary target of inflammation. In addition to inflammatory conditions, secondary cicatricial alopecia may result from exogenous insults (radiotherapy, burns), infections, developmental defects and neoplastic processes (Table 107.1).

Table 107.1 Causes of secondary cicatricial alopecia and developmental defects and hereditary disorders that present with hair loss.

Secondary cicatricial alopecia			
Traumatic	Radiodermatitis		
	Mechanical trauma		
	Postoperative (e.g. flap necrosis)		
	Burns		
	Accidental alopecia		
	Dermatitis artefacta		
	Traction alopecia		
	Hot comb alopecia		
Sclerosing disorders	Morphoea		
	Scleroderma		
	Lichen sclerosus		
	Sclerodermoid porphyria cutanea tarda		
	Chronic graft-versus-host disease		
Granulomatous	Sarcoidosis		
	Necrobiosis lipoidica		
	Infectious granulomas		
Infectious	Bacterial	Folliculitis	
		Carbuncle/furuncle	
	Fungal	Kerion	
		Favus	
		Tinea capitis (rarely scarring)	
	Viral	Shingles	
		Varicella	
		HIV	
	Protozoal	Leishmaniasis	
	Treponemal	Syphilis	
	Mycobacterial	Tuberculosis	
Neoplastic	Benign	Cylindroma	
		Other adnexal tumours	
	Malignant	Primary	Basal cell carcinoma
			Squamous cell carcinoma
			Cutaneous T-cell lymphoma
		Secondary	Renal, breast, lung, gastrointestinal
			Lymphoma, leukaemia
Developmental defects and hereditary disorders			
	Aplasia cutis		
	Facial hemiatrophy (Romberg syndrome)		
	Epidermal naevi		
	Hair follicle hamartomas		
	Incontinentia pigmenti		
	Focal dermal hypoplasia of Goltz		
	Porokeratosis of Mibelli		
	Ichthyosis		
	Epidermolysis bullosa		
	Polyostotic fibrous dysplasia		
	Conradi–Hünermann syndrome (chondrodysplasia punctata)		

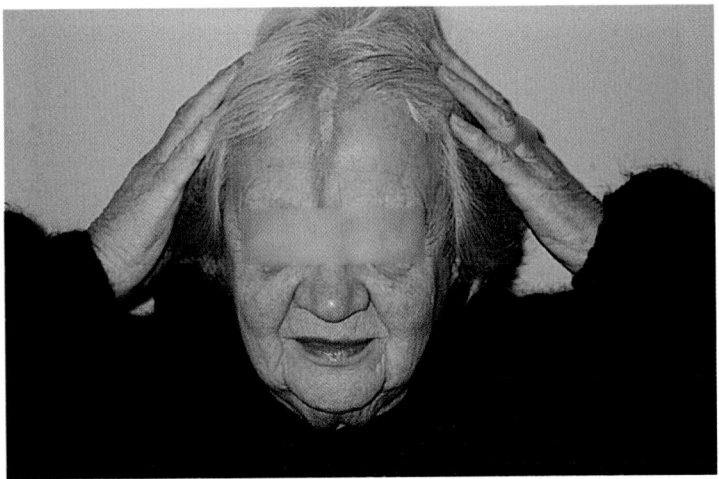

Figure 107.3 Linear morphoea (en coup de sabre). After having this lesion since adolescence, this woman later developed biopsy-proven lichen sclerosus of the vulva.

Scleroderma and morphoea

Introduction and general description

Scleroderma (see Chapter 56) can result from a number of localized or generalized connective tissue disorders. Morphoea (see Chapter 57) is a distinct autoimmune connective tissue disorder that can affect the scalp and produce localized areas of cicatricial alopecia. In early lesions of scalp morphoea, the centrifugally expanding lilac border is often obscured by hair. Well-established plaques of morphoea are white, smooth and hairless. Hair loss tends to be permanent. Lesional skin is thickened and indurated; as well as pallor there may be marginal hyperpigmentation. The lesions may be single or multiple.

Linear morphoea on the frontal scalp, also known as en coup de sabre, is characterized by a slowly progressive non-inflammatory linear alopecia (Figure 107.3). It has been suggested that lesions may follow the lines of Blaschko [1]. The line of morphoea may extend inferiorly into the cheek, nose or upper lip. Rarely it may involve the mouth and tongue.

Histological examination shows chronic inflammation of the upper and mid-follicle and prominent fibrosis [2].

The sclerodermatous phase of chronic graft-versus-host disease may involve the scalp to produce a cicatricial alopecia. Porphyria cutanea tarda may also produce scleroderma on the scalp.

Management

Potent topical steroids such as clobetasol propionate or intralesional triamcinolone may stop progression of morphoea, but systemic therapy is often required. Oral corticosteroids, penicillamine, sulfasalazine and chloroquine have all been used with varying success. Surgical excision of en coup de sabre may provide definitive treatment, although recurrences occur, especially if the lesion is enlarging at the time of excision.

Necrobiotic disorders

Both granuloma annulare and necrobiosis lipoidica have been described affecting the scalp but are uncommon presentations of these diseases. Lesions typically present as annular, red or yellow plaques, with or without atrophy and telangiectasia, and often involve the forehead and frontal scalp [1]. Necrobiotic disorders of the scalp result in secondary scarring alopecia. Distinguishing between necrobiosis lipoidica, granuloma annulare and sarcoidosis can be difficult on clinical grounds alone [2,3].

Sarcoidosis

Sarcoidosis is discussed in Chapter 98. Sarcoidosis occurs rarely in the scalp, but at this site can lead to both cicatricial and non-cicatricial alopecia (Figure 107.4) [1,2]. Initially, lesions may be papular or nodular and coalesce to form plaques, which flatten to leave areas of cicatricial alopecia showing variable degrees of erythema and scaling. These plaques may have a slightly raised annular border, but are otherwise non-descript. Affected areas may itch.

In the absence of characteristic lesions elsewhere on the skin or a known diagnosis of sarcoid, the diagnosis is made by demonstrating the characteristic naked, non-caseating, epithelioid granulomas on biopsy.

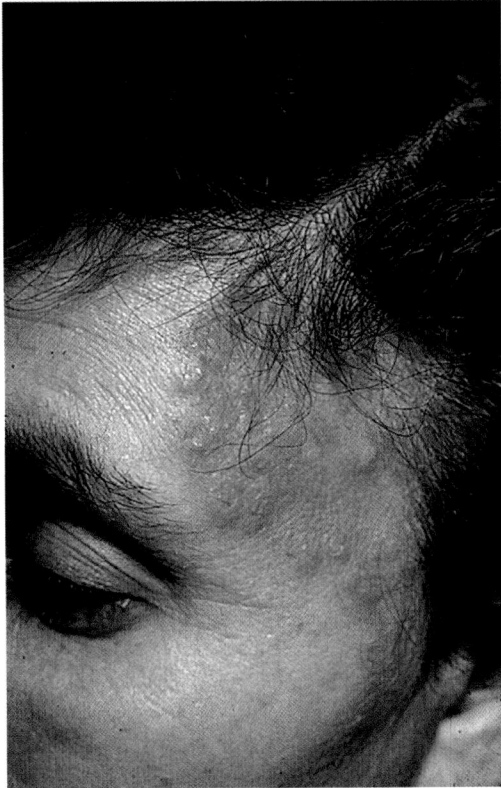

Figure 107.4 Sarcoidosis of the frontal hair line and forehead.

Topical or intralesional steroids should be tried first. Resistant cases will require systemic steroids to control the alopecia. Long-term maintenance therapy with low-dose methotrexate as a steroid-sparing agent is usually successful. The prognosis is variable, but treatment is required for at least 6 months in the majority of patients.

Follicular mucinosis

Introduction and general description
Follicular mucinosis occurs in two forms: a primary idiopathic form and a secondary form. The secondary form is most commonly associated with lymphoma, especially mycosis fungoides, but is also associated with chronic discoid lupus erythematous, angiolymphoid hyperplasia with eosinophilia, and with verruca vulgaris. The clinical features of primary and secondary cases are indistinguishable.

Epidemiology
Follicular mucinosis is a rare condition, with no reported racial predilection but is more common in males than females. Primary follicular mucinosis can occur at any age from early childhood onwards, but is most common between 10 and 40 years. Secondary follicular mucinosis tends to occur in an older age group.

Pathophysiology
All cases require a biopsy to confirm the diagnosis and to look for histological evidence of mycosis fungoides. The histology is characteristic and demonstrates degeneration of the hair follicles and sebaceous glands associated with copious mucin (hyaluronic acid), especially in the outer root sheath of the hair follicle. A variable dermal inflammatory infiltrate is present and should be studied carefully for evidence of mycosis fungoides. In many cases the features of mycosis fungoides are subtle and there is considerable overlap of features with the primary idiopathic type [1]. In such cases only regular follow-up of the patient will distinguish primary from secondary causes of follicular mucinosis.

Clinical features
Follicular mucinosis consists of grouped, sometimes itchy, follicular papules and erythematous, boggy plaques that occur mainly on the scalp and face, but can occur anywhere. Characteristically the plaques are devoid of hair; close inspection will reveal patulous follicular openings. Mucin can be expressed from the affected follicles. Sometimes the follicles are studded with horny plugs. Some lesions may ulcerate. Hair loss does not always occur and for this reason the name follicular mucinosis is preferred to the original name 'alopecia mucinosa'. Linear lesions following Blaschko's lines have been described.

In the secondary group the lesions may be widely disseminated on the trunk and limbs. Untreated, the plaques often resolve spontaneously within 2 months to 2 years, but in older patients they

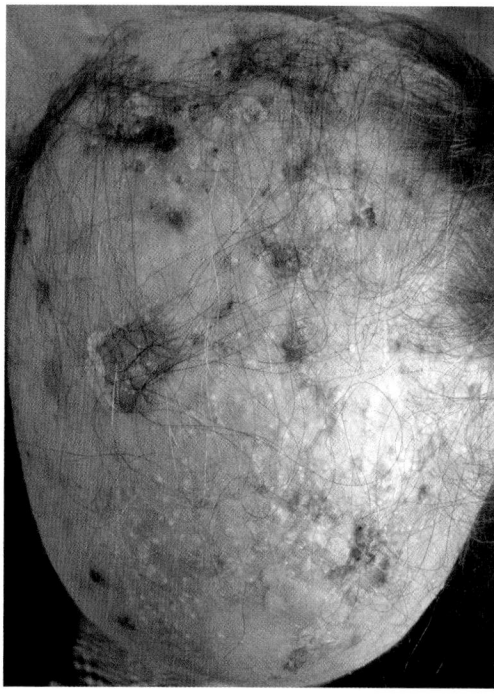

Figure 107.5 Cicatricial pemphigoid.

may be more persistent. Fifteen to 20% of chronic cases are associated with mycosis fungoides.

Management
Many cases spontaneously improve, however topical or intralesional steroids are generally effective. Superficial radiotherapy and phototherapy helps follicular mucinosis secondary to mycosis fungoides. Hydroxychloroquine has been reported as a successful treatment inducing rapid remission and hair regrowth in idiopathic follicular mucinosis [2]. Widespread pruritic lesions may benefit from low-dose systemic steroids or occasionally dapsone.

Cicatricial pemphigoid

Cicatricial pemphigoid is discussed in Chapter 50. It is an autoimmune, chronic, bullous disease that preferentially affects mucosal surfaces and heals with scarring. Cicatricial pemphigoid of the scalp is rare. It predominantly affects the elderly; women are more commonly affected than men [1,2].

Although the disease preferentially affects the ocular and/or genital mucous membranes, the skin is involved in 40–50% of cases, and skin lesions may precede the mucosal lesions by months or years [3]. The skin lesions repeatedly recur and leave scars. The favoured sites are the face and upper trunk, however the scalp is involved in approximately 10% of cases. Lesions typically present as erythematous plaques, with erosions, milia and cicatricial alopecia (Figure 107.5). Skin lesions, predominantly on the head and neck, are the major feature of the Brunsting–Perry variant.

PART 10: SITES, SEX, AGE

Mild to moderate disease may be controlled by topical therapy with super-potent topical steroids. Systemic corticosteroids and immunosuppressants may be required for more widespread and severe disease. As the condition is particularly chronic, therapy is often required long term.

Dissecting cellulitis of the scalp

Definition and nomenclature
Dissecting cellulitis manifests with a perifolliculitis of the scalp, deep and superficial abscesses in the dermis, sinus tracts formation and extensive scarring [1].

Synonyms and inclusions
- Dissecting folliculitis
- Perifolliculitis capitis abscedens

Epidemiology
Dissecting cellulitis of the scalp is rare and occurs predominantly in males aged between 18 and 40 years, and is seen most commonly in dark-skinned races. Familial cases are exceptional, as is childhood onset.

Pathophysiology
The aetiology of this inflammatory condition is unknown. Although staphylococci, streptococci and *Pseudomonas* may be cultured from various lesions, no specific causative organism has been isolated. Dissecting cellulitis is associated with hidradenitis suppurativa and acne conglobata in the follicular occlusion triad [2]. Other reported associations include pilonidal sinus and spondyloarthropathy.

Pathology [3]
Histology shows a perifolliculitis with a heavy infiltrate of lymphocytes, histiocytes and polymorphonuclear cells. Abscess formation results, and leads to destruction of the pilosebaceous follicles initially, and eventually the other cutaneous appendages. Keratin fragments induce a granulomatous reaction, with foreign body giant cells, lymphoid and plasma cells. Special stains for bacteria, fungi and mycobacteria are negative.

Clinical features
Painful, firm, skin-coloured nodules develop near the vertex of the scalp and later become softer and fluctuant (Figure 107.6). Confluent nodules form tubular ridges with an irregular cerebriform pattern, on an erythematous and oedematous background. Thin, blood-stained pus exudes from crusted sinuses, and pressure on one region of the scalp may cause discharge of pus from a neighbouring intercommunicating ridge. Cervical adenitis is present in some cases, but is more remarkable for its absence in many others. Progressive scarring and permanent alopecia occur. Characteristically, hair is lost from the summits of these inflammatory lesions

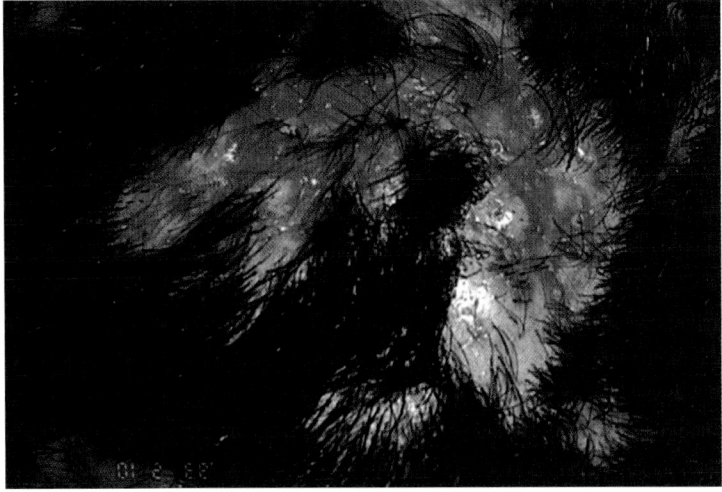

Figure 107.6 Dissecting cellulitis of the scalp. (From Dyall-Smith 1993 [7]. Reproduced with permission of Australasian Journal of Dermatology.)

and retained in the valleys. The condition is chronic, with frequent acute exacerbations.

Other disorders of the follicular occlusion triad may be present and there may be an associated pilonidal sinus (the follicular occlusion tetrad) or spondyloarthropathy. An asymmetrical peripheral and axial arthritis occurs with sacroiliitis in 73%. Activity of the arthritis parallels activity of the skin.

Differential diagnosis
Clinical differential diagnoses include kerion, pyoderma gangrenosum and erosive pustular dermatosis of the scalp.

Investigations
Culture from affected areas often grows bacterial organisms. Fungal cultures and a scalp biopsy for routine histology and direct immunofluorescence will exclude other causes of scarring alopecia.

Management
Although systemic antibiotics and topical or intralesional corticosteroids are sometimes helpful, relapses are frequent and the course is usually protracted. Isotretinoin (1 mg/kg daily), in combination with prednisolone (0.5–1 mg/kg daily) and erythromycin (500 mg four times daily), may induce a rapid remission and significant hair regrowth in areas not yet irreversibly damaged. Because the inflammation is predominantly perifollicular, a surprising amount of regrowth may occur. The antibiotics can be stopped after 4 weeks and the prednisolone gradually tailed off and replaced by topical steroids. The isotretinoin should be continued for at least 6 months, and reintroduced if the condition relapses. In recalcitrant cases, widespread excision and grafting may be considered. In older patients superficial radiotherapy has been used with success [4]. Improvement has also been noted following laser-assisted hair removal [5]. Antitumour necrosis factor biological agents have been used with success in resistant cases of dissecting cellulitis [6].

The benefit of isotretinoin in this condition contrasts with the frequent worsening seen with oral isotretinoin in folliculitis decalvans and suggests that these two conditions are distinct entities rather than different points along a spectrum of the same disease.

THICKENED SCALP DISORDERS

Cutis verticis gyrata

Introduction and general description

The term cutis verticis gyrata (CVG) describes a morphological syndrome in which there is hypertrophy and folding of the scalp skin producing a gyrate or cerebriform appearance. It can be divided into primary and secondary forms. The primary forms are subdivided into primary essential CVG, in which there are no associated features, and primary non-essential CVG, which is associated with a wide range of psychiatric, cerebral and ophthalmological abnormalities.

Primary CVG. The aetiology of primary CVG is not known. Most cases appear to be sporadic, although familial forms have been reported in the context of complex syndromes. The skin changes typically develop after puberty and usually before 30 years of age. It is more common in men, with a male to female ratio of 5 : 1. There is a strong association with learning difficulties. Akesson [1] found 47 cases (3.4%) of CVG in institutionalized subjects in Sweden, and CVG was observed in 22 out of 494 (4.5%) patients in an Italian psychiatric institution [2]. Cytogenetic analyses in the latter study showed chromosome fragile sites in nine subjects (chromosomes 9, 12 and X).

Secondary CVG. This has been described with a wide range of underlying causes. Congenital melanocytic naevi appear to be the most common but other naevoid abnormalities, such as naevus lipomatosus and connective tissue naevi, and acquired lesions such as neurofibroma, may also cause CVG. CVG has been described in association with a variety of endocrine and genetic disorders, including acromegaly, myxedema, insulin resistance, Turner syndrome and eczema. The age of onset is more variable than in primary CVG and, in the naevoid forms, it may be present at birth.

Pathophysiology

In CVG there is overgrowth of the scalp in relation to the underlying skull. In primary CVG, the histology appears normal in most cases. The histopathology in the secondary form depends on the nature of the underlying pathology.

Clinical features

Cutis verticis gyrata typically affects the vertex and occipital scalp but it may involve the entire scalp. The folds are usually arranged in an anteroposterior direction but may be transverse over the occiput. Hair density may be reduced over the convexities of the folds.

Differential diagnosis

The differential diagnosis includes pachydermoperiostosis and 'lumpy scalp syndrome'. The former is genetically determined and occurs mainly in men. It differs from CVG in several ways: (i) the scalp is folded but the skin of the face, hands and feet is also affected; (ii) the cutaneous changes are accompanied by thickening of the phalanges and long bones of the limbs; and (iii) skin involvement progresses for 10–15 years, then becomes static.

Management

Investigations are aimed at identifying the underlying causes. These may include neurological, endocrine, ophthalmological and cytogenetic studies. In early-onset CVG, a biopsy is advisable to identify those cases caused by a structural lesion, such as a melanocytic naevus. In the majority of cases treatment is symptomatic. Patients should be educated in scalp hygiene to avoid accumulation of skin debris and secretions in the furrows. Surgical correction can be helpful in selected cases [3], and may be indicated in cerebriform naevi.

Lipoedematous alopecia

Lipoedematous alopecia is a rare condition of unknown aetiology. It is characterized by a thick, boggy scalp with varying degrees of hair loss [1,2]. Although originally reported in black women, lipoedematous alopecia also occurs in white women [3,4] and in men [5]. There is slowly progressive, diffuse alopecia and boggy thickening of the scalp. There are no associated medical or physiological conditions. The fundamental pathological finding consists of an approximate doubling in scalp thickness resulting from expansion of the subcutaneous fat layer. There is associated atrophy and fibrous replacement of many hair follicles. Light and electron microscopy suggests that the increase in scalp thickness is caused by localized oedema, with disruption and degeneration of adipose tissue. In addition to thickening of the adipose tissue layer, dermal oedema, lymphatic dilatation and elastic fibre fragmentation are frequently seen which may suggest that the primary pathology is related to abnormal lymphatics [6]. Mucin is not seen [7]. Surgical debulking with scalp reduction has been described as a technique for managing a localized case [8].

TUMOURS OF THE SCALP

The scalp is a common location of tumours of the skin and these can be broadly categorized as benign, malignant or metastatic. Benign and malignant tumours can arise from the epidermis, the pilosebaceous unit or adnexal structures. Due to chronic sun exposure the scalp is a common site of squamous cell carcinoma, basal cell carcinoma, lentigo maligna, desmoplastic melanoma and angiosarcoma. Only tumours that have a particular predilection for the scalp are mentioned here.

Sebaceous naevus

Sebaceous naevus represents a common congenital hamartoma that presents as an orange-yellow hairless patch most commonly located on the scalp (see Chapter 75). They may be present at birth or may become more obvious through childhood and adolescence. From puberty it is common for the patch to become thickened and more verrucous in nature. The development of basal cell carcinomas and other adnexal tumours has been described and for that reason some dermatologists advocate surgical removal of sebaceous naevi as a preventative measure. In a large retrospective study of 706 patients and 707 specimens, the most common tumours found within a sebaceous naevus were trichoblastoma (7.4%), and syringocystadenoma papilliferum (5.2%). Malignant tumours were only found in 2.5% of cases (basal cell carcinomas 1.1% and squamous cell carcinomas 0.6%) and these did not occur in childhood, inferring that any removal can be planned for adolescence or adulthood [1].

Syringocystadenoma papilliferum

Syringocystadenoma papilliferum is a rare, benign, adnexal tumour of the apocrine or eccrine sweat ducts, which typically presents as a solitary, pink, dome-shaped nodule on the scalp (see Chapter 138). It may occur in association with a sebaceous naevus. They are usually present from birth or infancy. Malignant change has been described, heralded by ulceration, bleeding and rapid enlargement. Surgical excision is recommended as a preventative measure.

Tumours of the pilosebaceous unit

Trichoepitheliomas. Trichoepitheliomas are firm, red nodules that commonly occur on the scalp (see Chapter 138). Trichoepitheliomas can be solitary but typically multiple lesions coexist and can cover a large area of the scalp, which has led to the term 'turban tumour'. They are benign tumours, but they grow slowly and can cause considerable cosmetic issue. Trichoepitheliomas can be surgical excised.

Trichilemmal cysts. Trichilemmal cysts arise from the outer root sheath of the hair follicle (see Chapter 134). Ninety per cent of trichilemmal cysts are located on the scalp due to the increased density of follicles. Whilst lesions may be solitary, it is common for patients to have multiple lesions. Cysts can be surgically excised if treatment is required.

Scalp metastases

The scalp is a common site for cutaneous metastases, accounting for 12% of all skin metastases (see Chapter 147). They usually present as a single, smooth, bald nodule in the scalp and are often initially misdiagnosed as a benign cyst. Occasionally, they may be the first sign of an underlying malignancy. The primary tumour is commonly located in the lung, stomach, colon or kidney [1].

INFECTIONS OF THE SCALP

The scalp is a common site of skin infection and infestation. Hair loss can be a feature of this. Tinea capitis (see Chapter 32), infestations (see Chapter 34) and bacterial infections (see Chapter 26) are discussed elsewhere.

Syphilis

Hair loss occurs in approximately 2.9–7% of cases of secondary syphilis and may be the presenting feature [1,2,3] (see Chapter 29). The hair loss typically has a 'moth-eaten' appearance but may be diffuse in nature [4]. Other features of secondary syphilis are present in most cases, particularly lymph node enlargement and hepatomegaly, but hair loss has been reported as the only sign of the disease [4]. Histological features include an increase in catagen and telogen forms, and a peribulbar lymphocytic infiltrate, similar to the changes seen in alopecia areata [3]. Additional features in syphilis include lymphocytic infiltration of the isthmus region, parabulbar lymphoid aggregates and the presence of plasma cells within the infiltrate. Despite appropriate stains, *Treponema pallidum* is not usually seen. The alopecia is non-scarring and sometimes affects other hair-bearing areas [1,5]. The alopecia usually resolves within 3 months of appropriate treatment for syphilis [1].

The serpiginous nodulosquamous syphilide of tertiary syphilis may also affect the scalp. The syphilitic gumma is a cause of scarring alopecia.

Human immunodeficiency virus

A variety of alterations in hair growth have been described in patients with HIV infection (see Chapter 31). Telogen effluvium is common; causes include chronic HIV-1 infection itself, secondary infections, nutritional deficiencies and drugs [1]. Hair loss on the body as well as the scalp has been reported with several antiretroviral drugs, particularly indinavir [2] and other protease inhibitors. In one case, a 62-year-old man with HIV infection experienced alopecia totalis 18 months after initiating antiretroviral treatment, which included iopinavir/ritonavir. The alopecia reversed completely 2 months after stopping iopinavir/ritonavir [3]. There are also reports of alopecia areata occurring in patients with HIV infection [4–6]. Tinea capitis, psoriasis and seborrhoeic dermatitis are all more common in patients with HIV infection. Straightening of the hair is a common feature of HIV infection in black patients [7].

Various forms of folliculitis are seen in HIV infection, including acneform eruptions, staphylococcal folliculitis and eosinophilic pustular folliculitis.

PUSTULAR CONDITIONS OF THE SCALP

There are a large number of conditions that can present with pustules on the scalp. These vary from conditions where the pustules are isolated findings without hair loss, to those that are associated with localized cicatricial alopecia. Figure 107.7 shows a clinical diagnostic approach to pustules in the scalp.

Pustular conditions associated with cicatricial alopecia are discussed in Chapter 89. Other conditions are also covered elsewhere in this book:

- Scalp folliculitis: see Chapter 93.
- Pseudofolliculitis barbae: see Chapter 93.
- Necrotizing lymphocytic folliculitis of the scalp margin (acne varioliformis): see Chapter 93.
- Dissecting cellulitis/perifolliculitis capitis abscedens et suffodiens: see under secondary cicatricial alopecias earlier in this chapter.
- Folliculitis keloidalis/acne keloidalis nuchae: see Chapter 93.
- Folliculitis decalvans: see Chapter 89.

Erosive pustular dermatosis of the scalp

Introduction and general description

This clinical entity particularly affects the elderly [1,2]. Its cause is unknown but Grattan *et al.* [3], in their study of 12 cases, suggested that local trauma and sun damage are important. Surgery, cryosurgery, skin grafting and radiation therapy may all precipitate this condition [4].

Pathophysiology

Histological examination shows areas of epidermal erosion, a chronic inflammatory cell infiltration in the dermis consisting predominantly of lymphocytes and plasma cells, and sometimes small foci of foreign body giant cells where the hair follicles have been destroyed.

Clinical features

This condition almost always occurs in association with advanced pattern hair loss. Initially, a small area of scalp becomes red, crusted and irritable; crusting and superficial pustulation overlies a moist, eroded surface (Figure 107.8). As the condition extends, areas of activity coexist with areas of scarring. Squamous carcinoma has developed in the scars [5].

Differential diagnosis

Pyogenic and yeast infection is excluded by bacteriological examination and the lack of response to antibacterial or antifungal agents. Biopsy may be necessary to exclude pustular psoriasis, cicatricial pemphigoid, 'irritated' solar keratosis or squamous cell carcinoma.

Management

The stronger topical corticosteroids (e.g. 0.05% clobetasol propionate) will suppress the inflammatory changes. A gradual reduction in the potency of topical steroid over a 6-month period may result in cure. Maintenance therapy with sun protection and intermittent

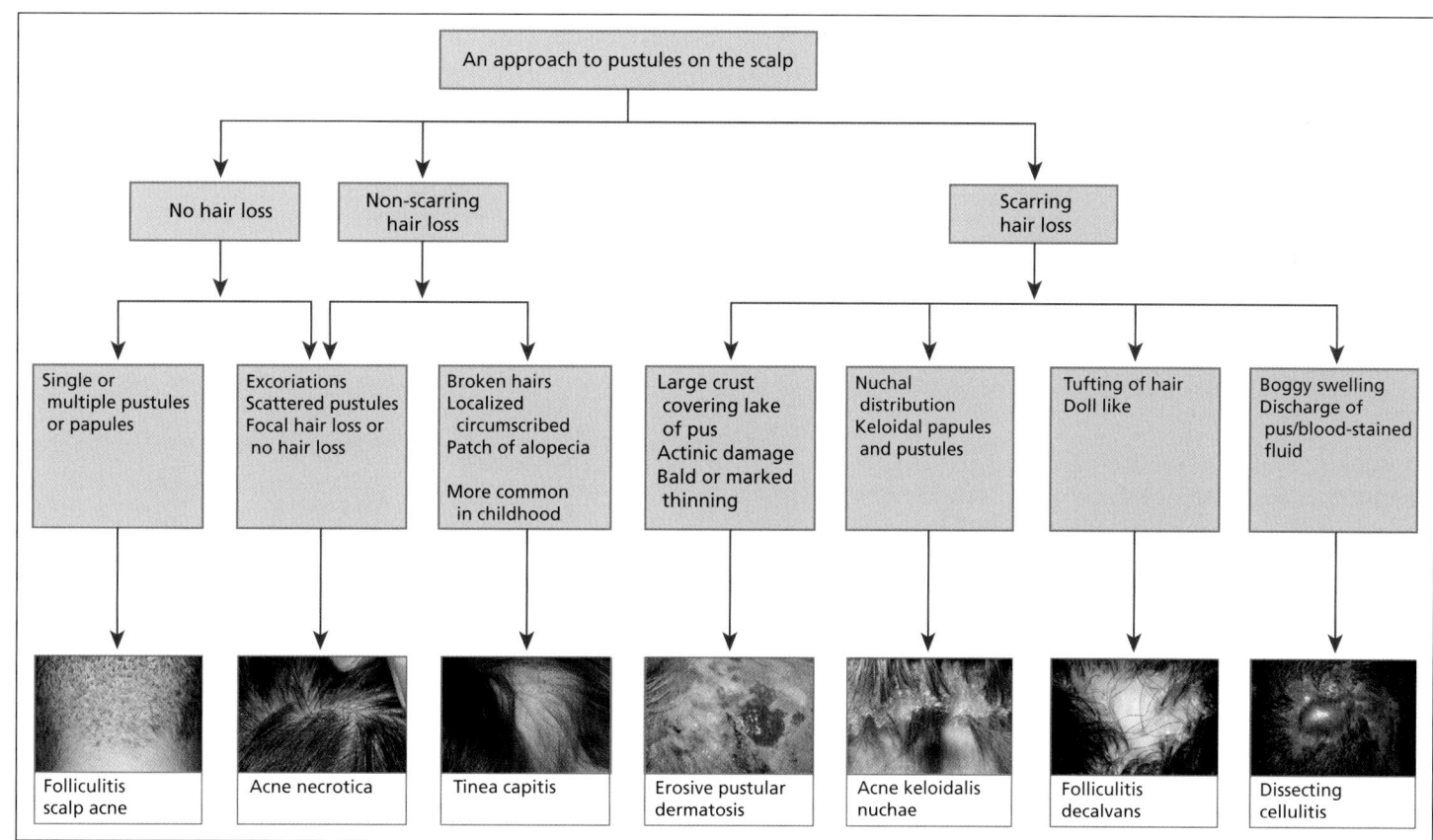

Figure 107.7 An approach to diagnosing pustules in the scalp.

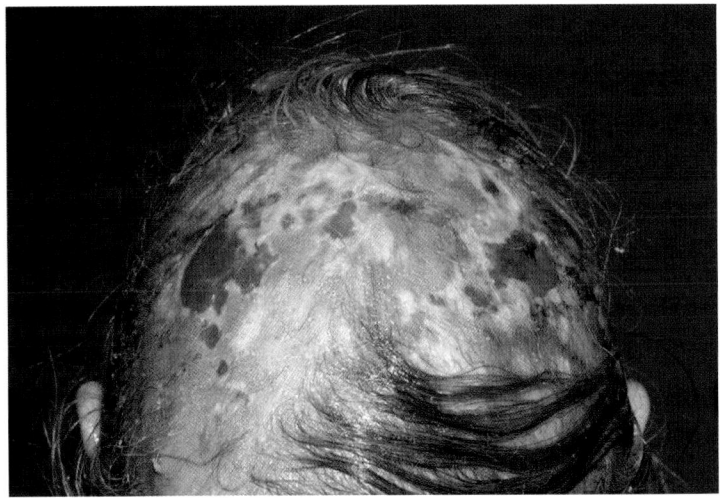

Figure 107.8 Erosive pustular dermatosis of the scalp.

moderate-potency steroid can provide long-term relief. Ikeda *et al.* [6] suggested that oral zinc sulphate, and Boffa [7] suggested that topical calcipotriol can be curative in some cases. Recently, topical dapsone 5% gel has been shown to be safe and efficacious [8].

Iatrogenic scalp pustulation

Scalp pustules in association with chemotherapy have been reported. Chiu *et al.* reported an 85-year-old man with lung cancer who developed a pustular eruption on the scalp following treatment with erlotinib [1]. Erlotinib is an epidermal growth factor receptor (EGFR) inhibitor. EGFR inhibitors are used to treat advanced malignancy, and they play an important role in skin and hair follicle metabolic signalling. Fifty to 70% of patients treated with EGFR inhibitors develop acneform eruptions or papulopustular rashes [2].

OTHER SCALP DISORDERS

Scalp pruritus

Introduction and general description
Scalp pruritus is a common symptom (see Chapter 83). It can be associated with a variety of conditions including dermatological, neurological and psychogenic diseases, as well as being a manifestation of a systemic problem, or being iatrogenically induced [1]. Scalp itch is distressing and causes significant morbidity. Often it can appear without any noticeable skin pathology. It can be both diagnostically and therapeutically challenging.

Epidemiology

Incidence and prevalence
Although scalp itch is recognized as common there is a lack of information published on its incidence and prevalence [2]. In an

epidemiological study conducted in a representative sample of the French population, 44% declared suffering from a 'sensitive scalp'. Of these subjects 25% complained of an itching sensation [3]. In 75 patients with generalized idiopathic pruritus without eruption, 14% described involvement of the scalp [4].

Age, sex and ethnicity
In 25% of patients within a French study population who had a 'sensitive itchy scalp' differences were noted according to age: 31% were under 35 years old, 27% 35–50 years old and 42% over 50 years old. Women suffered more frequently from a sensitive scalp than men. [3]. In 75 patients from Singapore with generalized idiopathic pruritus, there was no difference in gender or race affected. The mean age of those affected was 52 years.

Associated diseases
Scalp pruritus can be associated with a variety of conditions. These include dermatological disease, systemic disease, neurological disease and psychiatric/psychosomatic diseases (Table 107.2) [5].

Table 107.2 Diseases associated with scalp pruritus.

Type	Examples
Dermatological	Seborrhoeic dermatitis
	Psoriasis
	Urticaria
	Atopic eczema and lichen simplex chronicus
	Allergic contact dermatitis
	Alopecia areata
	Lichen planopilaris
	Central centrifugal cicatricial alopecia
	Discoid lupus erythematosus
	Dermatitis herpetiformis
	Acne necrotica
	Folliculitis decalvans
	Scalp folliculitis
	Infection and infestation
Systemic	Chronic renal failure
	Cholestatic liver disease
	Haematological malignancy, e.g. lymphoma or leukaemia
	Drug-induced pruritus
	Thyroid dysfunction
Neurological (diseases or disorders of the central or peripheral nervous system)	Diabetic neuropathy
	Postherpetic neuralgia
	Migraine
	Atypical facial neuralgia
	Scalp dysaesthesia
	Brain and spinal cord injury
	Wallenberg syndrome
	Brain tumour
Psychogenic/psychosomatic	Somatoform pruritus with co-morbidity of 'psychiatric and psychosomatic diseases'

Adapted from Goon *et al.* 2007 [4] and Ständer *et al.* 2007 [5].

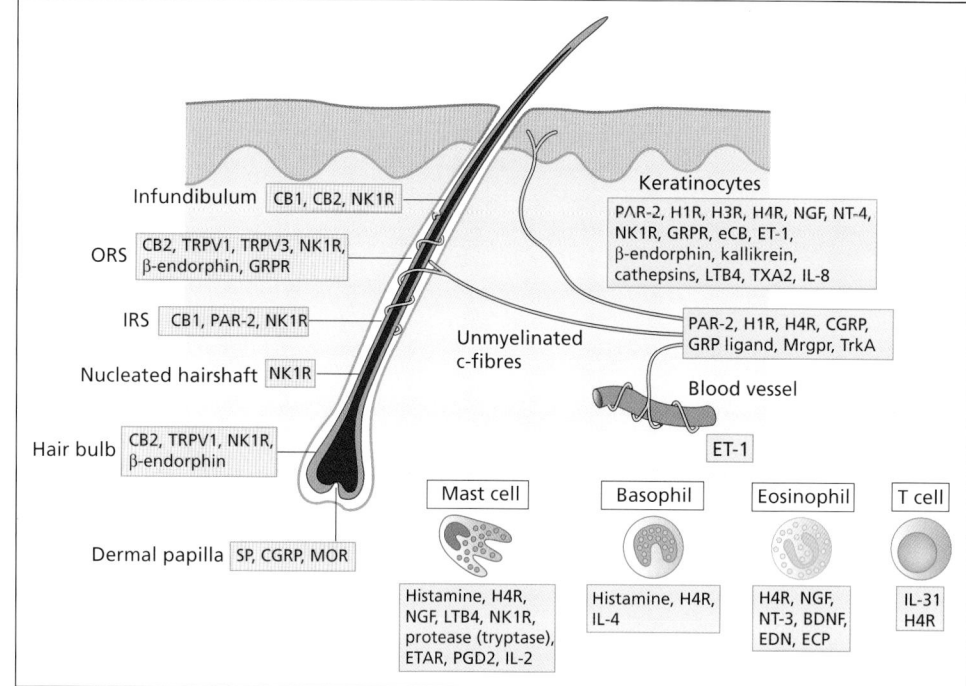

Figure 107.9 Cutaneous sensory receptors and mediators involved in the itchy scalp. BDNF, brain-derived neurotropic factor; CB, cannabinoid receptor; CGRP, calcitonin gene-related peptide; eCB, endogenous cannabinoids; ECP, eosinophil cationic protein; EDN, eosinophil-derived neurotoxin; ET-1, endothelin-1; ETAR, endothelin receptor A; GRP, gastrin-related peptide; GRPR, gastrin-related peptide receptor; H1R, histamine 1 receptor; H3R, histamine 3 receptor; H4R, histamine 4 receptor; IL, interleukin; IRS, inner root sheath; LTB4, leukotriene B4; MOR, mu opioid receptor; Mrgpr, Mas-related G-protein-coupled receptor; NGF, nerve growth factor; NK1R, neurokinin-1 receptor; NT, neurotrophin; ORS, outer root sheath; PAR-2, proteinase-activating receptor 2; PGD2, prostaglandin D2; SP, substance P; TrkA, high-affinity NGF receptor; TRPV, transient receptor potential vanilloid; TXA2, thromboxane A2. (Adapted from Bin Saif *et al.* 2011 [2].)

Pathophysiology

Pathology

Numerous different cells and mediators in the scalp are involved in scalp itch. Figure 107.9 illustrates the itch mediators and their sites of activity.

Mast cells release histamine, which induces pruritus via the H1 and H4 receptors on nerve fibres. Proteinase-activating receptor 2 (PAR-2) mediates chronic pruritus via calcitonin gene-related peptide (CGRP) and substance P. Exogenous activators of PAR-2 include serine proteases generated by bacteria, fungi and house dust. Transient receptor potential vanilloid type 1 receptor (TRPV1) can be activated by capsaicin, heat, acidosis and endogenous endovanilloids [6,7]. Mas-related G-protein-coupled receptor (Mrgpr) can be activated directly by peptides with common C-terminal motifs. The endogenous opioid system includes three opioid receptors: mu (MOR), delta (DOR), and kappa (KOR), and the opioid peptides enkephalins, endorphins, dynorphins and endomorphins. KOR signalling suppresses itch while MOR signalling stimulates itch. Activation of cannabinoid receptors CB1 and CB2 leads to the inhibition of pruritus. Substance P binds with high affinity to the neurokinin-1 receptor (NK1R) on keratinocytes, endothelial cells and mast cells. Degranulation of mast cells releases pruritogenic proinflammatory cytokines. CGRP promotes itch on release after C-fibre activity. Four members of the neurotrophin (NT) family are involved in the pathogenesis of itch: NGF, BDNF, NT-3 and NT-4. Gastrin-related peptide receptor (GRPR) is activated by histamine-independent mechanisms. Endothelin-1 (ET-1) evokes pruritus in humans and animals. Interleukins (ILs) are implicated in the pathogenesis of pruritus including IL-2, IL-31 and IL-8.

Causative organisms

Malassezia species are found in high concentrations on the scalp. In normal conditions, *Malassezia* yeast reduces the production of pro-inflammatory cytokines by keratinocytes. This is related to

the presence of a lipid-rich microfibrillar layer surrounding yeast cells [8]. A high quantity of lipid may prevent the yeast cell from inducing inflammation, whereas low lipid content may induce inflammation [9,10]. This may explain the aetiology of seborrhoeic dermatitis itch.

Staphylococcus aureus may also induce itch. Staphylococcal endotoxins lead to IL-31 expression, a known mediator of itch [11]. *Staphylococcus* can also mediate serine protease expression through PAR-2 receptor [12], this could explain why scalp folliculitis is itchy.

Clinical features

History

Pruritus is defined as an unpleasant sensation of the skin leading to the desire to scratch. This can be described as acute or chronic; the latter is defined as pruritus lasting 6 or more weeks.

Presentation

Pruritus of the scalp can be classified as that occurring on apparently normal skin, on diseased skin or on scratch-evoked lesions (Figure 107.10).

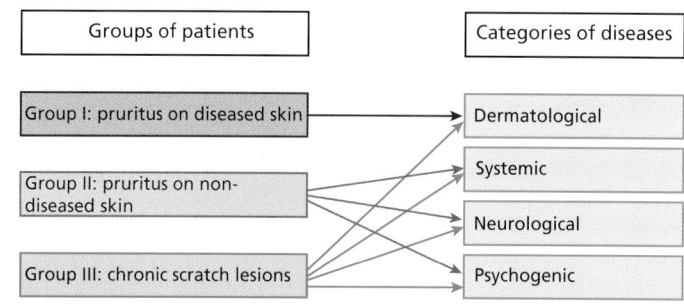

Figure 107.10 Clinical classification of scalp pruritus. (Adapted from [5].)

Table 107.3 Investigation of scalp itch [5].

Classification	Investigations
Pruritus on diseased skin	Microscopy and culture
	Skin biopsy for histology/immunofluorescence
Pruritus on non-diseased skin	Guided by medical history but may include:
	Full blood count
	Urea and electrolytes
	Thyroid function
	Liver function
	Ferritin
Pruritus with chronic scratch lesions	Often requires a combination of investigations for both pruritus on diseased skin and pruritus on non-diseased skin, e.g. biopsy and laboratory investigation

Adapted from Ständer *et al.* 2007 [5].

Complications and co-morbidities

Chronic pruritus can lead to scratching, rubbing and pinching. Scratching may induce skin damage such as excoriation, crusting, lichenification and excoriated papules and nodules. Lesions may coexist in different stages and secondary infection may occur. Lesions may resolve leaving atrophic, hyper- or hypopigmented scars.

Disease course and prognosis

The course and prognosis of scalp pruritus is dependent on the cause. Treatment of the underlying cause of pruritus should result in resolution. Chronic pruritus with no identifiable aetiology is more of a challenge and may persist for years despite supportive treatment.

Investigations

Grouping pruritus as that occurring on apparently normal skin, on diseased skin or on scratch-evoked lesions can aid selection of the most appropriate investigation, (Table 107.3).

Management

If there is evidence of a scalp dermatosis causing itch then that disorder should be treated. Coal tar shampoos, emollients (including oils, e.g. olive or arachis oil) and topical corticosteroids may offer some relief.

Scalp dysaesthesia

Introduction and general description

Hoss and Segal first described scalp dysaesthesia as chronic severe pain and/or pruritus of the scalp without objective findings [1]. The symptoms may be manifestations of an underlying psychiatric disorder or may represent a type of chronic pain syndrome (see Chapter 84).

Epidemiology and aetiology

In a study looking at the epidemiology of scalp sensitivity from a representative sample of the French population, 44% reported having a sensitive scalp. Women suffered more frequently from a sensitive scalp than men and no relationship with age was found. Prickling, itch and burning were the most common symptoms in those with a sensitive scalp. No link was found between scalp sensitivity and any specific scalp disease. Triggering factors of scalp sensitivity were heat, cold, pollution, emotions, dry or wet air, water and shampoos [2].

Hoss and Segal considered whether alopecia could have caused or contributed to scalp dysaesthesia and found that seven of 11 patients had mild androgenetic alopecia. It was concluded that this is not an increased incidence of androgenetic alopecia compared with the general population, therefore it was unlikely to be the sole cause of the scalp problems [1]. This study also considered the role of a psychiatric cause in scalp dysaesthesia. Five of the 11 patients studied had one or more physician-diagnosed psychiatric disorders; of these, four had problems that were present prior to the onset of scalp dysaesthesia. The symptoms in seven of the 11 intensified with psychological stress [1]. Hoss and Segal remain uncertain as to whether their patients have pain secondary to an underlying psychiatric condition, or if the psychiatric problems are unrelated or caused by the scalp dysaesthesia.

Other localized pruritic syndromes have been associated with pathological conditions of the spine. A retrospective review of 15 women with scalp dysaesthesia found that 14 patients had cervical spine disease confirmed by imaging [3]. The commonest finding on imaging was degenerative disc disease, with 10 out of 14 patients having changes at C5/C6. Fourteen patients had been recommended a topical or oral gabapentin regimen and of the seven followed up, four noted an improvement in symptoms when taking gabapentin. The authors postulated that chronic muscle tension placed on the pericranial muscles or scalp aponeurosis secondary to the underlying cervical spine disease may lead to the symptoms of scalp dysaesthesia [3].

Management

Pregabalin has also been used in the management of scalp dysaesthesia [4]. Nine of the 11 patients studied by Hoss and Segal experienced improvement or complete resolution of their scalp symptoms with low-dose antidepressants [1]. Mechanisms for the benefit of antidepressants in scalp dysaesthesia, and other localized pain syndromes, may include the following [5,6]:

• Antidepressant use may relieve depression associated with, or caused by, chronic pain and thereby relieve symptoms.
• The tricyclic antidepressants may have analgesic properties.
• Depression and pain may share a similar underlying biochemical mechanism.

Key references

The full list of references can be found in the online version at www.rooksdermatology.com.

Scaling disorders of the scalp

Seborrhoeic dermatitis

1 Gupta A, Bluhm R. Seborrhoeic dermatitis. *J Eur Acad Dermatol Venereol* 2004;18:13–26.

3 Gupta A, Richardson M, Paquet M. Systematic review of oral treatments for seborrhoeic dermatitis. *J Eur Acad Dermatol Venereol* 2014;28:16–26.

Psoriasis
2 Mason A, Mason J, Cork M, *et al.* Topical treatments for chronic plaque psoriasis of the scalp: a systematic review. *Br J Dermatol* 2013;169:519–27.

Pityriasis amiantacea
1 Knight AG. Pityriasis amiantacea: a clinical and histopathological investigation. *Clin Exp Dermatol* 1977;2:137–43.

Secondary cicatricial alopecia

Scleroderma and morphoea
2 Whiting DA. Cicatricial alopecia: clinico-pathological findings and treatment. *Clin Dermatol* 2001;19:211–25.

Necrobiotic disorders
2 Katta R, Nelson B, Chen D, *et al.* Sarcoidosis of the scalp: a case series and review of the literature. *J Am Acad Dermatol* 2000;42:690–2.

Sarcoidosis
2 Katta R, Nelson B, Chen D, *et al.* Sarcoidosis of the scalp: a case series and review of the literature. *J Am Acad Dermatol* 2000;42:690–2.

Follicular mucinosis
1 Rongioletti F, De Lucchi S, Meyes D, *et al.* Follicular mucinosis: a clinicopathologic, histochemical, immunohistochemical and molecular study comparing the primary benign form and the mycosis fungoides-associated follicular mucinosis. *J Cutan Pathol* 2010;37:15–19.

Cicatricial pemphigoid
3 Leenutaphong V, von Kries R, Plewig G. Localized cicatricial pemphigoid (Brunsting-Perry): electron microscopic study. *J Am Acad Dermatol* 1989;21:1089–93.

Dissecting cellulitis of the scalp
3 Whiting DA. Cicatricial alopecia: clinico-pathological findings and treatment. *Clin Dermatol* 2001;19:211–25.
6 Navarini A, Trueb R. Three cases of dissecting cellulitis of the scalp treated with adalimumab: control of inflammation within residual structural disease. *Arch Dermatol* 2010;146:517–20.

Thickened scalp disorders

Cutis verticis gyrata
2 Schepis C, Palazzo R, Cannavo SP, *et al.* Prevalence of primary cutis verticis gyrata in a psychiatric population: association with chromosomal fragile sites. *Acta Derm Venereol (Stockh)* 1990;70:483–6.

Lipoedematous alopecia
6 Yasar S, Gunes P, Serdar Z, *et al.* Clinicial and pathological features of 31 cases of lipedamtous scalp and lipedemtous alopecia. *Eur J Dermatol* 2011;21:520–8.
7 Fair KP, Knoell KA, Patterson JW, *et al.* Lipedematous alopecia: a clinicopathologic, histologic and ultrastructural study. *J Cutan Pathol* 2000;27:49–53.

Tumours of the scalp

Sebaceous naevus
1 Idriss M, Elston D. Secondary neoplasms associated with nevus sebaceus of Jadassohn: a study of 707 cases. *J Am Acad Dermatol* 2014;70:332–7.

Scalp metastases
1 Richmond H, Duvic M, Macfarlane D. Primary and metastatic malignant tumours of the scalp: an update. *Am J Clin Dermatol* 2010;11;233–46.

Infections of the scalp

Syphilis
1 Vafaie J, Weinberg J, Smith B, *et al.,* Alopecia in association with sexually transmitted disease: a review. *Cutis* 2005;76:361–6.
4 Lee JY, Hsu ML. Alopecia syphilitica, a simulator of alopecia areata: histopathology and differential diagnosis. *J Cutan Pathol* 1991;18:87–92.
5 Cuozzo DW, Benson PM, Sperling LC, *et al.* Essential syphilitic alopecia revisited. *J Am Acad Dermatol* 1995;32:840–3.

Human immunodeficiency virus
1 Smith KJ, Skelton HG, DeRusso D, *et al.* Clinical and histopathologic features of hair loss in patients with HIV-1 infection. *J Am Acad Dermatol* 1996;34:63–8.

Pustular conditions of the scalp

Erosive pustular dermatosis of the scalp
1 Caputo R, Veraldi S. Erosive pustular dermatosis of the scalp. *J Am Acad Dermatol* 1993;28:96–8.
2 Pye RJ, Peachey RD, Burton JL. Erosive pustular dermatosis of the scalp. *Br J Dermatol* 1979;100:559–66.
8 Broussard K, Berger, T, Rosenblum M, *et al.* Erosive pustular dermatosis of the scalp: a review with a focus on dapsone therapy. *J Am Acad Dermatol* 2012;66:680–6.

Iatrogenic scalp pustulation
2 Robert C, Soria JC, Spatz A, *et al.* Cutaneous side-effects of kinase inhibitors and blocking antibodies. *Lancet Oncol* 2005;6:491–500.

Other scalp disorders

Scalp pruritus
2 Bin Saif GA, Ericson ME, *et al.* The itchy scalp – scratching for an explanation. *Experimental Dermatology* 2011;20:959–68.
4 Goon AT-J, Yosipovitch G, Chan Y, *et al.* Clinical characteristics of generalized idiopathic pruritis in patients from a tertiary referral center in Singapore. *Int J Dermatol* 2007;46:1023–6.
5 Ständer S, Weissharr E, Mettang T, *et al.* Clinical classification of itch: a Position Paper of the International Forum for the Study of Itch. *Acta Derm Venereol* 2007;87:291–4.

Scalp dysaesthesia
1 Hoss D, Segal S. Scalp dysesthesia. *Arch Dermatol* 1998;143:327–30.
2 Misery L, Sibauld V, Ambronati M, *et al.* Sensitive scalp: does this condition exist? An epidemiological study. *Contact Dermatitis* 2008;58:234–8.

PART 10: SITES, SEX, AGE

CHAPTER 108

Dermatoses of the External Ear

Cameron Kennedy

Bristol Royal Infirmary and Bristol Royal Hospital for Children, Bristol, UK

Introduction

Anatomy and physiology [1,2,3]

The external ear consists of the auricle, the external auditory canal and the outer layer of the tympanic membrane.

The auricle, or pinna (Figure 108.1), is a convoluted, elastic and cartilaginous plate covered by skin which is continuous medially with the lining of the external auditory canal. Except on the non-cartilaginous lobe and at the back of the ear, the skin is bound firmly to the cartilage. The auricle is attached to the head by fibrous ligaments and three vestigial auricularis muscles. The size and general detail of the auricle can vary greatly between individuals, and may be characteristically affected in a number of congenital syndromes. In humans, the auricle is largely functionless and motionless.

The epidermis of the ear has a complex dermal–epidermal junction, a conspicuous stratum granulosum and a thick, compact stratum corneum. The dermis contains abundant elastic tissue. Sebaceous glands are numerous, particularly on the tragus and lobe, and fine vellus or terminal hairs occur over the entire surface, but are especially prominent on the helix and tragus. Coarser terminal hair is seen in some men, possibly as a Y-linked and androgen-dependent inherited trait (MIM 425500) (Figure 108.2). Eccrine sweat glands are sparsely and irregularly distributed except in the external auditory canal, which has, instead, a large number of modified apocrine or ceruminous glands. The pinna has a variably thick fatty layer that extends between the perichondrium and the reticular dermis and that also forms the main fibrofatty core of the lobe of the ear.

The blood supply to the auricle is provided by anastomosing branches of the superficial temporal and posterior auricular arteries, which drain via posterior auricular and superficial temporal veins into the external jugular vein and via the superficial temporal, maxillary and facial veins into the internal jugular vein. Lymphatic drainage is to the superficial parotid, retroauricular and superficial cervical lymph nodes. Embryonic fusion planes and minute deficiencies in the cartilaginous portion of the external

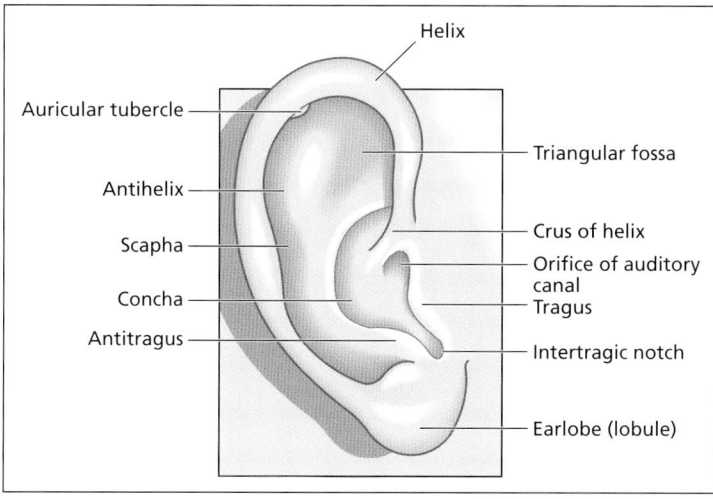

Figure 108.1 Anatomical landmarks of the auricle.

Labels: Helix; Auricular tubercle; Antihelix; Scapha; Concha; Antitragus; Triangular fossa; Crus of helix; Orifice of auditory canal; Tragus; Intertragic notch; Earlobe (lobule)

Rook's Textbook of Dermatology, Ninth Edition. Edited by Christopher Griffiths, Jonathan Barker, Tanya Bleiker, Robert Chalmers and Daniel Creamer.
© 2016 John Wiley & Sons, Ltd. Published 2016 by John Wiley & Sons, Ltd.
Companion website: www.rooksdermatology.com

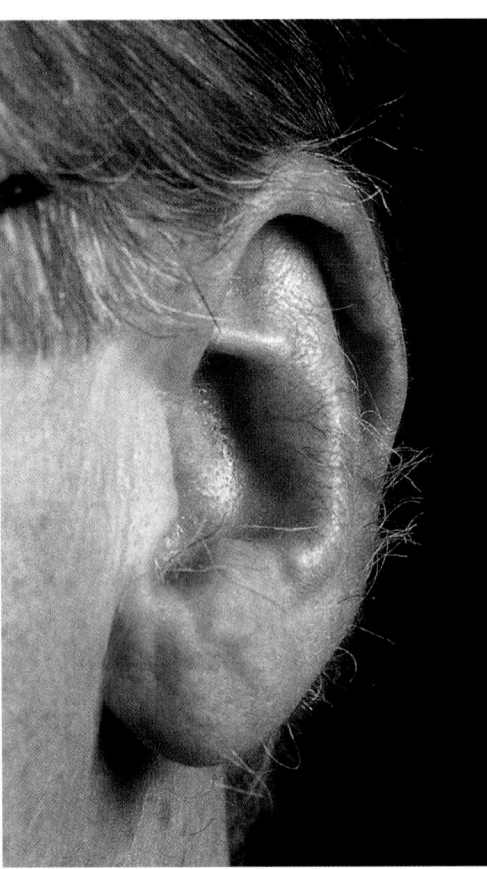

Figure 108.2 Coarse terminal hair on the auricle: a trait possibly associated with the Y chromosome.

auditory canal provide potential pathways for the spread of infection and tumours.

There is a complex nerve supply to the ear involving elements of the Vth, VIIth, IXth and Xth cranial nerves as well as cervical branches of the greater and lesser auricular nerves. The back of the ear is supplied by the greater auricular nerve (C2,3), the concha by the auricular branch of the vagus (Xth) and the anterior part of the pinna and the external auditory canal by the auriculotemporal branch of the Vth cranial nerve. Intercommunicating branches of the VIIth, IXth and Xth supply the deeper parts of the ear. With this complicated nerve supply, otalgia is more commonly due to referred pain than to disease in the ear itself [4]. Within the dermis, the nerve supply is abundant, especially around hair follicles where there are complicated basket-like networks of acetylcholinesterase and butyrylcholinesterase nerve fibres. Free nerve endings are also present, but there are no organized nerve endings as occur on glabrous skin elsewhere.

The external auditory canal extends upwards and backwards in an S-shaped curve from the concha to the tympanic membrane. The angle of curvature varies between races and individuals, being more marked in white people than in black people or Polynesians. This has a bearing on trauma, infection and the retention of moisture. The length of the canal is 2.5 cm as measured from the concha to the drum. The outer third of the canal is cartilaginous and is lined by a thicker layer of skin than the inner portion within the temporal bone. Anteroinferiorly there are two horizontal fissures in the cartilaginous canal, the fissures of Santorini. These can allow

infection or tumour to pass beyond the external auditory canal, for example to the parotid gland. Subcutaneous tissue is scanty, and the epithelium is firmly bound to the perichondrium. Sebaceous glands are plentiful, and open into the follicles of extremely fine vellus hairs. Occasionally, larger terminal hairs (tragi) arise in the canal or around the meatus and these, if they become matted with wax or debris, may interfere with normal epidermal 'migration' and ventilation of the ear and hence may play a part in the development of 'hot-weather ear'.

Eccrine sweat glands are not present in the auditory canal but modified apocrine (ceruminous) glands are numerous. They increase in size and activity at puberty. There is great individual and racial variability, and although concentrated in the cartilaginous part of the canal, they may also occur, albeit sparsely, in the osseous portion.

The inner osseous part of the acoustic canal constitutes two-thirds of its total length. The skin is firmly bound to the periosteum, subcutaneous tissue being nearly absent and only 30–50 μm thick. The epidermis here is thin and easily traumatized, and rete ridges are absent [1]. The skin of the external auditory canal and tympanic membrane is unique in that there is no frictional loss of stratum corneum; cerumen (wax) and epithelial debris have therefore to be removed by a special 'migratory' property of the external ear canal epithelium [5]. A slight narrowing of the canal, the isthmus, occurs at or just medial to the junction of the two parts. When marked, it may impede the flow of cerumen to the exterior. Just medial to the isthmus, inferiorly and anteriorly, is the tympanic sulcus. Debris often collects here, especially in patients with chronic external otitis.

The surface pH of the auditory canal varies from 5.6 to 5.8 at the concha to 7.3–7.5 at 5–10 mm within the canal. With inflammation, the pH becomes slightly more acid.

Microbiology

The skin of the external auditory canal in most healthy individuals supports the growth of multiple bacterial species, especially *Staphylococcus epidermidis*, *Corynebacterium* spp., *Bacillus* spp. and less often *Staphylococcus aureus*. *Pseudomonas aeruginosa*, often relevant to external otitis, and fungi are not normally found [2]. The normal flora can include organisms such as *Turicella otidis*, which can cause otitis media [6].

Cerumen (wax) [7]

Cerumen is the combined product of sebaceous and apocrine glands. It contains both squalene and insoluble fatty acids. Analysis by flash pyrolysis–gas chromatography/mass spectrometry has shown numerous diterpenoids [8]. Its main function is to waterproof the external auditory canal. Extrusion is aided by mastication and by the peripheral movement and desquamation of the epithelial cells of the canal. It is impeded if the ear canal is too narrow or tortuous, or when inflammation interferes with the normal process of 'migration'.

There are genetically determined differences in cerumen composition and character: so-called 'dry' ear wax is light grey, dry and flaky; 'wet' ear wax is golden brown and sticky. The former is very common in Asians. Wax phenotype is determined by a single gene pair, the wet wax allele being dominant [7]. Cerumen darkens with exposure to air.

Although not bactericidal, cerumen does not encourage bacterial or fungal growth. It is likely that antimicrobial peptides play a role [9,10]; other possible reasons include the presence of lysozyme, immunoglobulins and polyunsaturated fatty acids.

Two populations have been shown to have excessive production and/or impaction of cerumen: individuals with learning difficulties and the elderly [7]. An increased secretion of cerumen occurs in patients treated with aromatic retinoids [11].

If wax becomes impacted or adherent, it can cause various symptoms such as hearing loss, tinnitus, vertigo, pain and itching, and can be a contributory factor to external otitis. It may be removed by irrigation techniques or by suction under direct vision [12,13]. A systematic review found that on measures of wax clearance Cerumol®, sodium bicarbonate, olive oil and water are all more effective than no treatment; triethanolamine polypeptide (TP) is better than olive oil; wet irrigation is better than dry irrigation; sodium bicarbonate drops followed by irrigation by a nurse is more effective than sodium bicarbonate drops followed by self-irrigation; softening with TP and self-irrigation is more effective than self-irrigation only; and endoscopic de-waxing is better than microscopic de-waxing [14]. Regular use of an emollient liquid may have a role in prevention of impaction [15]. Inflammation interferes with normal epidermal migration and tends therefore both to induce and to encourage the retention of scale.

Examination [16]

As well as examining the pinna, the dermatologist may need to examine the ear canal. Equipment available should include a headlight or equivalent, otoscope, several sizes of ear speculae, ear curettes, metal applicators, bayonet forceps, ear irrigation apparatus and cotton.

General inspection of the auricles should take account of their symmetry, size, shape and position, and completeness of development.

The ear canal is best inspected when the auricle is pulled gently upwards, outwards and backwards, and the largest possible speculum is used. It is essential to avoid traumatizing the thin skin of the canal, particularly beyond the isthmus. If inspection reveals accumulation of cerumenous debris, this can sometimes be removed carefully using a curette or wire loop along the posterior wall. If the material is against the drum, gentle suction may be feasible. Irrigation should only be used if the drum is known to be intact.

Samples may need to be taken for bacteriology, mycology and histology. If a biopsy is required from the canal, this should be devolved to a surgeon with the necessary expertise.

Developmental defects

The auricle begins to develop at the end of the fifth week of embryonic life in the first branchial groove, contributed to by the first (mandibular) and second (hyoid) arches [1]. Six hillocks appear on these arches and later fuse to form the complex shape of the fully developed auricle. Inspection of the external ear at birth is important in the overall assessment of the neonate but interpretation can be complicated by the effects of birth trauma [2].

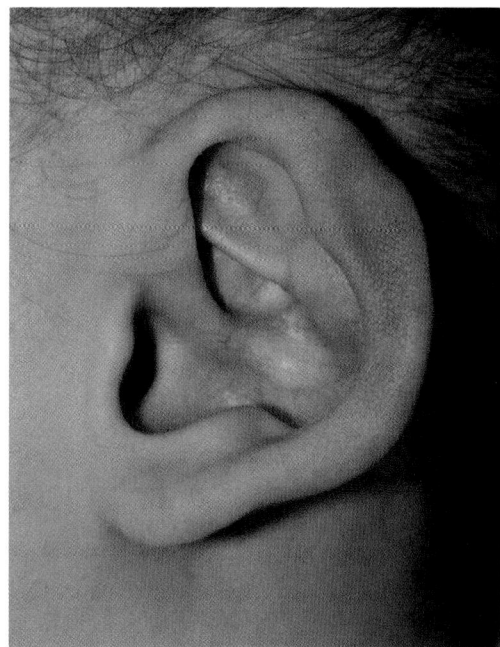

Figure 108.3 Coloboma of the eye, heart defects, atresia of the nasal choanae, retardation of growth and/or development, genital and/or urinary abnormalities, and ear abnormalities and deafness (CHARGE) syndrome – typical appearance of pinna with (i) almost triangular concha; (ii) discontinuity between the antihelix and antitragus; and (iii) 'snipped-off' appearance of the helical folds. (Source: Dr Michael Saunders, Consultant Paediatric Otolaryngologist, Bristol Royal Hospital for Children, UK.)

Those defects of the ear sufficiently common to constitute a part of general dermatological practice are therefore considered here, together with some general principles relating to congenital ear abnormalities and their more important medical and otological associations [3,4,5,6]. Pinna abnormalities are associated sufficiently often with conductive hearing loss that screening tests should be carried out [7].

About 30% of infants with external ear anomalies have a renal anomaly identifiable by ultrasound examination, and this combination is a strong pointer towards a multiple congenital anomaly syndrome, in particular Townes–Brocks, CHARGE (coloboma of the eye, heart defects, atresia of the nasal choanae, retardation of growth and/or development, genital and/or urinary abnormalities, and ear abnormalities and deafness) (Figure 108.3), branchio-oto-renal (Figure 108.4), Nager and diabetic embryopathy syndromes [8].

Many developmental defects are of unknown aetiology. Some, however, are associated with chromosomal abnormalities, for example those occurring in Down syndrome, or are associated with syndromes that have well-recognized Mendelian inheritance patterns, for example the ectrodactyly, ectodermal dysplasia and cleft lip–palate (EEC) syndrome. Environmental factors may be implicated as in fetal alcohol syndrome and fetal hydantoin syndrome, and maternal exposure to isotretinoin and thalidomide.

Congenital ear abnormalities exhibit great variability, even within syndromes or families, and any one aetiological factor may be associated with a variety of ear malformations. External ear malformations as part of a genetic syndrome account for less than 10% of all external ear abnormalities; isolated cases of ear malformation may either be non-genetic in origin or may have a genetic basis but with poor gene penetrance [9].

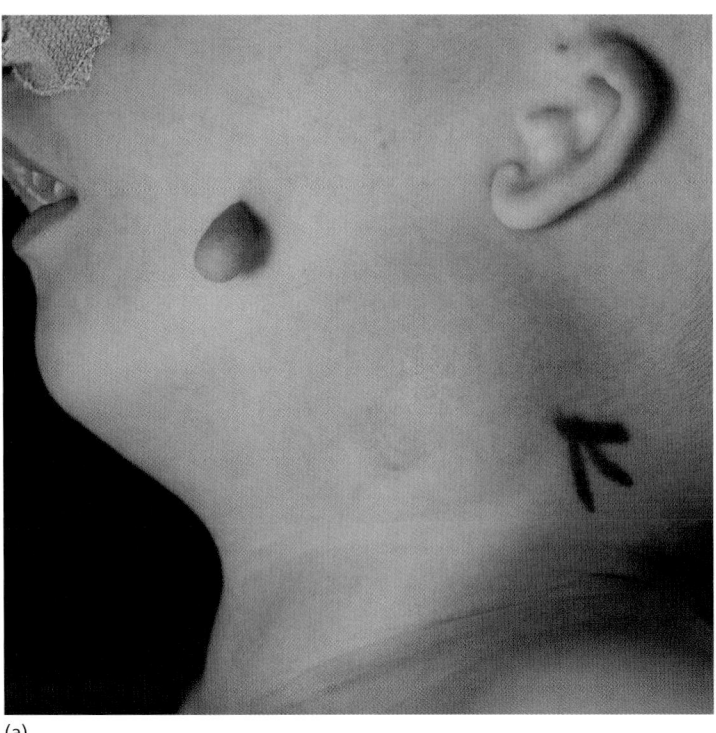
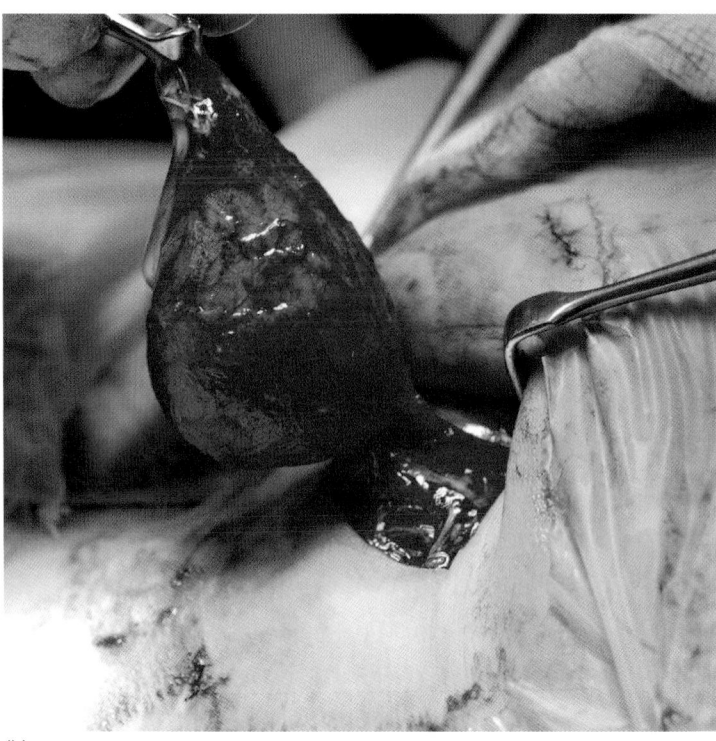

(a)   (b)

Figure 108.4 (a) Branchio-oto-renal syndrome: second arch branchial cyst (arrowed), pre-auricular skin tag, pre-auricular sinus and microtia with absent ear canal. (Source: Dr Michael Saunders, Consultant Paediatric Otolaryngologist, Bristol Royal Hospital for Children, UK.) (b) Branchio-oto-renal syndrome: surgical excision of second arch branchial cyst. (Source: Dr Michael Saunders, Consultant Paediatric Otolaryngologist, Bristol Royal Hospital for Children, UK.)

Microtia (small ears) [10]

Microtia designates a spectrum of underdevelopment of the pinna, from small ears to absence of an ear or ears (Figure 108.5). The prevalence varies between 1 and 17/17 000 in different populations [11]. Small ears are often associated with hearing deficit and may be a feature of many syndromes. In addition to being small, the pinna may be rudimentary, resembling the hillocks from which it is embryologically derived. The more primitive the appearance, the greater the likelihood of hearing abnormalities, in most cases due to defects or atresia of the ossicles. There may also be a narrowing or atresia of the auditory canal [10,11,12,13] and various abnormalities of the middle ear [14] and inner ear [15]. Small ears are a feature of many syndromes, including Down syndrome, Treacher Collins syndrome (Figure 108.6), Goldenhar syndrome, Apert syndrome, various first and second branchial arch and first branchial cleft syndromes, Mohr orofaciodigital syndrome, Duane retraction syndrome and thalidomide embryopathy [6,16].

Familial microtia inherited as an isolated autosomal dominant trait has been described [17]. Microtia is one of the birth defects that occurs more on the right than the left side [18].

Macrotia (large ears)

Macrotia is a developmental variation in which the amount of tissue between the helix and antihelix is increased, causing the ears to wing out. The ear may also be diffusely enlarged, or elongated. Such changes are common in Turner syndrome, and there may be associated sensorineural deafness. Large ears are well described in

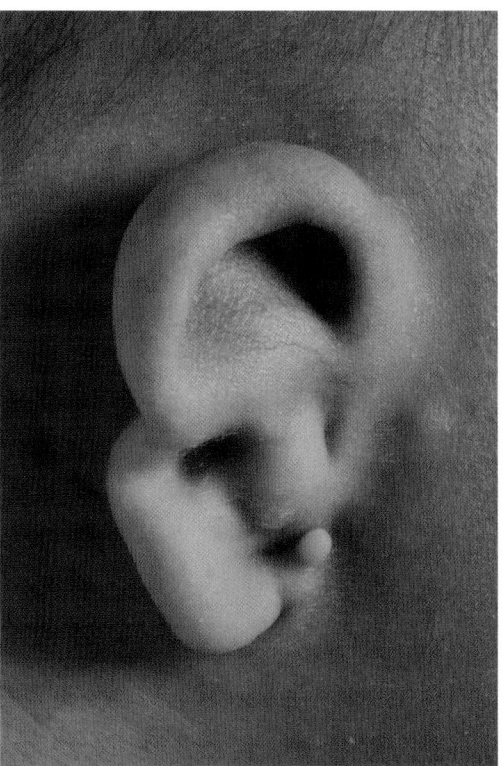

Figure 108.5 Microtia – absent ear canal, partly formed pinna and additional cartilage remnant and skin tag. (Source: Dr Michael Saunders, Consultant Paediatric Otolaryngologist, Bristol Royal Hospital for Children, UK.)

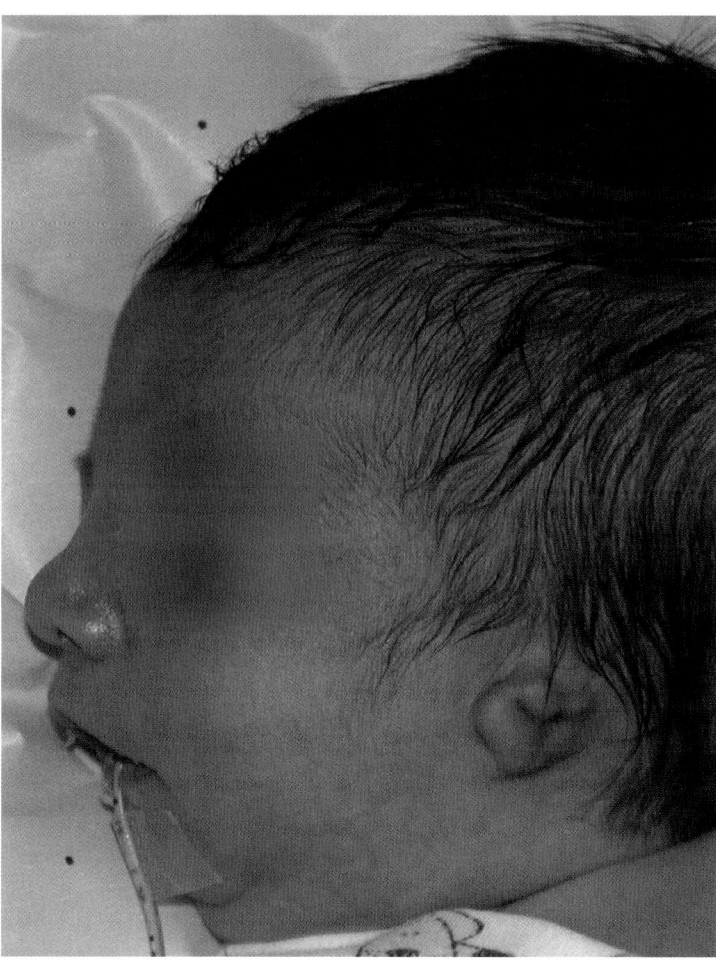

Figure 108.6 Treacher Collins syndrome – marked retrognathia, low set pinna with microtia. (Source: Dr Michael Saunders, Consultant Paediatric Otolaryngologist, Bristol Royal Hospital for Children, UK.)

fragile X syndrome [19] and Kabuki syndrome, although in the latter they may also be smaller than normal [20]. Generally enlarged ears are sometimes seen in patients with the XXXXY chromosome defect. The cartilaginous parts of the ears are enlarged and soft in Zimmermann–Laband syndrome [21,22]. In this rare disorder the ears are large and floppy, in association with a bulbous soft nose, gingival fibromatosis and a variety of other findings including absence or dysplasia of nails and/or of terminal phalanges, hyperextensibility of joints, hepatosplenomegaly, and rarely hypertrichosis and mental retardation.

Low-set ears

Normally, the top of the helix is at the same level as the eyebrow, the earlobe is above the angle of the mandible and the external auditory meatus is at the level of the ala nasi. Low-set ears may in addition be posteriorly rotated, and are often small. The condition is usually bilateral. Although it may be isolated, it is often associated with major middle-ear or systemic malformations, appearing for example in Turner, Noonan, Patau and Crouzon syndromes.

Peri-auricular anomalies

Pre-auricular pits, sinuses (Figure 108.7) and tags are relatively common, with an incidence of approximately 1% [10,23]. Lesions on or near the tragus are probably best termed 'accessory tragus' [24]. The term 'accessory auricle' is sometimes used for this, and for similar

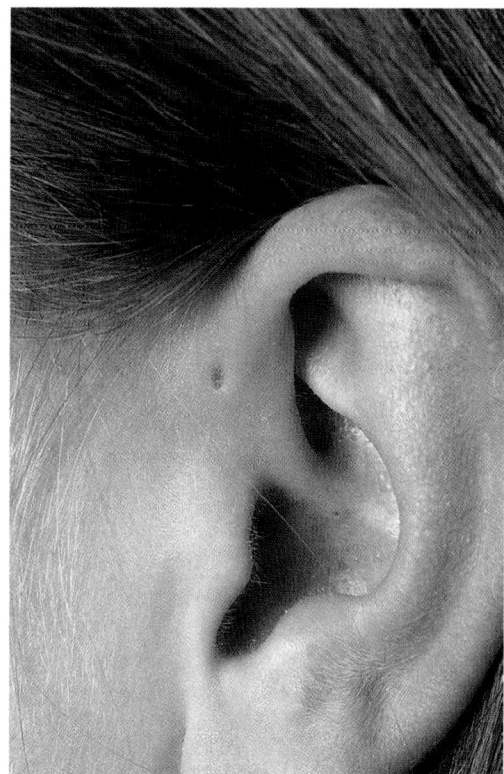

Figure 108.7 Pre-auricular sinus.

firm elevations of skin and cartilage just near the ascending crus of the helix. They may be single or multiple, and may occur anywhere in a line from the tragus to the angle of the mouth. Accessory auricles, congenital fistulae and other external ear manifestations may occur alone or may be associated with more widespread first and second branchial arch abnormalities, for example Treacher Collins and Goldenhar syndromes [4,5,9,23], or with developmental abnormalities of the genito-urinary tract [9,24], as well as with isolated hearing defects. Because of the association with renal abnormalities, it has been recommended that a renal ultrasound scan should be performed if there is a pre-auricular pit or sinus associated with one or more of the following: another malformation or dysmorphic feature, a family history of deafness, auricular and/or renal malformations, or a maternal history of gestational diabetes [25].

Variations in the shape of the pinna

Minor variations in size and shape are common and not usually associated with any other abnormality. These include *bat ear* or protruding ear, in which the antihelix lacks the usual bulge; *lop ear*, in which there is an unrolled helix, a poorly developed antihelix and scapha, and a large concha resulting in a somewhat floppy ear; and *prominent auricular (Darwin) tubercle*. Variations in the contour of the helix and antihelix to produce a bulge of the anterosuperior part of the pinna account for so-called *Mozart's ear*, and in *Wildemuth's ear* the antihelix is prominent and the formation of the helix is poor. These minor ear anomalies can be a syndromic feature or can be associated with conductive and occasionally sensorineural hearing loss, but in most instances they are isolated. They may, however, be inherited, as in the Mozart family. A distinctive *railroad track abnormality* with marked prominence of the crus of

PART 10: SITES, SEX, AGE

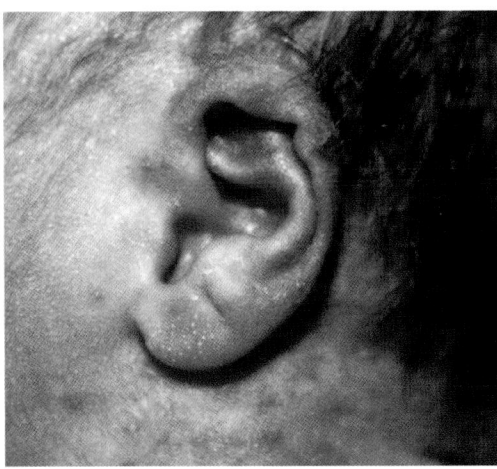

Figure 108.8 Diagonal earlobe crease in an infant with Beckwith–Wiedemann syndrome.

the helix is said to occur in up to 30% of children with fetal alcohol syndrome [12,16] and a protruding auricle may, rarely, be a sign of neuromuscular disease [26]. Various abnormalities of the configuration of the pinna have been described in the distinctive *lumpy scalp syndrome* [27], in which other features include absent or rudimentary nipples and dermal nodules on the scalp [28]. The lobule can show isolated abnormalities, for example pits and clefts. Absence of the lobule is, however, usually associated with a syndrome of a more serious nature [7]. Diagonal linear creases in the lobule are seen in Beckwith–Wiedemann syndrome (Figure 108.8), and in adult life in association with some degenerative diseases, although they are also a common finding in normal individuals.

Developmental anomalies of ear hair
Hypertrichosis of the pinnae (MIM 425500) was originally described as a Y-chromosome linked trait [29]. An autosomal dominant genetic basis for hairy ears has also been noted in South Indians [30] and Maltese [31]. Acquired hairy ears have been described in infants born of diabetic mothers [32,33] and in association with HIV infection [34].

Management
The infant with obvious malformation of the pinna that might have auditory system or other associations should be assessed by a paediatrician. The history may reveal exposure to a teratogen (e.g. isotretinoin) or family history of a syndrome and examination may show evidence of other anomalies. Investigations may include radiological evaluation [35], an auditory brainstem evoked response hearing test and a renal ultrasound. It may be appropriate for an ear, nose and throat (ENT) specialist and plastic surgeon to become involved with correction of complications and the physical deformity, respectively.

Ageing changes

Many changes seen on the skin of the pinna attributed to ageing are a result of its exposure to environmental factors, especially UV radiation, cold (perniosis) and infrared radiation. The elderly exposed pinna often shows varying degrees of dermal and epidermal atrophy, solar keratoses and lentigines, solar elastosis, telangiectasia and venous lakes. If the pinna is at least partially light

protected, as in many women, the skin may still appear somewhat thinned due to intrinsic ageing changes. It has long been observed that the pinna grows progressively throughout life, more so in males than females, and this has been confirmed in a large study [1].

Ear length
It is recognized in Chinese culture that length of the ear in men is a predictor for longevity [2]. Two studies would appear to confirm this: one from Kent, UK [3], and one from Japan [4]. The increase in length of the male ear from the age of 30 years onwards may have a 7-year periodicity [5].

Earlobe creases
First described in 1973 [6], and sometimes known as Frank's sign, a diagonal crease in the earlobes of adults has been associated in many studies with an increased risk for atherosclerotic coronary artery disease. A meta-analysis in 1983 gave a relative risk of 2.06 for heart disease if there are bilateral creases [7] and there is approximately double the risk for death from heart disease [8,9]. It has a greater positive predictive value in people under age 40 years [10]. The crease can be graded in terms of length and depth, and deeper, longer creases have the strongest association. The ear crease appears to be separate from other risk factors for coronary artery disease, and is not simply a function of age [11].

Diagonal earlobe creases are seen in other contexts, for example Beckwith–Wiedemann syndrome [12] (see Figure 108.8), and do not seem to be associated with coronary artery disease in Hawaiians [13], Native Americans [14] or Chinese [15].

Earlobe creases have also been associated with primary open-angle glaucoma [16].

Traumatic conditions

Contusion and haematoma
Bruises of the ear are usually due to blunt trauma and are common in contact sports, such as boxing, wrestling and rugby. In children, physical abuse may need to be excluded [1,2]. A distinctive condition known as *tin ear syndrome* has been considered pathognomonic of child abuse: a triad of isolated ear bruising, haemorrhagic retinopathy and a small, ipsilateral subdural haematoma [3].

Following trauma, blood and serum collects in the plane between the perichondrium and cartilage, and will undergo fibrosis if not removed early. The patient should be carefully examined for concurrent auditory canal, middle ear, parotid and central nervous system trauma.

Repeated trauma may result in the distorted nodular deformity known as *cauliflower ear*, which is due to varying degrees of cartilage necrosis, fibrosis and dystrophic calcification.

Treatment
Subperichondrial haematomas must be treated promptly, with full aseptic technique to avoid secondary perichondritis. Small collections of fluid can sometimes be aspirated by syringe, but usually need to be drained through a small incision and a laterally placed

pressure dressing applied to prevent reaccumulation [4,5]. Another useful technique is to use a through-and-through suture technique to maintain bolsters over the area where the haematoma has been evacuated [6]. Other approaches include a posterior incision and suction drainage [7], or fenestrations in the cartilage to promote adhesion of the opposing perichondrial layers [8]. Prophylactic antibiotics are sometimes given. Improvement of cauliflower ear usually requires multiple corrective procedures.

Ear piercing

Earrings have been worn by men and women since antiquity, and tend to follow the dictates of fashion. Current trends include using rings or studs in almost all parts of the body, the use of up to 10 or more in a single ear, and the piercing of cartilage. Body piercings other than earlobes represent a marker for risky behaviour [1,2,3].

Complications of ear piercing are very common, with rates of about 30% whether the procedure is carried out by medical personnel, a friend or a relative, or in a store; they are also independent of technique, there being little difference in frequency of complications from piercing by needle, staple gun or sharpened stud [4]. Minor infection is the most common adverse effect, with contact dermatitis, keloid and traumatic tear occurring less often [5]; other consequences occur occasionally. Although case series indicate that so-called 'high' ear piercing, that is through cartilage, has a significant risk for perichondritis [6,7] and chondritis [8], such events were not found in a population study of 1000 nurses [5]. Embedding of the earring seems to be a common problem in children [9].

The ear is also pierced in acupuncture as used in traditional medicine, and complications have been reported [10,11].

Complications

Bacterial infection

This is common and usually due to Gram-positive cocci. Predisposing factors include skin disease, such as atopic eczema or contact dermatitis. Life-threatening septicaemia has been described [12]. Infants with unsuspected immunodeficiency and individuals with valvular heart disease may be at particular risk [13]. Even in healthy individuals, infective endocarditis is a risk [14]. When cartilage is pierced the usual bacterial infection is with *Pseudomonas aeruginosa*, which causes perichondritis [6] or chondritis [8], and for which the best treatment is ciprofloxacin [7]. Any purulent material should be cultured, since other pathogens have been described (e.g. *Lactobacillus*) [14]. There is a report of pyogenic spondylitis [15]. Primary tuberculosis has been described [16].

Viral infection

Viral hepatitis may occasionally be a hazard [17,18].

Oedema and haematoma [1,19]

These commonly occur, and usually respond to cold compresses, pressure and removal of the earring. Haematoma may require incision and drainage [20].

Trauma

This can occur from pressure on the lobe and post-auricular skin, or from inaccurate insertion of the post of the earring. Heavy earrings can tear the earlobe, sometimes making it bifid. Repair of the latter is probably best by excision of the cleft and simple closure with eversion of the edges [21], although a staggered repair such as a Z-plasty may be appropriate in some cases.

Sensitization

Earrings remain a major source of sensitization to nickel, and ear piercing is one explanation for the higher incidence of nickel allergy in females [22]. Even stainless steel studs and clasps, which can produce irritant as well as allergic effects, may release sufficient nickel to elicit contact dermatitis [23]. Gold sensitization, although less common [24], can be a protracted cause of dermatitis even after the earrings are removed [25]. Contact dermatitis from other materials used in earrings, such as olive wood [26], copper [27], cobalt [28,29] and chromium [30], has been described, and may also occur from the use of topical antiseptics, antibiotics and dressings used to treat infection. When nickel in ear piercings has been banned, as in Denmark in 1992, there has been a substantial fall in nickel sensitization [31].

Granulomatous and lymphoid reactions

Reddish brown and purple papules and nodules at sites of ear piercing may denote a granulomatous response to gold [32,33] and a lymphocytoma cutis like reaction has been described [34–36]. Similar reactions have been associated with palladium [37] and titanium [38]. Sarcoidosis has presented after ear piercing [39,40].

Embedded earrings

The spring-loaded gun method of ear piercing can result in the earring backing becoming embedded in the back of the ear [41]. The 'vanishing earring' [42] can resemble a keloid [43]. The embedded metal can usually be pulled out, or if necessary an incision can be made to locate it.

Epidermoid cyst formation

Implantation epidermoid cysts due to ear piercing often present as tender, chronic, inflammatory swellings, sometimes with drainage. There is usually an epithelial lined track as well as cysts, and all epithelial tissue must be removed, for example with a skin punch [44].

Keloids

These quite commonly follow ear piercing, especially in those ethnic groups with a predisposition (Figure 108.9). Piercing before the age of 11 years is more likely to be followed by keloid than after that age [45]. The keloids seem to occur more on the back surface than the front of the earlobe [46]. As well as being unsightly, they can itch and be painful.

Treatment options include intralesional steroid, pressure [47], excision alone [48,49], with or without concurrent use of intralesional steroid [50] and radiotherapy [51] (see Chapter 10). Combinations of these methods are often advocated [52,53]. Prospective controlled trials are needed to assess these approaches. A relatively

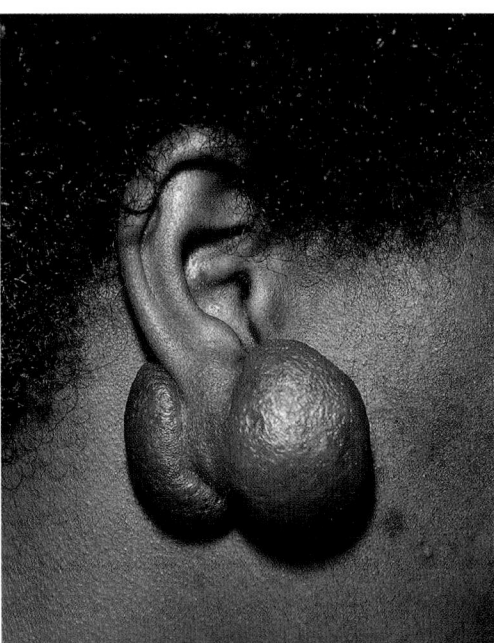

Figure 108.9 Keloids following ear piercing.

simple and safe method which has shown efficacy and acceptability is injection of intralesional steroid followed by Zimmer splints which can be decorated to look like earrings [54].

Localized argyria

This presents as bluish macules, usually on the posterior surface of the earlobe [55,56].

Frostbite

This has followed the use of ethyl chloride topical anaesthesia [57].

Relapsing polychondritis

A case of severe relapsing polychondritis following ear piercing has been reported [58].

Measures to prevent complications [59]

Many of the complications of ear piercing are avoidable. The procedure is best not carried out on children, or in those with immunodeficiency, valvular heart disease or sarcoidosis, and there is clearly a risk if the individual has a tendency to keloid formation. For a dermatologist who wishes to pierce ears or instruct others, a simple method with a low likelihood of complications has been described [**60**]. The use of a surgical-grade, stainless steel, one-piece earring with an interlocking groove has been recommended. Gold-plated or gold-alloy earrings should be avoided for at least 6 weeks after the ear has been pierced. Sterile technique is important. Piercing of cartilage should be avoided. Only nickel-free earrings should be used. Large or heavy earrings should be removed prior to activities that may result in tearing of the earlobes. A technique using a piece of intravenous catheter to avoid reactions in metal-sensitive individuals has been described [61].

Chondrodermatitis nodularis

Definition and nomenclature

Chondrodermatitis nodularis (CN) is a benign, usually painful condition of the parts of the ear containing cartilage, most commonly the superior portion of the helix, antihelix and tragus, and occasionally the antitragus and concha.

Synonyms and inclusions
- Chondrodermatitis nodularis chronica helicis and antihelicis (ante- is often used as an alternative to anti-)

Introduction and general description

Chondrodermatitis nodularis presents as an inflammatory condition involving cartilage and overlying skin, resulting in a firm nodule which often ulcerates and becomes crusted. It is usually painful. Most occur on the helix and antihelix. Males are more commonly affected than females, and most patients are middle aged or elderly. Pressure, such as sleeping predominantly on one side, is a common precipitating factor. It can mimic skin cancer and pre-cancerous conditions.

Epidemiology

Incidence

Although there are no good data on frequency, CN is common in older persons.

Age

Chondrodermatitis is most common in the middle aged and elderly. When it occurs in the younger patient [1] there is sometimes a structural abnormality and/or a pathological process in the cartilage, or use of an abnormally hard pillow.

Sex

There is a ratio of 10 males to 1 female in most series; it is relatively commoner in females in younger individuals.

Ethnicity

It occurs mainly in fair-skinned individuals.

Associated diseases

Weathering nodules and other skin diseases associated with outdoor exposure. Some cases are associated with diseases causing microvascular injury such as systemic sclerosis [2].

Pathophysiology

Arteriolar narrowing in the perichondrium may be the cause of the pathological changes seen in CN [3], with a number of predisposing contributory factors.

Predisposing factors

1 Pressure, e.g. from sleeping on one side, headgear or headphones results in compromised local blood supply.

2 Solar radiation.
3 Exposure to cold, wind.
4 Systemic sclerosis [4] and childhood dermatomyositis [5].
5 Abnormal structural variants of the pinna.

Pathology
A typical lesion of CN consists of a nodule of degenerate homogeneous collagen surrounded by vascular granulation tissue with an overlying acanthotic epidermis, and there may be a central ulcer through which the damaged collagen is extruded. In nearly all cases, there is inflammation and fibrosis of the underlying perichondrium, and degenerative changes may be seen in the cartilage. There is often transepidermal elimination of altered connective tissue [6]. There is an increased number of small nerves [7].

Genetics
Chondrodermatitis nodularis is not normally regarded as having a genetic basis, but simultaneous occurrence in monozygotic twins has been reported [8].

Environmental factors
These include pressure, previous weathering from exposure to solar radiation, cold, wind, etc.

Clinical features
The lesion usually begins as a globular or oval nodule, about 0.5–1 cm in diameter, raised above the often hyperaemic surrounding skin (Figure 108.10). The surface may be scaly or crusted, concealing a small ulcer. Sometimes the condition is first noticed as an ulcer. In men, nearly 90% of nodules are situated on the helix, usually at the upper pole and more frequently on the right, but may occur on the antihelix, tragus, concha and antitragus, in order of decreasing frequency. Occasionally, there are multiple nodules or lesions, and they may occur bilaterally. In women, the left and right ears are affected equally and the proportion of lesions on the antihelix and tragus is greater.

Presentation
The patient, usually a middle-aged to elderly man, seeks advice on account of pain. The more stoical may postpone consultation until the lesion interferes with sleep. The pain, which is sometimes severe, is initiated by pressure and occasionally by cold. It may be brief but can persist and throb for an hour or more. Occasionally, and particularly in women, there is little discomfort.

Differential diagnosis
Basal cell carcinoma (BCC), squamous carcinoma and actinic keratosis; weathering nodule of the ear [9].

Disease course and prognosis
If untreated, CN usually persists.

Investigations
Biopsy should be performed if there is any doubt about the diagnosis.

Management
For symptomatic CN, measures should be taken to relieve pressure over the ear where this is a contributory factor.

First line
Various interventions to provide relief of pressure during sleep include a doughnut-shaped pillow [10], protective hollowed-out foam [11], a moulded prosthesis and self-adhering foam [12].

Second line
Traditional medical measures include intralesional corticosteroid injection, e.g. triamcinolone 10 mg/mL [13], and liquid nitrogen cryotherapy.

Recently, promising results have been reported using twice-daily topical 2% nitroglycerin, a relaxant of arteriolar smooth muscle [14].

Surgical treatment can be curative. The most effective approach is to remove the abnormal cartilage and retain as much as possible of the overlying skin, ensuring that the edges of the cartilage are smooth [15,16,17]. A modification of this using a sutureless closure has been described [18]. Many other surgical techniques have been used, including curettage, shave excision, wedge excision, punch excision replacing the removed tissue with punch biopsy derived graft [19], and excision followed by flap repair [20].

Third line
Photodynamic therapy has been used successfully in a few cases [21,22]. Other treatments include cushioning from collagen injections and carbon dioxide laser treatment [23].

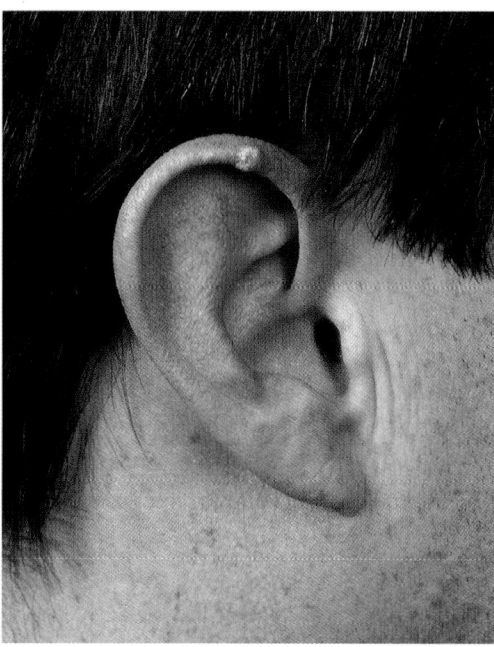

Figure 108.10 Chondrodermatitis nodularis of the helix. A superficially ulcerated, exquisitely tender nodule.

PART 10: SITES, SEX, AGE

Resources

Patient resources

http://www.patient.co.uk/doctor/chondrodermatitis-nodularis   (last   accessed
    October 2014).

Pseudocyst of the ear

Definition and nomenclature
A non-inflammatory fluid-filled cavity within the cartilage of the ear.

Synonyms and inclusions
- Pseudocyst of the auricle
- Endochondral pseudocyst
- Intracartilaginous cyst
- Cystic chondromalacia
- Benign idiopathic cystic chondromalacia

Introduction and general description
Pseudocyst of the ear is an uncommon fluid-filled swelling due
to the appearance of a space within the cartilage. It is probably a
result of trauma.

Epidemiology

Incidence and prevalence
Pseudocyst of the ear is uncommon. There are no data on the incidence or prevalence.

Age
It is most common in young men. It can occur over a wide age
range [1] including infants [2].

Sex
Males more than females.

Ethnicity
There may be a predilection for the Chinese, although this could
be due to reporting bias [3,4].

Pathophysiology
The exact pathophysiology is unknown. There is often minor
repetitive trauma, such as rubbing and ear twisting. It has been
suggested that trauma may induce a break in the cartilage [5]. It
has also been speculated that there might be an underlying malformation of the cartilage. A characteristic finding is elevation
of isoforms 4 and 5 of lactate dehydrogenase (LDH) – these are
released from chondrocytes [6]. It was once thought that cartilage degeneration was due to release of lysosomal enzymes from
the chondrocytes, but this has not been substantiated. A role for
cytokines has been suggested [7].

Predisposing factors
Circumstances which cause trauma include sporting injury, rubbing due to atopic eczema, habit-related twisting of the ears,
sleeping on hard pillows and wearing a motorcycle helmet and/
or earphones.

Pathology
There is a cavity within the cartilage. The walls of the cavity are
not lined by epithelium and within the cartilage there is eosinophilic amorphous material. There may be focal fibrosis, especially
in older lesions [8,9].

Clinical features

History
A painless swelling appears over a 1–3-month period.

Presentation
The swelling is typically fluctuant and non-tender. It is usually on
the upper outer aspect of the ear (Figure 108.11). The condition is
usually unilateral. If fluid is aspirated, it is clear or yellowish.

Clinical variants
Uncommonly, there may be some signs of inflammation and tenderness.

Differential diagnosis
Other swellings on the ear including haematoma, cysts, tumours,
perichondritis and relapsing polychondritis.

Disease course and prognosis
Untreated, the condition may lead to fibrosis causing deformity of
the pinna.

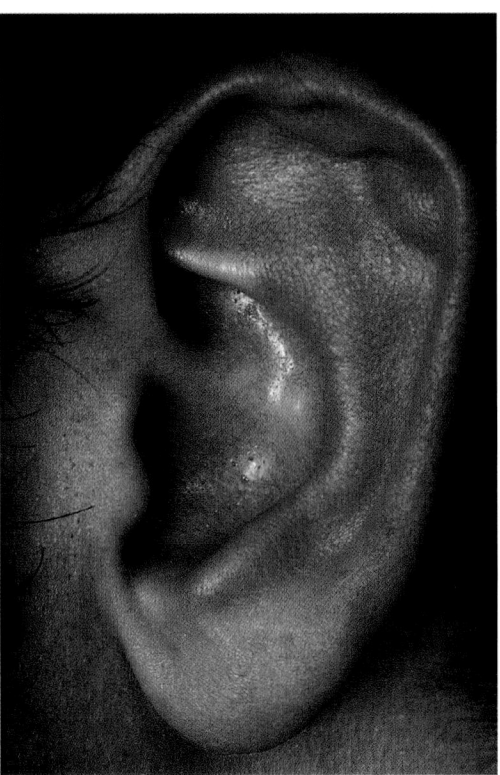

Figure 108.11 Pseudocyst. Asymptomatic fluctuant swellings on the upper pinna.

PART 10: SITES, SEX, AGE

Investigations
Biopsy may be needed to exclude other diagnoses.

Management
There are no adequate studies comparing the different modalities of treatment that have been described.

First line
Aspiration and local pressure for 3 weeks, e.g. from a thermoplastic material such as Aquaplast® [10] or a mastoid bandage.

Second line
De-roofing the anterior wall of the cyst through an incision along the antihelical line appears to be more successful than aspiration and dressing, or steroid injection [11].

Third line
Other treatments which have all been reported to be successful in small series include aspiration followed by intralesional triamcinolone [12], fibrin [13,14], minocycline or trichloracetic acid.

Manifestation of skin disease and systemic disease in the ear

The external ear is often the site for the manifestation of skin disease and systemic disease presenting in the skin. Some of these skin manifestations are shown in the Table 108.1, with cross references to other chapters where the condition is covered in more detail.

Infection

The anatomy of the ear, with its many folds and the semi-occluded nature of the external auditory canal, make it particularly susceptible to intertriginous infection, especially with Gram-negative organisms. The close anatomical relationship between the middle and external ear means that infections can pass relatively easily from one to the other, and the eardrum should always be examined. The cartilaginous and bony structures close to the skin are particularly vulnerable to infection. Although chondritis and perichondritis may have other causes, they are included in this section.

Infection of the pinna

Pyogenic infection
Staphylococcus aureus, alone or in association with group A β-haemolytic *Streptococcus*, may cause impetigo of the ear. This is a relatively common site for infection in infants and young children. *Staphylococcus aureus* is also the most common causative organism of furuncles (boils) and carbuncles, which are more common in the external auditory canal than on the pinna. Cracks and fissures around the auricle are often the portal of entry for β-haemolytic

streptococcal infection manifesting as erysipelas. This is more common in the elderly, the newborn and those suffering from malnutrition, disability, alcoholism, diabetes or immune deficiency states.

Staphylococcal furunculosis may occur on or near the auricle. Coalescence of adjacent infected follicles results in a carbuncle. In the ear canal furunculosis typically causes pain, which can be aggravated by chewing if there is involvement of the anterior wall of the canal. There may be sufficient swelling to obstruct the entrance to the canal. There is often regional lymphadenopathy and sometimes fever. Furunculosis is sometimes classified as acute localized otitis externa (OE).

Furunculosis can usually be distinguished from external otitis by the normal appearance of the canal epithelium and an absence of discharge; the two conditions can, however, coexist. If possible the tympanic membrane should be examined, in order to exclude otitis media and mastoiditis.

Erysipelas typically begins with high fever and constitutional upset, including malaise, vomiting and headache, and there is rapidly spreading erythema and oedema from the pinna on to the face. There is often lymphadenopathy. Recurrent attacks of cellulitis of the face may have the same predisposing factors as at other body sites. Recurrent attacks of cellulitis lead to fibrosis and lymphoedema. Treatment of erysipelas and cellulitis is discussed in Chapter 26. Necrotizing fasciitis has rarely been described arising from an initial infection of the pinna.

The term *infective eczematoid dermatitis* is still sometimes used for an oozing crusted eczematous condition occurring on and often below the pinna in association with chronic discharge from the ear. Coagulase-positive staphylococci are the most frequently isolated bacteria. The ear canal is oedematous and erythematous, and purulent discharge may be seen coming from a perforated tympanic membrane. The condition should be differentiated from impetigo, secondarily infected contact dermatitis, seborrhoeic dermatitis and atopic eczema.

Other bacterial infections
Mycobacterial infection can rarely involve the external ear. Lupus vulgaris can produce extensive destruction and may mimic other conditions. Secondary involvement from underlying lymph node disease (scrofuloderma) can present with hearing loss, tinnitus and periauricular lymphadenopathy, with only minimal secretion in the ear canal.

Atypical mycobacteria that may involve the ear include *M. marinum* acquired from swimming pool injuries. In leprosy, the ear is almost always involved in the lepromatous type, and there may be evident infiltration of the skin. The earlobe is often used for taking smears.

Syphilis may occasionally involve the ear, usually in the secondary stage.

Viral infections
Herpes simplex occasionally involves the ear. It is often transmitted during contact sports such as rugby and wrestling. Herpes zoster may present as an isolated herpetiform eruption of the external ear or may be associated with ipsilateral facial palsy

Table 108.1 Skin manifestations of the ear that may indicate other skin disease or systemic disease.

Diagnosis	Clinical features	Cross reference
Acne	Comedones frequently involve the concha, and are occasionally found on the helix, tragus or earlobe. Inflammatory cysts may be found on the lobe, at the entrance to the external auditory canal, or in both the pre- and post-auricular areas. Pressure from spectacle frames, telephone receivers or headsets can aggravate acne lesions	Chapter 90
Acromegaly	There may be enlargement of the auricular cartilage and coarsening of the overlying skin	Chapter 149
Addison disease	Pigmentary changes may involve the ear, and ossification of the auricular cartilage may occur in Addison disease [1]	Chapter 149
Alkaptonuria	This is typically associated with a bluish discoloration of the auricular cartilage due to oxidation of bound homogentisic acid (Figure 108.12). The cerumen in such patients may be very dark, a finding that can precede other clinical manifestations	Chapter 63
Amyloidosis, primary cutaneous	Asymptomatic papules on the helix and concha of the ear have been described as the sole manifestation of cutaneous amyloidosis [2]; such lesions can also occur with more generalized papular amyloid [3] and with macular amyloid of the back [4]	Chapter 58
Angiolymphoid hyperplasia with eosinophilia	This commonly affects the pinna, external auditory meatus (Figure 108.13) and post-auricular area. The lesions are red-brown papules or nodules. Occasionally, they itch and can be painful or pulsatile [5]. The condition mainly affects young to middle-aged adults, and in some series there is a female preponderance	Chapter 137
Asteatotic eczema	This common cause of a dry itchy ear is mainly seen in the elderly. Aggravating factors include overzealous cleansing, cold, windy weather, low humidity indoors and air-conditioned air during the summer. There may be little to see other than slight scaling. Similar changes can occur in the ear canal, where additional factors include drying vehicles used in ear drops, e.g. alcohol and acetone. Management will include avoidance of provocative factors, and use of emollients	Chapter 39
Atopic eczema	A crusted eczematous fissure at the junction of the earlobe and the face is a common finding in atopics, and can be regarded as a reliable feature of atopy [6]. In addition to involvement of the infra-auricular crease, the tragal notch and sometimes the whole of the pinna may be commonly involved	Chapter 41
Bazex syndrome	Bazex syndrome (acrokeratosis paraneoplastica) commonly affects the ears and is an important marker for internal malignancy [7]	Chapter 147
Bullous diseases	Pemphigus, pemphigoid, dermatitis herpetiformis and epidermolysis bullosa aquisita may all involve the ear, and occasionally the auditory canal. Blistering of the pinna and stenosis of the canal can occur in dystrophic epidermolysis bullosa [8]	Chapter 50
Calcification, dystrophic	Calcium deposition may occur in many circumstances and occasionally the ear is involved. Usually, calcium deposits in the ear occur for local reasons, e.g. degenerative changes in the cartilage. In infants, congenital nodular calcification of Winer should be considered [9] (Figure 108.14)	Chapter 61
Contact dermatitis	The external ear is commonly affected by both irritant and allergic contact dermatitis. Causes of contact allergy can be grouped as follows: • Products used for the hair and scalp • Items worn or placed in or on the ear: jewelry, especially nickel alloys • Plastic, rubber and metal ear appliances, e.g. hearing aids, spectacles, headphones, telephone receivers, earplugs, hairnets • Objects used to clean or scratch the ear • Topical medicaments • Transferred to the ear by fingers, e.g. nail varnish, plant resins, etc.	Chapters 128, 129
Crohn disease	Metastatic Crohn disease may rarely involve the ear [10]	Chapter 152
Cutis laxa	Cutis laxa may result in distinctive pendulous earlobes [11]	Chapter 96
Darier disease	Occasionally, Darier disease can present with involvement of the external ear as the principal affected site, with erythema, oedema and crusting mimicking an eczematous reaction [12]	
Drug reaction	Purpura of the ears has been described in a series of children receiving levamisole for nephritic syndrome [13]. Both vasculitis and thrombotic changes occurred, and there was an association with circulating autoantibodies Hypertrophy of the retroauricular folds may be seen as a consequence of phenytoin therapy [14] Hypertrichosis of the ear canal due to minoxidil therapy can be a predisposing factor for external otitis [15]	Chapter 66
Elephantiasis	Chronically red swollen ears may occur for a number of reasons, including longstanding eczema, psoriasis [16] and chronic streptococcal infection. Longstanding head louse infection has also been reported as a cause [17]	

Diagnosis	Clinical features	Cross reference
Gout	Gouty tophi frequently involve the pinna (Figure 108.15), and may antedate the onset of joint disease or appear decades after the initial attack. The helix and antihelix are typical sites. Histology is distinctive	Chapter 63
Granuloma annulare	Typical papular and annular dermal lesions of granuloma annulare may involve the pinna, sometimes in the absence of lesions elsewhere [18]	Chapter 97
Granuloma faciale	The ear is an occasional site for the brownish red plaques of this distinctive disorder [19]	Chapter 102
Granulomatosis with polyangiitis (Wegener granulomatosis)	Granulomatosis with polyangiitis can present with serous or suppurative otitis and conductive or sensorineural deafness [28]	Chapter 102
Jessner benign lymphocytic infiltration of the skin	This condition occasionally involves the ear and post-auricular region, and sunlight may precipitate or worsen the eruption	Chapter 135
Leprosy	In leprosy the earlobe is a valuable site for taking smears [20]	Chapter 28
Lichen planus	Lichen planus typically causes discharge and hearing loss due to stenosis of the external auditory canal. Pruritus, pain and bleeding may also occur. The canal appears red and there may be Wickham's striae [21]	
Lupus erythematosus	Discoid, subacute cutaneous and systemic lupus erythematosus can all involve the ears. The concha is a characteristic site for chronic discoid lupus erythematosus (Figure 108.16)	Chapter 37
Lymphoma	Systemic lymphoma can occasionally present as an isolated lesion on the ear [22], as can other haematological malignancies	Chapter 51
Mudi-chood	This distinctive dermatosis, which typically affects the nape of the neck and upper shoulders of girls and young women in the state of Kerala in South India, can occur on the ears. It is thought to be the result of the frictional and occlusive effects of moist oily hair in a hot and humid environment. Individual lesions are hyperpigmented papules with a thin surrounding rim of scale, occurring on the posterolateral aspects of the pinnae [23]	Chapter 140
Perforating disorders	The ear may occasionally be the site for lesions of Kyrle disease, elastosis perforans serpiginosa, perforating folliculitis and perforating papules of diabetic dialysis patients	
Photodermatoses	The ear is a common site for conditions provoked or aggravated by UV and/or visible radiation. A condition peculiar to the ear is juvenile spring eruption (Figure 108.17), a variant of polymorphic light eruption, typically found in young boys	Chapter 127
Porphyria	Porphyria cutanea tarda (Figure 108.18) may present with vesicles and bullae, often on a background of scarring, hyperpigmentation, milia, sclerodermoid plaques and hypertrichosis. Pseudocysts of the auricle and perichondritis may be simulated [24]	Chapter 60
Psoriasis	Both guttate and plaque psoriasis involve the external ear. Sometimes this is by extension from the scalp, face or neck. Like seborrhoeic dermatitis, psoriasis often involves the concha and distal part of the external auditory canal, but usually its colour, the nature of the scaling (Figure 108.19) and the presence of psoriasis elsewhere allow it to be differentiated. Sometimes both conditions appear to coexist	Chapter 35
Relapsing polychondritis	Relapsing polychondritis is characterised by redness, tenderness and swelling of the ear, but with sparing of the lobe	
Rheumatoid disease	Rheumatoid disease is characterized by nodules, which can occur on the ear, where they may ulcerate due to pressure from a pillow or spectacles	Chapter 154
Sarcoidosis	Cutaneous sarcoidosis [25] can involve the ear, especially the lupus pernio variety	Chapter 98
Seborrhoeic dermatitis	In its mildest form, seborrhoeic dermatitis simply causes a little scaling and inflammation at the entrance to the external auditory meatus, in the concha or in the auricular folds. When severe, the whole pinna may be affected and there may be infective eczematoid dermatitis both in and around the ear or post-auricularly.	Chapter 40
Systemic sclerosis	Scleroderma can produce pallor and telangiectasia of the auditory canal	Chapter 56
Verruciform xanthoma	This uncommon condition is typically found in the mouth but has been reported on the ear, where it can mimic squamous cell carcinoma [26]	Chapter 62
Weathering nodules	These asymptomatic histologically distinct nodules are found on the free edge of the helix (Figure 108.20). They are quite common, increasingly so with age in older men [27]	
Xanthogranuloma, adult	Symmetrical yellow-red nodular lesions with the same histology as juvenile xanthogranuloma have been described on the earlobes [29]	Chapter 136
Xanthoma	Xanthomas occasionally occur on the ears, presenting as yellow nodules	Chapter 62

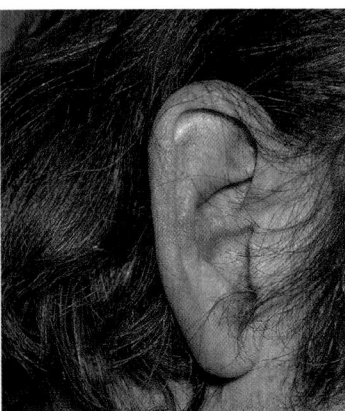

Figure 108.12 Alkaptonuria. The auricular cartilage has a distinctive blue colour. (Courtesy of Dr P. Hollingworth, Southmead Hospital, Bristol, UK.)

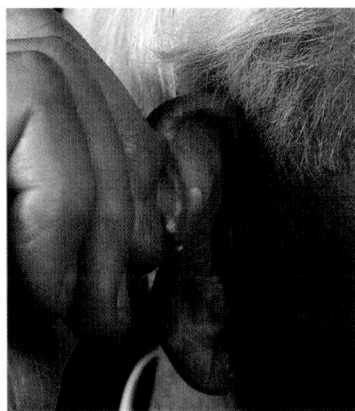

Figure 108.15 Gouty tophi. Yellowish dermal nodules.

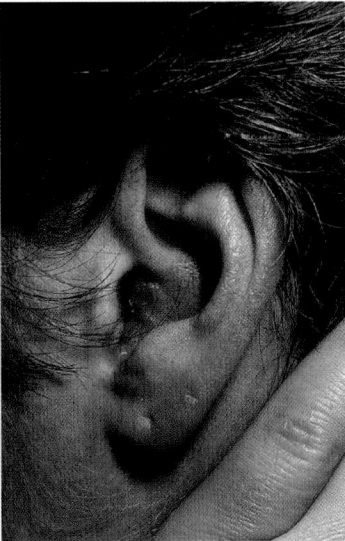

Figure 108.13 Angiolymphoid hyperplasia with eosinophilia. Firm red-brown nodules at the entrance to the external auditory canal.

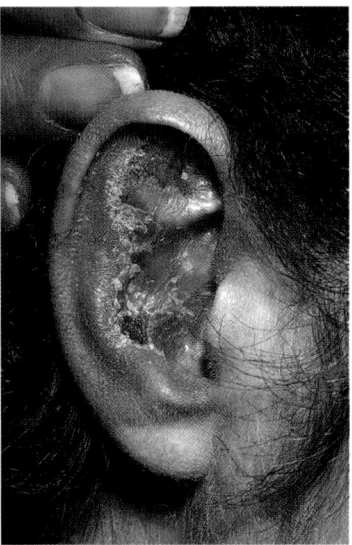

Figure 108.16 Cutaneous lupus erythematosus. Acute erythema and erosions following sun exposure.

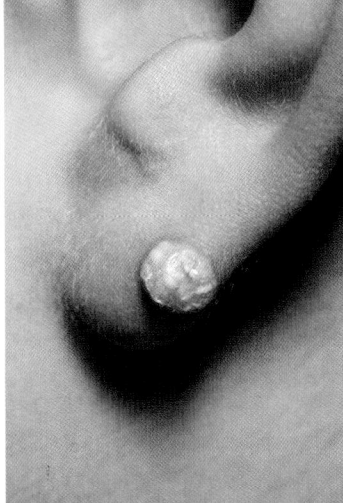

Figure 108.14 Subepidermal calcifying nodule. Hard whitish nodule with slight overlying scale.

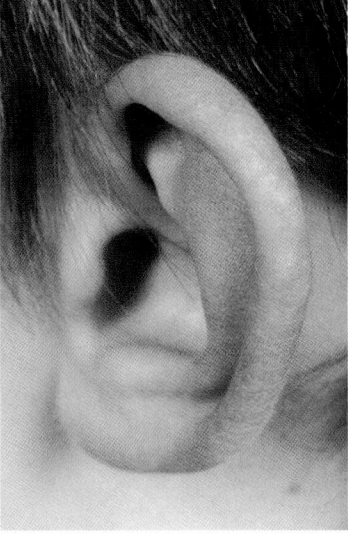

Figure 108.17 Juvenile spring eruption. Subtle oedematous plaques on helix of ear.

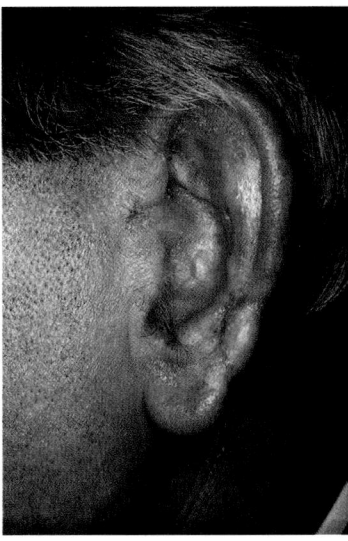

Figure 108.18 Porphyria cutanea tarda. Firm whitish sclerodermoid changes at the site of repeated blistering.

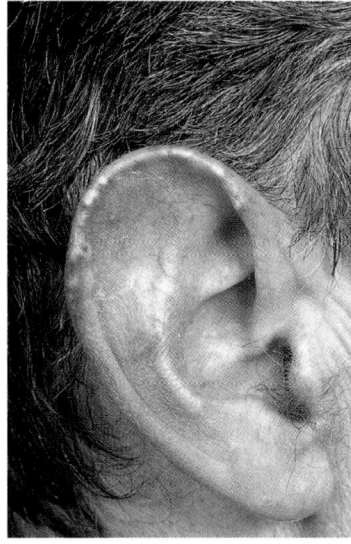

Figure 108.20 Several firm white 'weathering' nodules on the helical rim.

and auditory symptoms (Ramsay Hunt syndrome; geniculate herpes). The condition usually begins with pain and may initially be mistaken for erysipelas. Vesicles usually appear on about the fifth day and involve the pinna, the external auditory meatus and, rarely, the tympanic membrane. There is usually malaise, pyrexia and lymphadenopathy. Facial palsy, when it occurs, is usually transient, but more severe and persistent cases do occur. Taste and lacrimation may also be affected. Compression damage to the VIIIth cranial nerve may lead to tinnitus, vertigo, nystagmus, nausea and deafness. Management of herpes zoster is discussed in Chapter 25. Orf affecting the ear has been described, presenting as an inflammatory nodule on the tragus.

Superficial and deep mycoses

Dermatophyte fungi may rarely involve the ear, and when present can simulate granulomatous disease and chondritis. Pityriasis versicolor may involve the ears, but is usually easy to diagnose. In cases of ulcerative granulomatous disease of the ear, deep fungal infections, for example sporotrichosis, should be considered. Biopsy, examination of smears, cultures and serological studies should enable accurate diagnosis. Deep fungal infection may prompt an enquiry for underlying immune deficiency.

Otitis externa

Definition and nomenclature

Otitis externa is an inflammatory or infective condition of the skin of the auditory canal and often the adjacent pinna. It may cause varying degrees of pain, itch, deafness and discharge. Acute and chronic forms are recognized (Figure 108.21a,b).

> **Synonyms and inclusions**
> • External otitis
> • Swimmer's ear

Introduction and general description

The term OE may include a number of overlapping conditions:
• Acute localized OE – this term is sometimes used for furunculosis of the ear canal. It is not discussed further here.
• Acute diffuse OE – this has a rapid onset and is generally due to infection, often precipitated by trauma and/or excessive exposure to water or high humidity. Although the infective agent is usually bacterial, viral infection, e.g. herpes zoster, can present as OE.

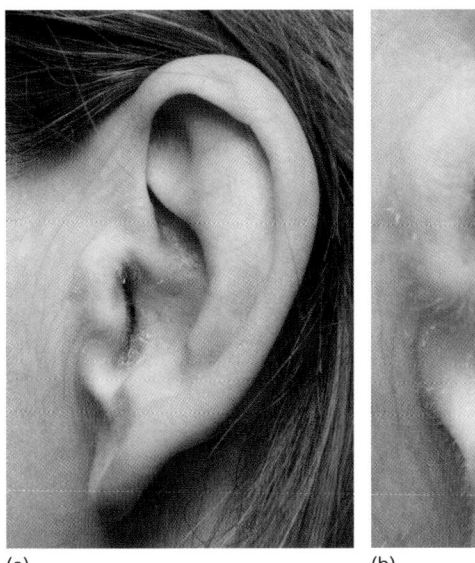
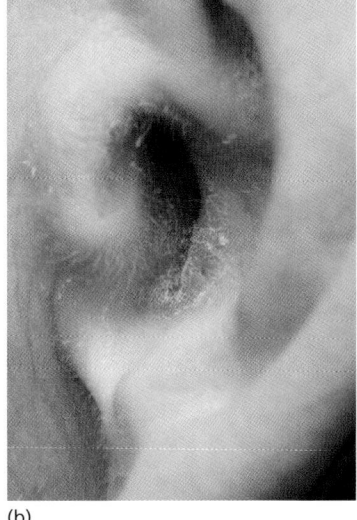

(a)   (b)

Figure 108.19 Psoriasis. (a) Well-defined erythema with prominent scaling at entrance to ear canal – close-up in (b).

PART 10: SITES, SEX, AGE

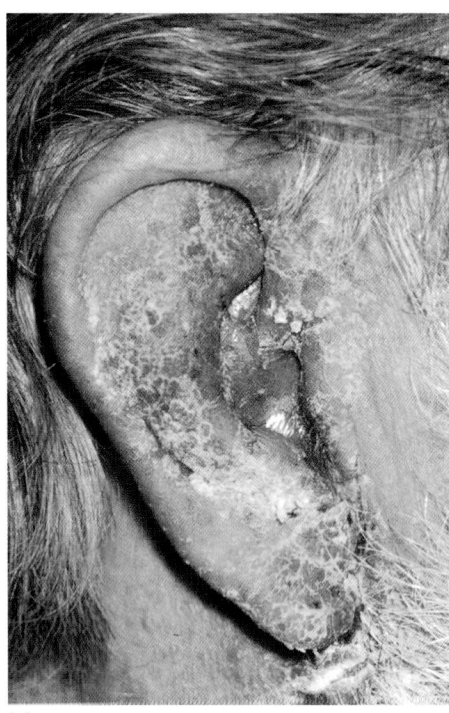

(a)

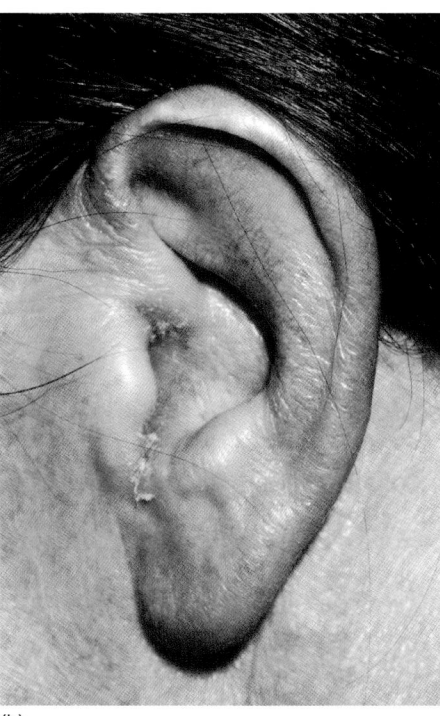

(b)

Figure 108.21 Otitis externa. (a) The pinna and skin nearby is erythematous with crusting and scaling. The entrance to the canal is narrowed. (b) The pinna is erythematous and oedematous. There is crusting at the entrance to a narrowed canal.

- Chronic OE – this lasts for 2 months or more [1]. Factors that contribute to this include an inflammatory dermatosis, trauma, microbial flora, alterations in cerumen and anatomical variations.
- Necrotizing (malignant) OE – this term is used for a more invasive and serious infection, and is discussed separately.

- Otomycosis – this is fungal infection of the external auditory canal; it is discussed separately below.

Epidemiology

Incidence and prevalence
Most data relate to acute diffuse OE, which is common, some studies indicating an annual incidence of about 1 : 250 [2] and appears to be commoner in the summer months, probably because of higher temperatures, humidity and more people engaging in swimming and other water sports [3]. By contrast, necrotizing OE is rare.

Age
Some studies indicate that acute diffuse OE is commoner in children, adolescents and young adults [4].

Sex
There is no sex predilection.

Ethnicity
There are significant racial and individual differences in susceptibility to OE. This may be due to anatomical differences in the curvature of the external auditory canal or narrowing of the isthmus, e.g. natives of New Guinea with wide straight canals only rarely suffer from external otitis [5].

Associated diseases
Chronic OE is often associated with an inflammatory dermatosis, particularly atopic eczema, seborrhoeic dermatitis, contact dermatitis or psoriasis, but occasionally other skin diseases such as discoid lupus erythematosus (Figure 108.22).

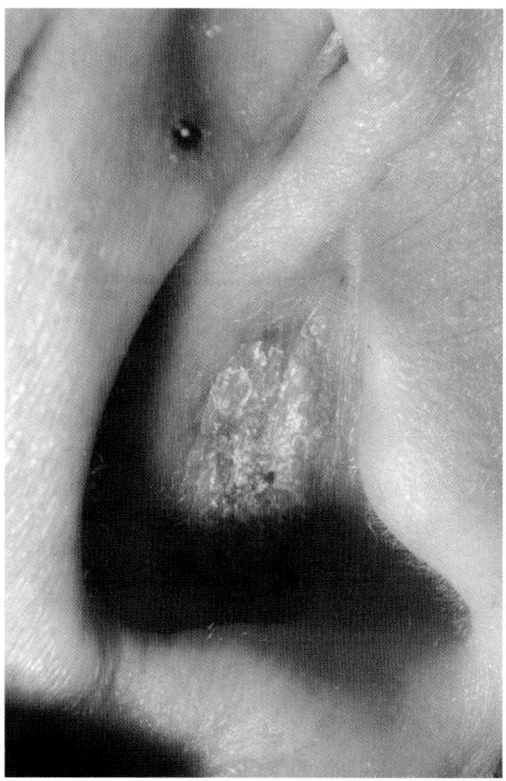

Figure 108.22 Discoid lupus erythematosus . Erythema with adherent scaling in the concha.

Necrotizing OE is likely to be associated with a co-morbidity, particularly diabetes, HIV or previous radiotherapy to the base of the skull.

Pathophysiology

Predisposing factors
Trauma is a common immediate precipitating factor. Examples include insertion of fingernails, paperclips, matches, hair grips and even hearing aid earpieces.

Water retention, e.g. from swimming, plugs of wax, a tortuous canal and abundant hair are also predisposing factors.

Absence of ear wax, e.g. from repeated water exposure or overzealous cleansing can contribute; some individuals may not produce enough cerumen.

Alkaline pH [6] may be associated with chronicity. Increased levels of proteases may also be associated with chronicity [7].

Variations in lectin binding may influence the likelihood of *Pseudomonas* infection – binding occurs more in individuals expressing blood group A on their epithelial cells [8].

Pathology
In most cases of external otitis, there is acanthosis, elongation of the rete ridges and an increase in orthokeratosis and parakeratosis. Spongiosis occurs in eczematous and seborrhoeic forms. The nature of the dermal infiltrate varies with both cause and chronicity. The histopathology is seldom diagnostic except when fungal mycelia are seen.

Causative organisms
Pseudomonas aeruginosa is the commonest infection, particularly in swimmers and in hot humid environments, and the organism probably comes from resident flora in the ear canal. Some strains may be more pathogenic [9]. In more temperate climates, *Staphylococcus aureus* is often isolated. This may be associated with evidence of skin disease elsewhere or with staphylococcal carriage. Meticillin-resistant *S. aureus* (MRSA) infections are becoming more common, especially when the patient has recently had hospital exposure [10].

In the tropics, mycotic infections of the external ear canal are relatively common. *Aspergillus*, *Candida*, *Penicillium* and *Mucor* spp. are the organisms most often incriminated. There is some debate, however, as to whether these fungi are pathogenic, opportunistic, saprophytic or simply commensal. Otomycosis is discussed later.

Environmental factors
Heat, humidity and moisture are undoubtedly important in hot-weather ear or swimmer's ear [11]. This condition is common, especially among white people in tropical and subtropical regions. High temperature, high relative humidity and swimming [12] all encourage maceration and secondary bacterial or fungal infections of the canal epithelium. Freshwater swimming appears to be a particular risk factor [13]. Failure to dry the ears completely after swimming, shampooing or showering may also be a factor in some cases [14].

Clinical features

History – acute otitis externa
Acute diffuse OE typically begins with pain in the ear, sometimes accompanied by itching, and soon there is also a sensation of fullness. There may be a variable degree of hearing loss and there may be clear or purulent discharge – which tends to be bluish-green when *Ps. aeruginosa* is the infective cause.

In chronic OE, the main symptoms are itch, variable pain and discharge, which have persisted for more than 3 months.

Presentation – acute otitis externa
Examination of acute diffuse OE shows erythema and swelling which may spread from the external auditory meatus to involve the concha or beyond. The external auditory canal shows erythema and oedema, and there is macerated debris and perhaps greenish pus present. In severe cases, inflammation can extend to involve the tympanic membrane. Hearing loss is due to oedema of the canal, and this may be sufficient to obscure vision of its full length. Traction on the pinna to examine the canal and pressure over the tragus characteristically elicit pain. There may be associated low-grade fever, malaise and regional lymphadenopathy. If there is a temperature of more than 38.5°C and/or obvious cellulitis, consider necrotizing OE.

In the process of a full examination, it is important to visualize the tympanic membrane to determine whether or not it is intact; if breached, the OE is secondary to otitis media, and drops containing aminoglycosides are best avoided. It may be necessary to gently remove debris by careful suction.

Presentation – chronic otitis externa
The term 'chronic external otitis' is used for cases who have had persistent symptoms for more than 2 months. Microbiological assessment demonstrated a significant organism in 82% of cases in one series [15]: *S. aureus* in one-third, *Pseudomonas* in one-third and various other Gram-negative and Gram-positive organisms in the remainder; in addition, 17 of the 99 patients had fungal disease alone. There is often a dry canal due to lack of cerumen. It is likely that in most cases of chronic OE, particularly when treatment has been used for the acute attack and symptoms have continued, concurrent dermatological disorders are present (Figure 108.23). In patients in whom the disorder behaves in a recalcitrant manner, it is important to consider the possibility that they may have an underlying systemic disease, such as HIV infection, malnutrition or uncontrolled diabetes; a poor therapeutic response is also seen in patients treated with high-dose steroids or chemotherapeutic agents [16].

Seborrhoeic dermatitis, atopic eczema and psoriasis usually occur only at the meatus but may sometimes extend further into the canal. Seborrhoeic OE is extremely common and has been regarded by some dermatologists as the basis for most cases of OE. The symptoms and signs, however, are normally mild unless complicated by secondary factors and usually consist of no more than superficial scaling and a little discomfort or itching. Signs of pityriasis capitis or seborrhoeic dermatitis elsewhere are usually present. The condition may deteriorate at times of stress or fatigue.

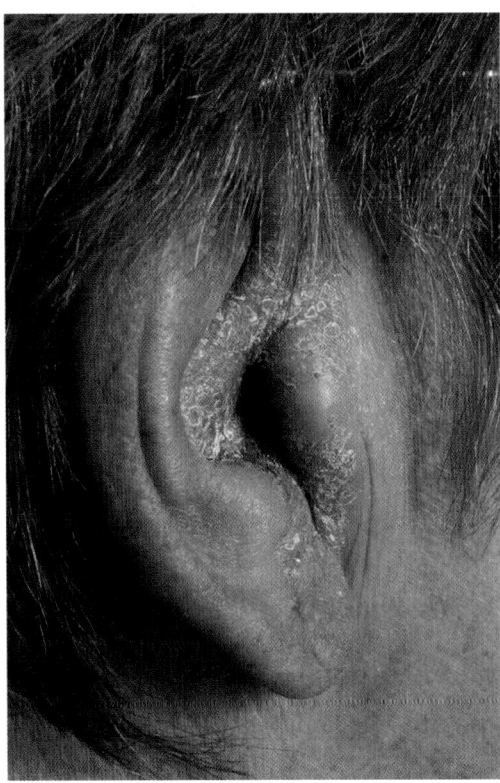

Figure 108.23 Chronic otitis externa. There is longstanding eczematous change, in part due to contact allergic reactions to ear drops, and induration causing narrowing of the canal.

Secondary bacterial infection is common. In this 'reactive' group the appearance is often that of a dermatitis spreading into the ear, in contrast with those cases with a primarily 'infective' aetiology where infection and/or inflammation often appears to be spreading out from the ear and where the entire length of the canal is commonly affected. The clinical appearance, however, is often non-diagnostic.

In infective eczema there is usually intense pruritus associated with exudate. The condition may complicate both otitis media and OE and is usually associated with some degree of otorrhoea. In others, it appears to develop from seborrhoeic dermatitis that has become secondarily infected. The condition may affect the meatus, concha, lobe and periauricular skin and often spreads widely. The post-auricular fold is commonly affected. The symptoms and signs are those of eczema with an accompanying or preceding aural discharge. In seborrhoeic individuals, other areas may be involved at the same time. Fissures and cellulitis are common complications.

Contact dermatitis is often occult and easily overlooked. It is both a complication (see below) and a contributory factor to chronicity. Sensitivity to topically applied medicaments is common in chronic external otitis. Neomycin and the related aminoglycosides are likely to be the commonest sensitizers [17–19]. As well as drops, medicated gauze should be considered [20]. Occlusion, the recurrent nature of the disease and frequent use of antibiotics on an already damaged skin probably account for the high incidence of contact dermatitis at this site. Other sensitivities include nickel from hair pins, metal implements, chromate and phosphorus

sesquisulfide in matches, and nail varnish. It is characteristic that the degree of itching and burning is often markedly out of proportion to the amount of erythema and oedema present. Contact dermatitis may also rarely occur with ear moulds [21]. Clinically, it is often difficult to differentiate neurodermatitis from contact dermatitis.

Lichen simplex (neurodermatitis) may be localized to one area of the meatus or may occur more diffusely over the tragus, triangular fossa and adjoining skin. The condition is usually diagnosed by the history rather than the signs. Itching is intense, but often intermittent. The need to scratch or rub is compulsive, although often denied. Signs of inflammation are often minimal, but some degree of oedema and scaling is common. Complications from trauma, infection and sensitization are frequent. Intermittent itching of the external auditory canal (non-specific external otitis) can also occur, irregularly and over a long period, without any obvious cause and with minimal signs of disease.

Whatever the primary aetiology, with the passage of time, chronic external otitis becomes an increasingly complex diagnostic and therapeutic problem.

Clinical variants
Bullous external otitis [22] is an uncommon variant in which there is a sudden onset of severe pain followed by discharge of blood from the ear canal. Bluish-red haemorrhagic bullae are visible on the osseous canal walls.

In granular external otitis, the lining of the meatus and canal is replaced in part or whole by granulation tissue, which can project inwards as pedunculated masses. These are usually found near the tympanic membrane, arising from the osseous end of the canal. Granular external otitis is associated with a severe or neglected course [23,24].

Differential diagnosis
The most important differential diagnosis is necrotizing OE. This should always be considered in a patient with significant fever and/or severe pain, especially if there is a co-morbidity such as diabetes or HIV. Careful examination of the canal should allow exclusion of OE secondary to otitis media. Other differentials include acute localized OE.

Classification of severity
With acute diffuse OE there is a spectrum. Mild cases have earache and or itching, some hearing loss and little or no discharge. At the severe end, the symptoms are more intense with swelling involving not only the ear canal but also the pinna; there may be low-grade fever and lymphadenopathy.

Complications and co-morbidities
Hypertrophic OE or localized elephantiasis nostra (lymphoedema) [25] of the ears may accompany recurrent OE, as a result of the effects of chronic lymphatic obstruction. The resultant narrowing of the external acoustic canal coupled with the underlying lymphoedema makes recurrent and repeated infections even more likely. Benign non-necrotizing OE presents as chronic non-painful otorrhoea with an ulcer present in the floor of the external canal.

Surgery may be a better alternative for this complication than long-term medical management [26]. Contact sensitization, discussed above as a contributory factor to chronic OE, is a common complication. Causes include the aminoglycosides, neomycin, framycetin and gentamicin, quinolines, corticosteroids, nail varnish, nickel, chromate and phosphorous sesquisulfide from match heads introduced into the ears.

Disease course and prognosis

Acute diffuse OE usually responds well to topical therapy. Recurrence is likely if there are background factors such as heat, humidity, frequent swimming, an abnormal ear canal, eczema, etc.

Once OE becomes chronic, it is less likely that it can be eradicated.

Investigations

When the presentation is with acute diffuse OE and there are no co-morbidities, investigations are probably not necessary.

For acute OE which has not responded to treatment a swab should be cultured for bacterial sensitivities, and microscopy and fungal culture are helpful to identify cases where fungal infection is a significant component.

Management

For acute diffuse OE, topical treatment of the ear canal together with appropriate analgesia is usually sufficient, and the condition can be expected to resolve in a week or so. Bacterial swabs are only recommended if there has been no response to treatment, if the patient is systemically unwell or if there is concern that the diagnosis is necrotizing external otitis.

Ideally, the eardrum should be visualized before deciding on a topical therapy because of the potential ototoxicity of topical aminoglycosides. Currently, there is a consensus that aminoglycoside in ear drops is safe even if the drum is perforated, provided it is used for not more than 2 weeks [27].

When there is marked swelling of the ear canal, ear drops will be more effective if there is an ear wick in place. If there is a lot of wax and keratinous debris in the canal, treatment will be more effective if this is removed regularly by gentle suction. If that is not available, advise patients with a swollen ear canal to lie on one side with the affected ear up and to keep this position for 10 min after the introduction of ear drops.

Recent systematic reviews and commentaries [27,28,29,30,31,32] of treatments for acute diffuse OE have established that:

- A topical antibiotic plus steroid ear drop is effective and probably better than either alone.
- There is little to choose in efficacy between aminoglycosides such as neomycin, framycetin and gentamicin, polymyxin B; fluoroquinolones, i.e. ciprofloxacin (currently only available in the UK as eye drops), ofloxacin (not available currently in the UK) and the antiseptic clioquinol.
- Treatment should be for 7 days, but longer (up to a further 7 days) if necessary.
- Acetic acid drops are as effective as an antibiotic–steroid combination in the short term, but less effective if longer treatment is needed.
- Aluminium acetate ear drops are probably as effective as antibiotic–steroid drops.

Apart from the possible risk of toxicity of aminoglycosides, other factors which may determine the choice of treatment are possible contact hypersensitivity (more likely a consideration when there is a history of recurrent episodes), availability, cost, dosing schedule (acetic acid and aluminium acetate require frequent administration) and possible bacterial resistance.

Acute diffuse OE. A topical antibiotic–steroid combination ear drop such as flumetasone–clioquinol or betamethasone–neomycin, together with ibuprofen and/or paracetamol for pain relief. Consider a systemic antibiotic if there is low-grade pyrexia and/or cellulitis. Review after 7 days. It may then be appropriate to take a swab and, while awaiting results, use a non-antibiotic treatment such as aluminium acetate solution.

Acute localized OE. Usually this can be treated with analgesia and application of warmth. If there are signs of severe infection, however, treat with an oral antibiotic, e.g. flucloxacillin, unless penicillin allergic, and consider the need for incision and drainage.

Chronic OE. Review the likely cause(s) for chronicity. These include a dermatosis such as atopic eczema or psoriasis, an anatomical problem causing canal stenosis, contact dermatitis and fungal overgrowth. Patch testing is recommended and, while awaiting results, aluminium acetate ear drops can be very useful. Topical 0.1% tacrolimus delivered via an ear wick is a useful alternative to topical steroids in chronic OE [33].

Occasionally, chronic OE is due to narrowing of the external auditory meatus. Surgical enlargement of the meatus can then bring about resolution [34–36].

Resources

Further information

http://emedicine.medscape.com/article/994550-treatment

Patient resources

http://www.patient.co.uk/doctor/otitis-externa-and-painful-discharging-ears#ref-11

(All last accessed October 2014.)

Necrotizing otitis externa

Definition and nomenclature

This is an infection of the skin of the external ear canal that spreads to deeper structures and causes necrosis.

Synonyms and inclusions
- Necrotizing external otitis
- Malignant OE
- Malignant external otitis
- Invasive OE
- Invasive externa otitis
- Skull base osteomyelitis

Introduction and general description

Necrotizing OE is an infection which begins in the external auditory canal and spreads into the temporal bone, causing osteomyelitis, and sometimes beyond, into the base of the skull, when cranial nerve palsies may occur. It is a serious and potentially fatal infection. The condition typically occurs in older diabetics and those who are immunosuppressed. The commonest cause is *Pseudomonas aeruginosa*, although occasionally other organisms are involved.

Epidemiology

Incidence and prevalence

Necrotizing external otitis is a rare disease. There are no good population frequency data.

Age

Necrotizing external otitis is commoner in the middle-aged and older patient, although it has been reported in children [1,2].

Sex

Necrotizing OE is commoner in males.

Ethnicity

There is no association with ethnicity.

Associated diseases

Most cases of necrotizing OE occur in diabetics, and other immunosuppressed patients, e.g. HIV-positive patients and renal transplant recipients.

Pathophysiology

Predisposing factors

Sometimes there is preceding OE. There is often a precipitating episode of water irrigation. Trauma, often minimal, can also be relevant. Heat and humidity can predispose. In diabetics, the higher pH of cerumen [3], poor clearance by neutrophils and macrophages [4,5] and microvascular impairment may all contribute to the association between the diabetic state and necrotizing OE.

Pathology

The epidermis may show hyperplastic changes, there is acute and chronic inflammation in the dermis and necrosis of the bone [6,7].

Causative organisms

Most cases are due to *Pseudomonas aeruginosa*. Many other organisms have been demonstrated, including *Staphylococcus aureus*, *Klebsiella* spp., commensals such as *S. epidermidis* and fungi such as *Mucor* spp., *Candida glabrata*, *Aspergillus*, *Malassezia* and *Scedosporium apiospermum*.

Genetics

There is no genetic predisposition.

Clinical features

History

The commonest presenting symptom is pain, which is usually very severe and persistent. It may spread from the region of the ear to the vertex, temporal or occipital areas, and there may be temporomandibular joint pain. Pain progresses more quickly in children than adults. The second most common symptom is discharge from the ear. In up to 50%, there is some degree of hearing loss. Systemic symptoms, including fever, are uncommon. There may be symptoms due to involvement of cranial nerves, particularly dysphagia.

Presentation

On examination, the external auditory canal is always abnormal, with varying degrees of oedema and erythema, and extensive granulation tissue formation is evident, particularly at the bone–cartilage junction. This is particularly seen on the posterior and inferior aspect of the wall at the junction between the bony and cartilaginous segments of the canal. There may be exposed bone in the floor of the canal and swelling of the soft tissues of the pinna and beyond. The tympanic membrane is frequently necrotic in children, but is characteristically spared in adults [2]. Cranial neuropathies may be found in up to 40% of patients. Facial palsy is the most common finding but involvement of other cranial nerves, particularly IX, X and XI, may be variably present. When such nerve involvement is found, the disease is more extensive.

Differential diagnosis

The main differential diagnosis is from severe OE, but this does not typically have granulations or exposed bone in the canal. The other uncommon entities which can be difficult to distinguish from necrotizing OE are erosive external otitis [8] and benign necrotizing OE [9]. Other differentials include carcinoma and granulomatous diseases, which can be excluded by taking samples for histology. Recently, there have been cases of bisphosphonate-induced osteonecrosis of the auditory canal mimicking some of the features of necrotizing external otitis [10].

Classification of severity

Involvement of the cranial nerves, associated meningitis and/or cerebral abscess constitute the severe end of a spectrum.

Complications and co-morbidities

Cranial nerve involvement may not recover, particularly in facial palsy. Other complications include temporomandibular joint osteomyelitis, dural sinus thrombosis, meningitis and cerebral abscess.

Disease course and prognosis

Mortality was around 50%, but now is usually 20% or lower. Adverse prognostic factors are skull base osteomyelitis, intracranial extension and involvement of multiple cranial nerves [11]. Concurrent *Aspergillus* infection may confer a poorer prognosis

[12]. The disease commonly recurs if the treatment time is too short.

Investigations
Establishing the organisms involved is important although sometimes difficult when antibiotic drops have already been given. Swabs, and if necessary, tissue should be sent for aerobic, anaerobic and fungal culture. Tissue should also be sent for histology. Imaging techniques can be helpful in distinguishing severe OE from necrotizing OE. A variety of methods have been evaluated for both diagnosis and monitoring treatment (plain radiographs, computed tomography (CT), magnetic resonance imaging (MRI) with and without enhancement, technetium and gallium scans), but all have some shortcomings [13]. MRI with or without gadolinium enhancement is useful for imaging soft-tissue involvement, and for the evaluation of the meninges and changes within the osseous medullary cavity, although CT is preferred for the initial diagnosis and recognition of cortical bone erosion [14,15]. When available, gallium scintigraphy may be the most useful for assessing response to treatment [16,17].

Management
Whenever possible, treatment should be guided by culture and sensitivities, and the antimicrobial therapy given for at least 6–8 weeks. As well as monitoring for clinical improvement, repeat imaging may be needed to assess whether the disease is responding.

First line
Pseudomonas is the usual cause, and provided the isolate is not resistant, ciprofloxacin 750 mg twice daily may be sufficient for the less severe end of the spectrum. If there is insufficient evidence of a response, IV ceftazidime 2 g 8 hourly should be added. If the *Pseudomonas* is resistant to ciprofloxacin, an aminoglycoside plus ceftazidime is likely to be the best choice. For other bacteria and fungi, the choice of treatment will be dictated by the microbial culture.

Second line
Rifampicin may worth adding to the antibiotic regimen [18].

Third line
Hyperbaric oxygen is sometimes used as an adjunct, but its role has not yet been established [19,20]. Surgical intervention is occasionally indicated, e.g. debridement of necrotic tissue and drainage of any abscess.

Resources

Further information
http://emedicine.medscape.com/article/845525-overview

Patient resources
There is a section on necrotizing OE in http://www.nhs.uk/Conditions/Otitis-externa/Pages/Complications.aspx
(All last accessed October 2014.)

Otomycosis

Definition and nomenclature
Otomycosis is an inflammatory condition of the ear canal in which yeast or fungal organisms play an essential part. It may occur as an isolated condition or as a complication of OE.

Synonyms and inclusions
• Otomycosis is sometimes included as a subtype of OE

Introduction and general description
Otomycosis is recognized clinically by visible growth of filamentous fungi on the skin of the ear canal. It is usually a chronic disorder. The use of topical corticosteroids and/or antibiotics in the treatment of OE predisposes to otomycosis; however, it can occur *de novo*. It is commoner in hot climates and when there is excessive exposure to water.

Epidemiology

Incidence and prevalence
There are little data on incidence or prevalence, but in tropical countries otomycosis constitutes about 10% of cases of OE.

Age
Otomycosis can occur at all ages but is commoner in middle age.

Sex
Otomycosis is approximately twice as common in males as in females.

Ethnicity
There is no ethnic or racial predilection recorded for otomycosis.

Associated diseases
Otomycosis is more common in patients with chronic OE treated with topical antibiotics and/or corticosteroids, and both diabetes and immunosuppression may make patients more susceptible.

Predisposing factors
Heat, humidity, trauma, frequent exposure to water, and prolonged use of antiobiotics and/or steroid drops in the ear canal may all be important predisposing factors. Otomycosis can follow acute otitis media [1].

Pathology
The fungal hyphae are in the stratum corneum. There may be little or no inflammatory change. Particularly in the immunosuppressed, the fungi can penetrate into the dermis and beyond.

Causative organisms
Most cases are due to *Aspergillus* and *Candida* species. In tropical regions, *Aspergillus* predominate whereas in more temperate

areas *Candida* isolates are more common [2]. *Candida* is also more common than *Aspergillus* in the immunocompromised [3]. Occasionally, other yeasts and fungi are found, including phycomycetes, *Rhizopus*, *Actinomyces* and *Penicillium*, and, rarely, dermatophytes. The fact that these organisms can be pathogenic as well as saprophytic has been confirmed in a number of studies [2,4,5].

Genetics
There is no recognized genetic predisposition.

Environmental factors
Otomycosis is probably commoner in hot and humid environments.

Clinical features

History
The usual symptoms are itching, earache, discharge, hearing loss, a sense of fullness and pain. Pain may be relatively more common in the immunocompromised [6].

Presentation
On examination, the dominant feature is the presence of wispy filamentous masses, which may be isolated or diffusely present in the canal. These masses are white, grey or stippled black if *Aspergillus* is present. Inflammation of the canal epithelium is usually mild. There may be some epithelial debris, which may be either moist or dry. Usually, only one ear is involved, but otomycosis is quite commonly bilateral in the immunosuppressed [6].

Differential diagnosis
The main differential diagnosis is from bacterial OE, with which it can coexist.

Classification of severity
The presence of cellulitis of the surrounding soft tissues without bacterial infection represents more severe infection, and is more likely in the immunocompromised.

Complications and co-morbidities
Perforation of the tympanic membrane can occur. Otomycosis can become an invasive disease with penetration into the temporal bone in the immunosuppressed.

Disease course and prognosis
Otomycosis is often a chronic disorder, but can be cured if adequately treated and any predisposing factors corrected.

Investigations
Fungal microscopy and culture are needed to establish the diagnosis.

Management
The ear canal should be carefully cleaned of debris and discharge and gentle suction used if available. Many agents have been advocated for otomycosis, but there is little evidence to promote one above the others. They include aluminium acetate, acetic acid, *m*-cresyl acetate, thiomersal, gentian violet, clioquinol, nystatin, amphotericin and the imidazoles.

Treatment ladder

First line
- 1% clotrimazole drops 2–3 times daily for at least 2 weeks

Second line
- If there is tympanic membrane perforation or a likelihood of invasive disease, a systemic agent, e.g. itraconazole, should be used

Third line
- If there is penetration into bone, voriconazole or posaconazole may be more effective systemic agents than itraconazole [7]

Tumours of the auricle and external auditory canal

Benign tumours
A wide variety of benign tumours have been described on the auricle. These will present as papules or nodules, sometimes with distinctive morphology.

In the external auditory canal, benign tumours tend to present with hearing loss and may predispose to infection. Benign mass lesions in the canal include exostosis and osteoma. Exostoses are usually bilateral, symmetrical, multiple, diffuse, broadly based growths of bone. Frequent exposure to cold water, such as from surfing, is an aetiological factor in nearly all cases. Somewhat similar are osteomas, although these can usually be differentiated by their solitary and unilateral distribution. Other benign lesions that may present in the canal are fibrous dysplasia – both monostotic and polyostotic (Albright syndrome), eosinophilic granuloma, cholesteatoma and keratosis obturans, benign ceruminous gland tumours, cartilaginous choristomas and temporomandibular joint herniation. Papillomatosis of the canal presents with multiple rounded papules; it has been associated with human papillomavirus (HPV) 6.

Glandular tumours
Tumours of the ceruminous glands are rare. It is often difficult to distinguish between adenoma and carcinoma on histological grounds [1,2]. The tumours comprise benign and pleomorphic adenomas, adenocarcinomas, adenoid cystic carcinomas and perhaps others including mucoepidermoid carcinomas. The glandular tissue of a ceruminous adenoma has myoepithelial basal cells which are positive for CK5/6, S100 and p63 and luminal ceruminous cells which stain for CK7 [3]. Tumours of the cerumen glands have been reported in association with other sweat gland tumours elsewhere [4].

Isolated cases of syringocystadenoma papilliferum, apocrine cystadenoma, benign eccrine cylindroma, hidradenoma papilliferum and carcinomas of eccrine and sebaceous origin have also been reported [5,6]. Extramammary Paget disease of the external ear and/or canal resembles Bowen disease or an inflammatory dermatosis [7].

Benign tumours produce symptoms of obstruction and hearing loss. Pain is the usual presenting feature of the more malignant tumours. They are usually seen as polypoid masses in the canal. Other symptoms include bleeding, otorrhoea and, with spread of the neoplasm, nerve palsies.

Treatment is in the province of the otorhinolaryngologist. Because of the potential for malignant behaviour, all ceruminous gland tumours should be fully excised with an adequate margin of normal tissue [8].

Pre-malignant epithelial neoplasms of the auricle

Because of its high level of exposure to UV radiation, especially in men, the auricle is a common site for pre-malignant and malignant lesions of epidermal origin. Other predisposing factors include prior ionizing radiation, a chronic dermatosis such as lupus vulgaris, and genetic factors such as xeroderma pigmentosum and Gorlin syndrome.

The commonest pre-malignant lesion is the solar keratosis, which can occur on all sun-exposed aspects of the auricle, but is especially common on the upper surface of the helix. The clinical presentations include an erythematous telangiectatic patch, a focal area of scaling or hyperkeratosis, or a cutaneous horn. Solar keratoses on the auricle are often multiple. Solar elastosis may be evident in the surrounding skin. On the auricle, progression to squamous carcinoma from solar keratosis may occur more readily than at other sites.

Other pre-malignant lesions include Bowen disease, radiation and tar keratoses and, rarely, keratoacanthoma.

Treatment

Several forms of treatment can eradicate pre-malignant lesions from the auricle, but there are no adequate data to compare them. They include excision, curettage, electrosurgery, cryotherapy, 5-fluorouracil and photodynamic therapy. The choice will depend on a number of factors, including the need for a tissue diagnosis, size and location of the lesion, likely cosmetic outcome and the available facilities. Follow-up is important for detection of recurrences and the appearance of new lesions. Lesions closely resembling squamous carcinoma, such as keratoacanthoma, should probably be totally excised to ensure accurate diagnosis.

Malignant tumours

Only squamous carcinoma is discussed in detail here. BCC is relatively less common than squamous cell carcinoma (SCC) on the auricle, and very uncommon in the external auditory canal (Figure 108.24). At the latter site, it can be difficult to eradicate. Malignant melanoma of the external ear is relatively uncommon, constituting about 1% of all cutaneous melanomas. Other malignant tumours involving the external ear or the external auditory canal are all rare. The dermatologist may encounter sebaceous carcinoma, atypical fibroxanthoma (Figure 108.25), trichilemmal

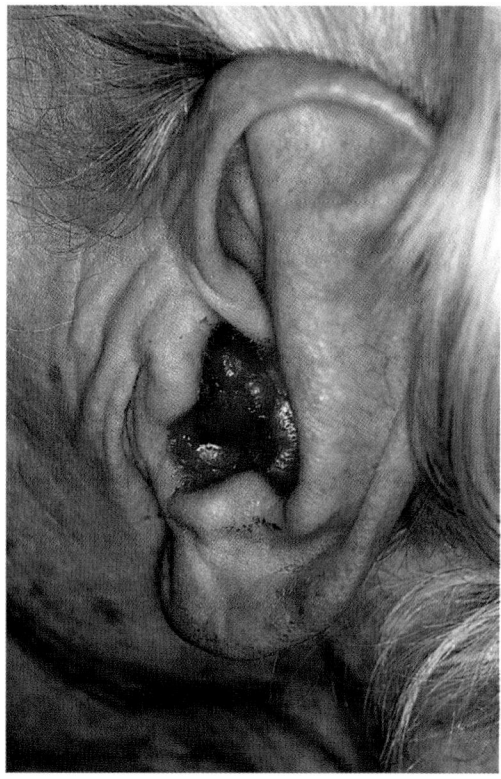

Figure 108.24 Basal cell carcinoma of the external auditory canal. An erythematous tumour presenting as obstruction at the entrance of the canal. (Courtesy of Mr M. Birchill, Southmead Hospital, Bristol, UK.)

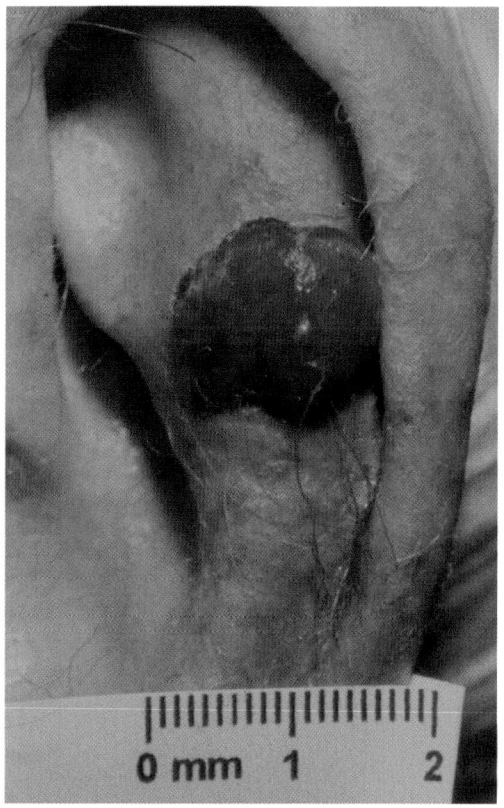

Figure 108.25 Atypical fibroxanthoma. A firm fleshy tumour of the pinna.

carcinoma, Merkel cell tumour, carcinosarcoma, Kaposi sarcoma, angiosarcoma and, mainly in children, rhabdomyosarcoma. Lymphomas may occur on the external ear (Figure 108.26). The ear may be involved by direct extension from tumours nearby, for example the parotid, and also by metastases from distant sites.

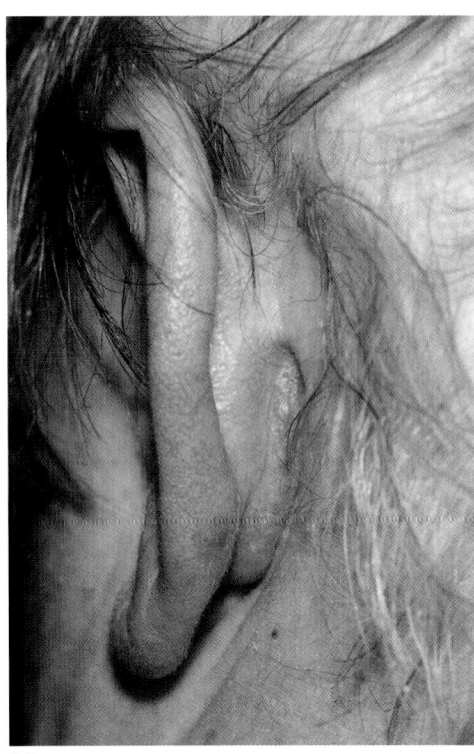

(a)

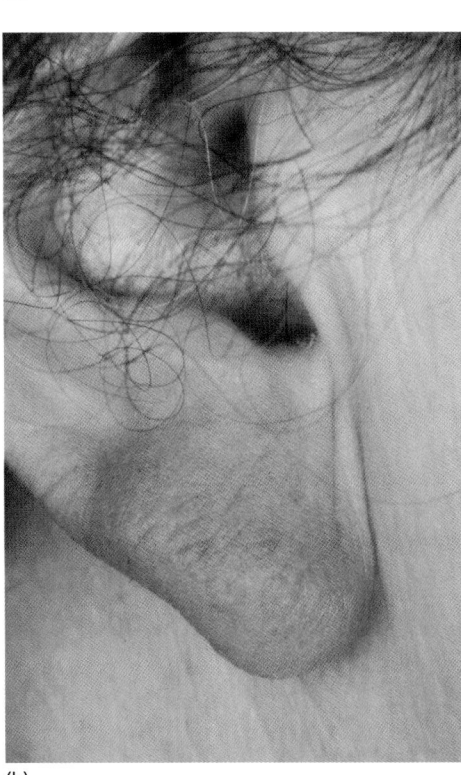

(b)

Figure 108.26 (a) B-cell lymphoma presenting as a purple nodular swelling in the retroauricular fold. (b) Erythematous swelling of the ear lobe due to infiltration by B-cell lymphoma.

Squamous cell carcinoma of the auricle (pinna)

Definition
A malignant keratinocyte neoplasm arising on the skin of the auricle (pinna).

Introduction and general description
In most instances, SCC evolves from a pre-malignant lesion, usually a solar keratosis, and occurs predominantly in elderly white men, although at a younger age in the immunosuppressed. The most common site is the helix [1]. Early SCC may be suspected when there is induration of the base of a scaly papule, nodule or cutaneous horn. With progression, SCC usually ulcerates and with invasion of the cartilage can become grossly destructive (Figure 108.27). Local spread along perichondrial, periosteal and neurovascular planes can make SCC of the auricle very difficult to control. With the exception of the lip, auricular SCC is more likely to metastasize than is SCC at any other sun-exposed site (11% compared with 2%) [2].

Epidemiology

Incidence and prevalence
Although the ratio of BCC to SCC is about 4 : 1 on the head and neck generally, on the ear SCC is relatively more common (BCC : SCC, 1.3 : 1) [3].

Age
Squamous cell carcinoma of the auricle is increasingly common with age.

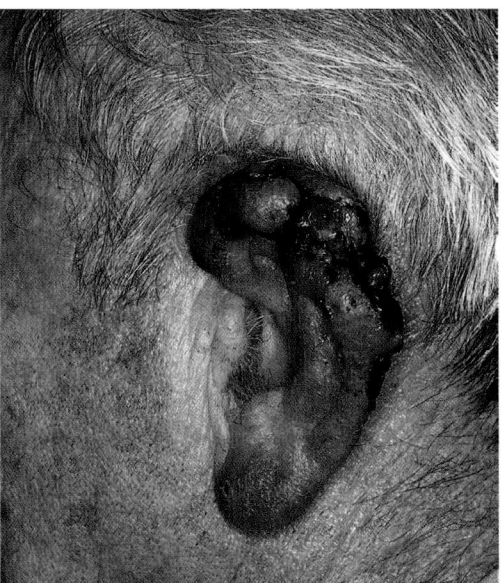

Figure 108.27 Squamous carcinoma of the auricle. An advanced tumour with extensive destruction of the ear cartilage. (Courtesy of Mr D. Baldwin, Southmead Hospital, Bristol, UK.)

Sex

Squamous cell carcinoma of the auricle is much commoner in males [3].

Ethnicity

Squamous cell carcinoma of the auricle is typically a disease of the fair skinned.

Associated diseases

Other UV exposure and age-related malignant and pre-malignant conditions.

Pathophysiology

Pathophysiology of squamous carcinoma is discussed in Chapter 142.

Predisposing factors

The predominant causative factor is chronic UV exposure. Other factors include exposure to ionizing radiation, HPV and chronic inflammation such as discoid lupus erythematosus.

Pathology

Pathology of squamous carcinoma is discussed in Chapter 142.

Causative organisms

Oncogenic HPV may be relevant to some cases of SCC in solid-organ transplant recipients.

Environmental factors

See above.

Clinical features

History

Squamous cell carcinoma of the auricle may become apparent as a change in a pre-existing lesion, e.g. a solar keratosis, or begin as a new growth or ulcer. Symptoms are sometimes present, and include pain and bleeding. Enlargement of the lesion is typically faster than that of a BCC.

Presentation

The appearance varies depending on whether an SCC evolves from a preceding lesion, i.e. a solar keratosis or Bowen disease, or appears *de novo*, and also with the degree of differentiation. Induration and a fleshy base are characteristic of an SCC evolving from a solar keratosis. A cutaneous horn may have an SCC at its base. There is often a keratinous core with well-differentiated SCCs, and keratoacanthoma can be closely mimicked. As an SCC grows, it typically becomes a nodular tumour, liable to be ulcerated and crusted. Poorly differentiated tumours tend to be friable and haemorrhagic, and do not show any evidence of keratinization.

Differential diagnosis

It can be impossible to differentiate keratoacanthoma. Some BCCs can resemble SCC. Amelanotic melanoma and Merkel cell tumour can be difficult to distinguish from poorly differentiated SCC. Sometimes a suspected SCC is found to be a hyperplastic solar keratosis after submission for histology. The differential diagnosis occasionally includes other benign or malignant conditions.

Classification of severity

For classification of SCC, see Chapter 142.

Complications and co-morbidities

Squamous cell carcinoma tends to metastasize locally, then to the regional lymph nodes.

Disease course and prognosis

Untreated, SCC of the auricle is often a destructive malignancy, with invasion of the cartilage. There is a risk for local, parotid and regional lymph node metastasis; perineural spread is relatively common. Adverse prognostic factors [4,5] for both local recurrence and metastasis of SCC include size; however, shallow lesions with large surface area (i.e. >2 cm diameter) do not seem to have a poor prognosis. There is an increased risk for a poor prognosis for SCC of the ear in renal transplant recipients [4,5,6]. If SCC recurs after primary treatment, there is a much greater risk for further recurrence and metastasis [8].

Investigations

The diagnosis should be confirmed by histology by excisional biopsy. For a larger lesion, and a tumour where there is clinical uncertainty, an incisional biopsy will guide further management. CT scanning may be appropriate to evaluate spread into bone. MRI and/or fine-needle aspirate cytology may be needed to evaluate the regional lymph nodes.

Management

First line

It is important to achieve control of the disease with the initial treatment for SCC. For small minimally invasive lesions, simple excision, cryotherapy or curettage with electrodesiccation may be adequate. Excellent results have been reported from the combination of curettage and cryotherapy for carefully selected cases [9]. For larger lesions, and especially for those with adverse prognostic factors, the choice is likely to be between wide margin excision and Mohs micrographic surgery.

The surgical procedure used will depend on the location and extent of the tumour. Smaller lesions can often be removed by wedge excision with primary repair by advancement flaps. Larger and ill-defined lesions are best closed by temporary grafts pending a histopathological assessment of the margins before definitive repair is carried out [10]. Partial or total amputation of the ear may be needed for large tumours. If there is spread beyond the auricle, resection of the parotid, temporal bone, temporomandibular joint or mandibular ramus may be required, with appropriate repair.

Several authors have recommended minimal resection margins, for example: 1 cm [11], 6 mm with frozen section control [12], 8 mm for 1 cm diameter tumours and 1.5 cm for 3 cm diameter tumours [13], all with removal of the underlying cartilage. Overall, there

PART 10: SITES, SEX, AGE

is an incidence of 18.7% recurrence during follow-up for 5 years or more with non-Mohs modalities compared with 5.3% for Mohs micrographic surgery, suggesting that the latter is the treatment of choice [4,14].

Squamous cell carcinomas in the tragal and pretragal location appear to have a greater tendency to spread along embryonic fusion planes and may only be curable by radical surgery, for example parotidectomy in association with removal of the tumour [15,16].

Various techniques are needed to reconstruct the ear after curative surgery [17–24].

Second line

Radiotherapy can be successful as a primary treatment for SCC of the auricle, megavoltage electron-beam therapy having therapeutic and cosmetic advantages over conventional orthovoltage X-ray treatment. Although results can be as good as from surgery [25], there may be a higher recurrence rate compared with surgery for large tumours. Radiation therapy can be complicated by damage to the cartilage and associated chronic infection; deformity of the auricle is another long-term consequence.

Third line

In renal transplant recipients, reducing the degree of immunosuppression can improve survival in poor prognosis SCC without necessarily jeopardizing the transplant [26].

For inoperable and metastatic tumours, local treatment will be palliative. Chemotherapy and epidermal growth factor inhibitors, such as erlotinib, may be of value.

Resources

Patient resources

http://www.patient.co.uk/doctor/squamous-cell-carcinoma-of-skin (last accessed October 2014).

Squamous carcinoma of the external auditory canal

Definition

Malignant or *in situ* malignant keratinocyte neoplasm of the epidermis lining the external auditory canal.

Introduction and general description

Squamous cell carcinoma of the external auditory canal is much less common than SCC of the pinna, and has a considerably worse prognosis.

Epidemiology

Incidence and prevalence

There are no accurate data on incidence and prevalence; 1 per million has been suggested [1].

Age

In most series, the mean age is 60 years.

Sex

Unlike SCC of the pinna, which is a predominantly male disease, the sex ratio is approximately equal.

Ethnicity

There is no association with an ethnic group.

Associated diseases

There is sometimes a concurrent history of chronic otitis.

Pathophysiology

See Chapter 142.

Predisposing factors

Factors identified include chronic suppurative otitis and previous radiotherapy [2].

Pathology

In most cases, there is an infiltrative growth pattern. It tends to grow along the canal, escaping anteriorly through Santorini's fissures in the cartilaginous segment and Huschke's foramen in the bony portion, into the temporomandibular joint and parotid. Spread also occurs posteriorly into the mastoid, and through the tympanic membrane into the middle ear and thence to the carotid canal, the apex of the petrous temple bone, the internal auditory canal, the base of the skull and the dura. Metastasis to lymph nodes may occur. Verrucous carcinoma of the external auditory canal is an uncommon variant that can appear cytologically banal but nevertheless invade bone, by a pushing rather than an infiltrative growth pattern [3,4]. Mucoepidermoid carcinoma is also encountered rarely [5]. Occasionally, SCC has been reported arising from benign papillomatosis [6].

Causative organisms

A subset of SCC of the external auditory canal is probably due to HPV. In a UK series, about 20% were associated with HPV 16 [7].

Clinical features

History

Symptoms include discharge, earache, hearing loss and facial palsy.

Presentation

Examination of the ear canal may reveal a mass (Figure 108.28).

Differential diagnosis

This includes chronic inflammatory disease of the ear canal and other tumours.

Classification of severity

The Pittsburgh classification [1] is a useful staging system:
- T1: tumour limited to the external auditory canal without bony erosion or evidence of soft-tissue extension

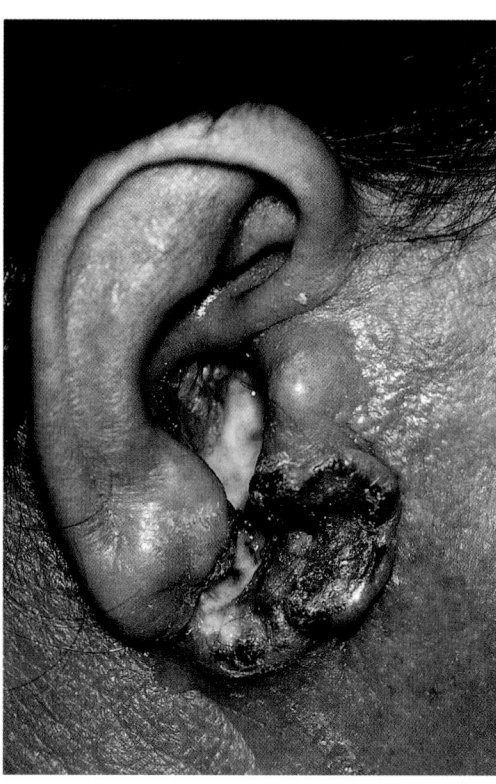

Figure 108.28 Squamous carcinoma of the external auditory canal. Purulent discharge, inflammation and destruction of the meatus. (Courtesy of Mr D. Baldwin, Southmead Hospital, Bristol, UK.)

- T2: tumour with limited external auditory canal bony erosion (not full thickness) or radiographic finding consistent with limited (<0.5 cm) soft-tissue involvement.
- T3: tumour eroding the osseous external auditory canal (full thickness) with limited (<0.5 cm) soft-tissue involvement, or tumour involving middle ear and/or mastoid, or patients presenting with facial paralysis.
- T4: tumour eroding the cochlea, petrous apex, medial wall of the middle ear, carotid canal, jugular foramen or dura, or with extensive (>0.5 cm) soft-tissue involvement.

The prognosis worsens with progression from T1 through to T4.

It was recognized that the presence of facial palsy confers a worse prognosis, and warrants classification as T4 – see Moody *et al.* for modified version [**8,9**].

Complications and co-morbidities
As well as facial nerve palsy, other cranial nerves palsies are likely to develop with disease progression.

Disease course and prognosis
The overall 5-year survival is 30–40%. With appropriate treatment, the 5-year survival for T1 disease can be 100%. By contrast, for T3 disease it is 25% and T4 disease only 16%. Lymph node involvement markedly worsens the prognosis. Adverse prognostic factors include facial palsy, extensive bony involvement [**10**] and both nodal and distant metastasis. Poor differentiation of the tumour is probably an independent adverse prognostic factor. The prognosis is much improved if the tumour is completely excised.

Investigations
Imaging is essential to staging and then planning appropriate treatment. CT gives the best information on the presence of tumour in bone, MRI the extent in soft tissue, and positron emission tomography (PET) scanning can help with whether nodes are involved and distant metastasis has occurred. Histological confirmation will be needed.

Management

First line
Management of SCC of the external auditory canal is not likely to be undertaken by a dermatological surgeon. The use of surgical techniques, radiotherapy and regional chemotherapy are reviewed [**11,12,13**].

Second line
Radiotherapy alone can be considered [**14**].

Miscellaneous conditions

Petrified ear
This is a rare clinical entity in which the cartilage of the ear is replaced by ectopic calcification or ossification [**1**]. When looked for on radiological images, it is much more commonly seen [**2**]. The clinical presentation is of a partially or wholly rigid auricle, which may be uncomfortable with pressure over it. One or both ears may be involved. Causes include frostbite, trauma, radiation therapy and several systemic diseases. Addison disease is the commonest; others include diabetes, hypopituitarism, acromegaly and hypothyroidism. It has been reported in pseudopseudohypoparathyroidism [**3**].

Cholesteatoma of the external auditory canal
Cholesteatoma of the middle ear space is accumulation of keratinous debris within a sac-like squamous epithelial lining. It can grow at the expense of normal structures and if it ruptures, the associated foreign body type inflammatory reaction can produce serious damage.

A similar condition occurs rarely in the external auditory canal, although its status as a true cholesteatoma is disputed [**1,2**]. The accumulation of stratum corneum occurs within a cyst-like penetration of the bony portion of the canal wall by the epithelial lining. There is localized ulceration of the skin of the floor of the canal, with underlying osteitis and sometimes necrosis of bone. A necrotic sequestrum may become incorporated into the cholesteatoma. Some cases are primary and several causes have been identified including previous trauma, operation and radiotherapy [**3**].

Cholesteatoma usually occurs in patients over the age of 40 years. Symptoms include a dull pain in one ear and otorrhoea. Examination shows a white cystic mass protruding into the canal. The main differential diagnosis is from neoplasms and keratosis obturans. External auditory canal cholesteatoma can occasionally behave aggressively, and may erode into the mastoid cavity, middle ear,

PART 10: SITES, SEX, AGE

temporomandibular joint and adjacent soft tissue. CT can be useful to assess the extent of the disease. Treatment is within the province of the otorhinolaryngologist.

Keratosis obturans

In this uncommon condition, there is a localized accumulation of desquamated keratin in the ear canal. It may be due to a defect in the normal epithelial migration [1]. It is usually bilateral and typically occurs in younger patients than those presenting with external auditory canal cholesteatoma, which it can resemble. There is conductive hearing loss, sometimes with otalgia. Keratosis obturans can be associated with paranasal sinus disease and bronchitis; it has also been described in association with the yellow nail syndrome [2]. Treatment consists of careful removal of the accumulated keratin. Irrigation with water should be avoided.

Referred pain [1]

Due to the complicated nerve supply to the ear, referred pain is commoner than pain due to lesions in the ear itself [2]. Non-otological causes of such pain include the otomandibular syndrome [3] due to dysfunction of the temporomandibular joint, cervical arthritis with involvement of the cervical nerves, tonsillitis and carcinoma of the pharynx. Hair in the ear canal is an occasional cause [4]. Psychogenic otalgia has also been reported [5].

Key references

The full list of references can be found in the online version at www.rooksdermatology.com.

Introduction, Anatomy and physiology, Microbiology, Cerumen, Examination

2 Kelly KE, Mohs DC. The external auditory canal: anatomy and physiology. *Otolaryngol Clin North Am* 1996;29:725–9.
6 Stroman DW, Roland PS, Dohar J, Burt W. Microbiology of normal external auditory canal. *Laryngoscope* 2001;111:2054–9.
7 Roeser RJ, Ballachanda BB. Physiology, pathophysiology, and anthropology/epidemiology of human ear canal secretions. *J Am Acad Audiol* 1997;8:391–400.
9 Stoeckelhuber M, Matthias C, Andratschke M, *et al.* Human ceruminous gland: ultrastructure and histochemical analysis of antimicrobial and cytoskeletal components. *Anat Rec* 2006;288:877–84.
10 Schwaab M, Gurr A, Neumann A, *et al.* Human antimicrobial proteins in ear wax. *Eur J Clin Microbiol Infect Dis.* 2011;30:997–1004.
14 Clegg AJ, Loveman E, Gospodarevskaya E, *et al.* The safety and effectiveness of different methods of earwax removal: a systematic review and economic evaluation. *Health Technol Assess* 2010;14:1–192.
15 Saloranta K, Westermarck T. Prevention of cerumen impaction by treatment of ear canal skin. A pilot randomized controlled study. *Clin Otolaryngol* 2005;30:112–4.
16 Lucente FE. Techniques of examination. In: Lucente FE, Lawson W, Novick NL, eds. *The External Ear*. Philadelphia: Saunders, 1995:18–24.

Developmental defects

3 Bellucci RJ. Congenital aural malformations: diagnosis and treatment. Symposium on Congenital Disorders in Otolaryngology. *Otolaryngol Clin North Am* 1981;14:95–124.
4 Melnick M. The etiology of external ear malformations and its relation to abnormalities of the middle ear, inner ear, and other organ systems. *Birth Defects* 1980;16:303–31.

6 Sakashita T, Sando I, Kamerer DB. Congenital anomalies of the external and middle ears. In: Bluestone CD, Stool SE, Kenna MA, eds. Pediatric *Otolaryngology*, 3rd edn. Philadelphia: Saunders, 1996:333–70.
8 Wang RY, Earl DL, Ruder RO, Graham JM. Syndromic ear anomalies and renal ultrasounds. *Pediatrics* 2001;108: E32.
9 Melnick M, Myrianthopoulos NC. External ear malformations: epidemiology, genetics and natural history. *Birth Defects* 1979;15:1–139.
10 Kelley PE, Scholes MA. Microtia and congenital aural atresia. *Otolaryngol Clin North Am* 2007;40:61–80.
11 Luquetti DV, Heike CL, Hing AV, *et al.* Microtia: epidemiology and genetics. *Am J Med Genet* A 2012;158A: 124–39.
13 Okajima H, Takeichi Y, Umeda K, Baba S. Clinical analysis of 592 patients with microtia. *Acta Otolaryngol (Stockh)* 1996;525:18–24.
25 Scheinfeld NS, Silverberg NB, Weinberg JM, Nozad V. The preauricular sinus: a review of its clinical presentation, treatment, and associations. *Pediatr Dermatol* 2004;21:191–6.

Ageing changes

1 Niemitz C, Nibbrig M, Zacher V. Human ears grow throughout the entire lifetime according to complicated and dimorphic patterns—conclusions from a cross-sectional analysis. *Anthropol Anz* 2007;65:391–413.
3 Heathcote JA. Why do old men have big ears? *BMJ* 1996;311:1668.
4 Asai Y, Yoshimura M, Nago N, Yamada T. Correlation of ear length with age in Japan. *BMJ* 1996;312:582.
5 Verhulst J, Onghena P. Circaseptennial rhythm in ear growth. *BMJ* 1996;313:1597–8.
8 Kirkham N, Murrells T, Melcher DH, Morrison EA. Diagonal earlobe creases and fatal cardiovascular disease: a necropsy study. *Br Heart J* 1989;61:361–4.
9 Patel V, Champ C, Andrews PS, et al. Diagonal earlobe creases and atheromatous disease: a post mortem study. *J R Coll Physicians Lond* 1992;26:274–7.
10 Edston E. The earlobe crease, coronary artery disease, and sudden cardiac death: an autopsy study of 520 individuals. *Am J Forensic Med Pathol* 2006;27:129–33.
11 Tranchesi B, Barbosa V, de Albuquerque CP, *et al.* Diagonal earlobe creases as a marker of the presence and extent of coronary atherosclerosis. *Am J Cardiol* 1992;70:1417–20.
12 Wiedemann HR. Earlobe creases, congenital and acquired. *N Engl J Med* 1979;301:111.

Traumatic conditions

Contusion and haematoma

1 Manning SC, Casselbrant M, Lammers D. Otolaryngolic manifestations of child abuse. *Int J Pediatr Otorhinolaryngol* 1990;20:7–16.
2 Willner A, Ledereich PS, de Vries EJ. Auricular injury as a presentation of child abuse. *Arch Otolaryngol Head Neck Surg* 1992;118:634–7.
3 Hanigan WC, Peterson RA, Njus G. Tin ear syndrome: rotational acceleration in pediatric head injuries. *Pediatrics* 1987;80:618–22.
4 Germon WH. The care and management of acute haematoma of the external ear. *Laryngoscope* 1980;90:881–5.
5 Lee D, Sperling N. Initial management of auricular trauma. *Am Fam Physician* 1996;53:2339–44.
6 Schuller DE, Dankle SD, Strauss RH. A technique to treat wrestler's auricular hematoma without interrupting training or competition. *Arch Otolaryngol Head Neck Surg* 1989;115:202–6.
7 Bull PD, Lancer JM. Treatment of auricular haematoma by suction drainage. *Clin Otolaryngol* 1984;9:355–60.
8 Tenta LT, Keyes GR. Reconstructive surgery of the external ear. *Otolaryngol Clin North Am* 1981;14:917–38.

Ear piercing

1 Deschesnes M, Fines P, Demers S. Are tattooing and body piercing indicators of risk-taking behaviours among high school students? *J Adolesc* 2006;29:379–93.
2 Laumann AE, Derick AJ. Tattoos and body piercings in the United States: a national data set. *J Am Acad Dermatol* 2006;55:413–21.
7 Hanif J, Frosh A, Marnane C, *et al.* 'High' ear piercing and the rising incidence of perichondritis of the pinna. *BMJ* 2001;322:906–7.
11 Davis O, Powell M. Auricular perichondritis secondary to acupuncture. *Arch Otolaryngol* 1985;111:770–1.

31 Jensen CS, Lisby S, Baadsgaard O, *et al.* Decrease in nickel sensitization in a Danish schoolgirl population with ears pierced after implementation of a nickel-exposure regulation. *Br J Dermatol* 2002;146:636–42.

50 Chowdri NA, Mattoo MMA, Darzi MA. Keloids and hypertrophic scars: results with intra-operative and serial post-operative corticosteroid injection therapy. *Aust N Z J Surg* 1999;69:655–9.

59 Hendricks WM. Complications of ear piercing: treatment and prevention. *Cutis* 1991;48:386–94.

60 Landeck A, Newman N, Breadon J, *et al.* A simple technique for ear piercing. *J Am Acad Dermatol* 1998;39:795–6.

Chondrodermatitis nodularis

3 Upile T, Patel NN, Jerjes, *et al.* Advances in the understanding of chondrodermatitis nodularis chronica helices: the perichondrial vasculitis theory. *Clin Otolaryngol* 2009;34:147–50.

10 Sanu A, Koppana R, Snow DG. Management of chondrodermatitis nodularis chronic helicis using a 'doughnut pillow'. *J Laryngol Otol* 2007;121:1096–8.

11 Moncrieff M, Sassoon EM. Effective treatment of chondrodermatitis nodularis chronica helicis using a conservative approach. *Br J Dermatol* 2004;150:892–4.

12 Travelute CR. Self-adhering foam: a simple method for pressure relief during sleep in patients with chondrodermatitis nodularis helicis. *Dermatol Surg* 2013;39:317–19.

13 Cox NH, Denham PF. Intralesional triamcinolone for chondrodermatitis nodularis: a follow-up study of 60 patients. *Br J Dermatol* 2002;146:712–13.

14 Flynn V, Chisholm C, Grimwood R. Topical nitroglycerin: a promising treatment option for chondrodermatitis nodularis helicis. *J Am Acad Dermatol* 2011;65:531–6.

15 Lawrence CM. The treatment of chondrodermatitis nodularis with cartilage removal alone. *Arch Dermatol* 1991;127:530–5.

16 Hudson-Peacock MJ, Cox NH, Lawrence CM. The long-term results of cartilage removal alone for the treatment of chondrodermatitis nodularis. *Br J Dermatol* 1999;141:703–5.

18 Hussain W, Chalmers RJG. Simplified surgical treatment of chondrodermatitis nodularis by cartilage trimming and sutureless skin closure. *Br J Dermatol* 2009;160:116–18.

21 Gilaberte Y, Frias MP, Pérez-Lorenz JB. Chondrodermatitis nodularis helicis successfully treated with photodynamic therapy. *Arch Dermatol* 2010;146:1080–2.

Pseudocyst of the ear

1 Lazar RH, Heffner DK, Hughes GB, Hyams VK. Pseudocyst of the auricle: a review of 21 cases. *Otolaryngol Head Neck Surg* 1986;94:360–1.

5 Grabski WJ, Salasche SJ, McCollough ML, Angeloni VL. Pseudocyst of the auricle associated with trauma. *Arch Dermatol* 1989;125:528–30.

6 Chen PP, Tsai SM, Wang HM, *et al.* Lactate dehydrogenase isoenzyme patterns in auricular pseudocyst fluid. *J Laryngol Otol* 2013;127:499–82.

7 Yamamoto T, Yokoyama A, Umeda T. Cytokine profile of bilateral pseudocyst of the auricle. *Acta Derm Venereol (Stockh)* 1995;76:92–3.

8 Glamb R, Kim R. Pseudocyst of the auricle. *J Am Acad Dermatol* 1984;11:58–63.

10 Salgado CJ, Hardy JE, Mardini S, *et al.* Treatment of auricular pseudocyst with aspiration and local pressure. *J Plast Reconstr Aesthet Surg* 2006;59:1450–2.

11 Patigaroo SA, Mehfooz N, Patigaroo FA, *et al.* Clinical characteristics and comparative study of different modalities of treatment of pseudocyst pinna. *Eur Arch Otorhinolaryngol* 2012;269:1747–54.

12 Myamoto H, Dida M, Onuma S, Uchiyama M. Steroid injection therapy for pseudocyst of the auricle. *Acta Derm Venereol (Stockh)* 1994;74:140–2.

13 Tuncer S, Basterzi Y, Yavuzer R. Recurrent auricular pseudocyst: a new treatment recommendation with curettage and fibrin glue. *Dermatol Surg* 2003;29:1080–3.

14 Oyama N, Satoh M, Iwatsuki K, *et al.* Treatment of recurrent auricle pseudocyst with intralesional injection of minocycline: a report of two cases. *J Am Acad Dermatol* 2001;45:554–6.

Manifestation of skin disease and systemic disease in the ear—Table 108.1.

1 Chadwick JM, Downham TF. Auricular calcification. *Int J Dermatol* 1978;17:799–801.

2 Hicks BC, Weber PJ, Hashimoto K, *et al.* Primary cutaneous amyloidosis of the auricular concha. *J Am Acad Dermatol* 1988;18:19–25.

3 Bakos L, Weissbluth ML, Pires AKS, Muller LFB. Primary amyloidosis of the concha (letter). *J Am Acad Dermatol* 1989;20:524–5.

4 Barnadas M, Perez M, Esquius J, *et al.* Papules in the auricular concha: lichen amyloidosus in a case of biphasic amyloidosis. *Dermatologica* 1990;181:149–51.

5 Olsen TG, Helwig EB. Angiolymphoid hyperplasia with eosinophilia. A clinico-pathologic study of 116 patients. *J Am Acad Dermatol* 1985;12:781–96.

6 Tada J, Toi Y, Akiyama H, Arata J. Infra-auricular fissures in atopic dermatitis. *Acta Derm Venereol (Stockh)* 1994;74:129–31.

7 Bazex A, Griffiths A. Acrokeratosis paraneoplastica: a new cutaneous marker of malignancy. *Br J Dermatol* 1980;102:301–6.

8 Kastanioudakis I, Bassioukas K, Ziavra N, Skevas A. External ear involvement in epidermolysis bullosa. *Otolaryngol Head Neck Surg* 2000;122:618.

9 Azon-Masoliver A, Ferrando J, Navarra E, Mascaro JE. Solitary congenital nodular calcification of Winer located on the ear: report of two cases. *Pediatr Dermatol* 1989;6:191–3.

10 McCallum DI, Gray WM. Metastatic Crohn's disease. *Br J Dermatol* 1976;95:551–4.

11 Ghigliotti G, Parodi A, Borgiani L, *et al.* Acquired cutis laxa confined to the face. *J Am Acad Dermatol* 1991;24:504–5.

12 Thompson AC, Shall L, Moralee SJ. Darier's disease of the external ear. *J Laryngol Otol* 1992;106:725–6.

13 Rongioletti F, Ghio L, Ginevri F, *et al.* Purpura of the ears: a distinctive vasculopathy with circulating autoantibodies complicating long-term treatment with levamisole in children. *Br J Dermatol* 1999;140:948–51.

14 Toriumi DM, Konior RJ, Berktold RE. Severe hypertrichosis of the external ear canal during minoxidil therapy. *Arch Otolaryngol Head Neck Surg* 1988;114:918–19.

15 Trunnell TN, Waisman M. Hypertrophied retroauricular folds attributable to diphenylhydantoin therapy. *Cutis* 1982;30:207–9.

16 Grant JM. Elephantiasis nostras verrucosa of the ears. *Cutis* 1982;29:441–4.

17 Mahzoon S, Azadeh B. Elephantiasis of external ears: a rare manifestation of pediculosis capitis. *Acta Derm Venereol (Stockh)* 1983;63:363–5.

18 Muhlbauer JE. Granuloma annulare. *J Am Acad Dermatol* 1980;3:217–30.

19 Foss MH. Granuloma faciale: report on a case. *Acta Derm Venereol (Stockh)* 1957;37:473–82.

20 Mansfield RE, Storkan MA, Cliff IS. Evaluation of the earlobe in leprosy. A clinical and histopathological study. *Arch Dermatol* 1969;100:407–12.

21 Sartori-Valinotti JC, Bruce AJ, Krotova Khan Y, Beatty CW. A 10-year review of otic lichen planus: the Mayo Clinic experience. *JAMA Dermatol.* 2013;149:1082–6.

22 Darvay A, Russell-Jones R, Acland KM, *et al.* Systemic B-cell lymphoma presenting as an isolated lesion on the ear. *Clin Exp Dermatol* 2001;26:166–9.

23 Sugathan P. Mudi-chood disease. *Dermatol Online J* 1999;5:5.

24 Bukachevsky R, Kimmelman CP. Otolaryngologic manifestations of porphyria cutanea tarda. *Otolaryngol Head Neck Surg* 1989;101:402–3.

25 Nova A. Sarcoidosis of the ear. *Ear Nose Throat J* 1981;60:307–8.

26 Jensen JL, Liao SY, Jeffes EW III. Verruciform xanthoma of the ear with coexisting epidermal dysplasia. *Am J Dermatopathol* 1992;14:426–30.

27 Kavanagh GM, Bradfield JW, Collins CM, Kennedy CT. Weathering nodules of the ear: a clinicopathological study. *Br J Dermatol* 1996;135:550–4.

28 Kornblut AD, Wolffs M, Fauci AS. Ear disease in patients with Wegener's granulomatosis. *Laryngoscope* 1982;92:713–17.

29 Sueki H, Saito T, Iijima M, Fujisawa R. Adult onset xanthogranuloma appearing symmetrically on the ear lobes. *J Am Acad Dermatol* 1995;32:372–4.

Infection

Otitis externa

2 Osguthorpe JD, Nielsen DR. Otitis externa: Review and clinical update. *Am Fam Physician* 2006;74:1510–16.

9 Matar GM, Harakeh HS, Ramlawi F, *et al.* Comparative analysis between *Pseudomonas aeruginosa* genotypes and severity of symptoms in patients with unilateral or bilateral otitis externa. *Curr Microbiol* 2001;42:190–3.

15 Hawke M, Wong J, Krajden S. Clinical and microbiological features of otitis externa. *J Otolaryngol* 1984;13:289–95.

26 Wormald PJ. Surgical management of benign necrotizing otitis externa. *J Laryngol Otol* 1994;108:101–5.

27 Hajioff D, Mackeith S. Otitis externa. *Clin Evid (Online)* 2010 Aug 3;0510 PMC3217807.

28 Kaushik V, Malik T, Saeed SR. Interventions for acute otitis externa. *Cochrane Database Syst Rev* 2010;(1):CD004740.

30 Burton MJ, Singer M, Rosenfeld RM. Extracts from The Cochrane Library: interventions for acute otitis externa. *Otolaryngol Head Neck Surg* 2010;143:8–11.

31 Rosenfeld RM, Singer M, Wasserman JM, Stinnett SS. Systematic review of topical antimicrobial therapy for acute otitis externa. *Otolaryngol Head Neck Surg* 2006;134(4 Suppl):S24–48.

33 Harth W, Caffeier PP, Mayelzadeh B, *et al*. Topical tacrolimus treatment for chronic dermatitis of the ear. *Eur J Dermatol* 2007;17:405–11.

Necrotizing otitis externa

8 Nguyen LT, Harris JP, Nguyen QT. Erosive external otitis: a novel distinct clinical entity of the external auditory canal in nonimmunosuppressed individuals. *Otol Neurotol* 2010;31:1409–11.

9 Tsikoudas A, Davis BC. Benign necrotizing otitis externa. *Ear Nose Throat J* 2009;88:E18.

10 Wickham N, Crawford A, Carney AS, Goss AN. Bisphosphonate-associated osteonecrosis of the external auditory canal. *J Laryngol Otol* 2013;127(Suppl. 2):S51–3.

11 Chen CN, Chen YS, Yeh TH, Hsu CJ, Tseng FY. Outcomes of malignant external otitis: survival vs mortality. *Acta Otolaryngol* 2010;130:89–94.

12 Franco-Vidal V, Blanchet H, Bebear C, *et al*. Necrotizing external otitis: a report of 46 cases. *Otol Neurotol* 2007;28:771–3.

13 Carfrae MJ, Kesser BW. Malignant otitis externa. *Otolaryngol Clin North Am* 2008;41:537–49.

15 Grandis JR, Curtin HD, Yu VL. Necrotizing (malignant) external otitis: prospective comparison of CT and MR imaging in diagnosis and follow-up. *Radiology* 1995;196:499–504.

16 Okpala NC, Siraj QH, Nilssen E, Pringle M. Radiological and radionuclide investigation of malignant otitis externa. *J Laryngol Otol* 2005;119:71–5.

19 Mahdyoun P, Pulcini C, Gahide I, *et al*. Necrotizing otitis externa: a systematic review. *Otol Neurotol* 2013;34:620–9.

20 Phillips JS, Jones SE. Hyperbaric oxygen as an adjuvant treatment for malignant otitis externa. *Cochrane Database Syst Rev* 2013;(5):CD004617.

Otomycosis

1 Ho T, Vrabec JT, Yoo D, Coker NJ. Otomycosis: clinical features and treatment implications. *Otolaryngol Head Neck Surg* 2006;135:787–91.

2 Lucente FE. Fungal infections of the external ear. *Otolaryngol Clin North Am* 1993;26:995–1006.

3 Viswanatha B, Sumatha D, Vijayashree MS. Otomycosis in immunocompetent and immunocompromised patients: comparative study and literature review. *Ear Nose Throat J* 2012;91:114–21.

4 Nielsen PG. Fungi isolated from chronic external ear disorders. *Mykosen* 1985;28:234–7.

5 Sood VB, Sinha A, Mohaoatra LN. Otomycosis: a clinical entity—clinical and experimental study. *J Laryngol Otol* 1988;81:999–1173.

6 Stern JC, Lucente FE. Otomycosis. *Ear Nose Throat J* 1988;67:804–10.

7 Vennewald I, Klemm E. Otomycosis: diagnosis and treatment. *Clin Dermatol* 2010;28:202–11.

Tumours of the auricle and external auditory canal

Glandular tumours

1 Lynde CW, McLean DI, Wood WS. Tumors of the ceruminous glands. *J Am Acad Dermatol* 1984;11:841–7.

2 Lassaletta L, Patron M, Oloriz J, *et al*. Avoiding misdiagnosis in ceruminous gland tumours. *Auris Nasus Larynx* 2003;30:287–90.

3 Thompson LD, Nelson BL, Barnes EL. Ceruminous adenomas: a clinicopathologic study of 41 cases with a review of the literature. *Am J Surg Pathol* 2004;28:308–18.

4 Habib MA. Ceruminoma in association with other sweat gland tumours. *J Laryngol Otol* 1981;95:415–20.

8 Mansour P, George MK, Pahor AL. Ceruminous gland tumours: a reappraisal. *J Laryngol Otol* 1992;106:727–32.

Squamous cell carcinoma of the auricle (pinna)

3 Ahmad I, Das Gupta AR. Epidemiology of basal cell carcinoma and squamous cell carcinoma of the pinna. *J Laryngol Otol* 2001;115:85–6.

4 Rowe DE, Carroll RJ, Day CL. Prognostic factors for local recurrence, metastasis and survival rates in squamous carcinoma of the skin, ear and lip. *J Am Acad Dermatol* 1992;26:976–90.

5 Veness MJ, Palme CE, Morgan GJ. High-risk cutaneous squamous cell carcinoma of the head and neck: results from 266 treated patients with metastatic lymph node disease. *Cancer* 2006;106:2389–96.

8 Lindelof B, Dal H, Wolk K, Malmborg N. Cutaneous squamous cell carcinoma in organ transplant recipients: a study of the Swedish cohort with regard to tumor site. *Arch Dermatol* 2005;141:447–51.

9 Nordin P, Stenquist B. Five-year results of curettage-cryosurgery for 100 consecutive auricular non-melanoma skin cancers. *J Laryngol Otol* 2002;116:893–8.

12 Kitchens GG. Auricular wedge resection and reconstruction. *Ear Nose Throat J* 1989;68:673–4, 677–9, 683.

13 Levine HL, Kinney SE, Bailin PL, Roberts JK. Cancer of the peri-auricular region. *Dermatol Clin* 1989;7:781–95.

25 Caccialanza M, Piccinno R, Kolesnikova L, Gnecchi L. Radiotherapy of skin carcinomas of the pinna: a study of 115 lesions in 108 patients. *Int J Dermatol*. 2005;44:513–17.

26 Moloney FJ, Kelly PO, Kay EW, *et al*. Maintenance versus reduction of immuno-suppression in renal transplant recipients with aggressive squamous cell carcinoma. *Dermatol Surg* 2004;30:674–8.

Squamous carcinoma of the external auditory canal

1 Arriaga M, Curtin H, Takahashi H, et al. Staging proposal for external auditory meatus carcinoma based on preoperative clinical examination and computed tomography findings. *Ann Otol Rhinol Laryngol* 1990;99:714–21.

2 Lim L H, Goh Y H, Chan Y M, *et al*. Malignancy of the temporal bone and external auditory canal. *Otolaryngol Head Neck Surg* 2000;122:882–6.

3 Stafford ND, Frootko NJ. Verrucous carcinoma in the external auditory canal. *Am J Otol*. 1986;7:443–5.

8 Moody SA, Hirsch BE, Myers EN. Squamous cell carcinoma of the external auditory canal: an evaluation of a staging system. *Am J Otol* 2000;21:582–8.

9 Higgins TS, Antonio SA. The role of facial palsy in staging squamous cell carcinoma of the temporal bone and external auditory canal: a comparative survival analysis. *Otol Neurotol*. 2010;31:1473–9.

10 Ito M, Hatano M, Yoshizaki T. Prognostic factors for squamous cell carcinoma of the temporal bone: extensive bone involvement or extensive soft tissue involvement? *Acta Otolaryngol*. 2009;129:1313–19.

11 Yamatodani T, Mineta H. Surgical approach for treatment of carcinoma of the anterior wall of the external auditory canal. *Otol Neurotol* 2012;33:450–4.

12 Gidley PW. Managing malignancies of the external auditory canal. *Expert Rev Anticancer Ther* 2009;9:1277–82.

13 Ogawa K, Nakamura K, Hatano K, et al. Treatment and prognosis of squamous cell carcinoma of the external auditory canal and middle ear: a multi-institutional retrospective review of 87 patients. *Int J Radiat Oncol Biol Phys*. 2007;68:1326–34.

14 Pemberton LS, Swindell R, Sykes AJ. Primary radical radiotherapy for squamous cell carcinoma of the middle ear and external auditory canal-an historical series. *Clin Oncol (R Coll Radiol)*. 2006;18:390–4.

Miscellaneous conditions

Petrified ear

1 Stites PC, Boyd AS, Zic J. Auricular ossificans (ectopic ossification of the auricle). *J Am Acad Dermatol* 2003;49:142–4.

2 Gossner J. Prevalence of the petrified ear: a computed tomographic study. *Eur Arch Otorhinolaryngol* 2014;271:195–7.

Cholesteatoma

1 Friedman I, Arnold W. *Pathology of the Ear*. Edinburgh: Churchill Livingstone, 1993:30–1.

2 Sismanis A, Williams GH, Abedi E. External auditory meatus cholesteatoma. In: Tos M, Thomas J, Peitersen E, eds. *Cholesteatoma and Mastoid Surgery*. Amsterdam: Kugler and Ghedini, 1984:577–82.

3 Owen HH, Rosborg J, Gaihede M. Cholesteatoma of the external ear canal: etiological factors, symptoms and clinical findings in a series of 48 cases. *BMC Ear Nose Throat Disord* 2006;6:16–25.

Keratosis obturans

1 Piepergerdes JC, Kramer BM, Behnke EE. Keratosis obturans and external auditory canal cholesteatoma. *Laryngoscope* 1980;90:383–90.

Referred pain

1 Shah RK, Blevins NH. Otalgia. *Otolaryngol Clin North Am* 2003;36:1137–51.

CHAPTER 109

Dermatoses of the Eye, Eyelids and Eyebrows

Valerie P. J. Saw[1] *and Jonathan N. Leonard*[2]

[1]Moorfields Eye Hospital NHS Foundation Trust and UCL Institute of Ophthalmology NIHR Biomedical Research Centre, London, UK
[2]Department of Dermatology, Imperial College Healthcare NHS Trust, London, UK

Introduction

This chapter is not intended to be a comprehensive account of all diseases that affect the skin and eyes, for which there are several reviews [1–5,6,7]. The main focus is on those conditions that commonly occur in clinical practice and that present a problem with management. It is also intended to alert the dermatologist to conditions that might threaten visual acuity and require urgent referral to an ophthalmologist. Also, many systemic diseases affect both the skin and eyes, and ophthalmic assessment will be of help in making the correct diagnosis and in the long-term management of such patients.

Anatomy and physiology of the eye [1,2]

The eye and skin share a common embryological origin. The structure of the lid, conjunctiva, lacrimal gland and associated drainage apparatus are of surface ectodermal origin while the remainder of the eye arises from epithelium of the ectodermal neural plate. The only mesodermal contribution to the eye is the myoblasts of the extraocular muscles. The anatomy of the eye is shown in Figure 109.1. The eye appendages are as follows.

Eyebrows

This hair-bearing area rests on a very mobile fat and muscle pad overlying the superior orbital ridge. Its mobility is important as a means of facial expression. The eyebrows help protect the eye from bright light and sweat.

Eyelids

The eyelids have distinct anatomical layers, comprising the skin with subcutaneous tissue and striated muscles that effect lid movement, the tarsal plate and conjunctiva (Figure 109.2). The grey line, an important anatomical landmark for surgical repair and pathological conditions of the lid margin such as blepharitis, divides the lid into an anterior lamella (skin and muscle) and a posterior lamella (tarsus and conjunctiva). The grey line represents the location of the marginal region of the orbicularis muscle (muscle of Riolan) seen through the lid skin.

The skin is thin and modified in several ways to protect the eyeball. It contains sebaceous glands associated with the fine hairs of

Rook's Textbook of Dermatology, Ninth Edition. Edited by Christopher Griffiths, Jonathan Barker, Tanya Bleiker, Robert Chalmers and Daniel Creamer.
© 2016 John Wiley & Sons, Ltd. Published 2016 by John Wiley & Sons, Ltd.
Companion website: www.rooksdermatology.com

PART 10: SITES, SEX, AGE

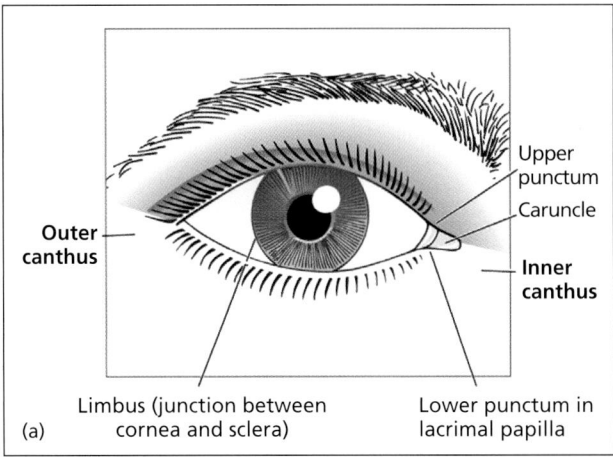

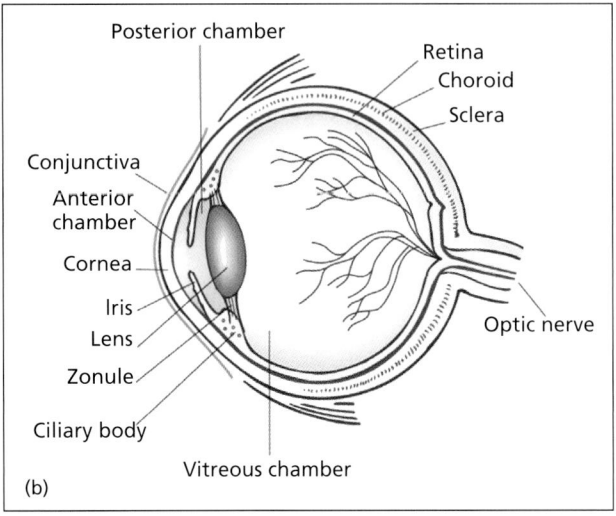

Figure 109.1 Anatomy of the normal eye. (a) The external appearance of the right eye. (b) Cross-section of the human eye.

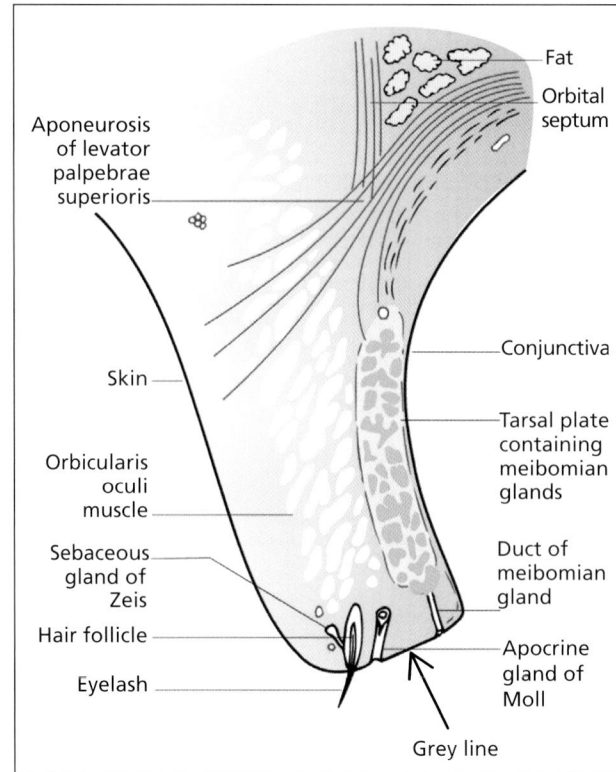

Figure 109.2 Cross-section of the upper eyelid.

the eyelashes (cilia) and both apocrine and eccrine sweat glands. There are about 300 eyelashes, arising in two rows along the eyelid margin, two-thirds of which are in the upper lid. They have no associated erector muscles, but rudimentary sebaceous glands (of Zeis) are present. Some lashes, particularly those of the lower lid, are associated with ancillary apocrine sweat glands (of Moll). The ducts of these glands open both into the lash follicles and directly onto the anterior lid margin between the lashes. The eyelashes help to protect foreign bodies from impinging on the eyeball. Each lash follicle has a rich nerve plexus, which is easily excited – light touch initiates reflex closure.

The tarsal plate of each eyelid gives the palpebral aperture shape and stability. They comprise dense, fibrous tissue surrounding modified sebaceous glands (meibomian glands). These secrete the outer lipid layer of the precorneal tear film through openings along the mucocutaneous junction of the eyelid margin. This lipid helps to stabilize the tear film and reduce evaporation. There are about 30 glands in the upper tarsal plate and 20 in the lower. Meibomian glands have up to 20 acini surrounding a central vertical duct and are visible through the conjunctiva.

The eyelids are lined by a mucous membrane called the palpebral conjunctiva. It is reflected over the anterior portion of the eyeball up to the edge of the cornea as the bulbar conjunctiva. The folds formed by the reflection of the conjunctiva from the lids onto the eyeball are called the superior and inferior palpebral fornices. The conjunctiva contains numerous goblet cells secreting mucin into the tear film. It also contains about 50 accessory lacrimal glands and its substantia propria contains neural tissue, mast cells, lymphocytes and lymphoid follicles, which are important in mediating local immunological reactions.

The striated muscle of the levator palpebrae superioris opens the eye, and the striated orbicularis oculi muscle closes it. Both are innervated by the facial nerve. Two divisions of the trigeminal nerve supply sensation to the eyelids; the upper lid and medial canthus are supplied by the ophthalmic division, and the remainder of the lower lid by the maxillary division.

The eyelid has a rich blood supply, mainly through the medial and lateral palpebral arteries, which are branches of the ophthalmic artery. There is also a rich anastomosis between adjacent arteries arising from the internal and external carotid. The blood drains through a network of veins to the facial and orbital veins and the cavernous sinus. Lymphatics drain the conjunctiva and tarsal plate to the post-tarsal plexus and the skin and orbicularis to the pretarsal plexus. The medial canthus and lower lid subsequently drain to the submandibular nodes whilst the lateral canthus and upper lid drain to the parotid and preauricular nodes.

Lacrimal glands

The main lacrimal gland is a modified sweat gland located in the lacrimal fossa, a bony depression just under the upper and outer margin of the orbit. It produces an aqueous secretion, which discharges through a network of ductules onto the conjunctiva of the palpebral conjunctiva. In addition, there are a variable number of accessory lacrimal glands in the upper and lower conjunctival fornices. The lacrimal gland is innervated whereas the accessory glands are not.

Precorneal tear film

The eyelids make a vital contribution to the composition and stability of the precorneal tear film. The precorneal tear film is now believed, based on tomographic, interferometric and reflectance spectral techinques, to be about 3 μm thick [3]. It is a layered structure consisting of a thin 50–100 nm outermost lipid layer secreted primarily by the meibomian glands with a lesser contribution from the eyelid glands of Moll and Zeiss (as discussed above) and a central aqueous-mucous layer secreted primarily by the main lacrimal gland and accessory lacrimal glands of Krause and Wolfring, with additional fluid and electrolytes secreted by ocular surface epithelial cells. The aqueous-mucin pool contains soluble gel-forming mucins secreted by conjunctival goblet cells. Anchored to the apical plasma membrane of the corneal and conjunctival epithelial cells are transmembrane mucins, which contribute to formation of a glycocalyx. Blinking consists of a lateral to medial movement of the eyelids, which enables resurfacing of the tear film of the cornea and propels the tears to the punctum of the tear duct; from here, they are actively removed by the lacrimal pump mechanism through the lacrimal canaliculi into the common canaliculus and lacrimal sac, and then via the nasolacrimal duct into the nose (Figure 109.3).

The tear film has a number of functions:
1 To supply oxygen and other nutrients to the cornea.
2 To remove particulate matter from the surface of the eye.
3 To prevent drying of the eye.
4 To act as a lubricant and prevent adhesion of the palpebral to the bulbar conjunctiva.

5 To protect the eye surface through its antibacterial role; it contains white blood cells, various proteins, lysozyme and immunoglobulins.

Glossary of ophthalmological terms

A glossary is provided in Table 109.1.

Disorders affecting the eyebrows and eyelashes

There is a wide variation in the colour, distribution and density of the eyebrow hairs. The inheritance of the appearance of the eyebrows is polygenic. Some hereditary variations are of no known significance, but others are associated with other development defects or are part of a recognized syndrome.

Disorders of the eyebrows [1]

Synophrys
This term is applied when the eyebrows are profuse with a tendency to meet in the centre of the face. Synophrys is a feature of some genodermatoses. The eyebrows also tend to become more bushy in the ageing male for reasons that are unknown. Bushy eyebrows may also occur in other acquired forms of hypertrichosis, for example due to drugs such as diazoxide, and fusion of the eyebrows has been reported in kwashiorkor.

Hypoplasia of eyebrows
Some inherited diseases are characterized by hypoplasia of the eyebrows. Acquired conditions can cause sparsity or sometimes complete loss of the eyebrows. They may be the only site affected in alopecia areata. Thinning of the eyebrows occurs in hypothyroidism, erythroderma, follicular mucinosis and secondary syphilis. Lepromatous leprosy causes thinning of the outer third of the

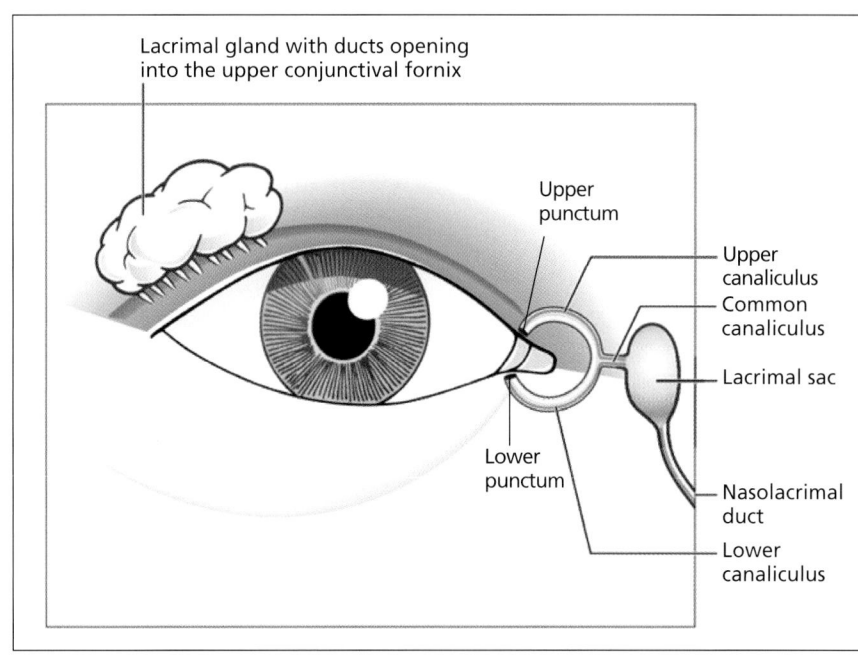

Figure 109.3 The lacrimal apparatus of the right eye.

Table 109.1 Glossary of ophthalmological terms.

Anophthalmia	Absence of eye
Astichiasis	Absence of lashes
Blepharitis	Inflammation of the eyelid margin
Blepharochalasis	Elastic tissue atrophy causing loose eyelid skin
Bruch membrane	The retinal layer sandwiched between the retinal pigment epithelium and the vascular choroid
Chemosis	Swelling or oedema of the conjunctiva, due to exudation from capillaries
Coloboma	Congenital cleft created by failure of development of a portion of the eye or adnexal structures
Dermatochalasis	Laxness of the skin of the eyelids
Distichiasis	Accessory row of eyelashes
Ectropion	Eversion of the eyelid
Entropion	Inversion of the eyelid
Epicanthal fold	Accessory fold of skin at the inner canthal region of the eye
Epicanthus inversus	Lower lid fold larger than upper lid fold
Epiphora	Excess tearing
Episcleritis	Inflammation of the superficial scleral tissues
Follicular inflammation	Inflammatory response of the conjunctiva characterized by discrete, round elevated lesions of the conjunctiva with a vascular network around the follicle, diameter 0.5–5.0 mm. Composed of lymphocytes, macrophages and plasma cells, may form lymphoid follicles. Usually located in the inferior palpebral conjunctiva, sometimes superiorly
Grey line	The grey line is an important anatomical landmark for surgical repair and pathological conditions of the lid margin such as blepharitis. The grey line divides the lid into an anterior lamella (skin and muscle) and a posterior lamella (tarsus and conjunctiva). The grey line represents the location of the marginal region of the orbicularis muscle (muscle of Riolan) seen through the lid skin
Hypertelorism	Increased distance between the two eyes measured radiologically
Hypopyon	The presence of pus in the anterior chamber
Keratitis	Inflammation of the cornea – various types are recognized, including: *filamentary keratitis* – the development of epithelialized mucous filaments on the corneal surface; *interstitial keratitis* – inflammation of the corneal stromal layer
Keratoconjunctivitis sicca	Corneal and conjunctival inflammation associated with impaired tear secretion and ocular dryness
Keratoconus	Conical distortion of the central cornea as a result of a degenerative process in the stroma
Keratopathy	Corneal abnormalities including: *exposure keratopathy* – from corneal exposure and drying of the cornea
Lagophthalmos	Persistent exposure of the eyeball despite closure of the eyelid
Limbus	Boundary between the cornea and sclera
Madarosis	Loss of the eyelashes
Pannus	Vascularized corneal scar
Papillary inflammation	Inflammatory response of the conjunctiva characterized by elevated polygonal hyperaemic areas each with a central fibrovascular core, separated by paler areas. Diameter of 0.3 mm (micropapillae) to 2.0 mm. 'Giant' papillae if >1.0 mm. Composed of polymorphonucelar leukocytes and other acute inflammatory cells, with epithelial hypertrophy. Typically occur on the tarsal conjunctiva and at the limbus
Phlyctenule	Wedge-shaped, peripheral corneal or conjunctival, nodule
Preseptal cellulitis	Cellulitis of the eyelids that has not penetrated through the orbital septum to involve the orbit
Symblepharon	Adhesions between the bulbar and palpebral conjunctiva resulting in complete or partial obliteration of the eyelid fornices
Telecanthus	Increased distance between the inner canthi
Trichiasis	Lashes that turn inward toward the cornea usually as a result of entropion
Uveitis	Inflammation of the uveal tract. It is subdivided into anterior uveitis, which is the most common, intermediate uveitis, posterior uveitis and pan uveitis. *Anterior uveitis* is subdivided into iritis, in which the inflammation predominantly affects the iris, and iridocyclitis, in which both the iris and the anterior part of the ciliary body (pars plicata) are equally involved. *Intermediate uveitis* involves the posterior part of the ciliary body (pars plana) and the extreme periphery of the choroid and retina. *Posterior uveitis* is inflammation located behind the vitreous base. *Pan uveitis* is involvement of the entire uveal tract

eyebrows in the early stages, often with depigmentation, progressing to total loss of the brows and lashes. Tuberculoid leprosy, by contrast, does not cause loss of the eyebrows. Plucking the eyebrows for cosmetic reasons is common, but true trichotillomania of the eyebrows is unusual.

Inflammatory disorders affecting the eyebrows

The eyebrows are often involved in seborrhoeic dermatitis and psoriasis. Post-inflammatory cicatricial alopecia from discoid lupus erythematosus, folliculitis decalvans, lupus vulgaris or tertiary syphilis

may cause loss of eyebrow hairs. Scarring with loss of eyebrows may also follow chemical and thermal burns or radiation. Loss of eyebrows can be camouflaged by the use of eyebrow pencils, permanent tattooing or by a hair prosthesis glued in place daily.

Disorders of the eyelashes

Trichomegaly [2–6]

This may be due to a genetic trait. Increased growth of the eyelashes has also been described in HIV infection and related to

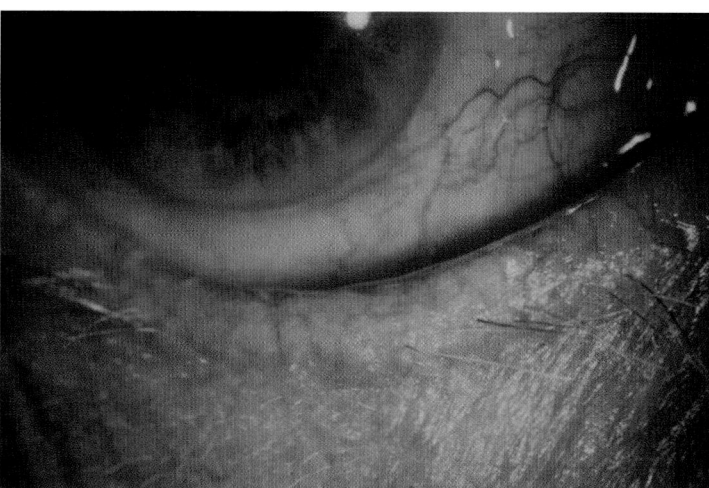

Figure 109.4 Madarosis due to staphylococcal blepharitis. (Courtesy of Mr J. Dart, Moorfields Eye Hospital, London, UK.)

various drugs including ciclosporin, zidovudine, interferon, epidermal growth factor receptor inhibitors and topical prostaglandin analogues such as bimatoprost. The latter can be used for the treatment of hypotrichosis of the eyelashes. Long lashes also occur in some patients with phenylketonuria.

Madarosis [1]
Madarosis is a decrease in the number or complete loss of lashes. A number of causes have been recognized and include alopecia areata, chronic anterior lid margin blepharitis (Figure 109.4), infiltrating tumours of the lid, burns, cryotherapy and radiotherapy, trichotillomania and discoid lupus erythematosus (see Figure 109.10e). Systemic diseases such as hypothyroidism and syphilis may also be responsible.

Abnormalities of the eyelids

These include dermatochalasis, blepharochalasis and lid laxity. Numerous developmental defects can affect the palpebral fissure or size and shape of the eyelids. A number of hereditary dermatoses affect the eyelids.

Ptosis
Drooping of the eyelids on one or both sides is a common genetic defect. Mild ptosis commonly develops in the elderly due to the laxity of the connective tissue. There are many important acquired causes, such as third nerve palsy, Horner syndrome and myasthenia gravis, which require neurological referral. Ptosis may be associated with other ocular abnormalities.

Skin diseases affecting the eyelids
A large number of dermatological conditions can affect the eyelids as part of a generalized process. Usually there is little diagnostic difficulty as the diagnosis is made by examination of the rest of the skin. Psoriasis and lichen planus can both involve the lids and cause considerable irritation. These are chronic diseases and

management can become a problem with use of potent topical corticosteroids on the eyelids over a prolonged period of time. Use of topical immunosuppressants tacrolimus and pimecrolimus is effective and can reduce topical corticosteroid exposure in facial psoriasis [1]. Unilateral involvement of an eyelid raises the possibility of infective conditions, including tinea and mycobacterial infections.

Psoriasis [2,3]
Eye involvement can occur in 10–58% of patients with psoriasis, mostly in those with psoriatic arthritis. Men are more susceptible to ocular disease. Involvement of the eyelid gives rise to blepharitis, madarosis and development of psoriatic plaques. Chronic non-specific conjunctivitis may occur over time and lead eventually to keratoconjunctivitis sicca with symblepharon formation and trichiasis. Conjunctivitis usually complicates eyelid margin involvement; white or yellow psoriatic plaques can spread from the lid on to the conjunctiva itself. Corneal changes are rare and are most commonly related to exposure and trichiasis. Anterior uveitis is rare but has been reported in patients with psoriatic arthritis and is similar to that seen in Reiter syndrome. Ocular psoriasis is treated with use of lubricants, topical corticosteroids and steroid-sparing topical calcineurin inhibitors where indicated. Patients with chronic eyelid involvement should be referred for ophthalmological assessment.

Contact dermatitis [4–10]
Contact dermatitis is the responsible cause in approximately half of patients with an eyelid dermatitis. The remainder have manifestations of atopic or seborrhoeic eczema. The eyelid skin is very sensitive to primary irritants. These can cause dermatitis in their own right or can aggravate an underlying constitutional tendency in patients with either atopic or seborrhoeic eczema.

Allergic contact dermatitis can present after many years of exposure to the culpable allergen. Clinically, it is characterized by severe itching, erythema and swelling of the eyelid, progressing to formation of vesicles. A large variety of allergens have been reported as causing an allergic contact dermatitis of the lid and include preservatives (used in cosmetics, topical medications (Figure 109.5) and contact lens cleaning solutions), fragrances and the resin used in nail polish. Patients with suspected contact dermatitis of the eyelids should be patch tested. Careful history taking is of paramount importance to make sure the relevant allergens are included in the test battery. The possibility of transferring antigen from the hands to the eyelids needs to be considered. Maibach described the upper eyelid dermatosis syndrome in which patients have discomfort of the eyelids with or without dermatitis; it is thought to be unrelated to the use of cosmetics.

Periorbital oedema [11,12]
The subcutaneous tissue of the eyelids is lax and prone to oedema. There are many systemic and dermatological causes of eyelid oedema that need to be considered. Systemic causes include glomerulonephritis, hypoalbuminaemia (especially nephrotic syndrome), cardiac failure, superior venocaval obstruction and thyroid disease. Some systemic infections, such as infectious mononucleosis and scarlatina, cause periorbital oedema. It may be the

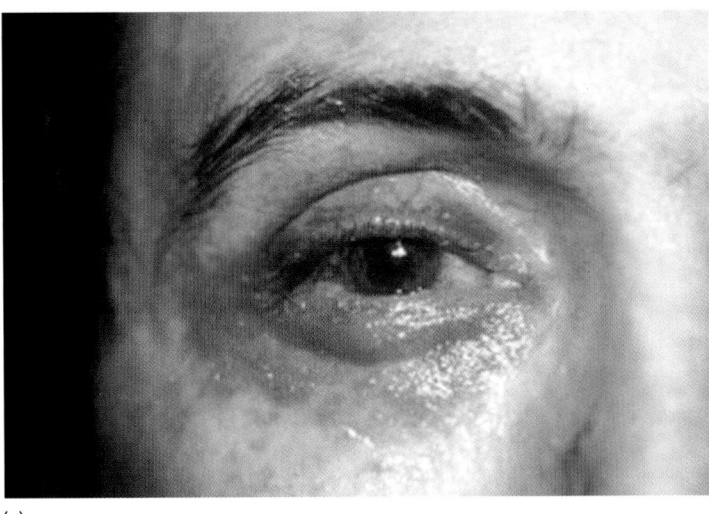

(a)

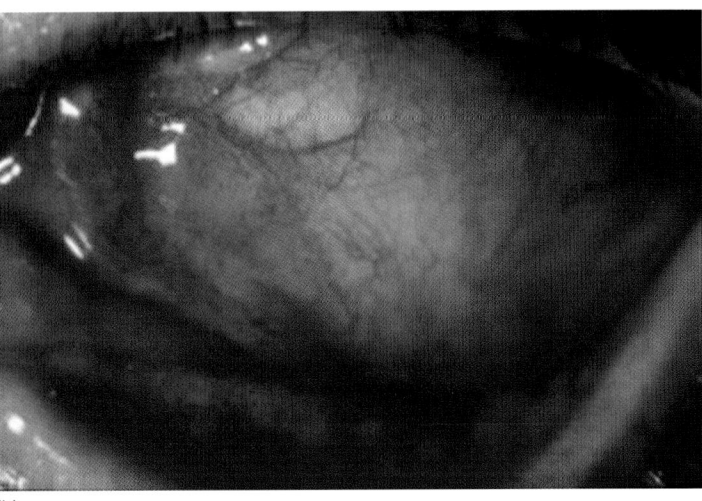

(b)

Figure 109.5 Allergic blepharoconjunctivitis due to topical medication toxicity. (a) Allergic eyelid skin reaction. (b) Follicular conjunctival inflammation accompanying allergic skin reaction. (Courtesy of Mr J. Dart, Moorfields Eye Hospital, London, UK.)

presenting feature of dermatomyositis and has been reported in systemic lupus erythematosus.

The most common dermatological causes of periorbital oedema are angio-oedema, lymphoedema, allergic contact dermatitis (Figure 109.6) and blepharochalasis; they are usually distinguished by the history. Angio-oedema is transient and often part of a more generalized urticarial eruption. Lymphoedema is permanent and tends to be worse first thing in the morning and improves during the day; it may be associated with underlying sinus disease or a chronic inflammatory condition such as granulomatous rosacea. Allergic contact dermatitis presents acutely with swelling, redness and itching. Blepharochalasis is an uncommon condition which may be inherited (autosomal dominant) or sporadic; it presents in the second decade with recurrent episodes of painless lid oedema, resulting in the development of excess skin and thickened subcutaneous tissue which may require treatment by blepharoplasty. Senile orbital fat prolapse through a deficient orbital septum may mimic periorbital oedema but is differentiated by the fact that

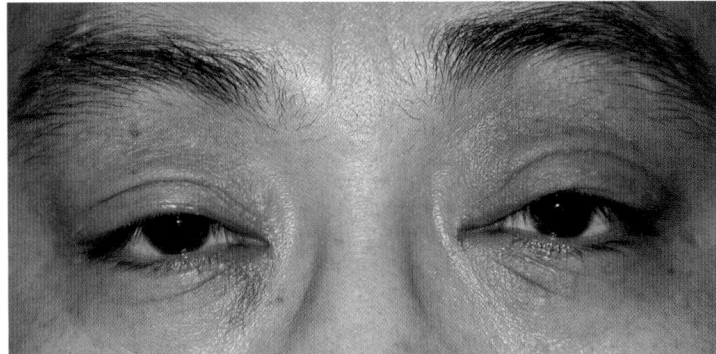

Figure 109.6 Periorbital oedema due to allergy.

there is minimal fluctuation in the associated swelling. Periorbital oedema may be the presenting feature of rosacea.

Changes in pigmentation [13–17]

There are considerable racial and familial variations of the degree of pigmentation of the eyelids. Marked periorbital melanosis is seen as a genetic trait. Pigmentation of the periorbital skin can also be post-traumatic, post-inflammatory or can accompany melanocyte-stimulating hormone-induced melanosis of any cause. Chemical pigmentation can occur from prolonged use of a mercurial or silver preparation, producing a slate-blue or grey-brown discoloration. Mauve discoloration of the eyelids and periorbital area is an early part of chrysiasis from parenteral gold therapy. A grey discoloration can complicate long-term treatment with minocycline. Local increase in pigmentation may also be due to cosmetics containing phototoxic agents, usually psoralens. Increased pigmentation can also follow inflammatory dermatoses such as eczema and lichen planus. The eyelids may be involved in vitiligo. Hypopigmentation can complicate the use of topical medications including thiotepa eye drops and mercurial ointments.

SKIN DISEASES AFFECTING THE EYE AND EYELIDS

Blepharitis, meibomian gland dysfunction, rosacea and seborrhoeic dermatitis [1–5]

Definition and nomenclature

A recent international workshop on meibomian gland dysfunction (MGD) has formalized definitions and terminology [2]. Blepharitis is a general term describing inflammation of the lid as a whole. Anterior blepharitis describes inflammation of the lid margin anterior to the grey line and concentrated around td he lashes. It may be accompanied by squamous debris or collarettes around the lashes, and inflammation may spill onto the posterior lid margin, resulting in posterior blepharitis. Posterior blepharitis describes inflammation of the posterior lid margin, which may have different causes, including MGD, conjunctival inflammation (allergic or infective) and/or other conditions, such as acne rosacea. MGD is a chronic, diffuse abnormality of the meibomian glands, commonly characterized by terminal duct obstruction and/or qualitative/quantitative changes in the glandular secretion. It may result in alteration of the tear film, symptoms of eye irritation, clinically apparent inflammation and ocular surface disease. MGD is further subcategorized into hyposecretory, obstructive and hypersecretory forms, as agreed by the recent international workshop.

Synonyms and inclusions

Contrary to some literature (including McCulley et al. [1]), the terms posterior blepharitis and MGD are not interchangeable or synonymous. MGD is only one cause of posterior blepharitis. Despite this, McCulley's clinical classification of 'chronic blepharitis' (Table 109.2) is still useful in that it identifies the main subtypes of MGD causing lid margin disease, as well as 'other' blepharitis, due to causes other than MGD. McCulley's study also correlated dermatological findings with the ocular classification. The MGD disorders in McCulley's classification (staphylococcal, seborrhoeic, meibomitis, meibomian seborrhoea) may occur simultaneously, and not all of them result in inflammation of the lid margin. They are frequently associated with conjunctivitis or keratoconjunctivitis. Chronic blepharitis may occur in the absence of any significant dermatological association, and its classification is further complicated both by the variable association of chronic blepharitis with rosacea and seborrhoeic dermatitis, and also by the term ocular rosacea, a condition which may occur in the absence of dermatological rosacea.

It is hardly surprising that this classification causes confusion amongst practitioners. This situation has arisen partly because the pathogenesis is poorly understood, with few unifying concepts.

Introduction and general description

Table 109.2 summarizes a clinical classification of blepharitis, its associations and features. It includes ocular rosacea amongst the meibomian gland disorders, with which it is always associated. Table 109.2 classifies the five types of common blepharitis (including ocular rosacea) into those that principally affect the anterior lid margin structures (cutaneous margin with lash-bearing skin and associated glands) and those affecting the posterior lid margin (mucocutaneous junction, meibomian orifices). This classification corresponds with, and simplifies understanding of, the treatment of the different conditions, which differs between the anterior-lid and posterior-lid margin disorders but not between the individual conditions within each of these two groups. The commoner clinical signs of staphylococcal blepharitis are shown in Figure 109.7. Ocular rosacea (see Table 109.3 and Figure 109.8) is an important condition because of its severity and wide spectrum of clinical features.

In addition to these very common types of blepharitis, there are other chronic causes in which the pathogenesis is clear. These are all uncommon and are often misdiagnosed as one of the types of chronic blepharitis described in Table 109.2. They include fungal infection (e.g. *Candida*), parasitic infection (e.g. phthiriasis), protozoal infection (e.g. leishmaniasis), some neoplasms and autoimmune conditions such as lupus erythematosus; some of these are illustrated in Figure 109.9. They should be considered when therapy for conventional blepharitis fails.

Acute blepharitis is a clearly defined group of conditions, for which the causes are summarized in Table 109.4.

The epidemiology of blepharitis has been hampered by difficulties of disease definition, lack of a standardized clinical assessment and the different perspectives of dermatologists and ophthalmologists.

Incidence and prevalence
Chronic blepharitis is one of the commonest disorders in both ophthalmic and general medical practice. In general medical practice it makes up about 70% of ophthalmic referrals, which themselves account for between 2 and 7% of all outpatient consultations. MGD is the commonest cause of blepharitis and affects 20–40% of all patients consulting ophthalmologists for routine eye examinations. The reported prevalence of MGD varies widely, with a suggested higher prevalence (>60%) in Asian populations compared with a prevalence of 3.5–20% in white people; however, there is significant variation in disease definition and the age of the study groups in these studies [6]. The incidence of ocular rosacea varies among ophthalmic and dermatological studies, ranging from 6 to 72%, being more prevalent in ophthalmology clinics [8]. Between 3 and 58% of patients with rosacea have ocular involvement; this wide variation in cited frequency largely reflecting differences in disease definition. Approximately half of patients with rosacea have signs of ocular rosacea, whilst one-quarter of patients with ocular rosacea have no dermatological disease. In participants with all types of blepharitis, the prevalence of acne rosacea ranges from 26.7 to 44%, and the prevalence of seborrhoeic dermatitis 32.9% [9,10].

Age
In a case–control study conducted in San Francisco and Texas [1,11], the average age of onset of staphylococcal blepharitis was 42 years, the mean age of participants with seborrhoeic blepharitis was 50 years, and that of MGD blepharitis patients was 50 years. Rosacea may be found in early childhood as well as in the elderly, but it is most often diagnosed at age 30–50 [12].

Sex
Whilst staphylococcal blepharitis occurs more commonly in women (80%), the prevalence of seborrhoeic blepharitis, MGD and ocular rosacea is equal between men and women [1,13].

Ethnicity
Asian ethnicity has been suggested to be a risk factor for MGD [6]; however, MGD is also more common in fair-skinned individuals due to its association with acne rosacea, which is more prevalent in this population [12].

Associated diseases
See Table 109.2.

There is some evidence to support hypotheses of pathogenesis in staphylococcal blepharitis and in meibomian dysfunction, but the pathogenesis is even more poorly understood in the other types of chronic blepharitis.

PART 10: SITES, SEX, AGE

Table 109.2 Classification of types of chronic blepharitis (lid margin disorders) [1,3].

	Anterior lid margin*		Posterior lid margin*			Anterior and/or posterior lid margin
	Staphylococcal blepharitis	**Seborrhoeic blepharitis**	**Meibomitis/ocular rosacea**	**Other meibomian gland dysfunction**	**Meibomian seborrhoea**	**Other blepharitis, e.g. atopic, psoriatic, fungal, protozoal, parasitic, neoplastic, lupus**
Associations with other types of blepharitis	Secondary meibomitis; Demodex blepharitis (cylindrical dandruff or sleeves on eyelashes)	Staphylococcal blepharitis; Any posterior lid margin condition	Staphylococcal and seborrhoeic blepharitis	Seborrhoeic blepharitis	Seborrhoeic blepharitis	
Associated skin disease	Atopic eczema; Impetigo; Rosacea (rare)	Seborrhoeic dermatitis; Rosacea (rare)	Acne rosacea in up to 50% of cases	Acne rosacea in up to 50% of cases		Atopy; Psoriasis; Lupus
Associated eye disease	Dry eye; Atopic keratoconjunctivitis	Dry eye	Scleritis and episcleritis in ocular rosacea	Scleritis and episcleritis in ocular rosacea		Variable according to aetiology
Main features *Symptoms*	Burning; Itching; Photophobia	Minimal	Foreign body sensation; Burning; Discomfort; Photophobia with ocular rosacea	Variable: Foreign body sensation; Burning; Discomfort	Variable: Foreign body sensation; Burning; Discomfort	Lack of resolution with standard MGD treatment; Variable according to aetiology
Lid signs	Unilateral/patchy lid margin involvement (Figure 109.7d); Brittle fibrinous scales bleed when detached, form collarettes at lash base (Figure 109.7a); Dilated vessels, styes (external hordeolum, Figure 109.24a); Poliosis, madarosis, eyelash misdirection (Figure 109.7b); Eyelid ulceration and scarring when severe; Chalazia (Figure 109.8b,f) and internal hordeolum (infected chalazion,Figure 109.24b) may occur	Bilateral greasy scales (not fibrinous)	Chalazia (Figure 109.8b); Irregular lid margins; Distorted meibomian orifices and meibomian gland drop-out; Inspissated secretions; Expression difficult; Surrounding inflammation; For lid signs in ocular rosacea see Table 109.3	Eyelash misdirection; Foamy discharge on eyelid margin; Poor quality meibum; Expression diff cult; Meibomian gland drop out; Chalazia; Irregular scarred lid margins in longstanding disease	Plugged and elevated orifices without inflammation	Variable according to aetiology
Conjunctival and corneal signs	Follicles, papillae and hyperaemia of lower tarsal conjunctiva and fornix (Figure 109.7c); Conjunctival and corneal phlyctenules may occur; Coarse punctate keratitis in lower third of cornea. Marginal keratitis (Figure 109.7e) typically at 10, 2, 4 or 8 o'clock and corneal vascularization and thinning. Conjunctival scarring (Figure 109.8a)	Mild conjunctival injection; Coarse punctate keratitis in lower third of cornea.	Early tear break up time; Foam/debris in tears; Punctate keratitis (dry eye); For conjunctival and corneal signs in ocular rosacea see Table 109.3	Early tear break up time; Foam/debris in tears; Punctate keratitis (dry eye); For conjunctival and corneal signs in ocular rosacea see Table 109.3	Minimal injection; Foamy tear film	Variable according to aetiology

*The anterior lid margin is the portion anterior to the meibomian gland orifices and the posterior lid margin is behind this, including the meibomian glands. Anterior and posterior lid margin disorders are commonly mixed, and there is often overlap in clinical features of these categories of blepharitis; frequent associations are shown in the table.
MGD, meibomian gland disease.

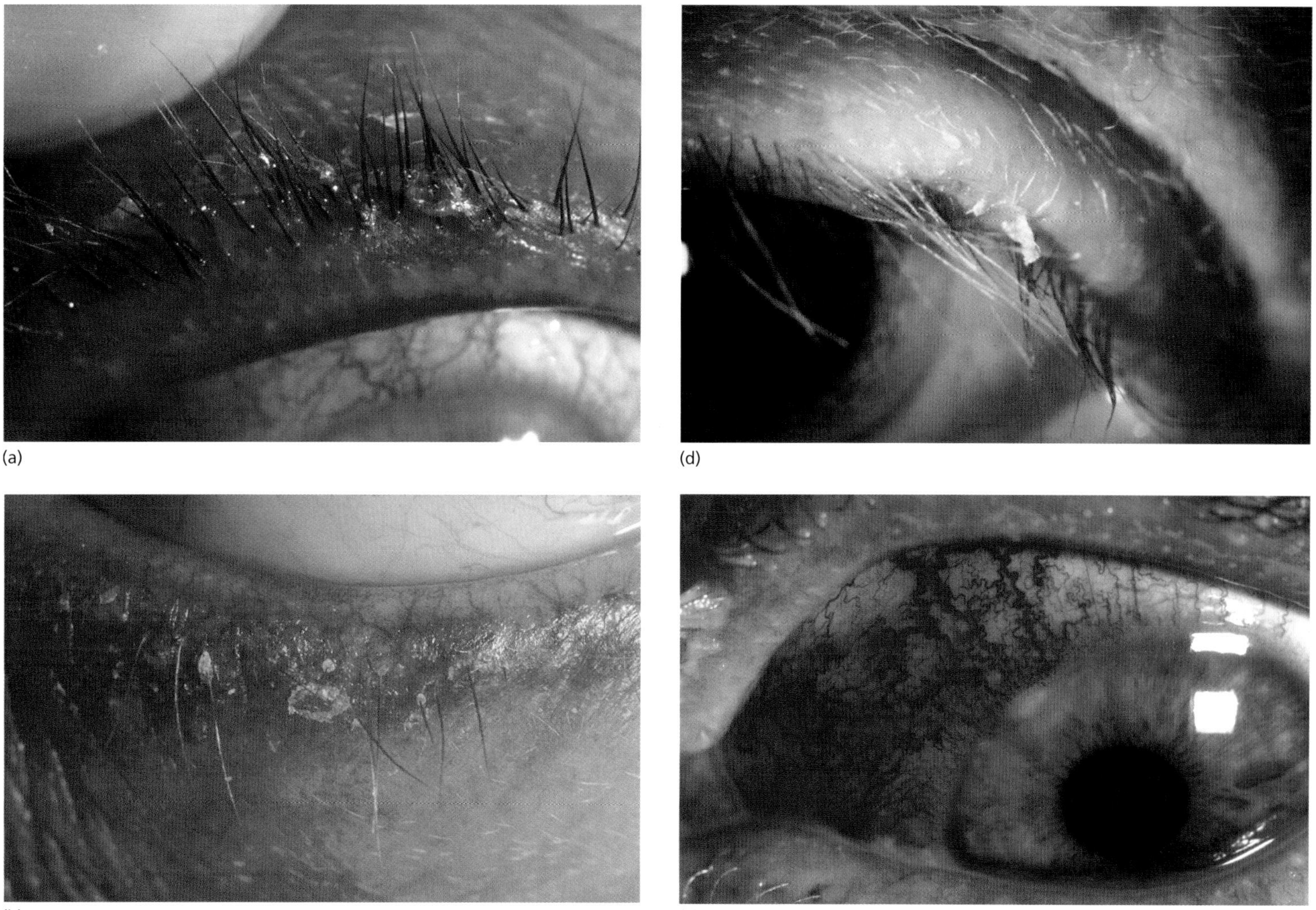

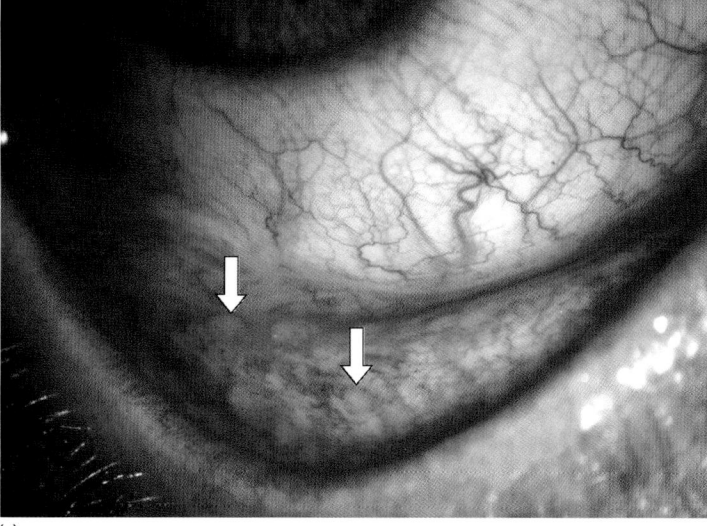

(a)

(b)

(c)

(d)

(e)

Figure 109.7 Staphylococcal blepharitis. (a) Fibrinous 'collarettes' lifting away from the skin as the lashes grow. (b) Fibrinous scales on the anterior lid margin with the madarosis (loss of lashes) and poliosis (white lashes) that accompanies chronic blepharitis. (c) Follicular conjunctivitis with arrows showing the white/yellow follicles. (d) Localized ulcerative blepharitis. Sectoral disease like this is quite common in staphylococcal blepharitis which can also be largely unilateral. (e) Marginal keratitis with ulceration, a common corneal complication of staphylococcal blepharitis. (Courtesy of Mr J. Dart, Moorfields Eye Hospital, London, UK.)

PART 10: SITES, SEX, AGE

Predisposing factors

Ophthalmic factors associated with MGD include contact lens wear, *Demodex folliculorum* and dry eye disease. Systemic factors that may promote MGD include, among others, androgen deficiency, menopause, ageing, Sjögren syndrome, hypercholesterol-aemia, psoriasis, atopy, rosacea, hypertension and benign prostatic hyperplasia (BPH). Medications associated with the pathogenesis of MGD include antiandrogens, medications used to treat BPH, postmenopausal hormone therapy (e.g. oestrogens and progestins), antihistamines, antidepressants and retinoids [6].

PART 10: SITES, SEX, AGE

Table 109.3 Clinical signs of ocular rosacea.

Signs	Common	Uncommon	Rare
Lid	Meibomitis (Figure 109.8a)	Entropion	
	Seborrhoeic blepharitis		
	Lid margin telangiectasia		
	Lid notching		
	Retroplacement of the mucocutaneous junction		
	Chalazia (Figure 109.8b,f)		
	Hordeoleum		
Conjunctiva	Conjunctival hyperaemia	Reticular and linear tarsal scarring and fornix shortening (Figure 109.8a)	
	Papillary conjunctivitis		
Cornea	Phlyctenular keratoconjunctivitis	Pseudopterygium (Figure 109.8d)	Corneal perforation
	Marginal corneal infiltration and ulceration (Figure 109.8d,e)		
Sclera and episclera		Episcleritis	Scleritis

Pathology

Staphylococcal blepharitis

In staphylococcal blepharitis there is an association with *Staphylococcus aureus* and *S. epidermidis* colonization of the lid margins, although colonization by *S. aureus* is often transient and the numbers of either organism are often no greater than in normal controls [14] (see also Chapter 26). Although folliculitis, styes and lid margin ulcers may be due to infection by *S. aureus*, the persistence of lid inflammation after treatment and the sterile marginal ulcers are not explained by infection alone. The importance of cell-mediated immunity in the pathogenesis of the disease was shown by experimental studies in rabbits; when these were immunized with either whole *S. aureus* or with cell wall ribitol teichoic acid, both ulcerative keratitis, phlyctenules and marginal corneal ulcers developed after secondary challenge, providing evidence for the hypothesis that these changes were due to the development of hypersensitivity to both viable and killed organisms [15,16]. These findings could not be reproduced for *S. epidermidis*. However, evidence for a similar pathogenesis in humans is lacking; the relationship between the clinical signs of staphylococcal blepharitis and hypersensitivity to subcutaneous injections of either whole *S. aureus* or of *S. aureus* cell wall protein A is poor. *Staphylococcus epidermidis* is more often isolated than *S. aureus* from the lids of patients with staphylococcal blepharitis, but the role of a hypersensitivity response is assumed and not supported by any firm data [17]. The pathogenesis of the, often severe, follicular and papillary conjunctivitis that accompanies this condition is assumed to be due to a combination of transient infection and hypersensitivity. Some researchers have hypothesized that toxins produced by the bacteria may cause irritation, but no specific toxin has been identified [18,19].

Demodex folliculorum are small parasitic mites that live in hair follicles, sebaceous glands and meibomian glands. They are found in 30% of chronic blepharitis patients, but are also found with nearly the same prevalence in patients without blepharitis [20]. They may have a role in both anterior and posterior blepharitis. It is theorized that the infestation and wastage of mites cause blockage of the follicles and glands and/or an inflammatory response. Patients with recalcitrant blepharitis have responded to therapy directed at eradicating *Demodex* mite, studies support its role in activation of immune mechanisms in subtypes of rosacea, e.g. papulopustular rosacea [21], and one study has found a correlation between serum immunoreactivity, ocular *Demodex* infestation, lid margin inflammation and facial rosacea [22].

Meibomian gland disease

The meibomian lipids (meibum) are a complex mixture of cholesterol esters and esterified unsaturated fatty acids. These lipids are responsible for maintaining a stable tear film, reducing tear film evaporation (and, therefore, preventing drying of the ocular surface) [23], preventing tear spill over the lid margins by lowering surface tension and reducing ocular surface contamination by sebum from the cutaneous surface of the lids, which otherwise forms dry spots. Three factors have been invoked as contributing to MGD: (i) keratinization of the meibomian ductules; (ii) the effect of bacterial lipases on the meibum at the lid margin; and (iii) primary abnormalities in the production of meibum by individuals with MGD [24].

Normal meibomian gland ducts open just anterior to the mucocutaneous junction. As the duct lining is partially keratinized, abnormalities of keratinization, analogous to those present in the sebaceous glands of patients with rosacea, may be important in the pathogenesis of MGD by altering gland function. Bacterial lipases are produced by all the bacteria that colonize the lid margin and have the potential to break down meibum into free fatty acids, which will destabilize the tear film [25]. These bacteria colonize the gland orifices and expression of lipid from deeper within the glands can stabilize the tear film. Meibomian lipids differ between individuals and, as analytical methods increase in sensitivity, the relative roles of primary abnormalities of meibum and those secondary to the effects of bacterial lipases in the pathogenesis of MGD are likely to become clearer [26]. Neither the pathogenesis of the conjunctival inflammation that is common in meibomitis (and which is a feature of ocular rosacea), nor that of the keratitis in ocular rosacea, has been explained.

Ocular rosacea

The precise aetiology and pathophysiology of ocular rosacea remains unknown, although different theories have been proposed [27] (see also Chapter 91). Recent molecular studies propose that abnormal recognition of common environmental stimuli leads to activation of pro-inflammatory systems as well as innate immune responses. Factors that trigger the innate immune system lead to increased expression of certain cytokines and antimicrobial molecules such as cathelicidin, which is vasoactive and pro-inflammatory [28]. Overreaction to environmental stimuli is believed in part to be due to elevated expression of toll-like receptor 2 in the epidermis of rosacea patients, which leads to increased serine protease and cathelicidin production. Furthermore, tetracyclines, which improve the signs and

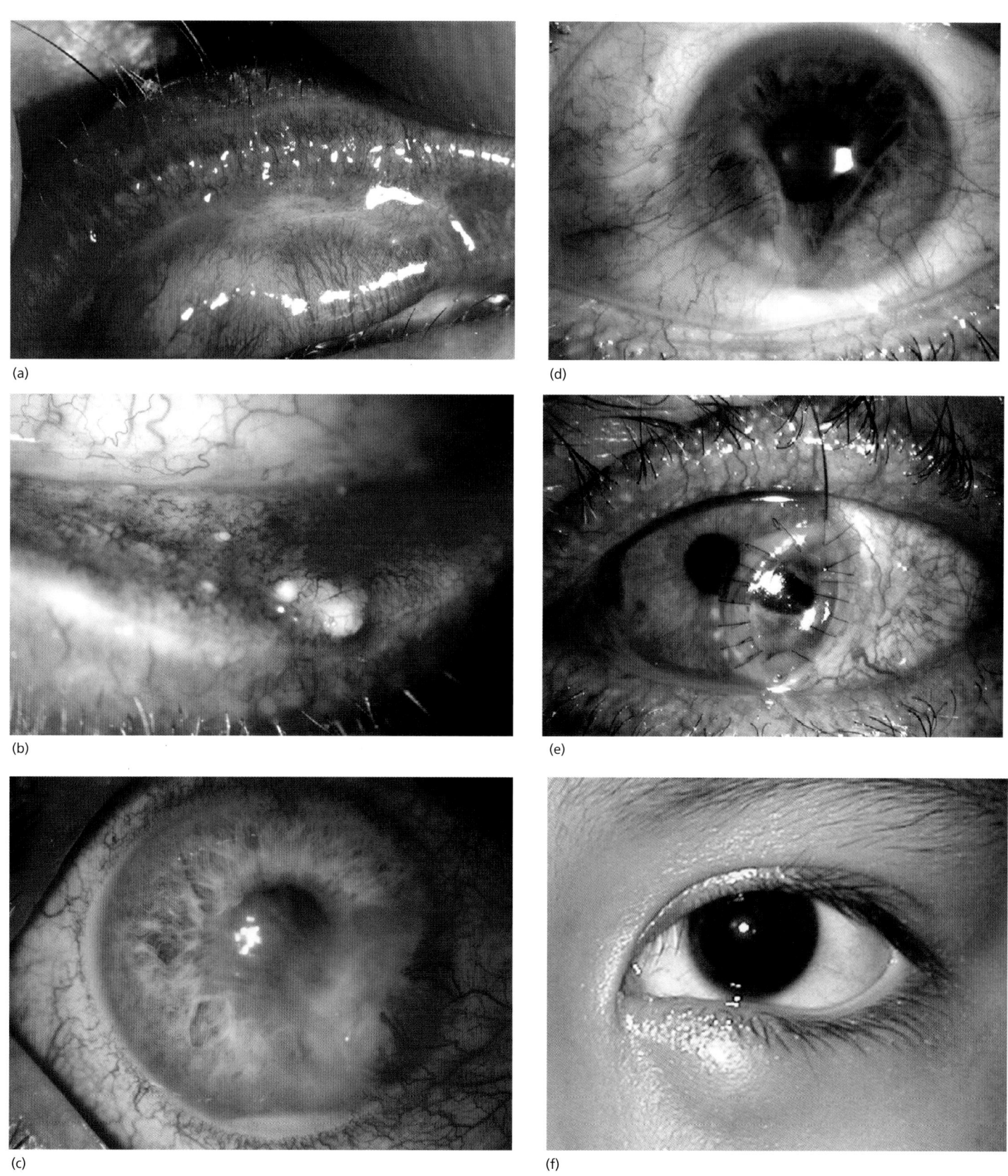

(a)

(b)

(c)

(d)

(e)

(f)

Figure 109.8 Ocular rosacea. (a) Scales on the anterior lid margin, meibomitis with posterior migration of the orifices associated with loss of the normal posterior lid margin architecture and scarring in the superior tarsal marginal sulcus. Entropion and trichiasis may result from this degree of scarring. (b) Meibomian dysfunction with blocked glands and small chalazia. (c) Marginal ulceration complicated by frank bacterial superinfection with an hypopyon ulcer. (d) Severe marginal ulcers with pseudopterygia. (e) Corneal transplant following perforation of a marginal ulcer; also shows meibomitis. (Courtesy of Mr J, Dart, Moorfields Eye Hospital, London, UK.) (f) Chalazion (meibomian gland cyst).

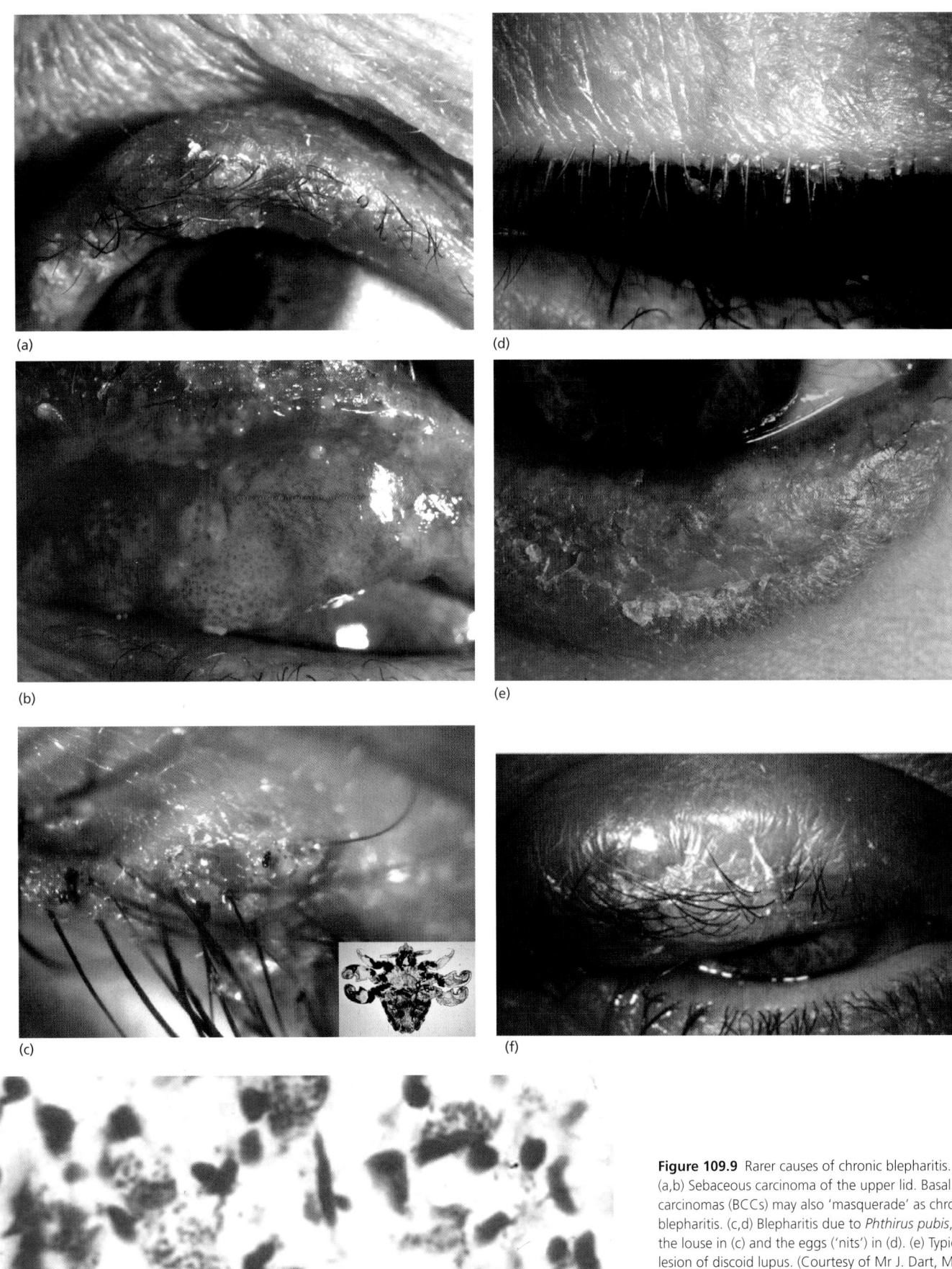

Figure 109.9 Rarer causes of chronic blepharitis. (a,b) Sebaceous carcinoma of the upper lid. Basal cell carcinomas (BCCs) may also 'masquerade' as chronic blepharitis. (c,d) Blepharitis due to *Phthirus pubis*, showing the louse in (c) and the eggs ('nits') in (d). (e) Typical lid lesion of discoid lupus. (Courtesy of Mr J. Dart, Moorfields Eye Hospital, London, UK.) (f) Cutaneous *Leishmania* infection of the upper eyelid. Diagnosis is by biopsy. (g) Histopathology of numerous *Leishmania* organisms distending histiocytes, giving a diagnostic morphology.

Table 109.4 Causes of acute blepharitis.

Acute anterior lid margin	Folliculitis (infected lash follicles)
	External hordeoleum (stye) (Figure 109.24a)
	Angular (at lateral canthus)
	Impetigo
	Pustular (herpes infections) (Figure 109.22a)
Acute posterior lid margin	Chalazion (Figure 109.8b,f)
	Internal hordeoleum (Figure 109.24b)
Generalized anterior and posterior	Necrotizing fasciitis

symptoms of rosacea, inhibit expression and activity of several matrix metalloproteinases, as well as a class of proteases that activate cathelicidin, thus supporting this theory.

Causative organisms

Staphylococcal blepharitis is believed to be associated with staphylococcal bacteria on the ocular surface, but there are likely to be additional contibuting factors, given that in some studies there is no difference in positive culture levels between controls and blepharitis patients.

Demodex mites have also been considered a causative factor in blepharitis and papulopustular rosacea. Another proposed mechanism is that *Demodex* mites may act as vectors for other organisms such as *Bacillus olenorius*, which may be responsible for initiating the inflammatory response via stimulation of toll-like receptor 2 and production of antigenic proteins [22].

Environmental factors

It has been postulated that staphylococcal blepharitis occurs more commonly in warmer climates, whilst MGD may be more common in cooler climates [29].

Clinical features

History
See Table 109.2.

Presentation
See Tables 109.2 and 109.3.

Clinical variants
See Tables 109.2 and 109.3.

Differential diagnosis
See Table 109.5.

Classification of severity
A severity grading for MGD, which can be used to guide treatment, has been described [30].

Complications and co-morbidities
See Tables 109.2 and 109.3.

In severe and longstanding staphylococcal blepharitis, trichiasis (misdirection of eyelashes towards the eye), poliosis (depigmentation of the eyelashes), madarosis (loss of eyelashes), eyelid ulceration, and eyelid and corneal scarring may occur [3].

Table 109.5 Differential diagnosis of blepharitis: other conditions associated with eyelid inflammation [3].

Condition	Entity
Bacterial infections	• Impetigo (due primarily to *Staphylococcus aureus*)
	• Erysipelas (due primarily to *Streptococcus pyogenes*)
Viral infections	• Herpes simplex virus
	• Molluscum contagiosum
	• Varicella zoster virus
	• Papillomavirus
	• Vaccinia
Parasitic infection	• Pediculosis palpebrarum (*Phthirus pubis*)
Immunological conditions	• Atopic eczema
	• Contact dermatitis
	• Erythema multiforme
	• Pemphigus foliaceus
	• Ocular mucous membrane pemphigoid
	• Stevens–Johnson syndrome
	• Connective tissue disorders
	• Discoid lupus
	• Dermatomyositis
	• Graft-versus-host disease
	• Crohn disease
Dermatoses	• Psoriasis
	• Ichthyosis
	• Exfoliative dermatitis
	• Erythroderma
Benign eyelid tumours	• Pseudoepitheliomatous hyperplasia
	• Actinic keratosis
	• Squamous cell papilloma
	• Sebaceous gland hyperplasia
	• Haemangioma
	• Pyogenic granuloma
Malignant eyelid tumours	• Basal cell carcinoma
	• Squamous cell carcinoma
	• Sebaceous carcinoma
	• Melanoma
	• Kaposi sarcoma
	• Mycosis fungoides
Trauma	• Chemical
	• Thermal
	• Radiation
	• Mechanical
	• Surgical
Toxic conditions	• Medicamentosa

Blepharitis due to MGD can be complicated by:
1 Ocular surface damage with conjunctival and corneal involvement, including meibomian keratoconjunctivitis and phlyctenular keratitis [31,32].
2 Evaporative dry eye [32]; and/or
3 Other ocular disorders including contact lens intolerance and recurrent corneal erosion syndrome [33].

Disease course and prognosis
The natural history of MGD is not precisely known, but it is regarded as a progressive but treatable disease, in which therapy may prevent irreversible damage [32]. Therapy to prevent progression is most important when the sight threatening complications of ocular rosacea and severe staphylococcal blepharitis including corneal

PART 10: SITES, SEX, AGE

PART 10: SITES, SEX, AGE

vascularization, corneal thinning, perforation, pseudopterygium and corneal phlyctenules are first detected. One of the most important aspects of caring for patients with blepharitis is educating them about the chronicity and recurrence of the disease process, and the likelihood that their symptoms can be improved but are rarely eliminated [3].

Investigations

There are no specific diagnostic tests for blepharitis, which depends on recognition of typical clinical signs and symptoms for diagnosis. However, cultures of the eyelid margins may be indicated for recurrent anterior blepharitis with severe inflammation, and for patients not responding to therapy. Microscopic examination of epilated lashes may reveal *Demodex* mites. A biopsy of the eyelid to exclude carcinoma should be considered in blepharitis unresponsive to therapy, especially if it is very asymmetrical, or unifocal recurrent chalazia which do not respond well to therapy. Consultation with the pathologist prior to taking biopsies for suspected sebaceous gland carcinoma is recommended, to discuss whether frozen sections and mapping is needed to search for pagetoid spread.

Meibomian gland disease may be diagnosed in isolation, or more commonly in association with dry eye or ocular surface damage. A proposed sequence of tests to perform in a general clinic, to first diagnose generic dry eye, and then to differentiate between MGD-related evaporative dry eye versus aqueous deficient dry eye include [32]:

1 Administration of a validated symptom questionnaire such as OSDI (Ocular Surface Disease Index).
2 Measurement of blink rate and blink interval.
3 Measurement of lower tear meniscus height.
4 Measurement of tear osmolarity (if available).
5 Instillation of fluorescein into the eye and measurement of tear film break up time (TBUT).
6 Grading of severity of fluorescein staining of the cornea and conjunctiva.
7 Schirmer test (or phenol red thread test).
8 Characterization of MGD by:
   • Quantification of morphological features.
   • Quantification of meibum expressibility/quality.
   • Quantification of meibomian gland dropout by meibography.

If testing suggests the diagnosis of a generic dry eye and tests of tear flow and volume (including tear meniscus height, Schirmer test) are normal, then evaporative dry eye is implied, and quantification of MGD will indicate the meibomian gland's contribution. This test sequence also allows a diagnosis of MGD, with or without ocular surface staining or dry eye, to be made. The grading scores for each test can be used to monitor the disease during treatment.

Management

The treatment of blepharitis is that of the underlying cause, if a specific cause can be identified. The blepharitis should initially be classified into either anterior or posterior lid disease or both (see Table 109.2). It is important to decide whether blepharitis is the cause of the symptoms; seborrhoea rarely causes symptoms and should not be used as a scapegoat to explain away symptoms possibly due to other, or undiagnosable, conditions. Other conditions that give rise to similar symptoms and signs (see Table 109.2) should be excluded or treated. Symptoms of dry eye, and associated skin disorders, should also be treated (Table 109.6).

Table 109.6 Treatment of chronic blepharitis.

Aims of treatment	Therapeutic guidelines
For anterior lid margin disease	
Treat infection	Staphylococcal and mixed staphylococcal/seborrhoeic groups
	Topical antibiotics (chloramphenicol or fucidic acid) 4 times daily to lid margins
	Oral oxytetracycline or erythromycin 500 mg twice daily for 10 days
	Tea tree oil lid scrubs for recalcitrant blepharitis due to *Demodex*
Clean lid margins	'Lid scrubs': 1–2 times daily with cotton wool bud dampened in boiled water or with proprietary lid cleaning pads, to remove debris
Lid hyperaemia and exudate	Topical chloramphenicol and hydrocortisone 0.5–1.0% to lid margins 2–4 times daily for 1 month
For posterior lid margin disease	
Mechanically unblock meibomian glands	Apply hot compresses for 3–5 min to liquefy meibomian secretions, followed by massage* of tarsal plate with cotton wool bud (or finger), to express lipid from glands, 1–2 times daily
Alter meibomian secretions	Oral tetracycline (e.g. doxycycline 100 mg once daily or lymecycline 300 mg daily) or erythromycin 250–500 mg twice daily for 12 weeks minimum
For the tear film	
Restore tear film	Artificial tears drops 2–4 hourly, or Viscotears 3–4 times daily
For associated conjunctivitis (papillary or mixed follicular and papillary)	
Reduce inflammation	Fluorometholone 0.1% four times daily for 1 week, progressively reducing to one time daily over a further 4 weeks
Treat associated skin disease	Seborrhoea – medicated soap and shampoo (ideally containing glycolic acid 10–15%)
	Rosacea – oral oxytetracycline (or doxycycline 100 mg) or erythromycin 250–500 mg twice daily for 12 weeks
For keratitis	
Coarse punctate keratitis and/or marginal keratoconjunctivitis and/or phlyctenules	Fluorometholone 0.1% four times daily for 1 week, progressively reducing to once daily over a further 4 weeks[†]
Corneal thinning and perforation	Exclude and treat any concomitant microbial keratitis and establish disease control by methods summarized above, apply tissue glue to perforations. Consider systemic immunosuppression (e.g. mycophenolate or azathioprine). Carry out tectonic corneal graft, if necessary, once the inflammation is controlled

*Lid scrubs, lid massage and low-dose systemic antibiotics take about 4–6 weeks to start to work. DO NOT assume treatment has failed until at least 8 weeks on treatment has elapsed, and continue the regime for a minimum of 2–3 months if benefit is shown. Then advise a maintenance regime of lid scrubs (for anterior lid margin disease), hot compresses and tarsal massage (for posterior lid margin disease), ± artificial tears. In the case of relapse, repeat a 3-month course of oral antibiotic treatment.

[†]More prolonged courses of corticosteroid or more potent corticosteroids may be needed under specialist ophthalmological supervision. Topical ciclosporin has recently been shown to be effective for controlling inflammation in posterior blepharitis in one randomized trial and another case series [24,25]. The author's experience with topical ciclosporin in ocular rosacea has been promising.

Diffuse folliculitis is generally caused by *S. aureus* and requires a course of an appropriate systemic antibiotic. Laboratory investigations are of limited value – bacteriology samples can be taken from lid margins using swabs dipped in trypsin digest broth, but are usually only performed for recurrent disease that has not responded to initial therapy.

Chalazion will resolve in time; approximately 60% of lesions will resolve in 6 months and the remainder will resolve spontaneously, given longer. Resolution of chalazia can be hastened by incision and curettage; the lid is incised, usually from the conjunctival surface, under local anaesthesia, and the necrotic granulomatous tissue in the centre of the lesion removed with a curette. This leaves a linear conjunctival and tarsal scar. It is only recommended for cosmetic reasons or to improve vision in large lesions affecting the upper lid, which can cause temporary astigmatism.

Practice points for dermatologists are that the association between blepharitis and skin disease is variable, that treatment with tetracyclines may be beneficial for both the ocular and dermatological manifestations of these disorders, and that ocular rosacea and staphylococcal blepharitis may produce sight-threatening complications.

First line (Figure 109.10) [30]

Inform patient about MGD, the potential impact of diet and environment on tear evaporation. Advise patient on improving ambient humidity, increasing dietary omega-3 fatty acid intake. Institute eyelid hygiene with eyelid warming (once or twice daily) followed by moderate to firm massage and expression of MG secretions.

Second line

First line management plus: artificial lubricants (for frequent use, non-preserved preferred). Consider topical azithromycin, topical emollient lubricant or liposomal lubricant.

Third line

Oral tetracyclines, lubricant ointment at bedtime, consider anti-inflammatory therapy (topical steroids, topical ciclosporin [34–36]) as indicated.

Atopy and atopic eye disease

Definition

The atopic eye diseases comprise a group of disorders that have in common a papillary conjunctivitis and evidence of a type I allergic mechanism (see also Chapter 41). They include the milder conditions of seasonal allergic conjunctivitis (SAC) and perennial allergic conjunctivitis (PAC) and the more severe atopic keratoconjunctivitis (AKC), atopic blepharoconjunctivitis (ABC) and vernal keratoconjunctivitis (VKC).

Introduction and general description

The atopic eye diseases all involve immunoglobulin E (IgE) mediated hypersensitivity responses although each disease has specific immunogenic pathways. Ocular involvement in atopic patients ranges from 15 to 40% but is generally mild with features of SAC or PAC. Only a very small proportion of patients with atopic eczema have significant ocular disease. Table 109.8 summarizes these disorders. Of these, only AKC and VKC can involve the cornea and threaten sight. They are often difficult to treat. The severity of symptoms is closely related to disease activity. Patients with minimal symptoms respond to simple topical measures and safe treatment with antihistamines and mast cell stabilizers. At the opposite extreme, acute exacerbations of AKC and VKC must be recognized and treated promptly as these may develop within hours and lead to blinding corneal complications within 1–2 days. ABC runs a similar course to AKC but has no corneal involvement and although infection with *Staphylococcus aureus* can be a significant complication the disease in itself is not a potentially blinding condition.

Epidemiology [1]

Incidence and prevalence

The incidence of allergic conditions has increased significantly over the past 40 years. It has been estimated that between 15 and 40% of atopic patients have some ocular involvement though this is usually mild. SAC is the commonest form of atopic eye disease (90%) followed by PAC (5%). The remaining 5% is accounted for by AKC, ABC and VKC.

Age

Seasonal allergic conjunctivitis and PAC can occur in any age group. AKC and ABC begin in the late teens or early twenties and persist often until the fifth decade of life. VKC occurs mainly in children and 90% resolve by adult life.

Sex

These diseases affect the sexes equally with the exception of VKC which is more common in boys than girls before puberty.

Ethnicity

These conditions affect all ethnic groups though VKC is more common in patients of African and Asian origin.

Associated diseases

Atopic keratoconjunctivitis is associated with a predisposition to staphylococcal lid and eye infections, and also herpes simplex lid and eye infections, such that bilateral herpetic eye disease is more frequently observed (usually herpetic eye disease is a unilateral condition). It is thought that susceptibility to these infections is related to impaired T-cell immunity in AKC patients.

Pathophysiology [1–5]

Predisposing factors

A personal or family history of atopy

Pathology

Recent advances in our understanding of the atopic eye diseases have come from investigation of the humoral mediators

PART 10: SITES, SEX, AGE

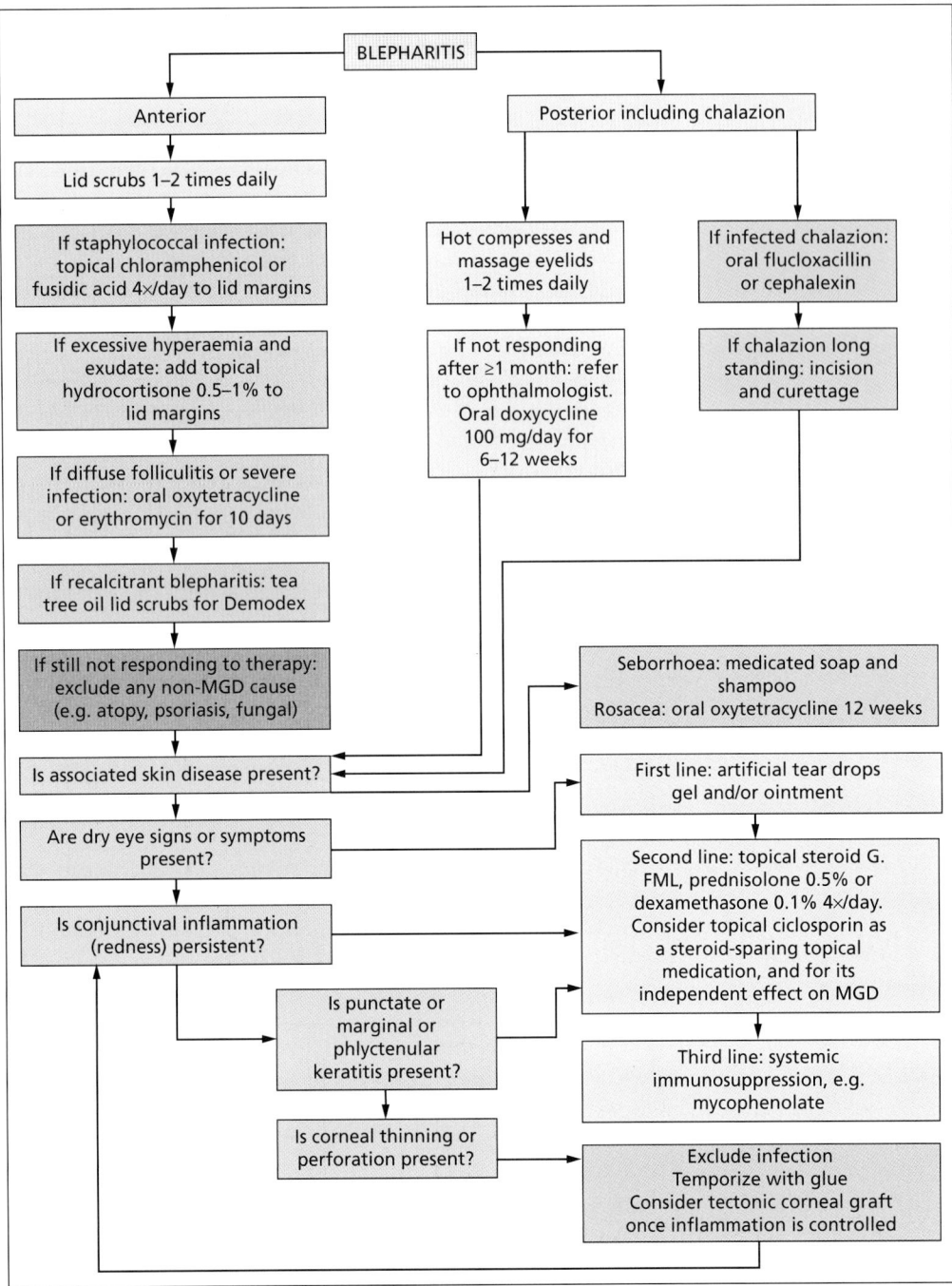

Figure 109.10 Management algorithm for Blepharitis. MGD, meibomian gland dysfunction; FML, fluoromethalone.

of inflammation in the tears and analysis of the cellular components by immunostaining and *in situ* hybridization of conjunctival biopsies. These techniques have shown that SAC and PAC are primarily type I IgE-mediated hypersensitivity responses whereas the others show varying degrees of a coexisting type IV hypersensitivity response and also involve the production of cytokines by various effector cells.

Seasonal allergic conjunctivitis and PAC show mast cells and eosinophils in the conjunctival mucosa and submucosa with high levels of locally produced IgE to specific allergens being present in the tears. Symptoms are due to release of histamine and other

inflammatory agents by mast cells which lead to dilatated blood vessels, irritated nerve endings and increased secretion of tears. The diseases can be mimicked by topical instillation of allergens and is blocked by drugs that are active against mast cells.

The pathogenesis of AKC and VKC involves both IgE-mediated type I and non-IgE-mediated type IV hypersensitivity responses, with the production of various cytokines by effector cells. These lead to the more severe inflammatory changes that cause corneal damage. AKC and VKC show the cellular components present in SAC and PAC but also increased fibroblast activity with connective tissue hyperplasia, CD4+ lymphocytes and plasma cells together with different subsets of mast cells. The T cells are probably important inducers of the cellular inflammatory response in these diseases. Differences in AKC and VKC phenotypes may be explained by differences in the predominance of T-helper subsets; the Th1 subset involved in delayed hypersensitivity responses and inactivated by ciclosporin is more predominant in AKC than VKC in which the Th2 subset predominate with a B-cell helper role. Mast cells and eosinophils are found in larger numbers in VKC than AKC and functional heterogeneity in their populations may also be determinants of disease phenotypes. Eosinophils play a central role in atopic eye diseases and it appears that the level of eosinophil activation rather than the absolute numbers is relevant to the development of corneal disease. Eosinophils elaborate a host of cytokines and release cationic proteins including major basic protein which is epitheliotoxic and has been identified in the tears of VKC. It is probably a major factor responsible for the development of corneal epithelial erosions and macroerosions. The presence of the latter, with the mucous and debris present in acute exacerbations of keratopathy, accounts for the formation of plaque. Basophils have also been found to contribute to the atopic eye diseases through IgE-induced release of chemical mediators.

Environmental factors

These are most relevant in SAC and PAC where airborne allergens play a causal role. Symptoms for many patients are worse when the weather is warm and dry.

Clinical features [1–12]

History

From the dermatologist's perspective these patients will be under their care primarily for the management of atopic eczema and develop or have developed ocular symptoms. The dermatologist needs to be aware that any sudden deterioration of vision may herald one of the blinding complications of these diseases and should be treated as an emergency.

Presentation

The initial symptoms are similar for all the atopic eye diseases. Patients complain of itching, watering and the production of a sticky white mucous discharge. In the more severe variants of AKC, ABC and VKC exacerbations lead to rapid deterioration in symptoms. The itching may be superseded by extreme discomfort with soreness with a foreign body sensation and vision deteriorates. The lids may be difficult to open in the morning because of a combination of discomfort and discharge.

Clinical variants

SAC is the commonest form of atopic eye disease often presenting with other features of hayfever – nasal and pharyngeal symptoms. The onset of symptoms is seasonally related to specific circulating aeroallergens most commonly grass and tree pollens. Ocular involvement is usually bilateral. The conjunctival surfaces are mildly injected and oedematous, lid oedema and papillary inflammation along tarsal conjunctival surfaces (Figure 109.11) are features. PAC is a variant of SAC that persists

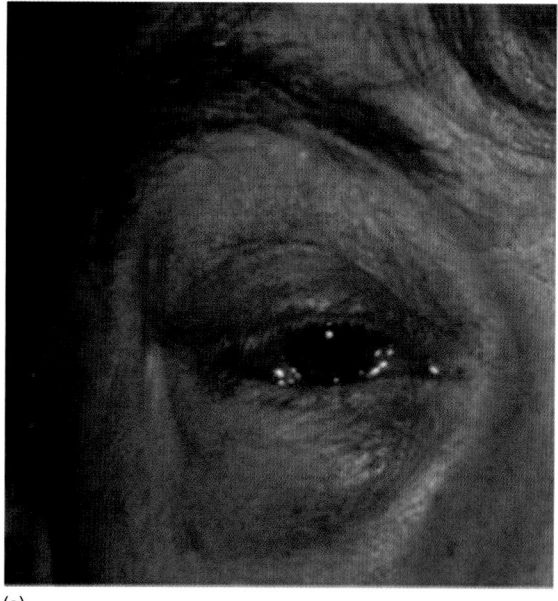

(a)

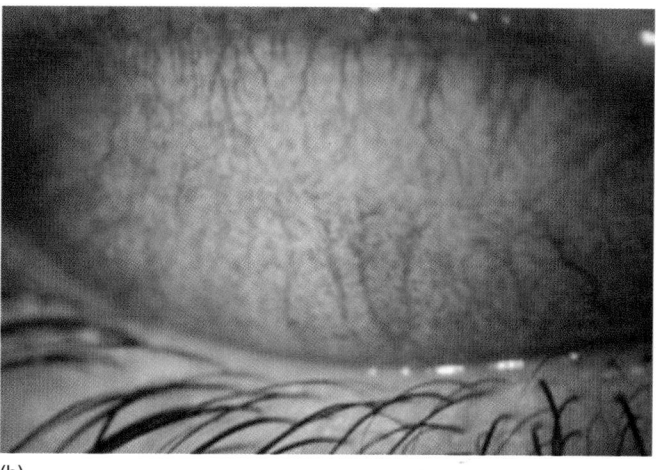

(b)

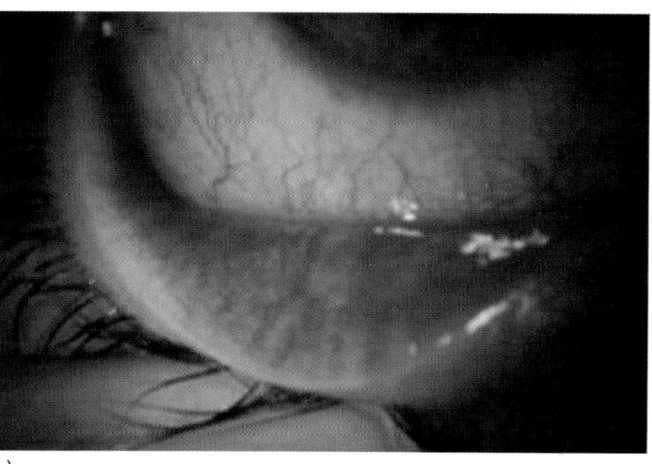

(c)

Figure 109.11 Seasonal and perennial allergic conjunctivitis (SAC and PAC) (a) Eyelid oedema and redness (b) Upper tarsal papillary inflammation (c) Lower tarsal papillary inflammation.

PART 10: SITES, SEX, AGE

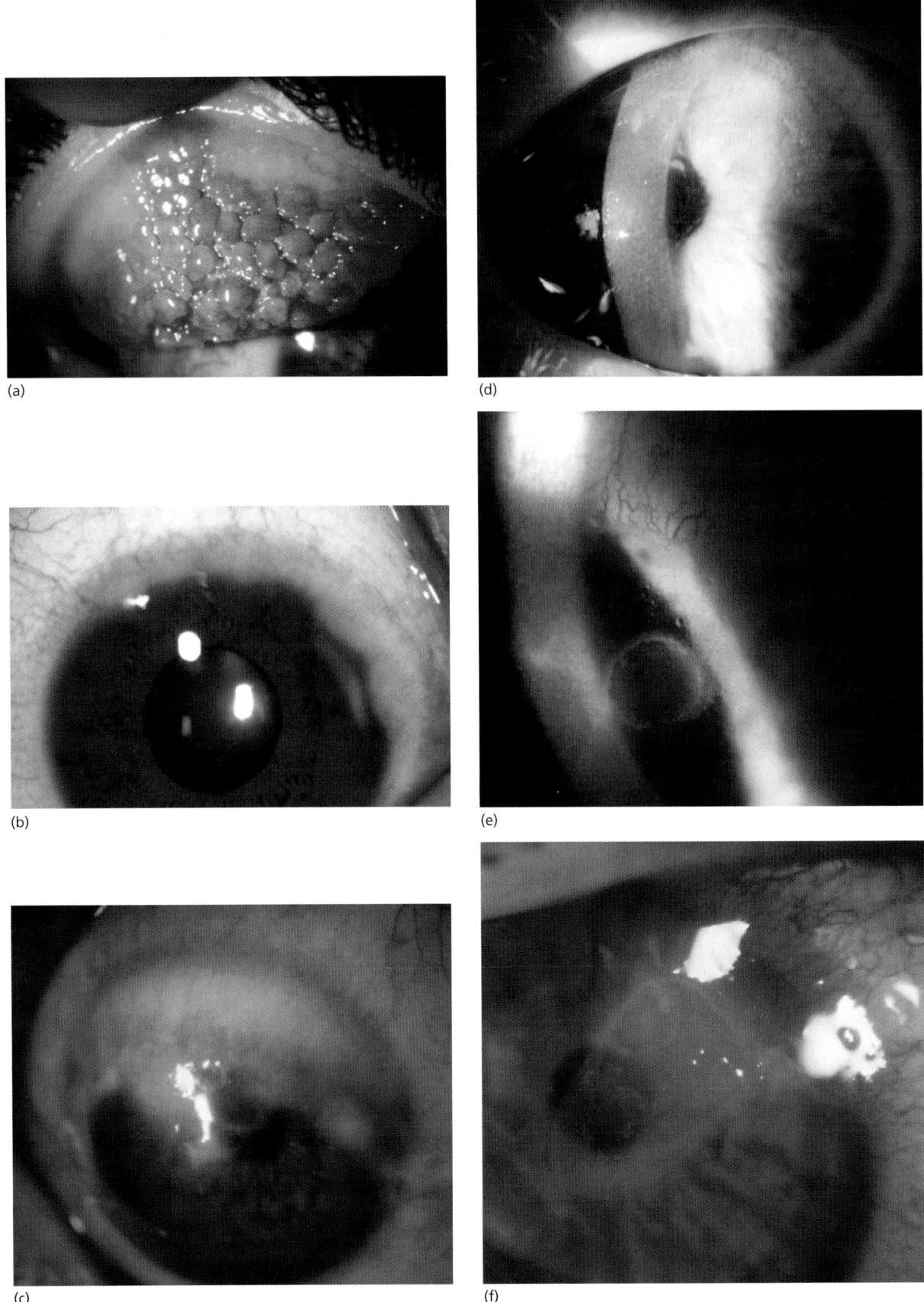

Figure 109.12 Vernal keratoconjunctivitis (VKC). (a) 'Giant' upper tarsal cobblestone papillae with mucous exudate in palpebral VKC. (b) Typical pale limbal papillae (Trantas dots) in limbal VKC. (c) Sclerosing variant of VKC. (d) Punctate keratopathy in VKC, predominantly affecting the upper half of the cornea. (e) Macroerosion. (f) Shield ulcer. (g) Fully developed vernal plaque. (h) Ring scar showing site of previous vernal plaque. (*Continued*)

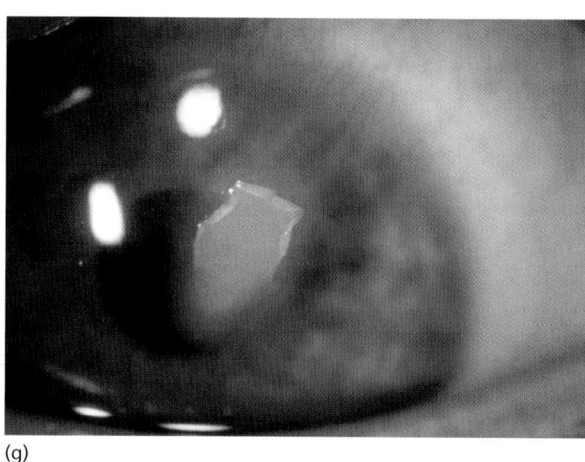

(g)

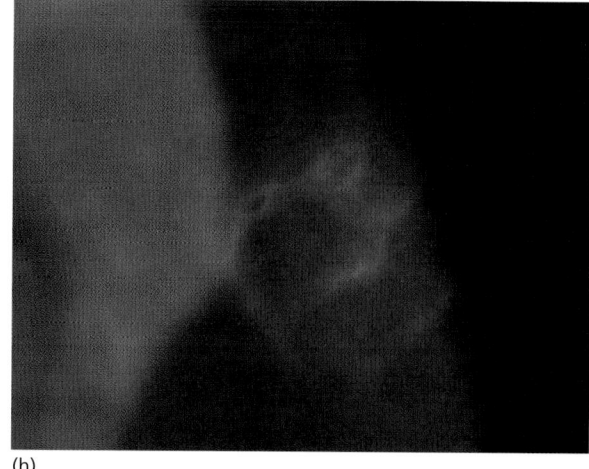

(h)

Figure 109.12 (*Continued*)

throughout the year though 80% of patients have seasonal exacerbations. Dust mites, animal dander and feathers are the most common allergic associations. SAC and PAC are mild and never affect the cornea. They are reversible upon removal of the causal allergen.

VKC is a severe chronic ocular inflammatory process affecting children, which typically manifests as cobblestone papillae in the upper tarsal conjunctiva (Figure 109.12a). The condition presents in children aged 5–15 years old who often have a history of seasonal allergy, asthma and eczema. Presenting symptoms include intense pruritus, eye watering and redness with mucus production. There is a marked seasonal incidence with the most frequent onset in spring. In VKC, involvement of one eye may be minimal when the other is severely affected. Lid margin signs are uncommon in VKC though an extra lower eyelid crease from oedema may be present (Dennie line). The lower tarsal conjunctiva is usually less involved than the upper lid, which can be seen to be thickened and velvety with papillary inflammation when the lid is everted. Persistent forms of VKC are associated with subepithelial fibrosis that appears as a white linear scar running parallel to the lid margin (Arlt line). Progressive fibrosis gives rise to giant upper tarsal papillae known as cobblestone papillae. This occurs more commonly in VKC than in AKC.

By definition, VKC affects children, not adults. The natural history of VKC is that it spontaneously resolves in 95% of children after 10 years. Children with VKC who continue to suffer actively inflamed atopic eye disease in adulthood, have disease which is then termed AKC. In burned out quiescent VKC there may be sheet-like scarring of the upper conjunctiva as evidence of previous fibrotic-inflammatory episodes. There are two clinical patterns of VKC: limbal and palpebral, depending on which part of the conjunctiva is mainly involved. Limbal VKC manifests with gelatinous macropapillae at the limbus (Trantas dots) (Figure 109.12b) and micropapillae on the upper tarsus. Palpebral VKC manifests with giant upper tarsal papillae (Figure 109.12a). Mixed forms show both limbal and palpebral disease. During exacerbations of VKC, the tarsal conjunctiva becomes very red and inflamed and covered with adherent mucous. In severe cases keratitis develops, most often in the upper cornea due to contact with cytokines released from the upper tarsal papillae, initially manifesting as punctate epitheliopathy (Figure 109.13d) and progressing to macroerosion (Figure 109.13e), shield ulcer (Figure 109.13f) and then a vernal plaque (Figure 109.12g). This results in severe discomfort to the patient with photophobia, tearing, pain and deterioration of vision. Central corneal scars may develop (Figure 109.12h). VKC will threaten sight if it involves the cornea. A sclerosing variant of VKC has been observed, where the limbus is sclerosed and vascularized (Figure 109.12c), most likely a long-term fibrotic sequel of limbal VKC. In the majority of cases, VKC burns out by the age of 30 (<10 years after onset).

Atopic keratoconjunctivitis affects patients in their early twenties to fifties. AKC usually presents with itching, burning and tearing which is more severe than with SAC and PAC. The disease is usually bilateral and symmetrical. AKC can recur at any time during the course of the associated atopic disease and is independent of its degree of severity. Patients with AKC may have prolonged exacerbations of the disease that are difficult to control which are associated with redness, severe photophobia, pain and blurring of vision. Examination of patients with AKC shows severe eczema affecting the eyelids and periorbital skin often extending onto the cheeks. The associated blepharoconjunctivitis gives rise to thickened and inflamed lid margins (Figure 109.13e). Excessive tearing can result in maceration of the eyelid skin and secondary staphylococcal infection. AKC patients have an increased susceptibility to staphylococcal infections as well as herpes simplex infections, which can involve the cornea (Figure 109.13d) and eyelid. The cornea infections are sight threatening, sometimes bilaterally, which is uncommon in non-AKC patients with herpes simplex keratitis. There may be absence of the lateral eyebrows from chronic rubbing. The conjunctivae are chronically inflamed. Papillary hypertrophy of both upper and lower tarsal conjunctiva is usual in the early years of the disease and giant (compound) upper tarsal papillae may occur in some patients (Figure 109.13c). The conjunctiva is often so thickened by infiltrate that the tarsal vessels are

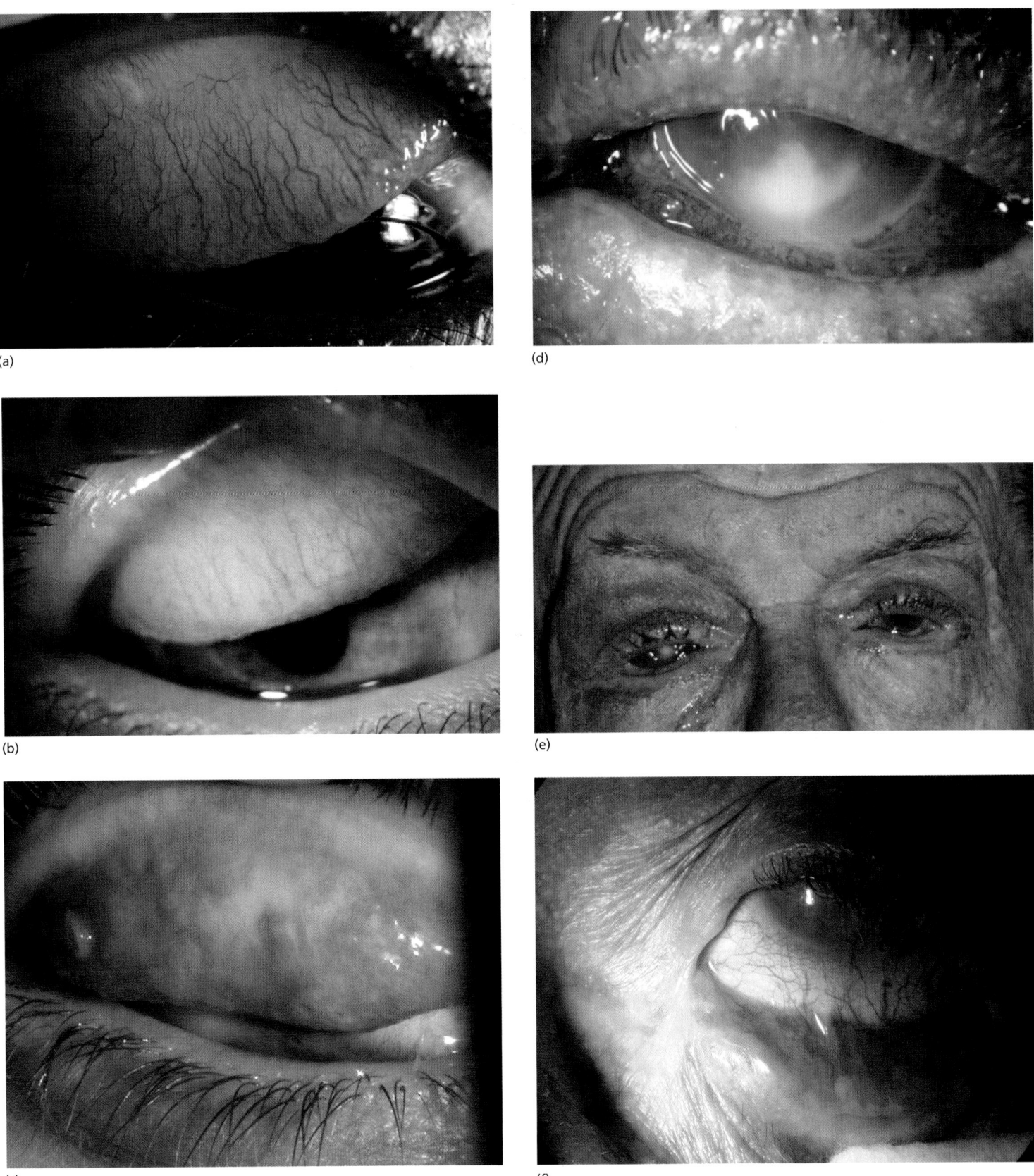

(a)

(b)

(c)

(d)

(e)

(f)

Figure 109.13 Atopic keratoconjunctivitis (AKC). (a) Normal upper tarsal conjunctiva; the tarsal vessels are clearly visible through the healthy conjunctival epithelium and substantia propria. (b) AKC with an infiltrated, papillary, upper tarsal conjunctiva. Compare with the normal tarsal conjunctiva in (a). (c) Giant upper tarsal papillae in AKC (d) Bacterial keratitis complicating AKC showing a corneal infiltrate. The eyes of this patient are shown in (e), with atopic eczema localized to the eyelids; the eczema is often generalized. The right eye shows the infection in (d). (f) Inferior fornix and plical scarring. (g) Limbitis in AKC. (h) Pseudogerontoxon. (i) AKC anterior subcapsular 'polar bear rug' cataract. (j) Herpes simplex viral ulcer in a corneal graft in AKC. (k) Corneal vascularization and opacification as a result of limbal stem cell damage in AKC. (l) Keratoconus associated with AKC. (*Continued*)

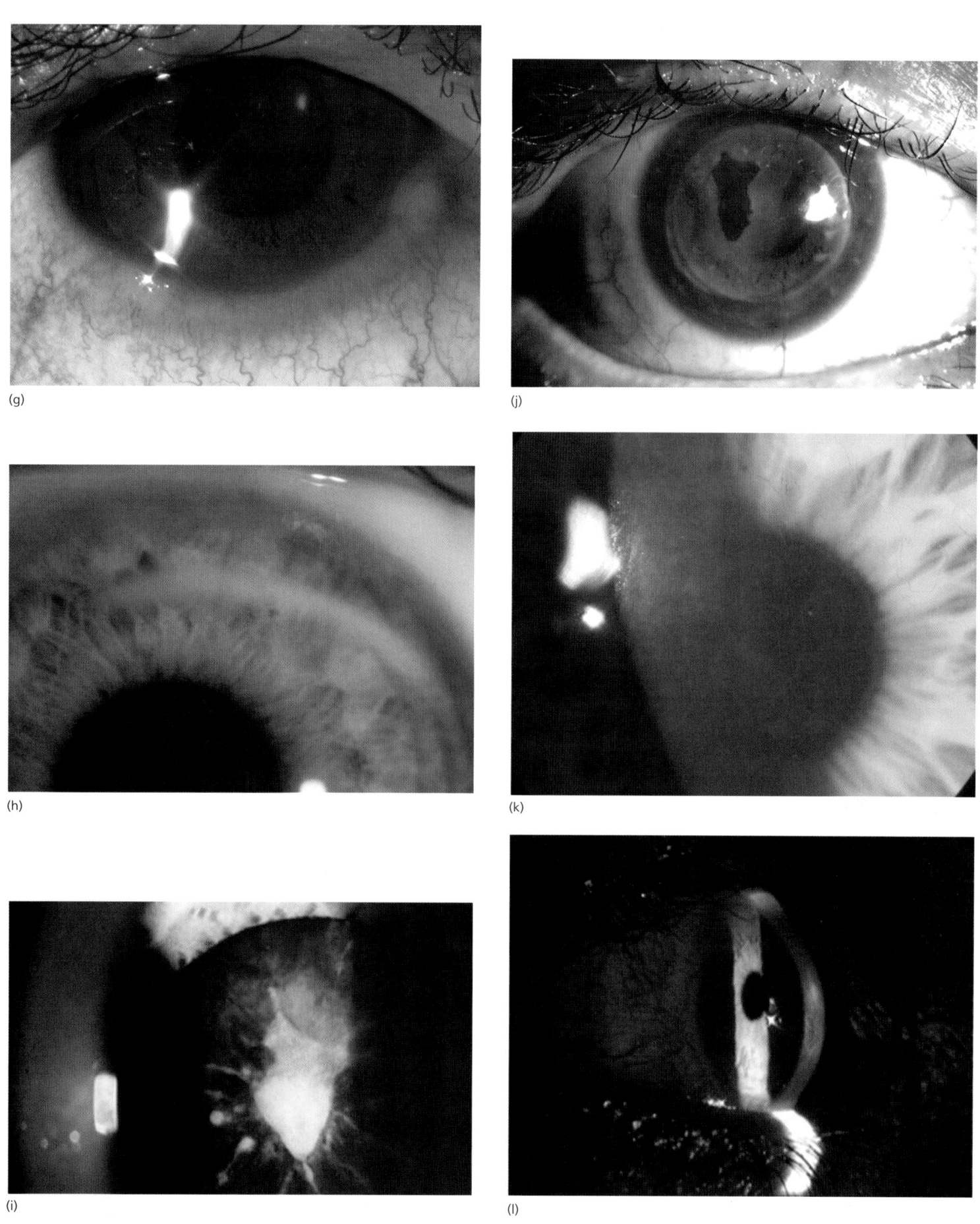

(g)

(j)

(h)

(k)

(i)

(l)

Figure 109.13 (*Continued*)

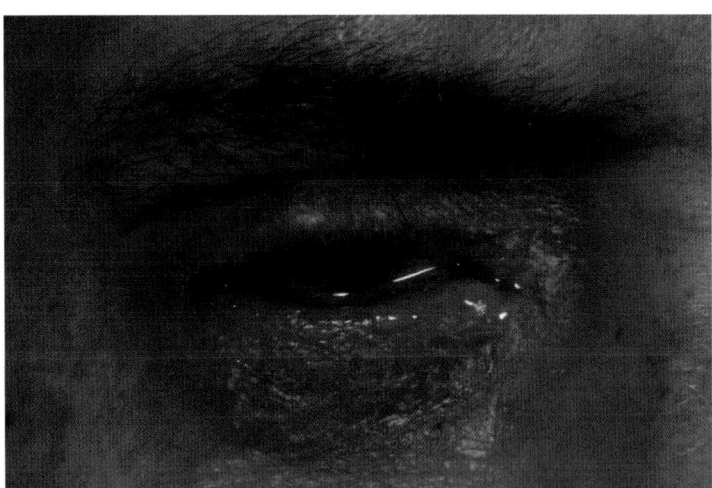

Figure 109.14 Atopic blepharoconjunctivitis (ABC).

obscured (Figure 109.13b) – later in the disease the papillae may be obscured by sheet scarring. Shortening of the inferior fornix develops in some patients and less often the medial and lateral fornices may be obliterated by scar tissue (Figure 109.13f). The bulbar conjunctiva is inflamed during exacerbations but otherwise grossly normal except for the limbal region which may be thickened and nodular with the presence of pinpoint Trantas dots at the apices of the nodules (Figure 109.13g). One of the more common corneal changes is pseudogerotoxon (Figure 109.13h), in which there is a limbal pannus giving rise to an arcus senilis like appearance.

Atopic blepharoconjunctivitis (Figure 109.14) runs a similar course to AKC but has no corneal involvement and therefore not potentially blinding. It can, however, be associated with chronic staphylococcal infection with the associated risk of long-term complications.

Key clinical features distinguishing the different variants of atopic eye disease are summarized in Table 109.8.

Differential diagnosis

The clinical features together with a personal or family history of atopy are usually sufficient for diagnosis. Diagnostic dilemmas usually occur in two settings. First, in those patients who do not respond to appropriate topical therapy as expected to control the disease process before starting systemic immunosuppression. Second, in cases of conjunctival scarring to differentiate AKC from other causes of cicatrization such as primary Sjögren disease, rosacea and mucous membrane pemphigoid (MMP) (see Table 109.11).

Classification of severity

There are no generally accepted or validated classifications of severity in these diseases; however, for the purposes of evaluating response to therapy in a treatment trial, severity grading scores have been used [16].

The more severely affected patients with AKC have associated blepharoconjunctivitis and corneal disease formation of

an atopic cataract (Figure 109.13i) and are particularly vulnerable to infection with *Staphylococcus aureus* and herpes simplex virus (Figure 109.13j). The corneal epithelium reveals punctate scarring with fluorescein and limbal inflammation with Trantas dots (Figure 109.13g). More severely affected patients can develop changes of a cicatrizing conjunctivitis with subepithelial fibrosis, shallowing of the conjunctival fornix obliterated by scar tissue and symblepharon formation (Figure 109.13f). Corneal scarring and neovascularization can lead to blindness (Figure 109.13k).

Complications and co-morbidities

Cataracts occur in 8–12% of patients with severe atopic eczema – young adults especially. They characteristically affect the anterior lens giving rise to a 'polar bear rug' appearance (Figure 109.13i). Posterior subcapsular cataracts are also present due to steroid usage. Keratoconus (Figure 109.13l) occurs in a small percentage of patients with AKC and VKC adding a further complexity to management – conversely, 16% of patients with keratoconus have atopic eczema. Patients with atopic eye disease are at risk of glaucoma because of the long-term use of topic steroid. It is difficult to treat, often requiring complex surgical procedures.

Disease course and prognosis

This is covered in the clinical variants section.

Investigations

Laboratory investigations may be required in patients who do not respond to therapy or who require topical or systemic immunosuppressive therapy for relief of symptoms or when the diagnosis is uncertain. Raised serum IgE levels may be helpful in supporting a diagnosis of atopy, but skin prick testing is of limited value as the results do not necessarily identify the causal allergens. Ophthalmic investigations (upper tarsal conjunctival punch biopsy, tear IgE evaluation, impression cytology of the upper tarsal conjunctiva) are the province of the ophthalmologist and are summarized in Table 109.7.

Management [5,13–20]

Most cases of atopic eye disease are managed with topical ocular therapy which has no effect on the dermatological aspects of the disorder. Because of the potential sight-threatening complications more severe atopic eye disease (VKC, AKC) is best managed by a specialist ophthalmologist with an interest in these conditions. Treatment with courses of systemic agents when needed either for the dermatological or ophthalmological aspects of atopy is clearly going to be beneficial to the management of both. The risk of cataract and glaucoma with the use of potent topical steroids in the periocular skin demands that regular screening is carried out. Use of steroid-sparing topical calcineurin inhibitors (tacrolimus, pimecrolimus) is therefore preferable.

First line (see Figure 109.15)

Simple measures of allergen avoidance, use of cold compresses, and lubrication with preservative-free artificial tears are helpful first line steps. Addition of a potent topical antihistamine

Table 109.7 Clinical characteristics and distinguishing features and diagnosis of the atopic eye diseases.

Disease	Disease course	Conjunctival signs	Corneal signs	Disease associations	Diagnostic tests
Seasonal allergic conjunctivitis (SAC)	Onset 5–20 years Spontaneous remissions common Rare in old age Strikingly seasonal	Hyperaemia. Stringy white discharge. Oedema Micropapillae if severe	None	Personal or family history of atopy including atopic eczema	*Cytology*: usually normal. Serum and tear IgE often elevated but not diagnostic
Perennial allergic conjunctivitis (PAC)	As for SAC but symptoms all year round with seasonal exacerbations	Hyperaemia, stringy white discharge, micropapillae common	None	Personal or family history of atopy including atopic eczema	
Atopic keratoconjunctivitis (AKC)	Onset between 20 and 50 years. Chronic course over many years (Figure 109.13e). Spontaneous resolution in old age Non-seasonal	Micropapillae with intense infiltrate (Figure 109.13b). Reticular and sheet scarring. Shortened fornices in some cases Trantas dots*	Punctate epithelial keratopathy, pannus, macroerosion[†] and plaque[‡] Pseudogerontoxon[§]. Herpes keratitis (Figure 109.13j) and bacterial keratitis (Figure 109.13d) common	*Systemic*: atopy and atopic eczema in all cases *Ocular*: staphylococcal lid disease, cataract, keratoconus, herpes simplex keratitis (often bilateral)	*Cytology*: shows eosinophils and mast cells. Serum IgE elevated. Skin prick tests positive to many allergens but not diagnostic *Upper tarsal conjunctival punch biopsy*: the gold standard for disease confirmation after a 2-week abstention from use of topical corticosteroids *Tear IgE*: useful unless the serum IgE is very high
Atopic blepharoconjunctivitis (ABC)	As for AKC	Micropapillae with intense infiltrate, reticular scarring	None	Personal or family history of atopy	
Vernal keratoconjunctivitis (VKC) – *palpebral, limbal and mixed forms*	Onset between 5 and 15 years. Spontaneous resolution in 95% after 10 years Seasonal exacerbations usual	*Palpebral form*: giant upper tarsal papillae (Figure 109.12a) often bilaterally asymmetrical *Limbal form*: micropapillae on upper tarsus but gelatinous macropapillae at limbus (Figure 109.12b). Trantas dots in both *Mixed form*: combines features of both diseases	*Palpebral form*: punctate epithelial keratopathy affecting upper half of cornea. Adherent mucus appearing as superficial syncytial opacity progressing to macroerosion, shield ulcer and then vernal plaque (Figure 109.12e–g) *Limbal form*: keratopathy extending in from limbus with associated epithelial dysplasia	*Ocular*: keratoconus (Figure 109.13l) and cataract (Figure 109.13i) *Systemic*: atopy in variable proportions from 0–100% depending on geographical location (atopy common in northern Europe but rare in Middle East)	

*Trantas dots: white, pinhead sized dots consisting of eosinophils and necrotic epithelial cells usually at the limbus.

[†]Macroerosion: large epithelial erosions usually in upper half of cornea.

[‡]Plaque (vernal plaque): laminated structure of protein and polysaccharide adherent to the anterior stroma with destruction of Bowman layer.

[§]Pseudogerontoxon: arcus-like appearance in relation to limbal pannus; may disappear in remissions.

(levocabastine or emadastine) or a systemic antihistamine may help relieve itch in some patients. Long-term systemic antihistamine intake can lead to dry eye, the clinical features of which can complicate the ocular allergy features. Topical cromones are mast cell stabilizers (sodium cromoglycate 2–4% or the more recently introduced nedocromil or lodoxamide), and are helpful as first line treatments given once to four times daily depending on symptoms. Topical olapatadine and ketotifen fumarate combine the effects of a cromone with that of an antihistamine and are probably used more widely than cromones as a first line

drug. These treatments are very safe and do not require ophthalmological supervision but are only effective for very mild disease. Cromones are often not tolerated until the inflammation is brought under control with high-dose topical steroids such as dexamethasone 0.1% or prednisolone 0.5%. Because of the attendant risk of glaucoma and steroid-induced cataract, a less potent topical steroid (e.g. fluoromethalone, rimexolone or clobetasone) should be substituted as soon as the disease is brought under safe control. Cromones are used topically wherever possible as corticosteroid-sparing drugs.

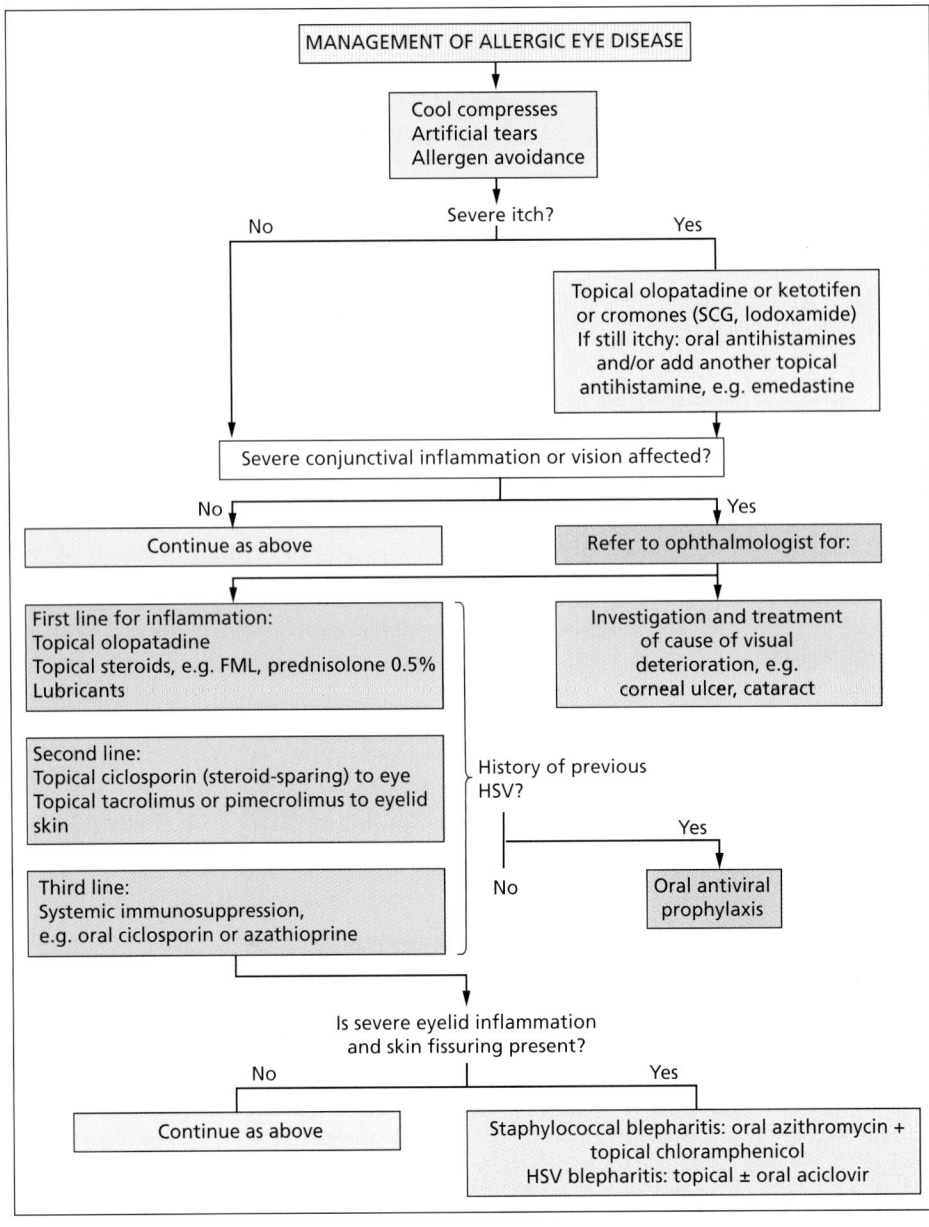

Figure 109.15 Management algorithm for allergic eye disease. FML, flouromethalone; HSV, herpes simplex virus; SCG, sodium cromoglycate.

Second line

Addition of topical calcineurin inhibitors is effective because T cells play a central role in the pathogenesis of the disease. Ciclosporin inactivates calcineurin which then inhibits T-cell activation and interleukin 2 (IL2) production. It also inhibits histamine release from mast cells. Unfortunately, topical ciclosporin is not yet available as a licensed preparation for any ocular condition in Europe although a preparation designed for use in dry eye is available in the USA (Restasis®, Allergan, USA). However, a veterinary preparation is available (Optimmune®, Schering), in addition to preparations made up in hospital pharmacies (through the NHS Medicines Manufacturing Service). These preparations can be made up in artificial tears but they are more soluble in an oily vehicle such as peanut or maize oil, both of which sting on application. A more tolerable preparation of topical ciclosporin has shown promise in two randomized trials for AKC and in both randomized trials and in one case series for VKC and is used by the authors for these indications. Adverse effects apart from stinging are infrequent and introduction of the drug as a corticosteroid-sparing agent for patients requiring high doses of topical corticosteroid has allowed reduction or complete withdrawal of corticosteroid in many cases. Topical ciclosporin is best tolerated if introduced during remissions. Topical ciclosporin 1% and 2% has been reported to be safely used in children with VKC for up to 4 years, with no reports of malignancy or infection.

Topical tacrolimus (0.03% and 0.1%) ointment and pimecrolimus cream are both commercially available and are very effective as steroid-sparing agents when applied to the eyelids. There is also some benefit from spreading onto the conjunctival surface in treating other aspects of the disease.

Severe staphylococcal blepharitis often accompanies AKC and ABC and can be treated with a course of azithromycin followed by local therapy with an antibiotic ointment to which the skin flora are sensitive, usually chloramphenicol together with a topical ophthalmic corticosteroid ointment such as hydrocortisone 0.5% or 1% applied to the lids. Combined preparations often contain aminoglycosides which frequently cause toxicity or allergy and should be avoided.

Herpetic blepharitis may require treatment with local aciclovir ointment, and corneal involvement may require systemic aciclovir therapy combined with appropriate topical steroid (see herpes infection section below).

Third line

Systemic immunosuppression is needed for severe exacerbations of disease; a 3–4-week course of systemic corticosteroids starting with prednisolone at a dose of 60 mg/day may be necessary to bring the disease under control while topical therapy is being introduced. Systemic steroids also carry a risk of glaucoma, but topical application of corticosteroid around the eyelids probably constitutes a higher risk.

Patients with a previous history of ocular herpes simplex virus or with serological evidence of previous exposure to herpes simplex virus, should be aware that they may develop herpes keratitis whilst on systemic or topical steroids. Patients who have had previous episodes of ocular herpes simplex virus should receive prophylaxis with oral aciclovir 400 mg bd (or valaciclovir 500 mg od); topical prophylaxis is unnecessary and may complicate the clinical signs in patients with complex keratoconjunctivitis. Patients with AKC are predisposed to bilateral herpes keratitis and prophylactic antivirals are advisable when they are using corticosteroids.

For a proportion of patients, systemic ciclosporin (usually starting at a dose of 5 mg/kg/day) can be very helpful. Patients who need systemic ciclosporin for management of their ocular eczema will usually obtain substantial collateral ocular benefits and vice versa. Other immunosuppressive agents such as azathioprine, mycophenolate mofetil and methotrexate can also be of value in the management of atopic eye disease.

Future therapeutic agents

New biologicals to modify T- and B-cell responses are all being trialed. Omalizumab, a humanized monoclonal anti-IgE molecule used in the management of asthma, looks promising acting downstream of IgE production by B cells that is characteristic of the atopic eye diseases.

Cicatrizing conjunctivitis associated with immunobullous disorders

Definition and nomenclature

Cicatrizing conjunctivitis is conjunctival inflammation with progressive scarring. The immunobullous disorder MMP is the commonest cause of progressive conjunctival cicatrization [1] (see also Chapter 50).

Introduction and general description

Although uncommon, cicatrizing conjunctivitis is one of the most difficult management problems in ophthalmology because of the widespread effects on the ocular surface, leading to corneal blindness in many patients. The classification of cicatrizing conjunctivitis follows the dermatological classification of immunobullous and other autoimmune mucocutaneous disorders; however, not all of the dermatological disorders are associated with conjunctivitis (Table 109.8). The severity of the conjunctival involvement varies but is mild, without scarring, in pemphigus vulgaris, with variable degrees of scarring and severity in the remainder.

As therapeutic options are limited, early diagnosis and treatment of progressive conjunctival cicatrization is important to try to prevent irreversible sequelae. Table 109.9 lists the different causes of progressive versus relatively static conjunctival cicatrization. Henceforth, this section will focus on the commonest causes of autoimmune cicatrizing conjunctivitis, first MMP, then erythema multiforme and graft-versus-host disease (GVHD).

Mucous membrane pemphigoid [2,3,4,5–7]

Introduction and general description

Mucous membrane pemphigoid is an immunologically heterogeneous group of systemic autoimmune disorders which share a cicatrizing clinical phenotype, affecting mucous membranes and skin. Disease may be localized to one site or may affect multiple sites (see Chapter 50). The proportion of patients with ocular involvement alone varies from 18 to 50%; these differences are likely to reflect differences in the referral base for each series. About 60% of patients presenting to a dermatology clinic will have conjunctival involvement, in addition to skin disease.

Table 109.8 Immunobullous diseases (those associated with cicatrizing conjunctivitis are shown in italics).

Immunobullous diseases	
Intraepithelial	**Subepithelial**
• Pemphigus	• Pemphigoid
Vulgaris	*Bullous*
Vegetans	*Mucous membrane* (Figure 109.15a–g)
• Pemphigus foliaceous	• Pemphigoid gestationis
• Pemphigus erythematosis	• *Epidermolysis bullosa aquisita*
• Brazilian pemphigus	• Bullous systemic lupus erythematosis
• *Paraneoplastic pemphigus*	• *Linear IgA disease*
• *Lichen planus*	• *Dermatitis herpetiformis*

Table 109.9 Differential diagnosis of cicatrizing conjunctivitis [22].

Static or very slowly progressive conjunctival scarring	Progressive conjunctival scarring
1 Trauma – physical, chemical, thermal, radiation injury, artefacta	**1** Neoplasia – squamous cell carcinoma, sebaceous cell carcinoma, lymphoma

2 Infection
Trachoma
Membranous streptococcal conjunctivitis
Adenoviral conjunctivitis
Corynebacterium diphtheria
Chronic mucocutaneous candidiasis
	2 Mucous membrane pemphigoid (MMP):
	  a Ocular MMP/ocular cicatricial pemphigoid
	  b Ocular MMP associated with other disorders:
	    Linear IgA disease
	    Epidermolysis bullosa acquisita
	    Paraneoplastic MMP (antilaminin-332 MMP)
	    Drug-induced ocular MMP
	    Stevens–Johnson syndrome

3 Allergic eye disease:
Atopic keratoconjunctivitis
Vernal keratoconjunctivitis
	3 Other mucocutaneous and immunobullous disorders:
	  a Mucocutaneous disorders: lichen planus
	  b Immunobullous disorders: paraneoplastic pemphigus

4 Drug-induced conjunctival cicatrization (DICC)[†‡]	
5 Mucocutaneous disorders: SJS/TEN[†] Graft-versus-host disease Discoid and systemic lupus erythematosus*	
6 Immunobullous disorders: Linear IgA disease[†] Epidermolysis bullosa acquisita[†] Bullous pemphigoid Pemphigus vulgaris Dermatitis herpetiformis	
7 Systemic disease: Rosacea Sjögren syndrome Sarcoidosis[‡] Scleroderma Granulomatosis with polyangiitis Inflammatory bowel disease Ectodermal dysplasia[†] Immune complex diseases Porphyria cutanea tarda Erythroderma ichthyosiform congenita	

*Rare cases can develop *progressive* scarring.
[†]A subset of patients with these diseases may develop autoantibody-positive *progressive* conjunctival scarring similar to ocular MMP.
[‡]Associated with granulomatous conjunctival inflammation.

Epidemiology

Incidence and prevalence
Unambiguous data on the epidemiology of MMP is difficult to obtain because studies have been based on the site of involvement. A recent UK ophthalmic surveillance study found the incidence of ocular MMP to be 0.8 per million UK population, and the overall incidence of cicatrizing conjunctivitis (including MMP, Stevens–Johnson syndrome and other causes) to be 1.3 per million UK population [1]. A French study of MMP patients presenting to dermatologists reported an incidence of 1.13 per million/year [8]. In ophthalmology centres, MMP affects between 1 : 8000 and 1 : 46 000 patients.

Age
The age range is 30–90 years with peak onset in the seventh decade, although patients may rarely present in childhood.

Sex
The male : female ratio is most commonly 1 : 3.

Ethnicity
No racial or geographical predilection to MMP is reported.

Associated diseases
Mucous membrane pemphigoid is associated with other autoimmune disorders including Sjögren syndrome, rheumatoid arthritis, systemic lupus erythematosus and polyarteritis nodosa. A subtype of MMP called antilaminin-332 (or antiepiligrin) MMP is associated with solid organ malignancies.

Pathophysiology

Predisposing factors
In the eye, drug-induced pemphigoid (pseudopemphigoid), Stevens–Johnson syndrome, toxic epidermal necrolysis (SJS/TEN) and ectodermal dysplasia [9–11] can also lead to the development of autoantibodies against basement membrane, and a clinical and immunopathological phenotype typical of ocular MMP, suggesting that chronic conjunctival damage can precipitate MMP in susceptible individuals, perhaps via epitope speading (the development of immune responses to endogenous epitopes secondary to the release of self-antigens during a chronic autoimmune or inflammatory response). Thus ocular MMP may be a final common pathway, following various conjunctival insults.

Pathology
Current evidence suggests that MMP develops as a consequence of the loss of immunological tolerance to structural proteins in the basement membrane. This results in the production of circulating autoantibodies which bind the basement membrane and weaken adhesion of the overlying epidermis or mucosal epithelium, via inflammatory mechanisms in the case of autoantibodies to bullous pemphigoid antigen 2 (BPAG2) [12] or via non-inflammatory mechanisms in the case of autoantibodies to laminin-332 [13,14]. Whilst the pathogenic activity of experimental or patient immunoglobulin G (IgG) versus the NC16A domain of BPAG2, and that of IgG versus laminin-332 have both been shown in passive transfer studies, the pathogenic activity of IgG versus integrin subunits α6 or β4 has not yet been shown. However, the latter IgGs against integrin subunits have been

shown to induce basement membrane separation in skin organ culture models.

Mucous membrane pemphigoid is a heterogeneous group of disorders, with different subtypes identified according to the autoantigens recognized by circulating autoantibodies. Autoantigens identified include: the NC16 and C-terminal regions of BPAG2 in oral and other forms of MMP (ocular, nasal, hypopharyngeal), the integrin subunit β4 in some ocular MMP patients, the integrin subunit α6 in some oral MMP patients, laminin-332 in antiepiligrin MMP, and the NC1 domain of collagen VII in mucosal-predominant epidermolysis bullosa acquisita [15].

In the eye, irreversible blinding consequences occur as a result of two main pathological processes: excessive inflammation (leading to limbal stem cell failure and/or corneal vascularization) and fibrosis (trichiasis and entropion leading to corneal ulceration and microbial keratitis and severe dry eye).

Inflammation

Immunohistology and cellular phenotyping studies have described the inflammatory cellular response in human ocular MMP, giving detailed phenotypic information but limited functional information [16]. In acute disease, subepithelial bulla formation is accompanied by inflammatory infiltration of the substantia propria by neutrophils, macrophages, dendritic antigen-presenting cells and some plasma cells, together with an increase in CD4 (helper) T cells, which probably reflects their role in recruiting other inflammatory cells. The cytokine profile observed in the acute phase of MMP indicates a mixed helper T-cell type 1 (Th1) interleukin 2 (IL-2), interferon γ (IFN)-γ and type 2 (Th2) IL-4, IL-5 and IL-13 response [17,18].

In chronic disease, macrophages and T cells are present, of which the Th1 subset is active, as demonstrated by the presence of the cytokines IL-2 and IFN-γ, as opposed to the Th2 subset that is involved in B-cell activation. This, coupled with the low numbers of B cells but increased number of plasma cells, suggests that B-cell activation must be occurring in the extraocular tissues with homing of mature plasma cells to the conjunctiva. MHC class II expression is increased, suggesting the potential for local antigen presentation to T-helper cells. There is a slight increase in activated T cells, which are involved in the recruitment of fibroblasts and macrophages.

Fibrosis

Growth factors including FGF (fibroblast growth factor), PDGF (platelet-derived growth factor) and TGF-β (transforming growth factor-β) are all present in MMP. PGDF upregulates the extracellular matrix component (ECM) thrombospondin which is itself important in activating latent TGF-β. PDGF is a powerful chemoattractant for macrophages and fibroblasts and is probably pivotal to the scarring response. However, only TGF-β is capable of stimulating fibroblasts to produce collagen and ECM components. It also blocks matrix degradation by decreasing protease synthesis and increasing protease inhibition. In acute disease, TGF-β is significantly increased and is produced by macrophages and fibroblasts in ocMMP conjunctiva. Once macrophages and fibroblasts are present in large numbers and activated they may become self-regulating; fibroblasts from

ocular MMP conjunctiva display a profibrotic phenotype in cell culture [19].

Implications of immunopathological findings for therapy

Inflammation is important in acute disease; severe inflammation is associated clinically with rapid scarring and therefore demands effective immunosuppression to reduce scarring. Inflammation may also play a role in chronic disease although scarring may continue even in the presence of minimal inflammation, suggesting that growth factor production by macrophages and fibroblasts may be relatively independent of the other inflammatory cells. Therefore, modulation of growth factor activity, collagen metabolism or fibroblast activity may be necessary to halt the disease process.

Genetics

A genetic predisposition to MMP has been found in an association with the HLA-DQB1*0301 haplotype [20].

Clinical features [4]

History

In most patients the onset is insidious, with non-specific conjunctival symptoms including irritation, hyperaemia and discharge due to what is often thought to be recurrent conjunctivitis. In other patients the first symptoms are due to trichiasis, or less commonly ptosis as a result of cicatricial entropion affecting the upper lid. Dry eye and mucous deficiency are late signs. Acute disease occurs in about 20% of new patients with severe inflammation and conjunctival ulceration; this presentation may follow failed lid surgery for entropion on undiagnosed cases.

Presentation

Signs, in order of progression, often start at the medial canthus with loss of the plica and later of the caruncle (Figure 109.16f), subepithelial reticular fibrosis of tarsal conjunctiva (Figure 109.16a), conjunctival infiltrate due to increased cellularity and collagen formation (Figure 109.16c,d), hyperaemia, shortening of the fornices (Figure 109.16a), symblepharon (Figure 109.16b), blepharitis, trichiasis and cicatricial entropion (Figure 109.16g), punctate keratopathy, limbitis (Figure 109.16d), conjunctival (Figure 109.16e) and corneal keratinization, and corneal surface failure (Figure 109.16e).

Clinical variants

Clinical variants of ocular MMP include:

1 Idiopathic autoimmune ocular MMP (most common).
2 Ocular MMP associated with other immunobullous disorders such as linear immunoglobulin A (IgA) disease, epidermolysis bullosa acquisita, antilaminin-332 MMP [21] (see Table 109.9).
3 Ocular MMP arising as a result of drug-induced conjunctival damage (also known as drug-induced conjunctival cicatrization (DICC), or drug-induced pseudopemphigoid).
4 Ocular MMP arising in association with Stevens–Johnson syndrome and other autoimmune conjunctival disorders.

PART 10: SITES, SEX, AGE

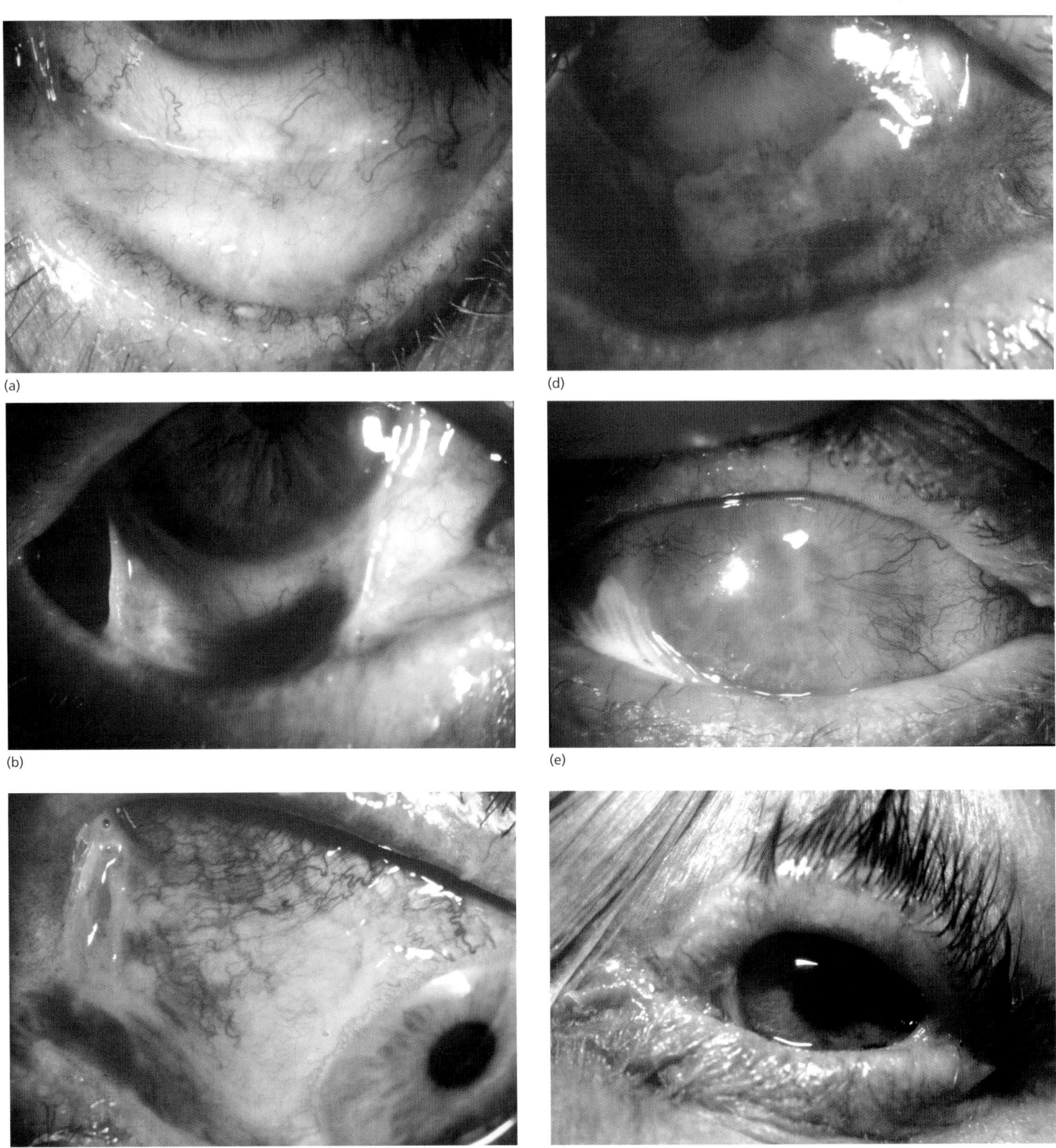

(a)

(b)

(c)

(d)

(e)

(f)

Figure 109.16 Ocular signs of mucous membrane pemphigoid (MMP). (a) Inferior fornix shortening and subconjunctival scarring. (b) Conjunctival symblepharon tethering the globe to the lower lid. (c) Acute exacerbation of conjunctival MMP showing conjunctival ulceration. This occurs in only 10% of patients presenting with MMP affecting the eye. (d) Severe conjunctival inflammation and limbitis. This leads rapidly to the ocular surface failure and corneal blindness shown in (e) unless it is promptly controlled with adequate immunosuppressive therapy. (e) Ocular surface failure and keratinization (the white area) in advanced pemphigoid. This eye is blind. (f) Advanced ocular pemphigoid showing loss of the medial canthal structures (plica and caruncle) with a reduced interpalpebral aperture secondary to shortening of the fornices (as in (a)) and fusion of the tarsal and bulbar conjunctivae. (Courtesy of Mr J. Dart, Moorfields Eye Hospital, London, UK.) (g) Upper and lower lid trichiasis due to cicatricial entropion. (h) Terminally dry keratinized blind eye with trichiasis and entropion. (i) Persistent epithelial defect (chronic corneal ulceration) in a corneal graft in an eye with advanced scarring due to ocular MMP. (*Continued*)

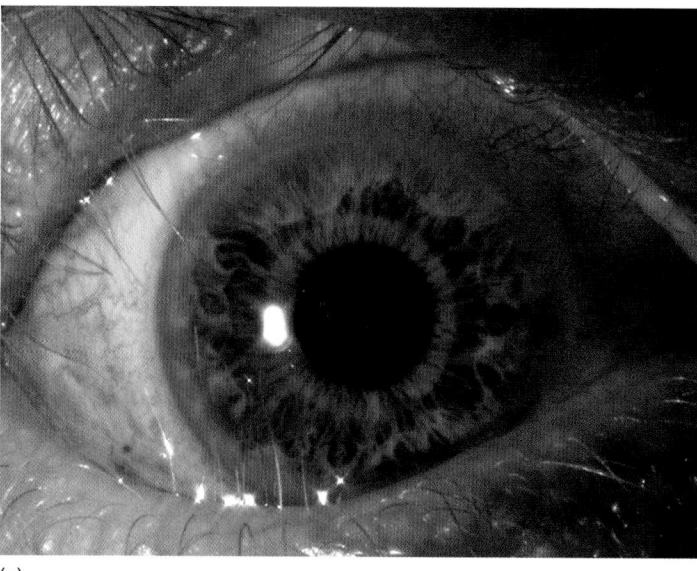

(g)

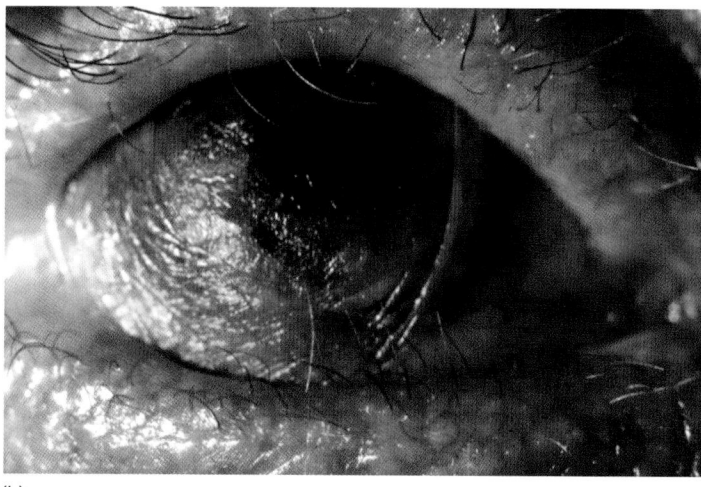

(h)

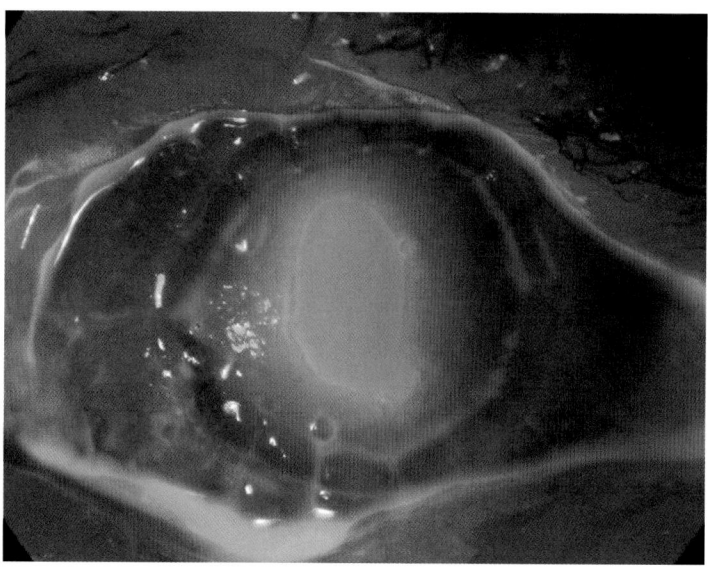

(i)

Figure 109.16 *(Continued)*

Differential diagnosis

The conjunctival signs in MMP may be identical to those produced by the other immunobullous disorders that are summarized in Table 109.10. However, in the latter conditions, the skin disease precedes the ocular disease, so that there is rarely any confusion. In erythema multiforme major, exacerbations of conjunctival inflammation can occur many years after the acute disease, leading to a condition indistinguishable from MMP both in terms of the clinical signs and immunopathology [22].

The principal problems in differential diagnosis relate to diseases other than the immunobullous disorders that may also cause cicatrizing conjunctivitis (Table 109.9). Patients with conjunctival cicatrization secondary to infective causes are sometimes referred for investigation of what has been longstanding conjunctival scarring, following a long-forgotten episode of infection, in whom the absence of a recent history of inflammation, or of progressive symptoms, usually indicates static disease. Patients with sarcoidosis or systemic sclerosis normally have a well-established diagnosis by the time conjunctival scarring develops. Sjögren syndrome may mimic early MMP, but can usually be differentiated by the presence of Sjögren-specific antibodies and/or a positive labial biopsy. AKC can occasionally be difficult to differentiate from slowly progressive MMP, but the history and clinical signs of severe eczema, and a tarsal conjunctival biopsy (performed after withdrawal of topical corticosteroids for 2 weeks) that shows

Table 109.10 Ocular effects of Stevens–Johnson syndrome and toxic epidermal necrolysis (SJS/TEN) [41].

Ocular effects	Resulting symptoms and signs
Loss of goblet cells Loss of accessory lacrimal glands Scarring of meibomian gland orifices	Disrupted tear film leading to poor vision and punctate keratopathy (Figure 109.20b)
Metaplasia of meibomian gland epithelium with development of metaplastic lashes	Trichiasis secondary to metaplastic lashes (Figure 109.20b)
Conjunctival scarring and obliteration of lacrimal gland ductules	Very dry eye with secondary conjunctival and corneal squamous metaplasia (Figure 109.20b)
Corneal and conjunctival keratinization due to squamous metaplasia	Exacerbates drying and discomfort
Conjunctival scarring with fornix shortening and symblepharon formation leading to lid shortening	May cause lagophthalmos and corneal exposure
Retroplacement of meibomian gland orifices and irregularity of mucocutaneous junction	Disrupts tear film
Entropion of upper and lower lids with trichiasis of both metaplastic and normal lashes	Corneal punctate keratopathy and ulceration
Corneal epithelial failure secondary to limbal inflammation causing loss of palisades of Vogt, conjunctivalization of cornea, corneal neovascularization and corneal opacification	Blindness

PART 10: SITES, SEX, AGE

excessive numbers of mast cells and eosinophils can confirm the diagnosis. Iatrogenic conjunctivitis is non-progressive, except in the case of drug-induced MMP, which is indistinguishable from classical MMP. Awareness that conjunctival scarring can occur in ocular rosacea and in staphylococcal blepharoconjunctivitis (see Figure 109.8a) is usually enough to distinguish these conditions from MMP. Factitious conjunctival trauma is rare and usually more focal than classical MMP but can mimic MMP while the self-trauma is active.

Classification of severity

The severity of conjunctival inflammation in ocular MMP is most commonly graded on a scale 0 (absent) to 4+ (severe) [1,5,23]. There are several grading schema for severity of conjunctival scarring in ocular MMP. The Tauber grading scheme incorporates aspects both the Foster and Mondino grading schemes [24]. At present there is no validated and accepted grading system for defining activity and severity of disease in ocular MMP as a whole.

Complications and co-morbidities

Late ocular MMP results in fusion of the lids and globe known as ankyloblepharon (Figure 109.16f), which may obscure the cornea completely. In these advanced cases the surface of the eye is extremely dry, keratinized, cicatrized and blind (Figure 109.16h). Persistent corneal epithelial defect (Figure 109.16i), microbial keratitis and corneal perforation are common in ocular MMP, either occurring as a result of trichiasis abrading the cornea, and/or severe cicatricial dry eye and/or exposure from scarred distorted eyelids. With the corneal surface failure, these corneal complications account for the management challenges posed by the disease.

Disease course and prognosis

Most patients with ocular MMP have progressive disease. Current aggressive treatment regimens with systemic immunosuppression, have been shown to reduce the rate of progression. Because patients can occasionally progress to blindness within months from the onset, both early diagnosis and effective treatment are critical in improving the prognosis. At presentation, between 25 and 38% of patients with ocular disease have significant visual loss and about 30% become legally blind.

Investigations

Diagnostic problems in predominantly ocular MMP [1,2,25–29]

The diagnosis of predominantly ocular MMP has been complicated by the definition of MMP used by the first International Consensus Statement on MMP [2] in which the disease is defined as 'a group of putative autoimmune, chronic inflammatory, subepithelial blistering diseases predominantly affecting mucous membranes that is characterized by linear deposition of IgG, IgA or C3 along the epithelial basement membrane zone'. Whilst it has done much to harmonize the various definitions of MMP in terms of the clinical and diagnostic characteristics, and also

to encourage both careful clinical phenotyping and the application of diagnostic immunopathology tests, the necessity of positive direct immunofluorescence (DIF) raises important issues for ocular MMP. It is well recognized that DIF is invariably positive from at least one site when MMP affects the oropharynx and skin as well as the eyes; compliance with a definition that requires positive DIF is therefore usually straightforward in such cases with multiple sites affected. However, from the perspective of clinicians caring for patients with MMP affecting the eyes alone, the Consensus Statement has resulted in a substantial proportion of patients (from 14 to 40% having negative DIF) failing to meet these immunopathological criteria for diagnosis. As a result, despite having a typical MMP phenotype and response to treatment, they fall outside the Consensus Statement diagnostic criteria. Subsequent to the publication of the Consensus Statement, peer reviewers of studies on ocular MMP have suggested that this group of patients be omitted from studies on MMP. Extending this to clinical settings, the resulting uncertainty about the diagnosis has meant that immunosuppressive therapy has been delayed or deferred in some patients.

Sensitivity and specificity of direct immunofluorescence for mucous membrane pemphigoid

However, DIF is not a specific test for MMP and a positive result does not exclude other immunobullous disorders as is made clear in the Consensus Statement. In effect, a positive DIF test is used as a surrogate to provide evidence for an autoimmune pathogenesis. For DIF to be integral to a diagnosis of ocular MMP, the test should ideally be both highly sensitive and specific. Not only is DIF of low sensitivity in ocular MMP, it is also of low specificity. Conjunctival biopsies may have a positive DIF result typical that found in MMP (linear IgG and/or IgA deposition along the basement membrane zone) in a range of disorders, including bullous pemphigoid, skin-dominated linear IgA bullous dermatosis, skin-dominated epidermolysis bullosa acquisita, drug-induced pemphigoid, Stevens–Johnson syndrome, rosacea and ulcerative colitis [2,27,28]; most of these are immunobullous disorders with an autoimmune basis, but not all. Furthermore, some must be differentiated from each other by the clinical phenotype or may require more sophisticated tests to reliably distinguish them from each other (such as indirect immunofluorescence (IIF) studies on salt-split skin, immunoblotting and immunoelectron microscopy. In addition, DIF may not be consistently positive and may change with time [26,29]. With regard to the low sensitivity of DIF, studies have shown that there is a well-recognized DIF-negative subgroup comprising up to 14–40% of patients with ocular MMP, these subjects having scarring conjunctival inflammation that is phenotypically indistinguishable from MMP, and which responds identically to immunosuppressive therapy.

Indirect immunofluorescence in mucous membrane pemphigoid

Indirect immunofluorescence was not included amongst the criteria for MMP in the Consensus Statement because this investigation is often negative in MMP. However, positive IIF also provides evidence for an underlying autoimmune pathology and may be positive in ocular MMP when DIF is negative.

Recommended criteria for the diagnosis of predominantly ocular mucous membrane pemphigoid

More workable, and clinically useful, criteria for ocular MMP used in our clinical service are as follows [1].

Predominantly ocular mucous membrane pemphigoid

This is a term that we use for those cases without any evidence of MMP affecting other systems. The term 'predominantly' is used to recognize the fact that, even with the most careful phenotyping, it is not possible to exclude asymptomatic involvement of, for example, the oesophagus.

Criteria for the diagnosis of ocular mucous membrane pemphigoid

1 Patients with positive conjunctival DIF or positive DIF from another site meet currently agreed criteria for the diagnosis of MMP and can be reported as such.
2 Patients with negative DIF from any site and positive IIF can be diagnosed as having MMP.
3 Patients with negative immunopathology can be diagnosed as 'presumed' ocular MMP, *providing that* they have a typical phenotype of progressive conjunctival scarring *and* providing that other diseases that may cause this same phenotype have been excluded (Sjögren syndrome, ocular rosacea, Stevens–Johnson syndrome, AKC, ectodermal dysplasia, sarcoidosis, scleroderma and drug-induced pseudopemphigoid).

When ocular cases are reported in studies, the authors believe that the detailed immunopathology findings should be recorded for each case so that the diagnosis can be interpreted in the light of future modifications to diagnostic criteria.

In ocular MMP patients (without extraocular disease), the laboratory investigations are outside the scope of many ophthalmology services and ideally such patients should be referred to specialist corneal and external eye disease departments. However, many patients are elderly, for whom distant referral is unwelcome. For such cases a diagnosis of 'presumed' ocular MMP, based on a history of progressive conjunctival scarring, the presence of the typical clinical signs and exclusion of other ocular causes, is adequate for clinical purposes.

Taking conjunctival biopsies for direct immunofluorescence

This has been described recently [21]. Conjunctival biopsies for DIF should be taken from the bulbar conjunctiva and the presence of IgA, IgG and the C3 component of complement confirm the diagnosis of MMP when positive. Fornix biopsies should be avoided as taking biopsies from this site may result in fornix contracture. The biopsy can be taken using topical anaesthesia with tetracaine, the conjunctiva is tented up and a piece about 2 mm in diameter cut off with spring scissors. This can be done in the outpatient department using magnification from the slit lamp microscope. Routine histopathology of conjunctival biopsies is of little value in the diagnosis because the conjunctiva is fragile and detection of basement membrane zone cleavage is unreliable. However, it should be done to exclude surface neoplasia, particularly in unilateral disease, as this can present with scarring and inflammation. Squamous metaplasia of the conjunctival epithelium and a reduction in goblet cells are non-specific findings, as is an increased inflammatory cell infiltrate. In acute disease, there is a neutrophil-rich infiltrate. In chronic disease, there is a lymphocytic cell infiltrate.

Management

General principles of management of cicatrizing conjunctivitis and its ocular complications [7,30–32]

The same strategies can be used to treat the ocular aspects of cicatrizing conjunctivitis due to any cause, whether it be due to ocular MMP or Stevens–Johnson syndrome. The aim of treatment is the successful management of each of five principal components of these diseases.

1 Treating any ocular surface disease present (for e.g. blepharitis, trichiasis, dry eye).
2 Excluding and treating any secondary infection.
3 Identifying any treatment toxicity.
4 Managing any underlying autoimmunity-driven inflammation.
5 Preventing and treating fibrosis.

These components of disease are present to variable degrees in different diseases. For example, in Stevens–Johnson syndrome, most patients have relatively little inflammation once the surface disease has been treated and any treatment toxicity eliminated, so it is the minority of these patients, with recurrent inflammation or progressive cicatrization [22], who require suppression of inflammation with systemic therapy. Conversely, most, but not all, MMP patients require management of all five components of disease, with 80% of patients requiring systemic immunosuppressive therapy to control the inflammation that persists once the surface disease, any infection or toxicity has been controlled. At present, there are no therapies available specifically targeting fibrosis. The only demonstrated means of slowing the progression of scarring is good control of inflammation, usually with systemic therapy. However, even with conventional immunosuppressive regimens in ocular MMP, fibrosis of the eye can still progress in 11–53% of patients [7].

The following management strategy is depicted as an algorithm in Figure 109.17.

Manage any ocular surface disease

Ocular surface disease is secondary to previous or current lid and conjunctival scarring and inflammation. This surface disease causes much of the damage to the cornea and is responsible for additional inflammation. Trichiasis and entropion, blepharitis, dry eye and filamentary keratitis, keratinization, persistent epithelial defect, microbial keratitis and corneal perforation may all result from a combination of a poor tear film, poor lid closure and corneal damage secondary to trichiasis. These are treated as follows.

• Trichiasis: epilate in the short term, use electrolysis or laser for odd lashes, cryotherapy for misdirected lashes and surgery for entropion (inferior retractor plication for lower lid and anterior lamellar reposition for upper lid, labial mucosal graft for conjunctival fornix reconstruction if indicated).

PART 10: SITES, SEX, AGE

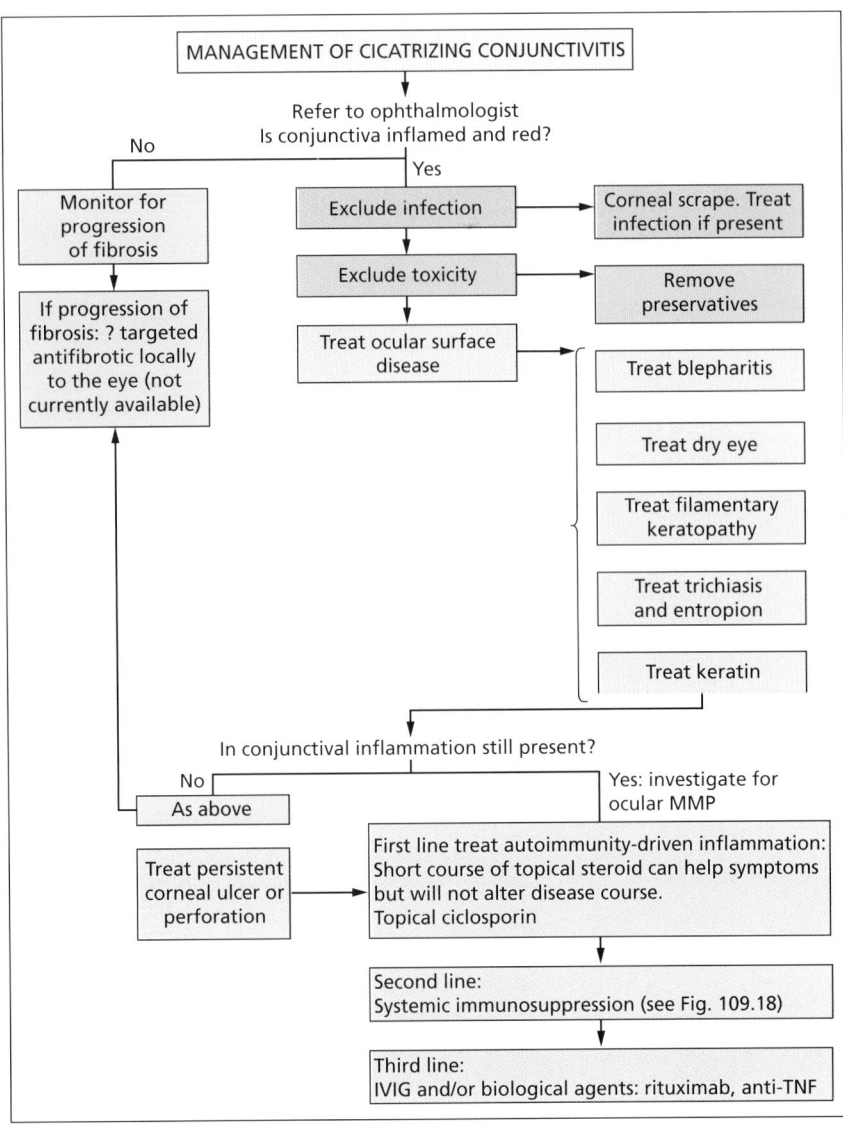

Figure 109.17 Management algorithm for the management of cicatrizing conjunctivitis. IVIG, intravenous immunoglobulin; MMP, mucous membrane pemphigoid; TNF, tumour necrosis factor.

- Blepharitis: use oral tetracyclines and institute a lid hygiene regimen (see section Blepharitis, meibomian gland dysfunction, rosacea and seborrhoeic dermatitis).
- Dry eye and filaments: use non-preserved lubricants, topical acetylcysteine 5–10% as a mucolytic, punctal occlusion to conserve tears (once any blepharitis has been controlled), courses of topical steroids and topical ciclosporin.
- Keratinization: topical retinoic acid is effective in 30% but is only available in specialized centres.
- Persistent corneal epithelial defect: exclude infection, treat ingrowing lashes, use non-preserved lubricants, therapeutic lenses (silicone hydrogel if the eyes are not too dry) and, if these measures are unsuccessful, close the eye with a botulinum toxin protective ptosis or with a temporary tarsorrhaphy. Other more specialized treatments may be needed.
- Corneal perforation: temporize with therapeutic contact lenses and/or corneal glue, followed by keratoplasty only if absolutely necessary.

Exclude and treat any secondary infection

The compromised environment of the cicatrized conjunctiva harbours more potentially pathogenic bacteria [33] and fungi such as yeasts. The index of suspicion for infection must be high, for example in the presence of any corneal epithelial defect, given that the typical clinical signs of a white cell mediated corneal infiltrate may be suppressed in an immunosuppressed host, and topical steroids may also contribute to lack of an infiltrate. Taking a small scrape from the edge of the corneal epithelial defect and sending it for microbiology will help confirm that an infection is present and whether it is likely to respond to the empirical treatment instituted.

Eliminate or minimize treatment toxicity

Treatment toxicity results principally from the preservative benzalkonium chloride, a component of most reusable bottles of eye drop preparations as well as of topical glaucoma medications and aminoglycoside eye drops. Unnecessary topical treatment should therefore be avoided and unpreserved drops or saline used as far as possible. The effects of topical treatment toxicity are hard to distinguish from those of the ocular surface disease. After withdrawal of toxic topical therapy, the mean recovery period is 2 weeks but may extend to 3 months.

Suppress inflammation/commence immunosuppressive therapy

Any inflammation on the upper bulbar conjunctiva which persists once any ocular surface disease has been treated and any infection and treatment toxicity excluded, is likely to be due to underlying autoimmune activity. The upper bulbar conjunctiva is a good location to assess underlying autoimmune disease activity because it is less susceptible to the effects of blepharitis and dry eye, given the protection of the upper eyelid. In some cases, conjunctival autoimmune activity can, however, manifest as a patchy distribution of inflammation, and this may not necessarily involve the upper bulbar conjunctiva. In these cases, persistence of inflammation despite maximal treatment of ocular surface disease is an indication that systemic immunosuppression is needed.

First line: anti-inflammatory therapy (Figure 109.18)

In *mild disease* (hyperaemia and oedema), low-dose topical corticosteroid may be helpful, particularly in the alleviation of the symptoms of very dry eye. Topical ciclosporin preparations are being widely used for dry eye in the USA where there is a well-tolerated preparation (Restasis®, Allergan) that has been licensed for use in dry eye. This preparation is not licensed in Europe, where less well-tolerated preparations are available from hospital pharmacies. The role of topical ciclosporin for the severe dry eye

associated with cicatrizing eye disease is currently uncertain but may provide benefits for this group of patients without the risks associated with topical steroid use [31]. Comparative studies or randomized controlled trials comparing topical ciclosporin and steroids for dry eye are not available.

Second line: systemic immunosuppressive therapy

For *moderate disease* (hyperaemia, intense infiltration), immunosuppressants used initially include a sulpha agent such as sulphapyridine or dapsone [7], or the antimetabolite methotrexate. The dose of sulphapyridine is 500 mg daily for 2 weeks then 1 g daily (sulfasalazine 1–2 g daily is an alternative); 55% of patients respond in 1–2 months, but 15% develop an allergic reaction. The dose of dapsone is 75 mg daily, increased each month by 25 mg daily to 125 mg but monitor haemoglobin levels and do not increase the dose if haemoglobin is less than 10 g/dL; there is a 70% response in 1–2 months, reducing to 50% after 1 year. Methotrexate (5.0–25.0 mg once weekly) is sometimes used as a first line immunosuppressant in ocular MMP (effective in about 80% depending on the severity of the disease) [32]. More recently, mycophenolate mofetil (1–2 g daily) has been used as a first line systemic immunosuppressant in ocular MMP, with a greater efficacy (effective in about 80% depending on the severity of the disease) than sulpha agents yet less frequent side effects [34]. Currently, this is the first line agent for ocular MMP in our clinic. Another agent that may be considered is azathioprine (1–2 mg/kg/day; effective in about 60%).

For *severe disease* (hyperaemia, limbitis, conjunctival ulceration), start oral prednisolone 1 mg/kg/day, reduce the dose after 2 weeks and tail off after 2–4 months. This is ineffective at low doses in the

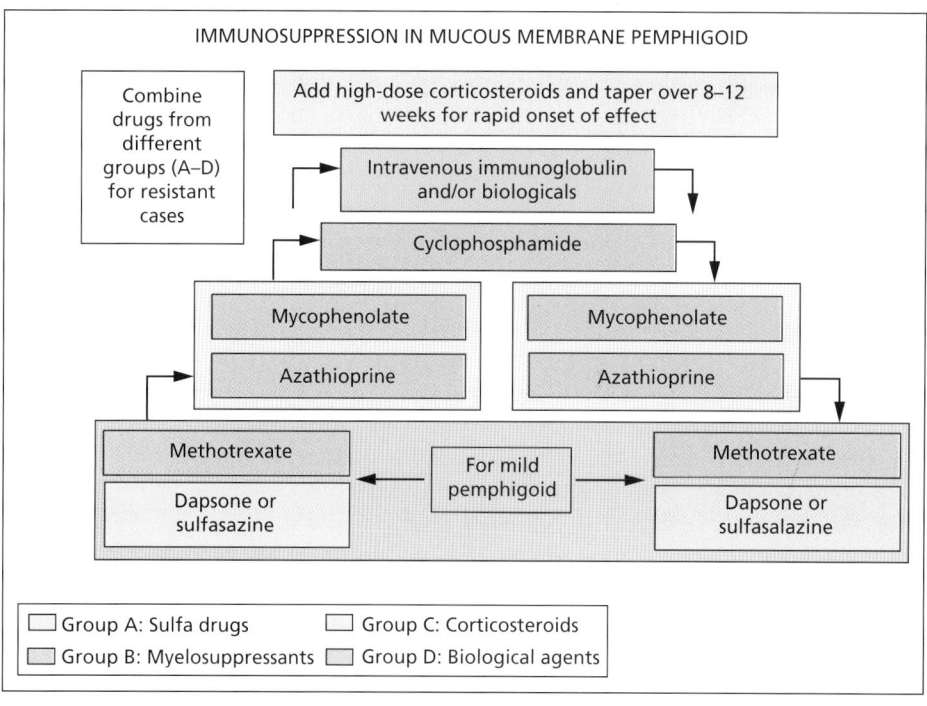

Figure 109.18 Systemic immunosuppression stepladder for ocular mucous membrane pemphigoid (MMP). Immunosuppression can be carried out using a 'stepladder' approach for the introduction of systemic drugs [7,39]. Dapsone or sulphapyridine (given as sulphasalazine) are only used in MMP and mild disease may respond well to these, or to methotrexate. If there is no response after 2–3 months, treatment is 'stepped up' to azathioprine or mycophenolate mofetil. If these drugs are not effective in another 2–3 months then cyclophosphamide is the drug of choice. For severe and rapidly progressive disease, cyclophosphamide is the drug of choice. Patients are started on this with a 2-month course of systemic steroids, which speeds up the control of inflammation, while the cyclophosphamide takes effect (2–3 months). When the disease has been controlled for several months, treatment can be 'stepped down' to a less toxic drug. Steroids, the sulphones (dapsone and sulphapyridine) and the bone marrow suppressive immunosuppressants (methotrexate, mycophenolate, azathioprine and mycophenolate) can be combined although the neutrophil count, in particular, must be monitored. About 10% of patients with severe disease will not be fully controlled with cyclophosphamide. For these patients, intravenous immunoglobulin or a biological agent (anti-tumour necrosis factor or rituximab) may be effective. Systemic ciclosporin has been little used in cicatrizing conjunctivitis because of lack of evidence of efficacy, concern about potential fibrogenic side effects as well as likely renal toxicity in the elderly subset of patients.

IMMUNOSUPPRESSION IN MUCOUS MEMBRANE PEMPHIGOID

Combine drugs from different groups (A–D) for resistant cases

Add high-dose corticosteroids and taper over 8–12 weeks for rapid onset of effect

Intravenous immunoglobulin and/or biologicals

Cyclophosphamide

Mycophenolate

Mycophenolate

Azathioprine

Azathioprine

Methotrexate

For mild pemphigoid

Methotrexate

Dapsone or sulfasazine

Dapsone or sulfasalazine

Group A: Sulfa drugs
Group B: Myelosuppressants
Group C: Corticosteroids
Group D: Biological agents

long term and a steroid-sparing immunosuppressive agent is usually added for long-term disease control. The most effective currently is cyclophosphamide 1 mg/kg/day. The dose is adjusted until the lymphocyte count is between 0.5 and 1.0×10^9/L; other haematological parameters should remain normal. Cyclophosphamide therapy is usually discontinued after 1 year and substituted by sulphonamides or immunosuppressive agents as described above.

Third line: biological therapies

For *severe or recalcitrant disease* which has not responded to cyclophosphamide, treatment with intravenous immunoglobulin, with or without rituximab (anti-CD20) [35,36], or anti-TNF-α agents [37] may be beneficial. Results of these therapies have been reported in non-randomized series or case reports.

Most of this therapy is empirical, and a sulphonamide (dapsone or sulphapyridine) is often used together with an alkylating agent (cyclophosphamide) or an antimetabolite (azathioprine, methotrexate or mycophenolate mofetil) to control inflammation. This immunosuppressive strategy is summarized in Figure 109.18 [38] and in a recent case series [7].

Preventing fibrosis

Currently, the only demonstrated means of slowing the progression of scarring is good control of inflammation with systemic immunosuppression. Therapy specifically targeted at fibrosis in MMP is limited. Mitomycin C has been delivered either subconjunctivally or applied intraoperatively following division of symblephara, but no controlled trials have been carried out. Adverse effects of mitomycin include tissue ischaemia, which may affect the success of mucous membrane graft reconstructive surgery and potential limbal stem cell damage. No currently available medical intervention is able to reverse the processes of cicatrization or ocular surface damage, once they have developed.

Other subepithelial disorders and conjunctivitis [39]

Other immunobullous disorders are much less frequently associated with conjunctival cicatrization. As a result, little is known about the pathogenesis of the conjunctival disease as opposed to the events in the skin. Bullous pemphigoid generally results in mild conjunctivitis although severe cicatrization has been reported. Epidermolysis bullosa aquisita, linear IgA disease, dermatitis herpetiformis and lichen planus may all be associated with progressive conjunctival scarring indistinguishable from that of MMP.

Erythema multiforme major and Stevens–Johnson syndrome/ toxic epidermal necrolysis. The ocular complications of erythema multiforme and Stevens–Johnson syndrome/toxic epidermal necrolysis (SJS/TEN) are identical (Table 109.10) [40] (see Chapters 47 and 119). About 70–80% of patients admitted for treatment of these diseases will develop eye disease. It is the eye disease which leads to the most profound, long-term morbidity in many such patients. In addition, the eye disease, unlike the lesions affecting the remaining mucosal surfaces, may progress years after the acute episode has resolved [22].

Acute ocular complications of SJS/TEN. These usually occur concurrently with the skin disease (Figure 109.19a) but may sometimes precede it by several days. The conjunctivitis varies from a papillary reaction with watery discharge (Figure 109.19b) to a membranous conjunctivitis with sloughing of the conjunctival epithelium. Corneal epithelial defects are common and may progress to corneal ulceration with or without bacterial superinfection. The morbidity of the disease may be due to the acute corneal complications but is more usually due to conjunctival scarring (Figure 109.19c).

Chronic ocular complications of SJS/TEN. These are numerous. The severe conjunctival inflammation leads to loss of goblet cells and the accessory conjunctival lacrimal glands as well as disruption of the meibomian gland orifices leading to MGD. This results in a disrupted tear film and a secondary punctate keratopathy. In mildly affected patients, this causes chronic mild discomfort, photophobia and slightly reduced vision. In more severely affected patients, the conjunctival inflammation leads to cicatrization of the lacrimal ductules, resulting in a severely dry eye accompanied by squamous metaplasia and keratinization (Figure 109.19d) of both the conjunctival and corneal components of the ocular surface, thereby causing more severe discomfort and loss of vision (Figure 109.19e). In addition, the meibomian gland ductal epithelium undergoes metaplasia, resulting in the development of fine metaplastic lashes which are not a feature of MMP. The conjunctival shortening leads both to entropion, resulting in ocular surface abrasion by normal as well as by metaplastic lashes, and may also cause lid shortening, leading to reduced eye closure (lagophthalmos), which is easily overlooked. Lash abrasion and trichiasis lead to the development of corneal epithelial defects which, as a result of the poor tear film, may persist. Persistent epithelial defect predisposes to corneal stromal melts and perforation, which are often precipitated by infection. This evolution of changes is not the direct consequence of the acute disease but is secondary to the effects on the tear film and lids. A grading system for the chronic ocular manifestations of Stevens–Johnson syndrome has been proposed [40].

The severe inflammation may also lead to blinding opacity of the corneal epithelium, not only as a result of squamous metaplasia, but also by loss of corneal epithelial progenitor cells (stem cells). Because of prolonged survival of transient amplifying cells, the progeny of stem cells, stem cell failure may not be manifest for 12–18 months after the onset of the disease.

An additional problem for patients with ocular complications of Stevens–Johnson syndrome is the development of severe conjunctival inflammation with progressive scarring that may be indistinguishable from MMP and may also be DIF positive. This can occur as a continuation of the acute episode or may occur many years after the onset of disease. Other inflammatory complications include recurrent conjunctival inflammation following Stevens–Johnson syndrome and necrotizing sclerokeratitis [22]. All of these severe inflammatory problems can precipitate stem cell failure and demand rapid control, usually requiring systemic immunosuppressive therapy. The cause of these late inflammatory complications is not understood.

Management of acute ocular SJS/TEN includes topical steroids [41] (see Chapter 119). Urgent amniotic membrane transplantation in acute disease with extensive ulceration can be helpful [42].

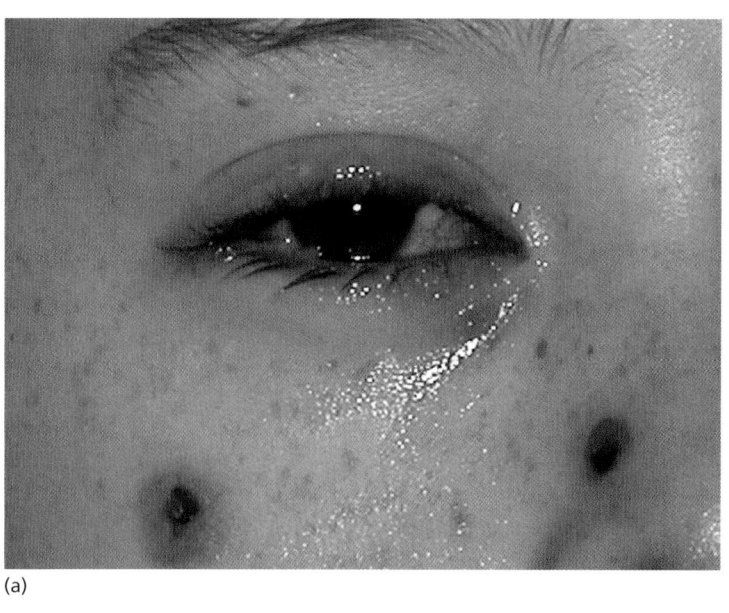

(a)

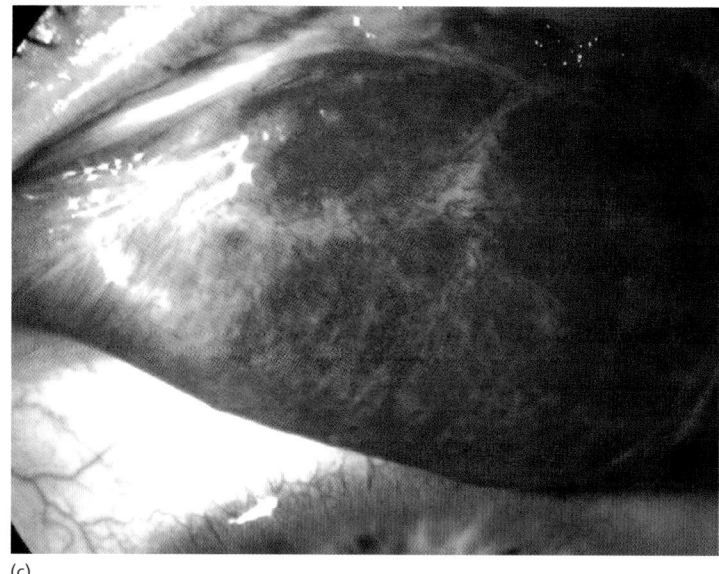

(c)

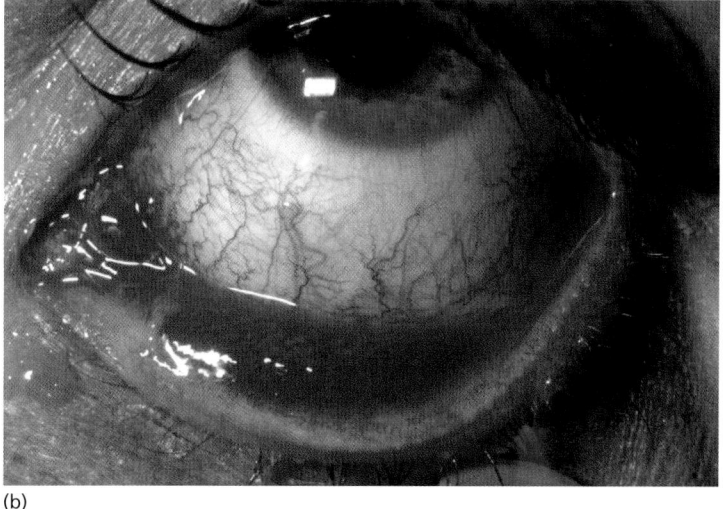

(b)

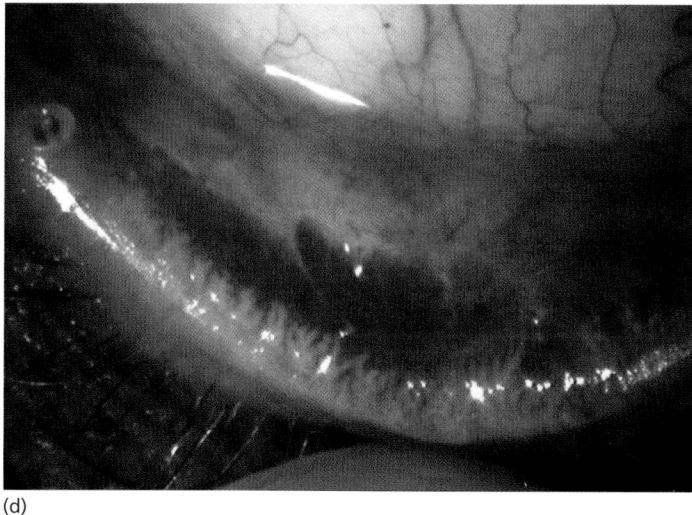

(d)

Figure 109.19 Ocular disease in Stevens–Johnson syndrome. (a) Acute conjunctivitis with mucus discharge occurring concurrently with typical erythema multiforme skin lesions. (b) Acute conjunctivitis in a patient with mild Stevens–Johnson syndrome. The conjunctiva is hyperaemic with a papillary reaction and mucopurulent discharge. (Courtesy of Mr J. Dart, Moorfields Eye Hospital, London, UK.) (c) Upper tarsal conjunctival scarring in Stevens–Johnson syndrome. (d) Lower tarsal conjunctival scarring with squamous metaplasia and keratinization adjacent to the mucocutaneous junction of the lower lid. A punctal plug is *in situ*, to conserve tears in a dry eye. (e) The late ocular complications of Stevens–Johnson syndrome showing entropion, a dry eye with ocular surface failure (in this case an opaque keratinized epithelium).

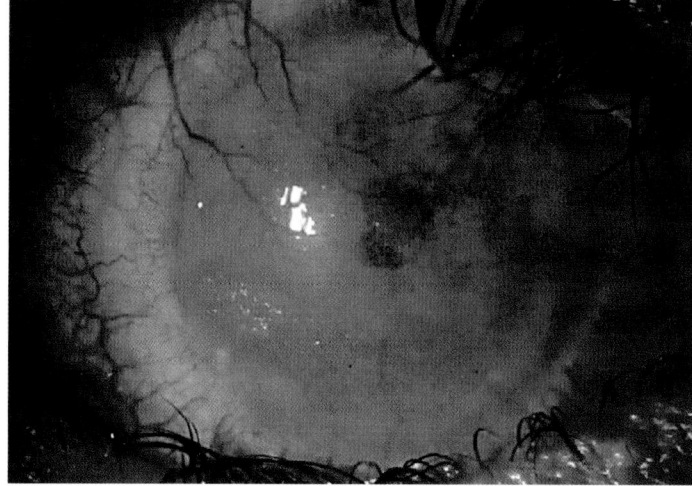

(e)

PART 10: SITES, SEX, AGE

Management of chronic ocular SJS/TEN includes management of severe dry eye, trichiasis and entropion [43], limbal stem cell deficiency and inflammation. Systemic immunosuppression may be needed if inflammatory complications of chronic disease (e.g. recurrent inflammation, secondary ocular MMP) do not respond to topical therapies. The immunosuppressive therapy strategy for ocular SJS/TEN is similar to that of cicatrizing conjunctivitis in MMP, apart from avoidance of sulpha agents which may precipitate SJS/TEN [38].

Graft-versus-host disease [44,45]. Ocular complications are common (60–90%) in patients with GVHD, and typically result from involvement of both the conjunctiva and the lacrimal gland (see also Chapter 38). The spectrum of chronic GVHD varies from dry eye to sight-threatening surface inflammation, scarring and, in rare cases, perforation, which may present many months after the bone marrow allograft. Notably, severe ocular disease can occur in the absence of systemic GVHD. Ocular GVHD can lead to loss of vision due to corneal involvement. In acute GVHD, conjunctivitis ranges from hyperaemia through chemosis to a pseudomembranous conjunctivitis, with or without corneal epithelial sloughing. Severe conjunctival involvement is a marker for the severity of acute GVHD, occurring in 12% of patients, and is a poor prognostic factor for mortality [44]. In chronic GVHD, conjunctival involvement has been observed in 11% of patients, for whom it was also associated with disease severity. Some of these patients develop a severe scarring response like that of MMP. Lacrimal gland involvement occurs in about 50% of patients with chronic GVHD who develop a Sjögren syndrome type picture of dry eyes. The pathogenesis of the conjunctival disease has been examined in a few cases and appears to be similar to that in the skin. Involvement of panophthalmic structures can sometimes be evident in chronic GVHD. Although dry eye and cicatrizing conjunctivitis are the commonest (90%) ocular findings in GVHD, choroiditis, retinitis and scleritis may also occur.

Anti-inflammatory treatments, particularly T-cell suppressants, can help manage GVHD. Topical anti-inflammatory therapy with steroids, and steroid-sparing calcineurin inhibitors such as ciclosporin and tacrolimus should be instituted early in the course of the disease [45]. Autologous serum eye drops have beneficial effects. Antifibrotic agents such as tranilast may also help.

Systemic diseases with skin and eye involvement

Some multisystem diseases affect both the skin and eye [1,2–23]. It is not possible to catalogue every complication of all these diseases but the most frequent are summarized in Table 109.11.

INFECTIONS

A number of infections involve the eyelids, but the following are important to recognize because they are common or require urgent therapy or referral to an ophthalmologist [1].

VIRAL INFECTIONS

Warts

Clinical features
These are common and found on the eyelid margins, often as a long thin (filiform) projection (Figure 109.20).

Management
Lesions in this site are best treated with careful cryotherapy and accurate application of liquid nitrogen to the tip of the lesion using a cotton wool bud rather than cryospray.

Molluscum contagiosum [2]

Clinical features
This condition mainly affects children and young adults (see Chapter 25). It is also prevalent in patients with AIDS, who may develop multiple lesions around the eyelids. As elsewhere on the skin, typical lesions arise as dome-shaped papules with a central umbilication. Lesions may grow in the lash line as well as on the lid skin and occasionally, on the mucocutaneous junction. Lesions can be easily overlooked or mistaken for an epidermoid cyst; this condition must always be considered in the differential diagnosis of patients with unilateral or bilateral follicular conjunctivitis. There is associated conjunctival discharge and a variable, often severe, follicular conjunctival response (Figure 109.21). A superficial epithelial keratitis may develop in longstanding cases which progresses to pannus formation across the cornea.

Management
Treatment involves removal of the lesions by curettage. Cryotherapy is also effective, but this may cause loss of pigment in pigmented skins. In a cooperative adult this can be done under local anaesthetic but for children a general anaesthetic is required.

Herpes simplex virus [3,4,5]

Clinical features
Primary herpes simplex virus infection is asymptomatic in many patients; in others it causes blepharoconjunctivitis (see Chapter 25). However, most of the ocular manifestations of herpes simplex virus infection are due to reactivation of latent infection in the trigeminal ganglion. Both the primary infection, and reactivation of latent disease, may be particularly severe in patients with atopic eczema or with immunodeficiency. The blepharoconjunctivitis of herpes simplex virus usually results in crops of small vesicles, which may be associated with mild oedema of the lids

Table 109.11 Systemic diseases with skin and eye involvement.

Systemic disease	Eye disease
Sarcoidosis *Epidemiology*: ocular involvement the presenting feature in 10%; 20–30% of patients have eye disease at some stage [1–7]	*Lids and orbital findings*: clusters of granulomatous eyelid swellings. Proptosis from orbital granulomas. Dry eye from lacrimal gland involvement *Heerfordt syndrome*: (uveoparotid fever) consists of uveitis and parotid gland enlargement, fever and facial nerve palsy. *Lofgren syndrome*: acute iritis, bilateral hilar lymphadenopathy, erythema nodosum and arthralgia. *Mikulicz syndrome*: bilateral swelling of lacrimal and salivary glands *Anterior segment findings*: conjunctivitis: occasionally a granulomatous conjunctivitis mimicking a follicular conjunctivitis. *Uveitis*: usually, but not always, bilateral granulomatous anterior uveitis in 80% of patients with eye manifestations with redness, pain, photophobia and blurred vision with floaters *Posterior segment findings*: rare
Systemic lupus erythematosus [8–10]	*Anterior segment findings*: dry eye, peripheral corneal ulcers. Scleritis is rare. Episcleritis occurs in 10% causing a red eye *Posterior segment findings*: retinal vasculitis common during exacerbations of systemic disease with flame shaped haemorrhages and cotton wool spots. May be associated with severe central nervous system vasculitis or lupus nephritis
Sjögren syndrome [11]	*Lids and orbital findings*: lacrimal gland inflammation causing dry eye *Anterior segment findings*: symptoms: often severe with chronic discomfort, foreign body sensation, dryness and blurred vision. Conjunctiva: conjunctivitis and scarring in some cases. *Cornea*: punctate keratopathy, persistent corneal epithelial defects leading to corneal ulceration and perforation or corneal infection
Reactive arthritis (formerly Reiter syndrome) *Epidemiology*: ocular involvement in about 30% of patients [1]	*Anterior segment findings (symptoms)*: red irritable eyes resolving spontaneously within 7–10 days *Conjunctiva*: bilateral mucopurulent conjunctivitis is the most frequent manifestation affecting approximately 30% of patients; this usually follows a urethritis by about 2 weeks and precedes the onset of arthritis. *Cornea*: keratitis may occur in isolation and is rare. *Uveitis*: anterior uveitis (iritis) occurs in about 20% of patients either with the first attack of Reiter syndrome or during a recurrence
Behçet syndrome *Epidemiology*: ocular involvement in 60–70% of patients [12,13]	*Anterior segment findings*: external eye diseases: conjunctivitis, keratitis and episcleritis may occur but are not specific for the condition. *Uveitis*: is the commonest manifestation of the disease *Posterior segment findings*: visual impairment or blindness is a frequent complication of Behçet syndrome as a result of the retinal ischaemia
Inflammatory bowel disease *Epidemiology*: ocular manifestations in about 5% of patients [14,15]	*Anterior segment findings*: external eye diseases: conjunctivitis, limbitis, peripheral corneal infiltrates and episcleritis may occur. *Uveitis*: acute iritis in about 5% of patients which may occur at the same time as exacerbation of colitis
AIDS *Epidemiology*: ocular complications occur in about 75% of patients [16,19]	*Common features*: (i) opportunistic infections with viruses, mycobacteria and fungi; (ii) malignancies, e.g. Kaposi sarcoma; (iii) retinal microangiopathy; and (iv) neuro-ophthalmic lesions with intracranial infections and tumours *Anterior segment findings*: external eye diseases: *Molluscum contagiosum* is a common ocular finding in patients with AIDS, they tend to be large and when located on the lid margin can give rise to follicular conjunctivitis. The lesions can be complicated by epithelial keratitis with associated pannus formation. *Kaposi sarcoma* may involve the lids and conjunctiva. *Herpes simplex* keratitis tends to be severe with more frequent relapses. The peripheral cornea is more often involved in contrast to central disease in immunocompetent patients. *Herpes zoster ophthalmicus* is common and may be a presenting feature of HIV infection, especially if severe disease presents in young patients *Posterior segment findings*: retinal microangiopathy is common and characterized by retinal haemorrhages, microaneurysms and cotton wool spots. *Cytomegalovirus* retinitis and *Pneumocystis carinii* choroiditis are serious ophthalmic complications signifying severe systemic involvement
Porphyria [20,21]	*Common feature*: ocular involvement results from either photosensitization and/or neurological dysfunction. Photosensitization can affect the eyelids, conjunctiva, cornea, sclera and possibly the retina *Lids and orbital findings*: inflammation can lead to vesicle and bulla formation, secondary infection scarring with ectropion and hyperpigmentation *Neuro-ophthalmic complications*: include optic neuritis, optic atrophy, ptosis and cranial nerve palsies
Granulomatosis with polyangiitis [22]	Episcleritis is very common in active stages. Also retinal vasculitis, optic neuritis, orbital pseudotumour
Polyarteritis nodosa	Episcleritis, scleritis and keratitis

with or without associated conjunctivitis (Figure 109.22a). As with herpes simplex virus elsewhere, the vesicles dry to a crust and heal within a few days. Neither the blepharitis nor conjunctivitis present a serious problem for most patients. The serious and sight-threatening ocular complications of herpes simplex virus infection of the eye are due to recurrent keratitis or keratouveitis. Herpetic keratitis may affect the epithelium alone (dendritic keratitis; Figure 109.22b), the stroma (in stromal herpetic keratitis (Figure 109.22c), geographical corneal ulceration and metaherpetic keratitis (Figure 109.22d) or the endothelium (disciform keratitis

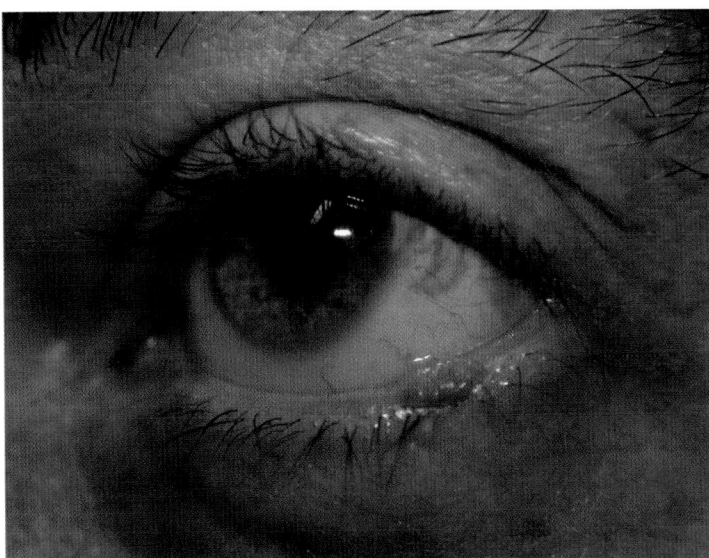

Figure 109.20 Wart on the eyelid.

or herpetic endotheliitis) Figure 109.22e). Dendritic keratitis is in itself a benign disease unless treated with topical corticosteroids when the disease will rapidly spread, resulting in geographical keratitis, which may cause destructive corneal disease. Most cases of corneal disease represent reactivation of latent herpes simplex virus and patients may develop any of the corneal manifestations. Stromal and endothelial disease can progress to blinding corneal vascularization, scarring (Figure 109.22f) and ulceration. Fortunately, the disease is normally unilateral, except in atopic individuals when it may often be bilateral.

Management

Because of the difficulties of managing the ocular manifestations of this disease, patients with suspected herpes simplex virus involvement of the eye should be referred for urgent ophthalmological assessment. The conjunctivitis can be treated with aciclovir ointment five times a day for 5 days or with oral aciclovir 400 mg five times per day for 5 days. Topical steroids must not be used alone

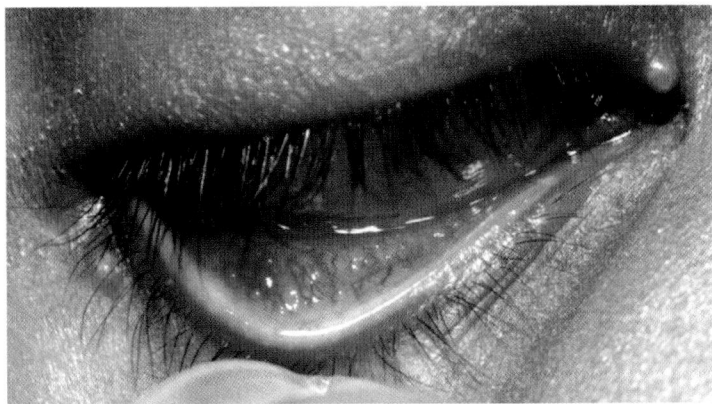

Figure 109.21 Molluscum contagiosum at the medial aspect of the upper lid margin with an associated follicular conjunctivitis. (Courtesy of Mr J. Dart, Moorfields Eye Hospital, London, UK.)

as these will mask the symptoms and signs, leading to spread of the ulcer and corneal perforation with disastrous consequences for the patient's vision. Dendritic keratitis may occur during treatment with topical corticosteroids. The management of the stromal and endothelial keratitis is beyond the scope of this review except to state that it involves the judicious use of topical corticosteroids with systemic or topical antivirals. Keratouveitis involves the endothelium and stroma and may be associated with secondary glaucoma.

Herpes zoster [6–10]

Clinical features

Herpes zoster of the ophthalmic division (HZO) of the trigeminal nerve (Figure 109.23a) is an important condition to recognize (see Chapter 25). As occurs when it affects other sites, it often presents with a non-specific flu-like illness with fever and malaise and symptoms of unilateral neuralgia. This develops over the distribution of the affected nerve and varies in severity from a mild tingling in the skin to a deep severe pain. The characteristic lesions of herpes zoster may appear up to a week after the initial symptoms. Erythematous macules develop into clusters of papules and vesicles becoming pustular and haemorrhagic after 3–4 days. The lesions then scab and are dry by 7–14 days, separating to leave pitted scars. Involvement of the nasociliary nerve, which supplies the skin on the side of the nose, occurs in about 35% of patients and vesicles at this site (Hutchinson sign) are associated with a high risk of ophthalmic complications. Ocular involvement may occur in the absence of nasociliary involvement but it is usually milder. Herpes zoster sine eruptione can cause ocular complications without the cutaneous eruption. It is rare but evidence of the infection can be found by polymerase chain reaction analysis of the aqueous fluid or sequential titres of varicella zoster virus antibodies. Patients whose eyes cannot be examined due to persistent lid oedema, or those with ocular signs and symptoms, should be referred for urgent ophthalmological assessment. The disease can affect any part of the eye, including the orbit, extraocular muscles, optic nerve and cornea, and may give rise to long-term complications including severe relapsing keratitis, glaucoma and cataract. The commonest ocular complications are dendritiform keratopathy (Figure 109.23b), stromal keratitis and uveitis (Figure 109.23c).

Management

Antiviral drugs reduce the duration and severity of acute herpes zoster but must be given within the first 3 days of the onset of the rash to be effective. Oral aciclovir has been the standard therapy at doses of 800 mg five times a day for 7–10 days. Valaciclovir (1000 mg three times per day) or famciclovir (500 mg three times per day for 7 days) are now preferred because of simpler dosing regimens and superior pharmacokinetics. Topical aciclovir is not indicated and unhelpful in almost all aspects of herpes zoster affecting the cornea, which respond to topical steroid treatment alone. One exception to this is late dendritiform lesions on the

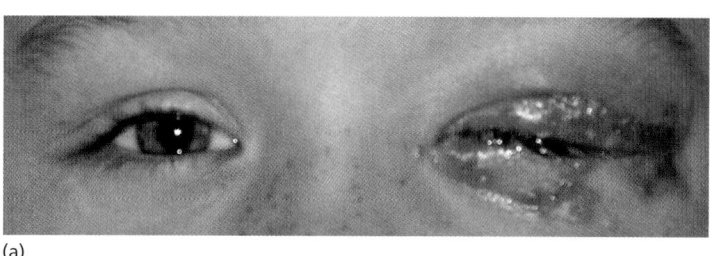

(a)

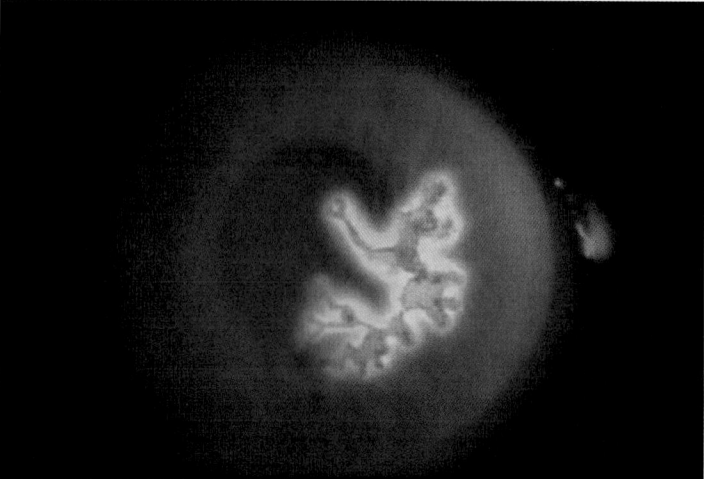

(b)

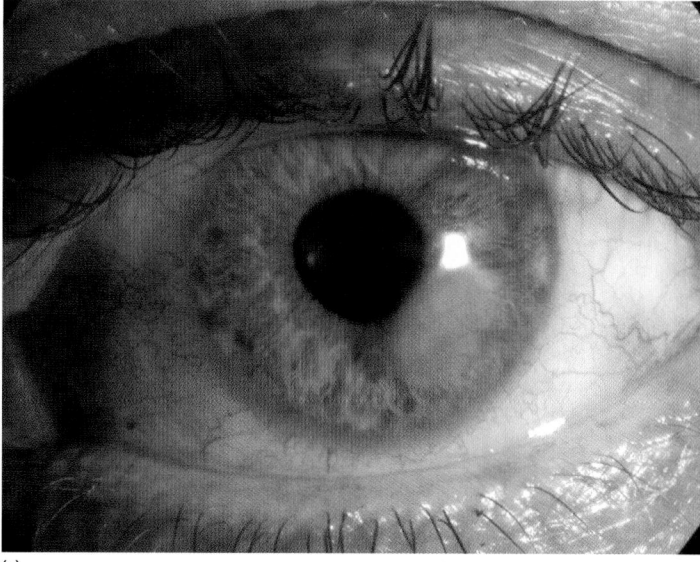

(c)

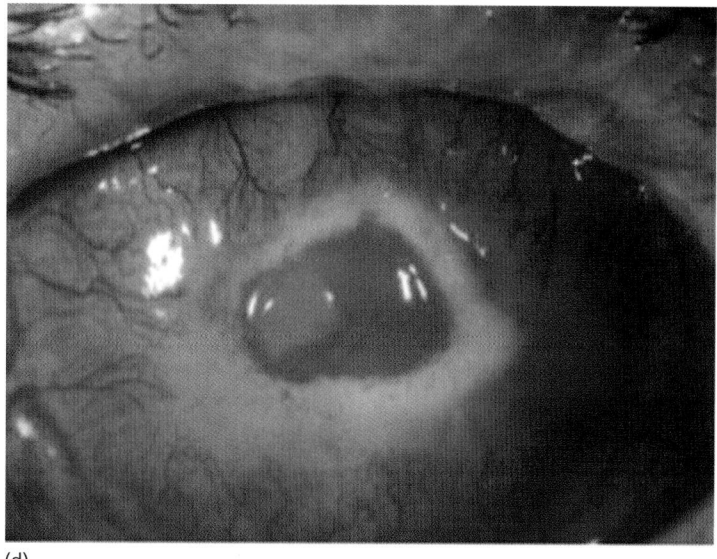

(d)

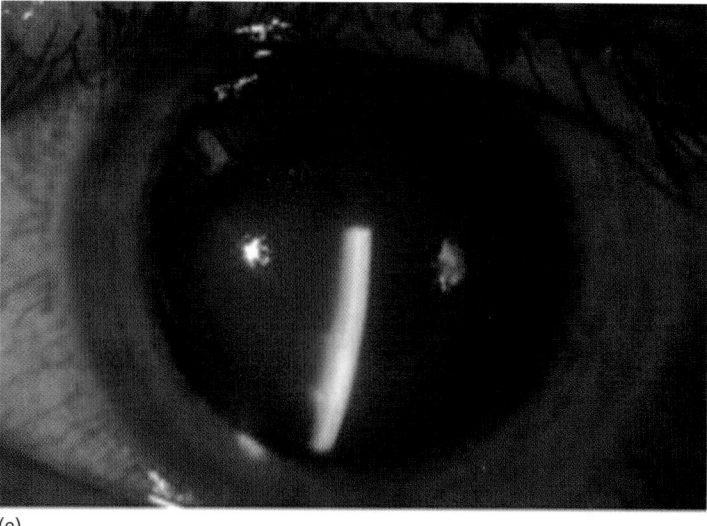

(e)

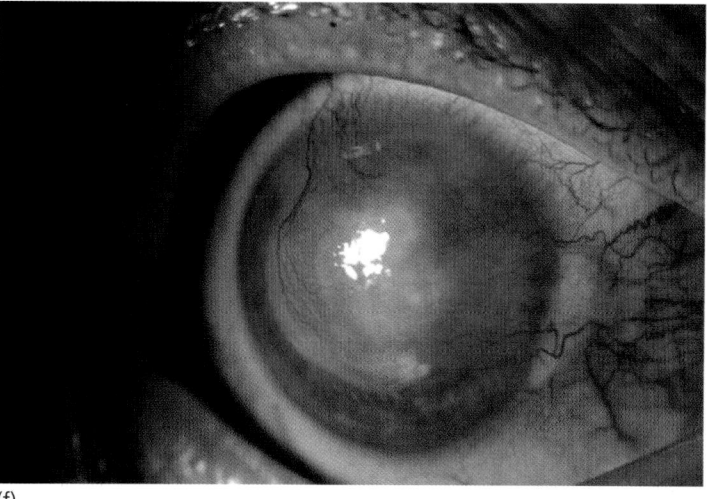

(f)

Figure 109.22 Herpes simplex virus. (a) Primary herpes simplex blepharoconjunctivitis in a child. (b) Dendritic epithelial keratitis. (c) Stromal herpetic keratitis. (d) Metaherpetic keratitis. (Courtesy of Mr J. Dart, Moorfields Eye Hospital, London, UK.) (e) Herpetic endotheliitis. (f) Herpetic corneal vascularization and scarring.

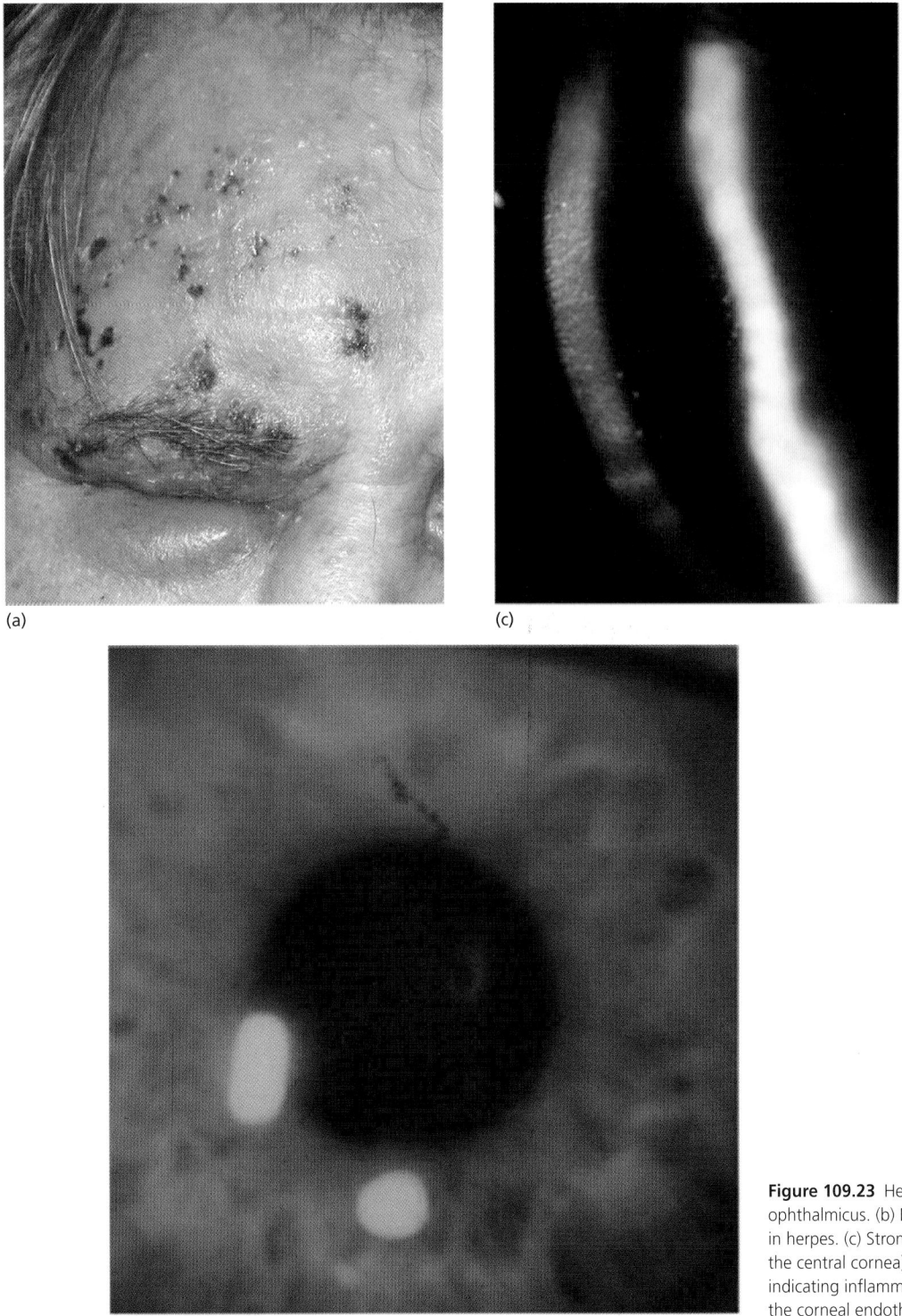

(a)

(c)

(b)

Figure 109.23 Herpes zoster. (a) Herpes zoster ophthalmicus. (b) Dendritiform keratopathy in herpes. (c) Stromal keratitis (opacity in the central cornea) and uveitis (white dots indicating inflammatory cells are deposited on the corneal endothelium, due to inflammation in the anterior chamber of the eye).

cornea in herpes zoster, which have been shown to be foci of productive varicella zoster virus [10], and thus require topical or systemic antiviral treatment in addition to topical steroids. Topical corticosteroid therapy is necessary control the numerous corneal manifestations of the disease and may need to be continued for several years. Some of these complications may be delayed and occur months after the initial skin eruption.

Prolonged or severe post-herpetic neuralgia is a painful and unpleasant sequel to herpes zoster infection. It occurs in about half of elderly patients but is rare in children. There is some evidence that the use of amitriptyline in the early stages of infection is helpful in reducing the incidence and severity. Oral corticosteroids given concurrently with the antivirals may reduce the severity of post-herpetic neuralgia in some patients.

BACTERIAL INFECTIONS

Staphylococcal infections

Impetigo

Clinical features

Impetigo is a common skin infection that mainly affects children (see Chapter 26). It can involve the eyelids, but usually as part of a general infection over the face. It presents as rapidly spreading erythematous macules, developing into flaccid vesicles that subsequently rupture to give rise to surface crusting.

Management

The lesions need to be swabbed for bacteriology and appropriate oral and topical antibiotics given.

Hordeolum

Clinical features

External hordeolum (stye) is caused by staphylococcal infection of an eyelash follicle and its associated glands. It presents with a tender red inflamed swelling on the lid margin, which subsequently points anteriorly and discharges close to the lash roots (Figure 109.24a).

Management

No treatment is usually required beyond the application of local soothing compresses and removal of the affected lash. If there is a local cellulitis then systemic antibiotics should be given. An internal hordeolum is a staphylococcal abscess of the meibomian glands (Figure 109.24b) and needs incision and drainage.

Streptococcal infections

Erysipelas [11]

Clinical features

This represents subcutaneous spreading cellulitis, usually caused by β-haemolytic *Streptococcus* (see Chapter 26). It usually presents with a rigor followed by a red raised erythematous plaque with a well-demarcated edge that spreads rapidly over the skin.

Management

Erysipelas is a serious skin infection that needs to be treated urgently with appropriate systemic antibiotics.

Necrotizing fasciitis [12]

Clinical features

This is a very rare condition, most commonly caused by *Streptococcus*, which mainly affects elderly or debilitated patients (see Chapter 26). A spreading purple discoloration of the eyelid rapidly progresses to gangrene. Unlike erysipelas, the periorbital tissue is not usually affected.

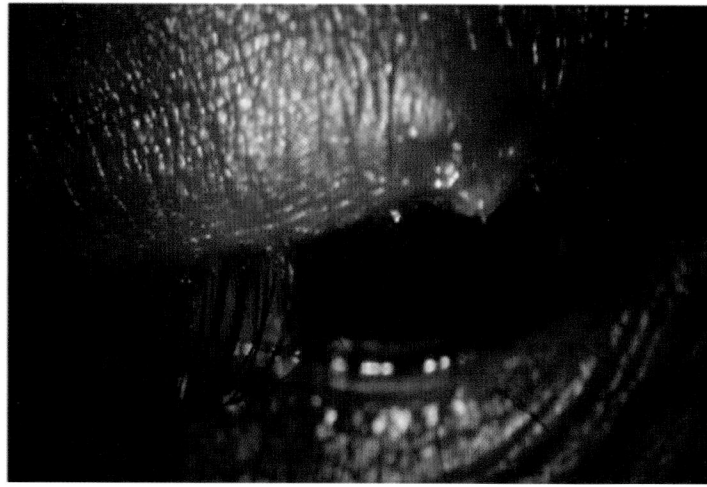

(a)

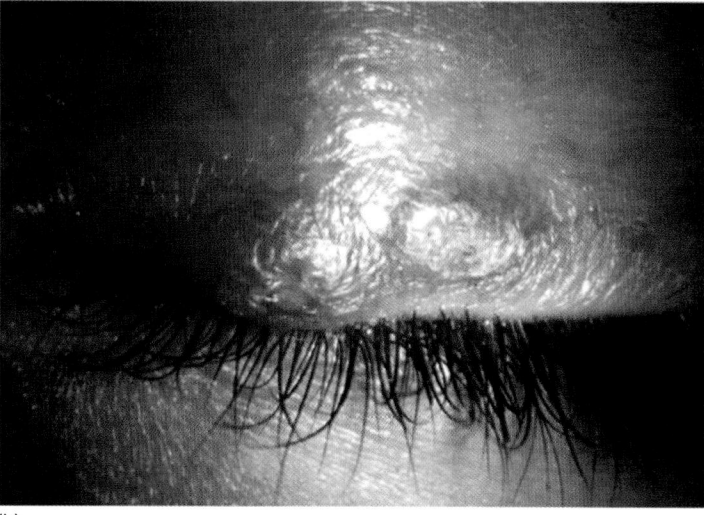

(b)

Figure 109.24 (a) External hordeolum (stye). (b) Internal hordeolum (infected chalazion) which has spontaneously discharged anteriorly through the skin, which is not uncommon. There is a large lesion on the left and a smaller lesion on the right.

Management

Early recognition, immediate institution of intravenous antibiotics and referral to an ophthalmic plastic surgeon for debridement of the necrotic tissue are mandatory as the condition carries a high mortality.

MYCOBACTERIAL INFECTIONS

Tuberculosis

Clinical features

There are no specific ocular findings in tuberculosis, and diagnosis is often based on indirect evidence such as intractable uveitis that is unresponsive to corticosteroid therapy, with negative findings for other causes of uveitis, and in the presence of tuberculosis at a distant body site (see Chapter 27). Chronic iridocyclitis, which is usually granulomatous, is the commonest feature. Choroiditis and retinal vasculitis may occur.

Management
Appropriate antituberculous chemotherapy should be given.

Leprosy [13,14]

Clinical features
Ocular complications of leprosy are common, most frequently madarosis, conjunctivitis, episcleritis or scleritis (see Chapter 28). Keratitis results from a combination of corneal anaesthesia, lagophthalmus, trichiasis and secondary infection. Iritis and its complications are the most common causes of blindness and leprosy. Lepromatous disease is more commonly associated with uveitis than is tuberculoid leprosy.

Management
Appropriate antilepromatous chemotherapy should be given.

TREPONEMAL INFECTIONS

Syphilis [15]

Clinical features
Ocular syphilis is very rare and there are no pathognomonic signs (see Chapter 29). Eye involvement mainly occurs during the secondary and tertiary stages, though primary chancre of the conjunctiva may occur. External features include madarosis, scleritis and interstitial keratitis. Uveitis and chorioretinitis are rare but serious complications of syphilis and lead to blindness. Neuro-ophthalmic features include Argyll Robertson pupils, optic nerve lesions, and palsies of the third and sixth cranial nerves. Gummatous involvement of the brain can cause visual field defects.

Management
Patients with suspected ocular syphilis should be referred to physicians for assessment and therapy. Their ophthalmic involvement should be treated by an ophthalmologist with expertise in managing the condition.

Lyme disease [16,17]

Clinical features
Ocular manifestations of Lyme disease involve all parts of the eye (see Chapter 26). As with syphilis, the ocular manifestations vary according to the stage of the disease. In stage 1, a localized conjunctivitis with photophobia occurs in 10% of patients. This is mild and brief, and ophthalmologists are rarely consulted. In stage 2, various ophthalmic complications have been described including cranial nerve palsies; these may occur within 1 month of the rash appearing. It is in the late stage 3 that most of the severe ocular complications are seen, including episcleritis, symblepharon, interstitial keratitis, uveitis, chorioretinitis and retinal vasculitis.

Management
Patients with suspected ocular involvement with Lyme disease should be referred to an ophthalmologist with a specific interest in the disease for assessment and management of the ocular complications.

PARASITIC INFECTIONS

Phthiriasis (lice) [18,19]

Clinical features
This is an infestation of the eyelashes by the pubic louse, *Phthirus pubis* (see Chapter 34). It mainly affects children and causes chronic itching, irritation and rubbing of the lids. As with louse infection elsewhere, the adult lice can be difficult to see, though nits (eggs) and their shells are visible, adhering to the eyelashes (see Figure 109.9c,d). The skin nearest to the base of the lashes may show small bluish spots due to the louse bites (maculae caeruleae).

Management
A number of measures have been used to treat louse infestation of the eyelids, including mechanical removal with forceps, epilation and trimming of infested lashes, and application of fluorescein, occlusive ointments (e.g. petrolatum) or aqueous malathion for 7–10 days.

Filariasis (onchocerciasis) [20]

Clinical features
Onchocerciasis or river blindness is caused by the filarial organism, *Onchocerca volvulus* (see Chapter 33). It is the second most common cause of preventable blindness in sub-Saharan Africa with an estimated prevalence of 500000 cases with visual impairment and 270000 with blindness. It appears that *Wolbachia endobacteria*, a bacterial symbiont, produces an endotoxin-like product which constitutes a major pro-inflammatory stimulus in the eye, causing corneal inflammation and sclerosing keratitis.

Management
Patients with suspected ocular onchocerciasis should be referred to an ophthalmologist with a special interest in tropical diseases for assessment and management.

OTHER INFECTIONS

Protozoal infections

Clinical features
Ocular disease may complicate leishmaniasis. In *Leishmania donovani* infection, bilateral retinal haemorrhages may be a feature (see Chapter 26). In *L. tropica* and *L. braziliasis* infection, eyelid (see Figure 109.9f,g) and corneal lesions occur, and subsequent destruction may lead to loss of the eye. In trypanosomiasis, unilateral oedema of the lids may occur.

Management
Patients with suspected ocular complications of leishmaniasis should be referred to an ophthalmologist with a special interest in the management of tropical diseases for assessment and management.

OTHER DISORDERS

Inherited disorders

A large number of inherited disorders affect the skin and eyes. Major reference texts are cited in [1–3]. The main ocular features are summarized in Table 109.12 [4–51].

Ocular complications of dermatological therapy

A number of drugs used by dermatologists have significant side effects on the eye and require careful monitoring.

Corticosteroids [1–15]
The use of corticosteroids can cause significant side effects on the eye. Both systemic and topical corticosteroids are responsible, though the greatest risk is to those receiving prednisolone at a dose of 10–15 mg/day for over a year. Continuous therapy is more likely to cause side effects than intermittent therapy.

Posterior subcapsular cataracts (Figure 109.25) are induced by long-term systemic corticosteroids in as many as 30% of patients. They rarely occur at doses less than 10 mg/day and for less than 1 year. Children are particularly vulnerable. Reversibility of cataracts is not common and progression of cataracts may occur in spite of reduction or discontinuation of corticosteroid therapy.

Patients also risk developing open angle glaucoma, particularly if genetically predisposed. The precise mechanism is unknown, though it is thought to be due to decreased aqueous outflow. Particular risk factors include type 1 diabetes, high myopia, connective tissue disorders and a family history of glaucoma. Topical corticosteroids induce a rise in intraocular pressure more quickly than systemic corticosteroids. Medium- or high-potency dermatological corticosteroids applied for long periods to, or near, the eyelids may spread over the lid margin and are absorbed through the cornea, reaching sufficient concentrations to elevate ocular pressures. Patients on long-term topical or systemic corticosteroids need to have their eye pressures monitored regularly at 1–6 monthly intervals depending on their degree of risk.

Topical corticosteroids predispose patients to cataract, glaucoma and secondary surface infection. Injudicious use in herpes simplex virus infection masks the clinical signs of dendritic ulcer and risks perforation. Wearing a soft contact lens is a contraindication to topical ocular corticosteroid usage. Other ocular complications from corticosteroids include angioneurotic oedema, papilloedema (Figure 109.25b) from raised intracranial pressure and toxic amblyopia. Systemic treatment with corticosteroids may cause serous chorioretinopathy or diffuse retinal pigment epitheliopathy.

Oral retinoids [16–21,22]
Both isotretinoin and acitretin can cause ocular side effects. The most common is dry eye with associated conjunctivitis and blepharoconjunctivitis, giving rise to blurred vision. The blepharoconjunctivitis is frequently associated with staphylococcal infection. Exposure keratopathy and corneal ulceration rarely occur; asymptomatic corneal opacities may develop but resolve after 6–8 weeks. Patients should be warned that they may be unable to tolerate contact lenses whilst on retinoid therapy. Use of tear substitutes, humidification of the environment and lid hygiene measures help. Retinal abnormalities may also occur, with poor night vision and increased sensitivity to glare, and can be a significant problem in those who drive at night; pilots are not allowed to fly whilst taking isotretinoin due to the potential effects on night vision. The cause is unknown but may be due to competitive inhibition of ocular retinol dehydrogenase causing local vitamin A deficiency and reduction in rhodopsin formation. More serious side effects include papilloedema from raised intracranial pressure, optic atrophy and cataract. Although these are rare, a history of visual disturbance should be asked for when patients come for follow-up. Severe headache early in the course of treatment is significant. The ocular manifestations are dose dependent and usually reversible, provided they are recognized and the treatment regimen adjusted. However, there have been reports of severe dry eye syndrome and night blindness persisting after retinoids have been discontinued.

Antimalarials [23–26,27]
The most serious potential side effect of antimalarial drugs is retinopathy. The mechanism is uncertain but seems to depend on the ability of the drug to bind the retinal pigment epithelium. Ocular side effects from antimalarials are much less common now that hydroxychloroquine rather than chloroquine is the drug of choice. However, both drugs should be used with caution in patients with hepatic or renal impairment. The Royal College of Ophthalmologists and American Academy of Ophthalmologists

Table 109.12 Inherited disorders affecting the skin and eyes.

Group	Condition	Inheritance	Ocular features
Bullous disorders	Acrodermatitis enteropathica [4]	AR (MIM 201100)	Loss of eyebrows and eyelashes, conjunctivitis, blepharitis, photophobia
Connective tissue disorder	Ehlers–Danlos syndrome [5]	Mainly AD (MIM 130000)	Lax eyelid skin with redundant folds, epicanthal folds, hypertelorism, strabismus, blue sclera, corneal abnormalities including keratoconus, angioid streaks, ectopic lens. Retinal detachments occasionally occur
	Marfan syndrome [6]	AD (MIM 154700)	Subluxation of lens – 60–80% of patients in early childhood. Amblyopia, myopia, cataract, corneal abnormalities, glaucoma. Retinal detachment is the most serious complication
	Pseudoxanthoma elasticum [7]	Types I and II AR (MIM 264800, 264810) Types III and IV AD (MIM 177850, 177860)	Angioid streaks (breaks in Bruch membrane) in majority. Haemorrhagic maculopathy after trauma may cause visual loss
Dysplasias, hyperplasia, atrophies and aplasias	Ablepharon macrostomia [8] syndrome	Unknown (MIM 200110)	Absent eyelids and ectropion
	Aplasia cutis congenita [9]	AD (MIM 107600) AR (MIM 207700)	Congenital absence of skin leading to eyelid colobomas, corneal opacities, scleral dermoids and lamellar cataracts
	Blepharophimosis ptosis epicanthus inversus syndrome [10]	AD (MIM 110100)	Blepharophimosis, ptosis, epicanthus inversus, telecanthus. Amblyopia in 50% of patients
	Cockayne syndrome [11]	AR (MIM 216400)	Corneal opacities, cataracts in 30%, retinitis pigmentosa, optic atrophy, strabismus, photophobia
	Dyskeratosis congenita [12]	XR (MIM 305000)	Obliteration of the lacrimal puncta in 80% of cases, conjunctivitis, blepharitis, ectropion, loss of eyelashes and eyebrows
	Ectodermal dysplasias – a complex group of disorders with various inheritance patterns and a variety of ocular findings [13] Examples are as follows:		
	(i) Christ–Siemens–Touraine syndrome	XR (MIM 305100)	Photophobia, dry eye
	(ii) Fischer–Jacobsen–Clouston syndrome	AD	Usually normal
	(iii) Ellis–van Creveld syndrome	AR (MIM 225500)	Coloboma of iris, microphthalmia, occasional cataract
	Focal dermal hypoplasia (Goltz syndrome) [14]	XD (MIM 305600)	40% have ocular abnormalities, the commonest being colobomas of iris, choroid, retina or optic nerve
	Fraser syndrome [15]	AR (MIM 219000)	Bilateral or unilateral absence of palpebral fissure with loss of eyebrows, anophthalmia, microphthalmia
	Frydman syndrome [16]	AR	Synophrys, blepharophimosis, weakness of extraocular and frontal muscles
	Hallermann–Streiff syndrome [17]	Unknown (MIM 264090)	Loss of hair of eyebrows and eyelashes, microphthalmos, cataracts, amblyopia and nystagmus
	MIDAS syndrome (MCOPS7) [18]	XD (MIM 309801)	Microphthalmia, sclerocorneal
	Pachyonychia congenita (PC) [19]	AD (PC1 MIM 167200) PC2 (MIM 167210)	Cataract and corneal dyskeratosis
Hair disorders	Brachmann–Lange syndrome [20]	AR	Synophrys, long thick eyelashes, narrow palpebral fissure, myopia, nystagmus and strabismus
	Monilethrix [21]	AD (MIM 158000)	Loss of eyebrows and lashes
	Pili torti [22]	AR (MIM 261900)	Loss of eyebrows and lashes
	Chondrodysplasia punctata [23]	AD (MIM 215105) XR (MIM 302950)	Cataracts Ocular albinism, cataracts, microphthalmia
Keratinization disorders	The ichthyoses [24]		
	(i) Ichthyosis congenita gravis	AR (MIM 242500)	Severe ectropion
	(ii) Ichthyosiform erythroderma	AD (MIM 242100)	Early development of ectropion is characteristic
	(iii) Lamellar ichthyosis	AR (various types)	Cicatricial ectropion with exposure keratitis Direct conjunctival involvement may occur
	(iv) X-linked ichthyosis	XI (MIM 308100)	Deep corneal opacities
	KID syndrome [25]	XD (MIM 148210)	Keratitis
	Refsum syndrome [26]	AR (MIM 266500)	Night blindness, posterior subcapsular cataracts develop in most cases
	Sjögren–Larsson syndrome [27]	AR (MIM 270200)	Blepharitis, conjunctivitis, punctate corneal erosions and pigmentary degeneration of the retina
	Ulerythema ophryogenes [28]	AD	Erythema and perifollicular papules on eye to eyebrows spreading medially causing thinning of eyebrows (occurs in keratosis pilaris, Noonan syndrome, cardiofaciocutaneous syndrome)

Group	Condition	Inheritance	Ocular features
Metabolic disorders	Alkaptonuria [29]	AR (MIM 203500)	Scleral pigmentation is early sign, eyelid pigmentation
	Angiokeratoma corporis diffusum [30]	XL (MIM 301500)	Angiokeratomas of conjunctiva, corneal opacities, posterior capsular cataracts
	Homocystinuria [31]	AR (MIM 236200)	Myopia, cataracts, subluxation of lens, secondary glaucoma, retinal detachment
	Hurler syndrome [32]	AR (MIM 252800)	Early clouding of cornea
Neurocutaneous syndromes	Richner–Hanhart syndrome [33]	AR (MIM 276600)	Corneal lesions vary from erosions to deep ulcers
			Nystagmus and lens opacities
	Neurofibromatosis type I [34]	AD (MIM 162200)	Neurofibromas of eyelid, corneal clouding, Lisch nodules of iris, optic nerve glioma, palsies from cranial nerve involvement
	Neurofibromatosis type II	AD (MIM 101000)	Cataract fundus lesions, extraocular motility abnormalities
	Tuberous sclerosis [35]	AD (MIM 191100)	Tumours of the lids or nodules on conjunctiva and retina
Photosensitive disorders	Basal cell naevus syndrome [36]	AD (MIM 109400)	Basal cell carcinoma of eyelid and periorbital area, hypertelorism, strabismus, colobomas of the choroid, cataracts, glaucomas in 5–10%
	Bloom syndrome [37]	AD (MIM 210900)	Telangiectasis on lower lids, blistering and scarring lower eyelids
	Rothmund–Thomson syndrome [38]	AR (MIM 268400)	Sparse eyebrows and eyelashes, degenerative changes in cornea, 50% of patients have bilateral cataracts which develop in childhood, strabismus
	Xeroderma pigmentosum [39]	AR (various types)	Angiomas, keratoses, papillomas, carcinomas develop on eyelids, sometimes extending on to conjunctiva and cornea, scarring and atrophy of lids with exposure keratitis leading to corneal ulceration symblepharon formation; ocular melanoma
Pigmentation disorders	Chediak–Higashi syndrome [40]	AR (MIM 214500)	Oculocutaneous albinism, corneal opacities
	Cross syndrome [41]	AR (MIM 257800)	Microphthalmia, small opaque cornea, coarse nystagmus
	Epidermal naevus syndrome [42]	Sporadic	Ocular melanocytic naevi, coloboma of the lids, iris and choroid; lipodermoid of conjunctiva or choroid
	Incontinentia pigmenti [43]	XD (MIM 308300)	35% of patients have eye abnormalities including strabismus, cataract and microphthalmia; retinal detachment may occur
	Hypomelanosis of Ito [44]	Sporadic (MIM 300337)	Hypertelorism, strabismus, myopia
	Oculocutaneous albinism [45]	AR (various types)	Total loss of pigment in eyes, nystagmus, absence of binocular vision
	Piebaldism [46]	AD (MIM 172800)	Absent pigmentation medially of eyebrows, eyelids and eyelashes, heterochromia of iris
	Waardenberg syndrome [47]	AD (MIM 193150)	Telecanthus, synophrys, partial albinism, heterochromia of iris
Vascular and haematological syndromes	Congenital telangiectatic cutis marmorata [48]	Unknown (MIM 219250)	Clouding of cornea, glaucoma
	Fanconi pancytopenia syndrome [49]	AR (MIM 227650)	Microphthalmia strabismus, nystagmus and colobomas
	Lymphoedema–distichiasis syndrome [50]	AD (MIM 153400)	Double row of eyelashes on upper and lower eyelids
	Sturge–Weber syndrome [51]	Sporadic (MIM 185300)	50% of patients have angiotomatous changes of the ipsilateral choroid causing glaucoma

AD, autosomal dominant; AR, autosomal recessive; KID, keratitis–icthyosis–deafness; MIDAS, microphthalmia, dermal aplasia and sclerocornea; XD, X-linked dominant; XL, X-linked; XR, X-linked recessive.

have issued clear guidelines on screening protocols for use of chloroquine and hydroxychloroquine. Baseline ophthalmic assessment of patients, for whom these drugs are proposed, is carried out by the dermatologist and requires questioning the patient about any known visual impairment (uncorrected by spectacles) and the recording of near visual acuity using a test type. If visual impairment is reported or detected then referral to an optometrist is advised; the optometrist will refer any patient with abnormal findings to an ophthalmologist. Patients should not be treated with more than the maximum daily dosage (hydroxychloroquine at a maximum dosage of 6.5 mg/kg or chloroquine phosphate not exceeding 4 mg/kg daily) and should have this visual screening repeated annually and recorded in their notes. Referral to an ophthalmologist is appropriate if visual impairment is detected at

baseline, if changes are detected on the annual screening or if the patient develops visual symptoms. The ophthalmologist will then carry out a range of tests, including visual acuity, colour vision, visual fields, Amsler fields, corneal and retinal examinations. If long-term treatment is required, for more than 5 years, the risks of ocular complications are increased; in this instance, individual arrangements for screening should be agreed with a local ophthalmologist. No screening is recommended for mepacrine as it is not associated with ophthalmological side effects.

Antibiotics for acne [28–32]
Oxytetracycline, minocycline and doxycycline can all cause raised intracranial pressure. The mechanism is unknown but is thought to be related to interference with energy-dependent

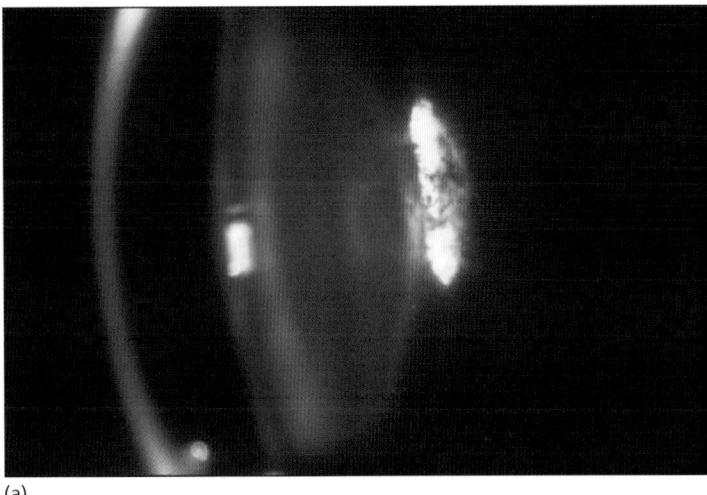

(a)

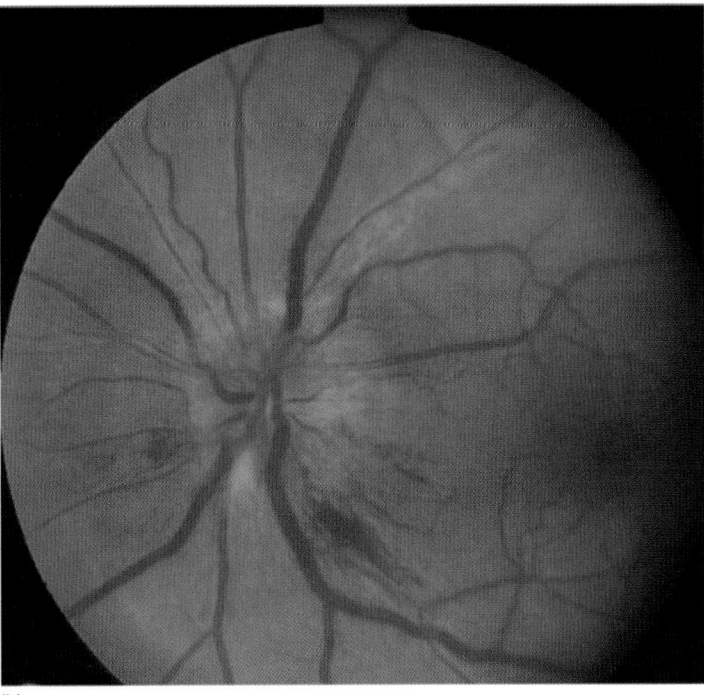

(b)

Figure 109.25 (a) Posterior subcapsular cataract typically induced by corticosteroid therapy. (b) Papilloedema (swollen optic disc) with accompanying retinal haemorrhages.

absorption mechanism of cerebrospinal fluid, which is mediated by cyclic adenosine monophosphate (AMP) at the arachnoid granulations. Patients who complain of headache should be examined carefully with fundoscopy through dilated pupils to look for papilloedema, and should have formal testing of visual acuity and of visual fields. The condition is far from benign; permanent visual field loss can occur if the condition is not recognized early and the drug stopped. Sometimes treatment with acetazolamide is required to reduce the pressure. Erythromycin or trimethoprim may cause erythema multiforme and associated ocular changes. Pigmentation due to minocycline can occur in the skin and has also been reported in the sclera.

Psoralens [33–46]

Psoralens have been shown to bind to the lens proteins, and some animal studies have shown induction of anterior cortical opacities though others have not. 8-Methoxypsoralen can be detected in the human lens 12 h after oral ingestion. There has been a long-standing concern about the risk of cataract in patients having psoralen and long-wave UV radiation (PUVA) therapy. Although PUVA has been used in treatment of skin diseases for 30 years, and clinical studies have not yet shown any convincing evidence of an increase in cataract as compared with the general population, it is still recommended that UV light A (UVA)-filtered spectacles are used for 12 h after ingestion of psoralens in case significant long-term sequelae eventually develop. Failure to do so may result in other signs of ocular toxicity such as conjunctival hyperaemia, decreased lacrimation and pinguecula formation, which represents elastotic degeneration of the cornea. Care must be taken to ensure that the spectacles are suitable for UV protection.

Botulinum toxin [47]

With the increased use of botulinum toxin for the treatment of facial wrinkling and eyebrow position, dermatologists need to be aware of the potential side effects. These include haematoma, ptosis, ectropion, diplopia and eyelid drooping, and are often related to poor injection technique.

Biological agents [48]

Potential ocular side effects of biological agents include (depending on the agent used) trichomegaly, blepharitis, conjunctivitis, cicatricial entropion, corneal erosion, reversible posterior leukoencephalic syndrome and possible optic neuritis. Further details are found in Hager and Seitz [48].

Tumours

Benign tumours of the eyelid

As would be expected of such complex tissue, the eyelid gives rise to a large number of skin tumours. Tumours can arise from the epidermis and dermis in addition to the adnexal structures, which include the meibomian and Zeis sebaceous glands, eccrine and Moll apocrine sweat glands, and the specialized hair follicles of the eyelashes. They may also originate from lymphoid neural and vascular tissue found in the preseptal tissues of the eyelid. Although optimal treatment of the tumours begins with accurate diagnosis, many are rather non-specific in their appearance and are only diagnosed with certainty by histology.

Keratoses

Both seborrhoeic and actinic keratoses occur on the eyelid. They have similar clinical features to those elsewhere on the skin and are treated in the same way with local destructive measures, using carefully applied cryotherapy, curettage and cautery or laser ablation under local anaesthetic. Recurrent actinic keratosis should be biopsied and sent for histological examination to make sure it is not a deceptive manifestation of an early skin cancer.

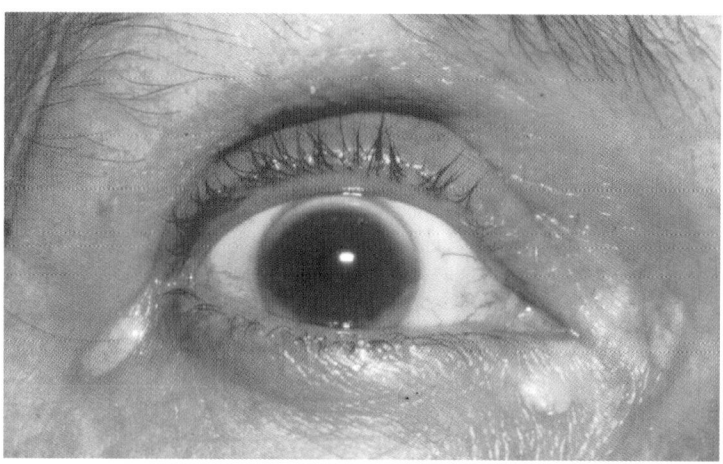

Figure 109.26 Xanthelasma. There are two lesions on the medial eyelid and one lesion on the temporal eyelid. The cornea shows arcus senilis, which is also associated with hypercholesterolaemia.

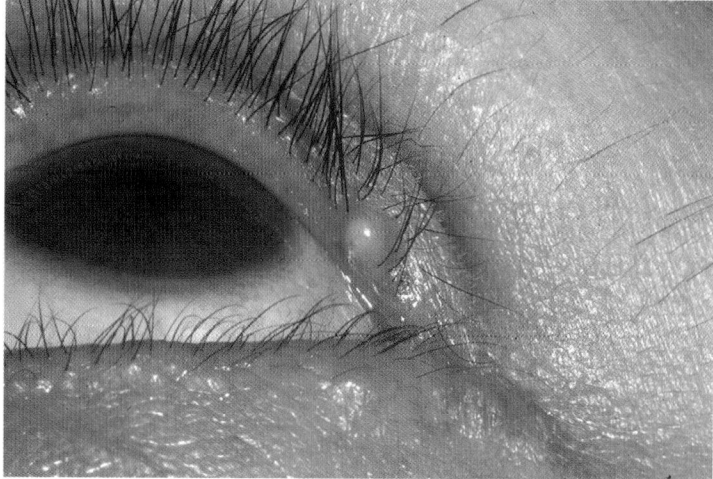

Figure 109.28 Cyst of Moll. Small translucent cyst on the anterior lid margin. (Courtesy of Mr N. Joshi, Chelsea and Westminster Hospital/Medical Illustration UK, London, UK.)

Xanthelasma [1,2]

These present as yellowish cutaneous plaques, most commonly located on the medial part of the eyelids (Figure 109.26). They are usually bilateral and are much more common in elderly patients. About 60% of patients have an associated hypercholesterolaemia and lipid levels should be measured. Patients often request treatment for cosmetic reasons. Although 90% trichloroacetic acid applied with a cotton wool bud is used there is a significant risk of spillage into the eye. More effective treatment is by surgical excision or ablation with carbon dioxide laser. Necrobiotic xanthogranuloma may look similar to xanthelasma but they are thicker and more nodular. These lesions may involve the conjunctiva and sclera. On the rare occasions that they infiltrate the orbit, they may cause proptosis.

Juvenile xanthogranuloma [3]

These lesions occasionally involve the eyelid, conjunctiva or uveal tract. They may be associated with glaucoma and threaten sight. Patients need screening by an ophthalmologist (Figure 109.27).

Adnexal tumours [4]

Syringomas, milia, trichoepitheliomas and tricholemmomas present as small papules around the eyelids. They can be very difficult to distinguish from each other. Syringomas are the most common, but histology from a biopsy is the only way to make a definite diagnosis. Treatment is by local destruction of the lesions. Eccrine hidrocystomas can present in an eruptive fashion on the face and eyelids; they may respond to topical atropine.

Benign cysts of the eyelid

Retention cysts may arise from either the glands of Moll or Zeis. A cyst of Moll usually presents as a small translucent lesion on the anterior lid margin close to the lacrimal punctum (Figure 109.28). Glands of Zeis are sebaceous glands and their retention cysts contain oily secretions and are more opaque than a cyst of Moll (Figure 109.29). An eccrine gland hidrocystoma is similar in appearance to a cyst of Moll but is not confined to the lid margin.

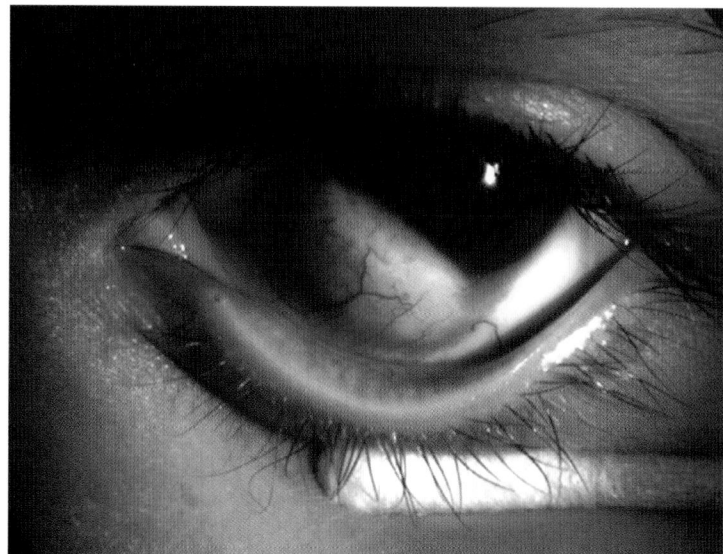

Figure 109.27 Juvenile xanthogranuloma.

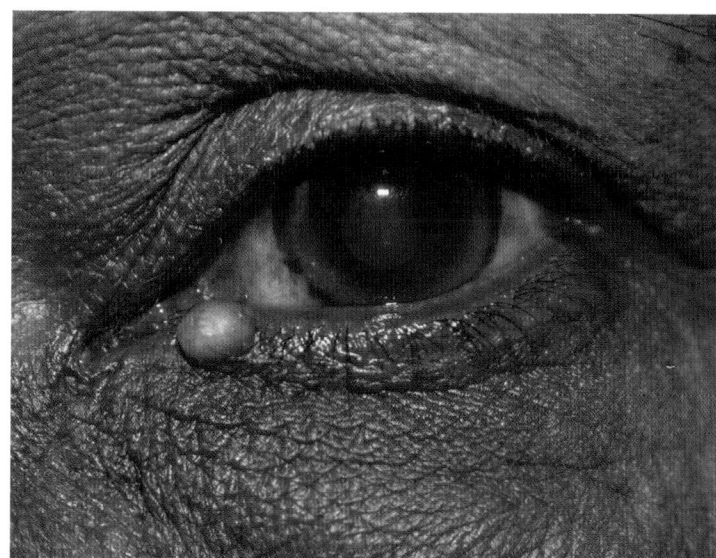

Figure 109.29 Cyst of Zeiss. Opaque sebaceous cyst.

These cysts are easily confused with a basal cell carcinoma clinically and are treated by excision and submission for histology.

Chalazion [5]

This lesion represents a chronic granulomatous inflammatory reaction around a blocked sebaceous gland. Patients with seborrhoeic dermatitis and rosacea are at increased risk of chalazion formation. A chalazion presents as a firm lump in the eyelid (see Figure 109.8b,f), which is clearly visible when the lid is everted; an association with chronic posterior blepharitis is common. Chalazia will usually resolve spontaneously but large and troublesome lesions can be treated by everting the lid with a special clamp, incising the cyst and curetting the contents through the tarsal plate. Patients who develop recurrent chalazion associated with seborrhoeic dermatitis and rosacea benefit from long-term antibiotic treatment using tetracyclines. Hot compresses reduce the inflammation.

Pigmented naevi [6,7]

The skin on the eyelid can develop pigmented naevi. Their appearance, classification and potential malignant change applies as elsewhere on the skin. Patients with dysplastic naevus syndrome should be referred to an ophthalmologist for ocular assessment (see Chapter 132). Melanocytic lesions of the conjunctiva extending onto the cornea or pigmented lesions of the conjunctiva, which change in character, should also be referred with a view to excision biopsy.

Naevus of Ota [8]

This lesion affects the eyelids, conjunctiva and sclera (see Chapter 75). Occasionally, the pigmentation is confined to the eye with no cutaneous involvement (Figure 109.30a,b). Naevus of Ota carries an increased risk of ocular melanoma and glaucoma and patients need to be referred for ophthalmic examination and long-term review.

Melanoacanthoma [9]

These are small shining black papules situated along the line of the lashes and are a form of dermatosis papulosa nigricans.

Vascular naevi [10–14]

Strawberry naevus (capillary haemangioma) can affect the eyelids (see Chapter 117). It is more common on the upper lid and presents as a unilateral red raised lesion, which grows quickly during the first year of life (Figure 109.31). Spontaneous involution occurs usually by age 9 years. Amblyopia is the main complication of larger periorbital lesions and results either from physical closure of the eye and occlusion of the pupil, giving rise to stimulus deprivation, or from refractive errors caused by corneal distortion due to lid pressure. Both systemic and intralesional corticosteroids can reduce the bulk of the haemangioma. Recently, systemic and topical β-blockers have been used to successfully treat infantile periocular haemangiomas. Surgical resection or laser therapy is helpful in certain cases.

Port-wine stain

This is a rare congenital vascular lesion, which may affect the eyelids (see Chapter 73). It presents as a sharply demarcated red patch. Extensive lesions involving the periocular region have a high risk

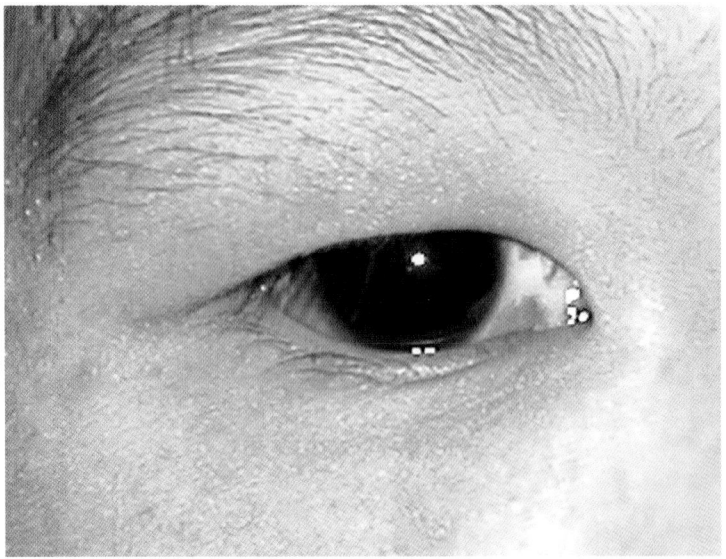
(a)

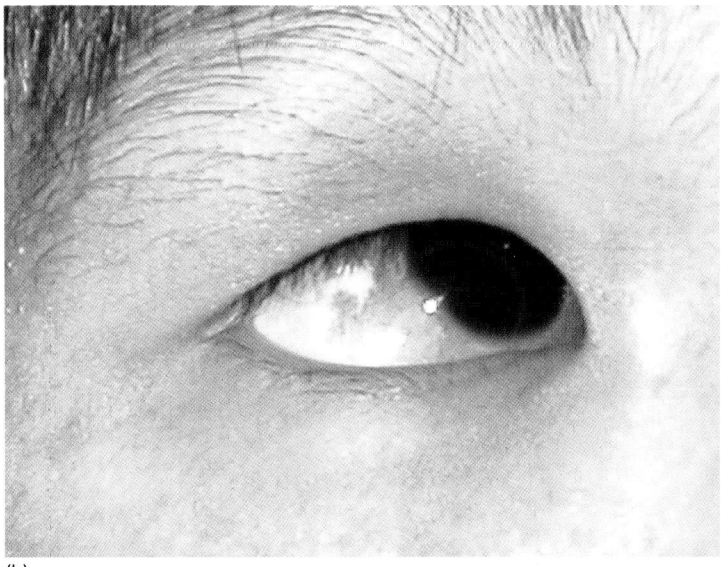
(b)

Figure 109.30 (a, b) Naevus of Ota. In this case the pigmentation is confined to the eye, with no cutaneous involvement. The yellow staining of the eyelid is due to fluorescein instillation into the eye to measure intraocular pressure.

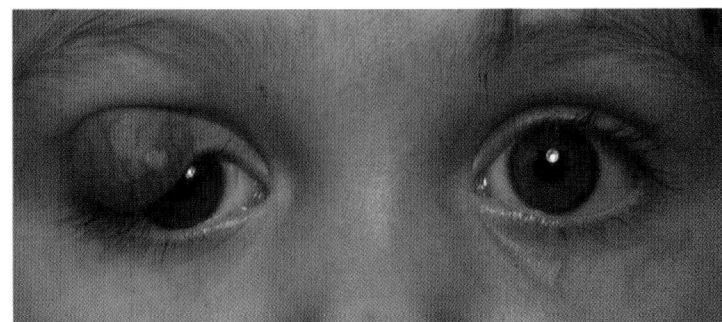

Figure 109.31 Capillary haemangioma. Enlarging lesion on the right upper lid, starting to occlude vision. (Courtesy of Mr N. Joshi, Chelsea and Westminster Hospital/ Medical Illustration UK, London, UK.)

PART 10: SITES, SEX, AGE

of central nervous involvement and of ipsilateral glaucoma (especially if the upper lid is involved), which may not develop until adult life. This combination of clinical features is called Sturge–Weber syndrome.

Keratoacanthoma

Keratoacanthomas may develop on the eyelid (see Chapter 142). They present as a small papule which grows rapidly, developing a characteristic keratin-filled crater and may reach up to 3 cm in diameter (Figure 109.32). The lesions then stop growing and remain static for 2 or 3 months before spontaneously involuting, which can lead to significant scarring of the eyelid. Because of this, the lesion should be excised at an early stage.

Malignant tumours of the eyelid [15–18]

Basal cell carcinomas (BCCs), squamous cell carcinomas (SCCs) and malignant melanomas all occur on the eyelid as on other areas of the skin (see Chapters 141 and 142). The same rules for management apply on the eyelid as at any site, but the eyelid poses specific problems in preserving good cosmesis and residual function. Clinical examination is an unreliable way of determining the extent of many of these lesions, particularly morphoeic BCC. Early referral to an oculoplastic surgeon is advisable with a view to Mohs micrographic surgery if appropriate.

Basal cell carcinomas [18–21]

These are the most common skin malignancy and in most series account for 90% of malignant tumours. They rarely metastasize but cause problems by local tissue destruction and invasion of periorbital tissue. Over 70% arise on the lower eyelid, followed in order of frequency by the medial canthus, upper eyelid and lateral canthus. Tumours located near to the medial canthus can invade the orbit and sinuses. They are more difficult to excise than those elsewhere, because of the high risk of damaging the tear duct. The majority of BCCs are solid or cystic and fairly straightforward to recognize (Figure 109.33). Sclerosing or morphoeic BCCs are less common and can be difficult to diagnose as they infiltrate beneath the epidermis,

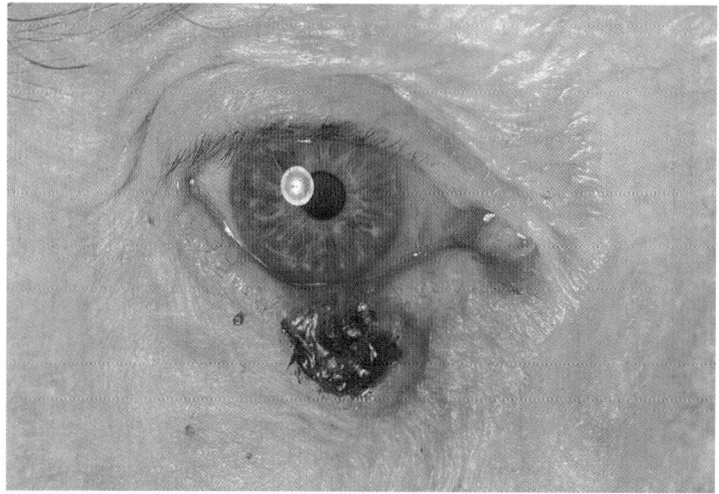

(a)

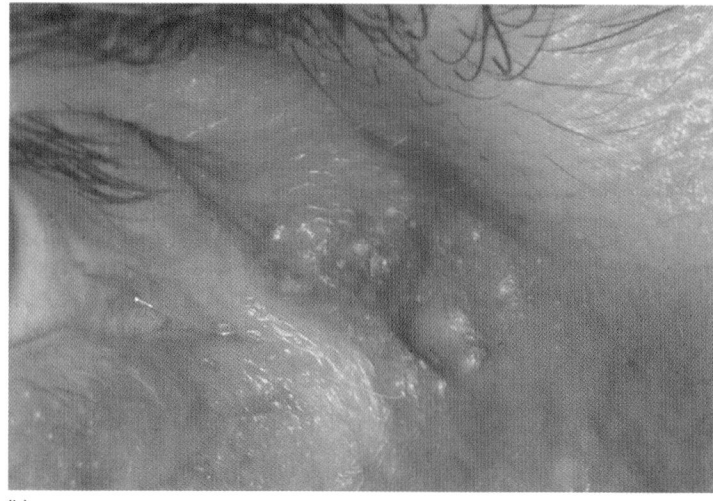

(b)

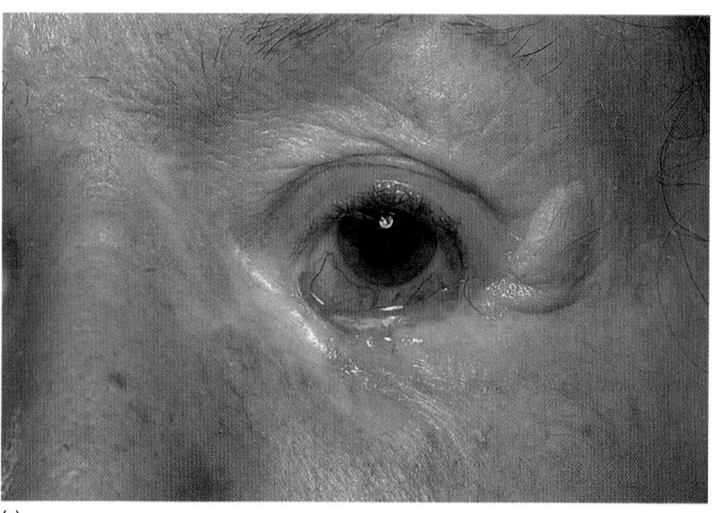

(c)

Figure 109.33 Basal cell carcinoma (BCC). (a) Ulcerated BCC on the lower lid. (b) Poorly defined BCC at medial canthus. (c) Morphoeic BCC along the lower lid. (Courtesy of Mr N. Joshi, Chelsea and Westminster Hospital/Medical Illustration UK, London, UK.)

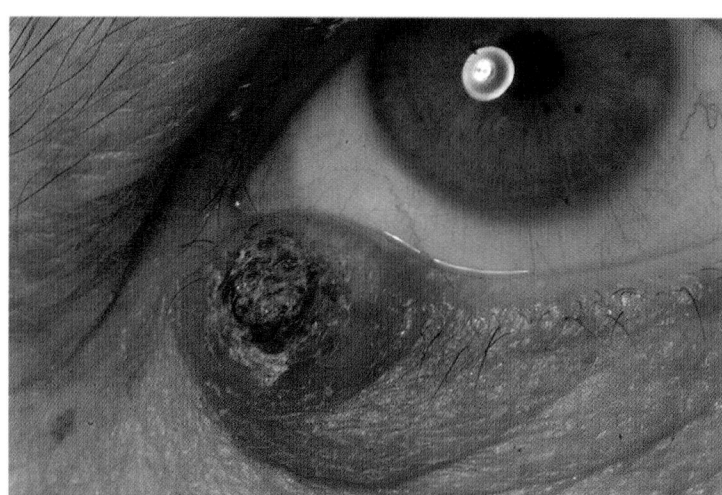

Figure 109.32 Keratoacanthoma. Keratin-filled crater on the lid margin. (Courtesy of Mr N. Joshi, Chelsea and Westminster Hospital/Medical Illustration UK, London, UK.)

PART 10: SITES, SEX, AGE

forming a flat indurated plaque with indistinct margins, which may simulate a localized area of chronic dermatitis. The paucity of reticular dermis and subcutaneous fat to resist deep invasion presents a particular problem with the eye. Once the orbital septum is penetrated the BCC can rapidly invade, threatening the orbit. At the medial canthus the lacrimal sac and the rich anastomosis of blood vessels offers little barrier. Curettage and cautery is generally not advised for the treatment of eyelid lesions. The skin is thin and tears easily and the sensitivity of the curette is lost in the soft tissue. Successful initial treatment with surgery and accurate margin assessment to ensure complete excision is mandatory in management of these tumours. Mohs micrographic surgery is usually the treatment of choice where margins are in doubt. Radiotherapy damages and scars the eyelid tissues and lacrimal system and should be reserved for situations when surgery is otherwise inappropriate. Cryotherapy is best avoided due to the risk of leaving residual tumour. Targeted therapy such as vismodegib, a hedgehog pathway inhibitor, shows particular promise in the management of patients with large infiltrating BCCs of the eyelid and in Gorlin syndrome who may have numerous bulky lesions of the eyelid.

Squamous cell carcinomas [22]

This is much less common than BCC, accounting for between 5 and 10% of eyelid malignancies. SCCs occur on a background of marked actinic damage. They mainly affect the lower eyelid and lid margin, and may arise *de novo* or from pre-existing actinic keratoses. SCC of the eyelids may be nodular, plaque-like or ulcerated (Figure 109.34). Excision with adequate margins is the treatment of choice. Tumours greater than 2 cm in diameter and those with deep penetration have a higher risk of metastasis. Histological evidence of poor differentiation or of perineural invasion are also poor prognostic factors requiring more aggressive treatment. Mohs micrographic surgery is indicated where the initial margins are not free of tumour, and offers a good long-term prognosis. As with BCC, cryotherapy and radiotherapy are reserved for situations where surgery is inappropriate. Targeted epidermal growth factor receptor (EGFR) inhibitor therapies have demonstrated clinical benefit in SCC.

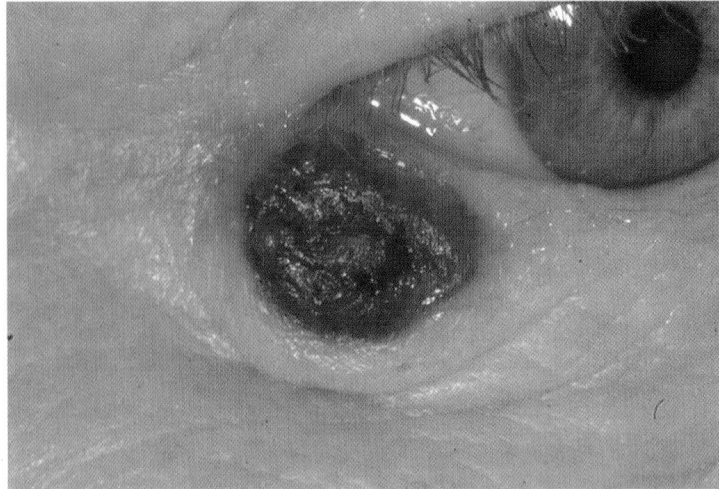

Figure 109.35 Malignant melanoma. Irregularly pigmented lesion on the lower lid. (Courtesy of Mr N. Joshi, Chelsea and Westminster Hospital/Medical Illustration UK, London, UK.)

Malignant melanoma

This may occur on the eyelids or conjunctiva (see Chapter 143). As elsewhere, melanomas are characterized by a change in size, shape or colour of a pigmented lesion (Figure 109.35). However, a significant proportion of lid melanomas are amelanotic and this may give rise to difficulties with clinical diagnosis.

Sebaceous gland carcinoma and epithelioma [23,24]

These are very rare tumours, accounting for less than 1–5% of malignant tumours of the eyelid (Figure 109.36). Sebaceous gland carcinoma usually arises from the meibomian glands, occasionally from the glands of Zeis. In contrast to BCC or SCC, the majority of lesions affect the upper lid. Most lesions are nodular and look very much like a chalazion (see Figures 109.5a,b and 109.18), causing delay in diagnosis; a sebaceous tumour should always be suspected if a 'chalazion' lasts for more than 6 months, and a 'chalazion' that recurs should be viewed with great suspicion,

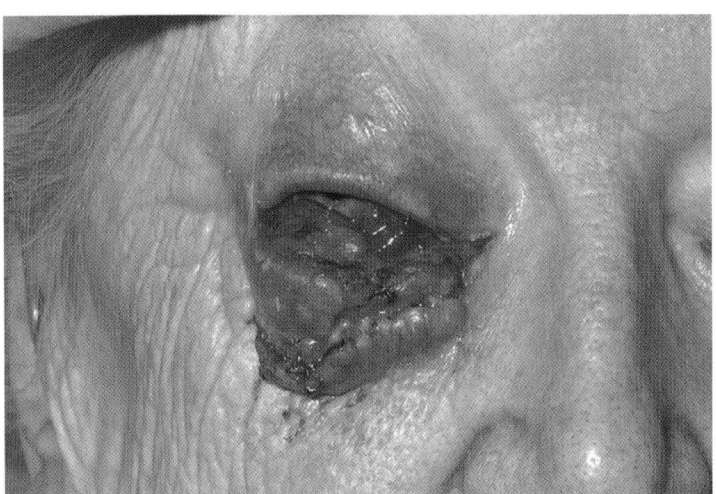

Figure 109.34 Squamous cell carcinoma (SCC). Infiltrating ulcerated SCC on the lower lid. (Courtesy of Mr N. Joshi, Chelsea and Westminster Hospital/Medical Illustration UK, London, UK.)

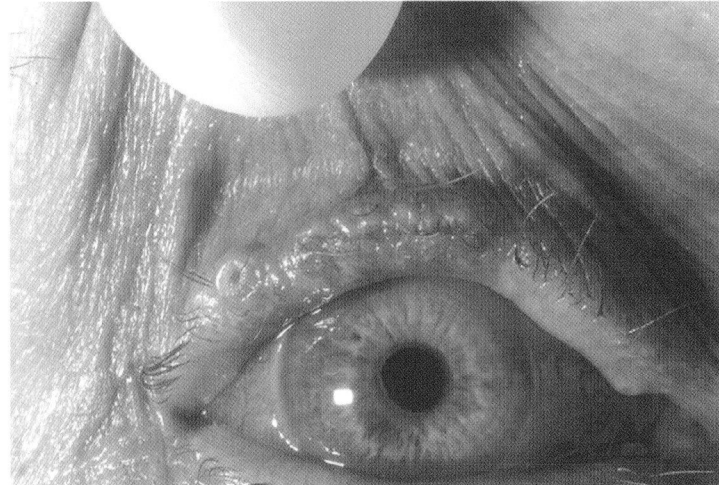

Figure 109.36 Sebaceous gland carcinoma. Infiltrating lesion on the upper lid. (Courtesy of Mr N. Joshi, Chelsea and Westminster Hospital/Medical Illustration UK, London, UK.)

excised and sent for histology. Because of late diagnosis, sebaceous gland carcinoma carries a significant mortality. Wide local excision is the treatment of choice. The multicentric nature of the tumour may limit the use of Mohs surgery.

Eccrine carcinoma [25]

These are rare cancers of the eye and may present as an indurated thickening of the lid or with a signet-ring appearance. They are commonest in middle-aged or elderly men and recur after excision.

Merkel cell carcinoma

A very rare tumour. It can also mimic a chalazion in its early stages, with delay in diagnosis (see Chapter 145). It is highly malignant and has often metastasized by the time of excision.

Kaposi sarcoma

A vascular malignancy, Kaposi sarcoma presents as a purple lesion on the eyelid or conjunctiva and can be mistaken for a benign hae-mangioma (see Chapter 137). However, it grows rapidly and may ulcerate and bleed. When it presents on the eyelid it is associated with HIV infection, of which it may be the sole manifestation at the time of presentation. These lesions are very radiosensitive, and this is the preferred mode of treatment once a biopsy has been taken to confirm the diagnosis.

Key references

The full list of references can be found in the online version at www.rooksdermatology.com.

Introduction
6 Mannis MJ, Macsai MS, Huntley AC, eds. *Eye and Skin Disease*. New York: Lippincott-Raven, 1996.

7 Ostler HB, Maibach HI, Hoko AW, Swab IR, eds. *Diseases of the Eye and Skin: a Color Atlas*. Philadelphia: Lippincott, Williams & Wilkins, 2004.

Skin diseases affecting the eye and eyelids

Blepharitis, meibomian gland dysfunction, rosacea and seborrhoeic dermatitis
6 Nichols KK, Foulks GN, Bron AJ, *et al*. The international workshop on meibo-mian gland dysfunction: executive summary. *IOVS* 2011;52(4):1922–9.

Cicatrizing conjunctivitis and the immunobullous disorders
4 Saw VP, Dart JK. Ocular mucous membrane pemphigoid: diagnosis and man-agement strategies. *Ocul Surf* 2008;6:128–42.
22 De Rojas MV, Dart JK, Saw VP. The natural history of Stevens–Johnson syn-drome: patterns of chronic ocular disease and the role of systemic immunosup-pressive therapy. *Br J Ophthalmol* 2007;91:1048–53.

Systemic diseases with skin and eye involvement
1 Callen JP, Mahl CF. Oculocutaneous manifestation observed in multisystem dis-orders. *Dermatol Clin* 1992;10:709–16.

Viral infections
4 Herpetic Eye Disease Study Group. Oral acyclovir for herpes simplex virus eye disease. Effect on prevention of epithelial keratitis and stromal keratitis. *Arch Ophthalmol* 2000;118:1030–6.

Other disorders

Ocular complications of dermatological therapy
22 Fraunfelder FT, Fraunfelder FW, Edwards R. Ocular side effects possibly associ-ated with isotretinoin usage. *Am J Ophthalmol* 2001;132:299–305.
27 Marmor MF, Carr RE, Easterbrook M, *et al*. Revised recommendations on screen-ing for chloroquine and hydroxychloroquine retinopathy. A report by the Ameri-can Academy of Ophthalmology. *Ophthalmology*. 2011;118(2):415-22.

CHAPTER 110

Dermatoses of the Oral Cavity and Lips

Crispian Scully
WHO Collaborating Centre for Oral Health-General Health, UK

PART 10: SITES, SEX, AGE

PART 10: SITES, SEX, AGE

Introduction

Oral and labial lesions are usually the result of local disease but may be the early signs of systemic disease, including dermatological disorders, and in some instances may cause the main symptoms. This chapter mainly discusses disorders of the periodontal and mucosal tissues that may be related to skin disease and that may present at a dermatology clinic. It should be borne in mind that the professionals most competent in diagnosing and treating oral diseases are those with formal dental training and who are therefore in a position to understand the full complexities of the region.

The chapter is an overview only and is divided into a brief discussion of the biology of the mouth, an overview of the more common signs and symptoms affecting specific oral tissues, discussion of the disorders of the oral mucosa of most relevance to dermatology and a tabulated review of oral manifestations of systemic diseases. Only the more classic oral lesions are illustrated. About 20 of the colour illustrations are from *Oral and Maxillofacial Diseases*, 2010 (reproduced by kind permission of C. Scully, S. Flint, J.V. Bagan *et al.*, Informa, London). More detail of histology is available elsewhere [1].

For reasons of space restrictions, diseases affecting the teeth, salivary glands, jaws or temporomandibular joints are not discussed in any depth.

BIOLOGY OF THE MOUTH

Oral epithelium

The oral epithelium consists of a *functional compartment* – the progenitor cells (basal and parabasal cells) – which is the site of cell division; a *maturation compartment* (spinous and granular cells) where the cells become more terminally differentiated; and a superficial *cornified compartment* of squames and areas of keratinization, either orthokeratotic or parakeratotic. In the non-keratinized regions such as the buccal (cheek) and floor-of-mouth mucosae, overt keratinization and granular cells are absent and the surface cells are flattened, with elongated nuclei [2].

Lips

The lips extend from the lower end of the nose to the upper end of the chin. They mainly consist of bundles of striated muscle, particularly the *orbicularis oris* muscle, with skin on the external surface and mucous membrane on the inner surface, which has a profusion of minor salivary glands.

The vermilion zone, the transitional zone between the glabrous skin and the mucous membrane, is found only in humans. The vermilion zone contains no hair or sweat glands but does contain sebaceous glands (Fordyce spots). The epithelium of the vermilion is distinctive, with a prominent stratum lucidum and a very thin stratum corneum. The dermal papillae are numerous at this site, with a rich capillary supply, which produces the reddish-pink colour of the lips in white people. Melanocytes are abundant in the basal layer of the vermilion of pigmented skin, but are infrequent in white skin.

The *oral commissures* are the angles where the upper and lower lip meet. The upper lip includes the *philtrum*, a midline depression, extending from the columella of the nose to the superior edge of the vermilion zone [3].

Oral mucosa

The mucosa is divided into masticatory, lining and specialized types. *Masticatory mucosa* (hard palate, gingiva) is adapted to the forces of pressure and friction and is keratinized, with numerous tall rete ridges and connective tissue papillae and little submucosa. *Lining mucosa* (buccal, labial and alveolar mucosa, floor of mouth, ventral surface of tongue, soft palate, lips) is non-keratinized, with broad rete ridges and connective tissue papillae and abundant elastic fibres in the lamina propria [4,5].

Specialized mucosa on the dorsum of the tongue, adapted for taste and mastication, is keratinized, with numerous rete ridges and connective tissue papillae, abundant elastic and collagen fibres in the lamina propria and no submucosa. The tongue is divided by a V-shaped groove, the *sulcus terminalis*, into an anterior two-thirds and a posterior third. Various papillae on the dorsum include the *filiform papillae*, which cover the entire anterior surface and form an abrasive surface to control the food bolus as it is pressed against the palate, and the *fungiform papillae*. The latter are mushroom-shaped red structures covered by non-keratinized epithelium. They are scattered between the filiform papillae and have taste buds on their surface. Adjacent and anterior to the sulcus terminalis are eight to 12 large *circumvallate papillae*, each surrounded by a deep groove into which open the ducts of serous minor salivary glands. The lateral walls of these papillae contain taste buds.

The *foliate papillae* consist of four to 11 parallel ridges, alternating with deep grooves in the mucosa, on the lateral margins on the posterior part of the tongue. There are taste buds on their lateral walls. The *lingual tonsils* are round or oval prominences with intervening lingual crypts lined by non-keratinized epithelium. They are part of *Waldeyer's oropharyngeal ring* of lymphoid tissue. The lingual tonsil is a mass of lymphoid tissue in the posterior third of the tongue, between the epiglottis posteriorly and the circumvallate papillae anteriorly. It is usually divided in the midline by a ligament.

Teeth

The teeth develop from neuroectoderm [6]. Tooth development begins in the fetus, at about 28 days *in utero*. Indeed, all the deciduous and some of the permanent dentition commence development in the fetus. At around the sixth week of intrauterine life, the oral epithelium proliferates over the maxillary and mandibular ridge areas to form primary epithelial bands that project into the mesoderm, and produce a dental lamina in which discrete swellings appear – the enamel organs of developing teeth. Each enamel organ eventually produces tooth enamel, and the mesenchyme, which condenses beneath the enamel organ (actually neuroectoderm), forms a dental papilla that produces the dentine and pulp of the tooth. The enamel organ together with the dental papilla constitute the tooth germ, and this becomes surrounded by a mesenchymal dental follicle, from which the periodontium forms, ultimately to anchor the tooth in its bony socket. Mineralization of the primary dentition commences at about 14 weeks *in utero* and all primary teeth are mineralizing by birth. Permanent incisor and first molar teeth begin to mineralize at, or close to, the time of birth; mineralization of other permanent teeth starting later. Tooth eruption occurs after crown formation when mineralization is largely complete but before the roots are fully formed.

Teeth comprise a crown of insensitive enamel, surrounding sensitive dentine, and a root which has no enamel covering. Teeth contain a vital pulp (nerve) and are supported by the periodontal ligament by which roots are attached into sockets in the alveolar process of the jaws (maxilla and mandible). The fibres of the periodontal ligament attach through cementum to the dentine surface. The alveolus is covered by the gingivae, or gums, which in health are pink, stippled and tightly bound down, and form a close-fitting cuff, with a small sulcus (gingival crevice), round the neck of each tooth.

The first or primary (deciduous or milk) dentition comprises two incisors, a canine and two molars in each of the four mouth quadrants (total 20 teeth). There are 10 deciduous (primary or milk) teeth in each jaw: all are fully erupted by the age of about 3 years (Table 110.1). The secondary or permanent teeth begin to

Table 110.1 Tooth eruption timings (average timings; there is a wide range).

	Upper	Lower
Deciduous (primary) teeth		
A Central incisors	8–13 months	6–10 months
B Lateral incisors	8–13 months	10–16 months
C Canines (cuspids)	16–23 months	16–23 months
D First molars	13–19 months	13–19 months
E Second molars	25–33 months	23–31 months
Permanent teeth		
1 Central incisors	7–8 years	6–7 years
2 Lateral incisors	8–9 years	7–8 years
3 Canines (cuspids)	11–12 years	9–10 years
4 First premolars (bicuspids)	10–11 years	10–12 years
5 Second premolars (bicuspids)	10–12 years	11–12 years
6 First molars	6–7 years	6–7 years
7 Second molars	11–13 years	11–13 years
8 Third molars	17–21 years	17–21 years

erupt at about the age of 6–7 years and the deciduous teeth are slowly lost by normal root resorption.

The normal permanent (adult) dentition comprises two incisors, a canine, two premolars and three molars in each quadrant (total 32 teeth). The full permanent dentition consists of 16 teeth in each jaw: normally most have erupted by about 12–14 years of age. However, some milk teeth may still be present at the age of 12–13 years. The last molars (third molars or wisdom teeth), if present, often erupt later or may impact and never appear in the mouth.

Junction of the mucosa with the teeth

The dentogingival junction represents a unique anatomical feature concerned with the attachment of the gingival (gum) mucosa to the tooth. Non-keratinized gingival epithelium forms a cuff surrounding the tooth, and at its lowest point on the tooth is adherent to the enamel or cementum. This 'junctional' epithelium is unique in being bounded both on its tooth and lamina propria aspects by basement membranes. Above this is a shallow sulcus or crevice (up to 2 mm deep), the gingival sulcus or crevice. Neutrophils continually migrate into the gingival crevice, and there is also a slow exudate of plasma (crevicular fluid).

Immunity in the oral cavity

Movement of the soft tissues during speech and swallowing, and salivation, ensures that much foreign material is swallowed. The need for this cleaning mechanism is clearly apparent in patients with facial paralysis, or in those with xerostomia, in whom there is accumulation of oral debris and subsequent infection.

Saliva also aggregates bacteria and deters their attachment to surfaces. Salivary lysozyme, thiocyanate, peroxides and various mucins and other components may be antimicrobial and saliva is inhibitory to various microbial agents including, for example, HIV.

Salivary tissue derives its B cells from the gut-associated lymphoid tissue (GALT) system [7]. Salivary acinar cells produce secretory component (transport piece) needed for transport of immunoglobulin A (IgA) into the saliva and its stability in the presence of salivary or gastric proteolytic enzymes. Although the exact contribution to oral defence made by salivary IgA antibodies is difficult to assess, some patients who have IgA deficiency suffer from oral infections, and in animals it is possible to induce protective salivary IgA antibodies to caries-producing organisms such as *Streptococcus mutans*.

Neutrophils and other leukocytes are particularly essential for oral health as shown by the fact that patients with HIV infection, neutropenia, agranulocytopenia, leukaemia or chronic granulomatous disease are predisposed to severe gingivitis and rapid periodontal breakdown, as well as mouth ulceration and infections.

EXAMINATION OF THE MOUTH AND PERIORAL REGION

Examination includes inspection under a good light, and palpation of the cervical lymph nodes, temporomandibular joints, jaws, salivary glands and oral cavity.

Lymph nodes (Table 110.2)

Lymph from the superficial tissue of the head and neck generally drains first to groups of superficially placed lymph nodes, then to the deep cervical lymph nodes.
- Systematically, each region needs to be examined lightly with the pulps of the fingers, trying to roll the lymph nodes against harder underlying structures.
- Parotid, mastoid and occipital lymph nodes can be palpated simultaneously using both hands.
- Superficial cervical lymph nodes are examined with lighter palpation as they can only be compressed against the softer sternomastoid muscle.
- Submental lymph nodes are examined by tipping the patient's head forward and rolling the lymph nodes against the inner aspect of the mandible.
- Submandibular lymph nodes are examined in the same way with the patient's head tipped to the side being examined.

Differentiation needs to be made between the submandibular salivary gland and submandibular lymph glands. Bimanual examination with one finger in the floor of the mouth may help.
- The deep cervical lymph nodes, which project anterior or posterior to the sternomastoid muscle, can be palpated. The jugulodigastric lymph node should be specifically examined, as this is the most common lymph node involved in tonsillar infections.
- The supraclavicular region should be examined at the same time as the rest of the neck; lymph nodes here may extend up into the posterior triangle of the neck on the scalene muscles, behind the sternomastoid.
- Parapharyngeal and tracheal lymph nodes can be compressed lightly against the trachea.

Table 110.2 Drainage areas of cervical lymph nodes.

Area	Draining lymph nodes
Scalp, temporal region	Superficial parotid
Scalp, posterior	Occipital
Scalp, parietal region	Mastoid
Ear, external	Superficial cervical over upper part of sternomastoid muscle
Ear, middle	Parotid
Over angle of mandible	Superficial cervical over upper part of sternomastoid muscle
Medial part of frontal region, medial eyelids, skin of nose	Submandibular
Lateral part of frontal region and lateral part of eyelids	Parotid
Cheek	Submandibular
Upper lip	Submandibular
Lower lip	Submental
Lower lip, lateral part	Submandibular
Mandibular gingivae	Submandibular
Maxillary teeth	Deep cervical
Maxillary gingivae	Deep cervical
Tongue tip	Submental; remainder drains to submandibular nodes
Tongue, anterior two-thirds	Submandibular; some midline cross-over of lymphatic drainage
Tongue, posterior third	Deep cervical
Tongue, ventrum	Deep cervical
Floor of mouth	Submandibular
Palate, hard	Deep cervical
Palate, soft	Retropharyngeal and deep cervical
Tonsil	Jugulodigastric

- Some information can be gained by the texture and nature of the lymphadenopathy.
- Tenderness and swelling should be documented. Lymph nodes that are tender may be inflammatory (lymphadenitis). Consistency should be noted. Nodes that are increasing in size and are hard or fixed to adjacent tissues may be malignant.
- Both anterior and posterior cervical nodes should be examined as well as other nodes, liver and spleen if systemic disease is a possibility.

Temporomandibular joints and muscles of mastication

Although disorders that affect the temporomandibular joint often appear to be unilateral, the joint should not be viewed in isolation but always considered together with its opposite joint, as part of the stomatognathic system. The area should be examined as follows.

Inspection
1 Facial symmetry.
2 Evidence of enlarged masseter muscles (masseteric hypertrophy) suggestive of clenching or bruxism.

3 Mandibular opening and closing paths.
4 Mandibular opening extent:
   - Measure the interincisal distance at maximum mouth opening.
   - Measure the amount of lateral excursions achievable.
   - Listen for joint noises (a stethoscope placed over the joint can help).

Palpation
- Both condyles: via the external auditory meatus to detect tenderness posteriorly, and by using a single finger placed over the joints in front of the ears to detect pain, abnormal movements or clicking within the joint.
- Masticatory muscles on both sides.

Masseters: by intraoral/extraoral compression between finger and thumb. Palpate the masseter bimanually by placing a finger of one hand intraorally and the index and middle fingers of the other hand on the cheek over the masseter over the lower mandibular ramus.

Temporalis: by direct palpation of the temporal region. Palpate the temporal origin of the temporalis muscle by asking the patient to clench the teeth. Palpate the insertion of the temporalis tendon intraorally along the anterior border of the ascending mandibular ramus.

Lateral pterygoid (lower head): by placing a little finger up behind the maxillary tuberosity (the 'pterygoid sign'). Examine the lateral pterygoid muscle, which cannot readily be palpated, indirectly by asking the patient to open the jaw against resistance and to move the jaw to one side while a gentle resistance force is applied.

Medial pterygoid muscle: intraorally lingually to the mandibular ramus. Some palpate using a pressure algometer to standardize the force used, and undertake range-of-movement measurements.
- Examination of the dentition and occlusion: this may require monitoring of study models on a semi-adjustable or fully adjustable articulator. Note particularly missing premolars or molars, and attrition.
- Examination of the mucosa: note particularly occlusal lines and scalloping of the tongue margins, which may indicate bruxism and tongue pressure.

Jaws

There is wide normal individual variation in morphology of the face. Most individuals have facial asymmetry but of a degree that cannot be regarded as abnormal.
- Maxillary, mandibular or zygomatic deformities or lumps may be more reliably confirmed by inspection from above (maxillae/zygomas) or behind (mandible). The jaws should be palpated to detect swelling or tenderness.
- Maxillary air sinuses can be examined by palpation for tenderness over the maxillary antrum, which may indicate sinus infection. Transillumination or endoscopy can be helpful.

PART 10: SITES, SEX, AGE

Salivary glands

Inspect and palpate the major salivary glands (parotid and sub-mandibular) for:

• Symmetry.
• Evidence of enlarged glands.
• Evidence of salivary flow from salivary ducts.
• Appearance of saliva.

Parotid glands. Palpate by placing fingers over the pre-auricular glands, to detect pain or swelling. Early enlargement of the parotid gland is characterized by outward deflection of the lower part of the earlobe, which is best observed by looking at the patient from behind. This simple sign may allow distinction from simple obesity. Swelling of the parotid sometimes causes trismus. Swellings may affect the whole or part of a gland or tenderness may be elicited. The parotid duct (Stensen's duct) is most readily palpated with the jaws clenched firmly since the duct turns medially at the front edge of masseter, pierces the buccinator muscle and opens at a papilla on the buccal mucosa opposite the upper molars.

Submandibular glands. Bimanually palpate using fingers inside the mouth and extraorally. The submandibular gland is best palpated with a finger of one hand in the floor of the mouth lingual to the lower molar teeth, and a finger of the other hand placed over the submandibular triangle. The submandibular duct (Wharton's duct) runs anteromedially across the floor of the mouth to open at the side of the lingual fraenum.

Intraoral examination

The examination should be conducted in a systematic fashion to ensure that all areas are included. If the patient wears any removable prostheses or appliances, these should be removed in the first instance, although it may be necessary later to replace the appliance to assess fit, function and relationship to any lesion.

Complete visualization with a good source of light is essential. All mucosal surfaces should be examined, starting away from the location of any known lesions or the focus of complaint. The lips should be inspected first. The labial mucosa, buccal (cheek) mucosae, floor of mouth and ventrum of tongue, dorsal surface of the tongue, hard and soft palates, gingivae and teeth should then be examined in sequence and lesions noted on a diagram of the oral cavity (Figure 110.1).

Lips. Features such as cyanosis are seen mainly in the lips in cardiac or respiratory disease; angular cheilitis (stomatitis) is seen mainly in oral candidosis or in iron, vitamin or immune deficiencies. Examination is facilitated if the mouth is gently closed at this stage, so that the lips can then be everted to examine the mucosa.

Labial mucosa. Normally appears moist with a fairly prominent vascular arcade. In the lower lip, the many minor salivary glands, which are often exuding mucus, are easily visible. The lips therefore feel slightly nodular and the labial arteries are readily felt. Many adults have a few yellowish pinhead-sized

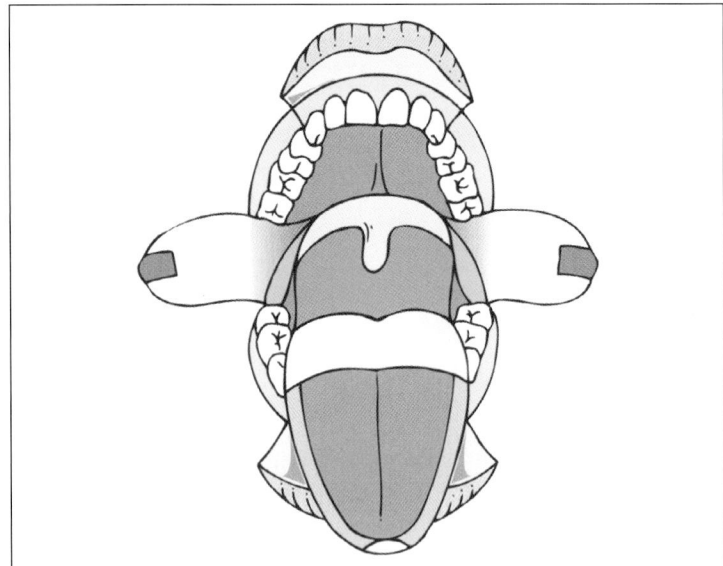

Figure 110.1 Diagram of the oral cavity.

papules in the vermilion border (particularly of the upper lip) and at the commissures; these are usually ectopic sebaceous glands (Fordyce spots), and may be numerous, especially as age advances.

Cheek (buccal) mucosa. This is readily inspected if the mouth is held half open. The vascular pattern and minor salivary glands so prominent in the labial mucosa are not obvious in the buccal mucosa but Fordyce spots may be conspicuous, particularly near the commissures and retromolar regions in adults. Place the surface of a dental mirror against the buccal mucosa. The mirror should lift off easily; if it adheres to the mucosa, then xerostomia is present.

Floor of mouth and ventrum of the tongue. These are best examined by asking the patient to push the tongue first into the palate then into each cheek in turn. This raises for inspection the floor of the mouth, an area where tumours may start (the 'coffin' or 'graveyard' area of the mouth). Its posterior part is the most difficult area to examine well and one where lesions are most easily missed. Lingual veins are prominent and, in the elderly, may be conspicuous (lingual varices). Bony lumps on the alveolar ridge lingual to the premolars are most often tori (torus mandibularis). During this part of the examination the quantity and consistency of saliva should be assessed. Examine for the normal pooling of saliva in the floor of the mouth; normally there is a pool of saliva in the floor of the mouth.

Dorsum of the tongue. This is best inspected by protrusion, when it can be held with gauze. This raises the floor of the mouth which aids inspection. The floor of the mouth and posterolateral margin of the tongue is an area where tumours may start. The posterior aspect of the floor of the mouth is the most difficult area to examine well and one where lesions are most likely to be missed.

The anterior two-thirds of the tongue is embryologically and anatomically distinct from the posterior third, and separated by a dozen or so large circumvallate papillae. The anterior two-thirds is coated with many filiform, but relatively few fungiform, papillae. Behind the circumvallate papillae, the tongue contains several large lymphoid masses (lingual tonsil) and the foliate papillae lie on the lateral borders posteriorly. These are often mistaken for tumours. The tongue may be fissured (scrotal) but this is usually regarded as a developmental anomaly. A healthy child's tongue is rarely coated but a mild coating is not uncommon in healthy adults. The voluntary tongue movements and sense of taste should be formally tested. Abnormalities of tongue movement (neurological or muscular disease) may be obvious from dysarthria or involuntary movements and any fibrillation or wasting noted. Hypoglossal palsy may lead to deviation of the tongue towards the affected side on protrusion. Taste sensation can be tested by placing the tongue across the terminals of a pocket torch battery when a metallic taste may be obvious. Formal testing with salt, sweet, sour and bitter should be carried out by applying solutions of salt, sugar, dilute acetic acid and 5% citric acid to the tongue on a cotton swab or cotton bud.

Palate and fauces. These consist of an anterior hard and posterior soft palate, and the tonsillar area and oropharynx. The mucosa of the hard palate is firmly bound down as a mucoperiosteum (similar to the gingivae) and with no obvious vascular arcades. Rugae are present anteriorly on either side of the incisive papilla that overlies the incisive foramen. Bony lumps in the posterior centre of the vault of the hard palate are usually tori (torus palatinus). Patients may complain of lumps distal to the upper molars that they think are unerupted teeth but the pterygoid hamulus or tuberosity is usually responsible for this complaint. The soft palate and fauces may show a faint vascular arcade. In the soft palate, just posterior to the junction with the hard palate, is a conglomeration of minor salivary glands. This region is often also yellowish. The palate should be inspected and movements examined when the patient says 'Aah'. Using a mirror, this also permits inspection of the posterior tongue, tonsils, oropharynx, and can even offer a glimpse of the larynx. Glossopharyngeal palsy may lead to uvula deviation to the contralateral side.

Anatomical variants

Patients sometimes become concerned after noticing various anatomical variants in the mouth. These include tori and exostoses [1–3], which are developmental bony lumps seen especially in Mongoloid and black races. Most common is torus palatinus, a slow-growing, asymptomatic, benign, bony lump in the midline of the palate (Figure 110.2). Tori mandibularis are bilateral, asymptomatic, benign, bony lumps lingual to the premolars.

The diagnosis is confirmed by radiography. Surgery is rarely indicated. These are excised or reduced only if causing severe difficulties with dentures. Rarely, there is a need to exclude other conditions such as Gardner syndrome and familial polyposis coli.

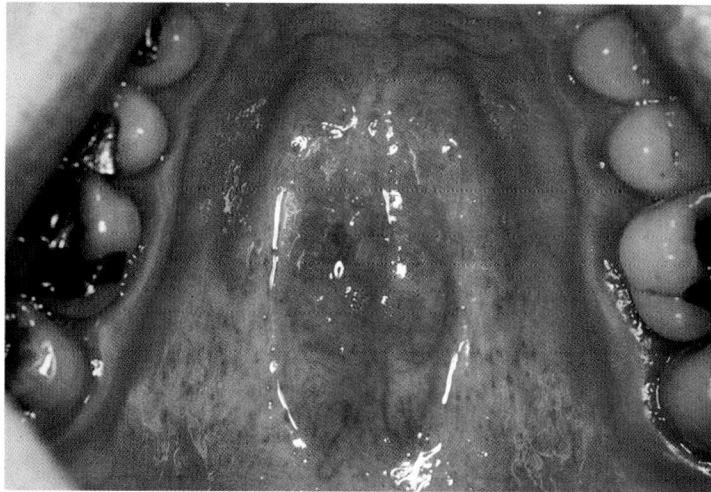

Figure 110.2 Torus palatinus.

DISORDERS AFFECTING THE ORAL MUCOSA OR LIPS

Blisters, erosions and ulcers

Blisters may be seen as a result of burns or mucocoeles. Most mucocoeles, caused by extravasation of mucus from minor salivary glands, produce isolated blisters, typically in the lower labial mucosa. Superficial mucocoeles can be seen there or on the soft palate and are sometimes associated with oral lichen planus. However, the most important vesiculobullous disorders affecting the oral mucosa are pemphigoid (including cicatricial pemphigoid) and pemphigus (Box 110.1). The bullae of mucous membrane pemphigoid may or may not be blood filled and, in the former case, a bleeding tendency must be excluded. Blood-filled blisters may also be caused by localized oral purpura (angina bullosa haemorrhagica) or amyloidosis. The bullae of pemphigus are rarely seen as they break down rapidly to produce ulcers. Epidermolysis bullosa and erythema multiforme (EM) may present with oral bullae or vesicles, although ulcers are more common. Vesicles may be seen in viral infections, especially in herpes simplex stomatitis, chickenpox, herpangina and hand, foot and mouth disease.

Oral ulcers are often caused by trauma or recurrent aphthae. Malignant neoplasms may present as ulcers. Various infections or systemic disorders, particularly those of the blood, gastrointestinal tract or skin, also produce mouth ulcers, as may drugs and irradiation (see Box 110.1).

Lumps and swellings

Mucosal swelling may be seen after trauma, from foreign bodies including cosmetic implants, and in angio-oedema, Crohn disease, orofacial granulomatosis, sarcoidosis, granulomatosis with polyangiitis (GPA) (previously termed Wegener's granulomatosis),

Box 110.1 Main causes of mouth ulcers associated with systemic disease

- Microbial disease
  - Herpetic stomatitis
  - Chickenpox
  - Herpes zoster
  - Hand, foot and mouth disease
  - Herpangina
  - Infectious mononucleosis
  - HIV disease
  - Tuberculosis
  - Syphilis
  - Fungal infections (rare)
- Malignant neoplasms
- Cutaneous disease
  - Erosive lichen planus and chronic ulcerative stomatitis
  - Pemphigus
  - Pemphigoid
  - Erythema multiforme
  - Dermatitis herpetiformis and linear IgA disease
  - Epidermolysis bullosa
  - Other dermatoses
- Blood disorders
  - Anaemia
  - Leukaemia
  - Neutropenia
  - Other white cell dyscrasias
- Gastrointestinal diseases
  - Coeliac disease
  - Crohn disease
  - Ulcerative colitis
- Rheumatic diseases
  - Lupus erythematosus
  - Behçet syndrome
  - Sweet syndrome
  - Reactive arthritis
- Drugs
  - Cytotoxic, NSAIDs, nicorandil, alendronate and other agents
  - Acrodynia
- Radiotherapy
- Disorders of uncertain pathogenesis
  - Angina bullosa haemorrhagica
  - Hypereosinophilic syndrome
  - Eosinophilic ulcer
  - Necrotizing sialometaplasia

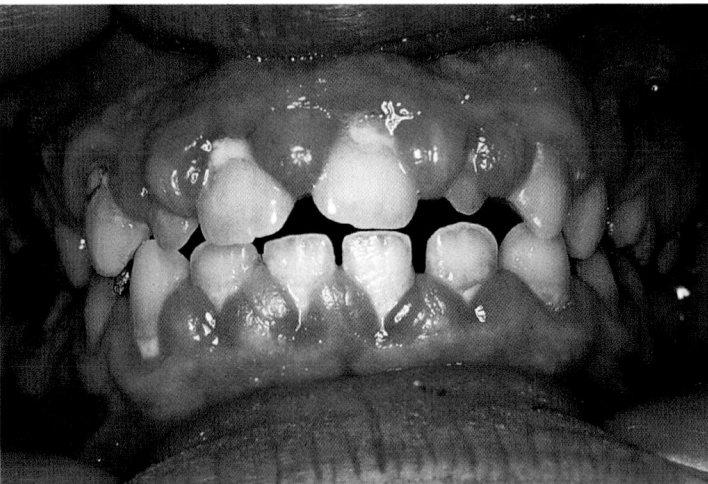

Figure 110.3 Gingival hyperplasia in phenytoin therapy. Concomitant folate deficiency in this patient also caused mouth ulcers, seen in the maxillary buccal vestibule.

Addison disease, Carney syndrome, Kaposi sarcoma, melanoma, Laugier–Hunziker syndrome, pigmentary incontinence and other causes must be excluded. Peutz–Jeghers disease is the association of circumoral and sometimes intraoral melanosis with small-intestinal polyposis (see Chapter 152). Oral petechiae are usually caused by trauma or suction. More widespread purpura is most frequently a manifestation of a bleeding tendency caused by thrombocytopenia/thrombocytopathy and may also be seen in infectious mononucleosis, rubella, HIV infection, leukaemia or scurvy. Petechiae may also occur in amyloidosis.

Redness

Red lesions may be inflammatory, or represent erythroplasia, haemangiomas or neoplasms such as carcinoma, GPA or Kaposi sarcoma [1,2]. Mucositis, with widespread erythema followed by

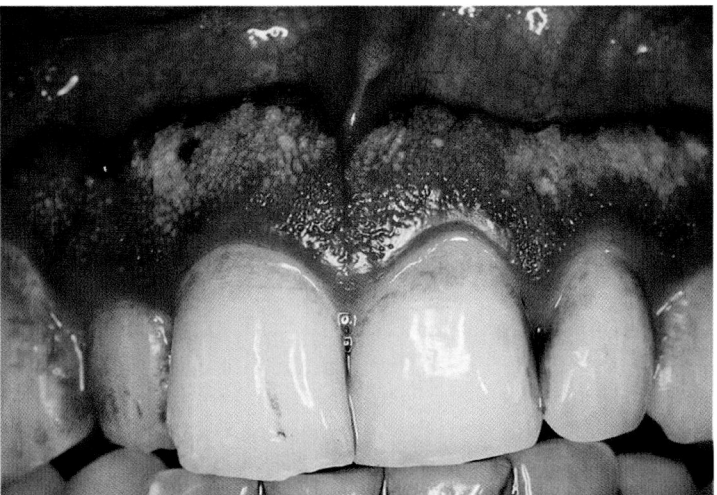

Figure 110.4 Gingival hyperpigmentation of racial origin. The white lesion is due to accumulated oral debris – oral hygiene is very poor.

amyloidosis and other disorders. Localized swellings may be of local aetiology (including cosmetic fillers) or can be manifestations of neoplasia, systemic disease or drugs (Figure 110.3).

Pigmentation

Mucosal pigmentation is usually seen in people of colour (but may be seen even in white people) (Figure 110.4). Other common causes include amalgam tattoo and melanotic macules.

erosions/ulcers can readily be induced by irradiation or chemotherapy.

Widespread erythema, particularly if associated with pain, is usually caused by primary herpes simplex stomatitis or a mucocutaneous disorder such as lichen planus or mucous membrane pemphigoid, rarely by pemphigus or other dermatoses and occasionally by allergic responses. Candidosis may cause red lesions, some of which may be painful.

Localized red areas may represent erythema migrans, erythroplasia, carcinoma, candidosis, lichen planus, lupus erythematosus or Kaposi sarcoma or epithelioid angiomatosis. Geographic tongue (erythema migrans) may cause red patches usually on the tongue dorsum and is often asymptomatic. Lingual depapillation in patches is seen in geographic tongue, and in deficiencies of iron, folate or vitamin B_{12} depapillation may produce the red tongue termed 'glossitis'. Kaposi sarcoma may present as a red, purple, brown or bluish macule or nodule, as may epithelioid angiomatosis. Hereditary mucoepithelial dysplasia is a rare cause of oral erythema.

Telangiectasia may be a manifestation of hereditary haemorrhagic telangiectasia, primary biliary cirrhosis or systemic sclerosis, or may follow radiotherapy. Haemangiomas are usually isolated but may occasionally extend deeply and rarely involve the ipsilateral meninges, producing a facial angioma and epilepsy, sometimes with learning disability (Sturge–Weber syndrome). Intraoral haemangiomas may be seen in Maffucci syndrome.

White patches (Box 110.2)

Thrush (acute candidosis) is a 'disease of the diseased' and produces oral white patches. HIV infection causes hairy leukoplakia, a white lesion on the tongue associated with Epstein–Barr virus (EBV) infection.

Box 110.2 Main causes of oral white lesions

- Local
  - Materia alba
  - Candidosis
  - Frictional keratosis
  - Smoker's keratosis
  - Idiopathic keratosis
  - Carcinoma
  - Burns (including snuff and cocaine)
  - Skin grafts
- Systemic
  - Candidosis
  - Lichen planus
  - Lupus erythematosus
  - Papillomas (some)
  - Hairy leukoplakia (mainly HIV disease)
  - Syphilitic keratosis
  - Chronic renal failure
  - Inherited lesions (e.g. white sponge naevus)

Leukoplakia is often associated with friction or smoking, occasionally with syphilis, candidosis or chronic renal failure, but most cases are idiopathic. Lichen planus and lupus erythematosus may present as white lesions. Rarely, lichenoid lesions are associated with various drugs, liver disease or graft-versus-host disease (GVHD). Carcinoma may present as a white lesion.

Inherited causes of white patches, such as white sponge naevus and dyskeratosis congenita, are rare [1–8].

GENETIC DISORDERS AFFECTING THE ORAL MUCOSA OR LIPS

This section discusses the main congenital causes of lumps and swellings pigmented lesions, red lesions, vesiculoerosive lesions, white or whitish lesions, and some orocutaneous disorders. These are alphabetically arranged to facilitate access.

LUMPS AND SWELLINGS

Angio-oedema (hereditary)

Synonyms and inclusions
- C1-esterase inhibitor deficiency

Hereditary angio-oedema (HANE) is a rare autosomal dominant disorder caused by C1-inhibitor deficiency. HANE mimics allergic angio-oedema (see Chapter 43), although it produces a more severe reaction, with oedema affecting the lips, mouth, face and neck region, the extremities and gastrointestinal tract after minor trauma [1,2–5].

Blunt injury is the most consistent precipitating event. The trauma of dental treatment is a potent trigger, and some attacks even follow emotional stress. Oedema may persist for many hours and even up to 4 days. Involvement of the airway is a constant threat. The mortality may be as high as 30% in some families but the disease is compatible with prolonged survival if emergencies are avoided or effectively treated.

Diagnosis
In 85% of cases plasma C1-esterase levels are reduced (type 1 hereditary angio-oedema) but in 15% the enzyme is present but dysfunctional (type 2 hereditary angio-oedema). In both types, plasma C4 levels fall but C3 levels are normal. Rarely, similar defects are acquired.

Management
C1-esterase concentrates are available for treatment [3,6–10]. Plasminogen inhibitors such as tranexamic acid have been used to mitigate attacks [3,11], more effective agents are the androgenic steroids danazol and stanozolol, which raise plasma C1-esterase inhibitor levels to normal [1,2–4], although current treatment is C1-esterase concentrate or ecallantide [12,13].

Focal dermal hypoplasia

Synonyms and inclusions
• Goltz–Gorlin syndrome

Focal dermal hypoplasia is a rare, presumably X-linked, genodermatosis [1–3] involving developmental anomalies of tissues and organs of mesoectodermal origin. Thus there are abnormalities of the eyes, skin, musculoskeletal system, central nervous system (CNS) and oral structures.

Papillomas, usually of the oral mucosae and lips, dental anomalies and occasional cleft lip and palate are the main oral features [2–6]. The dental anomalies, seen in about half of affected individuals, include hypodontia, enamel defects and taurodontism [7–10].

Acanthosis nigricans

Oral papillifcrous lesions may be a feature of both familial [1,2] and malignant [1,3–8] acanthosis nigricans. Between 30 and 50% of patients with acanthosis nigricans secondary to neoplasia (malignant acanthosis nigricans) have oral lesions, which involve the tongue and lips predominantly.

Lymphangioma

Lymphangioma is uncommon in the mouth. At least some are hamartomas and many are of similar structure to haemangiomas and can clinically resemble them, with a 'frog-spawn' appearance, but they contain lymph rather than blood (Figure 110.5).

Lymphangiomas are usually solitary and affect the tongue predominantly. They are occasionally associated with cystic hygroma [1–7]. One study has found blue domed lymphangiomas on the alveolar ridges of about 4% of newborn black children [3]. These lesions, which were usually bilateral, often regressed spontaneously.

Contrast-enhanced T_1-weighted magnetic resonance imaging (MRI) can be used to differentiate between lymphangiomas and deep haemangiomas [8]. Small lymphangiomas need no treatment. Larger lesions may require excision, although cryotherapy laser therapy and sclerotherapy can be useful and, more recently, radiofrequency ablation has been described [7,9].

A number of reports describe lymphangiomas presenting on the alveolar ridges of newborn children [3,10,11].

Dermoid cyst

Dermoid cyst is a hamartoma, a development lesion commonly arising in the midline of the neck, above the mylohyoid. It occasionally occurs elsewhere such as the tongue, antrum and rarely the parotid gland [1–7].

Dermoid cysts usually become clinically obvious in the second decade of life and cause elevation of the tongue. Occasionally, dermoid cysts become infected and then painful.

Treatment of dermoid cyst is by surgical excision.

Lingual tonsil

The lingual tonsil is a mass of lymphoid tissue in the posterior third of the tongue, between the epiglottis posteriorly and the circumvallate papillae anteriorly [1,2]. It is usually divided in the midline by a ligament (Figure 110.6). Although usually small and asymptomatic, it may become enlarged, especially in atopic individuals, in patients taking phenytoin or in some infections. It may be so prominent that it fills the vallecula and impinges against the epiglottis. If the lingual tonsil is large, it may cause a globus

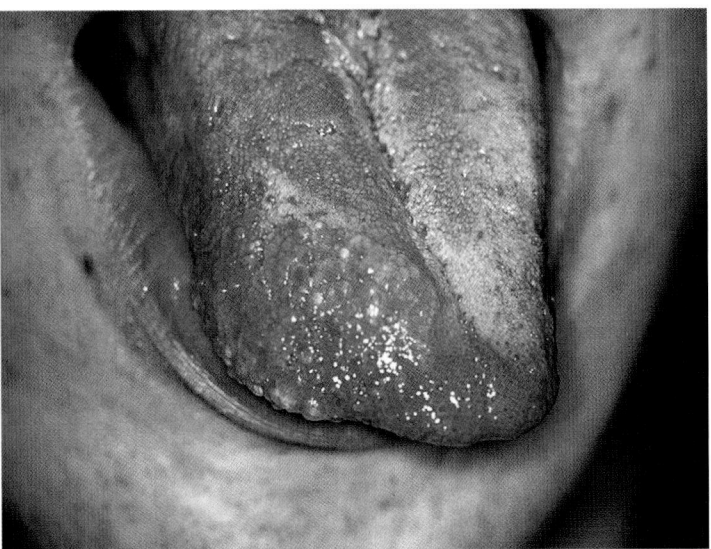

Figure 110.5 Lymphangioma of the tongue: a common site.

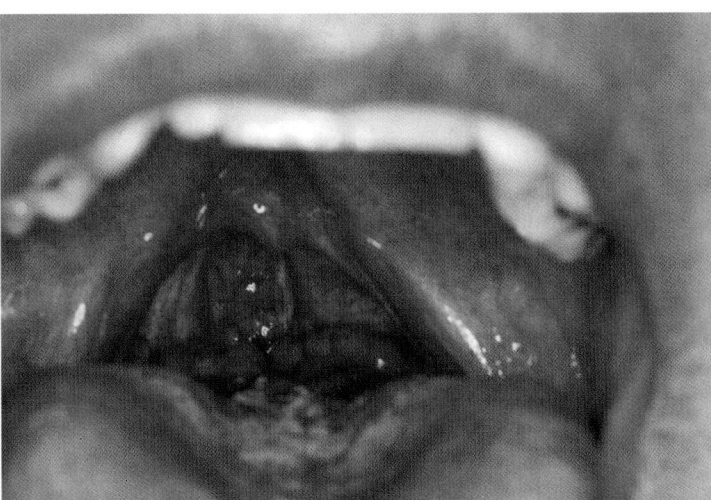

Figure 110.6 Lingual tonsil showing a well-demarcated midline groove. (Courtesy of Dr C.T.C. Kennedy, Bristol Royal Infirmary, Bristol, UK.)

sensation, alteration of the voice, obstructive sleep apnoea or airways obstruction [3–8]. It tends to involve with increasing age.

Occasionally, there may be lingual tonsillitis with a red, swollen, painful tongue, fever and neutrophilia [9].

The condition must be distinguished from benign and malignant tumours of the tongue, including lingual thyroid, but the symmetry of the lingual tonsil and its midline division are helpful diagnostic pointers.

Treatment may be required if the enlarged tonsil causes symptoms. Surgery may be hazardous because of the copious blood supply to the tongue base. Electrocautery and cryotherapy are generally regarded as the safer procedures [1,10,11].

Gastro-oesophageal reflux and body mass index may be associated with lingual tonsil hypertrophy in adults with sleep-disordered breathing [12].

Lingual thyroid

Ectopic thyroid tissue may rarely present clinically in the mouth, though some 10% of cadaver tongues contain thyroid tissue. Typically, an asymptomatic, smooth-surfaced lump in the midline of the base of the tongue, between the sulcus terminalis and epiglottis at the site of the foramen caecum [1–5], a lingual thyroid may occasionally produce dysphagia, cough, pain or, rarely, airways obstruction [1–11].

Not all lingual thyroid tissue is functional, and function tends to decline with age. Where thyroid-stimulating hormone levels are high, thyroid hormone supplements are indicated [1,12]. Malignant change is rare in lingual thyroid, although follicular carcinomas have been recorded. MRI and ^{99m}Tc pertechnate scintiscanning is important to ensure the presence of normal thyroid tissue in the neck [13–16] before considering treatment of a lingual thyroid by surgery or radioiodine [1,2,17,18]. If removal is deemed appropriate a total lingual thyroidectomy transoral approach with use of either a microscope or a robotic endoscope for optical assistance is recommended [19].

Multiple mucosal neuroma syndrome

The syndrome of multiple endocrine neoplasia (MEN) type 2b (also called type 3) is inherited as an autosomal dominant, although new cases often arise sporadically. The gene locus is on chromosome 10 with germline mutations in the RET proto-oncogene.

Multiple endocrine neoplasia type 2b is characterized by medullary carcinoma of the thyroid and phaeochromocytoma, in association with multiple mucosal neuromas and an abnormal phenotype – a striking facial appearance, with thick slightly everted lips that usually have a slightly bumpy surface due to multiple neuromas [1–4]. These are actually mucosal and submucosal hamartomatous proliferations of nerve axons, Schwann cells and ganglion cells.

Lesions may also involve the tongue and commissures but are less frequent on the buccal mucosa, gingivae, palate, pharynx or larynx (Figure 110.7).

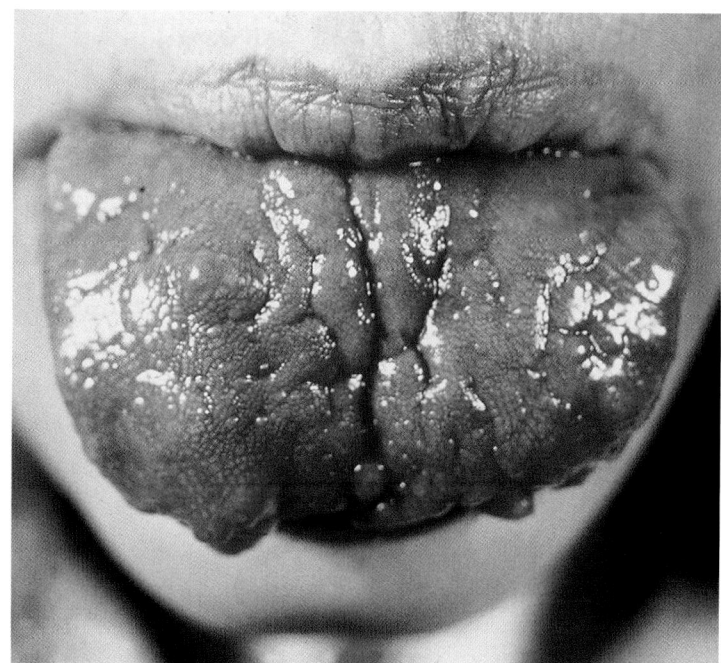

Figure 110.7 Multiple neuromas of the lips and tongue in a patient with multiple endocrine neoplasia syndrome (type 2). (Courtesy of Dr M. Hartog, Bristol Royal Infirmary, Bristol, UK.)

Most patients have an asthenic marfanoid habitus, with high arched palate, pectus excavatum, arachnodactyly and kyphoscoliosis, but the lens subluxation and cardiovascular abnormalities of Marfan syndrome are not present [5–12]. Differential diagnosis includes multiple idiopathic mucosal neuromas and PTEN hamartoma-tumour (Cowden) syndrome [13,14].

PIGMENTED LESIONS (Box 110.3)

Most oral hyperpigmentation is racial in origin (see Figure 110.4) but there are many other causes – especially various drugs – from antimalarials to imatinib. Seen mainly in people of African or Asian heritage, racial pigmentation can also be noted in patients of Mediterranean descent, sometimes even in some fairly light-skinned people. It is most obvious in the anterior labial gingivae and palatal mucosa and pigmentation is usually symmetrically distributed. Patches may be seen elsewhere. Pigmentation may be first noted by the patient in adult life and then incorrectly assumed to be acquired rather than congenital in origin.

Lentiginoses

The lentiginoses (or lentigenoses) include Peutz–Jeghers syndrome, LEOPARD syndrome (*l*entigines, *E*CG changes, *o*cular hyperteleorism, *p*ulmonary stenosis, *a*bnormal genitalia, *r*etardation of growth, *d*eafness), syndrome of arterial dissections with lentiginosis, Laugier–Hunziker–Baran syndrome, Cowden disease, Ruvalcaba–Myhre–Smith (Bannayan–Zonana) syndrome,

---

Box 110.3 Causes of mucosal pigmentation

- Localized
  - Amalgam tattoo
  - Ephelis (freckle)
  - Naevus
  - Malignant melanoma
  - Kaposi sarcoma
  - Peutz–Jeghers syndrome
  - Laugier–Hunziker syndrome
  - Melanotic macules
  - Complex of myxomas, spotty pigmentation and endocrine overactivity
- Generalized
  - Racial
  - Localized irritation, e.g. smoking
  - Drugs, e.g. phenothiazines, antimalarials, minocycline, contraceptives, mephenytoin
  - Addison disease
  - Nelson syndrome
  - Ectopic adrenocorticotrophic hormone (e.g. bronchogenic carcinoma)
  - Heavy metals
  - Albright syndrome
  - Other rare causes, e.g. haemochromatosis, generalized neurofibromatosis, incontinentia pigmenti
  - Malignant acanthosis nigricans

---

and the centrofacial, benign patterned and segmental lentiginoses, all of which can be associated with a variety of developmental defects.

Centrofacial lentiginosis syndrome

Synonyms and inclusions
- Touraine centrofacial lentiginosis

Centrofacial lentiginosis [1,2] is associated with bone abnormalities, malformations due to dysraphia, endocrine dysfunctions and neurological diseases.

Complex of myxomas, spotty pigmentation and endocrine overactivity

Synonyms and inclusions
- Carney syndrome
- Carney complex

This autosomal dominant trait, the Carney complex gene 1 is the regulatory subunit 1A of protein kinase A (PRKAR1A) located at 17q22-24. An inactivating heterozygous germ line mutation of PRKAR1A is observed in about two-thirds of Carney complex patients. Carney complex causes cardiac and cutaneous myxomas, with mammary myxoid fibroadenomas, spotty cutaneous hyperpigmentation, primary pigmented nodular adrenocortical disease, testicular Sertoli cell tumours and growth hormone-secreting pituitary adenoma. It may present with oral hyperpigmentation and myxomas [1–5].

The hyperpigmentation in Carney complex is facial and occurs on the vermilion of the lips in about 35%, although about 8% have pigmented lesions on the oral mucosa and about 2% have oral myxomas, usually on the palate or tongue [2]. Carney complex differs clinically from Peutz–Jeghers syndrome in that hyperpigmentation is less common intraorally but more common on the conjunctiva, and other manifestations are also present.

Cases previously described as NAME syndrome (*n*aevi, *a*trial myxoma, *m*yxoid neurofibromas, *e*phelides) and LAMB syndrome (*l*entigines, *a*trial myxoma, *m*ucocutaneous myxoma, *b*lue naevi) may represent this complex, which also has close similarities to LEOPARD syndrome and the syndrome of arterial dissections with lentiginosis.

Inherited patterned lentiginosis in black people

This autosomal dominant condition is characterized by small discrete hyperpigmented macules on the face, lips, extremities, buttocks and palmoplantar areas [1]. No series of patients have been reported with oral mucosal lesions or internal organ system abnormalities.

This condition can resemble other lentiginosis syndromes, especially Peutz–Jeghers syndrome, centrofacial lentiginosis syndrome and Carney complex.

Laugier–Hunziker syndrome [1–12]

Synonyms and inclusions
- Laugier–Hunziker–Baran syndrome

Laugier–Hunziker syndrome presents with labial, oral mucosal and nail hyperpigmentation. A possible variant of this or Peutz–Jeghers syndrome has been termed *idiopathic lenticular pigmentation* [1–8], in which there are oral, labial, perianal and digital hyperpigmented lenticular macules. Similar patients have been reported previously [9–11]. Treatment with the Q-switched Nd-Yag laser has been reported [12] as has recurrence after laser therapy [12].

Melanotic macule

The melanotic macule is an acquired, small, flat, brown to brown-black, asymptomatic, benign lesion, unchanging in character [1–4]. Oral melanotic macule is similar to the ephelis and lentigo.

Melanotic macules may be seen in up to 3% of normal persons, at any age. Melanotic macules are usually solitary, discrete, pigmented brown collections of melanin-containing cells. The macules are less than 2 cm in diameter, seen especially on the vermilion of the lips, gingiva, buccal mucosa or palate. Most on the lips are seen near the midline, on the lower lip vermilion. Most are solitary and seen in white adults and their colour ranges from brown to black [1,5,6]. Occasional cases are seen in HIV infection [7].

Clinically, the melanotic macule may resemble other lesions such as early melanoma and ephelides, although the latter tend to fade in winter and darken in summer. Histopathologically, the mucosal epithelium is normal apart from increased pigmentation of the basal layer, accentuated at the tips of rete ridges. There are no naevus cells or elongated rete ridges [3]. There is melanin in the epithelial basal layer and/or upper lamina propria. Occasionally they are seen along with melanonychia striata (Laugier–Hunziker syndrome, see below).

Melanotic macules can be excised to exclude melanoma or for cosmetic reasons, or removed by laser or hidden by lipstick [8–12].

Naevi

Pigmented naevi are much less common in the oral mucosa than in skin. Approximately half of naevi are histologically of the intradermal (intramucosal) type; one-third are blue naevi; many others are compound naevi; and some are junctional naevi.

Pathology. They are formed from increased melanin-containing cells, are flat or raised, do not change rapidly in size or colour, are painless and are seen particularly on the palate. The intramucosal type of naevus is most common (about 60%), while another 25% are blue naevi. Compound and junctional naevi and combined naevi are rare in the mouth. The intramucosal naevus consists of a collection of melanocytic cells in the lamina propria without involvement of the epithelium. The blue naevus consists of spindle cells at any level in the lamina propria. The junctional naevus consists of clusters of benign naevus cells at the epithelio–mesenchymal junction and the lamina propria is otherwise not involved.

Clinical features. Pigmented naevi are seen particularly on the vermilion border of the lip and on the palate or buccal mucosa [1,2]. These lesions are usually brown, macular, do not change rapidly in size or colour and are painless. The prognosis is good.

Management. Although there is no evidence that most pigmented naevi progress to melanoma [3], there has been concern expressed that junctional naevi may be a risk factor though evidence does not support this [4].

However, pigmented naevi may resemble melanomas and if early detection of oral melanomas is to be achieved, all pigmented oral cavity lesions should be viewed with suspicion. Therefore, excision biopsy is recommended to exclude malignancy [3] and may also be performed for cosmetic reasons. This is particularly important if the lesions are raised or nodular [2,3].

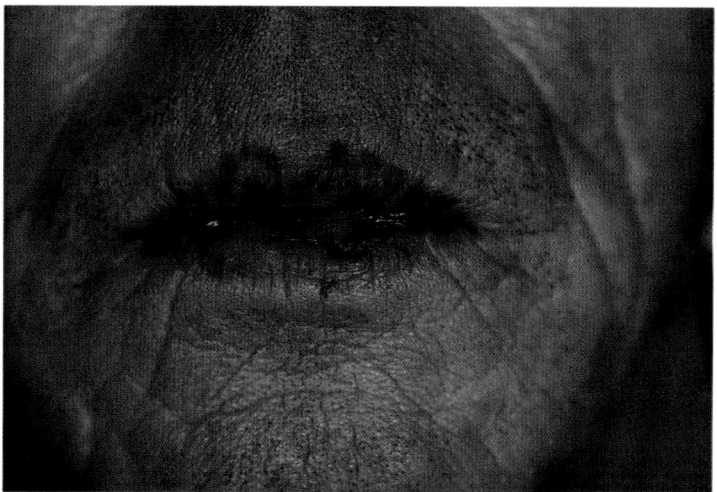

Figure 110.8 Peutz–Jeghers syndrome.

Peutz–Jeghers syndrome

Peutz–Jeghers syndrome is an autosomal dominant trait with mutations in serine/threonine kinase 11 (STK11) and characterized by gastrointestinal hamartomatous polyps, mucocutaneous pigmentation, especially circumorally, and an increased risk for specific cancers (see also Chapter 152). Those affected have discrete brown to bluish black macules mainly around the oral, nasal and ocular orifices. The lips, especially the lower, have pigmented macules in about 98% of patients (Figure 110.8). Oral brown or black macules, unlike the circumoral lesions, do not fade after puberty. Mucosal and facial hyperpigmentation may also be seen in relatives [1–3].

Intestinal polyps are found mainly in the small intestine and rarely undergo malignant change but if they produce intussusception, surgical intervention is required. There is a slightly increased risk of gastrointestinal carcinoma and carcinomas of the pancreas, breast and reproductive organs [4–9].

Ruby and argon lasers have been used to treat the pigmentation of the lips and oral mucosa [10] (see Chapter 160).

Pseudoxanthoma elasticum

See Chapter 96.

RED LESIONS

Benign migratory glossitis (geographic tongue)

Synonyms and inclusions
- Lingual erythema migrans
- Geographical tongue

A benign inflammatory condition of the tongue with map-like areas of erythema which are not constant in size, shape or location. Lingual erythema migrans is unrelated to cutaneous erythema migrans.

Introduction and general description

Geographic tongue is characterized by map-like red areas with increased thickness of intervening filiform papillae. Alternatively, there are rounded, sometimes scalloped, reddish areas with a white margin (Figures 110.9 and 110.10). These patterns change from day to day and even within a few hours.

Epidemiology

It is a common condition, affecting about 1–2% of the population [1–4].

Age

Patients of any age may be affected but why the condition sometimes gives rise to symptoms after it has been present asymptomatically for decades is unclear.

Pathophyslology

There is epithelial thinning at the centre of the lesion with an inflammatory infiltrate mainly of polymorphonuclear leukocytes [1,2].

Genetics

A positive family history may be obtainable. Human leukocyte antigen (HLA) findings have been equivocal, with reports of associations with B15 and DR7 [5].

Environmental factors

Some patients with lingual erythema migrans have atopic allergies such as hay fever and a few relate the oral lesions to a particular food, for example cheese, or to stress.

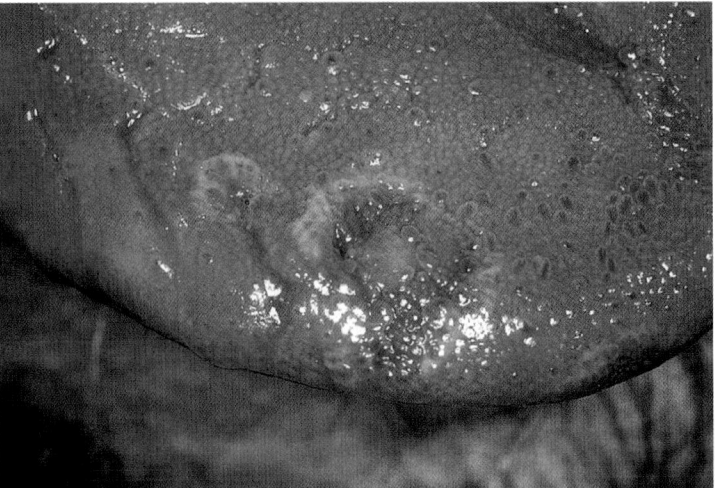

Figure 110.10 Somewhat less obvious signs of lingual erythema migrans.

Clinical features

Geographic tongue may be asymptomatic or cause a sore tongue [6,7–9]. Rarely, other sites, such as the labial or palatal mucosa, are affected. The tongue is usually, but not invariably, affected simultaneously with the other sites [10]. There are no complications.

Investigations

Clinical examination usually suffices to differentiate the condition from lichen planus, candidosis, psoriasis, reactive arthritis, larva migrans or deficiency glossitis. Many patients with a fissured tongue (scrotal tongue) also have lingual erythema migrans. Similar oral lesions may be seen in reactive arthritis (previously termed Reiter syndrome), generalized pustular psoriasis and acrodermatitis continua of Hallopeau [6,11–13]. Purported associations with diabetes [14,15] may be coincidental.

Management

In those with no systemic disorder, no effective treatment is available except reassurance but benzydamine hydrochloride 0.15% spray or mouthwash may provide symptomatic relief [16]. Topical 0.1% tacrolimus has been used [17] but there is an American Food and Drug Agency (FDA) advisory that may be relevant.

Hereditary haemorrhagic telangiectasia

Synonyms and inclusions
• Osler–Rendu–Weber syndrome

Hereditary haemorrhagic telangiectasia is predominantly caused by mutations in *ENG* and *ACVRL1*, which both belong to the transforming growth factor (TGF)-β signalling pathway. This syndrome is characterized by multiple telangiectasia on the lips, perioral skin, oral and nasal mucosae [1,2] as well as the gastrointestinal tract. Occasionally, there are colonic or hepatic complications [3–6]. Oral haemorrhage can be controlled by cryotherapy, cautery,

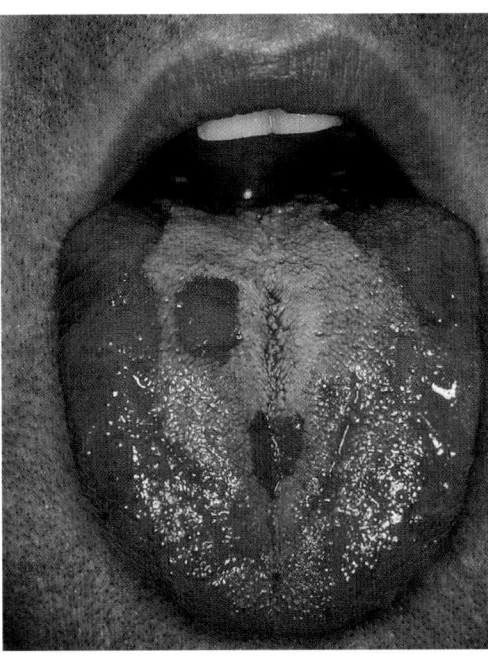

Figure 110.9 Classical geographic tongue (lingual erythema migrans).

infrared coagulation, Nd-Yag laser or intense pulsed light [7–9] or bevacizumab, a vascular endothelial growth factor (VEGF) inhibitor [10], which may reduce epistaxis, telangiectasias and iron deficiency anaemia.

Haemangioma

Haemangiomas are usually deep red or blue-purple, blanch on pressure, are fluctuant to palpation, and are level with the mucosa or have a lobulated or raised surface [1,2]. Most are small and of no consequence [1,3].

Most haemangiomas are seen in isolation but a few may be multiple and/or part of a wider syndrome, such as Maffucci syndrome [4,5]. Large facial haemangiomas, which can involve the lips, may be associated with Sturge–Weber syndrome (Figure 110.11) [4] or Dandy–Walker syndrome, or other posterior cranial fossa malformations [6,7].

Haemangiomas are at risk from trauma and prone to excessive bleeding if damaged (e.g. during tooth extraction). Occasionally, oral haemangiomas develop phlebolithiasis.

Oral lesions suspected of being haemangiomatous should not be routinely biopsied; aspiration is far safer. Kaposi sarcoma and epithelioid angiomatosis should be excluded. After intravenous administration of contrast medium, enhancement is observed in haemangiomas in areas corresponding to those with high signal on T_2-weighted MRI.

Oral haemangiomas are left alone unless causing symptoms, when they are best treated with cryosurgery or laser if small, or by ligation or embolization of feeding vessels if large.

Sturge–Weber–Krabbe syndrome

The haemangioma in the trigeminal area in Sturge–Weber syndrome is usually unilateral, may involve the mouth but fortunately rarely involves bone [1–7] (see Chapter 73). It may be associated

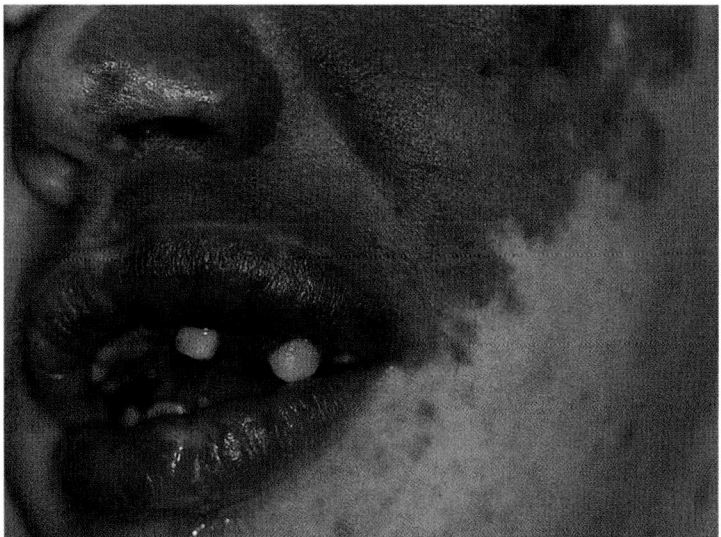

Figure 110.11 Haemangioma affecting the lip in Sturge–Weber syndrome.

with hypertrophy of affected tissues and, if the patient is treated with phenytoin, with gingival hyperplasia [3,4].

Klippel–Trenaunay–Weber syndrome (see Chapter 73)

Haemangiomas of the buccal mucosa and tongue, macroglossia, maxillary hyperplasia and an anterior open bite have been recorded in this syndrome [1–8]. Post-extraction bleeding can be a problem [8,9].

Blue rubber–bleb naevus syndrome (see Chapter 73)

Synonyms and inclusions
- Bean syndrome

Oral haemangiomas may be seen [1–5].

Glomovenous malformations

Glomovenous malformations are disseminated variants of cutaneous glomus tumours. Some have been treated successfully with sequential pulsed dye Nd-Yag laser [1].

Maffucci syndrome

Oral haemangiomas may be seen [1–5].

Mucoepithelial dysplasia

Hereditary mucoepithelial dysplasia is an autosomal dominant dyskeratotic epithelial syndrome affecting oral, nasal, vaginal, urethral, anal, bladder and conjunctival mucosae, causing cataracts, follicular keratosis, non-scarring alopecia and terminal lung disease [1–5].

Pathology. The condition is probably a pan-epithelial cell defect of desmosomal and gap junction structure. Histochemically, there is a lack of cornification and keratinization. Electron microscopy shows an abnormality in desmosomes and gap junctions, with a lack of keratohyalin granules, a paucity of desmosomes, intercellular accumulations, cytoplasmic vacuolization, and formation of bands and aggregates of filamentous fibres and structures in the cytoplasm resembling desmosomes and gap junctions. There is some acantholysis as well as benign dyskeratosis of individual cells [1,2]. Histologically, the mucosal epithelium shows dyshesion, thinning of the epithelial layer and dyskeratosis. Mucosal Papanicolaou smears show lack of epithelial maturation, cytoplasmic vacuoles and inclusions, and individual cell dyskeratosis.

Clinical features. Red periorificial mucosal lesions are typically noted during infancy and may persist throughout life. The oral lesions are painless red macules or maculopapules and are seen predominantly on the palate and gingiva [3–5].

Severe photophobia, tearing and nystagmus in infancy herald the development of keratitis, corneal vascularization and lens cataracts.

In addition, there may be various cardiorespiratory complications, especially potentially lethal bullous lung disease –

PART 10: SITES, SEX, AGE

spontaneous pneumothorax and bullous emphysema, terminating in cor pulmonale. Chronic rhinorrhoea and repeated upper respiratory infections frequently progress to bilateral pneumonia. Loss of hair, diarrhoea, melaena, enuresis, pyuria and haematuria may also be seen.

Venous mucocutaneous malformation

Venous mucocutaneous malformation are seen most commonly on mucous membranes, including the mouth, are lighter purple in colour than glomuvenous malformations, are compressible and not painful.

The oral location of the haemangiomas and lack of symptoms distinguish this from glomovenous malformations; lack of other gastrointestinal haemangiomas excluded blue rubber–bleb naevus syndrome; lack of limb hypertrophy differentiated from Klippel–Trenaunay syndrome; and lack of hyperhidrosis and normal D-dimer levels from Bean syndrome. Venous mucocutaneous malformation is a rare autosomal dominant condition with incomplete penetrance, reported in only about 20 families. Venous mucocutaneous malformations are associated with amino acid substitutions in the tyrosine-protein kinase endothelial cell receptor (TEK/TIE2; 9p21). Approximately 90% of individuals with a *TEK* gene mutation develop the venous mucocutaneous malformation by age 20; and ~10% are clinically unaffected.Treatment is with ethanol sclerotherapy. When D-dimers levels are raised, indicating coagulation activation, low-molecular-weight heparins can be used. Females should avoid using high oestrogen oral contraceptives in view of the coagulation tendency.

Resources

Further information

http://www.orpha.net/consor/cgi-bin/OC_Exp.php?lng=en&Expert=2451 (last accessed December 2014).

Wiskott–Aldrich syndrome

(see Chapter 82)

Oral petechiae and infections such as candidosis may occur in the Wiskott–Aldrich syndrome of thrombocytopenia, immune deficiency and eczema [1–4].

VESICULOEROSIVE DISORDERS

Acrodermatitis enteropathica

Acrodermatitis enteropathica is a rare autosomal recessive inborn error of metabolism resulting in zinc malabsorption and severe zinc deficiency seen mainly in premature babies [1–8].

Clinical features. Diarrhoea, mood changes, anorexia and neurological disturbance are reported, most frequently in infancy. Growth retardation, alopecia, weight loss and recurrent infections are prevalent in affected toddlers and schoolchildren. A vesiculobullous dermatitis with perioral involvement may be seen, often sparing the vermilion [2]. Zinc deficiency during growth periods results in growth failure and lack of gonadal development in males. Other effects of zinc deficiency include skin changes, poor appetite, mental lethargy, delayed wound healing, neurosensory disorders and cell-mediated immune disorders. Skin lesions and poor wound healing are observed in severe forms and the disorder can be lethal.

Diagnosis. Assays of zinc in granulocytes and lymphocytes provide better diagnostic criteria for marginal zinc deficiency than plasma zinc assays. In cases of doubt, zinc absorption tests using radioisotopes (^{65}Zn or ^{69m}Zn) may be performed. Levels of alkaline phosphatase are reduced.

Management. Management includes zinc sulphate 2 mg/kg daily, at least until adult life.

Epidermolysis bullosa (see Chapter 71)

Epidermolysis bullosa is characterized by blisters, sometimes preceded by white patches, which develop rapidly, particularly where there is trauma. Blisters rupture to produce ulcers, often with eventual scarring, particularly in the recessive dystrophic types [1–9]. Oral lesions are fairly common in dystrophic and lethal forms of epidermolysis bullosa but are rare in most simplex types except the superficial type, where they are found in 70% of patients [2,10–13]. Overall, oral mucosal lesions are found in about 30% of patients with epidermolysis bullosa [1–5]. There is a predisposition to oral squamous cell carcinoma, mainly in the Hallopeau–Siemens type.

Dental hypoplasia and other defects and delayed tooth eruption may also be a feature, especially in junctional epidermolysis bullosa (Table 110.3) and, with the difficulty in maintaining adequate oral hygiene, there is a predisposition to caries [4,7].

Patients with recessive dystrophic epidermolysis bullosa suffer from severe growth inhibition due to reduced food intake as a result of severe oropharyngeal and oesophageal blistering or scarring, with smaller maxillae and smaller mandibles than normal [8,14–17]. Treatment has improved with modalities such as implants [17–19].

The oral manifestations in the various inherited forms of this condition are summarized in Table 110.3 and epidermolysis bullosa acquisita is discussed in Chapter 50.

Felty syndrome

Oral ulceration may be seen in Felty syndrome [1–3]. Granulocyte colony-stimulating factor or rituximab may be effective therapy [3,4].

Table 110.3 Oral manifestations in epidermolysis bullosa (EB).

Type	EB subtype	Mucosal lesions	Dental hypoplasia
I Epidermolytic (simplex); autosomal dominant	Generalized (Koebner)	±	–
	Localized (Weber–Cockayne)	–	–
	Localized (Kallin)	–	Anodontia
	With mottled pigmentation and punctate keratoderma	+	–
	With bruising (Ogna)	–	±
	Herpetiform (Dowling–Meara)	+	–
	Superficial	+	–
II Junctional; autosomal recessive	Generalized, severe (Herlitz)	+	++
	Generalized, mild	+	+
	Localized	±	+
	Inverse	±	+
	Progressive	+	–
III Dermolytic (dystrophic)	Hyperplastic (Cockayne–Touraine)	±	–
Autosomal dominant	Albopapuloid (Pasini)	+	–
	Pretibial (Kuske–Portugal)	–	–
Autosomal recessive (Hallopeau–Siemens)	Localized	+	±
	Generalized	++	++
	Mutilating	+++	+++
	Inverse	+	–
VI Acquired type	Adult form	±	–
	Child form	+	–

–, Absent; +, mild; ++, moderate; +++, severe.

Immune defects

Mouth ulcers (and early-onset periodontitis) feature in congenital immune defects [1–7,8], including Chédiak–Higashi syndrome, Papillon–Lefèvre syndrome, familial neutropenia, cyclic neutropenia, Job syndrome, chronic granulomatous disease and glycogen storage disease type 1b.

WHITE OR WHITISH LESIONS

Chronic mucocutaneous candidosis

Chronic mucocutaneous candidosis includes a range of congenital disorders characterized by chronic candidosis involving mouth, nails and other sites (see also Chapter 32). Persistent adherent white lesions are seen in the mouth, often with angular stomatitis [1–4]; in candidosis–endocrinopathy syndrome, there may also be enamel hypoplasia [5,6] and, rarely, oral carcinoma [7,8]. *Candida* antigens may trigger a T-helper 2 (Th2) instead of Th1 cytokine response in patients with chronic mucocutaneous candidosis [9–12]. *STAT1* hyperphosphorylation and defective *IL12R/IL23R* signalling may underlie defective immunity in autosomal dominant chronic mucocutaneous candidosis [13].

Clouston syndrome

Hidrotic ectodermal dysplasia, Clouston type, is an autosomal dominant skin disorder most common in the French-Canadian population. Palmoplantar hyperkeratosis, hair defects, nail dysplasia and oral white lesions characterize this disorder. There may be diffuse white lesions in the buccal mucosa, palate, tongue and elsewhere but reports of malignancy are rare [1–3].

Darier disease (see Chapter 66)

Oral lesions are seen in up to 50% of patients with skin lesions of Darier disease. The oral changes are most marked in patients with the most severe skin changes and are typically flattish, coalescing, red plaques that eventually turn white and affect the keratinized mucosa of the dorsum of the tongue, palate and gingiva (Figure 110.12) and then may resemble nicotinic stomatitis clinically [1–6]. Salivary duct anomalies, including dilatations with periodic strictures and indentations, may affect the main ducts [7,8]. There are reports of carcinoma development [9].

Dyskeratosis congenita

Synonyms and inclusions
- Zinsser–Engman–Cole syndrome

Dyskeratosis congenita usually presents with oral lesions between the ages of 5 and 10 years, when the tongue and sometimes the

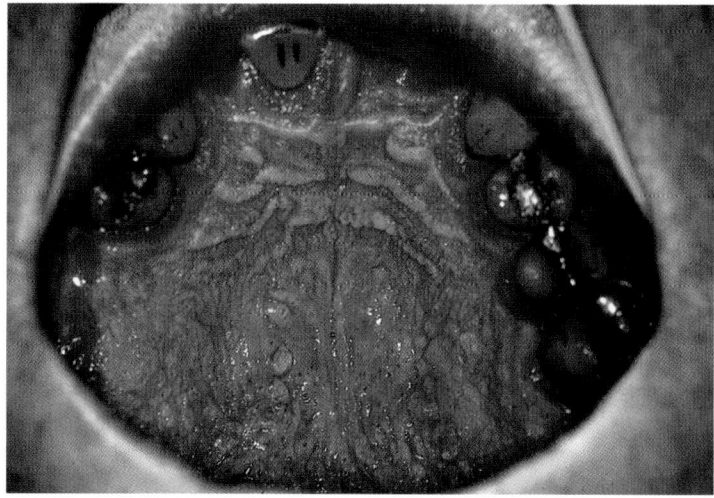

Figure 110.12 Darier disease: oral white lesions resemble those of nicotinic stomatitis.

PART 10: SITES, SEX, AGE

buccal mucosa and palate develop diffuse white lesions with a malignant potential [1,2]. The lesions resemble leukoplakia or lichen planus and show non-specific hyperkeratosis, a prominent granular cell layer and mild acanthosis [1–5].

Other manifestations include lesions of other mucosae, skin and appendages, and bone marrow dysfunction [6,7]. Other rare oral features include taurodont or hypocalcified teeth and mucosal hyperpigmentation.

Focal palmoplantar and oral hyperkeratosis syndrome

Synonyms and inclusions
• Keratosis palmaris et plantaris

Focal hyperkeratosis at weight-bearing areas of the palms and soles, with hyperkeratosis of the attached gingiva and occasionally other sites, is an autosomal dominant trait [1–4].

Fordyce spots

Definition and nomenclature
Fordyce spots are sebaceous glands containing neutral lipids similar to those found in skin sebaceous glands [1] but are not associated with hair follicles.

Synonyms and inclusions
• Fordyce granules

Introduction and general description
Fordyce spots are yellowish small grains seen beneath the buccal or labial mucosa.

Epidemiology
Incidence and prevalence
Fordyce spots are extremely common: probably 80% of the population have them.

Age
Fordyce spots are often not noticeable in children until after puberty (although they are present histologically), and they seem to be more obvious in male patients with greasy skin and the elderly.

Associated diseases
May be associated with genital Fordyce spots, or increased in some rheumatic disorders [6].

Clinical features
Usually seen in the buccal mucosa, particularly inside the commissures (Figure 110.13), and sometimes in the retromolar regions and upper lip [1–5].

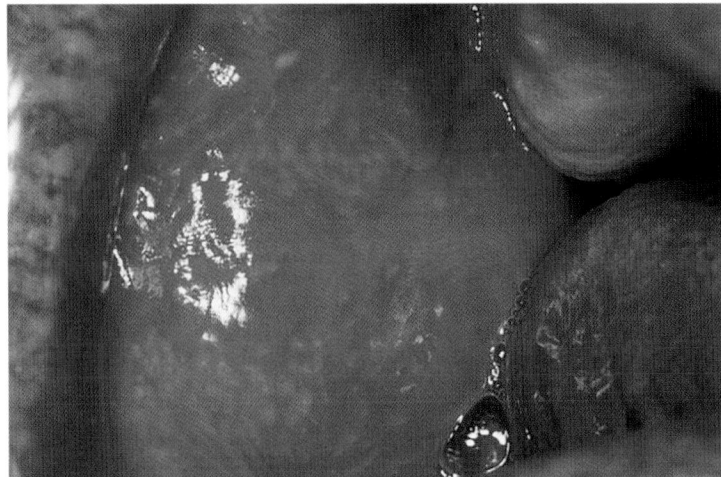

Figure 110.13 Fordyce spots: sebaceous glands in the buccal mucosa.

Management
Fordyce spots are totally benign, although the occasional patient or physician becomes concerned about them or misdiagnoses them as thrush or lichen planus. Occasionally, they may be mistaken for leukoplakia [7].

No treatment is indicated, other than reassurance. The spots may become less prominent if isotretinoin is given [8]. Carbon dioxide laser, electrodessication and curettage, and 5-aminolaevulinic acid photodynamic therapy have been reported as possible effective therapies [9–12].

Hereditary benign intraepithelial dyskeratosis

Synonyms and inclusions
• Witkop–von Sallmann syndrome

Aetiology. Hereditary benign intraepithelial dyskeratosis is a rare, benign, autosomal dominant condition associated with chromosome 4 anomalies, seen mainly in some groups of mixed ethnic origin, predominantly in North Carolina, USA [1–4].

Pathology. There is pronounced epithelial acanthosis, vacuolization in the stratum spinosum and eosinophilic cells apparently engulfed by normal squamous cells ('tobacco cells').

Clinical features. Oral milky white smooth somewhat translucent plaques appear in childhood and become more obvious by adolescence. These lesions affect predominantly the buccal mucosae, lips and ventrum of the tongue.

Ocular lesions include conjunctivitis with gelatinous conjunctival plaques, which become evident in infancy. There may be photophobia and eventual corneal involvement.

Oral biopsy is usually indicated for diagnosis.

Management. No treatment is required.

Keratitis, ichthyosis and deafness syndrome

Synonyms and inclusions
• KID syndrome

Dental dysplasia, persistent oral ulceration, chronic mucocutaneous candidosis and occasional carcinoma may be seen in the KID syndrome of keratitis, ichthyosiform dermatosis and deafness [1–3].

Leukoedema

Leukoedema is not a mucosal disease but simply the name given to the faint whitish lines seen in some normal buccal mucosae, often prominent in black people. The whitish lines disappear if the mucosa is stretched – a diagnostic test [1–4]. Confusion with lichen planus should thereby be avoided.

Naevus sebaceous of Jadassohn

Synonyms and inclusions
• Linear naevus syndrome

Oral manifestations may rarely occur as fibroepitheliomatous nodules in patients with a sebaceous naevus of the skin but are extremely rarely seen in isolation [1–3]. Patients have a 10–20% risk of development of cutaneous or adnexal neoplasia [4].

Olmsted syndrome [1–6]

Synonyms and inclusions
• Congenital palmoplantar and periorificial keratoderma with corneal epithelial dysplasia

Perioral keratoderma may be seen associated with palmoplantar keratoderma and corneal epithelial dysplasia [1–5]. Reported associations include haemangioma and melanoma [6,7].

Pachyonychia congenita

Synonyms and inclusions
• Jadassohn–Lewandowsky syndrome

Pachyonychia congenita is a benign disorder associated with mutations in keratin 16 [1–4]. A diagnostic triad of toenail thickening, plantar keratoderma and plantar pain was reported by 97% of patients with pachyonychia congenita by age 10 years [5].

Other clinical findings reported include fingernail dystrophy, oral leukokeratosis, palmar keratoderma, follicular hyperkeratosis, hyperhidrosis, cysts, hoarseness and natal teeth [5]. About 60% of patients have oral keratosis (sometimes with discomfort), 16% have natal or neonatal teeth and 10% have angular stomatitis [5–9]. There is a higher likelihood of oral leukokeratosis in individuals with KRT6A mutations, and a strong association of natal teeth and cysts in carriers of a KRT17 mutation [5].

The keratosis requires no treatment. Dental advice should be sought regarding natal or neonatal teeth.

Sebaceous adenoma

Sebaceous adenomas are exceedingly rare in the mouth, except in association with salivary glands but have been described in the buccal mucosa [1–6].

Tylosis

Tylosis is an autosomal dominant syndrome of palmoplantar hyperkeratosis that may predispose to oesophageal carcinoma but, although oral white lesions have also been described, there is little evidence that these are premalignant [1–5] (see Chapter 147).

Warty dyskeratoma [1–5]

Synonyms and inclusions
• Focal acantholytic dyskeratosis

Warty dyskeratoma, oral warty dyskeratoma or focal acantholytic dyskeratosis is considered to be associated with the pilosebaceous apparatus and is rare in the oral cavity but typically presents as a nodule or papule on the gingiva, palate or alveolar ridge. The histology is similar to that of Darier disease and transient acantholytic dermatosis, with suprabasal epithelial splits and corps ronds.

White sponge naevus

Synonyms and inclusions
• Cannon disease
• Pachydermia oralis
• White folded gingivostomatosis

Epidemiology

Incidence and prevalence
A rare familial disorder and inherited as an autosomal dominant trait [1,2].

Age
Usually first noticed in childhood.

Associated diseases
Similar lesions may also affect the upper respiratory tract, genitalia and anus.

Pathophysiology
There is hyperplastic acanthotic epithelium in which gross oedema causes a basket-weave appearance. The superficial epithelium has a 'washed-out' appearance as it stains only very lightly.

Genetics
Defects in keratins 4 and 13 with abnormal tonofilament aggregation [3–7,8].

Clinical features
The oral mucosa is almost invariably involved in white sponge naevus. Non-painful white plaques primarily involve the non-cornified buccal mucosae, gingiva and floor of the mouth. Painless, shaggy or folded white lesions typically affect the buccal mucosa bilaterally but may also involve other areas, although rarely the gingival margins [1,2].

Extraoral lesions most often occur in the oesophagus or anogenital area, but almost invariably follow the development of typical oral lesions.

Investigations
None. The family history and clinical examination are usually adequate to differentiate this from other more common causes of white lesions such as cheek biting, burns, lichen planus and candidosis.

Management
This is a benign condition with an excellent prognosis. Reassurance is all that is required, although some have suggested that tetracyclines might clear the lesions [9,10]. The family may be aware of the condition [11].

OTHER CONGENITAL ANOMALIES

Ankyloglossia

Definition and nomenclature
Ankyloglossia is an isolated anomaly in which the lingual fraenum is tight and the tongue cannot be fully protruded [1,2]. Ankyloglossia superior syndrome is a rare distinct malformation that consists of a fibrous or osseous connection between the tip of the tongue and the hard palate, and additional congenital anomalies such as cleft palate, gastrointestinal malformations and deformed limbs [3].

Synonyms and inclusions
• Tongue-tie

Epidemiology

Incidence and prevalence
Rare.

Age
From birth.

Pathophysiology

Genetics
The association of cleft palate with ankyloglossia is inherited as a semi-dominant, X-linked disorder previously described in several large families of different ethnic origins and related to chromosome Xq21: the T-box transcription factor gene *TBX22* is mutated [4–7].

Environmental factors
There are reports of cocaine use in some mothers.

Clinical features
The lingual fraenum is tight and the tongue cannot be fully protruded.

Complications and co-morbidities
There may be a family history and sometimes deviation of the epiglottis or larynx [4].

Speech is not usually affected in patients with ankyloglossia but the ability to suckle [8] and to cleanse the buccal sulcus with the tongue may be, and there can be effects on jaw development [9].

Investigations
None.

Management
If necessary, surgery to the fraenum will relieve ankyloglossia [2,**10**,11].

Fissured tongue

Synonyms and inclusions
• Plicated or scrotal tongue

Introduction and general description
Common fissures on the dorsum of the tongue.

Epidemiology

Incidence and prevalence
A common condition affecting more than 5% of the population [1].

Age
May be noted from childhood.

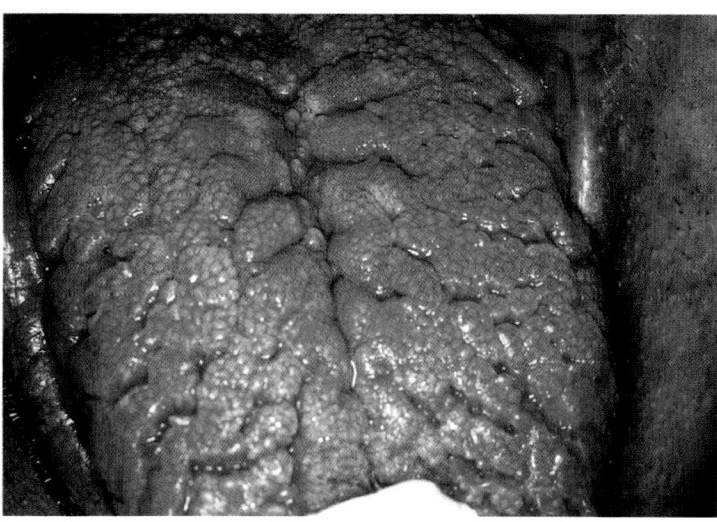

Figure 110.14 Fissured or scrotal tongue.

Genetics
One study of 69 individuals with fissured tongue and 125 healthy volunteers showed significantly increased frequencies of *HLA-DRB1*08*, *HLA-DRB1*14*, *HLA-DRB1*11* and *HLA-DRB1*16*, while *HLA-DRB1*03* and *HLA-DRB1*07* were decreased [2].

Associated diseases
Geographic tongue is commonly found in people with fissured tongues. Patients with Down syndrome often have a fissured tongue and it is a feature of the rare Melkersson–Rosenthal syndrome comprising recurrent orofacial swelling, facial palsy and plicated tongue. There is an occasional association with psoriasis and reports of improvement during infliximab treatment for psoriasis [3]. Conversely, it has been recorded as appearing in a patient with Melkersson–Rosenthal syndrome, in a psoriatic patient treated with etanercept – another antitumour necrosis factor (TNF)-α therapy [4]. Geographic tongue has also been recorded in four patients on treatment with bevacizumab [5] but this requires confirmation.

Clinical features
Fissures of various morphology on the dorsum of the tongue. Often accompanied by geographic tongue (Figure 110.14).

Investigations
None.

Management
Reassurance only.

Oral hair

Oral hair is a rare innocuous anomaly [1,2], not to be confused with hairy tongue or the hair on skin flaps used intraorally in reconstructions as, for example, after cancer resections.

VARIOUS OROCUTANEOUS SYNDROMES

Cleft lip/palate

Definition
The primary palate or premaxilla includes that portion of the alveolar ridge containing the four incisors. The secondary palate forms the remaining hard palate and all the soft palate. Cleft of the lip with or without cleft palate (CL/P) is one of the commonest congenital malformations in western countries. Based on their association with specific malformative patterns or their presence as isolated defects, CL/P can be classified as syndromic and non-syndromic, respectively. Both forms of CL/P are characterized by a strong genetic component. Syndromic forms are in many cases due to chromosomal aberrations or monogenic diseases. Non-syndromic CL/P is a multifactorial disease caused by the interaction between genetic and environmental factors.

Orofacial clefts result from an embryopathy in which there is failure of the frontonasal process and/or fusion of the palatal shelves. In the submucous cleft palate, the palatal shelves may fail to join, but the overlying mucous membranes are intact and the muscle attachments of the soft palate are abnormal, causing velopharyngeal insufficiency. Bifid uvula may signify a submucous cleft palate.

Introduction and general description
The common clefts are cleft lip with or without cleft palate (CL/P) and cleft palate only.

Epidemiology

Incidence and prevalence
The total incidence of facial clefting is between two and three per 1000 live births. A number of these do not develop as full-term fetuses. Cleft lip occurs in about 1/1000 white-skinned neonates. The prevalence is higher in Asian neonates (about 1.7/1000 births) and lower in black neonates (approximately 1/2500 births). Cleft palate as an isolated malformation behaves as an entity distinct from cleft lip with or without cleft palate. It has an incidence of 0.5/1000 births. The risk of recurrence in subsequent children is about 2% if one child has it, 6% if one parent has it, 15% if one parent and one child have it.

Age
Noted from birth.

Sex
Cleft palate is more prevalent in females, while cleft lip is more prevalent in males.

Ethnicity
There are racial differences with a high incidence of cleft palate in South-East Asia and a low incidence in Afro-Caribbean races.

Associated diseases

Facial clefts are associated with a syndrome in up to 15–60% of cases and are then termed syndromic clefts. More than 400 syndromes may include a facial cleft as one manifestation and cleft lip/palate may be associated with many congenital syndromes.

Not all cases of clefting are inherited; a number of teratogens (environmental agents that can cause birth defects) have been implicated, as well as defects in essential nutrients.

Pathophysiology

The development of the face and the upper lip takes place during the fifth to ninth week of pregnancy. Clefts of the lip with or without cleft palate and cleft palate alone result from the failure of the first branchial arches to complete fusion processes and are the most common of all craniofacial anomalies. The male to female ratio of cleft lip/palate is 2 : 1; the ratio for cleft palate alone is just the reverse, 1 : 2.

Failed fusion of the palatal shelves can be caused by different gene defects culminating in:
- A problem in the formation of the midline epithelial seam.
- Small size of the palatal processes.
- Unsynchronized timing of the elevation or growth of the palatal shelves with the growth of surrounding structures such as cranial base.
- A small mandible preventing the downwards relocation of the tongue which mechanically may prevent palatal fusion.

Predisposing factors

Cleft lip/palate is more prevalent in the lower socioeconomic classes. Environmental factors present during the first trimester of pregnancy and those which may generate cleft palate include maternal upper respiratory infection in the first trimester, smoking (especially when the mother has glutathione-S-transferase theta 1 (GSTT1) – null variants), obesity, diabetes, stress or exposure to various other agents. Paternal smoking has also been implicated. The teratogens incriminated include isotretinoin, which causes birth defects such as brain malformations, learning disability, heart problems, as well as facial abnormalities. Thalidomide given to pregnant mothers was, and anticonvulsants (phenytoin, valproic acid, lamotrigine, carbamazepine) and corticosteroids may be, associated with an increased incidence. Phenytoin may act via an effect causing fetal arrhythmias and hypoxia. Systemic corticosteroids have been reported to increase the risk (this is controversial) and there are also concerns about possible effects from topical steroids used in the first trimester. There has been concern about aspirin and diazepam as possible causes but there is no real evidence. Folic acid given periconceptually may lower the risk, but the evidence is weak [1–51].

Genetics

Clefts can be seen in over 300 different syndromes (Box 110.4) and mutations of the *IRF6* gene have also been found in popliteal pterygium syndromes (PPS), which can present with isolated cleft lip and palate. The cause of non-syndromic cleft lip with or without cleft palate (NSCLP) is unclear but there is a strong genetic component; there may be a family history of clefts and typically the same type of cleft is seen in affected members. In monozygotic twins,

there is nearly 40% concordance. No single gene defect appears responsible, however. Several loci have been identified. Candidate genes in cleft lip/palate include *TGF-α*, poliovirus receptor-related 1 (*PVRL1*), retinoic acid receptor alpha (*RARA*), T-box transcription factor-22 (*TBX22*), specific isoforms of glutamic acid decarboxylase (*GAD*), interferon regulatory factor 6 (*IRF6*), *MSX1* (formerly homeobox 7 – encodes a member of the muscle segment homeobox gene family) and fibroblast growth factor (FGF) genes.

Clinical features

Presentation

A person may have a cleft lip, cleft palate or both cleft lip and palate. A unilateral cleft lip occurs on one side of the upper lip. A bilateral cleft lip occurs on both sides of the upper lip. In its most severe form, the cleft may extend through the nose base. Cleft lip is not always complete (i.e. extending into the nostril). A cleft may involve only the upper lip or may extend to involve the nostril and the hard and soft palates. In about 9% of the cases, the cleft is associated with skin bridges or Simonart's bands. Isolated cleft lip may be unilateral or bilateral (approximately 20%). When unilateral, the cleft is more common on the left side (about 70%).

Lips are more frequently cleft bilaterally (approximately 25%) when combined with cleft palate. Cleft lip and palate is more common in men. Cleft lip and palate comprises about 50% of the cases, with cleft lip and isolated cleft palate each comprising about 25%. About 85% of bilateral cleft lips and 70% of unilateral cleft lips

---

Box 110.4 Syndromes which may include cleft lip/palate

- Apert syndrome
- Basal cell carcinoma naevoid syndrome
- Carpenter syndrome
- Cleidocranial dysplasia
- Craniosynostosis
- Crouzon syndrome
- Freeman–Sheldon syndrome
- Goldenhar syndrome
- Hallerman–Streiff syndrome
- Hemifacial microsomia
- Hydrocephalus
- Microtia
- Miller syndrome
- Moebius syndrome
- Nager syndrome
- Nasal encephalocoeles
- Neurofibromatosis (NF)
- Orbital hypertelorism
- Parry–Romberg syndrome
- Pfeiffer syndrome
- Pierre Robin sequence
- Saethre–Chotzen syndrome
- Shprintzen syndrome
- Stickler syndrome
- Treacher Collins syndrome
- Van der Woude syndrome
- Waardenberg syndrome

are associated with cleft palate. One subgroup have cleft lip and palate with median facial dysplasia and cerebrofacial malformations; others with laryngotracheal oesophageal clefts (Opitz–Firas or G syndrome) or cranial asymmetry (Opitz or B syndrome).

Clefts in the middle of the upper lip may be true or false. True median clefts have been described in association with bifid nose and ocular hypertelorism. Other cases of true median labial cleft are associated with polydactyly or other digital anomalies, constituting an autosomal recessive trait called *orofaciodigital syndrome II*.

Pseudocleft of the middle of the upper lip may occur in *orofaciodigital syndrome I*. A somewhat similar central defect, but of mild degree, is seen in chondroectodermal dysplasia (Ellis–van Creveld syndrome). Clefts in the lower lip are rare and usually median but may involve the mandible and sometimes the tongue. Management of cleft lip is discussed elsewhere.

Cleft palate may be incomplete involving only the uvula and the muscular soft palate (velum). A complete cleft palate extends the entire length of the palate. Cleft palates can be unilateral or bilateral. Clefts are often accompanied by impaired facial growth, dental anomalies, speech disorders, poor hearing and psychosocial problems.

Clinical variants

Submucous cleft palate can be recognized by a notched posterior nasal spine, a translucent zone in the midline of the soft palate and a bifid uvula, but not all these features are necessarily present and a bifid uvula may be seen in isolation. About 1/1200 births are affected and feeding difficulties, speech defects and middle-ear infections may develop in 90% of affected children. Adenoidectomy is contraindicated as it may reveal latent velopharyngeal insufficiency. A minority have other issues such as Loeys–Dietz syndrome (similar to Marfan syndrome), where there is a risk of arterial aneurysm and rupture.

Complications and co-morbidities

A high percentage of patients with cleft palate develop otitis media with effusion. Up to 20% have additional abnormalities that can affect management in various ways. Systemic disorders are more frequent in patients with cleft palate than in those with cleft lip alone, and include especially skeletal, cardiac, renal and CNS defects.

Investigations

Health care providers that frequently participate in a multidisciplinary cleft palate team include: audiologists; maxillofacial, ear, nose and throat, and plastic surgeons; geneticists; neurosurgeons; nurses; dentists (paediatric dentist/orthodontist/prosthodontist); paediatricians; social workers/psychologists, and speech and language pathologists.

Management [52–56]

Treatment of the airway takes priority and may be managed with positioning but, in severe cases, may need tracheostomy. Aesthetics is a major issue for parents. One of the problems for the child is feeding: a Rosti bottle with Gummi teat often helps. The timing of the initial cleft lip and palate repair is controversial. In general, when the lip alone is cleft, initial cosmetic repair is carried out at about 3–6 months of age, though earlier operations are becoming popular. Many repair cleft lip and palate within the first few days of life since, after repair, the appearance is dramatically improved, feeding difficulties are significantly minimized and speech develops better. If the palatal defect is too wide, it can be repaired 3 months later to allow for sufficient palatal growth. In any event, cleft palate is now usually repaired before the child speaks, between 6 and 18 months, typically at 6–12 months of age.

- *Age 1–5 years* is when it is important to have good hearing and normal appearance to avoid low self-esteem and help speech develop. These children need a hearing assessment, and if it is impaired, ear ventilation tubes (grommets) may be indicated.
- *Age 5–13 years* is when the orthodontist can help correct malocclusion and alveolar bone grafting may be needed. Speech, if poor despite the best efforts by the child and the speech pathologist, may be corrected with pharyngoplasty.
- *Age 13–18 years* is the time for final adjustments. Fine tuning such as scar revisions, rhinoplasty and orthognathic surgery is carried out to enable the child's appearance and speech to be restored to as near normal as possible.

Palatal ulcers seen in neonates with cleft lip and palate appear to result from trauma from the tongue and resolve if a palatal plate is fitted. Dental abnormalities include malocclusion (almost 100%), hypodontia (50%), hypoplasia (30%) and supernumerary teeth (20%). Children may have a higher prevalence of caries in both the primary and permanent dentitions, and significantly more gingivitis, especially in the maxillary anterior region. Adult cleft lip and palate patients may have poorer oral hygiene and more gingivitis. Prevention and continuity of care is essential and a high rate of success can be achieved.

Syndromic cleft palate

Current molecular epidemiology investigations have examined both syndromic and non-syndromic (isolated) cleft lip/palate and cleft palate. Linkage studies have identified a number of candidate genes, including *MSX1*, *RAR*, an X-linked locus, and the genes for TGF-β-3 and TGF-α. One of the common syndromic forms of cleft lip/palate, the Van der Woude syndrome, is caused by an autosomal dominant form of inheritance at a locus on chromosome 1.

Other examples include:
- Branchial arch syndromes.
- Craniosynostoses.
- Diseases associated with mutations in the Sonic Hedgehog (SHH) pathway.

Resources

Further information

http://www.bmj.com/specialties/otolaryngology-ent
http://www.entnet.org/healthinformation/
http://www.niaid.nih.gov/topics/Pages/default.aspx
http://www.entnet.org/
http://www.aaaai.org/home.aspx
http://www.medicine.ox.ac.uk/bandolier/booth/booths/ent.html
http://www.nhsdirect.wales.nhs.uk/encyclopaedia/c/article/cleftlipand palate/
    ghr.nlm.nih.gov/
(All last accessed December 2014.)

PART 10: SITES, SEX, AGE

Cowden syndrome (see Chapter 80)

Synonyms and inclusions
• Multiple hamartoma syndrome

Cowden syndrome may be associated with the *PTEN* gene [1] and multiple hamartomas [2,3]. Oral mucosal lesions may be found in the presence or absence of cutaneous stigma [3–9].

The oral lesions are typically smooth, pink or whitish benign fibromas found especially on the palatal, gingival and labial mucosae. Oral squamous carcinoma is a rare complication [10]. There may be overlap with Bannayan–Riley–Ruvalcaba syndrome [11–13] and the differential diagnosis includes multiple idiopathic mucosal neuromas and MEN2b syndrome.

Treatment with acitretin may lead to regression of the hypertrophic lesions of the lip and mouth [14]. The predisposition to thyroid and breast cancer necessitates referral [15].

De Lange syndrome

Synonyms and inclusions
• Amsterdam dwarf

Classical Brachmann or Cornelia de Lange syndrome presents with a striking face, pronounced growth and learning disability, and variable limb deficiencies. Most cases are sporadic [1,2]. About 50% of patients have been found to have heterozygous mutations in the *NIPBL* gene with some cases being caused by mutations in the X-linked *SMC1L1* gene [3]. A long philtrum and crescent-shaped mouth with down-turned corners is typical [4–7].

The characteristic face of classical de Lange syndrome is present at birth and changes little throughout life, although there is some lengthening of the face with age and the jaw becomes squared.

Double lip

Definition
Double lip is a developmental anomaly usually involving the upper lip.

Epidemiology

Incidence and prevalence
It is reported to be common among some groups of Africans [1].

Associated diseases
Double lip may occur alone or in association with other anomalies. The association with blepharochalasis (laxity of the upper eyelid skin) and sometimes non-toxic thyroid enlargement is known as *Ascher syndrome* [2]. Non-syndromic double lip has been reported [3]. A newly recognized syndrome with double upper and lower lip, hypertelorism, eyelid ptosis, blepharophimosis and third finger clinodactyly has been reported [4].

Clinical features
A fold of redundant tissue is found on the inner aspect of the involved lip [5,6].

Management
Double lip requires no treatment unless except for cosmetic purposes..

Down syndrome

The incidence of clefts, and of angular cheilitis is increased in people with Down syndrome, caused by an increased level of *Staphylococcus aureus* and *Candida albicans*, possibly because of immune defects [1–3]. Lip fissures may appear intermittently over a period of years or be intractable and longstanding.

Erythropoietic protoporphyria

Erythropoietic protoporphyria is an autosomal dominant disorder of ferrochelatase, resulting in inhibition of the conversion of protoporphyrin to haem.

Shallow elliptical or linear scars around the lips and linear perioral furrowing (pseudorhagades) are subtle changes that are pathognomonic when observed in children [1–3].

Focal mucinosis

Oral focal mucinosis is an uncommon clinicopathological entity considered to be the oral counterpart of cutaneous focal mucinosis and/or cutaneous myxoid cyst. The nature of the lesion is unclear but may be the result of fibroblastic overproduction of hyaluronic acid. It comprises a clinically elevated mass with a histological picture of localized areas of myxomatous connective tissue. Most of the lesions are swellings that affect the gingiva and alveolar mucosa [1–6].

All these diseases share distinct histological features. There is an increased number of fibroblast-like cells in early lesions, whereas these are diminished or predominantly at the margin in advanced ones. The myxomatous areas show slight to absent reticulum and elastic fibres, and collagen fibres are fragmented and replaced by variable amounts of mucin. Vimentin is consistently present and correlates with the number of fibroblast-like cells, these being negative for S-100 protein, Leu7, desmin and α-smooth muscle actin (α-SMA).

Gardner syndrome (see Chapter 80)

Multiple jaw osteomas are a feature of Gardner syndrome of familial adenomatous polyposis coli [1]. Some 80% of patients with familial adenomatosis polyposis coli have osteomas and 30% have dental anomalies such as supernumerary or impacted teeth, or odontomes [2–14,15].

Gorlin syndrome (see Chapter 80)

Synonyms and inclusions
• Naevoid basal cell carcinoma syndrome

Keratocystic odontogenic tumours (KCOT, odontogenic kerato-cysts or primordial cysts) of the jaws are a prominent feature of Gorlin syndrome [1–4] (see also Chapter 141). The syndrome is caused by mutations in the Sonic Hedgehog *patched* gene, a tumour suppressor gene [5]. A single point mutation in one *patched* allele may be responsible for the various malformations found in the syndrome [5–10]. Inactivation of both *patched* alleles results in the formation of tumours and cysts (basal cell carcinomas, odontogenic keratocysts and medulloblastomas) [5].

The keratocysts should be surgically removed but have a tendency to recur.

There are also occasional reports of oral neoplasms, notably fibrosarcoma, ameloblastoma, squamous carcinoma, basal cell carcinoma and B-cell lymphoma [6–15].

Jacob disease

Jacob disease is a rare condition consisting of new joint formation between the coronoid process of the mandible and the inner aspect of the zygomatic arch [1,2].

Kindler syndrome

Kindler syndrome (Weary–Kindler syndrome) is characterized by bulla formation, which starts at birth on areas of the skin that receive pressure and may lead to bilateral incomplete syndactylies involving all web spaces [1–3].

Oral lesions may include atrophy of the buccal mucosa, white patches on the gingiva and oral mucosa display, trismus (an inability to fully open the mouth), aggressive periodontitis and a form of desquamative gingivitis [4,5].

Histology shows classical features of poikiloderma, namely epidermal atrophy with flattening of the rete ridges, vacuolization of basal keratinocytes, pigmentary incontinence and mild dermal perivascularization. Ultrastructural studies demonstrate reduplication of the basal lamina with branching structures within the upper dermis and cleavage between the lamina densa and the cell membrane of the keratinocytes. Antibody against type VII collagen shows extensive broad bands with intermittently discontinuous and reticular staining at the dermal–epidermal junction.

Lip pits and sinuses

Congenital lip pits or sinuses are small blind fistulae on the vermilion border [1–5]. They are usually bilateral and symmetrical, often just to one side of the philtrum. The pits may be up to 3–4 mm in diameter and up to 2 cm deep. They may communicate with

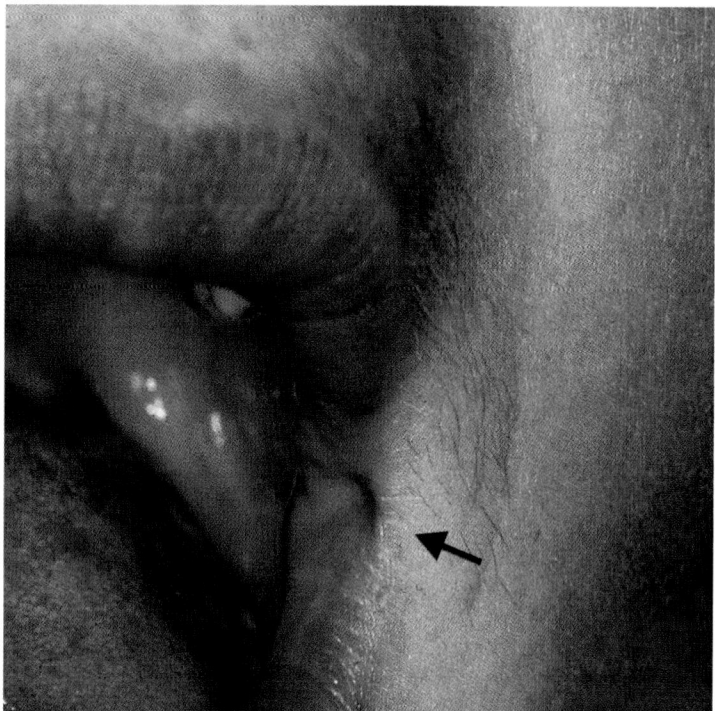

Figure 110.15 Angular sinus (lip-pit), a congenital anomaly.

underlying minor salivary glands. They may appear as isolated findings, but are often (67%) associated with cleft lip and/or palate (Van der Woude syndrome) [6–11] and caused by a DNA variation in *IRF6* [12]. This autosomal dominant syndrome has a frequency of 1/75 000 to 1/100 000 in white populations.

Dimples are common at the commissures. They should be distinguished from *commissural pits*, which are distinct definite pits ranging from 1 to 4 mm in diameter and depth [10,11] present from infancy, often showing a familial tendency and probably determined by a dominant gene (Figure 110.15). Their incidence is 1–20% in various population groups [13]; for example, in one series they were found in 12% of white people and 20% of black people [14]. Commissural pits are sometimes associated with aural sinuses or pits. Rarely, they may be infected and present as recurrent or refractory angular cheilitis.

Surgical removal may be indicated for cosmetic purposes.

Noonan syndrome

Synonyms and inclusions
• Ullrich–Turner syndrome

Ullrich–Turner syndrome is caused by monosomy X or a structural abnormality of the second X chromosome. It is seen in females with a syndrome of short stature, sexual infantilism and a pattern of characteristic minor anomalies including pterygium colli. This syndrome was later called Noonan syndrome, and it was shown that central giant cell lesions or cherubism of the jaws may be present [1–9]. Oral keratosis is sometimes seen [10].

Tuberous sclerosis

Synonyms and inclusions
- Epiloia
- Bourneville disease

Oral manifestations in tuberous sclerosis include pit-shaped enamel defects in both dentitions, and gingival fibromatosis [1–7] and rare instances of myxoma or desmoplastic fibroma [8,9].

Van der Woude syndrome

Van der Woude syndrome is a rare autosomal dominant syndrome [1] caused by a DNA variation in *IRF6* and mutations in *GRHL3* [2]. It is the most common syndromic form of cleft lip and palate, and in Van der Woude syndrome lower lip pits are associated with cleft lip and/or palate [2–5,6,7]. There is phenotypic and genotypic overlap between Van der Woude syndrome and isolated cleft of the lip and/or palate. Van der Woude syndrome is sometimes seen with syndactyly or talipes equinovarus, or cognitive dysfunction [8].

Von Recklinghausen neurofibromatosis

Neurofibromatosis consists of distinct variants due to *NF* gene mutations [1]: type I (NF-I), often referred to as von Recklinghausen disease or generalized NF; and type II (NF-II), a much less common disorder of bilateral acoustic schwannomas. The incidence of head and neck manifestations in patients with NF varies between 14 and 37%. Multiple neurofibromas may occur as a feature of NF; cosmetic lesions include pigmentary changes (café-au-lait spots) [2–6].

Neurofibromas may be seen mainly in NF-I. Neurofibromas may also be seen in NF-II, but bilateral acoustic neuromas are the hallmark of this disease and neurilemmomas and acoustic neuromas are the predominant neural tumours. Neurofibromas may also be part of the MEN syndrome (see Chapter 149).

Oral lesions are not uncommon in von Recklinghausen generalized NF [7–16]. About two-thirds of patients have intraoral neurofibromas affecting predominantly the tongue, lips, buccal mucosa or palate. Neurofibroma represents a benign overgrowth of all elements of a peripheral nerve (axon cylinder, Schwann cells and fibrous connective tissue), arranged in a variety of patterns. Enlarged fungiform papillae are found in about 50% of patients. About 60% of patients have radiographic evidence of disease, especially enlargement of the inferior alveolar canal or foramen, or branching of the canal.

Neurofibromas may occur multiply as a feature of NF but only rarely undergo sarcomatous change [17]. Other rare, malignant tumours include nerve sheath tumour [18], triton tumour [19] and Merkel cell carcinoma [20].

Xeroderma pigmentosum

Squamous cell carcinoma of the lip may arise in patients with xeroderma pigmentosum [1–3] and therefore it is crucial to institute sun protection. Oral retinoids such as etretinate or isotretinoin may be of prophylactic value [4–6]. Topical 5-fluorouracil or surgery may be used to treat potentially malignant lesions.

ACQUIRED DISORDERS OF THE ORAL MUCOSA OR LIPS

This section discusses the main acquired causes of mouth blisters, erosions and ulcers; loss of elasticity of mucosae; lumps and swellings; other causes of oral soreness, lumps and swellings; and pigmented, red or white lesions, arranged alphabetically for ease of reference. Further detail is available elsewhere.

Blisters, erosions and ulcers

Blisters may be of local cause such as a burn, due to mucocoeles, or associated with infections or vesiculobullous disease. Vesicles/blisters rapidly break down in the mouth as a result of trauma, moisture and infection to leave eosions or ulcers. The causes of mouth ulcers are thus diverse (Boxes 110.1 and 110.5), usually being caused by the following:
1 Systemic conditions:
 - Haematological.
 - Gastroenterological.
 - Dermatological.
 - Infective.
 - Vasculitis.
 - Iatrogenic.
 - Uncertain causes.
2 Malignant neoplasms.
3 Local factors.
4 Aphthae (recurrent aphthous stomatitis).
5 Drugs.

Box 110.5 Causes of mouth ulcers
(see also Table 110.6)

- Local causes (e.g. trauma)
- Recurrent aphthae (and Behçet syndrome)
- Malignant neoplasms
- Ulcers associated with systemic disease
- Drugs
- Irradiation of the oral mucosa
- Disorders of uncertain pathogenesis

Mouth ulcers of local aetiology

It is surprising that oral ulceration due to local factors is not more frequently seen but most resolve spontaneously and patients do not attend for health care.

Accidental cheek biting or facial trauma may cause ulceration in any individual; the history is usually quite clear and a single ulcer of short duration (5–10 days) is present. Ulceration due to biting an anaesthetized lower lip or tongue following a dental local analgesic injection is a fairly common problem in young children.

Orthodontic appliances or, more commonly, dentures (especially if new) are responsible for many traumatic oral ulcers. These ulcers are usually clearly related to the appliance and have been a problem in the care of cleft palate patients [1]. Chronic trauma may cause a well-defined ulcer with a whitish keratotic halo [2].

The possibility of some other aetiology for ulcers of apparently local cause should always be borne in mind. Riga–Fede disease consists of ulcers of the lingual frenum in neonates with natal lower incisors [3]. Child abuse may cause ulcers, especially over the upper labial fraena. Self-mutilation may be seen in some psychologically disturbed patients [4,5], patients with learning disability, individuals with sensory impairment and in Lesch–Nyhan syndrome [6–11]. Oral purpura or ulceration may be seen on the lingual fraenum or palate due to cunnilingus or fellatio, respectively [12]. Other local causes of ulceration include thermal burns, especially of the tongue and palate (e.g. 'pizza burn' – now more common with microwave oven use), chemical burns from the holding of medicaments or drugs (e.g. aspirin or cocaine) against the mucosa [13,14], and irradiation mucositis.

Prognosis. Most ulcers of local cause heal spontaneously within 7–14 days if the cause is removed.

Management. Maintenance of good oral hygiene and the use of hot saline mouthbaths and 0.2% aqueous chlorhexidine gluconate mouthwash aid healing. A 0.1% benzydamine mouthwash may help give relief. Occasionally, mechanical protection with a plastic guard may help [8]. Patients should be reviewed within 3 weeks to ensure healing has occurred. Any patient with a single ulcer lasting more than 2–3 weeks should be regarded with suspicion and investigated further, usually by biopsy – it may be a neoplasm or other serious disorder [15].

Eosinophilic ulcer of the oral mucosa [1–7,8,9]

Definition and nomenclature
A benign and self-limited lesion which typically affects the tongue.

> **Synonyms and inclusions**
> - Traumatic eosinophilic granuloma
> - Traumatic ulcerative granuloma with stromal eosinophilia (TUGSE)

Introduction and general description
Eosinophilic ulcers are unifocal, with a benign course.

Epidemiology

Incidence and prevalence
Rare.

Age
Children mainly.

Pathophysiology

Predisposing factors
The aetiology of the disease that affects older adults or children remains obscure and may be associated with traumatic factors.

Pathology
Pathological features show an extensive subepithelial inflammatory cell infiltration, with predominantly eosinophilic cells throughout the submucosa and histological similarities to CD30+ lymphoproliferative disorders [5]. Eosinophilic ulcer of the oral mucosa (EUOM) may be a reactive lesion showing overlapping features with entities such as atypical histiocytic granuloma, mucosal angiolymphoid hyperplasia with eosinophilia and Kimura disease [6] and sometimes a predominant oligoclonal CD3+ and CD30+ T lymphocyte infiltrate expressing EBV membrane protein, EBV possibly playing a role in triggering this reactive lymphoproliferative disorder [7]. The peripheral blood eosinophil count is normal.

Clinical features
Eosinophilic ulcer of the oral mucosa, also called traumatic eosinophilic granuloma or Rida–Fede disease (see above), is an uncommon, benign and self-limited lesion which typically affects the tongue, the lateral or dorsal surface. EUOM clinically manifests as a painful nodular inflammatory infiltration, usually with ulceration.

Management
Either a conservative excisional or incisional biopsy [8,9].

Recurrent mouth ulcers

Not all recurrent mouth ulcers are aphthae, but that is the most common cause.

Recurrent aphthous stomatitis

Definition and nomenclature
Recurrent aphthous stomatitis is characterized by recurring episodes of ulcers, typically from childhood or adolescence, each lasting from 1 to about 4 weeks before healing. Patients are otherwise apparently healthy.

> **Synonyms and inclusions**
> - Aphthae
> - Canker sores

Epidemiology

Incidence and prevalence
Recurrent aphthous stomatitis is a common disease that probably afflicts at least 20% of the population. There is a high prevalence in higher socioeconomic classes.

Age
Manifest initially in children.

Pathophysiology

The aetiology of recurrent aphthous stomatitis is not clear. There are identifiable predisposing factors in some patients (Table 110.4). There is no evidence that recurrent aphthous stomatitis is an auto-immune disease [1–4]. There is no known association with systemic autoimmune disorders, none of the common autoantibodies are found, and it tends to resolve or decrease spontaneously with increasing age. The serum immunoglobulin levels are usually normal, although IgA and IgG may be increased, and immune complexes may be found.

It now seems likely that there is a minor degree of immunological dysregulation underlying aphthae. Cell-mediated immune mechanisms appear to be involved in the pathogenesis of recurrent aphthous stomatitis. In the lesions, helper T cells predominate early on, with some natural killer cells. Cytotoxic cells then appear and there is evidence for an antibody-dependent cellular cytotoxicity reaction [1–4].

Causative organisms

Attempts to implicate a variety of viruses or bacteria in the aetiology of recurrent aphthous stomatitis have largely been unsuccessful, but there may be cross-reacting antigens between the oral mucosa and microorganisms such as *Streptococcus sanguis*, or heat-shock protein [10].

Genetics

A positive family history is found with about one-third of patients and there is an increased frequency of *HLA-A2*, *HLA-A11*, *HLA-B12* and *HLA-DR2*, supporting a genetic basis for susceptibility in some patients [1–4].

Environmental factors

Exacerbations with stress, trauma and cessation of tobacco smoking.

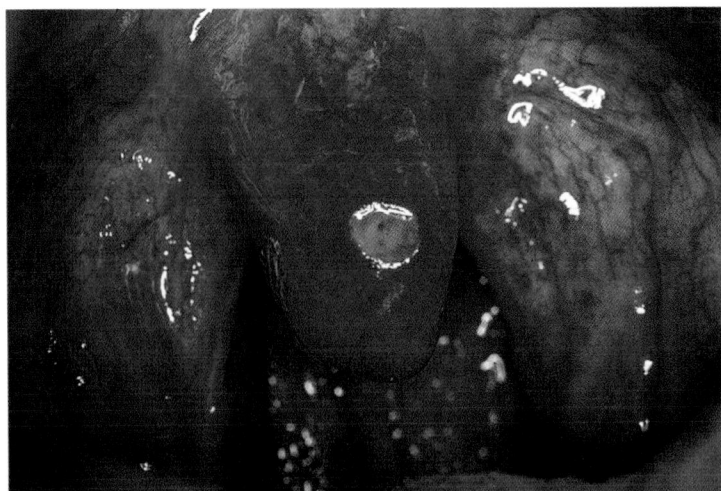

Figure 110.16 Recurrent aphthae.

Clinical features

History

Recurring episodes of mouth ulcers only, typically from childhood or adolescence.

Presentation

Aphthae typically are multiple round or ovoid ulcers with a circumscribed margin, erythematous halo and a yellow or grey floor (Figure 110.16). The term 'recurrent oral ulcer' is rather imprecise and should be avoided [1–4].

Clinical variants

There are three main clinical types of recurrent aphthous stomatitis. Most common are minor recurrent aphthous stomatitis (MiRAS), which account for 80% of all recurrent aphthous stomatitis. Some 10% of patients with recurrent aphthous stomatitis have major aphthous ulcers, and a further 10% suffer from a herpetiform type of ulceration (Table 110.5).

Table 110.4 Systemic and other factors that may occasionally underlie or be associated with recurrent aphthous stomatitis (RAS).

	Comments
Autoinflammatory disorders	Association of recurrent mouth ulcers with fevers and serositis
Behçet syndrome	Association of recurrent mouth ulcers with ocular lesions, genital ulcers and multisystem disease
Endocrine factors	In some women, RAS is clearly related to a fall in progestogens in the luteal phase of the menstrual cycle; hormone therapy may be beneficial
Gastrointestinal disease	Malabsorption states (pernicious anaemia, coeliac disease and Crohn disease) may precipitate RAS in a small minority
Haematinic deficiency	In some studies, 10–20% of patients with RAS have deficiencies of iron, folic acid or vitamin B_{12}
Immunodeficiency	A few patients have an immune defect such as HIV disease
Other factors	Trauma, certain foods, stress and cessation of smoking may play a part
Sweet syndrome	See Chapter 49

Table 110.5 Main features of recurrent aphthous stomatitis.

	Minor aphthae	Major aphthae	Herpetiform ulcers
Age of onset	Childhood or adolescence	Childhood or adolescence	Young adult
Ulcer size	2–4 mm	May be 10 mm or larger	Initially tiny but ulcers coalesce
Number of ulcers	Up to about 6	Up to about 6	10–100
Sites affected	Mainly vestibule, labial, buccal mucosa and floor of mouth; rarely dorsum of tongue, gingiva or palate	Any site	Any site but often on ventrum of tongue
Duration of each ulcer	Up to 10 days	Up to 1 month	Up to 1 month
Other comments	Most common type of aphthae	May heal with scarring	Affects females predominantly

Minor aphthous ulcers (synonym Mikulicz ulcers). MiRAS occur mainly in the 10–40-year age group, and often cause minimal symptoms. MiRAS are usually 2–4 mm in diameter and found mainly on the non-keratinized mobile mucosa of the lips, cheeks and floor of the mouth, sulci or ventrum of the tongue. They are uncommon on the gingiva, palate or dorsum of the tongue. Only a few ulcers (one to six) appear at a time; they heal in 7–10 days and recur at variable intervals. MiRAS are usually round or ovoid, but are often more linear when in the buccal sulcus, a common site. The ulcer floor is initially yellowish but becomes greyish as epithelialization proceeds. There is an erythematous halo and some oedema but MiRAS heal with little or no evidence of scarring.

Major aphthous ulcers (synonym Sutton ulcers). Previously known as periadenitis mucosa necrotica recurrens (PMNR), major recurrent aphthous stomatitis (MaRAS) are larger, recur more frequently, last longer and are more painful than MiRAS. They may reach a large size, even more than 1 cm in diameter. MaRAS are found on any area of the oral mucosa, including the dorsum of the tongue or palate. Usually only a few ulcers (one to six) occur at one time; they heal slowly over 10–40 days, and recur frequently. MaRAS are round or ovoid with an inflammatory halo, and may heal with scarring (Figure 110.17). Occasionally, a raised erythrocyte sedimentation rate or plasma viscosity is found.

Herpetiform ulceration (Figure 110.18). Herpetiform ulceration is found in a slightly older age group and there is a female predominance. Herpetiform ulcers are often extremely painful and recur so frequently that ulceration may be virtually continuous. Herpetiform ulceration begins with vesiculation, which passes rapidly into multiple, minute (2 mm), discrete ulcers at any oral site. The ulcers increase in size and coalesce to leave large ragged ulcers that heal in 10 days or longer. Their similarity to herpetic stomatitis gives herpetiform ulcers their name, but there is no evidence that herpes simplex virus (HSV) is involved.

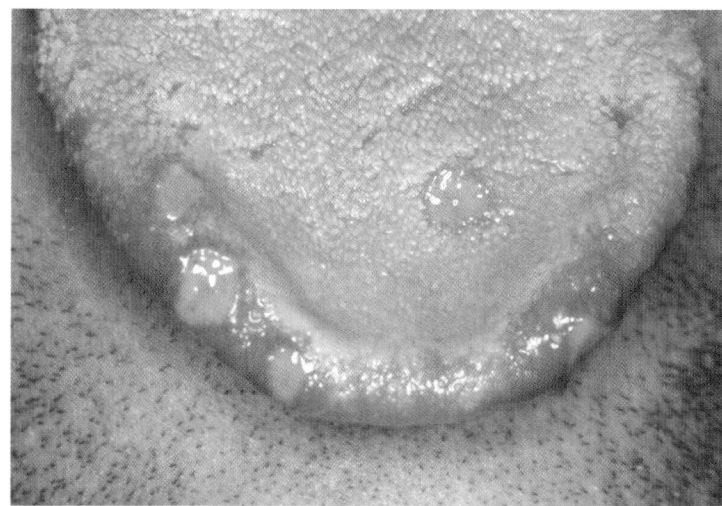

Figure 110.17 Major aphthous ulcers.

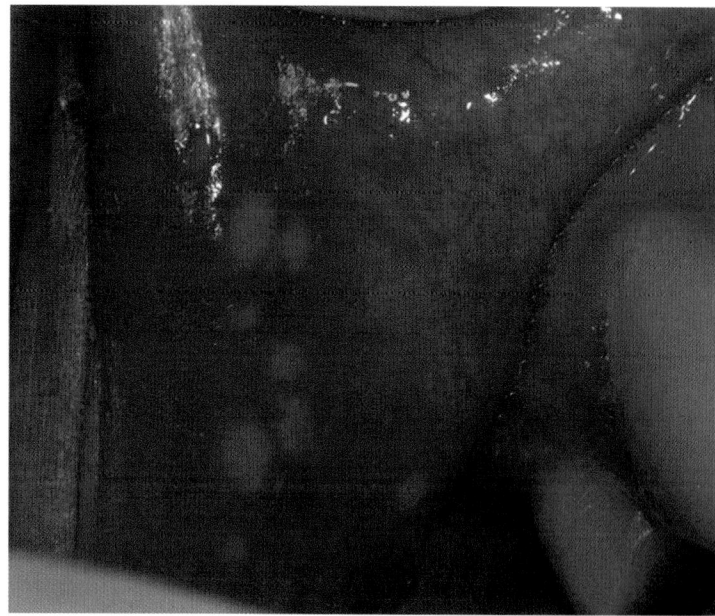

Figure 110.18 Herpetiform ulceration

Differential diagnosis

The diagnosis is not infrequently misapplied to similar ulcers (aphthous-like ulcers), which may be seen in a range of systemic conditions such as immune deficiencies, Behçet syndrome, coeliac disease, Crohn disease and autoinflammatory conditions. A minority (about 10–20%) of patients attending outpatient clinics with recurrent ulcers have an underlying haematological abnormality, usually a low serum iron or ferritin, or deficiency of folate or vitamin B_{12}. A few have multiple deficiencies [5,6]. Up to 3% of patients with recurrent ulcers have coeliac disease but in others a gluten-free diet is of no value [7]. Patients with deficiency states often, but not always, have gastrointestinal symptoms, and their ulceration is often of recent onset. Other aetiological factors in patients with recurrent ulcers can include Behçet syndrome; Sweet syndrome; HIV infection, cyclic neutropenia and other immunodeficiencies; autoinflammatory disorders; and, rarely, in children in association with fever and pharyngitis (periodic fever, aphthous stomatitis, pharyngitis and cervical adenitis; PFAPA) [8,9]. However, the diagnostic criteria for PFAPA have low specificity and this diagnosis is rarely confirmed.

Investigations

Diagnosis of recurrent aphthous stomatitis is based on the history and clinical features; no specific tests are available. Biopsy is indicated only where some other cause of ulceration is suspected. To exclude relevant systemic predisposing factors it is often useful to perform:

- Full blood count.
- Haemoglobin assay.
- White cell count and differential.
- Red cell indices.
- Iron studies.
- Red cell folate level.
- Serum vitamin B_{12} measurements.

- Serum antiendomysial antibodies and IgA antitissue transglutaminase antibodies.

The relevance of HLA studies for differentiating recurrent aphthous stomatitis from Behçet syndrome is discussed below.

Management

Recurrent aphthous stomatitis in most patients resolves or abates spontaneously with age. An underlying, identifiable predisposing cause is particularly likely where ulceration commences or worsens in adult life [5–10] and these patients are better classified as suffering aphthous-like ulcers.

Few patients have spontaneous remission until after several years and thus treatment is often indicated [11–13]. Fortunately, the natural history of recurrent aphthous stomatitis is one of eventual remission in most cases.

Predisposing factors should be corrected. If there is an obvious relationship to certain foods, the causal food should be excluded from the diet [14]. Good oral hygiene should be maintained: chlorhexidine or triclosan mouthwashes help to achieve this and may help reduce ulcer duration [1–4]. Topical minocycline and tetracycline mouthrinses may be of benefit [15].

Topical corticosteroids are the primary therapeutic agents used. Ulcer pain can usually be reduced, and the time to healing reduced, with hydrocortisone hemisuccinate pellets (Corlan®) 2.5 mg or triamcinolone acetonide in carboxymethylcellulose paste (Adcortyl® in Orabase®) used four times daily; failing the success of these, a stronger topical corticosteroid (e.g. betamethasone, beclomethasone, fluticasone, mometasone, clobetasol) [16–18] or systemic corticosteroid (e.g. prednisolone) may be required.

Other therapies for recurrent aphthous stomatitis, such as sucralfate [19], colchicine and pentoxifylline (oxpentifylline), may have a role in individual cases but are not generally very effective or have adverse effects [3,20–23].

Thalidomide, in doses from 50 mg up to 300 mg daily, can frequently induce remission, especially in major aphthae, but its important teratogenic effects and the risk of neuropathy must be considered [22,24–26]. Topical tacrolimus may be effective but randomized trials are awaited.

There are multiple other therapies available, including carbenoxolone, benzydamine, dapsone, cromoglicate, levamisole and many others, but generally their efficacy has not been well proven or they have unacceptable adverse effects [3]. Vitamin B_{12} may be of benefit [27]. In severe cases, biologicals may be indicated [28–33].

Resources

Further information

http://emedicine.medscape.com/article/867080-overview (last accessed December 2014).

Behçet syndrome

Synonyms and inclusions
- Adamantiades syndrome

Definition

Behçet syndrome is the association of recurrent aphthous stomatitis with genital ulceration and eye disease (especially iridocyclitis and retinal vasculitis) [1,2–5]. There may be a number of other systemic or cutaneous manifestations (Table 110.6).

Aetiology

The aetiology of Behçet syndrome is uncertain but it appears to be becoming more common (see also Chapter 48). There is a genetic background and, as in recurrent aphthous stomatitis, there are occasional familial cases and associations with HLA types, in Behçet syndrome particularly with HLA-B5 (Bw51 split). HLA-B51 or its B101 allele is significantly associated with Behçet syndrome in Japan, Korea, Turkey and France, as well as with the ocular manifestations in Britain. The MICA6 allele, a member of the polymorphic major histocompatibility complex (MHC) class I-related gene A (MICA) family, is thought to be in linkage disequilibrium with HLA-B51 and has been shown to be significantly associated with Behçet syndrome in Japan and France [6,7]. HLA-DR/DQ haplotypes are more important than individual HLA-DR and HLA-DQ phenotypes for the development of mucocutaneous type of Behçet syndrome and for disease shift from recurrent aphthous stomatitis to mucocutaneous type of Behçet syndrome [8].

The aetiopathogenesis of Behçet syndrome is still unclear [5,9–11]. It does not appear to be infectious, contagious or sexually transmitted. The disease is found worldwide but is most common in the eastern Mediterranean countries and eastern Asia, along the Silk Road taken by Marco Polo. In these countries, it is a leading cause of blindness though this is not the case in resource-rich countries.

There are many immunological findings in Behçet syndrome:
- Circulating autoantibodies against a number of components, including intermediate filaments found in mucous membranes, cardiolipin and neutrophil cytoplasm.

Table 110.6 Behçet syndrome.

	Features	Incidence (%)
Major criteria		
Oral	Aphthae	90–100
Genital	Ulcers	64–88
Neuro-ocular	Iridocyclitis	10–90
	Retinal vasculitis	
	Optic atrophy	
	Syndromes resembling disseminated sclerosis, pseudobulbar palsy or neurosyphilis	
	Meningoencephalitis	
	Others	
Dermatological	Pustules	48–88
	Erythema nodosum	
	Pathergy	
Minor criteria	Proteinuria and haematuria	
	Thrombophlebitis	
	Aneurysms	
	Arthralgias	

- Circulating immune complexes and changed levels of complement.
- Immunoglobulins and complement deposition within and around blood vessel walls.
- Decreased ratio of T-helper (CD4) cells to T-suppressor (CD8) cells.

These immunological changes mimic those seen in patients with recurrent aphthous stomatitis – various T-lymphocyte abnormalities (especially T-suppressor cell dysfunction), changes in serum complement and increased polymorphonuclear leukocyte motility. There is also evidence that mononuclear cells may initiate antibody-dependent cellular cytotoxicity to oral epithelial cells, and evidence of disturbance of natural killer cell activity.

The common denominator in all systems is vasculitis, usually leukocytoclastic vasculitis. Many of the features of Behçet syndrome (erythema nodosum, arthralgia, uveitis) are common to established immune complex disease and, indeed, immune complexes (usually antigen–antibody complexes) are found in the sera. The antigen responsible has not been reliably identified but may include HSV or streptococcal antigens [12,13–15]. As in recurrent aphthous stomatitis, heat-shock proteins have been implicated. TLR (Toll-like receptor) expression and single nucleotide polymorphisms (SNPs) in *TLR* genes showed no difference in tissue from patients with Behçet syndrome compared with either disease or healthy controls but there is an association with the increased function variant of TIRAP (Toll-interleukin 1 receptor (TIR) domain containing adaptor protein) suggesting that encounters with a pathogen at mucosal sites will lead to increased cytokine production and tissue damage with persistence of mucosal lesions [16].

Clinical features

Behçet syndrome is a chronic multisystem disorder, most patients being male, usually in their third or fourth decade.

Because Behçet syndrome is rare and symptoms of the disease overlap symptoms of other diseases, it can be very difficult to diagnose. Spontaneous remission is common for patients with Behçet syndrome; this can add to the difficulty in diagnosis.

Behçet syndrome is characterized mainly by a triad of recurrent aphthous stomatitis [6,17,18], genital ulcers [15,16] and ocular lesions [19,20]. The CNS, heart and intestinal tract may be involved.

One variant of Behçet syndrome (MAGIC syndrome) is associated with *m*outh *a*nd *g*enital ulcers and *i*nflamed *c*artilage [21,22]. Other oculomucocutaneous syndromes (Table 110.7) may cause similar manifestations [23,24].

Diagnosis

Behçet syndrome is usually diagnosed on clinical grounds, although findings of HLA-B5101 and pathergy are supportive, as are antibodies to cardiolipin and neutrophil cytoplasm. Disease activity may be assessed by serum levels of acute phase proteins or antibodies to intermediate filaments, or by erythrocyte sedimentation rate; all are raised in active Behçet syndrome.

Table 110.7 Oculomucocutaneous syndromes.*

Disease	Oral and genital	Ocular	Skin
		Main lesions	
Behçet syndrome	Aphthae	Uveitis	Erythema nodosum
Sweet syndrome	Aphthae	Conjunctivitis, episcleritis	Inflamed papule or nodule
Erythema multiforme	Erosions	Erosions	Target lesions
Cicatricial pemphigoid	Bullae	Erosions	Occasional dome-shaped bullae
	Erosions	Scarring	
Pemphigus	Erosions	Erosions	Multiple, flaccid bullae
Reactive arthritis	Ulcers	Conjunctivitis	Keratoderma blenorrhagica

*Ulcerative colitis, herpes simplex, syphilis, lupus erythematosus, mixed connective tissue disease and other disorders may also cause oral, cutaneous and ocular lesions.

Differential diagnosis is mainly from the following:
- Sweet syndrome: aphthae, conjunctivitis, episcleritis, inflamed tender papule or nodule.
- Erythema multiforme: erosions, target (iris) lesions.
- Pemphigoid: bullae, erosions.
- Pemphigus: erosions, multiple flaccid bullae.
- Reactive arthritis: ulcers, conjunctivitis, keratoderma blenorrhagica.
- Ulcerative colitis.
- Herpes simplex.
- Syphilis.
- Lupus erythematosus.
- Mixed connective tissue disease.

The diagnosis is often made on the basis of recurrent aphthous stomatitis plus two or more of recurrent genital ulceration, eye lesions, skin lesions and pathergy [6,25,26]. Major criteria are:

1 Recurrent aphthous stomatitis: in 90–100% of cases.
2 Recurrent painful genital ulcers that tend to heal with scars in 64–88% of cases. Genital ulcers are especially common in females with Behçet syndrome, and resemble recurrent aphthous stomatitis.
3 Ocular lesions: uveitis with conjunctivitis (early) and hypopyon (late), retinal vasculitis (posterior uveitis), iridocyclitis and optic atrophy. The most common ocular manifestation is relapsing iridocyclitis but uveitis, retinal vascular changes and optic atrophy may occur. Both eyes are eventually involved and blindness may result.
4 Central nervous system lesions: meningoencephalitis, cerebral infarction, psychosis, cranial nerve palsies, cerebellar and spinal cord lesions, hemiparesis and quadriparesis.
5 Skin lesions: erythema nodosum, papulopustular lesions and acneform nodules. Venepuncture is, in some patients, followed by pustulation (pathergy).

Minor criteria are:
1 Arthralgia: large joint arthropathies that are subacute, non-migratory, self-limiting and non-deforming.

2 Superficial or deep migratory thrombophlebitis, especially of the lower limbs.
3 Intestinal lesions: inflammatory bowel disease with discrete ulcerations.
4 Lung involvement: pneumonitis.
5 Haematuria and proteinuria.

However, very non-specific signs and symptoms, which may be recurrent, may precede the onset of the mucosal membrane ulceration by 6 months to 5 years. These include malaise, anorexia, weight loss, generalized weakness, headache, perspiration, decreased or elevated temperature, lymphadenopathy and pain in the substernal and temporal regions.

A history of repeated sore throats, tonsillitis, myalgias and migratory erythralgias without overt arthritis is also common.

Management

Unlike recurrent aphthous stomatitis, Behçet syndrome is not self-limiting. It causes morbidity (especially in terms of ocular and neurological disease) and mortality. Most patients present with oral and ocular disease but there follows a relapsing and remitting but variable course. CNS involvement, thromboses of major vessels and gastrointestinal perforation result in a poor prognosis. Few patients with Behçet syndrome have spontaneous remission and thus treatment is indicated [6,27,28].

Chronic morbidity is usual; the leading cause is ophthalmic involvement, which can result in blindness. The effects of the disease may be cumulative, especially with neurological, vascular and ocular involvement. Mortality is low but can occur from neurological involvement, vascular disease, bowel perforation, cardiopulmonary disease or as a complication of immunosuppressive therapy. In the face of the serious potential complications, patients with suspected Behçet syndrome should be referred early for specialist advice.

Topical treatment for oral ulcers. Oral ulcers may respond to topical corticosteroids or 5-aminosalicylic acid [6,29]. Even nicotine patches may have some success [30].

Systemic treatment includes mainly colchicine 0.5–1.5 mg daily. Other systemic treatments include corticosteroids, azathioprine, ciclosporin, chlorambucil, cyclophosphamide, dapsone, interferon-α, levamisole, thalidomide and anti-TNF-α biologicals. Ocular lesions usually respond to ciclosporin, but tend to relapse when treatment is stopped. Thalidomide at a dose of up to 400 mg daily may be of value in recalcitrant orogenital ulceration, although it must be used with caution in view of the adverse effects of teratogenicity and neuropathy [31–34, 38–41]. Biologicals such as infliximab have been successfully used [35–38,42–45].

Sweet syndrome (see Chapter 49)

Pustular lesions leading to aphthous-like ulcers may be found in Sweet syndrome and there are occasional associations with Behçet syndrome and Sjögren syndrome, each of which has oral manifestations. About 5% of patients in the UK with Sweet syndrome have oral aphthous-like ulcers, although up to 30% of Japanese patients suffer these [1–5].

Malignant neoplasms

More than 90% of malignant neoplasms in the mouth are squamous cell carcinomas (oral squamous cell carcinoma) (see also Chapter 142).

Oral squamous cell carcinoma

The mouth is the most common site for cancer in the head and neck. Cancers can develop on the lips, tongue, floor of the mouth (beneath the tongue), buccal mucosae, palate, gingivae or oropharynx. Head and neck cancers can also affect the throat, and there are rarer cancers of the nose, sinuses, salivary glands, skin and middle ear, or arising in other tissues. Oral cancer is a significant world health problem, being overall the sixth most common malignant neoplasm. In parts of South-East Asia for example, particularly India, some 40% of all malignancy is oral cancer [1,2–11]. High levels are also seen in resource-poor countries such as Brazil, but also in parts of Europe such as areas of northern France and eastern Europe.

Nearly 30% of all squamous cell carcinomas affect the lip; some 25% affect the tongue, the most common intraoral site [1–9]. Most intraoral cancers involve the posterolateral border of the tongue and/or the floor of the mouth (the 'graveyard' area). In betel chewing, the buccal mucosa is a common site for carcinoma [10]. Mouth cancers mostly include:
- Lip cancer; most occur on the lower lip (Figure 110.19).
- Intraoral cancer; most develop on the lateral tongue and the floor of the mouth (Figure 110.20).
- Oropharyngeal cancer; arise in the fauces/posterior tongue.

Oral squamous cell carcinoma was the eleventh most common cancer in the world in 2008, accounting for an estimated 263 000 new incident cases and 127 700 deaths annually. Oral squamous cell carcinoma is generally a disease affecting the middle ages and

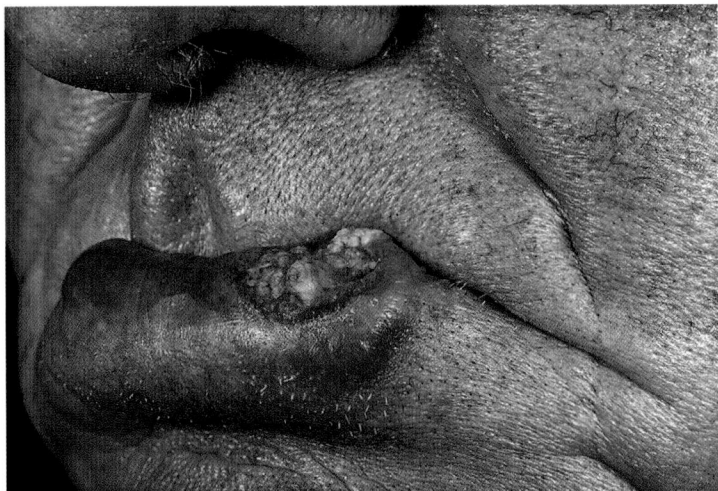

Figure 110.19 Squamous cell carcinoma of the lip.

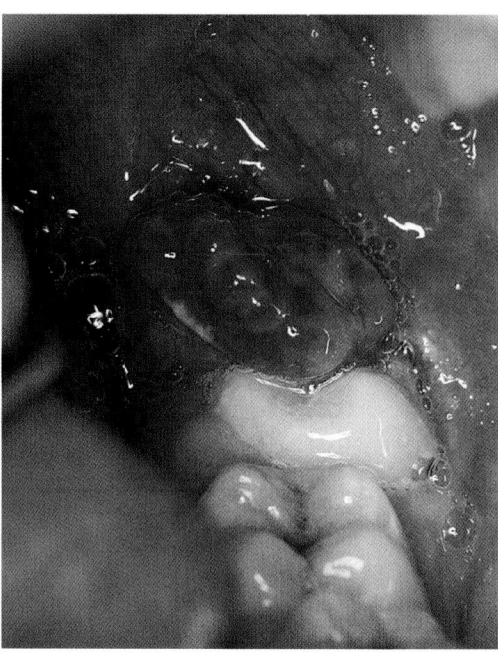

Figure 110.20 Oral squamous cell carcinoma.

the elderly with a mean age of onset in the sixth decade of life. However, an increased incidence of tongue cancer and oropharyngeal carcinoma in both genders below 45 years of age has been documented over recent decades.

Epidemiology

Worldwide, approximately 500 000 new cases of head and neck cancer are diagnosed annually which includes an estimated incidence of 378 500 new cases of intraoral cancer. Oral squamous cell carcinoma is the eighth most common form of cancer overall in people in developed countries. The incidence is generally higher in ethnic minorities in developed countries.There is concern about an ongoing increase in younger patients and in women. More than 1 in 10 cases is now diagnosed in people below age 50.

Mouth cancer is particularly common in people from the developing world. Oral and pharyngeal cancers, when considered together, are the sixth leading cancers in the world and rank in the top three in high incidence areas. In parts of India, oral cancer can represent more than 50% of all cancers. There is a wide geographical variation but two-thirds of the cases occur in people from resource-poor countries such as in South Asia (including Sri Lanka, India, Pakistan, Taiwan); Latin America (Brazil, Uruguay, Puerto Rico and Cuba); and Papua New Guinea, and other pacific islands in Melanesia. In certain countries, such as Sri Lanka, India, Pakistan and Bangladesh, oral cancer is the most common cancer.

Pathophysiology

Predisposing factors

Factors important in mouth cancer include especially lifestyle modifiable risk factors and the following:
- *Age.* Mouth cancer is more common in people over 45.
- *Gender.* Mouth cancer is generally more common in men than women, attributable to heavier indulgence in risk associated

habits (tobacco and alcohol intake) by men and exposure to sunlight (for lip cancer) as a part of outdoor occupations.
- *Social class.* Oral cancer is a problem particularly of people of lower social and economic status, especially in males.

The International Agency for Research on Cancer (IARC) and the World Cancer Research Fund/American Institute for Cancer Research (WCRF/AICR) are the gold standard in cancer epidemiology, and their conclusions about cancer risk factors are shown in Table 110.8.

The main modifiable risk factors are as follows:
- Tobacco use.
- Betel use.
- Alcoholic beverages.
- A diet poor in fresh fruit and vegetables.
- In the case of lip carcinoma, exposure to sunlight.
- In the case of oropharyngeal carcinoma, exposure to human papillomavirus (HPV).

Tobacco is a major risk factor for mouth cancer. All forms of tobacco both smoked and smokeless are carcinogenic. There is for mouth cancer a 20-fold higher risk in heavy smokers (dark tobacco is worst) and a strong dose–response relationship.

Smoking cessation leads to a fall in mouth cancer risk; by 1–4 years after smoking cessation, the risk of mouth cancer is 35% lower than that of a current smoker, and by 20 years or more after cessation the risk is reduced to that of a never-smoker. The risk of oropharynx/hypopharynx cancer risk reduces by around half by 5–9 years of smoking cessation, and is almost that of a never-smoker by 20 years.

Table 110.8 International Agency for Research on Cancer (IARC) and World Cancer Research Fund/American Institute for Cancer Research (WCRF/AICR) evaluations of mouth and head and neck cancer risk factors.

Increases risk ('sufficient' or 'convincing' evidence)	May increase risk ('limited' or 'probable' evidence)	May decrease risk ('limited' or 'probable' evidence)
Alcoholic beverages (oral cavity, tonsil, pharynx)	Hydrochlorothiazide (lip)	Non-starchy vegetables (not salted or pickled) (mouth, pharynx and larynx)
Betel quid with tobacco (oral cavity, tonsil, pharynx)	Solar radiation (lip)	
Betel quid without tobacco (oral cavity)	Human papillomavirus type 18 (oral cavity)	
Human papillomavirus type 16 (oral cavity, tonsil, pharynx)	Radioiodines, including Iodine-131 (salivary gland)	Fruits (not salted or pickled) (mouth, pharynx and larynx)
Tobacco, smokeless (oral cavity)	Asbestos (all forms) (pharynx)	Foods containing carotenoids (mouth, pharynx and larynx)
Tobacco smoking (oral cavity, tonsil, pharynx, nasopharynx)	Mate drinking, hot (pharynx)	
X-radiation, γ-radiation (salivary gland)	Printing processes (pharynx)	
Epstein–Barr virus (nasopharynx)	Tobacco smoke, secondhand smoke (pharynx)	
Formaldehyde (nasopharynx)		
Salted fish, Chinese-style (nasopharynx)		
Wood dust (nasopharynx)		

Alcohol (ethanol or ethyl alcohol) may be carcinogenic. There is for mouth cancer a 20-fold risk with heavy alcohol drinkers (spirits are the worst), and a strong dose–response relationship.

The more alcohol a person drinks, and the greater number of years they drink for, the higher the risk. Genetic variations in the activities of alcohol-metabolizing enzymes (alcohol dehydrogenase, ADH, and acetaldehyde dehydrogenase, ALDH) may influence the outcome of exposure to alcohol, and thus its carcinogenicity in any individual. Risk of a secondary primary tumour (SPT) in the upper aerodigestive tract (UADT) is increased by 9% for every 1.25 units of alcohol consumed per day. Some studies have suggested that mouthwashes with a high alcohol content could increase the risk of mouth cancer but other studies have found that this is not the case and the controversy continues.

Tobacco plus alcohol contribute to a multiplicative carcinogenic effect. Heavy tobacco smokers have a 20-fold greater risk; heavy alcohol drinkers a fivefold greater risk and those who do both have a 50-fold greater risk. People who both smoke and drink heavily over several years have the highest risk of developing head and neck cancers. Smokeless tobacco in conjunction with alcohol also increases the mouth cancer risk.

Betel quid chewing, common in parts of Asia and in some immigrant groups in Europe, North America and Australia, increases rates of mouth cancer. Betel quid *with* tobacco increases the risk of mouth cancer in those who neither smoke nor drink by around seven times. People who smoke tobacco, drink alcohol and chew betel have over 30 times the mouth cancer risk compared with those who abstain from these habits. Betel quid *alone* (with no tobacco) increases the risk of mouth cancer in tobacco non-smokers by around 3.5 times, and in those who neither smoke nor drink alcohol by around 15 times. Betel may cause oral submucous fibrosis.

Various other chewing habits, usually combinations that contain tobacco, are used in different cultures (e.g. khat, Shammah, toombak). Khat (*Catha edulis*) is commonly used especially by young males in and from South Arabia/Eastern Africa. Often tobacco is also smoked. The carcinogenicity of other psychotropic products such as marijuana is controversial.

Other possible risk factors for mouth cancer include:
1 Diseases:
  • Chronic candidosis.
  • Diabetes.
  • Discoid lupus erythematosus.
  • HIV/AIDS.
  • Plummer–Vinson syndrome.
  • Scleroderma.
2 Genetic causes:
  • Dyskeratosis congenital.
  • Fanconi anaemia.
  • Xeroderma pigmentosum.
3 Iatrogenic causes:
  • Deep X-ray (DXR) (radiotherapy).
  • Drugs, etc. including:
    – Antihypertensives.
    – Immunosuppressives.
    – Marijhuana.

People who have had mouth or oropharyngeal cancer have an increased risk of getting a second one. Women have a higher risk of a second oral cancer than men. People who have had some other types of cancer also have an increased risk of mouth cancer. These include the following:
• Cancer of the oesophagus.
• Lung cancer.
• Squamous cell skin cancer.
• Cervical, anal or genital cancer in women.
• Cancer of the rectum in men.

Causative organisms
Human papillomavirus infection is increasingly implicated, particularly in *oropharyngeal* cancer. Other infective agents may be implicated in some other cases. HPV-related tumours tend to be seen in younger patients, in the fauces and have usually a better prognosis. HPV-positive oropharyngeal cancers are associated with oral sex and marijhuana use. High-risk (oncogenic) HPV subtypes have been identified in a significant fraction of oropharyngeal tumours, including HPV-16, -18, -31 and -33. Greater numbers of sexual partners, early age of first sexual intercourse and high-risk sexual behaviour are emerging as risk factors for HPV-related disease independent of tobacco and alcohol abuse. Nevertheless, smoking also increases the risk of HPV infection in the mouth.

Oral cancer is also increased in:
• Patients with anogenital cancer.
• Patients with cervical cancer.
• Partners of women with cervical cancer.

Anal, genital and skin cancers are increased in patients with mouth cancer. IARC classifies HPV-16 as a cause of oral cavity, tonsil and pharynx cancers, and HPV-18 as a probable cause of oral cancer. HPV infection causes around 8% of mouth cancers and around 14% of oropharyngeal cancers in the UK. Around 4/10 (40%) oropharyngeal cancer cases in Europe are HPV-positive.

The HPV vaccines now administered to young people in an effort to prevent cervical cancer afford protection against other HPV-related lesions, including oral lesions, but there is no hard evidence yet as to a significant protective effect against mouth cancer.

Genetics
There are a few familial cases, and people with certain syndromes have a high risk of mouth and throat cancer. There may be a higher risk of developing a head and neck cancer if a close relative (a parent, brother, sister or child) has had head and neck cancer. A family history of oral and pharyngeal cancer and laryngeal cancer is a strong determinant of oral and pharyngeal cancer risk, independent of tobacco and alcohol use. A family history of head and neck cancer, particularly in a sibling, may be associated with almost doubling (70% increase) of head and neck cancer risk. Syndromes with a predisposition to mouth cancer include mainly:
• Dyskeratosis congenita.
• Fanconi anaemia.
• Xeroderma pigmentosum.

Environmental factors
Lip cancer is an issue mainly in older men exposed over long periods to sunlight, as these areas are often exposed to UV light.

Occupations with an increased risk of mouth cancer mostly involve blue collar workers, and may include:
- Benzene exposure.
- Blacksmithing.
- Building industry.
- Carpet installation.
- Construction work.
- Driving.
- Electricity working.
- Fossil fuel exposure.
- Furniture industry.
- Grain production.
- Machinery operation.
- Masonry.
- Metal working.
- Painting.
- Pesticide exposure.
- Petroleum industry.
- Plumbers.
- Railway working.
- Textile industry.
- Woodworkers.

Other causes

There is an increased risk of mouth cancer following a previous cancer diagnosis. People with a previous head and neck cancer (including of the tongue, mouth, pharynx, and larynx) have between 12- and 16-fold increased risk of subsequent head and neck cancer. Survivors of oesophageal squamous cell carcinoma have an almost sevenfold increase in risk of mouth and pharynx cancers. People with a previous lung cancer have between 1.5 and 5.7 times the general population risk of developing head and neck cancer.

Socioeconomic deprivation has been linked to an increased risk of oral cancer, but many other explanations (e.g. habits, oral health, diet, nutrition) may be responsible. A diet high in animal fats and low in fresh fruit and vegetables may increase the risk of developing head and neck cancer.

Since the onset of the HIV epidemic, there have been many case reports of mouth cancer in people with HIV/AIDS. Meta-analyses have shown people with HIV/AIDS have around double the risk of mouth, oropharyngeal and pharyngeal cancers, compared with the general population. There is a positive association between HIV and HPV infection, which might be relevant.

Factors that may reduce mouth cancer risk

WCRF/AICR classifies consumption of non-starchy vegetables and fruits (not salted or pickled), and foods containing carotenoids, as possibly protective against mouth, pharynx and larynx cancers. A significant protective effect of diet against mouth cancer has generally been shown in persons who consume β-carotene-rich vegetables and citric fruits. There is an inverse association between caffeinated coffee drinking and risk of mouth and pharynx cancer. Tea and decaffeinated coffee do not appear to be associated with oral cancer risk. Recreational physical activity is associated with a 26–47% reduction in mouth cancer risk, and a 33–42% reduction in pharyngeal cancer risk [11–26,**27**,28–109].

Box 110.6 Features suggestive of oral squamous cell carcinoma

Any persistent:
- Red lesion (erythroplasia or erythroplakia)
- Mixed red/white lesion (erythroleukoplakia)
- Nodular white lesion (verrucous leukoplakia)
- Lump
- Ulcer with fissuring or raised exophytic margins
- Pain or numbness
- Abnormal blood vessels supplying a lump
- Loose tooth
- Extraction socket not healing
- Induration, i.e. a firm infiltration beneath the lesion
- Fixation of lesion to deeper tissues or to overlying skin or mucosa
- Regional lymph node enlargement
- Dysphagia
- Weight loss

History

Oral cancer in the initial clinically detectable stage is a red or red and white (erytholeukoplastic) area without symptoms – difficult to differentiate from potentially malignant disorders (PMD) and early cancers are rarely painful. The initial lesions are usually solitary and asymptomatic when they are small and thus, in the early stages, it is quite possible to make a misdiagnosis. Lesions of oral cancer can range from a few millimetres to several centimetres in diameter in the more advanced cases (Box 110.6). In advanced cancers, there is often a red or red and white single lesion, ulcer or lump with irregular margins which are rigid to touch (indurated) and there may be pain especially in the tongue and floor of the mouth lesions. The *rule* is that a single lesion of 3 or more weeks' duration, especially a red and/or white lesion; an ulcer; a lump; or especially a combination of these; or if indurated (firm on palpation), it should be regarded with suspicion, and a biopsy arranged.

Presentation

Some mouth cancers arise in clinically apparently normal mucosa, but some are preceded by clinically obvious PMD. There is range of PMD; the most important are erythroplakia (erythroplasia), leukoplakia and lichenoid lesions. Others, such as actinic cheilitis, submucous fibrosis, Fanconi anaemia (syndrome), are less common (Table 110.9).

Table 110.9 Potentially malignant disorders.

Entities	Approximate malignant potential over 10 years		
	Very high (70-85%)	High (10–30%)	Low (1–5%)
Main	Erythroplakia (erythroplasia)	Candidal leukoplakia	Leukoplakia (homogeneous)
		Leukoplakia (non-homogeneous)	Lichenoid lesions/ lichen planus
Less common		Actinic cheilitis	Discoid lupus erythematosus
		Dyskeratosis congenita	Fanconi syndrome
		Submucous fibrosis	

The risk of malignant transformation in the PMDs is approximately as shown in Table 110.9.

Potentially malignant lesions are initially usually symptomless, but any symptoms should raise the index of suspicion of malignant change.

The most common sites of mouth cancer include the lower lip, the lateral margin of the tongue and the floor of the mouth. Most lip cancers manifest on the lower lip at the mucocutaneous junction as a chronic small lump, ulcer or scabbed lesion. Intraoral cancer can have a highly variable clinical appearance – mainly an ulcer, red or white area, lump or fissure. Most intraoral cancers manifest on the middle third of the lateral margins of the tongue with an erythroplastic component and, sometimes, induration. Late tongue cancer may manifest as an exophytic lesion, an ulcer or an area of superficial ulceration with induration. The floor of the mouth is the second most common intraoral site for cancer and more commonly is associated with leukoplakia. Most cancer arises in the anterior floor of the mouth as an indurated mass that soon ulcerates, resulting in slurring of speech. The sump area or 'coffin corner' at the posterior tongue/floor of the mouth is a common site for cancer but may be missed by cursory inspection; special care is needed to ensure close examination. Carcinomas of the alveolus or gingiva are mostly seen in the mandibular premolar and molar regions, usually as a lump (epulis) or ulcer. The underlying alveolar bone is invaded in 50% of cases, even in the absence of radiographic changes, and adjacent teeth may be loose. Carcinomas of the buccal mucosa are mostly seen at the commissure or in the retromolar area. Most are ulcerated lumps, and some arise in candidal leukoplakias. A typical malignant ulcer is hard with heaped-up and often everted or rolled edges and a granular floor.

The presenting features of mouth cancer usually relate to the local effects of the primary tumour, occasionally to regional spread, metastatic disease or paraneoplastic phenomena. Oral squamous cell carcinoma predominantly metastasizes locally and to draining regional lymph nodes, primarily in the anterior neck. Mouth cancer spreads by haematogenous dissemination only late in its natural history.

Extraoral examination should therefore include cervical lymph node examination. Mouth cancer often spreads to the submental and submandibular nodes. A painless enlarged cervical lymph node may be the only presenting symptom. Lymph node examination is of paramount importance; from 30 to 80% of patients with oral squamous cell carcinoma have metastases in the cervical lymph nodes at presentation. A systematic and thorough examination of the cervical lymph nodes, mouth and fauces should be performed by a clinician trained in the diagnosis of oral diseases, and a general physical examination is indicated.

Differential diagnosis
Other causes of mouth lumps or ulcers.

Classification of severity
Grading is used as a prognostic indicator; well-differentiated or low-grade cancers have the better prognosis (Box 110.7). Low-grade tumours will usually grow more slowly and be less likely to spread than a high-grade tumour. High grade means the cells look more abnormal and the tumours metastasize more readily.

> **Box 110.7 Grades of carcinoma**
>
> **Well differentiated**
> - Elongated rete pegs invading lamina propria, with keratin pearls
>
> **Moderately differentiated**
> - Irregular invading rete pegs; loss of cellular cohesion
>
> **Poorly differentiated**
> - Sheets of invading epithelium with no obvious architecture, but severe cellular abnormalities such as pleomorphism and hyperchromatism

The most important prognostic factors are site and TNM stage (tumour, node, metastasis) which describes:
- Tumour size (T).
- Whether the cancer has spread to the nodes (N).
- Whether the cancer has metastasized (M).

TNM classification
- Primary tumour:
  - T0: no primary tumour.
  - Tis: carcinoma *in situ*.
  - T1: tumour 2 cm or smaller.
  - T2: tumour 4 cm or smaller
  - T3: tumour larger than 4 cm.
  - T4: tumour larger than 4 cm and deep invasion to muscle, bone or deep structures (e.g. antrum).
- Lymphatic node involvement:
  - N0: no nodes.
  - N1: single homolateral node smaller than 3 cm.
  - N2: nodes(s) homolateral smaller than 6 cm.
  - N3: nodes(s) larger than 6 cm and/or bilateral.
- Tumour metastasis:
  - M0: no metastasis.
  - M1: metastasis noted.

Staging
- Stage I: T1, N0, M0.
- Stage II: T2, N0, M0.
- Stage III:
  - T3, N0, M0.
  - T1, T2, T3, N1, M0.
- Stage IV:
  - T4, N0, M0.
  - Any T, N2 or N3, M0.
  - Any T, any N, any M.

There is also a number stage system for mouth and oropharyngeal cancers which uses four main stages but some also refer to stage 0 as follows.
- **Stage 0 or carcinoma *in situ*:** this is a very early stage cancer.
- **Stage 1:** this is the earliest stage of invasive cancer; it is <2 cm across and has not spread to nearby tissues, lymph nodes or other organs.
- **Stage 2:** this is >2 cm across, but <4 cm and has not spread to lymph nodes or other organs.

- **Stage 3**: either the cancer is >4 cm but has not spread to any lymph nodes or other parts of the body, or the tumour is any size but has spread to one lymph node on the same side of the neck as the cancer. In this case, the lymph node involved is no more than 3 cm across. Stage 3 cancer may be subdivided into stage 3a, stage 3b and stage 3c. A stage 3b cancer may differ from a stage 3a cancer in either the tumour size or if the cancer has spread to lymph nodes.
- **Stage 4**: this is advanced; it is divided into three:
  - Stage 4a: this has grown through the tissues around the lips and mouth – lymph nodes in the area may or may not contain cancer cells.
  - Stage 4b: this is any size and has spread to more than one lymph node on the same side of the neck, *or* to lymph nodes on both sides of the neck, *or* any lymph node is bigger than 6 cm.
  - Stage 4c: this has spread to other parts such as the lungs or bones.

The number stages are made up of different combinations of the TNM stages. So, a stage 1 cancer may be described as either T1, N0, M0 or T2, N0, M0.

Disease course and prognosis

The quality of life during and after mouth cancer treatment has steadily improved over the years but survival rates have increased at a slower pace. The stage at which mouth cancer is diagnosed has a significant effect on overall survival and quality of life: early diagnosis reduces mortality and also minimizes:
- Morbidity.
- Disfigurement.
- Treatment duration.
- Costs.

Thus while localized cancer (confined to the primary site) and small tumours (stage I: <2 cm), have ~90% 2-year survival rate, most cancers are found at a late stage, larger than 2 cm (stages III and IV disease – when survival is about half as good. Indeed, about 60% of patients with mouth cancer present with late stage (stages III and IV) disease. The reasons for a patient to be diagnosed with advanced disease can be due to patient delays, doctor delays and system delays and are longer in:
- Heavy smokers.
- Heavy alcohol drinkers.
- People with lower socioeconomic status.

Investigations

A conventional oral examination (COE) with white light ('incandescent light') (visual and palpation examination), constitutes the gold standard for the diagnosis of oral precancer and cancer. There is no doubt that clinician education improves the diagnostic skills and that experience counts.

A range of diagnostic aids is appearing on the market, or in the scientific literature, but analysis of the evidence has shown that there is insufficient evidence that:
- Commercial devices based on autofluorescence enhance visual detection beyond a conventional visual and tactile examination.
- Commercial devices based on tissue reflectance enhance visual detection beyond a conventional visual and tactile examination.

- Commercial devices can assess the validity of transepithelial cytology of seemingly innocuous mucosal lesions.

The diagnosis is often arrived at by a biopsy from the primary lesion or site. The principles are to confirm the diagnosis histopathologically. Then, if it is oral squamous cell carcinoma, patients may benefit from a range of investigations. The principles are to:
- Confirm the cancer diagnosis histopathologically.
- Determine if there is malignant disease elsewhere:
  - Local invasion (e.g. bone, muscles or cervical regional lymph nodes).
  - Metastases, which initially are to lymph nodes and later to liver, bone and brain. Imaging may detect abnormalities that escape clinical examination.
  - Second primary tumours: there is controversy as to the cost-effectiveness for endoscopy in all cases.

Usually examination under general anaesthesia (EUA), is indicated to carefully delineate the primary tumour extent, palpate for cervical lymph nodes and identify synchronous primary lesions – typically located in the upper aerodigestive tract (e.g. the mouth, nose, pharynx, larynx, oesophagus). EUA may particularly be indicated, particularly for patients with:
- Tumours in the posterior tongue.
- Tumours where the margins cannot be readily defined
- An enlarged cervical node but no visible primary neoplasm.

When a cervical lymph node is positive without any primary site evident, a meticulous EUA might reveal the primary tumour. If a primary site is not determined by visual inspection or palpation, random biopsies of the nasopharynx, base of the tongue, hypopharynx and an ipsilateral tonsillectomy are often performed. These are the areas for most occult primary sites.

Whether endoscopy is warranted to detect such second primary tumours in all cases remains controversial. Metastasis initially occurs to regional lymph nodes and later to the liver, bones and brain. Imaging and other studies may help detect abnormalities missed during the clinical examination. Positron emission tomography (PET) scan, when combined with computed tomography (CT) imaging, may be useful in detecting occult lymph node involvement and metastatic disease. Investigations – particularly node biopsy – are commonly performed usually using fine-needle aspiration (FNA). Ultrasound-guided FNA cytology (US-FNAC) is now favoured. A sentinel lymph node biopsy (SLNB) can be used to help determine the extent, or stage, of spread of the cancer.

Jaw radiography, MRI or CT scanning and PET scanning, panendoscopy and chest radiography are valuable for excluding synchronous second primary tumours and as pre-anaesthetic checks.

Management

If mouth cancer can be diagnosed at an early stage, when the lesions are small, treatment is generally less complicated and more effective. The treatment of mouth cancer requires a multispecialty approach. Surgery and radiation are the only definitive treatment modalities for both early and locally advanced disease (Box 110.8). Surgical resection, wherein the tumour is completely removed with uninvolved resection margins, is challenging and can involve sacrificing critical structures. Radiation, when used as definitive therapy, circumvents this difficulty, but often produces

---

Box 110.8 Treatments for mouth cancer

Beneficial
• Surgery
• Radiotherapy

Likely to be beneficial
• Chemotherapy
• Robotic surgery
• Conformal radiotherapy

Emergent treatments
• Targeted therapies (mainly cetuximab)

---

significant acute and late toxicity. Chemotherapy alone is not a curative therapeutic modality, but may improve outcomes when used in conjunction with radiation for locally advanced disease.

Lip cancer
This is treated mainly surgically.

Intraoral cancers
• T1 tumours are generally treated equally effectively by surgery or radiotherapy.
• Most others are treated largely by surgery and/or radiation therapy to control the primary tumour and metastases in the draining cervical lymph nodes with a considered balance between length of survival and the quality of remaining life.
• T2 tumours: generally managed surgically. However, tumours of the lateral margin of the tongue may be treated by radiotherapy using external beam (40 Gy) plus radioactive iridium implants (25–30 Gy). For many patients, this must include treatment of the neck lymph nodes and thus often the treatment of choice is surgery (tumour excision with neck dissection), together with radiotherapy.
• T3 tumours: generally treated by surgery followed by radiotherapy if there is extracapsular spread or multiple lymph node involvement. For many patients, the treatment is often surgery (tumour excision with neck dissection), together with radiotherapy.
• T4 tumours: may be treated with chemoradiotherapy.

A 2010 Cochrane review found that adding chemotherapy to surgery or radiotherapy for oropharyngeal cancer can work better than one of these treatments alone [110].

Verrucous carcinoma

Verrucous carcinoma (Ackerman tumour) is an uncommon warty white neoplasm that is rarely ulcerated [1–6], sometimes called carcinoma cuniculatum. It may develop from proliferative verrucous leukoplakia. Risk factors include a possible association with HPV and some verrucous carcinomas develop as a result of the local use of snuff or tobacco. Confirmation of the diagnosis by biopsy is particularly important because verrucous carcinoma responds well to excision but, if irradiated, may undergo anaplastic change, with subsequent acceleration of growth and

invasiveness [7]. Methotrexate, methisoprinol, imiquimod and laser may be of value [8–12].

Florid oral papillomatosis

Florid oral papillomatosis is a rare but well-defined clinical entity of unknown pathogenesis. Risk factors include possible association with HPV, tobacco, and chronic inflammation or irritation.

Florid oral papillomatosis is essentially a verrucous carcinoma, a clinicopathological variant of squamous cell carcinoma also known by a confusing array of names such as Ackerman tumour, Buschke–Loewenstein tumour, epithelioma cuniculatum, carcinoma cuniculatum and cutis papillomatosis carcinoides of Gottron.

Clinical features
The papillomatous lesions are exuberant, warty or verrucous, and characterized by their benign appearance on histology, although this is usually associated with a marked capacity for recurrence and a tendency for carcinomatous change. Its apparent clinical benign nature may lead to lengthy periods of misdiagnosis, during which it slowly but relentlessly destroys and extends into underlying tissue but rarely metastasizes to the lymph nodes [1,2]. It may be associated with malignant canthosis nigricans.

Diagnosis
Biopsy is required, although to those unfamiliar with the diagnosis the relatively bland histological features are often more suggestive of verruca vulgaris or pseudoepitheliomatous hyperplasia than of squamous cell carcinoma. Alternatively, when it extends into underlying tissues, it may be mistaken for a benign adnexal tumour or even a cyst.

Management
Treatment in the early stage of the disease is usually successful. Etretinate therapy (200 mg/day) or chemotherapy with bleomycin may reduce the lesion bulk [3,4]. Treatment can also be with photodynamic therapy, laser, interferon α or imiquimod [3–9].

Surgical or laser excision is favoured. The use of radiotherapy is controversial since in numerous reported cases this has produced an anaplastic squamous cell carcinoma.

Other oral malignant primary neoplasms

The following comprise up to 10% of all oral malignant tumours.
1 Salivary gland tumours.
2 Malignant melanoma.
3 Lymphomas: non-Hodgkin lymphomas are increasingly seen in the fauces in HIV disease and immunocompromised persons.
4 Sarcomas.
5 Kaposi sarcoma: oral Kaposi sarcoma is typically seen in HIV disease or other immunocompromised persons and especially in the posterior palate as a brown or purple macule that becomes nodular and ulcerates.
6 Some odontogenic tumours.
7 Maxillary antral carcinoma (or other neoplasms).
8 Langerhans cell histiocytosis.

9 Neoplasms of bone and connective tissue.
10 Other neoplasms.

Granular cell tumours

Congenital granular cell epulis is a rare lesion of unknown histogenesis with a predilection for the maxillary alveolar ridge of newborn girls. Microscopically, there are nests of polygonal cells with granular cytoplasm, a prominent capillary network and attenuated overlying squamous epithelium. The lesion lacks immunoreactivity for S-100, laminin, chromogranin and most other markers except neuron-specific enolase and vimentin [1–4]. This lesion should be distinguished from the more common adult granular cell tumour as well as other differential diagnoses.

Adult granular cell tumour (Abrikossoff tumour) develops between the second and sixth decades of life, more frequently among women and people of African heritage. The head and neck area is affected in 45–65% of cases and, of these, 70% are located intraorally (tongue, oral mucosa, hard palate) [5]. The benign form shows polygonal cells with granular eosinophilic cytoplasm and small nuclei. The malignant form, however, is associated with a high mitotic index and pleomorphic cellular tissue.

The clinical feature of either is a swelling covered by mucosa of normal clinical appearance. Histological examination is required. The treatment is surgery.

Metastatic oral neoplasms

Metastases to the oral cavity are rare. Most appear in the bone, especially the mandibular premolar or molar area or condyle. Metastases may occasionally appear as an alveolar or gingival swelling or ulcer.

Most oral metastases originate from carcinomas of the breast, lung, kidney, thyroid, stomach, liver, colon or prostate [1–12]. Tumour deposits may arise from lymphatic or haematogenous spread.

In one large study [13], 25% of cases, oral metastases were found to be the first sign of metastatic spread and in 23% it was the first indication of an undiscovered malignancy. The mandible was more frequently affected than the oral soft tissues (2 : 1). In the oral soft tissues, the attached gingiva was the most commonly affected site (54%). The major primary sites presenting oral metastases were the lung, kidney, liver and prostate for men, and the breast, female genital organs, kidney and colorectum for women. The primary site differs according to oral site colonization: in men, the lung was the most common primary site affecting both the jaw bones and oral mucosa (22% and 31.3%, respectively) followed by the prostate gland in the jaw bones (11%) and kidney in the oral soft tissues (14%). In women, the breast was the most common primary tumour affecting the jaw bones and soft tissues (41% and 24.3%, respectively), followed by the adrenal and female genital organs in the jaw bones (7.7%) and female genital organs in the soft tissues (14.8%).

Clinical features. Metastases usually present as a lesion in the jaw, sometimes only revealed coincidentally by imaging, at other times causing symptoms. In up to one-third of patients, the jaw lesions are the first manifestation of the tumour. Non-Hodgkin lymphomas are frequently gingival or faucial in location.

Many metastases are asymptomatic but others manifest with:
- Pain.
- Paraesthesia or hypoaesthesia.
- Swelling.
- Tooth mobility.
- Non-healing extraction sockets.
- Pathological fracture.
- Radiolucency or radio-opacity.

Diagnosis. Early manifestation of metastases may resemble a hyperplastic or reactive lesion, such as pyogenic granuloma, peripheral giant cell granuloma or fibrous lump. Diagnosis is from history and clinical features supplemented by radiography and histopathology. In any case, where the clinical presentation is unusual especially in patients with known malignant disease, biopsy is mandatory.

Management. Radiotherapy, surgery or chemotherapy.

Ulcers in association with systemic disease

Aphthous-like ulcers may be associated with systemic disease. However, a wide range of systemic diseases, especially haematological, gastrointestinal and dermatological disorders, may cause other oral lesions which, because of the moisture, trauma and infection in the mouth, tend to break down to leave ulcers or erosions. Oral ulceration is also frequently caused by infections and can be caused by iatrogenic problems such as drugs or irradiation or GVHD (see Box 110.5).

Haematological diseases

Deficiency states

Low iron, folate or vitamin B_{12} levels may predispose to mouth ulcers. A few of these patients also have anaemia, sometimes with other oral features such as glossitis or angular stomatitis, but many have a deficiency state with no established anaemia [1–3]. Occasionally, patients with deficiency of B vitamins may develop other types of oral ulcer, and sometimes epithelial dysplasia [4].

Leukopenias and agranulocytosis

White cell dyscrasias and HIV infection are also often complicated by oral ulceration (Figure 110.21). Oral ulceration may be a major symptom in patients with leukopenias, and may be the first manifestation of drug-induced agranulocytosis. Painful deep irregular ulcers, often with only a minimal inflammatory halo, involve the mouth and/or pharynx and tend to extend and penetrate slowly. In cyclic neutropenia, ulcers appear episodically at 21-day intervals in association with the neutropenic episodes. Severe periodontitis is often also a feature of leukocyte and other immune defects and the patients may suffer from recurrent infections elsewhere [1–5]. Methotrexate can cause oral ulceration in the absence of leukopenia.

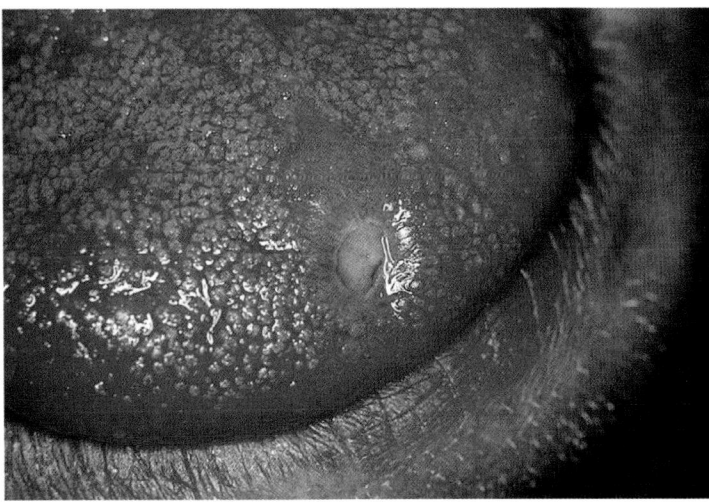

Figure 110.21 Aphthous-like ulceration in HIV disease.

Leukaemias

Oral ulceration may be a prominent feature, especially in the acute leukaemias. Other oral manifestations of leukaemia include mucosal pallor, gingival haemorrhage, gingival swelling, petechiae and ecchymoses [1–7]. Oral infections with *Candida albicans* and Gram-negative bacteria including *Pseudomonas* spp., *Escherichia coli*, *Proteus*, *Klebsiella* and *Serratia* spp. are common, especially in acute leukaemias, and may act as a portal for septicaemia [8]. Herpes simplex or zoster-varicella virus ulcers are also common (Figure 110.22). Chemotherapy complicates the situation because it too can produce oral ulceration [1,7,9], as can bone marrow transplantation.

Other occasional findings include paraesthesia (particularly of the lower lip), facial palsy, extrusion of teeth or bone, painful swellings over the mandible and parotid swelling (Mikulicz syndrome) [10,11].

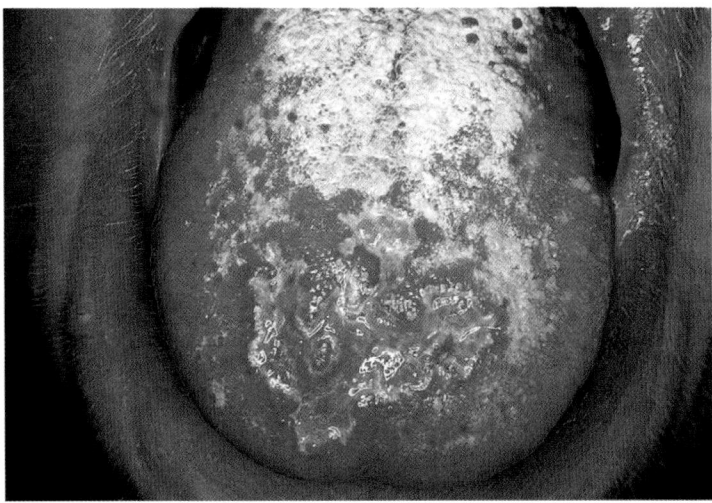

Figure 110.22 Herpes simplex lingual recurrence, and candidosis in leukaemia: similar lesions may be seen in HIV infection.

Granulocytic sarcoma

Synonyms and inclusions
• Chloroma

Granulocytic sarcomas are rare in the oral cavity. Most present with swelling or symptoms related to skeletal involvement [1–4]. The maxilla is particularly involved [1,5–7].

Myelodysplastic syndromes

Oral manifestations in myelodysplastic syndrome include particularly ulceration but also paraesthesiae, petechiae, burning mouth, gingival swelling, xerostomia and herpes labialis [1–4].

Lymphomas

Some 2–10% of lymphomas present first in the oral cavity. Of these oral lymphomas, 80% are composed of follicular centre cells or post-follicular cells [1–6]. Lymphomas usually occur on the pharynx or palate, but occasionally on the tongue, gingivae or lips; they may appear as oral swellings, which sometimes ulcerate and may cause pain or sensory disturbance. Oral herpes zoster and herpes simplex infections are common in patients with lymphomas.

There is an increased incidence of oral lymphomas in HIV disease [7,8] including oral plasmablastic lymphomas [9–11].

Lethal midline granuloma

This is the term sometimes used to include a spectrum of conditions including GPA, polymorphic reticulosis (lymphomatoid granulomatosis) and idiopathic midline destructive disease.

Granulomatosis with polyangiitis

Oral manifestations are common and may be the first sign of GPA [12–26]. A painless, progressive swelling of the gingiva in a previously healthy mouth, particularly associated with swollen inflamed papillae, should arouse suspicion of GPA. The gingival enlargement may have a fairly characteristic 'strawberry-like' appearance [25]. GPA may also present with oral ulceration, failure of an extraction socket to heal or occasionally swelling of the lip or salivary gland.

Lymphomatoid granulomatosis (synonym polymorphic reticulosis)

Lymphomatoid granulomatosis may present with orofacial angio-oedema, palatal, gingival or buccal ulceration but usually no lymphadenopathy [20,27–30].

Idiopathic midline destructive disease [31–34]

Downward spread from nasal disease can lead to palatal necrosis and ulceration in idiopathic midline destructive disease. Occasionally, the disease presents with delayed healing of an extraction socket.

Mycosis fungoides

Oral lesions in mycosis fungoides typically are red or white areas on the tongue but are usually late manifestations of this disease [1–6].

Pseudolymphoma

Rare tumour-like lymphoproliferative infiltrates that lack the malignant potential of lymphomas may be seen intraorally, notably in the palate [1–3].

Histiocytoses

The histiocytoses typically produce lytic bone lesions but gingival swelling, periodontal destruction with loosening of teeth, non-healing extraction sockets and mouth ulceration may be seen. ^{111}In-pentetreotide imaging may be useful in diagnosis of Langerhans cell histiocytosis [1–9].

Multicentric reticulohistiocytosis

Oral lesions are seen in up to 50% of patients with multicentric reticulohistiocytosis [1,2]. Lesions are collections of histiocytes that form nodular or granular lesions, particularly in the labial or buccal mucosa. The temporomandibular joint may also be involved as part of the polyarthropathy.

Hypereosinophilic syndrome

Oral erosions affecting buccal, gingival or labial mucosae may be a feature of the hypereosinophilic syndrome [1–6] and may herald cardiac involvement [2]. Etoposide, interferon-α and hydroxyurea (hydroxycarbamide) may be effective therapy [4,5].

Hypoplasminogenaemia

Gingival swelling and ulceration are features of hypoplasminogenaemia.

Gastrointestinal diseases

Crohn disease

Crohn disease lesions are indistinguishable from orofacial granulomatosis.

Orofacial granulomatosis

Crohn disease can affect the mouth but some patients appear to develop similar oral lesions in the absence of detectable Crohn disease; these are termed orofacial granulomatosis. It is unclear where in the spectrum of Crohn disease/sarcoidosis/allergy/infection these lesions (and related conditions such as Melkersson–Rosenthal syndrome and granulomatous cheilitis) lie [1,2–5].

Age. Lesions are most commonly seen in children and adolescents

Pathophysiology. Crohn disease can affect the mouth but some patients appear to develop similar oral lesions because of an adverse reaction to various food additives, such as cinnamaldehyde or benzoates, butylated hydroxyanisole or dodecyl gallate (in margarine), or to menthol (in peppermint oil) or cobalt, although these reactions are by no means always relevant [1,6–20]. For example, the lesions in only one of nine patients in one study had any relationship to food intake [19]. Nevertheless,

cinnamon and/or benzoate-free diets may produce improvement [20].

Pathology. Non-caseating granulomas and lymphoedema may be seen but the granulomas tend to be sparse and deep, close to the muscle.

Genetics. The genetic background [21], any role of allergy [22] and diverse possible other aetiological factors such as *Mycobacterium paratuberculosis* [23] is unclear.

Clinical features. Ulcers classically involve the buccal sulcus where they appear as linear ulcers, often with granulomatous masses flanking them.

Mucosal lesions also include thickening and folding of the mucosa to produce a 'cobblestone' type of appearance and mucosal tags. Purple granulomatous enlargements may appear on the gingiva. The lips or face may swell (Figure 110.23) and there may be splitting of the lips and angular stomatitis [24–26].

Investigations. The oral history is not specific, and investigation of the gastrointestinal tract is mandatory. Investigations such as chest radiography, serum angiotensin-converting enzyme and a gallium scan may be required to exclude sarcoidosis. Patch tests may be indicated to exclude reactions to various foodstuffs or additives.

Management. Elimination diets may be warranted in patients with orofacial granulomatosis if allergy is suspected [15,20]. Topical or intralesional corticosteroids may effectively control the oral lesions [11]. Intralesional corticosteroid injections may also reduce the swelling. The injection of up to 10 mL triamcinolone (10 mg/L) into the lips after local analgesia may be effective [19,27–30]. The injections may have to be repeated every 4–6 months once a response plateau has been reached.

Clofazimine appears to be effective during the early stages and works by clearing granulomas. In a dose of 100 mg twice daily for

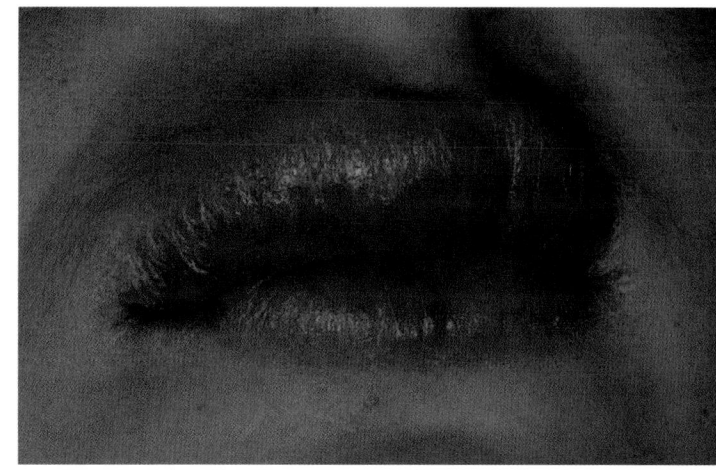

Figure 110.23 Orofacial granulomatosis.

10 days, then twice weekly for 4 months, clofazimine appears to help the majority of patients [31,32,33].

Systemic corticosteroids are rarely indicated and in any event not all patients respond [29,31]. Metronidazole [8] or sulfasalazine [31] may be of value in some cases. Thalidomide has also been reported as beneficial [34].

Pyostomatitis vegetans

The oral lesions termed pyostomatitis vegetans are deep fissures, pustules and papillary projections. Less than 50 cases have been recorded and most patients have had inflammatory bowel disease, that is ulcerative colitis or Crohn disease [1–14]. The course of these lesions tends to follow that of the associated bowel disease [1–5,13].

Although the oral lesions may respond at least partially to topical therapy (e.g. corticosteroids), systemic treatment is often needed [1–5,13].

Dermatological diseases

Several dermatoses can be associated with oral ulcers or erosions; lichen planus is the most common, pemphigus the most serious and pemphgoid is intermediate.

Chronic ulcerative stomatitis with epithelial antinuclear antibodies

Chronic erosive or ulcerative stomatitis often presents as desquamative gingivitis with or without lesions on buccal or lingual mucosa and sometimes resembles lichen planus, and may be associated with lichenoid histology, but is associated with antinuclear antibodies directed against stratified squamous epithelia [1–4]. These autoantibodies are directed against a 70 kDa epithelial nuclear protein homologous to the p53 tumour suppressor and the p73 putative tumour suppressor, and shown to be a splicing variant of the KET gene [5,6].

The lesions may respond to hydroxychloroquine [1–4].

Chronic bullous dermatosis of childhood (see Chapter 50)
Oral ulceration and desquamative gingivitis have been reported [1–6].

Dermatitis herpetiformis and adult linear IgA disease
(see Chapter 50)
Oral lesions may occur in dermatitis herpetiformis and in most patients with linear IgA disease. Macules, papules, petechiae, vesicles, bullae and erosions or desquamative gingivitis are the usual manifestations [1–13]. These disorders must be differentiated, especially from pemphigoid, angina bullosa haemorrhagica, superficial mucocoeles and lichen planus.

Salivary IgA antigliadin antibodies may be found but this is not useful diagnostically. Dapsone and sulfapyridine are the most effective therapeutic agents along with a gluten-free diet in dermatitis herpetiformis. Mycophenolate mofetil may be of benefit in the treatment of linear IgA disease [13].

Epidermolysis bullosa acquisita (see Chapter 50)
Blisters or ulcers may be seen in the oral mucosa in epidermolysis bullosa acquisita, with antibodies directed against collagen VII [1].

Lesional biopsy shows IgG and C3 in the sublamina densa zone of the epithelial basement membrane using immunoelectron microscopy [2–5].

Erythema multiforme (see Chapter 47)

Aetiology. The aetiology of EM is unclear in most patients, but appears to be an immunological hypersensitivity reaction with the appearance of cytotoxic effector cells (CD8+ T lymphocytes) in the epithelium, inducing apoptosis of scattered keratinocytes and leading to satellite cell necrosis.

Erythema multiforme has been classified into a number of variants – EM minor affecting one mucosa and EM major affecting two or more mucous membranes. In Stevens–Johnson syndrome there is extensive skin involvement, multisite mucositis and an associated mortality rate of 10% [1,2].

Predisposing factors. There may be a genetic predisposition, with associations of recurrent EM with HLA-B15 (B62), HLA-B35, HLA-A33, HLA-DR53 and HLA-DQB1*0301. HLA-DQ3 has been proven to be especially related to recurrent EM and may be a helpful marker for distinguishing this herpes-associated EM from other diseases with EM-like lesions. Patients with extensive mucosal involvement may have the rare HLA allele DQB1*0402 [3].

The reaction is triggered by the following:
* Infective agents, particularly HSV (herpes-associated EM), which is implicated in 70% of recurrent EM. Bacteria (Mycoplasma pneumoniae, and many others), other viruses, fungi or parasites are less commonly implicated [1,2,4–10].
* Drugs such as sulphonamides (e.g. co-trimoxazole), cephalosporins, aminopenicillins, quinolones, barbiturates, oxicam non-steroidal anti-inflammatory drugs, anticonvulsants, protease inhibitors, allopurinol and many others may trigger severe EM or toxic epidermal necrolysis in particular [1,2,11,12].
* Food additives or chemicals such as benzoates, nitrobenzene, perfumes, terpenes.
* Immune conditions such as bacille Calmette–Guérin (BCG) or hepatitis B immunization, sarcoidosis, GVHD, inflammatory bowel disease, polyarteritis nodosa or systemic lupus erythematosus (SLE).

Clinical features. Most patients with EM (70%), of either minor or major forms, have oral lesions. The oral mucosa may be involved alone or in association with skin lesions. Mucosal lesions begin as erythematous areas that blister and break down to irregular extensive painful erosions with extensive surrounding erythema. The labial mucosa is often involved, and a serosanguinous exudate leads to crusting of the swollen lips [1,2,13–18].

Mucosal erosions plus typical or raised atypical targets and epidermal detachment involving less than 10% of the body surface and usually located on the extremities and/or the face characterize herpes simplex-induced EM major.

Mucosal erosions plus widespread distribution of flat atypical targets or purpuric macules and epithelial detachment involving less than 10% of body surface on the trunk, face and extremities are characteristic of drug-induced Stevens–Johnson syndrome [19].

Diagnosis. A diagnosis of EM can be difficult to establish easily, and there may be a need to differentiate from viral stomatitides, pemphigus, toxic epidermal necrolysis and the subepithelial immune blistering disorders (pemphigoid and others). There are no specific diagnostic tests.

The diagnosis is mainly clinical; the Nikolsky sign is negative. It may be helpful to undertake serology for *Mycoplasma pneumoniae* or HSV, or other microorganisms. Biopsy of perilesional tissue with immunostaining and histological examination may help, although pathology can be variable and immunostaining is not specific.

Management. Spontaneous healing can be slow, up to 2–3 weeks in EM minor and up to 6 weeks in EM major. Treatment is thus indicated but controversial. No specific treatment is available but supportive care is important; a liquid diet and intravenous fluid therapy may be necessary. Electrolytes and nutritional support should be started as soon as possible. Oral hygiene should be improved with 0.2% aqueous chlorhexidine mouthbaths.

The use of corticosteroids is controversial [1,2,20–22].

- EM minor may respond to topical corticosteroids, although systemic corticosteroids may still be required.
- EM major should be treated with systemic corticosteroids (prednisolone 0.5–1 mg/kg/day tapered over 7–10 days) and/or azathioprine or other immunomodulatory drugs [1,2].

  Levamisole [22,23] and thalidomide have occasionally been used to some effect [24,25]. Plasmapheresis possibly has a place in the management of severe disease.

  Antimicrobials may be indicated [1,2,26,27].
- Aciclovir in EM related to HSV. Give a 5-day course at the first sign of lesions, or give 400 mg three times daily for 6 months for prophylaxis in EM related to HSV [10]. Continuous therapy with valaciclovir 500 mg twice a day has also been reported to be effective [1,2,10,27].
- Tetracycline is indicated in EM related to *Mycoplasma pneumoniae*.

Lichen planus (see Chapter 37)

Oral lichen planus may affect up to 1–2% of the population and is probably about eight times more common than cutaneous lichen planus. The oral mucosa may be involved alone or in association with lesions on skin or other mucosa, and oral lesions may precede, accompany or follow lesions elsewhere [1–7]. The association of oral lichen planus with gingival involvement, together with vulvovaginal lesions, has been termed the *vulvovaginal–gingival syndrome*.

Aetiology. Most oral lichen planus is idiopathic but significantly greater anxiety and depression are observed among patients with oral lichen planus compared with controls [8,9]. Lesions clinically and histologically similar, termed 'lichenoid lesions', are sometimes caused by dental restorative materials, chronic GVHD or hepatitis C virus (HCV).

Some lichenoid lesions may be related to dental materials: the prevalence of positive reactions to potential allergens in the North American Contact Dermatitis Group (NACDG) is higher in oral lichen planus for chromate, gold and thimerosal [10]. Other lichenoid reactions may be caused by GVHD, drug use (e.g. non-steroidal anti-inflammatory agents), diabetes [11] or liver

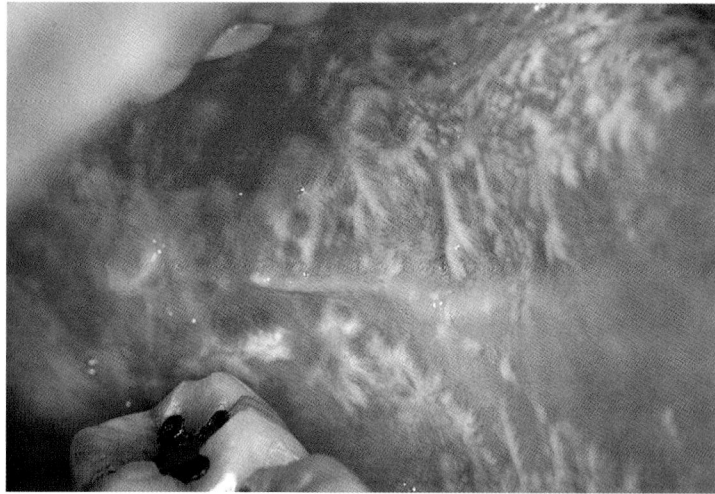

Figure 110.24 Lichen planus: reticulopapular lesions in the common oral site, the buccal mucosa.

disease. Chronic liver disease, especially chronic active hepatitis and HCV infection, may be associated with erosive lichen planus in persons of southern European, Japanese or some other extractions [12–14] and there may be anticardiolipin antibodies [15]. In persons of northern European extraction, oral lichen planus is only rarely associated with liver disease or with hepatitis C, hepatitis G or transfusion-transmitted virus [16–18]. Evidence from three meta-analyses indicates that HCV is associated with lichen planus and might be involved in its pathogenesis.

Pathology. The pathology is similar to that of cutaneous lichen planus, although sawtooth rete ridges are rarely seen in oral biopsies, and other epithelial changes may be less distinct.

Clinical features. The common oral lesions of lichen planus are bilateral white lesions in the buccal and/or lingual mucosa. They may be reticular, papular or plaque-like (Figures 110.24, 110.25, 110.26, 110.27 and 110.28). They are often symptomless but may cause soreness [1–6].

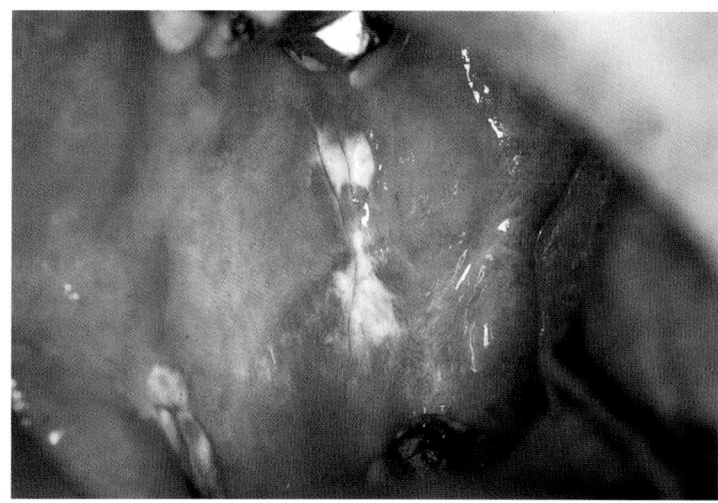

Figure 110.25 Lichen planus: plaque-like lesions resemble leukoplakia.

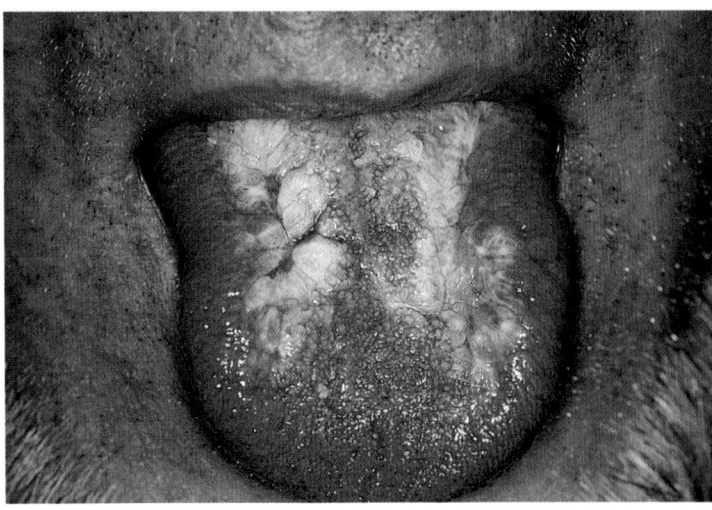

Figure 110.26 Lichen planus on the tongue.

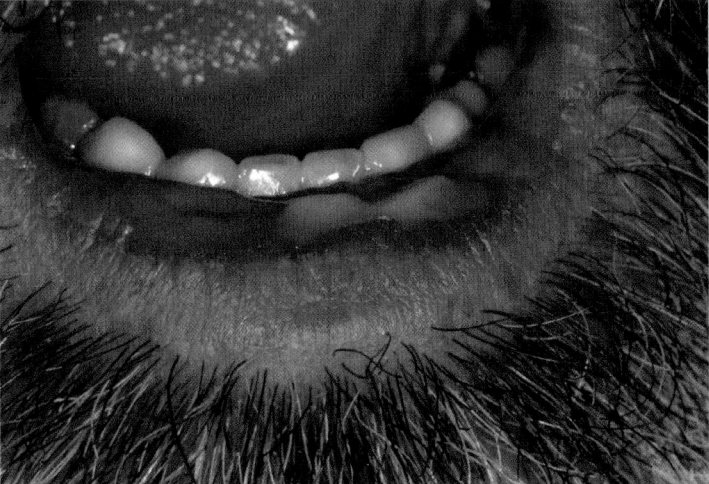

Figure 110.27 Erosive lichen planus.

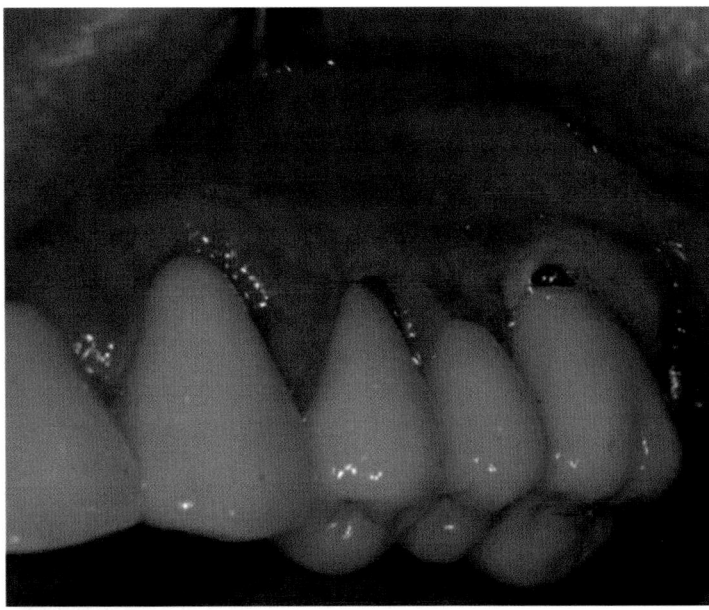

Figure 110.28 Lichen planus on the gingivae

Erosive lichen planus, which frequently affects the dorsum and lateral borders of the tongue or the buccal mucosae on both sides, is uncommon. The erosions are often large, slightly depressed or raised with a yellow slough, and have an irregular outline (Figure 110.27), but they are not always as painful as might be imagined. The surrounding mucosa is often erythematous and glazed in appearance, with loss of filiform papillae of the tongue, and there are often pathognomonic whitish striae. Lichen planus may also produce a desquamative gingivitis. Candidosis may complicate oral lichen planus.

Reticular lichen planus is the most frequent clinical presentation in both HCV-positive and HCV-negative patients. HCV-positive patients particularly have lip, tongue and gingival lesions [19].

Prognosis. There appears to be a predisposition for some oral lichen planus, particularly the non-reticular forms, to develop carcinoma – possibly a risk of up to 5% over 10 years [1–6,20].

Diagnosis. Biopsy with immunofluorescence is often indicated to exclude keratosis, chronic ulcerative stomatitis with stratified epithelium-specific antinuclear antibodies, lichen sclerosus, lupus erythematosus, malignancy and other disorders.

Management. Treatment is not always necessary, unless there are symptoms. Unfortunately, although the natural history of cutaneous lichen planus is one of remission in most cases, oral lichen planus rarely remits, and thus treatment is indicated for symptomatic oral lichen planus [1–6,21].
- Predisposing factors should be corrected. It may be wise to consider removal of dental amalgams if the lesions are closely related to these, or are unilateral [22], but there are no tests (e.g. patch tests) that will reliably indicate which patients will benefit from this. There is no evidence that either lichen planus or lichenoid lesions patients would routinely benefit from having all their amalgam restorations replaced. Weak evidence from potentially very biased, small non-randomized unblinded studies suggests that a small fraction of patients may benefit from targeted amalgam replacement.
- If drugs are implicated, the physician should be consulted as to possible changes in therapy.
- If there is diabetes or HCV infection, this should be treated by a physician.
- Improvement in oral hygiene may result in some subjective benefit. Thus good oral hygiene should be maintained. Chlorhexidine or triclosan mouthwashes may help.
- Antifungals may help, especially where there is candidal superinfection. Symptoms can often be controlled with topical medication: corticosteroids, such as betamethasone sodium phosphate mouthwash and fluticasone propionate spray, cream or mouthwash or pastes containing fluocinonide, fluocinolone, triamcinolone, betamethasone valerate or clobetasol [23–26]. Topical tacrolimus has been used [27,28] but does not have FDA approval. Topical aloe vera, topical pimecrolimus and oral curcuminoids are the most promising new treatment modalities. Other interesting topical modalities are topically applied thalidomide and amlexanox.

Mild lichen planus

Topical corticosteroids are the mainstay of therapy (e.g. triamcinolone acetate, betamethasone or fluocinolone). Erosive and gingival lesions are often recalcitrant. Next, high-potency corticosteroids such as clobetasol, fluocinonide or fluticasone may be employed initially and then changed to a lower potency drug.

Moderate lichen planus

If there is severe or extensive oral involvement, topical ciclosporin or tacrolimus may be of significant benefit, often being used with a high-potency or super-potent topical steroid such as clobetasol, fluticasone or mometasone. Topical creams or pastes can be applied in a suitable customized tray or veneer to be worn at night. This regimen is useful in the management of lichen planus-related desquamative gingivitis recalcitrant to other therapies.

Severe lichen planus

In severe lichen planus in multiple sites, patients may require systemic corticosteroids, azathioprine, cyclophosphamide, hydroxychloroquine, acitretin, thalidomide or ciclosporin. Dapsone is occasionally effective. Other therapies for lichen planus include retinoids, low-molecular-weight heparin [29,31–41] and many others including biologicals [42–47], but either their efficacy has not been well proven or they have unacceptable adverse effects.

Non-reticular lichen planus

Patients with non-reticular lichen planus should be monitored to exclude development of carcinoma; tobacco and alcohol use should be minimized.

Overlap syndromes

Lichen planus pemphigoides. Oral lesions in lichen planus pemphigoides may be similar to those of lichen planus or pemphigoid [1–5], clinically and histologically with direct immunofluorescence demonstrating linear deposits of immunoglobulin G and complement component C3 along the basement membrane [3].

Lichen planus/lichen sclerosus overlap syndrome. This may involve the oral and/or genital mucosa [6–8].

Lichen sclerosus (see Chapter 57). Oral lichen sclerosus et atrophicus is uncommon but since it presents with whitish plaques, papules or a reticular pattern, or erosions, all features of lichen planus [1–13], it may be underdiagnosed. Histologically, however, lichen sclerosus is characterized by epithelial atrophy with hyperkeratosis, oedema in the papillary corium but the lymphocytic infiltrate is not as closely associated to the epithelium as seen in lichen planus.

It has been suggested that mucosal lichen sclerosus is more common than formerly thought and may even cause dysplasia [5].

Lupus erythematosus (see Chapter 51). Almost 50% of patients with SLE suffer from oral lesions, which begin as red patches that break down to irregular slit-like ulcers which often heal with scarring [1–4]. Lesions particularly affect the palate. Sjögren syndrome may occur in SLE. Oral petechiae and herpetic infections are also common. Rarely, dental surgery has been followed by facial swelling [5].

Similar erosions, with a white border, occur in discoid lupus erythematosus (DLE) (Figure 110.29). DLE may predispose to oral carcinoma [6,7]. Oral ulceration has also been described in drug-induced lupus.

Systemic corticosteroids, often with an immunosuppressant, may be required in severe cases of SLE; topical steroids for DLE.

Pemphigoid (subepithelial immune bullous diseases). A spectrum of immune-mediated subepithelial bullous diseases can present with oral blisters and/or erosions and/or desquamative gingivitis, and with immune deposits at the epithelial basement membrane zone. Several distinct groups, and probably several overlap syndromes, are now recognized to exist.

Mucous membrane pemphigoid (see Chapter 50). Mucous membrane pemphigoid is a mucocutaneous, immune-mediated, subepithelial blistering disease characterized by autoantibodies to different molecules in the basement membrane zone [1,2,3,4–10]. The mouth may be involved as part of a wider disease, though in many patients only oral lesions are seen [9]. Sera of oral pemphigoid patients selectively and specifically bind to human α6 integrin, a 120 kDa protein BP180 ectodomain that appears to be a target antigen in this particular variant [3,8,11]. 75% of patients without the scarring phenotype possessed circulating autoantibodies against the BP180 molecule. The IL-4RA-1902 A/A genotype has been associated with a reduced response to IL-4 and has been found in 90% and can partially explain the low likelihood of scarring.

Mucous membrane pemphigoid involves the oral mucosa in more than one-third of cases, commonly causing gingival lesions [1,2,3,10]. The usual lesion, desquamative gingivitis, is characterized by erythematous glazed sore gingivae (Figure 110.30). Bullae are less common, and are seen particularly on the soft palate. They rupture to form erosions [1,2,3,7,11–13].

The bullae in mucous membrane pemphigoid are subepithelial and tend to persist for longer than those of pemphigus. Oral

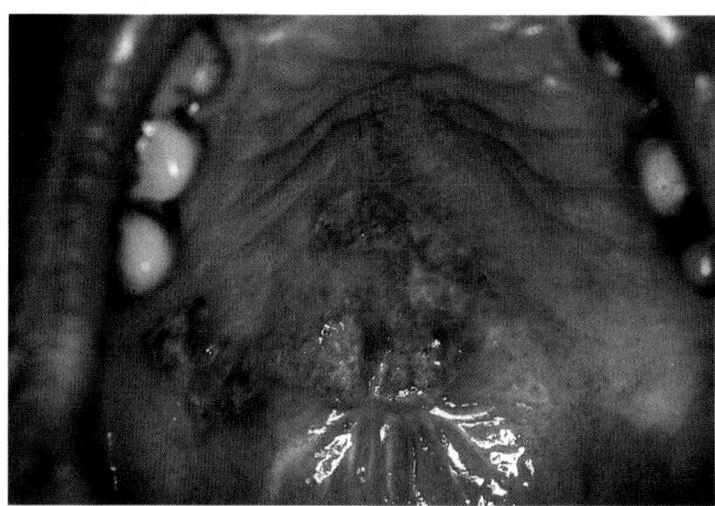

Figure 110.29 Chronic oral lesions in discoid lupus erythematosus.

PART 10: SITES, SEX, AGE

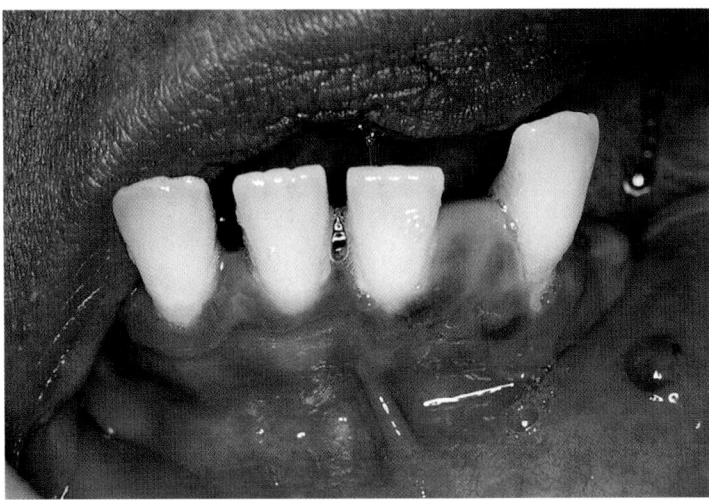

Figure 110.30 Pemphigoid: vesicles and desquamative gingivitis.

Table 110.10 Immunostaining in oral mucosal vesiculobullous disorders.

Disease	DIF	Oral mucosal deposits mainly:	Pattern of IF	IIF	Autoantibodies against:
Pemphigus	+	IgG	Epithelial intercellular	+	Epithelial intercellular cement
		C3			
Mucous membrane pemphigoid	+	C3	Linear epithelial basement membrane	±	Epithelial basement membrane
		IgG			
Bullous pemphigoid	+	IgG	Linear epithelial basement membrane	+	Epithelial basement membrane
		C3			
Dermatitis herpetiformis	+	IgA	Granular epithelial basement membrane	–	Reticulin
		C3			
Linear IgA disease	+	IgA	Linear epithelial basement membrane	–	–
		C3			
Erythema multiforme	±	C3	Vessel walls in lamina propria	–	–
		IgM			
Lichen planus*	±	Fibrin†	Globular epithelial or lamina propria and in Civatte bodies	–	–
		IgM, IgG, IgA, C3			
Discoid lupus erythematosus*	+	IgG, IgA	Granular epithelial basement membrane	±	None, or antinuclear
		IgM, C3			
Angina bullosa haemorrhagica	–	–	–	–	–
Superficial mucocoeles	–	–	–	–	–

DIF, direct immunofluorescence (biopsy); IF, immunofluorescence; IIF, indirect immunofluorescence (serology).

+, Present; –, absent; ±, sometimes.

*Rarely vesiculobullous; †non-specific deposits.

lesions may scar but this is uncommon. The bullae are typically filled with serous fluid and should be distinguished from superficial mucocoeles, epidermolysis bullosa acquisita, dermatitis herpetiformis and linear IgA disease. Occasionally, blisters are blood filled, and then must be differentiated from angina bullosa haemorrhagica.

A biopsy is required for diagnosis [3,7,13]. Serum autoantibodies to epithelial basement membrane may be detected in a few patients (Table 110.10) but many have immune deposits at the epithelial and mucous gland basement membrane zone.

Most patients respond to topical corticosteroids or tacrolimus. In 'high-risk' patients or if pemphigoid fails to respond to these measures, systemic immunomodulators may be required. Topical corticosteroids usually help if the lesions are restricted to the oral mucosa; azathioprine may be an alternative [1,14–17]. Systemic corticosteroids may occasionally be required but tetracyclines with or without nicotinamide may help [17–21]. Dapsone may be useful, especially in the treatment of desquamative gingivitis [2,3,21–23]. Recalcitrant mucous membrane pemphigoid may respond to tacrolimus, mycophenolate mofetil [7,24–26], intravenous immunoglobulins infliximab or other biologicals [27–30,31,32–38].

There may be associated autoimmune disorders, and associations with parkinsonism, cerebrovascular events and disseminated sclerosis. Internal malignancy such as lymphoma may be present in some patients with antiepiligrin (antilaminin 322) pemphigoid but patients with antibodies to α 6 integrin may have a possible reduced relative risk for developing cancer [8].

Vegetating cicatricial pemphigoid (synonym pemphigoid vegetans). A subset of bullous pemphigoid, although clinically indistinguishable from pemphigus vegetans and sometimes producing oral blisters and erosions, vegetating cicatricial pemphigoid shows linear deposits of IgG and C3 at the epithelial basement membrane zone on oral biopsy but no circulating basement membrane antibodies [1,2].

Palate and gingiva have been especially involved in the rare cases described [2–4].

Pemphigus (see Chapter 50)

Oral lesions are the rule in pemphigus vulgaris [1,2–9], but rare in the superficial forms of pemphigus [1].

Pemphigus vulgaris

Pemphigus vulgaris is caused by a variety of autoantibodies to keratinocyte self-antigens, which concur to cause blistering by acting synergistically. The concept of apoptolysis distinguishes the unique mechanism of autoantibody-induced keratinocyte damage in pemphigus vulgaris from other known forms of cell death. The main antigen in pemphigus vulgaris is desmoglein (Dsg) 3. However, 50% of patients with pemphigus vulgaris also have autoantibodies to Dsg1 (the main antigen in pemphigus foliaceus) and the proportion of Dsg1 and Dsg3 antibodies appears to be related to clinical severity. Those cases of pemphigus vulgaris which are predominantly oral have only Dsg3 antibodies. Dsg1 autoantibodies are found in over 50% of cases of pemphigus vulgaris, and the frequency may differ with race since they are found in a significantly greater proportion of patients of Indian origin than white northern Europeans [1,10–14]; such variations may be HLA related [5,15,16].

Typically, an individual patient develops a single variant of pemphigus, although cases have been described of transition to another variant, presumably through epitope spread, and the clinical manifestations of a single variant can change over time, possibly related to changes in the proportions of Dsg1 and Dsg3 autoantibodies.

The oral mucosa is almost invariably involved in pemphigus vulgaris and oral lesions are commonly the presenting feature (Figure 110.31). Bullae appear on any part of the oral mucosa including the palate, but break so rapidly that they are rarely seen [1,5,9,17–23]. Usually, the patient presents with large, painful, irregular and persistent red lesions which, by the time they become secondarily infected, can be difficult to differentiate clinically from those of other erosive conditions, such as pemphigoid and other immune blistering disorders, although intact bullae are more commonly seen in these, whereas the Nikolsky sign is more often positive in pemphigus. Oral lesions of pemphigus vulgaris are typically seen in adults, rarely in childhood.

The prevalence of oral involvement varies: one multicentre study involving patients from several countries showed that Bulgarian patients with pemphigus vulgaris had oral mucous membrane lesions less frequently (66%) than Italian (83%) or Israeli (92%) patients [9]. Rarely in pemphigus vulgaris there can be an acquired macroglossia [22] or desquamative gingivitis [23–25].

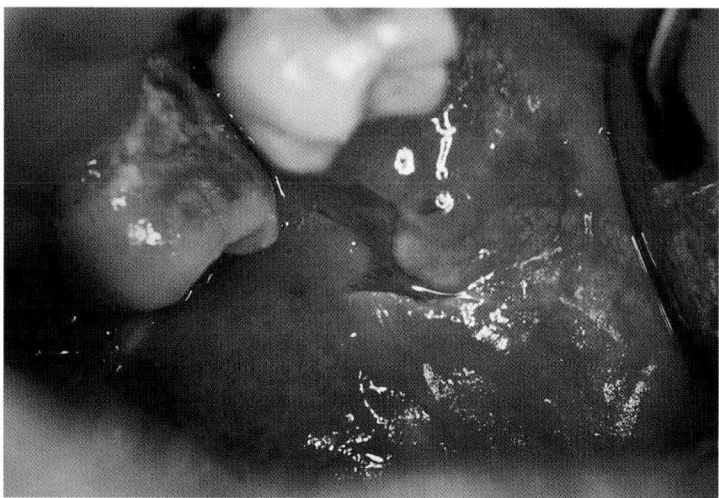

Figure 110.31 Pemphigus vulgaris: irregular persistent oral erosions.

Diagnosis should be confirmed by biopsy and immune studies. A biopsy of perilesional mucosa should be taken for haematoxylin and eosin stained sections and immunostaining (see Table 110.10) and serum collected for autoantibody titres, which can help diagnosis and monitoring of disease activity. Differential binding of anti-Dsg antibodies suggests that both human skin and monkey oesophagus should be used in the diagnosis of pemphigus vulgaris, since patients with predominantly oral disease may only have Dsg3 antibodies, which are not always detectable using human skin [5,26]. Enzyme-linked immunoadsorbent assay (ELISA) may help [27].

Oral cytology is of little practical diagnostic value. Treatment is largely based on systemic immunosuppression using corticosteroids, with azathioprine, dapsone, methotrexate, cyclophosphamide, gold or ciclosporin as adjuvants or alternatives; this has significantly reduced the mortality [1,8,23–30]. Adverse effects of these drugs are common, though deflazacort may have fewer adverse effects compared with prednisolone [31].

Mycophenolate mofetil offers safer immunosuppression with possibly less nephrotoxicity and hepatotoxicity [32–35].

Mucosal lesions are recalcitrant, often only healing after skin lesions have resolved when immunosuppressive therapy is given, and they may persist even though skin lesions are controlled. Topical corticosteroids may then help, or possibly prostaglandin E_2 [36,37]. Tacrolimus topically may well prove to have a place in the control of oral lesions [38–40].

Anti-CD20 monoclonal antibody, rituximab, may be an effective alternative therapy for the treatment of refractory pemphigus vulgaris [41–45,**46**,47–52].

Paraneoplastic pemphigus

Apart from pemphigus vulgaris, the other important pemphigus variant affecting the mouth is paraneoplastic pemphigus, usually associated with lymphoproliferative disease or thymoma [1–6], although one case associated with oral squamous cell carcinoma has been reported [7]. Oral lesions may be the sole manifestation [8] and have been seen in all reported cases of paraneoplastic pemphigus [4,9–13]. Oral lesions may be seen in isolation [1].

Painful extensive stomatitis, painful paronychia and lichenoid papules may be seen, and histology may show lichenoid changes, acantholytic blister formation and apoptotic keratinocytes. Direct immunofluorescence is positive for IgG both in the epidermal intercellular spaces and along the basement membrane zone. Indirect immunofluorescence is similarly positive in a pemphigus vulgaris pattern.

There is often only a partial response to intravenous corticosteroids. Recent therapeutic advances include the use of anti-CD20 monoclonal antibody (rituximab) [14–16] and mycophenolate [17–19].

Pemphigus vegetans

Oral lesions in pemphigus vegetans are hyperplastic masses which, on the tongue, can give a cerebriform appearance [1–3].

Other pemphigus variants

Oral lesions may be seen in less common pemphigus variants, especially in most cases with IgA pemphigus (intraepithelial IgA pustulosis or intraepidermal neutrophilic IgA dermatosis) [1–3], and in some cases of pemphigus associated with inflammatory bowel disease [4–10].

Stevens–Johnson syndrome/toxic epidermal necrolysis (see Chapter 119)

> **Synonyms and inclusions**
> • Lyell disease

Toxic epidermal necrolysis is a rare clinicopathological entity, with a high mortality, characterized by extensive detachment of full-thickness epithelium. Toxic epidermal necrolysis and Stevens–Johnson syndrome appear to be severity variants of the same disease, which differs from EM. The distinction from EM is unclear, however, but most cases of toxic epidermal necrolysis are drug induced and the lesions are extremely widespread [1–6].

Recently, an increased number of cases in patients with HIV/AIDS has been recorded [7–9].

Clinical features. Toxic epidermal necrolysis presents with cough, sore throat, burning eyes, malaise and low fever, followed after about 1–2 days by skin and mucous membrane lesions. Oral lesions can be seen in over 95% of patients with toxic epidermal necrolysis. The entire skin surface and oral mucosa may be involved, with up to 100% sloughing off. Gingival lesions are common and clinically are inflamed, with blister formation leading to painful widespread erosions. The blisters and erosions may precede the skin lesions by a day or so and may persist [3–7,10–12].

Diagnosis. Sheet-like loss of the epithelium and a positive Nikolsky sign are characteristic. Biopsy of perilesional tissue with immunostaining and histological examination are essential to the diagnosis. Histopathological examination is characteristic, showing necrosis of the whole epithelium detached from the lamina propria.

Management. Patients must be admitted to an intensive care unit as soon as possible for management [4,5,13–18]. There is no specific therapy for oral lesions but 2% lidocaine (lignocaine) and 0.2% aqueous chlorhexidine mouthbaths may provide symptomatic relief. Intravenous immunoglobulin (IVIG) has been proposed as a treatment for toxic epidermal necrolysis with varying effects reported [4,17].

Collagen–vascular diseases

Dermatomyositis and mixed connective tissue disease may be associated with non-specific mucosal erosions [1].

Oral involvement in reactive arthritis may include red patches or superficial painless mucosal erosions which may resemble erythema migrans (geographic tongue) both clinically and histologically.

Infective diseases

Oral ulceration is common worldwide in some viral infections, typically in the herpesvirus or enterovirus infections seen in childhood. It can also be seen in HIV/AIDS and several bacterial diseases, notably acute necrotizing gingivitis (but also in tuberculosis and syphilis), but is rare in fungal infections in the resource-rich countries, although the deep mycoses may be responsible for infection in resource-poor countries, in travellers or in the immunocompromised. Parasitic infections may occasionally cause ulceration.

Chikungunya

This togavirus (RNA), transmitted in areas around the Indian Ocean by the Asian tiger mosquito (*Aedes albopictus*) and now spread to Europe and the Americas, has an incubation period of 2–4 days. Similar to dengue and o'nyong'nyong, it features oral ulceration, central maculopapular rash, headache, malaise, arthraliga and fever up to 39 degrees [1,2]. No cures or drug treatments are available.

Dengue

Gingival bleeding and taste changes have been reported, but ulceration is not a prominent feature [1–4].

Enteroviruses

Herpangina

Aetiology. Herpangina is caused by Coxsackieviruses mainly. The incubation period is 3–7 days and young children are predominantly affected.

Clinical features. Many infections are subclinical but features of the clinical syndrome include malaise, anorexia, irritability, low fever, slightly enlarged and tender anterior cervical lymph nodes and mouth ulcers, predominantly on the soft palate [1,2].

Diagnosis. There may be a contact history. It is possible to culture Coxsackieviruses in suckling mice if absolutely necessary. The main differential diagnosis is primary herpetic stomatitis, but in herpangina there is less fever, no acute gingivitis and ulceration is mainly restricted to the soft palate.

Management. The condition is self-limiting and treatment is supportive only.

Hand, foot and mouth disease (see Chapter 117)

Aetiology. Hand, foot and mouth disease is caused particularly by Coxsackie A viruses but sometimes by Coxsackie B viruses or enteroviruses [1,2].

Clinical features. The incubation period is 3–10 days and, although young children are predominantly infected, there are occasional outbreaks in adults. Many infections are subclinical but features of the clinical syndrome include the following:
• General features: malaise, anorexia, irritability and fever may be present but usually only in severe cases.
• Anterior cervical lymph nodes may occasionally be slightly enlarged and tender.

- Mouth ulcers are round or ovoid, usually sparse and may affect any site [3–8].
- Rash: painful, sometimes deep-seated vesicles may appear, usually on the hands and/or feet, particularly on digits or at the base of the phalanges.

Hand, foot and mouth disease is self-limiting and only rarely complicated by systemic illness such as encephalitis [9,10]. The condition tends to be more severe when it occurs in adults.

Diagnosis and management. As for herpangina.

Herpesviruses
All herpesviruses can affect the oral cavity [1].

Herpes simplex stomatitis
Oral infection is common with the herpesviruses, which thereafter remain latent, are often excreted in saliva (especially in immuno-compromised persons), and are sometimes implicated in clinical recurrences and malignant complications [1].

Incidence and prevalence. HSV infection is a very common oral infection.

Age. Predominantly children and adolescents. With improving soci-oeconomic circumstances and standards of hygiene, a larger number of children are not exposed to HSV and enter adult life without immunity. Cases of primary herpetic stomatitis are therefore now seen occasionally in adults, and the manifestations can be severe. HSV is usually transmitted in saliva and can be shed in asympto-matic individuals [2–4,5]. Oral sex is more of an issue for HSV-1 transmission: HSV-1 is a fast-growing cause of genital herpes.

HSV-1 infection possibly lowers the risk of acquiring HSV-2 sexually.

Pathology. Cellular protein Med23 binds to HSV transcription factor IRF7, inducing type III interferons (IFN lambda) as part of innate immune response.

Causative organisms. Herpes simplex viruses. In general, HSV-1 causes primary herpetic stomatitis (and the secondary infection of recurrent herpes labialis). There are no precise distinctions now in the type of HSV causing oral herpes. With more frequent orogeni-tal and oroanal sexual practices, oral infection with HSV-2 is more frequently seen [6–11].
- 80% of adults are infected with HSV-1.
- 20% of adults are infected with HSV-2.
- 50% of adults have HSV-1 or HSV-2.
- 10% of adults have both HSV-1 and HSV-2.

It is possible to have genital outbreaks of HSV-1 and HSV-2 at different times.

Infection with one strain is *not* protective against infection with the other HSV.

Clinical features. The incubation period is 3–7 days. Many infec-tions with HSV occur in childhood and are subclinical and, where there is disease, it varies greatly in severity. In many, it is trivial and misdiagnosed or passed off as 'teething' [8,11–14].

Primary herpetic stomatitis typically presents with malaise, anorexia, irritability, fever, enlarged and tender anterior cervical lymph nodes, and a diffuse, purple, boggy gingivitis (hence the alternative term *herpetic gingivostomatitis*), especially anteriorly, with multiple vesicles followed by round or ovoid ulcers 1–3 mm in diameter scattered across the oral mucosa and gingiva (Figure 110.32) in an acute illness lasting only up to about 14 days [6,7,11,14]. In immunocompromised persons, diagnosis can be dif-ficult since herpes may manifest with chronic ulcers [14–18].

Differential diagnosis. The main differential diagnoses of herpetic stomatitis in otherwise healthy persons are chickenpox and other viral causes of mouth ulcers, and acute leukaemia. In immuno-compromised persons, the differential is wider.

Disease course and prognosis. Spontaneous resolution in other-wise healthy people; protracted course in immunocompromised patients. Herpetic stomatitis resolves spontaneously in 7–14 days but HSV remains latent in the trigeminal ganglion. The most obvi-ous sequel is that about one-third of patients are thereafter pre-disposed to recurrences [19]. HSV is shed intermittently into the saliva [2–4,5]. HSV is implicated in many instances of EM and may cause chronic ulcers in the immunocompromised (see below) or occasionally ulcers following trauma to the mouth. HSV can be dangerous in neonates and the immunocompromised, when it can spread to the skin, eyes and brain (encephalitis).

Investigations. Usually a clinical diagnosis. A full blood picture, white cell count and differential, and viral studies may be prudent [6,7,11,14,20,21]. The latter include the following:
- Nucleic acid studies. Polymerase chain reaction detection of HSV DNA: this is sensitive but expensive.
- Immunodetection: detection of HSV antigens is of some value. Direct fluorescent antigen (DFA). Conventional ELISA for serum antibodies have poor sensitivity and specificity; newer assays based on HSV glycoproteins are comparable with Western blot assays. A rising titre of serum antibodies is confirmatory but only gives the diagnosis retrospectively.
- Rising antibody titre is confirmatory.

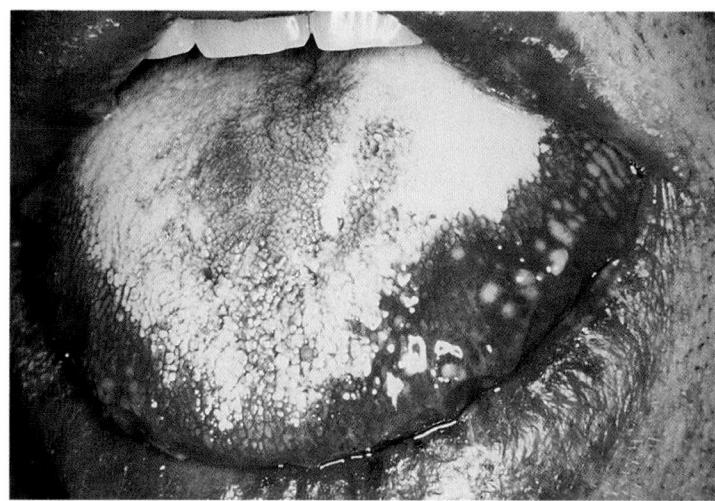

Figure 110.32 Scattered ulcers and a furred tongue in primary herpetic stomatitis.

Management

- Encourage patient not to touch lesions.
- Encourage patient not to transmit.
- Avoid sharing eating utensils, or toys.
- Wash utensils by dishwasher, or by hand.
- Wash hands frequently.
- Blisters and sores should be kept dry.
- Antiviral medications can shorten outbreaks.
- Aciclovir, famciclovir or other antivirals used systemically are essential to control infection in immunocompromised patients.

For most, management is supportive with antipyretic analgesics (e.g. acetaminophen/paracetamol), sponging with tepid water and a high fluid intake. Analgesics (as elixirs or syrups for children) and, in adults, lidocaine mouthbaths help ease discomfort and 0.2% aqueous chlorhexidine mouthbaths aid resolution. An antihistamine such as promethazine may help sedate an irritable child.

Specific antiviral agents are most useful in the very early stages of disease (though most patients present later) and for immunocompromised patients who may otherwise suffer severe infection [22–28].

Recurrent labial HSV infection (RHL). Primary oral infection by HSV may produce perioral lesions (Figure 110.33). However, recurrent herpes labialis involving the lip is the more common cause of blisters at the mucocutaneous junction (Figure 110.34) [6–9,11,19]. Part of the innate antiviral immune response is deficient due to single nucleotide polymorphism (SNP) – the most common type of genetic variation – in IFN-lambda 3 promoter. The lesions arise at the mucocutaneous junction as itching papules which progress to vesicles, pustules and then scab. They are unsightly and occasionally become infected with *Staphylococcus* or *Streptococcus*, resulting in impetigo (Figure 110.35). In immunocompromised persons, extensive and persistent lesions may result. In atopic persons, the lesions may spread to produce eczema herpeticum (Figure 110.36). Aciclovir has been the standard treatment used as a 5% cream, although penciclovir 1% is reportedly more effective [29,30]. Hydrocolloid patches may be beneficial.

Prevention may be achieved with prophylactic antivirals; a meta-analysis reviewed 2683 papers, 10 met inclusion criteria and of these, only one had a low bias risk; oral aciclovir (800–1600 mg daily) and valaciclovir (500 mg daily for 4 months) were effective prevention of RHL when taken prior to symptoms or exposure to triggers [31]. The efficacy of the helicase–primase inhibitor pritelivir on RHL has yet to be reported.

Recurrent intraoral HSV infection. Chronic oral herpetic ulcers, often with a raised white border and sometimes with a dendritic appearance, may occasionally affect apparently healthy individuals, especially at sites of trauma, for example following palatal infiltration of a local anaesthetic. Chronic indolent lesions, usually ulcerative or nodular, may be seen in patients with neutropenia or chronic leukaemia; in patients with more severe immunosuppression, such as acute leukaemia or HIV infection, more aggressive chronic ulcers may be seen [14–18,32,33]. Aciclovir or other antivirals may be indicated systemically [15,34,35].

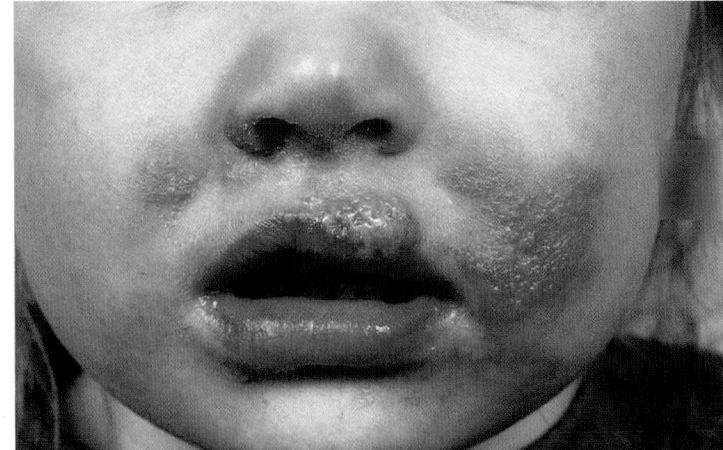

Figure 110.33 Primary herpetic stomatitis with extraoral lesions.

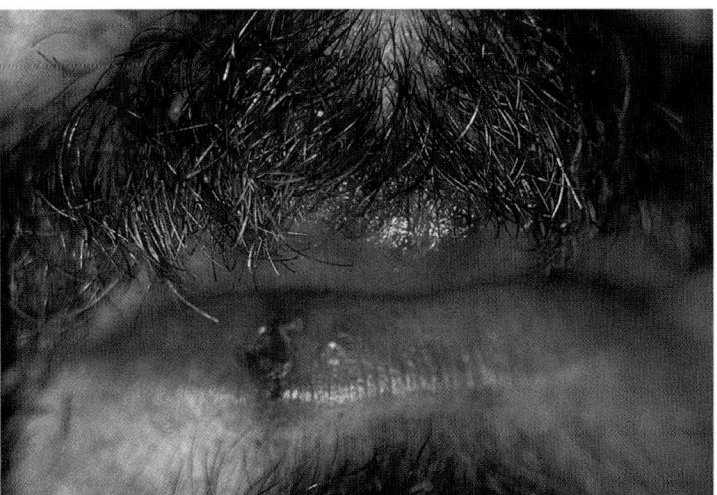

Figure 110.34 Herpes labialis.

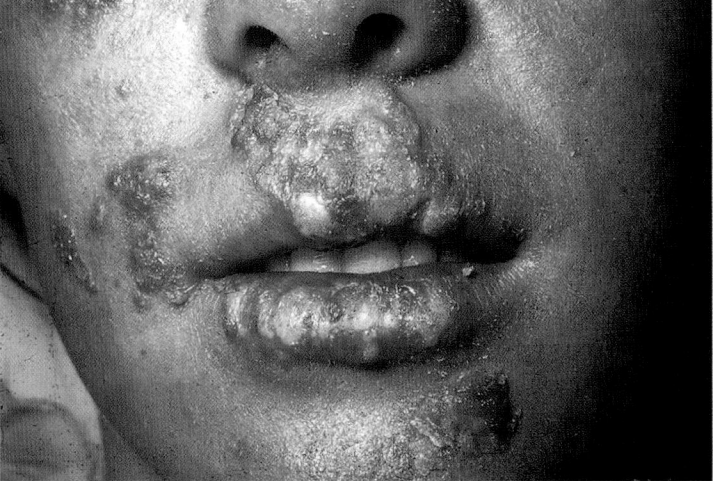

Figure 110.35 Impetigo.

mandibular division of the trigeminal nerve is involved. One side of the palate, the upper gingiva and buccal sulcus are involved in maxillary zoster. Rarely, mandibular or maxillary zoster may disturb the formation of developing teeth [5–7] or cause jaw necrosis [6,7].

If the geniculate ganglion of the facial nerve is affected, there may be unilateral facial palsy, with vesicles in the ipsilateral ear and ulcers in the soft palate ipsilaterally (Ramsay–Hunt syndrome) [8–14].

Occasionally, there is misdiagnosis of toothache, leading to extraction, the true diagnosis becoming apparent only when the rash appears. Zoster resolves spontaneously but postherpetic neuralgia can be distressing.

Management. An underlying immune defect, such as AIDS or malignancy, should be excluded in patients with zoster, although most zoster is related simply to lesser problems in advanced age.

Treatment is mainly supportive but antivirals such as aciclovir can be useful. Analgesics are indicated in zoster, although the pain may prove refractory to even potent analgesics [15,16], when antidepressants such as amitriptyline and fluphenazine may have a place [17,18]. Treatment advances include lidocaine patches, opioid analgesics and gabapentin. Early recognition and treatment of high-risk herpes zoster patients with antiviral and analgesic therapies is mandatory [18].

Epstein–Barr virus infections (see Chapter 25)

Epstein–Barr virus is responsible for infectious mononucleosis and is found in pharyngeal epithelium and appears in the saliva of patients and for several months after clinical recovery. Infection appears to be spread by close oral contact, especially kissing. It is typically a disease of the student population.

Infection is often subclinical. Infectious mononucleosis is also protean in its clinical manifestations, which include particularly lymphadenopathy, sore throat, fever, malaise and rashes. In the anginose type (sore-throat type), the throat is sore with soft-palate petechiae and a whitish exudate on oedematous tonsils [1–3]. There may be non-specific oral ulceration or pericoronitis [1]. The glandular type of infectious mononucleosis is characterized by generalized lymph node enlargement and splenomegaly; the febrile type is characterized by fever.

Similar syndromes may be caused by cytomegalovirus, human herpesvirus (HHV)-6, toxoplasmosis and HIV. Characteristic of infectious mononucleosis are large numbers of atypical mononuclear cells in the blood and a wide variety of serological changes, particularly heterophil antibodies, which are detectable by the Paul–Bunnell or Monospot tests, usually during the first or second week of illness [4]. Several other antibodies against EBV appear during the course of infectious mononucleosis, but the most frequent is the antibody to viral capsid antigen, the titre of which reaches a peak at about 4 weeks.

No specific treatment is available for infectious mononucleosis, but supportive care is important, not only because of the potential for airways obstruction but also because of the associated lassitude. Systemic corticosteroids are required if there is pharyngeal oedema severe enough to hazard the airway.

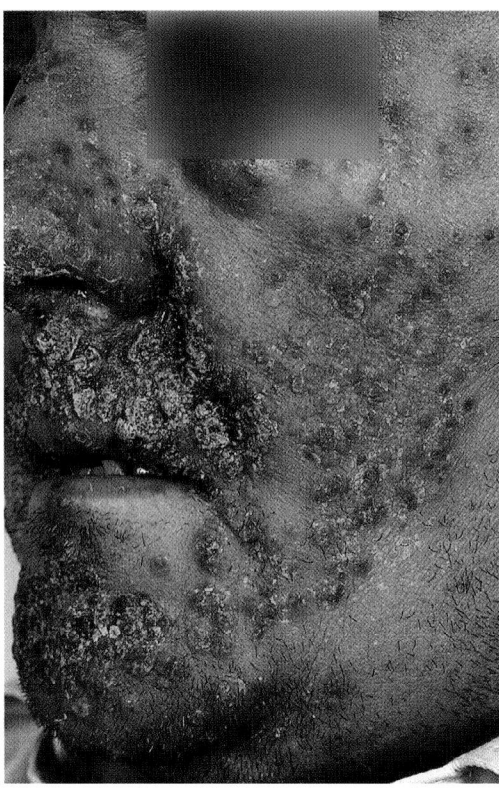

Figure 110.36 Eczema herpeticum.

Chickenpox (see Chapter 25)

Synonyms and inclusions
- Varicella

Chickenpox affects children predominantly and may present with mouth ulcers that resemble those of herpetic stomatitis, but there is no gingivitis [1]. There may be a contact history. Many primary infections with varicella-zoster virus are subclinical or produce so few lesions as to pass almost unnoticed. Varicella-zoster virus remains latent in sensory ganglia and may be reactivated to produce shingles.

Herpes zoster (see Chapter 25)

Synonyms and inclusions
- Shingles

If shingles affects the maxillary or mandibular divisions of the trigeminal nerve, mouth ulcers are usually seen [2–4].

Clinical features. The pain of trigeminal zoster may simulate toothache. Severe pain often precedes, accompanies and follows the rash, and postherpetic neuralgia may persist for months or years.

The rash is restricted to a dermatome and is unilateral, but sometimes a few chickenpox-type lesions can be found elsewhere. Oral ulcers appear in the distribution of the involved nerve division [3]. There is ulceration of one side of the tongue, floor of the mouth and lower labial and buccal mucosa if the

EBV is also commonly found in the mouths of immunocompromised patients [5–12] and is implicated in oral hairy leukoplakia, oral ulceration, advanced periodontal disease [13,14] and some oral lymphomas [15–18] although any relationship with other malignancies such as oral squamous cell carcinoma is controversial [19,20].

Cytomegalovirus infection

Cytomegalovirus may cause a glandular fever type of syndrome, and rarely causes oral ulceration. Indolent cytomegalovirus-induced oral ulcers may be seen in immunosuppressed patients and in AIDS [1–7]. Cytomegalovirus has been implicated in the pathogenesis of periodontal disease [8].

Herpesviruses 6, 7 and 8

Oral lesions have yet to be demonstrated in infections with HHV-6 or HHV-7. However, HHV-8 is implicated in oral Kaposi sarcoma [1–8]. Treatment with highly active antiretroviral therapy (HAART) may reduce HHV-8 infection [8,9], however, Kaposi sarcoma-associated immune reconstitution following commencement of HAART has been reported [10–12].

Bacterial infections

Acute necrotizing (ulcerative) gingivitis and noma

Synonyms and inclusions
- ANUG: trench mouth
- Noma: cancrum oris or gangrenous stomatitis

Acute necrotizing (ulcerative) gingivitis (ANUG) is typically an acute gingival ulceration, rarely complicated by gangrenous stomatitis (when it is called noma), although this is increasingly reported in HIV disease.

Incidence and prevalence. ANUG is uncommon, typically seen in students, malnutrition or in conflict situations. Noma is a serious destructive necrosis affecting the soft tissues and bones of the mouth and adjoining orofacial areas. Noma is seen predominantly in sub-Saharan Africa, where the estimated frequency in some communities varies from 1 to 7 cases per 1000 population.

Age. ANUG is typically seen in children or adolescents, but may occur in young adults [1,2].

Associated diseases. ANUG and noma are increased in HIV/AIDS or other immune defects

Predisposing factors. Viral respiratory infections, overwork and fatigue, smoking or immune defects may precede the onset of disease, suggesting depression of immunity as a predisposing cause. A similar lesion may be a feature of HIV infection and related diseases [3,4–7].

Pathology. There is no firm evidence of communicability of ANUG, although it may occur in epidemic form, especially in institutions or in the military (trench mouth).

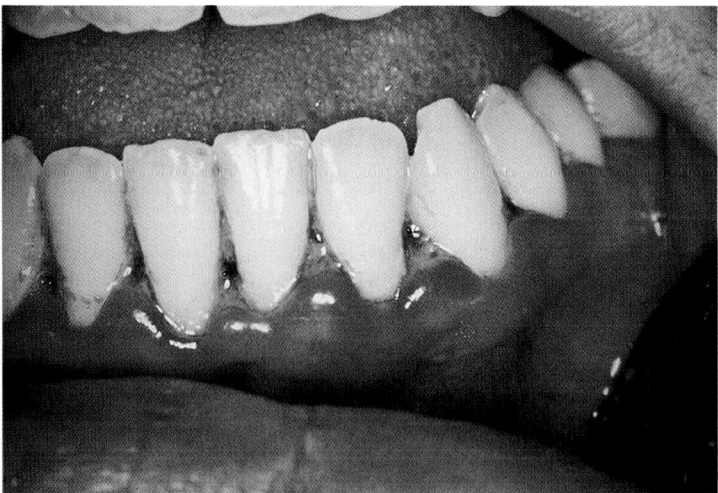

Figure 110.37 Acute necrotizing gingivitis showing typical ulceration of interdental gingival papillae. This was in HIV infection.

Causative organisms. A mixed, mostly anaerobic, flora (the fusospirochaetal complex), consisting mainly of *Fusobacterium nucleatum* (*F. fusiformis* or *Bacillus fusiformis*) and *Borrelia vincentii*, is associated with this infection [8–10].

Presentation. The mouth ulceration is usually initially restricted to the gingiva, specifically the interdental papillae, which appear blunted (Figures 110.37 and 110.38). The history is characteristic, with an acute onset of gingival soreness, bleeding and halitosis. Acute necrotizing gingivitis occurs especially in the anterior part of the mouth where the affected gingiva are extremely tender to touch and readily bleed on minimal pressure. Occasionally, the ulceration extends elsewhere on the gingiva, or onto the adjacent mucosa. There is often enlargement of the cervical lymph nodes and there may be pyrexia and malaise.

Differential diagnosis. Diagnosis is mainly from gingival lesions in primary herpetic stomatitis, leukaemias and HIV disease.

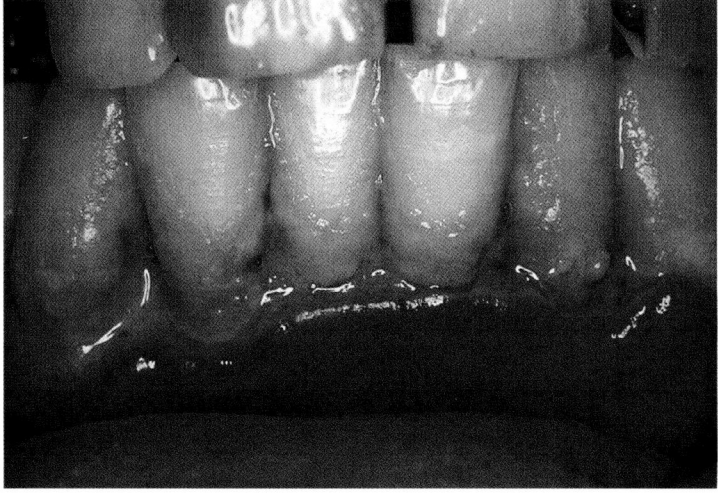

Figure 110.38 Untreated acute necrotizing gingivitis can lead to extensive gingival ulceration and irreparable damage.

Failure to adequately treat acute necrotizing gingivitis may predispose to recurrence and, in malnourished or immunocompromised individuals, may lead to noma (cancrum oris, orofacial gangrene) [5–15].

Investigations. A full immunological/haematological work-up is needed in noma; bacteriological smear may be helpful.

Management. Gentle cleansing with a hydrogen peroxide mouthwash and a soft toothbrush is remarkably effective. Oral metronidazole 200 mg should be given three times daily for 3–7 days to limit the tissue destruction in ANUG. Penicillin is equally effective. The patient should also be referred for dental advice [3]. Noma requires attention also to nutrition, and antimicrobials and sometimes reconstructive surgery.

Resources

Further information
http://www.nlm.nih.gov/medlineplus/ency/article/001342.htm
http://emedicine.medscape.com/article/763801-overview
(All last accessed December 2014.)

Epithelioid (bacillary) angiomatosis (see Chapter 26)
Oral lesions clinically and, to some extent, histologically reminiscent of Kaposi sarcoma have been seen in HIV disease [1–4], sometimes as the first manifestation of HIV infection [3].

Gonorrhoea
Oral mucosal erythema, sometimes with oedema and ulceration, is occasionally seen in oropharyngeal gonorrhoea. Oropharyngeal asymptomatic carriage of gonococci is more common, found in around 4% of those attending clinics for sexually transmitted diseases [1–5].

Leprosy
Leprosy can manifest orofacially with swellings, hyperpigmented skin macules and neurological sequelae such as a palpable supraorbital branch of the trigeminal nerve and greater auricular nerve and facial palsy [1,2].

Syphilis
Oral ulcers may be seen at any stage but particularly in secondary syphilis [1–9]. In primary syphilis, a primary chancre (hard or Hunterian chancre) may involve the lips, tongue or palate. A small firm pink macule changes to a papule which ulcerates to form a painless round ulcer with a raised margin and indurated base [4,10]. Chancres heal spontaneously in 3–8 weeks but are highly infectious and are associated with enlarged painless regional lymph nodes.

Secondary syphilis follows after 6–8 weeks, with oral lesions in about one-third of patients [1,3,7]. These are highly infectious and are usually fairly painless ulcers (mucous patches and snail-track ulcers).

The most characteristic oral lesion of tertiary syphilis is a localized granuloma (gumma) that varies in size from a pinhead to several centimetres, affecting particularly the palate, or the tongue.

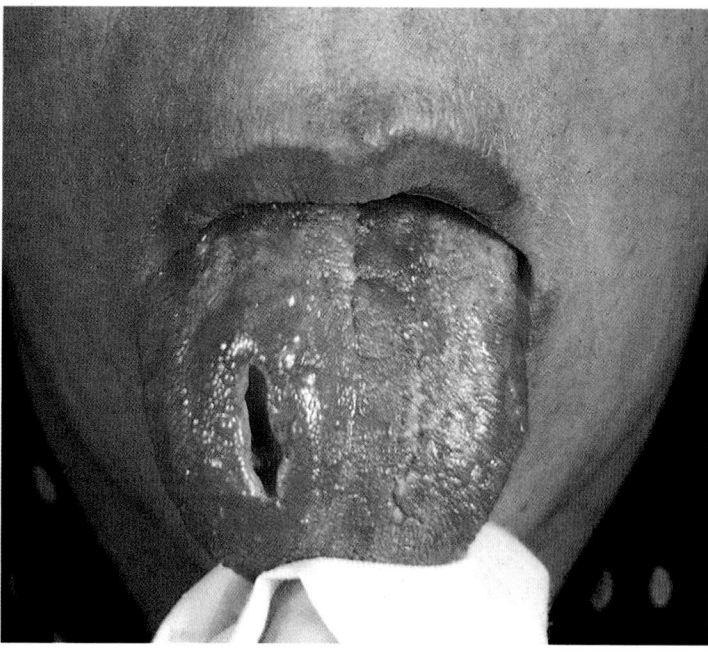

Figure 110.39 Gumma.

Gummas break down to form deep chronic punched-out ulcers that are not infectious (Figure 110.39). However, the most common oral manifestation of tertiary syphilis is leukoplakia, which particularly affects the dorsum of the tongue and has a high potential for malignant change [9].

Exudate from a suspected oral lesion of syphilis should be examined for treponemes by dark-ground microscopy; however, since the diagnosis can be confused by oral commensal treponemes, lesions should first be thoroughly swabbed with a sterile gauze or cotton wool and then gently scraped with a sterile spatula, the scraping being examined immediately by dark-ground microscopy. Serology is indicated. Biopsy is not usually indicated, but lesions are characterized by a dense plasma cell infiltrate [7].

Tuberculosis
Oral lesions can develop in pulmonary tuberculosis but are not common. A chronic ulcer, usually of the dorsum of the tongue, is the most common oral presentation but jaw lesions or cervical lymph node involvement may be seen [1–12]. Atypical mycobacteria are not uncommonly involved.

Mycobacterial oral ulcers, particularly caused by *Mycobacterium avium–intracellulare*, have been reported as a complication of AIDS and occasionally in apparently healthy individuals [13–17]. Cervicofacial infection is occasionally caused by *M. chelonei*, usually in the form of lymph node abscesses, or occasionally as intraoral swellings [18–21].

Fungal infections

Oral fungal infections, apart from candidosis, rarely causes mouth ulcers in resource-rich countries, where they are usually seen only in immunocompromised or debilitated patients, including those with AIDS. However, they may be seen occasionally in otherwise healthy persons from the tropics (Table 110.11).

Table 110.11 Rare orofacial fungal infections.

Infection	Oral manifestations
Aspergillosis	Aspergilloma
	Rhinocerebral type causes palatal necrosis
	Disseminated in immunocompromised patients
Blastomycosis	
North American	Oral ulcers or suppurating granulomas
South American (paracoccidioidomycosis)	Oral ulcers and lymphadenopathy
Coccidioidomycosis	Rarely oral ulcers
Cryptococcosis	Oral ulcers
Histoplasmosis	Lumps or ulcers in mouth
Phycomycosis (mucormycosis, zygomycosis)	Antral involvement with palatal ulceration in immunocompromised patients, especially diabetics
Sporotrichosis	Oral lesions rare

Aspergillosis

Rhinocerebral aspergillosis may ulcerate through to the mouth. This is a rare event, except in the severely immunocompromised [1–3]. Mandibular aspergillosis has also been reported [4].

Occasionally, solitary aspergillosis arises as a consequence of endodontic treatment where root canal filling material enters the antrum [5–7] but this does not cause oral ulceration. Surgical debridement is usually indicated.

Blastomycoses

Blastomycoses may produce oral lesions which are typically mulberry-like ulcerated swellings especially seen on the gingiva and alveolus [1–3].

Candidosis

See p. 110.68.

Cryptococcosis

Cryptococcus neoformans may occasionally produce indolent oral ulcers in immunocompromised patients [1–4].

Geotrichosis

Geotrichosis is a rare livid sharply defined enanthema of the oral mucosa with ulcerations seen in immunocompromised persons, such as those with leukaemia or HIV infection. *Geotrichum capitatum* is responsible and there may also be pneumonic lung infiltrates [1]. Treatment includes amphotericin, 5-fluorocytosine and itraconazole.

Histoplasmosis

Oral lesions of histoplasmosis are uncommon. They are typically seen in chronic disseminated histoplasmosis, usually as a non-specific lump or ulcer on the tongue, palate, buccal mucosa or gingiva [1–8], sometimes in AIDS [9–15].

Mucormycosis

Rhinocerebral mucormycosis typically commences in the nasal cavity or paranasal sinuses and invades the palate to produce a black necrotic ulcer, although it might occasionally commence in the palate [1–4]. Most cases are seen in diabetics or in immunocompromised patients such as those with AIDS [4,5]. Biopsy and radiography are required for diagnosis. Treatment is surgical debridement together with amphotericin intravenously and/or azoles.

Protozoal infestations

Leishmaniasis

Leishmaniasis is rare in northern Europe and the USA; it is not uncommon, however, in hotter climes and may cause ulcers in the mouth or more commonly on the lips [1–5], and is seen increasingly in HIV disease [6–10] or in other immunocompromised persons.

Immune defects

HIV infection (see Chapter 31)

HIV/AIDS has become predominantly a chronic condition with those infected experiencing a fairly normal life expectancy, albeit with increased tendencies to long-term complications. Oral lesions include three types of oral and pharyngeal candidiasis (pseudomembranous, erythematous and angular cheilitis), hairy leukoplakia due to EBV infection, other herpes-group virus infections including herpes simplex and herpes zoster, papillomavirus warts, severe periodontal disease, Kaposi sarcoma and AIDS lymphoma [1–7]. Oral lesions are seen less often in those undergoing antiretroviral treatment, the exception being oral warts which seem to be more common in those patients. Oral lesions of HIV infection can serve as early markers of the disease and indicators of disease progression in the untreated, and their presence correlates with HIV load and CD4 cell depletion.

Oral ulceration in patients infected with HIV may be due to any of the causes of mouth ulceration, and aphthous-like ulcers are also seen. However, it is important to exclude infections, mainly herpesviruses. There are also occasional examples of mouth ulcers due to mycobacteria, *Rochalimaea*, syphilis, *Histoplasma*, *Cryptococcus*, leishmaniasis and others. Malignant disease (mainly Kaposi sarcoma or non-Hodgkin lymphoma) may result in lumps that can ulcerate.

Aphthous-like ulcers in HIV may respond to local treatment or, failing that, thalidomide at a dose of 200 mg/day has been shown in randomized double-blind placebo-controlled trials to be effective in the treatment of HIV-related recurrent aphthous ulceration [8].

Other mouth ulcers should be treated as appropriate.

Resources

Further information

http://emedicine.medscape.com/article/211316-overview (last accessed December 2014).

Vasculitides

Giant cell arteritis

Synonyms and inclusions
- Horton disease

PART 10: SITES, SEX, AGE

Patients may suffer ischaemic pain during mastication, intermittent claudication of the tongue [1,2] or, rarely, facial palsy [3] or lumps [2,4,5]. Ulceration and necrosis of the tongue [6–18] or occasionally the lip [19] have also been observed [2,3].

Periarteritis (polyarteritis) nodosa

Transient submucosal oral nodules may occur singly or in crops along the path of vessels and especially in the tongue. Other mucosal lesions include erythema, papules, haemorrhages, ulceration or necrosis [1–4].

Iatrogenic conditions

Mucositis

Aetiology. Mucositis, sometimes called *mucosal barrier injury*, is the term given to the widespread oral erythema, ulceration and soreness that is a common complication of a number of therapeutic procedures involving chemotherapy, radiotherapy or chemoradiotherapy, used largely in the treatment of cancer but also in the conditioning prior to bone marrow transplantation (i.e. haematopoietic stem cell transplantation) [1–3,4]. Mucositis appears 3–15 days after cancer treatment, earlier after chemotherapy than after radiotherapy.

Mucositis invariably follows external beam radiotherapy involving the orofacial tissues, and is also common in upper mantle head and neck radiation, and particularly in total body irradiation.

Some 40–90% of patients on chemotherapy develop mucositis. Patients on fluorouracil and cisplatin in particular develop mucositis, while etoposide and melphalan cause particularly severe mucositis. Oral mucositis is particularly severe after haemopoietic stem cell transplantation, because of radiation damage and myeloablation, and the course follows the polymorphonuclear leukocyte count.

The impaired mucosal barrier in mucositis predisposes to life-threatening septic complications; the prevalence of an oral focus in febrile neutropenia has been reported in up to 30% of cases [1–3,5,6].

Clinical features. Mucositis typically presents with pain (which can be so intense as to interfere with eating and significantly affect the quality of life), erythema, ulceration and sometimes bleeding.

Diagnosis. This is clinical and it is helpful to score the degree of mucositis in order to monitor progression and therapy.

Management. The basic strategies in the management of mucositis aim at pain relief, efforts to hasten healing and prevention of infectious complications. However, prophylaxis is the goal.

Pain relief is usually achieved with opioids given by patient-controlled analgesia and benzydamine can aid relief. Oral cooling with ice chips ameliorates chemotherapy-induced mucositis [7–12].

Other treatments currently used but for which hard data for reliable efficacy are unavailable include the following:

- Medications to reduce salivation and thus exposure of the mucosa to chemotherapeutic drugs that are secreted in saliva.
- Anti-inflammatory medications.

- Cytokines such as IL-1, IL-11, TGF-β-3 and keratinocyte growth factor.
- Granulocyte–macrophage colony-stimulating factor (GM-CSF) and granulocyte colony-stimulating factor (G-CSF) [13].
- Thalidomide: an angiogenesis-inhibiting drug.
- Amifostine: a cytoprotector.
- Melatonin: the pineal hormone.
- Protegrin antimicrobial peptides, which possess activity against Gram-positive and Gram-negative bacteria and yeasts.
- Low-energy lasers.
- Other agents such as sucralfate, tretinoin, glutamine, vitamin E and misoprostol [1–3,5,10–12,13].

Monitoring microbial colonization and the institution of antiviral prophylaxis and antifungal prophylaxis, to avoid colonization and superinfection, is particularly important in patients with low neutrophil counts.

Invasive fungal infections of the oral cavity can be associated with systemic fungal infection and are indications for the use of liposomal amphotericin.

Bone marrow transplantation (haematopoietic stem cell transplantation)

Oral complications are common and can be a major cause of morbidity following bone marrow transplantation. Mucositis, infections, bleeding, xerostomia and loss of taste result from the effects of the underlying disease, chemotherapy or radiotherapy, and GVHD. The ventrum of the tongue, buccal and labial mucosa and gingiva may be affected by ulceration or mucositis [1–8].

Graft-versus-host disease

The oral manifestations of acute GVHD consist of painful mucosal desquamation and ulceration, and/or cheilitis, and the presence of lichenoid plaques or striae. Small white lesions affect the buccal and lingual mucosa early on, but clear by day 14 [1,2]. Erythema and ulceration are most pronounced at 7–11 days, and may be associated with obvious infection. Candidosis is common, as is herpes simplex stomatitis (occasionally zoster) and oral purpura may occur, especially in adults [1,3–7]. *Bartonella*-related pseudomembranous angiomatous papillomatosis of the oral cavity has been reported secondary to bone marrow transplantation and oral chronic GVHD [8].

The oral lesions in chronic GVHD are coincident with skin lesions, and include generalized mucosal erythema, lichenoid lesions, mainly in the buccal mucosa, and xerostomia. There may be depressed salivary IgA levels in minor gland saliva [9]. Xerostomia is most significant in the first 14 days after transplant and is a consequence of drug treatment, irradiation and/or GVHD. There may be an increased risk of developing oral squamous cell carcinoma in chronic GVHD patients [10,11].

Lip biopsy is useful in the diagnosis of chronic GVHD and should include both mucosa and underlying minor salivary glands [12]. Histology shows changes similar to those seen in Sjögren syndrome.

Drugs

A wide range of drugs can occasionally induce mouth ulcers, by a variety of effects [1]. Oral local use of caustics or agents such as cocaine can cause erosions or ulcers [2,3]. Oral ulcers are regularly produced by cytotoxic agents [4,5] (see Mucositis above). Aphthous-like ulcers may follow the use of the potassium channel blocking cardioactive agent nicorandil [6,7].

Drugs may also cause mucocutaneous lesions; ulcers of a lichenoid type may follow exposure to non-steroidal anti-inflammatory drugs and other agents, erythema multiforme may follow the use of a range of drugs and drug-induced ulcers may also resemble toxic epidermal necrolysis or may have features reminiscent of other dermatological disorders.

The ulcers usually resolve in 10–14 days if the offending drug can be identified and withdrawn.

Oral and perioral ulceration, hypersalivation, gingivitis and early tooth loss are features of acrodynia caused by mercury poisoning, now rarely seen [8].

Miscellaneous causes

Glucagonoma
Oral ulceration can be a severe manifestation in glucagonoma [1,2] but cheilitis is usually more prominent [3].

Monoclonal plasmacytic ulcerative stomatitis
Ulcerative stomatitis may occasionally appear with a lichenoid rash, related to a plasmacytic infiltrate [1,2].

Mucha–Haberman disease
Erythematous and ulcerative oral lesions have been reported in pityriasis lichenoides et varioliformis acuta (Mucha–Haberman disease) [1,2].

Mucocutaneous lymph node syndrome

> **Synonyms and inclusions**
> • Kawasaki disease (see Chapters 102 and 117)

Mucocutaneous lymph node syndrome is a disorder of uncertain, but possibly infectious, aetiology. Male children are predominantly affected. At least one oral feature should be present for the diagnosis to be made. The oral and pharyngeal mucosa become generally red and sore and the lips dry and fissured. There may be oral ulceration and a 'strawberry tongue' appearance [1–4]. Cervical lymphadenopathy, conjunctivitis and fever also occur, followed later by the characteristic desquamation of the skin of the hands and feet. Early therapy with immunoglobulin is essential to avoid cardiac complications.

Necrotizing sialometaplasia
Necrotizing sialometaplasia is an uncommon benign self-limiting condition seen predominantly in the posterior hard palate of young adult males, most of whom smoke tobacco [1–5] but has been reported at other oral sites, such as the tongue, floor of the mouth and salivary glands [6,7]. Hypoxia-inducible factor (HIF)-1α, VEGF and epidermal growth factor receptor (EGFR) have been implicated in the pathogenesis [8]. An association with bulimia has been reported [9–13].

A painless deep ulcer persists for several weeks before spontaneously healing. This benign lesion must be differentiated from malignancy; indeed occasionally it is found in association with neoplasms, especially salivary [14,15]. Biopsy is usually indicated and reveals necrosis and pseudoepitheliomatous changes probably resulting from squamous metaplasia following infarction of minor salivary glands [16].

Superficial mucocoeles
Superficial extravasation mucocoeles of the intraoral minor salivary glands in the palate, buccal mucosa or labial mucosa are not uncommon, especially associated with oral lichen planus in middle-aged or elderly women and rarely with chronic GVHD [1]. This benign self-limiting condition may cause confusion with vesiculobullous disorders [2–8]. No treatment is available or required.

LOSS OF ELASTICITY OF ORAL TISSUES

Fibrosis of oral tissues leads to restricted oral opening, and can follow burns or irradiation. It may also be associated with habits such as the chewing of betel nut (*Areca*), which predisposes to oral submucous fibrosis and may be caused by a connective tissue disorder such as scleroderma. Rarely, it is occupational (polyvinylchloride workers). Epidermolysis bullosa commonly, and mucous membrane pemphigoid and lichen planus occasionally, may cause scarring and the orofacial region can be involved in multiple idiopathic fibrosis [1].

Oral submucous fibrosis

Definition
Oral submucous fibrosis is a chronic disease of the oral mucosa that appears to be caused by exposure to constituents of the *Areca* nut.

Epidemiology

Incidence and prevalence
The rate varies from 0.2 to 2.3% in males and 1.2 to 4.57% in females in Indian communities.

Age
Any.

Sex
Females more than males.

Ethnicity
It is found virtually exclusively in persons from the Indian subcontinent; most of those affected chew *Areca* nut with tobacco, betel leaf and lime [1,2,3–11] and may be related to copper, possibly through dietary copper or copper sulphate, a constituent of Bordeaux mixture, the fungicide sprayed on *Areca* plantations in monsoon regions.

Associated diseases
Betel use may be associated with the following:
- Cancers: hepatocellular, oesophageal, oral, pancreatic.
- Adverse birth outcomes.
- Chronic kidney disease.
- Contact dermatitis.
- Liver cirrhosis.
- Hearing impairment.
- Hypertension.
- Metabolic syndrome.
- Periodontitis.

Pathophysiology

Predisposing factors
Chewing betel quid, which is available in various forms both in the countries of Asia and in peoples from those areas living in resource-rich countries [1,2,3–7]:
- Betel quid without tobacco; mostly used by South-East Asians (i.e. China, Guam, Myanmar, Papua New Guinea, Taiwan, Thailand).
- Gutka (gutkha, guttkha or guthka): a manufactured version of betel quid with tobacco sold as a single-use sachet. Mainly used by peoples in or from the Indian subcontinent (i.e. India, Pakistan, Bangladesh).
- Mainpuri tobacco: a mixture of *Areca* nut, tobacco, lime and various condiments used in parts of northern India. Sweeteners or spices (i.e. anise seed, cardamom, clove, mustard, saffron, turmeric) may also be added.
- Mawa (kharra): a combination of *Areca* nut, tobacco and lime.
- Pan: freshly prepared betel quid (with or without tobacco).
- Pan masala: a commercially manufactured powdered version of betel quid without tobacco used by people from the Indian subcontinent.
- Pan Parag: a brand name of pan masala and gutka used by people from the Indian subcontinent.

Commercially freeze-dried products such as pan masala, gutka and mawa have higher concentrations of *Areca* nut per chew and appear to cause oral submucous fibrosis more rapidly than self-prepared conventional betel quid.

Pathology
Arecoline, an active alkaloid in betel nuts, stimulates fibroblasts to increase collagen production, while flavanoid, catechin and tannin cause collagen fibres to cross-link. There is a subepithelial chronic inflammatory reaction with fibrosis extending to the submucosa and muscle. Epithelial changes range from atrophy to keratosis and there may be dysplasia.

Genetics
Patients with oral submucous fibrosis have an increased frequency of HLA-A10, HLA-B7 and HLA-DR3. A6 of *MICA* (major histocompatibility complex class I chain-related gene A) is significantly higher in people with oral submucous fibrosis. *CYP1AI* and *CYP2E1* gene polymorphisms may increase susceptibility, and TGF-β may be involved [8–10].

Environmental factors
A hypersensitivity reaction to chilies used by some, may contribute to oral submucous fibrosis.

Clinical features
The buccal mucosa is the most commonly involved site, but any part of the mouth can be involved, and the pharynx. Oral submucous fibrosis develops insidiously, often initially presenting with oral dysaesthesia (burning sensation) and a non-specific vesicular stomatitis [11–20].

Oral submucous fibrosis appears to be restricted to the mouth, although many patients are also anaemic.

Complications and co-morbidities
Later there may be symmetrical fibrosis of the cheeks, lips or palate, which may be symptomless and noted only as bands running through the mucosa. This can, however, become so severe that the affected site becomes white and firm, with severely restricted opening of the mouth.

Disease course and prognosis
Oral submucous fibrosis may predispose to the development of leukoplakia, and oral carcinoma, which occurs in 2–10% of patients over a period of 10 years. There may be mutations in the *APC* gene and low expression of the wild-type *TP53* tumor suppressor gene product.

Investigations
The diagnosis can be confirmed by biopsy.

Management
Management is difficult. Intralesional corticosteroids and jaw exercises may be useful in the early stages, but surgery may be needed to relieve the fibrosis. Pentoxyfylline, spirulina, salvianolic acid B, aloe vera, isoxsuprine and lycopene have each been used with some effect [21–32].

Systemic sclerosis (see Chapter 56)

Oral features are common in systemic sclerosis and are generally more obvious in those with diffuse than localized scleroderma. Decreased mouth opening is the main feature and most patients have restricted oral opening with linear wrinkles of the lips. Decreased oral opening is correlated to oesophageal involvement. About 70% of patients have hyposalivation, most commonly in anticentromere antibodies positive cutaneous limited forms of systemic sclerosis, and there is an increase in both caries and periodontal disease. A characteristic finding is of increased width of the periodontal ligament space of all teeth on radiography [1–23]. There are mandibular erosions in the angle particularly, but also in the condyle, coronoid or digastric regions. Calcifications within the periodontal ligament space and pulp calcifications have been reported. Telangiectasia may be seen. The dropped head sign and tongue atrophy, are rare manifestations in systemic sclerosis associated myopathy. Systemic sclerosis patients are at increased risk of developing cancer, especially of the lung, oral cavity and pharynx.

Specific mouth-opening rehabilitation programmes, connective tissue massage, Kabat's technique, kinesitherapy and home-based exercises may help oral opening. Autologous fat tissue grafting has been successfully used [1–23].

LUMPS AND SWELLINGS

Lumps and swellings in the mouth range from simple anatomical variants, which can cause the patient considerable concern, to pathological lumps caused by inflammatory, cystic (Figure 110.40), neoplastic and other disorders (Box 110.9).

Abscesses

Most intraoral abscesses are odontogenic in origin, as a final consequence of dental caries. Most abscesses discharge in the mouth on the buccal gingiva but occasionally discharge palatally, lingually, on the chin or submental region (Figure 110.41), or elsewhere. Very occasionally, abscesses follow trauma or a foreign body, or rarely are related to unusual oral infections such as actinomycosis [1–3], nocardiosis or botryomycosis [4,5].

Drainage and appropriate antimicrobials are indicated [6–10]. Dental attention is required; dental abscesses are drained by tooth extraction, incision and drainage, or through the root canal (endodontics).

Amyloidosis (see Chapter 58)

In primary amyloidosis the tongue is enlarged and firm or hard. There may also be yellowish submucosal nodules, lumps or

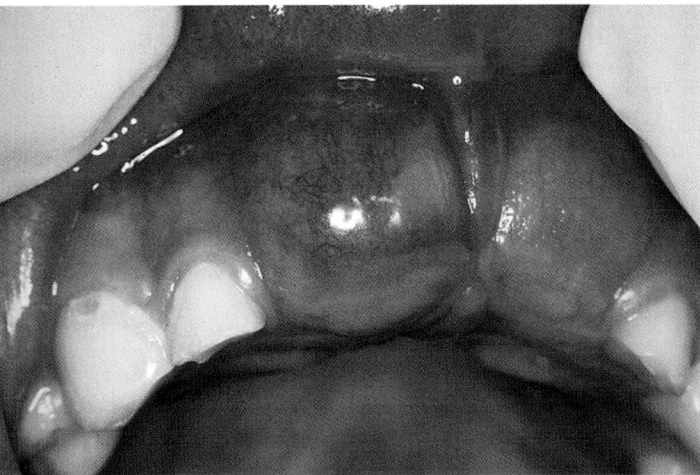

Figure 110.40 Bluish, fluctuant swelling of an oral cyst, in this case an eruption cyst over an erupting maxillary permanent incisor. (The lesion on the maxillary canine is early dental caries.)

Box 110.9 Lesions that may cause the complaint of lumps or swellings in the mouth

- Normal anatomical features
  - Pterygoid hamulus
  - Parotid papillae
  - Foliate or other lingual papillae
  - Unerupted teeth
- Developmental
  - Haemangioma
  - Lymphangioma
  - Maxillary and mandibular tori
  - Hereditary gingival fibromatosis
  - Von Recklinghausen neurofibromatosis
  - Cysts of developmental origin
  - Odontomes
- Inflammatory
  - Abscess
  - Pyogenic granuloma
  - Oral Crohn disease
  - Orofacial granulomatosis
  - Pulse granuloma
  - Sarcoidosis
  - Granulomatosis with polyangiitis
  - Others
- Traumatic
  - Epulis
  - Fibroepithelial polyp
  - Denture-induced granuloma
  - Mucocoele
  - Herniation of buccal fat pad
- Infective
  - Various papillomatous lesions
- Cystic
  - Cysts of odontogenic origin (e.g. dental cysts)
- Deposits
  - Amyloidosis
  - Hyalinosis
  - Hypoplasminogenaemia
- Drug therapy (gingival swelling only)
  - Oral contraceptive (pill gingivitis)
  - Phenytoin
  - Calcium-channel blockers
  - Ciclosporin
- Hormonal
  - Pubertal gingivitis
  - Pregnancy epulis/gingivitis
- Blood dyscrasias
  - Leukaemia, lymphoma and myeloma
- Benign neoplasms
  - Various
- Malignant neoplasms
  - Primary and secondary
- Others
  - Angio-oedema
  - Fibro-osseous diseases
  - Acanthosis nigricans

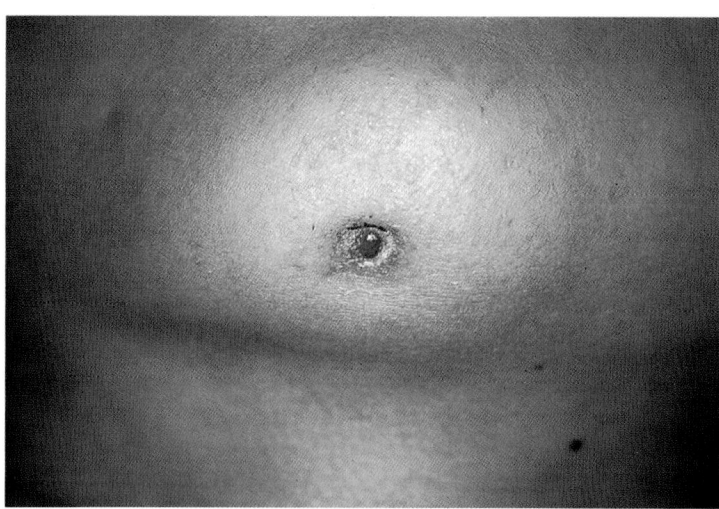

Figure 110.41 Sinus on the chin related to a dental abscess on a mandibular incisor tooth.

petechiae (Figure 110.42). Rarely, there are similar deposits elsewhere (e.g. in the soft palate), and jaw claudication, salivary gland swelling or hyposalivation [1–15] and sometimes burning sensations.

Secondary amyloidoses rarely involve the mouth except in the case of multiple myeloma or haemodialysis-associated amyloid, which may occasionally produce oral nodules or ulceration. Bullous amyloidosis may cause oral blistering.

Solitary intraoral amyloid is rare. Localized tongue amyloidosis does not appear to increase the risk of developing systemic involvement.

Hereditary gelsolin amyloidosis (also known as AGel amyloidosis), a rare dominantly inherited systemic disease caused by c.654G>A or c.654G>T gelsolin gene mutation may cause oral dryness and cranial polyneuropathy. Labial salivary gland biopsies

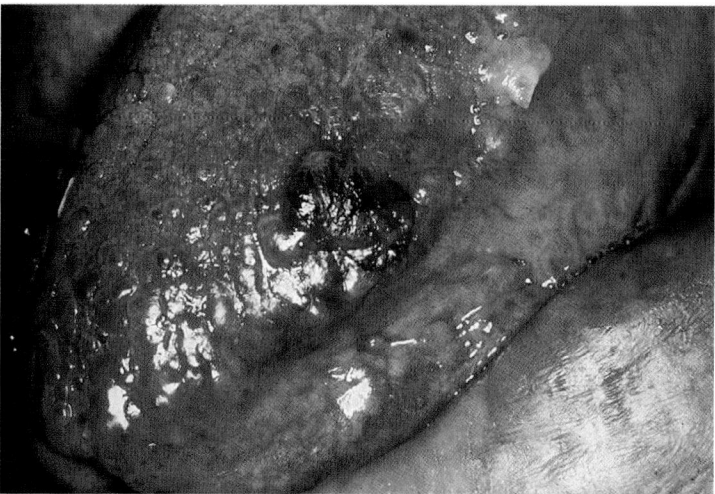

Figure 110.42 Macroglossia and oral petechiae in amyloidosis.

showed deposition of gelsolin amyloid, atrophy and inflammation [16–25].

In amyloidosis, Congo red or thioflavine T staining of a biopsy usually confirms the diagnosis, although in extreme cases the deposits are seen on haematoxylin and eosin staining. Treatment is unsatisfactory but the underlying disease, where present, should be treated.

Angio-oedema

Oral swelling may be a feature of allergic angio-oedema and angio-oedema due to Cl-esterase inhibitor deficiency. Allergic angio-oedema can occur secondary to antibiotic therapy, exposure to latex or ingestion of certain food substances and may be life threatening. Angio-oedema due to C1-esterase inhibitor deficiency may be hereditary, first occurring in childhood, or acquired, with onset usually in adulthood. Type I hereditary angio-oedema exhibits low levels of functionally normal C1-esterase inhibitor while in the type II variant C1-esterase inhibitor is dysfunctional. The swelling may affect the lips, tongue or other areas and is often only mild and transient, although there is the potential for obstruction of the airway. Local anaesthetics [1] or more commonly angiotensin-converting enzyme inhibitors [2–12] may cause angio-oedema, which can occasionally be lethal [4]. It may respond to a sympathomimetic such as epinephrine or to antihistamines. Synthetic androgens have proven useful in reducing the frequency and duration of attacks [1,2].

Buccal fat-pad herniation

Trauma may rarely cause the buccal pad of fat to herniate through the buccinator muscle, producing an intraoral swelling [1–3]. This usually occurs in males under the age of 4 years. Surgery is indicated.

Denture-induced hyperplasia

Synonyms and inclusions
- Denture granuloma
- Epulis fissuratum

Where a denture flange is overextended and irritates the vestibular mucosa, a linear reparative process may result, eventually producing an elongated fibroepithelial enlargement known as denture-induced hyperplasia [1–5]. Firm leaf-like painless swellings are seen, usually in the buccal or labial vestibule. The pathology is that of a fibrous lump. A denture-induced granuloma should be excised and examined histologically to exclude more serious pathology, if modification of the denture does not induce regression [2]. Rarely, denture-induced hyperplasia arises because some other lesion develops beneath a denture and causes the mucosa to be irritated.

PART 10: SITES, SEX, AGE

Focal epithelial hyperplasia (multifocal epithelial hyperplasia)

Synonyms and inclusions
- Heck disease

Focal epithelial hyperplasia is a rare benign familial disorder with no sex predisposition, characterized by multiple, soft, circumscribed, sessile, nodular elevations of the oral mucosa [1–8].

Heck disease occurs particularly in Native Americans, in Inuits in Greenland and in Chinese but has been reported rarely from many other countries. The prevalence in Greenland and Venezuela approaches 35% [1,9,10].

Aetiology. The papillomaviruses HPV-13 and HPV-32 appear to be causal in patients with the genetic predisposition to focal epithelial hyperplasia [5–8,11–16]. Household transmission of HPV through saliva and the shared use of contaminated objects may be implicated.

Pathology. The characteristics of focal epithelial hyperplasia are local epithelial hyperplasia, acanthosis and elongated 'Bronze Age axe' rete ridges, together with a ballooning type of nuclear degeneration. Epithelial cells have a pseudomitotic appearance.

Clinical features. Among Native Americans, focal epithelial hyperplasia mainly affects children and usually involves the lower lip, whereas in the Inuit and in white people the lesions are found mainly in the fourth decade and later and often affect the tongue.

Management. This is a benign asymptomatic condition, requiring only reassurance.

Foliate papillitis [1]

The foliate lingual papillae may become inflamed and swell. Because of their location on the posterolateral tongue this may give undue concern about malignancy. The condition resolves spontaneously.

Franklin disease

Synonyms and inclusions
- Heavy-chain disease

Palatal oedema and oral ulceration have been described in a few patients with heavy-chain disease, but the former feature is not as invariable as initially described [1,2].

Leiomyoma

This benign tumour of smooth muscle is rare in the oral cavity but if present usually affects the tongue or palate [1–5]. Sometimes it is an angioleiomyoma [6–8] and rarely multiple [9]. Excision is the usual management.

Lipoma (see Chapter 100)

Lipomas are uncommon in the mouth, comprising less than 5% of oral benign tumours [1–8]. They present as slow-growing, spherical, smooth and soft semi-fluctuant lumps with a characteristic yellowish colour. Most involve the buccal mucosa or floor of the mouth. Occasionally, lipomas can develop within the tongue [9]. Although benign, they may rarely infiltrate [10]. Histology shows adult fat cells gathered into lobules by vascular septa of fibrous connective tissue. Angiolipomas, spindle cell lipomas and liposarcomas are in the differential diagnosis. Surgery is rarely indicated for lipomas except for infiltrating lipomas [11,12].

Macroglossia

The tongue may be congenitally enlarged (macroglossia) in Down syndrome or Beckwith–Wiedemann syndrome or where there is an angioma. It may also enlarge in angio-oedema, gigantism, acromegaly or amyloidosis [1–7].

Mucocoele (mucous cyst)

Synonyms and inclusions
- Mucous retention cyst
- Ranula
- Mucocele
- Myxoid cyst of lip

Mucocoeles are common and usually seen in the lower labial mucosa (Figure 110.43), resulting from the escape of mucus into the lamina propria from a damaged minor salivary gland duct.

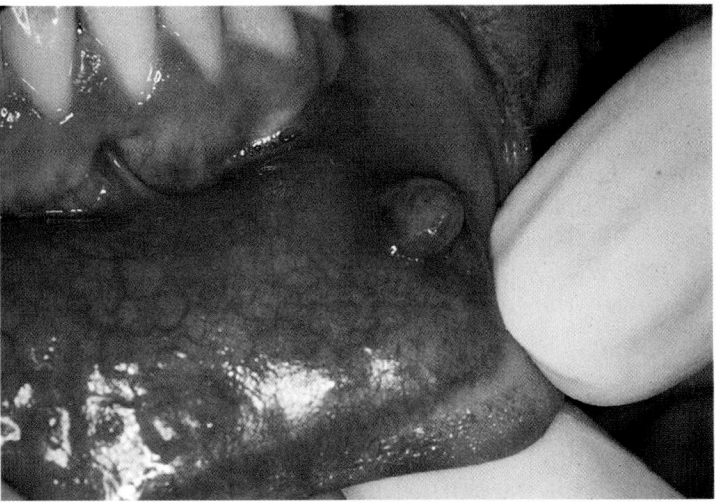

Figure 110.43 Mucocoele.

Mucocoeles appear usually as solitary, painless, dome-shaped, translucent, whitish blue papules or nodules [1–7]. Care should be taken to ensure that the lesion is not a salivary gland tumour with cystic change, especially when dealing with an apparent mucous cyst in the upper lip [8] or other lesions such as cysticercosis or mycetoma. Mucocoeles can be seen in GVHD [6]. Mucocoeles can be excised but they also respond well to cryosurgery, using a single freeze–thaw cycle [9,10] or sclerotherapy.

Superficial mucocoeles are seen mainly in lichen planus [11,12]; palatal lesions may be seen [13]. Treatment is rarely indicated.

Myeloma and paraproteinaemias

Multiple myeloma very occasionally presents with an intraoral mass or oral bleeding. Osteolytic bone lesions are more common. Solitary plasmacytomas may also be seen; indeed, some 80% of these rare tumours are found in the head and neck region but typically in the nasal cavity or pharynx rather than in the mouth [1–8].

Patients with myeloma treated with intravenous bisphosphonates are at risk from jaw osteonecrosis.

Myxoma

Myxomas are rare in the oral cavity [1–5] mainly as odontogenic or soft tissue myxomas [6]. Neurothekeoma (nerve sheath myxoma [7]) may also affect the oral cavity. Myxomas arise in bone or soft tissue and, although benign, are aggressive and difficult to eradicate because of the tendency to infiltrate normal tissue [8,9].

Nodular fasciitis

Nodular (pseudosarcomatous) fasciitis affects the head and neck in 20% of cases but rarely involves the mouth [1–7]. In the mouth, most cases involve the lips and buccal mucosae [7]. The spindle cells are positive for smooth muscle actin and muscle-specific actin (HHF-35) antibodies. Treatment typically involves conservative excision, but the lesion may regress spontaneously [8].

Oral allergy syndrome

Oral allergy syndrome is the combination of oral pruritus, irritation and swelling of the lips, tongue, palate and throat, sometimes associated with other allergic features such as rhinoconjunctivitis, asthma, urticaria–angio-oedema and anaphylactic shock, precipitated mainly by fresh foods such as fruits and vegetables (e.g. apple, peach, kiwi and melon), and sometimes by cross-reacting pollen allergens [1–6], particularly oak and birch. Patients with nasal pollinosis frequently have oral allergy syndrome [7]. Cooking often destroys food allergens.

Oral allergy syndrome may respond to antihistamines or to a sympathomimetic agent such as ephedrine taken by mouth.

Osteoma mucosae

Synonyms and inclusions
- Osseous choristoma

There are rare cases of osteoma of the oral mucosa, usually in the tongue. Most have been in females in the third and fourth decades and have arisen as pedunculated hard painless lumps on the dorsum of the tongue immediately posterior to the foramen caecum [1–5]. They may arise from thyroid anlages. Simple excision suffices.

Papillary hyperplasia

Papillary hyperplasia may be seen in the vault of the palate, typically in otherwise healthy persons with chronic denture-related stomatitis though occasionally in its absence, and may be related to *Candida* infection [1–10]. Other papilliferous lesions should be excluded, such as HPV-related lesions in organ transplant recipients [11] and therefore biopsy may be prudent. Papillary hyperplasia may require treatment with antifungals, excision or laser removal.

Papilloma

Aetiology. These are caused by HPV [1–5].

Pathology. Histology includes acanthotic and sometimes hyperkeratotic epithelium with occasional koilocytosis.

Clinical features. Papillomas can appear anywhere in the mouth, but are most common at the junction of the hard and soft palate. The papilloma is a white or pink, cauliflower-like lesion that may resemble a wart. Papillomas of normal colour may be confused with the commoner fibroepithelial polyps, although the latter are commonest at sites of potential trauma. Papillomas are common in HIV-infected people and have increased with the introduction of HAART [3].

Prognosis. Unlike some papillomas of the larynx or bowel, oral papillomas are generally benign although some are dysplastic [3,6].

Diagnosis. Oral papillomas should be removed and examined histologically to establish a correct diagnosis.

Management. Excision must be total, deep and wide enough to include any abnormal cells beyond the zone of the pedicle.

Pulse granuloma

Synonyms and inclusions
- Lewar disease
- Hyaline ring granuloma

Pulse or hyaline ring granulomas are rare well-defined oral lesions due to implantation of the cellulose moiety of plant foods. Embedded vegetable matter causes chronic mandibular periostitis, typically presenting as a submucosal lump over the lower alveolus. Histology shows amorphous hyaline material and a granulomatous inflammatory reaction [1–4]. Excision suffices.

Extraoral pulse or hyaline ring granulomas may affect lungs, stomach and intestines [5].

Rhabdomyoma

Rhabdomyomas are rare but most extracardiac rhabdomyomas present in the mouth, typically as lumps in the floor of the mouth, tongue or soft palate [1–5]. Most are seen in the sixth decade, predominantly in males, most are solitary but cases with multiple lesions have been reported [6,7]. Surgery is effective provided total excision is achieved.

Rhabdomyosarcoma

Some 45% of soft-tissue sarcomas in the head and neck region are rhabdomyosarcomas. Individuals with Costello syndrome have an approximately 15% lifetime risk for malignant tumours including rhabdomyosarcoma and neuroblastoma [1]. The most common oral presentation is a progressively enlarging mass; some 20% have enlarged regional lymph nodes [2–8]. In advanced disease there may be pain, paraesthesia, trismus or loosening of teeth. Intraosseous lesions have been reported [5].

The prognosis is poor. Treatment includes cytotoxic chemotherapy, surgery and radiotherapy.

Sarcoidosis

Isolated nodules [1,2], gingival lesions [3], facial or labial swelling [4] and salivary gland involvement are the main oral or perioral lesions of sarcoidosis [5–11], but are uncommon. However, even where the mucosa is clinically normal, patients with sarcoidosis may have characteristic changes in palatal or labial salivary gland biopsies [9,12]. Intraosseous lesions are rare [13,14]. Orofacial and lip lesions are often isolated with no systemic manifestations, may occasionally precede systemic involvement, and are found mainly in younger patients, with more frequent lacrimal or salivary gland and upper respiratory tract sarcoidosis [15,16].

Thrombotic thrombocytopenic purpura

This may present with oral purpura and/or spontaneous gingival haemorrhage [1–3]. Gingival biopsy is a recommended investigation [4,5].

Verruciform xanthoma

Although verruciform xanthoma was originally described as a distinct oral entity but is now also known occasionally to affect skin and non-oral mucosae [1,2]. The lesion is usually found in the fifth decade, the aetiology is unknown but may be a reaction to some irritant.

The lesions consist of parakeratotic verruciform epithelium, with large foamy xanthoma cells containing slightly PAS-positive granules and abundant lipid in the lamina propria between the epithelial pegs [3–10].

Verruciform xanthoma is usually a solitary symptomless lesion, typically on the gingiva, with a normal, pale, reddish or keratotic surface [1–10]. Excision is only rarely followed by recurrence.

Verruciform xanthoma has been reported in GVHD [11].

Waldenström macroglobulinaemia

Oral manifestations in Waldenström macroglobulinaemia include purpura, ulceration and occasional mental nerve anaesthesia [1–4].

Warts (see Chapter 25)

Both common warts (verrucae vulgaris) and venereal warts (condyloma acuminatum) are caused by HPV [1–8]. They are rare in the mouth (Figure 110.44) but are more common in HIV disease, especially after long-term antiretroviral therapy [9]. None is known to be premalignant. Most can be treated by podophyllum or imiquimod, or excision, cryosurgery or laser.

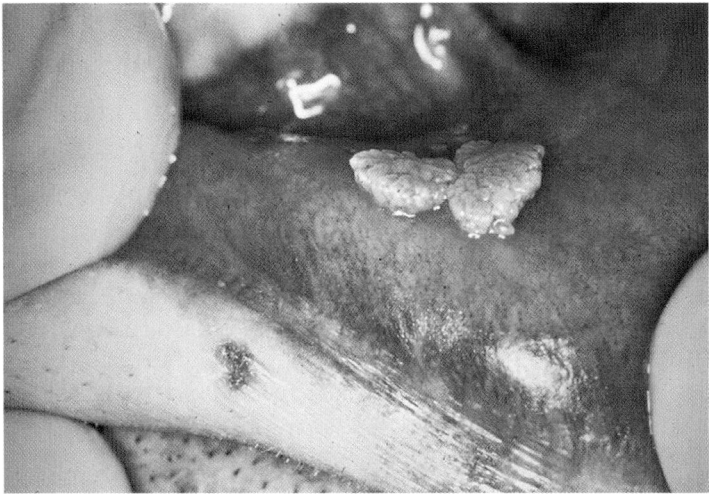

Figure 110.44 Warts on the lower lip in HIV infection. (There is also a healing herpes simplex lesion on the lip.)

ORAL SORENESS WITHOUT ULCERATION

Most oral pain is of local aetiology, usually resulting from odontogenic infections. Neurological, vascular and referred causes are less common, but must also be excluded. Psychogenic pain is all too frequent and this is discussed below.

Chronic oral soreness may be particularly caused by ulceration, or by mucosal lesions in geographic tongue, lichen planus or deficiency states. Geographic tongue and burning mouth syndrome are the common causes of a sore tongue. Lichen planus is the most common cause of chronic soreness in the buccal mucosae. Desquamative gingivitis is the common cause of persistently sore gingivae.

Burning mouth syndrome

Definition and nomenclature
A chronic burning sensation in the mouth, typically the tongue (see also Chapter 84).

Synonyms and inclusions
- Oral dysaesthesia
- Glossopyrosis
- Glossodynia

Introduction and general description
A chronic burning sensation in the mouth may be due to organic lesions such as geographic tongue or candidosis, or may arise with no evident cause, when it is termed burning mouth syndrome.

Epidemiology

Incidence and prevalence
The overall prevalence is roughly 4%.

Age
Burning mouth syndrome most frequently affects middle-aged and older patients [1–4].

Sex
Females more than males.

Associated diseases
A burning sensation may have defined causes. Several organic lesions, for example haematinic deficiency states, erythema migrans, ulcers, mucositis, lichen planus and candidosis, can cause oral soreness or burning sensation. However, burning mouth syndrome is often a medically unexplained symptom.

Pathophysiology
Idiopathic burning mouth syndrome is considered 'primary' (or 'true') burning mouth syndrome, whereas 'secondary' burning mouth syndrome has an identifiable cause.

- Type 1 : no symptoms upon waking, with progression throughout the day. Night-time symptoms are variable. Nutritional deficiency and diabetes may produce a similar pattern.
- Type 2: continuous symptoms throughout the day and frequently asymptomatic at night. This type is associated with chronic anxiety.
- Type 3: intermittent symptoms throughout the day and symptom-free days. Food allergy is suggested as a potential mechanism.

Burning mouth syndrome has long been considered a psychogenic illness but a neuropathic mechanism with changes in nociceptive fibres may be implicated. Anxiety is associated with burning mouth syndrome but whether it is a cause or the effect is unclear.

Pathology
Burning mouth syndrome with a tongue of normal clinical appearance may be seen in deficiency states, drugs (e.g. angiotensin-converting enzyme inhibitors such as captopril, enalapril, lisinopril; protease inhibitors; cytotoxic agents; clonazepam), with psychogenic causes and diabetes. A monosymptomatic hypochondriasis or an underlying anxiety about cancer or a sexually transmitted infection with perhaps excessive tongue activity appear to be the basis for the complaint of burning mouth syndrome in many patients (Box 110.10) [1–15]. More recently, evidence for a neuropathic basis has emerged [12,14,16].

Uncommon causes that may need to be considered include hypothyroidism, lupus erythematosus, hypersensitivity (to sodium metabisulphite, nuts, dental materials and other substances) and galvanic reactions to metals in the mouth [17–21].

Clinical features
Although the tongue is most frequently involved, the patient may also occasionally complain of burning lips, gums or palate. The burning sensation is usually bilateral and often relieved by eating

---

Box 110.10 Causes of burning mouth

- Local
  - Candidosis
  - Other infections
  - Geographic tongue
  - Lichen planus
  - Oral submucous fibrosis
  - Dentures
- Systemic
  - Psychogenic
    - Cancerophobia
    - Depression
    - Anxiety states
    - Hypochondriasis
  - Deficiency states
    - Pernicious anaemia and other vitamin B deficiencies
    - Folate deficiency
    - Iron deficiency
  - Diabetes
  - Drugs (captopril)

and drinking [1,11,12]. In contrast, oral discomfort associated with inflammatory lesions is typically aggravated by eating.

Investigations

Oral examination very occasionally reveals an organic cause. Hyposalivation should be excluded as this may predispose to candidosis. Laboratory screening for anaemia, diabetes, a deficiency state or candidosis should be undertaken.

Management

Few patients with burning mouth syndrome have spontaneous remission in the short term, and thus an attempt at treatment is indicated. Reassurance, treatment of any defined underlying organic abnormality and, occasionally, psychological treatment, antidepressants or psychiatric care are indicated, but active dental or oral surgical treatment, or attempts at 'hormone replacement', in the absence of any specific indication, should be avoided. However, treatment is rarely completely successful, although the condition only infrequently becomes severe. Fortunately, about 50% remit spontaneously over 6 or 7 years.
- Patients should avoid anything that aggravates symptoms, such as sparkling wines, citrus drinks and spices.
- Reassurance and attention to any factors such as dentures or haematinic deficiencies may be indicated. There are few treatments of proven benefit [12–21,**22**].
  - Cognitive–behavioural therapy or a specialist referral may be indicated [14,23].
- Some patients respond to medication:
  - Effects of vitamin B are controversial [24–26].
  - Topical benzydamine 0.01% rinse or spray [27,**28**].
  - Although antidepressants must be given for at least 2–3 weeks to achieve any antidepressive effect, most patients with medically unexplained symptoms show benefit within 1 week [29–32].
  - Topical capsaicin cream 0.025% (Zacin®) or 0.075% (Axsain®) [11].
  - Clonazepam tablet sucked locally [14].
  - α-lipoic acid systemically [14,33].

Treatment with placebos, however, may produce a response 72% as large as the response to active drugs [34].

Deficiency glossitis

Aetiology. Deficiency glossitis may be related particularly to deficiency of iron, folate or vitamin B_{12}, and may then be associated with angular stomatitis and/or mouth ulcers. Deficiencies of other B-group vitamins occasionally cause glossitis, usually in chronic alcoholics or in those with malabsorption [1–8].

Pathology. Epithelial atrophy, rarely with some dysplasia, is seen.

Clinical features. In anaemic glossitis the tongue is red, sore and smooth (Figure 110.45). Occasionally, pernicious anaemia can also produce red areas or patterns of red lines. In many other patients, the tongue can become sore but appear clinically completely

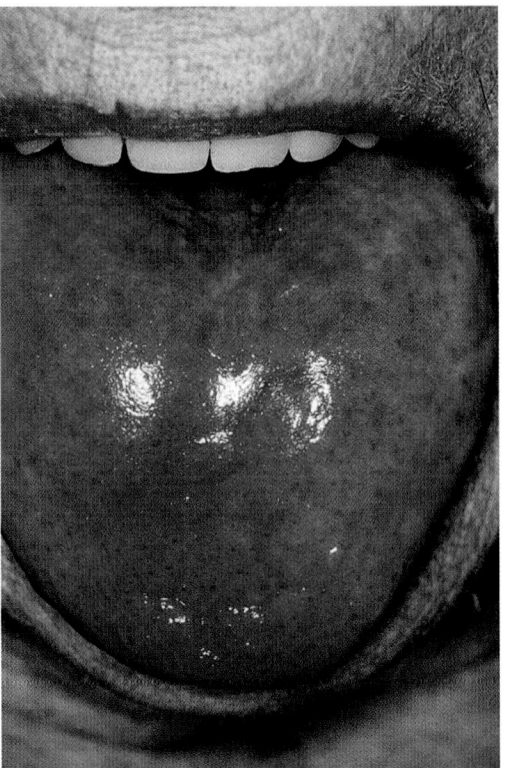

Figure 110.45 Atrophic glossitis in vitamin B_{12} deficiency.

normal and such patients' complaints are liable to be mislabelled as psychogenic.

Diagnosis. A full blood picture and assays of iron, folate and vitamin B_{12} are essential in management, as sore tongue can be the initial symptom of a deficiency and can precede any fall in the haemoglobin level.

Management. The cause of the deficiency should be sought before replacement treatment is given.

Geographic tongue

See p. 110.13.

Lichen planus

See Chapter 37 and p. 110.43.

PIGMENTED LESIONS

The tongue is often discoloured due to superficial staining from foods, drinks or habits such as tobacco or betel use.

Localized hyperpigmented lesions are usually due to pigmentary incontinence, amalgam tattoos, melanotic macule or naevi,

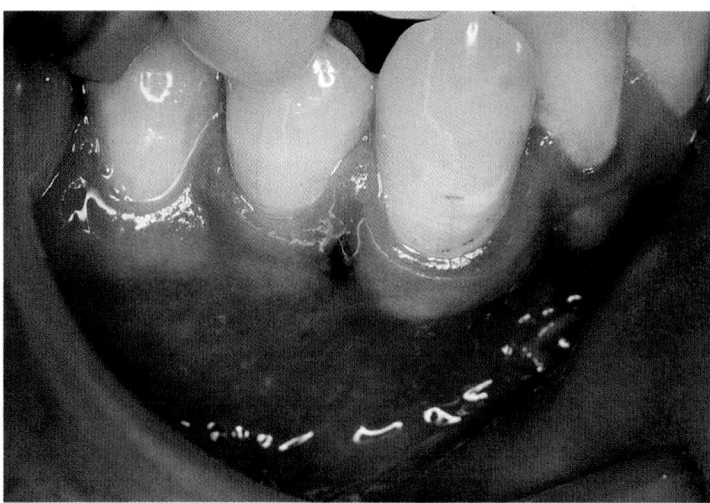

Figure 110.46 Amalgam tattoo in a common site. This was presumably related to filling of the deciduous predecessor.

although melanomas, Kaposi sarcoma and epithelioid angiomatosis must be excluded.

Generalized oral mucosal hyperpigmentation is usually racial in origin and only occasionally has a systemic cause, such as Addison disease.

Amalgam tattoos

Amalgam tattoos are common causes of blue-black pigmentation, usually seen in the mandibular gingiva or at least close to the teeth (Figure 110.46), or in the scar of an apicectomy where there has been a retrograde root filling with amalgam used as root-end filling material [1–6]. The amalgam associates with elastin fibres [7]. Radio-opacities may or may not be seen on radiography. Similar lesions can result if, for some reason, pencil lead or other similar foreign bodies become embedded in the oral tissues [8,9].

Radiography may help to confirm the diagnosis. Biopsy may be indicated to exclude a melanoma but otherwise these innocuous lesions require no treatment.

Body art

Extraoral tattoos are common after the incorporation of foreign material as after trauma such as road traffic accidents, and are deliberately placed in many cultures.

Tattooing of the lower lip may occasionally be seen. A tattooed lower lip in a Sudanese woman, for example, signifies that she is married. The Wodaabe people of Nigeria and Cameroon may tattoo on the skin surface at the angle of the mouth, a practice which has its basis in ritual warding-off of the 'evil eye'. Similar tattoos may be seen on Bedouin women of North Africa. The vermilion may be tattooed red in some people in the Western countries. Tattooing of the chin is seen increasingly in

Maoris ('Moki') and tattooing inside the lip may now be seen in resource-rich countries.

Intraoral tattooing is less common. Deliberate gingival tattooing is a rare cause of oral pigmentation [1,2].

The practice of piercing oral and facial soft tissues and then placing foreign objects/ornaments in the defects on a more or less permanent basis is one which has also been largely confined, historically, to certain tribal groups in continental Africa and isolated Amazon regions of South America, for example the Suia and Txukahamei tribes of Brazil.

Piercing is now common in resource-rich countries [3] where adolescents are characterized by a compulsive tendency to distinguish themselves in clothes, hairstyle or 'decorative' details. The prevalence of oral and/or perioral piercings is unclear, but in one study ranged from 0.8% to 12%, with a mean prevalence of 5.2%. The most common sites are the tongue (a prevalence of 5.6%), followed by the lip (1.5%). Oral piercings are four times more prevalent in women (5.6%) than men (1.6%) [4].

Oral piercing injuries treated in US hospital emergency departments (EDs) are most prevalent in teenagers and young adults. An estimated 24 459 oral piercing injuries presented to US EDs during one recent 7-year period. Patients 14–22 years old accounted for 73% of the ED visits. Injuries to lips (46%), tongue (42%) and teeth (10%) predominated. Infections (42%) and soft-tissue puncture wounds (29%) were most common. Hospitalization was rarely required (<1%) [5]. Dental defects prevalence is greater for tongue than lip piercing. Gingival recession is similar for tongue and lip piercing. Complications secondary to oral and facial piercings include pain, bleeding, dental fractures and gingival damage [6–12].

Coated, furred, brown or black hairy tongue

Aetiology and pathology. Children rarely have a furred (coated) tongue in health but it may be coated with off-white debris in febrile and other illnesses.

Adults, however, not infrequently have a coating on the tongue in health, particularly if they are edentulous, are on a soft non-abrasive diet, have poor oral hygiene or are fasting. The coating appears more obvious in ill patients or those with hyposalivation, especially those who cannot maintain oral hygiene.

The coating in most cases consists of epithelial, food and microbial debris; indeed, the tongue is the main oral reservoir of some microorganisms, such as *Candida albicans* and viridans streptococci. The filiform papillae are excessively long and stained by the accumulation of squames and chromogenic microorganisms.

Poor oral hygiene, or habits such as alcohol, tobacco and betel use, various medicaments such as chlorhexidine or iron, and confectionary or beverages can cause a black or brown superficial staining of the tongue (and teeth).

Occasionally, a brown or black hairy tongue may be caused by GVHD, lansoprazole, EGFR inhibitors, drugs that induce hyposalivation, or antimicrobials, when it may be related to overgrowth

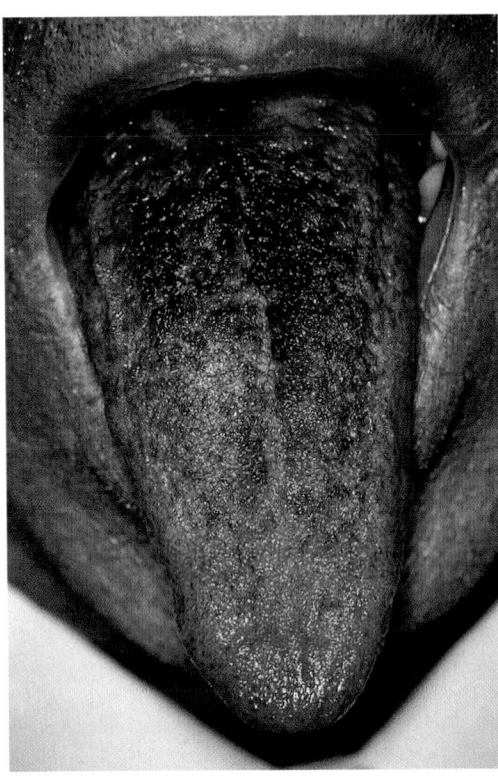

Figure 110.47 Black hairy tongue.

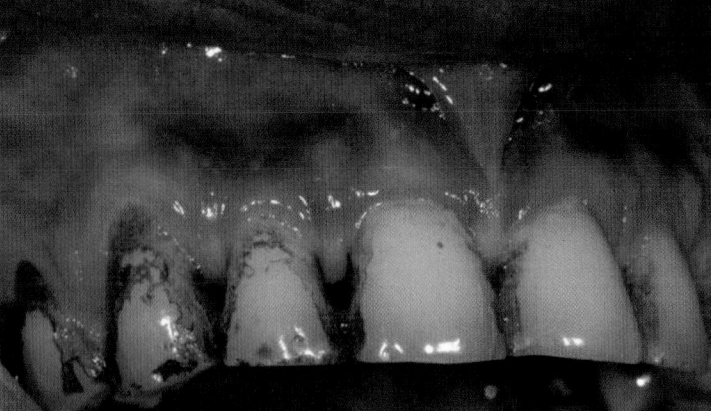

Figure 110.48 Betel staining of teeth.

of microorganisms such as *Candida* species and may respond to withdrawal of the drug [1–5].

Clinical features. Black hairy tongue affects mainly the posterior part of the dorsum of the tongue, especially centrally (Figure 110.47) [3–7].

Management. Patients with black hairy tongue may find the condition improves if they avoid habits or drugs that stain the tongue, increase their standard of oral hygiene, brush the tongue with a hard toothbrush, use sodium bicarbonate mouthwashes, chew gum or suck a peach stone. Topical tretinoin may be effective [8].

Drug, food, habits and heavy metal induced hyperpigmentation

Causes (see Box 110.3) [1–4] can include:
- Foods and beverages (such as beetroot, red wine, coffee and tea).
- Confectionery (such as liquorice).
- Smoking tobacco – a fairly common cause (smoker's melanosis) and this may produce extrinsic discoloration but also intrinsic pigmentary incontinence, with pigment cells increasing and appearing in the lamina propria. This is especially likely in persons who smoke with the lighted end of the cigarette within the mouth (reverse smoking), as practised mainly in some Asian communities [5–7].

- Chewing betel may cause superficial brownish-red discoloration, mainly in the buccal mucosa (and on the teeth), with an irregular epithelial surface that has a tendency to desquamate, seen mainly in women from South and South-East Asia [8,9] (Figure 110.48). The epithelium in betel chewer's mucosa is often hyperplastic, and brownish amorphous material from the betel quid may be seen on the epithelial surface and intracellularly and intercellularly, with ballooning of epithelial cells [8]. Betel chewer's mucosa is not known to be precancerous but betel use predisposes to submucous fibrosis and squamous cell carcinoma.
- Drugs such as chlorhexidine, iron salts, griseofulvin, crack cocaine, minocycline, bismuth subsalicylate, lansoprazole, and hormone replacement therapy. Drugs that cause intrinsic staining include the following [10–23]:
  - Antimalarials produce a variety of colours in the mucosa, ranging from yellow with mepacrine to blue-black with amodiaquine.
  - Minocycline may cause blackish discoloration of teeth, gingivae and bone, skin, sclera and even breast milk. Minocycline can, in a minority of patients, produce blue-grey gingival pigmentation caused by staining of the underlying bone, and some intrinsic faint bluish-grey staining, mainly near the anterior teeth.
  - Busulphan, hydroxyurea, some other cytotoxic drugs, oral contraceptives, phenothiazines and anticonvulsants may also occasionally produce, or increase, brown pigmentation, as may zidovudine and clofazimine.
  - Gold may produce purplish gingival discoloration. Many of the heavy metals formerly implicated in producing oral hyperpigmentation (such as mercury, lead and bismuth) are not used therapeutically now, although industrial or accidental exposure is still occasionally seen [24]. Metallic sulphides deposited in the tissues were seen especially where oral hygiene was poor, with bacteria producing sulphides that resulted in pigmentation at the gingival margin (e.g. lead line).

Oral hyperpigmentation may be seen in ACTH therapy, Addison disease, Nelson syndrome or ectopic adrenocorticotrophic hormone production (e.g. by bronchogenic carcinoma) [25–31].

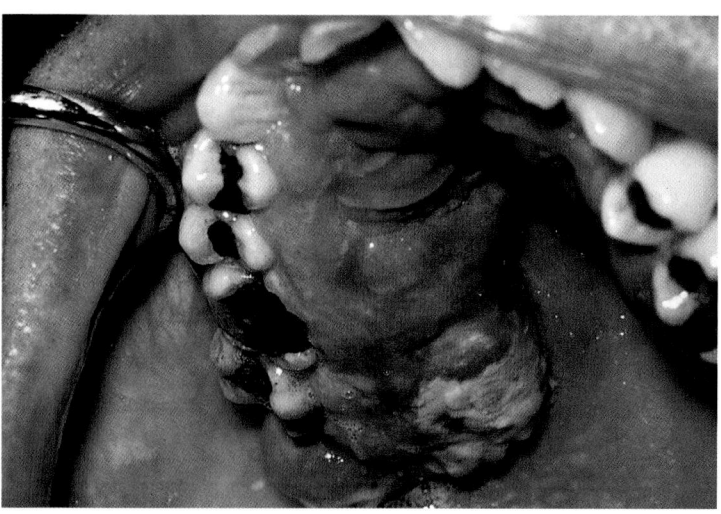

Figure 110.49 Kaposi sarcoma in a typical site with a characteristic purplish appearance. (Courtesy of Dr J.B. Epstein, Cancer Control Agency, Vancouver, Canada.)

The brown or black pigmentation is variable in distribution but is seen typically on the soft palate, buccal mucosa and at sites of trauma.

Management. Some drug-induced hyperpigmentation resolves on cessation of exposure to the drug and improved oral hygiene, although resolution can take months or years.

HIV infection

Oral hyperpigmentation may be seen in HIV infection, sometimes related to adrenal hypofunction or drug use [1–5].

Kaposi sarcoma (see Chapter 137)

Kaposi sarcoma is seen predominantly as a consequence of HIV infection, mainly in men who have sex with men. It appears to be associated with HHV-8 [1–9]. Up to 50% of male homosexual AIDS patients have developed oral Kaposi sarcoma, although it appears to be declining in frequency and is rare in other HIV-infected patients.

Oral Kaposi sarcoma is the first presentation of HIV in 20–60% of affected patients, often associated with oral candidosis. Kaposi sarcoma affects the hard-palate mucosa in particular (Figure 110.49). Up to 95% of lesions are seen in the palate, 23% in the gingiva and others on the tongue or buccal mucosa. A red-purple macule is the early lesion, progressing to a purple nodular swelling that may be extensive and ulcerated. Multiple lesions are common [3–6]. Lesions are often asymptomatic but more than 25% are painful and about 8% bleed. Oral Kaposi sarcoma is also occasionally seen in other non-HIV-infected immunocompromised patients.

Occasionally, oral Kaposi sarcoma may regress spontaneously, or with HAART, zidovudine or systemic vinca alkaloids, etoposide or interferon, but the more usual treatment is local radiotherapy, laser removal or intralesional vinblastine. The latter produces fewer adverse effects than radiotherapy [10–19].

Melanoma (see Chapter 143)

Oral melanoma is rare. Most patients are over 50 years of age and there is a male preponderance.

Malignant melanoma may arise in apparently normal oral mucosa or in a pre-existent pigmented naevus, most commonly in the palate or maxillary alveolus [1–10]. Features suggestive of malignancy include a rapid increase in size, change in colour, ulceration, pain, bleeding, the occurrence of satellite pigmented spots, or regional lymph node enlargement. The prognosis is poor unless detected very early [2,3]. Metastatic melanoma is rare [4]. The optimal treatment is surgery [6,8].

The histology may show anaplastic spindle-shaped or squamoid cells. However, the histology is quite varied and staining with dopa or antibodies may be required to help the diagnosis. Most cases are positive for S-100, tyrosinase and Mart-1/melana-A. Lesions suspected to be melanoma should not be biopsied until the time of definitive surgical excision [11–15]. Proton therapy (PT) and carbon ion therapy (CIT) are of equal efficacy [16].

Melanocanthoma

Oral melanoacanthoma, is a rare reactive melanocytic lesion with solitary or multifocal diffuse pigmentation, found mainly in children: most reported cases have been in black people. A hyperpigmented symptomless macule appears over a course of days or weeks. There is a female predominance amongst the patients with solitary oral melanoacanthoma, whereas multifocal oral melanoacanthoma showed an equal gender distribution. Multifocal lesions tended to occur on the palate, and solitary lesions on the buccal mucosa. The sudden appearance and rapid radial growth often mimics melanoma. Biopsy shows increased number of dendritic melanocytes in an acanthotic epithelium. The course is benign, and some cases resolve spontaneously within 6 months [1–10]. No specific treatment is required but argon plasma coagulation is a relatively safe and effective modality.

Melanotic macule

A melanotic macule is a small well-circumscribed melanocytic benign lesion. It can occur on the lips and intraorally and ranges in colour from brown to black (Figure 110.50). Microscopically, it is characterized by elevated levels of melanin production by basal melanocytes, which appear normal in number, morphology and distribution. Pigment-filled dendritic cells that appear to be melanocytes are found in the stratum malpighii but, in contrast to melanoma, basal layer melanocytes are not increased [1–9].

Melanotic macules occasionally appear suddenly as reactive lesions following trauma.

Excision biopsy may be indicated to exclude melanoma.

PART 10: SITES, SEX, AGE

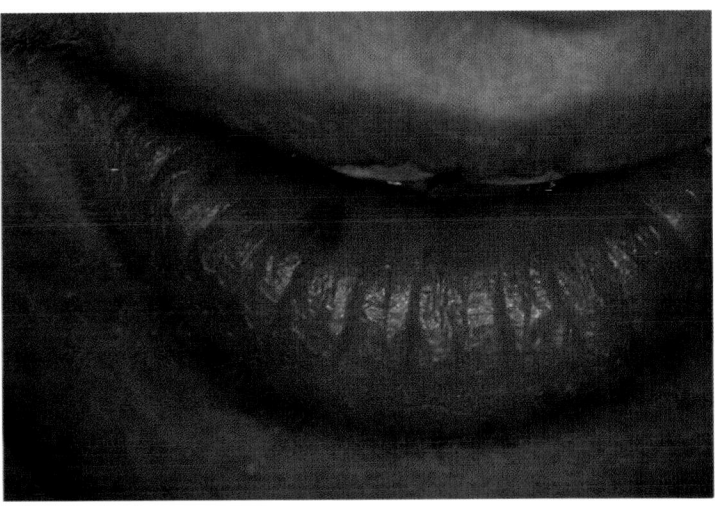

Figure 110.50 Melanotic macule of the lower lip.

Pigmentary incontinence [1]

Melanin pigment ingested by macrophages in the upper lamina propria (pigmentary incontinence) may give rise to hyperpigmentation in lichen planus, especially in dark-skinned people [1].

Purpura

Petechiae are usually caused by trauma, often from suction, but senile purpura or a thrombocytopathy (as in chemotherapy, infectious mononucleosis, HIV infection or leukaemia) must be excluded [1,2] (Figure 110.51). Petechiae may be seen in parvovirus-related papular-purpuric 'gloves and socks' syndrome [3,5].

Blood-filled blisters may be seen in localized oral purpura (angina bullosa haemorrhagica) and pemphigoid, and occasionally

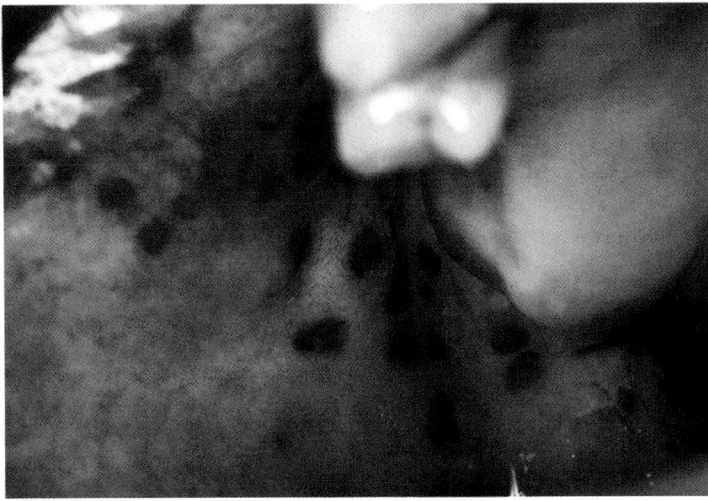

Figure 110.51 Oral purpura in thrombocytopenia.

in amyloidosis [3,4,7]. Rarely a purpuric lesion may be seen in pigmented purpuric stomatitis [6].

RED LESIONS

Some oral red lesions are due to superficial staining with, for example, betel, but most are inflammatory in nature, although epithelial thinning (in geographic tongue) and desquamation (in desquamative gingivitis) are fairly common, and epithelial atrophy is an important cause, especially in deficiency glossitis and erythroplasia. Tattoos may be red. Telangiectases are usually red and haemangiomas purplish in colour.

Angina bullosa haemorrhagica

Synonyms and inclusions
• Localized oral purpura

This is the term given to a benign fairly common condition of unknown aetiology that usually presents in the elderly with oral blood blisters. These subepithelial blisters are seen mainly in the soft palate and after a few hours rupture to leave ulcers (Figure 110.52). The patients appear well otherwise, with no detectable immunological or bleeding disorder [1–3,4,5]. Occasional cases are related to the use of corticosteroid inhalers. Only symptomatic care is available.

Candidosis

Candidosis often presents with oral white lesions but red variants are increasingly recognized. The overall prognosis is typically good, and rarely is the condition life threatening with invasive or recalcitrant disease.

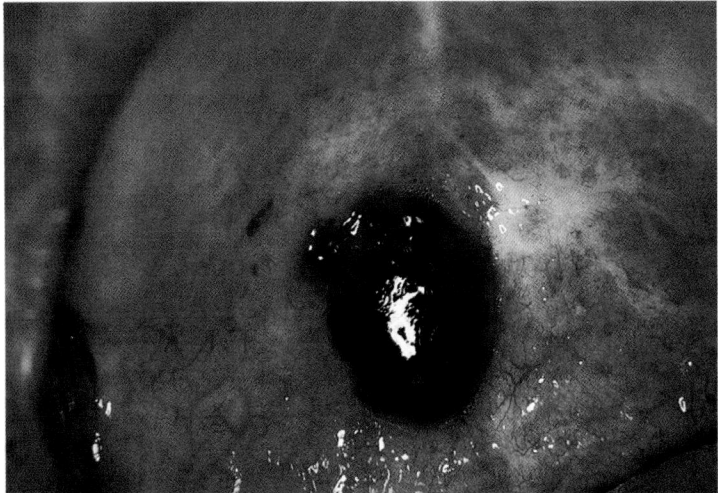

Figure 110.52 Angina bullosa haemorrhagica: a large blood blister in a typical site on the soft palate. The adjacent whitish lesions are from scarring after a previous biopsy.

Acute candidosis

Acute oral candidosis may complicate corticosteroid or antibiotic therapy, particularly with long-term broad-spectrum antimicrobials such as used in transplant or terminally ill patients [1–5]. There is widespread erythema and soreness of the oral mucosa, particularly noticeable on the tongue, sometimes with associated thrush. Topical antifungals usually suffice [6].

Denture-related stomatitis

Synonyms and inclusions
- Denture sore mouth

This common form of mild, chronic, atrophic oral candidosis occurs only beneath a denture, usually a complete upper denture, and is not often sore despite its name.

Incidence and prevalence. In some studies of institutionalized older patients, as many as 70% have been found to have denture-related stomatitis but overall it is considerably less common, particularly in normal healthy subjects.

Age. Older.

Associated diseases. Dentures worn throughout the night, or with a dry mouth, favour development of this infection with *Candida* species mainly. It is not caused by allergy to the denture material and it is not clear why only some denture wearers develop the condition. It is a disease mainly of the middle-aged or elderly and is more prevalent in women than men. Patients appear otherwise healthy.

Denture-related stomatitis consists of mild inflammation and erythema of the mucosa beneath a denture (Figure 110.53).

Pathology. Dentures can produce a number of ecological changes, including the following:
- Changes in the oral flora.
- Plaque accumulation between the mucosal surface of the denture and the palate.

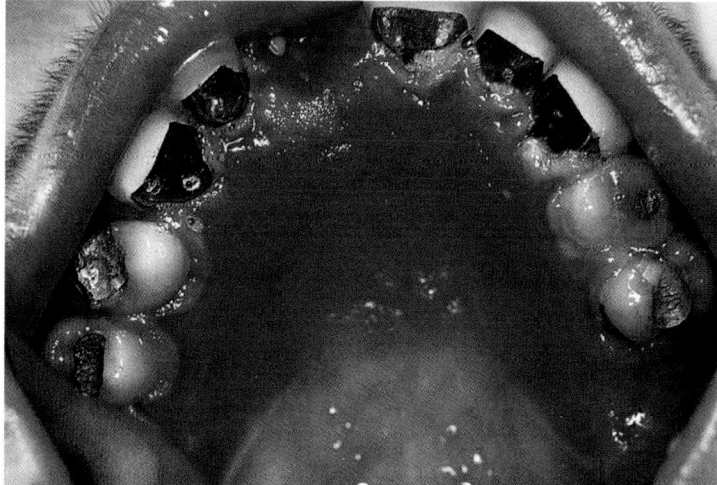

Figure 110.53 Denture-induced stomatitis showing diffuse erythema in the denture-bearing area.

- Saliva present between the maxillary denture and the mucosa may have a lower pH than usual.
- Accumulation of microbial plaque (bacteria and/or yeasts) on and in the fitting surface of the denture and the underlying mucosa.

In some persons, the cause appears to be related to a non-specific plaque. This plaque undergoes sequential development, and is colonized by *Candida* organisms mainly. Mycelial adhesion increases with surface roughness of the resin because mycelia infiltrate the minute protuberances on rough surfaces. Although there is no increased aspartyl proteinase production from the *Candida* involved, the decreased salivary flow and a low pH under the denture probably results in a high *Candida* enzymatic activity, which can cause inflammation.

Yeasts such as *Candida* are isolated from up to 90% of persons with denture-related stomatitis and even 66% of all denture wearers. The most frequently isolated species is *Candida albicans*. Of the *C. albicans* isolates, 75% are serotype A and 25% serotype B, a significant increase in serotype B compared with a control group of non-denture-wearing HIV-seronegative individuals with oral candidosis. Resistogram strain C is the most predominant (24% of total isolates), while strain A-CDE is the least (1.5% of total isolates). Adherence of *C. albicans* to denture-base materials *in vitro* is related to the hydrophobicity of the organism. When *Candida* is involved in denture-related stomatitis, the more common terms 'Candida-associated denture stomatitis', 'denture-induced candidosis' or 'chronic atrophic candidosis' are used. However, denture-related stomatitis is not exclusively associated with *Candida* and, occasionally, other factors such as bacterial infection or mechanical irritation are at play [16]. *C. albicans* is the most frequently isolated species, followed by *C. tropicalis* and *C. glabrata*.

C. dubliniensis. S. aureus, S. epidermidis and *Klebsiella pneumonia* may also be present. The association between *Candida* spp. and bacteria suggests that these microorganisms may play important roles in the establishment and persistence of the disease. Histological examination of the soft tissue beneath dentures has shown proliferative or degenerative responses with reduced keratinization and thinner epithelium.

However, it is not clear why only some denture wearers develop denture-related stomatitis, since most patients appear otherwise healthy. There have been few studies. Patients with denture-related stomatitis have no serious, cell-mediated immune defects but they may sometimes be deficient in migration inhibition factor and may have overactive suppressor T cells or other T-lymphocyte/phagocyte defects. Mean concentrations of serum IL-6 and TNF-α are statistically significantly higher and soluble TNF receptors lower in denture wearers compared with controls but there are no differences when stomatitis is present [1,2–26].

Predisposing factors. Dental appliances (mainly maxillary dentures), especially when worn throughout the night, or with a dry mouth, are the major predisposing factor. Diabetes, immunosuppressive therapy or a high-carbohydrate diet occasionally predispose and HIV is a rare underlying factor.

Factors that are usually *not* significant include allergy to the dental material (if it were, denture-related stomatitis would affect mucosae other than just that beneath the appliance), trauma (the condition is more common beneath maxillary dentures than mandibular dentures, yet trauma is more common with the latter), pharmacological agents and smoking.

Clinical features. The characteristic presenting features of denture-related stomatitis are:
- Chronic erythema and oedema of the mucosa that contacts the fitting surface of the denture (usually a complete upper denture).
- The mucosa below lower dentures is rarely involved.
- Erythema is restricted to the denture-bearing area.
- Usually there are no symptoms.
- Uncommon complications include angular stomatitis, and papillary hyperplasia in the vault of the palate.

Clinical variants. The lesions have been classified into three clinical types (Newton's types), increasing in severity.
- Type 1: a localized simple inflammation or a pinpoint hyperaemia.
- Type 2: an erythematous or generalized simple type presenting as more diffuse erythema involving a part of, or the entire, denture covered mucosa.
- Type 3: a granular type (inflammatory papillary hyperplasia) commonly involving the central part of the hard palate and the alveolar ridge.

Investigations. Denture-related stomatitis is a clinical diagnosis.

Management. Any underlying systemic disease should be treated where possible. The oral biofilm must be removed regularly. The denture plaque and fitting surface is infested, usually with *C. albicans* and dentures acts as a reservoir for microbial colonization.

Therefore, to treat (and prevent recurrence of) denture-related stomatitis, dentures should be removed from the mouth at night, cleaned and disinfected, and stored in an antiseptic. Disinfection modalities, antifungal medications, antiseptic mouthwashes, natural antimicrobial substances and photodynamic therapy could be adjuncts or alternatives.

Cleansing is crucial to therapeutic success. Microwave irradiation in combination with soaking in denture cleanser and brushing effectively disinfects dentures and removes denture biofilm. Microwave disinfection, at once per week for two treatments, can be as effective as topical antifungal therapy for treating denture stomatitis. Sodium hypochlorite 0.5% can help disinfect denture liners and tissue conditioners. Hypochlorite is an effective anticandidal agent but can turn chrome cobalt dentures black. The incorporation of nystatin in those materials is also able to treat or prevent oral candidosis. Denture cleansers also include chlorhexidine gluconate, alkaline peroxides, alkaline hypochlorites, acids, Brazilian green propolis, melaleuca oil, proteolytic enzymes, *Ricinus communis*, *Salvia officinalis* L. and yeast lytic enzymes.

The mucosal infection is eradicated by brushing the palate and using antifungals for at least 4 weeks. Effective agents include nystatin pastilles or suspension, amphotericin lozenges, miconazole gel or fluconazole suspension or tablets, administered concurrently with an oral antiseptic such as chlorhexidine, which itself has antifungal activity [26–67].

Surgery may occasionally be needed to excise papillary hyperplasia [68].

Resources

Further information

http://emedicine.medscape.com/article/1075227-overview (last accessed December 2014).

HIV-associated candidosis

Fungal infections in and around the mouth have increased greatly, especially candidosis, particularly as the HIV epidemic has spread, and now other species (especially *C. krusei*) and antifungal resistance are serious clinical realities [1–10]. There may be transmission of *Candida* species from HIV-infected persons [9] and new species and clades are being recognized [10,11]. Low CD4 counts, and denture-wearing predispose to candidosis.

The most dominant oral fungal species, in decreasing order of frequency, are:
- *C. albicans.*
- *C. glabrata.*
- *C. tropicalis.*
- *C. parapsilosis* (*C. parapsilosis sensu stricto*, *C. metapsilosis* and *C. orthopsilosis*).
- *C. krusei.*
- Other *Candida* species such as *C. dubliniensis*, *C. africanus* and *C. inconspicua.*
- Other genera (*Rhodotorula, Saccharomyces,* etc.), which are rare and transient.

Erythematous or atrophic candidosis may arise as a consequence of persistent acute pseudomembranous candidosis when the pseudomembranes are shed, may develop *de novo*, or in HIV infection may precede pseudomembranous candidosis. The clinical presentation is of erythematous areas generally on the dorsum of the tongue, palate or buccal mucosa. Lesions on the dorsum of the tongue present as depapillated areas. Red areas are often seen in the palate in HIV disease. There can be an associated angular stomatitis and/or thrush.

Thrush is a well-recognized feature of T-cell immunodeficiencies, particularly after the severe T-cell immunosuppression necessary for organ transplantation and in other secondary immunodeficiencies, such as leukaemia, diabetes or HIV/AIDS. It is a common and early feature of AIDS [1–19].

Furthermore, with increasing use of antimycotic therapy, especially in HIV disease, there is a shift towards not only resistant *C. albicans*, as well as the appearance of novel species, but also other species such as *C. glabrata* and *C. krusei*. Thrush is characterized by white patches on the surface of the oral mucosa, tongue and elsewhere. The lesions develop to form confluent plaques that resemble milk curds, and can be wiped off to reveal a raw, erythematous and sometimes bleeding base. Complications of oropharyngeal thrush may sometimes present as lesions of the adjacent mucosa, particularly in the upper respiratory tract and the oesophagus. The combination of oral and oesophageal candidosis is particularly prevalent in HIV-infected patients.

Antifungal therapy is indicated [20–22]. Gentian violet solution at the concentration of 0.00165% does not stain the oral mucosa, is stable and possesses potent antifungal activity. HAART reduces the frequency of candidosis [13]. The therapeutic benefits of HAART are: immune reconstitution; reduction of the HIV/AIDS-related oral diseases; prevention and cure of AIDS-related neoplasms; and reduction in maternofetal transmission of HIV. The negative effects of HAART are: increase in oral lesions from HPV; xerostomia; dysgeusia/ageusia, hyposmia, perioral paraesthesia; hyperpigmentation of oral mucosa; facial lipodystrophy; and ulceration.

Median rhomboid glossitis

Synonyms and inclusions
- Central papillary atrophy of the tongue

This red, depapillated, rhomboidal, flat maculate or mamillated and raised benign lesion is seen almost invariably in the midline of the dorsum of the tongue, just anterior to the sulcus terminalis.

Incidence and prevalence. Uncommon.

Age. Mainly older patients.

Associated diseases. There is a significant association between median rhomboid glossitis, *Candida* and diabetes, but the other possible risk factors, such as gender, smoking and denture, wearing may not be present. Occasionally, immune defects (including HIV) and diabetes predispose to this lesion [1–9].

Pathophysiology. Histology shows irregular pseudoepitheliomatous epithelial hyperplasia that may resemble a carcinoma but it is not a malignant condition.

Clinical features. There is typically a red central lesion of somewhat rhomboidal shape anterior to the sulcus terminalis on the dorsum of the tongue (Figure 110.54) sometimes with discomfort. Occasionally, there is a nodular component. Multiple oral lesions may occasionally be present, especially a 'kissing' lesion in the palatal vault. There may also sometimes be a coexistent erythematous candidosis in the palate, which some have termed 'chronic oral multifocal candidosis'.

Investigations. Median rhomboid glossitis is usually diagnosed on clinical grounds. Long disease duration and no benefit from topical steroids are suggestive of this condition. The differential diagnosis may include haemangioma, pyogenic granuloma, amyloidosis, granular cell tumour, Kaposi sarcoma and neoplasms [10–12]. Since some lesions are nodular and may simulate a neoplasm or other pathology, biopsy may be indicated.

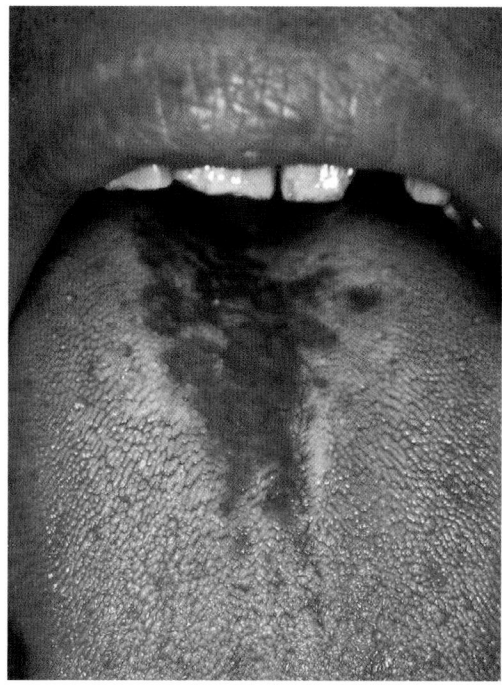

Figure 110.54 Median rhomboid glossitis.

Management. Median rhomboid glossitis may respond to cessation of smoking and to the use of antifungals [13]. After antifungal treatment, tongue pain disappears or improves markedly in most.

Desquamative gingivitis

This is an erosive condition, usually caused by pemphigoid or lichen planus but is also seen in patients with pemphigus vulgaris and lupus erythematosus [1,2,3].

Erythroplasia

Erythroplasia (erythroplakia) is a red velvety lesion level with, or depressed below, the surrounding mucosa. It is uncommon and affects patients of either sex in their sixth and seventh decades [1,2,**3**,**4**]. Erythroplasia usually is solitary and involves the floor of the mouth, the ventrum of the tongue or the soft palate (Figure 110.55) [1,2,**3**,4,5]. Risk factors for erythroplasia are as for carcinoma, mainly tobacco, alcohol and betel. A more than additive interaction has been found between tobacco chewing and low vegetable intake, whereas a more than multiplicative interaction has been found between alcohol drinking and low vegetable intake, and between drinking and low fruit intake [6].

Some 75–90% of cases of erythroplasia prove to be carcinoma or carcinoma *in situ* or show severe dysplasia. The incidence of malignant change in erythroplasia is 17 times higher than in leukoplakia.

Areas of erythroplasia should be removed by surgery, either by cold knife (scalpel) or by laser excision, and sent for histological

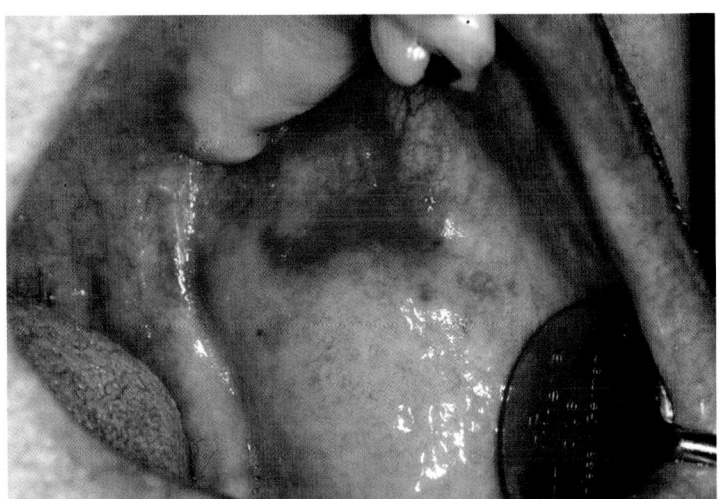

Figure 110.55 Erythroplasia.

examination but there are no reliable data about the prognosis or recurrence rate.

Resources

Further information

http://emedicine.medscape.com/article/1840467-overview (last accessed December 2014).

Glossitis

See p. 110.64.

Larva migrans (see Chapter 33)

Cutaneous larva migrans is rarely seen in the mouth, where it presents as irregular linear lesions with an inflammatory border resembling erythema migrans [1,2].

Strawberry tongue

Prominence of the lingual papillae may be seen in scarlet fever, Kawasaki disease and Riley–Day syndrome (familial dysautonomia), giving rise to an appearance similar to a strawberry [1].

Telangiectasia (see Chapter 103)

Oral telangiectases occur mainly in hereditary haemorrhagic telangiectasia, CREST (calcinosis, Raynaud, esophageal, sclerodactyly, telangiectasia) syndrome [1–3] (see Chapter 56), chronic liver disease, pregnancy [4] and after irradiation.

Varicosities

Bluish oral varicosities may often be seen in elderly patients, particularly in the ventrum and lateral margin of the tongue. They are benign and inconsequential.

Vascular proliferative lesions

Benign atypical vascular lesions may exhibit cytological or architectural features that simulate angiosarcoma such that considerable caution is required in diagnosis [1]. The head and neck region is a common location, particularly for lobular capillary haemangioma (pyogenic granuloma), while the lip is an especially common site for lobular capillary haemangioma [2–5] and intravascular papillary endothelial hyperplasia (Masson haemangioma or pseudoangiosarcoma) [5,6]. Intravascular papillary endothelial hyperplasia is a benign non-neoplastic vascular lesion characterized histologically by papillary fronds lined by proliferating endothelium and probably represents an organizing thrombus. Seen mainly in the lip or tongue in females, it may simulate angiosarcoma histologically [7]. Excision suffices.

Vascular lesions such as epithelioid haemangioma, epithelioid haemangioendothelioma, spindle cell haemangioendothelioma, acquired progressive lymphangioma or angiosarcoma and Kaposi sarcoma may need to be excluded.

Venous lake

Synonyms and inclusions
- Venous varix
- Senile haemangioma of lip

This is a bluish-purple soft swelling, 2–10 mm in diameter, usually seen on the lower lip of an elderly person, due to a venous dilatation (Figure 110.56). The lesion is lined by a single layer of

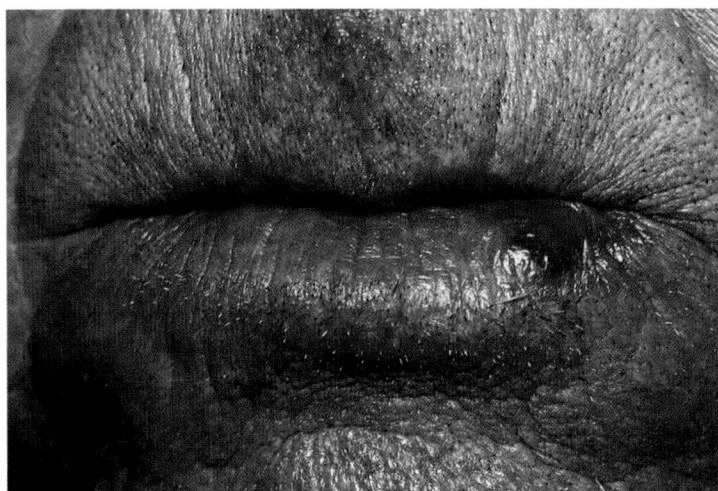

Figure 110.56 Venous lake of the lip. (Courtesy of Addenbrooke's Hospital, Cambridge, UK.)

flattened endothelial cells with a thick wall of fibrous tissue. The lesion empties on prolonged pressure [1–4].

A venous lake may be only a trivial cosmetic problem or it can bleed severely after trauma. It can be excised, but careful cryotherapy, electrocautery, infrared coagulation or treatment with an argon laser [2–4] can also give good results.

WHITE LESIONS

Congenital lesions are discussed on p. 110.17.

Acquired white lesions in the mouth are usually caused by materia alba (Figure 110.57), cheek biting or chemical burns, but keratoses, infections (mainly candidosis), dermatoses (usually lichen planus), neoplastic disorders and other conditions must be excluded (see Box 110.2).

Burns

Chemical burns (due, for example, to holding mouthwashes in the mouth or drugs against the buccal mucosa) or burns caused by heat, cold or irradiation can cause white sloughing lesions of the mucosa [1–11]. Such lesions typically heal spontaneously within 1–3 weeks.

Candidosis

Up to 50% of the healthy population harbour *Candida albicans* as an oral commensal. Carriage is more common in cigarette smokers. *Candida* resides particularly on the posterior dorsum of the tongue [1–8].

Infection is likely to result from xerostomia, local disturbances in salivary flora such as occurs during broad-spectrum antimicrobial treatment, or depressed immune responses [1–4,9–13]. Of the several clinical presentations of oral candidosis, only thrush,

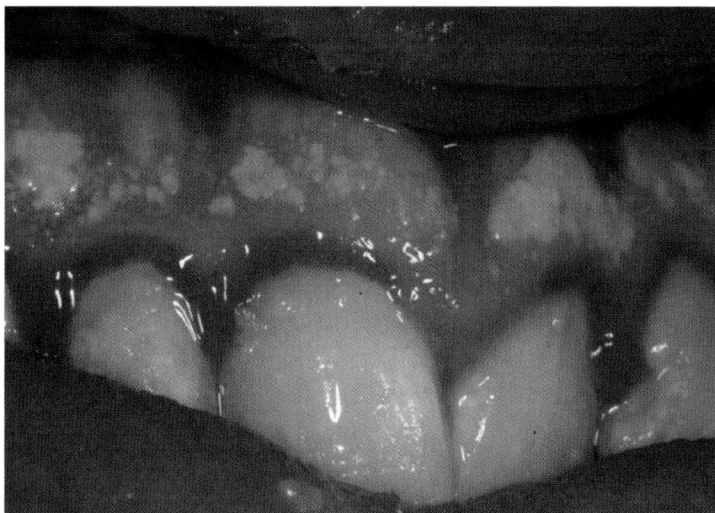

Figure 110.57 Materia alba.

Table 110.12 Intraoral candidosis.

Type of candidosis	Usual age at onset	Predisposing factors*
Acute pseudomembranous candidosis (thrush)†	Any	Local: dry mouth, antimicrobials General: corticosteroids, leukaemia, HIV
Acute atrophic candidosis ('antibiotic mouth'; antibiotic sore mouth)	Any	Broad-spectrum antibiotics or corticosteroids
Erythematous candidosis		Any, HIV especially
Chronic atrophic candidosis (denture-related stomatitis)	Adults	Denture wearing, especially at night
Chronic hyperplastic candidosis (candidal leukoplakia)†	Usually middle aged or elderly	Tobacco smoking, denture wearing, immune defect
Median rhomboid glossitis	Third or later decades	Tobacco smoking, denture wearing, HIV
Chronic mucocutaneous candidosis†	Usually first decade	Often immune defect; rarely endocrinopathy

*Immune defects can predispose to any form.
†White lesions.

candidal leukoplakia and chronic mucocutaneous candidosis present as white lesions; the other types, acute and chronic atrophic candidosis, are red (Table 110.12).

Thrush

Synonyms and inclusions
- Acute pseudomembranous candidosis

Aetiology. Healthy neonates, who have yet to develop immunity to *Candida* species, may develop thrush. In other patients, predisposing factors include antibiotic or corticosteroid use, xerostomia and severe T-cell immune defects associated with immunosuppression (e.g. given to prevent graft rejection in organ transplantation) or immunodeficiencies such as leukaemia or HIV disease. Thrush is a common and early feature of HIV infection and may be a portent of developing AIDS [1–4,10,12,13].

Clinical features. The soft creamy patches of thrush, which resemble milk curds, can be wiped off the oral mucosa with gauze, leaving an area of erythema (Figure 110.58).

Chronic candidosis

Aetiology. The aetiology of chronic oral candidosis is unclear and in only a few patients can either a local cause or underlying immune defect be identified [1–3]. HIV/AIDS and chronic mucocutaneous candidosis syndromes are rare causes (see Chapter 32).

Clinical features. Longstanding oral candidosis may produce tough adherent white patches (chronic hyperplastic candidosis or candidal leukoplakias) which can have a malignant potential,

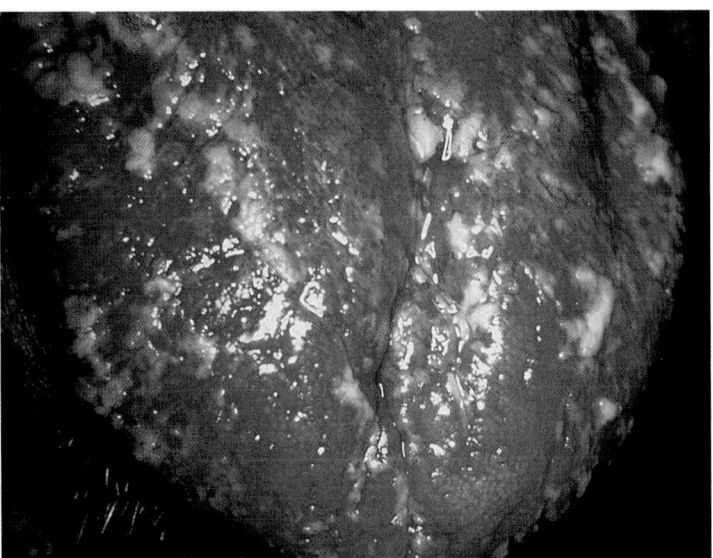

Figure 110.58 Thrush: scattered white lesions on an erythematous background.

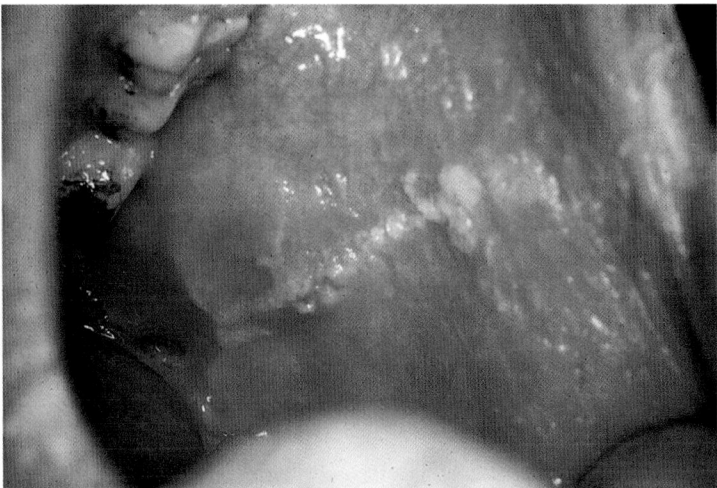

Figure 110.59 Frictional keratosis and cheek biting (morsicatio buccarum) at the occlusal line.

and may be indistinguishable from other leukoplakias except by biopsy. Candidal leukoplakias may, however, be speckled.

Diagnosis of candidosis. The diagnosis of oral thrush is usually clinical but it tends to be overdiagnosed by physicians. In contrast, erythematous candidosis is probably underdiagnosed. In immunosuppressed patients, a Gram-stained smear should be taken to distinguish thrush from the plaques produced by opportunistic bacteria. Hyphae seem to indicate that the *Candida* organisms are acting as pathogens and not simple commensals. However, there is no convincing evidence of any test able to discriminate the transition from candidal saprophytism to pathogenicity.

Suspected candidal leukoplakia should be biopsied, both to distinguish it from other non-candidal plaques and also because of possible dysplasia. Although candidal hyphae and a neutrophil infiltrate may be seen on haematoxylin and eosin staining, PAS will demonstrate the purple staining of the hyphae.

Management
- **Acute candidosis.** Except in healthy neonates, possible predisposing causes should be looked for and treated. Topical polyenes such as nystatin or amphotericin, or imidazoles such as miconazole are often indicated but, in HIV infection, antiretroviral agents and fluconazole may be required.
- **Chronic hyperplastic candidosis.** The oral lesions of chronic hyperplastic candidosis may respond poorly to the polyenes [6]. These cases, and some cases of chronic mucocutaneous candidosis, may respond only to flucytosine, ketoconazole, fluconazole, itraconazole, voriconazole or caspofungin [1,14–19].

Cheek biting

Synonyms and inclusions
- Morsicatio buccarum

A horizontal white line may be seen in the buccal mucosa of healthy people (linea alba) but can be exaggerated in tense individuals. Cheek biting causes a whitish shredded appearance usually of the buccal or lower labial mucosa at the occlusal line (adjacent to where the teeth meet) (Figure 110.59) [1–8]. The habit is most common in tense or anxious individuals who may also show bruxism, mandibular (myofascial) pain dysfunction or other oral features of psychogenic disorders. The lesion is benign but may simulate white sponge naevus (see p. 110.19), leukoplakia or lichen planus.

Cheilitis (actinic)

See p. 110.78.

Hairy leukoplakia

Aetiology. Hairy leukoplakia is seen in severe immune defects, especially HIV/AIDS, and occasionally in the apparently immunocompetent [1–6]. HIV is not found within the genome of epithelial cells in hairy leukoplakia and it is more likely that the features are a consequence of an opportunistic infection with EBV. It is now clear that normal human oral mucosa from HIV-negative and HIV-positive individuals may contain latent EBV [7–10]. A decreased frequency of HIV-related oral manifestations including oral hairy leukoplakia has been associated with the introduction of HAART [5].

Epstein–Barr virus has been shown to be present in hairy leukoplakia, especially in the upper layers of the epithelium. The oral site of predilection for hairy leukoplakia appears to relate to the presence of EBV receptors only on the parakeratinized mucosae such as the lateral margin of the tongue. Hairy leukoplakia regresses on treatment with antivirals but fails to resolve with antifungals, despite the frequent presence of *Candida* species.

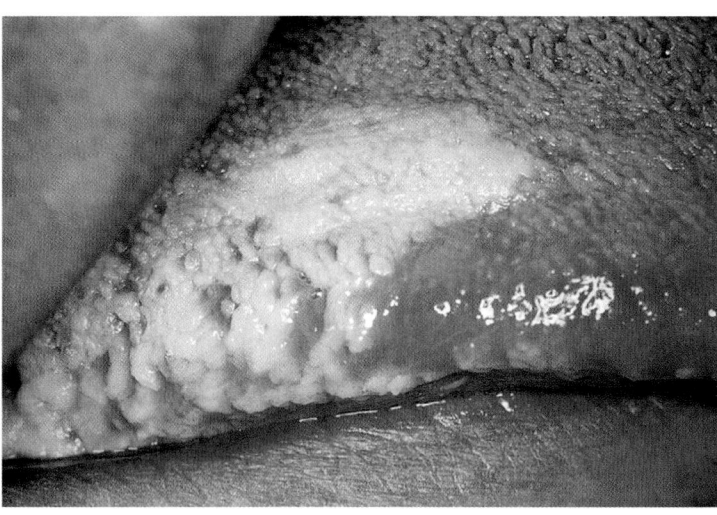

Figure 110.60 Hairy leukoplakia. Found mainly in HIV infection, vertical white ridges on the lateral margin of the tongue.

Pathology. Histological features include hyperparakeratosis, hyperplasia and ballooning of prickle cells, few or absent Langerhans cells, and only a sparse inflammatory cell infiltrate in the lamina propria.

Clinical features. Hairy leukoplakia is a white patch, usually seen on the parakeratinized mucosa of the tongue, frequently bilaterally (Figure 110.60). The lesions are corrugated or have a shaggy or hairy appearance, are mostly symptomless and, unlike some oral keratoses, have no known premalignant potential [1,4,10,11]. The majority of the affected patients who are HIV-positive appear eventually to develop AIDS. Hairy leukoplakia also occurs in HIV-negative persons [6,12–19].

Diagnosis. Some of the histological features typical of hairy leukoplakia, especially the hyperparakeratosis, can be seen in oral white lesions other than hairy leukoplakia in HIV-infected persons [20]. Not only are there oral lesions that mimic hairy leukoplakia in HIV infection, but lesions similar to hairy leukoplakia can be seen in other immunocompromised persons and even in some apparently healthy individuals. However, most cases can be distinguished from the hairy leukoplakia of HIV infection by the absence of EBV DNA on histology and, of course, by the presence of HIV serum antibody.

Management. Hairy leukoplakia really needs no treatment but in HIV/AIDS antiretroviral agents, aciclovir or ganciclovir may cause resolution.

Keratoses

Aetiology. The cause of most keratoses is unknown (idiopathic keratoses) but some are caused by chronic irritation, particular lifestyle habits or infective agents as follows.
- *Tobacco-induced keratoses.* Consumption of tobacco products has long been causally connected with oral cancer and is a common cause of keratosis. Tobacco use also predisposes to cancers elsewhere in the upper aerodigestive tract, bladder and other sites. Tobacco use should thus be discouraged; the drug amfebutamone or varenicline may help users break the habit.
- *Tobacco chewing.* Tobacco is chewed in many parts of the world and may induce keratosis. In many communities from resource-poor countries, tobacco is a component of betel quid, along with *Areca* nut and betel leaf, and sometimes slaked lime and spices. Sometimes betel is used without tobacco (pan or paan), though others use paan with tobacco. Oral carcinoma can result.
- *Reverse smoking (bidi).* In some communities, especially in Asia, cigarettes are smoked with the lit end within the mouth. Palatal or other oral carcinoma can result.
- *Cigarette-induced keratoses.* Mild keratosis may be seen especially on the palate, lip (occasionally nicotine-stained) and at the commissures, along with nicotine-stained teeth. Malignant change is uncommon.
- *Pipe smoking.* Diffuse whiteness over the palate is termed 'smoker's keratosis' or 'stomatitis nicotina'. The palatal minor salivary gland orifices appear red against this white background. Malignant change is uncommon.
- *Cigar smoking.* Cigar smokers may develop stomatitis nicotina and nicotine-stained teeth. Malignant change is uncommon.
- *Snuff dipper's keratosis and other smokeless tobacco lesions.* Snuff may produce keratosis – white hyperkeratotic lesions caused by snuff-dipping (holding flavoured tobacco powder in the oral sulcus or vestibule), together with gingival recession at the site of use. Malignant change is rare.

Koplik spots (see Chapter 25)

White specks may be seen in the buccal mucosa in early measles.

Leukoplakia

Definition
The World Health Organization defines leukoplakia as a white patch or plaque on the mucosa that cannot be rubbed off and that is not recognized as a specific disease entity [1–4], which implies a diagnosis of exclusion (e.g. of lichen planus, candidosis). By definition, the term excludes entities such as frictional keratosis or smoker's keratosis. The term is also used irrespective of the presence or absence of epithelial dysplasia, although there is a small malignant potential to some lesions [1–6].

Epidemiology

Incidence and prevalence
Leukoplakia is common in adults: around 1% are affected, although some populations show higher prevalences.

Age
Most cases are seen in the 50–70 age group.

Sex
Males more than females.

Pathophysiology

Predisposing factors
Risk factors for leukoplakia are as for carcinoma, mainly tobacco, alcohol and betel. Other factors may include:
- Proliferative verrucous leukoplakia – often associated with HPV. Malignant change is uncommon.
- Candidal leukoplakias – may be associated with an increased risk of malignant change, although it is uncommon.
- Syphilitic leukoplakia – rarely seen now. Malignant change is common.

Pathology
Leukoplakias show, to a varying degree, increased keratin production, change in epithelial thickness and disordered epithelial maturation. Mild dysplasia is not usually regarded as of serious significance. The presence of severe epithelial dysplasia is thought to indicate a considerable risk of malignant development. Pagetoid dyskeratosis is considered a selective keratinocytic response in which a small part of the normal population of keratinocytes is induced to proliferate in response to friction. Pagetoid dyskeratosis has been found in 42.2% of lip biopsies, more frequent in younger patients and in women. Pagetoid cells are more common in suprabasal location and in the labial mucosa. These cells show positivity for high-molecular-weight cytokeratin and negative reaction for low-molecular-weight cytokeratin, epithelial membrane antigen, carcinoembryonic antigen and HPV. The immunohistochemical profile is different from the surrounding keratinocytes, indicating premature keratinization. The morphological features of dyskeratotic pagetoid cells are distinctive and easily recognized as an incidental finding, thus preventing confusion with other important entities including an intraepidermal tumour.

The main differential diagnoses include white sponge naevus, leukoedema, oral koilocytoses, hairy leukoplakia, pagetoid squamous cell carcinoma *in situ* and extramammary Paget disease of the oral mucosa.

Clinical features
Leukoplakias vary in size: some are small and focal, others more widespread, occasionally involving very large areas of the oral mucosa; in other patients several discrete separate areas of leukoplakia can be seen. Leukoplakia has a wide range of clinical presentations, from homogeneous white plaques that can be faintly white or very thick and opaque, to nodular white lesions or lesions admixed with red lesions [1–4]. The malignant potential depends on the following.

Homogeneous leukoplakia, the most common, presents with uniformly white plaques, common in the buccal (cheek) mucosa and usually of low premalignant potential (Figure 110.61).

Non-homogeneous or heterogeneous leukoplakias are nodular, verrucous and speckled leukoplakias that consist of white patches or nodules in a red, often eroded, area of mucosa (Figure 110.62). They have a high risk of malignant transformation and are therefore far more serious.

High-risk sites for malignant transformation include the soft palate complex and ventrolateral tongue and floor of the mouth (where sublingual keratosis has a particularly high risk of

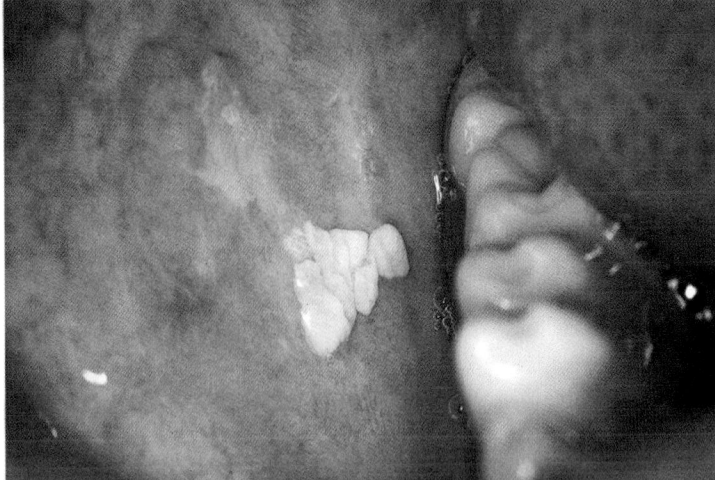

Figure 110.61 Homogeneous leukoplakia in the buccal mucosa.

malignant change; Figure 110.63). Sublingual keratosis is more common in women than men, has a typical 'ebbing-tide' appearance clinically and has a high malignant potential.

Disease course and prognosis
Leukoplakia can be totally benign or sometimes can be precancerous or a marker for cancer elsewhere in the upper aerodigestive tract. The prevalence of malignant transformation in leukoplakias ranges from 3 to 33% over 10 years; homogeneous leukoplakias are only very occasionally premalignant, but speckled or verrucous leukoplakias are more likely to be premalignant.

Leukoplakia is much more common than erythroplakia and it also is associated mainly with tobacco and alcohol. Leukoplakia can appear as:
- Homogeneous leukoplakia (flat, thin, uniform white in colour).
- Non-homogeneous leukoplakia, either:
  - A white-and-red lesion ('erythroleukoplakia'), that may be either irregularly flat (speckled), or
  - Nodular, or

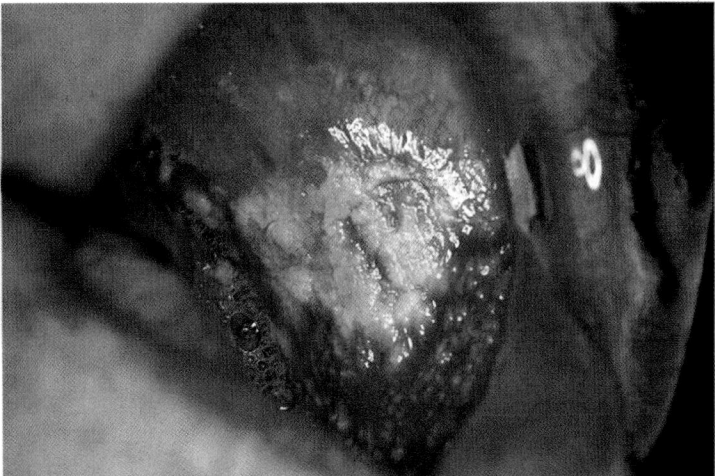

Figure 110.62 Speckled leukoplakia.

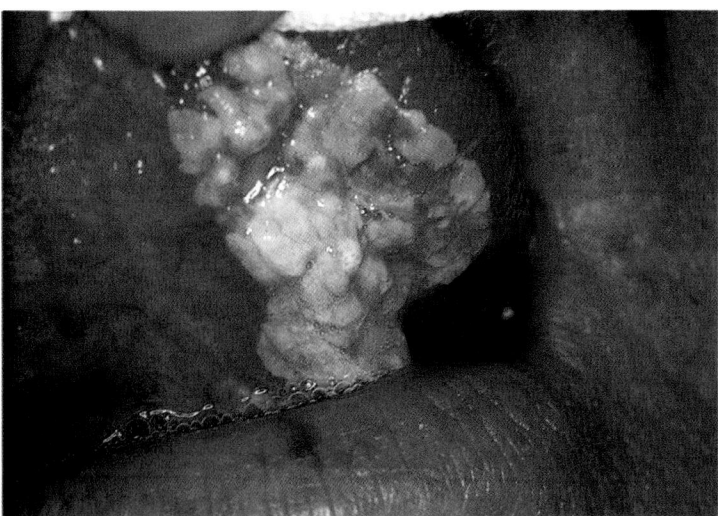

Figure 110.63 Sublingual keratosis.

- Verrucous. Proliferative verrucous leukoplakia (PVL) is a special subtype of verrucous leukoplakia, characterized by multifocal lesions, and a high malignant transformation rate.

There is clear evidence of the malignant potential of some oral leukoplakias. An annual malignant transformation rate of about 1–2% over 10 years is probably a realistic figure for leukoplakias overall. In dysplastic leukoplakias, however, the malignant transformation may reach 30%. Biomarkers such as DNA ploidy, and changes in the tumour suppressor gene p53, and loss of heterozygosity (LOH) in chromosomes 3 and 9 that might predict malignant change and other indicators are shown in Boxes 110.11 and 110.12, but it is not possible at present reliably to predict which lesions will progress to carcinoma nor to be absolutely certain that a lesion has malignant potential or not.

Overall, around 2–5% of leukoplakias become malignant in 10 years and 5–20% of leukoplakias are dysplastic. Of leukoplakias with dysplasia, 10–35% proceed to carcinoma. Malignant change to carcinoma is most frequent in women older than 50 years and in large lesions. Interestingly, leukoplakias developing in nonsmokers have a higher rather than lower risk of malignant change. However, some leukoplakias (15–30%) regress clinically, not only when supposed aetiological factors have been removed but also sometimes spontaneously, and there is concern over observer and interobserver variation in the diagnosis of dysplasia [7–11].

Investigations

There are no signs or symptoms that reliably predict whether a leukoplakia will undergo malignant change, and thus histology must be used to detect dysplasia. Scalpel or punch biopsy is therefore generally indicated and is mandatory for those leukoplakias that exhibit the following characteristics:

- Are found in patients with previous or concurrent head and neck cancer.
- Are non-homogeneous, i.e. have red areas and/or are verrucous and/or are indurated.
- Are in a high-risk site such as the floor of the mouth or tongue.
- Are focal.
- With symptoms.
- Without obvious aetiological factors.

Many would advise biopsy of all keratoses and leukoplakias.

Management

Management can be difficult, not least because of the wide extent of some lesions, their frequent admixture with areas of erythroplasia (speckled leukoplakias), and controversy as to the prognosis and long-term benefit and effects of various therapies. There is also no scientific evidence that treatment truly prevents the possible future development of a carcinoma.

Possible aetiological factors should be removed, and an observation of 2–4 weeks seems acceptable to observe any possible regression.

Since some potentially malignant lesions which on initial biopsy have shown no serious pathology have, on excision, been shown to contain cancers in up to 10%, it is probably best to remove all oral leukoplakias if feasible, especially if there is epithelial dysplasia on biopsy, rather than so-called 'watchful waiting'. The efficacy of continuous follow-up of oral leukoplakia patients is virtually unknown. Nevertheless, recurrence rates after any form of treatment may be up to 30%, probably mainly depending on the duration of follow-up.

The most commonly used treatments are surgical excision or carbon dioxide laser therapy and the specimen must be sent for histopathological examination [12–17]. For widespread leukoplakias, photodynamic therapy may be considered [18]. The evidence from systematic reviews is that medical therapies are not reliably effective: topical anticancer agents such as podophyllin or bleomycin or retinoids have only temporary efficacy, and perhaps their best indication is when the location or extent of the lesion prevent adequate surgical removal.

Since oral dysplasia predicts a significant rate of transformation to cancer, and was decreased significantly but not eliminated by excision, excision and continued surveillance are prudent. Surgery may thus have a beneficial effect, but there is little evidence that this will reliably reduce the risk of later recurrence, nor malignant transformation of PMD, at the same or another site. Fully informed consent is crucial, all the uncertainties being discussed with the patient.

Resources

Further information
http://emedicine.medscape.com/article/853864-overview (last accessed December 2014)

Lichen planus

See Chapter 37 and p. 110.43.

Psoriasis (see Chapter 35)

The oral mucosa appears to be rarely involved in psoriasis, with less than 100 cases reported, although there are occasionally lip lesions or white oral lesions, especially in the buccal mucosa, or lesions clinically indistinguishable from geographic tongue (sometimes termed 'annulus migrans' or 'erythema circinatum'), particularly in generalized pustular psoriasis [1–15].

ACQUIRED LIP LESIONS

Lip lesions can be seen in many of the disorders described earlier in this chapter; this section covers conditions that manifest mainly or exclusively on the lips alone.

Actinic cheilitis (solar cheilosis)

Definition and nomenclature
This is a premalignant keratosis of the lip caused by exposure to solar irradiation.

Synonyms and inclusions
- Actinic keratosis
- Solar cheilosis
- Sailor's lip

Epidemiology

Age
Most actinic cheilitis is seen on the lower lip of fair-skinned men in their fourth to eighth decade of life.

Sex
Males more than females.

Ethnicity
Caucasian mainly.

Associated diseases
Other UV-related issues.

Pathophysiology

Predisposing factors
UV light. Actinic cheilitis is most common in hot dry regions, especially in outdoor workers and in fair-skinned people (skin types I and II). The vermilion of the lower lip in particular receives a high dose of UV irradiation because it is almost at right angles to the rays of the midday sun and is poorly protected by keratin and melanocytes [1,2–7,8,9]. Tobacco smoking may aggravate. Voriconazole therapy may predispose [10]. In view of an increased risk of lip cancer in non-Hispanic whites receiving treatment for hypertension with long-term use of photosensitizing drugs, these people should take extra care [11].

Pathology
Histology shows a flattened or atrophic epithelium, beneath which is a band of inflammatory infiltrate in which plasma cells may predominate [2]. Nuclear atypia and abnormal mitoses may be seen in the more severe cases, and some develop into invasive squamous carcinoma [3–5]. The collagen generally shows basophilic (elastotic) degeneration [6].

Clinical features (Figure 110.64)
Actinic cheilitis tends to affect the lower lip of adults who have had prolonged exposure to sunlight [1,7]. In the early stages there may be redness and oedema, but later the lips become dry and scaly. Later still, the epithelium becomes palpably thickened with small greyish-white plaques and, eventually, warty nodules may form. Eventually, these may undergo malignant change, the possibility

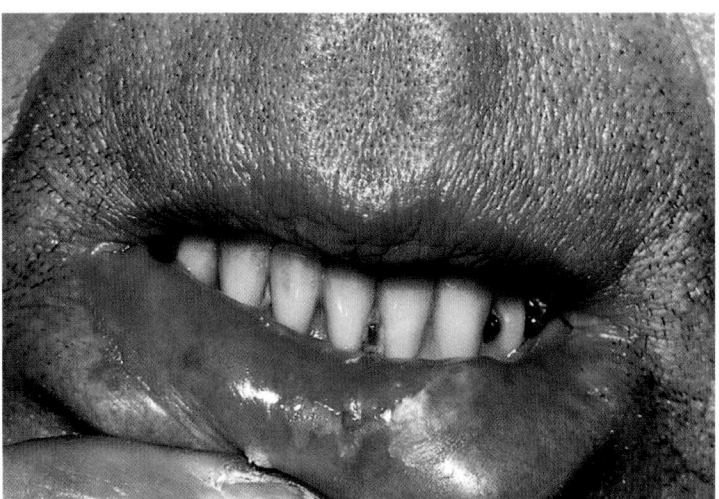

Figure 110.64 Chronic actinic cheilitis with leukoplakia. (Courtesy of Addenbrooke's Hospital, Cambridge, UK.)

of which must always be considered when ulceration develops or when there are other suspect features such as:

- A red and white, blotchy appearance with an indistinct vermilion border.
- Generalized atrophy with focal areas of whitish thickening.
- Persistent flaking and crusting [8,9].
  Ulceration and nodularity may indicate malignant progression.

Investigations
Biopsy may be prudent.

Management
Treatment of actinic cheilitis is required to relieve symptoms and to endeavour to prevent development of squamous carcinoma. Therapies include:

- Topical agents: 5% fluorouracil three times daily for 10 days is suitable [12]. Topical tretinoin [12], trichloracetic acid [13] or diclofenac gel [14] may also be effective.
- Vermilionectomy (lip shave) [15–17].
- Laser ablation [18–24].
- Photodynamic therapy [25–29] sometimes also with imiquimod [30].
  Following treatment, the regular use of a sunscreen lipsalve containing *p*-aminobenzoic acid probably gives the best protection [31–34]. Particular care should be taken to protect the vermilion of the lips with adequate sunscreens in patients with photosensitivity disorders such as xeroderma pigmentosum, in those whose exposure to UVB is high, such as in farmers, fishermen, mountaineers, windsurfers and skiers and those using photosensitizing agents.

Resources

Further information
http://www.dermnetnz.org/site-age-specific/solar-cheilitis.html (last accessed December 2014)

Actinic prurigo (see Chapter 127)

Definition
Actinic prurigo is a photodermatosis characterized by symmetrical involvement of sun-exposed areas of the skin, lips and conjunctivae.

Epidemiology

Incidence and prevalence
Rare, probably <5% of referrals to photodermatology clinics.

Age
Usually manifests during childhood.

Sex
Predominates in women.

Ethnicity
Seen mainly in native populations living at high altitudes especially in Latin America, and in Asia, including in India, Thailand and China. The absence of mucosal involvement is a distinguishing feature between Asian and Caucasian populations.

Associated diseases
Commonly associated with cheilitis and conjunctivitis.

Pathophysiology

Pathology
Histological examination shows acanthosis, mild spongiosis, oedema of the lamina propria, moderate-to-dense in a band-like lymphocytic inflammatory infiltrate, eosinophils and, occasionally, lymphoid follicles.

Genetics
HLA subtype DRB1*0407, is found in actinic prurigo patients in England, Scotland, Ireland, Mexico and Colombia [1–4,**5**,6–14].

Environmental factors
Sun exposure (UV-A and UV-B).

Clinical features
Facial skin and lips are involved in two-thirds of cases with an intensely itchy, excoriated papular and nodular skin eruption, and lip pruritus, oedema, scales, fissures, crusts and ulceration. Polymorphic light eruption (PLE) is usually present in the actinic prurigo of Native Americans. It commonly presents in young women as a photosensitive facial rash with pruritic lower lip cheilitis, and it may be associated with conjunctivitis, eyebrow alopecia and pterygion. HLA-DR4 (DRB1*0407) could be used as a marker to distinguish PLE from actinic prurigo.

Investigations
Biopsy. Actinic prurigo is distinguished from actinic cheilitis, which is due to prolonged and excessive exposure to UV irradiation, by the relative absence of epidermal dysplasia and solar elastosis.

Management
Actinic prurigo treatment is with sunscreens, β-carotene, psoralen and UVA (PUVA), and antihistamines. Oral thalidomide or pentoxifylline may be tried [15–17].

Resources

Further information
http://emedicine.medscape.com/article/1120153-overview (last accessed December 2014)

Angular cheilitis

Definition and nomenclature
Angular cheilitis is an acute or chronic inflammation of the skin and contiguous labial mucous membrane at the angles of the mouth [**1**,**2**,3].

Synonyms and inclusions
- Perleche

Epidemiology

Incidence and prevalence
Common.

Age
Older.

Associated diseases
Denture-related stomatitis

Pathophysiology

Predisposing factors
Most cases are due to mechanical and/or infective causes or dry mouth but nutritional or immune defects are also causes.
- *Infective agents* are the major cause.
- *Immune deficiency*, such as diabetes and HIV infection, may present with angular stomatitis [4–7]. Outbreaks of acute pustular and fissured cheilitis may occur in children, particularly if they are malnourished, and in some cases streptococci or staphylococci have appeared to be causative [8].
- *Mechanical factors* in edentulous patients who do not wear a denture or who have inadequate dentures, and also as a normal consequence of the ageing process, produce an oblique curved fold and keep the small area of skin constantly macerated. The recurrent trauma of dental flossing is a very rare cause of angular cheilitis [9].
- *Nutritional deficiencies*, particularly deficiencies of riboflavin, folate, iron and general protein malnutrition, may produce smooth shiny red lips associated with angular stomatitis, a combination called *cheilosis* [1,10–12]. Crohn disease or orofacial granulomatosis may be found in some [13,14].
- *Hyposalivation*, such as after drug therapy, irradiation or in Sjögren syndrome may predispose [15].

Pathology
Inflammation.

Causative organisms
Candida and/or staphylococci are isolated from most patients [16–19], especially if there is HIV infection. Permanent cure can be achieved only by eliminating the *Candida* beneath the upper denture [20,21]. Candidosis was probably responsible for some of the cases of cheilitis attributed to allergy to denture materials, since contamination of denture material by *Candida* may cause false-positive patch-test reactions [22]. Agents causing hyposalivation (e.g. irradiation, chemotherapy or anticholinergic drugs) can predispose to infections.

Clinical features
Angular cheilitis presents as a roughly triangular area of erythema and oedema at one, or more commonly both, angles of the mouth (Figure 110.65). Linear furrows or fissures radiating from the angle

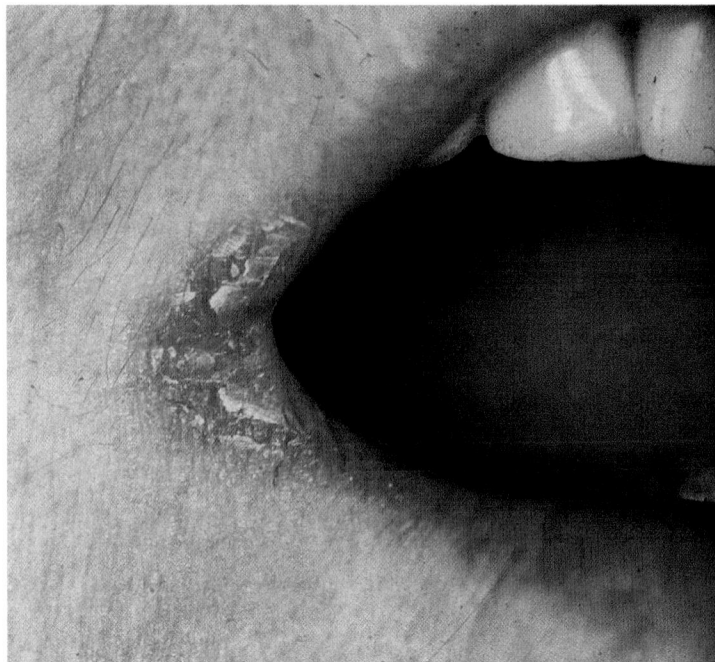

Figure 110.65 Angular cheilitis.

of the mouth (rhagades) are seen in the more severe forms, especially in denture wearers.

Complications and co-morbidities
Denture-related stomatitis.

Investigations
Diagnosis is usually obvious though trauma from activities such as dental flossing may mimic angular stomatitis. *Candida* should be sought not only in the lesions but also beneath the denture.

Management
Dentures should be removed from the mouth at night and stored in a candidacidal solution such as hypochlorite. Denture-related stomatitis should be treated with an antifungal. Miconazole may be preferable treatment for candidosis (cream applied locally, together with the oral gel) as it has some Gram-positive bacteriostatic action. New dentures that restore facial contour may help. The skin lesions should be swabbed and staphylococcal infection treated with fusidic acid ointment or cream at least four times daily.

Resources

Further information
http://emedicine.medscape.com/article/1075994-overview
http://www.dermnetnz.org/site-age-specific/angular-cheilitis.html
(Both last accessed December 2014.)

Blisters on the lips

Blistering is commonly due to recurrent herpes labialis but may be caused by various forms of cheilitis; trauma; burns from irradiation, heat or chemicals; solvent abuse ('huffing'); infections such as impetigo; mucocoeles; allergies; lupus erythematosus; amyloidosis; or vesiculobullous disorders [1–9].

Cancer of the lip

Carcinoma of the lip

Squamous cell carcinoma is the most common malignancy to affect the vermilion zone and, as with squamous carcinoma of the glabrous skin, usually due to actinic damage [1–3] but there are occasional cases of sebaceous carcinoma, and other variants.

Like actinic cheilitis squamous cell carcinoma is most common on the lower lip of fair-skinned outdoor workers in sunny climates, and is relatively rare in pigmented skin [4–6]. Lip cancer is common in certain population groups in the UK, Romania, Hungary, Poland, Spain, Finland, Israel, Canada, the USA and Australia, but in most areas reported the incidence is falling.

Squamous cell carcinomas occur on the lower lip in 89%, with 3% on the upper lip and 8% at the commissures. The buccal mucosa may also be involved, particularly in association with betel quid chewing. Facts that support a relationship to actinic radiation include the following:

- Lip cancer involves the more exposed lower lip, rather than the upper lip.
- There is a higher incidence of lip cancer in outdoor workers such as farming and fishing and rural populations than in office workers or urban populations.
- Fair-skinned more than dark-skinned people tend to develop lip cancer (as well as skin cancer and melanoma) in sunny climates.

Other risk factors may include low social class, tobacco smoking, syphilis, poor dentition, infection with HSV or HPVs and immune suppression [2,3,6–23]. Several large cohort studies and a meta-analysis have shown that organ transplant patients (who of course are chronically immunosuppressed) have between 17 and 46 times an increased risk of lip cancer and 2–5 times increased risk of mouth and pharyngeal cancers, compared with the general population. Lip cancer risk is particularly raised in kidney, heart or lung transplants, possibly due to persistent HPV infection and increased sensitivity to UV radiation.

A US cohort study showed white people who were taking the photosensitizing antihypertensive hydrochlorothiazide for 5 or more years had a fourfold increased risk of lip cancer. IARC classifies hydrochlorothiazide as a probable cause of lip cancer.

The initial features are a keratinous growth or swelling of the lip (see Figure 110.19), soreness and ulceration. Most lesions are amenable to surgical excision, with more than 70% surviving for 5 years.

Basal cell carcinoma of the lip

Actinic radiation is a major aetiological factor in the development of basal cell carcinoma, greater than 85% occurring on the sun-exposed areas of the head and neck [1,2]. Fair-skinned individuals who burn and those whose occupations require excessive exposure to sunshine are at greatest risk; the tumour is rare in dark-skinned persons, and 95% occur after the age of 40 years [3].

Other significant risk factors for the development of basal cell carcinoma include prior burns, vaccinations, irradiation, exposure to inorganic arsenic, genetic syndromes (e.g. xeroderma pigmentosum, naevoid basal cell carcinoma syndrome, albinism and Bazex syndrome) and immunosuppression [4–9]. Rare cases have a familial background [10].

Clinical features. On the lip these manifest as a pearly, sometimes ulcerated, nodule or papule. Unlike squamous cell carcinomas, basal cell carcinomas only rarely originate on the vermilion but commonly occur periorally [11–14]. In contrast to squamous cell carcinomas, basal cell carcinomas more commonly arise on the upper than the lower lip. The lesions can also arise *de novo* on the vermilion [15] or occasionally the mucosa of the lip, although spread of a tumour from an adjacent site may rarely occur.

Basal cell carcinoma has multiple forms that can be divided as follows:
- Nodular: the most frequent type around the lips presents as a waxy translucent nodule with fine telangiectasias, often ulcerated.
- Morphoeic: an atrophic plaque resembling a scar, with an aggressive infiltrative growth pattern and high rate of recurrence after excision.
- Superficial: appears as an erythematous plaque with elevated borders and central atrophy or ulceration. It is rare around the lips.

Although the tumour rarely metastasizes, it is responsible for considerable functional and cosmetic morbidity.

Multiple lesions are commonly encountered and the various forms have overlapping clinical features. Basal cell carcinoma can be frequently pigmented, resembling melanomas and other melanocytic lesions. Basal cell carcinoma may, of course, be a feature of naevoid basal cell carcinoma syndrome (Gorlin–Goltz syndrome, see Chapter 141). Furthermore, in addition to having a significantly increased risk for new skin cancers, patients with basal cell carcinoma have been shown to have an increased risk of developing non-cutaneous cancers, including respiratory cancers, testicular cancer, breast cancer and non-Hodgkin lymphoma [16–18].

Diagnosis. Basal cell carcinoma of the lips must be differentiated from other nodules, including squamous cell carcinoma, keratoacanthoma, trichoepithelioma and sebaceous adenoma. Since lesions that arise periorally are often aggressive, early detection and confirmation by biopsy will prevent infiltration and destruction of the underlying structures.

Management. Various treatment modalities for basal cell carcinoma include scalpel, electrosurgery, cryosurgery and laser surgery, radiation, curettage and intralesional chemotherapy or α-interferon [19–21]. Selection of the treatment modality depends on the size, site and histological pattern of the tumour as well as the age of the patient.

Since lip lesions are often of the nodular or morphoeic types, Mohs micrographic surgery [22], utilizing microscopically controlled excision, potentially offers the highest cure rate with the greatest preservation of tissue. The cure rate for basal cell carcinoma is over 90%.

PART 10: SITES, SEX, AGE

Keratoacanthoma of the lip

Keratoacanthoma is a rapidly growing lesion that probably arises from the supraseboglandular part of a sebaceous gland. Keratoacanthomas are common self-limiting proliferative tumours that arise most frequently in men after the sixth decade of life [1,2]. The lesions mimic squamous cell carcinoma both clinically and microscopically. Although some believe keratoacanthomas represent well-differentiated squamous cell carcinomas, significant differences between the two entities have been demonstrated [3]. A number of well-documented variants, many with generally distributed eruptive keratoacanthomas, have been described. One variant, Ferguson–Smith syndrome, is a familial trait.

Aetiology. The role of actinic damage is strongly supported by the fact that the majority of lesions occur on sun-exposed skin (90%), with up to 10% occurring periorally or on the vermilion border of the lips, often on the lower lip. HPV has also been suggested as an aetiological agent [4], and increased numbers of keratoacanthomas have been reported in immunocompromised patients.

Clinical features. Keratoacanthomas often manifest at the vermilion border, as indurated dome-shaped nodules displaying a characteristic central, keratin-filled, crusted and frequently darkened crater. While cutaneous lesions are asymptomatic, labial and oral lesions are frequently painful [5–12].

Intraoral keratoacanthomas are rare. They usually appear as an ulcer with a rolled margin, usually on the anterior or maxillary gingiva, clinically indistinguishable from squamous cell carcinoma. It is unclear whether intraoral keratoacanthomas regress spontaneously, as all have been excised for diagnosis.

Keratoacanthomas grow rapidly, attaining a size typically greater than 1 cm, may be locally invasive and result in significant tissue damage but, if left untreated, many undergo spontaneous involution after 1–2 months [13].

Diagnosis. Keratoacanthomas require differentiation from squamous cell carcinoma. When lesions develop intraorally or on the lips, they should immediately be subjected to biopsy for confirmation, since squamous cell carcinomas at these sites frequently metastasize.

Management. Management is often by surgical excision. Intralesional therapy with methotrexate or 5-fluorouracil can also be employed with excellent results [14,15]. Other suggested medical therapies include intralesional interferon α-2a and systemic isotretinoin [16–18].

'Chapping' of the lips

Chapping is a reaction to adverse environmental conditions usually caused by exposure to freezing cold or to hot dry winds. The keratin of the vermilion loses its plasticity, so that the lips become sore, cracked and scaly. The affected person tends to lick the lips, or to pick at the scales, which may aggravate the condition.

Treatment is by application of petroleum jelly and avoidance of the adverse environmental conditions.

Cheilitis

Synonyms and inclusions
• Inflammation of the lips

Cheilitis may arise as a primary disorder of the vermilion zone or the inflammation may extend from nearby skin or, less often, from the oral mucosa (Box 110.13) [1].

Contact cheilitis

Contact cheilitis is an inflammatory reaction provoked by the irritant or sensitizing action of chemicals. Most cases are caused by the deliberate application of lipsticks or lipsalves but many substances have been incriminated, sometimes from accidental contact with an offending substance (Box 110.14), as follows.

• *Lipsticks and lipsalves* (Table 110.13). Lipsticks are composed of mineral oils and wax (which form the stick), castor oil as a solvent for the dyes, lanolin as an emollient, preservatives, perfumes and colours [1–7]. The dyes may include azo dyes and eosin, a bromofluorescein derivative. An eosin impurity used to be an important sensitizer [8] but is now rarely if ever used. Other ingredients occasionally incriminated include azo dyes, carmine, oleyl alcohol [9], lanolin, perfumes, azulene, propyl gallate [10], sesame oil [11], stearates [12], shellac and colophony [13,14]. Sunscreens in lipstick or lipsalve (e.g. cinnamic aldehyde) can also cause contact cheilitis [15]. Phenyl salicylate and antibiotics have also been incriminated [16,17]. Petrolatum chapsticks may cause an unusual form of acne with a single row of large open comedones along the cutaneous margin of the upper lip [18].
• *Mouthwashes and dentrifices* [19–23]. Sensitizers used in some toothpastes include essential oils, such as peppermint, cinnamon, clove and spearmint; carvone along with imonene, pinene, phellandrene, dipentene, cineole, linalool, and esters of dihydrocuminyl

> **Box 110.13 Causes of cheilitis**
>
> • Chapping due to cold and wind
> • Eczematous cheilitis
> • Contact cheilitis
> • Drug-induced cheilitis (retinoids, voriconazole)
> • Infective cheilitis
> • Angular cheilitis
> • Ultraviolet irradiation
>   • Actinic cheilitis
>   • Actinic prurigo of the lip
> • Glandular cheilitis
> • Granulomatous cheilitis
> • Exfoliative (factitious) cheilitis
> • Plasma cell cheilitis
> • Nutritional cheilitis
> • Dermatoses
> • Trauma

Box 110.14 Substances incriminated in contact cheilitis

- Aciclovir
- *Agaricus blazei* Murill mushroom extract
- Amalgam
- Anethole
- Artichoke
- Aspargagus
- Benzophenone-3
- Benzydamine
- Betel quid
- Bisabolol
- C_{18} aliphatic compounds
- Candelilla wax
- Cane reed
- Carnauba wax
- Carvone
- Cinnamon
- Citral
- Cocamidopropyl betaine
- Colophony
- D&C Yellow No. 11
- D&C Red No. 7
- Dental metals
- Diisostearyl maleate
- Dipentaerythritol fatty acid ester
- Ditrimethylolpropane triethylhexanoate

- Dodecyl gallate
- Epimine containing dental materials
- Essential oils
- Ester
- Ethylene glycol
- Exocarp of sweet oranges
- Garlic
- Geraniol
- Glyceryl isostearate
- Green tea
- Hydroxyisoflavans in cocus wood *Brya ebenus* DC (Fabaceae)
- Iodoform
- Isopalmityl diglyceryl sebacate
- Lampol 5
- Latex
- Lip balms
- Lip salves
- Lipsticks
- Lithol Rubine BCA
- Mango
- Methylmethacrylate
- Mint flavoured toothpaste
- Mouthwashes

- *Myroxylon pereirae* (Balsam of Peru) in papaw ointment
- Nuts
- Oleyl alcohol
- Olive oil
- Osage orange
- Oxybenzone
- Pentaerythritol rosinate
- Peppermint oil
- Phenyl salicylate
- Pineapple
- Polysilicone-15
- Polyvinylpyrrolidone/hexadecene copolymer
- P-phenylenediamine
- Procaine
- Propolis
- Propyl gallate
- Ricinoleic acid
- Sesame oil
- Shellac
- Tartar control dentifrices
- Thiuram
- Titanium
- Toothpastes

alcohol and dehydrocarveol; bactericidal agents; propolis, derived from resin collected by bees [24–26]; and tartar-control dentifrices, which contain pyrophosphate compounds [27].

- *Dental materials.*
- *Foods and confectionary* (possible fruit and vegetable allergens are listed in Table 110.14).
- *Miscellaneous objects.* Metal hair clips, metal pencils, the cobalt paint on blue pencils, nail varnish, and the metal, wooden, nickel and reed mouthpieces of musical wind instruments [15] may be implicated.

Clinical features. Lipstick cheilitis is sometimes confined to the vermilion but more often extends beyond. There may be persistent irritation and scaling or a more acute reaction with oedema and vesiculation.

The other forms of cheilitis vary greatly in their clinical appearance. Those caused by foods commonly also involve the skin around the mouth. If a small sucked object is responsible, the reaction may be confined to one part of the lips. Hyperpigmentation is an occasional complication.

Table 110.13 Possible allergens in lipsticks and lipsalves.

Azo dyes	Azulene	Benzoic acid
Carmine	Castor oil	Cinnamon
Colophony	Eosin	Ester gum
Eusolex	Lanolin	Oleyl alcohol
Oxybenzone p-tertiary-butylphenol	Phenyl salicylate	Propolis
Propyl gallate	Ricinoleic acid	Salol
Sesame oil	Shellac	Vanilla
Wax		

Table 110.14 Possible fruit and vegetable allergens.

Apple	Artichoke	Asparagus
Banana	Carrot	Celery
Cherry	Fennel	Garlic
Kiwi fruit	Lemon	Lime
Mango	Onion	Orange
Parsley	Parsnip	Peach
Pear	Pineapple	Plum
Potato	Tomato	

Diagnosis. If acute eczematous changes are obviously present, the diagnosis of contact cheilitis presents no difficulty. If the changes are confined to irritation and scaling, the various forms of exfoliative cheilitis must be excluded.

If an allergic reaction is suspected, patch tests should be carried out.

Management. Topical corticosteroids or pimecrolimus will often give symptomatic relief but the offending substance should be identified and avoided.

Drug-induced cheilitis

Haemorrhagic crusting of the lips (Figure 110.66) is a feature of erythema multiforme (particularly in Stevens–Johnson syndrome) (see Chapter 47), but cheilitis can also occur as an isolated feature of a drug reaction.

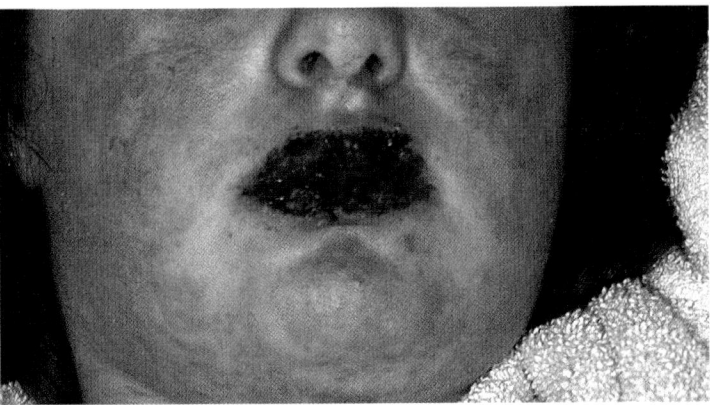

Figure 110.66 Haemorrhagic crusting of the lips in Stevens–Johnson syndrome.

Aromatic retinoids such as etretinate and isotretinoin cause cheilitis, dryness and cracking of the lips in many patients [1,2]. Similar effects may follow use of voriconazole [3–6].

Eczematous cheilitis

The lips are often involved secondarily to atopic eczema (see Chapter 41). The treatment is with emollients and topical corticosteroids. A potent steroid such as fludrocortisone may be required.

Exfoliative cheilitis

Synonyms and inclusions
- Tic de lèvres
- Morsicatio laborum

Exfoliative cheilitis is a chronic superficial inflammatory disorder of the vermilion borders of the lips characterized by persistent scaling (Figures 110.67 and 110.68). The diagnosis is now restricted to those few patients whose lesions cannot be attributed to other causes, such as contact sensitization or light (see Actinic cheilitis, p. 110.78).

Incidence and prevalence. Uncommon.

Age. Adolescents or adults.

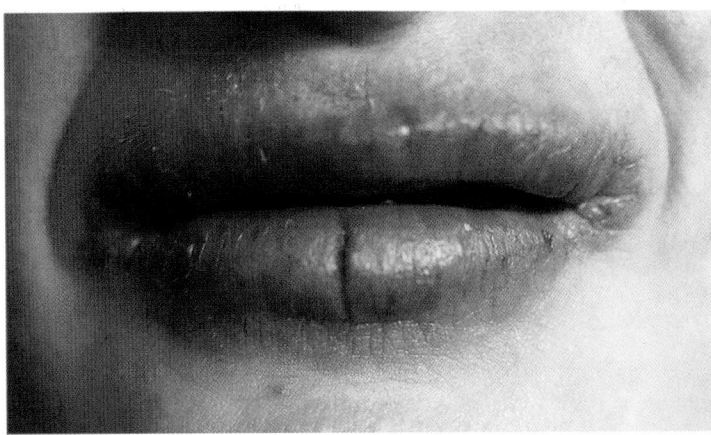

Figure 110.67 Factitious cheilitis due to repeated lip sucking.

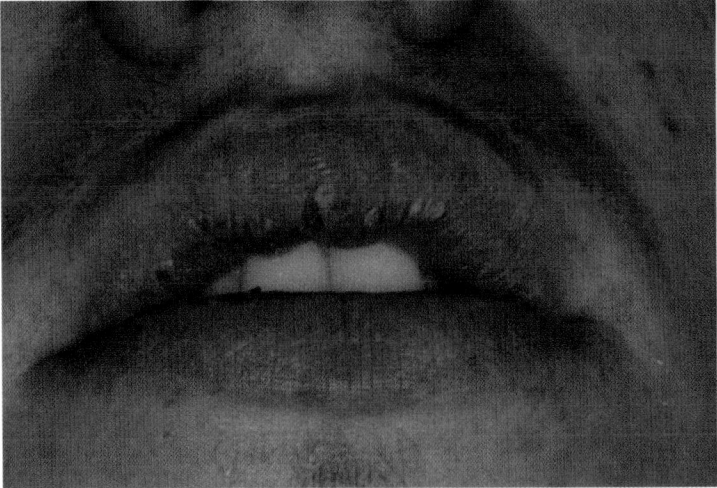

Figure 110.68 Exfoliative cheilitis.

Sex. Females more than males.

Associated diseases. In a large Russian series, almost half the cases had associated thyroid disease [1], but this observation has not been confirmed.

Pathophysiology. Many cases are now thought to be factitious, owing to repeated lip sucking, chewing or other manipulation of the lips [2–6]. There is no association with dermatological or systemic disease, although rare cases are seen in HIV infection. Some are infected with *Candida* species [7,8].

Clinical features. Most cases occur in girls or young women, and the majority have a personality disorder [9,10]. The process, which often starts in the middle of the lower lip and spreads to involve the whole of the lower or both lips, consists of scaling and crusting, more or less confined to the vermilion border, and persisting in varying severity for months or years. The patient often complains of irritation or burning, and can be observed frequently biting or sucking the lips. In some cases, the condition appears to start with chapping or with atopic eczema, and develops into a habit tic.

Differential diagnosis. Contact and active cheilitis must be carefully excluded. Chronic exfoliative cheilitis is readily contaminated by *Candida*. In such cases, the clinical features are variable and may simulate carcinoma, lichen planus or lupus erythematosus.

Management. Some cases resolve spontaneously [3,11] or with improved oral hygiene [12]. Reassurance and moisturizing agents and topical corticosteroids [2], or tacrolimus [5,**13**] may be helpful in some cases as may *Calendula* [14] but others require psychotherapy, antidepressants or tranquillizers [4,6,11,15].

Resources

Further information
http://www.dermnetnz.org/site-age-specific/exfoliative-cheilitis.html (last accessed December 2014).

Table 110.15 Some lip/facial fillers.

Origin	Material	Source
Natural	Collagen	Human or bovine natural skin protein
	Fat (free fat transfer, autologous fat transfer/transplantation, liposculpture, lipostructure micro-lipoinjection)	Human typically from inner thigh or abdomen
	Hyaluronic acid	Human or animal
	Hydroxyapatite	Mineral suspended in a gel-like formulation
Synthetic*	Polyacrylamide	Hydrophilic polyacrylamide gel (HPG)
	Poly-L-lactic acid	
	Polymethylmethacrylate	20–25% PMMA microspheres in collagen gel
	Silicone	Dimethylsiloxane

*Usually non-resorbable.

Foreign body cheilitis

Injectable fillers used in cosmetic procedures may include dimethylpolysiloxane (silicone), bovine collagen, polylactic acid, polymethylmethacrylate (PMMA) and polyethylene (Table 110.15), any of which may induce foreign body reactions [1–9]. Complications may include temporary pain, bleeding, bruising, swelling, seromas (fluid collections), infection or allergy. Clinically, patients may present with painless or painful, diffuse lip/facial swellings, usually of a firm elastic consistency. MRI shows signs of intense inflammatory reactions in the affected areas. The histology reveals foreign body granulomas with multinucleated giant cells. The patients may need treatment with systemically administered corticosteroids. PMMA filler complications, despite being rare, are often permanent and difficult or even impossible to treat.

Glandular cheilitis

Definition. Glandular cheilitis is characterized by inflammatory changes and swelling of salivary glands in the lips [1–3].

Aetiology. This is an uncommon idiopathic condition which in a few cases has apparently been familial [4]. Although it was originally thought that the condition was due to inflammation of enlarged heterotopic salivary glands, the glands are often normal in size, depth and histology [5]. It is possible that the excessive salivary secretion from minor salivary glands in this condition might be an unusual clinical response to irritation of the lip from some other cause such as actinic damage or repeated licking.

Pathology. In the milder forms there is some fibrosis surrounding the salivary glands, while in the more severe forms there may be a dense chronic inflammatory infiltrate. Only rarely do patients show genuine hyperplasia of the salivary glands or duct ectasia.

Clinical features. The onset is at any age from childhood onwards. Clinically, three variants have been described: cheilitis glandularis simplex, cheilitis glandularis suppurativa, and cheilitis glandularis apostematosa (*Volkmann cheilitis*).

In simple glandular cheilitis, the lower lip is slightly thickened and bears numerous pinhead-sized orifices, from which mucous saliva can readily be squeezed. The upper lip is rarely involved [6].

In the more severe suppurative form the lip is considerably and permanently enlarged, and subject to episodes of pain, tenderness and increased enlargement. The surface is covered by crusts and scales, beneath which the salivary duct orifices may be discovered. In the most severe forms there may be deep-seated infection with abscess formation and fistulous tracts.

The condition may be premalignant; in some series 20–30% of cases progress to squamous carcinoma. This does, of course, support the suggestion that in many cases glandular cheilitis is a consequence of actinic cheilitis [5].

Management. Cheilitis granulomatosa, cheilitis exfoliativa, and self-induced changes (Munchausen syndrome) should be considered in the differential diagnosis [7]. Actinic cheilitis, if identified, should be treated appropriately. If the lips are grossly enlarged, excision of an elongated ellipse of tissue may be required; in other cases shave vermilionectomy may be all that is necessary.

Granulomatous cheilitis

Definition and nomenclature
This is a chronic swelling of the lip due to granulomatous inflammation of unknown cause. It is clinically and histologically indistinguishable from orofacial granulomatosis – in which there may be orofacial lesions in addition to labial swelling.

Melkersson in 1928 [1] described labial oedema in association with recurrent facial palsy. Rosenthal in 1930 emphasized the role of genetic factors and added fissured tongue to the syndrome. The full syndrome has since been called Melkersson–Rosenthal syndrome [2–4].

In Miescher cheilitis, the granulomatous changes are confined to the lip, and this is generally regarded as a monosymptomatic form of Melkersson–Rosenthal syndrome, although the possibility remains that these may be two separate diseases.

Synonyms and inclusions
- Miescher cheilitis
- Melkersson–Rosenthal syndrome

Introduction and general description
Chronic swelling of the lip due to granulomatous inflammation.

Epidemiology

Incidence and prevalence
Uncommon.

Age
The earliest manifestations usually develop in childhood or adolescence but may be delayed until middle or old age.

Sex
The condition affects the sexes equally.

Pathophysiology

Predisposing factors
There is no convincing evidence that granulomatous cheilitis is due to an infective agent. Some cases may represent a localized form of sarcoidosis [6,7] or ectopic Crohn disease [7–9] or orofacial granulomatosis. There is increasing evidence that some patients with granulomatous cheilitis are predisposed to Crohn disease [9–11]. In some cases, granulomatous cheilitis is followed some years later by regional ileitis [12–16].

A few patients react to cobalt [17] or to food additives such as cinnamic aldehyde [18–21] and have no extra oral lesions, although these reactions are by no means always relevant; for example, in one study only one of nine patients had a relationship between cheilitis and food intake [22]. Other precipitants may include:
- Other dietary antigens.
  - Butylated hydroxyanisole.
  - Dodecyl gallate.
  - Menthol.
  - Monosodium glutamate.
- Contact antigens (e.g. cobalt, gold, mercury).

Some cases have been reported in patients treated with anti-TNF biologicals.

Pathology
Biopsy of the swollen lip or facial tissues during the early stages of the disease shows only oedema and perivascular lymphocytic infiltration. In some cases of long duration no other changes are seen, but in others the infiltrate becomes more dense and pleomorphic and small focal granulomas are formed, indistinguishable from sarcoidosis or orofacial granulomatosis/Crohn disease. Similar changes may be present in cervical lymph nodes [23–26]. In some cases, small granulomas occur in the lymphatic walls [27].

Genetics
Melkersson–Rosenthal syndrome may have a genetic predisposition [5]; siblings have been affected and a fissured tongue may be present in otherwise normal relatives.

Clinical features
The earliest cutaneous manifestation is sudden diffuse or nodular swellings [10,11,28,29] involving the upper lip, the lower lip and one or both cheeks in decreasing order of frequency [8,26,30]. Labial swelling occurs in about 75% and facial swelling in 50% of patients [31]. Less commonly, the forehead, eyelids or one side of the scalp may be involved. The attacks are sometimes accompanied by fever and mild constitutional symptoms, including headache and even visual disturbance. At the first episode the oedema typically subsides completely in hours or days, but after recurrent attacks the swelling may persist, and slowly increases in degree (Figure 110.69). It gradually becomes firmer and eventually acquires the consistency of firm rubber. After some years, the swelling may very slowly regress.

A fissured or scrotal tongue is seen in 20–40% of cases [11]. It is present from birth in some, which may indicate genetic susceptibility. There may be loss of sense of taste and decreased salivary gland secretion [26].

The regional lymph nodes are enlarged in 50% of cases [5] but not usually very greatly.

Facial palsy of the lower motor neurone type occurs in some 30% of cases. It may precede the attacks of oedema by months or years, but more commonly develops later. Although intermittent at first, the palsy may become permanent. It may be unilateral or bilateral, and partial or complete [26]. Other cranial nerves (olfactory, auditory, glossopharyngeal and hypoglossal) may occasionally be involved [32]. Involvement of the CNS has also been reported, but the significance of the resulting symptoms is easily overlooked as they are very variable, sometimes simulating disseminated sclerosis but often with a poorly defined association of psychotic and neurological features. Autonomic disturbances may occur.

Differential diagnosis
The essential feature is the granulomatous swelling of lip or face. In the early attacks clinical differentiation from angio-oedema may be impossible in the absence of either scrotal tongue or facial palsy. Persistence of the swelling between attacks should suggest the diagnosis. Sarcoidosis, tuberculosis or orofacial granulomatosis/Crohn disease are the main differential diagnoses. In established cases, other causes of macrocheilia (Table 110.16) must be excluded. Lymphoma is a rare differential diagnosis [33]. Ascher

PART 10: SITES, SEX, AGE

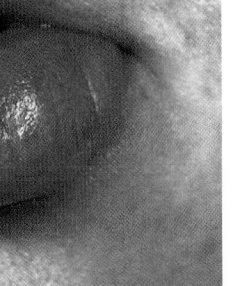

(a)

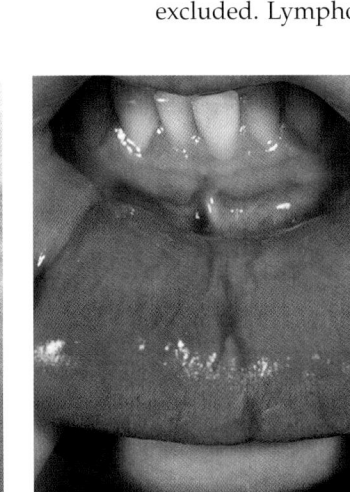

(b)

Figure 110.69 Granulomatous cheilitis of the lower lip. (Courtesy of Addenbrooke's Hospital, Cambridge, UK.)

Table 110.16 Macrocheilia: acute or chronic enlargement of one or both lips.

Acute	Chronic
Traumatic	Developmental
Infective	Familial idiopathic
• Pyococcal	• Double lip
• Anthrax	• Ascher syndrome
• Diphtheria	• Lymphangioma
• Primary syphilis	• Haemangioma
• Trichophytosis	• Neurofibroma
• Leishmaniasis	• Mucopolysaccharidoses
• Herpes simplex	• Fucosidosis
• Trichiniasis	Coffin–Siris syndrome
Angio-oedema	Acquired
Erythema multiforme	Post-traumatic
Actinic cheilitis	Postinfective on basis of developmental
Other forms of cheilitis	Lymphatic defect
	• Infective
	• Tuberculosis
	• Leprosy
	• Rhinoscleroma
	• Leishmaniasis
	Neoplastic
	Meischer cheilitis
	Melkersson–Rosenthal syndrome
	Cheilitis glandularis
	Sarcoidosis
	Crohn disease
	Orofacial granulomatosis

syndrome associated with blepharochalasia rarely causes a confusion, as the swelling of the lip is caused by redundant salivary tissue and is present from childhood.

Investigations

Diagnosis can sometimes be confirmed by biopsy. However, the histological changes are not always conspicuous or specific. Reactions to dietary components should be sought.

Management

Possible antigens should be avoided.

The injection of a corticosteroid such as up to 10 mL triamcinolone (10 mg/L) into the lips after local analgesia may be effective [22,29,34–39,53–56]. The injections may have to be repeated every 4–6 months once a response plateau has been reached. The injections must be continued periodically after the surgery or there may be an exaggerated recurrence of the condition. Intralesional triamcinolone acetonide in combination with topical pimecrolimus 1% has also been used. Systemic corticosteroids are rarely indicated [44] since adverse effects may be a problem and not all respond [41,45]. Metronidazole may also produce resolution in granulomatous cheilitis [37,49,50,57,58]. Other treatments which have occasionally been helpful include penicillin, erythromycin, and sulfasalazine (sulphasalazine). Clofazimine appears to help the majority of patients [36,46–48,59–64], in a dose of 100 mg twice daily for 10 days, then twice weekly for 4 months. However, pink to brownish skin pigmentation in 75–100% of patients within a few weeks upon exposure to the sun, as well as similar

discoloration of most bodily fluids and secretions and gastrointestinal intolerance in 40–50% of patients do not encourage this regimen. Rarely, patients have also died from bowel obstructions and intestinal bleeding, or required surgery. More recently, methotrexate, ketotifen, thalidomide, adalimumab, etanercept or infliximab have been used [51,52,65–72].

Surgical reduction (cheiloplasty) is rarely used [40–42]. Surgery alone is relatively unsuccessful [36,43,73].

Resources

Further information

http://emedicine.medscape.com/article/1075333-overview (last accessed December 2014).

Infective cheilitis

Types of infective cheilitis are as follows.
• *Viral.* Lip infections with HSV are common, and varicella-zoster virus and HPV may also affect the lips. Rare viral infections such as orf [1–4] and vaccinia [5] can affect the lips.
• *Bacterial.* Dental infection or occasionally a furuncle or carbuncle may cause swelling of the lip. Impetigo may mimic herpes labialis (see Chapter 26). Cancrum oris (fusospirochaetal infection) may cause labial and buccal necrosis [6–8].
  • The lip is the most common extragenital site for a primary syphilitic lesion. Most lip chancres in males tend to occur on the upper lip, in females on the lower lip. In secondary syphilis, moist flat papulonodular lesions (condylomata lata) often appear at the mucocutaneous junctions and on mucosal surfaces especially at the commissures [9,10]. The tropical treponematoses may present similarly to syphilis.
  • Tuberculosis or leprosy may cause chronic lip swelling or ulceration [11,16].
  • Rhinoscleroma initially affects the nasal mucosa but may spread slowly to the upper lip, producing plaques or nodules with sunken centres. The extreme hardness of the infiltrations is characteristic. The lip can appear to fuse to the alveolar process but the overlying skin and mucosa remain normal.
• *Protozoal.* Cutaneous or mucocutaneous leishmaniasis typically causes swellings on the upper lip with later enlargement and destruction of the lip [12–14,17], reflecting the three stages of oedema, granulomatous proliferation and then necrosis.
• *Fungal.* Blastomycosis and paracoccidioidomycosis are uncommon causes of chronic ulceration affecting the lip, producing very similar clinical lesions to leishmaniasis [15].
• *Others.* Red swollen lips with fissuring and exfoliation are prominent in mucocutaneous lymph node syndrome (Kawasaki disease).

Plasma cell cheilitis

Synonyms and inclusions
• Plasma cell orificial mucositis

Plasma cell cheilitis is an idiopathic benign inflammatory condition, characterized by dense plasma cell infiltrates in the lips and other mucosae close to body orifices [1–5]. The condition has been reported (under a wide variety of names) to affect the penis, vulva, lips, buccal mucosa, palate, gingiva, tongue, epiglottis and larynx.

Plasma cell cheilitis is the counterpart of Zoon plasma cell balanitis (see Chapter 111). It presents as circumscribed flat or elevated patches of erythema, usually on the lower lip in an elderly person. The cause is unknown, but it responds to the application of powerful topical corticosteroids such as clobetasol, or to the intradermal injection of triamcinolone [5–7], or to systemic griseofulvin [4,8] or to topical tacrolimus [9–12].

A similar lesion, which tends to form a tumorous mass with a hyperkeratotic surface and needs to be differentiated from extramedullary plasmacytoma [13], has been called *plasma-acanthoma* [14,15].

Other lesions of the lip

Calibre-persistent artery

A calibre-persistent artery is defined as an artery with a larger than normal diameter near a mucosal or external surface. When such arteries occur in the gut wall (Dieulafoy malformation) they may bleed, but in the lip they tend to cause chronic ulceration that can be mistaken for a mucocoele or a squamous cancer [1–4]. Intraoral examples have been reported [5].The ulcer is attributed to continual pulsation from the large artery running parallel to the surface, although the exact mechanism is obscure [1,2]. Ultrasound may assist diagnosis [6]. Ligation of the artery appears successful [3].

Lip fissure

A lip fissure may develop when a patient, typically a child, is mouth-breathing (Figure 110.70). Otherwise the aetiology may be obscure, though sun, wind, cold weather and smoking are thought to predispose. A hereditary predisposition for weakness in the first branchial arch fusion seems to exist.

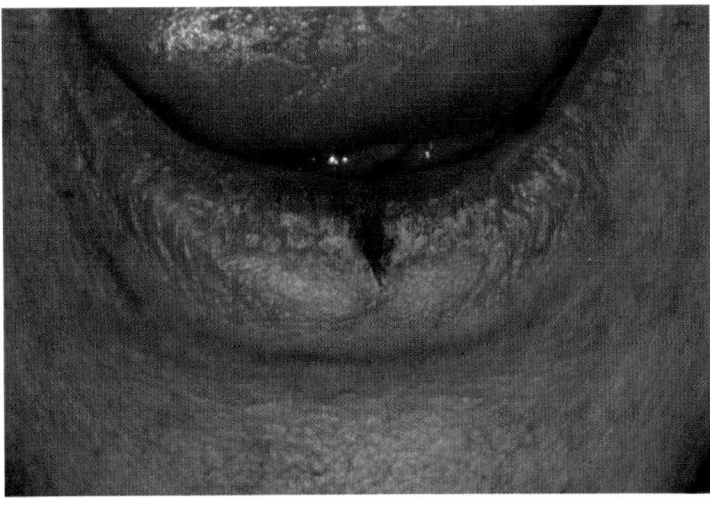

Figure 110.70 Lip fissure.

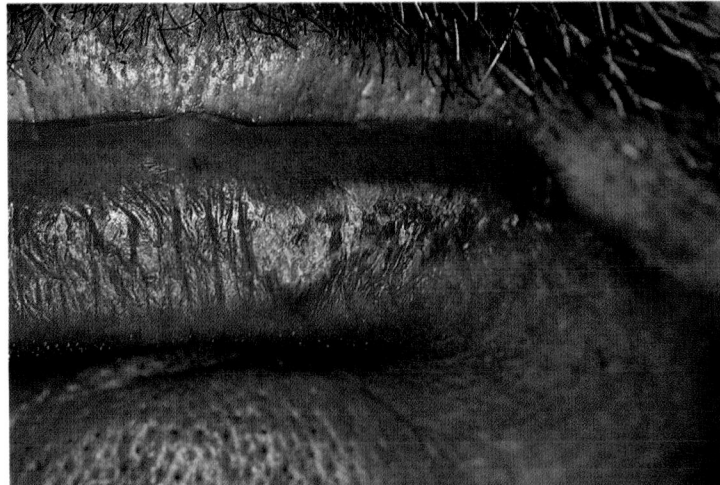

Figure 110.71 Discoid lupus erythematosus of the lower lip.

Lip fissures are common in Down syndrome and the lips may also crack in this way if swollen, for example in cheilitis granulomatosa [1–6].

Clinical features. Most lip fissures are seen in males, typically median in the lower lip and chronic, causing discomfort and possibly bleeding from time to time. Contrary to the clinical impression that fissures are seen only in the lower lip, there is also a high prevalence in the upper lip.

Diagnosis. The diagnosis is clinical.

Management. Predisposing factors should be managed. Bland creams may help the lesion heal spontaneously. Otherwise, local applications of 1–2% silver nitrate, 0.5% Balsam of Peru, salicylic acid and topical antimicrobials seem less effective than excision, preferably with a Z-plasty [7–10], cryosurgery [11] or carbon dioxide laser [12].

Lupus erythematosus (see Chapter 51)

Involvement of the vermilion zone is quite common in both discoid erythematosus and SLE [1–14]. The cheilitis of SLE tends to be more severe, with erosions and haemorrhagic crusts. Lupus erythematosus can be very difficult to distinguish from lichen planus of the lips, both clinically and by histology (Figure 110.71). Discoid lupus can be premalignant [4–6], and should be treated vigorously with topical steroid ointments and sunscreens [7,8]. Microinvasive squamous carcinoma arising in DLE lesions have been successfully treated with imiquimod 5% cream [14].

Reactive perforating collagenosis (see Chapter 96)

Crateriform papules of the lower lip have been reported in reactive perforating collagenosis [1].

Sarcoidosis (see Chapter 98)

Sarcoidosis may cause chronic violaceous lesions on, or swelling of, or in, the lips [1–8].

ORAL MANIFESTATIONS OF SYSTEMIC DISEASES

Oral manifestations can occasionally be seen in a range of systemic diseases (Tables 110.17, 110.18, 110.19, 110.20, 110.21, 110.22, 110.23, 110.24, 110.25, 110.26, 110.27, 110.28, 110.29, 110.30 and 110.31). Space precludes all but a brief tabular synopsis here. Further details can be found elsewhere [1–5].

Table 110.17 Endocrine disorders.

Disease	Oral manifestations
Pituitary dwarfism	Microdontia
	Retarded tooth eruption
Congenital hypothyroidism	Macroglossia
	Retarded tooth eruption
Congenital hypoparathyroidism	Dental hypoplasia
	May be chronic candidosis if associated immune defect
Gigantism/acromegaly	Spaced teeth
	Mandibular prognathism
	Macroglossia
	Megadontia (in gigantism)
Hyperparathyroidism	Bone rarefaction
	Brown tumours
Addison disease	Mucosal hyperpigmentation
Diabetes	Periodontal disease
	Xerostomia
	Candidosis
	Sialosis
	Lichen planus
Pregnancy	Gingivitis
	Epulis
Precocious puberty	Accelerated tooth eruption (fibrous dysplasia in Albright syndrome)

Table 110.18 Liver diseases.

Disease	Oral manifestations
Most liver diseases with jaundice	Bleeding tendency
	Jaundice
Alcoholic cirrhosis	Bleeding tendency
	Sialosis
Chronic active hepatitis	Lichen planus
Primary biliary cirrhosis	Sjögren syndrome
	Lichen planus
Hepatitis C	Lichen planus
	Sjögren syndrome

Table 110.19 Psychiatric disease.

Disease	Oral manifestations
Depression, hypochondriasis and various psychoses	Various complaints such as dry mouth, discharges, pain, disturbed taste and sensation
	Drug reactions
	Often multiple complaints
	Artefactual ulcers
Anxiety states	Cheek biting
	Bruxism (teeth grinding)
Bulimia	Tooth erosion

Table 110.20 Drug effects.

Tissue	Drug effect	Drugs commonly implicated
Gingiva	Swelling	Phenytoin
		Ciclosporin
		Nifedipine
		Diltiazem
Salivary glands	Dry mouth	Tricyclic antidepressants
		Phenothiazines
		Antihypertensives
		Lithium
Taste	Disturbed	Metronidazole
		Penicillamine
Facial movements	Dyskinaesias	Phenothiazines
		Metoclopramide
Mucosa	Thrush	Broad-spectrum antimicrobials
		Corticosteroids
		Cytotoxic drugs
	Ulcers	Cytotoxic drugs
		Non-steroidal anti-inflammatory agents
	Lichenoid lesions	Non-steroidal anti-inflammatory agents
	Erythema multiforme	Barbiturates
		Sulphonamides
	Cheilitis	Retinoids
		Voriconazole

Table 110.21 Gastrointestinal diseases.

Disease	Oral manifestations
Pernicious anaemia	Ulcers
	Glossitis
	Angular stomatitis
	Red lesions
Any cause of malabsorption	Ulcers
	Glossitis
	Angular stomatitis
Any cause of regurgitation	Tooth erosion
	Halitosis
Tylosis	Leukoplakia
Crohn disease (and orofacial granulomatosis)	Facial swelling
	Mucosal tags
	Gingival hyperplasia
	Cobblestoning of mucosa
	Ulcers
	Glossitis
	Angular stomatitis
Coeliac disease	Ulcers
	Glossitis
	Angular stomatitis
	Dental hypoplasia
Peutz–Jeghers syndrome (small intestinal polyps)	Melanosis
Chronic pancreatitis	Sialosis (rarely)
Cystic fibrosis	Salivary gland swelling
Gardner syndrome (familial colonic polyposis)	Osteomas

Table 110.22 Renal diseases.

Disease	Oral manifestations
Chronic kidney disease of any cause	Hyposalivation
	Halitosis/taste disturbance
	Leukoplakia
	Dental hypoplasia in children
	Renal osteodystrophy
Post organ transplant (immunosuppressed)	Bleeding tendency (especially if anticoagulated)
	Infections, particularly herpetic and candidal
	Bleeding tendency if anticoagulated
	Gingival hyperplasia if on ciclosporin
	Kaposi sarcoma (rarely)
	Hairy leukoplakia (rarely)
Nephrotic syndrome	Dental hypoplasia
Renal rickets (vitamin D resistant)	Delayed tooth eruption
	Dental hypoplasia (rarely)
	Enlarged pulp

Table 110.23 Haematological diseases.

Disease	Oral manifestations
Deficiency of the haematinics (iron, folic acid or vitamin B$_{12}$)	Burning mouth sensation
	Ulcers
	Glossitis
	Angular stomatitis
Sickle cell anaemia	Jaw deformities
	Osteomyelitis or pain
Thalassaemia major	Jaw deformities
Aplastic anaemia	Ulcers
	Bleeding tendency
Haemolytic disease of newborn	Tooth pigmentation
	Enamel defects
Any leukocyte defect	Infections, especially herpetic and candidal
	Ulcers
Any cause of purpura	Bleeding tendency
	Purpura
Leukaemia/lymphoma	Infections
	Ulcers
	Bleeding tendency and purpura (in leukaemias only)
	Gingival swelling in myelomonocytic leukaemia
Multiple myeloma	Bone pain
	Tooth mobility
	Amyloidosis
Amyloid disease	Enlarged tongue
	Purpura

Table 110.25 Primary and secondary immunodeficiencies.

Disease	Oral manifestations
Severe combined immunodeficiency	Candidosis
	Viral infections
	Ulcers
	Absent tonsils
	Recurrent sinusitis
Sex-linked agammaglobulinaemia	Ulcers
	Recurrent sinusitis
	Absent tonsils
Common variable immunodeficiency	Recurrent sinusitis
	Candidosis
Selective IgA deficiency	Tonsillar hyperplasia
	Ulcers
	Viral infections
	Parotitis
DiGeorge syndrome	Abnormal facies
	Candidosis
	Viral infections
	Bifid uvula
Ataxia-telangiectasia	Recurrent sinusitis
	Ulcers
	Telangiectasia
Wiskott–Aldrich syndrome	Candidosis
	Viral infections
	Purpura
Hereditary angio-oedema	Swellings
Chronic benign neutropenia	Ulcers
	Severe periodontitis
Cyclic neutropenia	Ulcers
	Severe periodontitis
	Eczematous lesions of the face
Chronic granulomatous disease	Candidosis
	Enamel hypoplasia
	Acute gingivitis
	Ulcers
Myeloperoxidase deficiency	Candidosis
Chédiak–Higashi syndrome	Ulcers
	Periodontitis
Job syndrome	Abnormal facies
Secondary immune defects	Ulcers
	Periodontitis
	Candidosis
	Viral infections
	Malignant neoplasms
	Hairy leukoplakia

Table 110.24 Cardiovascular diseases.

Disease	Oral manifestations
Any disorder causing right-to-left shunt, e.g. Fallot tetralogy	Cyanosis
Angina pectoris	Pain referred to jaw
Hereditary haemorrhagic telangiectasia	Telangiectasis and bleeding
Giant cell arteritis (cranial or temporal arteritis)	Tongue pain or necrosis
Polyarteritis nodosa	Ulcers
Any disorder in which anticoagulants are used	Bleeding tendency
Hypertension	Dry mouth and other problems caused by some antihypertensives, e.g. gingival hyperplasia (nifedipine or diltiazem), lichenoid lesions (angiotensin-converting enzyme inhibitors, methyldopa and others)

Table 110.26 Metabolic disorders.

Disease	Oral manifestations
Congenital hyperuricaemia (Lesch–Nyhan syndrome)	Self-mutilation
Mucopolysaccharidoses	Spaced teeth
	Retarded tooth eruption
	Cystic radiolucencies
	Temporomandibular joint anomalies
	Enamel defects
	Gingival hyperplasia
Niemann–Pick disease	Retarded tooth eruption
	Loosening of teeth
	Mucosal pigmentation
Mucolipidoses	Gingival hyperplasia
Hypophosphatasia	Loosening and loss of teeth
Erythropoietic porphyria	Reddish teeth
	Bullae/erosions
	Dental hypoplasia
Amyloidosis	Macroglossia
	Purpura
Vitamin B_{12} or folic acid deficiency	Ulcers
	Glossitis
	Angular stomatitis
Scurvy	Gingival swelling
	Purpura
	Ulcers
Rickets (vitamin D dependent)	Dental hypoplasia
	Large pulp chambers
	Large tooth eruption

Table 110.27 Collagen–vascular diseases.

Disease	Oral manifestations
Any collagen–vascular disease	Sjögren syndrome
Rheumatoid arthritis	Temporomandibular arthritis
	Drug reaction (e.g. lichenoid)
	Ulcers in Felty syndrome
	Temporomandibular ankylosis in juvenile arthritides
Lupus erythematosus	White lesions
	Ulcers
Systemic sclerosis	Stiffness of lips, tongue, etc.
	Trismus
	Telangiectasia
	Mandibular condylar resorption
	Periodontal ligament widened on radiography

Table 110.28 Miscellaneous disorders.

Disease	Oral manifestations
Sarcoidosis	Hyposalivation
	Salivary gland swelling
	Heerfordt syndrome (parotid swelling, lacrimal swelling, facial palsy)
	Gingival swelling
Behçet syndrome	Aphthous-like ulcers
Sweet syndrome	Aphthous-like ulcers
Reactive arthritis	Ulcers
Langerhans cell histiocytosis	Loosening of teeth
	Jaw radiolucencies
Granulomatosis with polyangiitis	Gingival swellings
	Ulcers
Kawasaki disease (mucocutaneous lymph node syndrome)	Sore tongue
	Cheilitis
Ellis–van Creveld syndrome (chondroectodermal dysplasia)	Multiple fraena
	Short roots
	Hypodontia
Tuberous sclerosis	Enamel defects
	Gingival fibromatosis

Table 110.29 Other infections.

Disease	Oral manifestations
Syphilis	Chancre
	Mucous patches
	Ulcers
	Gumma
	Pain from neurosyphilis
	Leukoplakia
	Lymph node enlargement
	Hutchinson teeth and Moon molars in congenital syphilis
Gonorrhoea	Pharyngitis (occasionally)
	Gingivitis (occasionally)
	Temporomandibular arthritis (rarely)
Tuberculosis (including atypical mycobacteria)	Ulcers (rarely)
	Cervical lymphadenopathy
Leprosy	Cranial nerve palsies (rarely)
	Swellings
Lyme disease	Facial palsy
Candidosis	White lesions
	Red lesions
	Angular stomatitis
Cryptococcosis	Ulcers
Coccidioidomycosis	Ulcers
Histoplasmosis	Ulcers (especially in immune defects)
Blastomycosis	Ulcers
Paracoccidioidomycosis	Ulcers
Mucormycosis, aspergillosis	Antral infections or ulcers (especially in immune defects)

Table 110.30 Viral infections.

Disease	Oral manifestations
Chikigungya	Ulcers
Coxsackieviruses and ECHO viruses	Ulcers in herpangina and hand, foot and mouth disease
Dengue	Gingival bleeding
	Taste anomalies
Epstein–Barr virus (in infectious mononucleosis)	Sore throat
	Tonsillar exudate
Herpes simplex	Ulcers in primary infection
	Gingivitis in primary infection
	Vesicles on lips in recurrence (rarely oral ulcers)
	Erythema multiforme
	Facial palsy
Herpes zoster–varicella	Ulcers in chickenpox, or in zoster of maxillary or mandibular divisions of the trigeminal nerve
	Pain in maxillary or mandibular zoster
	Palatal petechiae
	Recurrent parotitis (possibly)
	Hairy leukoplakia
	Lymphomas
	Nasopharyngeal carcinoma
Measles	Koplik spots
Mumps	Salivary gland swelling
Papillomaviruses	Warts
	Papillomas
	Focal epithelial hyperplasia
	Oropharyngeal carcinoma
HIV common	Candidosis
	Hairy leukoplakia
	Gingival and periodontal disease
	Herpes simplex infection
	Herpes zoster infection
	Papillomavirus infection
	Kaposi sarcoma
	Lymphoma
	Aphthous-like ulcers
	Hyposalivation
HIV uncommon	Infections
	• *Cryptococcus*
	• Mycobacteria
	• *Histoplasma*
	• Cytomegalovirus
	• Others
	Salivary gland swelling
	Sjögren syndrome-like disease
	Cranial neuropathies
	Fetal AIDS syndrome

Table 110.31 Neurological disorders.

Disease	Oral manifestations
Facial palsy of any cause	Palsy and poor natural cleansing of mouth on same side
Trigeminal neuralgia	Pain
Bulbar palsy	Fasciculation of tongue
Parkinsonism	Drooling/hypersalivation
	Tremor of tongue
	Dysarthria
Neurosyphilis	Pain (rarely)
	Dysarthria
	Tremor of tongue
Cerebral palsy	Spastic tongue
	Dysarthria
	Attrition
	Periodontal disease
Choreoathetosis	Green staining of teeth in kernicterus
	Hypoplasia of deciduous dentition in congenital rubella
Epilepsy	Trauma to teeth/jaws/mucosa
	Gingival hyperplasia if taking phenytoin
Down syndrome	Delayed tooth eruption
	Macroglossia
	Scrotal tongue
	Maxillary hypoplasia
	Anterior open bite
	Hypodontia
	Periodontal disease
	Cleft lip or palate in some

Key references

The full list of references can be found in the online version at www.rooksdermatology.com.

Disorders affecting the oral mucosa or lips

1 Scully C. *Handbook of Oral Disease: Diagnosis and Management*. London: Martin Dunitz, 1999.
2 Scully C. *ABC of Oral Health*. London: BMJ Books, 2000.
3 Felix D, Luker J, Scully C. *Oral Medicine – Update for the Dental Team*. London: Dental Update Books, 2015.
4 Scully C, Flint S, Bagan JV, et al. *Oral and Maxillofacial Diseases*. London: Informa, 2010.
5 Scully C, Almeida ODP, Bagan J, Diz PD, Mosqueda A. *Oral Medicine and Pathology at a Glance*. Oxford: Wiley- Blackwell, 2010.
6 Bloch-Zupan A, Sedano H, Scully C. *Dento/Oro/Craniofacial Anomalies and Genetics*. London: Elsevier, 2012.
7 Scully C, Bagan JV, Carrozzo M, Flaitz C, Gandolfo S. *Pocketbook of Oral Disease*. London: Elsevier, 2012.
8 Scully C. *Oral and Maxillofacial Medicine*. 3rd edn. Edinburgh: Churchill Livingstone, 2013.

Genetic disorders affecting the oral mucosa or lips

Lumps and swellings

1 Cicardi M, Aberer W, Banerji A, *et al*. Classification, diagnosis, and approach to treatment for angioedema: consensus *report* from the Hereditary Angioedema International Working Group. *Allergy* 2014 May;69(5):602–16.

Naevi

4 Meleti M, Mooi WJ, Casparie MK, van der Waal I. Melanocytic nevi of the oral mucosa – no evidence of increased risk for oral malignant melanoma: An analysis of 119 cases. *Oral Oncol* 2007;43:976–81.

Red lesions

Benign migratory glossitis (geographic tongue)
6 Pass B, Brown RS, Childers EL. Geographic tongue: literature review and case reports. *Dent Today* 2005;24:54, 56–7.

Vesiculoerosive disorders

Immune defects
8 Atkinson JC, O'Connell A, Aframian D. Oral manifestations of primary immunological diseases. *J Am Dent Assoc* 2000;131:345–56.

White or whitish lesions

White sponge naevus
8 Zhang JM, Yang ZW, Chen RY, Gao P, Zhang YR, Zhang LF. Two new mutations in the keratin 4 gene causing oral white sponge nevus in Chinese family. *Oral Dis* 2009 Jan;15(1):100–5.

Other congenital abnormalities

Ankyloglossia
10 Messner AH, Lalakea ML. Ankyloglossia: controversies in management. *Int J Pediatr Otorhinolaryngol* 2000;54:123–31.

Cleft lip/palate
4 Ghassibe M, Bayet M, Revencu N, *et al.* Orofacial clefting: update on the role of genetics. *B-ENT* 2006;2 Suppl. 4:20–4.

Gardner syndrome
15 de Oliveira Ribas M, Martins WD, de Sousa MH, *et al.* Oral and maxillofacial manifestations of familial adenomatous polyposis (Gardner's syndrome): a report of two cases. *J Contemp Dent Pract* 2009 Jan 1;10(1):82–90.

Van der Woude syndrome
6 Ziai MN, Benson AG, Djalilian HR. Congenital lip pits and van der Woude syndrome. *J Craniofac Surg* 2005;16:930–2.

Acquired disorders of the oral mucosa or lips

Eosinophilic ulcer of the oral mucosa
8 Chawla O, Burke GA, MacBean AD. The eosinophilic ulcer revisited. *Dent Update* 2007;34:56–7.

Recurrent aphthous stomatitis
1 Scully C. Aphthous ulceration. *N Engl J Med* 2006;355:41–8.
2 Chattopadhyay A, Shetty KV. Recurrent aphthous stomatitis. *Otolaryngol Clin North Am* 2011;44:79–88.
3 Jurge S, Kuffer R, Scully C, Porter SR. Recurrent aphthous stomatitis. *Oral Dis* 2006;12;1–21.
4 Baccaglini L, Lalla RV, Bruce AJ, *et al.* Urban legends: recurrent aphthous stomatitis. *Oral Dis* 2011 Nov:17(8):755–70.

Behçet syndrome
1 Escudier M, Bagan J, Scully C. Behcet's syndrome (Adamantiades syndrome). *Oral Dis* 2006;12:78–84.
12 Webb CJ, Moots RJ, Swift AC. Ear, nose and throat manifestations of Behçet's disease: a review. *J Laryngol Otol* 2008;Dec;122(12):1279–83.

Oral squamous cell carcinoma
1 Scully C. Rule for cancer diagnosis. *Br Dent J* 2013;215(6):265–6.

27 International Agency for Research on Cancer. List of Classifications by cancer sites with sufficient or limited evidence in humans, Volumes 1–105. http://monographs.iarc.fr/ENG/Classification/index.php (last accessed December 2014).

Orofacial granulomatosis
1 Scully C, Eveson JW. Orofacial granulomatosis. *Lancet* 1991;338:20–1.
31 Van der Waal RI, Schulten EA, van der Mehj EH, *et al.* Cheilitis granulomatosa: overview of 13 patients with long-term follow-up – results of management. *Int J Dermatol* 2002;41:225–9.

Erythema multiforme
1 Farthing P, Bagan JV, Scully C. Mucosal disease series. Number IV. Erythema multiforme. *Oral Dis* 2005;11:261–7.

Acute necrotizing (ulcerative) gingivitis and noma
3 Enwonwu CO, Falkler WA Jr, Phillips RS. Noma (cancrum oris). *Lancet* 2006;368:147–56.

Mucositis
4 Lalla RV, Saunders DP, Peterson DE. Chemotherapy or radiation-induced oral mucositis. *Dent Clin North Am* 2014 Apr;58(2):341–9.
13 Scully C, Sonis S, Diz Dios P. Oral mucositis. *Oral Dis* 2006;12:229–41.

Graft-versus-host disease
2 Kuten-Shorrer M, Woo SB, Treister NS. Oral graft-versus-host disease. *Dent Clin North Am* 2014 Apr;58(2):351–68.

Loss of elasticity of oral tissues

Oral submucous fibrosis
1 Arakeri G, Brennan PA. Oral submucous fibrosis: an overview of the aetiology, pathogenesis, classification, and principles of management. *Br J Oral Maxillofac Surg* 2013 Oct;51(7):587–93.
2 Dionne KR, Warnakulasuriya S, Binti Zain R, Cheong SC. Potentially malignant disorders of the oral cavity: Current practice and future directions in the clinic and laboratory. *Int J Cancer* 2014; Jan 31.

Oral soreness without ulceration

Burning mouth syndrome
22 Buchanan J, Zakrzewska J. Burning mouth syndrome. *Clin Evidence* 2003;9:1506–11.
28 Zakrzewska JM, Forssell H, Glenny AM. Interventions for the treatment of burning mouth syndrome: a systematic review. *J Orofac Pain* 2003;17:293–300.

Lichen planus
31 Baccaglini L, Thongprasom K, Carrozzo M, Bigby M. Urban legends series: lichen planus. *Oral Dis* 2013 Mar;19(2):128–43.

Mucous membrane pemphigoid
3 Bagan J, Lo Muzio L, Scully C. Mucosal disease series. Number III. Mucous membrane pemphigoid. *Oral Dis* 2005;11:197–218.
31 Di Zenzo G, Carrozzo M, Chan LS. Urban legend series: mucous membrane pemphigoid. *Oral Dis* 2014 Jan;20(1):35–54.

Pemphigus
1 Scully C, Challacombe SJ. Pemphigus vulgaris: update on etiopathogenesis, oral manifestations and management. *Crit Rev Oral Biol Med* 2002;13:397–408.
46 Cirillo N, Cozzani E, Carrozzo M, Grando SA. Urban legends: pemphigus vulgaris. *Oral Dis* 2012 Jul;18(5):442–58.

Herpesviruses
1 Grinde B. Herpesviruses: latency and reactivation – viral strategies and host response. *J Oral Microbiol* 2013;5:10.

PART 10: SITES, SEX, AGE

Herpes simplex stomatitis

5 Gilbert SC. Oral shedding of herpes simplex virus type 1 in immunocompetent persons. *J Oral Pathol Med* 2006;35:548–53.

Pigmented lesions

HIV infection

8 Patton LL, Ramirez-Amador V, Anaya-Saavedra G, Nittayananta W, Carrozzo M, Ranganathan K. Urban legends series: oral manifestations of HIV infection. *Oral Dis* 2013 Sep;19(6):533–50.

Red lesions

Angina bullosa haemorrhagica

4 Giuliani M, Favia GF, Lajolo C, Miani CM. Angina bullosa haemorrhagica: presentation of eight new cases and a review of the literature. *Oral Dis* 2002;8:54–8.

Denture-related stomatitis

1 Figueiral MH, Azul A, Pinto E, Fonseca PA, Branco FM, Scully C. Denture-related stomatitis:Identification and characterization of aetiological and predisposing factors – a large cohort. *J Oral Rehabil* 2007;34:448–55.

Median rhomboid glossitis

13 McCullough MJ, Savage NW. Oral candidosis and the therapeutic use of antifungal agents in dentistry. *Aust Dent J* 2005;50:S36–9.

Desquamative gingivitis

3 Leao JC, Ingafou M, Khan A, Scully C, Porter SR. Desquamative gingivitis; retrospective analysis of disease associations of a large cohort. *Oral Dis* 2008;14:556–60.

Erythroplasia

3 Reichert PA, Philipsen HP. Oral erythroplakia – a review. *Oral Oncol* 2005;41:551–61.

4 Villa A, Villa C, Abati S. Oral cancer and oral erythroplakia: an update and implication for clinicians. *Aust Dent J* 2011 Sep;56(3):253–6.

White lesions

Candidosis

12 Manfredi M, Polonelli L, Aguirre-Urizar JM, Carrozzo M, McCullough MJ. Urban legends series: oral candidosis. *Oral Dis* 2013 Apr;19(3):245–61.

Acquired lip lesions

Actinic cheilitis

1 Markopoulos A, Albanidou-Farmaki E, Kayavis I. Actinic cheilitis: clinical and pathologic characteristics in 65 cases. *Oral Dis* 2004;10:212–16.

8 Lim GF, Cusack CA, Kist JM. Perioral lesions and dermatoses. *Dent Clin North Am* 2014 Apr;58(2):401–35.

Actinic prurigo

5 Vega-Memije ME, Mosqueda Taylor A, Irigoyen Camacho ME, *et al*. Actinic prurigo cheilitis: clinicopathologic analysis and therapeutic results in 116 cases. *Oral Surg Oral Med Oral Pathol Oral Radiol Endod* 2002;94:83–91.

Angular cheilitis

1 Park KK, Brodell RT, Helms SE. Angular cheilitis, part 1: local etiologies. *Cutis* 2011 Jun;87(6):289–95.

2 Park KK, Brodell RT, Helms SE. Angular cheilitis, part 2: nutritional, systemic, and drug-related causes and treatment. *Cutis* 2011 Jul;88(1):27–32.

Exfoliative cheilitis

13 Almazrooa SA, Woo SB, Mawardi H, Treister N. Characterization and management of exfoliative cheilitis: a single-center experience. *Oral Surg Oral Med Oral Pathol Oral Radiol* 2013 Dec;116(6):e485–9.

15 Crotty CP, Dicken CH. Factitious lip crusting. *Arch Dermatol* 1981;117:338–40.

Granulomatous cheilitis

52 Van der Waal RI, Schulten EA, Van der Meij EH, *et al*. Cheilitis granulomatosa: overview of 13 patients with long-term follow-up-results of management. *Int J Dermatol* 2002;41:225–9.

CHAPTER 111

Dermatoses of the Male Genitalia

Christopher B. Bunker[1] *and William M. Porter*[2]

[1]University College London Hospitals and Chelsea & Westminster Hospitals, London, UK
[2]Gloucestershire Hospitals NHS Foundation Trust, Gloucester, UK

PART 10: SITES, SEX, AGE

Rook's Textbook of Dermatology, Ninth Edition. Edited by Christopher Griffiths, Jonathan Barker, Tanya Bleiker, Robert Chalmers and Daniel Creamer.
© 2016 John Wiley & Sons, Ltd. Published 2016 by John Wiley & Sons, Ltd.
Companion website: www.rooksdermatology.com

Introduction

Male patients with non-venereological and non-urological skin problems commonly present to genito-urinary or urology clinics where the training and expertise are not orientated to adequate dermatological diagnosis and treatment [1].

Careful dermatological evaluation, including a full history and complete examination, usually allows confident clinical differential diagnosis. A biopsy and other investigations are sometimes indicated. It is important to consider the possibility of sexually transmitted disease or a urological disorder and refer accordingly; combined clinics are useful.

Itching, rashes and tumours are the major components of general dermatology and the genito-crural area is not spared. The pruritic diseases that may affect the region are listed in Boxes 111.1, 111.2 and 111.3 and the causes of genito-crural intertrigo are listed in Boxes 111.4 and 111.5. Itch occurring in the absence of specific diagnostic skin lesions is not usually confined to the genito-crural area, but if so it should not be labelled as psychogenic until all possible causes have been excluded. The intensity with which itch can be perceived in the ano-genital area may be a result of the vagaries of cortical representation afforded the region in the sensorium as well as anxiety about exposure to sexually transmitted disease and genital cleanliness.

History and examination

The symptomatology of genital dermatology is more extensive than the standard symptomatic presentation of skin disease. This obliges the clinician to elicit symptoms resulting from sexual

> **Box 111.1 Common causes of genital pruritus**
>
> - Pruritus ani
> - Eczema/dermatitis
>   - Exogenous
>   - Contact
>   - Irritant
>   - Allergic
>   - Endogenous
>   - Atopic
>   - Seborrhoeic
>   - Lichen simplex
> - Psoriasis
> - Lichen sclerosus
> - Lichen
> - Perianal streptococcal dermatitis
> - Erythrasma
> - Herpes simplex
> - Candidosis
> - Tinea
> - Onchocerciasis (in developing countries)
> - Phthiriasis
> - Scabies
>
> Reproduced from Bunker CB. *Male Genital Skin Disease*.
> London: Saunders, 2004. © 2004, with permission from the author.

> **Box 111.2 Rare causes of genital pruritus**
>
> - Insect bites/papular urticaria
> - Radiodermatitis
> - Hirsutism
> - Hyperhidrosis
> - Fox–Fordyce disease
> - Urticaria and dermographism [2]
> - Dermatitis herpetiformis
> - Chlamydia
> - Gonorrhoea
> - Syphilis
> - Other sexually transmitted diseases
> - Trichosporosis
> - Larva currens
> - Cutaneous larva migrans
> - Onchocerciasis (in Western practice)
> - Bowen disease
> - Extramammary Paget disease
> - Langerhans cell histiocytosis
> - Drugs
> - Foods
> - Senile pruritus
> - Dysaesthesia syndromes
>
> Reproduced from Bunker CB. *Male Genital Skin Disease*.
> London: Saunders, 2004. © 2004, with permission from the author.

dysfunction (e.g. soreness, pain, bleeding or tearing on intercourse) [2] and the components of sexual function (erection, lubrication, libido, ejaculation, orgasm, fertility), urinary dysfunction (frequency, discharge, dysuria) or colorectal symptomatology (pain, bleeding, discharge).

Complete examination is mandatory to elicit important signs at extragenital sites. The physical examination of the male at any age is incomplete without examination of the genitals and scrotum (but this is frequently not carried out in general clinical settings)

> **Box 111.3 Causes of genital itching in the absence of fixed clinical findings**
>
> - Symptomatic dermographism
> - Contact urticaria
>   - Non-immunological (e.g. mechanical friction of pubic hair, topical substances)
>   - Immunological (latex, body fluids)
> - Contact dermatitis
> - Incognito disease
>   - Psoriasis
>   - Candidosis
>   - Scabies
> - Drugs and foods
> - Senile pruritus
> - Delusions of parasitosis
> - Dermatological non-disease
> - Dysaesthesia syndromes
> - Psychosexual
>
> Reproduced from Bunker CB. *Male Genital Skin Disease*.
> London: Saunders, 2004. © 2004, with permission from the author.

Box 111.4 Common causes of genito-crural intertrigo

- Eczema
  - Exogenous
    - Irritant contact
  - Endogenous
    - Seborrhoeic
- Psoriasis (inverse pattern/flexural)
- Erythrasma
- Candidosis
- Tinea
- Trichosporosis (in India)
- Pseudoacanthosis nigricans

Box 111.6 Causes of phimosis

- Non-specific balanoposthitis (e.g. in diabetes)
- Lichen sclerosus
- Lichen planus
- Hidradenitis suppurativa
- Crohn disease
- Cicatricial pemphigoid
- Chronic penile lymphoedema
- Cutaneous lymphoma
- Kaposi sarcoma

Reproduced from Bunker CB. *Male Genital Skin Disease*. London: Saunders, 2004. © 2004, with permission from the author.

and urologists teach that there are three primary reasons for careful examination of the scrotum: pain, swelling and absence of contents. The presence or absence of the prepuce, phimosis or paraphimosis should be sought and the foreskin retracted gently (if present). The gluteal and crural folds should be parted to allow adequate inspection. Sometimes it is useful to elicit dermographism of the inner thighs. Urinalysis completes the physical examination.

Findings specific to the male genitalia include phimosis, paraphimosis, balanitis and posthitis. Phimosis ('muzzling') refers to a non-retractable foreskin. The literature can be confusing; Rickwood *et al.* [3] have defined it as scarring of the tip of the foreskin. There are many possible causes of phimosis (Box 111.6). In adults, phimosis is usually the consequence of a number of disease processes, including titanium balanitis attributed to titanium formulated in proprietary topical preparations [4]. In one report, diabetes was diagnosed in 36% of men between 17 and 59 years of age presenting with phimosis of less than 2 years' duration, with no specific

preputial pathology identified histologically [5]. In boys, the histological findings may be normal in nearly half of those circumcised [6]. This finding does not exclude lichen sclerosus or other dermatoses, since the prepuce may not be the seat of the disease, but might contribute to it.

Paraphimosis refers to a foreskin fixed in retraction. Although some authors have used the term to describe a foreskin that is tight in retraction around the flaccid penile shaft, 'waisting' or 'constrictive posthitis' may be better terms [7]. Rickwood [8] has said that paraphimosis results from abuse not disease of the foreskin, but some medical causes can be identified (Box 111.7).

Balanitis is inflammation of the glans penis; posthitis is inflammation of the prepuce [9]. Balanoposthitis means inflammation of the glans and prepuce, and can be regarded as a special form of intertrigo (Boxes 111.8 and 111.9). By definition, therefore,

Box 111.7 Causes of paraphimosis

- Acute contact urticaria
- Acute allergic contact dermatitis
- Lichen sclerosus

Reproduced from Bunker CB. *Male Genital Skin Disease*. London: Saunders, 2004. © 2004, with permission from the author.

Box 111.5 Rare causes of genito-crural intertrigo

- Eczema
  - Exogenous
    - Allergic contact
  - Endogenous
    - Atopic
- Reactive arthritis
- Lichen sclerosus
- Hailey–Hailey disease
- Darier disease
- Streptococcal dermatitis
- Gonorrhoea
- Secondary syphilis
  - Part of a syphilide
  - Mucous patch
- Congenital syphilis (in the infant)
- Trichosporosis (in industrialized countries)
- Extramammary Paget disease
- Kaposi sarcoma
- Langerhans cell histiocytosis
- Carcinoma erysipeloides

Reproduced from Bunker CB. *Male Genital Skin Disease*. London: Saunders, 2004. © 2004, with permission from the author.

Box 111.8 Common causes of balanoposthitis

- Eczema
  - Exogenous
    - Allergic contact
    - Irritant contact
  - Endogenous
    - Seborrhoeic
- Psoriasis
- Reactive arthrtitis
- Zoon plasma cell balanitis
- Lichen sclerosus
- Gonorrhoea
- Human papillomavirus
- Herpes simplex
- Candidosis

Reproduced from Bunker CB. *Male Genital Skin Disease*. London: Saunders, 2004. © 2004, with permission from the author.

Box 111.9 Rare causes of balanoposthitis

- Crohn disease
- Streptococcal dermatitis
- Staphylococcal cellulitis
- Gonorrhoea
- Syphilis
  - Chancre with balanitis of Follmann
  - Mucous patch
- *Mycoplasma*
- *Trichomonas vaginalis*
- Lymphogranuloma venereum
- Non-syphilitic spirochaetal ulcerative balanoposthitis
- Tinea
- Amoebiasis
- Myiasis
- Scabies
- Eccrine syringofibroadenomatosis
- Erythroplasia of Queyrat
- Kaposi sarcoma
- Chronic lymphatic leukaemia
- Fixed drug eruption

Reproduced from Bunker CB. *Male Genital Skin Disease*. London: Saunders, 2004. © 2004, with permission from the author.

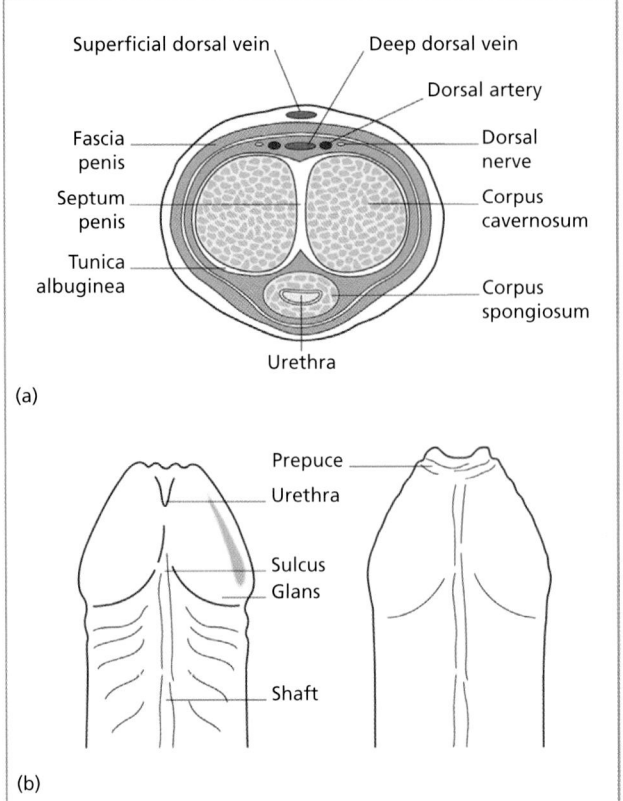

Figure 111.1 (a) Cross-section of the body of the penis. (b) Circumcised and uncircumcised glans penis. (Adapted from *Last's Anatomy*, 9th edn. Reproduced from Bunker CB. *Male Genital Skin Disease*. London: Saunders, 2004. © 2004, with permission from the author.)

balanoposthitis cannot normally occur in the circumcised male, but with age and obesity men may acquire a 'pseudo' foreskin, with attendant risks. Generally, dermatologists feel that balanitis, posthitis and balanoposthitis are probably more commonly caused by inflammatory and pre-cancerous dermatoses than do genito-urinary physicians, who teach that most cases are caused by infection, usually with *Candida* [10,11]. However, the evidence for *Candida* as a primary cause of balanoposthitis is not strong [12].

The principal causes of male genital ulceration are sexually transmitted and non-sexually transmitted infection, cancer and artefact [13]. Several causes can co-present, especially in HIV/AIDS. Dorsal perforation of the prepuce is a recently highlighted complication of several ulcerative penile diseases, sexually and non-sexually acquired, as listed in Box 111.10 [14,15]. Penile necrosis is a rare but devastating presentation with an important differential diagnosis.

Investigations

In genito-urinary clinics, application of 3–5% acetic acid to the penis is used as an aid to the clinical diagnosis of viral warts and is held to reveal subclinical infection [16], but is not in routine use in

Box 111.10 Causes of dorsal perforation of the prepuce

- Hidradenitis suppurativa
- Pyoderma gangrenosum
- Florid condylomata
- Podophyllin
- Chancroid
- Herpes simplex

dermatological practice. Human papillomavirus (HPV) polymerase chain reaction (PCR) screening suggests that the acetowhite test is not very specific [17–20]. Penoscopy is not generally practised by dermatologists. A penis biopsy is not often necessary but can be informative in carefully selected cases of suspected neoplasia rather than the differential diagnosis of the inflammatory dermatoses [21,22]. It is safe to use small amounts of epinephrine (adrenaline) with the local anaesthetic. Beware of the distal ventral midline area where the urethra is very close to the skin surface. It is often not necessary to suture a punch biopsy site.

Structure and function of the male genitalia

The penis is the male organ of urinary elimination and sexual function (for the insemination of the female). The prepuce and its secretions provide physical and immunological protective functions, and it has erogenous properties (e.g. the penile dartos muscle and the corpuscular receptor-rich ridged band), but none of these is indispensable for erogenous function in copulation or other sexual activity [1]. The scrotum maintains the testes at the ideal temperature for spermatogenesis. The male genital structures are illustrated in Figure 111.1. The *anatomical* position is that of full penile erection.

The anatomy is explained by the embryology [2]. At about the third week of fetal development, mesenchymal tissue from the primitive streak forms cloacal folds around the cloacal membrane, joined anteriorly and cranially to form the genital tubercle, posteriorly and caudally to form an annulus. The cloacal membrane is thus divided into uro-genital and anal membranes craniocaudally, and lateral genital swellings appear as precursors of either the scrotum or labia majora.

Fetal and testicular androgens then induce lengthening of the genital tubercle to form first an urethral groove and then the urethral canal. The urethral epithelium of the penis is therefore derived from endoderm. Initially, it is incomplete cranially where the glans has developed from the genital tubercle. The glandular urethra and the meatus form from an invading canalizing cord of ectoderm. The scrotal swellings fuse posteriorly at about 14 weeks but are empty until birth.

The prepuce [1] is formed by a midline fusion of ectoderm, neuroectoderm and mesenchyme, resulting in a pentalaminar structure consisting of (from the inner layer outwards) squamous mucosal epithelium, lamina propria, dartos muscle, dermis and glabrous skin. The preputial fold progressively extends, but there is also an ingrowth of a cellular lamella. It then fuses with the mucosa of the glans. The female analogue is the clitoral hood.

The ano-genital area is densely endowed with eccrine and apocrine sweat glands. Also in plentiful number are holocrine sebaceous glands, usually in association with hair follicles but also occurring as free glands at some sites such as the anal rim or around the coronal sulcus (Tyson glands). These secretions exist to lubricate hair, lubricate the mucocutaneous junctions to assist in the voiding of excreta and protect the epithelia from irritation, and to lubricate the penis for sexual activity (probably mainly the retraction of the foreskin rather than the penetration of the introitus and vagina).

Pubic hair appears in puberty as vellus hair that is focally replaced by terminal hair. The pattern of pubic hair in men is different from that in women, and its distribution varies widely between men. McGregor [3] defined three patterns (Figure 111.2). Generally, the abdominal wall, pubic mound, groins, scrotum and perineum are hairy but the natal cleft, perianal skin, distal penile shaft, prepuce and glans are hairless.

The pattern of keratinization of the epithelium is different throughout the ano-genital area, particularly at the mucosal junctions, the prepuce and distal penile shaft and the glans in the circumcised male. The spectrum of differentiation of the male uro-genital tract is manifest in the expression of differing epithelial cytokeratins [4].

Normal variants

Normal male genital variants include pigmentary variation, hair variation (as discussed earlier), skin tags, pearly penile papules, sebaceous prominence, melanocytic naevi, prominent veins, angiomas and angiokeratomas, common congenital abnormalities and circumcision.

Skin tags are common in the groins, especially of obese men. They may catch on clothing, bleed and become infected. Treatment is by electrocautery or scissor amputation and cautery. Fibrosed haemorrhoids result in perianal skin tags. Larger, fleshier, more oedematous skin tags should arouse the suspicion of Crohn disease. They can predate gastrointestinal disease by several years. Sigmoidoscopy and biopsy should be considered [1].

Pearly penile papules are common; they may be found in up to 50% of men [2,3]. They present as flesh-coloured, pink, smooth, rounded, 1–3 mm papules, occurring predominantly around the coronal margin of the glans, rarely on the glans, in rows or rings (Figure 111.3). Ectopic lesions on the penile shaft have been reported [4]. They are frequently mistaken for warts and misdiagnosed as Tyson glands or ectopic sebaceous glands of Fordyce. The patient is often an anxious adolescent. The histology is that of angiofibroma. The lesion is analogous to other acral angiofibromas such as adenoma sebaceum, subungual and periungual fibromas, fibrous papule of the nose, acquired acral angiofibroma and oral fibroma [5]. Reassurance is usually sufficient but cryotherapy and laser treatment can be effective [6,7].

Sebaceous gland prominence, Tyson glands, sebaceous hyperplasia and ectopic sebaceous glands of Fordyce are all virtually synonymous, common, normal variants of the skin of the scrotal sac and penile shaft, but they may cause concern to the patient

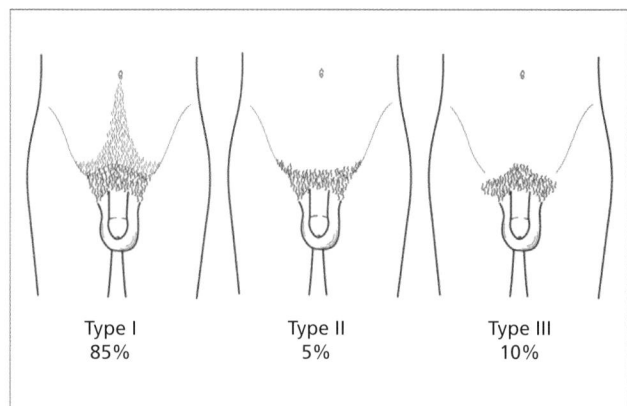

Figure 111.2 Normal distribution of pubic hair in men (three types). (After McGregor [3]. Reproduced from Bunker CB. *Male Genital Skin Disease*. London: Saunders, 2004. © 2004 with permission from the author.)

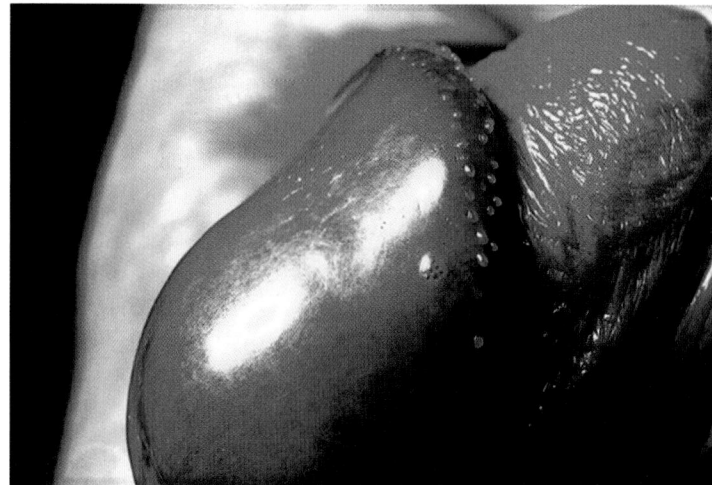

Figure 111.3 Pearly penile papules. (Courtesy of Dr D. A. Burns, Leicester, UK.)

PART 10: SITES, SEX, AGE

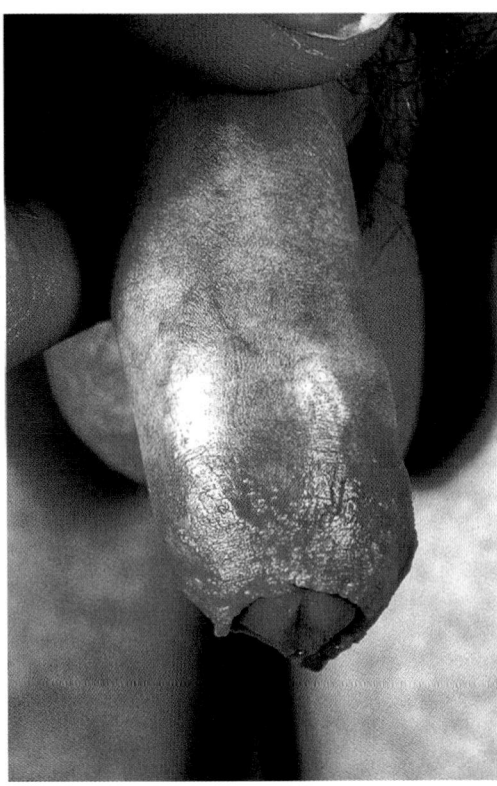

Figure 111.4 Prominent sebaceous glands on the penis. (Courtesy of Dr F. A. Ive, Durham, UK.)

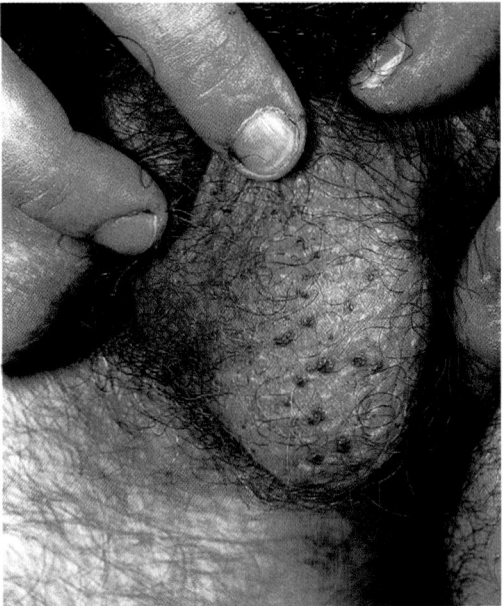

Figure 111.5 Scrotal angiokeratoma of Fordyce. (Courtesy of Dr D. A. Burns, Leicester, UK.)

(Figure 111.4). They have been held to be very rare or their presence doubted at all [8]. Fordyce's condition also commonly affects the vermilion border of the lips. Naevoid linear lesions on the penile shaft have been seen [9–11]. The glans can be affected [12]. Reassurance is usually all that is required, but dysmorphophobia can occur.

Congenital and acquired melanocytic naevi are common. It is possible that naevi on the penis occur more frequently in patients with the atypical naevus syndrome, but this has not been formally documented. Genital epithelioid blue naevus is very rare [13]. A man who developed multiple blue naevi on the glans penis has been described [14]. Spitz naevus has been described [15]. Divided or 'kissing' naevus (analogous to the entity recognized on the eyelids) has been reported, with one component located on the glans and the other on the distal penile shaft or prepuce, separated by uninvolved skin across the coronal sulcus [16–18]; melanoma developed in one case [19]. Large 'bathing trunk' naevi frequently involve the ano-genital area and pose significant management problems, including the risk of melanoma.

Prominent veins are common, if not universal, and occasionally give rise to concern. Vascular white spots are sometimes seen on the glans, and are possibly analogous to Bier spots seen on the palms and forearms.

Cherry Campbell de Morgan angiomas may, unusually, be confined to the genitalia. Angiokeratomas on the genitalia have also confusingly been given the Fordyce eponym (Figure 111.5). They are usually multiple, blue to purple, smooth, 2–5 mm papules on the scrotum; angiokeratomas occur rarely on the penile shaft [20] and glans [10,21]. The role of local venous hypertension in the causation of these lesions is controversial [22]. Angiomas and angiokeratomas may bleed following trauma. The differential diagnosis includes angiokeratoma corporis diffusum, acquired capillary and cavernous haemangiomas, Masson tumour, glomus tumour, epithelioid haemangioma, bacillary angiomatosis, Kaposi sarcoma and epithelioid haemangioendothelioma. One case of florid genital angiokeratomatosis has been associated, perhaps coincidentally, with corporeal papular xanthomatosis [23]. Hyfrecation, electrocautery or laser ablation [24] can be offered, but lesions recur. Appearing in some contexts, such as HIV infection or follow-up for genital cancer, they can cause alarm [25]. Most patients are content with reassurance, and a biopsy is not usually necessary.

The foreskin

The prepuce has been present in primates for 65–100 million years and its function is controversial [1,2,3,4]. It is usual for it to be adherent to the glans at birth. Four per cent of boys have a retractable foreskin at birth, 15% at 6 months, 50% at 1 year and 80–90% at 3 years; the process should be complete by 17 years [5]. The foreskin varies in length and retractability: 'short' and 'long' variants are seen.

Circumcision

Circumcision has been performed for religious, cultural or medical reasons throughout history [1] and a variety of techniques or alternative surgical procedures are now employed [2,3]. Worldwide, it has been estimated that approximately 25% of men have been circumcised [4]. Routine neonatal circumcision is controversial [5,6–8]. The UK General Medical Council (GMC) undertook a review of infantile circumcision in 1997, which 'demonstrated widely conflicting views in society that neither doctors nor the GMC can resolve' [9]. The debate still rages although some policy makers now endorse the procedure for derived health benefits [10]. The effects of circumcision on male sexual function and sensitivity are also disputed [11,12].

During infancy, circumcised boys have a higher incidence of penile problems than the uncircumcised, but after infancy the situation is significantly reversed [13,14]. Circumcision reduces the retrieval of pathogenic microorganisms from the penis [15,16]. Many have concluded that circumcision protects men from HPV infection, cancer of the penis and urinary tract, and sexually transmitted infections including HIV [17,18–20]. However, the incidence of penis cancer is low in countries where circumcision is uncommon [21], so other factors are important in penile carcinogenesis. Also, the effects of circumcision on the other outcomes may be small [22] (e.g. urethritis may be more common in the circumcised, whereas ulcerative disease is more common in the uncircumcised). Circumcision protects men from inflammatory genital dermatoses including psoriasis, seborrhoeic dermatitis, lichen planus and lichen sclerosus [23]. This fact may be related to the occlusion and moisture consequent on the presence of the prepuce. O'Farrell *et al.* observed penile wetness in hardly any circumcised men, yet it is present in 40% of uncircumcised men with 'balanitis' [24].

Circumcision is important in the management of disorders of the penis and the foreskin, including dermatological disease. However, variability exists between clinicians in the indications for circumcision, especially in children. They include true phimosis, recurrent balanoposthitis, lichen sclerosus, penile lymphoedema, intraepithelial neoplasia and carcinoma.

The consensus is that circumcision has insignificant adverse effects on health, but it is not risk free or complication free: bleeding, infection, necrosis, adhesions, bridges, fistula, keloid, concealed or buried penis, amputation, necrosis, excessive excision of penile skin, meatal stenosis, meatitis and meatal ulcer, cysts, chordee, hypospadias and epispadias, amputation neuromas, abnormal sexual behaviour, psychological distress and dysmorphophobia [25–36]. In some developing world settings, the complication rate can be very high [35], implying that better training is required if circumcision is going to become more commonly adopted as part of HIV-prevention strategies [18]. 'Uncircumcision' describes preputial restoration performed throughout history for various reasons [37,38].

As circumcised men age and become obese the penis may retract into the pubic mound – the 'vanishing penis syndrome'. This phenomenon can create a 'pseudoforeskin', especially if the initial circumcision was inadequate or incomplete, and this favours the development of dermatoses found characteristically only in uncircumcised men, such as Zoon balanitis and lichen sclerosus [39].

Congenital and developmental abnormalities

Congenital and developmental anomalies are common, reflecting the complicated embryogenesis and subsequent sexual differentiation of the ano-genital region. The dermatologist may not be called upon to make a primary diagnosis, but needs to be aware of syndromic associations as well as anatomical and functional abnormalities because these additionally predispose the area to dermatoses and infections. Naevi are discussed earlier. Other common abnormalities include meatal pit, sacral pit, hypospadias, median raphe cysts, canals and sinuses, and ambiguous genitalia [1,2,3].

Rarer anomalies include hypospadias variants, epispadias, penile hypoplasia, mucoid or urethral cysts, dermoid cyst, juvenile xanthogranuloma, buried penis, urethral atresia, penoscrotal transposition, congenital lymphoedema, lymphangiectasia, lymphangioma, giant preputial sac, megaprepuce, accessory scrotum, haemangiomas, strawberry naevus, white sponge naevus, os penis, true aposthia and faun tail [2,4,5,6].

This is not the place exhaustively to catalogue all of the syndromes that may be associated with one or other of the above common or rarer anomalies; however, examples include anogenital haemangiomas in the PELVIS syndrome (perineal haemangioma, external genitalia malformations, lipomyelomeningocele, vesicorenal abnormalities, imperforate anus and skin tag) [7], ano-genital lymphoedema in Hennekam syndrome [8], the micropenis of the MORM syndrome (mental retardation, truncal obesity, retinal dystrophy and micropenis) and Kabuki make-up syndrome [9,10], the cribriform scrotal atrophy associated with an unusual form of ectodermal dysplasia [11] and genital leukoplakia associated with dyskeratosis congenita [12].

TRAUMA AND ARTEFACT

Definition

Exogenous causes of penile trauma.

Introduction and general description

This is a rarely encountered phenomenon in male genital dermatology clinics.

Penile haematoma and rupture

The genitals may be readily traumatized, including by sexual activity. The penis is very vascular but haematoma formation and 'fracture' (penile rupture) are quite rare [1,2]. Pain, swelling and deformity associated with the history of a cracking noise during strenuous or contorted intercourse characterize the diagnosis. Splitting of the tunica albuginea of the corpus cavernosum can result in urethral damage, haematoma and retention. The prognosis is generally good but Peyronie disease can occur [3]. Injection of drugs for erectile dysfunction can be complicated by haematoma.

Sclerosing lymphangitis

Non-venereal sclerosing lymphangitis/penile venereal oedema/ Mondor phlebitis/localized penile (venereal) lymphoedema/ penile lymphocele presents with a serpiginous mass in the coronal sulcus. The lesion usually arises after prolonged or frequent sexual intercourse with a passive or unenthusiastic partner; subsequent sexual activity may result in tenderness and enlargement. The circumferential scar left by circumcision may be a predisposing factor. There may be spontaneous resolution, or surgical excision may be needed [4]. It is not known whether lymphangitis or phlebitis is the cause [5]. True phlebitis of penile and scrotal veins has been reported in three patients, of whom one had been injured by a golf ball, but the other cases were idiopathic [6]. Its occurrence after taking tadalafil for erectile dysfunction has been used to argue for an anatomical variation in the distal draining subcoronal venous emissary arcade [7]. Thrombophlebitis of superficial penile and scrotal veins is analogous to Mondor phlebitis of the chest wall, but it may be associated with polyarteritis nodosa and thromboangiitis obliterans [8]. Penile thrombophlebitis has been misdiagnosed as Peyronie disease, and has also been the initial manifestation of a paraneoplastic migratory thrombophlebitis resulting from pancreatic cancer [9]. Given the circumstances that usually create the problem patients should be screened for underlying sexually transmitted infection, despite the appellation [10].

Strangulation of the penis

The penis may be strangulated by ring devices [11,12], including vacuum erection equipment [13], condom rings [14], rubber bands, string, rings (washers), nuts, bushes and sprockets, which are placed deliberately on the penis by the patient for masturbation or to prolong erection [15,16]. In boys, strangulation can occur following experimental use of rubber bands, string or thread to control enuresis, or can result from encoiled hair after circumcision [17]. Penile strangulation – the tourniquet syndrome – causes pain, swelling, urethral fistula, pseudoainhum, gangrene, amputation and even death [18].

Foreign body

Self-instrumentation of the external genitalia may have an autoerotic, psychiatric, therapeutic (relief of itch [19], aiding voiding, cleaning) or accidental aetiology [20]. Complications include frequency, haematuria, abscess, retention, fistulae and calculi. The diagnosis is made by palpation and radiography. Endoscopic removal is usually possible for foreign bodies below the uro-genital diaphragm.

Glass beads, spheres of plastic or small round smooth stones (even pearls) may be introduced under the skin of the penis for erotic reasons, causing clinical and radiographical confusion. In the Philippines, this practice is called 'bulleetus', in Sumatra 'persimbraon', in Korea 'chagan ball' and in Thailand 'mukhsa' or 'tancho' [21,22,23]. Extrusion of a testicular prosthesis has been reported as a cause of scrotal ulceration [24].

If oil, petroleum jelly or silicone is used then a paraffinoma, silicone granuloma or (sclerosing) lipogranuloma can result.

Lipogranuloma

Patients may take it upon themselves to inject various substances with the aim of maintaining erection or enlarging the penis. The consequences may not be desirable. Infection is an obvious risk [25]. Mineral oil, petroleum jelly and silicone introduced into the genital skin can elicit lipogranuloma or paraffinoma. Most cases are self-induced, either to increase penile size or enhance sexual pleasure, but some may be accidental [26,27]. One patient injected his penis with an industrial high-pressure pneumatic grease gun [28]. Idiopathic cases attributed to endogenous fat liberation have been reported, predominantly from Japan [29]. The psychological consequences may be debilitating [30].

Dermatitis artefacta and mutilation

Dermatitis artefacta of the genitalia does occur. Lesions are typically geometrical, angulated and rectilinear. Sometimes they are induced by needles, knives or cigarette burns, and extraneous foreign material may be introduced into the skin (lipogranuloma and silicone granuloma are discussed earlier).

Psychotic patients may mutilate their genitalia, as may transvestites [30], but non-psychotic genital self-mutilation can also occur. Australian aborigines create a slit in the penis by opening the urethra ventrally, thereby creating hypospadias; this is called subincision [31,32,33]. Biopsy and other investigations may be necessary to exclude penile cancer. It is important also to consider pyoderma gangrenosum, which is rare but frequently omitted from the differential diagnosis of penile ulceration by non-dermatologists.

Child abuse

Physical and sexual child abuse should be considered in the differential diagnosis of cutaneous disease of the ano-genital area in children (Box 111.11), but signs should be interpreted with caution and re-examination should be avoided [34,35–38]. Child abuse may be erroneously suspected (Box 111.12) when the ano-genital area is involved by a dermatosis or a diarrhoeal illness [39].

Box 111.11 Ano-genital signs of child abuse

- Overall context
- Emotional disturbance
- Passivity on ano-genital examination
- Anal relaxation/dilatation
- Purpura, bruising, tearing
- Signs of sexually transmitted disease

Reproduced from Bunker CB. *Male Genital Skin Disease*. London: Saunders, 2004. © 2004, with permission from the author.

Box 111.12 Ano-genital mimics of child abuse

- Nappy rash
- Innocent skin tags and fissures
- Threadworms
- Eczema
- Phytophotodermatitis
- Lichen sclerosus
- Henoch–Schönlein purpura
- Acute haemorrhagic oedema of childhood
- Ano-genital streptococcal dermatitis
- Causes of diarrhoea
  - Haemolytic–uraemic syndrome
  - Crohn disease
- Causes of constipation
  - Hirschsprung disease

Reproduced from Bunker CB. *Male Genital Skin Disease.* London: Saunders, 2004. © 2004, with permission from the author.

The significance of ano-genital warts in suggesting possible child sexual abuse is controversial. However, early recognition as a marker for child sexual abuse is in the child's long-term best interest [40].

Other traumatic and artefactual conditions

Sometimes the penis is bitten by another individual or an animal [41]. Purpura and ecchymoses may develop after oral sex ('love bites') or the use of vacuum erection devices [13]. Post-traumatic neuromas may be encountered and be mistaken for genital warts or pearly penile papules [42]. Degloving injuries can occur in accidents with industrial or agricultural equipment [43]. Electrical burns are rare [44]. Sex aids can result in abrasions, eczema and ulceration. Self-circumcision might be attempted, with adverse consequences [45]. Ano-genital tattoos are commonplace [46].

Localized gangrene of the scrotum and penis resulting from arterial embolization with particulate matter complicating accidental femoral self-injection of heroin in an addict has been reported [47]. Scrotal gangrene from a snake bite has been described [48].

INFLAMMATORY DERMATOSES

Psoriasis

Introduction and general description
This is a common condition that can affect the male genital region in isolation or as part of widely distributed disease. Reactive arthritis (part of the same continuum as psoriasis in genetically predisposed individuals) is discussed elsewhere. Characteristic, sometimes severe, involvement of the penis (circinate balanitis) occurs. The penile lesions have the same histopathology as psoriasis.

Epidemiology
Approximately 2% of the population are said to have psoriasis but it is possible that many more than 2% of men may have or have had ano-genital psoriasis at some time; it is certainly a common ano-genital diagnosis in isolation.

Pathophysiology
Psoriasis and its clinical manifestations and the relationship of psoriasis to HIV/AIDS are discussed in other chapters (see Chapters 35 and 31).

Clinical features

Presentation
Ano-genital presentations of psoriasis may be vague in symptomatology and non-specific on examination. It is not usually itchy; significant itch should arouse suspicions of another dermatosis such as an eczematous dermatitis or tinea. Soreness occurs with superinfection, especially with *Candida*. Other typically affected sites should be examined for signs of the disease. Genital appearances may be challenging to interpret, especially in the uncircumcised patient, because a mucosal site is affected rather than keratinized skin. The diagnosis is usually easier in the circumcised male where the morphology is similar to extragenital lesions.

Inverse pattern psoriasis refers to the manifestation of the disease on intertriginous skin in the axillae, natal cleft, gluteal folds, groins and in the preputial sac and on the glans of the uncircumcised male, where its occurrence is probably brought about by the Koebner phenomenon.

Differential diagnosis
Eczema, fixed drug eruption, lichen planus, carcinoma *in situ*, extramammary Paget disease.

Investigations
Usually, the diagnosis of psoriasis is clinical, but a biopsy may be necessary (e.g. of a solitary mucosal lesion in an uncircumcised individual) to distinguish psoriasis from Zoon balanitis, lichen planus, carcinoma *in situ* (Bowen disease, erythroplasia of Queyrat) or Kaposi sarcoma. Carcinoma *in situ* and extramammary Paget disease may be misdiagnosed as psoriasis when there are single or several foci on the penile shaft and/or in the groins.

Management
Topical treatment includes emollients, soap substitutes, corticosteroids combined with antibiotic and antifungal agents or weak tar solutions. Strong crude tar preparations should be avoided at this site given that ano-genital skin has a propensity to increased absorption of topical agents and because of the risk of genital cancer; one of the first occupational diseases described was scrotal carcinoma in chimney sweeps. Dithranol is usually avoided in this region. The vitamin D analogue calcipotriol can be helpful. Topical ciclosporin (100 mg/mL in wet dressings three times daily) has been advocated [1]. Topical calcineurin inhibitors may be helpful [2,3,4] and appear to be well tolerated but should be used with circumspection in the uncircumcised because of the squamous cancer risk. Phototherapy is contraindicated because of the risk of

ano-genital cancer. Severe ano-genital psoriasis can be an indication for systemic treatment. Circinate balanitis responds to topical calcineurin inhibitors.

Eczema

Introduction and general description

This is a very common presentation and is covered in more detail in other chapters (see Chapters 39, 40 and 41). It has several clinical manifestations and causes, and may present with male genital involvement in isolation.

Clinical variants and presentation

Eczematous dermatoses

Itching and lichenification, particularly around the scrotum, are common presenting problems. Contributory factors include pre-existing dermatoses such as xerosis, atopy and psoriasis, sedentary occupations, motor car and aeroplane travel, and tight underclothing and trousers.

Irritation is a key adverse exogenous influence to which ano-genital sites are vulnerable, and sweat, sebum, desquamated corneocytes, dirt, excreta, sexual secretions, clothing, detergents, toiletries, cosmetics, contraceptives and some therapeutic topical treatments are all potential irritants.

Frequently underrated are the effects of overwashing and the excessive use of soap and toiletries, especially in the presence of skin symptoms or urinary or bowel problems, and particularly if patients feel that they might have been exposed to a sexually transmitted disease.

Lichen simplex

Lichen simplex is common around the male genitalia. It is not usually a flexural condition but can be seen on the penile shaft and scrotum (Figure 111.6). Giant forms (of Pautrier) occur, giving a

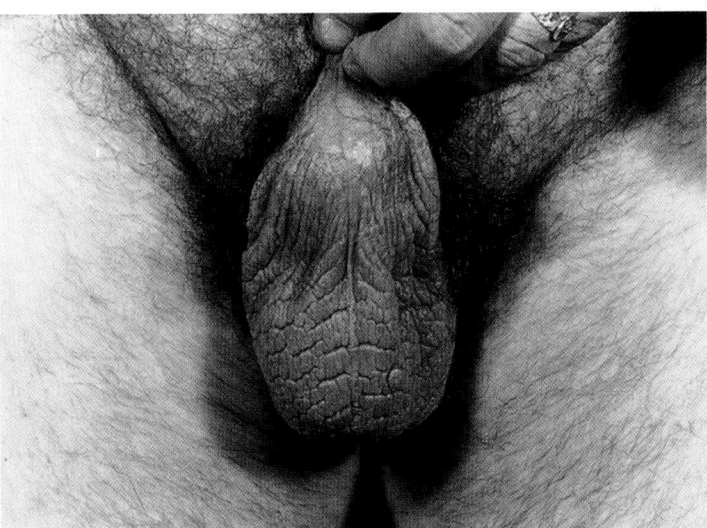

Figure 111.6 Scrotal lichen simplex. (Courtesy of Dr F. A. Ive, Durham, UK.)

> **Box 111.13 Ano-genital irritants**
>
> - Sweat
> - Sebum
> - Desquamated corneocytes
> - Dirt
> - Excreta
> - Sexual secretions
> - Clothing
> - Soap and detergents
> - Toiletries
> - Toilet paper
> - Cosmetics
> - Contraceptives
> - Therapeutic agents
> - Friction
> - Maceration
>
> Reproduced from Bunker CB. *Male Genital Skin Disease*. London: Saunders, 2004. © 2004, with permission from the author.

---

pineapple appearance [1]. The skin may be broken by excoriations and become secondarily impetiginized or colonized by *Candida*.

Irritant contact dermatitis

Ano-genital irritants are discussed earlier and listed in Box 111.13. Friction [2], maceration, overwashing, and concomitant anorectal or urological disease are the chief influences. There may be an association with atopy; Birley *et al.* [3] diagnosed irritant dermatitis in 72% of patients presenting to a genito-urinary clinic with 'balanitis' (probably meaning balanoposthitis) of whom a possible 67% had a history of atopy, but none of these patients was patch tested. An irritant scrotal dermatitis in cellists has been described [4]. Topical 5-fluorouracil used to treat keratoses at extragenital sites has caused genital irritant dermatitis [5]. Acute or chronic, sterile or superinfected (with staphylococci or *Candida*, or both), eroded or hyperkeratotic presentations are seen, depending on the scenario. A good example is nappy (diaper) rash.

Allergic contact dermatitis

The risks of allergic contact dermatitis of the genital skin come about from: (i) direct contact with the allergen (e.g. medicaments – even coal tar allergy has been reported [6]), contraceptive usage and prosthetic limbs in amputees [3,7]; or, very rarely, (ii) transfer of allergen (e.g. urushiol as in poison oak, poison ivy and poison sumac dermatitis) to the genitalia [8] and possibly subsequent exposure to sunlight (e.g. psoralens from fig or citrus plants, as in phytodermatitis); and (iii) involvement in a more generalized eczematous response (e.g. to a medicament or dressing used on venous eczema or ulceration, as in the autosensitization/secondary spread/secondary generalization syndrome).

Eczematous symptomatology can appear approximately 1 week after first contact with the allergen if previously unsensitized, or within a few hours if already allergic. The patient may present with pruritus ani [9] or paraphimosis [10]. More immediate symptomatology and acute erythema and angio-oedema suggest a contact urticaria, which can occur with some of the rubber constituents of condoms and gloves [4,5,**11**,12,13,**14**].

The most common relevant sensitivities are to rubber, contraceptives, preservatives and fragrances in toiletries and medicaments, and the active agents (antibiotics, steroids, anaesthetics) in medicaments. Allergy to methylisothiozolinone, an ubiquitous preservative, is becoming an often reported phenomenon [6,15].

Genital rubber dermatitis is not confined to young sexually active male condom users and their partners [16–18,19]. Incontinent men who use external urinary collection devices (Paul's tubing) are also at risk. Latex allergy may be a problem in patients with spinal cord injury using rubber products for the management of urinary difficulties; life-threatening anaphylactic reactions have occurred [20]. Condoms made from lamb caecum are available for rubber-allergic patients, but they may provide less protection against sexually transmitted disease than latex. Creating hypoallergenic condoms by washing in an ammonium solution to remove the residues of the accelerator chemicals that actually cause the hypersensitivity has proved unsuccessful [21]. Patients may become sensitized to the spermicide [15].

Celandine juice [10] and clothing dye dermatitis of the scrotum [22] have been reported.

Atopic eczema

Genital skin disease caused by atopic eczema is not uncommon but rarely occurs in isolation, unlike other common chronic dermatoses such as seborrhoeic dermatitis and psoriasis. It is not known how genital atopic eczema is related to circumcision, sexual activity and sexually transmitted disease. Evidence of atopy was found in a possible 67% of a total of 72% of patients diagnosed as having irritant dermatitis from a consecutive series of men presenting to a genito-urinary clinic with 'balanitis' – probably balanoposthitis [8,22].

Radiodermatitis

Radiodermatitis is not usually a diagnostic challenge or a therapeutic problem in the acute stage after radiotherapy to the ano-genital skin for skin disease or internal cancer. In the chronic state, there may be pruritus together with the typical poikiloderma. Radiotherapy has been used for the treatment of numerous ano-genital dermatoses over the years, including Bowen disease, erythroplasia of Queyrat, squamous carcinoma, psoriasis, Peyronie disease and pruritus ani [8,22]. Radiotherapy confers a long-term increased risk of skin cancer, especially basal cell carcinoma. There is concern that radiotherapy for Bowen disease or erythroplasia of Queyrat may increase the subsequent risk of invasive carcinoma.

Seborrhoeic dermatitis

Genital involvement is frequent with this common dermatosis. The groins and penis may be the only sites involved. A good history (including family history) and careful examination of other sites typically affected aid the diagnosis. On the scalp, the face, in the flexures and at ano-genital sites seborrhoeic dermatitis and psoriasis may be indistinguishable.

Investigations

The diagnosis is usually clinical. Biopsy is rarely required. Patch testing may be suggested for cases suspicious of a contact precipitant.

Box 111.14 Allergens of particular relevance to genital contact dermatitis

- Euxyl® K 400 (methyldibromoglutaronitrile)
- Kathon® CG (isothiazolinones)
- Lidocaine (lignocaine) and other topical anaesthetics
- Neomycin
- Nystatin
- Steroid moieties
- Thiuramdisulphide: rubber
- Latex condoms
- Spermicides
- Mitomycin C

Reproduced from Bunker CB. *Male Genital Skin Disease*. London: Saunders, 2004. © 2004, with permission from the author.

Management

The broad principle of managing allergic contact dermatitis on genital skin is the identification of the potential allergen (Box 111.14) and its likely source, and then its elimination. There may be clues to these factors at presentation but subsequent patch testing is often required. Following patch testing, Shelley and Shelley [5] and Bauer *et al.* [14] made a final diagnosis of allergic contact dermatitis in 35% of patients with ano-genital skin problems. Allergic contact dermatitis can persist even after withdrawal of the trigger allergen. Management is otherwise as for irritant contact dermatitis, lichen simplex and pruritus ani.

Treatment of male genital lichen simplex follows the lines of management relating to irritants, with emphasis on the relief of scratching, soap substitution and moisturization, and occlusion of the area if possible with a bland dressing – wet if the skin is fiercely eczematized. A potent topical corticosteroid ointment can be used for a few days and then tailed off. Preparations containing tar or combinations of antibacterial, anticandidal and antifungal agents are also useful. Two cases of extensive giant lichen simplex of the scrotum have been successfully treated by hemiscrotectomy [1,9,23].

Management of irritant dermatitis follows lines similar to those for pruritus ani. Irritants should be identified and eliminated or reduced. Advice is given about soap substitutes, moisturizers, towels and toilet paper. Topical corticosteroid ointments, with or without antibiotic and anticandidal agents, are employed to control the dermatitis. Oral antihistamines are useful. Topical local anaesthetics should be avoided because of the risk of sensitization. Occasionally, secondary infection may be severe; a swab should be taken and oral antibiotics and oral antifungals prescribed.

A more acute picture (itch, burning or pain, swelling, erythema, vesiculation) may occur if highly irritant chemicals in high concentration are accidentally or deliberately used on the genitalia. Patients with a genital rash who are frightened that it may have been sexually acquired will sometimes self-treat with unsuitable preparations and in the process increase their morbidity and conceal an underlying sexually transmitted disease or a dermatosis. Treatment is with potassium permanganate soaks, very potent topical corticosteroid creams (sometimes systemic corticosteroids) and systemic antibiotics.

PART 10: SITES, SEX, AGE

No treatment of seborrhoeic dermatitis may be required other than reassurance that it is not sexually transmitted or related to poor hygiene. However, treatments that diminish the *Malassezia* load and reduce irritation and eczematization can be successfully and safely used long term. These include topical antifungals (such as clioquinol, nystatin and imidazoles) as ointments, creams, lotions or shampoos, and mixtures of the same agents with mild and moderately potent topical corticosteroids used alongside emollients and soap substitutes. In severe cases, patients with concomitant seborrhoeic folliculitis, or in patients with HIV/AIDS, treatment with an oral imidazole and/or an oral tetracycline may be suitable.

Zoon balanitis

Introduction and general description
An asymptomatic, inflammatory and irritant condition of the glans and mucosal prepuce that is probably overdiagnosed.

Epidemiology
Zoon plasma cell balanitis is a disorder of the middle-aged and older uncircumcised male [1,2], although an analogous condition has been reported to afflict the vulva, mouth, lips [3] and epiglottis [3,4].

Pathophysiology
Since Zoon's original reports, there have been many accounts in the literature, but the aetiology remains uncertain. The evidence suggests that Zoon balanitis is a chronic, reactive, principally irritant dermatosis brought about by a dysfunctional prepuce. Retention of urine and squames between two tightly apposed and infrequently and inadequately separated and/or inappropriately bathed, commensally hypercolonized, desquamative, secretory epithelial surfaces leads to a disturbed 'preputial ecology' and excessive frictional trauma (Zoon balanitis is often located on the dorsal aspect of the glans and/or the adjacent prepuce, sites of maximal friction on foreskin retraction), and irritation by urine [5,6,7,8]. There is no evidence of an infectious cause, and immunohistochemical findings suggest that Zoon balanitis represents a non-specific polyclonal tissue reaction [9,10], consistent with an irritant dermatosis.

Pathology
The classic histology is of epidermal attenuation with absent granular and horny layers, and diamond- or lozenge-shaped basal cell keratinocytes with sparse dyskeratosis and spongiosis. There is a band of dermal infiltration with plasma cells of variable density. Extravasated erythrocytes, haemosiderin and vascular proliferation are also seen. Although Zoon stressed the presence of the plasma cell infiltrate in this condition, the plasma cell numbers can be very variable [7,8,11].

Clinical features
The presentation is classically indolent and asymptomatic, although staining of the underclothes with blood has been reported [12]. Well-

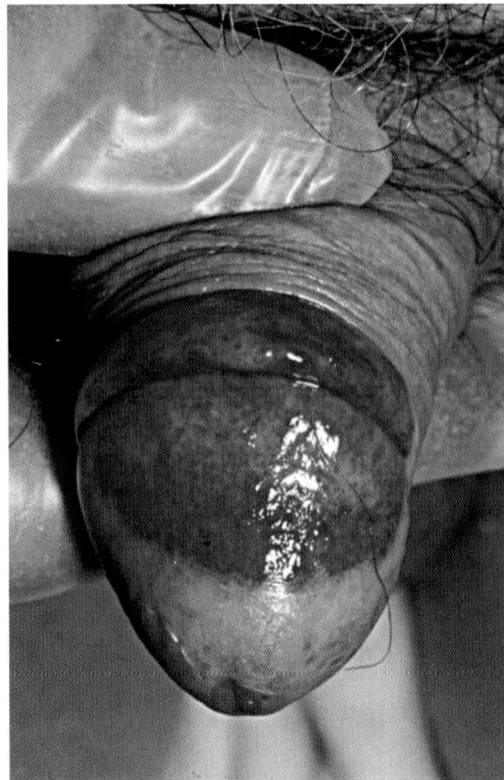

Figure 111.7 Zoon balanitis. Symmetrical moist erythema of the glans and prepuce. (Courtesy of Professor C. B. Bunker, with permission from Medical Illustration UK, Chelsea & Westminster Hospital, London, UK.)

demarcated, glistening, moist, bright red or autumn brown patches involve the glans and visceral prepuce, with sparing of the keratinized penile shaft and foreskin (Figure 111.7). The navicular fossa may be involved. Other signs include dark red stippling – 'cayenne pepper spots' – and purpura with haemosiderin deposition, solitary or multiple lesions of differing sizes (guttate or nummular), characteristically symmetrical about the axis of the coronal sulcus and 'kissing'. Although vegetative and nodular presentations have been recorded, atypical or unusual morphology should be viewed with great suspicion and biopsied [7,8].

Differential diagnosis
The differential diagnosis includes lichen sclerosus, erosive lichen planus, psoriasis, seborrhoeic dermatitis, contact dermatitis, fixed drug eruption, secondary syphilis, histoplasmosis [13], erythroplasia of Queyrat [14] and Kaposi sarcoma. A confident clinical diagnosis is not always possible or safe [6,8,15], so a biopsy is advisable, and the pathologist should be asked to look for concomitant disease. Frank cases of lichen sclerosus, lichen planus, bowenoid papulosis (BP) and penile cancer often appear to have Zoon balanitis-like changes on clinical examination and on histology [8,15]. In other words, the signs of Zoon balanitis may be secondary to underlying preputial disease [8]. It is likely that some of the clinical and histological variants that have been reported [16–18], and a recent claim that Zoon balanitis per se is a pre-malignant condition in a single case report [19], are a consequence of this phenomenon. Zoon balanitis indicates a dysfunctional foreskin

and a more common or more sinister dermatosis may be concealed [8]. Most patients diagnosed with Zoons balanoposthitis probably have clinically subtler underlying lichen sclerosus.

Investigations
The diagnosis is usually clinical.

Management
Although Zoon balanitis can improve with altered washing habits and the intermittent application of a mild or potent topical corticosteroid (with or without an antibiotic and anticandidal agent), it usually persists or relapses [7,8]. Case reports concerning the use of topical calcineurin inhibitors have appeared [20,21,22] but these agents should be used with circumspection in the setting of a dysfunctional foreskin and the attendant risk of penis cancer, long term. It has been claimed that erbium : YAG or carbon dioxide laser treatment is effective [8,23–26]. There have been reports of efficacy with topical imiquimod 5% [27,28]. Circumcision is curative [7,8]. Again, the pathologist should be asked to examine the whole specimen for signs of another underlying dermatosis.

Lichen sclerosus

Definition and nomenclature
Lichen sclerosus is a common inflammatory dermatosis with a predilection for ano-genital skin.

Synonyms and inclusions
• Lichen sclerosus et atrophicus

Introduction and general description
Lichen sclerosus is a common dermatosis of the penis. The diagnosis and management of lichen sclerosus is a frequent reason for patients to be referred to a male genital dermatology clinic.

Epidemiology
Genital lichen sclerosus is more common than extragenital or oral disease, but there may (rarely) be concomitant involvement of these sites. In adults, ano-genital lichen sclerosus is said to be about 10 times more common in women than men. Perianal disease is very rare in the male. The age of presentation is bimodal [1]. The first report of genital lichen sclerosus in boys appeared only in 1977 [2]. Lichen sclerosus may be much more frequent than is generally supposed in young boys, being diagnosed histologically in 14–95% of prepuces removed for phimosis [3,4].

Pathophysiology
The aetiopathogenesis of male genital lichen sclerosus has become clearer in recent years. A credible unifying mechanism must explain key clinical features and the results of prior investigative research: the predilection for the genitalia generally and in males, the uncircumcised [1,5]; the rarity of perianal involvement in men compared with women [1]; the inconsistent association with organ-specific autoimmune disease [1,6,7–13] and atopy [14]; an

association with *ECM1* autoreactivity (probably an epiphenomenon) [15]; the association with squamous carcinoma [6,7–10]; the bimodal pattern of prevalence [1,2,3,16]; the relationship with obesity [17] anatomical abnormality and trauma [9,18]; specifically, lichen sclerosus occurs in hypospadias and complicates its repair [4,19]; it recurs in grafts from unrelated sites, especially skin grafts compared with mucosal grafts [20–24]; it complicates genital piercing and occurs around ureterostomies and urethrostomies [25,26]; and it is common in the bariatric patient. HPV has been reported to be present in 70% of cases of childhood penile lichen sclerosus (types 6, 16 and 18) [27,28], and in 17.4% of adult cases (types 16, 18 and 45) compared with 8.7% of normal males [29] in one study, and in 33% of adult cases (types 16, 18, 33 and 51) in another [30]; recent work suggests that these are not pathogenic associations but represent a 'bystander' phenomenon [2,8,31,32]. Topical steroid treatment of lichen sclerosus may lead to HPV reactivation [33]. Borreliosis [34] and hepatitis C [35] have been implicated and refuted. But the epidemiology and clinical tenor of lichen sclerosus are not those of an infectious or sexually transmitted disease: it is never seen in sexual partners [9,36]. The presence of the histopathological features of lichen sclerosus in a percentage of acrochordons (skin tags) suggests that occlusion of flaccid skin is a pathogenic factor [37]. All the evidence points to male genital lichen sclerosus being due to chronic occluded exposure of susceptible epithelium to urine [1,38–40,41]. Careful interrogation of patients elicits symptoms of post micturition micro-incontinence ('dribbling') in 90–100% [42] and meticulous physical examination often reveals very variable naviculo-meatal anatomy to account for this dysfunction of the putative naviculomeatal valve. Nuclear magnetic resonance spectroscopy of urine has not identified a single culpable chemical constituent of urine [43].

Pathology
The epidermis is atrophic with basal cell hydropic degeneration. The superficial dermis is oedematous and hyalinised. Deep to the hyalinzed zone is a band-like lymphohistiocytic infiltrate. In early cases, the inflammatory infiltrate may be found superficially. Plasma cells are seen in addition to lymphocytes and histiocytes. Telangiectatic vessels are common, as is purpura. The occasional association of endarteritis led originally to the usage of the term 'obliterans' [44]. In two cases in boys, a dermal lymphohistiocytic and granulomatous phlebitis has been found, and one also had evidence of HPV [45]. A 'garland-like' basal lamina has been found ultrastructurally [46]. Sometimes, lichen sclerosus may be difficult to differentiate from lichen planus, and criteria to assist, in the vulva, have been proposed by Fung and LeBoit [47]. The histological features may simulate mycosis fungoides [48].

Clinical features
The development of secondary phimosis in school-age boys is highly suggestive of lichen sclerosus [14]. In the older male, persistent primary phimosis or the secondary development of phimosis in a previously retractable foreskin may be related to lichen sclerosus [9]. Lichen sclerosus of the penis may be asymptomatic, but diverse, sometimes vague, symptomatology is usually encountered at rest or during or after sexual congress. Patients may describe itching, burning, bleeding, tearing, splitting, rash,

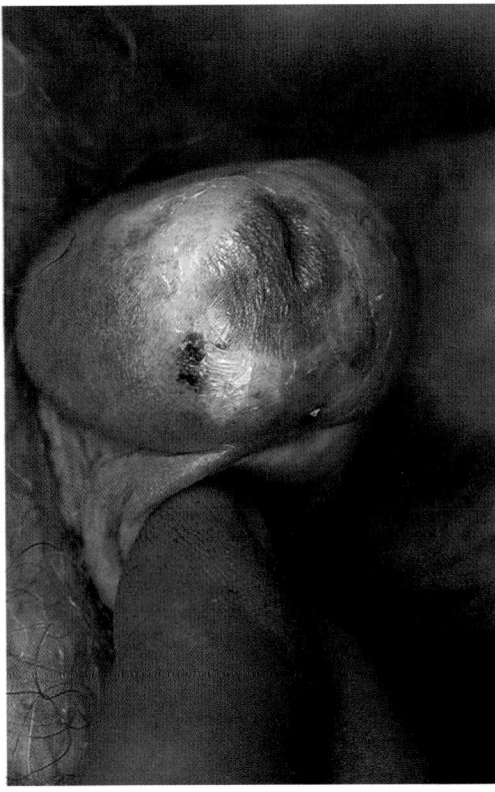

Figure 111.8 Lichen sclerosus. White plaques and haemorrhagic areas on the glans. (Courtesy of Dr D. A. Burns, Leicester, UK.)

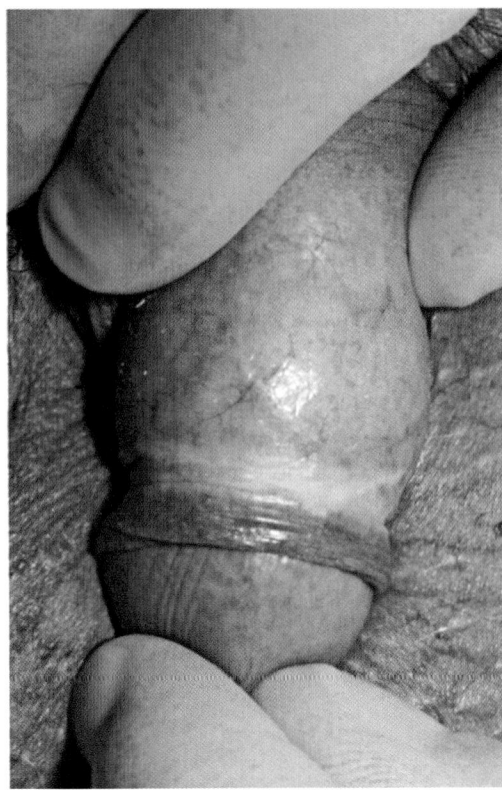

Figure 111.9 Lichen sclerosus. Sclerotic band of the prepuce causing 'waisting'. (Courtesy of Professor C. B. Bunker, with permission from Medical Illustration UK, Chelsea & Westminster Hospital, London, UK.)

haemorrhagic blisters, any manner of symptoms signifying sexual dysfunction or dyspareunia, discomfort with urination and narrowing of the urinary stream, and/or they may be concerned about the changing anatomy of their genitalia. Genital, just like extragenital, lichen sclerosus can manifest as atrophic leukodermic patches or plaques, or lilac, slightly scaly patches with telangiectasia and sparse purpura (Figure 111.8). There may be subtle or florid mixed lichenoid and zoonoid balanoposthitis. Predominant purpura, angiokeratomas, bullae, erosions and ulceration may be encountered. Signs may be subtle, with meatal 'pin hole' narrowing, slight tightening of the retracted prepuce because of sclerotic plaques, bands and adhesions, with or without difficulty in retraction – incomplete paraphimosis or 'waisting' due to a constrictive posthitis (Figure 111.9). Alternatively, the clinical features may be florid with severe inflammation, gross adhesions, loss of anatomical definition and dissolution or effacement of the normally sharply defined architectural features, especially of the frenulum and the coronal sulcus and rim: pearly penile papules may be destroyed. The arrangement of the naviculo-meatal fossa and meatus may be abnormal, as above. Post-inflammatory hyper- and hypopigmentation are often seen. There may be evident signs of dysplasia, carcinoma *in situ* or of a frank cancer.

Posthitis xerotica obliterans refers to chronic damage to the prepuce by lichen sclerosus, whereas balanitis xerotica obliterans properly describes involvement of the glans penis (although the term has been used imprecisely). Balanitis xerotica obliterans can be a consequence of other scarring dermatoses such as lichen planus and cicatricial pemphigoid. The involvement of the anterior

urethra can be serious; 29% of patients undergoing urethroplasty for urethral stricture had pathological evidence of lichen sclerosus [25]. Other recognized clinical presentations include non-retractile foreskin (phimosis) (Figure 111.10), foreskin fixed in retraction (paraphimosis), urinary retention (even renal failure), chronic penile oedema [49], pseudoepitheliomatous and micaceous hyperkeratotic balanitis [50], pre-cancer (usually erythroplasia of Queyrat) and squamous carcinoma. Most cases of genital lichen sclerosus can be diagnosed clinically.

Lichen planus, Zoon balanoposthitis, non-specific balanoposthitis and very rarely mucous membrane pemphigoid are in the differential diagnosis. A biopsy might be performed if there is clinical doubt or if the result might impact on management decisions. There should be a low threshold for biopsying lesions that are eroded, ulcerated or verrucous. The site and timing of a biopsy is critical. Non-specific or zoonoid histology do not exclude lichen sclerosus.

Investigations
A biopsy is rarely required.

Management
Guidelines for the management of lichen sclerosus have been published by the British Association of Dermatologists [51,52] not to general approbation [53]. The aims are early diagnosis and effective treatment to obtain normalization of sexual function, reverse or check urinary dysfunction and limit urethral disease and reduce, if not abolish, the risk of penis cancer [1,53,54]. Contact

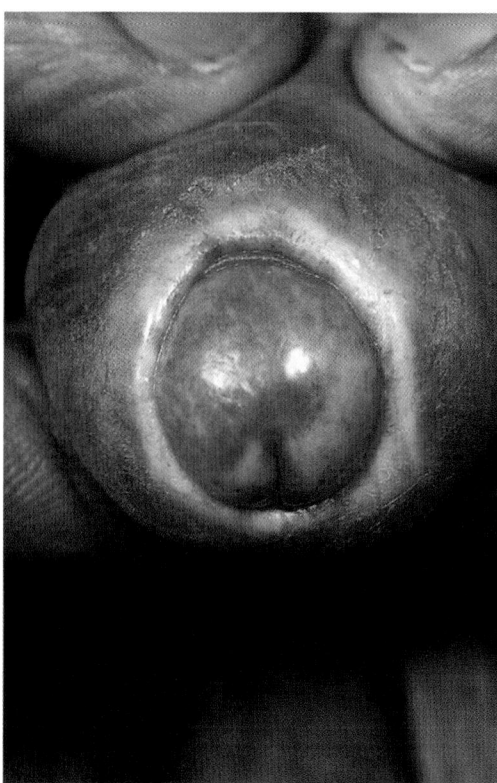

Figure 111.10 Lichen sclerosus causing phimosis. (Courtesy of Dr D. A. Burns, Leicester, UK.)

with soap, urine and pubic hair should be avoided by use of a soap substitute and a barrier preparation. An ultrapotent topical corticosteroid (usually clobetasol propionate) used under supervision for a finite course is effective [6,55–57] and usually problem free, but herpes simplex and wart reactivation do occur [33,**51**,52]. Patients with a history of genital herpes simplex virus (HSV) should be prescribed prophylactic aciclovir. The plasticity of the male genital epithelium seems to allow significant remodelling, with the relief of phimosis, improvement of incomplete phimosis or constrictive posthitis, improvement in the histological changes and avoidance of circumcision [1,9,56,58]: 50–60% of patients will achieve a durable remission. Topical clobetasol propionate has been shown to relieve undifferentiated 'phimosis' in many boys and so obviate the need for circumcision [57]. Secondary candidal and bacterial infection should be treated. There are reports of the efficacy of long-term systemic antibiotic therapy (penicillin and azithromycin) in cases of lichen sclerosus thought to be associated with *Borrelia* infection [59,60]. Topical testosterone propionate, oral stanozolol, freezing with ethyl chloride, liquid nitrogen cryotherapy, carbon dioxide laser and adrenocorticotrophic hormone (ACTH) have been used but are not recommended [9]. A recent trial of oral acitretin has shown some benefit [**61**]. The exhibition of topical calcineurin inhibitors is to be deprecated because of the risk of accelerated carcinogenesis [1,53,62,**63**]. If medical treatment with ultrapotent topical steroid is not possible or fails, then surgery is indicated. Circumcision (including by carbon dioxide laser), frenuloplasty, meatotomy, glans resurfacing and sophisticated plastic repair, depending upon the clinical presentation, can be offered [64–66]. In boys, complete circumcision is the treatment

of choice because all affected tissue is removed and any secondary involvement of the glans probably regresses or resolves [16]; it is the unproven impression that this phenomenon also occurs in most adult patients. Surgery works in male genital lichen sclerosus if it relieves susceptible epithelium from chronic occluded exposure to urine. Surgery fails if it does not achieve this goal or if the damage to urethral structural and functional integrity is beyond intervention and if skin rather than mucosal grafts are used (if a graft is needed). Surgery may inadvertently worsen the problem by increasing the overall incontinence of the distal urinary system. Fundamental to planning of penile surgery for lichen sclerosus is the recognition of the pernicious role in the initiation and progression of male genital lichen sclerosus played by the chronic occluded exposure of genital skin to urine [67]. In the long term, about 40% of patients will respond to medical treatment: the majority of the remainder will be cured by surgery, usually circumcision [1].

Persistent disease requires individualized follow-up and management. Residual burnt-out disease on the glans may improve with long-term topical retinoid treatment. Subdermal injection of polydeoxyribonucleotide (a mitogen for fibroblasts, endothelial cells and adipocytes) is an interesting new approach [68]. Squamous carcinoma of the penis is the most serious potential complication of lichen sclerosus [1,9]. Carcinoma *in situ* and early microinvasive disease can be difficult to diagnose clinically against a background of lichen sclerosus [1,9,69]. Squamous hyperplasia (SH) and the basal and parabasal dysplasia of the differentiated penile intraepithelial neoplasia (PeIN) seen histologically in association with lichen sclerosus–associated squamous carcinoma can be subtle and underappreciated by pathologists and clinicians [70]. The risk of squamous carcinoma complicating male genital lichen sclerosus suggested by the literature is 0–12.5%, depending on size of study, length of follow-up; the latent period may be one to three decades [1,9,10,69–72,**73**,74–77]. Involvement of the glans penis confers a greater risk [71]. The types of squamous carcinoma associated with lichen sclerosus are the 'usual' and verrucous subtypes [70,78]. One third to one half of all established penile cancer is associated with lichen sclerosus [76,79,80]. The effect of medical and surgical treatment on the subsequent incidence of penile cancer is not precisely known [81,82]. Liatsikos *et al.* [75] report squamous carcinoma of the glans developing in one of eight patients followed-up after circumcision for lichen sclerosus. However, of the large cohort of patients reported by Edmonds *et al.* not one patient has developed squamous carcinoma: compared with the published figures this implies that accurate diagnosis and effective medical and surgical management abolish or significantly attenuate the risk [1]. Some patients may need to be followed-up long term especially if circumcision has not been performed or if symptoms persist or recur after any form of treatment.

Resources

Further information
British Association of Dermatologists Guidelines
http://www.bad.org.uk/

Patient resources
Worldwide Lichen Sclerosus Support www.lichensclerosus.org/
http://issvd.org/wordpress/wp-content/uploads/2012/04/LS2010.pdf
http://issvd.org/wordpress/wp-content/uploads/2012/04/LSchildren2010.pdf
All last accessed August 2015.

Lichen planus

Introduction and general description
It is a common inflammatory dermatosis with a particular predilection for the oro-genital epithelium [1] (see also Chapter 37).

Pathophysiology
The aetiopathogenesis of lichen planus is not known. Drugs can cause a generalized lichenoid eruption; a case of a lichenoid drug eruption confined to the penis resulting from propranolol has been reported [2].

Clinical features
Lichen planus can present in, and remain localized to, the ano-genital area, including the groins and perianal skin. Like the classical disease at other sites, it presents as itchy red-purple papules, patches, plaques and annular lesions (Figure 111.11). It may also present as phimosis [3,4]. The male genitalia represent the commonest site for the annular subtype of lichen planus [5]. The Koebner phenomenon may partly explain the oro-genital predilection [6]. Occasionally, an erosive form is encountered. There is a male equivalent of the

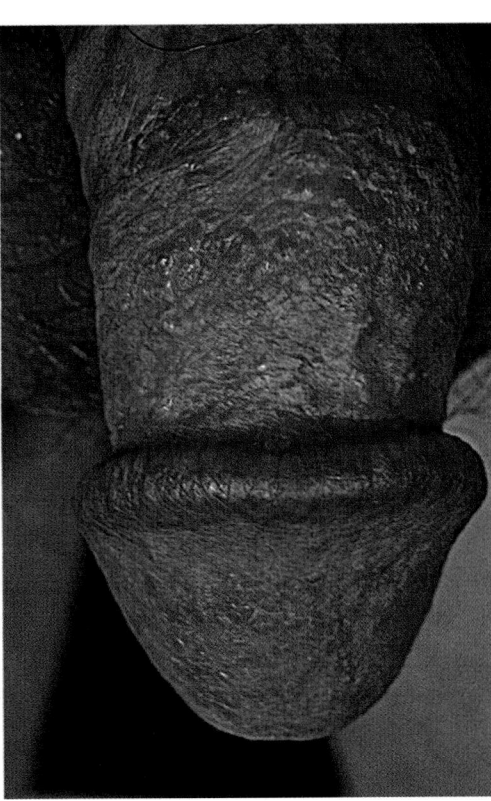

Figure 111.11 Lichen planus. Papules and annular lesions with striae of Wickham on the glans and shaft. (Courtesy of Professor C. B. Bunker, with permission from Medical Illustration UK, Chelsea & Westminster Hospital, London, UK.)

vulvovaginal syndrome of Hewitt – the genitogingival syndrome – with chronic erosive gingival and genital lesions [7]. In most cases, ano-genital lichen planus is self-limiting, although some patients remit and relapse. Adhesions can form and contribute to phimosis. Post-inflammatory hyperpigmentation can persist for months or years. A case of paraneoplastic lichen planus with oro-genital and cicatrizing conjunctival involvement in a patient with thymoma has been reported [8]. Chronic mucosal erosive lichen planus is associated with a risk of progression to squamous carcinoma, but most reports of this concern oral lichen planus. There are rare reports of squamous carcinoma eventuating from chronic penile dermatoses thought to be lichen planus [9,10,**11,12**].

Lichen nitidus has an affinity for the penis; it is sometimes seen on penile skin in isolation in young Asian males. Lichen nitidus can be difficult to diagnose because the signs may be subtle, even when the lesions are widespread.

Differential diagnosis
The differential diagnosis of ano-genital lichen planus includes psoriasis, Zoon balanitis, lichen sclerosus, viral warts, BP and porokeratosis.

Complications and co-morbidites
In the follow-up of cases of chronic ano-genital lichen planus, erosive, ulcerative or verrucous features arouse concern about the development of squamous carcinoma.

Investigations
A biopsy is frequently necessary for diagnostic purposes.

Management
Potent and ultrapotent topical corticosteroids usually suffice for treatment. Patients are told to continue with the treatment until the lesions are non-itchy and flat; they are warned about post-inflammatory hyperpigmentation. Reactivation of genital warts may occur [13]. Topical and oral ciclosporin have been used [14,**15**], but there has been a report of squamous carcinoma arising in lichen planus of the penis treated with topical ciclosporin [**16**]. Topical calcineurin inhibitors should be used with caution [**16**,17,18]. Circumcision may be necessary for phimosis [19] and should be considered in refractory erosive disease [**20**], the rationale being that the abolition of koebnerization influences and facilitates resolution of the lichen planus. Photodynamic therapy was used inadvertently in one patient with lichen planus of the glans penis, to good effect [**21**]. Pulsed dexamethasone therapy has been used for erosive disease [**22**].

MISCELLANEOUS INFLAMMATORY DERMATOSES

Non-specific balanoposthitis

Clinical experience and histological evidence indicate that non-specific balanoposthitis is a real entity [**1,2**]; however, in practice it is a diagnosis of exclusion. Sexually transmitted disease, eczematous dermatoses, psoriasis, Zoon balanitis, lichen planus, lichen sclerosus, cicatrizing pemphigoid and penile carcinoma *in situ* need to be considered and eliminated by special investigations, including biopsy. There is usually a failure to respond to specific rational treatments. Non-specific balanoposthitis is a manifestation of a dysfunctional foreskin. Patients generally present with dyspareunia, and may have variable signs, including eczematous, lichenoid and Zoon-like inflammation, and even scarring. *Candida* and other organisms may be retrieved, but they probably represent secondary opportunistic infection. Diabetes should be excluded. Specific and non-specific interventions may be tried, such as avoidance of contact with soap and urine and other irritants, treatment for candidosis and other infections, and medical treatment for lichen sclerosus and lichen planus. Invariably these treatments fail and the patient is cured by circumcision. A prior clinical diagnosis may be overturned at this stage by foreskin histology showing lichen sclerosus, lichen planus or carcinoma *in situ*, but there will always be cases where a thorough histological examination of the excised prepuce fails to reveal more than non-specific chronic inflammatory changes.

Ulcerative disease and penile necrosis

The causes of genital ulceration are listed in Boxes 111.15 and 111.16, and the causes of penile necrosis in Box 111.17. Many of the causes are discussed in this or other sections.

Aphthous ulceration of the penis and scrotum can occur, including in HIV/AIDS, but specific exclusion of sexually transmitted diseases and consideration of other causes of genital ulceration, especially Behçet syndrome, is necessary. The causes are obscure and the histology is non-specific.

Rare cases of spontaneous scrotal ulceration in young, previously fit men have been described – juvenile gangrenous vasculitis of the scrotum [1]. Histology shows non-specific vasculitis, and spontaneous resolution can occur. This entity may be related to idiopathic scrotal panniculitis and fat necrosis. It is distinct from other causes of the acute scrotum in prepubertal boys. It presents

---

Box 111.15 Common causes of genital ulcers

- Trauma
- Pressure sores
- Aphthae
- Pilonidal sinus
- Anal fistula
- Anal fissure
- Erythema multiforme/Stevens–Johnson syndrome
- Hidradenitis suppurativa
- Crohn disease
- Chancroid
- Donovanosis/granuloma inguinale
- Lymphogranuloma venereum
- Syphilis: primary chancre
- Squamous carcinoma

Reproduced from Bunker CB. *Male Genital Skin Disease*.
London: Saunders, 2004. © 2004, with permission from the author.

Box 111.16 Rare causes of genital ulcers

- Extrusion of testicular prosthesis
- Embolization
- Dermatitis artefacta
- Penile necrosis
- Spontaneous scrotal ulceration
- Sarcoid
- Autoimmune bullous diseases
  - Bullous pemphigoid
  - Cicatricial pemphigoid
  - Linear IgA disease
- Necrobiosis lipoidica
- Pyoderma gangrenosum
- Erythema elevatum diutinum
- Necrotizing vasculitis
  - Granulomatosis with polyangiitis
  - Polyarteritis nodosa
  - Systemic lupus erythematosus
  - Idiopathic systemic vasculitis
  - Hereditary spherocytosis with vascular necrosis
- Degos malignant atrophic papulosis
- Calciphylaxis
- Hypereosinophilic syndrome
- *Pseudomonas*
  - Ecthyma gangrenosum
  - Necrotizing anorectal ulcer in leukaemia
- Gonorrhoea
- Chancroid
- Donovanosis (granuloma inguinale)
- Lymphogranuloma venereum
- Fournier gangrene
- Tuberculosis and tuberculides
- Atypical mycobacteria, e.g. *Mycobacterium ulcerans*
- Syphilis: snail track ulcers
- Yaws
- Non-syphilitic spirochaetal ulcerative balanoposthitis
- Herpes simplex
- Herpes zoster
- HIV
- Chikongunya
- Deep fungal infections
  - Histoplasmosis
  - Blastomycosis
  - Cryptococcosis
- Actinomycosis
- Paracoccidioidomycosis
- Leishmaniasis
- Amoebiasis
- Filariasis
- Langerhans cell histiocytosis
- Extramammary Paget disease
- Basal cell carcinoma
- Squamous carcinoma
- Verrucous carcinoma
- Sweat gland carcinoma
- Melanoma
- Kaposi sarcoma
- Leukaemia
- Lymphoma
- Drug reaction

Reproduced from Bunker CB. *Male Genital Skin Disease*.
London: Saunders, 2004. © 2004, with permission from the author.

PART 10: SITES, SEX, AGE

> **Box 111.17 Causes of penile necrosis**
>
> - Decubitus ulcer
> - Spider bite
> - Priapism
> - Embolism
> - Strangulation and tourniquet syndromes
> - Vacuum erection device
> - Systemic vasculitis [46]
>   - Lupus erythematosus
>   - Polyarteritis nodosa [47]
>   - Granulomatosis with polyangiitis
> - Diabetes [48,49]
> - Chronic renal failure [50]
> - Thrombocytopenia
> - Polycythaemia
> - Cryoglobulinaemia
> - Coagulopathy [51]
> - Pyoderma gangrenosum
> - Calciphylaxis
> - Ecthyma gangrenosum
> - Fournier gangrene
> - Herpes simplex
> - Leukaemia
> - Mucormycosis (in acute myeloblastic leukaemia) [52]
> - Warfarin
> - Fixed drug eruption
>
> Reproduced from Bunker CB. *Male Genital Skin Disease.*
> London: Saunders, 2004. © 2004, with permission from the author.

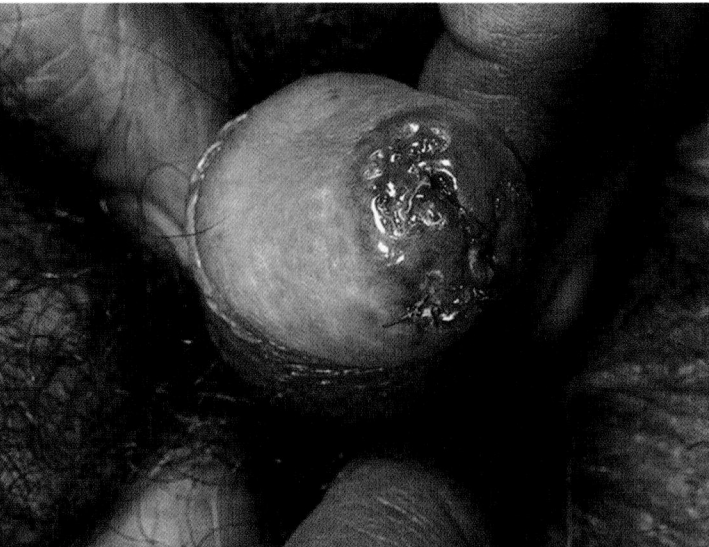

Figure 111.12 Pyoderma gangrenosum in a patient with severe seronegative arthropathy. (Courtesy of Dr F. A. Ive, Durham, UK.)

as acute, tender, sometimes painful, swelling (classically, but not always, after swimming in cold water). Masses may be palpable in the scrotal wall. Otherwise, the boy is well, with no fever or leukocytosis. Idiopathic scrotal necrosis in a 2-month-old boy has been documented by Sarihan [2], where trauma, extreme cold and Fournier gangrene were excluded. Management is expectant and conservative [3,4]. In adults, one case of idiopathic scrotal panniculitis has been reported [5] and another associated with pancreatitis [6].

Subtle or severe oro-genital ulceration can occur in erythema multiforme or the Stevens–Johnson syndrome.

Behçet disease is discussed in another chapter (see Chapter 48). Recurrent genital ulceration is not mandatory for the diagnosis; if patients do not have genital ulceration then they must have ophthalmic and dermatological involvement or a positive pathergy test [7]. In practice, there are many patients who have an incomplete syndrome. Other ano-genital manifestations include epididymitis and urethritis [8], spontaneous haematocele from venous rupture resulting from lymphocytic venulitis [9] and erectile dysfunction [10]. The genital ulcers in men can be very painful and occur anywhere in the ano-genital area, including the perianal skin. Generally, they are larger, deeper, fewer and less recurrent than those in the mouth. Patients with relapsing polychondritis and Behçet disease have been reported, and the acronym MAGIC (mouth and genital ulcers with inflamed cartilage) syndrome has been proposed [11,**12**]. The histology of Behçet disease is usually non-specific and does not enable it to be distinguished from idiopathic aphthae, although sometimes necrotizing vasculitis can be present.

Scrotal involvement can occur in Hailey–Hailey disease [**13**].

Degos malignant atrophic papulosis can cause painful penile ulceration, that may precede the development of the eruption elsewhere and be associated with fatal involvement of other organs, despite aggressive treatment [**14**,15].

The hypereosinophilic syndrome involves the skin in up to 50% of cases, with oro-genital ulceration, erythroderma and urticaria. It may occur in HIV infection [16].

Granulomatosis with polyangiitis may present with glans penis ulceration and necrosis; repeated antineutrophil cytoplasmic antibodies (ANCA) estimation may be needed and it may be some time before systemic manifestations declare themselves [17–20,**21**].

There has been one case report of a patient with erythema elevatum diutinum causing penile ulceration [22]. Three cases of necrobiosis lipoidica have been reported presenting as erythematous ulcerated lesions of the glans penis. One patient was diabetic and also had lesions on the legs [23]; the others had penile lesions only, and were treated with oral pentoxifylline [24,25].

There are a number of case reports of pyoderma gangrenosum, including the variant superficial granulomatous pyoderma [26], involving the penis and scrotum in adults and children (where the ano-genital area is a site of predilection as well as the head and neck) (Figure 111.12) [27,28]. Genital pyoderma gangrenosum may occur following local trauma such as urological surgery [29,30] or treatment for cancer [31], or complicate ulcerative colitis [32] or chronic lymphocytic leukaemia, or it may be idiopathic [33–36]. Pyoderma gangrenosum is a diagnosis made when other causes of purulent ulceration, such as infection (sexually acquired and exotic or rare, including Fournier gangrene), malignancy and artefact have been excluded. Systemic treatment is usually required but one case has responded to topical tacrolimus [**37**].

Calciphylaxis is a rare and serious complication of chronic renal failure in which extending ischaemic gangrenous necrosis affects acral tissues and sometimes the thighs, buttocks and genitals [38,39,**40**,**41**,42,43].

Ulcers in the peno-scrotal region have been reported to appear 2–4 weeks after chikungunya, a novel togavirus arboviral infection that causes fever, headache and arthralgia [44].

There has been one case report of primary cutaneous T-cell lymphoma of the penis presenting with a 2-year history of 'recurrent balanitis', a preputial ulcer and phimosis [45]. Other reports include genital ulceration due to amoebiasis, meticillin-resistant *Staphylococcus aureus* (MRSA) infection, tuberculosis and in association with leukaemias [46–50].

Penile necrosis is rare but has been reported with polyartertitis nodosa, systemic lupus, hyperparathyroidism, calciphylaxis, diabetes, vena caval thrombosis and opportunistic fungal infection [51–60].

Pilonidal sinus

Pilonidal sinus very rarely affects the penis [1], but when it does it usually occurs in the coronal sulcus [2,3]. Some of the reported cases have been complicated by actinomycosis [2,4], and one has been associated with a dermoid cyst [5].

Penile acne

There is no literature on this condition but it is occasionally encountered. Patients have comedones, papules, pustules and inflammatory nodules of the proximal shaft of the penis. The differential diagnosis should include chloracne. Patients respond to conventional treatment for acne.

Peyronie disease

Peyronie disease [1,2], which affects middle-aged and older men, is a localized fibrotic disorder involving tissue immediately adjacent to the erectile tissues. It presents with pain and curvature on erection, a sensation of a cord within the penis, palpation of a lump or knot, decreased erection distal to the plaque, interference with intercourse and progressive impotence. It may be subclinical in many men, given that 23% of autopsies have shown histological evidence of the condition [1]. Psychological complications and marital difficulties occur. The penis curves towards the lesion, with dorsal curvature being most common. Peyronie (a physician to Louis XIV) described nodules as 'rosary beads' but plaques vary in size. It has been associated with systemic sclerosis [3,4], and such patients may have penile Raynaud phenomenon [5]. It has occurred as a complication of the use of a vacuum erection device [6], but in most men the cause is unknown. Some evidence has been advanced for an autoimmune pathogenesis [7]. A case complicating chronic graft-versus-host disease has been reported [8].

The differential diagnosis includes congenital curvature, fibrosis secondary to trauma or urethritis and abscess, syphilitic gumma, lymphogranuloma venereum, and infiltrative tumours (e.g. lipogranuloma). Penile thrombophlebitis as the initial presentation of a paraneoplastic migratory thrombophlebitis resulting from pancreatic cancer has been misdiagnosed as Peyronie disease [9].

In some men, there may be spontaneous regression. Treatments include intralesional corticosteroid injection [10], including delivery by Dermojet® [11]. Surgery is avoided, but some specialized techniques are available [12]. Symptomatic relief has been claimed following iontophoresis of drugs such as dexamethasone, lidocaine (lignocaine), *para*-aminobenzoic acid and verapamil [13,14].

Drug reactions

The penis is a site of predilection for fixed drug eruption. The symptoms are itch or burning. The eruption is acute, with an erythematous plaque, sometimes with central blister formation, erosion and ulceration. Cases have occurred in men after congress with sexual partners who have taken the drug to which they were known to be sensitive: co-trimoxazole, diclofenac, isosorbide and aspirin are the drugs cited [1,2]. The differential diagnosis of penile fixed drug eruption includes herpes simplex and erythema multiforme.

Ulceration has been reported following the inadvertent subcutaneous injection of papaverine for the treatment of erectile impotence [3]. Dequalinium is a topical antibacterial that was used for the treatment of impetigo and moniliasis in the 1950s and 1960s, but it caused a necrotizing balanitis with ulceration when used for the treatment of balanitis in uncircumcised men [4]. All-*trans*-retinoic acid has been reported to induce scrotal ulceration in a patient with acute promyelocytic leukaemia [5]. Foscarnet is a recognized cause of genital ulceration in HIV-infected patients [6,7–9]. Nicorandil is a newly recognized cause of ano-genital and peristomal ulceration [10,11]. Erosion following the use of topical steroids has been seen. Penile argyria due to chronic application of silver sulfadiazine has been reported [12], as has necrosis following warfarin administration [13,14].

Other inflammatory dermatoses

Bottomley and Cotterill [1] have described an acutely tender erythematous scrotum associated with zinc deficiency in a patient with Crohn disease. Necrolytic migratory erythema can be localized to the genitalia [2]. Skin fragility and ulceration in the ano-genital area are features of prolidase deficiency [3].

Autoimmune bullous diseases such as pemphigus can involve the penis (the glans is the usual site) (Figure 111.13), but very rarely in isolation [4]. Pemphigus vegetans presenting with a 4-year history of indolent tender balanitis has been reported [5]. In this case, the glans penis was involved with a moist vegetative plaque with beefy red erosions separating irregular hyperkeratotic mounds [5]. Linear immunoglobulin A (IgA) disease commonly involves the mucosae. Mucosal lesions of bullous pemphigoid are uncommon; their presence suggests another diagnosis or an underlying neoplasm.

Cicatricial pemphigoid (or 'benign') mucous membrane pemphigoid is a rare variant of bullous pemphigoid in which blisters affect the skin and the mucous membranes. Skin lesions are usually less

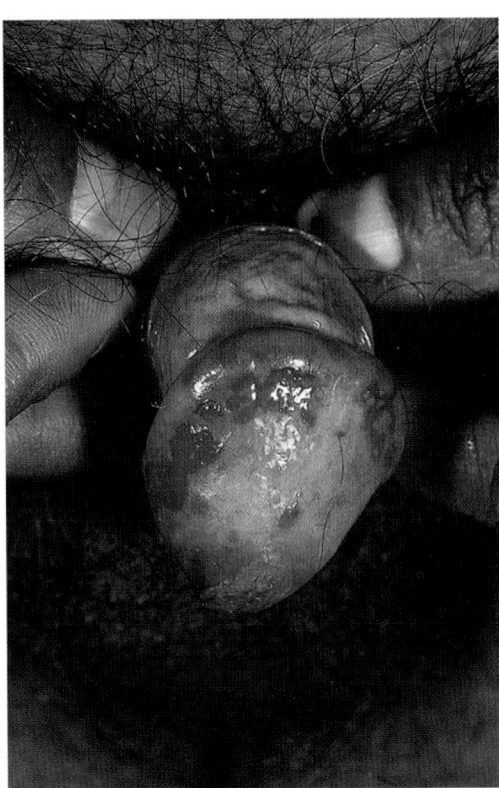

Figure 111.13 Pemphigus of the penis. (Courtesy of Dr F. A. Ive, Durham, UK.)

widespread than in bullous pemphigoid and they may heal with scarring. Oral lesions predominantly involve the palate and gingivae, but there may be oesophageal involvement with dysphagia, and conjunctival disease can lead to blindness. Involvement of the penis may be with blisters, erosions, ulcers, transcoronal adhesions, scarring and phimosis [6,7,8]. Although direct immunofluorescence is usually positive, circulating antibodies to the basement membrane zone are rarely found. The disease often responds poorly to oral steroids, but dapsone or other sulpha drugs such as sulphamethoxypyridazine can be effective. Regular haematology screening is mandatory with dapsone because of the risk of agranulocytosis.

One patient with Darier disease developed a HPV-16 associated squamous carcinoma of the scrotum during oral isotretinoin treatment; he had not previously had radiotherapy to the genito-crural area [9]. Genito-crural papular acantholytic dermatosis can involve the penis, as can granuloma annulare. Erythematous smooth, round and linear nodules are described in the latter. Most patients are uncircumcised. Extragenital granuloma annulare is uncommon in these patients.

Occasionally, patients with generalized cutaneous sarcoid present with genital lesions [10]. Tender erythematous induration of the distal shaft of the penis and yellowish subcutaneous nodules on the glans have been described [11]. A case presenting with penile ulceration has been reported [12]. Importantly, sarcoid can masquerade as testicular malignancy [12,13–15].

A granulomatous lymphangitis may be found histologically in the investigation of penile lymphoedema [16]. It can be a rare feature of the Melkersson–Rosenthal syndrome. Crohn disease can involve the penis and scrotum, presenting as peno-scrotal lymphoedema or erosions and ulcers [17–20,21,22,23].

Primary cutaneous amyloidosis of the penis is a rare entity. Nodular cutaneous amyloid is associated with systemic disease and up to 10% of cases with associated paraproteinaemia progress to systemic disease [24]. A soft-tissue mass in the penis associated with systemic amyloid has been reported [25]. True penile-limited cutaneous amyloidosis is highly associated with nodular amyloidosis. Primary cutaneous penile amyloidosis has a low incidence of systemic progression [24]. Primary amyloid of the urethra is very rare indeed, but accurate diagnosis is essential, as its presentation simulates carcinoma, with dysuria, bloody discharge and tender induration of the penis [26], or as an obstructive voiding syndrome, with tender periurethral masses and irregular urethral strictures [27].

One case each of eccrine syringofibroadenomatosis with penile involvement manifesting as a balanoposthitis [28], benign mucinous metaplasia with a preputial 0.6 cm papule replacing the superficial epidermis [29], and mucinous syringometaplasia with an ulcerated papule on the shaft of the penis [30] have been reported.

Acute scrotum is a clinical syndrome defined as acute painful swelling of the scrotum or its contents, usually in boys, accompanied by local signs and general symptoms [31]. The critical differential diagnosis is torsion of the testis or spermatic cord. Other causes include idiopathic scrotal oedema, epididymitis, orchitis, hernia and haematocele. Thromboangiitis obliterans has been found in two cases [32]. Acute scrotal swelling may be a physical sign of primary peritonitis in children and infants [33] or secondary peritonitis resulting from appendicitis, healed meconium peritonitis in the neonate, haemoperitonitis (ruptured spleen) and pseudotorsion resulting from ventriculoperitoneal shunts inserted for hydrocephalus that have migrated into the scrotum from the peritoneum. Acute idiopathic scrotal oedema usually affects children aged 4–12 years old. Allergy, infection (umbilical sepsis), trauma, insect bites, urinary extravasation and Henoch–Schönlein purpura have all been considered as causes. It is rare in adults, but cases in association with septic diabetic foot have been reported [34].

Henoch–Schönlein purpura/anaphylactoid purpura/allergic vasculitis may affect the genitalia. Ureteritis, renal pelvic haemorrhage and pain and swelling of the spermatic cord have been reported. The incidence of scrotal involvement ranges from 2% to 38%. Penile shaft involvement is less common and involvement of the glans very rare [35]. In some cases, the presentation has masqueraded as testicular torsion, resulting in unnecessary surgical exploration. Ultrasonography can help to distinguish between them [36]. However, testicular torsion can also be a real and serious complication of Henoch–Schönlein purpura [36].

Acute haemorrhagic oedema of childhood may present as tenderness, redness and swelling of the penis and scrotum with the development of more widespread haemorrhagic lesions [37]. The differential diagnosis includes acute febrile neutrophilic dermatosis, erythema multiforme, Henoch–Schönlein purpura and child abuse. The prognosis for complete recovery is excellent. Acute inflammation of the scrotum in patients with familial Mediterranean fever can occur [38]. It is manifested by pain, erythema and swelling, fever, leukocytosis and elevated erythrocyte sedimentation rate (ESR). It may occur in isolation or accompanying peritonitis. The differential diagnosis includes torsion, orchitis and epididymitis in boys.

Polyarteritis nodosa may be associated with testicular and epididymal involvement, with scrotal pain and swelling. In one case these were the sole presenting features and testicular biopsy provided the diagnosis [39–41].

There has been one patient who presented with 'inaugural' painless erythematous papules on the penis that histologically showed granulomatous vasculitis, leading to the diagnosis of Churg–Strauss syndrome (eosinophilic granulomatosis with polyangiitis) [42].

NON-SEXUALLY TRANSMITTED INFECTIONS

Staphylococcal cellulitis

Cellulitis may affect the penis. Piercing and genital jewellery predispose to infection. Cellulitis and abscess formation can complicate cysts, sinuses and fistulae, and sexually transmitted infections. The exact relationship between episodes of acute infection and chronic penile oedema, which often is complicated by cellulitis, is uncertain.

Ano-genital infection is a serious complication in patients with malignant disease, and potentially life-threatening necrotizing fasciitis and Fournier gangrene may occur.

Streptococcal dermatitis/perianal cellulitis

This syndrome in children [1] probably also has a corollary in adults [2], but it is much more common in boys in whom, if the penis is involved, there may be dysuria, erythema and swelling of the penis and balanoposthitis. Bullous necrotic erysipelas of the penis due to *Streptococcus pyogenes* has been reported [3].

Chronic penile oedema

Chronic penile lymphoedema is a relatively rare, reactive, disfiguring condition that causes sexual dysfunction and phimosis (see also Chapter 105) [4]. It has been called tumorous lymphoedema or elephantiasis verrucosa nostra [5]. Evidence of streptococcal infection may be present, and this could lead to irreversible lymphatic damage. Other cases seem to be idiopathic and are perhaps brought about by primary hypoplastic lymphatics. Other reported causes include compulsive masturbation, chronic strangulation, circumcision and hidradenitis suppurativa [6,7,8,9]. Some patients have a coexistent penile dermatosis. Few cases and series of chronic penile oedema have been reported [4,10,11] and the aetiopathogenesis may have been misunderstood.

Peno-scrotal oedema has also been attributed to continuous ambulatory peritoneal dialysis [12], amputation of septic limbs in diabetes [13], acute necrotizing pancreatitis [14], streptococcal infections [15] and, most importantly, Crohn disease, which may be occult and asymptomatic, metachronous or synchronous, and be present in up to one third of patients [11,16,17]. Filariasis and pelvic mass lesions should be excluded. Penile venereal oedema has been associated with gonococcal and herpes infection, and scabies infestation, and resolves after treatment of the underlying disease [18]. Similarly, childhood penile oedema is self-limiting [19]. It is possible that some cases of chronic penile oedema are related to any of the above factors and/or to repetitive sexually transmitted disease. A persistent lymphatic insult from whatever cause could result in an inflammatory process affecting genital and pelvic lymphatic vessels and nodes. Imaging of lymphatic channels is not particularly helpful [20].

Patients with chronic penile oedema present with chronic swelling of the penis, foreskin, scrotum, pubic mound, buttocks and thighs, which may be warm and red [11]. There may be intercurrent attacks of cellulitis and/or erysipelas with systemic upset. Acute attacks require admission to hospital and treatment with systemic broad spectrum antibiotics; a short course of prednisolone may also be helpful. Investigations should be directed at elucidating possible underlying causes (such as streptococcal infection (ASOT), Crohn disease and sarcoid, pelvic cancer and filariasis) and predisposing factors, as discussed earlier (Boxes 111.18, 111.19 and 111.20). All cases of peno-scrotal oedema should be treated aggressively at first presentation, because the more chronic the genital lymphoedema the more difficult it is to treat, both medically and surgically [11,21]. Aims of management of chronic penile oedema must be prophylaxis against further infective episodes and aggressive treatment of relapses.

Long-term treatment with erythromycin, clarithromycin, clindamycin, clindamycin plus rifampicin, trimethoprim, sulphamethoxazole plus trimethoprim or ciprofloxacin appears to ameliorate and stabilize the process. Antibiotics together with short intermittent courses of oral prednisolone should improve both the appearance and function of the penis. Success of this approach supports the importance of infection as a factor in the perpetuation, if not

---

Box 111.18 Causes of genital lymphoedema

- Idiopathic congenital lymphoedema (Milroy disease)
- Lipogranuloma and silicone granuloma
- Strangulation of the penis
- Iatrogenic
- Radical abdominopelvic surgery
- Radiotherapy
- Granulomatous lymphangitis
  - Crohn disease
  - Sarcoid
- Post-infectious
  - Cellulitis and erysipelas
  - Chronic penile lymphoedema
  - Chancroid
  - Lymphogranuloma venereum
  - Tuberculosis
  - Leprosy
  - Syphilis
  - Filariasis/onchocerciasis
- Carcinomatosis
  - Lymphatic involvement
  - Lymphatic blockage
- Lymphoma

Reproduced from Bunker CB. *Male Genital Skin Disease.* London: Saunders, 2004. © 2004, with permission from the author.

PART 10: SITES, SEX, AGE

Box 111.19 Commoner causes of penoscrotal swelling

- Paraphimosis
- Foreign body
- Strangulation of the penis
- Iatrogenic
  - Contact dermatitis
  - Continuous ambulatory peritoneal dialysis
  - Genital oedema resulting from raised right heart filling pressure in ITU
  - Postoperative
  - Post-radiotherapy
- Varicocele
- Hydrocele
- Strangulated hernia
- Priapism
- Peyronie disease
- Epididymitis and orchitis
- Cellulitis
- Idiopathic chronic penile oedema
- Testicular tumours

Reproduced from Bunker CB. *Male Genital Skin Disease*. London: Saunders, 2004. © 2004, with permission from the author.

Box 111.20 Rarer causes of penoscrotal swelling

- Idiopathic congenital lymphoedema [6]
- Lymphangiectasia (with chylous reflux) [7]
- Giant haemangioma
- Urethral diverticulum
- Segmental urethral hypospadias
- Accessory scrotum [8,9]
- Herniation of scrotal contents into penile shaft
- Foreign body
- Haematocele
- Lipogranuloma and silicone granuloma
- Aortic aneurysm [10]
- Scrotal fat necrosis
- Henoch–Schönlein purpura
- Familial Mediterranean fever
- Acute haemorrhagic oedema of childhood
- Granulomatous lymphangitis
  - Crohn disease
  - Sarcoid
- Pancreatitis
- Infected cyst
- Abscess of corpus cavernosum [11]
- Fournier gangrene
- Tuberculosis
- Paracoccidioidomycosis
- Amputation of septic limbs in diabetics
- Giant scrotal tumours (e.g. neurilemmoma)
- Epithelioid haemangioma
- Kaposi sarcoma
- Epithelioid haemangioendiothelioma
- Lymphoma
- Sarcoma
- Drugs (e.g. angio-oedema caused by lisinopril)

Reproduced from Bunker CB. *Male Genital Skin Disease*. London: Saunders, 2004. © 2004, with permission from the author.

---

initiation, of the process. Medical control with antibiotics then allows surgical intervention in the form of circumcision. Plastic repair may be necessary after excision of affected tissue [11,22,23] and may lead to improvement in quality of life [11,24].

Ecthyma gangrenosum

Ecthyma gangrenosum has a predilection for the acral and ano-genital regions, and may affect the penis in isolation, leading to gangrene [1]. The prognosis is poor. A case has been reported that was probably caused by direct arterial septic embolization of the penis from femoral heroin injection [2].

Fournier gangrene

Fournier gangrene is analogous to necrotizing fasciitis and Meleney gangrene. In 1883, the Parisian dermatologist Jean Alfred Fournier described five cases of spontaneous genital gangrene and ulceration, but Baurienne (1764) probably first reported this condition [3]. The disease begins with urethral or appendageal polybacterial infection. Most of the organisms isolated are resident urethral or lower gastro-intestinal flora, and most patients have mixed infections. In children, staphylococci and streptococci are most commonly isolated [4]. A necrotizing vasculitis, possibly exotoxin mediated, ensues with devastating consequences for involved skin, subcutis, fascia and muscle. It is held to be the human counterpart of the local Shwartzman phenomenon [5,6]. A typical presentation is characterized by painful, erythematous, non-suppurative swelling of the genital skin (particularly the scrotum [7], where a dark red or a black spot may appear [8]), or the perianal zone or lower abdominal skin, accompanied by crepitus [9], marked systemic toxicity (may be absent in children [4]) and urinary retention. Necrosis of skin and deeper tissues can occur rapidly, and there is a very high mortality unless the diagnosis is made promptly and radical management undertaken. Plain X-rays may show soft-tissue gas [10]. Predisposing factors are listed in Box 111.21. Preceding surgery, including vasectomy and instrumentation, including genital piercing [11], especially in patients with the listed risk factors, is particularly important. The differential diagnosis is given in Box 111.22.

If a diagnosis of Fournier gangrene is made, radical surgical debridement of all affected tissue is undertaken and broad spectrum systemic antibiotic therapy initiated. Plastic repair can be undertaken if the patient survives [7]. Hyperbaric oxygen, high-dose systemic steroids and unprocessed honey treatment have been used [6,12,13,14,15]. In adults, the mortality is approximately 25%. Children can be treated with more conservative surgery, and their mortality rate is lower [4,16].

Trichomycosis pubis

Trichomycosis pubis causes asymptomatic yellow, red or black micronodules around hair shafts [1]. Pubic and axillary hair may be involved. The skin is normal but the sweat may be discoloured.

Box 111.21 Risk factors for Fournier gangrene

- Diabetes
- Alcoholism
- Ano-genital infection
- Chemotherapy
- HIV
- Post-instrumentation (especially in the immunocompromised)
- Postoperative (urological and colorectal)
- Heroin addiction
- Trauma
- Unconventional sexual practices

Box 111.22 Differential diagnosis of Fournier gangrene

- Trauma
- Herpes simplex
- Cellulitis (streptococcal, staphylococcal)
- Streptococcal necrotizing fasciitis
- Gonococcal balanitis and oedema
- Ecthyma gangrenosum
- Allergic vasculitis
- Polyarteritis nodosa
- Necrolytic migratory erythema
- Vascular occlusion syndromes
- Warfarin necrosis

Reproduced from Bunker CB. *Male Genital Skin Disease.* London: Saunders, 2004. © 2004, with permission from the author.

Trichomycosis pubis is rare in Western dermatological practice but is common in the Middle East [2], and may occur concomitantly with trichosporosis in India [3]. It is caused by *Corynebacterium* spp. The differential diagnosis includes true mycoses such as white or black piedra. Treatment is with topical benzoic acid, salicylic acid, clindamycin or naftifine [1].

Tuberculosis

Tuberculosis of the penis is rare [4] but important given the resurgence of the disease. Primary penile ulceration (solitary and multiple), with or without inguinal lymphadenopathy, caused by sexual infection or contact with infected clothing may occur [5], or the ulceration may be secondary to tuberculosis elsewhere (e.g. the lung) [6]. A cold abscess (presenting as erectile impotence) has been reported [7]. Tuberculides have involved the penis, including in isolation [8]. Penile manifestations have also followed immunotherapy [9,10].

Non-syphilitic spirochaetal ulcerative balanoposthitis

This condition is recognized in the Tropics and South Africa, presenting as large serpiginous foul-smelling ulcers in uncircumcised men, associated in some with non-tender inguinal lymphadenopathy. Treatment is with penicillin or metronidazole [11].

Yaws

An ulcerated, crusted and papillomatous lesion has been reported on the prepuce as part of disseminated early yaws (with other skin lesions elsewhere) in a patient in an endemic region. Several family members were also infected. The genital lesion probably arose from autoinnoculation [12].

Candidosis

Genito-urinary physicians maintain that *Candida* can be the cause of urethritis and balanoposthitis [13] and cause erosive disease of the glans and prepuce. The glans penis and prepuce may be eroded. *Candida* of the penis (with a prevalence of approximately 10% of that of vaginal candidosis) has attracted very little research interest [14]. However, *Candida* may be more often a secondary pathogen than a sexually acquired infection. Observing the signs of candidosis, or demonstrating the presence of the organism, does not prove that it is the cause of all the symptoms and signs. An underlying dermatological or medical cause should be excluded. The symptoms and signs of *Candida* may be more florid than the underlying predisposing cause. Medical causes include diabetes, iatrogenic immunosuppression and systemic antibiotic treatment. Although oropharyngeal candidosis is almost invariably found in HIV infection, candidal balanoposthitis is not generally associated, perhaps because it is overlooked or because many patients take long-term imidazole antifungals orally.

Candida albicans is such a ready opportunist organism because it is a part of the resident flora of the gastrointestinal tract and may be retrieved from intertriginous areas, including the preputial folds, in the absence of symptoms and signs. Candidal balanoposthitis could be a sexually transmitted disease that may have an affinity for the anatomically or physiologically abnormal penis, or in individuals predisposed by other factors or disease, and where there is chronic vaginal or anal carriage in a partner. Screening should be performed for other sexually transmitted diseases.

Underlying disease should be identified and treated, and predisposing factors rectified. Treatment includes topical nystatin, clioquinol or an imidazole, often usefully combined with hydrocortisone or a moderately potent corticosteroid. In severe disease, an oral imidazole may be indicated.

Tinea

Tinea of the penis or scrotum is uncommon and when it occurs it is usually associated with crural disease. Rarely encountered is the occurrence of tinea on the glans penis as a seat of itch or pain, and producing an erythematous patch or a crop of scaly papules [15–19,20]. Penile tinea in India has been associated with occlusion resulting from the wearing of a langota – a T-shaped piece of cloth tied over the genitalia [17].

Deep fungal infections

Although histoplasmosis is a common cause of disseminated fungal infection in the USA, urological and ano-genital disease (usually ulceration and adenopathy in an ill patient) is rare [21,22]. An otherwise well man with a small warty nodule on the glans penis has been reported [23]. One patient with a penile ulcer transmitted the disease venereally to his wife [24]. Another report documents a phimosis at presentation [25]. In blastomycosis, although the genito-urinary tract (prostate and epididymis) is involved in 20–30% of cases [26], involvement of the genital skin is rare. However, lesions of the prepuce and perianal skin have been recorded [27,28]. Paracoccidioidomycosis can be the cause of scrotal swelling and genital nodules and erosions [29]. Zygomycosis is usually regarded as rhinocerebral infection but a diabetic with purulent lesions of the penis has been described [30].

Other non-sexually transmitted infections

Bacillary angiomatosis is important in the differential diagnosis of AIDS-related Kaposi sarcoma. A case in which the presenting tender red nodules affected the scrotum and groins has been published [1].

Buruli ulcer of the penis and scrotum due to *M. ulcerans* is a rare disease. Medical treatment is disappointing and lesions need excision and grafting [2].

Male genital involvement with leprosy is uncommon, but there are reports, and it may occur in isolation [3,4,5].

The penis is rarely affected by pityriasis versicolor and probably almost never in isolation [6,7]. However, *Malassezia* yeasts may colonize both the circumcised and uncircumcised penis [8]. Occasionally, the anterior pelvic girdle is the site involved.

One case only of superficial phaeohyphomycosis manifesting as multiple, 1–3 mm, pigmented papules, resembling seborrhoeic keratoses, on the scrotum of an HIV-positive patient has been described. Microscopy showed a mass of mycelia, and two dematiaceous fungi were cultured [9].

Genital herpes simplex may be acquired non-sexually (e.g. during contact sports such as rugby football [10]). A phenomenon of chronic erosive and verrucous herpes as part of immunoreconstitution disease has been described in HIV infection [11].

Sacral herpes zoster lesions may be found on the scrotum and penis [12], and urinary retention and constipation can occur.

It is not unusual for the herald patch of pityriasis rosea (thought now to be due to human herpesvirus (HHV)-6/7) to appear on suprapubic skin or in the groin. Incomplete or limited presentations (e.g. affecting the pelvic girdle) are not rare, although careful examination may elicit another patch on the neck or in the axilla.

A distinctive sequel of chikungunya may be ulcers in the peno-scrotal region [13]. Amoebiasis can rarely present as a painful ulcerative balanitis, with swelling, frequency, dysuria and retention [14]. Self-inoculation from concomitant intestinal infection, by heterosexual intercourse where the female partner has amoebic vaginitis, or by sodomy, are the putative mechanisms. Amoebiasis as the cause of genital ulceration should lead to the suspicion of underlying HIV infection [15].

Cutaneous leishmaniasis can affect the genitalia [16,17]. An erythematous scaly plaque [18] and a giant hyperkeratotic nodule on the glans [19], as well as a sporotrichoid distribution on the shaft of the penis [20] have been reported. Post-kala-azar dermal leishmaniasis of the penis and scrotum has been described. Rarely, genital skin lesions may lead to the diagnosis of schistosomiasis. They occur because ova shed by worms enter the perineal vessels [21]. The papules and nodules may be skin coloured, pink or brown, scattered or grouped, affecting the penis and scrotum. They can spread onto the perineum and around the anus, and may develop into soft, warty, vegetating lesions. Ulceration is rare and, even more rarely, concomitant carcinoma has been reported [21].

The ano-genital consequences of onchocerciasis are 'leopard skin' hypopigmentation (the scrotum is commonly involved), ileal crest and scrotal nodules, 'hanging groin', and scrotal enlargement [22,23]. The differential diagnosis of the scrotal enlargement includes bancroftian filariasis [24]. Other filarial infections can lead to mild hydrocele or gross elephantiasis. Filariasis can cause secondary lymphangiectasis. Excision, grafting and genital reconstruction can be undertaken [25].

Primary penile cryptococcal infection has been reported [26,27] and treated successfully with oral azoles and amphotericin.

DERMATOLOGICAL ASPECTS OF SEXUALLY TRANSMITTED DISEASE

MRSA

MRSA presents increasing challenges in general dermatology. There is emerging evidence that community-associated MRSA can be a sexually transmitted disease [1].

Syphilis

Syphilis is endemic throughout the world. It is enjoying a resurgence in both heterosexual and homosexual populations [2]. All manifestations of syphilis can affect the genital region [3]. In 1899, primary syphilis was reported in New York to be a complication of Mosaic circumcision rites in newborn Jewish boys where rabbis used the mouth as a means of stopping haemorrhage [4]. Balanoposthitis can complicate and obscure penile chancre. The granulomatous gumma may affect the genital area as an ulcer, a white plaque or as an atrophic scar. Pseudochancre redux describes gummatous (tertiary stage) recurrence at the site of the primary chancre [5]; it is very rare.

Viral warts

The burden of genital infection with HPV is enormous (see also Chapter 25) [6]. Circumcised men are more likely to have genital warts than the uncircumcised, but when warts are present in uncircumcised men they are more likely to be distally situated [7]. The risk of acquiring genital warts is significantly reduced by using condoms [8]. Clinically inapparent disease may present as balanoposthitis [9]. Subclinical or latent genital HPV infection may be 100 times more common than classical condylomas [10]. The prevalence of HPV in the genital tract of men is similar to that in women, and is between 3% and 45% depending on the age and population [11]. The estimated lifetime risk of acquiring HPV sexually is greater than 50%, and may be 80% [10]. Only 25% of the population of the USA were thought to have no prior or current genital HPV infection in 1997 [12]. The 5% acetic acid test is not a very specific aid to the identification of warts or dysplastic lesions [13]. Accurate diagnosis of HPV infection can probably only be achieved by molecular methods [14]. Congenital and acquired immunosuppression increases the susceptibility of the ano-genital region to HPV infection and reactivation and progression to dysplasia and frank malignancy [15]. There is a growing argument for vaccination of males, as well as females, against oncogenic HPV subtypes [16,17] but as yet efficacy and cost-effectiveness remain unproven. Topical steroid treatment of genital dermatoses may reactivate genital warts [18].

The clinical diagnosis of HPV infection is usually certain, but condylomata lata (secondary syphilis), lichen planus, molluscum contagiosum, bowenoid papulosis and pearly penile papules enter the differential diagnosis. Solitary lesions have a wider differential diagnosis, including giant condyloma, squamous carcinoma and transitional cell carcinoma of the distal urethra, which can present as a warty lesion at the urethral meatus [19]. Biopsy should be performed if there is diagnostic doubt. Patients with ano-genital warts and their partners may require full sexually transmitted disease and sometimes colorectal assessment. Treatment can be challenging [3,6].

Molluscum contagiosum

Young men are commonly seen with penile and pubic lesions and it is assumed that this is a sexually transmitted infection, but this may not always be the case.

HIV infection

Ulcerative genital disease is a risk factor for HIV [20,21], but ano-genital ulceration may be a consequence of HIV infection [22]. Box 111.23 lists the main causes. Biopsy, with special stains and culture, is mandatory. Other genital problems in HIV, such as

---

Box 111.23 Causes of penile and scrotal ulcers in HIV infection

- *Pseudomonas*
- Syphilis
- Chancroid
- Herpes simplex
- Penicilliosis
- Amoebiasis
- Fournier gangrene
- Squamous cell carcinoma
- Kaposi sarcoma
- Drugs (e.g. foscarnet)

psoriasis, warts, intraepithelial neoplasia, squamous carcinoma and Kaposi sarcoma, are discussed elsewhere.

Phthiriasis

Phthiriasis can present with marked genital and pubic itching with few overt physical signs, or as an infected genito-crural and pubic eczema that conceals the underlying primary signs. In hirsute men, the abdomen, chest, axillae and thighs may also be involved. Screening for other sexually transmitted diseases should be offered to the patient and partner(s).

Scabies

Scabies may present with ano-genital itch, 'folliculitis' (including of the buttocks) and penile, scrotal and pubic nodules (Figure 111.14). An AIDS patient with single non-pruritic, 'crusted' lesion

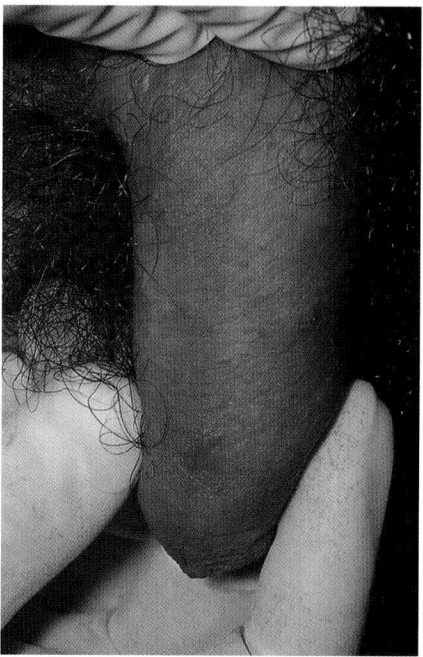

Figure 111.14 Papules on the penis in scabies. (Courtesy of Dr C. White, University Hospital of North Durham, Durham, UK.)

on the glans penis has been described [23]. Topical pimecrolimus has been used with benefit in the treatment of steroid-resistant post-scabies nodules [24].

Other infections

Human bite injuries acquired during oro-genital contact usually heal well but a penile ulcer infected with the oral flora organism *Eikenelia corrodens* has been reported [25].

BENIGN TUMOURS

The following entities are all encountered in the male genital area: pearly penile papules (angiofibromas); angiomas and angiokeratomas, and angiokeratoma corporis diffusum; basal cell papillomas (may be mistaken for viral warts [1] or bowenoid papulosis); melanocytic naevi; inguinogenital epidermoid or (much rarer) pilar (including giant forms) cysts; these may become infected, and lesions containing molluscum contagiosum have been described [2,3].

Median raphe cysts

Congenital cystic median raphe anomalies may remain unobtrusive until adulthood. Cystic or nodular and linear swellings of the ventral penis occur near the glans. In adolescence or adulthood they may become traumatized or infected with staphylococci, gonococci or *Trichomonas* and present as tender, erythematous, purulent nodules [4]. Histologically, they are either dermoid or mucoid, depending on their embryology or epithelial lining [5]. Very rarely, the basal epithelial lining of the cysts may contain melanocytes, imparting a brown-black pigment to the lesion [6].

Mucoid cysts

These are rare lesions that are present at birth or develop in childhood as small, flesh-coloured, mobile cystic papules or nodules with no punctum, commonly on the ventral glans or foreskin, rarely in the perineum. They can be asymptomatic, become infected or interfere with intercourse. The histological features suggest that they arise from ectopic urethral tissue during embryological development [7].

Scrotal calcinosis

Scrotal calcinosis is a relatively common, benign, idiopathic disorder presenting as solitary or multiple, hard, smooth, white papules or nodules on the scrotum, rarely the penis (Figure 111.15). Interestingly, these lesions are much rarer on the vulva [8]. Occasionally, they may become secondarily inflamed or infected following trauma. Their occurrence was first described by Hutchinson [9]. Their origin has been debated: they have been said to arise from epidermoid cysts, eccrine duct milia, eccrine epithelial cysts, dystrophy

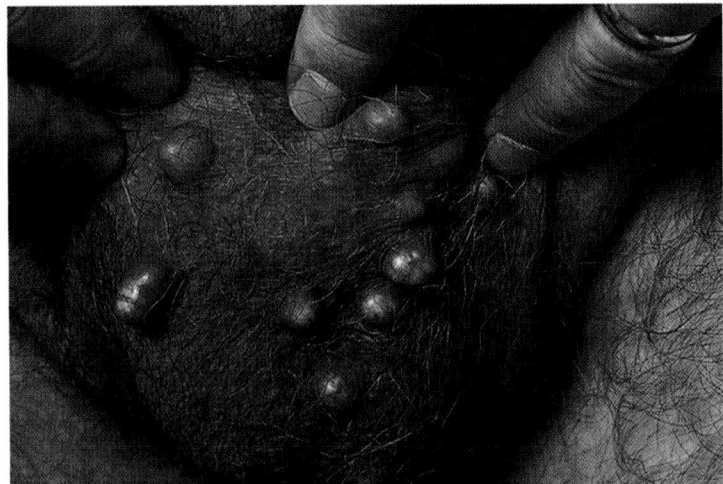

Figure 111.15 Scrotal calcinosis. (Courtesy of Dr D. A. Burns, Leicester, UK.)

of the dartos muscle, trauma and the presence of foreign bodies [10–20]. Scrotal calcinosis may occur after meconium peritonitis, with leakage of meconium through the processus vaginalis, and in testicular tumours such as teratomas, gonadoblastomas and Leydig cell tumours [17]. In endemic areas of onchocerciasis, calcified scrotal cysts may be caused by the living or dead nematodes, and patients have evidence of the disease elsewhere [21,22]. Onchocercal nodules are more common on the iliac crests and the rib cage. The unsightly and embarrassing lesions can be treated by incision and eventration under local anaesthesia. Idiopathic calcinosis of the penis is very rare [23,24]. A man who presented with a dome-shaped nodule on his glans has been described; the dystrophic calcinosis here was thought to derive from syringoma [25]. Other associations are trauma, self-injection with papaverine, Peyronie disease and cytotoxic chemotherapy [23]. Metastatic calcinosis is due to renal failure and secondary hyperparathyroidism.

Verruciform xanthoma

Verruciform xanthoma mainly affects the mouth. The genitalia are the next most frequently involved area, where it presents as a painless, yellow-brown or red, verrucous, sessile or papillary plaque. Fewer than 20 cases have been reported [26]. The histological findings are hyperkeratosis, focal parakeratosis, acanthosis and fat-filled foam cells in the papillary dermis. Verruciform xanthoma is thought to represent epidermal degeneration, with keratinocyte lipid then taken up by dermal macrophages [27] or fibroblasts to form the foam cells. HPV infection and lymphoedema have been proposed as crucial cofactors in the pathogenesis [28,29]. Treatment is by surgical excision.

Other benign tumours

Naevus comedonicus of the glans penis, generally devoid of pilosebaceous structures, has been reported [30]. Keloid is rare, but can complicate circumcision [31,32,33], and other surgery and trauma [34,35]. Keloid has been simulated on the dorsum of the penis by chronic oedema caused by a condom catheter [36]. Dermoid cyst affecting the penis, presenting with pain, swelling and suppuration from abscess formation, has been reported [37]. Acanthosis nigricans almost always affects the groins. In pseudoacanthosis nigricans, the associated obesity is almost always responsible for intertrigo and skin tags. Penile colloid degeneration has been described, presenting as a dermal plaque of the dorsal shaft [38]. Some cases of multiple syringomata localized to the penis have been described, mimicking genital warts or lichen planus [39–42]. Other benign tumours that have been reported rarely to affect the genital area include apocrine cystadenoma [43,44], syringocystadenoma papilliferum [45], mixed syringocystadenoma papilliferum and papillary eccrine adenoma occurring in a scrotal condyloma [46], composite adnexal tumour [47], dermatofibroma [48], reticulohistiocytoma [49], giant cell fibroblastoma [50], connective tissue naevi (scrotum) [51], fibrous hamartoma of infancy [52], leiomyoma [48,53], genital smooth muscle hamartoma (scrotum) [54,55], traumatic neuroma [56], neurofibroma, neurilemoma, granular cell myoblastoma [48,57–59], varicosities/venous lakes, acquired capillary and cavernous haemangioma [48] (other angiomatous lesions are very much rarer, and controversy exists as to whether they represent a true neoplasm, herniation of the corpus spongiosum or vascularization of a haematoma or thrombus [60]), Masson vegetant intravascular haemangioendothelioma [61], angiokeratoma circumscriptum of Mibelli [62], glomus tumour [51,63], port-wine stain, strawberry naevus [64–66], haemangiomas and PELVIS syndrome [67], epithelioid haemangioma [68], epithelioid haemangioendothelioma [48,69], pyogenic granuloma [70], angiolymphoid hyperplasia with eosinophilia/Kimura disease (penis and spermatic cord) [71,72,73] and lymphangioma circumscriptum [74,75].

PRE-CANCEROUS DERMATOSES AND CARCINOMA *IN SITU*

Erythroplasia of Queyrat, Bowen disease of the penis and bowenoid papulosis

Definition
Erythroplasia of Queyrat, Bowen disease of the penis (BDP) and bowenoid papulosis (BP) are three clinical variants of carcinoma *in situ* of the penis.

Introduction and general description
There is a heterogenous spectrum of clinical and histological presentations of the three clinical variants of carcinoma *in situ* of the penis: erythroplasia of Queyrat, BDP and BP [1,2,3]. These entities are ultimately defined histologically. PeIN (corresponding to cervical, vulval and anal intraepithelial neoplasia; CIN, VIN and AIN) is a histological umbrella term. The terms squamous hyperplasia (SH) and squamous intraepithelial lesion (SIL: squamous, basaloid or warty, high or low grade) are also in use

[4]. Distinct morphological subtypes of PeIN, differentiated and undifferentiated (bowenoid), are recognized, and the latter can be subdivided into warty, basaloid and warty-basaloid: mixed types can be encountered. Differentiated PeIN manifests basal and parabasal atypia (and this can be subtle) and is associated with SH and lichen sclerosus and the 'usual' and verrucous keratinizing subtypes of squamous carcinoma of the penis. Undifferentiated (or 'usual' type PeIN) has bowenoid histology (two thirds to full thickness PeIN type 3) koilocytic change and high-grade SIL and is associated with HPV and the warty, condylomatous, basaloid and 'mixed' subtypes of penile squamous carcinoma [5,6].

Although erythroplasia of Queyrat and BDP are synonymous in describing carcinoma *in situ* of the penis, BD is used to refer to squamous carcinoma *in situ* at other cutaneous sites. Erythroplasia of Queyrat should be used to describe red shiny patches or plaques of the 'mucosal' penis (glans and prepuce of the uncircumcised), although erythroplasia of Queyrat has been recorded in a partially circumcised man [7]. BDP should be used to describe red, sometimes slightly pigmented, scaly patches and plaques of the keratinized penis. These distinctions have not always been made in the literature. BP is analogous to, but clinically different from, erythroplasia of Queyrat and BDP. The term should be used to describe multiple warty lesions, which are often pigmented in keratinized sites, and more numerous and more inflamed at 'mucosal' sites (Figure 111.16). BP lesions are less papillomatous, smoother topped, more polymorphic and more coalescent than common genital viral condylomata acuminata, and occur in younger, sexually active men, as opposed to the patches or scaly plaques of erythroplasia of Queyrat and BDP, respectively, seen in older men. BP may be associated with a lesser risk of squamous carcinoma than erythroplasia of Queyrat and BDP. It is particularly associated with HPV infection (especially HPV-16) and HIV infection. Voltz *et al.* [8] found ano-genital warts in 16% of all HIV-positive males, nearly half of whom showed histological signs of intraepithelial neoplasia.

Aetiology and pathophysiology
The exact aetiology of erythroplasia of Queyrat, BDP and BP is not known. Local carcinogenic influences in uncircumcised men such as poor hygiene, smegma, trauma, friction, heat, maceration,

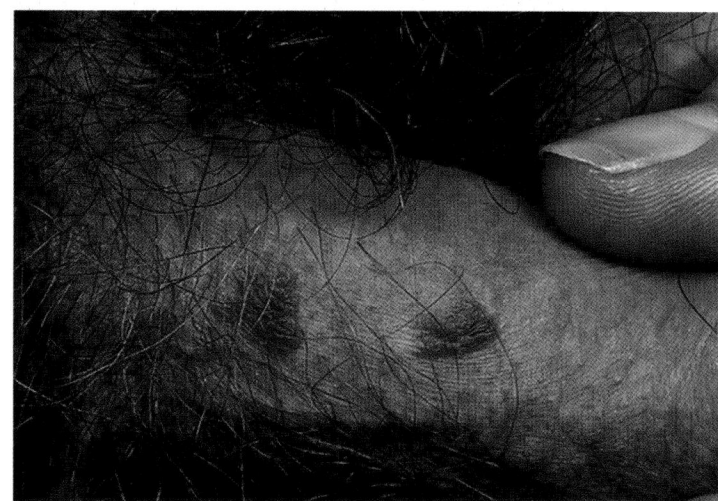

Figure 111.16 Bowenoid papulosis. (Courtesy of Dr D. A. Burns, Leicester, UK.)

inflammation, phimosis, dermatoses such as lichen sclerosus and smoking (tar metabolites in urine) are acknowledged associations [9]. PeIN can be found in men being screened for HPV infection [10], and HPV (commonly types 16, 18, 39 and 51) is probably the most important factor in 70–100% of cases of carcinoma *in situ* [11], particularly in BP [12]. Indeed, BP is probably virus-induced epithelial dysplasia associated mainly with HPV-16, but other types have been found [13–15]. Erythroplasia of Queyrat has been shown to be associated with co-infection with the rare epidermodysplasia verruciformis-associated HPV-8 and the genital high-risk HPV-16 [16]. There is a high prevalence of PeIN in male sexual partners of women with CIN [17,18], but many patients with PeIN have consorts with no evidence of warts or CIN. Immunosuppression is an important risk; 50% of HIV patients with ano-genital warts had carcinoma *in situ* on histology in one study [8]. Nothing is known about the influence of immunogenotype. The evidence confirming that erythroplasia of Queyrat/BDP may result in squamous carcinoma has been reviewed comprehensively [9,19]. The risk of progression to invasive squamous cell carcinoma is cited at 10–33% [11] with erythroplasia of Queyrat probably being more dangerous than BDP. The risk of progression of BP to invasive squamous carcinoma is not known, but is probably low in the absence of other risk factors, especially immunocompromise. Spontaneous regression can occur [11] including with restitution of immunocompetence in the treatment of HIV [20]. The grade of the intraepithelial neoplasia and the development of invasive carcinoma are related to age [21]. *p53* mutations do not appear to be important in male genital carcinogenesis [22].

The histology is of an intraepithelial carcinoma [23] and the histological subtypes have been described earlier: it is not possible reliably to separate them macroscopically [6]. In some cases, especially those associated with lichen sclerosus, it can be very difficult to distinguish SHs from differentiated PeIN and immunohistochemistry for *p53* and *Ki-67* may be helpful [6,14].

Clinical features

Some patients with these lesions may be quite young [24]. There may be several foci of BDP or erythroplasia of Queyrat and they may occur concomitantly. The non-specificity of the clinical appearances makes for an important differential diagnosis, which includes psoriasis, lichen sclerosus, lichen planus, Zoon balanitis and extramammary Paget disease. The differential diagnosis of BP includes lichen planus, common warts, seborrhoeic warts, naevi and condylomata lata. A biopsy is indicated in instances where the clinical diagnosis is uncertain. Aynaud *et al.* [25] have shown that shrewd clinical interpretation predicts which lesions will show carcinoma *in situ* histologically and which will contain oncogenic HPV. Reflectance confocal microscopy shows promise [26]. Secondary amyloid deposition has been reported histologically in one case of BP [27].

Investigations

Occasionally, it may be necessary to perform several biopsies.

Management

Treatment choice depends on many factors [2,3,11] Circumcision removes a major risk factor for cancer and provides extensive tissue

for histology. Topical 5-fluorouracil as a 5% cream is a well-established conventional option for the treatment of BDP, erythroplasia of Queyrat and BP [1,2,3,28]. Other treatments include cryosurgery, curettage and electrocautery, excisional surgery, glans resurfacing, Mohs micrographic surgery, laser and photodynamic therapy [1,2,3,11,29,30]. Radiotherapy should be avoided. Topical imiquimod may help some patients [31,32,33]. Topical cidofovir has been used [34,35,36]. There have been no trials. A recent retrospective review of patients with penile carcinoma *in situ* using topical 5-fluorouracil as first line therapy, and topical imiquimod as second line treatment, demonstrated a complete response in 57%, partial response in 13.6%, and no response in 29.5% [11,37]. HPV vaccination may have a part to play in prevention and treatment. Patients with these conditions should be counselled and screened for HPV and other sexually transmitted diseases, including HIV infection. They should stop smoking. Sexual partners should be advised to seek assessment. Follow-up may need to be long term depending on individual circumstances [2,3,21].

Miscellaneous pre-cancerous conditions

Squamous hyperplasia and squamous intraepithelial lesion(s)

SH lesions consist of white patches and plaques (Box 111.24). Although SH is the most common epithelial abnormality found in association with invasive squamous carcinoma of the penis, histologically there is *no* cytological atypia. Acanthosis and orthokeratotic hyperkeratosis are found; it is associated with differentiated PeIN, underlying lichen sclerosus and penile carcinoma of the 'usual' and verrucous subtypes. SIL presents clinically as redder or more pigmented papules and plaques; it is classified histologically into squamous, basaloid or warty, high- or low-grade subtypes; it is associated with undifferentiated (or 'usual' type) bowenoid PeIN, HPV and the warty, condylomatous, basaloid and 'mixed' subtypes of penile squamous carcinoma [1,2].

Box 111.24 Causes of white patches and plaques

- Post-traumatic or surgical scar
- Lichen simplex
- Lichen sclerosus
- Vitiligo
- Mucous membrane (cicatricial) pemphigoid
- Peyronie disease
- Syphilis
  - Leukoderma: post-secondary syphilide
  - Gumma
  - Post-gummatous atrophic scar
- Viral warts
- Pityriasis versicolor
- Pseudoepitheliomatous micaceous and keratotic balanitis
- Intraepithelial neoplasia
- Squamous cell carcinoma

Reproduced from Bunker CB. *Male Genital Skin Disease*. London: Saunders, 2004. © 2004, with permission from the author.

Penile horn

It is rare for cutaneous horn to affect the penis [3]. Multiple lesions have been described in a 70-year-old man [4]. The underlying causes include pseudoepitheliomatous micaceous and keratotic balanitis [5], verrucous carcinoma [6,7,8,9] and squamous carcinoma [10]. Chronic inflammation and recent circumcision for long-standing phimosis are said to be important predisposing factors. The lesion is pre-malignant or, in one-third of cases, malignant at presentation, with squamous carcinoma the underlying pathology. Treatment should be dictated by precise diagnosis achieved by adequate excision and histology of the whole lesion. Follow-up is mandatory because recurrence may occur.

Porokeratosis

Genital porokeratosis of Mibelli is rare, but classical lesions have been reported on the penis and scrotum. It may be commoner in Asian populations [11]. Pruritus and ulceration may occur [12]. Porokeratosis may be confused with psoriasis, Bowen disease, granuloma annulare or lichen planus; biopsy differentiates these conditions [13]. Topical 5-fluorouracil and imiquimod have been used for treatment [14,15].

Pseudoepitheliomatous micaceous and keratotic balanitis

Pseudoepitheliomatous micaceous and keratotic balanitis (PEMKB) is a rare penile condition. It presents as thick scaly micaceous patches (possibly a cutaneous horn) on the glans penis in older uncircumcised men [5,16]. Perimeatal hyperkeratosis may cause multiple urinary streams on micturition – a 'watering-can penis' [17]. Histological examination shows hyperkeratosis, parakeratosis, acanthosis, prolongation of the rete ridges and mild lower epidermal dysplasia, with a non-specific dermal inflammatory infiltrate of eosinophils and lymphocytes. PEMKB is a variant of lichen sclerosus unassociated with HPV but strongly associated with verrucous carcinoma [18,19,20]. Metastatic spread has not occurred except where there was a penile horn [21], and in one patient who developed an aggressive soft-tissue sarcoma of the penis [22]. Recurrence is common. Topical 5-fluorouracil, radiotherapy and surgery have been the principal treatment choices [5] but contemporaneous thinking is that lichen sclerosus should be identified and treated and that radiotherapy should be avoided.

SQUAMOUS CARCINOMA AND OTHER MALIGNANT NEOPLASMS

Carcinoma of the penis

Introduction and general description

The earliest stages of penis cancer and pre-cancer form a heterogenous spectrum of disease as discussed in detail earlier [1,2]. Although some penile cancers arise *de novo*, others develop from

pre-malignant situations, which may be misdiagnosed or may be difficult to diagnose and there are the issues of multifocality, field change and the temporal dynamic to acknowledge. The precise aetiologies of the types of PeIN and squamous carcinoma of the penis are unknown, but the picture has become much clearer in recent years: there is a dichotomous pathway, HPV related or lichen sclerosus related, as in the vulva.

Epidemiology

Of the approximately 500 new cases per year, carcinoma of the penis causes about 100 deaths per annum in the UK and accounts for less than 1% of deaths from cancer in the USA. It constitutes 10–20% of tumours seen in males in either developing countries or in areas where early circumcision is not commonly practised; overall, the highest incidence is in Africa, South America and Asia (2–4/100 000 inhabitants) and lowest in the USA and Europe (0.3–1/100 000) [1,3].

Pathophysiology

Risk factors for penis cancer are listed in Box 111.25. The presence of a foreskin, HPV infection and lichen sclerosus are the most important considerations [1–3,4].

Neonatal circumcision protects against penile carcinoma [1,5,6]. Circumcision in later life may reduce the risk but does not abolish it, especially if the circumcision was performed for penile disease [1,4,7,8,9]. However, there have been very rare cases in Jews and others circumcised at birth [4,10–12]. The incidence of penis cancer is low in Japan and Denmark, where circumcision is rare [13,14], so other factors are important in carcinogenesis [1,4].

Although penile cancer is associated with multiple sexual partners and previous sexually transmitted disease, including HIV, the epidemiological features are not those characteristic of

---

Box 111.25 Risk factors for squamous carcinoma of the penis

- Uncircumcised
- Phimosis
- Long foreskin
- Poor hygiene
- Chronic irritation, inflammation, scarring
- Smoking
- Many sexual partners
- Lichen sclerosus
- Lichen planus
- Human papillomavirus
- HIV
- Squamous hyperplasia/squamous intraepithelial lesion
- Bowen disease
- Erythroplasia of Queyrat
- Bowenoid papulosis
- Pseudoepitheliomatous micaceous and keratotic balanitis
- Giant condyloma/verrucous carcinoma
- Photochemotherapy
- Iatrogenic immunosuppression
  - Renal transplantation
  - Systemic lupus erythematosus
- Radiotherapy

a sexually transmitted disease [15] – unlike carcinoma of the cervix and, to a lesser extent, anal carcinoma. In cervical cancer, the evidence is that it is a sexually transmitted disease and that HPV is the aetiological agent. Yet penile cancer puts female sexual partners at risk of cervical cancer and there is a high prevalence of HPV, condylomas, SIL and PIN in sexual partners of women with CIN. In India, the incidence of cervical cancer is lower in Muslim women than in Hindus and Christians. HPV is certainly implicated in penis cancer [1,3,4,16], but many patients have no evidence of HPV [13,16,17]. Oncogenic HPV, particularly types 16 and 18 (but also types 31, 33, 35, 39, 45, 51, 52, 54, 56, 58, 59, 66, 68 and 69), have been incriminated in 22–45% of penile squamous cell carcinoma and in 70–100% of penile squamous cell carcinoma *in situ* [1,3].

Phimosis and balanitis are known risk factors for penile cancer [14]. The possession of a 'long' foreskin may be important. Poor personal and sexual hygiene [14] and phimosis may lead to the retention of smegma and development of balanitis. However, the carcinogenicity of human smegma has not been ascertained [18], and it is not widely appreciated that phimosis is a physical sign and not a diagnosis. Hence, there may be more in the carcinogenic propensity of phimosis than simply physical retention of smegma.

Lichen sclerosus is a common cause of phimosis in males and it predisposes to penile carcinoma [1,17–21]. Powell *et al.* [22] found that half of patients with penis cancer had a clinical history and/or histological evidence of lichen sclerosus.

Regarding other chronic dermatoses, chronic erosive and hypertrophic lichen planus are pre-malignant conditions, and lichen planus is a cause of phimosis [4]. Chronic irritation and inflammation or scarring are all risk factors for squamous carcinoma of the skin generally and the penis is no exception; penis cancer complicating a burn scar and a chronic sinus tract have been reported [4]. Quantifying the malignant potential of the precancerous dermatoses, BDP, erythroplasia of Queyrat and PIN is difficult, but they are acknowledged risks for penile cancer and HPV is found in 70–100% of penile squamous cell carcinoma *in situ* cases [1,4,23,24].

Smoking is a risk factor, independent of phimosis, for penile carcinoma [4,15], and is also a recognized risk factor for anal and cervical cancer. Smoking may cause squamoepithelial cancer, not only in parts of the body in contact with smoke but also at distant sites by dissemination of carcinogens in the circulation or in secretions. The presence of tobacco-specific nitrosamines in the preputial secretions of rats has been demonstrated [4].

Penile carcinoma is a complication of psoralen and UVA therapy (PUVA) [4,25], and possibly other treatments for psoriasis The photodye treatment of genital herpes simplex ceased in the 1970s because of the occurrence of BDP in young men who did not have other risk factors for carcinoma *in situ* [4]. However, increased UV exposure of the genitals from sunlamps and sunbeds had not led to an increase in genital skin cancer in the USA by 1986 [4].

Penis cancer complicates immunosuppression in solid organ transplantation [4,26] and HIV infection [4] (risk increased five– to sixfold). It is also seen in men with psoriasis treated with immunosuppressive drugs [4,27,28]. Topical immunosuppressive agents such as the calcineurin inhibitors should be used with extreme caution for genital dermatoses, especially in the uncircumcised,

Table 111.1 Classification and frequency of squamous cell carcinomas of the penis [3].

Subtype	Frequency (%)
Usual squamous cell carcinoma	48–65
Basaloid carcinoma	4–10
Warty carcinoma	7–10
Verrucous carcinoma	3–8
Papillary carcinoma	5–15
Sarcomatoid carcinoma	1–3
Mixed carcinomas	9–10
Adenosquamous carcinoma	1–2
Pseudohyperplastic carcinoma	<1
Carcinoma cuniculatum	<1
Pseudoglandular carcinoma	<1
Warty–basaloid carcinoma	9–14

After Chaux and Cubilla 2012 [3].

because of the risk of squamous carcinoma [29–31]. There is no evidence for a risk attributable to topical steroids [32].

In summary, as in vulval cancer, all the evidence points to there being a pathogenetic dichotomy with two largely independent pathways to the development of penile squamous cell carcinoma: HPV related and lichen sclerosus related. The HPV-dependent pathway leads predominantly to basaloid and warty subtypes and the lichen sclerosus–related pathway leads mainly to usual and verrucous subtypes [1,3,16].

Pathology

There is a spectrum of histological subtypes of penile squamous cell carcinoma [1,3,23,24]. Histological signs of SH, SIL, CIS, PeIN, lichen sclerosus and HPV are commonly found. HPV typing and immunohistochemistry, for example for p16INK 4a (as a co-factor for HPV), are emerging as adjunctive diagnostic tools [3,24]. Chaux and Cubilla [3] have classified penile squamous cell carcinoma as detailed in Table 111.1.

Clinical features

Itch, irritation, pain, bleeding, discharge, ulceration or the discovery of a mass are the presenting symptoms of squamous carcinoma. There is often a long history of preceding problems with the penis and foreskin, manifest as dyspareunia, balanoposthitis or phimosis and dysuria. Irregular nodular and ulcerative morphology is found on examination (Figures 111.17 and 111.18) and there may be background BDP, erythroplasia of Queyrat and BP, lichen sclerosus or lichen planus. Undiagnosed, untreated disease is destructive and mutilating. Phimosis should be regarded as a sinister situation, not least because it impedes complete inspection and palpation of the glans and coronal sulcus. The inguinal lymph glands must be palpated, although in penile cancer only 50% of enlarged glands will be found to contain tumour [33]. The concomitant presence of sexually transmitted diseases and immunocompromise should be excluded. The differential diagnosis includes the manifestations of intraepithelial neoplasia (and the differential diagnosis of these), erosive or ulcerative sexually transmitted disease, basal cell carcinoma, Kaposi sarcoma, pyoderma gangrenosum and artefact. Genito-urinary and urological assessment should be sought.

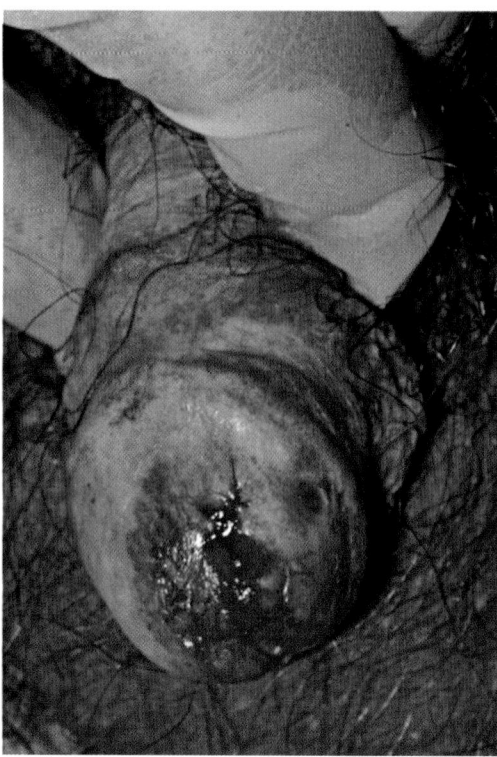

Figure 111.17 High-grade dysplasia and invasive squamous carcinoma. (Courtesy of Professor C. B. Bunker, with permission from Medical Illustration UK, Chelsea & Westminster Hospital, London, UK.)

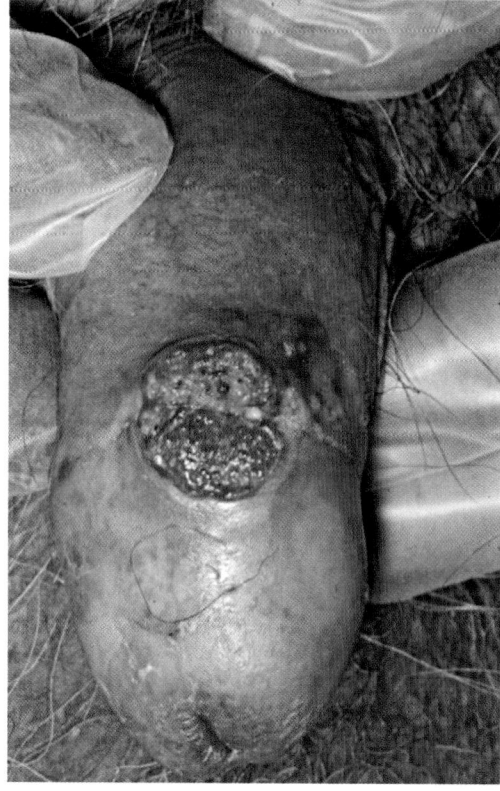

Figure 111.18 Squamous carcinoma. Severe background lichen sclerosus. (Reproduced from Bunker CB. Skin conditions of the male genitalia. *Medicine* 2001;29:9–13, by kind permission of the Medicine Publishing Company.)

Investigations

Diagnosis is confirmed histologically by incisional or excisional biopsy. An incisional biopsy should be of adequate size and depth, and it may be necessary to sample several sites. The biopsy(ies) may need to be performed by a urologist under general anaesthesia. Patients who have negative or equivocal biopsies, but who have risk factors or in whom there is a high index of suspicion, should be followed up closely and rebiopsied if indicated. Staging should not be based on incisional biopsies.

Management [34]

The treatment of ano-genital squamous carcinoma is not generally the province of the dermatologist. The overriding general principles are to stage the disease clinically, histologically and by imaging to offer adequate surgical excision, including circumcision, for disease of the penis. The penile surgery may need to be radical, total or partial, depending on location and extent. To conserve tissue and minimize residual sexual dysfunction, conservative techniques are increasingly used, with narrow excisional margins and innovative plastic repair, as are laser treatment and Mohs micrographic surgery for squamous carcinoma of the penis. The concepts of field change, multifocality, and the temporal dynamic and implications of infection by HPV must also be considered. Fundamental to the planning of penile surgery for penile carcinoma associated with lichen sclerosus is the recognition of the pernicious role in the initiation and progression of lichen sclerosus played by the chronic occluded exposure of genital skin to urine [35]: the laudable goals of organ–saving surgery in penis cancer should include the avoidance of new or, more likely, recurrent lichen

sclerosus, because of the ensuing morbidity and risk of second squamous cancers There are established indications for sentinel node biopsy and inguinal and pelvic lymphadenectomy. Radiotherapy may be offered as an adjunct to surgery or as definitive alternative treatment. Combination chemotherapy has been used for palliation and adjuvant treatment of carcinoma of the penis, but remains under evaluation. Lymphatic or haematogenous dissemination of genital cancer dictates individualized expert multidisciplinary treatment, in the UK, by a multidisciplinary team.

The prognosis of penis cancer relates to the extent of inguinal lymphadenopathy and involvement of the corpus. It does not correlate with HPV status [36]. Penile cancer puts female sexual partners at risk of cervical cancer [37]. In black men who develop penile cancer there is a substantial risk (18%) of the later development of a second primary malignancy.

The prognosis for scrotal carcinoma is not good, despite apparently adequate primary surgical treatment: the 5-year mortality is 50–60%.

Carcinoma of the scrotum

Squamous carcinoma of the scrotum has been recognized in chimney sweeps (exposed to carcinogens in soot) [1], mule spinners (exposed to carcinogens in lubricating oils for the spinning jenny in the cloth industry), Persian nomads (who travelled with pots of burning charcoal between their legs) and Indian jute oil processors [2–5,6]. Oil-mist exposure in industry continues to be widespread

PART 10: SITES, SEX, AGE

and, apart from scrotal cancer, has been associated with other cutaneous problems (such as contact dermatitis and oil acne) and respiratory diseases, including cancer [7].

Other individuals at risk of scrotal squamous carcinoma include those with a history of psoriasis treated with arsenic, coal tar, UVB and PUVA, radiotherapy [8,9,10,11,12,13], scrotal HPV infection, hidradenitis suppurativa, Bowen disease and multiple cutaneous keratoses and epitheliomas [14,15,16,17,18]. Rarely, black men may be affected [19].

The presentation of scrotal carcinoma is similar to that of penis cancer, with itch, irritation, pain, bleeding, discharge, ulceration or the discovery of a lump, and irregular nodular and ulcerative clinical features. A pigmented squamous carcinoma of the scrotum has been reported [20]. The differential diagnosis includes the manifestations of intraepithelial neoplasia (and the differential diagnosis of these), erosive or ulcerative sexually transmitted disease, basal cell carcinoma, Kaposi sarcoma, metastasis, extramammary Paget disease, pyoderma gangrenosum and artefact. The diagnosis is confirmed by biopsy [21].

Verrucous carcinoma/giant condyloma/ Buschke–Löwenstein tumour

These terms have been used interchangeably for large verruciform tumours of the penis presenting with an exophytic and papillomatous pattern of growth. They are well differentiated, with low metastatic rate and better survival compared with usual squamous cell carcinoma. It is perhaps more accurate and more clinically useful to consider giant condyloma and the Buschke–Löwenstein tumour as synonymous or overlapping HPV-related entities. Verrucous carcinoma is HPV unrelated but associated with lichen sclerosus and more dangerous. Dramatic polypoid or cauliflower-like clinical lesions are encountered (Figure 111.19).

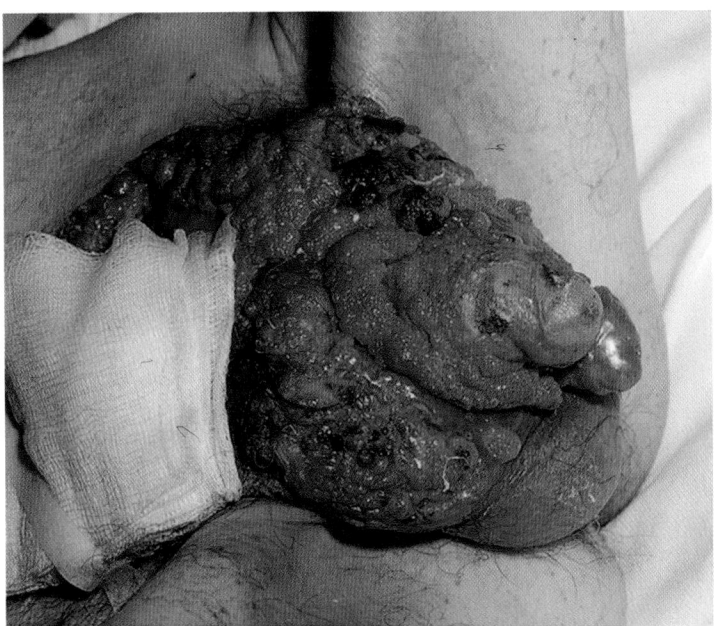

Figure 111.19 Gross condylomas of Buschke–Löwenstein of the penis. (Courtesy of Professor R. M. MacKie, Glasgow University, Glasgow, UK.)

As well as lichen sclerosus [1], tumours occurring on background hidradenitis suppurativa and very rarely lichen planus have occurred [2,3,4]. A deep surgical biopsy is necessary because the histological differential diagnosis can be challenging. Surgical excision is the treatment usually recommended (e.g. glansectomy [5] or penectomy). Mohs micrographic surgery [6,7,8], cryotherapy [9], laser treatment [10,11], interferon-α [12,13,14,15], radiotherapy [16] or bleomycin [17] have been deployed.

The prognosis can be poor because verrucous carcinoma might continue to grow and invade locally, causing death by exsanguination from femoral arterial invasion or cachexia [18]. Even with treatment, recurrence and progressive malignant transformation do occur so follow-up is necessary.

Extramammary Paget disease

Definition
Extramammary Paget disease is a malignant skin condition in which there is intraepidermal infiltration by neoplastic cells showing glandular differentiation.

Introduction and general description
Clinically, extramammary Paget disease presents as a unilateral erythematous patch or plaque affecting the ano-genital skin, or other sites rich in apocrine glands. It tends to progress slowly over a number of years so that a delay in diagnosis is not uncommon. Extramammary Paget disease is often associated with an underlying malignancy [1]. In a large series, 24% of patients had a proximate cutaneous adnexal adenocarcinoma, 12% were found to have a concurrent, and another 17% to have a non-concurrent internal malignancy [2].

Although properly regarded as a type of carcinoma *in situ*, extramammary Paget disease may itself become invasive and metastatic. There may be subjacent carcinoma (e.g. in periurethral glands) or distant carcinoma (e.g. prostate or bladder), or both (e.g. in periurethral glands and bladder). Pagetoid epidermal invasion of inguinal cutaneous metastatic mesothelioma of the tunica vaginalis of the testis has been reported.

Epidemiology
Extramammary Paget disease presents in men aged 60–70 as irritating, itchy, burning, red scaly patches or plaques that may be solitary or multifocal.

Pathophysiology
Immunohistochemical and enzyme histochemical evidence points to sweat gland epithelium as the source of Paget cells in extramammary Paget disease. The distribution along the 'milk line' has led to the suggestion that the 'clear cells of Toker' are the histogenic precursors of both clear cell papulosis and mammary and extramammary Paget disease, respectively. HPV is not present [3], but the c-erbB-2 oncoprotein may have a role in the pathogenesis of extramammary Paget disease.

Pathology

Histological examination shows nests of large vacuolated cells with circular nuclei and foamy pale cytoplasm in the epidermis (Paget cells). Dermal involvement signifies a poor prognosis. Pagetoid dyskeratosis can be found in a number of benign lesions such as naevi, skin tags and lentigines [1]. Pale cells resembling Paget cells can be seen incidentally in benign papular intertriginous conditions, and in nearly 40% of prepuces sent for histological examination following circumcision for phimosis [1,2,3,4,5]. Ano-genital Paget disease can be accompanied by epidermal hyperplasia similar to fibroepithelioma of Pinkus.

Clinical features

Extramammary Paget disease can occur anywhere in the ano-genital area, including the glans penis [1,3,4]. Penile extramammary Paget disease is frequently misdiagnosed as psoriasis, eczema, tinea or Bowen disease [3,4]. An 'underpants' pattern of erythema has been reported in a number of patients. Subclinical extramammary Paget disease has been documented, where the skin looks normal macroscopically but is involved microscopically. Extramammary Paget disease behaves indolently, spreading by local extension and metastasis [1].

The concurrence of genital and extragenital extramammary Paget disease is extremely rare, but overt and latent axillary extramammary Paget disease can coexist and change daily in association with penile and pubic extramammary Paget disease. Also very rare is depigmented extramammary Paget disease of the genitalia, evoking the differential diagnosis of vitiligo, hypopigmented mycosis fungoides and lichen sclerosus. A focus of cutaneous squamous carcinoma has been reported complicating genital extramammary Paget disease [5].

Investigations

Diagnosis is by biopsy. A search for an underlying adenocarcinoma should be undertaken.

Management

Wide excisional surgery is the treatment of choice. Other treatments used for extramammary Paget disease [3] include cryotherapy and topical 5-fluorouracil, micrographic surgery, radiotherapy, and photodynamic therapy. Topical imiquimod has been promising. A combination of treatments is often required. Recurrence is common. Excision of an underlying neoplasm, if present, can cause regression of the extramammary Paget disease.

Malignant melanoma

This is a rare condition of the penis. It is estimated to account for 1–1.5% of all malignancies of the penis [1,2] and less than 0.15% of all melanomas [3]. Melanoma is even rarer on the scrotum, with only four cases appearing in the literature [4,5].

Genital melanoma presents as a pigmented macule or as a pigmented or amelanotic papule or nodule, possibly developing from a lentiginous area or pre-existing dysplastic naevus or 'kissing' naevus, that may ulcerate or bleed [1,2,6–9]. Multifocal melanoma of the glans penis has been reported [10]. Patients are usually middle-aged or older, although it has been reported in a boy [11]. It is exceedingly rare in Asians and has not been reported in black people (although a case of melanoma of the urethra has been seen) [12]. The diagnosis is often delayed [2].

Between 60% and 70% of lesions occur on the glans. There may be a family history of melanoma and other atypical or 'dysplastic' naevi on examination. The inguinal and other nodes, as well as the abdomen, should be palpated. Between 40% and 50% of patients have lymphatic or other metastatic dissemination at the time of presentation. Clinically, atypical lesions should be biopsied and the histology critically reviewed [13,14]. Malignant melanoma of any histological subtype may be encountered [15].

Treatment is by primary excision. Subsequent management depends on the Breslow thickness of the lesion and complete clinical staging. Radical surgery and chemotherapy may be needed, but the prognosis is poor for all melanomas that have already metastasized [1,11,16].

Kaposi sarcoma

Solitary Kaposi sarcoma of the penis was very rarely seen before the HIV epidemic and cases are still occasionally seen in HIV-negative patients [1,2,3,4], but genital KS is essentially an HIV-associated problem. It presents on the penis or scrotum, perineum or perianal skin in one of its classic forms: purple, slightly scaly patches or plaques, nodules or ulcerative lesions [5]. More atypical presentations that have been seen include engorgement with hypervascularity [6], penile lymphoedema [7] and phimosis. The differential diagnosis includes cellular naevus, histiocytoma, angioma, angiokeratoma, pseudo-Kaposi sarcoma [8], bacillary angiomatosis and melanoma.

Other malignant neoplasms

Although basal cell carcinoma is the most common type of skin cancer, it is rare in the ano-genital area [1], including one case report of fibroepithelioma of Pinkus affecting the base of the penis [2]. A case of multiple erosive scrotal basal cell carcinomas with metastasis has been described [3].

Fibrosarcoma, haemangiopericytoma, leiomyosarcoma, malignant fibrous histiocytoma, epithelioid sarcoma, dermatofibrosarcoma protuberans and spindle cell sarcoma may occur, presenting as painful or painless nodules, masses or swelling with dysuria and erectile difficulties (e.g. masquerading as Peyronie disease) [4,5,6]. Other rarities include Merkel cell carcinoma [7], malignant eccrine poroma [8], malignant schwannoma [4,9] and solitary reticulohistiocytic granuloma of the scrotum [10]. Scrotal angiosarcoma complicating oedema following surgery and radiotherapy for carcinoma of the rectum has been described [11].

Involvement of the penis with Langerhans cell histiocytosis is very rare; fleshy papules on the dorsal penis, a painful nodule of the prepuce and penile ulceration have been reported [12,13].

Mycosis fungoides can be confined to, or concentrated in, the genital region. Localized perianal involvement [14], a solitary plaque on the penis [15] and response to treatment with imiquimod have been described [15,16].

Although lymphoma is the most frequent secondary tumour of the testis, it is rare in other parts of the male uro-genital tract [4]. Penile lymphoma can present as painless subcutaneous nodules, erythematous swelling, phimosis and ulceration [17–21,22]. There may be no evidence of systemic lymphoma. Ulcerating scrotal lymphoma has been reported [23], as have scrotal and penile ulceration resulting from leukaemic infiltration [24,25].

Metastases to the penis are rare, but several hundred cases have been reported [26,27]. They are usually secondary to cancer of the uro-genital tract [28] or gastrointestinal system, or other common cancers such as of the lung [29], and present with pain, swelling, priapism, urinary symptoms or haematuria. A very rare cause is secondary melanoma [26,30] and primary cholangiocarcinoma [31].

MISCELLANEOUS CUTANEOUS MALE GENITAL CONDITIONS

Penile melanosis

Causes of ano-genital hypo- and hyperpigmentation are listed in Boxes 111.26 and 111.27.

Pigmented macules are not uncommon on the glans and shaft of the penis [1,2]. They are benign but, because they may be large or enlarging, with irregular edges and multifocal and variegated pigmentary patterns, they arouse concern about atypical melanocytic proliferation and acral lentiginous melanoma. Such clinical concerns should lead to biopsy [3]; it is important to decolorize slides from deeply pigmented lesions because large quantities of melanin can obscure cytological detail [2]. Post-inflammatory hyperpigmentation (e.g. lichen sclerosus, lichen planus) may be the cause in many patients. Some cases have been associated with previous treatment with dithranol, PUVA therapy or diabetes [4,5]. The eruptive appearance of melanotic macules and papules in the ano-genital region may be associated with advanced metastatic adenocarcinoma [6].

Penile melanosis is the term for lesions without lentiginous hyperplasia [5,7]. Revuz and Clerici [7] proposed the grouping of penile melanosis, vulvovaginal melanosis and the predominantly oral mucosal hyperpigmentation of the Laugier–Hunziker syndrome under the umbrella of essential melanotic hyperpigmentation of the mucosa. Lenane et al. [8] used the term genital melanotic macules. On histological examination there may be increased basal epidermal pigmentation, with or without benign lentiginous melanocytic hyperplasia, or an increase in basal melanocyte number. Breathnach et al. [9] have proposed

Box 111.26 Causes of genital post-inflammatory hypopigmentation

- Following cryotherapy
  - Electrotherapy
  - Chemocautery
  - Laser surgery
- Contact dermatitis
- Lichen sclerosus
- Systemic sclerosis
- Lichen planus
- Cicatricial pemphigoid
- Gonococcal dermatitis
- Syphilis
  - Leukoderma: post-secondary syphilide
  - Gumma
  - Post-gummatous atrophic scar
- Herpes simplex
- Pityriasis versicolor
- Onchocerciasis 'leopard skin'
- Peyronie disease
- Pseudoepitheliomatous micaceous and keratotic balanitis

Reproduced from Bunker CB. *Male Genital Skin Disease*. London: Saunders, 2004. © 2004, with permission from the author.

that depigmentation is an essential element of penile melanosis and demonstrated melanocytic hyperplasia in areas of hyperpigmentation. Harmelin et al. have reported vitiligo-like macules in penile melanosis, speculatively due to local antimelanocyte autoimmunity [10].

Patients ask for treatment of penile melanosis as it is unsightly and embarrassing, but options are limited [2]. Laser treatment or topical depimenting agents may help [11].

Acral lentiginous melanoma is very rare but important [12,13].

Hypopigmentation

Striae as a consequence of growth or weight surges are common around the pelvic girdle, or represent a complication of topical corticosteroid application [14]. Initially, they are often purple-red in colour. Vitiligo is a commonly observed affliction of the male genitalia, although patients may be unaware of it and clinicians might not always observe it [15]. Penile vitiligo attributed to the use of topical imiquimod for the treatment of genital warts has been described [16].

Box 111.27 Causes of genital post-inflammatory hyperpigmentation

- Post-traumatic
- Lichen planus
- Herpes simplex
- Fixed drug eruption

Reproduced from Bunker CB. *Male Genital Skin Disease*. London: Saunders, 2004. © 2004, with permission from the author.

Pain and swelling

Some presentations of many entities can be painful but generally pain is an unusual presentation for a dermatosis. Swelling is more common and may be painful or not. A common factor in many but not all causes of swelling may be oedema or lymphoedema. Rigorous clinical evaluation is important [1,2]. Causes of ano-genital lymphoedema and penoscrotal swelling are listed in Boxes 111.18, 111.19 and 111.20.

Iatrogenic swelling and lymphoedema

Congenital defects of the inguinal canal and other non-inguinal peritoneal leaks can lead to scrotal and penile swelling as a manifestation of dialysate oedema in patients with end-stage renal failure treated by continuous ambulatory peritoneal dialysis [3]. Genital oedema is commonplace in intensive care units, because of the practice of maintaining a raised right heart filling pressure. Radical cancer surgery and/or radiotherapy to the ano-genital area and the lymphatics can cause swelling because of lymphoedema, early or delayed [4]. Chronic oedema, resembling keloid, of the penis has been caused by a condom catheter for neurogenic bladder [5].

Increasingly, patients seek plastic surgery to the penis [6] for psychosexual reasons (e.g. dysmorphophobia), but surgery can result in significant complications (Box 111.28).

Idiopathic lipogranuloma

Cases of characteristic, spontaneously resolving, painless, Y-shaped swelling of the scrotum embracing the penile root, with sclerosing eosinophilic lipogranuloma on histology and electron microscopy (but no exogenous lipids) and associated with blood eosinophilia (one patient had arthralgia), have been reported from Japan [7].

Priapism

Priapism is defined as the prolonged, painful erection of the penis, unassociated with sexual desire and not relieved by ejaculation. Although not predominantly a dermatological concern,

---

Box 111.28 Complications of plastic surgery to the penis

- Hypertrophic scars
- Wide scars
- Proximal penile hump (thick hair-bearing Y flap)
- Low-hanging penis
- Loss of fat
- Nodules
- Deformed shaft

Reproduced from Bunker CB. *Male Genital Skin Disease*. London: Saunders, 2004. © 2004, with permission from the author.

Box 111.29 Causes of priapism

- Idiopathic
- Os penis
  - Congenital
  - Acquired
    - Ageing
    - Trauma
    - Metabolic disorder
- Perineal trauma
- Strangulation
- Hypertension
- Nephrotic syndrome
- Neurological causes
- Quadriplegia
- Spinal canal stenosis
- Cauda equina compression
- Sickle cell disease
- Coagulopathy
  - Protein C deficiency
  - Factor V Leiden
  - Warfarin necrosis
- Peyronie disease
- Rheumatoid arthritis
- Vasculitis
- Tuberculosis
- Pelvic tumours
- Leukaemia
- Lymphoma
- Penile metastases
- Drugs
  - Papaverine
  - Antipsychotics
    - Chlorpromazine
    - Trazodone
  - Antihypertensives
    - Hydralazine
    - Guanethidine, prazosin
  - Marijuana
  - Adrenal corticosteroids
  - Warfarin necrosis

After Levine *et al.* 1991 [1]. Reproduced from Bunker CB. *Male Genital Skin Disease*. London: Saunders, 2004. © 2004, with permission from the author.

---

it has an important differential diagnosis. The principal causes [1,2] are listed in Box 111.29. It results in impotence in more than 50% of those affected [3,4] and can lead to gangrenous penile necrosis [5].

Veno-occlusive priapism can be distinguished from arterial priapism [1]. Veno-occlusive priapism results from persistent obstruction to venous outflow from the lacunar spaces. It is a potential vascular emergency because, as the corporeal bodies expand to maximal volume, an obstructed outflow causes decreased arterial inflow, with the potential for ischaemia, pain, fibrosis and hence impotence. Arterial priapism is usually secondary to trauma, such that a damaged cavernosal artery causes unregulated blood flow to the lacunar spaces; it is thus non-ischaemic [1].

Dermatological non-disease, dysaesthesia and chronic pain syndromes

'Dermatological non-disease' may be the diagnosis where there is a paucity or even absence of primary dermatological signs to account for florid symptomatology. Genital symptoms include itching, excessive redness, burning and discomfort – in some cases so severe that it prevents the patient from sitting down. Dysmorphophobia, depression and psychosis may be present, and attempted suicide is a real risk in such patients [1,2].

Itching of the urethra may lead to insertion of a foreign body in an attempt to relieve the sensation [3], or this might be done for sexual gratification.

Patients with symptoms of itching, burning and pain localized to the penis or scrotum are not uncommonly encountered. The skin is usually completely normal. The situation is analogous to vulvodynia in women, and terms such as penodynia and scrotodynia have been coined to describe the syndrome in men. Doxepin, dosulepin amitriptyline and paroxetine can afford some relief.

Fisher [4] has defined the red burning scrotum syndrome as 'persistent redness of the anterior half of the scrotum that may involve the base of the penis usually accompanied by a persistent itching or burning sensation and hyperalgesia'. It is a chronic condition that is resistant to treatment and its cause is unknown [4,5]. Accompanying the erythema there may be telangiectasia. It is related to idiopathic penile and scrotal pain syndromes [6]. Prednisolone and antidepressants have given some relief to some patients. There are reports of successful treatment with doxycycline [7].

Localized dermographism should be sought by stroking the inside of the thigh, because such patients may be helped by oral antihistamine treatment.

The possibilities of zinc deficiency and necrolytic migratory erythema should be entertained.

Chronic uro-genital and rectal pain syndromes include penile pain (penodynia), scrotodynia, orchialgia, prostatodynia, coccygodynia, proctalgia fugax, perineal pain, the descending perineum syndrome and vulvodynia [8,9,10]. The neuroanatomy of the pelvis is complicated and the neurophysiological basis of the pathogenesis of these syndromes is poorly understood, but their clinical presentations are well recognized. The differential diagnosis is addressed above. Cohen *et al.* have cautioned that 'idiopathic' anogenital pruritus may be attributable to lumbosacral radiculopathy so recommend neurological evaluation [11].

The koro syndrome is a psychiatric disorder characterized by fear of genital retraction (i.e. the penis shrinking, retracting or disappearing into the abdomen), acute anxiety and fear of death and genital pain. There is rarely real associated genital pathology. Although originally thought to be a culture-specific condition in South-East Asia and China, it has been observed in the West, without fear of death [12].

A diagnosis of a chronic pain syndrome implies the prospect of considerable psychological morbidity. Treatment is challenging and only empirical at best. Most agree that invasive and irreversible procedures should be avoided if at all possible. If lumbosacral radiculopathy is found then paravertebral blockade can be offered [11]. Multidisciplinary management is often necessary [6].

Key references

The full list of references can be found in the online version at www.rooksdermatology.com.

Introduction
3 Rickwood AM, Hemalatha V, Batcup G, Spitz L. Phimosis in boys. *Br J Urol* 1980;52:147–50.
5 Chopra R, Fisher RD, Fencel R. Phimosis and diabetes mellitus. *J Urol* 1982;127:1101–2.
6 Clemmensen OJ, Krogh J, Petri M. The histologic spectrum of prepuces from patients with phimosis. *Am J Dermatopathol* 1988;10:104–8.
7 Bunker CB. *Male Genital Skin Disease*. London: Saunders, 2004.
8 Rickwood AM. Medical indications for circumcision. *BJU Int* 1999;83(Suppl. 1):45–51.
9 Waugh MA. Balanitis. *Dermatol Clin* 1998;16:757–62.
10 Edwards S. Balanitis and balanoposthitis: a review. *Genitourin Med* 1996;72:155–9.
11 English JC III, Laws RA, Keough GC, et al. Dermatoses of the glans penis and prepuce. *J Am Acad Dermatol* 1997;37:1–24.
21 Mallon E, Ross JS, Hawkins DA, et al. Biopsy of male genital dermatosis. *Genitourin Med* 1997;73:421.
22 Rao A, Bunker CB. Male genital skin biopsy. *Int J STD AIDS* 2011;22:418–19.

Structure and function of the male genitalia
1 Cold CJ, Taylor JR. The prepuce. *BJU Int* 1999;83(Suppl. 1):34–44.
2 Ammini AC, Sabherwal U, Mukhopadhyay C, et al. Morphogenesis of the human external male genitalia. *Pediatr Surg Int* 1997;12:401–6.
3 McGregor D. Distribution of pubic hair in sample of fit men. *Br J Dermatol* 1961;73:61–4.
4 Achtstätter T, Moll R, Moore B, Franke WW. Cytokeratin polypeptide patterns of different epithelia of the human male urogenital tract: immunofluorescence and gel electrophoretic studies. *J Histochem Cytochem* 1985;33:415–26.

Normal variants
3 Sonnex C, Dockerty WG. Pearly penile papules: a common cause of concern. *Int J STD AIDS* 1999;10:726–7.
4 Neri I, Bardazzi F, Raone B, et al. Ectopic pearly penile papules: a paediatric case. *Genitourin Med* 1997;73:136.
5 Ackerman AD, Kornberg R. Pearly penile papules. *Arch Dermatol* 1973;108:673–5.
6 Porter W, Bunker CB. Treatment of pearly penile papules with cryotherapy. *Br J Dermatol* 2000;142:847–8.
13 Izquierdo MJ, Pastor MA, Carrasco L, et al. Epithelioid blue naevus of the genital mucosa: report of four cases. *Br J Dermatol* 2001;145:496–501.
14 de Giorgi V, Massi D, Brunasso G, et al. Eruptive multiple blue nevi of the penis: a clinical dermoscopic pathologic case study. *J Cutan Pathol* 2004;31:185–8.
15 Aoyagi S, Sato-Matsumura KS, Akiyama M, et al. Spitz naevus of the glans penis: an unusual location. *Acta Derm Venereol* 2004;84:324–5.
18 Phan PT, Francis N, Madden N, Bunker CB. Kissing naevus of the penis. *Clin Exp Dermatol* 2004;29:471–2.
22 Erkek E, Basar MM, Bagci Y, et al. Fordyce angiokeratomas as clues to local venous hypertension. *Arch Dermatol* 2005;141:1325–6.
23 Caputo R, Passoni E, Cavicchini S. Papular xanthoma associated with angiokeratoma of Fordyce: considerations on the nosography of this rare non-Langerhans cell histiocytoxanthomatosis. *Dermatology* 2003;206:165–8.

The foreskin
1 Whitfield H. Circumcision. *BJU Int* 1999;83(Suppl. 1):1–113.
2 Porter WM, Bunker CB. The dysfunctional foreskin. *Int J STD AIDS* 2001;12:216–20.

3 Taves DR. The intromission function of the foreskin. *Med Hypotheses* 2002;59:180–2.
4 Bunker CB. *Male Genital Skin Disease*. London: Saunders, 2004.
5 Cold CJ, Taylor JR. The prepuce. *BJU Int* 1999;83(Suppl. 1):34–44.

Circumcision

5 Whitfield H. Circumcision. *BJU Int* 1999;83(Suppl. 1):1–113.
9 Anonymous. *Guidance for Doctors who are Asked to Circumcise Male Children*. London: General Medical Council, 1997.
10 American Academy of Paediatrics Task Force on Circumcision. Circumcision policy statement. *Pediatrics* 2012;130;585–86.
11 Morris B, Kreiger J. Does male circumcision affect sexual function, sensitivity or satisfaction? A systematic review. *J Sex Med* 2013; 10: 2644–57.
13 Fergusson DM, Lawton JM, Shannon FT. Neonatal circumcision and penile problems: an 8 year longitudinal study. *Pediatrics* 1988;81:537–41.
16 Ladenhauf H, Ardelean M, Schimke C, *et al.* Reduced bacterial colonization of the glans penis after male circumcision in children – a prospective study. *J Ped Urol* 2013; 9 (6 pt B); 1137–44.
17 O'Farrell N, Egger M. Circumcision in men and the prevention of HIV infection: a 'meta-analysis' revisited. *Int J STD AIDS* 2000;11:137–42.
22 Laumann EO, Masi CM, Zuckerman EW. Circumcision in the United States: prevalence, prophylactic effects, and sexual practice. *JAMA* 1997;277:1052–7.
23 Mallon E, Hawkins D, Dinneen M, *et al.* Circumcision and genital dermatoses. *Arch Dermatol* 2000;136:350–4.
39 Toker SC, Baskan EB, Tunali S, *et al.* Zoon's balanitis in a circumcised man. *J Am Acad Dermatol* 2007;57:S6–7.

Congenital and developmental abnormalities

1 Baskin LS, Ebbers MB. Hypospadias: anatomy, etiology and technique. *J Pediatr Surg* 2006;41:463–72.
2 Bunker CB. *Male Genital Skin Disease*. London: Saunders, 2004.
3 Park CO, Chun EY, Lee JH. Median raphe cyst on the scrotum and perineum. *J Am Acad Dermatol* 2005;55:S114–15.
4 Browne WG, Izatt MM, Renwick JH. White sponge naevus of the mucosa: clinical and linkage data. *Ann Hum Genet* 1969;32:271–81.
5 Jorgenson RJ, Levin LS. White sponge nevus. *Arch Dermatol* 1981;117:73–6.
6 Shah A, Meacock L, More B, Chandran H. Lymphangioma of the penis: a rare anomaly. *Pediatr Surg Int* 2005;21:329–30.
7 Girard C, Bigorre M, Guillot B, Bessis D. Pelvis syndrome. *Arch Dermatol* 2006;142:884–8.
8 Musumeci ML, Nasca MR, De Pasquale R, *et al.* Cutaneous manifestations and massive genital involvement in Hennekam syndrome. *Pediatr Dermatol* 2006;23:239–42.
9 Hampshire DJ, Ayub M, Springell K, *et al.* MORM syndrome (mental retardation, truncal obesity, retinal dystrophy and micropenis), a new autosomal recessive disorder, links to 9q34. *Eur J Hum Genet* 2006;14:543–8.
10 Vaccaro M, Salpietro DC, Briuglia S, *et al.* Cutis laxa in Kabuki make-up syndrome. *J Am Acad Dermatol* 2005;53:S247–51.

Trauma and artefact

1 Nouri M, Koutani A, Tazi K, *et al.* Fractures of the penis: apropos of 56 cases. *Prog Urol* 1998;8:542–7.
21 George WM. Papular pearly penile pearls. *J Am Acad Dermatol* 1989;20:852.
25 Al-Mutairi N, Sharma AK, Zaki A, *et al.* Penile self-injections: an unusual act. *Int J Dermatol* 2004;43:680–2.
29 Matsuda T, Shichiri Y, Hida S, *et al.* Eosinophilic sclerosing lipogranuloma of the male genitalia not caused by exogenous lipids. *J Urol* 1988;140:1021.
31 Greilsheimer H, Groves JE. Male genital self-mutilation. *Arch Gen Psychiatry* 1979;36:441–6.
34 McCann J, Voris J. Perianal injuries resulting from sexual abuse: a longitudinal study. *Pediatrics* 1993;91:390–3.
39 Vickers D, Morris K, Coulthard MG, Eastham EJ. Anal signs in haemolytic uraemic syndrome. *Lancet* 1998;1:998.
40 Hobbs CJ, Wynne JM. How to manage warts. *Arch Dis Child* 1999;81:460.
43 Hrbaty J, Molitor M. Traumatic skin loss from the male genitalia. *Acta Chir Plast* 2001;43:17–20.
45 Sagar J, Sagar B, Shah DK. Penile skin necrosis – complication following self-circumcision. *Ann R Coll Surg Engl* 2005;87:W5–7.

Inflammatory dermatoses

1 Wiskemann A. X-ray irradiation of dermatoses in the genital area. *Hautarzt* 1977;28:219–23.
2 Lebwohl M, Freeman AK, Chapman MS, *et al.* Tacrolimus ointment is effective for facial and intertriginous psoriasis. *J Am Acad Dermatol* 2004;51:723–30.
3 Gribetz C, Ling M, Lebwohl M, *et al.* Pimecrolimus cream 1% in the treatment of intertriginous psoriasis: a double-blind, randomized study. *J Am Acad Dermatol* 2004;51:731–8.
4 Bissonnette R, Nigen S, Bolduc C. Efficacy and tolerability of topical tacrolimus ointment for the treatment of male genital psoriasis. *J Cutan Med Surg* 2008;12;230–4.

Eczema

1 Porter WM, Bewley A, Dinneen M, *et al.* Nodular lichen simplex of the scrotum treated by surgical excision. *Br J Dermatol* 2001;144:915–16.
3 Birley HDL, Walker MM, Luzzi GA, *et al.* Clinical features and management of recurrent balanitis; association with atopy and genital washing. *Genitourin Med* 1993;69:400–3.
7 Lyon CC, Kulkarni J, Zimerson E, *et al.* Skin disorders in amputees. *J Am Acad Dermatol* 2000;42:501–7.
11 Turjanmaa K, Alenius H, Makinen-Kiljunen S, *et al.* Natural rubber latex allergy. *Allergy* 1996;51:593–602.
14 Bauer A, Geier J, Elsner P. Allergic contact dermatitis in patients with anogenital complaints. *J Reprod Med* 2000;45:649–54.
15 Garcia-Gavin J, Vansina S, Keree S, *et al.* Methylisothiozolinone, an emerging allergen in cosmetics. *Contact Dermatitis* 2010;63:96–101.
19 Harmon CB, Connolly SM, Larson TR. Condom-related allergic contact dermatitis. *J Urol* 1995;153:1227–8.
22 Wiskemann A. X-ray irradiation of dermatoses in the genital area. *Hautarzt* 1977;28:219–23.
23 Bunker CB. *Male Genital Skin Disease*. London: Saunders, 2004.

Zoon balanitis

2 Zoon JJ. Balanoposthite chronique circonscrite benigne a plasmocytes. *Dermatologica* 1952;105:1–7.
3 Baughman RD, Berger P, Pringle WM. Plasma cell cheilitis. *Arch Dermatol* 1974;110:725–6.
7 Bunker CB. Topics in penile dermatology. *Clin Exp Dermatol* 2001;26:469–79.
8 Bunker CB. *Male Genital Skin Disease*. London: Saunders, 2004.
9 Nishimura M, Matsuda T, Muto M, Hori Y. Balanitis of Zoon. *Int J Dermatol* 1990;29:421–3.
10 Farrell AM, Francis N, Bunker CB. Zoon's balanitis: an immunohistochemical study. *Br J Dermatol* 1996;135(Suppl. 47):57.
14 Davis-Daneshfar A, Trueb RM. Bowen's disease of the glans penis (erythroplasia of Queyrat) in plasma cell balanitis. *Cutis* 2000;65:395–8.
15 Weyers W, Ende Y, Schalla W, Diaz-Cascajo C. Balanitis of Zoon: a clinicopathologic study of 45 cases. *Am J Dermatopathol* 2002;24:459–67.
20 Moreno-Arias GA, Camps-Fresneda A, Llaberia C, Palou-Almerich J. Plasma cell balanitis treated with tacrolimus 0.1%. *Br J Dermatol* 2005;153:1204–6.
28 Marconi B, Campanati A, Simonetti A, *et al.* Zoon's balanitis treated with imiquimod 5% cream. *Eur J Dermatol* 2010;20;134–5.

Lichen sclerosus

1 Edmonds EVJ, Hunt S, Hawkins D, Dinneen M, Francis N, Bunker CB. Clinical parameters in male genital lichen sclerosus: a case series of 329 patients. *J Eur Acad Dermatol Venereol* 2011;26(6):730–7.
6 Ridley CM. Lichen sclerosus et atrophicus. *BMJ* 1987;295:1295–6.
15 Edmonds EVJ, Oyama N, Chan I, Francis N, McGrath JA, Bunker CB. Extracellular matrix protein 1 autoantibodies in male genital lichen sclerosus. *Br J Dermatol* 2011;165(1):218–19.
32 Shim T, de Koning M, Muneer A, *et al.* HPV in male genital lichen sclerosus, penile carcinoma in situ and penile squamous carcinoma. *J Invest Dermatol* 2013;133(Suppl. 1):S195.
41 Bunker CB. Atopy, the barrier, urine and genital lichen sclerosus (LS). *Br J Dermatol* 2013;169:953.
43 Edmonds EVJ, Bunker CB. Nuclear magnetic resonance spectroscopy of urine in male genital lichen sclerosus. *Br J Dermatol* 2010;163(6):1355–6.
49 Bunker CB, Shim TN. Male genital edema in Crohn's disease. *J Am Acad Dermatol* 2014;70:385.

51 Neill SM, Tatnall FM, Cox NH. Guidelines for the management of lichen sclerosus. *Br J Dermatol* 2002;147:640–9.

61 Ioannides D, Lazaridou E, Apalla Z, Sotiriou E, Gregoriou S, Rigopoulos D. (2010). Acitretin for severe lichen sclerosus of male genitalia: a randomized, placebo controlled study. *J Urol* 2010;183:1395–9.

63 Bunker CB, Neill S, Staughton RCD. Topical tacrolimus, genital lichen sclerosus and risk of squamous cell carcinoma. *Arch Dermatol* 2004;140:1169.

73 Nasca MR, Innocenzi D, Micali G. Penile cancer among patients with genital lichen sclerosus. *J Am Acad Dermatol* 1999;41:911–14.

Lichen planus

3 Itin PH, Hirsbrunner P, Buchner S. Lichen planus: an unusual cause of phimosis. *Acta Dermatol Venereol* 1992;72:41–2.

4 Bunker CB. *Male Genital Skin Disease*. London: Saunders, 2004.

6 El-Gadi S. Biopsy before excision. *J Eur Acad Dermatol Venereol* 1996;7:87–90.

11 Leal-Khouri S, Hruza GJ. Squamous cell carcinoma developing within lichen planus of the penis: treatment with Mohs micrographic surgery. *J Dermatol Surg Oncol* 1994;20:272–6.

12 Hoshi A, Usui Y, Terachi T. Penile carcinoma originating from lichen planus on glans penis. *Urology* 2008;71;816–17.

15 Schmitt EC, Pigatto PD, Boneschi V, *et al.* Erosiver lichen planus der glans penis: behandlung mit cyclosporin A. *Hautarzt* 1993;44:43–5.

16 Cox NH. Squamous cell carcinoma arising in lichen planus of the penis during topical cyclosporin therapy. *Clin Exp Dermatol* 1996;21:323–4.

20 Porter WM, Dinneen M, Hawkins DA, Bunker CB. Erosive penile lichen planus responding to circumcision. *J Eur Acad Dermatol Venereol* 2001;15:266–8.

21 Kirby B, Whitehurst C, Moore JV, Yates VM. Treatment of lichen planus of the penis with photodynamic therapy. *Br J Dermatol* 1999;141:765–6.

22 Weyandt G, Vetter-Kauczok C, Becker J, *et al.* Successful dexamethasone pulse therapy for widespread erosive perianal lichen planus. *Hautarzt* 2007;58;241–2.

Miscellaneous inflammatory dermatoses

Non-specific balanoposthitis

1 Bunker CB. *Male Genital Skin Disease*. London: Saunders, 2004.

2 Alessi E, Coggi A, Gianotti R. Review of 120 biopsies performed on the balano-preputial sac. *Dermatol* 2004;208:120–4.

Ulcerative disease and penile necrosis

2 Sarihan H. Idiopathic scrotal necrosis. *Br J Urol* 1994;74:259.

12 Orme RL, Nordlund JJ, Barich L, Brown T. The magic syndrome (mouth and genital ulcers with inflamed cartilage). *Arch Dermatol* 1990;126:940–4.

13 Chan C-C, Thyong H-Y, Chan Y-C, Liao Y-H. Human papillomavirus type 5 infection in a patient with Hailey–Hailey disease successfully treated with imiquimod. *Br J Dermatol* 2007;156:579–81.

14 Thomson KF, Highet AS. Penile ulceration in fatal malignant atrophic papulosis (Degos' disease). *Br J Dermatol* 2000;143:1320–2.

21 Bories N, Becuwe C, Marcilly MC, *et al.* Glans penis ulceration revealing Wegener's granulomatosis. *Dermatology* 2007;214:187–9.

29 Farrell AM, Black MM, Bracka A, Bunker CB. Pyoderma gangrenosum of the penis. *Br J Dermatol* 1998;138:337–40.

37 Lally A, Hollowood K, Bunker CB, Turner R. Penile pyoderma gangrenosum treated with topical tacrolimus. *Arch Dermatol* 2005;141:1175–6.

40 Boccaletti VP, Ricci R, Sebastio N, *et al.* Penile necrosis. *Arch Dermatol* 2000;136:261, 264.

41 Woods M, Pattee SF, Levine N. Penile calciphylaxis. *J Am Acad Dermatol* 2006;54:736–7.

45 Thorns C, Urban H, Remmler K, *et al.* Primary cutaneous T-cell lymphoma of the penis. *Histopathology.* 2003;42:513–14.

Pilonidal sinus

1 Al-Qassim Z, Reddy K, Khan Z, Reddy I. Pilonidal sinus cyst of the penis. *BMJ* 2013;21.

2 Val-Bernal JF, Azcarretazabal T, Garijo MF. Pilonidal sinus of the penis: a report of two cases, one of them associated with actinomycosis. *J Cutan Pathol* 1999;26:155–8.

3 O'Kane HF, Duggan B, Mulholland C, Crosbie J. Pilonidal sinus of the penis. *Sci World J* 2004;4(Suppl. 1):258–9.

4 Rashid AMH, Menai Williams R, Parry D, Malone PR. Actinomycosis associated with pilonidal sinus of the penis. *J Urol* 1992;148:405–6.

5 Tomasini C, Aloi F, Puiatti P, Caliendo V. Dermoid cyst of the penis. *Dermatology* 1997;194:188–90.

Peyronie disease

2 Billig R, Baker R, Immergut M, Maxted W. Peyronie's disease. *Urology* 1975;6:409–18.

3 Simeon CP, Fonollosa V, Vilardell M, *et al.* Impotence and Peyronie's disease in systemic sclerosis. *Clin Exp Rheumatol* 1994;12:464.

5 Mooradian AD, Viosca SP, Kaiser FE, *et al.* Penile Raynaud's phenomenon: a possible cause of erectile failure. *Am J Med* 1988;85:748–50.

8 Grigg AP, Underhill C, Russell J, Sale G. Peyronie's disease as a complication of chronic graft versus host disease. *Hematology* 2002;7:165–8.

9 Horn AS, Pecora A, Chiesa JC, Alloy A. Penile thrombophlebitis as a presenting manifestation of pancreatic carcinoma. *Am J Gastroenterol* 1985;80:463–5.

10 Desanctis PN, Furey CA Jr. Steroid injection therapy for Peyronie's disease: a 10-year summary and review of 38 cases. *J Urol* 1967;97:114–16.

11 Winter CC, Khanna R. Peyronie's disease: results with dermo-jet injection of dexamethasone. *J Urol* 1975;114:898–900.

12 Chun JL, McGregor A, Krishnan R, Carson CC. A comparison of dermal and cadaveric pericardial grafts in the modified Horton–Devine procedure for Peyronie's disease. *J Urol* 2001;166:185–8.

13 Riedl CR, Plas E, Engelhardt P, *et al.* Iontophoresis for treatment of Peyronie's disease. *J Urol* 2000;163:95–9.

14 Paullis G, Cavallini G, Brancato T, Alvaro R. Peironimev-Plus in the treatment of chronic inflammation of tunica albuginea. Results of a controlled study. *Inflamm Allergy Drug Targets* 2013;12:61–7.

Drug reactions

1 Gruber F, Stasic A, Lenkovic M, Brajac I. Postcoital fixed drug eruption in a man sensitive to trimethoprim-sulphamethoxazole. *Clin Exp Dermatol* 1997;22:144–5.

2 Zawar V, Kirloskar M, Chuh A. Fixed drug eruption – a sexually inducible reaction? *Int J STD AIDS* 2004;15:560–3.

3 Borgstrom E. Penile ulcer as complication in self-induced papaverine erections. *Urology* 1988;32:416–17.

4 Coles RB, Wilkinson DS. Necrosis and dequalinium. I. Balanitis. *Trans St John's Hosp Dermatol Soc* 1965;51:46–8.

5 Esser AC, Nossa R, Shoji T, Sapadin AN. All-*trans*-retinoic acid-induced scrotal ulcerations in a patient with acute promyelocytic leukaemia. *J Am Acad Dermatol* 2000;43:316–17.

6 Evans LM, Grossman ME. Foscarnet-induced penile ulcer. *J Am Acad Dermatol* 1992;27:124–6.

11 Ogden S, Mukasa Y, Lyon CC, Coulson IH. Nicorandil-induced peristomal ulcers: is nicorandil also associated with gastrointestinal fistula formation? *Br J Dermatol* 2007;156:575–612.

12 Griffiths MR, Milne JT, Porter WM. Penile argyria. *Br J Dermatol* 2006;154:1074–5.

13 Harmanyeri Y, Taskapan O, Dogan B, *et al.* A case of coumarin necrosis with penile and pedal involvement. *J Eur Acad Dermatol Venereol* 1998;10:248–52.

14 Chang I, Ha M, Chi B, *et al.* Warfarin-induced penile necrosis in a patient with heparin-induced thrombocytopenia. *J Kor Med Sci* 2010;25:1390–3.

Other inflammatory dermatoses

2 Bewley AP, Ross JS, Bunker CB, Staughton RC. Successful treatment of a patient with octreotide-resistant necrolytic migratory erythema. *Br J Dermatol* 1996;134:1101–4.

4 Sami N, Ahmed AR. Penile pemphigus. *Arch Dermatol* 2001;137:756–8.

8 Fueston JC, Adams BB, Mutasim DF. Cicatricial pemphigoid-induced phimosis. *J Am Acad Dermatol* 2001;46:S128–9.

12 Mahmood N, Afzal N, Joyce A. Sarcoidosis of the penis. *Br J Urol* 1997;80:155.

21 Slaney G, Muller S, Clay J, *et al.* Crohn's disease involving the penis. *Gut* 1986;27:329–33.

24 Merika EE, Darling MI, Craig P, *et al.* Primary cutaneous amyloidosis of the glans penis. Two case reports and a review of the literature. *Br J Dermatol* 2014 Mar;170(3):730–4 (review).

31 Melekos MD, Asbach HW, Markou SA. Aetiology of acute scrotum in 100 boys with regard to age distribution. *J Urol* 1988;139:1023.

33 Udall DA, Drake DJ, Rosenberg RS Acute scrotal swelling: a physical sign of primary peritonitis. *J Urol* 1981;125:750–1.

35 David S, Schiff JD, Poppas DP. Henoch–Schönlein purpura involving the glans penis. *Urology* 2003;61:1035.

42 Rivollier C, Martin L, Machet L, *et al.* Genital papules revealing a Churg–Strauss syndrome. *Ann Dermatol Venereol* 2002;129:1049–52.

Chronic penile oedema

2 Neri I, Bardazzi F, Marzaduri S, Patrizi A. Perianal streptococcal dermatitis in adults. *Br J Dermatol* 1996;135:796–8.

4 Porter WM, Dinneen M, Bunker C. Chronic penile lymphoedema. *Arch Dermatol* 2001;137:1108–10.

6 Baughman S, Cespedes R. Unusual presentation of hidradenitis suppurativa with massive enlargement of the penis. *Urology* 2004;64:377–8.

8 Calabro R, Gali A, Marino S, Bramanti P. Compulsive masturbation and chronic penile lymphedema. *Arch Sex Behav* 2012;41:737–9.

11 Bunker CB, Shim TN. Male genital edema in Crohn's disease. *J Am Acad Dermatol* 2014;70:385.

14 Choong KK. Acute penoscrotal oedema due to acute necrotizing pancreatitis. *J Ultrasound Med* 1996;15:247–8.

16 Saha M, Edmonds E, Martin J, Bunker CB. Penile lymphoedema in association with asymptomatic Crohn's disease. *Clin Exp Dermatol* 2009;34:88–90.

21 Malloy TR, Wein AJ, Gross P. Scrotal and penile lymphedema: surgical considerations and management. *J Urol* 1983;130:263–5.

22 Morey AF, Meng MV, McAninch JW. Skin graft reconstruction of chronic genital lymphoedema. *Urology* 1997;50:423–6.

24 Modolin M, Mitre A, da Silva J, *et al.* Surgical treatment of lymphedema of the penis and scrotum. *Clinics (Sao Paulo)* 2006;61:289–94.

Non-sexually transmitted infections

Ecthyma gangrenosum and Fournier gangrene

1 Rabinowitz R, Lewin EB. Gangrene of the genitalia in children with *Pseudomonas* sepsis. *J Urol* 1980;124:431–2.

3 Smith GL, Bunker CB, Dineen MD. Fournier's gangrene. *Br J Urol* 1998;81:347–55.

4 Adams JR Jr, Mata JA, Venable DD, *et al.* Fournier's gangrene in children. *Urology* 1990;35:439–41.

6 Schultz ES, Diepgen TL, von den Driesch P, Hornstein OP. Systemic corticosteroids are important in the treatment of Fournier's gangrene: a case report. *J Dermatol* 1995;133:633–5.

7 Ferreira PC, Reis JC, Amarante JM, *et al.* Fournier's gangrene: a review of 43 reconstructive cases. *Plast Reconstr Surg* 2007;119:175–84.

8 Bubrick MP, Hitchcock CR. Necrotizing anorectal and perineal infection. *Surgery* 1979;86:655–62.

9 Chang I-J, Lee C-C, Chen S-Y. Fulminant gangrenous and crepitating scrotum. *Arch Dermatol* 2006;142:797–8.

10 Fisher JR, Conway ML, Takeshita RT, *et al.* Necrotizing fasciitis: importance of roentgenographic studies for soft-tissue gas. *JAMA* 1979;241:803–6.

14 Tahmaz L, Erdemir F, Kibar Y, *et al.* Fournier's gangrene: report of thirty-three cases and a review of the literature. *Int J Urol* 2006;13:960–7.

16 Bunker CB. *Male Genital Skin Disease*. London: Saunders, 2004.

Trichomycosis pubis, TB, non-syphilitic spirochaetal ulcerative balanoposthitis, yaws, candidosis, tinea and deep fungal infections

3 Kamalam A, Senthamilselvi G, Ajithadas K, Thambiah AS. Cutaneous trichosporosis. *Mycopathologia* 1988;101:167–75.

4 Minkin W, Frank SB, Cohen HJ. Penile granuloma. *Arch Dermatol* 1972;106:756.

5 Rossi R, Urbano F, Tortoli E, *et al.* Primary tuberculosis of the penis. *J Eur Acad Dermatol Venereol* 1999;12:174–6.

11 Piot P, Duncan M, van Dyck E, *et al.* Ulcerative balanoposthitis associated with non-syphilitic spirochaetal infection. *Genitourin Med* 1986;62:44–6.

12 Engelkens HJ, Judanarso J, van der Sluis JJ, *et al.* Disseminated early yaws: report of a child with a remarkable genital lesion mimicking venereal syphilis. *Pediatr Dermatol* 1990;7:60–2.

14 Odds FC. Genital candidiasis. *Clin Exp Dermatol* 1982;7:345–54.

20 Pielop J, Rosen T. Penile dermatophytosis. *J Am Acad Dermatol* 2001;44:864–7.

22 Preminger B, Gerard PS, Lutwick L, *et al.* Histoplasmosis of the penis. *J Urol* 1993;149:848–50.

28 English JC III, Laws RA, Keough GC, *et al.* Dermatoses of the glans penis and prepuce. *J Am Acad Dermatol* 1997;37:1–24; quiz 25–6.

30 Cohen-Ludmann C, Kerob D, Feuilhade M, *et al.* Zygomycosis of the penis due to *Rhizopus oryzae* successfully treated with surgical debridement and a combination of high dose liposomal and topical amphotericin B. *Arch Dermatol* 2006;142:1657–8.

Other non-sexually transmitted infections

4 Mukhopadhyay AK. Primary involvement of penile skin in lepromatous leprosy. *Indian J Lepr* 2005;77:317–21.

11 Fox PA, Barton SE, Francis N, *et al.* Chronic erosive herpes simplex virus infection of the penis: a possible immune reconstitution disease. *HIV Med* 1999;1:10–18.

12 Spray A, Glaser DA. Herpes zoster of the penis: an unusual location for a common eruption. *J Am Acad Dermatol* 2002;47:S177–9.

14 Cooke RA, Rodriguez RB. Amoebic balanitis. *Med J Aust* 1964;5:114–17.

15 Gbery IP, Dheja D, Kacou DE, *et al.* Chronic genital ulcerations and HIV infection: 29 cases. *Med Trop* 1999;59:279–82.

16 Cain C, Seabury-Stone M, Thieburg M, Wilson ME. Non-healing genital ulcers. *Arch Dermatol* 1994;130:1311–16.

18 Grunwald MH, Amichai B, Trau H. Cutaneous leishmaniasis on an unusual site: the glans penis. *Br J Urol* 1998;82:928.

20 Masmoudi A, Boudaya S, Bouzid L, *et al.* Penile sporotrichoid cutaneous leishmaniasis. *Bull Soc Pathol Exot* 2005;98:380–1.

22 Zawahry ME. Cutaneous amoebiasis. *Indian J Dermatol* 1966;11:77–8.

26 Narvaez-Moreno B, Bernabeu-Wittel J, Zulueta-Dorado T, *et al.* Primary cutaneous crytococcosis of the penis. *Sex Transm Dis* 2012;39:792–3.

Dermatological aspects of sexually transmitted disease

2 Angus J, Langan SM, Stanway A, *et al.* The many faces of secondary syphilis: a re-emergence of an old disease. *Clin Exp Dermatol* 2006;31:741–5.

6 Fox PA, Tung M-Y. Human papillomavirus: burden of illness and treatment cost considerations. *Am J Clin Dermatol* 2005;6:365–81.

8 Wen LM, Estcourt CS, Simpson JM, Mindel A. Risk factors for the acquisition of genital warts: are condoms protective? *Sex Transm Infect* 1999;75:312–16.

12 Koutsky L. Epidemiology of genital human papilloma virus infection. *Am J Med* 1997;102(5A):3–8.

13 Voog E, Ricksten A, Olofsson S, *et al.* Demonstration of Epstein–Barr virus DNA and human papillomavirus DNA in acetowhite lesions of the penile skin and the oral mucosa. *Int J STD AIDS* 1997;8:772–5.

15 Daneshpouy M, Socic G, Clavel C, *et al.* Human papillomavirus infection and anogenital condyloma in bone marrow transplant recipients. *Transplantation* 2001;71:167–9.

16 Luyten J, Engelen B, Beutels P. The sexual ethics of HPV vaccination for boys. *HEC Forum.*2014;26:27–42.

17 Lawton M, Nathan M, Asboe D. HPV vaccination to prevent anal cancer in men who have sex with men. *Sex Transm Infect* 2013;89:342–3.

18 Von Krogh G, Dahlman-Ghozlan K, Syrjänen S. Potential human papillomavirus reactivation following topical corticosteroid therapy of genital lichen sclerosus and erosive lichen planus. *J Eur Acad Dermatol Venereol* 2002;16:130–3.

21 Sardana K, Sehgal VN. Genital ulcer disease and human immunodeficiency virus: a focus. *J Dermatol* 2005;44:391–405.

Benign tumours

7 Cole LA, Helwig EB. Mucoid cysts of the penile skin. *J Urol* 1976;115:397–400.

17 Swinehart JM, Golitz LE. Scrotal calcinosis. *Arch Dermatol* 1982;118:985–8.

22 Akogun OB, Akoh JI, Hellandendu H. Non-ocular clinical onchocerciasis in relation to skin microfilaria in the Taraba River Valley, Nigeria. *J Hyg Epidemiol Microbiol Immunol* 1992;36:368–83.

30 Abdel-Aal H, Abdel-Aziz AM. Naevus comedonicus: report of three cases localized on glans penis. *Acta Derm Venereol* 1975;55:78–80.

32 Gürünlüoglu R, Bayramicli M, Dogan T, Numanoglu A. Unusual complications of circumcision. *Plast Reconstr Surg* 1999;104:1938–9.

48 Dehner LP, Smith BH. Soft tissue tumours of the penis. *Cancer* 1970;25:1431–47.

63 Macaluso JN, Sullivan JW, Tomberlin S. Glomus tumor of the glans penis. *Urology* 1985;25:409–10.

68 Srigley JR, Ayala AG, Ordóñez NG, van Nostrand AW. Epithelioid hemangioma of the penis: a rare and distinctive vascular lesion. *Arch Pathol Lab Med* 1985;109:51–4.

PART 10: SITES, SEX, AGE

73 Sezer E, Erbil H, Koseoglu D, *et al.* Angiolymphoid hyperplasia with eosinophilia mimicking Bowenoid papulosis. *Clin Exp Dermatol* 2007;32:281–3.

74 Osborne GE, Chinn RJ, Francis ND, Bunker CB. Magnetic resonance imaging in the investigation of penile lymphangioma circumscriptum. *Br J Dermatol* 2000;143:467–8.

Pre-cancerous dermatoses and carcinoma *in situ*

Erythroplasia of Queyrat, Bowen disease of the penis and bowenoid papulosis

1 Bunker CB. Topics in penile dermatology. *Clin Exp Dermatol* 2001;26:469–79.

2 Porter WM, Francis N, Hawkins D, *et al.* Penile intraepithelial neoplasia: clinical spectrum and treatment of 35 cases. *Br J Dermatol* 2002;147:1159–65.

9 Graham JH, Helwig EB. Erythroplasia of Queyrat: a clinicopathologic and histochemical study. *Cancer* 1973;32:1396–414.

10 Zabbo A, Stein BS. Penile intraepithelial neoplasia in patients examined for exposure to human papilloma virus. *Urology* 1993;41:24–6.

11 Brady KL, Mercurio MG, Brown MD. Malignant tumors of the penis. *Dermatol Surg* 2013;39:527–47.

12 Griffiths TRL, Mellon JK. Human papillomavirus and urological tumours: basic science and role in penile cancer. *BJU Int* 1999;84:579–86.

24 McAninch JW, Moore CA. Precancerous penile lesions in young men. *J Urol* 1970;104:287–90.

25 Aynaud O, Ionesco M, Barrasso R. Penile intraepithelial neoplasia: specific clinical features correlate with histologic and virologic findings. *Cancer* 1994;74:1762–7.

33 Micali G, Masca MR, De Pasquale R. Erythroplasia of Queyrat treated with imiquimod 5% cream. *J Am Acad Dermatol* 2006;55:901–3.

36 Calista D. Topical cidofovir for erythroplasia of Queyrat of theglans penis. *Br J Dermatol* 2002;147:399–400.

Miscellaneous pre-cancerous conditions

4 Tewari M, Gupta SK, Kumar M. Multiple cutaneous horns of the penis: a case report. *Indian J Pathol Microbiol* 2003;46:53–4.

5 Bart RS, Kopf AW. Tumor conference No. 14: on a dilemma of penile horns – pseudoepitheliomatous, hyperkeratotic and micaceous balanitis. *J Dermatol Surg Oncol* 1977;3:580.

6 Willsher MK, Daley KJ, Conway JF, *et al.* Penile horns. *J Urol* 1984;132:1192–3.

7 Yeager JK, Findlay RF, McAleer IM. Penile verrucous carcinoma. *Arch Dermatol* 1990;126:1208–10.

10 Ponce De Leon J, Algaba F, Salvador J. Cutaneous horn of the glans penis. *Br J Urol* 1994;74:257–8.

13 Levell NJ, Bewley AP, Levene GM. Porokeratosis of Mibelli on the penis, scrotum and natal cleft. *Clin Exp Dermatol* 1994;19:77–8.

14 Porter WM, Du P, Menagé H, Philip G, Bunker CB. Porokeratosis of the penis. *Br J Dermatol* 2001;144:643–4.

16 Ganem JP, Steele BW, Creager AJ, Carson CC. Pseudo-epitheliomatous keratotic and micaceous balanitis. *J Urol* 1999;161:217–18.

20 Bunker CB, Francis N. Pseudoepitheliomatous keratotic and micaceous balanitis: comment. *Clin Exp Dermatol* 2012;37(4):434–5.

22 Irvine C, Anderson JR, Pye RJ. Micaceous and keratotic pseudoepitheliomatous balanitis and rapidly fatal fibrosarcoma of the penis occurring in the same patient. *Br J Urol* 1987;116:719–25.

Squamous carcinoma and other malignant neoplasms

Carcinoma of the penis

1 Brady KL, Mercurio MG, Brown MD. Malignant tumors of the penis. *Dermatol Surg* 2013;39:527–47.

2 Porter WM, Francis N, Hawkins D, *et al.* Penile intraepithelial neoplasia: clinical spectrum and treatment of 35 cases. *Br J Dermatol* 2002;147:1159–65.

4 Bunker CB. *Male Genital Skin Disease.* London: Saunders, 2004.

9 Rempelakos A, Bastas E, Lymperakis CH, Thanos A. Carcinoma of the penis: experience from 360 cases. *J Balkan Union Oncol* 2004;9:51–5.

11 Boczko S, Freed S. Penile carcinoma in circumcised males. *NY State J Med* 1979;79:1903–4.

18 Van Howe RS, Hodges FM. The carcinogenicity of smegma: debunking a myth. *J Eur Acad Dermatol Venereol* 2006;20:1046–54.

27 Fryrear RS II, Wiggins AK, Sanguesa O, Yosipovitch G. Rapid onset of cutaneous squamous cell carcinoma of the penis in a patient with psoriasis on etanercept therapy. *J Am Acad Dermatol* 2004;51:1026.

28 Kreuter A, Meyer MF, Wieland U. Occurrence of penile intraepithelial neoplasia following adalimumab treatment for psoriatic arthritis. *Arch Dermatol* 2011;147:1001–2.

33 Droller MJ. Carcinoma of the penis: an overview. *Urol Clin North Am* 1980;7:783–4.

Carcinoma of the scrotum

1 Potts P. Cancer scroti. *Chirurgical Works* 1779;3:225–9.

6 Murthy KVN. Primary cutaneous carcinoma of the scrotum. *J Occup Med* 1993;35:888–9.

9 McGarry GW, Robertson JR. Scrotal carcinoma following prolonged use of crude coal tar ointment. *Br J Urol* 1989;63:211–19.

12 Gross DJ, Schosser RH. Squamous cell carcinoma of the scrotum. *Cutis* 1991;47:402–4.

13 Loughlin KR. Psoriasis: association with two rare cutaneous urological malignancies. *J Urol* 1997;157:622–3.

14 Dean AL. Epithelioma of the scrotum. *J Urol* 1948;60:508–18.

15 Black SB, Woods JE. Squamous cell carcinoma complicating hidradenitis suppurativa. *J Surg Oncol* 1982;19:25–6.

16 Andrews PE, Farrow GM, Oesterling JE. Squamous cell carcinoma of the scrotum: long-term follow-up of 14 patients. *J Urol* 1991;146:1299–304.

19 Lowe FC. Squamous cell carcinoma of scrotum. *Urology* 1985;25:63–5.

21 Azike JE. A review of the history, epidemiology and treatment of squamous cell carcinoma of the scrotum. *Rare Tumors* 2009 Jul 22;1(1):e17.

Verrucous carcinoma/giant condyloma/Buschke–Löwenstein tumour

1 Weber P, Rabinovitz H, Garland L. Verrucous carcinoma in penile lichen sclerosus et atrophicus. *J Dermatol Surg Oncol* 1987;13:529.

2 Micali G, Nasca MR, Innocenzi D. Lichen sclerosus of the glans is significantly associated with penile carcinoma. *Sex Transm Infect* 2001;77:226.

3 Cosman BC, O'Grady TC, Pekarske S. Verrucous carcinoma arising in hidradenitis suppurativa. *Int J Colorectal Dis* 2000;15:342–6.

4 Bain L, Geronemus R. The association of lichen planus of the penis with squamous cell carcinoma in situ and with verrucous squamous carcinoma. *J Dermatol Surg Oncol* 1989;15:413–17.

7 Brown MD, Zachary CB, Grekin RC, *et al.* Penile tumours: their management by Mohs micrographic surgery. *J Dermatol Surg Oncol* 1987;13:1163–7.

8 Brown MD, Zachary CB, Grekin RC, Swanson NA. Genital tumours: their management by micrographic surgery. *J Am Acad Dermatol* 1988;18:115–22.

11 Ayer J, Matthews S, Francis N, Walker NP, Dinneen M, Bunker CB. Successful treatment of Buschke–Lowenstein tumour of the penis with carbon dioxide laser vaporisation. *Acta Derm Venereol* 2012;92:656–7.

14 Geusau A, Heinz-Peer G, Volc-Platzer B, *et al.* Regression of deeply infiltrating giant condyloma (Buschke–Löwenstein tumor) following long-term intralesional interferon alfa therapy. *Arch Dermatol* 2000;136:707–10.

16 Sobrado CW, Mester M, Nadalin W, *et al.* Radiation-induced total regression of a highly recurrent giant perianal condyloma: report of case. *Dis Colon Rectum* 2000;43:257–60.

18 South LM, O'Sullivan JP, Gazet JC. Giant condylomata of Buschke and Löwenstein. *Clin Oncol* 1977;3:107–15.

Extramammary Paget disease

1 Helwig EB, Graham JH. Anogenital (extramammary) Paget's disease: a clinicopathological study. *Cancer* 1963;16:387–403.

2 Chanda JJ. Extramammary Paget's disease: prognosis and relationship to internal malignancy. *J Am Acad Dermatol* 1985;13:1009–14.

3 Brady KL, Mercurio MG, Brown MD. Malignant tumors of the penis. *Dermatol Surg* 2013;39:527–47.

4 Bunker CB. *Male Genital Skin Disease.* London: Saunders, 2004.

5 Tanabe H, Kishigawa T, Sayama S, Tanaka T. A case of giant extramammary Paget's disease of the genital area with squamous cell carcinoma. *Dermatology* 2001;202:249–51.

Malignant melanoma

2 Brady KL, Mercurio MG, Brown MD. Malignant tumors of the penis. *Dermatol Surg* 2013;39:527–47.

3 Cascielli N. Melanoma maligno del pene. *Tumori* 1969;55:313–15.
15 Lucia MS, Miller GJ. Histopathology of malignant lesions of the penis. *Urol Clin North Am* 1992;19:227–46.

Kaposi sarcoma

1 Dehner LP, Smith BH. Soft tissue tumours of the penis. *Cancer* 1970;25:1431–7.
2 Kavak A, Akman RY, Alper M, Büyükbabani N. Penile Kaposi's sarcoma in a human immunodeficiency virus-seronegative patient. *Br J Dermatol* 2001;144:207–8.
3 Micali G, Nasca MR, De Pasquale R, Innocenzi D. Primary classic Kaposi's sarcoma of the penis: a report of a case and review. *J Eur Acad Dermatol Venereol* 2003;17:320–3.
4 Cecchi R, Troiano M, Ghilardi M, Bartoli L. Karposi sarcoma of the penis in an HIV-negative patient. *J Cutan Med Surg* 2011;15:118–20.
5 Schwartz JJ, Dias BM, Safari B. HIV-related malignancies. *Dermatol Clin* 1991;9:503–15.
6 Bayne D, Wise GJ. Kaposi sarcoma of the penis and genitalia: a disease of our times. *Urology* 1988;31:22–5.
7 Schwartz RA, Cohen JB, Watson RA, et al. Penile Kaposi's sarcoma preceded by chronic penile lymphoedema. *Br J Dermatol* 2000;142:153–6.
8 Kapdagli H, Gunduz K, Ozturk G, Kandiloglu G. Pseudo-Kaposi's sarcoma (Mali type). *Int J Dermatol* 1998;37:223–5.

Other malignant neoplasms

1 Brady KL, Mercurio MG, Brown MD. Malignant tumors of the penis. *Dermatol Surg* 2013;39:527–47.
3 Staley TE, Nieh PT, Ciesielski TE, Cieplinski W. Metastatic basal cell carcinoma of the scrotum. *J Urol* 1983;130:792–4.
4 Dehner LP, Smith BH. Soft tissue tumours of the penis. *Cancer* 1970;25:1431–7.
11 Chiu LS, Wong KH, Lam WY, et al. Angiosarcoma of the scrotum after treatment of cancer of the rectum. *Clin Exp Dermatol* 2006;31:706–7.
13 Hagiuda J, Ueno M, Ashimine S, et al. Langerhans cell histiocytosis on the penis: a case report. *BMC Urol* 2006;6:28.
16 Chiam LY, Chan YC. Solitary plaque mycosis fungoides on the penis responding to topical imiquimod therapy. *Br J Dermatol* 2007;156:560–2.
22 Thorns C, Urban H, Remmler K, et al. Primary cutaneous T-cell lymphoma of the penis. *Histopathology* 2003;42:513–14.
23 Doll DC, Diaz-Arias AA. Peripheral T-cell lymphoma of the scrotum. *Acta Haematol* 1994;91:77–9.
27 Chaux A, Amin M, Cubilla A, Young R. Metastatic tumours to the penis: a report of 17 cases and review of the literature. *Int J Surg Path* 2010;19:597–606.
31 Pastore A, Palleschi G, Manfredonia G, et al. Penile metastasis from primary cholangiocarcinoma: the first case report. *BMC Gastroenterol* 2013;13;149.

Miscellaneous cutaneous male genital conditions

Penile melanosis and hypopigmentation

1 Kaporis A, Lynfield Y. Penile lentiginosis. *J Am Acad Dermatol* 1998;38:781.
3 Kopf AW, Bart RS. Tumor conference 43: penile lentigo. *J Dermatol Surg Oncol* 1982;8:637–9.
4 Rhodes AR, Harrist TJ, Momtaz TK. The PUVA-induced pigmented macule: a lentiginous proliferation of large, sometimes cytologically atypical, melanocytes. *J Am Acad Dermatol* 1983;9:47–58.
5 Barnhill RL, Albert LS, Sharma SK, et al. Genital lentiginosis: a clinical and histopathologic study. *J Am Acad Dermatol* 1990;22:453–60.
7 Revuz J, Clerici T. Penile melanosis. *J Am Acad Dermatol* 1989;20:567–70.
8 Lenane P, Keane CO, Connell BO, et al. Genital melanotic macules: clinical, histologic, immunohistochemical, and ultrastructural features. *J Am Acad Dermatol* 2000;42:640–4.

9 Breathnach AS, Balus L, Amantea A. Penile lentiginosis: an ultrastructural study. *Pigment Cell Res* 1992;5:404–13.
11 Delaney TA, Walker NPJ. Penile melanosis successfully treated with the Q-switched ruby laser. *Br J Dermatol* 1994;130:663–4.
14 Stankler L. Striae of the penis. *Br J Dermatol* 1982;107:371–2.
16 Stefanaki C, Nicolaidou E, Hadjivassiliou M, et al. Imiquimod-induced vitiligo in a patient with genital warts. *J Eur Acad Dermatol Venereol* 2006;20:755.

Pain and swelling, iatrogenic swelling and lymphoedema, and idiopathic lipogranuloma

1 Bunker CB. *Male Genital Skin Disease*. London: Saunders, 2004.
2 Weinberger LN, Zirwas MJ, English JC III. A diagnostic algorithm for male genital oedema. *J Eur Acad Dermatol Venereol* 2007;21:156–62.
3 Kopecky RT, Funk MM, Kreitzer PR. Localized genital oedema in patients undergoing continuous ambulatory peritoneal dialysis. *J Eur Acad Dermatol Venereol* 2007;21:156–62.
4 Horinaga M, Masuda T, Jitsukawa S. A case of scrotal elephantiasis 30 years after treatment of penile carcinoma. *Hinyokika Kiyo* 1998;44:839–41.
5 Bang RL. Penile oedema induced by continuous condom catheter use and mimicking keloid scar. *Scand J Urol Nephrol* 1994;28:333–5.

Priapism

1 Levine FJ, de Tejada IS, Payton TR, Goldstein I. Recurrent prolonged erections and priapism as a sequela of priapism: pathophysiology and management. *J Urol* 1991;145:764–7.
2 Bunker CB. *Male Genital Skin Disease*. London: Saunders, 2004.
3 Nelson JH III, Winter CC. Priapism: evolution of management in 48 patients in a 22-year series. *J Urol* 1977;117:455–8.
4 O'Brien WM, O'Connor KP, Lynch JH. Priapism: current concepts. *Ann Emerg Med* 1989;18:980–3.
5 Khoriaty N, Schick E. Penile gangrene: an unusual complication of priapism. How to avoid it. *Urology* 1980;16:280.

Dermatological non-disease, dysaesthesia and chronic pain syndromes

1 Cotterill JA. A dermatological non-disease: a common and potentially fatal disturbance of cutaneous body image. *Br J Dermatol* 1981;104:611–19.
2 Bunker CB, Bridgett CK. Depression and the skin. In: Robertson MM, Katona CLE, eds. *Depression and Physical Illness*. London: John Wiley, 1997:225–53.
3 Al-Durazi M, Saleem I, Mohammed AA. Urethral foreign body. *Br J Urol* 1992;69:434.
4 Fisher BK. The red scrotum syndrome. *Cutis* 1997;60:139–41.
5 Markos AR. The male genital skin burning syndrome (dysaesthetic peno/scroto-dynia). *Int J STD AIDS* 2002;13:271–2.
6 Wesselmann U, Burnett AL, Heinberg LJ. The urogenital and rectal pain syndromes. *Pain* 1997;73:269–94.
7 Abbas O, Kibbi A, Chedraoui A, Ghosen S. Red scrotum syndrome: successful treatment with oral doxycycline. *J Dermatol Treat* 2008;19;1–2.
10 Neill ME, Swash M. Chronic perianal pain: an unsolved problem. *J R Soc Med* 1982;75:96–101.
11 Cohen AD, Vander T, Medvendovsky E, et al. Paravertebral blockade may be used for alleviation of symptoms in patients with anogenital pruritus. Neuropathic scrotal pruritus: anogenital pruritus is a symptom of lumbosacral radiculopathy. *J Am Acad Dermatol* 2005;52:61–6.
12 Cabellero JM, Avila A, Cardona X, et al. Genital pain without urogenital pathology: the koro-like syndrome. *J Urol* 2000;163:243.

PART 10: SITES, SEX, AGE

CHAPTER 112

Dermatoses of the Female Genitalia

Fiona Lewis

Wexham Park Hospital, Frimley Health; and St John's Institute of Dermatology, Guy's and St Thomas' NHS Foundation Trust, London, UK

PART 10: SITES, SEX, AGE

Introduction

Common dermatoses that are easily recognized elsewhere may have a modified appearance on the vulva, where the typical clinical features are often altered significantly. The ano-genital skin is vulnerable, with the local environmental influences of heat, moisture and friction all acting as irritants; changes in the normal bacterial flora are also important.

There has been some confusion regarding the terminology used for vulval disease. The classification of vulval disorders has been clarified and older terms such as vulval dystro-phy, leukoplakia and kraurosis vulvae should no longer be used [1].

The development of vulval clinics has helped to improve the management of women with vulval disease. A multidisciplinary approach is needed as the management of many vulval disorders will require the expertise of different specialties including dermatology, gynaecology and genito-urinary medicine, and clinicopathological correlation involving discussion with a histopathologist is vital [2]. Clear pathways of care and links with other specialites including plastic surgery, urology, paediatrics, psychology and psychosexual medicine are important in the management of specific conditions.

Rook's Textbook of Dermatology, Ninth Edition. Edited by Christopher Griffiths, Jonathan Barker, Tanya Bleiker, Robert Chalmers and Daniel Creamer.
© 2016 John Wiley & Sons, Ltd. Published 2016 by John Wiley & Sons, Ltd.
Companion website: www.rooksdermatology.com

History and examination

An accurate diagnosis depends on a thorough history, examination of the genital and extragenital skin, and relevant investigations. The history must include the nature and duration of the presenting complaint, how the problem changes (e.g. variation with menstrual cycle) and the type, regimen and effectiveness of any prescribed or over-the-counter treatment used. The complaint of 'irritation' should be defined since the patient may use the term to describe the sensation of itch, dryness, pain or burning. This is important as a patient with itch will scratch or rub the skin, and the response will be lichen simplex or lichenification, whereas with discomfort or pain there will be no such change as the patient avoids touching the area.

A personal and family history of autoimmune disease, atopy or psoriasis should be established, together with any known skin sensitivities. The patient should also be asked about vaginal discharge, urinary symptoms and bowel function. It is helpful to know if there have been any abnormalities with cervical cytology and also whether the patient smokes cigarettes, as this is a major risk factor for intraepithelial neoplasia. Finally, as the vulva is important for normal sexual function, relevant questions should be included where appropriate.

The examination is often embarrassing for the patient, so must be carried out sympathetically. Good lighting and a means of magnification are needed. A methodical approach will ensure that all areas of the vulva and perianal skin are examined fully. It is important to know the normal anatomy of the vulva as some dermatoses result in scarring and therefore architectural changes can give diagnostic clues. The examination must also include inspection of other flexural sites and mucosae, the scalp and nails. It is also useful to determine if the patient exhibits dermographism [3]. The vagina and cervix should be examined in patients who have dermatoses that affect the mucosal surfaces and in patients with symptoms of dyspareunia, vaginal discharge or postcoital bleeding.

Investigations

Investigations are determined by the specific problem. If an unusual or sexually transmitted infection is high on the differential diagnosis, it is important to involve a genito-urinary physician in the investigation and work-up of these patients and their sexual partners.

Vulval biopsy is often required and very useful in the diagnosis of ano-genital dermatoses. However, careful clinicopathological correlation and discussion with a dermatopathologist is vital.

Some investigations are not the usual remit of the dermatologist but are necessary in patients with ano-genital dermatoses, for example cervical smear and proctoscopy.

Structure and function of the female genitalia

The vulva is the collective term used for the structures that comprise the female external genitalia. Anatomically, it is the region known as the uro-genital triangle, bounded anteriorly by the symphysis pubis, the pubic rami laterally and the transverse perineal body posteriorly. The vulval structures included within this area are the mons pubis, labia majora and labia minora, clitoris, vulval vestibule and hymen (Figure 112.1a). It is recognized that there can be a wide variety in size and appearance of these components [1,2]. The epithelia that cover the vulva change from skin on the outer aspects to mucosa on the inner aspects of the labia minora.

The mons pubis lies in front of and above the upper part of the symphysis pubis. The densely hair-bearing epithelium covers a thick cushion of subcutaneous fat.

The labia majora are paired, rounded folds of skin and are the homologue of the scrotum. They extend downwards and backwards from the mons pubis and meet posteriorly in the midline to form the posterior commissure, which lies approximately 2 cm anterior to the anus. The structure is similar to that of the mons pubis in that there is a thick layer of adipose tissue and a dense distribution of hair on the outer surfaces of the labia. Hair is absent from the inner surfaces but numerous sebaceous glands remain. The inner aspects of the labia majora fuse into the outer aspects of the labia minora laterally, forming the interlabial sulci.

The labia minora are the equivalent of the male prepuce, and are paired pendulous folds, which lie between the labia majora and the vulval vestibule. Anteriorly they split into two folds on each side, which fuse in the midline. The superior folds form the clitoral hood, and the lower folds fuse on the inferior aspect of the clitoris,

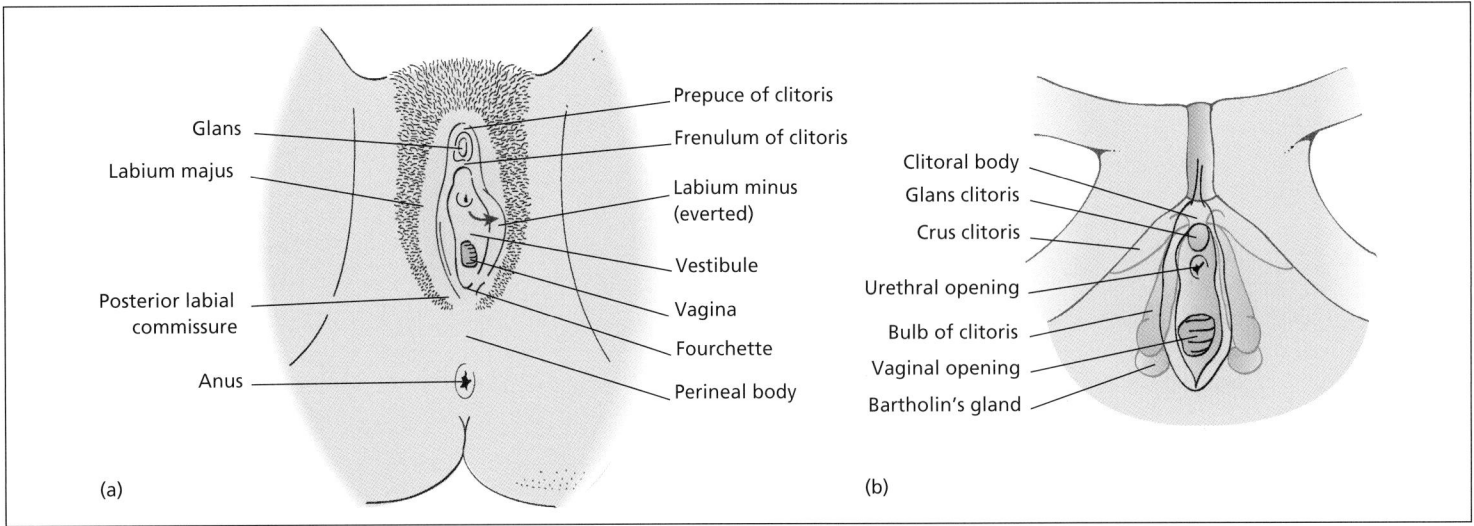

Figure 112.1 (a) The vulva. (b) The clitoris. (From Neill and Lewis 2009 [**2**]. Reproduced with permission of John Wiley & Sons.)

forming the clitoral frenulum. Posteriorly, the labia minora fuse to form the fourchette, and sometimes form a depression in the midline – the fossa navicularis. The labia minora possess little subcutaneous fat. Their epithelium lacks hair but there are numerous sebaceous glands and sweat glands. The epithelium is cornified but its barrier function is not as effective as skin elsewhere.

The clitoris is the homologue of the penis and contains all the vascular and muscular structures found in its male counterpart. The end of the clitoris is surmounted by a small rounded tubercle, the glans clitoris (Figure 112.1b).

The vestibule is the area that lies between the labia minora and contains the openings of the urethra and vagina. The vaginal opening is partially closed by the hymen. When the hymen is ruptured, its remnants form rounded crenulations, the hymenal caruncle. Sometimes a clear line of demarcation between the keratinized epithelium of the labia minora and the non-keratinized mucosa of the vestibule can be seen (Hart's line). The vestibule is a mucosal epithelium and lacks hairs and sebaceous glands. On each side, the duct of the Bartholin glands can be seen sited between the hymenal ring and posterior part of the labium minus. The ducts of the minor vestibular glands, Skene's glands, open on either side of the urethral orifice.

Labial and clitoral variations

There may be a persistence of the most caudal elements of the milk line in the labia majora, and there is great variation in the size and symmetry of normal labia minora. There may be very marked hypertrophy of the labia minora, some cases of which are examples of neurofibromatosis.

Labial adhesions may occur as an inherited familial trait [3] or in association with abnormal sexual differentiation. In general, most occur in the neonatal period and early infancy, and usually divide spontaneously by the time the child is 6 years old. No intervention is necessary unless there is a problem with urination. Some cases of labial adhesions result from lichen sclerosus.

Accessory labio-scrotal folds are well described in males, usually in association with a perineal lipoma. They are extremely rare in women and only two cases have been reported [4].

The clitoris may be absent because of a failure of the genital tubercle to fuse, it may remain hypoplastic [5] or it may be enlarged because of congenital adrenal hyperplasia. The Lawrence–Seip syndrome, which is a congenital generalized lipodystrophy with the onset of insulin-resistant diabetes around the time of puberty, may also result in clitoral hypertrophy. Clitoral tumours may mimic genital sexual ambiguity [6–8]. A pseudocyst of the clitoris, caused by a build up of keratinous debris under clitoral hood adhesions, can occur in lichen sclerosus.

Virilization of the external genitalia may also occur with maternal ingestion of testosterone or synthetic progestogens in the first trimester, and if taken later in pregnancy there may be clitoral hypertrophy alone.

An imperforate hymen is usually discovered at puberty and is caused either by failure of the epithelial cells of the hymen to degenerate or by scarring after an inflammatory reaction in the hymen at birth.

Normal flora

The skin of the perineal area has a higher pH, temperature and degree of humidity than skin elsewhere and, because of its proximity to the vagina and rectum, harbours many of the flora from these sites. The main resident organisms are micrococci, diphtheroids and lactobacilli. Lactobacilli are probably the most common organisms, particularly on the mucosal surfaces, as the glycogenated epithelium of the vagina, under the influence of oestrogen, encourages colonization by them. The lactobacilli in turn metabolize the glycogen to lactic acid, which keeps the vaginal pH at approximately 4.5, restricting the growth of many organisms.

Normal variants

Angiokeratomas

Angiokeratomas are small (1–4 mm) vascular papules found on the labia majora. They vary in colour from red to blue-black and are normally asymptomatic, but can become quite large and bleed if traumatized, particularly in pregnancy.

Fordyce spots

These are sebaceous glands seen on the inner aspects of the labia majora and labia minora where the glands do not usually have an associated hair unit. They open directly onto the surface, and may be very prominent and numerous. The yellow, uniform papules are often best seen when the skin is stretched (Figure 112.2). They may be associated with pruritus and sometimes become inflamed and painful in the week prior to the menses. Rarely, they become very large and can be mistaken for a sebaceous gland adenoma [9].

Vestibular papillomatosis

Vestibular papillomatosis is the term used to describe the occasional normal finding of multiple, tiny filiform or soft, frond-like projections on the vestibular epithelium and inner aspects of the labia minora. Vestibular papillae are symmetrically distributed

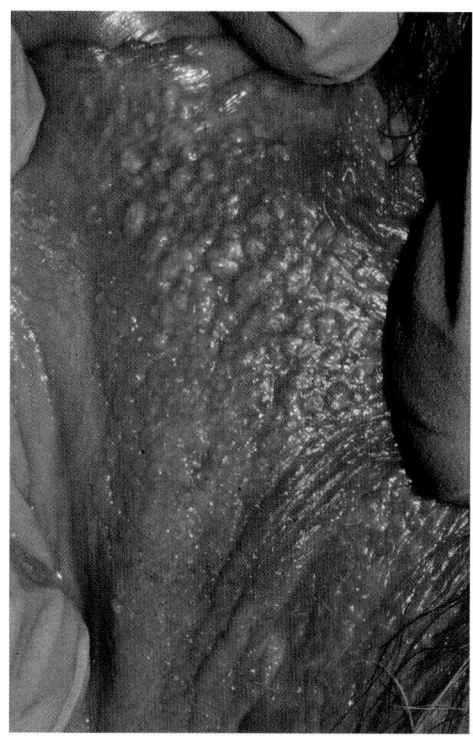

Figure 112.2 Fordyce spots.

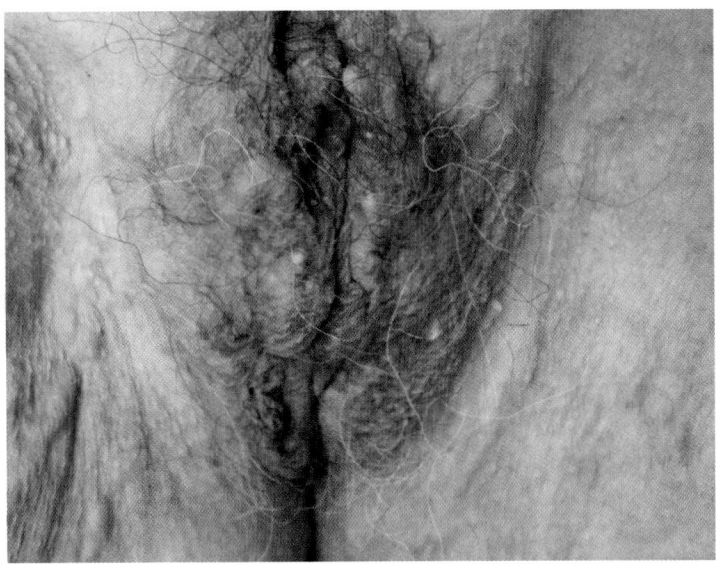

Figure 112.3 Vulval varicosities.

and each papilla has a solitary base. Previously, there was some confusion as the vestibule has heavily glycogenated epithelial cells that become vacuolated on processing and may resemble koilocytes. It is now known that human papillomavirus infection is not associated with these papillae [10] and that they are a normal entity and probably the female equivalent of pearly penile papules.

Varicosities
Varicosities of the labial veins (Figure 112.3) may occur unilaterally in association with limb varicosities, or appear in pregnancy. Other changes in pregnancy include a fall in the pH and increased pigmentation. At the menopause vascularity decreases and the sebaceous glands become less active.

CONGENITAL ABNORMALITIES

Disorders of sexual development

Definition and nomenclature
This group of disorders relates to those where there is an abnormality in gonadal development or sexual differentiation.

Synonyms and inclusions
- Ambiguous external genitalia
- Intersex disorders

Introduction and general description
In a newborn, the external genitalia may not be phenotypical of either a male or female. Evaluation and management of these infants requires an expert multidisciplinary team. The disorders

Table 112.1 Classification of disorders of sexual development.

Chromosome abnormality	Example disorder
Sex chromosome DSD	Klinefelter syndrome
	Turner syndrome
46XY DSD	
46XX DSD	
Disorders of gonadal development	Gonadal dysgenesis
	Ovotesticular DSD
	Testicular DSD
Androgen excess	
Others	

of sexual development (DSD) have been reclassified [1] as shown in Table 112.1.

The 46XX is the most common type of DSD encountered and 60% will be due to congenital adrenal hyperplasia. The ovaries are normal but the masculinization of the external genitalia results from androgen exposure in utero.

GENODERMATOSES

Epidermolysis bullosa

Definition
Epidermolysis bullosa (EB) is a group of disorders characterized by skin fagility and blister formation.

Introduction and general description
The forms of EB that specifically involve the vulva are junctional EB inversa and recessive dystrophic EB inversa (see also Chapter 71).

Clinical features

Presentation
Extensive erosion and ulceration can affect the ano-genital area and may heal with scarring. In junctional EB inversa, blistering and erosions occur in the flexures, vulva and vagina and oesophagus. There may be nail dystrophy and atrophic scarring elsewhere.

In recessive dystrophic EB inversa, oral lesions are always present and oesophageal involvement may be severe. Vaginal strictures have been reported [1].

Complications and co-morbidities
A case of vulval squamous cell carcinoma (SCC) has been reported [2].

Management
The management depends on expert nursing care and follows the principles used for other sites.

Hailey–Hailey disease

Definition and nomenclature

Hailey–Hailey disease (HHD) is an autosomal dominant inherited disorder of keratinization with incomplete penetrance (see also Chapter 66).

Synonyms and inclusions
• Benign familial chronic pemphigus

Epidemiology

Age

The clinical features usually start in the teenage years but may present at any time up to the fourth decade.

Pathophysiology

Pathology

Acantholysis is seen throughout the epidermis, giving rise to the 'delapidated brick wall' appearance. Direct immunofluorescence will be negative.

Clinical features

History

Patients complain of painful erosions in flexural sites, particularly the axillae and inguinal folds.

Presentation

Erythematous, moist plaques are seen in the flexures and these may be eroded and crusted. The vulva and perineum are frequently involved. Heat, friction and pregnancy may exacerbate the symptoms.

Differential diagnosis

Hailey–Hailey disease is often misdiagnosed as intertrigo initially. Flexural psoriasis, Darier disease, pemphigus erythematosus and extramammary Paget disease can have similar clinical features.

Complications and co-morbidities

Secondary infection with bacteria (most commonly *Staphylococcus aureus*), viruses (herpes simplex) and *Candida* is a common complication and needs appropriate management. Squamous cell carcinoma has also been described [1,2].

Investigations

A skin biopsy will confirm the diagnosis.

Management

First line

Reduction in friction, with the use of emollients and a moderately potent topical steroid.

Second line

Topical tacrolimus may be of benefit [3] but a case of SCC developing after treatment has been reported [4]. Long-term antibiotics may be required for those where secondary infection is a major issue.

Third line

There is one case report of a patient with perineal disease responding to alefacept [5]. Photodynamic therapy [6] and CO_2 laser [7] have been used. Botulinum toxin has been used in axillary HHD but is not reported for vulval disease.

Resources

Patient resources
Hailey–Hailey Disease Society: www.haileyhailey.com (last accessed June 2014).

Darier disease

Definition

Darier disease is an acantholytic disorder of keratinization, usually with autosomal dominant inheritance (see also Chapter 66).

Epidemiology

Age

Lesions develop in childhood and adolescence and tend to fluctuate in severity.

Clinical features

History

Patients complain of uncomfortable lesions on the vulva and in the inguinal folds. The lesions can weep and become macerated.

Presentation

All areas of the vulva can be affected, and rarely it may be the only site affected [1,2].

Differential diagnosis

There can be considerable overlap with Hailey–Hailey disease and genital papular dyskeratosis.

Complications and co-morbidities

Secondary bacterial and viral infections are common on ano-genital lesions. There is one case report of a SCC developing in vulval Darier disease [3].

Management

The management of vulval Darier disease is the same as for other sites but topical preparations may be more irritant in the ano-genital area. Prompt treatment of any infection is important.

INFLAMMATORY DERMATOSES OF THE VULVA

Lichen sclerosus

Definition and nomenclature

Lichen sclerosus (LS) is a common inflammatory dermatosis with a predilection for ano-genital skin (see also Chapter 57).

Synonyms and inclusions
• Lichen sclerosus et atrophicus

Introduction and general description

Lichen sclerosus is one of the common dermatoses to affect the ano-genital skin [1]. The aetiology is still unknown but there is some evidence in women that LS is a genetically determined autoimmune disorder, and antibodies to extracellular matrix protein 1 have been identified in about 75% of women with the disease [2].

Epidemiology

Incidence and prevalence

It is estimated to occur in 1 in 30 older women [3]. The prevalence in children is unknown.

Age

Lichen sclerosus can affect females of any age, but there are two peaks of incidence, in prepubertal girls and postmenopausal women.

Sex

Lichen sclerosus is 6–10 times more common in females than males.

Associated diseases

There is a link with other autoimmune disorders in 21% of patients [4], with thyroid disease being the commonest association. However, this link is not as great in males [5]. It is also observed that there is often concomitant psoriasis in patients with LS [6,7].

Pathophysiology

Predisposing factors

Lichen sclerosus is known to exhibit the Koebner phenomenon and is sometimes seen in episiotomy scars. The Koebner phenomenon has also been reported at sites of radiotherapy [8], scar tissue [9], vaccination [10] and congenital haemangioma [11].

Pathology

The classic histology is a thinned epidermis with flattening of the rete pegs. The underlying dermis is hyalinized and there are

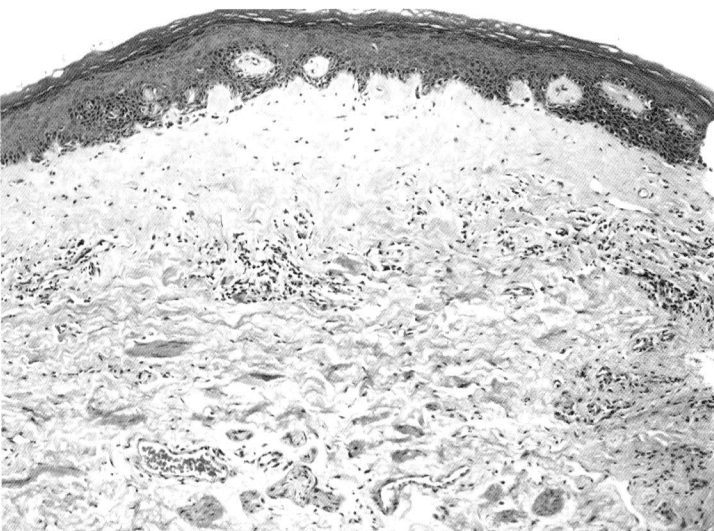

Figure 112.4 Histological features of lichen sclerosus.

often extravasated red cells. Below the hyalinized area is a band-like zone of chronic inflammatory cells (Figure 112.4). There is an absence of elastic fibres in the upper dermis. There have been attempts to grade the histological appearances but there is probably little correlation between the timing of a lesion and its histological appearance [12]. In some cases the epidermis is thickened, and this is LS with squamous cell hyperplasia. It is found in approximately 30% of cases of LS in association with vulval SCC [13].

There are abnormalities of the basement membrane, but it is uncertain whether these are a primary or secondary event [14]. Immunofluorescence studies are usually negative or demonstrate non-specific fibrin deposition at the dermal–epidermal junction. There is also an alteration of the elastin and fibrillin in the affected dermis [15]. Studies of cell kinetics show active regeneration of collagen [16] and there is altered p53 expression and epidermal cell proliferation [17]. Increased numbers of CD1+ Langerhans cells are found at all stages of disease [18].

Causative organisms

The role of *Borrelia burgdorferi* is controversial but there is no consistent evidence that it is causative.

Genetics

A positive family history is recognized in 12% of patients [19] and the disorder has been described in twins, both identical [20] and non-identical [21]. There is an increased incidence of DQ7 in both adults [22] and girls [23].

Clinical features

History

The presenting symptom is usually itching, which is often severe and distressing. Patients may also complain of discomfort and dyspareunia if there is introital narrowing. Constipation is a common feature in girls with prepubertal disease.

Presentation

Ano-genital disease tends to be characterized by flat, atrophic, whitened epithelium (Figure 112.5), which may become confluent, extending around the vulval and perianal skin in a figure-of-eight configuration. There may also be oedema, purpura, bullae, erosions, fissures (Figure 112.6) and ulceration. Sometimes the epithelium can become thickened (Figure 112.7). The sites most commonly affected are the genito-crural folds, the inner aspects of the labia majora, labia minora, clitoris and clitoral hood. Vestibular involvement is rare and vaginal lesions do not occur, as LS seems to spare mucosal epithelium. The one exception to this is when significant prolapse causes the skin to keratinize, which may then become affected by lichen sclerosus [24,25]. Perianal lesions occur in approximately 30% of female patients, in contrast with men who do not seem to develop perianal involvement. The classic lesions seen on the extragenital skin are ivory white papules and plaques with follicular delling. These occur in 10% of women with vulval disease. The extragenital areas may be truncal, at sites of pressure, or on the upper back, wrists, buttocks and thighs. Facial [26], lip [27], scalp [28] and nail involvement [29] have all been recorded.

Lesions of LS in the oral cavity are extremely rare but are reported on the tongue [30]. Many of the reports of oral involvement in the literature have often not been confirmed histologically [31] and may have been examples of lichen planus. It is not uncommon for patients with vulval LS to have coexistent oral lichen planus [32].

LS is a scarring dermatosis and the changes that can occur on the vulva include loss of the labia minora and sealing over of the clitoral hood, burying the clitoris (Figure 112.8a,b). Introital narrowing resulting from anterior and posterior labial fusion,

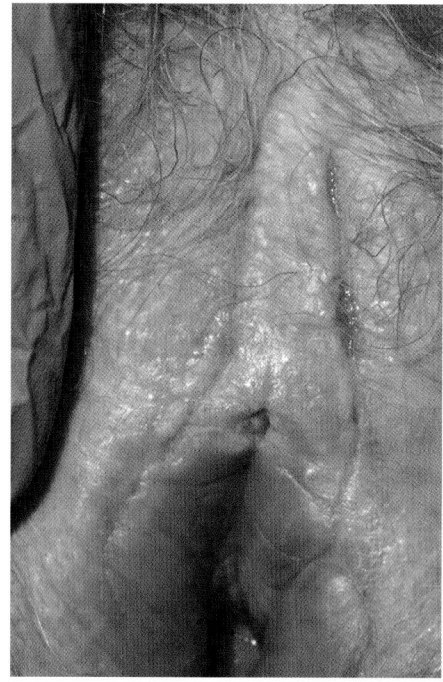

Figure 112.6 Fissuring in lichen sclerosus.

sometimes resulting in a tiny opening into the vestibule. Milia may occur.

Differential diagnosis

Vitiligo, mucous membrane pemphigoid, lichen planus and morphoea may present with a similar clinical appearance. There can be

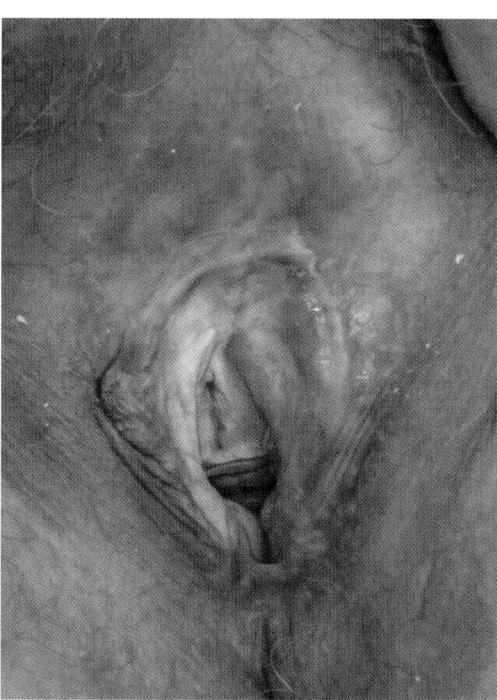

Figure 112.5 Lichen sclerosus showing white sclerotic plaques and architectural change.

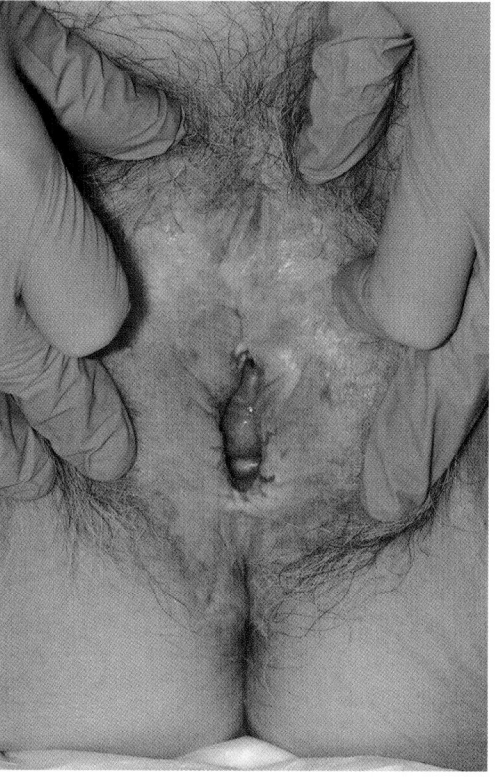

Figure 112.7 Thickened epithelium in acanthotic lichen sclerosus.

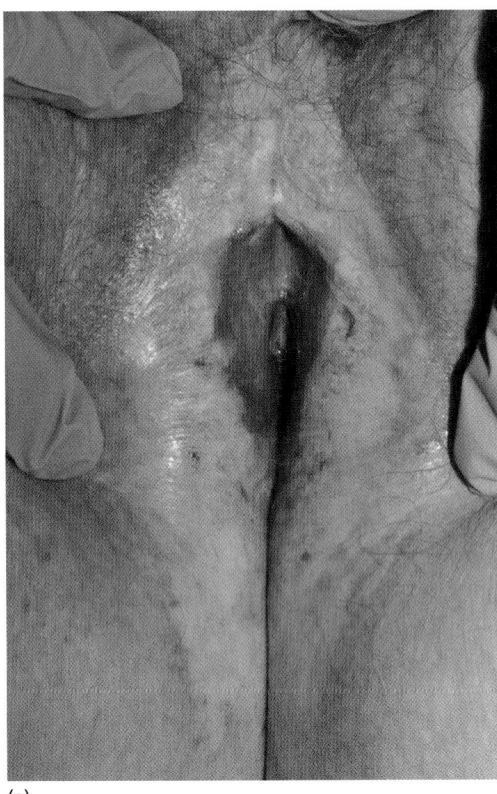

(a)

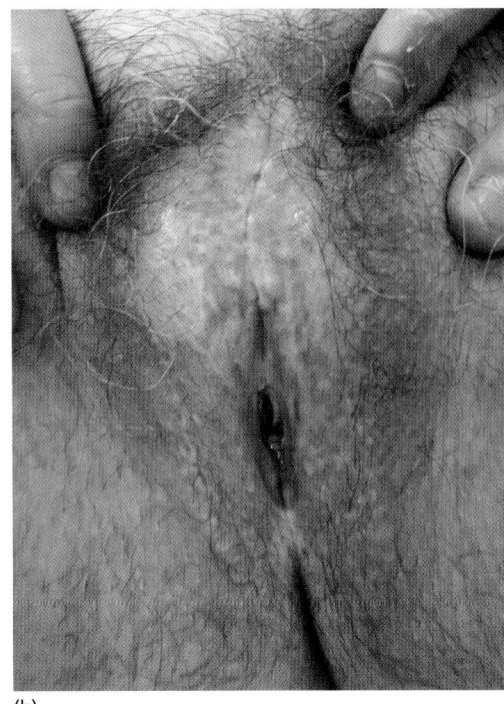

(b)

Figure 112.8 (a) Scarring in lichen sclerosus with ecchymosis. (b) Scarring in lichen sclerosus with loss of the labia minora and sealing of the clitoral hood.

clinical and histological overlap between morphoea, lichen planus and LS, and they may represent a spectrum of disease rather than three distinct conditions [33].

Lichen sclerosus and other dermatoses can be mistaken for sexual abuse [34–37], but sometimes the sexual abuse may be the initiating or exacerbating factor of the dermatological condition [38]. The possibility of sexual abuse sometimes has to be considered in a child whose lichen sclerosus, despite appropriate treatment and compliance, has not responded as expected.

Complications and co-morbidities

There is undoubtedly an association between vulval SCC and LS (Figure 112.9) but the incidence is less than 4% [39]. However, in retrospective reviews of pathological specimens of vulval carcinoma, histological evidence of LS is found in approximately half of the cases [40,41,42]. These series included patients presenting with SCC as well as those on long-term follow-up for LS. A longitudinal cohort study of 211 patients showed that the number of invasive SCCs significantly exceeded that in an age-matched group [43]. The oncogenic human papillomavirus types do not appear to be implicated in the development of SCC on LS [44,45]. It is not yet known whether good control of LS reduces the risk of neoplastic change.

The histological patterns associated with SCC arising on LS include epithelial hyperplasia and differentiated intraepithelial neoplasia (dysplastic changes that are confined to the basal layers). Several studies have looked at markers to predict possible progression to SCC [46].

LS has been reported in association with verrucous carcinoma [47,48], basal cell carcinoma [49] and melanoma [50–52]. However, malignant melanoma and atypical genital naevi are known to be difficult to diagnose in the presence of LS [53,54].

Disease course and prognosis

There is generally a good response to a super-potent topical steroid [55] but some patients have a relapse of symptoms requiring

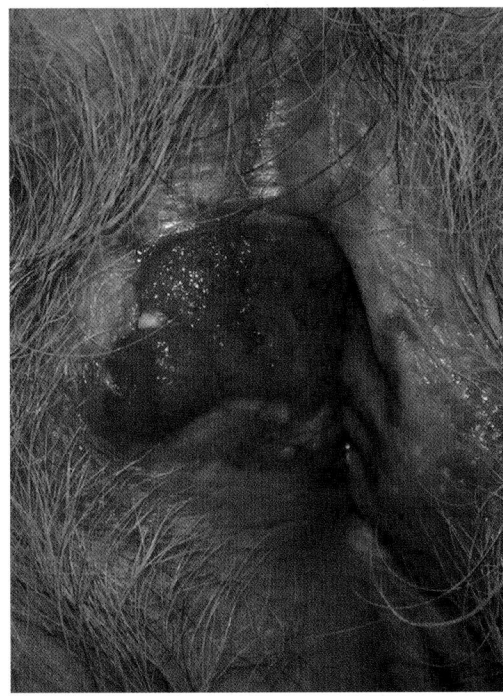

Figure 112.9 Squamous cell carcinoma arising on a background of lichen sclerosus.

repeated treatment. There is still uncertainty whether LS in prepubertal girls remits spontaneously at puberty [56].

Investigations
A biopsy can confirm the diagnosis and is essential in atypical disease or if there is a failure to respond to treatment.

Management
The super-potent topical corticosteroid, clobetasol propionate 0.05%, is first line treatment [57]. There are no randomized controlled trials providing evidence for any particular corticosteroid or treatment regimen being more effective than any other. The regimen currently recommended for a newly diagnosed case is initially clobetasol propionate ointment once nightly for 4 weeks, then alternate nights for 4 weeks, and twice a week for a further month [58]. A 30 g tube of clobetasol propionate should last 12 weeks, and the patient is then reviewed. The clobetasol propionate is then used as and when required to control itching. Most patients seem to require 30–60 g annually. Some patients go into complete remission and do not require further treatment. Others will continue to have flares and remissions and they are advised to use clobetasol propionate ointment as required. A soap substitute is also recommended such as emulsifying ointment.

Topical testosterone has no role in the management of LS. It is expensive and is not as effective as clobetasol propionate [59]. Recent reports have suggested the use of the calcineurin inhibitors tacrolimus [60] or pimecrolimus [61] as steroid-sparing alternatives. The use of these topical immunosuppressants should be limited to the treatment of the rare cases of LS that prove unresponsive to a potent topical steroid. The treatment should be a short course and it should not be used long term as the safety of these immunosuppressants is still unknown, particularly as the condition carries a risk of neoplastic change. Ciclosporin [62] and UVA1 [63] have also been used to treat recalcitrant disease.

Surgery is only indicated for the management of functional problems caused by postinflammatory scarring, premalignant lesions and malignancy [64].

Resources

Further information
British Association of Dermatologists Guidelines: http://www.bad.org.uk/library-media/documents/Lichen_sclerosus_2010.pdf (last accessed June 2014).

Patient resources
International Society for the Study of Vulvo-vaginal Disease information sheets: http://issvd.org/wordpress/wp-content/uploads/2012/04/LS2010.pdf; http://issvd.org/wordpress/wp-content/uploads/2012/04/LSchildren2010.pdf
Worldwide Lichen Sclerosus Support: www.lichensclerosus.org/.
(Both last accessed June 2014.)

Lichen planus

Synonyms and inclusions
- Syndrome of Hewitt and Pelisse
- Desquamative vaginitis

Introduction and general description
Lichen planus (LP) is an inflammatory dermatosis that can affect the skin and mucous membranes. It may affect the anogenital skin and mucosa without involvement elsewhere but can also present at multiple sites, requiring multidisciplinary management [1] (see also Chapter 37).

Epidemiology

Incidence and prevalence
The incidence in the general population is unknown but in one study of 3350 women attending a vulval clinic, 3.7% had vulval lichen planus [2]. Vulval LP was also found in 57% of patients with oral LP [3] and in 51% of those presenting with cutaneous lesions. Many were asymptomatic [4].

Age
The symptoms usually start in the fifth and sixth decades of life [5].

Associated diseases
There is an association of LP with autoimmune diseases including alopecia areata, vitiligo and thyroid disease. An association with hepatitis C infection has been reported in some Mediterranean and Japanese populations but not in northern Europe [6].

Pathophysiology
Lichen planus is probably a T-cell-mediated inflammatory disorder but no causative antigen that may trigger the T-lymphocyte response has been found. Antibasement membrane antibodies have been reported [7].

Pathology
On a cornified epithelium there is hyperkeratosis, irregular acanthosis with a typical saw-tooth appearance of the rete pegs, an increased granular layer, and disruption of the basal layer with a closely apposed, dermal band-like lymphocytic infiltrate (Figure 112.10). The acanthosis and hyperkeratosis are marked in

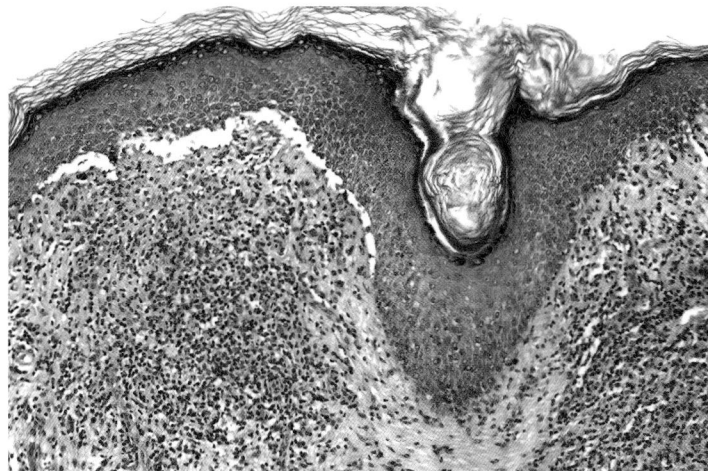

Figure 112.10 Histological features of lichen planus.

the hypertrophic form, and the characteristic band-like infiltrate may be focal. Eosinophilic colloid bodies may be seen. The classic histological features in the epidermis may not be seen in erosive disease, and mucosal lesions may show many plasma cells, which is where the diagnosis of Zoon's vulvitis is often made incorrectly. Immunofluorescence studies reveal uneven staining of the basement membrane zone for fibrinogen and immunoglobulin M (IgM), cytoid bodies and, on occasion, IgG or IgA.

Genetics

Familial cases have been described and although HLA findings are conflicting, an association with HLA-DR1 is postulated [8]. Different HLA subtypes may occur in the vulvo-vaginal–gingival syndrome form of erosive LP [9].

Clinical features

History

The symptoms will depend on the clinical type of LP. Itching may be predominant in the classic and hypertrophic variants, whereas soreness, pain and dyspareunia are the common complaints in erosive LP. If vaginal disease is present, a sero-sanguinous discharge and postcoital bleeding may occur.

Presentation

The clinical features vary with clinical type.

Clinical variants

Three clinical forms are recognized but there may sometimes be overlap features.

1 *Classic/papular lichen planus.* This type can occur with cutaneous lesions. The typical violaceous papules are seen on the outer labia majora, interlabial sulci and clitoral hood. These may coalesce into small plaques or annular lesions (Figure 112.11a). The hallmark Wickham striae may be present (Figure 112.11b). Hyperpigmentation is common and may affect other flexural sites including the inguinal and inframammary folds and axillae. Lichen plano-pilaris has also been described on the vulva [10].

2 *Hypertrophic lichen planus.* This is the least common form of LP seen on the genital skin. Thickened, intensely pruritic plaques, sometimes with a violaceous edge, are seen on the labia majora, perineum and perianal skin.

Vaginal lesions do not occur in classic or hypertrophic LP.

3 *Erosive lichen planus.* Erosive LP is the commonest type to affect the female genital area. On the vulva, symmetrical erosions are most commonly seen at the fourchette and vestibule. These may have an irregular lacy edge with Wickham striae. Diagnostic criteria have been put forward for the diagnosis of erosive LP [11], with the suggestion that three supportive citeria should be present to make the diagnosis.

• *Vulvo-vaginal–gingival syndrome (VVG).* This distinctive erosive subtype of LP principally affects the inner aspects of the labia minora, vestibule and vagina (Figure 112.12), together with a characteristic gingival erythema (Figure 112.13), which may be asymptomatic [12,13,14]). In the past, many cases labelled desquamative vaginitis were probably this entity [15]. The mucosa is eroded and there may be marked loss of architecture (Figure 112.14). The anal margin, external urethral meatus and cervix may also be involved.

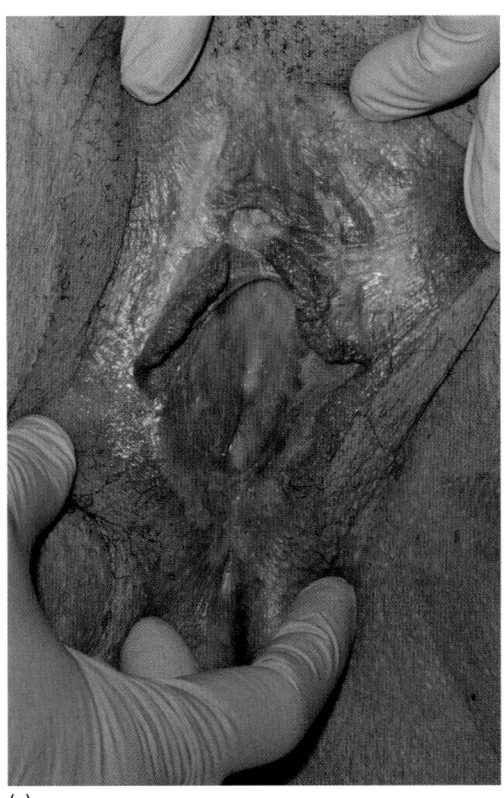
(a)

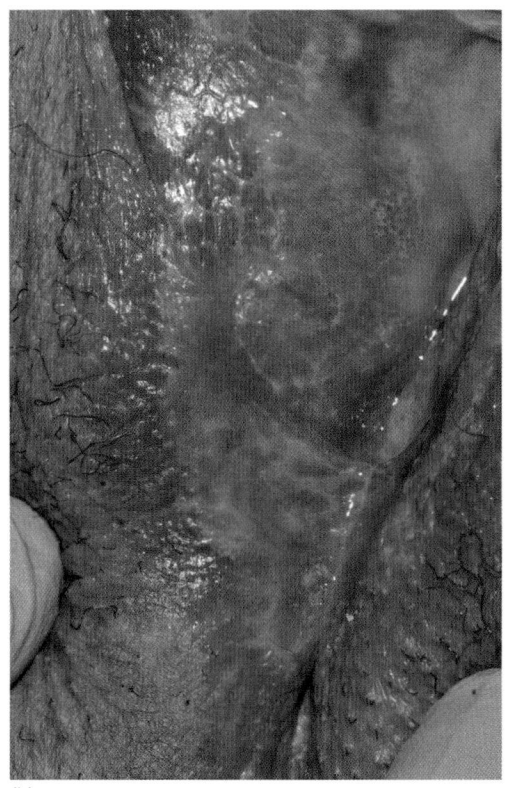
(b)

Figure 112.11 (a) Classic vulval lichen planus showing plaques in the interlabial sulci. (b) Classic vulval lichen planus with Wickham striae.

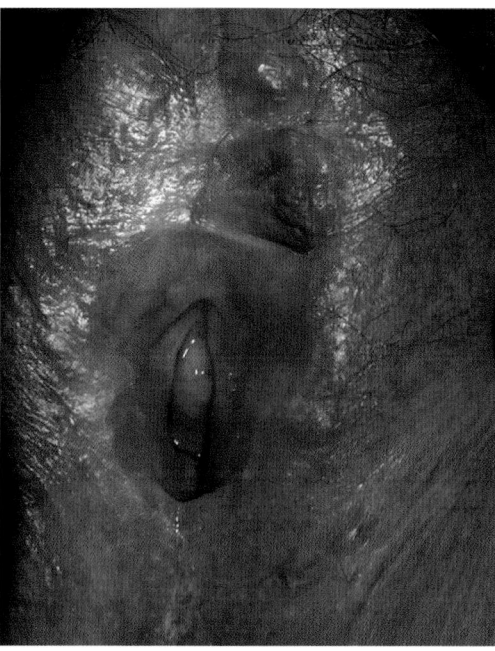

Figure 112.12 Lichen planus: vulval aspect showing glazed erythema and distortion of the architecture, with a remnant of the left labium minus and buried clitoris above it.

The vaginal lesions are velvety red erosions or bright red, glazed erythema, which is friable and bleeds when touched. Vaginal synechiae and adhesions develop, which may rapidly lead to vaginal stenosis and unfortunately many patients present at this stage. Vaginal examination is therefore mandatory in these patients.

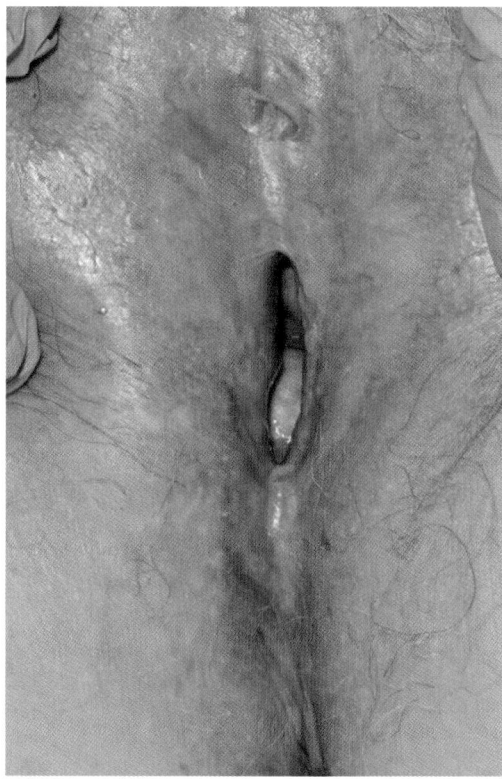

Figure 112.14 Scarring in erosive vulval lichen planus.

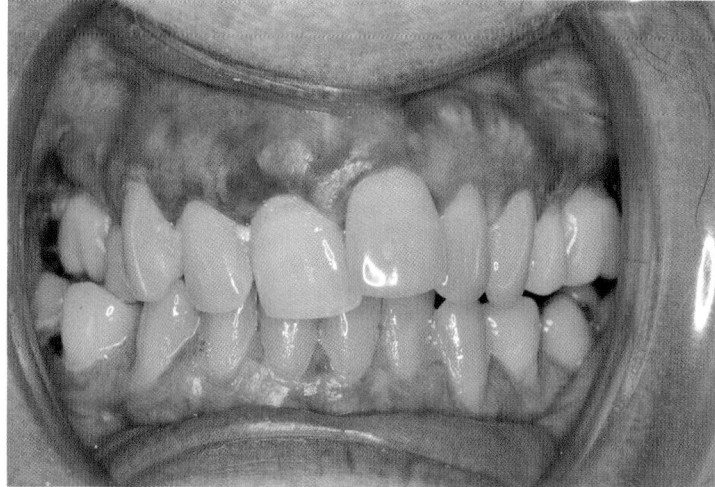

Figure 112.13 Gingival erythema in vulvo-vaginal–gingival syndrome.

This is increasingly recognized as a multisite disease with lesions described on the conjunctiva [16], lacrimal duct (Figure 112.15) [17], oesophagus [18,19] and external auditory canal [20]. The manifestations of this syndrome do not necessarily all occur synchronously.

Differential diagnosis

The main differential diagnosis is usually lichen sclerosus, but mucous membrane pemphigoid, morphoea and lichenoid drug eruptions should also be included. In some cases, the differentiation between LS and LP can be extremely difficult as the two diseases share so many features in common [21,22]. The lichenoid form of graft-versus-host disease has clinical features that may be indistinguishable from erosive LP but this diagnosis should be clear from the history. Frequently, there are cases of LP misdiagnosed as Zoon's vulvitis. Some hypertrophic lesions can mimic malignancy and histology is vital.

Complications and co-morbidities

Scarring is a major issue, particularly in erosive LP, and early diagnosis and appropriate management is important.

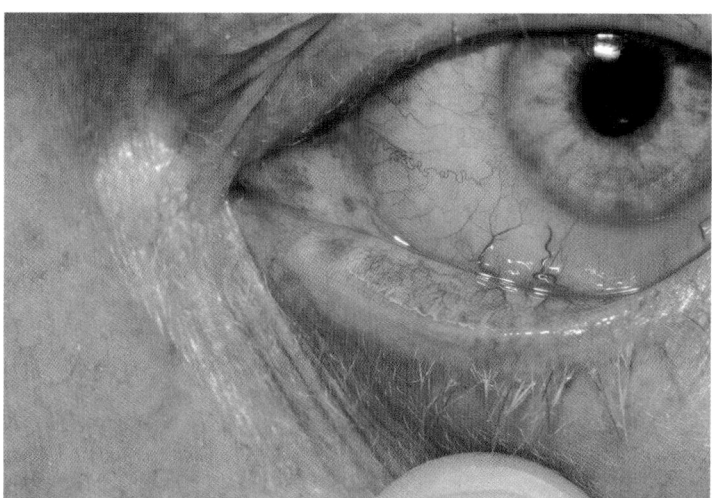

Figure 112.15 Lacrimal duct scarring in erosive lichen planus.

Malignancy is not thought to occur in erosive LP but SCC and SCC *in situ* have been reported in other forms of the disease [23–25]. Studies of patients with vulval SCC have shown that LP is present in the surrounding tissue in about 15% of patients [26,27].

In addition to the sites mentioned above which may be involved in the VVG syndrome, oral manifestations may be seen in all forms of genital LP on the buccal mucosa, tongue and palate. Nail changes are sometimes seen and scarring alopecia may occur in any form of genital LP. Frontal fibrosing alopecia was the commonest association in one series [28].

Disease course and prognosis

Classic LP often clears completely with little or no scarring. Hyperpigmentation may take months to resolve. Erosive and hypertrophic disease tends to pursue a chronic course with flares of disease.

Investigations

The clinical diagnosis can be confirmed on biopsy. The use of topical anaesthesia may obscure the true histological diagnosis [29].

Management

There are no randomized controlled trials of treatment in genital LP and most therapy is based on small case series and single case reports [30]. A recent Cochrane review of treatments for mucosal erosive LP did not include studies of genital disease [31].

First line

Super-potent topical steroid ointment for vulva and intravaginal foam preparations for vaginal disease [32,33].

Emollients are also used as first-line treatment.

Second line

There are reports about the use of calcineurin inhibitors [34–36] but these must be used with caution, as in lichen sclerosus, as there have been concerns about malignant change after their use [37,38].

Third line

Oral retinoids, dapsone, ciclosporin and hydroxychloroquine have been used anecdotally but there is little evidence for their use [39]. Low-dose methotrexate together with topical. steroids and tacrolimus has been reported to be useful [40].

Surgery to release vulval and vaginal adhesions may be required [41,42] but the use of super-potent topical steroids in the early postoperative phase is vital to prevent re-stenosis.

There are single case reports of the use of biologics to treat widespread erosive LP [43], but lichenoid eruptions may be a side effect [44,45], so they should be used with caution.

Resources

Patient resources

International Society for the Study of Vulvo-vaginal Disease information sheet: http://issvd.org/wordpress/wp-content/uploads/2012/04/VULVARLI-CHENPLANUS2010.pdf
UK Lichen Planus: www.uklp.org.uk/.
(Both last accessed June 2014.)

Zoon's vulvitis

Synonyms and inclusions
- Vulvitis circumscripta
- Plasma cell vulvitis

Introduction and general description

Although Zoon's balanitis is well described, true Zoon's vulvitis is rare. The criteria needed to make the diagnosis have varied in the literature, and there is some doubt whether plasma cell vulvitis is a distinct clinicopathological entity, as many of the reports of vestibular Zoon's are probably LP [1]. It is likely that it represents a reaction pattern to another inflammatory condition. A plasma cell-rich infiltrate in a vestibular biopsy may be a misleading finding, because plasma cells are commonly found in inflammatory conditions of the vestibule. Many of the cases are examples of unrecognized dermatoses such as LP, or a chronic postinflammatory phenomenon.

Pathophysiology

Pathology

The essential features are epidermal thinning, absent horny and granular layers and distinctive lozenge-shaped keratinocytes with widened intercellular spaces. In the dermis there is a dense, inflammatory, infiltrate composed largely of plasma cells, with dilated blood vessels and usually a lot of haemosiderin. Russell bodies and dermal–epidermal splitting have also been described [2].

Clinical features

History

Patients may complain of pruritus or discomfort, but it can be asymptomatic.

Presentation

The original description was of erythematous patches with a glazed appearance, usually on the labia minora or vestibule [3]. The clitoris is rarely, if ever, affected.

Clinical variants

It is not uncommon to find patients with purpuric patches, often at the vestibule (Figure 112.16), in which haemosiderin and plasma cells are found without any specific epidermal change, and the term *chronic vulval purpura* may be a more accurate description [4]. An association with lichen aureus has been suggested, as pressure factors are thought to be relevant in the extravasation of blood [5].

Differential diagnosis

Lichen planus, postinflammatory pigmentation and vulval adenosis have similar features.

Disease course and prognosis

It follows a chronic but benign course.

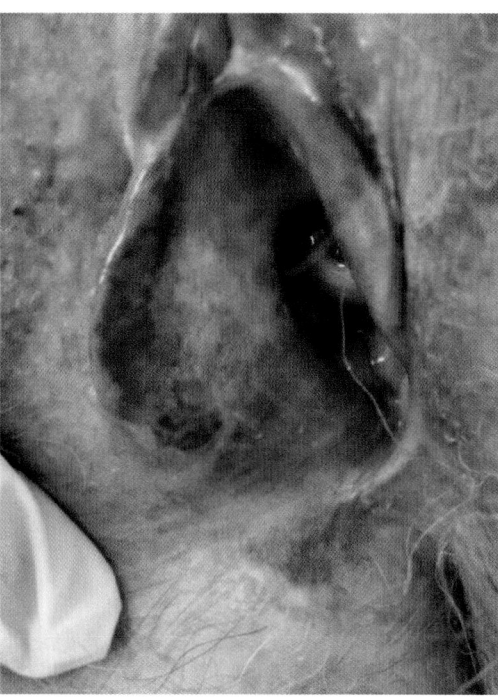

Figure 112.16 Chronic vulval purpura.

Investigations
A vulval biopsy will show the above features.

Management

First line
Emollients and a potent topical steroid are used as first line treatment.

Second line
Lidocaine 5% is useful if there are symptoms for burning in the absence of any inflammatory disease.

Third line
There are case reports of the use of misoprostol [6] and intralesional interferon α [7]. Topical tacrolimus has not been found to be useful [8].

Seborrhoeic eczema

Introduction and general description
This is a common type of eczema in younger people and may affect the vulva (see also Chapter 40).

Pathophysiology

Pathology
Histological examination is not always helpful as there may be features of both eczema and psoriasis. There is moderate acanthosis with slight spongiosis and a mild dermal inflammatory infiltrate.

Clinical features

History
Patients describe intermittent itching and soreness if fissures occur.

Presentation
The signs may be subtle, but scaling and erythema are seen on the inguinal folds, labia majora, perineum and perianal skin. Keratin debris may build up in the interlabial sulci and sometimes under the clitoral hood.

Vulval involvement may be associated with skin changes on the scalp and changes at other flexural sites.

Differential diagnosis
This condition has both eczematous and psoriasiform features, sometimes making differentiation between it and psoriasis difficult. In psoriasis, the lesions are usually better defined and thickened.

Disease course and prognosis
Vulval lesions may recur and require intermittent treatment until resolution.

Investigations
The diagnosis is usually clinical.

Management

Treatment ladder

First line
- Emollients
- Mild topical steroid once daily as needed

Second line
- Topical calcineurin inhibitors may be used but are not always well tolerated on the vulva

---

Irritant eczema

Synonyms and inclusions
- Irritant contact eczema
- Irritant contact dermatitis

Introduction and general description
If the barrier function of the vulval skin is impaired, as measured by transepidermal water loss, there is an increased susceptibility to irritant contact eczema [1,2] (see also Chapter 129).

Epidemiology

Age
An irritant contact eczema is common in children and in older women, particularly those who are incontinent.

Pathophysiology

Predisposing factors
The problem may occur because of the dampness and maceration secondary to a heavy vaginal discharge, or increased contact with urine in the incontinent patient. Contact with irritant chemicals in topical agents, particularly cleansers, bubble baths, lubricants, perfumed products, deodorants and medicaments, may all be responsible for an irritant dermatitis.

Clinical features

History
Soreness is often more common than pruritus in an irritant contact eczema. If severe, it can be painful, especially with micturition.

Presentation
Erythema is most pronounced on the convex areas – the outer labia majora, perianal skin and buttocks – which are the sites most in contact with external irritants.

Differential diagnosis
There are some features in common with seborrhoeic eczema but extravulval involvement is unlikely. There is less scaling in irritant dermatitis compared with seborrheoic eczema.

Complications and co-morbidities
In severe cases of irritant dermatitis, most commonly in older women with urinary incontinence, ulcerative lesions similar to those seen in infantile gluteal granuloma may occur. These are often on the outer labia majora [3].

Investigations
The diagnosis is clinical.

Management

> **Treatment ladder**
>
> **First line**
> - Removal of irritants
> - Referral to a uro-gynaecologist can be helpful to improve urinary incontinence
> - Emollients as soap substitute
> - Barrier preparations
>
> **Second line**
> - Mild topical steroid, with antibacterial/antifungal if appropriate

Allergic contact dermatitis

Introduction and general description
Allergic contact dermatitis is a type IV delayed hypersensitivity reaction. It is rare as a primary cause of vulval symptoms but can complicate other dermatoses (see also Chapter 128).

Epidemiology

Incidence and prevalence
A high incidence of vulval contact dermatitis has been described [1,2,3,4] but this may be explained by many patients who also have perianal involvement. One study has shown a higher incidence of positive patch tests in patients with ano-genital dermatoses if both the genital and perianal areas are involved, compared with dermatoses affecting the genital skin alone [5].

Pathophysiology

Predisposing factors
There are reports of allergy to vaginal preparations and an intrauterine device [6–8], sanitary wear [9] and condoms [10]. Oestradiol may rarely cause a localized allergic contact dermatitis at a transdermal patch site, or generalized contact dermatitis with oral therapy [11].

Clinical features

Presentation
An allergic contact dermatitis most commonly presents with pruritus but, if acute, an erosive eruption may be seen which frequently extends down the thighs.

Differential diagnosis
Other forms of eczema and ano-genital psoriasis may have similar features.

Disease course and prognosis
Once the causative allergen is established and then avoided, the problem should resolve.

Investigations
A detailed history is vital; patch testing is needed in patients where an allergic contact dermatitis is suspected. It is important to include allergens that may be important in the genital area, and vulval/perianal allergen series are widely available. It may also be helpful to include patient's own products.

Management

> **Treatment ladder**
>
> **First line**
> - Remove relevant allergens
> - Emollients
> - Moderately potent topical steroid ± an antibacterial or antifungal
>
> **Second line**
> - Potassium permanganate soaks (1 : 10 000 dilution applied on gauze) if weeping and eroded
> - Antibiotics if secondary infection

Resources

Patient resources
International Society for the Study of Vulvo-vaginal Disease information sheet: http://issvd.org/wordpress/wp-content/uploads/2012/04/ContactDermatitis.pdf (last accessed June 2014).

Allergic contact urticaria

Introduction and general description
This is a type I immediate hypersensitivity reaction; the two most common causes of contact urticaria in the vulvo-vaginal area are latex and semen (see also Chapter 42). Seminal fluid usually induces an urticarial immediate type I reaction and rarely produces a type IV contact allergy. There are reports of mixed sensitivities; one patient was allergic to semen and latex and another to her husband's semen and sweat [1,2]. However, semen itself may not be the responsible allergen, the problem being caused by a medication or other allergen carried in the seminal fluid [3–5].

Epidemiology

Associated diseases
There is often a history of atopy.

Clinical features

History
The history is helpful diagnostically since immediate swelling of the vulva will occur. A condom will abolish the symptoms if the patient is allergic to semen but will cause the problem if latex is the relevant allergen.

Presentation
Immediate swelling occurs during or just after intercourse.

Differential diagnosis
Pressure urticaria can cause identical clinical features but occurs with or without a condom and dermographism elsewhere is usually seen.

Investigations
Intradermal testing with appropriate precautions can be done for semen allergy. Serological tests for latex can be used.

Management
Remove the cause – for instance, use non-latex condoms if the patient is latex allergic. Antigenic treatment of semen before artificial insemination has resulted in successful pregnancy if there is semen allergy [6]. Patients need referral to a specialized allergy or immunology centre.

Lichen simplex

Synonyms and inclusions
- Lichen simplex chronicus
- Lichenification
- Neurodermatitis

Introduction and general description
Lichen simplex is used to describe the changes seen on apparently normal skin secondary to rubbing the skin in response to itch, although the provoking symptom of itch may be initiated by a low-grade dermatosis. The term lichenification is used for similar changes arising on a background of a visible dermatosis (see also Chapter 83).

Epidemiology

Associated diseases
Lichen simplex occurs more commonly in patients who have a background of psoriasis or eczema.

Pathophysiology

Pathology
There is hyperkeratosis, acanthosis, a prominent granular layer, lengthened rete ridges and a chronic inflammatory dermal infiltrate. In addition, lamellar thickening of the papillary dermis and perineural fibrosis can be seen. Twelve cases of what was termed multinucleated atypia of the vulva have been reported [1], but this is thought to be a non-specific change found in lichenified skin [2,3].

Clinical features

History
The patient describes intense itching which may keep them awake at night. This often starts on the vulva but frequently spreads to involve the perineum and perianal skin.

Presentation
There are localized, thickened plaques, most commonly affecting the outer labia majora (Figure 112.17). The perianal skin is frequently

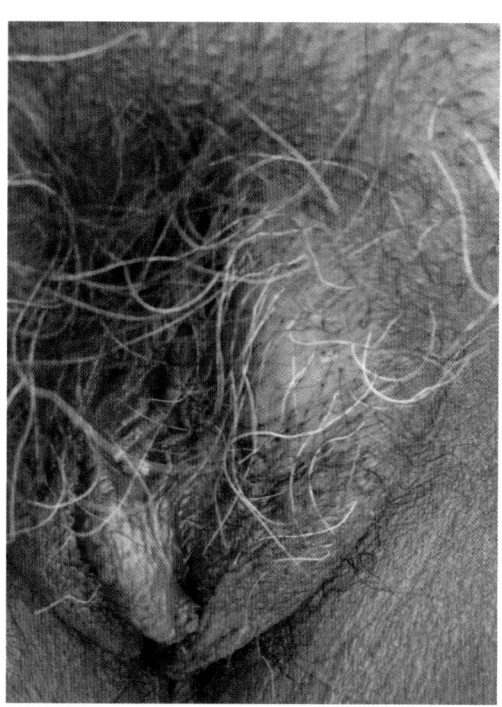

Figure 112.17 Lichen simplex.

involved. The epidermis becomes ridged and the trauma of continued rubbing can lead to hair loss in hair-bearing skin.

Differential diagnosis

It is always important to exclude an underlying dermatosis where the lichenification may be a secondary phenomenon.

Disease course and prognosis

In many cases, patients respond well to appropriate treatment but some enter a chronic itch–scratch–itch cycle that is more challenging to treat. Dysaesthesia may develop when the lichenification has resolved.

Investigations

The diagnosis is usually made on clinical grounds but if there are atypical features or a failure to respond to treatment, a biopsy will be helpful.

In cases where an allergic contact dermatitis trigger is suspected, patch testing is useful, but is not done routinely.

Management

Treatment ladder

First line

- Emollients and a potent topical steroid on a reducing regimen over 2–3 months. The symptoms may improve quickly but there is often relapse if the treatment is stopped before the lichenification has resolved

Second line

- Sedative antihistamines at night, e.g. hydroxyzine 25–50 mg

Third line

- Doxepin, low-dose tricylics in increasing doses, e.g. 10 mg nocte and increasing by 10 mg increments every 3–4 weeks

---

Psoriasis

Synonyms and inclusions
- Flexural psoriasis
- Inverse psoriasis
- Intertriginous psoriasis

Introduction and general description

Psoriasis may affect the ano-genital area as part of generalized disease but can occur in isolation (see also Chapter 35).

Epidemiology

Incidence and prevalence

Vulval psoriasis is said to account for up to 5% of patients who present with persistent vulval symptoms [1]. In one study, 64.9%

of patients presenting with vulval psoriasis were found to have psoriasis elsewhere [2]. Patients often find the problem embarrassing and do not consult readily about the issues [3].

Associated diseases

Many patients with lichen sclerosus are also noted to have psoriasis [4,5].

Pathophysiology

Pathology

Flexural psoriasis does not always have the typical histological features of psoriasis seen elsewhere and there may be marked spongiosis and papillary oedema.

Environmental factors

Friction and occlusion are important aggravating factors in vulval psoriasis.

Clinical features

History

Most patients complain of itching but soreness and pain can occur, particularly if the lesions become fissured. Dyspareunia may also be a feature, which can have an impact on sexual function [6].

Presentation

Well-demarcated erythematous plaques are seen on the labia majora, and extension on to the mons pubis, inguinal folds, perianal skin and gluteal cleft is common (Figure 112.18). The typical silvery scale seen elsewhere is lost but may be seen on the mons. Rarely, there may be some scarring associated with vulval psoriasis, with loss of the labia minora [7].

Differential diagnosis

Seborrhoeic eczema and intertrigo can have very similar clinical features. Extramammary Paget disease occasionally has psoriasiform features.

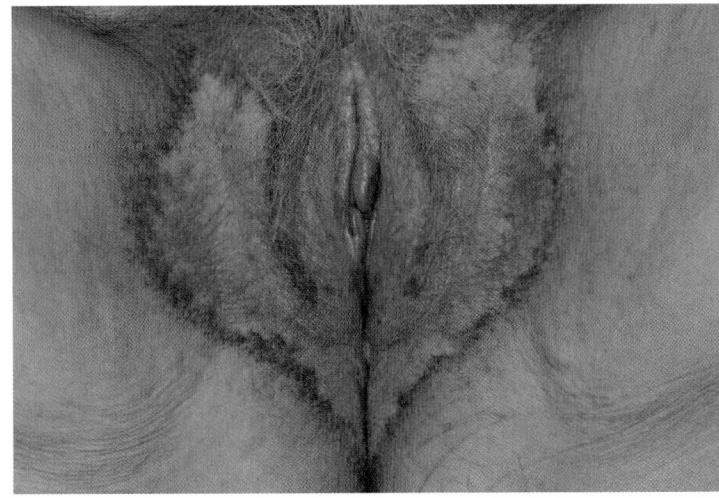

Figure 112.18 Vulval psoriasis.

Disease course and prognosis

Ano-genital psoriasis generally runs a chronic course. It is reported that over 90% of adult and children respond to treatment but this may need to be used intermittently to control the disease [2].

Investigations

Psoriasis is usually diagnosed clinically and a biopsy is rarely needed. Swabs may be required if there is extensive fissuring and evidence of secondary infection.

Management

Treatment ladder

First line
- Emollients and moderately potent topical steroid once daily on a reducing regimen [8]

Second line
- Calcineurin inhibitors
- Calcipotriol (but with care because of irritancy)
- Weak coal tar preparations

Third line
- Systemic agents and biologics may be used if severe, but these are rarely necessary for isolated genital disease. There is one report of the successful use of dapsone in flexural psoriasis [9]

Resources

Patient resources

International Society for the Study of Vulvo-vaginal Disease information sheet: http:// issvd.org/wordpress/wp-content/uploads/2012/04/VulvarPsoriasis2010. pdf.

Psoriasis Association: www.psoriasis-association.org.uk.

(Both last accessed June 2014.)

Reactive arthritis

Definition and nomenclature

Reactive arthritis is the triad of polyarthritis (of over a month's duration following gastrointestinal or lower genital tract infection), urethritis and non-gonococcal conjunctivitis. A scaly and erosive dermatosis of the vulva may accompany the above features.

Synonyms and inclusions
- Circinate vulvo-vaginitis
- Reiter syndrome

Epidemiology

Sex

Genital lesions are rare in women.

Pathophysiology

Pathology

Histology shows hyperkeratosis and parakeratosis, an absent granular layer and prominent neutrophil epidermal microabscesses.

Causative organisms

Shigella dysentery (*Shigella flexneri* and *S. dysenteriae*) were the first infections to be associated with reactive arthritis, but species of *Salmonella*, *Yersinia*, *Campylobacter*, *Streptococcus* and *Mycoplasma* have all been associated with the disease. Sexually transmitted infections with *Chlamydia trachomatis* may also lead to reactive arthritis.

Genetics

It is more likely to occur in HLA-B27-positive individuals and also those with HLA-B51 positivity.

Clinical features

Presentation

Scaling, crusting and erosions are seen and the whole vulva may be involved including the mucosa [1]. A rash on the hands and feet that is indistinguishable from psoriasis is often present.

Differential diagnosis

The vulval lesions in reactive arthritis may resemble psoriasis and candidiasis.

Complications and co-morbidities

Cervicitis may develop.

Disease course and prognosis

The disease may follow a relapsing course. It is more difficult to control in patients with HIV infection.

Investigations

Associated infection must be sought. A biopsy may also be informative.

Management

Management should be shared with rheumatology, especially in complex cases. Any infection should be treated and this may require the input of a genito-urinary specialist.

Treatment ladder

First line
- Potent topical steroids

Second line
- Systemic agents such as methotrexate may be needed

ULCERATIVE AND BULLOUS DISORDERS

The differential diagnosis of genital ulceration is wide and an accurate diagnosis involves careful history taking, clinical examination and appropriate microbiological and histological investigation. The major causes of vulval ulceration are listed in Table 112.2 and many are discussed fully elsewhere in this book.

Aphthous ulcers

Introduction and general description
Aphthous ulcers are recurrent, often multiple, small ulcers affecting the oral and genital mucosa.

Table 112.2 Causes of vulval ulcers.

1 Genetic
Epidermolysis bullosa
Acantholytic dermatoses

2 Infective

Non-sexually transmitted	*Sexually transmitted*
Herpes simplex/zoster	Chancroid
Epstein–Barr virus, HIV	Lymphogranuloma venereum
Tuberculosis, actinomycosis, amoebiasis	Granuloma inguinale
Leishmaniasis, schistosomiasis	Syphilis

3 Inflammatory

Bullous	*Non-bullous*
Autoimmune bullous disorders	Aphthae
Erythema multiforme	Lichen sclerosus/lichen planus
Stevens–Johnson syndrome/toxic epidermal necrolysis	Crohn disease
	Behçet disease
	Lupus erythematosus
	Graft-versus-host disease
	Pyoderma gangrenosum
	Hidradenitis suppurativa
	Drug reactions, fixed drug eruptions, foscarnet, nicorandil
	Rheumatoid nodule
	Reactive arthritis

4 Tumours

Malignant	*Benign*
Squamous cell carcinoma/vulval intraepithelial neoplasia	Capillary haemangioma
Extramammary Paget disease	
Basal cell carcinoma	
Cutaneous lymphoma/leukaemia	
Langerhans cell histiocytosis	
Melanoma	

5 Trauma
Blunt/sharp accidental/non-accidental trauma
Chemical – irritant contact dermatitis
Dermatitis artefacta
Radiation damage
Nympho-hymenal tears

Epidemiology

Age
The age of onset is in childhood, and there may be a family history.

Clinical features

History
There is acute onset of painful ulcers, and oral ulcers may be concurrent. Sometimes there are premenstrual exacerbations once the menarche is reached.

Presentation
The lesions are usually multiple, small (2–10 mm), superficial and painful. They are sited most frequently on the labia minora. They have a yellow base surrounded by a red rim and tend to heal quickly. Less commonly aphthous ulcers are solitary or few in number. Larger ulcers are referred to as giant aphthae.

Differential diagnosis
Herpes simplex and Behçet's ulcers are similar.

Disease course and prognosis
Lesions frequently recur in some patients.

Investigations
The diagnosis is clinical.

Management
Topical steroids and local anaesthetic preparations are helpful.

Lipschutz ulceration

Synonyms and inclusions
• Ulcus vulvae acutum

Introduction and general description
These are acute vulval ulcers presenting in young girls, usually as a reactive phenomenon to infection. They were first described by Lipschutz in 1913 [1].

Epidemiology

Age
These ulcers typically occur in teenagers and young adults [2].

Pathophysiology

Causative organisms
They have been most commonly linked with Epstein–Barr virus infection, which has been isolated from the ulcers in some cases [3,4]. Typhoid, paratyphoid fever and mumps have also been associated [5].

Clinical features

History

The onset is acute with rapidly expanding, and very painful, vulval ulcers. There may be a history of preceding systemic illness or sore throat.

Presentation

The lesions start as haemorrhagic blisters and then enlarge and ulcerate. The base is covered by thick slough. They are usually located on the lower inner labia majora amd may be bilateral ('kissing' ulcers).

Differential diagnosis

Major aphthae and Behçet's ulcers can have similar features. One case mimicked a lymphoma [6].

Disease course and prognosis

The ulcers heal spontaneously over a few weeks. Recurrence is uncommon.

Investigations

Viral serology may be helpful. The diagnosis is usually clinical.

Management

Small ulcers can be treated with a moderately potent topical steroid. 5% lidocaine ointment and oral analgesia are helpful in relieving symptoms. Larger lesions may require a short course of oral prednisolone (e.g. 15–20 mg/day for 10 days).

Behçet disease

Definition

Behçet disease is a multisystem disease with ulceration affecting the mucous membranes and is associated with systemic features (see also Chapter 48).

Clinical features

Presentation

The vulval ulcers seen in Behçet disease are recurrent, deep and heal with scarring after a few weeks. They can occur on the labia minora and majora and may be accompanied by some oedema. Vaginal ulcers have been reported [1].

Differential diagnosis

Initially, the genital ulcers can have similar features to simple aphthae and herpes simplex, but are larger and more persistent.

Investigations

Patients need full investigation for manifestations at other sites.

Management

Topical steroids are helpful initially for the genital ulcers. Management requires a multidisciplinary approach and is discussed elsewhere.

Immunobullous disease

Synonyms and inclusions
- Mucous membrane pemphigoid
- Cicatricial pemphigoid
- Linear IgA disease of children
- Chronic bullous disease of childhood

Introduction and general description

The features of those diseases that commonly affect the genital area in females will be covered here – bullous pemphigoid (BP), mucous membrane pemphigoid (MMP), pemphigus vulgaris (PV), epidermolysis bullosa acquisita (EBA) and linear IgA disease.

Epidemiology

Incidence and prevalence

Genital involvement is common in BP and MMP, where 50% of adults with these conditions will have vulval involvement [1]. In those with linear IgA disease, 50% of adults and 80% of children will have vulval lesions.

Clinical features

Presentation

See Table 112.3 for the clinical presentations of immunobullous diseases on the vulva.

Differential diagnosis

Erosive lichen planus and lichen sclerosus can show similar scarring to MMP. It is also important to exclude herpes simplex in the early stages.

Complications and co-morbidities

Scarring of the vulva and vagina can occur in mucous membrane pemphigoid.

Investigations

Investigations are the same as for autoimmune bullous disease on extragenital skin.

Table 112.3 Clinical presentation of immunobullous disease on the vulva.

	Bullous pemphigoid	Mucous membrane pemphigoid	Pemphigus vulgaris	Linear IgA	Epidermolysis bullosa acquisita
Age	Elderly	Adults, uncommon in children	Usually middle aged	Children and adults	Rare; adults and children
Clinical features	Tense fluid-filled bullae	Vaginal lesions common with scarring	Flaccid bullae, painful erosions. Vaginal disease can cause a discharge [2]	Tense bullae, may be clustered in children	Tense bullae

Management

Topical steroids and potassium permanganate soaks for open, eroded areas are helpful, but most patients will require systemic therapy as for diseases at other sites.

PIGMENTARY DISORDERS

Vitiligo

Definition

This is an acquired disorder characterized by loss of pigmentation in the skin and hair (see also Chapter 88).

Clinical features

History

Asymptomatic areas of hypopigmentation are noticed.

Presentation

There is complete depigmentation of the skin, which is otherwise normal. The edge is well defined and the outer labia majora are usually affected. There may be extension into the inguinal folds and perianal skin. In hair-bearing skin, the hair may also lose its colour (poliosis).

Differential diagnosis

The major differential diagnosis is lichen sclerosus but there is no architectural change in vitiligo and the texture of the skin is normal. The pallor sometimes seen in lichenification can also mimic vitiligo.

Complications and co-morbidities

Vitiligo and lichen sclerosus can coexist.

Management

No treatment is needed and treatment modalities used at other sites (e.g. psoralen and UVA) are inappropriate on the genital skin.

Vulval melanosis

Definition and nomenclature

Vulval melanosis is characterized by hyperpigmented lesions in the absence of any previous cause. There is no increase in melanocytes [1].

Synonyms and inclusions
• Idiopathic lenticular mucocutaneous pigmentation

Epidemiology

Age

Vulval melanosis is seen more commonly in young women.

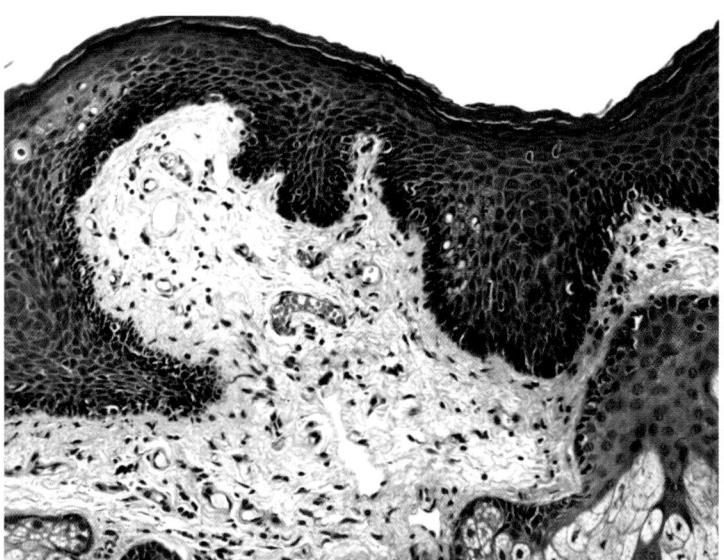

Figure 112.19 Histological features of vulval melanosis.

Pathophysiology

Pathology

There is basal cell layer hyperpigmentation but no increase in the number of melanocytes. Pigmentary incontinence and pigment-rich macrophages may be seen in the dermis (Figure 112.19).

Clinical features

History

Melanosis is asymptomatic and usually an incidental finding.

Presentation

The lesions are usually multifocal (a single lesion would be termed a genital melanotic macule) and often irregular and asymmetrical (Figure 112.20). The colour may vary. They are most common on the inner labia minora and vestibule but the vagina and cervix may also be involved [2]. There may be similar lesions on the oral mucosa.

Differential diagnosis

The main differential diagnosis is from genital lentigines, but this term is used when there are increased numbers of melanocytes. The clinical appearance can mimic melanoma. Melanosis is often darker than postinflammatory hyperpigmentation.

Disease course and prognosis

Melanoma has not been reported in vulva melanosis and the accepted view is that vulval melanosis is a benign condition, but there are no long-term follow-up studies.

Investigations

The diagnosis is easily confirmed on vulval biopsy.

Management

Most clinicians advise continuing observation, using photographs or diagrams as an aid.

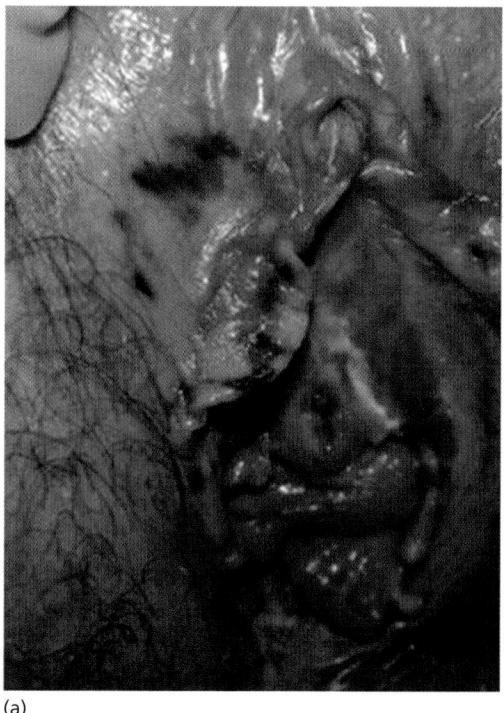
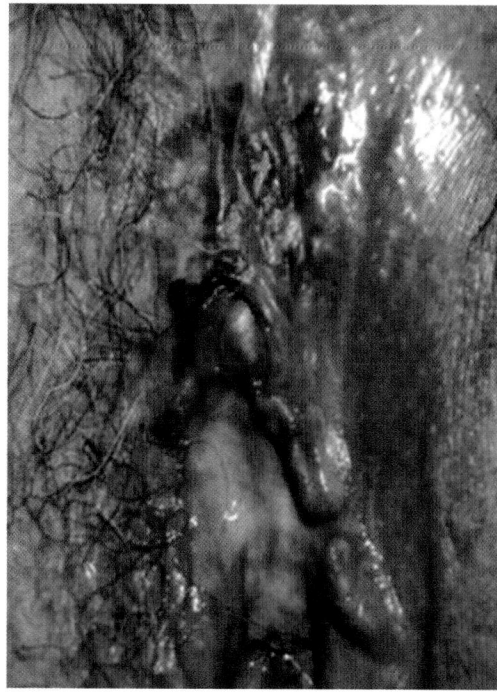

Figure 112.20 (a) *In situ* melanoma. (b) Vulval melanosis.   (a)   (b)

Acanthosis nigricans

Definition

Acanthosis nigricans is characterized by hyperpigmentation and thickening of the skin, particularly in the flexures.

Epidemiology

Associated diseases

Acanthosis nigricans is associated with insulin resistance in almost all cases. In adults, it can be a cutaneous sign of an underlying malignancy, usually an adenocarcinoma. If linked with malignancy, the onset and progression is rapid and unusual sites such as the eyelids, lips and palms (tripe palms) may be involved.

Clinical features

Presentation

The genital area is almost always involved [1] and velvety, dark plaques are seen on the labia majora, extending into the inguinal folds. These then develop a warty texture and skin tags are common on the plaques.

Differential diagnosis

Pseudo acanthosis nigricans may be seen in obese patients and is related to moisture, friction and subsequent maceration. Epidermal naevi may have similar clinical and histological features but are unlikely to occur at several sites.

Investigations

The diagnosis can be made clinically and confirmed on biopsy. Referral for endocrine investigation is important to investigate insulin resistance. If there is a rapid onset or unusual features in an adult, then a potential associated malignancy should be sought.

Management

Keratolytics, retinoids and laser treatment have all been tried. These may be irritant in the genital skin.

Dowling–Degos disease

Definition and nomenclature

This condition is characterized by reticulate pigmentation in the flexures.

Synonyms and inclusions
• Reticulated pigmented anomaly of the flexures

Epidemiology

Age

Lesions typically appear in the third or fourth decade of life.

Pathophysiology

Pathology

Irregular elongation of the rete ridges is seen with melanin at the tips. The number of melanocytes is not increased.

Genetics
It is probably inherited in an autosomal dominant pattern.

Clinical features

History
Dowling–Degos disease is asymptomatic.

Presentation
Reticulate pigmentation is seen on the vulva, which may be involved in isolation rarely [1] or as part of more widespread disease [2].

Clinical variants
Galli–Galli disease has acantholysis as a feature.

Differential diagnosis
Simple lentigines and the postinflammatory pigmentation seen with lichen planus have similar clinical features. Multiple genital lentigines are occasionally features of Laugier–Hunziker disease, Carney's complex or LAMB syndrome (lentigines, atrial myxoma, mucocutaneous myxomas, blue naevi).

Investigations
A skin biopsy will show typical histological features.

Management
Depigmenting agents, adapalene and laser treatment have been reported to be successful in individual cases [3].

VULVAL OEDEMA

The causes of vulval oedema are generally classified into acute and chronic (Table 112.4) [1], and most cases are due to leakage through the capillaries. The skin of the vulva is lax and fluid easily accumulates.

Table 112.4 Causes of vulval oedema.

Acute causes	Chronic causes
Inflammatory dermatoses, e.g. acute eczema	Primary lymphoedema secondary to congenital lymphatic hypoplasia
Infections, e.g. candidiasis	Crohn disease
Urticaria – pressure urticaria after intercourse	Hidradenitis suppurativa
Type 1 allergy (see allergic contact urticaria)	Infections, e.g. filariasis
Ovarian hyperstimulation syndrome	Lymphangioma – lymphangioma circumscriptum [2] and cavernous lymphangioma [3]
Pre-eclampsia	Malignancy
	Post-radiotherapy or lymphadenectomy
	Cyclist's vulva [4]

Crohn disease

Definition
Crohn disease is an inflammatory disease of the gastrointestinal tract.

Introduction and general description
Vulval disease may present many years before intestinal involvement, and in some cases there is vulval oedema only, with no evidence of granulomatous inflammation [1,2,3].

Epidemiology

Incidence and prevalence
Ano-genital lesions may occur in about 30% of patients with gastrointestinal Crohn disease. This may either be by direct extension or by so-called 'metastatic' disease. However, it can occur in patients without any bowel involvement and the cutaneous lesions may precede it.

Age
The average age of presentation is in the fourth decade but it has been reported in children [4].

Associated diseases
Crohn disease may be associated with pyoderma gangrenosum, erythema nodosum and a leukocytoclastic vasculitis.

Pathophysiology

Pathology
Initially only dermal oedema and lymphangiectasia may be seen. Non-caseating granulomas occur later with features of ulceration in more severe disease.

Clinical features

History
The patient may simply complain of vulval oedema initially but soreness, pain and discharge occurs in more severe disease.

Presentation
Oedema may be the initial finding, which may be unilateral and generally affects the labia majora first. Ulceration, erosions, abscesses, sinuses and fistulae can form and the classic feature is that of deep linear fissures (knife cut sign) along the skin creases.

Clinical variants
A separate form of vulval granuloma akin to the oro-facial lesions seen in Melkersson–Rosenthal syndrome has been described [5,6].

Differential diagnosis
Hidradenitis suppurativa is the main differential diagnosis and there are some patients with features of both conditions.

Complications and co-morbidities
Bowen disease has been reported to occur in Crohn disease [7] and rarely squamous cell carcinoma [8].

Disease course and prognosis

The disease follows a chronic course with secondary infection being a common feature. The oedema may become firm and fixed.

Investigations

A biopsy may be helpful, but may show only oedema.

Management

If genital Crohn disease is the presenting problem it is important to involve a gastroenterologist in management, as these patients need a full work-up to assess if there is intestinal disease as well. In ulcerative disease it is essential to exclude any fistulous tracts. In patients who have no systemic disease, topical measures may be sufficient to control the cutaneous lesions, that is the use of an super-potent topical steroid or topical tacrolimus [9]. Severe disease may respond to oral steroids but recalcitrant ulcerative ano-genital lesions and fistulous tracts may require infliximab [10].

NON-SEXUALLY TRANSMITTED INFECTIONS

The majority of infections in the ano-genital area are sexually acquired and these are dealt with elsewhere. Non-sexually acquired routes of infection include transfer by touch, fomites or contact with contaminated water. Threadworms and *Candida* species may spread from the anus.

DIAGNOSIS OF VAGINAL DISCHARGE

The diagnosis usually falls into one of the categories seen in Table 112.5. If an infective cause is suspected, the patient shoud be referred to a genitourinary clinic for full evaluation and management.

Table 112.5 Causes of vaginal discharge.

Cause	Example	Clinical features
Physiological	Excess physiological secretion of mucus, usually resulting from cervical erosion or an increase in the amount of vaginal transudate	The discharge is thick, with a grey-white appearance, and is odourless and non-irritant. Vaginal pH is normal
Iatrogenic	Tamoxifen, oral contraceptive pills, danthron [1]	
Infective	Bacterial vaginosis	pH usually >6. Grey, watery discharge with fishy odour
	Infective cervicitis (gonorrhoea, Chlamydia, herpes simplex, trichomonas)	Associated with deep pelvic pain
	Threadworms [2]	
Inflammatory	Erosive lichen planus, pemphigus	Chronic odourless discharge, which may be blood-tinged. Postcoital bleeding may occur
Neoplastic	Tumours of fallopian tubes, uterus, cervix and vagina	

Resources

Patient resources

International Society for the Study of Vulvo-vaginal Disease information sheets: http://issvd.org/wordpress/wp-content/uploads/2012/04/VaginalDischarge2010.pdf; http://issvd.org/wordpress/wp-content/uploads/2012/04/Vaginitis2010.pdf (both last accessed June 2014).

BACTERIAL INFECTIONS

Staphylococcal infections

Introduction and general description

Staphylococcus aureus is usually the causative agent in infective folliculitis, boils and abscesses of the vulva (see also Chapter 26). Panton–Valentine leukocidin *S. aureus* infection [1] can cause infection in the ano-genital skin.

Epidemiology

Associated diseases

Staphylococcal infection is often associated with diabetes and immunosuppression.

Pathophysiology

Predisposing factors

Shaving and waxing to remove hair can predispose to folliculitis.

Pathology

The impetiginous lesion shows subcorneal pustules filled with neutrophils and some spongiosis, with a moderate inflammatory response in the papillary dermis. Acute folliculitis may be superficial, with a subcorneal pustule present at the follicular opening, or be deep and associated with a perifollicular abscess and destruction of the follicle wall and sebaceous gland. Chronic deep intrafollicular abscesses may have the additional features of fibrosis and foreign body giant cells.

Causative organisms

Staphylococcus aureus is the most common bacteria to cause folliculitis and furunculosis.

Clinical features

Clinical variants

A staphylococcal folliculitis on the buttocks may occur secondary to the pruritus induced by intestinal infestation with pinworm.

Menstrual toxic shock syndrome is caused by *S. aureus* superantigenic toxins and is associated with fever, hypotension and macular erythema. In the 1980s, retained tampons were a common focus of infection but this is now rare.

Staphylococcal scalded skin syndrome is a toxin-mediated infection and the flexural areas may often be the first to be involved.

An abscess of the Bartholin gland caused by acute infection of the duct may be caused by *S. aureus*.

PART 10: SITES, SEX, AGE

Differential diagnosis

Pseudofolliculitis is a sterile folliculitis that may follow shaving or waxing and is caused by the newly regrowing hairs inducing an inflammatory reaction. It is a foreign body reaction and results in changes from mild inflammation to the formation of abscesses and sinuses.

Investigations

Microscopy and culture of lesional swabs will confirm the diagnosis. If recurrent, exclude staphylococcal carriage at other body sites.

Management

Topical antibiotics may be sufficient for mild folliculitis with antibacterial washes. Oral or intravenous antibiotics are required for more severe or widespread infection.

Streptococcal infections

Introduction and general description

Group B haemolytic streptococcal species are commonly found as commensals in the vulva and vagina, and do not cause symptoms [1]. Group A species can cause cellulitis and more severe infections such as necrotizing fasciitis (see also Chapter 26).

Pathophysiology

Causative organisms

Streptococcus pyogenes and other β-haemolytic Lancefield group A bacteria are the usual cause of vulval cellulitis. *Streptococcus faecalis* may cause Bartholin abscesses.

Clinical features

Clinical variants

- *Vulval cellulitis.* The erythema and oedema may be extreme, and vesicles and bullae develop. There are usually associated systemic features. The infection arises at sites of trauma and is most commonly seen following a vulvectomy with lymphadenectomy. If there is residual lymphoedema then further attacks of cellulitis are more common.
- *Streptococcal dermatitis.* This usually affects the ano-genital area of children.
- Necrotizing fasciitis (synergistic bacterial gangrene). This severe, rapidly extending and life-threatening disease is caused by the synergistic effect of a microaerophilic *Streptococcus* and *Staphylococcus aureus.* Anaerobes and Gram-negative bacilli may also be involved.

Differential diagnosis

It is important to distinguish more severe infection from pyoderma gangrenosum.

Investigations

Microscopy and culture of the lesion confirms the diagnosis. In severe infection, blood cultures may be positive.

Management

Appropriate antibiotic therapy and supportive care is needed in severe infections. Immediate surgical debridement is needed in necrotizing fasciitis.

Mycobacterial infections

Synonyms and inclusions
- Genital tuberculosis
- Leprosy

Introduction and general description

Tuberculosis of the female genital tract is not uncommon in endemic areas (see also Chapter 27). Vulval lesions are rare and the upper genital tract is most commonly affected [1].

Pathophysiology

Predisposing factors

Genital tuberculosis is more common in HIV-positive patients and has been reported in a renal transplant patient [2].

Causative organisms

Mycobacterium tuberculosis is the cause of tuberculosis and occurs by haematogenous spread from foci outside the genital tract, by distal spread from the upper genital tract, or as a primary exogenous infection contracted from sputum or sexual intercourse.

Mycobacterium leprae causes leprosy.

Clinical features

Presentation

In a primary infection the initial lesion may be inconspicuous, the main feature being a caseating lymphadenopathy. In other cases the lesions are masses or nodules that may ulcerate and lead to lymphoedema. Bartholin's gland may be involved.

Vulval lesions are rare in leprosy [3] and may present with loss of pubic hair.

Investigations

Investigation is similar to that at other sites.

Management

Management of both tuberculosis and leprosy requires specialist input from infectious disease specialists.

Malakoplakia

Definition

Malakoplakia results from an atypical inflammatory response to *Escherichia coli* or other pathogens.

Epidemiology

Associated diseases
There is often underlying immunosuppression, the aetiology of which may include malignancy, dermatomyositis [1], lupus erythematosus, rheumatoid arthritis and organ transplantation [2].

Pathophysiology

Predisposing factors
Malakoplakia is due to macrophage dysfunction, and primary or acquired immunodeficiency is common [3].

Pathology
There are confluent sheets of histiocytes with eosinophilic granular cytoplasm and small eccentric nuclei. Round, sometimes laminated, structures are found with these cells and are known as Michaelis–Gutmann bodies. The histiocytic infiltrate may be mixed with neutrophils, lymphocytes and plasma cells, with associated granulation tissue. Electron microscopy of malakoplakia shows that the histiocytes contain numerous phagolysosomes within which there may be occasional intact and partly digested bacteria.

Causative organisms
It is not usually caused by one specific agent but the organisms involved include *Escherichia coli*, *Pseudomonas* and *Staphylococcus aureus*.

Clinical features

Presentation
Malakoplakia most often affects the urinary or gastrointestinal tract but cutaneous lesions may occur on the vagina, vulva and perineum. Involvement of Bartholin's gland has been described [4]. The lesions include persistent plaques, ulcers, nodules and sinuses. Vaginal lesions may bleed.

Differential diagnosis
Crohn disease, hidradenitis supurativa and malignancy may have similar features.

Investigations
A culture of lesions and histology will confirm the diagnosis.

Management
Long-term antibiotics are needed and surgery may be required for the sinuses.

Other bacterial infections

Synonyms and inclusions
- Actinomycosis
- *Mycoplasma* infection

Introduction and general description
Some higher bacteria will cause genital infections, primarily actinomycosis species and *Mycoplasma* organisms.

Pathophysiology

Predisposing factors
Genital infection usually arises from bowel disease [1], but isolated lesions of the vulva have been reported.

Causative organisms
The Gram-positive acid-fast organisms responsible for actinomycosis are predominantly *Actinomyces israelii* and *A. gerencseriae*.
Mycoplasma hominis and *Ureaplasma urealyticum* are found in the vagina and rarely cause disease. There are rare reports of *M. hominis* being isolated from cases of Bartholin abscess [2,3].

Clinical features

Presentation
Actinomycosis organisms may colonize intrauterine devices and are usually asymptomatic, but invasion of the genital tract can occur [4,5].

Investigations
Culture of lesional skin and histology are needed.

Management
Penicillin is the treatment of choice, and treatment may need to be prolonged. Tetracyclines, clindamycin and erythromycin are alternative agents.

FUNGAL INFECTIONS

Candidal vulvo-vaginitis

Synonyms and inclusions
- Thrush infection
- Yeast infection

Introduction and general description
Candida albicans causes vulvo-vaginitis and 75% of women will experience at least one episode (see also Chapter 32).

Epidemiology

Incidence and prevalence
Vulvo-vaginal candidiasis is the second most common genital infection (bacterial vaginosis being the commonest) in the western world [1].

Age
It is rare before menarche and is most prevalent in the third and fourth decades.

Pathophysiology

Predisposing factors

Pregnancy, diabetes, possibly oral antibiotics, high-dose oestrogen oral contraceptive pills and immunosuppression may all be predisposing factors.

Causative organisms

Candida and *Torulopsis* are both yeasts that can infect the vulva and vagina. *Torulopsis* accounts for very few infections, whereas *Candida albicans* is the most frequently isolated and accounts for 90% of symptomatic episodes. It is a non-pathogenic commensal in the gastrointestinal tract in 30% of the normal population.

Changes in host factors and cell-mediated immunity are important in the transition to pathogenicity.

Clinical features

History

The major symptom is pruritus. Some patients may report vulval swelling.

Presentation

The primary infection arises in the vagina, causing inflammation and a heavy, white, curdy discharge, which then leads to a secondary vulvitis with well-demarcated sheets of erythema on the outer aspects of the vulva, sometimes extending on occasions into the genito-crural folds and perianally. There may be a scaly or vesiculopustular edge. Beyond this edge lie grouped or isolated superficial small pustules, which rupture rapidly, leaving a slightly scaly periphery.

Differential diagnosis

Eczema and flexural psoriasis may have similar appearances.

Complications and co-morbidities

In some cases of vulval eczema and psoriasis, *Candida* is cultured from skin swabs but the candidal overgrowth is a secondary problem arising on a background of an inflamed epithelium. Treating the dermatosis alone with a topical steroid will usually resolve the problem, without the addition of anticandidal agents.

Investigations

The diagnosis is confirmed by direct microscopy and culture. In resistant and recurrent infection, swabs for species and sensitivities are indicated.

Management

Treatment of vulvo-vaginal candidiasis requires vaginal pessaries or creams and/or oral imidazoles. In those patients with recurrent infection, it is always important to consider diabetes.

Resources

Further information

British Association for Sexual Health and HIV guidelines on the management of vulvo-vaginal candidiasis: http://www.bashh.org/documents/1798.pdf (last accessed June 2014).

Patient resources

International Society for the Study of Vulvo-vaginal Disease information sheet: http://issvd.org/wordpress/wp-content/uploads/2012/04/Candidiasis2010.pdf (last accessed June 2014).

Tinea cruris

Definition

Tinea cruris is a dermatophyte infection affecting the inguinal folds, which may extend to the vulva and perianal area (see also Chapter 32).

Epidemiology

Sex

Fungal infection in the genital area is more common in men.

Pathophysiology

Predisposing factors

Heat, occlusion and humidity predispose to this infection.

Causative organisms

The causative agents are *Trichophyton rubrum* and *Epidermophyton floccosum*.

Clinical features

History

The rash is usually itchy.

Presentation

The lesions are erythematous and scaly, with a spreading serpiginous edge (Figure 112.21). Folliculitis is also seen, particularly in the perianal area. Tinea incognito may also occur perianally following the inappropriate use of a topical steroid in the presence of an unrecognized dermatophyte infection.

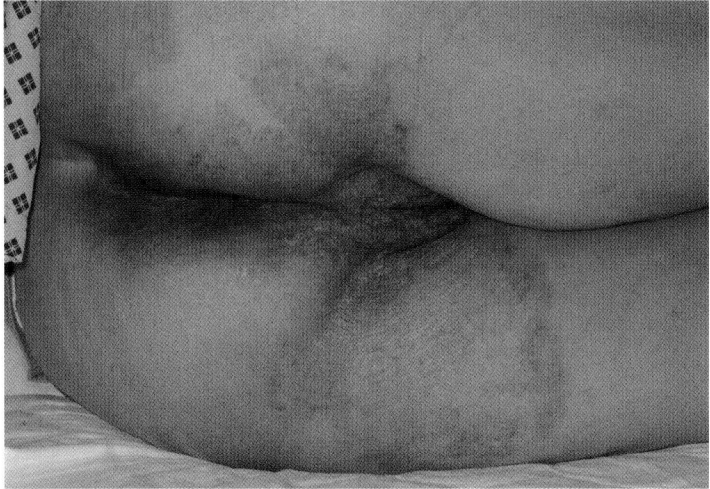

Figure 112.21 Tinea cruris.

Differential diagnosis

Flexural psoriasis, eczema, erythrasma and candidiasis are the major differential diagnoses.

Pityriasis versicolor classically occurs on the trunk, but in severe widespread infection there may be vulval involvement [1,2].

Complications and co-morbidities

Deep fungal infections are rare but have been reported with *Microsporum canis* infection [3]. Vulval phycomycosis has been described [4]. Subcutaneous infections occur in children and young adults. Histologically, the epidermis is unremarkable but subcutaneously there are deep granulomatous masses containing hyphae. There is one case report of chromomycosis (chromoblastomycosis) affecting the vulva [5]. *Cryptococcus neoformans* can induce painless ulceration of the vulva in the immunosuppressed patient [6].

Investigations

The diagnosis is usually made by direct microscopy and the culture of skin scrapings.

Management

> **Treatment ladder**
>
> **First line**
> - Topical azoles if non-hair-bearing skin
>
> **Second line**
> - Oral terbinafine 250 mg/day for 4 weeks or itraconazole 200 mg b.d. for 2 weeks

VIRAL INFECTIONS

Three groups of viruses are important causes of infection in the genital area: the poxviruses, papillomaviruses and herpesviruses (see also Chapter 25). Other viruses seldom give rise to distinctive clinical pictures, although vulval lesions may occur as part of a generalized viral infection.

Poxvirus infections

Synonyms and inclusions
- Molluscum contagiosum
- Orf
- Cowpox

Introduction and general description

The most common poxvirus infection of the vulva is molluscum contagiosum but isolated reports of orf [1] and cowpox [2] infection exist (see also Chapter 25).

Epidemiology

Age

Molluscum infection can occur in adults and children.

Pathophysiology

Predisposing factors

Atopic eczema, immunodeficiency, HIV infection and Darier disease can all predispose to mollusum contagiosum.

Causative organisms

Molluscum contagiosum virus (MCV) has four subtypes. MCV I usually causes childhood infection, whereas MCV II is a common cause in adults and is the major type seen in HIV-positive individuals.

Clinical features

Presentation

Lesions are often found on the mons pubis and labia majora, and the typical lesions are small pearly papules with an umbilicated centre. Lesions of molluscum contagiosum can be profuse and large in immunosuppressed women.

Clinical variants

Giant molluscum lesions may occur and these can be mistaken for large genital warts.

Differential diagnosis

They may resemble genital warts and other infections and, if inflamed, mimic folliculitis.

Complications and co-morbidities

Adults with gential molluscum should be offered screening for other sexually transmitted infections.

Disease course and prognosis

The lesions regress spontaneously but may take many months to do so.

Investigations

The diagnosis is usually made clinically. If there is any doubt, then a biopsy will show the classic histological features.

Management

No treatment is needed as lesions will resolve. However, podophyllotoxin [3] and imiquimod [4] have shown cure rates of over 90% in controlled trials. Cryotherapy, curettage and extirpation of the core are other treatments used.

Resources

Further information

British Association for Sexual Health and HIV guidelines on the management of molluscum contagiosum: http://www.bashh.org/documents/26/26.pdf (last accessed June 2014).

Herpes simplex

Epidemiology

Incidence and prevalence
Ninety-five per cent of infections are acquired sexually and the rest are cases of auto-inoculation or non-sexual contact (see also Chapter 25).

Pathophysiology

Causative organisms
Once this sexually transmitted DNA virus is acquired it lies dormant in the dorsal root ganglia and can give rise to recurrent symptomsatic lesions. It exists in two types: I and II. Type I usually affects non-genital sites and type II is responsible for 50–80% of genital infections.

Clinical features

History
There may be prodromal symptoms of tingling or tender, enlarged inguinal nodes. Paraesthesiae may occur, affecting S2–S4, which may lead to urinary retention. Pain and oedema may also lead to retention, particularly in primary infections.

Presentation
The lesions are typically painful vesicles or ulcers, which are often multiple in primary infection but are fewer and usually localized to one side with recurrences. Cervical ulceration may be seen.

Clinical variants
Hypertrophic herpes simplex virus (HSV) infection in immuno-suppressed patients can mimic tumours [1].

Differential diagnosis
Varicella-zoster virus may also affect the vulva if the third sacral dermatome is involved. It may be accompanied by bowel and bladder dysfunction [2].

Cytomegalovirus infection can sometimes resemble herpes simplex. This has been reported in an infant with congenital HIV disease who presented with pustular and ulcerative lesions on the perineum [3].

Complications and co-morbidities
HSV infection is an important co-factor in the transmission of HIV. Autonomic dysfunction can lead to constipation and hyperaesthesia of the perineal and sacral region. Aseptic meningitis is reported in up to 36% of women [4].

Investigations
It is important to obtain a definite diagnosis with a positive culture of HSV, and it is necessary to perform the test as soon as the blisters arise as the virus is harder to culture from older lesions. Polymerase chain reaction (PCR) techniques are increasingly used in diagnosis [5].

Patients should also be screened for other sexually transmitted infections.

Management
The treatment is either oral aciclovir 200 mg five times daily for 5 days, valaciclovir 500 mg twice daily for 5 days or famciclovir 250 mg three times daily for 5 days. Suppressant therapy is sometimes required for patients with frequent recurrences (six or more in a year).

Resources

Further information
British Association for Sexual Health and HIV guidelines on the management of genital herpes: http://www.bashh.org/documents/115/115.pdf (last accessed June 2014).

Patient resources
International Society for the Study of Vulvo-vaginal Disease information sheet: http://issvd.org/wordpress/wp-content/uploads/2012/04/GENITALHerpes2010.pdf (last accessed June 2014).

Human papillomavirus infection

Introduction and general description
Human papillomavirus (HPV) is a small DNA virus, and the types that most commonly infect the vulval skin are HPV 6, 11, 16 and 18 (see also Chapter 25).

Epidemiology

Incidence and prevalence
HPV is the commonest sexually transmitted infection and up to 85% of people will be infected with at least one type in their lifetime.

Age
Warts are more common in the younger age groups after sexual activity starts. If seen in children, this must always raise the possibility of sexual abuse [1].

Associated diseases
Immunosuppressed patients often have more florid infection with lesions that are difficult to treat. They are also at greater risk of developing HPV-related ano-genital cancers.

Pathophysiology

Predisposing factors
There is an increased risk of acquiring genital warts with a higher number of sexual partners, the presence of other sexually transmitted infections and a history of smoking.

Pathology
The histology of genital warts is characterized by the koilocyte, a vacuolated squamous cell with a basophilic and pyknotic nucleus

in the upper part of the epidermis. It is important not to confuse it with the heavily glycogenated clear cells of vestibular epithelium. Other histological features are elongated dermal papillae, acanthosis, a prominent granular layer often containing koilocytes, and a stratum corneum of variable thickness.

Clinical features

Presentation
The warty lesions are known as condylomata acuminate (Figure 112.22). Extensive vegetating masses can cover the vulva and perianal area, particularly in diabetes, pregnancy and immunocompromised patients.

Differential diagnosis
Secondary syphilis may also present with extensive papulosquamous lesions.

Complications and co-morbidities
HPV types 16 and 18 are associated with ano-genital intraepithelial neoplasia and SCC.

Disease course and prognosis
Warts may resolve spontaneously, but may persist and be resistant especially in the immunosuppressed.

Investigations
The diagnosis is usually clinical, but if there are atypical features it is important to exclude vulval intraepithelial neoplasia with histological examination. Patients with genital warts should also be screened for other sexually transmitted infections.

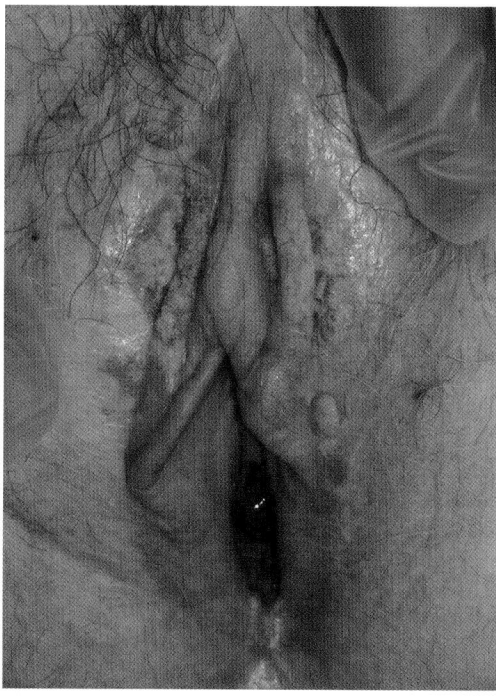

Figure 112.22 Vulval warts with plaques in the interlabial sulci.

Management
Treatment of genital warts is usually undertaken in the setting of a genitourinary clinic. Podophyllotoxin, cryotherapy and destructive treatments are used.

The new immune response modulating cream, imiquimod, is now used for resistant cases or patients with extensive lesions. This has to be used with care as it also induces an inflammatory response in patients who have latent or active dermatitis. It should not be used in patients who have benign vulval aphthous ulcers.

In pregnancy, only cryotherapy or destructive techniques with cautery or hyfrecation can be used safely.

Prophylactic vaccination prior to exposure is now available for HPV types 6, 11, 16 and 18 and has been shown to reduce the incidence of warts and gential intraepithelial neoplasia [2].

Resources

Further information
British Association for Sexual Health and HIV guidelines on the management of ano-genital warts: http://www.bashh.org/documents/86/86.pdf (last accessed June 2014).

BENIGN TUMOURS

The main benign tumours are discussed in this section, with Table 112.6 giving details of some others [1,2,3,4]. Nodular fasciitis [5] and glomus tumours [6,7] are rarely reported.

Mucinous cysts

Introduction and general description
Mucinous cysts occur at the site if there is obstruction of the duct of a minor vestibular gland.

Epidemiology

Age
These occur in adult women and rarely in adolescence.

Pathophysiology
The cysts are of uro-genital sinus origin and not, as was once thought, of Müllerian origin [1,2].

Pathology
The cysts are lined by a layer of mucinous epithelium

Clinical features

Presentation
The lesions present as single or multiple lesions in the vestibule.

Management
Simple excision is curative.

Table 112.6 Other benign tumours of the vulva.

	Fibroma	Fibroepithelial polyps	Epidermal cyst	Lipomas	Verruciform xanthoma [1]	Granular cell myoblastoma [2,3]	Urethral caruncle	Neurofibroma	Leiomyoma	Syringoma [4]
Origin	Deeper connective tissue structures, e.g. introitus, perineal body		Epithelial implants after surgery or at fusion sites during embryogenesis	Fatty tissue of labia majora			Inflamed eversion of urethral mucosa	Solitary or part of generalized neurofibromatosis	Smooth muscle of erectile tissue, round ligament or myoepithelial cells of the Bartholin duct. Not associated with uterine lesions	Adenoma of eccrine sweat glands
Sites	Labia majora		Labia majora		Labia majora usually		Urethral meatus	Labia majora	Labia, clitoris	Labia majora
Clinical features	Penduculated	Soft polypoidal nodules	Single or multiple		Solitary plaque or warty lesion	Flesh coloured, sometimes pedunculated or ulcerated solitary lesion		Painless nodules, can mimic intersex problems	Painless nodules. Can enlarge during pregnancy	Multiple, may be pruritic
Pathology		Fibrovascular core covered by epithelium. Cellular atypia occasionally seen			Acanthosis, papillomatos is and foamy macrophages in papillary dermis		Vascular connective tissue with glardular structures or islands of urethral mucosa in inflamed stroma			Small ducts with comma like tails

Bartholin's cyst

Introduction and general description
Bartholin's cysts are common and arise as a result of obstruction of the main duct of the Bartholin gland.

Epidemiology

Age
These are most common in women of child-bearing age.

Pathophysiology

Pathology
The cyst is lined by transitional epithelium which may exhibit squamous metaplasia.

Clinical features

History
Simple cysts are asymptomatic and the patient may simply notice a lump.

Presentation
The lesions present as swellings 1–3 cm in size on the lower third of the inner labium majus.

Differential diagnosis
Benign or malignant tumours can present in a similar way.

Complications and co-morbidities
If the cysts become infected, then this abscess leads to painful swelling. There is a case report of a squamous cell carcinoma arising within a cyst [1].

Management
The treatment is enucleation of the cyst but if incompletely removed they can recur.

Papillary hidradenoma

Definition and nomenclature
This sweat gland adenoma with apocrine differentiation occurs almost exclusively in the ano-genital region of middle-aged white women [1].

Synonyms and inclusions
• Hidradenoma papilliferum

Epidemiology

Age
These occur in middle-aged women.

Pathophysiology

Pathology
A well-demarcated nodule is seen that is composed of papillary processes that extend into cystic spaces. Periodic acid–Schiff stain (PAS) positive cytoplasmic granules are common.

Clinical features

History
The lesions are often asymptomatic but may be painful.

Presentation
The lesions are 1–2 cm nodules and occur most commonly on the labia majora, interlabial sulcus, lateral surfaces of the labia minora or perineal region [2]. Although usually single, there are occasionally multiple lesions. Curiously, when they are multiple, all the lesions tend to develop on one side of the vulva. In most patients, the covering epidermis remains intact, but in a proportion the elevated epithelium may become ulcerated [3]. Larger lesions are described [4]. They are rarely described on the nipple, eyelid and external auditory meatus.

Complications and co-morbidities
Malignant change within a papillary hidradenoma has been reported, producing apocrine carcinoma [5] and adenosquamous carcinoma [6].

Management
Simple excision is curative.

Cutaneous endometriosis

Introduction and general description
Endometrial deposits on the vulva are rare [1].

Pathophysiology

Pathology
Endometrial glands and stroma are seen.

Clinical features

History
The lesions may be painful and patients may report a variation in size with the menstrual cycle. They may bleed at the same time as menstruation.

Presentation
The lesions present as small, bluish nodules and common sites are the perineum or episiotomy scars and the umbilicus.

Management
Surgical excision is usually curative.

Atypical genital naevi

Synonyms and inclusions
• Atypical melanocytic naevi of genital type

Introduction and general description
All types of naevi can occur on the genital skin but they may show atypical and concerning features, and it is important to be aware of the entity to avoid aggressive treatment (see also Chapter 132).

Epidemiology

Incidence and prevalence
The prevalence of vulval naevi has been estimated as 2.3% in one series [1].

Age
These are most commonly seen in young women, but children and teenagers can be affected as well.

Pathophysiology

Pathology
The histological features of these lesions can be difficult to interpret [2]. They may be asymmetrical with the junctional component often involving the adnexae and exhibiting large nests of cells. The naevoid cells are atypical with this cytological atypia visible in both junctional and dermal parts. Dermal mitoses may be evident.

Clinical features

History
The naevi are asymptomatic and often an incidental finding.

Presentation
The most common sites where naevi develop are the inner aspects of the labia majora, the labia minora and the clitoris.

Differential diagnosis
Melanoma is usually seen in elderly women.

Disease course and prognosis
There are no long-term follow-up studies but these naevi are thought to be benign [3].

Investigations
Histological examination reveals the above findings.

Management
Complete excision is recommended.

PRE-MALIGNANT CONDITIONS

Vulval intraepithelial neoplasia

Synonyms and inclusions
• Bowen disease
• Bowenoid papulosis
• Carcinoma *in situ*
• Carcinoma simplex

Introduction and general description
Vulval intraepithelial neoplasia (VIN) is a non-invasive, premalignant disease that may progress to vulval squamous cell carcinoma. There are two forms (undifferentiated and differentiated) with different aetiologies and prognostic factors. (Table 112.7).

Epidemiology

Incidence and prevalence
The incidence of VIN has been increasing, with an estimated doubling of incidence in undifferentiated VIN (uVIN) to 2.1 per 100 000 population in 2005 [1].

Pathophysiology

Predisposing factors
Smoking is a known risk factor in uVIN. HIV-positive women have an increased incidence and prevalence of both uVIN and vulval cancer [2].

Pathology
Undifferentiated VIN has been divided into warty, basaloid or mixed variants. There is two-thirds to full-thickness loss of cellular stratification throughout the epidermis, with large hyperchromatic cells, dyskeratosis, multinucleated cells and numerous typical and atypical mitoses (Figure 112.23). In warty uVIN, the appearance may be condylomatous, whereas basaloid uVIN has a thickened epithelium with a non-papillomatous surface.

Table 112.7 Differences between types of vulval intraepithelial neoplasia (VIN).

	Undifferentiated VIN	Differentiated VIN
Age	Younger women	Older women
HPV infection	Types 16 and 18 strongly associated	Very rare
Lichen sclerosus	Not generally associated	Usually associated
Lesions	Often multifocal	Usually unifocal
Risk factors	Smoking, immunosuppression	None known
Progression to SCC	Low risk (9% within 1–8 years)	High risk
Treatment	Responds to medical treatment	Surgical excision is treatment of choice

HPV, human papillomavirus; SCC, squamous cell carcinoma.

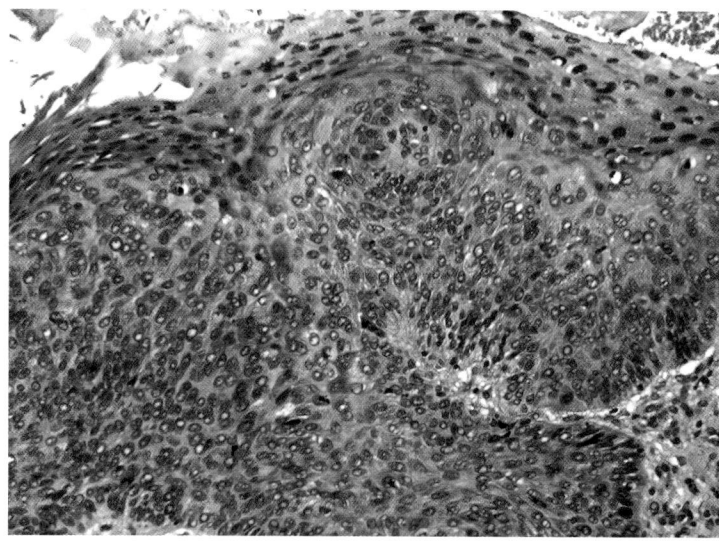

Figure 112.23 Histological features of undifferentiated vulval intraepithelial neoplasia.

Features of both types may be seen in the same lesion, when it is then referred to as 'mixed'.

A rare histological variant of VIN, which resembles extramammary Paget disease, is known as pagetoid VIN or pagetoid Bowen disease. Pagetoid Bowen disease has been reported extragenitally and genitally in males. There is one report of vulval involvement [3]. Unexpectedly, the abnormal cells in pagetoid VIN are CK7-positive, like true Paget cells of extramammary Paget disease, but mucin stains and cam5.2 are negative.

In differentiated VIN (dVIN), the histology may be mistaken for a benign dermatosis as there may be subtle abnormalities in the basal layers with normal keratinocyte differentiation above this (Figure 112.24). In addition to the basal changes, the rete ridges may be long and forked with keratin pearls. This change on a background of LS/LP represents either very early invasive disease or heralds its imminent onset.

Causative organisms

Multifocal ano-genital uVIN is strongly associated with the oncogenic papillomaviruses, particularly HPV types 16 and 18 [4,5].

Clinical features

History
The main symptom is pruritus but some patients are asymptomatic.

Presentation
The lesions of uVIN can be solitary or multiple. The morphology of the lesions is also diverse, with lesions that resemble viral warts, plaques that may be shiny and smooth, skin-coloured, red or white, or others that are warty and pigmented and resemble seborrhoeic keratoses (Figure 112.25). Less commonly, the lesions may be large and papillomatous, particularly perianally, where they may be polypoid. Vaginal involvement is uncommon.

Differentiated VIN is often subtle but erythematous, hyperkeratotic or irregular lesions on a background or lichen sclerosus should be biopsied early and subjected to good clinicopathological correlation to confirm the diagnosis.

Differential diagnosis
The warty lesions of uVIN need to be distinguished from simple condylomas. The erythematous lesions can resemble dermatoses and extramammary Paget disease.

Classification of severity
The previous three tier grading of VIN is misleading as there is interobserver variation in the grading and in clinical practice

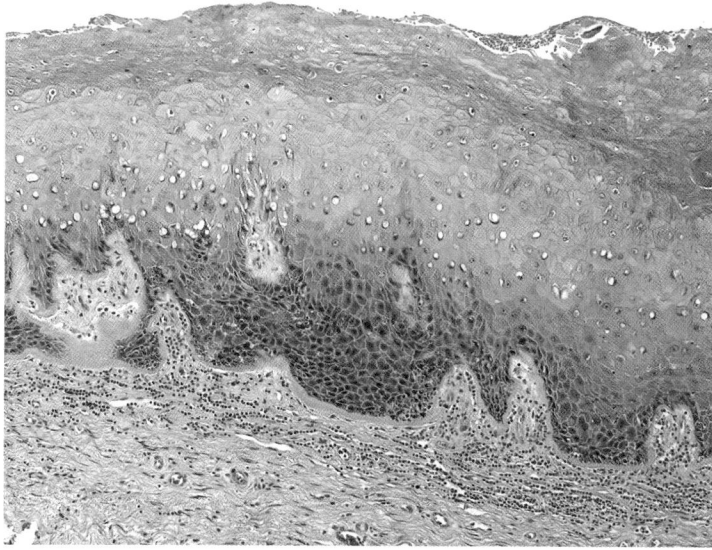

Figure 112.24 Histological features of differentiated vulval intraepithelial neoplasia.

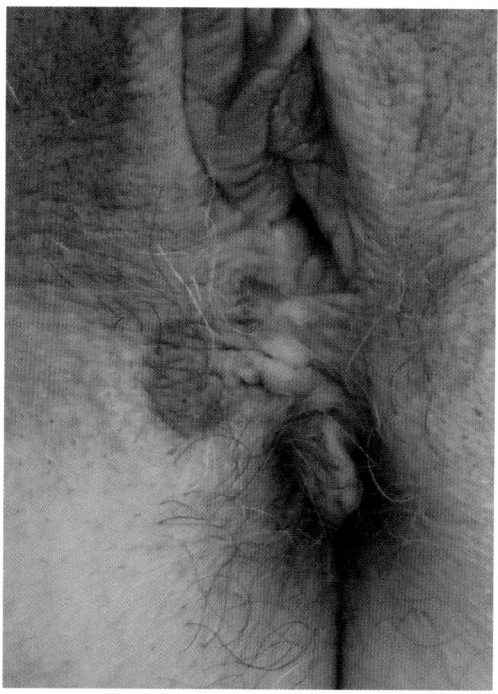

Figure 112.25 Vulval intraepithelial neoplasia.

many cases of VIN 1 with basal atypia are not truly pre-malignant but reparative (e.g. LP), or proliferative as in a benign condyloma. Therefore, in 2004, the International Society for the Study of Vulvo-vaginal Disease (ISSVD) proposed replacing the three tier grading system with two types of VIN, undifferentiated and differentiated. This classification eliminates the term VIN 1 and replaces the terms VIN 2 and 3 with 'undifferentiated VIN'. 'Differentiated VIN' remains as the term reserved for the severe atypia confined to the basal layers, most often seen on a background of a chronic scarring dermatosis. This classification does not include extramammary Paget disease or melanoma *in situ* [6].

Complications and co-morbidities

Undifferentiated VIN occurs almost exclusively in smokers. The condition is caused by a failure of the host to mount an immune response to HPV. Patients who are immunocompromised have a higher incidence of this problem, but the majority of young women with this problem do not have an identifiable immunodeficiency. In addition to being multifocal, VIN may be associated with multicentric disease, with lesions of intraepithelial neoplasia involving the cervix, vagina and perianal skin. Up to two-thirds of patients with uVIN have a current or past history of cervical intraepithelial neoplasia.

Disease course and prognosis

The risk of progression to invasive disease is estimated as 10% or less in multifocal uVIN, but this risk is likely to be higher in immunocompromised patients, those with perianal disease and in the older woman with a solitary plaque. Patients with dVIN are much more likely to develop an invasive tumour and in fact dVIN is rarely diagnosed prior to the development of an SCC [7].

Investigations

VIN is a multicentric problem, and other sites that need to be monitored are the cervix, vagina and perianal area. If there is perianal disease, anoscopy should be performed to exclude involvement of the anal canal.

Management

This is tailored to the individual but the patient should be managed in a specialized vulval clinic. In the case of a solitary lesion that is amenable to simple excision, this is the treatment of choice; surgical excision is always needed for areas of dVIN. In the woman with extensive undifferentiated disease, surgery would be mutilating physically and distressing psychologically, and does not guarantee a cure as the risk of recurrence is significant. Such patients require regular and long-term follow-up, with biopsies of suspicious areas. Thick or polypoid lesions should be excised, as early invasive changes are difficult to detect in these areas [8].

Cryotherapy is not effective, but 5-fluorouracil can be used successfully for lesions of the labia minora, vestibule and clitoral area. It is not effective on the hair-bearing parts of the vulva, probably because of the deep adnexal structures, which can all be involved. Laser vaporization has a high recurrence rate, particularly if the hair-bearing parts of the vulva are involved, and there is the additional danger that early invasive disease may be missed and therefore inappropriately treated. It is also extremely painful postoperatively.

Imiquimod has proved very effective in the treatment of multifocal uVIN in younger patients and recurrent disease after surgical excision [9]. Lower recurrence rates compared with surgery have also been confirmed [10]. This is now being used more frequently for first line treatment.

The development of HPV vaccines, which became licensed in Europe for preventative management in 2006, will have an impact on HPV-related VIN.

Resources

Patient resources
International Society for the Study of Vulvo-vaginal Disease information sheet http://issvd.org/wordpress/wp-content/uploads/2012/04/VIN2010.pdf.
Macmillan Cancer Support information sheet: http://www.macmillan.org.uk/Cancerinformation/Cancertypes/Vulva/Pre-cancerousconditions/Vin.aspx. (Both last accessed June 2014.)

MALIGNANT NEOPLASMS

Squamous cell carcinoma

Introduction and general description

SCC is the most common malignancy occurring on the female genitalia (see also Chapter 142).

Epidemiology

Incidence and prevalence

SCC accounts for 90% of all vulval malignancies. The incidence of vulval SCC is 1–2 per 100 000.

Pathophysiology

Predisposing factors

Aetiologically, there appear to be two types of vulval SCC [1,2]. The first and largest group occurs in elderly women on a background of a chronic dermatosis such as LS or LP. The second type, which accounts for approximately 40% of cases, occurs in younger women and is associated with intraepithelial neoplasia associated with oncogenic-type HPV infection. There is, however, some overlap, and SCC arising in lichen sclerosus may be HPV positive [3].

Pathology

In the older age group, the tumours are usually well to moderately differentiated and keratinizing, whereas in the younger HPV-associated group, they are poorly differentiated and often non-keratinizing.

There is also an adenoid variant of SCC with acantholysis in the centres of some of the infiltrating nests, producing cystic spaces lined by cubocolumnar nests. These pseudocysts do not contain mucin, which differentiates them from adenosquamous cell carcinoma.

Causative organisms

High-risk oncogenic HPV types 16 and 18 are associated with VIN and the development of SCC in the younger age group.

Clinical features

History

The common symptoms are soreness and pruritus. The patient may present because of the presence of a nodule or plaque that causes few symptoms. Bleeding can occur if the tumour has ulcerated.

Presentation

Tumours can occur on any area of the vulva but common sites are the labia majora, clitoris, perineal body and fourchette.

Differential diagnosis

Some forms of ulcerated exophytic infection can mimic SCC.

Classification of severity

There are combined TNM (tumour size, lymph nodes, distant metastasis) and FIGO (Federation of Gynaecology and Obstetrics) staging systems based on clinical examination and histological criteria. The depth of stromal invasion is measured from the epithelial–stromal junction of the adjacent dermal papilla to the deepest point of invasion by the tumour [4].

Disease course and prognosis

The overall 5-year survival is approximately 75%, which rises to 90% or greater in those with no nodal metastases. The main reason for failure of treatment is the inability to control lymphatic and distant metastases, lymphatic spread being the most important factor.

Investigations

A biopsy can confirm the diagnosis, and multiple mapping biopsies may be needed in multifocal disease. The patient must also be assessed for other sites of disease with cervical cytology, colposcopy and anoscopy if appropriate.

Management

Surgical excision is tailored to the individual, and is determined by the size and site of the tumour. Less radical surgery has not reduced survival rates but has significantly improved morbidity [5,6]. These patients are managed in a multidisciplinary setting with gynaecology oncologists and clinical and medical oncologists.

The vulval lymphatics drain to the inguinal and femoral nodes and from there to the pelvic nodes. Central lesions (those placed near the clitoris, urethra, vagina, fourchette and perianal area) have a bilateral lymphatic drainage, and it is important in these cases that the inguino-femoral nodes on both sides are excised. Radiotherapy is used as an adjuvant in patients with positive nodes and in those with inoperable tumours. It is also sometimes used as a primary treatment, together with chemotherapy, in tumours of the anus and urethra, to reduce their size before surgery and to try to preserve sphincter function.

Sentinel lymph node biopsy techniques are now being used in the management of these patients.

Resources

Further information
International Federation of Gynecology and Obstetrics staging: www.figo.org/docs/staging_booklet.pdf.
Royal College of Obstetricians and Gynaecologists guidelines on the management of vulva cancer: http://www.rcog.org.uk/files/rcog-corp/uploaded-files/WPRVulvalCancerFull2006.pdf.
(Both last accessed June 2014.)

Patient resources
International Society for the Study of Vulvo-vaginal Disease information sheet: http://issvd.org/wordpress/wp-content/uploads/2012/04/VulvarCancer.pdf.
Macmillan Cancer Support information sheet: http://www.macmillan.org.uk/Cancerinformation/Cancertypes/Vulva/Vulvalcancer.aspx.
(Both last accessed June 2014.)

Verrucous carcinoma

Definition and nomenclature

A verrucous carcinoma is a low-grade and slowly growing form of squamous cell carcinoma (see also Chapter 142).

> **Synonyms and inclusions**
> - Well-differentiated epidermoid squamous cell carcinoma
> - Epithelioma cuniculatum
> - Carcinoma cuniculatum
> - Buschke–Löwenstein tumour
> - Giant condyloma of Buschke–Löwenstein

Epidemiology

Age

These tumours occur in older women.

Associated diseases

Verrucous carcinomas can arise on a background of lichen sclerosus [1].

Pathophysiology

Pathology

The histological changes include epidermal acanthosis, with large bulbous rete ridges which compress and push down the underlying stroma. There is very little cellular atypia and the few, if any, mitoses are confined to the basal layers. The upper keratinocytes are often paler and there is a loss of the granular layer. Lymph node and distant metastases occur rarely.

Causative organisms

A proportion of cases may harbour HPV [2,3].

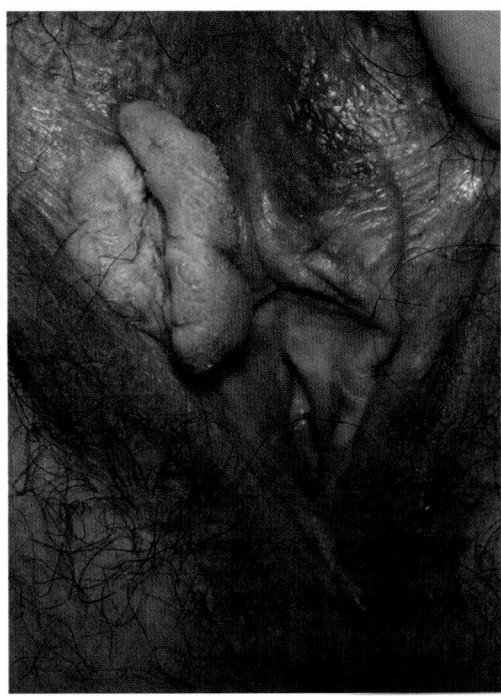

Figure 112.26 Verrucous carcinoma on a background of lichen sclerosus.

Clinical features

Presentation
Clinically, the lesions appear as a warty plaque or cauliflower-like tumour (Figure 112.26) which can ulcerate and become extremely large.

Differential diagnosis
Verrucous carcinomas are often misdiagnosed as squamous papillomas or condylomas because of the benign histological features.

Investigations
Multiple biopsies may be required to reach a firm diagnosis.

Management
Treatment is wide, local excision. Radiotherapy is not used as it is associated with a worse prognosis, probably because it can induce anaplastic transformation [4]. Oral retinoids may also be helpful [5].

Extramammary Paget disease

Definition
Primary extramammary Paget disease (EMPD) is an intraepithelial adenocarcinoma arising in the epidermis or skin appendages. Secondary EMPD is epidermal involvement from an internal neoplasm, either by direct extension or metastasis.

Introduction and general description
The proposed classification for EMPD is shown in Table 112.8 [1]. In contrast to Paget disease of the nipple, the association with malignancy is only about 30% [2].

Table 112.8 Classification of extramammary Paget disease (EMPD).

Primary EMPD	Secondary EMPD
Primary intraepithelial neoplasm	Secondary to anal or rectal carcinoma
Intraepithelial neoplasm with invasion	Secondary to urothelial neoplasia
Manifestation of primary adenocarcinoma of a skin appendage or subcutaneous gland	Secondary to adenocarcinoma or related tumours of other sites

From Wilkinson and Brown 2002 [1]. Reproduced with permission of Elsevier.

The differentiation between primary and secondary disease is not always straightforward clinically and sometimes relies on immunohistological investigations (Table 112.9) [3–5].

Epidemiology

Incidence and prevalence
The true prevalence is unknown but it accounts for 1–2% of all vulval malignancies.

Age
It generally affects women over 50 years [6,7].

Pathophysiology

Pathology
There is frequently epidermal hyperplasia. The epidermis is infiltrated with pale-staining Paget cells. The Paget cells are PAS positive and diastase resistant, and stain with Alcian blue and markers for the simple keratins.

Clinical features

History
The lesions may be asymptomatic initially and patients may report a longstanding eruption. Itching and burning are common symptoms.

Presentation
The lesions are typically moist, erythematous plaques (Figure 112.27). The site of the lesions is important as disease involving the urethra and perianal skin is more likely to be associated with an underlying malignancy of the urinary or gastrointestinal tract, respectively.

Table 112.9 Immunocytochemical markers in extramammary Paget disease (EMPD).

	Primary EMP	Secondary EMP	Bowen	Malignant melanoma
PAS	+	+	−	−
CK7	+	+	−	−
CK20	Usually −	Usually +	−	−
CEA	+	+	−	−
CAM5.2	+	+	−	−
GCDFP-15	+	+	−	−
S100	−	−	−	+
Melan A	−	−	−	+
Uroplakin III		+if urothelial Ca		

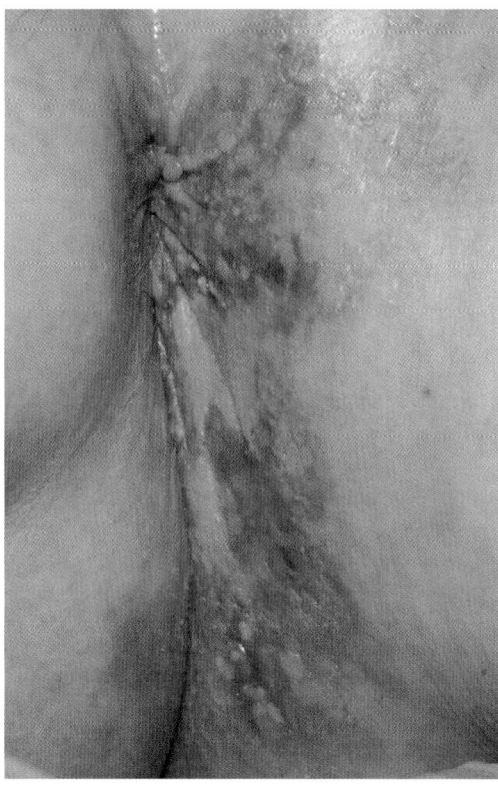

Figure 112.27 Extramammary Paget disease

Differential diagnosis

The clinical differential diagnosis includes psoriasis and eczema. Vulval intraepithelial neoplasia can have similar features. The important histological differential diagnoses are VIN, melanoma and Bowen disease.

Complications and co-morbidities

The two most common tumours associated with secondary vulval EMPD are ano-rectal adenocarcinoma and urothelial carcinoma of the bladder or urethra. Other associated tumours reported include the cervix, endometrium and ovary [2,6].

Disease course and prognosis

Recurrence is common with all currently available treatment modalities. Regular monitoring and evaluation for invasion are important. The prognosis for primary intraepithelial disease is excellent. Invasive disease has an estimated 5-year survival of 72% [8].

Investigations

The diagnosis is confirmed histologically. Patients should have a full clinical examination and cervical cytology and mammography should be up to date. Further urological and bowel investigation should be undertaken if appropriate.

Management

In primary EMPD, excision of visible disease is often recommended for treatment and to exclude underlying appendageal adenocarcinoma. Sometimes in the very elderly, with extensive disease or recurrence after vulvectomy, this is not always an option. Patients should be regularly monitored, and topical steroids can be used if there is troublesome pruritus. Recurrence rates of over 40% are reported after surgery, and even with Mohs micrographic surgery, the disease can recur in up to 27% and large margins are required [9,10].

Topical 5-fluorouracil, bleomycin and oral retinoids have been used, with some success. The recurrence rates are high after carbon dioxide laser and radiotherapy. Photodynamic therapy is reported to be of some benefit [11] but long-term results have not been evaluated.

There has been interest in the use of 5% imiquimod and although it is not licensed to treat EMPD, it can be useful in widespread disease and in recurrence after surgery [7,12].

Overexpression of the HER-2/neu protein is found in about 30% of cases, and in recurrent disease there are reports of the use of trastuzumab as targeted therapy [13].

In secondary disease, the treatment is directed predominantly at the associated carcinoma.

Resources

Patient resources
International Society for the Study of Vulvo-vaginal Disease information sheet: http://issvd.org/wordpress/wp-content/uploads/2012/04/EMPfinal.pdf (last accessed June 2014).

Basal cell carcinoma

Introduction and general description
Basal cell carcinomas account for 2–5% of all vulval malignancies (see also Chapter 141).

Epidemiology

Age
These tumours generally occur in the elderly but can be seen in younger women.

Clinical features

Presentation
Vulval basal cell carcinomas present as an eroded plaque, which may be pigmented. Less commonly, the tumour may form a nodule or ulcer. They occur most frequently on the labia majora or mons pubis [1,2].

Disease course and prognosis
Inadequate excision accounts for a high recurrence rate and metastases to regional lymph nodes [3]. Patients with vulval basal cell carcinomas frequently develop basal cell carcinomas at other sites [4].

Management
Adequate excision is vital and Mohs micrographic surgery is the treatment of choice [5].

Vulval melanoma

Introduction and general description

Vulval melanoma is rare. All types of melanoma may occur on the vulva [1] (see also Chapter 143).

Epidemiology

Incidence and prevalence

Vulval melanoma accounts for about 2–10% of vulval malignancy. About 3% of all melanomas are found on the genital tract and the estimated annual incidence is about one per 1 million women.

Age

It is more usually found in the sixth and seventh decades of life. It has been reported in children but is extremely rare [2].

Genetics

Mutations in the KIT pathway are more common in vulval melanomas than other mucosal lesions [3].

Clinical features

History

Vulval melanoma is often asymptomatic until it ulcerates, or becomes nodular. Bleeding may occur.

Presentation

The labia majora and clitoris are most common sites involved (Figure 112.28). The vagina is rarely involved and the cervix even less

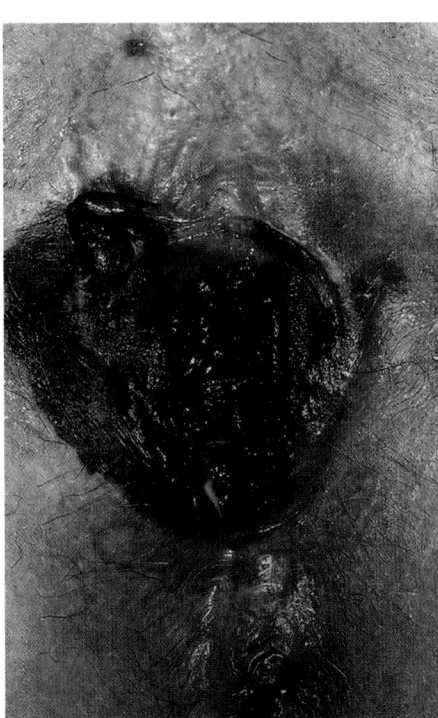

Figure 112.28 Melanoma of the vulva. (Courtesy of Dr F. A. Ive, Durham, UK.)

so. The clinical features are similar to melanoma elsewhere but in one study of 219 patients, 27% were amelanotic [4].

Differential diagnosis

Amelanotic variants can mimic SCC and other tumours. Melanosis can have similar features to early lentigo maligna melanoma.

Disease course and prognosis

There is often a delay in diagnosis and a poorer prognosis for vulval and vaginal melanoma in particular. A 5-year survival rate of 11.4% is estimated for female genital tract melanoma [5].

Investigations

The diagnosis is made histologically.

Management

The primary management is wide, local excision, with input from a specialist multidisciplinary team. Adjuvant treatment may be needed [6].

Resources

Patient resources

Cancer Research UK information sheet: http://www.cancerresearchuk.org/cancer-help/about-cancer/cancer-questions/vaginal-melanoma (last accessed June 2014).

Langerhans cell histiocytosis

Definition

Langerhans cell histiocytosis is a systemic disease with growth and proliferation of the Langerhans cells (see also Chapter 136). It can affect many organs and its presentation is variable.

Epidemiology

Age

Vulval Langerhans cell histiocytosis can present from childhood to old age. Primary or isolated involvement of the genitalia is uncommon [1,2].

Pathophysiology

Pathology

Large histiocytic cells with coffee bean nuclei are seen. Langerhans cells stain positively with S100 and characteristic Birkbeck granules are seen on electron microscopy.

Clinical features

Presentation

In infants, it may present as a resistant napkin eruption with yellowish and sometimes purpuric lesions. In adults, the lesions are papular, and scarring and ulceration may be prominent.

Box 112.1 Other vulval neoplasms

• Adenocarcinoma	Present as painless subcutaneous nodules that can invade deeply. The mucinous carcinomas may be of cloacal origin [1]
• Lymphoma	Non-Hodgkin lymphoma is more common than Hodgkin's [2] and has been reported post-transplantation [3] and in HIV-positive individuals [4]
• Bartholin's duct tumours	These may be better regarded as hyperplasia or hamartomas [5,6]
• Bartholin's gland carcinoma [7]	
• Dermatofibrosarcoma protuberans [8]	
• Liposarcoma [9]	
• Epithelioid sarcoma [10]	
• Merkel cell carcinoma [11]	
• Myofibroblastic tumours	Angiomyofibroblastoma, cellular angiofibroma and aggressive angiomyxoma have a predilection for vulva soft tissues [12]
• Metastatic tumours	These are uncommon and may be from malignancies of the cervix, endometrium, vagina, ovary, urethra, kidney, breast and lung [13,14]

Differential diagnosis
The differential diagnosis is wide as it can mimic dermatoses and malignancy.

Management
Small localized lesions can be excised but for more extensive disease this is impractical and radiotherapy, chemotherapy and thalidomide have been used [3].

Other malignant vulval neoplasms

There are some other tumours that are seen on the vulva but these are uncommon. These are detailed in Box 112.1.

PAIN DISORDERS

Vulval pain

Definition and nomenclature
Vulvodynia is defined as vulval discomfort, most often described as burning pain, occurring in the absence of relevant visible findings or a specific, clinically identifiable neurological disorder [1] (see also Chapter 84).

Box 112.2 International Society for the Study of Vulvo-vaginal Disease (ISSVD) terminology and classification of vulval pain 2003 [1]

A. Vulval pain related to a specific disorder
  1 Infection
  2 Inflammatory
  3 Neoplastic
  4 Neurological

B. Vulvodynia
  1 Generalized
    a Provoked
    b Unprovoked
    c Mixed, provoked and unprovoked
  2 Localized
    a Provoked
    b Unprovoked
    c Mixed, provoked and unprovoked

Synonyms and inclusions
• Previously termed dysaesthetic vulvodynia, essential vulvodynia, vestibulitis

Introduction and general description
There has been much confusion in the literature about the terminology used for vulval pain and a simplified system has been established by the ISSVD (Box 112.2). A diagnosis of vulvodynia should be strictly reserved for those patients who have the symptoms of pain or in the absence of any visible abnormality or explanation that would account for their symptoms. If any active dermatosis or dermographism is found that could account for the symptoms then that condition is the diagnosis rather than vulvodynia.

The two common types seen are vestibulodynia (localized provoked vulval pain) and generalized vulvodynia (generalized spontaneous vulval pain). There is often overlap between the two types.

It is also important to remember that a form of dysaesthetic vulvodynia probably more accurately labelled postinflammatory vulval hyperaesthesia is a frequent problem following inflammatory conditions of the vulva, particularly the vestibule. It is seen most frequently following LP, when the patient still has symptoms despite the fact that the dermatitis has responded to treatment.

Epidemiology

Incidence and prevalence
The exact prevalence is not known but 16% of women in one study reported vulval pain lasting more than 3 months [2].

Age
Vestibulodynia occurs in young women, whereas the generalized form is more common in older postmenopausal women.

Associated diseases
There is frequently a history of other pain issues such as fibromyalgia, migraine and back pain. There is a 6.9 relative risk for vulvodynia in patients with interstitial cystitis [3].

Depression is a common feature in chronic pain but it is difficult to determine if this is a primary cause or a secondary effect of the symptoms.

Pathophysiology
The pathophysiology of vulvodynia is unknown but the existence of complex regional pain syndromes is now well recognized. Chronic pain syndromes are rarely caused by primary psychiatric disorders as originally thought, but are the result of peripheral and/or central neuronal sensitization.

Predisposing factors
The majority of patients affected by vestibulodynia are psychologically normal but they do have higher anxiety and somatization scores [4].

Pathology
There is now good evidence that inflammation is not a feature in vulvodynia [5].

Causative organisms
There is no evidence to support an association with chronic infection with either *Candida* or HPV.

Clinical features

History
In vestibulodynia, the classic history is of pain with penetration at intercourse. This can also occur with the use of tampons or speculum examination. Patients will sometimes relate the onset of symptoms to a particular event such as a severe episode of candidiasis or urinary tract infection. They frequently complain of increased sensitivity at other sites.

In the generalized form, the history is of constant pain with no obvious trigger factors. The pain may vary in intensity and patients may complain of shooting pain into the pelvis, thighs or anal area. Dyspareunia is not generally a feature.

Presentation
The vulva looks completely normal on examination. In vestibulodynia, there will be touch-provoked tenderness over the vestibule when pressure is applied with a cotton-tipped swab (the touch test). This is usually at a maximum between 5 and 7 o'clock, which is where the Bartholin glands open. In some patients, the pain is localized to the clitoris and this is then termed clitorodynia.

Differential diagnosis
Dermatoses, infections and malignancy can cause pain but the signs are evident. Dermographism, nympho-hymenal tears and vestibular fissures can cause pain with intercourse and sometimes it is helpful to examine the patient soon after intercourse to assess these. Pudendal neuralgia can be confused with generalized vulvodynia but here the pain is alleviated by standing.

Disease course and prognosis
Spontaneous resolution may occur but is unusual. As with any chronic pain problem, most patients show a steady but slow response to treatment and sometimes combination therapies are needed. Treatment outcomes are summarized in guidelines [6,7].

Investigations
The diagnosis is clinical and investigation is unhelpful.

Management [6,7]

First line
Lidocaine 5% ointment can be applied regularly to the maximum points of tenderness. This is particularly helpful for vestibulodynia.

Second line
Low-dose tricyclics, e.g. amitriptyline 10 mg nocte increasing by 10 mg increments to a maximum of 100 mg/day. Pregabalin and gabapentin are alternatives. Physiotherapy is particularly useful for associated vaginismus.

Third line
Referral to a pain clinic and expert psychosexual counselling is helpful. Vestibulectomy has been used for vestibulodynia but is only suitable for a small minority and there are few long-term results of efficacy. Psychological issues must be dealt with as these have an impact on outcome. It is not advocated as a routine procedure and surgery is rarely used for other neuropathic pain problems.

There is often a need for combination therapies [8].

Resources

Patient resources
British Vulval Pain Society: www.vulvalpainsociety.org.
International Society for the Study of Vulvo-vaginal Disease information sheets: http://issvd.org/wordpress/wp-content/uploads/2012/04/Generalized-Unprovoked-VD-final.pdf; http://issvd.org/wordpress/wp-content/uploads/2012/04/Vestibulodynia2010.pdf.
National Vulvodynia Association: www.nva.org.
(All last accessed June 2014.)

TRAUMATIC LESIONS

There are various causes of vulval trauma, including accidental injury, obstetrical tears and self-induced lesion [1,2]. Sclerosing lipogranuloma [3] is a granulomatous response induced artefactually.

Nympho-hymenal tears

Synonyms and inclusions
• Postcoital fissures
• Hymeneal fissures

Introduction and general description
Nympho-hymenal tears are a cause of dyspareunia and occur in nulliparous women on each intercourse.

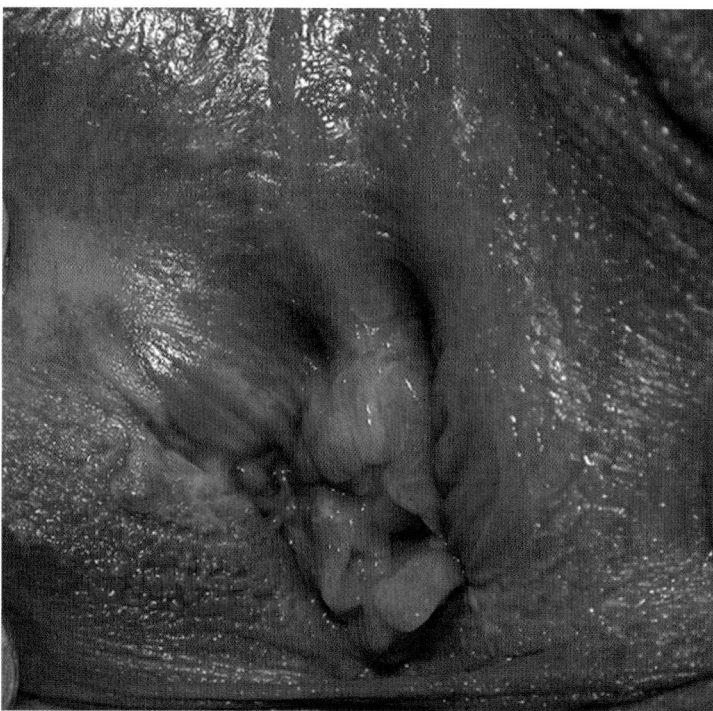

Figure 112.29 Tear of the right inferior aspect of the nymphohymenal sulcus.

Clinical features

History
Postcoital bleeding and pain at the site of the tear are the main symptoms. Abstinence, even for long periods of time, does not prevent recurrence.

Presentation
Fissures occur radially at 3 and 9 o'clock (Figure 112.29). They can be bilateral and extend from the hymenal ring into the vagina.

Differential diagnosis
The symptoms of vestibulodynia may be similar.

Disease course and prognosis
They heal rapidly within a few days but recur at the same site with each intercourse. They may leave a pale scar.

Investigations
The diagnosis is clinical. It is important to examine the patient after intercourse or the signs may be missed.

Management
Excision of the fissure with re-suturing usually resolves the problem.

Female genital mutilation

Synonyms and inclusions
• Female circumcision
• Cutting

Introduction and general description
Female genital mutilation (FGM), although banned in most European countries, is still forced on many women worldwide. Many cases are now being seen in the UK because of the rise in immigration of women who have had previous FGM. It involves a variety of procedures to remove parts of the female genitalia for non-medical reasons [1].

Epidemiology

Incidence and prevalence
It may affect up to 140 million women worldwide.

Age
Most FGM occurs before the age of 1, but in Egypt girls are likely to be circumcised between 5 and 15 years old.

Clinical features

Presentation
There are four types of operation performed, which vary according to the country and culture:
1 Clitoridectomy: removal of the clitoris and/or the clitoral hood (Sunna circumcision).
2 Excision: removal of the clitoris and part or all of the labia minora.
3 Narrowing of the introitus by cutting and apposing the labia minora and/or the labia majora, with or without excision of the clitoris (infibulation), leaving a tiny opening for urination and menstruation.
4 All other practices, which might involve cauterization, applying corrosive material, and piercing or cutting of the clitoris, surrounding skin or vagina.

Complications and co-morbidities
There may be immediate damage to the urethra and vagina but the later complications are often only seen during delivery in those who have had infibulation. Many of the women who have had FGM experience difficulties with sexual intercourse, urination and pregnancy.

Management
Referral to a specialist clinic for further management is recommended.

Resources

Further information
Royal College of Obstetricians and Gynaecologists guidelines 2009:
http://www.rcog.org.uk/files/rcog-corp/GreenTop53FemaleGenitalMutilation.pdf.
World Health Organization information:
www.who.int/topics/female_genital_mutilation/en/.
(Both last accessed June 2014.)

Patient resources
Foundation for Women's Health Research and Development: www.forwarduk.org.uk (last accessed June 2014).

PART 10: SITES, SEX, AGE

MISCELLANEOUS

Graft-versus-host disease

Definition
Graft-versus-host disease (GVHD) occurs with acute followed by chronic features after allogeneic stem cell transplant, and is due to the donor cells reacting against host tissue (see also Chapter 38).

Epidemiology

Incidence and prevalence
Genital GVHD can occur in up to 49% of patients after transplant [1].

Clinical features

Presentation
Vulval and vaginal erythema and erosions are seen.

Differential diagnosis
The clinical features are indistinguishable from erosive lichen planus. This is sometimes difficult to differentiate histologically as there may be a lichenoid infiltrate present.

Complications and co-morbidities
Vaginal involvement leads to the development of synechiae and complete stenosis, hence early recognition is vital [2]. It may be associated with cutaneous and oral GVHD.

Management

> **Treatment ladder**
>
> **First line**
> • Super-potent topical steroids [3]
>
> **Second line**
> • Systemic steroids or immunosuppressive agents as guided by transplant physicians [4]. Patients also respond to ciclosporin [5]
>
> **Third line**
> • Extracorporeal photophoresis. Those with vaginal stenosis need expert surgical intervention to open the adhesions. Potent topical steroids must be used immediately postoperatively to maintain patency of the vagina

Vulvo-vaginal adenosis

Definition
Vulvo-vaginal adenosis is the presence of metaplastic cervical or endometrial epithelium.

Epidemiology

Associated diseases
Vulval adenosis may follow severe erosive disease such as toxic epidermal necrolysis.

Pathophysiology
The pathogenesis is unknown but it is postulated that it develops from remnant tissue of paramesonephric origin.

Predisposing factors
Prolonged use of the oral contraceptive pill and trauma can predispose to adenosis. Upper vaginal disease is well recognized to occur after *in utero* exposure to diethyl stilboestrol taken during pregnancy.

Clinical features

Presentation
The lesions are erythematous and very friable.

Complications and co-morbidities
Vaginal adenosis has been associated with vaginal adenocarcinoma [1].

Investigations
Histology is typical.

Management
Laser treatment has been used successfully.

Necrolytic migratory erythema

> **Synonyms and inclusions**
> • Glucagonoma syndrome

Introduction and general description
This dermatosis is usually seen in patients with the glucagonoma syndrome, but it is possible for it to occur in the absence of a glucagonoma or increased levels of glucagon [1] (see also Chapter 149).

Pathophysiology
The aetiology is unknown and even though there is a vey strong link with high levels of glucagon in the glucagonoma syndrome, they do not appear to cause it. The eruption is not reproduced by application or injection of glucagon and does not occur in other conditions where increased levels of glucagon are found such as diabetes and renal failure.

Pathology
Keratinocytes are vacuolated and pale; necrosis leads to intraepidermal clefting. Subcorneal pustules may be a feature.

Environmental factors
Moisture, friction and trauma may precipitate fresh lesions.

Clinical features

History

The lesions are pruritic, and flaccid bullae occur which then rupture and crust over. This may occur in cycles.

Presentation

The lesions occur on the vulva, perineum and perianal skin and extend onto the thighs and lower abdomen. The central face and limbs may rarely be involved. Extensive eroded erythema with crusting and a desquamative, serpiginous edge, which spreads out centrifugally, gives rise to the characteristic annular lesions.

Differential diagnosis

A similar clinical picture is seen with zinc and protein deficiency and there are now a number of reports of necrolytic migratory erythema occurring with liver diseases in the absence of a glucagonoma [2]. Acrodermatitis and pellagra have similar histological features.

Disease course and prognosis

The eruption may relapse and remit and postinflammatory hyperpigmentation can last for a few weeks. The eruption resolves rapidly after surgery or medical treatment of the glucagonoma.

Investigations

A skin biopsy will show the features described, and further endocrinological and imaging investigations are required to confirm any associated glucagonoma.

Management

Expert advice form an endocrinologist is needed for management. Topical steroids are helpful.

Genital papular acantholytic dyskeratosis

Introduction and general description

This was first described in 1984 [1], and is characterized by the presence of multiple papules or, less frequently, a single papule or plaque-like lesion on genital skin [2–5].

Epidemiology

Age

Middle-aged females are most affected.

Pathophysiology

Pathology

Histology shows hyperkeratosis and acantholysis.

Clinical features

History

The main symptom is pruritus.

Presentation

Multiple, small papules up to a few millimeters in size appear in the inguinal folds and may extend to the thighs and perineum. They may coalesce into nodules and small plaques.

Clinical variants

Cases with disseminated lesions have been described [6]. A case with positive immunofluoresence has been reported [7].

Differential diagnosis

The histological changes are similar to those seen in Darier disease or Hailey–Hailey disease, but there is no family history or evidence of these diseases at other sites.

Investigations

The diagnosis is made on histology.

Management

Laser treatment has been reported to be useful in those who are unresponsive to topical steroids or retinoids [8].

Key references

The full list of references can be found in the online version at www.rooksdermatology.com.

Introduction

1 Lynch PJ, Moyal-Barracco M, Scurry J, Stockdale C. 2011 ISSVD terminology and classification of vulvar dermatological disorders; an approach to clinical diagnosis. *J Lower Gen Tract Dis* 2012;16:339–44.

Structure and function of the female genitalia

1 Lloyd J, Crouch NS, Minto CL, Liao L, Creighton SM. Female genital appearance: 'normality' unfolds. *Br J Obstet Gynaecol* 2005;112:643–6.
2 Neill SM, Lewis FM. Basics of vulval embryology, anatomy and physiology. In: Neill SM, Lewis FM, eds. *Ridley's The Vulva*, 3rd edn. London: Wiley Blackwell, 2009:13–33.

Congenital abnormalities

Disorders of sexual development

1 Hughes IA. Disorders of sexual development: new definition and classification. *Best Pract Res Clin Endocrinol Metab* 2008;22:119–34.

Inflammatory dermatoses of the vulva

Lichen sclerosus

5 Kreuter A, Kryvosheyeva Y, Terras S et al. Association of autoimmune diseases with lichen sclerosus in 532 male and female patients. *Acta Derm Venereol* 2013;93:238–41.
6 Simpkin S, Oakley A. Clinical review of 202 patients with vulval lichen sclerosus: a possible association with psoriasis. *Austral J Dermatol* 2007;48:28–31.
40 Zaki I, Dalziel KL, Solomons FA, *et al.* The under-reporting of skin disease in association with squamous cell carcinoma of the vulva. *Clin Exp Dermatol* 1997;21:334–7.
55 Cooper S, Gao X-H, Powell JJ, Wojnarowska F. Does treatment of lichen sclerosus influence its prognosis? *Arch Dermatol* 2004;140:702–6.
57 Chi CC, Kitschig G, Baldo M, Brackenbury F, Lewis F, Wojnarowska F. Topical interventions of genital lichen sclerosus [Review]. *Cochrane Database Syst Rev* 2011;Dec. 7(12):CD008240.

58 Neill SM, Lewis FM, Tatnall FM, Cox NH. British Association of Dermatologists' guidelines for the management of lichen sclerosus 2010. *Br J Dermatol* 2010;163:672–82.

Lichen planus

4 Lewis Boyd AS, Neldner KH. Lichen planus. *J Am Acad Dermatol* 1991:25;593–619.
5 Lewis FM, Shah M, Harrington CI. Vulval involvement in lichen planus: a study of 37 women. *Br J Dermatol* 1996;135:89–91.
9 Setterfield JF, Neill SM, Shirlaw PJ, et al. The vulvovaginal gingival syndrome: a severe subgroup of lichen planus with characteristic clinical features and a novel association with the Class II HLA DQB1*0201 allele. *J Am Acad Dermatol* 2006;55;98–113.
12 Pelisse M, Leibowitch M, Sedel D, Hewitt J. Un nouveau syndrome vulvo-vagino-gingival. Lichen plan erosive plurimuqueux. *Ann Dermatol Vénéréol* 1982;109:797–8.
26 Zaki I, Dalziel KL, Solomons FA, et al. The under-reporting of skin disease in association with squamous cell carcinoma of the vulva. *Clin Exp Dermatol* 1997;21:334–7.
27 Derrick EK, Ridley CM, Kobza-Black A, et al. A clinical study of 23 cases of female anogenital carcinoma. *Br J Dermatol* 2000;143:1217–23.
30 Cooper SM, Haefner H, Abrahams-Gessel S, Margesson LJ. Vulvovaginal lichen planus treatment: a survey of current practices. *Arch Dermatol* 2008;144:1520–1.
32 Cooper SM, Wojnarowska F. Influence of treatment of erosive lichen planus of the vulva on its prognosis. *Arch Dermatol* 2006;142:289–294.
39 Panagiotopoulou N, Wong CSM, Winter-Roach B. Vulvovaginal-gingival syndrome. *J Obstet Gynaecol* 2010;30:226–30.

Zoon's vulvitis

1 Scurry J, Dennerstein G, Brennan J. Vulvitis corcumscripta. A clinico-pathological entity? *J Reprod Med* 1993;38:14–18.

Allergic contact dermatitis

1 O'Gorman SM, Torgerson RR. Allergic contsct dermatitis of the vulva. *Dermatitis* 2013;24:64–72.
4 Haverhoek E, Reid C, Gordon L, et al. Prospective study of patch tests in patients with vulval pruritus. *Australas J Dermatol* 2008;49:80–5.
5 Goldsmith PC, Rycroft RJ, White IR, et al. Contact sensitivity in women with anogenital dermatoses. *Contact Dermatitis* 1997;36:174–5.

Allergic contact urticaria

6 Lee-Wong M, Collins JS, Nozad C, Resnick DJ. Diagnosis and treatment of human seminal plasma hypersensitivity. *Obstet Gynecol* 2008;111:538–9.

Psoriasis

2 Kapila S, Bradford J, Fischer G. Vulvar psoriasis in adults and children: a clinical audit of 194 cases and review of the literature. *J Lower Gen Tract Dis* 2012;16:108.
4 Simpkin S, Oakley A. Clinical review of 202 patients with vulval lichen sclerosus: a possible association with psoriasis. *Aust J Dermatol* 2007;48:28–31.
7 Albert S, Neill S, Derrick EK, Calonje EJ. Psoriasis associated with vulval scarring. *Clin Exp Dermatol* 2004;29:354–6.
8 Meeuwis K, de Hullu J, Massuger L, et al. Genital psoriasis: a systematic literature review on this hidden skin disease. *Acta Derm Venereol* 2011;91:5–11.

Reactive arthritis

1 Edwards L, Hansen R. Reiter's syndrome of the vulva. The psoriasis spectrum. *Arch Dermatol* 1992;128:811–14.

Ulcerative and bullous disorders

Lipschutz ulceration

2 Barnes CJ, Alio AB, Cunningham BB, et al. Epstein–Barr virus associated genital ulcers: an under-recognised disorder. *Paediatr Dermatol* 2007;24:130.
3 Portnoy J, Arontheim GA, Ghibu F, et al. Recovery of Epstein–Barr virus from genital ulcers. *N Engl J Med* 1984;311:966–8.

4 Halvorsen JA, Brevig T, Aas T, et al. Genital ulcers as initial manifestation of Epstein–Barr virus infection: two new cases and review of the literature. *Acta Derm Venereol* 2006;86:439–42.

Immunobullous disease

1 Marren P, Wojnarowska F, Venning V, Wilson C, Nayar M. Vulvar involvement in auto-immune bullous diseases. *J Reprod Med* 1993;38:101–7.
2 Batta K, Munday PE, Tatnall FM. Pemphigus vulgaris localized to the vagina and presenting as a chronic vaginal discharge. *Br J Dermatol* 1999;140:945–7.

Pigmentary disorders

Vulval melanosis

1 Barnhill RI, Alber LS, Shama SK, et al. Genital lentiginosis: a clinical and histopathological study. *J Am Acad Dermatol* 1990;22:453–60.

Dowling–Degos disease

3 Ong Kang H, Hur J, Woo Lee J, et al. A case of Dowling–Degos disease on the vulva. *Ann Dermatol* 2011;23:205–8.

Vulval oedema

1 Neill SM, Lewis FM. Non-infective cutaneous conditions of the vulva. In: Neill SM, Lewis FM, eds. *Ridley's The Vulva*, 3rd edn. London: Wiley Blackwell, 2009:129–30.

Crohn disease

2 Foo WC, Papalas JA, Robboy SJ, Selim MA. Vulvar manifestations of Crohn's disease. *Am J Dermatopathol* 2011;33:588–93.
3 Martin J, Holdstock G. Isolated vulval oedema as a feature of Crohn's disease. *J Obstet Gynecol* 1997;17:92–3.
10 Preston W, Hudson N, Lewis FM. Treatment of vulval Crohn's disease with infliximab. *Clin Exp Dermatol* 2006;31:378–80.

Non-sexually transmitted infections

Viral infections

Herpes simplex
4 Lautenschlager S, Eichmann A. The heterogenous clinical spectrum of genital herpes. *Dermatology* 2001;202:211–19.
5 Gupta R, Warren T, Wald A. Genital herpes. *Lancet* 2007;370:2127–37.

Human papillomavirus infection
2 Garland SM, Hernandez-Avila M, Wheeler SM, et al. Quadrivalent vaccine against human papilloma virus to prevent ano-genital diseases. *N Eng J Med* 2007;356:1928–43.

Benign tumours

1 Fite C, Plantier F, Dupin N, Anil MF, Moyal-Barracco M. Vulvar verruciform xanthoma: ten cases associated with lichen sclerosus, lichen planus or other conditions. *Arch Dermatol* 2011;147:1087–92.
4 Juang YH, Chuang YH, Kuo TT, et al. Vulvar syringoma: a clinicopathologic and immunohistologic syudy of 18 patients and results of treatment. *J Am Acad Dermatol* 2003;48:735–9.

Papillary hidradenoma

4 Duhan N, Kalra R, Singh S, Rajotia N. Hidradenoma papilliferum of the vulva: a case report and review of the literature. *Arch Gynecol Obstet* 2011;284:1015–17.

Cutaneous endometriosis

1 Agarwal A, Fong YF. Cutaneous endometriosis. *Singapore Med J* 2008;49:704–9.

Atypical genital naevi

1 Rock B, Hood AF, Rock JA. Prospective study of vulvar nevi. *J Am Acad Dermatol* 1990;22:104–6.
2 Brenn T. Atypical genital naevus. *Arch Pathol Lab Med* 2011;135:317–20.

3 Ribé A. Melanocytic lesions of the genital area with attention given to atypical genital nevi. *J Cutan Pathol* 2008;35(Suppl. 2):24–7.

Pre-malignant conditions

Vulval intraepithelial neoplasia

1 Terlou A, Blok LJ, Helmerhorst TJM, van Beurden M. Premalignant epithelial disorders of the uvlva: squamous vulvar intra-epithelial neoplasia, vulvar Paget's and melanoma in situ. *Acta Obstet Gynecol* 2010:89:741–8.
2 Gormley RH, Kovarik CL. Human papillomavirus-related genital disease in the immunocompromised host. *J Am Acad Dermatol* 2012;66:1–14.
6 Sideri M, Jones RW, Wilkinson EJ, *et al.* Squamous vulvar intraepithelial neoplasia: 2004 modified terminology, ISSVD Vulvaroncology Subcommittee. *J Reprod Med* 2005;50:807–10.
9 Van Seters M, van beurden M, ten Kate FJW, *et al.* Treatment of vulvar intraepithelial neoplasia with topical imiquimod. *N Engl J Med* 2008;358:1465–73.

Malignant neoplasms

Squamous cell carcinoma

2 Crum C. Carcinoma of the vulva: epidemiology and pathogenesis. *Obstet Gynecol* 1992;79:448–58.
3 Van Seters M, ten Kate FJ, van Beurden M, *et al.* In the absence of (early) invasive carcinoma, vulvar intraepithelial neoplasia associated with lichen sclerosus is mainly of undifferentiated type: new insights in histology and aetiology. *J Clin Pathol* 2007;60:504–9.
4 Benedet JL, Hacker NF, Ngan HYS, *et al.* Staging classifications and clinical practice guidelines of gynaecologic cancers. *Int J Gynecol Obstet* 2000;70:209–62.
5 Ghurani GB, Penalver MA. An update on vulval cancer. *Am J Obstet Gynaecol* 2001;185:294–99.
6 Rouzier R, Paniel BJ. Management of vulval cancers In: Neill SM, Lewis FM, eds. *Ridley's The Vulva*, 3rd edn. London: Wiley Blackwell, 2009:239–54.

Extramammary Paget disease

1 Wilkinson EJ, Brown HM. Vulvar Paget disease of urothelial origin: a report of three cases and a proposed classification of vulval Paget disease. *Hum Pathol* 2002;33:549–54.
2 Preti M, Micheletti L, Massobrio M, *et al.* Vulvar Paget disease: one century after first reported. *J Lower Gen Tract Dis* 2003;7:122–35.
6 Maclean AB, Makwana M, Ellis PE, Cunnington F. The management of Paget's disease of the vulva. *J Obstet Gynecol* 2004;24:124–8.
7 Delport ES. Extramammary Paget's disease of the vulva: an annotated review of the current literature. *Aust J Dermatol* 2013;54:9–21.
12 Wang LC, Blanchard A, Judge DE, *et al.* Successful treatment of recurrent extramammary Paget's disease of the vulva with 5% topical imiquimod cream. *J Am Acad Dermatol* 2003;49:769–72.
13 Karam A, Berek JS, Stenson A, *et al.* HER-2/neu targeting for recurrent vulvar Paget's disease. A case report and literature review. *Gynecol Oncol* 2008;111:568–71.

Basal cell carcinoma

1 Gibson GE, Ahmed I. Perianal and genital BCC: a clinic-pathological review of 51 cases. *J Am Acad Dermatol* 2001;45:68–71.
2 De Girogi V, Salvini C, Massi D, Raspollini MR, Carli P. Vulvar basal cell carcinoma: retrospective study and review of the literature. *Gynecol Oncol* 2005;97:192–4.
5 Brown MD, Zachary CB, Grekin RC, Swanson N. Genital tumors: their management by micrographic surgery. *J Am Acad Dermatol* 1998;18:115–22.

Vulval melanoma

1 Postow MA, Hamid O, Carvajal RD. Mucosal melanoma: pathogenesis, clinical behaviour and management. *Curr Oncol Rep* 2012;14:441–8.

2 Egan CA, Bradley RR, Logsdon VK, *et al.* Vulvar melanoma in children. *Arch Dermatol* 1997;133:345–8.
3 Omholt K, Grafstrom E, Kanter-Lewensohn L, *et al.* KIT pathway alterations in mucosal melanomas of the vulva and other sites. *Clin Cancer Res* 2011;15:3933–42.
6 Janco JM, Markovic SN, Weaver AL, Cliby WA. Vulvar and vaginal melanoma: case series and review of current management options including neoadjuvant chemotherapy. *Gynecol Oncol* 2013;129:533–7.

Langerhans cell histiocytosis

1 Santillan A. Vulvar Langerhans cell histiocytosis: a case report and review of the literature. *Gynecol Oncol* 2003;91:241–6.
2 Jiang W, Li L, He Y, Yang K. Langerhans cell histiocytosis of the female genital tract: a literature review with additional thress case studies in China. *Arch Gynecol Obstet* 2012;285:99–103.
3 El-Safadi S, Dreyer T, Oehmke F, Muenstedt K. Management of adult primary vulvae Langerhans cell histiocytosis: review of the literature and a case history. *Eur J Obstet Gynecol Reprod Biol* 2012;163:123–8.

Pain disorders

Vulval pain

1 Moyal-Barracco M, Lynch PJ. 2003 ISSVD terminology and classification of vulvodynia: a historical perspective. *J Reprod Med* 2004;49:772–7.
6 Mandal D, Nunns D, Byrne M, *et al.* Guidelines for the management of vulvodynia. *Br J Dermatol* 2010;162:1180–5.
7 Haefner HK, Collins ME, David GD, *et al.* The vulvodynia guideline. *J Lower Gen Tract Dis* 2005;9:40–51.

Traumatic lesions

2 Neill SM, Lewis FM. Traumatic lesions In: Neill SM, Lewis FM, eds. *Ridley's The Vulva*, 3rd edn. London: Wiley Blackwell, 2009:131.

Female genital mutilation

1 Simpson J, Robinson K, Crieghton SM, Hodes D. Female genital mutilation: the role of health professionals in prevention assessment and management. *BMJ* 2012;344:37–41.

Miscellaneous

Graft-versus-host disease

1 Zantomio D, Grigg AP, MacGregor L, *et al.* Female genital tract graft versus host disease:incidence, risk factors and recommendations for management. *Bone Marrow Transplant* 2006;38:567–72.
2 Hirsch P, Leclerc M, Rybojad M, *et al.* Female genital chronic graft-versus-host disease: importance of early diagnosis to avoid severe complications. *Transplantation* 2012;93:1265–9.
3 Stratton P, Turner ML, Childs R, *et al.* Vulvovaginal graft versus host disease with allogeneic haemopoetic stem cell transplantation. *Obstet Gynecol* 2007;110:1041–9.

Vulvo-vaginal adenosis

1 Yaghsezian H, Palazzo JP, Finkel GC, *et al.* Primary vaginal adenocarcinoma of the intestinal type associated with adenosis. *Gynecol Oncol* 1992;45:62–5.

Genital papular acantholytic dyskeratosis

7 Güneş AT, Ilknur T, Pabuççuoglu U, *et al.* Papular acantholytic dyskeratosis of the anogenital area with positive direct immunofluorescence results. *Clin Exp Dermatol* 2007;32:301–3.
8 Dittmer CJ, Hornemann A, Rose CJ, *et al.* Successful laser therapy in a papular dyskeratosis of the vulva: case report and review of the literature. *Arch Gynecol Obstet* 2010;281:723–5.

CHAPTER 113

Dermatoses of Perineal and Perianal Skin

Eleanor Mallon

Croydon University Hospital, Croydon; and St John's Institute of Dermatology, Guy's and St Thomas' NHS Foundation Trust, London, UK

Introduction

History and examination

The correct diagnosis of skin disease affecting the perineum and perianal skin depends on detailed history taking, thorough methodical examination including of extragenital skin and relevant investigations. The history should include a history of topical treatments that have been used including over-the-counter remedies and wet wipes. Examination using Wood's light can be helpful in the diagnosis of conditions including erythrasma and vitiligo.

Investigations in perineal and perianal dermatology

Investigations are determined by history and clinical findings. Clinicopathological correlation is essential through discussion with a dermatopathologist. Clinicians should have a low threshold to take bacterial and viral swabs, or scrapings for fungal culture. Diagnostic imaging techniques such as pelvic magnetic resonance imaging (MRI) and endoanal ultrasound are utilized in the investigation of conditions such as anal fistula and anal malignancy.

Structure and function of the ano-genital region

The perineum is a diamond-shaped region that lies below the pelvic floor and corresponds to the outlet of the pelvis (Figure 113.1). The anterior boundary is formed by the symphysis pubis, the posterior

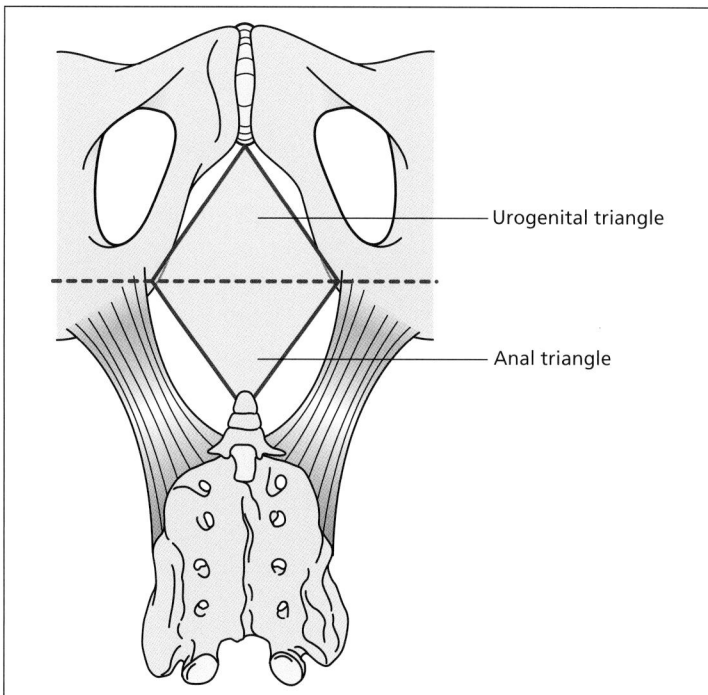

Figure 113.1 The perineum is a diamond-shaped region that lies below the pevic floor. A transverse imaginary line drawn between the ischial tuberosities divides the perineum into an anterior urogenital triangle and posterior anal triangle. (Adapted from Snell 2012 [9]. Reproduced with permission of Lippincott Williams & Wilkins/Wolters Kluwer.)

Rook's Textbook of Dermatology, Ninth Edition. Edited by Christopher Griffiths, Jonathan Barker, Tanya Bleiker, Robert Chalmers and Daniel Creamer.
© 2016 John Wiley & Sons, Ltd. Published 2016 by John Wiley & Sons, Ltd.
Companion website: www.rooksdermatology.com

PART 10: SITES, SEX, AGE

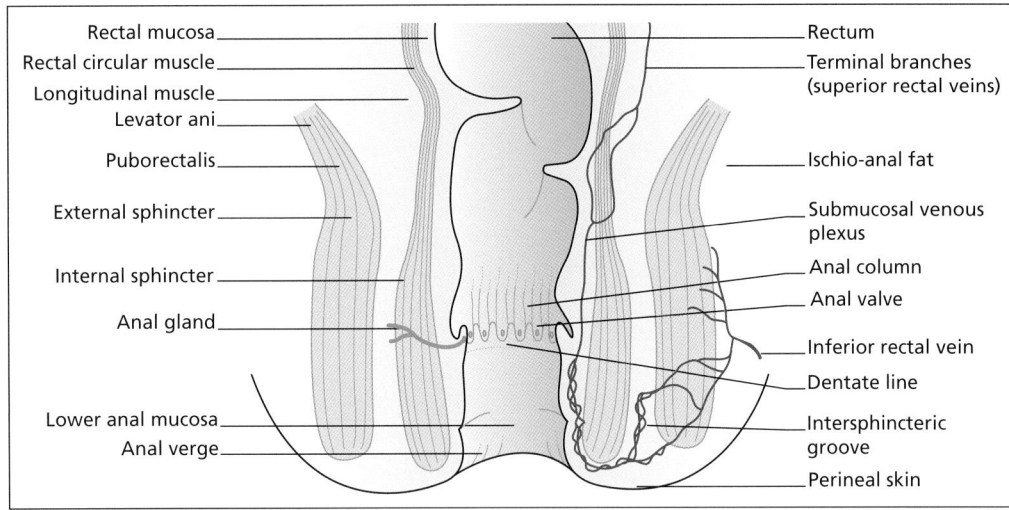

Rectal mucosa
Rectal circular muscle
Longitudinal muscle
Levator ani
Puborectalis
External sphincter
Internal sphincter
Anal gland
Lower anal mucosa
Anal verge

Rectum
Terminal branches (superior rectal veins)
Ischio-anal fat
Submucosal venous plexus
Anal column
Anal valve
Inferior rectal vein
Dentate line
Intersphincteric groove
Perineal skin

Figure 113.2 Coronal section through the anal canal. (From Standring 2008 [1].)

boundary by the coccyx, the anterolateral boundary by the ischio-pubic rami and ischial tuberosities and the posterolateral boundary by the sacrotuberous ligaments. The deep limit of the perineum is the inferior surface of muscles forming the pelvic diaphragm and the superficial limit is the skin, which is continuous with the skin of the groins and lower abdomen. An imaginary line drawn transversely joining the ischial tuberosities divides the perineum into an anterior uro-genital triangle and a posterior anal triangle. The perineal body is the central point between the uro-genital and anal triangles. The anal triangle contains the anal canal and its sphincters and the ischio-anal fossae, a horse shoe-shaped region filling the majority of the anal triangle. The uro-genital triangle contains the male or female genitalia.

The anal orifice lies in the midline approximately 2–3 cm in front of and slightly below the tip if the coccyx. The anus is principally for the evacuation of faeces, but may also be an organ of sexual utility. The anal canal is the terminal portion of the large intestine and is anatomically defined as extending from the dentate line to the anal verge (Figure 113.2) [1]. The anal verge is a narrow band of tissue that separates the anal canal from perianal skin. It extends from the intersphincteric groove onto the skin surrounding the anus. It is covered by thin squamous epithelium that can be identified by the lack of hair follicles. It is marked by a sharp turn where the squamous epithelium lining the lower end of the anal canal becomes continuous with the skin of the perineum (Figure 113.2). The skin of the anal verge is pigmented and is puckered due to the contraction of fibres of the conjoint longitudinal layer. Identification of the anal verge may be difficult, particularly in males in whom the perineum may funnel upwards towards the lower anal canal. The distinct border between the anal verge and perianal skin, as identified by the appearance of hair follicles and keratinizing epithelium, is called the anal margin. The anal margin extends for 5 cm in circumference distal to the anal verge.

The anal canal measures approximately 2.5–5 cm in length and consists of an epithelial lining, vascular subepithelium and anal sphincters, and has a dense neuronal network of autonomic and somatic origin. The anal glands originate within either the internal anal sphincter or the intersphincteric plane between the internal and external anal sphincter (Figure 113.2) and open into small depressions, anal crypts, in the anal valves [2]. The ducts carry mucous from the glands to the valves. The glands are branched and lined by stratified columnar epithelium. Cystic dilatation of the glands may extend through the internal sphincter and further into the external sphincter. Infection of the anal glands is the main cause of anal sepsis, including anal abscesses.

The upper portion of the anal canal is lined by columnar epithelium similar to that of the rectum and contains secretory and absorptive cells. The columnar epithelium in the mid anal canal is thrown into 6–10 vertical folds, the anal columns. Each column contains a terminal radicle of the superior rectal artery and vein. The columns are expanded in three areas in the anal canal to form the anal cushions. The lower end of the columns form semilunar folds, called the anal valves, between which lie small recesses referred to as anal sinuses. The anal valves and sinuses together form the dentate line. The dentate line represents an important landmark because the blood supply and innervation of the anal canal transition at this point. Proximal to the dentate line, the anus is innervated by parasympathetic and sympathetic nerves with an absence of pain fibres. Distal to the dentate line, the anal canal has numerous somatic nerve endings derived from the inferior rectal nerve and is sensitive to pain, temperature, touch and pressure.

The columnar epithelial cells of the upper anal canal transition to non-keratinized squamous epithelial cells approximately 1–1.5 cm proximal to the dentate line in an area referred to as the anal transition zone. Mucosa below the dentate line lacks sweat and sebaceous glands and hair follicles. It extends to the intersphincteric groove, a depression at the lower border of the internal sphincter. The canal below the intersphincteric groove is lined by hair-bearing, keratinizing, stratified epithelium that is continuous with perianal skin.

The smooth muscle of the internal anal sphincter is innervated by sympathetic and parasympathetic nerves and is in a state of tonic contraction. The striated muscle of the external anal sphincter is innervated by the inferior rectal nerve. The external anal sphincter is also in a state of tonic contraction, but has a component of voluntary control. The anal canal remains closed at rest as a result of tonic circumferential contraction of the sphincters and the presence of the anal cushions.

The ischio-anal fossa is a wedge-shaped space on each side of the anal canal filled with loose adipose tissue. The base of the wedge is formed by perianal and buttock skin. Infections, tumours and fluid collections may spread relatively freely within the ischio-anal space to the side of the anal canal and across the midline to the opposite side. The inferior rectal nerve supplies the perianal skin.

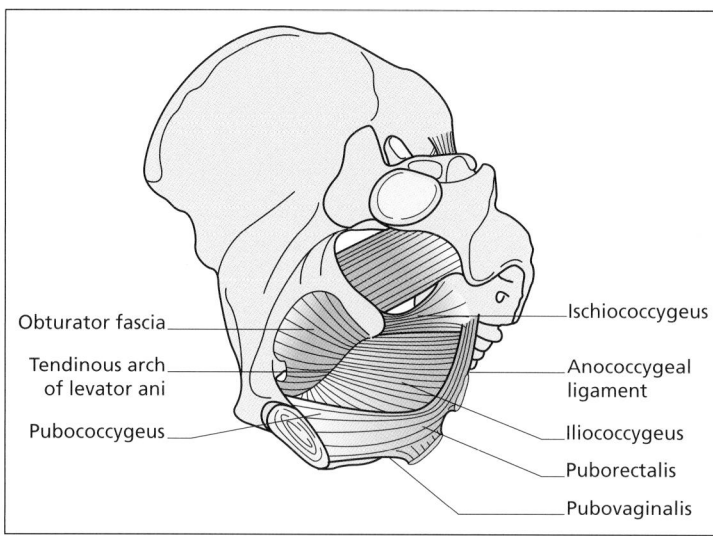

Figure 113.3 Muscles of the pelvic floor in a female. The levator ani muscle complex is composed of the ischiococcygeus, iliococcygeus and pubococcygeus muscles. The levator ani forms a large part of the pelvic floor, dividing the abdominal cavity from the perineum. (From Standring 2008 [1].)

The lymphatic vessels of the perianal skin and the lower anal canal (below the dentate line) drain into inguinal lymph nodes. Lymphatic drainage above the dentate line is to the mesorectal, lateral pelvic and inferior mesenteric nodes. Lymphatic spread of malignant disease from the lower half of the anal canal is to the inguinal lymph nodes.

The deep natal cleft (gluteal cleft), the inguinal (crural) folds and the infragluteal folds are intertriginous sites because they are areas where two layers of skin come into close apposition. The natal cleft is deep and firmly fixed to the underlying fibrous and fascial tissues, and its sides are steep and closely apposed. Mucous discharges, excreta and moisture are retained easily within this cleft.

The levator ani muscle complex forms the pelvic diaphragm and divides the abdominal cavity from the perineum (Figure 113.3).

Embryogenesis of the ano-genital region

In the early embryo, the blind ending diverticulum called the allantois and the hindgut open into a common cavity called the cloaca [3]. The cloaca is partitioned into the uro-genital sinus anteriorly and the ano-rectal canal posteriorly (Figure 113.4). The

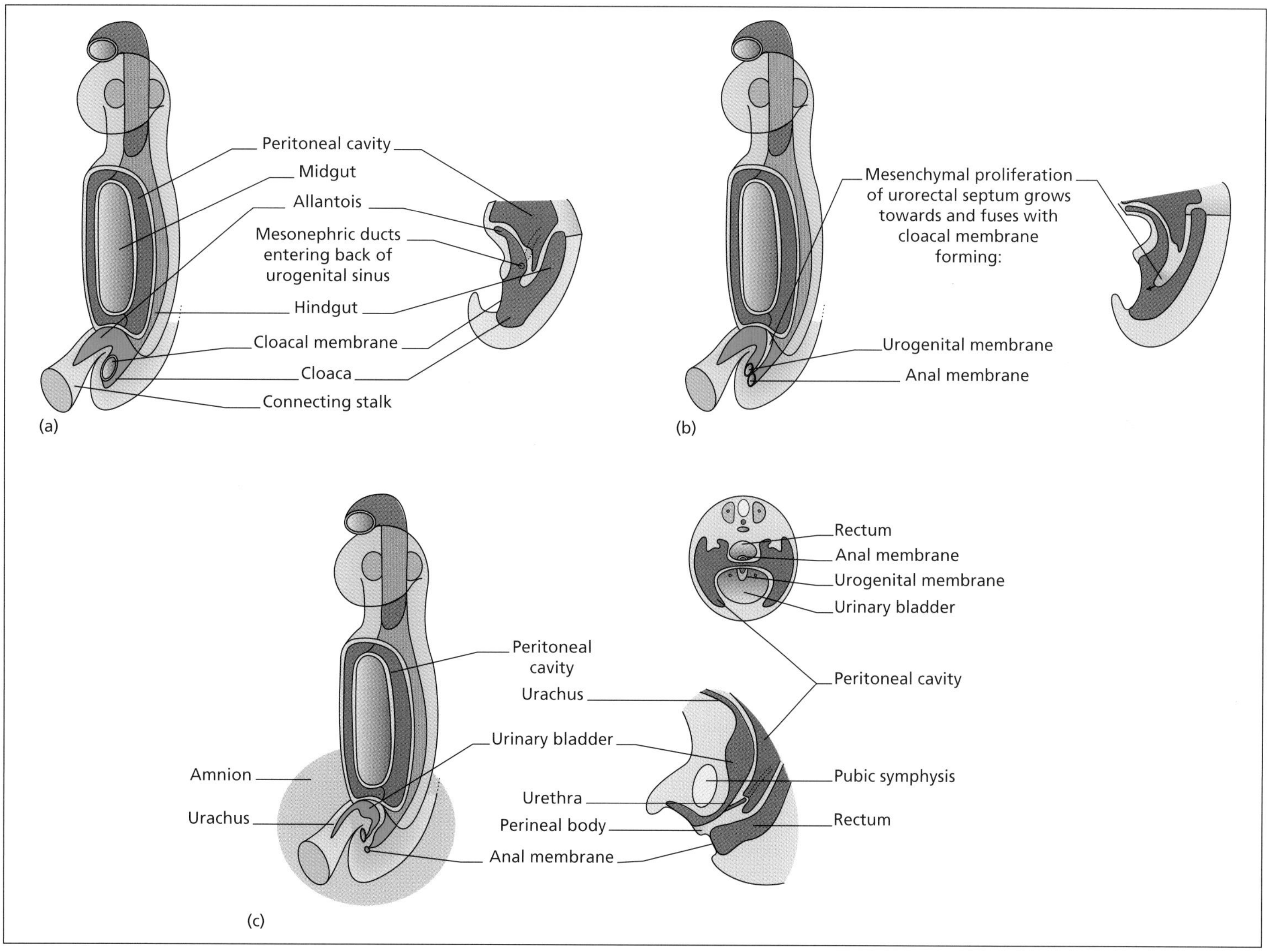

Figure 113.4 Partitioning of the cloacal membrane into the uro-genital membrane and anal membrane with the formation of the perineum occurs at 5–7 weeks' gestation. It is brought about by the separation of the cloacal portion of the hindgut by the uro-rectal septum growing caudally between the allantois anteriorly and the hindgut posteriorly to fuse with the cloacal membrane. The area of fusion becomes the perineal body and separates the dorsal anal membrane from the larger ventral uro-genital membrane. (a) Early cloaca. (b) Proliferation of the urorectal septum. (c) Separation of the urethra and the anal canal. (From Standring 2008 [1].)

anal membrane disintegrates at about 9 weeks to open into an ectodermal anal pit formed in the posterior cloacal folds. The mucosa of the upper half of the anal canal is derived from hindgut endoderm and is lined by columnar epithelium, it is innervated by autonomic nerves and the lymphatics and veins drain towards the portal system in the abdomen. The lower half of the anal canal is derived from ectoderm, is lined by stratified squamous epithelium, has a somatic nerve supply and venous drainage is towards the external iliac system while the lymphatics drain to the inguinal lymph nodes.

Congenital and developmental abnormalities

Complete or partial failure of the anal membrane to resorb during embryogenesis can result in anal stenosis. Other congenital abnormalities resulting from defective embryogenesis of the cloacal region include imperforate anus, anal agenesis, anal duplication, perineal groove and perineal fistulae.

Dermoid cysts are ectodermal growths that occur at embryonic fusion lines. They can occur on or adjacent to the perineal raphe and sacral area.

Congenital hypertrichosis over the midline in the lumbosacral area (the faun tail) is a sign of underlying spinal dysraphism (e.g. spina bifida). Other skin lesions presenting in the sacral region that can be associated with spinal dysraphism include congenital melanocytic naevi and hamartomas.

Infantile haemangiomas may involve the perianal skin (Figure 113.5). Large perineal infantile haemangiomas may

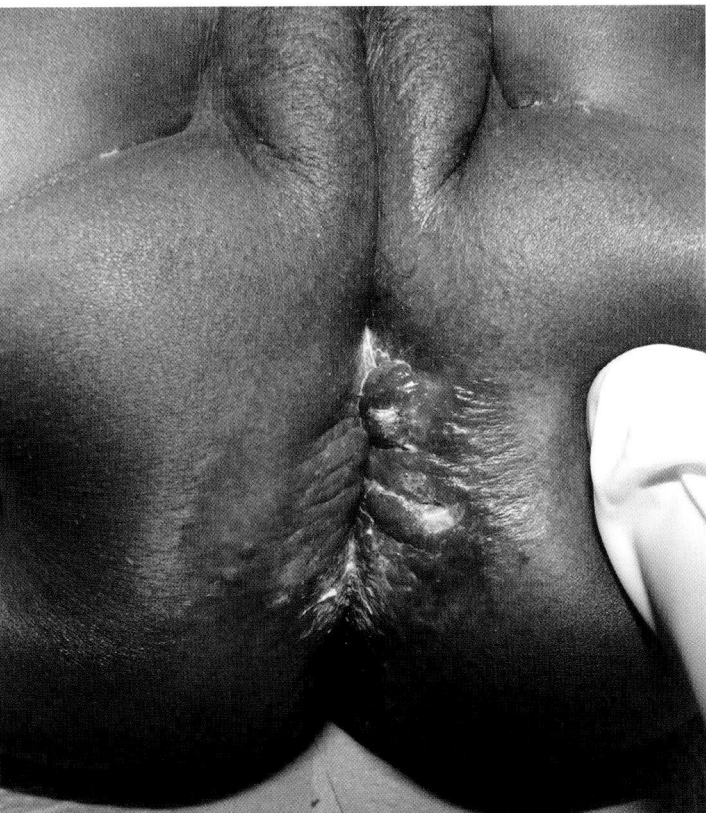

Figure 113.5 A 4-month-old female child with a perianal infantile haemangioma.

be associated with structural abnormalities including lipomyelomeningocele and imperforate anus [4].

Chordomas arise from the embryonic precursor of the axial skeleton, the notochord. They can involve the skin of the perineum, sacral area and buttocks by direct extension, recurrence or metastasis [5]. They present as single or multiple, smooth, skin-coloured, non-tender nodules. Persistent sacrococcygeal pain including coccygodynia may precede the diagnosis by many years.

Perianal keratotic plaques may occur in Olmsted syndrome [6]. Inflammatory linear verrucous epidermal naevi can affect the anogenital region [7]. Hereditary mucoepithelial dysplasia is associated with perineal intertriginous plaques [8].

PERIANAL ITCHING

Pruritus ani

Definition
This is the symptom of perianal itch or burning. Pruritus ani can be primary (idiopathic) or secondary and is not a diagnosis unless qualified as constitutional or idiopathic.

Introduction and general description
The symptom of pruritus ani has many causes. Management requires detailed assessment to determine whether there is an underlying cause. Pruritus ani can be associated with most forms of ano-rectal disease or perianal skin disease.

Pruritus ani is considered idiopathic when no dermatological or ano-rectal cause can be found. Idiopathic pruritus ani is responsible for 50–90% of all cases of pruritus ani [1]. The pathogenesis of idiopathic pruritus ani is thought to be primarily the consequence of faecal contamination or possibly the intake of certain food or drinks. The discussion below primarily deals with idiopathic pruritus ani. See Box 113.1 for secondary causes.

Epidemiology

Incidence and prevalence
It affects 1–5% of the general population [2].

Age
It most commonly presents in the fourth to sixth decade.

Sex
It is four times commoner in men than women.

Ethnicity
It is commoner in middle-aged white males [2].

Pathophysiology

Predisposing factors
The common factor linking most cases of idiopathic pruritus ani is faecal contamination. Faeces contain potential irritants

Box 113.1 Secondary causes of pruritus ani

Inflammatory skin disease
- Endogenous eczema including seborrhoeic and atopic
- Allergic or irritant contact dermatitis
- Psoriasis
- Lichen planus
- Urticaria
- Lichen sclerosus (females only)
- Hidradentitis suppurativa

Infections
- Candidiasis and dermatophytes
- Erythrasma (*Corynebacterium minutissimum*)
- *Staphylococcus aureus*, β-haemolytic streptococci
- Gonorrhoea, syphillis
- Human papillomavirus, herpes simplex virus
- Human immunodeficiency virus

Infestations
- Threadworms (*Enterobius vermicularis*)
- Pubic lice (*Phthiriasis pubis*)

Perianal premalignant or malignant disease
- Anal intraepithelial neoplasia, anal carcinoma
- Extramammary Paget disease

Ano-rectal disease
- Haemorrhoids, anal fissure
- Perianal fistula, perianal abscess
- Inflammatory bowel disease

Systemic disease
- Metabolic including diabetes, renal, thyroid and liver disease
- Iron deficiency anaemia
- Malignancy including leukaemia and lymphoma

3 Loose frequent stools. These will cause faecal soiling and an increase in perianal trauma from frequent wiping of the skin. Underlying conditions include irritable bowel syndrome.

Other contributing factors include the following:

1 Food and drink. The role of food and drinks is uncertain but those implicated include coffee, tea, cola, beer, chocolate, tomatoes, spices and citrus fruits. The mechanisms proposed include effects on anal sphincter tone, production of loose stools and undigested food components irritating or sensitizing the perianal skin.

2 Psychological factors. Idiopathic pruritus ani has been attributed to stress and anxiety. Patients are often tense individuals in whom everyday problems induce a profound colonic reflex, resulting in defecation and soiling.

Clinical features

History

The complaint is of itching, stinging or soreness that may be chronic and recurrent. Symptoms may be triggered by a bowel movement or wiping with toilet paper, but may occur at night.

Presentation

Physical signs result from the effects of rubbing, scratching (Figure 113.6), secondary infection or contact dermatitis. There may be no visible abnormality at the time of examination.

Differential diagnosis

Fungal infection often causes intense pruritus, and diabetes must be excluded in all severe or persistent candidal infection. See Box 113.1 for other secondary causes.

Complications and co-morbidities

Lichenification, excoriation and secondary infection can occur. A contact dermatitis can result from overwashing and treatment.

and allergens, demonstrated by positive skin patch tests to autologous faeces and enzymes of bacterial origin, that are capable of inducing itch and inflammation. Patients with idiopathic pruritus ani have a high incidence of loose stools and are rarely constipated. Patients with a colostomy do not suffer from pruritus ani. Any factor that increases faecal contamination exposes perianal skin to irritants. A sedentary lifestyle has been implicated.

Causes of faecal contamination include the following (more than one factor may be operative):

1 Difficulty cleaning the perianal area:
- Obesity leads to poor ventilation and maceration.
- Anatomical factors including deeply placed 'funnel anus' and hirsuitism can cause mechanical problems in the maintenance of hygiene.

2 Anal leakage:
- Local causes that alter anal morphology or function such as haemorrhoids, perianal tags or fissures can lead to anal incontinence.
- Primary anal sphincter dysfunction. Exaggerated recto-anal inhibitory refex and anal sphincter dysfunction may result in faecal soiling. Caffiene can lower anal resting pressure.

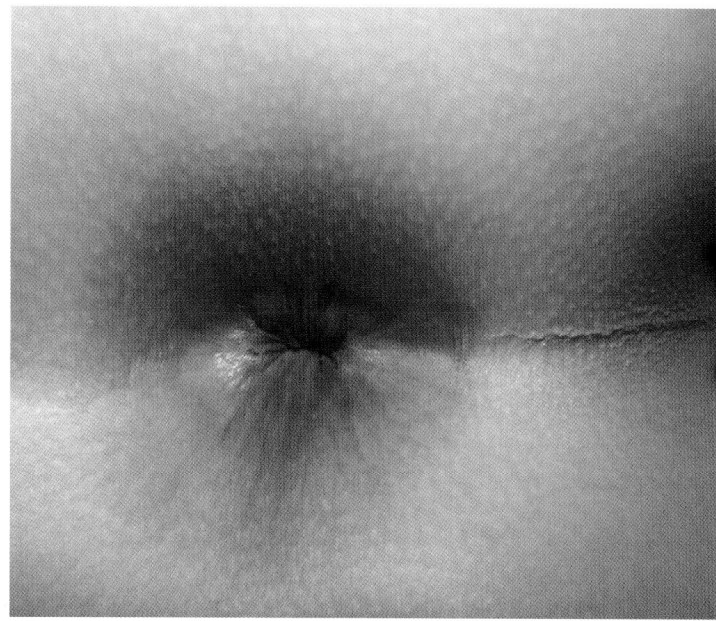

Figure 113.6 Excoriations secondary to idiopathic pruritus ani in a 6-year-old boy. It is important to exclude threadworms at this age.

Patients with pruritus ani are at high risk of sensitization from topical medicaments, toiletries and wet tissue wipes. Common allergens include neomycin, fragrance mix, Balsum of Peru [3] and methylisothiazolinone [4]. Chronic pruritus ani can lead to disruption in quality of life, irritability and depression [5].

Disease course and prognosis
Generic measures usually improve symptoms in 90% of patients [2]. Many patients who undergo surgery for potentially implicated causes such as haemorrhoids continue to have symptoms.

Investigations
In the young, threadworms should be sought with the Sellotape test or by stool examination. Skin patch testing should be considered at an early stage [3].

Management
Specific secondary causes should be addressed. Management includes attention to the patient's washing habits. It is important to maintain cleanliness and to ensure that the perianal area is dried after washing. Soap substitutes should be used and shampoo residues washed off. An emollient should be applied after each wash. A barrier preparation can be preapplied to the perianal skin before the bowels are opened. Washing in a bidet after defecation is preferable to wiping with toilet paper. Rubbing with toilet paper should be discouraged and dabbing recommended. Premoistened toilet paper or wet wipes should be avoided. Underwear should be loose and preferably made of cotton. Topical anaesthetic preparations should be avoided as sensitization commonly occurs. Fingernails should be kept short.

A reduction of coffee consumption or elimination of food or drinks implicated may help. A high-fibre diet should be encouraged if there is any history of constipation or haemorrhoids.

Referral to a colo-rectal specialist is indicated if ano-rectal disease is suspected.

First line
The aim of treatment is to break the compulsive itch–scratch cycle. Local applications should be soothing and as mild as possible. Use of a twice daily liquid cleanser can be as effective as twice daily potent topical steroid application [6]. Mild steroid ointments (1% hydrocortisone) can be helpful [7] and these can be combined with antibacterials or antifungals. Caution should be exercised with topical steroids because perianal skin is occluded and atrophy may occur.

Second line
Other treatments that have been advocated include zinc paste with 1–2% phenol, 0.006% capsaicin ointment [8], 0.1% tacrolimus ointment [9], oral antihistamines, intralesional corticosteroids and corticosteroid suppositories.

Third line
Successful treatment of refractory pruritus ani with intradermal injection of 1–2% methylene blue alone or in combination with 0.5% lidocaine has been reported [10]. Cryotherapy has also been used.

INFLAMMATORY DERMATOSES

The microenvironment of the ano-genital and genito-crural region may alter the usual morphology of skin conditions easily recognized elsewhere. Skin disease may take on a vegetating appearance, especially in hot humid climates and in the presence of infection (Figure 113.7). Specific inflammatory dermatoses that commonly affect the perineum and perianal region are briefly described. The reader is referred to detailed description of specific diseases in relevant chapters.

In adults, inflammation may result from the coexistence of several factors such as haemorrhoids, anal discharge and the effects of scratching. In all cases of perianal and perineal inflammation, the urine should be tested for glucose and swabs and scrapings tested for organisms. Inflammatory skin conditions can cause diagnostic difficulties as clinical features may be altered by the perianal microenvironment.

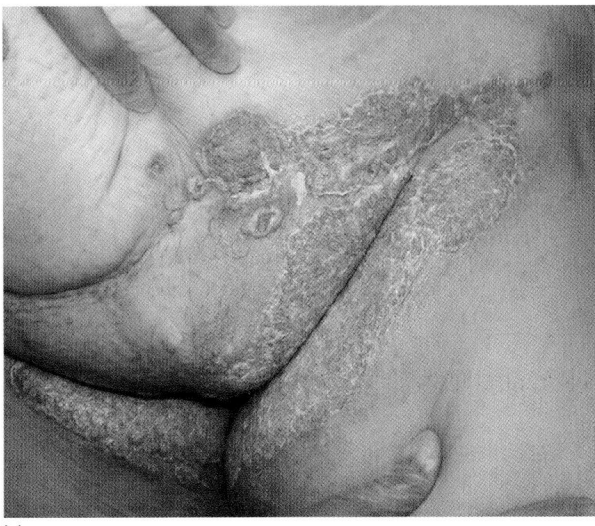

(a)

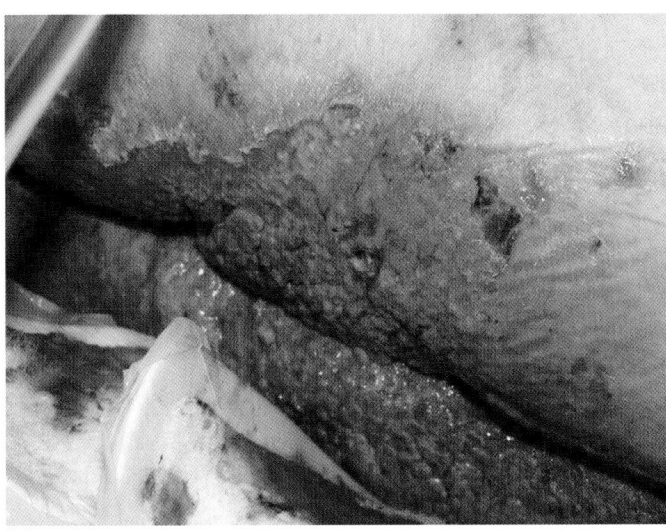

(b)

Figure 113.7 Vegetative pemphigus foliaceous. (a) Affecting the genito-crural region and lower abdomen. (b) Affecting the perianal region and buttocks in the same patient.

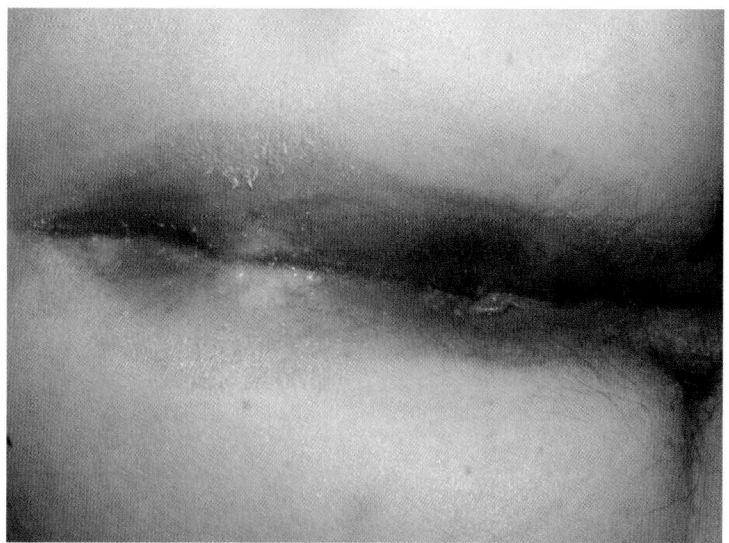

Figure 113.8 Seborrhoeic dermatitis affecting the natal cleft and perianal skin.

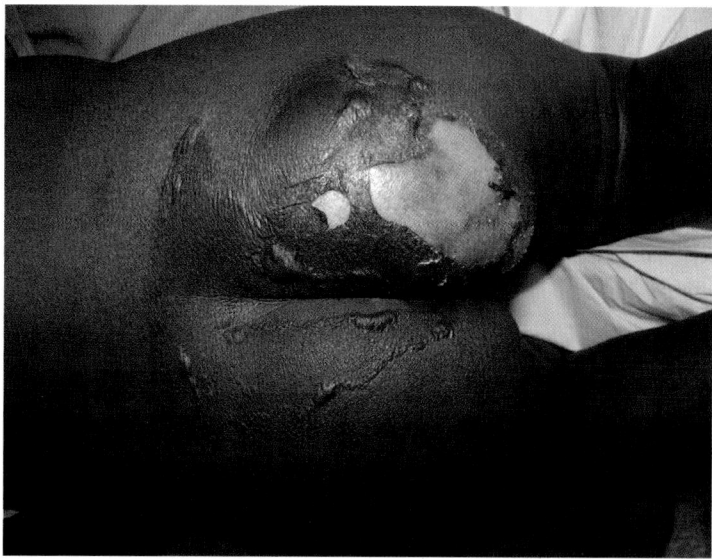

Figure 113.10 Contact dermatitis causing blistering in an infant due to the use of wet wipes.

Seborrhoeic dermatitis. This causes a brownish red inflammation with large greasy scales towards the edge, extending beyond and outside the natal cleft (Figure 113.8). Other areas may be involved including the scalp and other flexures.

Psoriasis. Psoriasis has a smooth glazed surface, dull red hue and is often fissured (Figure 113.9). Other signs of the disease are usually present including scalp and nail changes.

Lichen simplex. This simulates psoriasis but is usually unilateral, except when it involves the perianal area. It may occur as a small, intensely irritable area, localized to the edge of the anus.

Fungal infection. This should be suspected particularly if there has been prior use of topical corticosteroids.

Allergic contact dermatitis. Allergic contact dermatitis is markedly inflamed and may have an ill-defined spreading border. Blistering may occur (Figure 113.10). Patients with chronic perianal dermatoses are at a higher risk of developing sensitization

to topical medicaments than patients with genital dermatoses [1]. Common contact allergens in the ano-genital region include neomycin, fragrance and Balsam of Peru. Methylisothiazolinone currently present in wet wipes is a common cause of allergy in patients presenting with perineal eczema [2]. Carers may present with a hand dermatitis. Condom or spermicide allergy may develop in those practising ano-receptive sex.

Irritant contact dermatitis. Perineal dermatitis can commonly arise as a result of contact with urine or faeces. Danthron erythema is a form of irritant contact dermatitis caused by the use of laxatives containing danthron.

Lichen sclerosus. This extends from the vulval skin to the perianal skin in 30% of women, producing a typical figure-of-eight distribution (Figure 113.11). Perianal lichen sclerosus occurs in 30% of women with genital lichen sclerosus and its occurrence has been associated with urinary incontinence. This pattern reflects the areas of ano-genital skin that come into contact with urine. Men rarely if ever have perianal lichen sclerosus, probably because the male perineum is rarely exposed to urine [3]. The development of perineal lichen sclerosus on previously healthy perineal skin has been described in men following perineal urethrostomy for anterior urethral stricture (4). It is possible that chronic occluded contact of urine with susceptible epithelium is involved in the pathogenesis of ano-genital lichen sclerosus. The barrier function of wet skin is diminished and it is more permeable to irritants. In addition, wet skin has an increased frictional coefficient and higher microbial content (5).

Lichen planus. Lichen planus affecting the perianal region is typically very pruritic and may become excoriated or hypertrophic. Solitary involvement of the perianal region may occur (Figure 113.12).

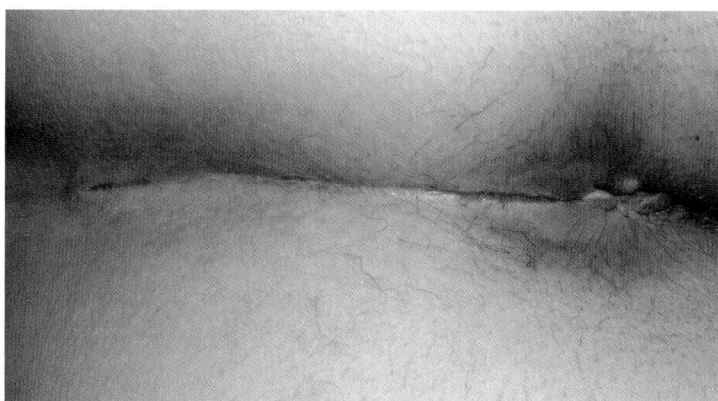

Figure 113.9 Perianal and natal cleft psoriasis causing fissures in a 42–year-old woman.

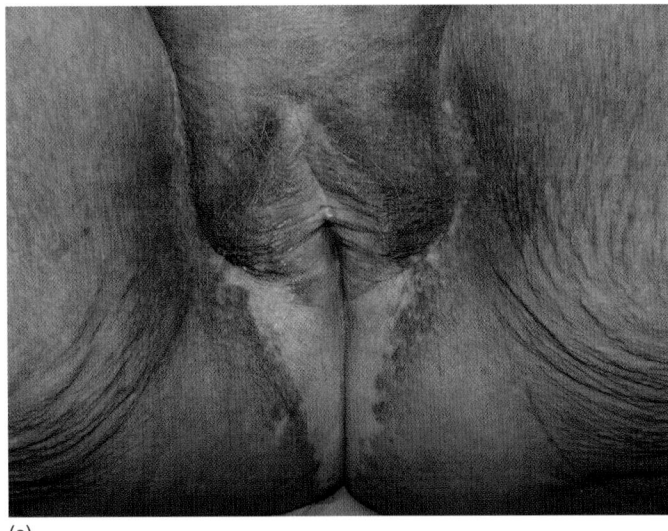

(a)

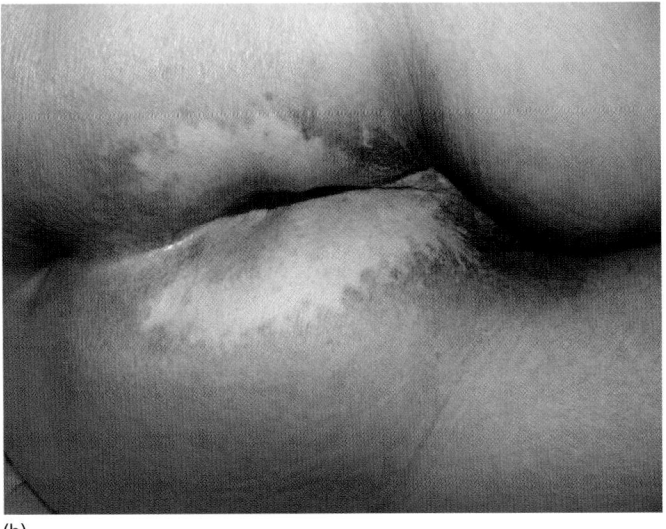

(b)

Figure 113.11 Lichen sclerosus. (a) Ano-genital lichen sclerosus in a female in a typical figure-of-eight configuration. (b) Perianal lichen sclerosus.

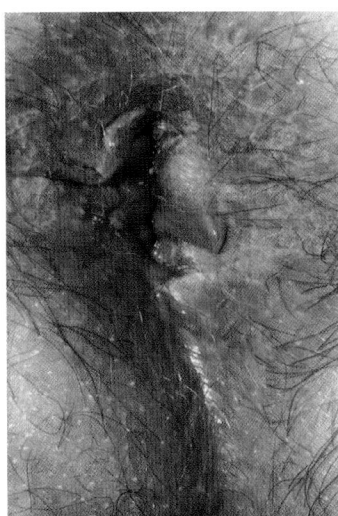

Figure 113.12 Perianal lichen planus showing Wickham's striae. (Courtesy of Dr F. Ive, Durham, UK.)

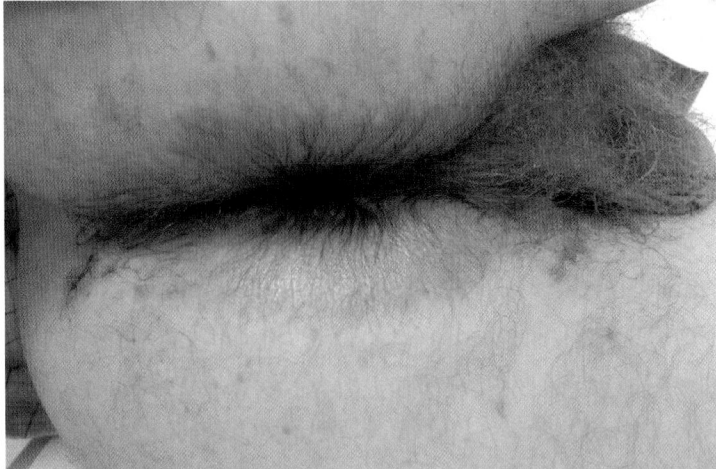

Figure 113.13 Hailey–Hailey disease affecting the ano genital region and causing inflammation and superficial blistering. A skin biopsy has been taken for histology and direct immunofluorescence.

Hailey–Hailey disease. Heat, friction, infection and contact dermatitis can predispose to exacerbations in the ano-genital region (Figure 113.13). It is frequently misdiagnosed as other skin diseases such as seborrhoeic dermatitis. Histology and negative direct immunofluorescence are required to confirm the diagnosis.

Acrodermatitis enteropathica. This should be considered in the differential diagnosis of perianal inflammation in children or adults resulting from malnutrition or malabsorption.

Cicatricial pemphigoid and Stevens–Johnson syndrome. These may cause perianal inflammation, ulceration and scarring and lead to anal stenosis.

Behçet disease. Behçet disease can present with multiple shallow ulcers and fissures of the anal margin.

Radiodermatitis. This may be encountered following treatment for anal carcinoma.

DRUG REACTIONS

Fixed drug eruption. Fixed drug eruptions may produce striking pigmentation.

Cutaneous atrophy. Prolonged use of topical steroids can cause dusky erythema, telangiectasiae, atrophy and induration. Acneform lesions and comedomes may occur.

Perianal contact dermatitis. Topical treatments such as imiquimod cream may cause a contact dermatitis that can be irritant or allergic in nature (Figure 113.14).

Perianal ulceration. Perianal ulceration is a well-recognized complication of nicorandil (Figure 113.15).

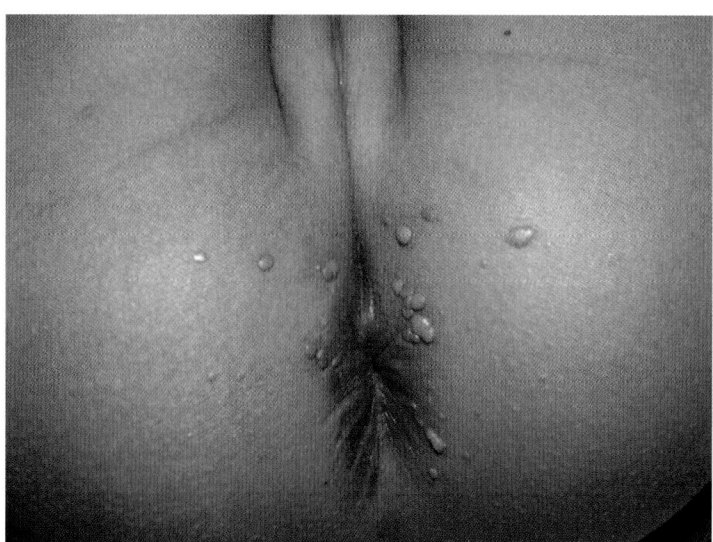

Figure 113.14 Perianal contact dermatitis caused by imiquimod cream used to treat perianal warts.

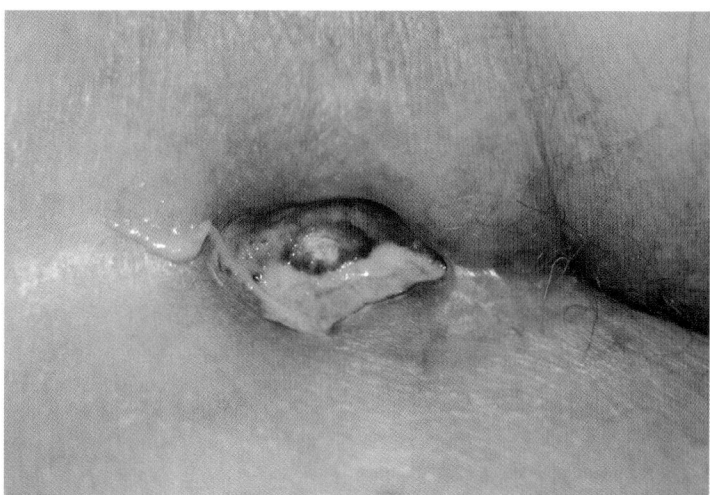

Figure 113.15 Perianal ulceration due to nicorandil. (Courtesy of Dr S. Baron and Dr E. Kulakov, Kent, UK.)

INFECTIONS

BACTERIAL INFECTIONS

Folliculitis and furunculosis

Definition and nomenclature

Folliculitis is an inflammatory or infective process occurring in the hair follicle. Furunculosis is a deep infection of the hair follicle and can lead to abscess formation and is usually caused by *Staphylococcus aureus*.

Synonyms and inclusions
- Boils

Introduction and general description

The ano-genital area, particularly the buttocks and thighs of men, can be susceptible to infection particularly with *S. aureus*. Severe involvement with furunculosis and abscesses suggests an overlap with hidradenitis suppurativa.

Epidemiology

Incidence and prevalence
These infections are common.

Age
All age groups are affected.

Sex
Both sexes are affected equally.

Associated diseases
Diabetes, immunodeficiency, anaemia and atopic eczema are all associated. Eosinophic folliculitis is associated with immunosuppression, including HIV infection [1].

Pathophysiology

Predisposing factors
The high temperature and humidity of the ano-genital area, combined with pressure and friction, encourage colonization with *S. aureus*. Poor personal hygiene, hyperhidrosis, obesity, anaemia, family history and skin conditions such as atopic eczema are also predisposing factors. Nasal carriage of *S. aureus* is the primary risk factor for recurrent furunculosis and occurs in 60% of individuals [2]. Recurrent furunculosis may be a manifestation of underlying immunodeficiency including HIV infection, diabetes and malnutrition. Neutrophil dysfunction may contribute to recurrent furunculosis including iron deficiency-associated reduction in myeloperoxidase activity [3].

Folliculitis is a side effect of drugs including epidermal growth factor receptor inhibitors (e.g. cetuximab).

Pathology
An inflammatory infiltrate occurs within the follicle and may rupture through the follicular epithelium. Organisms may be identified within the follicle.

Causative organisms
Staphylococcus aureus is the commonest pathogen. Meticillin-resistant *S. aureus* (MRSA) and *S. aureus* possessing the Panton–Valentine leukocidin (PVL) virulence factor are common causes of recurrent furunculosis (Figure 113.16) [2]. PVL consists of two proteins that cause lysis and cell death of neutrophils, leading to tissue necrosis and abscess formation. Other organisms include *Pseudomonas* species (hot tub or wet suit folliculitis), *Malassezia furfur* (*Pityrosporum*

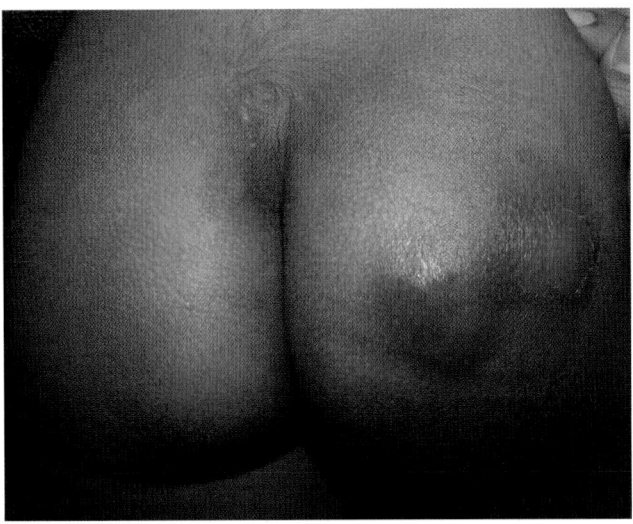

Figure 113.16 Panton–Valentine leukocidin *Staphylococcus aureus* infection affecting the buttock of a 3-year-old female.

folliculitis), *Klebsiella* (Gram-negative folliculitis) and herpes simplex virus.

Clinical features

History
Symptoms include pruritus, painful nodules and purulent discharge.

Presentation
Papules, pustules and suppurative nodules are seen (Figure 113.17). Scarring and hair loss may occur. PVL infection is associated with larger, more erythematous, painful furuncules and may affect other family members [2].

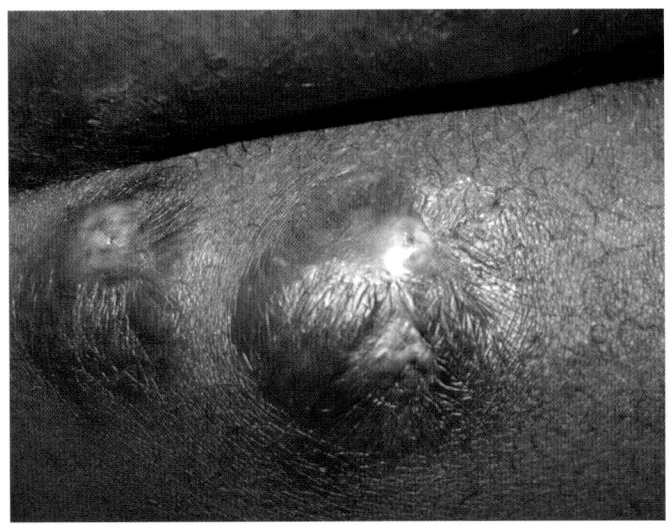

Figure 113.17 Furunculosis affecting the buttocks of a 22-year-old female.

Differential diagnosis
This includes hidradentitis suppurative, pilonidal sinus and Crohn disease.

Complications and co-morbidities
These include bacteraemia, infective endocarditis and necrotizing pneumonia.

Disease course and prognosis
Most patients present with a few boils that resolve with first line treatment. Colonization with *S. aureus* may lead to recurrent furunculosis.

Investigations
Bacterial, fungal or viral swabs or scrapings should be taken. Swabs of nasal and other carrier sites including of close contacts should be considered.

Management
Antibacterial soaps and good personal, interpersonal and environmental hygiene should be advised. Incision and drainage may be required. A topical decolonization regimen should be considered in recurrent furunculosis and where MRSA or PVL *S. aureus* infection has been identified.

First line
Topical antibiotics may be helpful in superficial folliculitis. Systemic antibacterial therapy is usually required for furunculosis based, if possible, on the results of culture.

OTHER BACTERIAL INFECTIONS

Streptococcal dermatitis/perianal cellulitis. Group A β-haemolytic streptococcal perianal dermatitis is most common in children between the ages of 6 and 10 months [1] but may occur in adults [2]. The child may present with pruritus, perianal soreness and painful defecation. Examination reveals a sharply demarcated, boggy erythema. Satellite pustulosis may be present on the buttocks. It is commoner in boys. β-haemolytic streptococci are frequently cultured from the pharynx [1], and streptococcal perianal dermatitis may trigger guttate psoriasis [3]. Treatment includes systemic antibiotics.

Ano-genital cellulitis. Cellulitis and abscess formation can complicate cysts, sinuses and fistulae. The differential diagnosis is given in Box 113.2.

Perianal tuberculosis. Perianal tuberculosis can cause indolent, irregular, painful ulcers, fistulae and abscesses and may be difficult to distinguish from Crohn disease. Lupus vulgaris may spread widely over the buttocks and perianal region or assume a fungating, vegetating appearance. Perineal scrofuloderma (secondary skin involvement from underlying lymph node disease) may cause diagnostic difficulty.

PART 10: SITES, SEX, AGE

Box 113.2 Differential diagnosis of ano-genital cellulitis

- Staphylococcal cellulitis
- Streptococcal cellulitis
- Hidradenititis suppurativa
- Crohn disease
- Gonococcal cellulitis
- Necrotizing soft-tissue infections, e.g. necrotizing fasciitis
- Extramammary Paget disease
- Carcinoma erysipeloides (bladder, prostate, colon)

Adapted from Bunker 2004 [4]. Reproduced with permission of Elsevier.

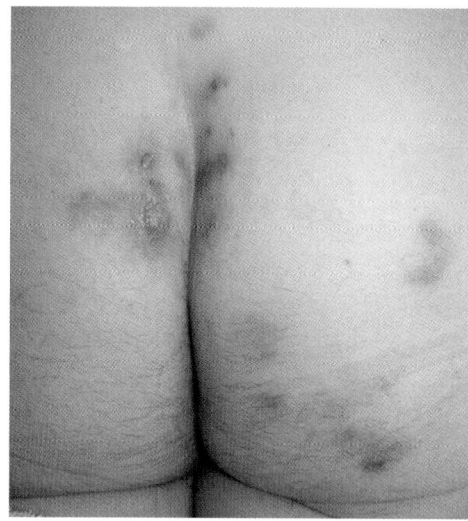

Figure 113.18 Ulcerated and inflamed skin affecting the natal cleft and buttock secondary to herpes simplex type II virus infection.

Necrotizing soft-tissue infections. A number of overlapping, severe, gangrenous, necrotizing conditions may affect the ano-rectal and perineal skin and subcutaneous tissues including muscle. Previously known by names such as clostridial and non-clostridial gangrene, gas gangrene and Fournier gangrene they are now referred to by the generic term of necrotizing soft-tissue infection [5]. Pathogens such as *Streptococcus* and *Clostridium* species are usually involved. Early recognition and intervention is crucial as delay in diagnosis increases mortality. Necrotizing fasciitis is one of these infections.

Necrotizing fasciitis most often affects middle-aged and elderly subjects but all ages can be affected. Risk factors include diabetes, intravenous drug use, trauma and haematological malignancy. Pain – often severe and out of proportion to physical signs – fever and cellulitic skin changes usually develop first. A distinct, dusky red to black spot may appear on affected skin. Tenderness and dusky red erythema extend with extreme rapidity to involve wide areas of the perineum. Crepitus is an important feature, as is the presence of a dark brown, turbid fluid without pus. Deterioration and septicaemia may occur rapidly. Swift surgical intervention with exploration and debridement of affected tissue is essential to improve outcome.

Ecthyma gangrenosum. Ecthyma gangrenosum is usually caused by *Pseudomonas aeruginosa* and occurs in the critically ill or immunosuppressed. It has a predeliction for the ano-genital region and may cause severe, painful, necrotizing, ano-rectal ulceration and septicaemia. The mortality is high.

FUNGAL INFECTIONS

The possibility of fungal infection should be considered in all unusual forms of perianal dermatitis. Microscopy and culture should be performed.

Candidiasis. This causes a bright red, glazed area, often with outlying small pustules and may spread to the groins or natal cleft.

Dermatophyte infection. Dermatophye infection (e.g. with *Trichophyton rubrum*) produces a well-defined, scaly patch with a circinate edge. Prior treatment with corticosteroids may disguise the appearance.

Histoplasmosis and blastomycosis. These can produce perianal lesions.

VIRAL INFECTIONS

Herpes simplex virus infection. This commonly affects the buttocks and perianal skin (Figure 113.18).

Human papillomavirus infection. See the section on human papillomavirus later in this chapter.

Cytomegalovirus infection. This may cause perianal ulceration. It is rare in the immunocompetent but may occur in HIV infection.

Kawasaki disease. The cause is unknown but of possible viral aetiology. An erythematous, desquamating, perineal eruption occurring in the first week of the disease may be the first cutaneous feature in up to two-thirds of children [1].

HELMINTH INFECTIONS

Strongyloides stercoralis. Strongyloides stercoralis usually presents with cutaneous or gastrointestinal symptoms but may be asymptomatic in over 60% of cases and indicated only by a raised blood eosinophil count [1]. In chronic infection, filiform larvae passed in the stool can attach to the perianal skin and lead to autoinfection by migrating through the skin at this site (exoautoinvasion). Rapid intradermal migration of these infectious larvae causes the rash of larva currens and usually presents with very itchy erythematous papules and serpiginous tracts on perianal, buttock and upper thigh skin. Larva currens is pathognomonic for strongyloidiasis [2].

Cutaneous larva migrans. This results from migration of infective larvae from the dog or cat hookworms *Ancylostoma brasiliense* or *A. caninum* after percutaneous invasion and may occur on perineal skin.

Schistosomiasis (bilharziasis). Perineal granulomatous lesions are a rare manifestation presenting as pruritic papules in the ano-genital region in endemic countries.

MISCELLANEOUS INFECTIONS

Scabies infection. Infection with *Sarcoptes scabiei* var *hominis* can cause nodules on the buttocks and perineum.

Amoebiasis. This is caused by the protozoan *Entamoeba histolytica*. The spectrum of disease includes proctocolitis, liver and perianal abscess and perianal ulceration. Transmission usually occurs by the faecal–oral route but direct inoculation of abraded perianal skin may occur. The highest prevalence is in developing countries. Ulcers typically extend slowly but may progress rapidly until a phagedenic ulcer completely destroys the perianal and sacral tissue [1].

OTHER DISEASES AND INFECTIONS

Sexually transmitted diseases

Introduction and general description
Clinical descriptions pertinent to perineal/perianal skin only are discussed. The reader is directed to detailed description of specific sexually transmitted infections elsewhere.

In female patients perianal symptoms may be caused by the posterior spread of genital infections such as candidiasis or trichomoniasis. An irritant perianal dermatitis may occur due to vaginal or anal discharge.

Clinical features

Gonorrhoea. This may cause anal inflammation and discharge or an oedematous perianal dermatitis with multiple fissures and erosions.

Syphilis. This should always be considered as a cause of perianal and anal ulceration, especially in men who have sex with men (MSM). Primary chancres can be mistaken for anal fissures. In secondary syphilis, papular lesions may coalesce in moist areas such as the perianal region to form highly contagious condylomata lata (Figure 113.19). These can be mistaken for genital warts

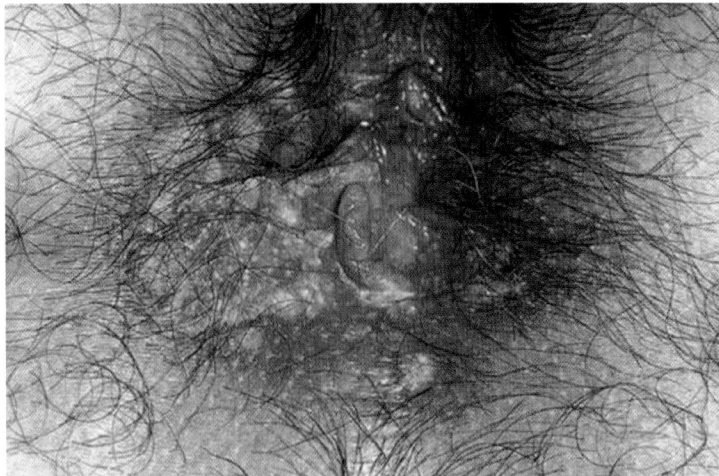

Figure 113.19 Condylomata lata. (Courtesy of Dr S. Gold, London.)

(condylomata acuminata). A granulomatous gumma of tertiary syphilis may affect the perianal area and present as an ulcer, white plaque or atrophic scar. Congenital syphilis may cause perianal rhagades.

Lymphogranuloma venereum (LGV). LGV is a sexually transmitted infection endemic in tropical areas including West Africa. It is caused by one of three invasive serovars (L1, L2 or L3) of *Chlamydia trachomatis* and usually presents with an inguinal syndrome. Infection has become endemic in the UK since 2004 in MSM, particularly HIV-positive men [1]. Similar outbreaks have been reported across Europe and the USA [2]. An ano-rectal LGV syndrome is the usual presentation in industrialized countries with the development of ulcerative haemorrhagic proctitis that can mimic Crohn's colitis. Perianal ulcers and fissures may occur [1]. If untreated, LGV may progress to cause widespread vegetating and scarring lesions of the genito-perineal area.

Human papillomavirus (HPV) infection. HPV infection is the commonest viral sexually transmitted disease. Anal warts are common in young adults but are not always sexually transmitted.

Herpes simplex virus infection. Herpes simplex virus type 2 infection is a common cause of acute painful perianal and anal ulceration in MSM. Proctitis can occur often without visible perianal ulceration [3].

Granuloma inguinale (Donovanosis). This is an infection caused by *Klebsiella granulomatis* and is most frequently seen in tropical countries and is rare in temperate climates. It usually affects perineal skin, causing relatively painless papules and nodules that ulcerate. Ulcers may be phagedenic. Nodules may be mistaken for lymph nodes (pseudobubo). Perianal lesions can scar leading to anal stenosis and squamous cell carcinoma can occur.

Chancroid. Chancroid is an infection caused by *Haemophilus ducreyi* and is characterized by painful ano-genital or perianal ulceration and inguinal lymphadenopathy. The prevalence of chancroid has decreased worldwide.

Infestations. Infestations including *Phthiriasis pubis* (pubic lice) should be considered.

Management
Patients should be managed by a genito-urinary medicine specialist.

Human immunodeficiency virus infection

Introduction and general description
Many skin conditions can affect perianal skin, including seborrhoeic dermatitis and flexural psoriasis, and are associated with HIV infection. The reader is referred to Chapter 31. Ano-rectal disease is common in HIV infection. Up to 66% of patients may have more than one condition [1]. Anal warts are the commonest disorder. There is a higher risk of progression to anal intraepithelial neoplasia and frank malignancy in HIV-positive men and women [2].

Painful perianal and intra-anal ulcers are also common, occurring in 32% of patients in a cohort of 180 HIV-positive men and women with ano-rectal symptoms [3]. Most of the ulcers were idiopathic; 12% were due to herpes simplex virus infection and 7% due to cytomegalovirus reactivation.

Ano-genital ulceration can increase the risk of HIV acquisition per sexual exposure by a factor 10–50 for male to female transmission and of 50–300 for female to male transmission [4].

Severe, painful recrudescence of ulcerated herpes simplex infection type 2 may occur including as a manifestation of immune reconstitution after initiation of antiretroviral therapy [5].

Box 113.3 lists the main causes of anal ulceration associated with HIV infection.

Box 113.3 Causes of anal/perianal ulceration in HIV infection

- Herpes simplex virus infection
- Syphilis (primary chancre)
- Lymphogranuloma venereum
- Idiopathic (aphthous)
- Anal fissures
- Anal sepsis (perianal abscess, perianal fistula)
- Haemorrhoids
- Cytomegalovirus infection
- Kaposi sarcoma
- Non-Hodgkin lymphoma
- Squamous cell carcinoma
- Pruritus ani
- Trauma
- Amoebiasis

Human papillomavirus infection

Definition and nomenclature
Human papillomaviruses are DNA viruses that infect squamous epithelia or cells with the potential for squamous maturation, including the skin and mucosae of the ano-genital region.

Synonyms and inclusions
- Condylomata acuminata
- External genital warts.

Introduction and general description
Infection with HPV of the ano-genital region is the commonest viral sexually transmitted disease. Perianal and intra-anal HPV infection is common. Approximately 40 out of the 180 known HPV genotypes have been associated with ano-genital lesions. The majority of HPV-associated diseases are caused by HPV types 6, 11, 16 and 18. HPV genotypes are divided into low-risk types such as HPV-6 and -11 that predominantly cause benign ano-genital warts and high-risk types such as HPV-16 and -18 that may cause neoplasia including anal intraepithelial neoplasia (AIN) and anal cancer. At least 13 of the known HPV genotypes have oncogenic potential.

Epidemiology

Incidence and prevalence
The annual incidence of clinically visible ano-genital HPV infection has been estimated to be 1–2% in sexually active individuals. Many other patients may have subclinical or latent infection. The estimated lifetime risk of ano-genital wart infection is 10% [1].

Age
The peak prevalence of genital HPV infection occurs in females in their late teens and twenties and prevalence declines in subsequent decades. Men acquire infection in their late teens but prevalence does not decline with age [2]. The rate of acquiring a new genital HPV infection decreases with age in women but does not vary by age in men.

Sex
Genital HPV prevalence is higher in men than women. Anal HPV infection has been studied more frequently in men than women. Anal HPV prevalence among MSM is twice that of women and anal HPV prevalence in women is twice that of men who have sex with women [2]. The prevalence of anal HPV in men who have sex with women has been shown to be 12% [2] and up to 70% in MSM [3]. Anal HPV prevalence is higher in women with HPV-related cervical disease and women at risk of HPV infection [2].

Pathophysiology

Predisposing factors

Warts in the anal canal are associated with anoreceptive sex. An increased number of lifetime sexual partners and immunosuppression are risk factors for HPV infection.

Pathology

Histology is characterized by papillomatosis, acanthosis, hyperkeratosis and parakeratosis (Figure 113.20a). Koilocytes in the granular cell layer as well as coarse keratohyaline granules are characteristic (Figure 113.20b, c).

Causative organisms

Viral gene expression is confined to the keratinocytes. HPV infects and replicates in differentiating squamous epithelium only and is effective at evading host recognition and immunity [4]. HPV-6 and -11 are low-risk HPVs and are responsible for over 90% of ano-genital warts [5]. The presence of low-risk HPV infection may be a marker for the carriage of high-risk genotypes such as HPV-16.

Clinical features

History

Symptoms include pruritus ani, discomfort, bleeding and palpable lesions.

Presentation

Warty papules, plaques and nodules are seen and may be profuse and extend into the anal canal.

Clinical variants

Perianal viral warts may occur in infants and young children (Figure 113.21). Sexual abuse needs to be considered in all cases, particularly in children older than 2 years where vertical transmission is less likely. The upper age limit for vertical transmission is uncertain as latent infection may occur. Furthermore, HPV genotypes do not seem to show the same degree of tropism for either mucosal or cutaneous sites, as occurs in adults [6]. The presence of warts or HPV DNA alone is not sufficient to make a diagnosis of sexual abuse and social, behavioural and other supporting clinical information is required.

Differential diagnosis

Molluscum contagiosum, condylomata lata, lichen planus, AIN and anal carcinoma should all be considered as possible diagnoses.

Complications and co-morbidities

Diagnosis of ano-genital warts is associated with a long-term risk of ano-genital neoplasia and other malignancies including oropharygeal carcinoma. There is a higher risk of progression to AIN and anal carcinoma in the immunosuppressed.

   MSM with ano-genital HPV infection have a significantly higher risk of acquiring HIV infection [7].

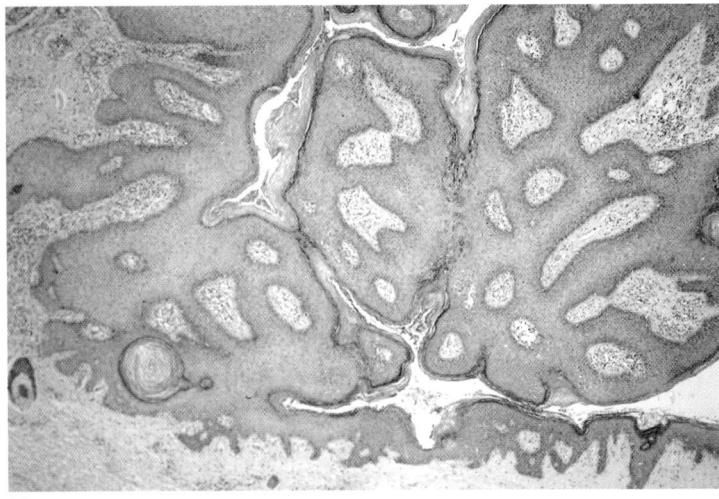

(a)

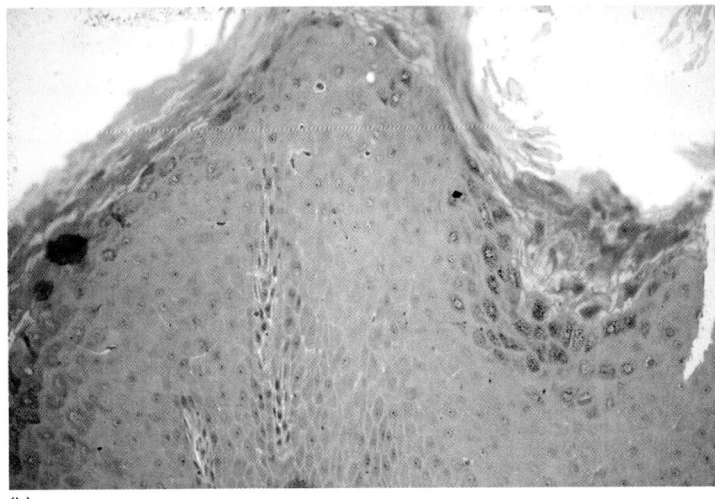

(b)

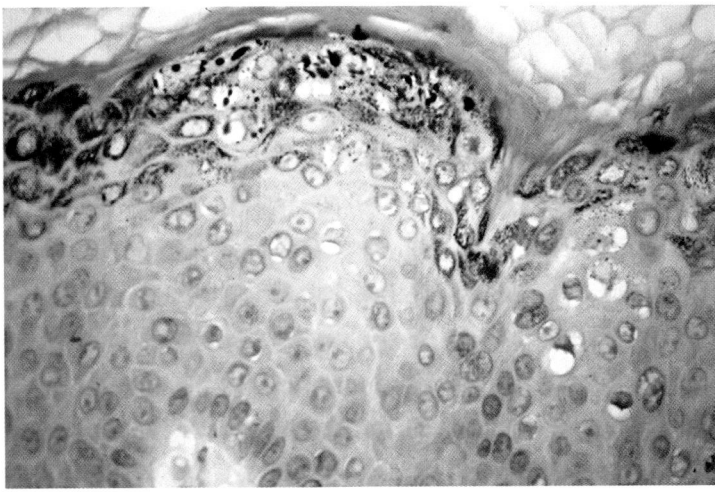

(c)

Figure 113.20 Perianal wart. (a) Low power histological features of a perianal wart showing hyperkeratosis, acanthosis and papillomatosis. Magnification 40×. (b) Higher power view of a perianal wart showing papillomatosis, hyperkeratosis, coarse keratohyaline granules and koilocytosis. Magnification 200×. (c) High power view of a perianal viral wart showing keratohyaline granules and koilocytes; there is also low-grade dysplasia. Magnification 400×. (Courtesy of Dr Nick Francis, London, UK.)

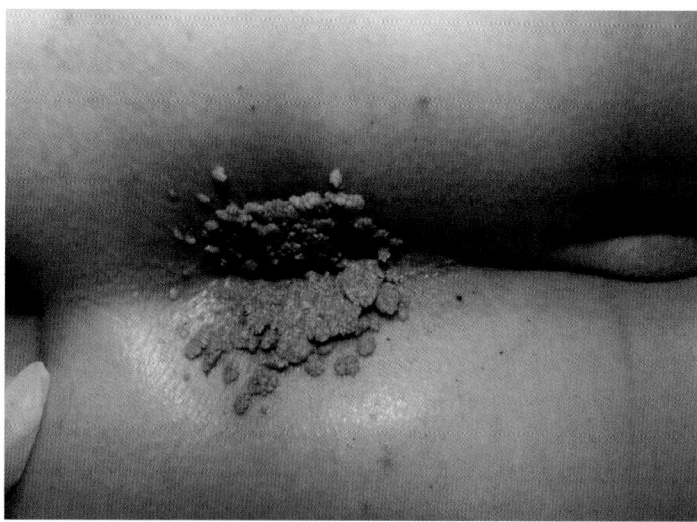

Figure 113.21 Florid perianal warts in a 5-year-old male.

Disease course and prognosis

The average incubation period from sexual exposure to HPV and development of ano-genital warts in young adults is 3 months. Approximately 80–90% of ano-genital HPV infections regress due to a successful cell-mediated immune response. Persistent HPV infection with high-risk oncogenic genotypes able to evade host immunity can lead to the expression of potent oncogenes E6 and E7, with subsequent neoplastic transformation and progression to high-grade AIN or anal carcinoma [4].

Investigations

Infection with HPV can be investigated using molecular hybridization to detect HPV DNA in biopsy specimens, swabs or scrapings obtained from the mucosa or skin.

Management

Patients should be managed by a genito-urinary medicine specialist. A full sexual health screen is required and colo-rectal assessment if intra-anal disease is suspected. A biopsy should be performed if diagnosis is in doubt or dysplasia suspected. The treatment choice depends on the morphology, number of lesions and patient preference. Relapse is common.

HPV vaccination

The quadrivalent HPV vaccine consists of virus-like particles assembled from major capsid proteins (L1) of HPV-16, -18, -6 and -11. It has been shown to reduce ano-genital HPV infection prevalence in young females by more than 90%, as well as reducing high-grade cervical intraepithelial neoplasia in the same population [8]. Randomized controlled trials with the quadrivalent HPV vaccine have also demonstrated high efficacy against the development of ano-genital warts in men who have sex with women and MSM [9]. Currently, only a few countries including Australia and the USA recommend vaccination of adolescent boys. A gender-neutral vaccination programme has been advocated to induce true herd immunity and prevent all HPV-associated disease including anal cancer and oropharyngeal cancer in men and women [10].

First line

Options include imiquimod cream 5%, podophyllin, podophyllotoxin or trichloroacetic acid solution.

Second line

Options include ablative therapy with cryotherapy or electrocautery, surgical excision or laser therapy.

Third line

Topical, intralesional or systemic interferon treatment has been described. Interferons are not recommended for routine management of anogenital warts. Various regimens have been described using interferons α, β and γ as creams and as intralesional or systemic injection [11].

Resources

Further information

British Association for Sexual Health and HIV: www.bashh.org/guidelines (last accessed August 2015).

Anal intraepithelial neoplasia

Definition and nomenclature

This is an intraepidermal, non-invasive, squamous neoplasia that can affect the anal canal and perianal skin.

> **Synonyms and inclusions**
> - Anal intraepithelial dysplasia
> - Carcinoma *in situ*
> - Anal squamous intraepithelial lesion
> - Bowen disease
> - Bowenoid papulosis

Introduction and general description

The clinical presentation of AIN is variable. Perianal lesions are often referred to as Bowen disease. The high-risk HPV genotypes HPV-16 and -18 are strongly associated with the development of AIN. Early diagnosis and management of AIN is important to prevent progression to invasive squamous cell carcinoma.

Epidemiology

Incidence and prevalence

The incidence of high-grade AIN is estimated to be 0.45 per 100 000 of the general population. The prevalence is higher in high-risk groups and is estimated to occur in 52% of HIV-positive MSM and 5% of renal transplant recipients [1].

Age

It is commoner in older women and younger men.

Sex

Anal intraepithelial neoplasia is commoner in women and in MSM.

Associated diseases

Anal intraepithelial neoplasia can be part of multicentric disease affecting other genital sites including the vulva, cervix and penis.

Pathophysiology

Predisposing factors

Predisposing factors include receptive anal sex, a history of anogenital warts, smoking, lifetime number of sexual partners and immunosuppression including renal transplant recipients. The highest risk group for AIN is HIV-positive MSM.

Pathology

Cytological atypia is confined to the epidermal layer. AIN is characterized by varying degrees of loss of stratification and nuclear polarity, dyskeratosis, nuclear pleomorphism and hyperchromatism and increased mitotic activity with the presence of mitoses high in the epithelium. Koilocytes may be present. Atypia can be graded into low grade (Figure 113.22) or high grade (Figure 113.23) depending on severity. Expression of proliferative biomarkers such as p16 can be a useful diagnostic tool to confirm the grade of disease.

Causative organisms

There are approximately 15 recognized high-risk oncogenic anogenital HPV genotypes. HPV-16 and -18 are predominantly associated with AIN in men and women [2].

Clinical features

History

Anal intraepithelial neoplasia is often asymptomatic. Symptoms include pruritus ani and bleeding.

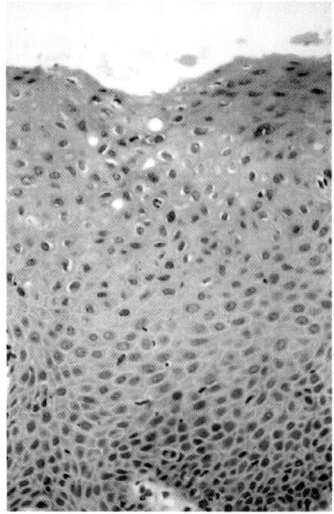

Figure 113.22 Histopathology of low-grade anal intraepithelial neoplasia. Koilocytes are present high in the upper half of the epidermis. Magnification 200×. (Courtesy of Dr Nick Francis, London, UK.)

Presentation

Lesions can be solitary or multifocal. Intra-anal AIN when visible macroscopically may present as papillomatous papules or plaques that can appear erythematous, white, pigmented or fissured. Induration or ulceration may indicate invasion. Intra-anal AIN can be identified after the application of 3% acetic acid during high-resolution anoscopy. AIN is often an incidental finding on surgical specimens.

Clinical variants

Perianal Bowen disease presents as relatively asymptomatic red, shiny or scaly plaques (Figure 113.24). There may be continuity with dysplastic lesions in the anal canal. HPV-16 has been

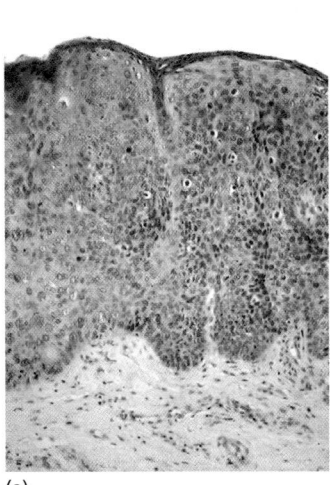

(a)

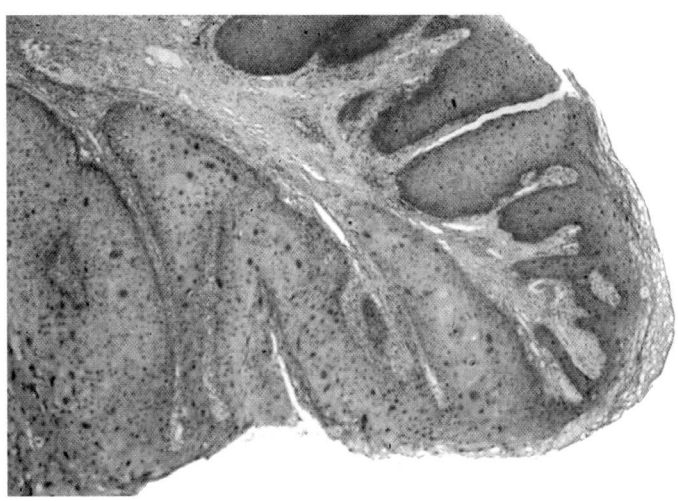

(b)

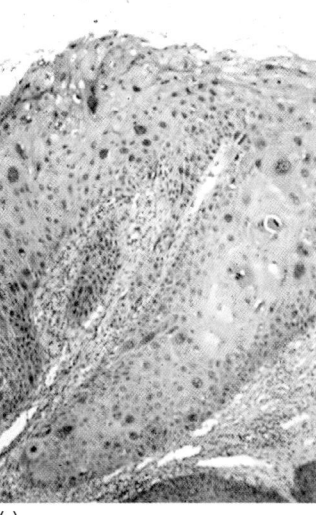

(c)

Figure 113.23 Histopathology of high-grade anal intraepithelial neoplasia (AIN). (a) High-grade, full-thickness AIN. Magnification 100×. (b) High-grade AIN occurring within a perianal wart. There is marked nuclear atypia, dyskeratosis and basal crowding of the nuclei. Magnification 40×. (c) High-grade AIN occurring within a perianal wart. Magnification 100×. (Courtesy of Dr Nick Francis, London, UK.)

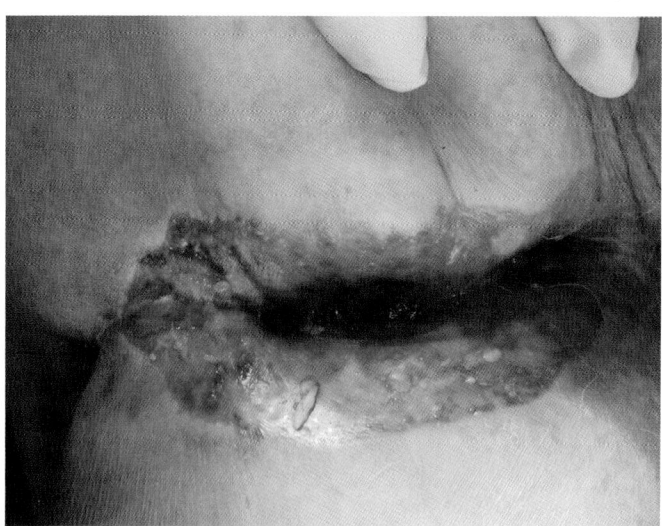

Figure 113.24 Eroded patch of perianal high-grade intra-epithelial neoplasia (Bowen disease) in a 75-year-old female.

identified in 60–80% of cases [3]. Perianal Bowen disease is estimated to progress to invasive squamous cell carcinoma in 2–6% of cases [3].

Bowenoid papulosis is a distinct clinical entity presenting as solitary or multiple, reddish brown, pigmented or flesh-coloured papules with a flat or verrucous surface that can merge into plaques. It typically occurs in the ano-genital region or groin of young, sexually active individuals. Histology is of full-thickness epithelial dysplasia. HPV-16 is usually implicated. The risk of progression to invasive carcinoma is unknown.

Differential diagnosis
Anal carcinoma, HPV infection, psoriasis and lichen planus should be considered.

Classification of severity
Anal intraepithelial neoplasia is commonly defined as low or high grade based on the degree of cytological atypia.

Disease course and prognosis
The risk of progression to anal or perianal squamous cell carcinoma is poorly understood, partly because there are relatively few trained experts in anoscopy and few and limited published data. The risk of progression of high-grade AIN to invasive anal carcinoma in immunocompetent patients over 5 years is approximately 10% [4]. The risk of progression to anal carcinoma in HIV-positive patients is currently unknown but invasive disease can develop quickly [5].

Investigations
Histological assessment of the suspected area of AIN is required to confirm the diagnosis and investigate whether there is evidence of invasive disease. Screening for AIN includes anal cytology and high-resolution anoscopy with mapping biopsies of suspicious areas.

Management
Multidisciplinary specialist management is essential. Digital rectal examination and anoscopy is required to determine if there is intra-anal disease. Genital skin should be examined for evidence of associated diseases. All females with AIN require gynaecological assessment in view of the high prevalence of concomitant cervical intraepithelial neoplasia.

The aims of management are to alleviate symptoms and prevent progression to anal cancer. Management of AIN is not standardized. Some advocate close follow-up for low-grade intra-anal disease. Recurrence is common following intervention especially in the immunosuppressed.

First line
Topical 5% imiquimod or 5-fluorouracil cream are therapeutic options for perianal or intra-anal disease and can be self-applied [6]. Targeted ablation options include CO_2 laser, electrocautery or infrared coagulation. Solitary, small perianal lesions may be amenable to surgical excision. Risks of surgery include anal stenosis and faecal incontinence.

Second line
Photodynamic therapy can be considered.

Screening and prevention
The utility of screening for AIN using anal cytology and high-resolution anoscopy is currently controversial in terms of cost effectiveness and there are no national screening programmes in place, but it has been recommended for high-risk populations including MSM and HIV-positive patients [7].

HPV vaccination has been shown to reduce the prevalence of AIN in MSM [8]. HPV vaccination is also being explored as a therapeutic option to prevent recurrence of AIN.

Anal and perianal malignancy

Synonyms and inclusions
- Anal cancer
- Squamous cell carcinoma
- Epidermoid carcinoma

Introduction and general description
Malignancies of the anal region are relatively uncommon, comprising 2–4% of all ano-rectal malignancies. Tumours of the anal region include tumours of the anal canal and anal margin. Distinction between tumour location at the anal margin or anal canal is important as there are differences in management and prognosis. Unfortunately the literature has often grouped these two anatomical sites together, leading to difficulties in interpreting the results of interventions.

Squamous cell carcinoma is the most common type of anal cancer, comprising approximately 80% of cases [1]. Anal adenocarcinoma accounts for less than 10% of all anal cancers [2]. Other rarer malignancies affecting the anal region include melanoma, lymphoma and Kaposi sarcoma. Ano-genital Kaposi sarcoma is essentially HIV related.

Squamous cell carcinoma of the anal region is usually preceded by AIN. Most cases are a result of sexually acquired infection with oncogenic HPV subtypes, predominantly HPV-16 and -18. Prevention may be possible through the use of HPV vaccination.

The following discussion will be limited to squamous cell carcinoma (SCC).

Epidemiology

Incidence and prevalence

Anal SCC is rare but the incidence is increasing worldwide in men and women. The rise in incidence in women is thought to be due to more women having ano-receptive sex with a resultant increased risk of exposure to high-risk HPV types. The rise in incidence in men is attributed to prolonged survival of patients with HIV infection, enabling progression of persistent high-risk HPV infection to AIN and subsequent invasive malignancy. The incidence of SCC of the anal canal is approximately 1.5 cases per 100 000 per year globally [3]. Anal cancer is not an AIDS defining diagnosis but the incidence is 40–70 times higher in HIV-positive patients, and highest in MSM who practice anoreceptive sex [4].

Age

Women older than 50 years have a higher incidence rate. Men have a higher incidence rate in the 20–49-year age group [5].

Sex

It is commoner in women and HIV-positive men.

Associated diseases

Associated diseases include ano-genital HPV infection and other sexually transmitted diseases, vulval, penile and cervical intraepithelial neoplasia and carcinoma.

Pathophysiology

Predisposing factors

Factors that increase the risk of ano-genital HPV infection or modulate the host immune response to HPV are associated with anal SCC. These include anoreceptive sex, lifetime number of sexual partners, immunosuppression (including organ transplant recipients) and smoking. Anal SCC is also increased in autoimmune disease including psoriasis and granulomatosis with polyangiitis [6]. The highest risk group is HIV-positive MSM. HIV control as measured by the per cent of time with undetectable HIV viral load has been reported to decrease the risk of anal SCC [7]. Optimizing antiretroviral therapy and control of HIV viral load may decrease the risk of anal SCC.

Perianal SCC can also develop on a background of chronic dermatoses including lichen planus, lichen sclerosus and hidradenitis suppurativa.

Pathology

Anal intraepithelial neoplasia is thought to be the precursor of invasive SCC (Figure 113.25). Histological features of anal

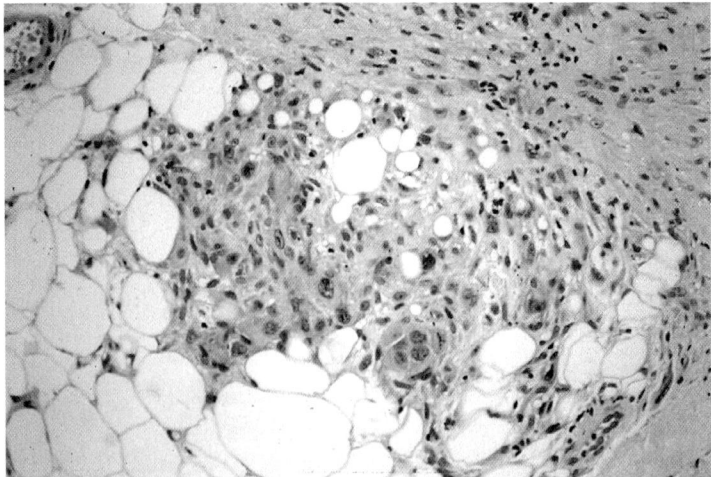

Figure 113.25 Squamous cell carcinoma infiltrating adipose tissue that has developed from adjacent high-grade anal intraepithelial neoplasia. Magnification 400×. (Courtesy of Dr Nick Francis, London, UK.)

SCC include hyperkeratosis, acanthosis, ectopic keratinization, nuclear pleomorphism and mitoses. Cells can vary from large, pale eosinophilic cells to small, basaloid or spindle-shaped cells. Tongues of atypical keratinocytes invade the dermis. The invasive margin can vary from well circumscribed to irregular. A lymphocytic infiltrate of varying degrees may be present. No significant association between histological subtype and prognosis has been established.

Causative organisms

Anal SCC is associated with high-risk HPV infection, including HPV-16, in more than 96% of cases [8].

Clinical features

History

Symptoms include pruritus ani, bleeding, pain, tenesmus, faecal incontinence, discharge, change in bowel habit, ulceration and presence of a mass. History may include ano-genital HPV infection, HIV infection, anoreceptive sex or smoking.

Presentation

Presentation includes an ulcer or a hard mass that can be flat, raised or polypoid (Figures 113.26 and 113.27). SCC of the anal margin is at least fivefold less common than of the anal canal [9], but is the commonest tumour of the anal margin. Anal margin SCC is commoner in men [10]. It can be difficult to determine from the outset whether the tumour originated in the anal canal or anal margin as often both areas are involved at the time of diagnosis.

Locally advanced disease may present with perianal infection, fistula formation and inguinal lymphadenopathy. Lymph node involvement at diagnosis occurs in 30–40% of cases with distant extrapelvic metastases recorded in 5–8% at diagnosis. Rates of metastatic progression after primary treatment vary between 10% and 20% [10]. Tumours distal to the dentate line drain to the inguinal and femoral nodal chains.

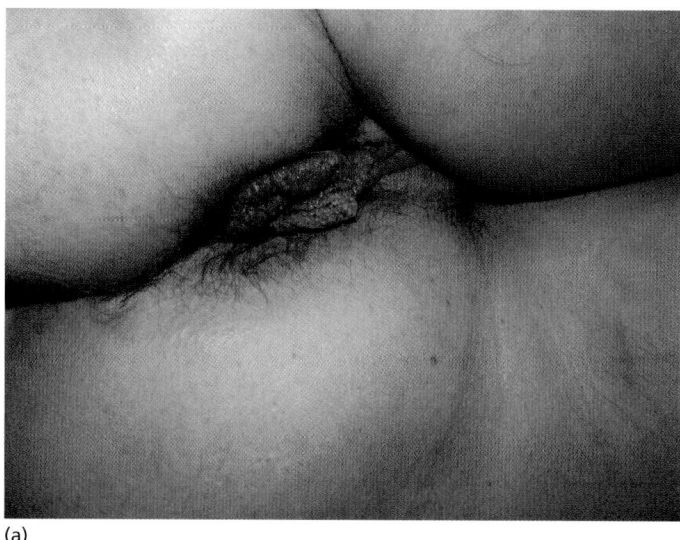

(a)

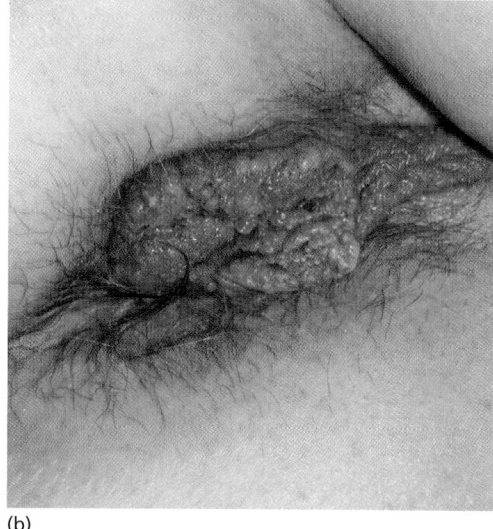

(b)

Figure 113.26 (a) Large polypoid mass of perianal carcinoma in a 56-year-old female. (b) Close-up view of the same carcinoma.

Clinical variants

Buschke–Löwenstein tumour (also called giant condyloma acuminatum or verrucous carcinoma) is a rare, slow-growing, cauliflower-like exophytic tumour of the ano-genital region caused by HPV and characterized by invasive growth (Figure 113.28). HPV-6 and -11 are the most common HPV genotypes identified. HPV-16 and -18 can also be detected, especially in cases with foci of invasive SCC. The histological features are similar to those of condyloma acuminatum. The Buschke–Löwenstein tumour is thought to exhibit intermediate biological behaviour towards malignancy. Wide local excision or abdomino-perineal resection are considered the treatment of choice. Adjuvant chemoradiotherapy may be necessary if there is an invasive component. Malignant transformation to SCC can occur in 40–60% of cases.

Differential diagnosis

Anal carcinoma should be considered in all nodulo-ulcerative anal and perianal disease, including when there is a history of perianal chronic inflammatory skin disease such as lichen planus, lichen sclerosus, hidradentitis suppurativa or a background of immunodeficiency. The diagnosis of anal cancer is often delayed and is mistaken for benign disease such as haemorrhoids or anal tags.

Classification of severity

Anal and perianal SCC can be staged according to the American Joint Committee on Cancer TNM classification, which includes assessment of the tumour, lymph nodes and distant metastasis [11].

Disease course and prognosis

Tumour size (≥5 cm), nodal involvement and male sex are associated with a less favourable prognosis. Anal margin tumours have

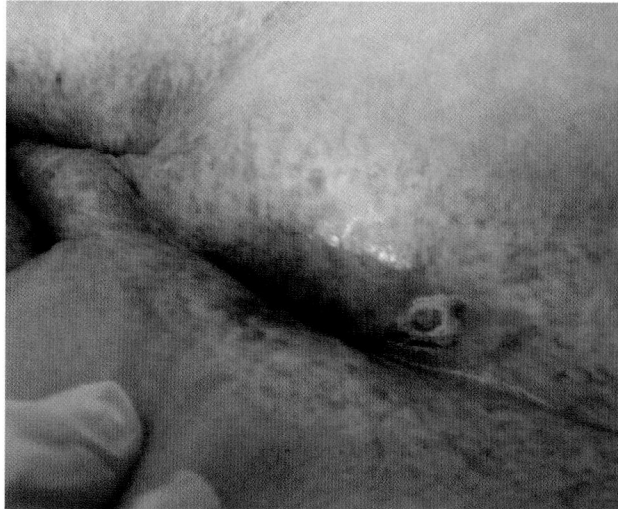

Figure 113.27 Poorly differentiated, eroded, perianal nodule of squamous cell carcinoma present at the anal margin occurring in a 50-year-old HIV-negative man within the radiotherapy treatment field 10 years after treatment of anal carcinoma with chemoradiotherapy. The patient subsequently had an abdomino-perineal resection and perineal reconstruction for the recurrent disease.

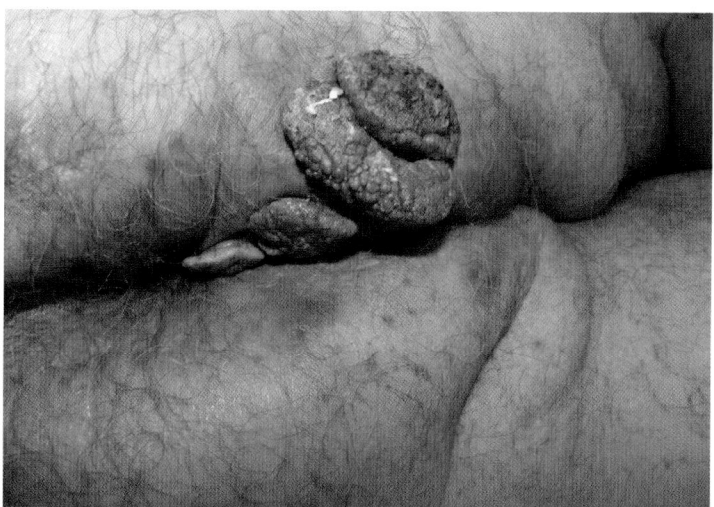

Figure 113.28 Buschke–Löwenstein tumour affecting the perianal skin of a 56-year-old male.

a better prognosis. Overall 5-year survival rates for localized disease, disease with regional lymph node involvement and disease with distant metastases are 80%, 58% and 31%, respectively [12]. Chemoradiation leads to complete tumour regression in 80–90% of patients. HIV-positive patients on highly active antiretroviral therapy have been shown to have similar clinical response and tolerability to chemoradiation as HIV-negative patients [13].

Anal margin SCC has a slightly better prognosis.

Investigations

Histological diagnosis is required and imaging undertaken for tumour staging. MRI of the pelvis and endoanal ultrasound enable assessment including of tumour size and anal sphincter involvement. Distant metastatic spread is assessed by computed tomography of the thorax, abdomen and pelvis.

Management

A multidisciplinary approach is essential including involvement of an ano-rectal surgeon, radiotherapist and medical oncologist.

The aim of treatment is to achieve cure with preservation of faecal continence. Chemoradiotherapy using a combination of 5-fluorouracil and mitomycin C have been established as first line treatment for invasive anal canal disease [10]. Small, well-differentiated anal margin tumours without nodal involvement can be treated with wide local excision if anal sphincter function can be preserved.

The main role for surgery in anal cancer is for residual or recurrent disease after failure of chemoradiotherapy and is referred to as salvage surgery. Abdomino-perineal resection with perineal reconstruction is the most frequently performed operation. This operation involves resection of the anus and rectum, end colostomy formation and reconstruction of the perineum.

Miscellaneous malignancies

Extramammary Paget disease (EMPD). EMPD is a rare but important diagnosis. Primary EMPD is an intraepithelial adenocarcinoma arising possibly from intraepidermal cells of the apocrine gland ducts or from pluripotent keratinocyte stem cells, and is the commonest form of EMPD [1]. Secondary EMPD arises from an underlying malignancy in a dermal adnexal gland or a local organ with contiguous epithelium. Perianal EMPD represents approximately 20% of cases of extramammary disease [2]. The association between EMPD and malignancy is variable, ranging from 38% to 70% [2]. The commonest tumours are ano-rectal adenocarcinoma and adenocarcinoma of the bladder or urethra, but distant tumours including breast may be responsible. Perianal EMPD is strongly associated with ano-rectal adenocarcinoma, with up to 80% of patients having an underlying ano-rectal adenocarcinoma [1,2].

Common symptoms are pruritus ani and perianal bleeding [3]. Lesions are typically red plaques or erosions that are moist or hyperkeratotic. Perianal lesions can extend into the anal canal.

Management of primary disease is tailored to the extent of the EMPD and can include imiquimod cream, surgery (including Mohs micrographic surgery) or photodynamic therapy. Recurrence is common. Management of secondary disease is primarily directed towards the associated malignancy.

Basal cell carcinoma. This very common cancer rarely affects the ano-genital area. Predisposing factors include radiation, trauma or burns [4].

Melanoma. Anal margin melanoma is rare, accounting for 2–4% of all ano-rectal malignancies [4].

Langerhans cell histiocytosis. This condition can cause perianal ulceration.

Carcinoma erysipeloides. Infiltration of the skin with neoplastic cells produces the clinical appearance of cellulitis or erysipelas. Infiltrative papules can be seen on close inspection. It has been reported in the perineum and on the thigh in carcinoma of the bladder and prostate [5] and in the genito-crural region secondary to adenocarcioma of the colon (Figure 113.29) (E. Mallon, personal observation).

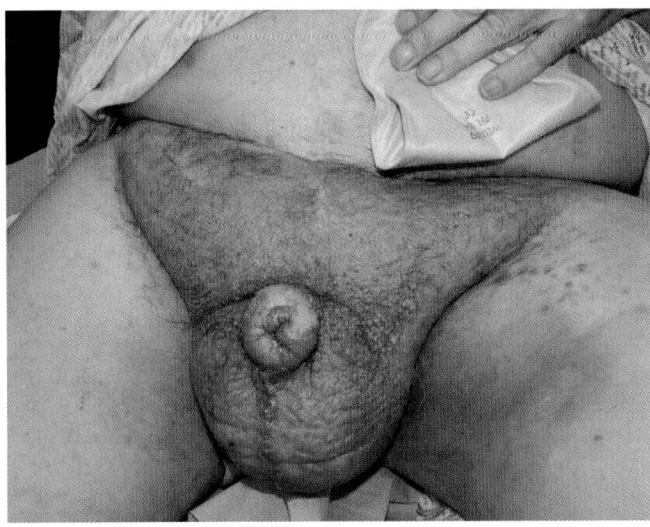

(a)

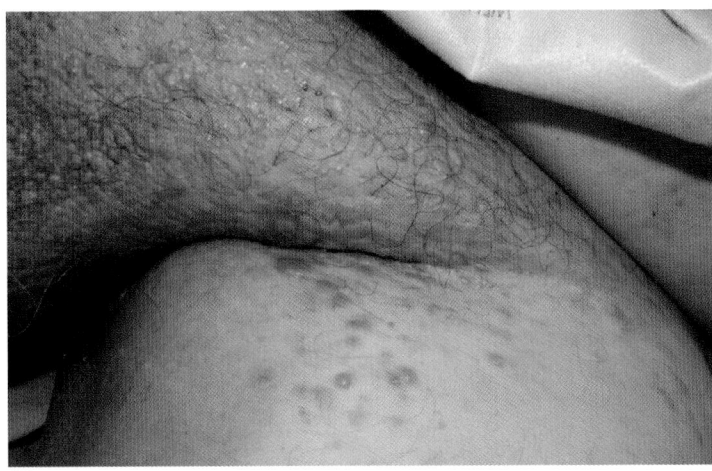

(b)

Figure 113.29 (a) Infiltrative carcinoma erysipeloides affecting the genito-crural region and lower abdomen in a man with adenocarcinoma of the colon. A colostomy bag is visible. (b) Close-up view showing a cellulitis-like appearance and infiltrated papules of cutaneous metastatic adenocarcinoma.

Hidradentitis suppurativa

Definition and nomenclature
Hidradenitis suppurativa is a chronic, follicular, occlusive, inflammatory skin disease that affects the hair follicles in apocrine gland-bearing skin of the axillae, ano-genital and perianal region, buttocks, groin and inframammary region. It is characterized by recurrent abscesses, sinuses and scarring (see also Chapter 92).

Synonyms and inclusions
- Acne inversa
- Verneuil disease
- Chronic perianal proderma

Introduction and general description
It is characterized by recurrent, painful, deep-seated nodules and abscesses that progress to the development of bridged comedomes, sinus tracts and scars. It typically affects the ano-genital region in men and the axillae in women. Follicular occlusion is the primary event.

Epidemiology

Incidence and prevalence
Prevalence is up to 4% [1].

Age
The average age of onset is the early twenties. Peak prevalence is in the fourth decade and declines with age [2].

Sex
There is a female to male ratio of 3 : 1.

Ethnicity
It is commoner in Afro-Carribeans [3].

Associated diseases
These include other follicular occlusive disorders that form the follicular occlusion tetrad, namely acne conglobata, dissecting cellulitis of the scalp and sacrococcygeal pilonidal sinus disease. Other disease associations include inflammatory bowel disease, pyoderma gangrenosum, spondyloarthropathies and non-melanoma skin carcinoma.

Pathophysiology

Predisposing factors
These include obesity, smoking, friction and pressure.

Pathology
Features include follicular hyperplasia, ductal hyperkeratosis, chronic inflammation, fibrosis and sinus tract formation.

Genetics
There may be a positive family history.

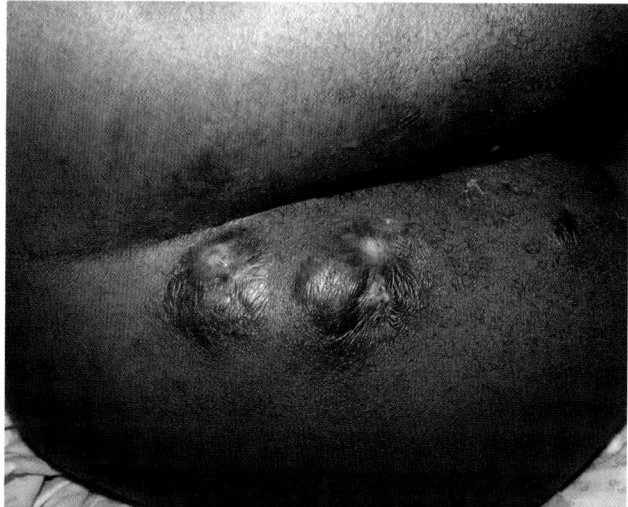

Figure 113.30 Hurley stage I hidradenitis suppurativa presenting as chronic furunculosis on the buttocks.

Clinical features

History
There is usually a history of painful recurring lumps with a discharge that is often malodourous and blood stained. Quality of life can be severly impaired; activities such as sitting, walking and defaecation can be impaired.

Presentation
There is a clinical spectrum overlapping with chronic furunculosis (Figure 113.30) through to severe disease. Mild or localized forms are frequently misdiagnosed as furunculosis or infected cysts. Recurrent deep-seated nodules occur at the same site.

Groin disease is common (Figure 113.31a). Women are more likely to have upper torso and axillary involvement (Figure 113.31b), while men are more likely to have perineal or perianal disease (Figure 113.32). In established hidradenitis suppurativa, fluctuant abscesses, bridged comedomes and deep, burrowing, discharging sinuses occur as well as scarring, including keloid scars (Figure 113.32a). Men tend to have more severe disease and a history of severe acne [4]. Inflammation can invade fat and extend widely over the buttocks and thighs (Figure 113.32b). Persistent perineal sinuses are frequent and deep-seated lesions may lead to anal fistulae.

Differential diagnosis
Crohn disease can coexist with and may simulate hidradenitis suppurativa. Acne conglobata, lymphogranuloma venereum, developmental fistulae and chloracne should all be considered as well.

Classification of severity
The Hurley staging system can be used (Table 113.1) [5]. Males and smokers are more likely to have higher stage disease severity [2,4].

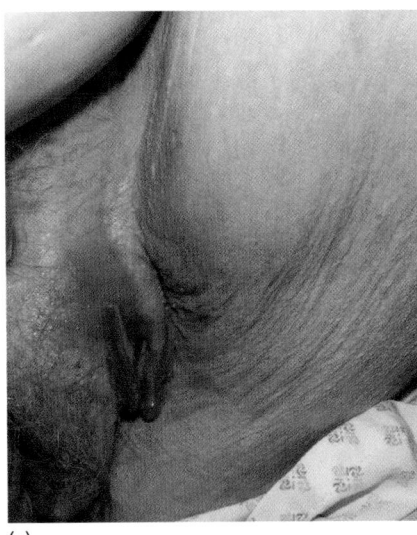

(a)

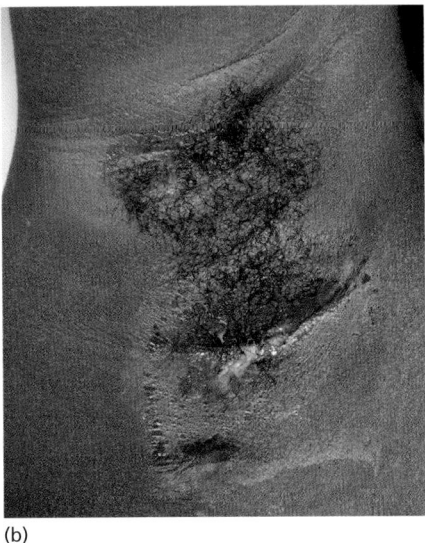

(b)

Figure 113.31 Hurley stage II hidradentitis suppurativa. (a) Affecting the groin of a female causing sinus track formation and scarring. (b) Affecting the axilla of a female causing sinus track formation and scarring.

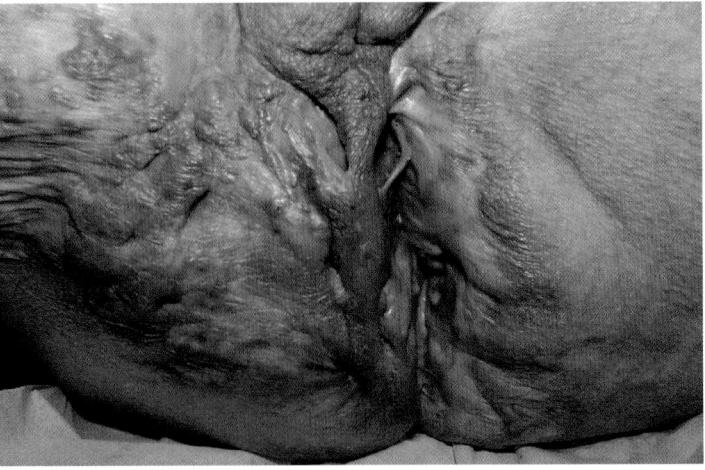

(a)

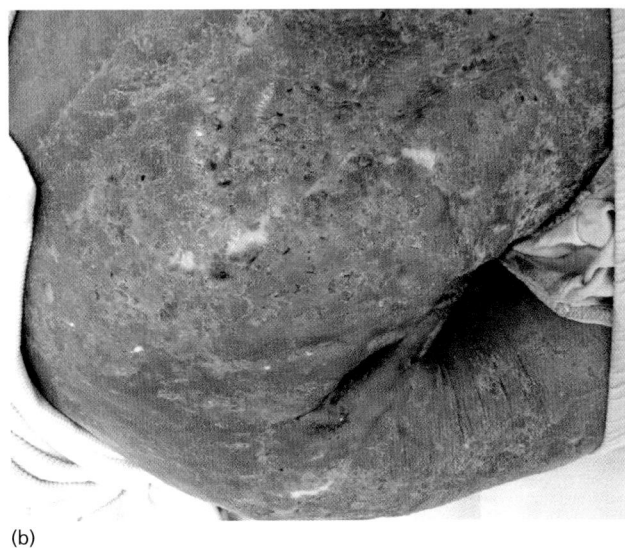

(b)

Figure 113.32 Hurley stage III severe hidradentitis suppurativa. (a) Affecting the perineum and causing extensive keloid scar formation in a 75-year-old male patient. (b) Affecting the buttocks and thighs causing extensive sinus formation and scarring.

Complications and co-morbidities
Secondary bacterial infection is an important complicating factor. Complications of severe disease include anaemia, SCC, genital lymphoedema, contractures and reactive arthritis.

Disease course and prognosis
The disease course is chronic and recurrent. Prevalence decreases with age.

Investigations
Swabs should be taken for culture.

Management
Hidradentitis suppurativa can be a difficult condition to treat. A combination of different treatment modalities is often required.

First line
Topical antibiotics and long-term combination oral antibiotic therapy should be used. Oral antibiotic therapy is seldom of lasting value, although the elimination of specific secondary infection organisms such as *Streptococcus milleri* may be effective.

Small localized sinuses may be phenolized successfully, and early lesions may respond to intralesional corticosteroids. Surgical

Table 113.1 Hurley severity stages [5].

Stage	Definition
Stage I	Solitary or multiple abscesses occurring without formation of sinus tracks or scarring
Stage II	Recurrent abscesses with sinus track formation and scarring occurring within an anatomical region but separated by areas of normal skin
Stage III	Confluent involvement of an entire anatomical region with multiple interconnected abscesses, nodules, sinus tracks and scarring

and laser therapy are useful adjuncts for early disease. Marsupialization and diathermy of the affected tissue have been successful in some cases. Wide local excision for severe disease has been advocated [6]. Disease recurrence rates are high.

Second line
Oral retinoids have been used with mixed results [7].

Third line
Biological drugs such as infliximab and adalimumab have been shown to be effective [7].

Resources

Further information
Hidradentitis Suppurativa Trust: www.hstrust.org (last accessed October 2014).

Pilonidal sinus

Definition and nomenclature
Pilonidal sinus is an acquired midline sinus due to entrapment of hairs in the pilosebaceous unit of the sacrococcygeal region.

Synonyms and inclusions
- Pilonidal disease
- Sacrococcygeal pilonidal disease
- Pilonidal cyst
- Jeep driver's disease

Introduction and general description
Pilonidal disease is commonest in the sacrococcygeal region but can also occur on the pubis, anterior perineum or on the hands of people with certain occupations such as dog groomers or hairdressers. The word pilonidal is derived from the latin pilus (hair) and nidus (nest).

Epidemiology

Incidence and prevalence
The incidence was determined to be 26 per 100 000 in a study from Norway [1].

Age
The peak is in the second to third decades.

Sex
The male to female ratio is 2.2 : 1 [1].

Associated diseases
Other diseases involving follicular occlusion, namely hidradenitis suppurativa, dissecting cellulitis and acne conglobate, are associated.

Pathophysiology

Predisposing factors
The disease was previously thought to be congenital due to failure of fusion in the dorsal midline resulting in entrapment of hair follicles in the sacrococcygeal region, but is currently considered an acquired disorder [2].

Trauma, obesity, hirsuitism, sedentary lifestyle and family history are predisposing factors. Hair follicles altered by pressure and maceration become occluded and hairs continue to grow beneath the surface, leading to a foreign body inflammatory reaction.

Clinical features

History
Symptoms include itch, pain (including coccygodynia), recurrent abscess, purulent discharge and persistent nodules in the natal cleft. It may be asymptomatic.

Presentation
A midline pit/sinus may be visible in the natal cleft (Figure 113.33) but may be obscured by a suppurative discharging nodule. Hairs

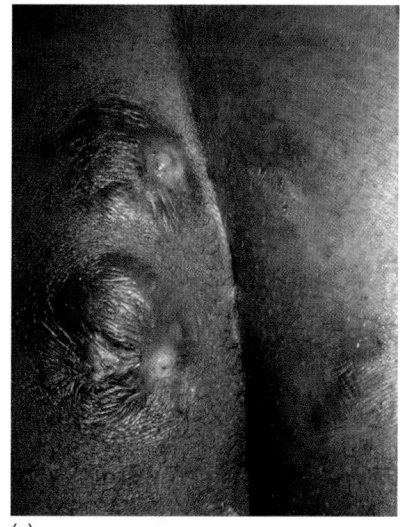
(a)

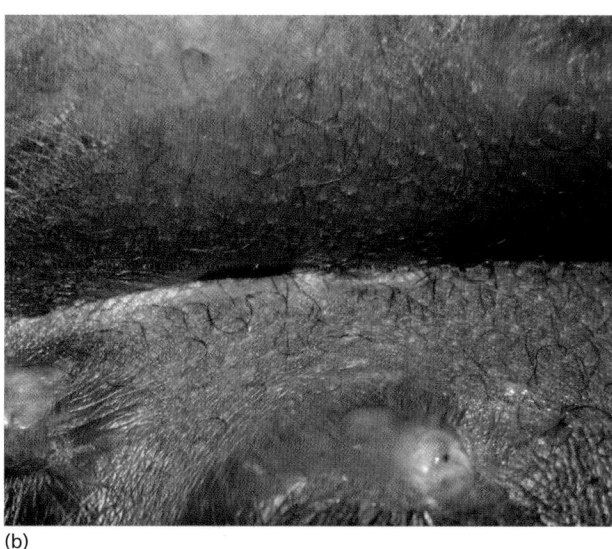
(b)

Figure 113.33 (a) Pilonidal sinuses in a natal cleft with buttock abscesses. (b) Close-up view of the same pilonidal sinus.

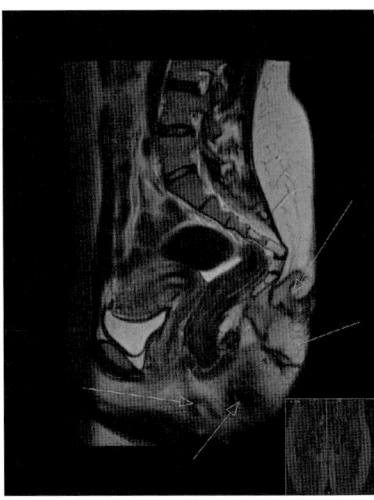

Figure 113.34 MRI scan of the patient with sacrococcygeal pilondal disease shown in Figure 113.33 A sagittal T$_2$-weighted small field of view image showing multiple sinus tracks (arrows) extending from the natal cleft and buttock skin into the subcutaneous tissue, almost reaching the coccyx. (Courtesy of Dr John Rendle, Department of Imaging, Croydon University Hospital, UK.)

may protrude from the sinuses. The sinus may extend to the sacrum. Secondary tracks and sinuses may develop off the midline in chronic disease (Figure 113.34).

Differential diagnosis
Perianal abscess, perianal fistula, Crohn disease and hidradenitis suppurativa should all be considered.

Complications and co-morbidities
Chronic inflammation over many years can lead to SCC.

Investigations
An MRI scan of the pelvis can define the sinus tracks (Figure 113.34).

Management
Depilation of hair in the natal cleft (e.g. by shaving) has been advocated [2]. The treatment of symptomatic disease is surgical. Various procedures ranging from excision, incision and marsupialization or phenol injections to complex flaps to remove the natal cleft have been described. Asymptomatic pits do not require treatment [3].

Crohn disease

Definition and nomenclature
Crohn disease is an idiopathic, chronic, granulomatous, inflammatory disease that can affect any part of the gastrointestinal tract from mouth to anus.

Synonyms and inclusions
• Regional enteritis

Introduction and general description
Mucocutaneous manifestations of Crohn disease occur in up to 44% of patients [1] and can be categorized as granulomatous (contiguous or non-contiguous with the gastrointestinal tract), non-granulomatous reactive (e.g. pyoderma gangrenosum) or nutritional. Granuloumatous disease non-contiguous with the gastrointestinal tract is referred to as metastatic Crohn disease. Crohn disease affects the perianal skin in 20–30% of cases, with the majority of patients having fistulae or abscesses.

Epidemiology

Incidence and prevalence
Prevalence in the UK is estimated to be 50–100 per 100 000.

Age
The peak age of onset is the second to fourth decade.

Sex
It is commoner in females.

Pathophysiology

Predisposing factors
The aetiology is unknown. Smoking and a diet high in fatty foods may be risk factors.

Pathology
Histology is of non-caseating granulomas.

Clinical features

History
Perianal symptoms include pruritus ani, discharge and pain. Symptoms of inflammatory bowel disease include diarrhoea, abdominal pain and ano-rectal bleeding.

Presentation
Approximately 25% of patients with large or small bowel disease have perianal manifestations [2]. Perianal disease can precede symptoms of intestinal disease. The perianal manifestations are listed in Box 113.4.

Box 113.4 Perianal features of Crohn disease

• Pruritus ani
• Maceration
• Erosions
• Ulceration
• Fissures
• Abscesses
• Fistulae
• Secondary infection
• Skin tags
• Anal stenosis
• Metastatic granulomatous ulcers, nodules or plaques

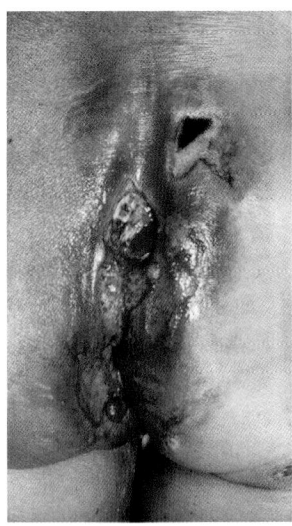

Figure 113.35 Crohn disease: perianal and buttock involvement. (Courtesy of Dr D. I. McCallum, Inverness, UK.)

The commonest perianal lesions are ulcers, anal fissures, abscesses and fistulae (Figure 113.35) [2]. Up to 50% of patients with Crohn disease develop fistulae [3], of which 54% are perianal [4]. The fistulae are often complex and multiple with severe impairment of quality of life.

Metastatic Crohn disease is rare. Lesions may present as ulcers, nodules or plaques and have been reported to occur on the face, retroauricular area, limbs, inframammary area, abdomen and genital skin.

Cutaneous disease activity does not correlate consistently with intestinal activity. Mucocutaneous manifestations of Crohn disease are listed in Box 113.5.

Differential diagnosis

This includes the causes of pruritus ani, anal fissures, fistulae and perianal ulceration. Other possible diagnoses include ulcerative colitis, diverticulitis, hidradenitis suppurativa and pyoderma gangrenosum.

Box 113.5 Mucocutaneous features of Crohn disease

- Erythema nodosum
- Pyoderma gangrenosum
- Polyarteritis nodosa
- Granulomatous cheilitis
- Oral apthous ulceration
- Anal and perianal lesions (see Box 113.4)
- Epidermolysis bullosa aquisita
- Genital disease including balanitis, chronic penile or vulval lymphoedema and contiguous granulomatous disease of the vulva
- Erosions and ulceration around ileostomies and colostomies
- Metastatic Crohn disease
- Ulceration of the perineum and buttocks after colectomy
- Skin changes secondary to malabsorption including pallor

Granulomatous nodules, with or without ulceration, create a differential diagnosis that includes sarcoidoisis, tuberculosis, atypical mycobacterial infection, deep fungal infection, foreign body reaction, granuloma inguinale, lymphogranuloma venereum, chanchroid, amoebiasis and syphilis.

Complications and co-morbidities

These include anal stenosis, faecal incontinence and anal carcinoma.

Disease course and prognosis

The course can be chronic and relapsing. Prognosis is variable.

Investigations

Endoscopic visualization and biopsy are needed. Histological confirmation of non-caseating granulomas of both the skin and bowel should be sought. Endoanal ultrasound and MRI will assist in defining fistula tracks.

Management

A multidisciplinary approach is required. Management options include topical and intralesional steroids, oral prednisolone, oral antibiotics, sulfasalazine and immunosuppressive therapy including antitumour necrosis factor (anti-TNF) agents [5]. Surgical intervention may be required including for management of fistulae and drainage of abscesses.

First line

Local measures include soaks with potassium permanganate and the use of an antiseptic soap substitute. Potent or very potent topical steroid/antibiotic combinations and oral antibiotics (as for hidradenitis suppurativa) may be effective for localized perianal disease.

Anti-TNF agents should be considered as first line treatment in patients with fistulae [6] and can lead to clinical remission of trans-, supra- and extrasphincteric fistulae [2].

Resources

Further information

Crohn's and Colitis UK: www.crohnsandcolitis.org.uk (last accessed October 2014).

Anal abscess

Definition and nomenclature

Anal abscess is a form of ano-rectal sepsis. Pus formation occurs in the connective tissue around the anus and rectum.

Synonyms and inclusions
- Perianal abscess
- Ano-rectal abscess

Introduction and general description

Anal abscesses are common in healthy individuals but may occur in patients with inflammatory bowel disease including Crohn

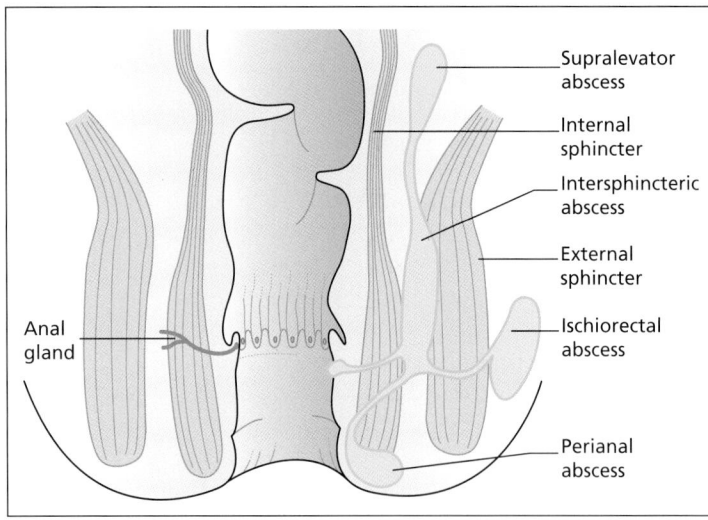

Figure 113.36 Classification of ano-rectal abscesses based on the relation of the abscess to the internal and external anal sphincters.

disease. Anal abscesses are classified based on their location in relation to the anal sphincters and anatomical spaces of the ano-rectal region (Figure 113.36).

Epidemiology

Incidence and prevalence
They are common.

Sex
Anal abscesses are twice as common in men as in women [1].

Age
Anal abscess is primarily a disease of the young to middle aged.

Pathophysiology

Predisposing factors
Anal gland infection in the intersphincteric space is the likely cause secondary to impaction with faecal debris (cryptoglandular hypothesis). Anal glands tend to atrophy with age, perhaps explaining why anal abscesses are less common in the elderly. Predisposing factors include trauma (e.g. impacted fish bone), constipation, sedentary occupation, immunodeficiency (including leukaemia and HIV infection), diabetes and anal cancer.

Clinical features

History
Symptoms include pain, swelling, discharge, fever and malaise.

Presentation
Perianal abscesses are common and superficial infections that extend between the internal and external sphincter and reach the anal verge (Figure 113.36). If the abscess penetrates the external anal sphincter, it becomes an ischio-rectal abscess. Intersphincteric

abscesses develop in the space between the internal and external sphincters [1].

Perianal abscess may cause an eythematous, fluctuant, tender, indurated swelling.

Clinical variants
See Figure 113.36.

Differential diagnosis
Crohn disease, hidradenitits suppurativa, tuberculosis, thrombosed external haemorrhoids, perianal cellulitis, threadworm infection and malignancy should all be considered.

Complications and co-morbidities
Fistula formation following perianal abscess occurs in 26–37% of cases [2].

Disease course and prognosis
Risk factors for recurrence include diabetes, Crohn disease, immunosuppression and ischio-anal location.

Management
Incision and drainage is required.

First line
Antibiotics are not required unless there are signs of cellulitis or the patient is at risk from underlying co-morbidities such as diabetes or immunosuppression. Antibiotic therapy after surgical drainage does not seem to protect against fistula formation [3].

Anal fistula

Definition and nomenclature
A fistula is an abnormal communication between two epithelial surfaces. An anal fistula is a communication between the ano-rectal canal and perianal skin that is lined with granulation tissue.

Synonyms and inclusions
- Fistula-in-ano
- Ano-rectal fistula

Introduction and general description
Anal fistula is part of the spectrum of perianal sepsis. An anal fistula may present *de novo* or after an acute ano-rectal abscess. A high index of suspicion of anal fistula is necessary when examining patients with a perianal abscess.

Epidemiology

Incidence and prevalence
The prevalence of anal fistulae is 1–2 per 10 000 of population in European studies [1]. This may be an underestimate as many patients do not seek medical advice because of embarrassment.

Box 113.6 Conditions associated with anal fistulae

- Crohn disease
- Tuberculosis
- Hidradenitis suppurativa
- Pilonidal disease
- HIV infection
- Trauma: obstetric or ano-rectal
- Foreign bodies
- Surgery
- Radiotherapy
- Malignancy
- Lymphogranuloma venereum
- Perianal actinomycosis
- Bridging of anal fissure
- Sacrococcygeal teratoma
- Ano-rectal duplication
- Presacral dermoid cysts

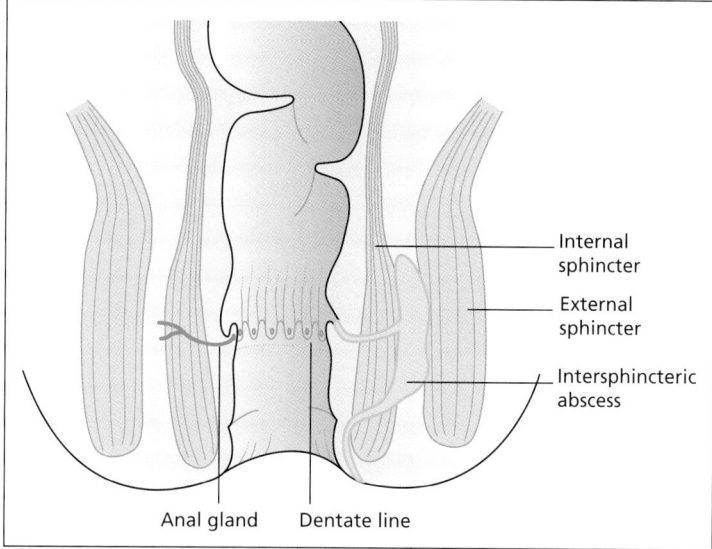

Figure 113.37 Cryptoglandular hypothesis of the development of an intersphincteric fistula.

Age
It most commonly presents at around 40 years.

Sex
Men are twice as likely to be affected.

Associated diseases
See Box 113.6.

Pathophysiology

Predisposing factors
Approximately 90% of anal fistulae are idiopathic [2]. Infection of anal glands in the intersphincteric space of the anal canal is thought to underlie both acute ano-rectal abscesses and anal fistulae [2,3]. This is called the cryptoglandular hypothesis (Figure 113.37).

It is not clear why certain cases of perianal sepsis are limited to abscess formation whereas others are associated with fistula track formation. The rate of formation of fistula following perianal abscess is 26–37% [4].

See Box 113.6 for diseases associated with anal fistulae. The prevalence of fistulae in patients with Crohn disease is up to 50% [5], of which most are perianal (see Figure 113.35). The transmural inflammation characteristic of Crohn disease predisposes patients to fistula formation. Fistulae in Crohn disease are often complex and multiple.

Clinical features

History
Patients may complain of pruritus ani, discharge, pain and constipation. In severe cases faecal material may pass through the fistula, leading to soiling of underwear and skin irritation. There is often a history of an abscess that failed to heal after surgical drainage or recurred at the same site.

Presentation
An anal fistula may appear as a pit in the skin with a surrounding rim of granulation tissue, and discharge may be noted. Surrounding skin may be indurated and tender and there may be scarring from previous abscess formation.

Fistulae have a primary track but there may be secondary extensions. Most occur on the midline posteriorly, but there may be multiple openings. The fistula may harbour chronic infection that may discharge onto the skin. Intermittent discharge is usually caused by cyclical accumulation of an abscess with associated discomfort and pain before some relief from discharge [2].

Differential diagnosis
Underlying diseases associated with anal fistula should be considered, including Crohn disease and infections such as tuberculosis (see Box 113.6). Tuberculosis should always be suspected and excluded, especially in patients who fail to respond to treatment or who have recurrent disease.

Classification of severity
Fistulae are classified based on their relation to the anal sphincter complex and whether the track is low or high. A low fistula track passes through few or no sphincter muscle fibres and is relatively close to the skin. A high fistula describes a track that passes through or above large amounts of muscle (Figure 113.38).

After considering whether a fistula track is low or high, additional complexity arises from the presence of secondary tracks or residual abscess cavities.

Complications and co-morbidities
Squamous cell carcinoma is a rare complication that may arise in chronic complex fistulae.

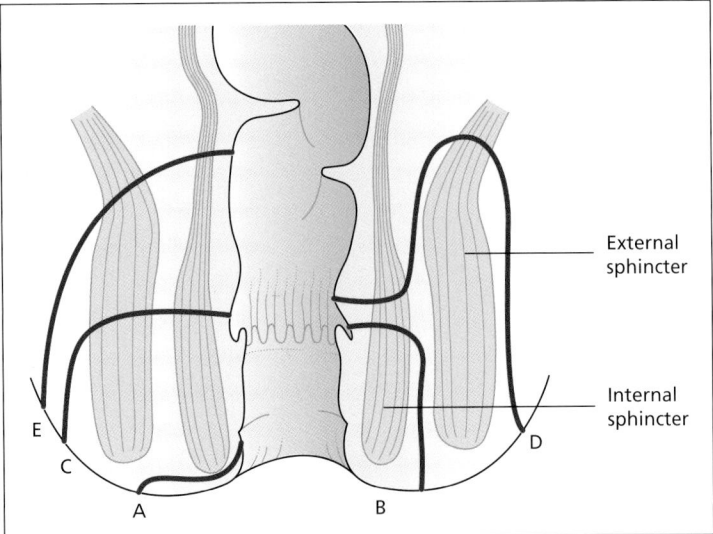

Figure 113.38 Parks classification of anal fistulae. A: superficial fistula track beneath the internal and external sphincters. B: intersphincteric fistula track between the internal and external sphincters in the intersphincteric space. C: transsphincteric fistula track crossing both the external and internal anal sphincters. D: suprasphincteric fistula passing outside the internal and external anal sphincters over the top of the puborectalis muscle and penetrating the levator muscle before tracking down to the skin. E: extrasphincteric fistula tracking outside the external anal sphincter and penetrating the levator muscle into the rectum. (Adapted from Parks *et al.* 1976 [3].)

Disease course and prognosis

Anal fistulae will not heal without intervention and if left untreated are at risk of recurrent perianal abscess and development of a complex fistula network [2]. The consequences may include chronic pain, bleeding, incontinence, cellulitis and systemic sepsis. In some cases, treatment may require stoma formation.

Investigations

Endoanal ultrasound and MRI improve the charcterization of the fistula anatomy and are the most useful imaging techniques in complex cases [6].

Management

Referral to a colo-rectal specialist is required. The aims of management are to eradicate the fistula and prevent recurrence while maintaining continence. Successful management of an anal fistula requires that all primary and secondary tracks are drained and eradicated [2]. Antibiotics are not usually effective in treating perianal abscess or infection associated with anal fistula, but are recommended in patients who have cellulitis [3].

First line

Surgical procedures performed by a colo-rectal specialist include fistulotomy and seton insertion (see below) [7]. Fistulotomy entails the division of superficial tissue to lay open the fistula track and is an effective way to treat low fistulae. Fistulotomy should be avoided where there is significant anal sphincter involvement to avoid the risk of postoperative faecal incontinence. A seton is a thread (usually a non-absorbable suture or vascular sling) placed

through the fistula track and tied to form a continuous ring between the internal and external openings of the fistula. Setons maintain the patency of the fistula track, acting as a wick and allowing the drainage of pus and healing to occur. Secondary treatment is usually required to close the track.

Second line

Fibrin glue can be injected into the fistula track and is a sphincter-sparing technique.

Third line

Other surgical options include the insertion of a fistula plug derived from porcine small intestine and an endo-rectal advancement flap. Formation of a colostomy is considered a last resort in non-healing anal fistula [2]. Defunctioning colostomy is more frequently utilzed in Crohn disease where wound healing is poor following other surgical procedures.

Resources

Further information

Crohn's and Colitis UK: www.crohnsandcolitis.org.uk.
Patient.co.uk:www.patient.co.uk.
(Both last accessed October 2014.)

Anal fissure

Definition and nomenclature

An anal fissure is a longitudinal ulcer occurring in the squamous epithelium of the anal canal located distal to the dentate line.

> **Synonyms and inclusions**
> • Fissure-in-ano

Introduction and general description

Primary anal fissures are idiopathic and usually affect the posterior midline. Secondary anal fissures usually occur in the lateral aspect of the anal canal and are associated with underling diseases such as Crohn disease.

Epidemiology

Incidence and prevalence

The exact incidence is unknown and probably underreported as it is likely that many patients do not seek medical advice as the fissure heals without intervention. It is has been suggested that the lifetime incidence is 11% [1].

Age

Anal fissures are commonly encountered in young adults but may affect extremes of age [2].

Sex

There is an equal prevalence in males and females.

Associated diseases

Atypical fissures (large, irregular, multiple and non-midline) are associated with underlying disease such as Crohn disease, HIV infection, syphilis, tuberculosis and malignancy.

Pathophysiology

Predisposing factors

The aetiology is poorly understood. Trauma causing pressure or necrosis by the passage of hard stools is thought to be an initating factor. Pregancy-associated anal fissures are thought to arise due to shearing forces during labour.

Pathology

Histology in idiopathic cases is of non-specific ulceration. In secondary anal fissures, specific pathology such as anal carcinoma or Crohn disease will be identified.

Clinical features

History

Painful defecation occurs, often described as a tearing sensation. Blood may be present on the surface of the stool. Other symptoms include mucous discharge and constipation. Anal fissures result in significant morbidity and reduction of quality of life [3].

Presentation

The tear can usually be visualised in the distal anal canal [2]. Acute fissures are usually superficial with well-delineated mucosal edges and granulation tissue at the base. Chronic fissures may have a fibrotic rolled edge, sentinel tag at the anal pole of the fissure and visible transverse fibres of the internal anal sphincter.

Fissures are usually single and occur in the posterior midline in 80–90% of cases [2]. Anterior midline fissures are usually found in women. Fissures occurring in patients older than 65 are usually secondary and appropriate investigations are required to exclude underlying disease.

Clinical variants

Although not true anal fissures, erosions and fissures may occur in the sulcus beneath odematous haemorrhoids or in any area of perianal skin disease including the natal cleft. These fissures, which are secondary to inflammatory skin disease such as psoriasis or lichen simplex, or to trauma, are sometimes referred to as anal rhagades. The presence of even a small fissure in an area of cutaneous inflammation maintains the pruritus and may predispose to infection.

Differential diagnosis

Sexually transmitted diseases including primary syphillis, Crohn disease, tuberculous and HIV infection should be considered and excluded by appropriate investigations. Trauma is also a possible cause. Behçet disease occasionally presents with multiple shallow ulcers and fissures of the perianal skin.

Complications and co-morbidities

Constipation is frequently found. Perianal tags may result when an anal fissure has healed. Squamous cell carcinoma is a rare complication of chronic anal fissure.

Disease course and prognosis

More than 50% of acute fissures heal spontaneously with conservative management [2]. Only 10% of chronic fissures will heal spontaneously and either surgical or medical intervention is required to achieve healing.

Investigations

Proctoscopy and histological assessment is mandatory if the aetiology is in doubt.

Management

Management is the domain of the ano-rectal specialist. Conservative management, including advice on high-fibre diet, is advisable. Warm sitz baths (a shallow bath used for cleansing the perineal and perianal skin) can help with symptomatic relief [4]. The aim of management of chronic fissures is to treat the triad of anal pain, spasm and ischaemia. Medical treatment should be pursued prior to surgical intervention.

First line

The use of topical nitrate (e.g. glyceryl trinitrate 0.4% ointment) may be considered. Topical calcium channel blockers (e.g. diltiazem 2% gel) can be tried in patients unresponsive to topical nitrates.

Second line

Surgery is the mainstay of treatment for chronic anal fissures unresponsive to first line measures. Lateral internal sphincterotomy results in cure rates of up to 98% but may compromise anal continence in up to 30% [2].

The relatively high risk of anal incontinence following surgical intervention has led to the search for medical therapy to reduce anal pressure. Options that may be tried prior to surgery include oral calcium channel blockers (e.g. nifedipine) or injection of botulinum neurotoxin A into the internal anal sphincter.

Third line

Fissurectomy and endoanal advancement flap are surgical options [2].

Haemorrhoids

Definition and nomenclature

Haemorrhoids are dilatations in the venous system draining the anus.

Synonyms and inclusions
- Piles (Latin *pila*, a ball)
- Varicose veins of the anus

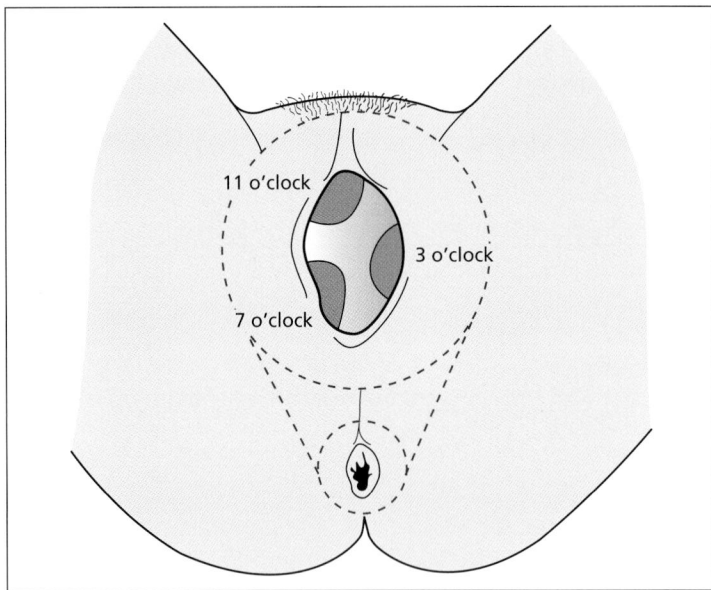

Figure 113.39 Typical positions of development of internal haemorrhoids in the anal canal at 3, 7 and 11 o'clock seen with the patient in the dorsal lithotomy position. The anal column blood vessels are largest at the left lateral, right posterior and right anterior quadrants of the anal canal where the subepithelial tissues expand to form three anal cushions. The cushions help to seal the anal canal to maintain continence to faeces and flatus, and are also important in the pathogenesis of internal haemorrhoids. (Adapted from Snell 2012 [4]. Reproduced with permission of Lippincott Williams & Wilkins/Wolters Kluwer.)

Introduction and general description

Internal haemorrhoids typically develop from three anal cushions present in the anal canal (Figure 113.39). Anatomically, an internal haemorrhoid is a fold of mucous membrane and submucosa containing a varicosed tributary of the superior rectal vein and a terminal branch of the superior rectal artery (Figure 113.40). Internal haemorrhoids are proximal to the dentate line and have visceral innervation with an absence of pain fibres. External haemorrhoids are varicosities of tributaries of the inferior rectal vein and are

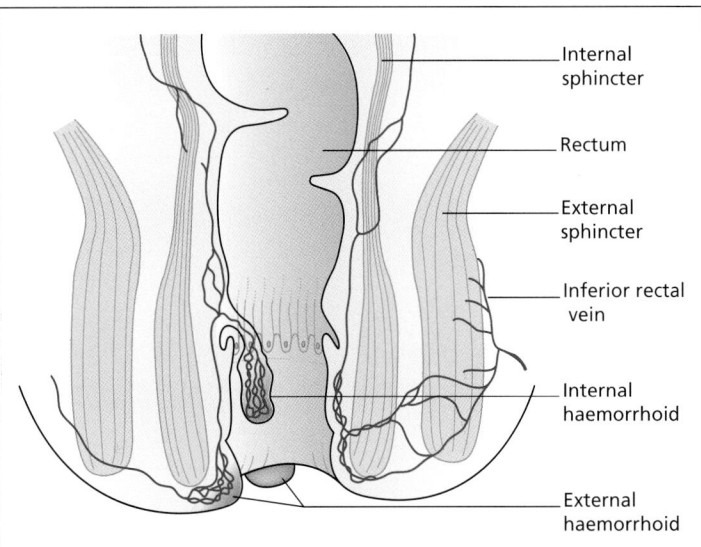

Figure 113.40 Origin of internal and external haemorrhoids. (Adapted from Snell 2012 [4]. Reproduced with permission of Lippincott Williams & Wilkins/Wolters Kluwer.)

located below the dentate line in the distal third of the anal canal (Figure 113.40). They are covered by squamous epithelium and have somatic pain fibre innervation. External haemorrhoids are commonly associated with internal haemorrhoids.

Epidemiology

Incidence and prevalence
Symptomatic haemorrhoids affect up to 36% of the population [1].

Age
Prevalence increases with age.

Sex
They are common in both men and women.

Pathophysiology

Predisposing factors
Factors that increase intra-abdominal pressure, including pregnancy, obesity and straining at stool due to constipation, contribute to the incidence of haemorrhoids. Other predisposing factors include portal hypertension due to liver cirrhosis and malignancy causing compression of the superior rectal vein. Haemorrhoids are often familial and there may be a family history of leg varicose veins. Age-related loss of anal canal muscle support may explain the increase in prevalence with age [2].

Clinical features

History
Symptoms are bleeding, mucous or faecal discharge, pruritus ani and the sensation or awareness of prolapse. Typically, uncomplicated internal haemorrhoids cause painless bleeding. Pain may arise if thrombosis, ulceration or infection occurs. External haemorrhoids are more likely to cause pain. Haemorrhoidal bleeding consists of bright red blood on the stool or toilet paper or dripping into the toilet. The symptoms of haemorrhoidal disease do not correlate with the size of the haemorrhoids.

Presentation
Prolapsed internal haemorrhoids with an overlying columnar mucosal surface may be visible on inspection of the perianal skin (Figure 113.41). External thrombosed haemorrhoids can be differentiated as they are covered by squamous epithelium. A perianal dermatitis may occur secondary to skin irritation resulting from faecal leakage, or a contact dermatitis (irritant or allergic) secondary to overwashing or medicaments. Examination should include digital rectal examination to exclude the presence of a mass and proctocopy to evaluate if there is any other ano-rectal pathology.

Clinical variants
Perianal skin tags (anal tags) can result from thrombosed external haemorrhoids and are common (Figure 113.42). In contrast to external haemorrhoids, perianal skin tags do not swell with blood when the patient strains or reduce with pressure. Perianal tags are

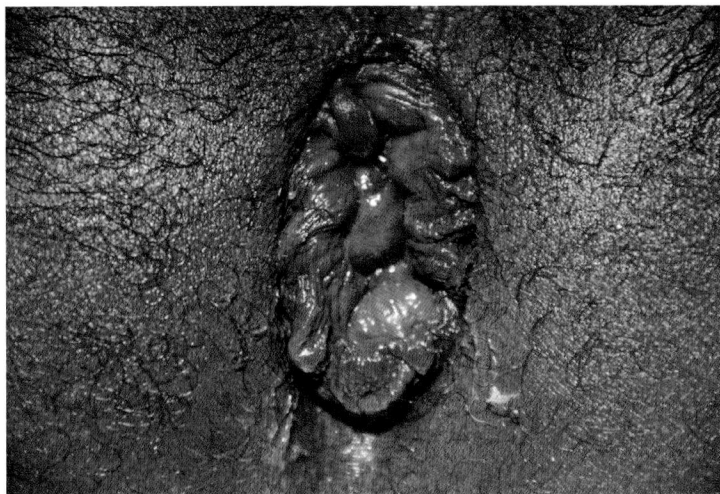

Figure 113.41 Second degree prolapsed internal haemorrhoids with surrounding anal tags. (Courtesy of Mr M. Abulafi, Croydon University Hospital, UK.)

usually asymptomatic but large or multiple lesions can interfere with perianal hygiene and predispose to perianal dermatitis.

Perianal haematoma (perianal thrombosis) is caused by the rupture of tributaries of the inferior rectal vein as a result of coughing or straining, with the appearance of a haematoma affecting perianal skin (incorrectly called a thrombosed haemorrhoid). The history is of sudden onset of pain and swelling. A blue-black nodule that can be multilocular can be seen on inspection of the anal margin region. If the overlying skin perforates, a clot of blood is extruded leading to pain relief. A perianal skin tag can result when the haematoma resolves. Many perianal haematomas are associated with haemorrhoids.

Differential diagnosis

The differential diagnosis includes ano-rectal malignancy, Crohn disease, perianal metastases and Kaposi sarcoma.

Classification of severity

See Table 113.2.

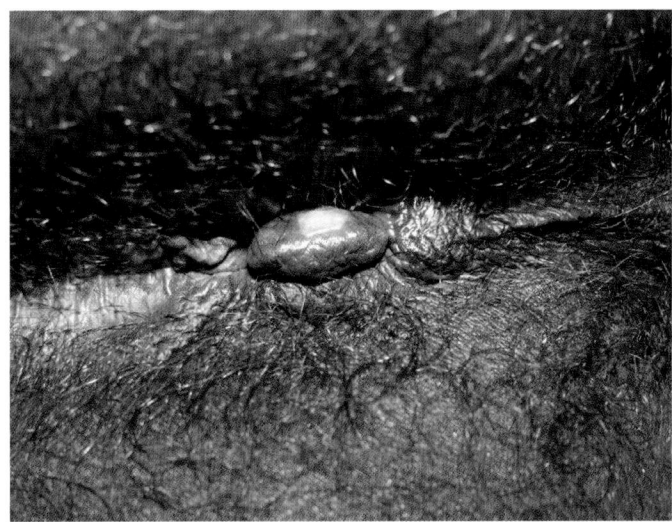

Figure 113.42 Perianal skin tag.

Table 113.2 Classification of haemorrhoid severity.

Severity	Definition
First degree	Contained within the anal canal
Second degree	Prolapse on straining and defecation but reduce spontaneously
Third degree	Prolapse on straining but remain outside the anus and require manual reduction
Fourth degree	Prolapsed and incarcerated

Complications and co-morbidities

The complications of haemorrhoids include pain, thrombosis, strangulation, ulceration, fibrosis, infection and abscess and incarceration of a prolapsed haemorrhoid.

Management

Management of symptomatic haemorrhoids is the domain of the ano-rectal specialist. First and second degree disease (Table 113.2) can usually be treated conservatively without the need for operative intervention. The aims of management include addressing any predisposing factors such as constipation or diarrhoea. Symptomatic relief for perianal symptoms can be achieved with topical agents including lubricants and mild topical steroids. Dietary fibre should be increased and there should be adequate water intake.

Third degree haemorrhoids usually require surgical intervention. First line options include injection sclerotherapy, rubber band ligation, infrared coagulation and cryotherapy. These techniques result in tissue destruction, subsequent fibrosis and resultant resolution of the haemorrhoid.

Fourth degree haemorrhoids require urgent surgical intervention. Surgical procedures include excisional haemorrhoidectomy, stapled haemorrhoidopexy and Doppler-guided transanal haemorrhoid devascularization [3].

Resources

Further information

www.pilesadvice.co.uk (last accessed October 2014).

Trauma and artefact

Definition

Trauma includes accidental, or self-induced, or iatrogenic injury, as well as sexual abuse.

Introduction and general description

Anal, perianal and perineal trauma is not uncommon. Trauma can lead to anal stenosis.

Clinical features

Clinical variants

Pressure sores (synonym decubitus sores) in the sacral area are common. Reported prevalence rates range from 4.7% to 32% in hospital populations, and 22% in nursing homes [1]. In elderly

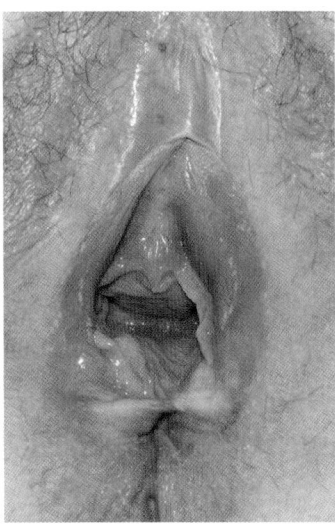

(a)

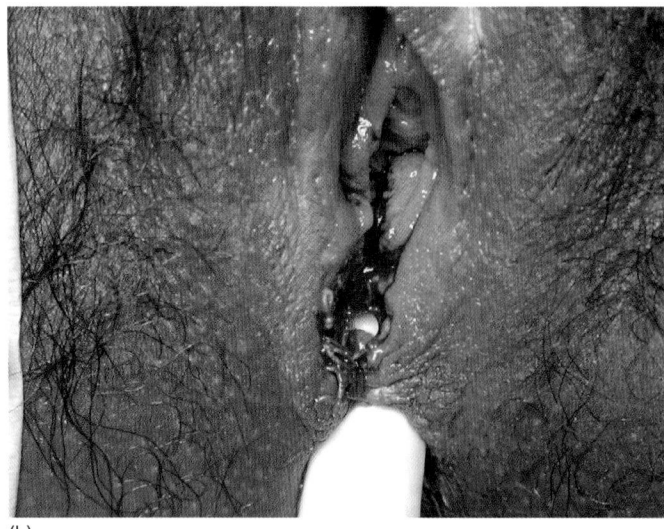

(b)

Figure 113.43 Obstetric perineal trauma. (a) Cloacal-like defect following a missed third degree tear. The perineal body is absent and there is minimal tissue separating the anus from the vagina. (b) Break down of a wound following the repair of a fourth degree tear has occurred, leading to a recto-vaginal fistula. Suture threads from the perineal tear closure are visible. (Courtesy of Mr A. Sultan, Department of Obstetrics and Gynaecology, Croydon University Hospital, UK.)

Table 113.3 Classification of obstetric perineal trauma [5].

Degree of trauma	Definition
First degree	Laceration of vaginal mucosa or perineal skin only
Second degree	Involvement of perineal muscles but not anal sphincter
Third degree	Disruption of anal sphincter muscles:
	3a: <50% of external anal sphincter torn
	3b: >50% of external anal sphincter torn
	3c: internal anal sphincter also torn
Fourth degree	Third degree tear with disruption of anal epithelium

or bed-ridden patients, a persistent patch of non-blanchable erythema on the sacral or ischial region is a sign of impending ulceration. Oedema, induration or pain may also be present. Progression to ulceration can be prevented if this early stage is identified promptly [2].

Clinical signs of perianal and anal trauma following sexual abuse in children include gaping of the anus and anal fissures [3]. Perianal skin diseases can be mistaken for sexual abuse including lichen sclerosus and perianal *Streptococcus* infection. The presence of definitive skin disease does not exclude sexual abuse.

Obstetric perineal trauma is sustained in more than 85% of women during vaginal delivery in the UK and up to 69% will require sutures [4]. Injury may occur spontaneously or be iatrogenic (Figure 113.43). Prevalence is dependent on variations in obstetric practice. Prospective studies using endoanal ultrasound scanning have identified that occult anal sphincter injury is common [4]. See Table 113.3 for a classification of obstetric trauma [5].

Perineal and perianal pain

Functional ano-rectal pain occurs in the absence of any underlying discernable organic disease. Functional disorders of the perineum causing pain include proctalgia fugax, levator ani syndrome and idiopathic coccygodynia [1].

Proctalgia fugax is characterized by severe, self-limiting, fleeting, episodic ano-rectal pain. Attacks tend to be infrequent, averaging once monthly [2]. Sudden-onset cramp-like pain occurs and lasts from a few seconds up to 20 min. Patients usually cannot identify any triggers. The prevalence is 4–18% and it is commoner in females [3]. The pathogenesis is unknown but may be due to spasm of the internal anal sphincter or compression of the pudendal nerve.

Chronic proctalgia (chronic idiopathic anal pain) can be defined as chronic or recurrent episodes of ano-rectal pain lasting more than 20 min in the absence of organic cause. Levator ani syndrome causes recurrent or persistent pain, pressure or discomfort in the perineal region and is commoner in females [4]. It is thought to be due to spasm of the levator ani muscles. Digital rectal examination distinguishes between levator ani syndrome and unspecified functional ano-rectal pain. Tenderness occurs on palpation of the puborectalis muscle in levator ani syndrome but not in patients with unspecified functional ano-rectal pain.

Coccygodynia is the symptom of pain in and around the coccyx. It is usually precipitated by prolonged sitting and rising from the seated position. Idiopathic coccygodynia is commoner in females and is associated with obesity. Secondary causes of coccygodynia include trauma, arthritis or rare tumours such as chordoma, intradural schwannoma, perineural cyst or intraosseous lipoma [5].

Descending perineum syndrome is commoner in females and is associated with multiparity. Clinical features include poorly localized deep perineal discomfort, faecal incontinence, constipation, rectal prolapse and perineal descent [6].

Precipitating factors of pain in chronic pain syndromes include sitting, defecation and psychological stress. Treatment is usually unnecessary for the transient symptoms of proctalgia fugax. Treatment options for chronic pain include analgesia, biofeedback, sitz baths, tricyclic antidepressants, botulinum toxin injections and sacral nerve stimulation. Coccygectomy has been advocated for refractory coccygodynia [7].

Key references

The full list of references can be found in the online version at www.rooksdermatology.com.

Introduction
1 Standring S, ed. in chief. *Grays Anatomy. The Anatomical Basis of Clinical Practice*, 40th edn. London: Churchill Livingston, Elsevier, 2008.

Perianal itching

Pruritus ani
2 Markell KW, Billingham R. Pruritus ani: etiology and management. *Surg Clin North Am* 2010;90(1):125–35.

Other diseases and infections

Sexually transmitted diseases
1 Singhrao T, Higham E, French P. Lymphogranuloma venereum presenting as perianal ulceration: an emerging clinical presentation? *Sex Transm Infect* 2011;87:123–4.

Human immunodeficiency virus infection
1 Barrett W, Callahan T, Orkin B. Perianal manifestations of human immuno-deficiency virus infection: experience with 260 patients. *Dis Colon Rectum* 1998;41:606–11.
3 Yuhan R, Orsay C, Del Pino A, *et al.* Anorectal disease in HIV-infected patients. *Dis Colon Rectum* 1998;41:1367–70.

Human papillomavirus infection
2 Giuliana A, Nyitray A, Kreimer A, *et al.* EUROGIN 2014 roadmap: differences in human papillomavirus infection, natural history, transmission and human papillomavirus-related cancer incidence by gender and anatomic site of infection. *Int J Cancer* 2014, doi: 10.1002/ijc.29082.
4 Stanley M. Epithelial cell responses to infection with human papillomavirus. *Clin Microbiol Rev* 2012;25:215–22.
11 Yang J, Pu YG, Zeng ZM, Yu ZJ, Huang N, Deng QW. Interferon for the treatment of genital warts: a systematic review. *BMC Infect Dis* 2009;9:156.

Anal intraepithelial neoplasia
2 Stanley M, Winder D, Sterling J, *et al.* HPV infection, anal-intraepithelail neoplasia (AIN) and anal cancer: current issues. *BMC Cancer* 2012;12:398.
5 Wieland U, Kreuter A. One step towards standardized management of anal dysplasia. *Lancet Oncol* 2013;14:273–4.
8 Palefsky J, Giuliano A, Goldstone S, *et al.* HPV vaccine against anal HPV infection and anal intraepithelial neoplasia. *N Eng J Med* 2011;365:1576–85.

Anal and perianal malignancy
6 Sunesen K, Norgaard M, Thorlacius-Ussing O *et al.* Immunosuppressive disorders and risk of anal squamous cell carcinoma: a nationwide cohort study in Denmark, 1978–2005. *Int J Cancer* 2009;127:675–84.
8 Hillman R, Garland S, Gunathilake M, *et al.* Human papillomavirus (HPV) genotypes in an Australian sample of anal cancers. *Int J Cancer* 2014;135:996–1001.
9 Newlin H, Zlotecki R, Morris C, *et al.* Squamous cell carcinoma of the anal margin. *J Surg Oncol* 2004;86:55–62.

Hidradentitis suppurativa
4 Schrader A, Deckers I, Van der Zee H, *et al.* Hidradenitis suppurativa: a retrospective study of 846 Dutch patients to identify factors associated with disease severity. *J Am Acad Dermatol* 2014;71:460–7.

CHAPTER 114

Cutaneous Complications of Stomas and Fistulae

Calum Lyon

York Hospital NHS Trust, York; and Salford Royal Hospital NHS Trust, Salford, UK

Introduction

An abdominal stoma (ostomy) is a surgically created opening from the gastrointestinal or urinary tract onto the skin in order to drain the effluent from that system. This typically involves a collection device worn on the skin, usually held in place by an adhesive material. Approximately 21 000 people have an abdominal stoma formed each year in the UK, with a large proportion intended as temporary or palliative procedures rather than a long-term therapeutic solution. There are no exact figures available and although estimates vary, at any one time there are probably over 100 000 people in the UK with a chronic abdominal stoma. Skin problems are the commonest longer term complications and figures from several studies suggest that between one-third and two-thirds will experience a skin problem around their stoma at some time that will interfere with normal appliance use [1]. In theory, most dermatoses could affect peristomal skin but in practice the majority fall into one or more of a few groups that are predictable because of the occluded nature of the peristomal skin, prolonged contact with the appliance and any medicaments or cleansers, leakage of urine or faeces onto the skin and the underlying abdominal disease itself. The common cutaneous complications are: irritant reactions (including dermatoses exacerbated by trauma), allergic reactions, infections, common generalized inflammatory dermatoses (e.g. pemphigoid) and disorders associated with the reason for surgery (especially Crohn disease) [2].

Types of stomas and appliances

Most ostomates use modern stoma appliances that consist of a polythene or vinyl bag attached to a firm thermoplastic armature, which is itself fixed to an adhesive system that is intended to contact the abdominal skin (Figure 114.1) [3]. Patients with a short or buried stoma may use an appliance with a convex skin barrier to effectively lengthen the stoma spout. The types of stomas covered in this chapter and the appliances used are described in Table 114.1.

Assessment of the patient

The involvement of an experienced stoma nurse specialist is invaluable, particularly as they may know the patient well. The stoma nurse can advise the patient on how to manage their stoma, including advice on appliance modifications and the use of accessory adhesives, filler pastes, etc. In this way many irritant reactions can be resolved without further dermatological input. Specific points to consider when assessing a stoma patient – in addition to a general dermatological consultation – are listed in Table 114.2.

General aspects of treatment for stomas

Inflammatory dermatoses can usually be managed with topical therapies as at other body sites. However these topical therapies need to be chosen carefully, particularly with regard to the vehicles used in order to minimize greasiness that would interfere with appliance adhesion (see Table 114.4). Progression to systemic therapy should be considered earlier for more severe inflammatory dermatoses, such as psoriasis or pemphigoid, as such disorders themselves will diminish adhesion and the resulting leakage may worsen the skin disease. Avoidance of irritants or allergens is dealt with in the sections on allergic contact dermatitis and irritant skin reactions.

Allergic contact dermatitis

Introduction and epidemiology

Allergic contact dermatitis (ACD) affecting the skin around stomas is relatively uncommon [1], being less than 1% of the skin

PART 10: SITES, SEX, AGE

Rook's Textbook of Dermatology, Ninth Edition. Edited by Christopher Griffiths, Jonathan Barker, Tanya Bleiker, Robert Chalmers and Daniel Creamer.
© 2016 John Wiley & Sons, Ltd. Published 2016 by John Wiley & Sons, Ltd.
Companion website: www.rooksdermatology.com

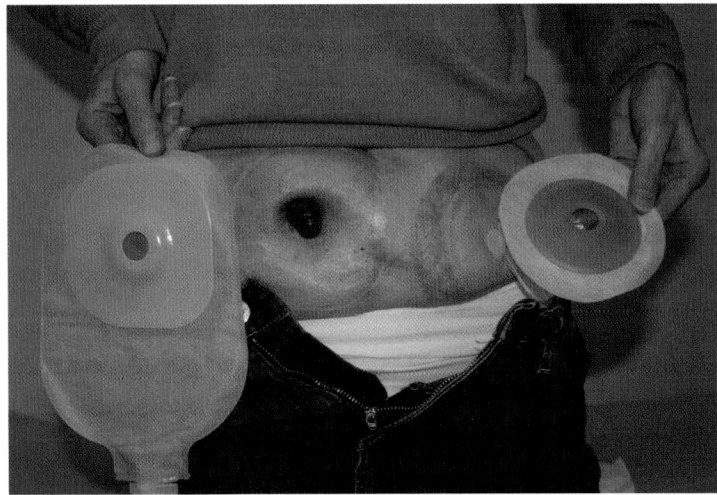

Figure 114.1 Patient with a urostomy for bladder carcinoma who has reacted to the tape border of a two-piece appliance on a 5-day skin test (right of picture). She has not reacted to the hydrocolloid central portion or the all-hydrocolloid one-piece appliance on the left. The product on the left is a typical drainable urostomy bag with a nylon tap at the bottom of the device. Similar bags with different drain systems are used by ileostomy patients and some with colostomies of the ascending colon.

problems seen in almost 1000 patients attending a dedicated dermatology and joint stoma care clinic. Despite this, many patients and stoma nurses suspect allergy to a stoma appliance as the cause of an otherwise unexplained dermatitis before considering any other aetiology. This can be partly explained by the number of individual case reports published in the last 30 years detailing sensitivities to individual components many of which, such as epoxy resin systems, are no longer used in appliance manufacture. These reports have been eloquently summarized by Martin *et al.* [2]. Where ACD occurs it is usually to biocides in cleansers, fragrances in deodorizers or resin systems in pastes used to fill irregularities in the peristomal skin (Gantrez® PMV/MA co-polymers).

Pathophysiology
See Chapter 128 for pathogenetic information on allergic contact dermatitis.

Clinical features
The symptoms and clinical appearances of ACD and irritant dermatitis are similar in the occluded peristomal environment and are therefore difficult to distinguish on clinical grounds alone. The patient experiences an itchy, sometimes burning, eczematous

Table 114.1 Types of stoma and appliance.[a]

Type of stoma	Description	Indications	Appliance types used	Specific associated skin problems
Ileostomy	Placed usually in right iliac fossa with an ideal spout length of at least 2 cm. Produces liquid contents output which increases in inverse proportion to the amount of functioning ileum remaining	Inflammatory bowel disease (IBD) either as a permanent or temporary end ileostomy. Loop ileostomies (double-barrelled) intended to protect the distal bowel pending re-anastomosis or pouch formation. Other indications include bowel carcinoma and ischaemic bowel	One-piece and occasionally two-piece drainable pouches changed every 2–3 days	Irritant reactions, particularly with high-output stomas. Short or imperfectly placed stomas, e.g. in an abdominal fold, and loop ileostomies are especially prone to leakage onto skin Disorders associated with the underlying bowel pathology
Colostomy	Placed typically in left iliac fossa with a minimal spout	Large bowel carcinoma and IBD including temporary stomas to rest diseased distal bowel or perineum	One-piece closed appliance changed daily or more frequently depending on output	Irritant reactions are relatively uncommon unless stool is not formed Bleeding over-granulating papules
Urostomy (ileal conduit)	A length of ileum with a spout similar to an ileostomy into which one or usually both ureters drain. Can be on right or left	Bladder carcinoma, incontinence and iatrogenic damage to urological tract either due to radiotherapy or surgical trauma	One- or two-piece drainable appliances changed every 2–3 days	Irritant reactions particularly with short or poorly positioned stomas
Abdominal fistula	Opening of an abdominal viscus directly onto the skin	Usually results from dehiscence of a surgical abdominal wound especially in IBD, fistulating diverticular disease or carcinoma	A variety of appliances together with dressings may be used	Irritant reactions
Others	A gastrostomy is placed in the left upper quadrant and nephrostomy on either flank	A gastrostomy is typically used for nutritional support. A nephrostomy is usually temporary and is used to divert urine from a distal obstruction often secondary to carcinoma	Drainable appliance is used for a nephrostomy	Nephrostomies are occasionally associated with irritant reactions Gastrosomies develop exuberant granulation tissue that can bleed and be painful

[a] The appliances usually attach to the skin by means of a hydrocolloid material. These are commonly composed of polyisobutylene (PIB), which provides 'dry tack' adhesion to the skin, and a mixture of carboxymethylcellulose and fruit pectins, which serve to preserve the acidic pH of the skin and to absorb water, thereby maintaining the dry skin adhesion. The polymer's adhesion is not optimal until warmed so most barriers incorporate an immediate adhesive tackifier on the surface, traditionally rosin based (pentaerythritol ester of rosin), but increasingly non-allergenic, synthetic hydrocarbon materials are used. A range of accessories may be used including belts, additional adhesive tapes, cleansers, adhesive removers, deodorizers and barrier preparations including acrylic adhesive materials.

Table 114.2 Dermatological assessment: aspects specific to peristomal skin.

Aspect	Problems	Actions
Patient's technique	Appliance may no longer be appropriate size or shape	Stoma nurse input is essential
	Patient may be inappropriately rough when cleaning skin or may be using the wrong accessory fillers, medicants, etc.	
Patient anxiety or acceptance of the stoma	Usually fear of leaks or noise leads patients to change appliances too frequently, wear excessively tight belts or use too much unnecessary additional adhesive tapes	Stoma nurse input is essential
Stoma itself	Stoma may be short, in the wrong place or contractile causing it to shorten and leak. Parastomal hernias are common and cause bag failures	Stoma nurse input may help but surgical referral may be necessary
Bowel contents	Liquid motions are more likely to cause leaks	Consider codeine phosphate or loperamide
Infection	Local skin infection may not present in a typical manner under occlusion, and broken skin may become secondarily infected	Always swab rashes and consider *Candida* infection
Underlying bowel disease	Extraintestinal manifestations of Crohn disease and metastatic Crohn disease	Consider biopsy early
	Complications of antineoplastic therapy	Liaise with stoma nurse for advice
Other skin diseases	These may present atypically under occlusion, e.g. bullae in localized pemphigoid may not be apparent	Consider biopsy early

rash affecting the skin in contact with the material responsible and spreading out from the area.

Investigations

Patch testing (see Chapter 128) is carried out to a standard series, a specific stoma series (Table 114.3) and samples of the appliance and any accessory products used. It is also useful for the patient to undertake a usage test. This involves applying a stoma bag together with accessories such as additional hydrocolloid washers or skin pastes to the non-stoma side of the abdomen. The appliances are changed at the same time as that on their stoma and the test continues for 5–7 days. The test, if positive (see Figure 114.1), can confirm which part of an appliance or which accessory product is likely to be causing a skin reaction, although this may or may not be an allergic reaction.

Management

As confirmation of the allergy requires clearance of ACD on avoidance of the culprit product, further management is usually unnecessary. Topical corticosteroid is, however, useful for relief of symptoms and to speed resolution of the dermatitis.

Infections

Introduction and epidemiology

The moist, occluded environment of the peristomal skin is ideal for microbiological growth. Despite this, significant infections are relatively uncommon, accounting for approximately 7% of patients that seek help for skin problems [1]. The most frequent infections are *Candida* overgrowth (Figure 114.2) and folliculitis (staphylococcal), usually from shaving or plucking the hairs with bag adhesive. Secondary bacterial infection, particularly cellulitis (Figure 114.3), affecting ulcerating conditions occurs occasionally. Synergic gangrene (Figure 114.4) and other serious infections are rare, as is tinea corporis.

Pathophysiology

See Chapter 26 for pathogenetic information on specific bacterial infections and Chapter 32 for *Candida* skin infection.

Clinical features

Bacterial infection presents either as a typical folliculitis or a patchy dermatitis with moist, superficial erosions. The latter is non-specific with psoriasiform or eczematous features and can occur with a variety of pathogens [1]. A swab should therefore be taken in all cases of unexplained rash. Bacterial cellulitis presents typically and can complicate pre-existing skin disorders (Figure 114.3).

Table 114.3 Suggested stoma patch test series.

No.	Agent	No.	Agent
1	Cinnamyl alcohol	21	Tetrahydrofurfuryl methacrylate
2	Cinnamaldehyde	22	Tetraethyleneglycol dimethacrylate
3	Eugenol	23	N,N-dimethylaminoethyl methacrylate
4	Alpha-amyl-cinnamaldehyde		
5	Hydroxycitronellal	24	Ethyl cyanoacrylate
6	Geraniol	25	Diazolidinyl urea
7	Isoeugenol	26	Propylene glycol 20% in aqueous
8	Oak moss absolute	27	Chlorhexidine digluconate 0.5% in aqueous
9	Sorbitan sesquioleate		
10	Methyl methacrylate	28	2-Ethylhexyl acrylate 0.1% in petrolatum
11	n-Butyl methacrylate		
12	2-Hydroxypropyl methacrylate	29	Isopropyl 10% in aqueous
13	2-Hydroxyethyl methacrylate	30	Cetrimide 0.1% in aqueous
14	Ethyleneglycol dimethacrylate	31	Polyvinyl pyrrolidone in 1% aqueous
15	Triethyleneglycol dimethacrylate		
16	1,4-Butanediol dimethacrylate	32	Gantrez ES225/gantrez ES425
17	Urethane dimethacrylate	33	Cavilon foam applicator
18	BIS-MA (bisphenol A dimethacrylate)	34	Karaya 10% in aqueous
		35	Benzoyl oeroxide
19	BIS-GMA (bisphenol A glycerolate dimethacrylate)	36	1H-benzotriazole 1% in petroleum
		37	D-Limonene 10% in petroleum
20	1,6-Hexanediol diacrylate	38	Propyl gallate 1% in petroleum

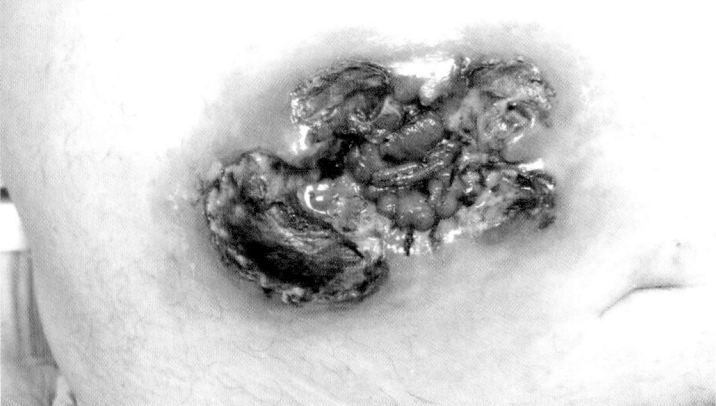

Figure 114.4 Synergic gangrene affecting a recently formed ileostomy. The patient required surgical debridement in addition to systemic antibiotics.

Synergic gangrene occurs in the weeks after surgery, usually following surgical wound breakdown (mucocutaneous separation [2]).

Investigations
A swab should be taken from all rashes for bacteriology and skin scrapings where appropriate for mycology.

Management
Antibiotic prescribing should be guided by microbiology findings. Systemic treatment is preferable as topical creams interfere with appliance adhesion. Patients who shave their abdomen are advised to do this no more than once per week. An adhesive remover spray is helpful if strong adhesion is causing hair plucking.

Other skin conditions presenting near stomas

Introduction and epidemiology
Theoretically almost any dermatosis could involve the peristomal skin, and a dermatologist will be able to diagnose such disorders based upon features both locally and beyond the stoma. In practice a few skin diseases warrant special mention either because they are more common than expected or because they can present atypically. The isomorphic (Koebner) phenomenon might be expected to make certain disorders more likely in the potentially traumatized peristomal skin although in the author's experience, with the exception of psoriasis, these are uncommon.

Psoriasis is more than twice as common in patients with inflammatory bowel disease (IBD) compared with the population as a whole [1], and is the most frequent generalized dermatosis seen around stomas as a result of this and probably also the Koebner phenomenon [2]. Around stomas it presents like flexural psoriasis (Figure 114.5). Features of psoriasis elsewhere may be limited and subtle so that diagnosis may not be immediately obvious.

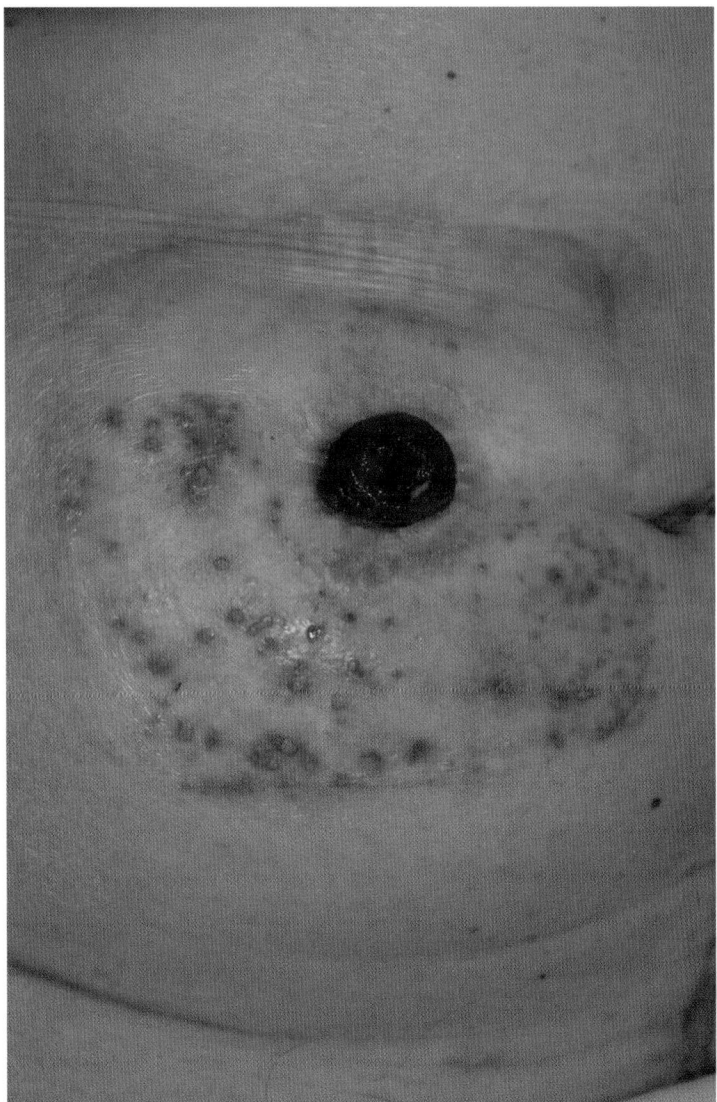

Figure 114.2 *Candida* infection presenting as an itchy, non-follicular pustular rash affecting an immunosuppressed woman with an ileostomy for Crohn disease.

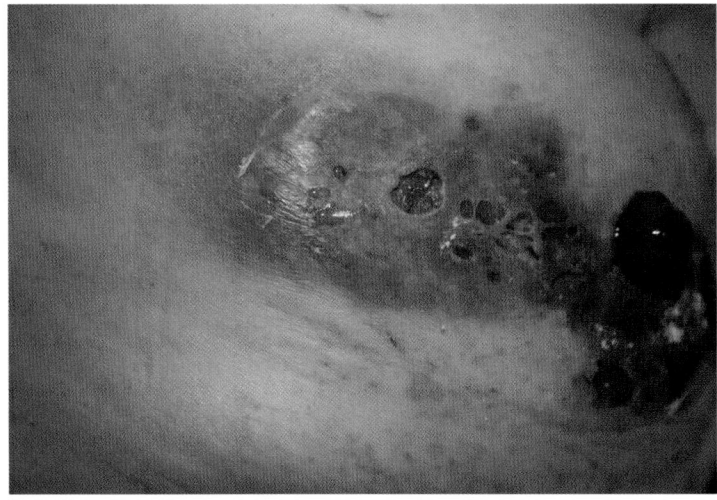

Figure 114.3 Streptococcal cellulitis complicating healing pyoderma gangrenosum in a 65-year-old woman with inflammatory bowel disease.

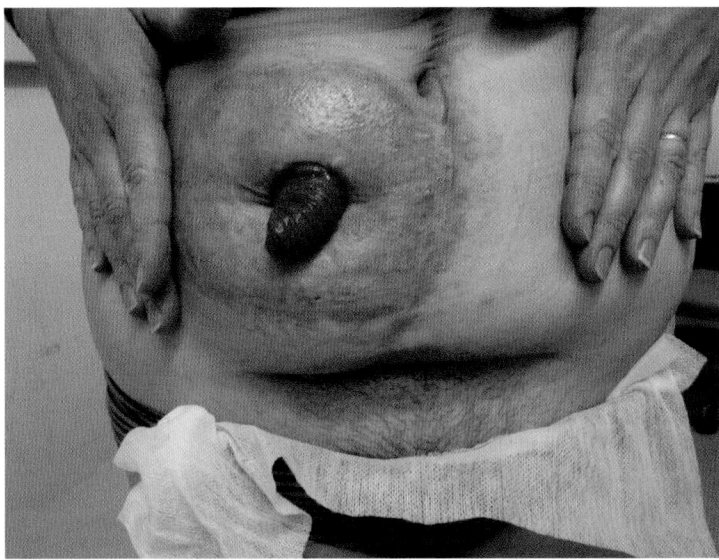

(a)

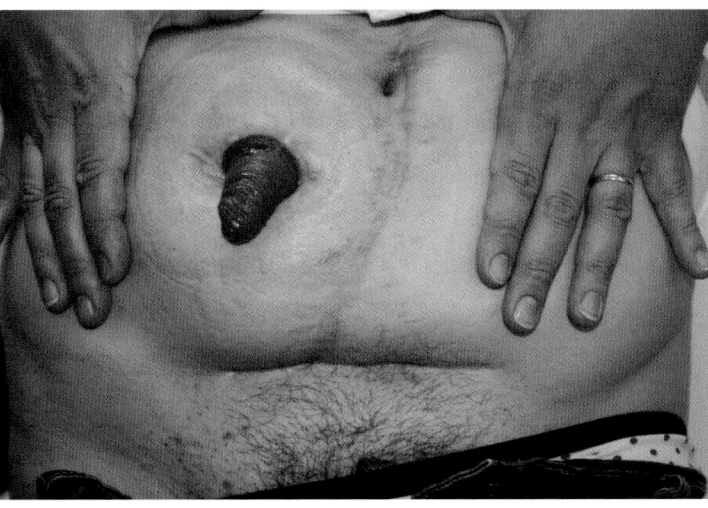

(b)

Figure 114.5 (a) Psoriasis affecting an ileostomy in a woman with Crohn disease; this was confirmed histologically. She had a history suggestive of scalp psoriasis in the past and had flexural psoriasis in the abdomen and natal cleft. (b) The flexural psoriasis cleared within 1 month using clobetasol propionate scalp foam 2–3 times per week at appliance changes.

Lichen sclerosus has been described involving peristomal skin [3,4] where it can present acutely with features similar to active genital lichen sclerosus (Figure 114.6). It particularly affects urostomies and can appear without associated genital involvement [4,5].

The antianginal nitrate drug nicorandil is known to cause oral aphthous ulceration [6], perianal ulcers [7], peristomal ulceration (Figure 114.7) [8] and bowel perforation [9] or fistula formation, particularly in patients with diverticular disease [10,11]. It accounted for up to 2% of referrals to one specialist stoma care/dermatology clinic [10]. This drug is rarely used in the Americas and is currently not approved by the US Food and Drug Administration.

Localized bullous pemphigoid occasionally involves peristomal skin (Figure 114.8). It can cause diagnostic confusion as the typical

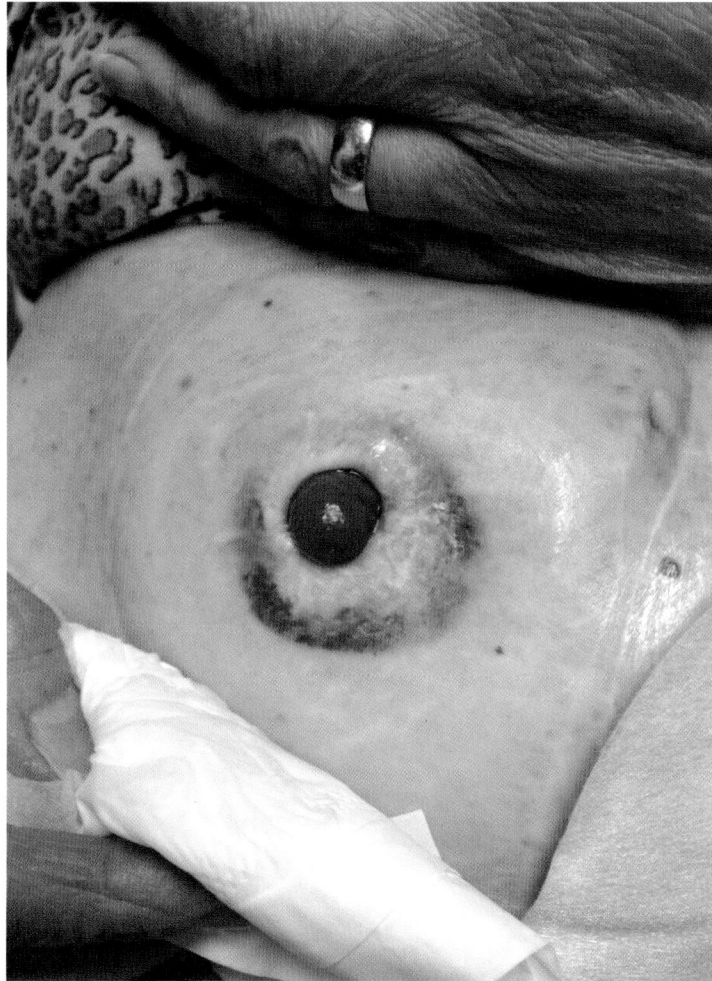

(a)

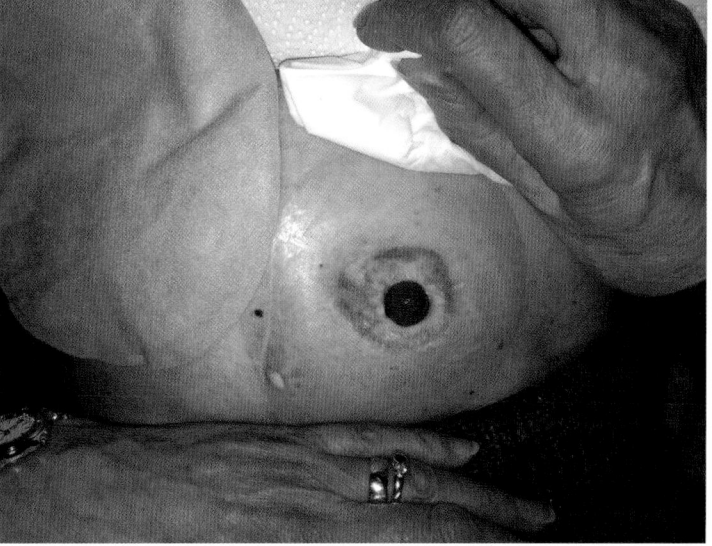

(b)

Figure 114.6 (a) Lichen sclerosus affecting a urostomy in a woman with a history of genital lichen sclerosus presenting some years prior to stoma formation for bladder carcinoma. (b) The inflammation settled rapidly within 1 month after administration of triamcinolone acetonide 20 mg intralesionally.

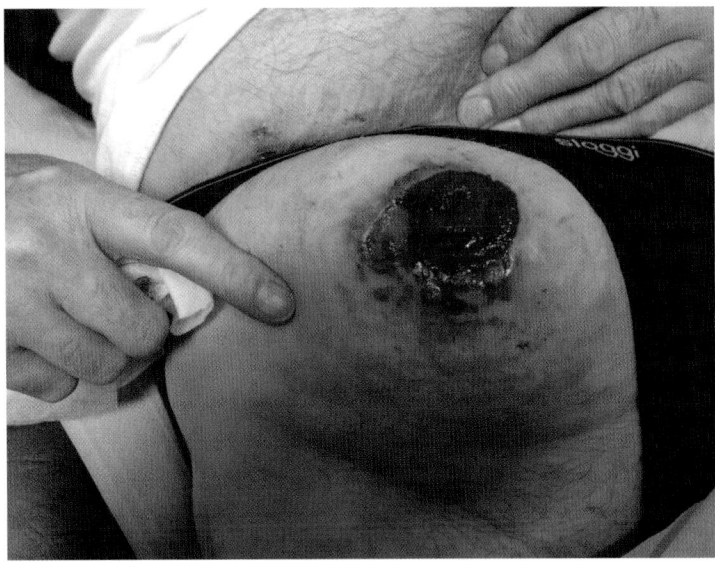

(a)

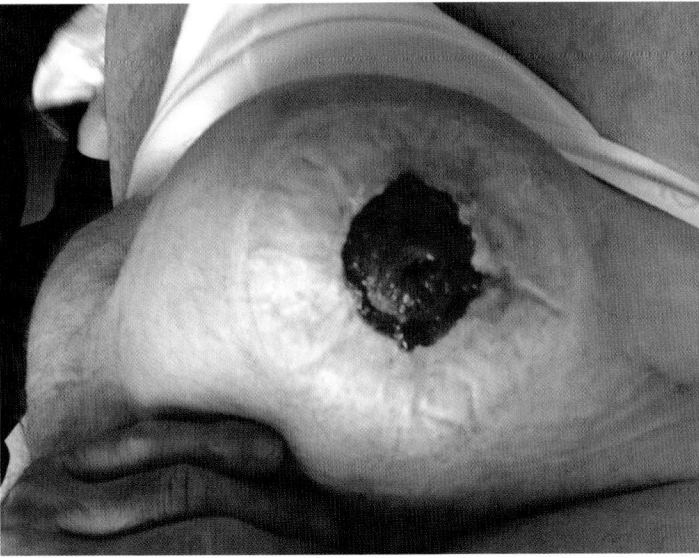

(b)

Figure 114.7 (a) Nicorandil ulceration affecting an ileostomy for ulcerative colitis. (b) This healed completely within 6 weeks of stopping the drug.

blisters are not seen, having been de-roofed by the action of the appliance adhesive [12].

Other congenital or acquired bullous or hyperkeratotic disorders are surprisingly rare around abdominal stomas.

Pathophysiology

Refer to specific disease chapters.

Clinical features

Psoriasis presents typically outside the area covered by the appliance and will only cause diagnostic confusion if the features of psoriasis elsewhere are scant or subtle. Under an appliance it has the features of flexural psoriasis.

Lichen sclerosus may present as an asymptomatic papery, atrophic plaque of typical extragenital lichen sclerosus, but more

usually presents as painful, purpuric plaques often associated with ulceration.

Nicorandil ulcers are sometimes painful but rarely inflamed and tend to look rather bland. Ulceration appears to be mostly associated with higher doses of 40 mg or more per day. The differential diagnosis includes superficial, traumatic ulcers such as those associated with parastomal hernias.

Localized pemhigoid affecting stomas presents as painful and often itchy denuded areas.

Investigations

For all these conditions a skin biopsy is indicated if there is any doubt about the diagnosis. However, for nicorandil ulceration histology is non-specific, typically with mild, chronic inflammation.

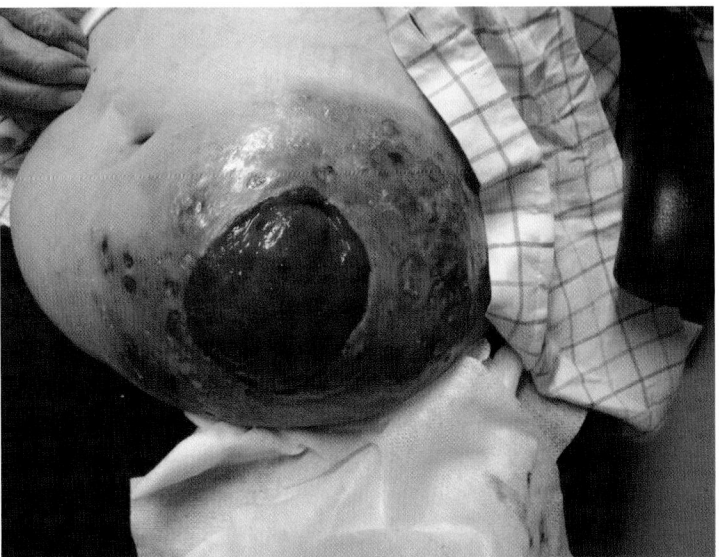

(a)

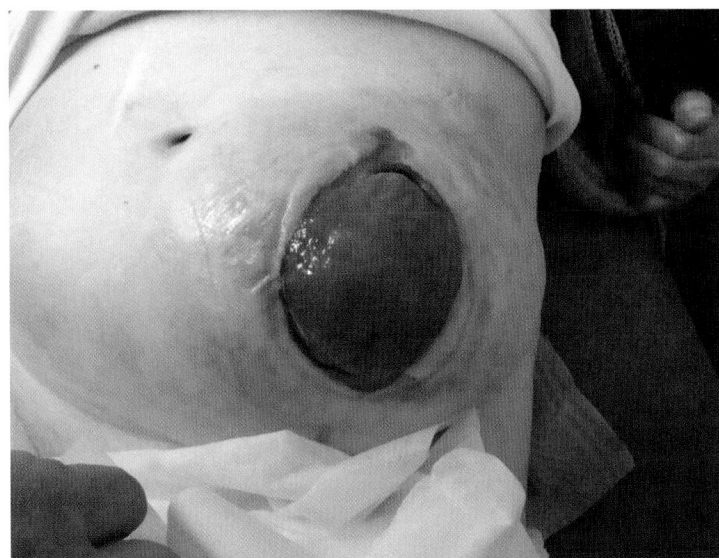

(b)

Figure 114.8 (a) Localized bullous pemphigoid affecting a large colostomy in a 90-year-old man. At presentation denuded areas of skin were seen, but there were no obvious blisters. (b) The skin healed 1 month later on a reducing dose of oral prednisolone (average 20 mg per day).

The diagnosis is therefore largely clinical and improvement on cessation of the drug corroborates this.

Management

The principles of topical treatments are detailed in the note under Table 114.4. Topical treatment alone is usually effective for psoriasis. If the patient is not using a mostly or wholly hydrocolloid barrier it is worth changing to one as psoriasis may clear under occlusion with a hydrocolloid but not a thin fabric dressing [2,13]. UV phototherapy can be used; the patient should hold a cardboard tube (from a toilet roll or similar) filled with gauze over the stoma to protect it from UV exposure and leakage. Systemic treatment may be required early because the psoriasis reduces bag adhesion and irritation from leaks can exacerbate the dermatosis. The clinician should be aware that the nephrotoxic effects of certain drugs, particularly ciclosporin, can be enhanced by the haemodynamic changes that result from even moderate output ileostomies.

Lichen sclerosus, particularly if ulcerated, usually requires intralesional corticosteroids to gain control (e.g. triamcinolone acetonide 20 mg).

Nicorandil ulceration around stomas responds to cessation of the drug. This can usually be stopped immediately and the nitrate effect replaced by an increased dose of an alternative such as isosorbide mononitrate.

Bullous pemphigoid responds to the usual treatments and, although topical treatments may suffice, systemic treatments may be required at an earlier stage.

Dermatoses associated with underlying bowel disease

Introduction and epidemiology

Superficial ulceration secondary to trauma is relatively common near stomas, particularly if there is an associated parastomal hernia. Such ulcers typically settle rapidly with conservative treatment from the stoma nurse specialist. Where they persist or worsen one should consider other diagnoses and the possibility of secondary infection or progression to pyoderma gangrenosum via the pathergy phenomenon.

In the author's speciality clinic, perineal and genital Crohn disease (CD) are common referrals, whilst CD affecting peristomal skin is rare. Where it does occur it is usually contiguous with the stoma itself and may be associated with fistulation (Figure 114.9). As a result most patients require gastro-enterological and/or colorectal surgical management.

Pyoderma gangrenosum (PG), by contrast, is commoner than expected. Whereas an average dermatologist might be expected to see no more than two new cases per year, PG accounts for over 4% of the patients presenting with peristomal skin problems [1]. This high prevalence is partly explained by the association with IBD, but PG also occurs in stoma patients with no IBD and can also affect urostomies suggesting other pathogenic mechanisms may be involved.

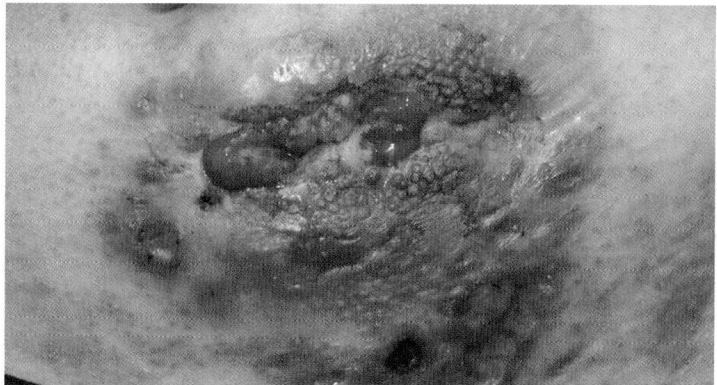

Figure 114.9 Fistulating Crohn disease affecting an ileostomy in a teenage girl. The original stoma on the left was partly destroyed by the inflammatory process and faeces emerged from this and three other fistulous openings. There was associated irritant dermatitis in which papule formation is prominent.

Pathophysiology

See Chapter 49 for pathogenetic information on PG and Chapters 113 and 152 for CD of the skin.

There is some evidence that PG is more likely where underlying IBD is currently active [2–5] but this is not universal [6]. PG should not be considered an indication for further bowel resection unless otherwise indicated.

Pathergy (e.g. from skin stripping on appliance removal) probably contributes to the prevalence of peristomal PG. Convex appliances (see Figure 114.1) put pressure on the peristomal skin and are associated with PG. In the author's experience [7], in the early 2000s, 14% of our stoma patients were using convex appliances. Of those with a first episode of PG, 30% were using these appliances, and in patients with recurrent episodes the figure rose to 74%.

Clinical features

The clinical features of a Crohn ulcer near a stoma (Figure 114.10) are similar to PG and a biopsy may be necessary to distinguish them if there is no mucosal involvement. PG itself almost never involves the stoma mucosa.

The clinical features of peristomal PG are essentially the same as for PG elsewhere (see Chapter 49) although patients may not recall a pustular or papular stage and this is only occasionally observed by the clinician. The ulceration is typically very painful (Figure 114.11) and this is worsened by stoma leaks. Some ulcers are not painful at all because of surgical damage to local sensory nerves. Figure 114.12 demonstrates the typical features of an overhanging, purple and perforated edge that results in cribriform scarring. Irregular scarring itself will impair appliance adhesion. Although some stoma patients have concurrent PG at more typical sites, like the leg [8], the great majority in the author's experience are restricted to the peristomal area.

Investigations

A biopsy is required to differentiate a Crohn ulcer from a PG ulcer if there are no other features of Crohn disease.

Investigations for peristomal PG are as the same as for PG elsewhere, and directed at finding a potential underlying disease and

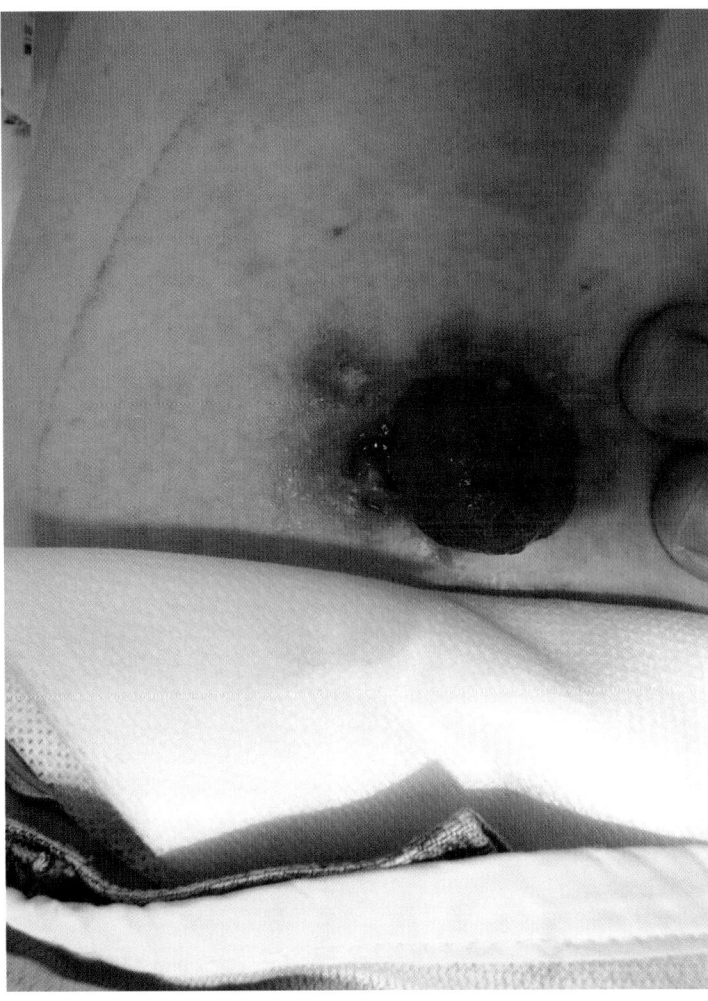

(a)

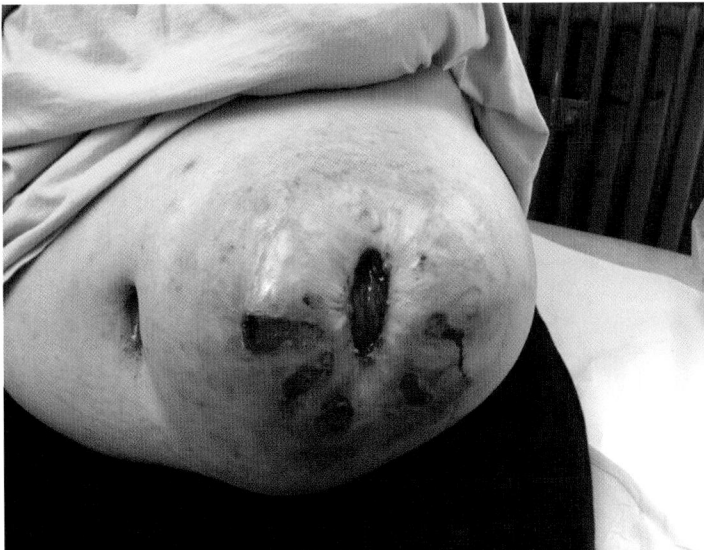

(b)

Figure 114.10 (a) Crohn ulcer near a recently formed ileostomy. The ulceration was painful and slowly expanded. (b) Crohn ulceration affecting a colostomy site. A biopsy from the umbilical ulceration also demonstrated the granulomatous inflammation of Crohn disease.

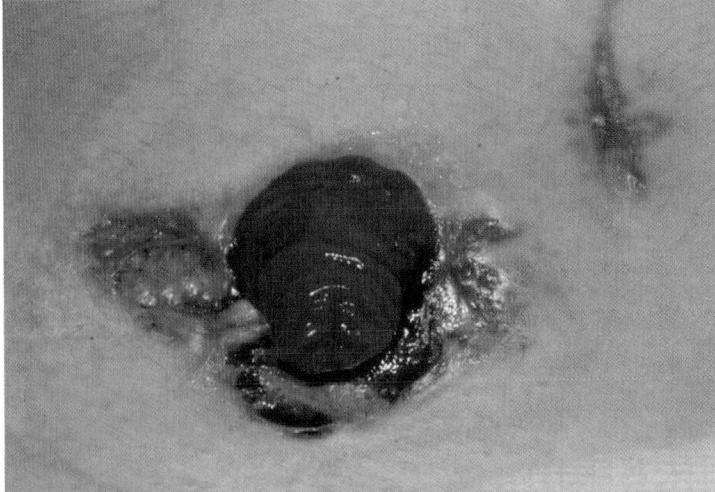

Figure 114.11 Pyoderma gangrenosum (PG) affecting an ileostomy in a teenage girl with a permanent end-ileostomy for Crohn disease. There is active PG at the 5 to 7 o'clock position, healed PG at the 3 o'clock position and partly healed PG with skin bridging at the 9 o'clock position. The healed midline surgical scar has become inflamed and a sterile pustule is evident. This type of inflammation in scars is typical and can be recurrent over many years in Crohn disease.

ruling out other differential diagnoses. An ulcer biopsy is usually recommended for this purpose. However, there is a risk of worsening the ulceration via pathergy, therefore in the presence of a typical peristomal clinical picture, in association with underlying bowel disease, this author recommends a trial of topical treatment for up to 2 weeks before considering a skin biopsy. The possibility of infection causing or complicating the ulcerative processes on the occluded peristomal skin should be borne in mind and a biopsy for microbiological examination as well as histology may be indicated.

Management

For both PG and the much rarer Crohn ulcer, the deleterious effect on normal stoma appliance use of both the active disease and the resultant scarring warrants early introduction of effective treatments. The majority of cases respond satisfactorily to topical therapy alone [9]; corticosteroid preparations that can be used are detailed in Table 114.4. There is no perfect preparation applicable to stomas that is available 'off the shelf' and getting medicaments manufactured can be problematic and expensive. An ideal preparation for ulcerated lesions was triamcinolone in carboxymethylcellulose paste (Adcortyl-in-Orabase™) but this was taken off the market in the UK in 2009; it may be available under other trade names in other parts of the world. If one of the topical corticosteroid preparations is not effective, or well tolerated, within 14 days, then a suitable second-line agent is tacrolimus 0.3% in Orabase™ paste applied once daily for up to 1 month. The addition of fludroxycortide tape applied over the paste reduces healing time and appears to minimize the overgranulation that can occur during healing [10]. If topical treatments are ineffective or PG is very severe at presentation (Figure 114.13), the systemic treatment approach is as for PG in general (see Chapter 49). In patients with

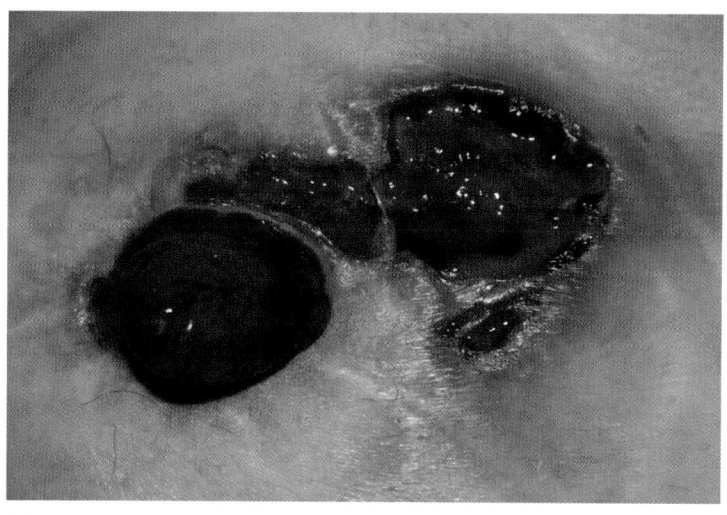

(a)

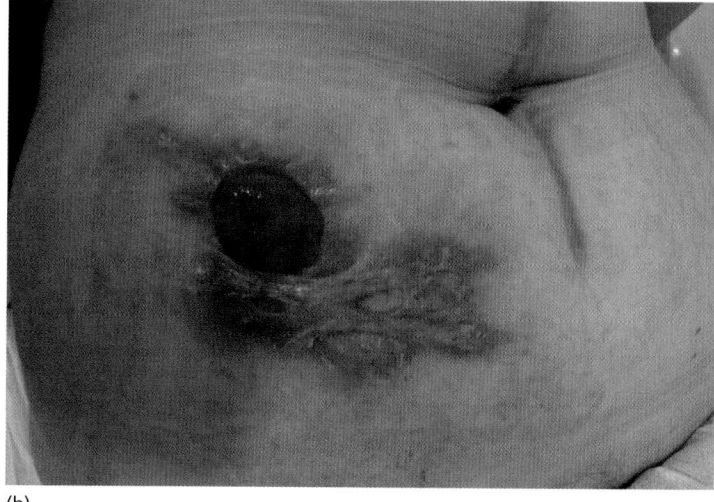

(b)

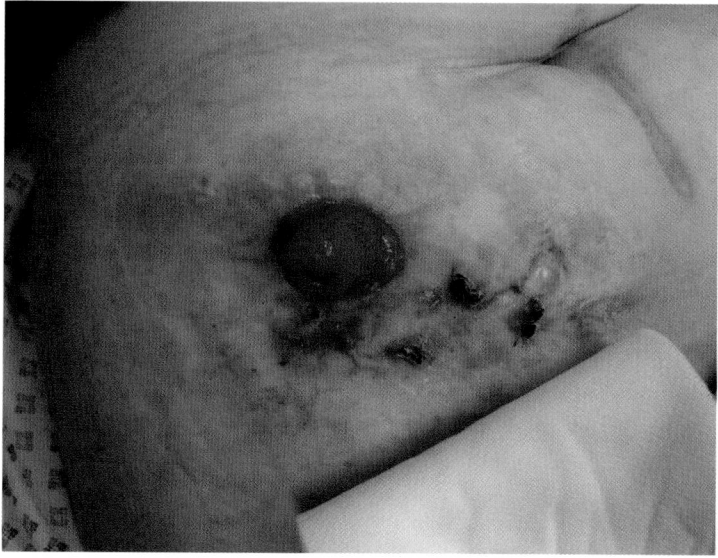

(c)

Figure 114.12 (a) Pyoderma gangrenosum (PG) affecting a permanent ileostomy in a man with a history of ulcerative colitis. The perforated edge is typical and results, in severe cases, in very irregular cribriform scarring which can interfere with appliance adhesion. (b) This shows an example in 30-year-old woman with Crohn disease where the PG has healed. (c) The skin bridging was removed under local anaesthetic to prevent trauma and maceration to the underlying skin that could have triggered further PG. This minor surgery should be delayed until after PG has healed completely to minimize the risk of further ulceration via the pathergy phenomenon.

Table 114.4 Topical corticosteroids useful for inflammatory peristomal skin diseases.[a]

Active ingredient	Trade name	Other ingredients
Betamethasone valerate 0.1%: scalp lotion	Betnovate™ (Glaxo-Smith Kline)	Carbomer, sodium hydroxide and water
Betamethasone dipropionate 0.05%: scalp lotion	Diprosone™ (Schering-Plough)	Carbomer, sodium hydroxide and water
Clobetasol propionate 0.05%: scalp lotion	Dermovate™ (Glaxo-Smith Kline)	Carbomer, sodium hydroxide and water
Clobetasol propionate 0.05%: spray scalp foam	Clarelux™ (Fabre)	Cetyl alcohol, propylene glycol and stearyl alcohol
Fluocinolone 0.025%: scalp gel	Synalar™ (GP Pharma Ltd)	Benzoates and propylene glycol
Betamethasone and calcipotriol: scalp gel	Dovobet™ gel (Leo Laboratories)	Paraffin, liquid polyoxypropylene-15, stearyl ether, castor oil and butylhydroxytoluene (E321)
Beclometasone dipropionate 200 μg: metered dose asthma inhaler	Clenil modulate™ (Chiesi)	None
Fludroxycortide 4 μg/cm²: tape	Haelan™ (Typharm)	None

[a] Lotions containing oils should be avoided and the patient should be warned that preparations containing propylene glycol and Dovobet gel should be left to dry for 10 min before placing their bag. Alcoholic scalp lotions can sting when applied to broken skin and can be applied to the bag directly and left to dry before fitting. Potency of steroid is increased under occlusion. Continuous daily treatment should be for no more than 4 weeks and thereafter no more than three times per week to avoid skin atrophy. Haelan tape is useful for small ulcerated lesions, particularly pyoderma gangrenosum.

PART 10: SITES, SEX, AGE

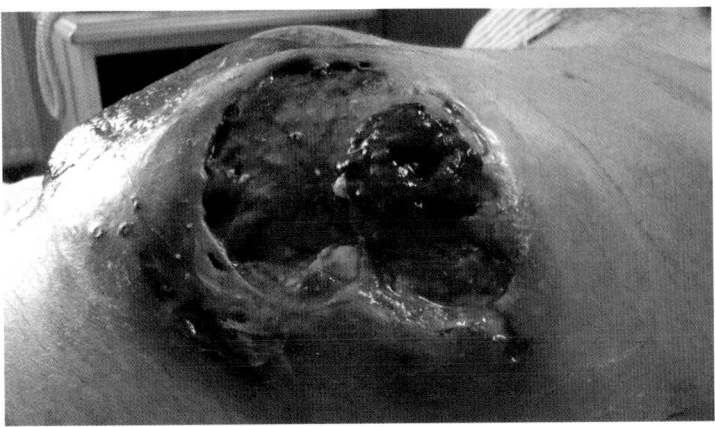

Figure 114.13 Severe pyoderma gangrenosum (PG) in a middle-aged man with acute onset of Crohn disease requiring a pan-proctocolectomy and ileostomy. He received adalimumab (40 mg SC every 2 weeks) which controlled the ileal Crohn disease and settled the PG over 3 months.

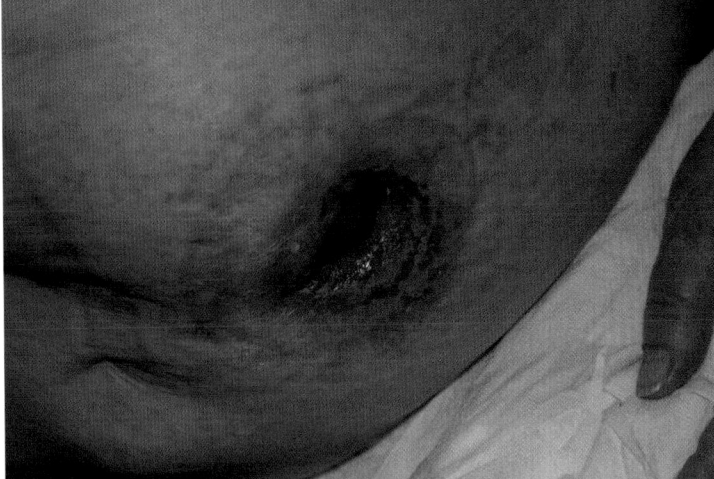

Figure 114.14 A short ileostomy buried in a skin fold near the umbilicus. This stoma was undertaken as an emergency procedure and siting is suboptimal. The eroded dermatitis is due to the corrosive faecal contents.

any active IBD, particularly Crohn disease, anti-TNF therapy with infliximab [11] or adalimumab is usually highly effective.

Irritant skin reactions

Introduction and epidemiology

Irritant reactions account for more than 50% of the skin problems experienced by stoma patients [1,2]. They may present with a dermatitis or one of a range of distinctive papular reactions [3]. In most cases the patient's stoma nurse specialist will have diagnosed the problem and arranged effective management, usually by modification of the appliance system to prevent leaks or adhesive reactions. The causes and types of these disorders are detailed in Tables 114.1 and 114.2. Most patients presenting to dermatologists will therefore be those that require further investigations or treatments that cannot be undertaken or prescribed by the nurse.

Pathophysiology

See Chapter 129 for pathogenetic information on irritant contact dermatitis.

Damage to the skin barrier producing irritant reactions results from repeated exposure to stoma contents which, in the case of faeces, is corrosive. Repeated microscopic skin stripping when changing appliances may also contribute to dermatitis reactions [4]. When all potential causes of peristomal dermatitis have been excluded (including allergy, infection and psoriasis, etc.) there remain approximately 10% of stoma patients with what is regarded as idiopathic dermatitis [2].

Clinical features

Faecal or urinary irritant dermatitis may result from wearing an appliance that is too large so that it exposes skin to effluent, either because the stoma is buried or in a skin fold (Figure 114.14), or

because the stoma is short (Figure 114.15) and faeces track under the barrier. Occasionally ileostomies or urostomies are very contractile such that they spasmodically shorten with the same result (Figure 114.16). Some patients develop persistent reactions to portions of the adhesive barrier with no demonstrable allergic component. This is particularly the case with adhesive tape borders similar to the dressings used for patch testing (Figures 114.1 and 114.17). A proportion of patients (up to 10%) have persistent or recurrent dermatitis affecting the whole of the occluded skin for which no cause can be found (Figure 114.18).

Three patterns of papular reaction deserve particular mention. All are the probable consequence of exposure to stoma effluent.
1 Hypergranulating polyps or 'granulomas' occur, particularly around colostomies, as cherry red papules at the

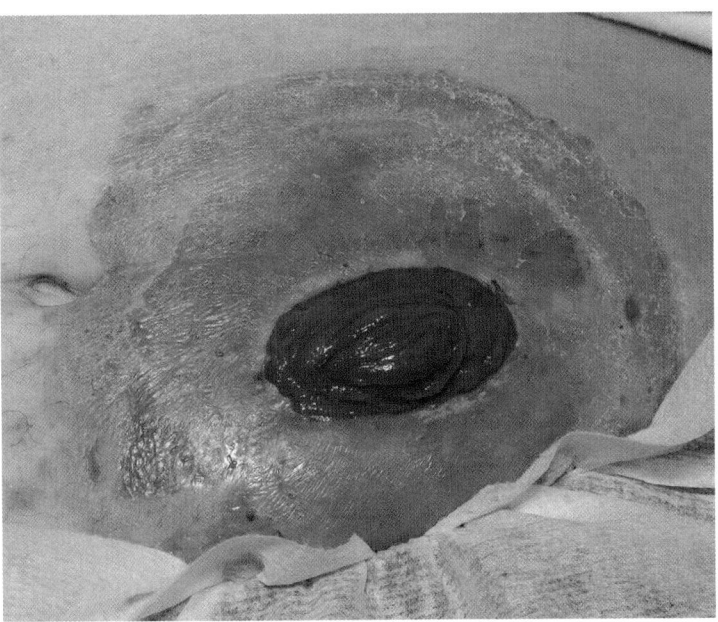

Figure 114.15 A proximal colostomy with liquid effluent that leaked onto the skin because the stoma is short. This results in an eroded faecal dermatitis.

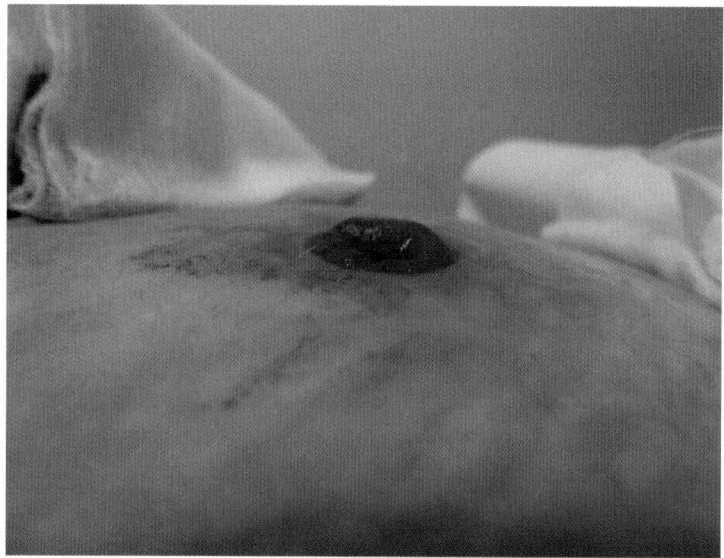

Figure 114.16 A highly contractile ileostomy that varies in length from flush (pictured) to 3 cm long.

mucocutaneous junction. They may proliferate into normal skin if exposed to faeces (Figure 114.19) [5]. A similar process can affect ileostomies, where it presents as flat, red, bleeding areas in which bowel metaplasia of the skin is relatively common (Figure 114.20). Either case may be symptomatic from bleeding or leakage. Occasionally, hypergranulating polyps are painful (Figure 114.21). The metaplastic lesions may very rarely develop primary adenocarcinoma [6]. Rarely the metaplastic process affects urostomies (Figure 114.22).

2 Multiple hyperkeratotic and acanthotic papules occur around shortileostomies and particularly abdominal fistulae (Figure 114.23).

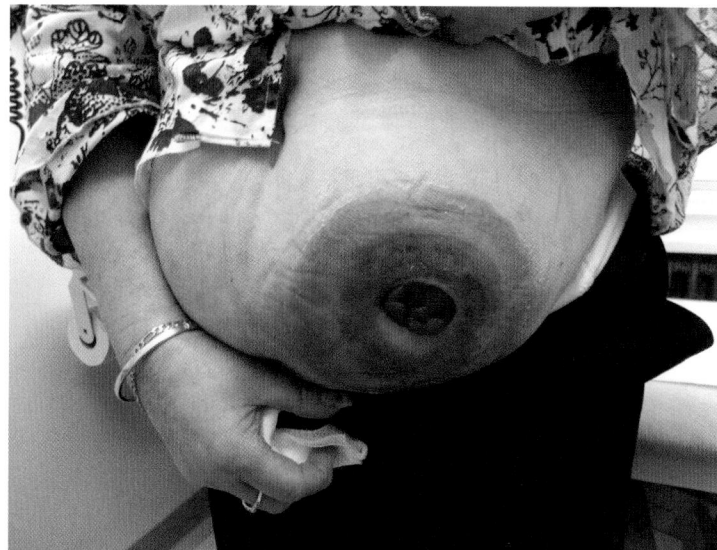

Figure 114.17 A short colostomy demonstrating faecal dermatitis. The patient also has a persistent reaction to the tape border of her appliance (outer ring of dermatitis).

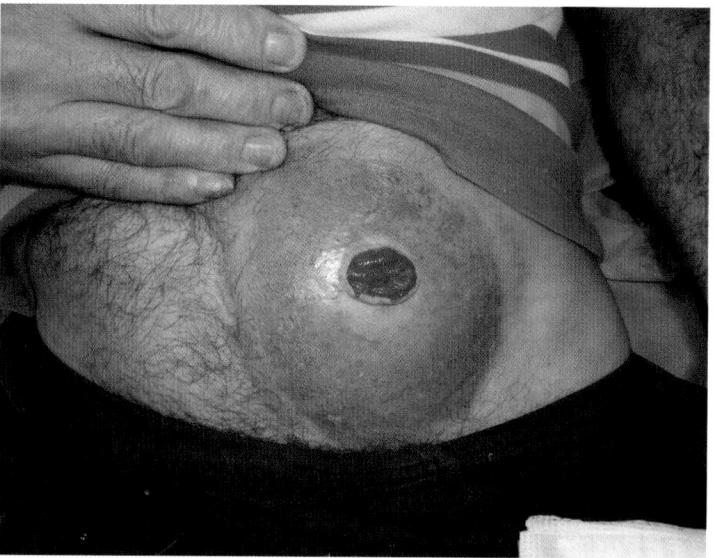

Figure 114.18 Idiopathic dermatitis affecting the whole skin covered by the stoma barrier. The patient did not develop a reaction to the appliance when it was worn for 7 days on a normal piece of skin.

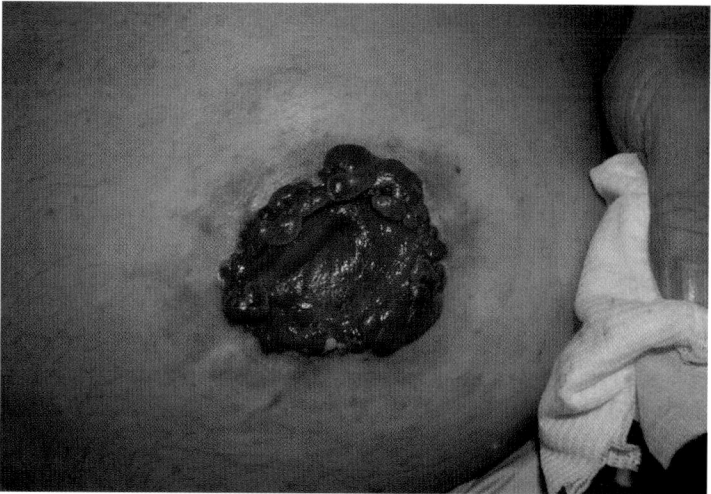

(a)

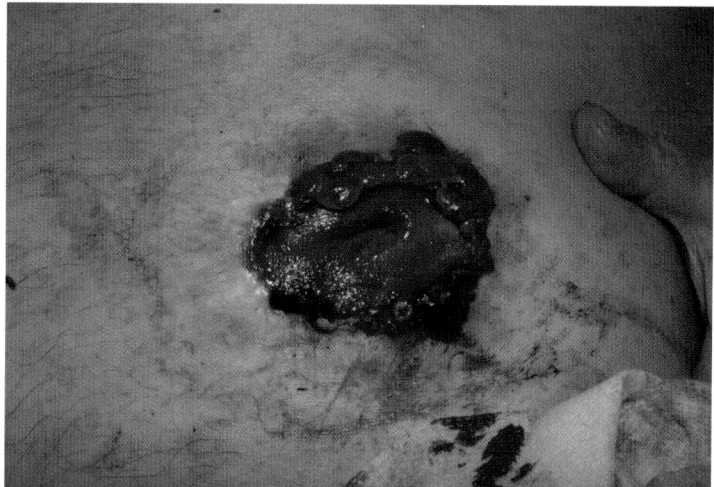

(b)

Figure 114.19 (a) Inflammatory polyps affecting a colostomy where the skin has been exposed to faeces. (b) Where these bleed, proliferate, cause pain or otherwise result in appliance failure, they can be removed under local anaesthetic by curettage and cautery.

PART 10: SITES, SEX, AGE

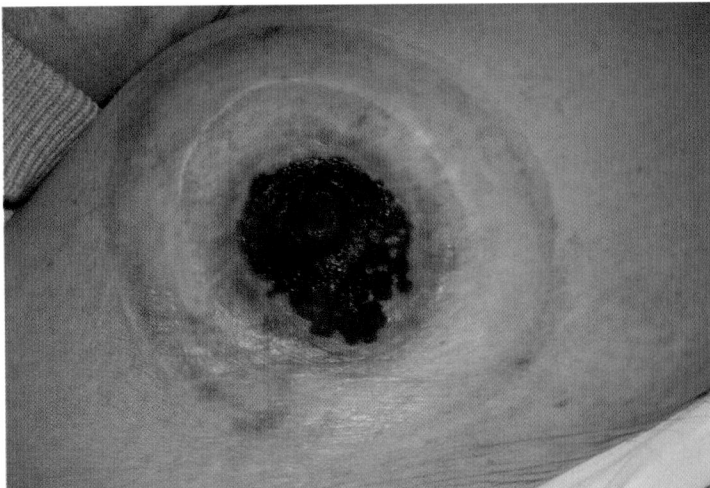

Figure 114.20 Granulation tissue with bowel metaplasia affecting an ileostomy. These lesions cause bag failures, especially by bleeding. Because of this, and in particular in the presence of metaplasia, the skin should be resurfaced under local anaesthetic with light cautery or, if available, laser.

3 Chronic papillomatous dermatitis is a term used by Bergman *et al.* [7] to describe a distinctive hyperkeratotic irritant skin reaction affecting leaking urostomies. The term has been used by subsequent authors to refer to lesions near ileostomies, but it is probably best reserved for urostomies as the clinical presentation is distinct (Figure 114.24). Small hyperkeratotic papules can lead to massive and progressive hyperkeratotic plaques that may impinge on the stoma resulting in stenosis in some cases if the leaking onto the skin is not corrected.

Investigations

In most cases the diagnosis is clinically obvious and response to measures taken to prevent further skin damage will confirm the underlying irritancy. A biopsy may be undertaken in the remaining cases to look for other diagnoses (see the section on other diseases

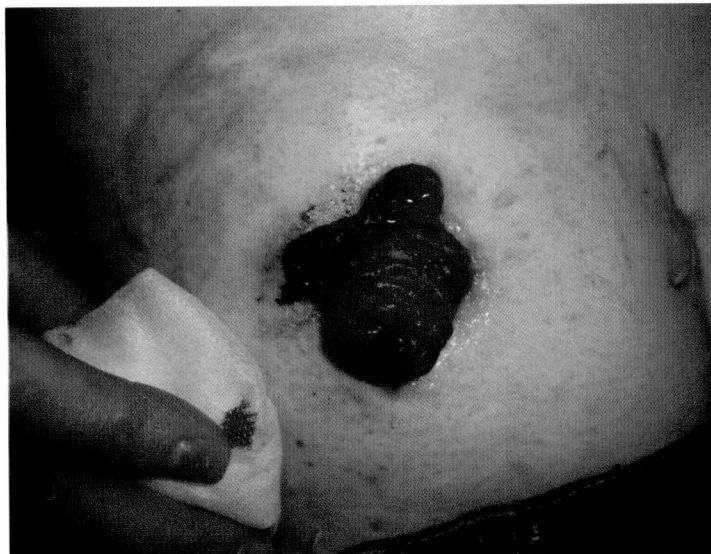

Figure 114.21 Pain is occasionally prominent and sometimes severe as in this young woman with an ileostomy for ulcerative colitis. Treatment is as for Figure 114.20.

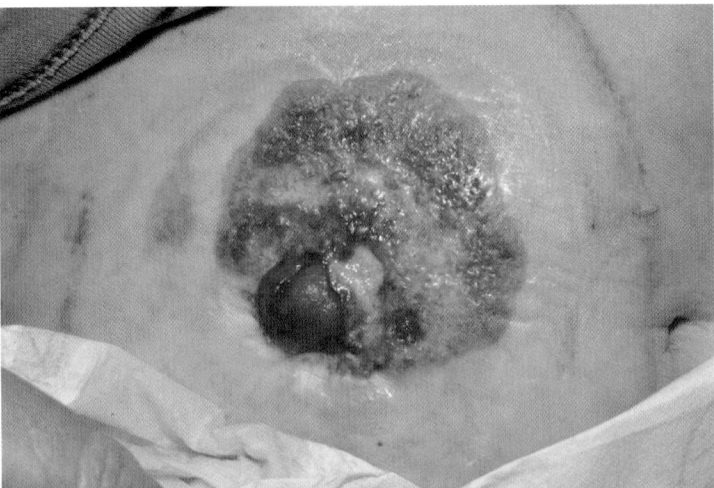

Figure 114.22 Ileal metaplasia affecting a longstanding urostomy and covering a wide area of skin. This was treated with laser resurfacing.

earlier in this chapter). The histological features of all the irritant reactions, including an idiopathic dermatitis, are essentially the same, comprising various degrees of acanthosis, hyperkeratosis, erosion, mixed inflammatory infiltrate and capillary dilatation. Patients with longstanding stomas, usually ileostomies for ulcerative colitis, may very rarely develop carcinoma in the surrounding skin, such that a biopsy is indicated for any unusual or persistent lesions.

Management

The general management for all irritant reactions is to avoid exposure to the irritant wherever possible. It is therefore essential to liaise with a stoma nurse specialist in the management of these patients. Chronic papillomatous dermatitis in particular responds rapidly to measures to prevent leaks. Patients presenting to a dermatologist will, in most cases, have already seen their nurse and will require specific dermatological intervention as well. Where the stoma is short, suboptimally placed or associated with a hernia, surgical refashioning might seem the most appropriate

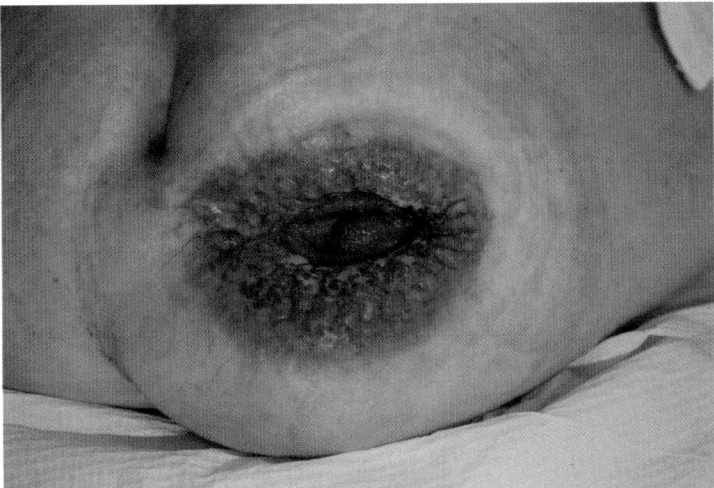

Figure 114.23 A short and buried ileostomy where leaks are inevitable. The mottled appearance of the hyperkeratotic papules is typical.

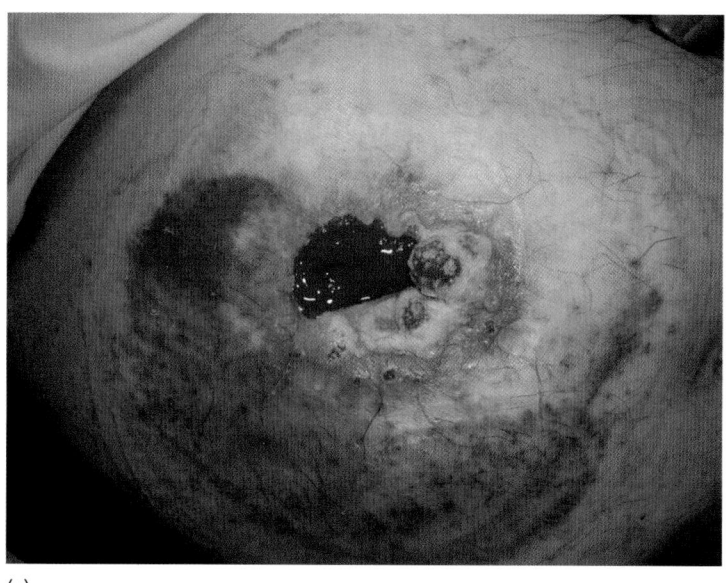

(a)

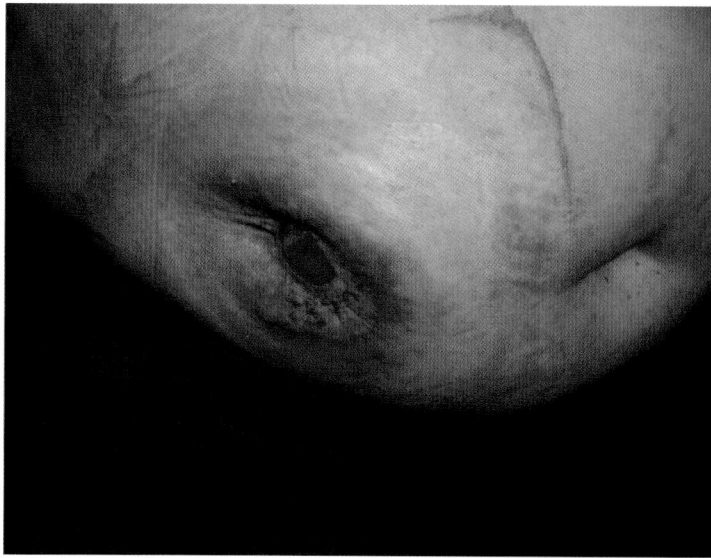

(b)

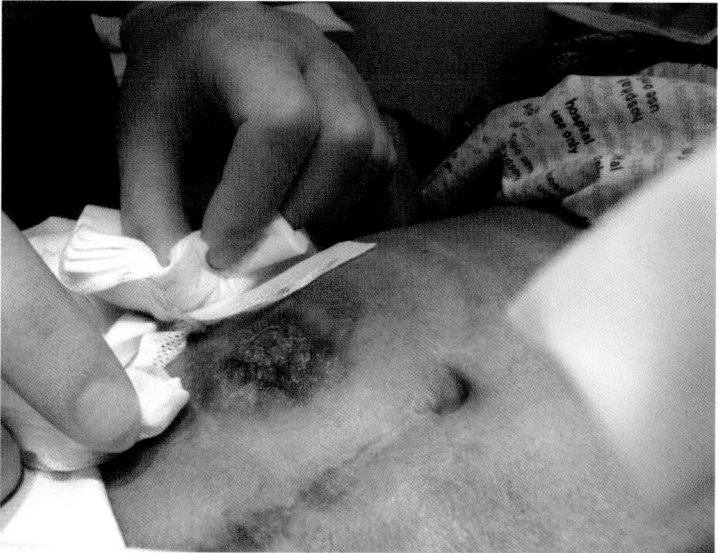

(c)

Figure 114.24 (a) Chronic papillomatous dermatitis (CPD) and irritant dermatitis associated with a leaking urostomy. The papules are typical. (b) These may proliferate and are occasionally blue due to bacterial degradation of the tryptophan in urine producing an indigo-like substance. (c) These hyperkeratotic papules can encroach on the urostomy, as in this Asian woman with a urostomy for neurological incontinence. Squamous epithelium encroaching onto the urostomy mucosa is seen in severe cases. Surgical removal under local anaesthetic may be necessary as in this case to prevent stoma stenosis.

step. However, surgical considerations such as the amount of available remaining bowel or medical considerations such as anaesthetic risk may make this too hazardous for the patient.

For dermatitis, short-term topical corticosteroid is usually all that is needed in order to settle inflammation and enhance appliance adhesion (see Table 114.4). This may be required intermittently in the longer term, particularly for idiopathic dermatitis.

Chronic papillomatous dermatitis responds very well to attempts to prevent urine leakage, which is typically more achievable than for leaking ileostomies, colostomies or fistulae. One effective, additional measure for early chronic papillomatous dermatitis is to apply 20% domestic vinegar (diluted in tap water) to the skin, using soaked gauze, for 10 min each day after cleaning [8]. It probably works by reducing the corrosive effects of ammonia produced by urea-splitting bacteria as well as maintaining the physiological pH of the skin. Papular irritant reactions that do not respond to the prevention of leaks can be removed surgically

under local anaesthetic, usually by cautery with or without prior curettage or shaving off of the lesions (see Figures 114.19, 114.20, 114.21, 114.22, 114.23 and 114.24). This may need to be repeated periodically – as often as every 3–4 months in the case of granulomas as they tend to recur.

Gastrostomies are sometimes complicated by painful bleeding and exuberant granulation tissue that is difficult to address surgically [9].

Key references

The full list of references can be found in the online version at www.rooksdermatology.com.

Introduction

1 Jemec GB, Nybaek H. Peristomal skin problems account for more than one in three visits to ostomy nurses. *Br J Dermatol* 2008;159(5):1211–12.

2 Lyon CC, Smith AD, Griffiths CE, Beck MH. The spectrum of skin disorders in abdominal stoma patients. *Br J Dermatol* 2000;143(6):1248–60.

3 Al-Niaimi F, Almaani N, Samarasinghe V, Williams J, Lyon C. The relevance of patch testing in peristomal dermatitis. *Br J Dermatol* 2012;167:103–9.

Allergic contact dermatitis

1 Al-Niaimi F, Almaani N, Samarasinghe V, Williams J, Lyon C. The relevance of patch testing in peristomal dermatitis. *Br J Dermatol* 2012;167:103–9.

Infections

1 Lyon CC, Smith AD, Griffiths CE, Beck MH. The spectrum of skin disorders in abdominal stoma patients. *Br J Dermatol* 2000;143(6):1248–60.

Other skin conditions presenting near stomas

2 Lyon CC, Smith AD, Griffiths CE, Beck MH. The spectrum of skin disorders in abdominal stoma patients. *Br J Dermatol* 2000;143(6):1248–60.

Dermatoses associated with underlying bowel disease

6 Hughes AP, Jackson JM, Callen JP. Clinical features and treatment of peristomal pyoderma gangrenosum. *JAMA* 2000;284(12):1546–8.

10 Lyon CC, Stapleton M, Smith AJ, Mendelsohn S, Beck MH, Griffiths CE. Topical tacrolimus in the management of peristomal pyoderma gangrenosum. *J Dermatolog Treat* 2001;12(1):13–17.

Irritant skin reactions

1 Herlufsen P, Olsen AG, Carlsen B, *et al.* Study of peristomal skin disorders in patients with permanent stomas. *Br J Nurs* 2006;15(16):854–62.

2 Lyon CC, Smith AD, Griffiths CE, Beck MH. The spectrum of skin disorders in abdominal stoma patients. *Br J Dermatol* 2000;143(6):1248–60.

7 Bergman BFK, Lincoln K, Lowhagen GB, Mobacken H, Wahlen P. Chronic papillomatous dermatitis as a peristomal complication in conduit urinary diversion. *Scand J Urol Nephrol* 1979;13:201–14.

CHAPTER 115

Dermatoses of Pregnancy

Samantha Vaughan Jones

Department of Dermatology, St Peter's Hospital, Ashford; St Peter's Foundation Trust, Chertsey, UK

PHYSIOLOGICAL SKIN CHANGES IN PREGNANCY

During pregnancy there are marked changes in the levels of sex hormones, particularly oestrogen and progesterone, and this can lead to profound changes in the skin. It is important to be able to recognize these physiological skin changes and to distinguish them from true skin disease (Box 115.1).

Pigmentation

Most women notice a generalized increase in skin pigmentation during pregnancy and the change is more marked in women with darker skin types [1]. Areas that are already pigmented become darker, in particular the nipples, areolae, genital areas and midline of the abdominal wall (linea nigra) (Figure 115.1). This pigmentation usually fades after delivery, but seldom to its previous level. Many women also notice an increase in the size, activity and number of melanocytic naevi [2].

In approximately 70% of women, especially those of dark complexion, melasma (or chloasma) pigmentation also develops during the second half of pregnancy. Irregular, sharply marginated areas of pigmentation develop in a symmetrical pattern, either on the forehead and temples or on the central part of the face. Melasma usually fades completely after parturition, but may persist and require treatment post-delivery.

The extent to which human pigmentary changes are brought about by oestrogen and progesterone, or by melanocyte-stimulating hormone (MSH) derived from pro-opiomelanocortin and other factors is uncertain.

Hair and nail changes

Many women notice that hair growth on the scalp is more pronounced during pregnancy. In the third trimester, the proportion of hair follicles retained in the anagen phase rises. Following delivery there is a noticeable compensatory decrease in hair growth associated with shedding of hair postpartum, known as telogen effluvium [1]. Spontaneous recovery within 6–12 months is usual. Mild frontoparietal recession may also occur [3].

Minor degrees of hypertrichosis are not uncommon. Hirsutism, accompanied by acne and, in severe cases, by other evidence of virilization, occurs rarely, usually during the second half of pregnancy. It may result from an androgen-secreting

Rook's Textbook of Dermatology, Ninth Edition. Edited by Christopher Griffiths, Jonathan Barker, Tanya Bleiker, Robert Chalmers and Daniel Creamer.
© 2016 John Wiley & Sons, Ltd. Published 2016 by John Wiley & Sons, Ltd.
Companion website: www.rooksdermatology.com

PART 10: SITES, SEX, AGE

PART 10: SITES, SEX, AGE

Box 115.1 Physiological skin changes in pregnancy

Pigmentation
- Areola
- Linea nigra
- Melasma
- Changes in melanocytic naevi

Hair changes
- Hypertrichosis
- Postpartum telogen effluvium
- Postpartum androgenetic alopecia (rare, typically male-pattern balding)

Nail changes
- Increased brittleness
- Distal onycholysis
- Subungual hyperkeratosis
- Transverse grooving
- Longitudinal melanonychia

Glandular function
- Increased eccrine gland activity
- Decreased apocrine gland activity
- Increased sebaceous gland activity

Vascular changes
- Peripheral oedema
- Varicosities
- Spider naevi/angioma
- Palmar erythema
- Gingival hyperaemia and oedema
- Pregnancy epulis
- Pyogenic granuloma

Striae distensae
- Abdomen, thighs and buttocks

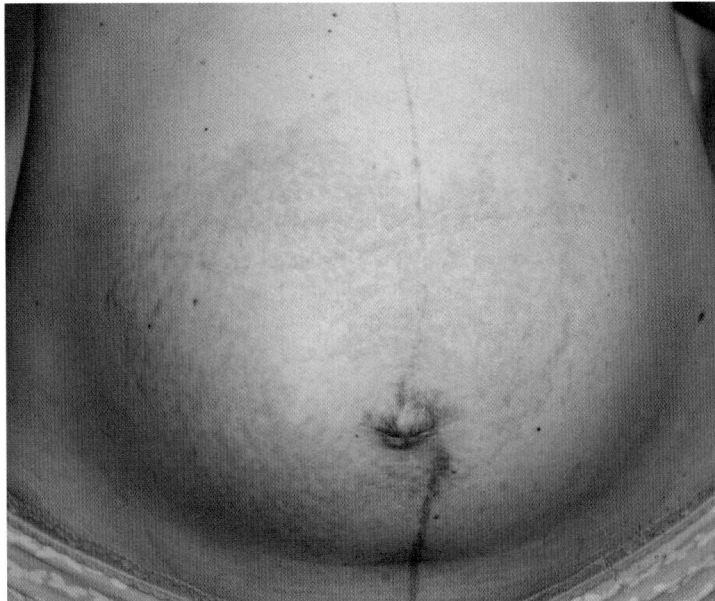

Figure 115.1 Physiological skin changes in pregnancy showing a prominent linea nigra and striae distensae at 28 weeks' gestation.

---

tumour, luteoma, lutein cysts or polycystic ovary disease [1,4]. All cases should be thoroughly investigated. A female fetus may be masculinized. In the absence of a tumour that can be eradicated, the problem tends to recur in subsequent pregnancies. Hirsutism may regress between pregnancies, but this is not always complete.

Pregnant women often report brittleness of the nail plate and some develop distal onycholysis, similar to that seen occasionally in thyrotoxicosis [3]. Other nail changes such as subungual hyperkeratosis, transverse grooving and longitudinal melanonychia have also been reported to occur during pregnancy.

Eccrine, apocrine and sebaceous gland activity

Eccrine activity may be noticeably increased during pregnancy, although palmar sweating diminishes [1,3]. This may be responsible for the recognized increased frequency of miliaria. There is no increase in apocrine sweating immediately postpartum, but

Fox–Fordyce disease usually improves in pregnancy, which suggests that apocrine activity is reduced [1].

The rate of sebum excretion tends to increase during pregnancy and return to normal after delivery [5] and this is due to rising maternal progesterone and androgen levels in the third trimester. Sebaceous gland activity therefore increases towards the end of pregnancy.

Vascular changes

The vascular changes of pregnancy are similar to those in hyperthyroidism or cirrhosis. All are thought to be due to sustained high levels of circulating oestrogen. Vascular 'spider naevi' are very common in pregnancy and usually disappear postpartum. Palmar erythema is also common, affecting at least 70% of women with skin types I and II and 30% of women with darker skin types.

Less commonly, pregnant women develop small haemangiomas or pyogenic granulomas. These can occur in approximately 5% of pregnancies and often present on the head and neck or digits [1].

Varicose veins of the legs and haemorrhoids are frequent complications of pregnancy. A rarer but more serious event is the development of deep vein thrombosis, which can lead to permanent damage to the veins of the legs and, occasionally, death from pulmonary embolism. Many pregnant women (up to 50%) also develop non-pitting oedema of the face, eyelids, feet and hands. The swelling is usually most pronounced in the early morning and disappears during the course of the day. There is no known treatment, but it is important to recognize and differentiate the condition from oedema seen in cardiac, renal disease or pre-eclampsia.

Eighty per cent or more of pregnant women also develop some gingival oedema and redness [6]. This can become painful and ulcerative, especially if oral hygiene is poor. In approximately 2%, the gingival changes are associated with the appearance of a small vascular lesion similar to a pyogenic granuloma, known as a pregnancy epulis or granuloma gravidarum [1]. This may bleed profusely on contact. These phenomena, like palmar erythema and vascular spider naevi, are probably brought about by the general increase in vascularity associated with high oestrogen levels. In most women, gum changes resolve after parturition.

Striae distensae

Striae distensae are extremely common in the second and third trimester of pregnancy and can arise in up to 90% of pregnant women. They are linear pink or purple atrophic bands that develop at right angles to the skin tension lines on the abdomen, breasts, thighs and buttocks (Figure 115.1). They are similar to the striae seen in patients with Cushing syndrome, corticosteroid therapy and rapid changes in body weight. They are uncommon in Afro-Caribbean or Asian women and there may be a familial predisposition [7].

Immune system changes

In order to prevent fetal rejection there is a profound change in a woman's immune system during pregnancy, with a shift from a predominantly T_H1 lymphocyte profile to a T_H2 profile. This changes the cytokines that are produced by the placenta, so that levels of interleukin 12 and γ-interferon are reduced, while levels of interleukins 4 and 10 are increased. This influences a woman's susceptibility to skin disease, thus increasing autoimmune disease and reducing her cell-mediated immunity (causing an increased risk of skin infections). Diseases that are T_H1-driven such as psoriasis tend to improve while T_H2-driven diseases such as atopic eczema and systemic lupus erythematosus (SLE) are exacerbated [8,9].

Reduced cell-mediated immunity during normal pregnancy probably accounts for the increased frequency and severity of certain infections such as candidiasis, herpes simplex and varicella zoster [10]. *Candida* infection, genital warts and herpes simplex virus (HSV) can all be transmitted to the baby during childbirth.

SKIN INFECTIONS

Human papillomavirus infection

Synonyms and inclusions
• Condyloma acuminata

Condyloma acuminata (due to human papilloma virus (HPV) infection) can be exacerbated, growing very rapidly particularly in the second trimester and occasionally obstructing the birth canal. Infants born through an infected cervix are at increased risk

Box 115.2 Treatment of human papillomavirus infection

Physical treatments
• Cryotherapy
• Electrocautery

Avoid
• Podophyllin
• Imiquimod
• 5-fluorouracil

for laryngeal papillomatosis, usually associated with HPV types 6 and 11. Therefore, genital HPV infections should be treated during pregnancy and if necessary a caesarean section performed. However, there is doubt whether this practice prevents neonatal infection [1] either by herpesvirus or by genital warts. Podophyllin, imiquimod and 5-fluorouracil should never be used in the treatment of warts during pregnancy because of potential maternal and fetal toxicity; physical treatments such as crythotherapy or electrocautery are preferable (Box 115. 2) [1]. With the advent of the two new vaccines against HPV – a bivalent vaccine (Cervarix®) containing HPV types 16 and 18 and a quadrivalent vaccine (Gardasil®) containing HPV types 6, 11, 16 and 18 – there should be a significant reduction in the prevalence of these viruses in future. Both vaccines offer protection against the HPV types that cause 70% of cervical cancers.

Herpes simplex virus infection

Primary herpetic infection (HSV-1 or HSV-2) occurs in 2% of pregnancies and is often more severe than in the non-pregnant state. In babies of very low birth weight, infection with herpes simplex (see Chapter 25) can be life threatening [2]. Primary or recurrent genital HSV infection (identified clinically or with culture at the time of delivery) is an indication for a caesarean section and drug therapy. Systemic aciclovir, although rated as US Food and Drug Administration (FDA) pregnancy category C is considered safe in pregnancy as it has been used extensively without adverse effects.

Varicella zoster virus infection

Herpes zoster (see Chapter 25) in pregnancy (reactivation of latent varicella zoster virus (VZV) infection) is not associated with viraemia and therefore does not put the fetus at risk. Primary VZV infections occur in up to 1 : 2000 pregnancies (Figure 115.2) and may put both mother and child at risk of pneumonia and encephalitis. Infections during weeks 1–20 (with highest risk from weeks 13 to 20) (see Chapter 25) can lead to fetal varicella syndrome in a small percentage of cases (1–2%) with significant neurological and growth defects. Passive

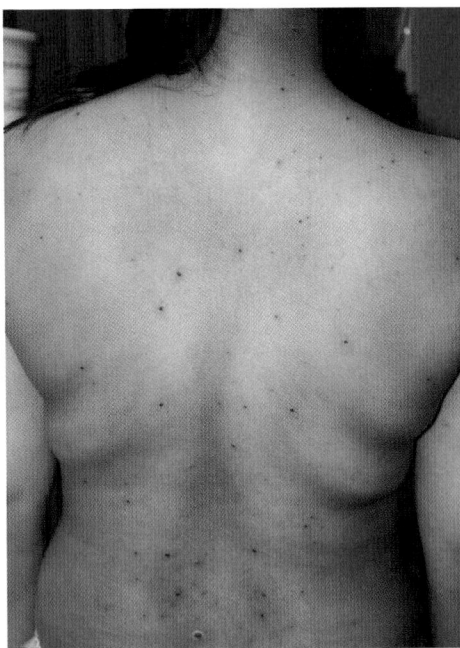

Figure 115.2 Chicken pox (primary herpes zoster infection) presenting in pregnancy with multiple excoriated papules on the back in the second trimester.

immunization with varicella zoster immunoglobulin to seronegative mothers within 72 h post exposure may prevent or ameliorate maternal infection. Confirmed varicella should be treated early with aciclovir either orally or intravenously for pneumonia or other complications. Perinatal VZV infections pose considerable risk to the development of neonatal varicella, particularly if the infant is exposed to infection at or just after birth (Box 115.3). The infant will then develop widespread cutaneous and visceral disease, usually with severe pneumonia and a 30% mortality rate. Treatment of neonatal varicella is with high-dose intravenous aciclovir [3].

HIV infection

With the widespread implementation of routine antenatal screening for HIV-1, transmission of HIV-1 from mother to child is now a rare occurrence in the UK. The prevalence of HIV infection among women giving birth in the UK is monitored through an unlinked anonymous survey based on residual neonatal dried blood spots. The prevalence of HIV in 2009 was approximately 2.2 per 1000 women giving birth [4]. HIV infection is often associated with dermatological manifestations, although to a lesser extent since the advent of highly active antiretroviral therapy (HAART) [5,6]. In HIV-positive pregnant women, antiretroviral therapy can be given and continued during labour and delivery. Normal vaginal delivery can still occur if there is a low viral load, but caesarean section must be considered if the viral load is high [4]. All mothers known to be HIV positive should be advised to avoid breastfeeding and to use formula feeding exclusively from birth. Infants born to HIV-positive mothers should follow the routine national primary immunization schedule and

---

HIV-positive infants must be given pneumocystis prophylaxis with co-trimoxazole (Box 115.4) [4].

Scabies

Infestation with scabies (caused by *Sarcoptes scabiei*) is common during pregnancy and this diagnosis should always be considered when assessing a pregnant woman with an itchy skin eruption (see Chapter 34). First line treatment should be topical permethrin 5% and second line treatment benzoyl benzoate 25% [7]. It is important to repeat the treatment after a week to kill eggs and persistent mites as cell-mediated immunity is reduced. All potentially infectious close contacts must also be treated. Antihistamines and mild to moderately potent topical steroids may be needed to control the marked irritant dermatitis that often results when the mites are destroyed in the skin. Oral antihistamines can be given to help aid sleep if pruritus is severe. Lindane has now been withdrawn from the market and oral ivermectin is not safe to use during pregnancy.

Management

Treatment ladder

First line
- Topical permethrin 5%
- Antihistamines to reduce itch, e.g. chlorphenamine, loratadine, cetirizine

Second line
- Benzoyl benzoate 25%

Lindane and ivermectin must be avoided in pregnancy

Leprosy

The immune alterations of pregnancy, childbirth and the puerperium with a reduction in cell-mediated immunity may have an adverse effect on leprosy [8] (see Chapter 28). Most studies on leprosy and pregnancy were done in the days before multidrug therapy and results are therefore difficult to interpret [9]. Erythema nodosum leprosum in pregnancy is associated with an early loss of nerve function compared with non-pregnant individuals. Without treatment there is a significant risk of nerve damage and disability, so regular neurological examinations must be carried out in pregnant and newly delivered women and early treatment given.

Leprosy reactional states are more common and the decline in immune reactivity may also lead to an increase in drug resistance [8]. Leprosy reactions can be treated with prednisolone 40–60 mg daily for 2 weeks followed by a steady reduction in the dose. There are specific problems with some anti-leprosy drugs: thalidomide cannot be used because of its teratogenicity and clofazimine crosses the placenta and has been associated with mild pigmentation in the infant and unexplained fetal death [10]. When possible, patients should plan their pregnancy for when the disease is well controlled.

AUTOIMMUNE SKIN DISEASES

Systemic lupus erythematosus

About 60% of women with pre-existing SLE have a flare during pregnancy or the puerperium compared with 40% of non-pregnant women over the same time period [1] (see Chapter 51). Cutaneous flares are the most common, followed by joint symptoms. Corticosteroids are the drug of choice, but do not prevent flares. SLE in pregnancy can cause spontaneous abortion, fetal loss, pre-eclampsia, preterm delivery and intrauterine growth restriction (IUGR) (Box 115.5). It can also be associated with antiphospholipid syndrome with an increased risk of venous thromboembolism. A recent, large retrospective review of 396 pregnancies in women with SLE over a 27-year period found a higher risk of adverse pregnancy outcome associated with the presence of antiphospholipid antibodies, lupus nephritis, Raynaud phenomenon, hypertension and either active disease at the time of conception or a first presentation of SLE during pregnancy [2].

Neonatal lupus erythematosus

About 30% of women with SLE have anti-Ro antibodies. They are most common with subacute cutaneous lupus erythematosus and Sjögren syndrome. These antibodies cross the placenta and can cause immune damage in the fetus leading to neonatal lupus. Cutaneous neonatal lupus erythematosus occurs in the first 2 weeks of life with a scaly, annular eruption on the face and scalp. The rash disappears spontaneously within 6 months and scarring is unusual. There is a risk of congenital

---

Box 115.5 Potential complications of SLE in pregnancy

- Flare of LE activity (60%)
- Spontaneous abortion
- Fetal loss
- Antiphospholipid syndrome – venous thromboembolism
- Pre-eclampsia
- Preterm delivery
- Intrauterine growth restriction
- Neonatal lupus erythematosus – annular rash face and scalp
- Congenital heart block (2–3%)

---

heart block due to fibrosis of the conducting system (2–3% risk if anti-Ro positive) usually detected *in utero* at around 18–20 weeks. Twenty per cent of affected babies will die in the early neonatal period, and those who survive may need a pacemaker [3].

Management

Corticosteroids are the drug of choice, but do not prevent flares. Hydroxychloroquine is safe to continue in pregnancy and while breastfeeding and should not be stopped in women who have active SLE at time of conception. Pre-pregnancy counselling may be helpful to advise those women with pre-existing SLE on the management of their disease during pregnancy.

Treatment ladder

First line
- Topical corticosteroids
- Hydroxychloroquine
- Prednisolone

Second line
- Azathioprine

Pemphigus vulgaris and foliaceus

Pemphigus vulgaris and foliaceus can both develop or worsen during pregnancy and can also be transmitted to the fetus (see Chapter 50). In the literature there are many well-documented pregnancies in women with pemphigus vulgaris (Figure 115.3). Fetal skin shares the same desmoglein 3 profile as adult oral mucosa so that neonatal pemphigus is more likely to occur if the mother has oral disease. Fetal prognosis is variable and there are three possible scenarios:
- Normal delivery with birth of a healthy infant.
- Transient neonatal pemphigus with erosions and blistering in the neonate lasting a few weeks (Box 115.6). This is due to transplacental passage of immunoglobulin (IgG4) antibodies across the placenta.
- Fetal demise with stillbirth or spontaneous abortion [4].

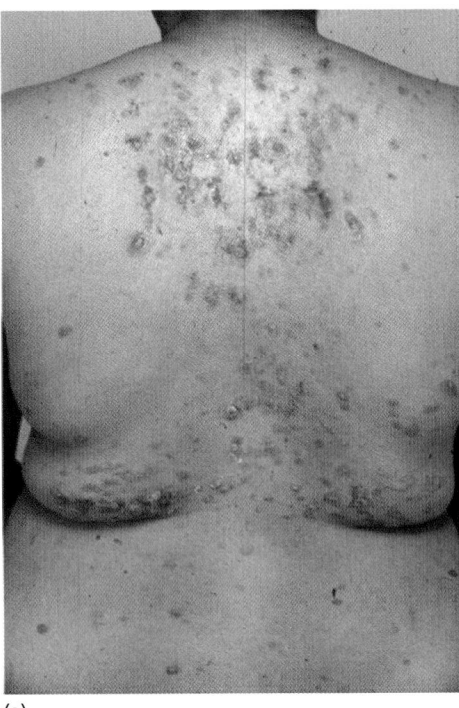

(a)

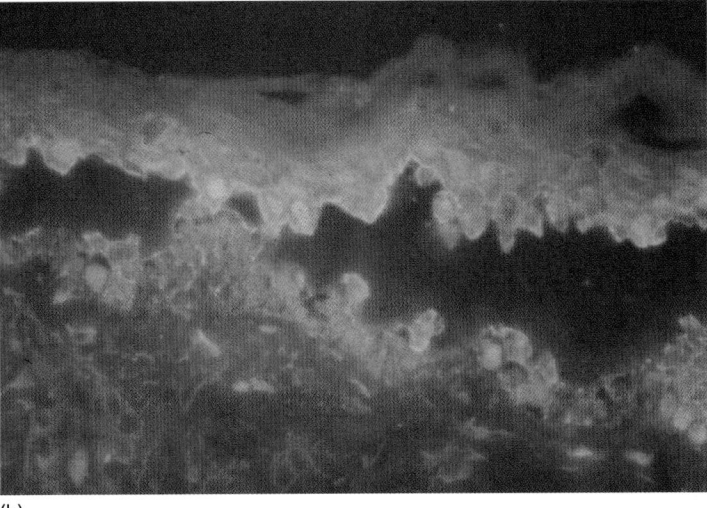

(b)

Figure 115.3 Pemphigus vulgaris. (a) New disease onset in the second trimester showing erosions on the back. (b) Indirect immunofluorescence using the patient's serum and showing intercellular IgG with intraepidermal split.

There is no direct correlation between the severity of the mother's disease and the extent of neonatal involvement. Women in remission have given birth to neonates with extensive disease and, conversely, women with active pemphigus have delivered disease-free babies [4–7]. Disease activity may improve in the third trimester due to rising maternal endogenous cortisol levels and consequent immunosuppression. Treatment with immunosuppressant therapy is normally required. The clinical presentation with blistering and erosions can be very similar to pemphigoid gestationis so a skin biopsy including direct immunofluorescence is required for an accurate diagnosis. Enzyme-linked immunosorbent assay (ELISA) using recombinant desmoglein 3 can also confirm the diagnosis [8].

A review in 2009 looked at 38 reports of pregnancies from 49 women with pemphigus vulgaris. Among the 40 women in whom clinical profiles were provided, 33 had active disease and seven were disease-free. Prednisolone was used in 75% of cases and other treatments included plasmapheresis, plasma exchange, dapsone (one case) and azathioprine (five cases). Of the 44 live births, 20 had neonatal involvement with pemphigus vulgaris lesions at birth and 24 were disease-free. Five stillbirths were reported. In all cases with neonatal pemphigus vulgaris, skin lesions resolved within 4 weeks' postpartum. The perinatal mortality rate was 12% (six out of 49 cases) [4].

In a further study of 48 women with pemphigus vulgaris in pregnancy, 28 women (54%) had an exacerbation of pemphigus, 15 cases (31%) had no change in disease activity and nine cases (17%) improved [5]. In conclusion, careful monitoring of high-risk mother and fetus is mandatory. In the management of pemphigus vulgaris, close collaboration between the obstetricians and dermatologists is essential to reduce perinatal mortality.

There have been two reports of pemphigus foliaceus in pregnancy causing neonatal involvement although this happens less frequently than in pemphigus vulgaris [9].

Management

> **Treatment ladder**
>
> **First line**
> - Prednisolone
>
> **Second line**
> - Azathioprine
>
> **Third line**
> - Plasma exchange
> - Plasmapheresis

> **Box 115.6 Potential complications of pemphigus vulgaris in pregnancy**
>
> - Spontaneous abortion
> - Exacerbation of disease (T_H-2 mediated)
> - Stillbirth
> - Caesarean section needed if there is severe vulvo-vaginal disease
> - Neonatal pemphigus with transient blistering
> - Perinatal mortality of 12% with placental dysfunction [4]

Other connective tissue disorders

Women with Ehlers–Danlos syndrome types I and IV often have major problems, including bleeding, uterine lacerations and wound dehiscence [10]. Some patients with pseudoxanthoma elasticum have suffered major gastrointestinal bleeds necessitating blood transfusion [10].

SKIN TUMOURS

Benign melanocytic naevi

Pre-existing naevi may darken in pregnancy due to increased circulating levels of MSH and high circulating levels of sex hormones. This can lead to anxiety and concern about possible malignant melanoma. The advent of dermoscopy and digital mole mapping has increased our ability to define and monitor mole changes more clearly. Several studies document that the dermoscopic appearance of moles may change during pregnancy, causing diagnostic concern. There can be an increase in total dermoscopic score on the Stolz ABCD scoring system (*a*symmetry, *b*order change, *c*olour change, *d*iameter change) [1] and vascularity at the end of pregnancy. These changes may reverse following delivery. Early biopsy should be recommended in any woman presenting with a suspicious pigmented lesion during pregnancy, as melanoma may present in young women of child-bearing age. A recent study of 56 women with 97 naevi showed a significant increase in mean diameter of the naevi and in total dermoscopic score between the first and third trimester [2]. The authors commented that some of the changes observed may be due to expansion of the skin during pregnancy (especially on the anterior trunk). However, an earlier study of naevi in pregnancy demonstrated no significant changes [3].

Malignant melanoma

Malignant melanoma represents the fourth commonest cancer in pregnancy, accounting for about 8% of all malignant tumours arising in gestation (Figure 115.4) (see Chapter 143). There has been much debate as to whether pregnancy influences prognosis and outcome in patients with melanoma. Several well-controlled studies have now demonstrated similar survival rates between pregnant and non-pregnant women, and concluded that early reports of advanced melanoma in pregnancy in the 1950s were probably

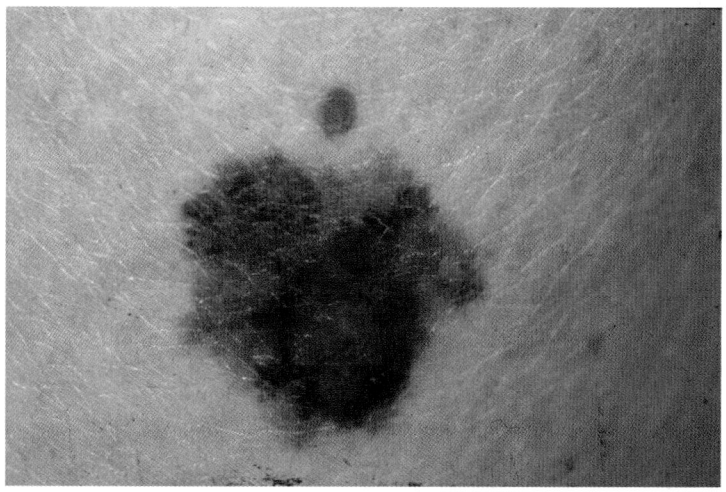

Figure 115.4 Superfical spreading melanoma on the abdomen (see Chapter 132).

Table 115.1 Summary of recent studies of melanoma in pregnancy.

Study	Findings
Driscoll and Grant-Kels 2006 [5]	No effect of pregnancy on prognosis
Silipo *et al.* 2006 [6]	No effect of pregnancy on prognosis
Miller *et al.* 2010 [4]	Increased Breslow thickness (4.28 mm versus 1.69 mm) and worse prognosis versus controls (11 cases) $P = 0.15$
Pages *et al.* 2010 [8]	No effect of pregnancy on prognosis (22 cases) but one case with placental metastases

due to late diagnosis. One review of pregnant women with melanoma over a 9-year period (1997–2006, $n = 11$) compared prognosis and outcome with 65 controls. The mean Breslow thickness was 4.28 mm compared with 1.69 mm in the controls ($P = 0.15$). Sentinel nodes were metastatic in five pregnant women compared with four controls ($P < 0.0001$). These results conclude a negative effect of pregnancy on the course of malignant melanoma, suggesting that melanomas present with increased thickness in pregnancy [4]. Two further reports showed no significant difference in outcome or survival rate between pregnant and non-pregnant women with melanoma [5,6]. This subject is still debated (Table 115.1).

Close follow-up of pigmented lesions during pregnancy with clinical and dermoscopic documentation is vital during pregnancy with careful assessment of other risk factors for skin cancer. In more advanced cases of melanoma, transplacental metastatic spread can occur so the placenta should be examined closely after delivery to exclude placental metastases. A recent murine study showed that pregnancy appeared to promote melanoma metastasis through enhanced lymphangiogenesis [7]. A retrospective study of 22 women with AJCC (American Joint Committee on Cancer) stage III and IV melanoma in 2010 found no cases with neonatal involvement but placental metastases were found in one case. The 2-year maternal survival rates for pregnant women with stage III melanoma were 56% and 17% for stage IV disease. Mortality rates did not support a worsened prognosis due to pregnancy [8].

Box 115.7 lists some important aspects of the management of melanoma during pregnancy.

Box 115.7 Guidance for the management of melanoma in pregnancy

- Most studies show no adverse effect of pregnancy on prognosis
- Melanoma may have increased Breslow thickness at presentation in pregnancy
- A low threshold is recommended for excising changing pigmented lesions
- Transplacental metastatic spread can occur – examine the placenta closely
- Ultrasound or magnetic resonance imaging scanning is preferable to computed tomography scanning
- Sentinel node biopsy can be done (avoid methylene blue dye as there is a risk of intestinal atresia)
- There is a 56% 5-year survival rate for stage II melanoma
- There is a 17% 5-year survival rate for stage IV melanoma

INFLAMMATORY SKIN DISEASES

Psoriasis and generalized pustular psoriasis

The effect of pregnancy on psoriasis is variable (see Chapter 35). Psoriasis typically improves during pregnancy (due to the immune changes described previously) but in up to 10–20% of women it can worsen, requiring increased treatment (Figure 115.5) [1]. A previous population study of 1463 pregnant women in

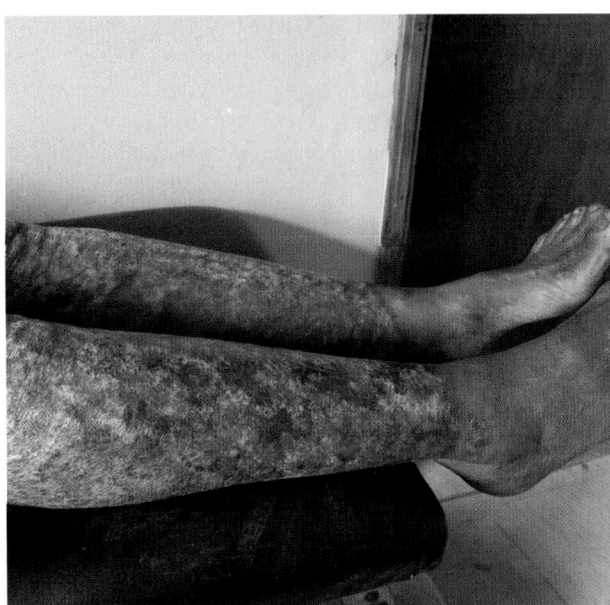

(a)

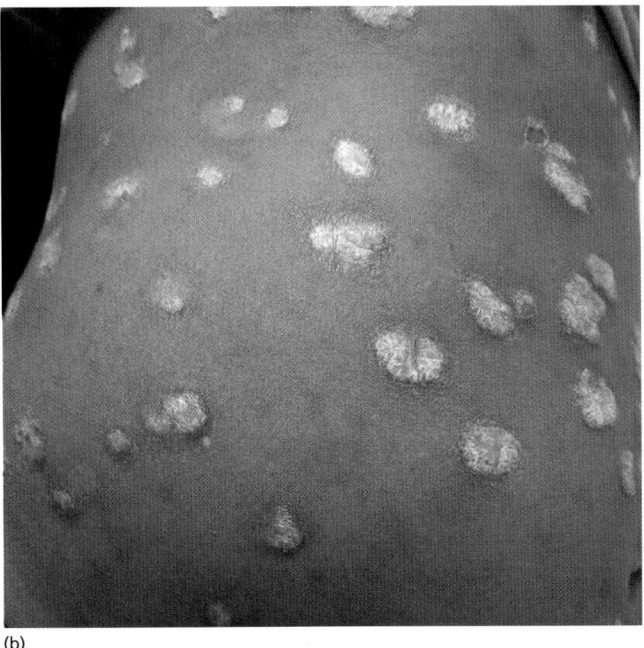

(b)

Figure 115.5 Chronic plaque psoriasis in pregnancy on (a) the lower legs and (b) the trunk showing marked silver scaling and underlying erythema.

Taiwan with psoriasis showed that those women with severe psoriasis had an increased risk of delivering low birth weight infants, whereas mild psoriasis was not associated with excess risk of adverse birth outcomes [2]. Yoon-Soo *et al.* recently published a proposed treatment algorithm for treating psoriasis in pregnant women [3]:

Generalized pustular psoriasis (GPP) can present in pregnancy, often requiring systemic treatment. The term impetigo herpetiformis has been used to describe a severe variant of GPP occurring in pregnant women. It presents with flexural erythema and pustules, along with periumbilical pustulation, and can be associated with fever, tetany and hypocalcaemia. Recurrence in subsequent pregnancies is characteristic with earlier onset and increased severity. A recent case was treated effectively with prednisolone and narrow-band UVB [4]. There is debate as to the validity of using a separate name, impetigo herpetiformis, for GPP in pregnancy.

Management

Treatment ladder

First line
- Emollients
- Topical corticosteroids (low to mid potency)

Second line
- Narrow-band UVB (TL-01)
Or
- Broad-band UVB

Third line
- Ciclosporin
- Systemic corticosteroids in impetigo herpetiformis (second and third trimesters only)
- Tumour necrosis factor inhibitors (adalimumab, etanercept, infliximab)

Acne vulgaris and rosacea

Acne vulgaris (see Chapter 90) often improves in early pregnancy but worsens in the third trimester as maternal androgen levels increase. Systemic and topical retinoids should be avoided because of their known teratogenic potential [5] but oral erythromycin and azithromycin appear safe (after the first trimester). Severe acne conglobata may require treatment with systemic corticosteroids in addition to oral antibiotics. Acne neonatorum may occur due to the passive transfer of maternal androgens across the placenta during the third trimester. This is usually a transient eruption in the young infant that does not require ongoing treatment.

Rosacea (see Chapter 91) often worsens during pregnancy as oestrogen levels increase, and may require systemic treatment. Rosacea fulminans is a rare variant of rosacea that may flare severely in pregnancy.

This is characterized by numerous pustules, marked facial erythema, cystic swellings and coalescing sinuses. Rosacea fulminans normally requires treatment with oral erythromycin and oral corticosteroids. A study of three cases reviewed therapeutic options and differing obstetric outcomes [6]. Azithromycin has also been used with good success in treating this condition during pregnancy [7].

Oral erythromycin would normally be the first choice of antibiotic for acne vulgaris or rosacea in pregnancy as oral tetracyclines are contraindicated after the first trimester due to their effect on fetal bone and teeth development. However, two recent Swedish studies demonstrated a risk of cardiovascular defects in the neonate in patients taking erythromycin so this treatment should be avoided if possible in the first trimester [8,9]. Narrow-band UVB can also be used as second line therapy for more severe acne vulgaris during pregnancy [10].

Management of acne vulgaris and rosacea

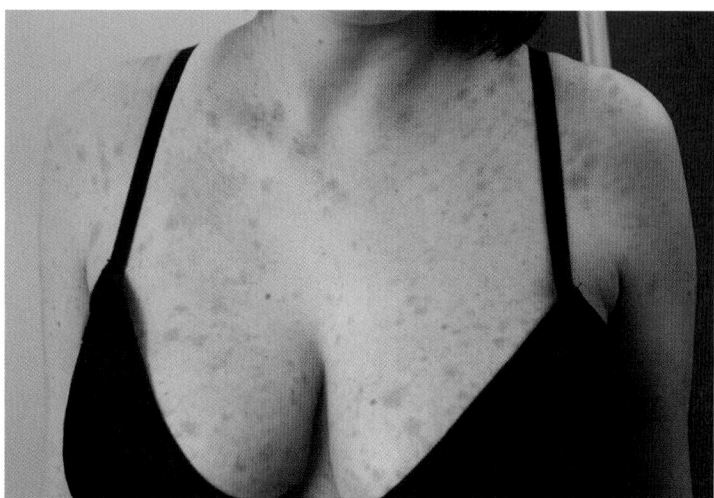

Figure 115.6 Pityriasis rosea in pregnancy with a macular eruption on the upper trunk and upper limbs.

Treatment ladder

First line
- Topical therapy: azelaic acid 10–15%
- Benzoyl peroxide gel 2.5–10%
- Oral erythromycin (avoid in first trimester)
- Oral azithromycin

Second line
- Narrow-band UVB (TL-01)

Third line
- Prednisolone (can be combined with oral antibiotic therapy)

Topical and oral retinoids must be avoided in pregnancy

Pityriasis rosea

Pityriasis rosea is another inflammatory skin condition that can present during pregnancy and often causes confusion in differential diagnosis (as it can mimic psoriasis or tinea corporis). It classically presents with oval, scaly plaques on the trunk, often preceded by a 'herald patch' (Figure 115.6). It has been associated with human herpesvirus 6 (HHV-6) infection. A study of 38 women presenting with pityriasis rosea in pregnancy showed that nine women had a premature delivery and five miscarried. Neonatal hypotonia, weak motility and hyperactivity were noted in six cases. In this small case series the authors concluded that pityriasis rosea may be associated with active HHV-6 infection, and this may be implicated with fetal demise in the first trimester [11]. Treatment is normally conservative as the rash fades rapidly within a few weeks in most cases. However, screening for HHV-6 infection and close fetal surveillance is recommended.

Urticaria

Urticaria can mimic other pregnancy dermatoses, particularly the pre-bullous phase of pemphigoid gestationis or polymorphic eruption of pregnancy. Urticaria presents frequently during pregnancy and can be difficult to control effectively (Figure 115.7) (see Chaper 42). Oral antihistamines are the treatment of choice; the second generation antihistamines loratadine and cetirizine are safe to use from the second trimester onwards.

Management

Treatment ladder

First line
- Topical emollients: aqueous cream + 1–2% menthol
- Oral antihistamines: loratadine and cetirizine

Second line
- Prednisolone

Erythema nodosum

Erythema nodosum (see Chapter 99) is a reactive inflammation of the subcutaneous fat, secondary to a wide variety of underlying conditions including streptococcal infections, tuberculosis, leprosy, sarcoidosis and inflammatory bowel disease. Pregnancy and oral contraceptive therapy can also trigger this eruption, which presents with tender erythematous nodules or plaques over the anterior lower legs. Fever, malaise and arthralgia often occur and the eruption typically lasts up to 6–8 weeks. Supportive treatment is normally all that is required – rest, leg elevation, compression hosiery and analgesia can all help to improve symptoms.

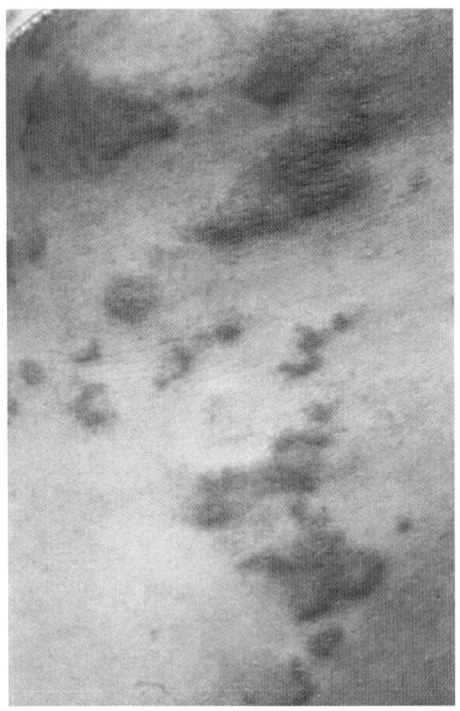

(a)

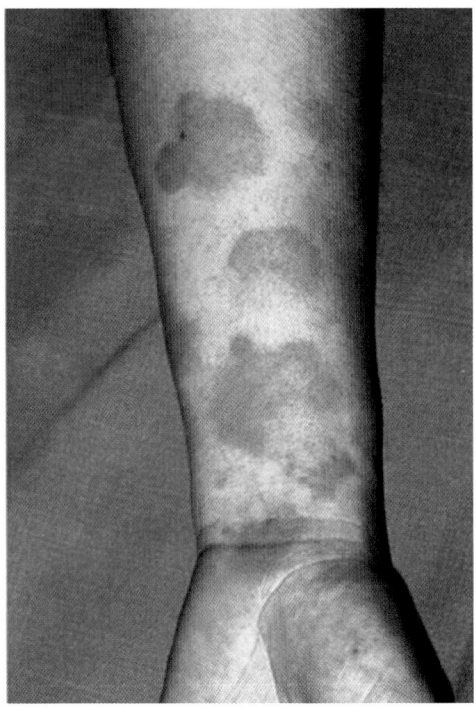

(b)

Figure 115.7 Urticaria showing classic urticarial weals on (a) the trunk and (b) the forearm. (Courtesy of St John's Institute of Dermatology, London, UK.)

ITCHING

Pruritus gravidarum

Itching in pregnancy (or pruritus gravidarum) occurs in up to one-fifth of all pregnancies [1]. In most cases, this is due to an underlying skin disorder such as eczema, urticaria, or one of the specific pregnancy-related inflammatory dermatoses. However, there is also a small group of women who experience intense pruritus without evident primary cutaneous changes and it is to these patients that the term pruritus gravidarum applies.

Pruritus gravidarum is considered to be a mild variant of recurrent intrahepatic cholestasis of pregnancy (see Chapter 83), occurring in 0.02–2.4% of pregnancies [2].

Intrahepatic cholestasis of pregnancy

Synonyms and inclusions
- Obstetric cholestasis
- Cholestasis of pregnancy
- Jaundice of pregnancy
- Pruritus/prurigo gravidarum

Clinical features

Presentation
The itching begins in the second or third trimester and is often localized to the abdomen, or the palms and soles, although it may also be widespread. In about 10% of cases the patient may be mildly jaundiced. Secondary skin lesions develop due to scratching and range from subtle excoriations to severe prurigo nodules as pruritus persists.

Disease course and fetal prognosis
The prognosis for the mother is generally good. After delivery, pruritus disappears spontaneously within days to weeks, but may recur with subsequent pregnancies and oral contraception [3]. In cases of jaundice and vitamin K deficiency, there is an increased risk for intra- and postpartum haemorrhage in both the mother and child [3]. However, more significantly fetal prognosis can be impaired with an increased risk of prematurity, fetal distress and stillbirth [3,4]. Therefore, prompt diagnosis, specific therapy, close obstetric monitoring and maternal counselling are essential.

Pathophysiology
Intrahepatic cholestasis of pregnancy is a reversible form of hormonally triggered cholestasis that typically develops in genetically predisposed individuals in late pregnancy. The cause is thought to be multifactorial [5].

Investigations
Liver function tests are usually normal, while alkaline phosphatase may be raised (which is normal for pregnancy due to placental production) [6]. Serum bile acids are elevated.

Management
Ursodeoxycholic acid (UDCA) is the treatment of choice and is effective in reducing itch and reducing serum bile acid levels [7].

Other drugs including antihistamines, S-adenosyl-L-methionine, dexamethasone and cholestyramine have not been shown to improve fetal prognosis [3]. Of note, cholestyramine and other bile acid exchange resins may contribute to malabsorption of vitamin K with possible bleeding complications, and should therefore be avoided [8]. In addition to UDCA treatment, close obstetric surveillance is indicated with weekly fetal heart rate cardiotocographic monitoring from 34 weeks' gestation onwards. Early delivery (as soon as fetal lung maturity is achieved at 36–37 weeks) is recommended by several authors [9].

Treatment ladder

First line
- Topical emollients: aqueous cream + 1–2% menthol
- Oral antihistamines: loratadine and cetirizine
- Oral UDCA 15 mg/kg/day (off licence)

Second line
- S-adenosyl-L-methionine
- Dexamethasone
- Cholestyramine

Other recommendations
- Weekly fetal cardiotocography to monitor fetal heart rate and detect early signs of fetal distress
- Maternal vitamin K replacement (if jaundice is present)
- Early delivery (36–37 weeks)
- Dexamethasone may be needed for fetal lung maturity

SPECIFIC DERMATOSES

The specific dermatoses of pregnancy have been renamed and reclassified many times over the last 50–100 years, with several names for each disease, leading to confusion. Table 115.2 gives the most up-to-date classification, with previous synonyms included.

A retrospective study of over 500 pregnant women with pruritus demonstrated considerable overlap in clinical presentation and histopathology between pregnant women with atopic eczema, prurigo of pregnancy and pruritic folliculitis of pregnancy (together accounting for 50% of the patient database) [2,3]. This led to the disorders being grouped together under the term 'atopic eruption of pregnancy' [2,3]. Consequently a new classification of specific dermatoses of pregnancy has emerged: pemphigoid gestationis, polymorphic eruption of pregnancy, intrahepatic cholestasis of pregnancy and atopic eruption of pregnancy [2,3].

Whereas in the USA the terms herpes gestationis and pruritic urticarial papules and plaques of pregnancy (PUPPP) are still preferred, in Europe the names pemphigoid gestationis (indicating the autoimmune pathogenesis and avoiding any association with herpesvirus) and polymorphic eruption of pregnancy

Table 115.2 Classification of the specific dermatoses of pregnancy.

Classification	Synonyms
Pemphigoid gestationis	Herpes gestationis
	Gestational pemphigoid
Polymorphic eruption of pregnancy (PEP)[a]	Pruritic urticarial papules and plaques of pregnancy (PUPPP)
	Toxaemic rash of pregnancy
	Late onset prurigo of pregnancy
	Toxic erythema of pregnancy
Intrahepatic cholestasis of pregnancy	Cholestasis of pregnancy
	Pruritus/prurigo gravidarum
	Obstetric cholestasis
	Jaundice of pregnancy
Atopic eruption of pregnancy	Prurigo of pregnancy[a]
	Prurigo gestationis
	Early onset prurigo of pregnancy
	Papular dermatitis of pregnancy
	Pruritic folliculitis of pregnancy*
	Eczema in pregnancy

[a] Previous classification by Holmes and Black [1].

(highlighting the morphological spectrum) are now widely accepted.

Polymorphic eruption of pregnancy

Synonyms and inclusions
- Pruritic urticarial papules and plaques of pregnancy (PUPPP)
- Toxaemic rash of pregnancy
- Late-onset prurigo of pregnancy
- Toxic erythema of pregnancy

Introduction and general description
Polymorphic eruption of pregnancy (PEP) is the term favoured in the UK, as proposed by Holmes and Black [1]. Elsewhere, the lengthy descriptive phrase 'pruritic urticarial papules and plaques of pregnancy' or PUPPP still finds favour, especially in the USA [2].

Epidemiology
Polymorphic eruption of pregnancy is a benign, self-limiting pruritic inflammatory disorder that usually affects primigravidae in the last few weeks of pregnancy or immediately postpartum (15%) [3]. Its incidence is about 1 : 160 pregnancies and it is associated with excessive maternal weight gain and multiple pregnancy [3,4].

Pathophysiology
The pathogenesis of PEP remains unclear. The main theories proposed focus on abdominal distension and hormonal and immunological factors [3,5]. The fact that PEP starts within

PART 10: SITES, SEX, AGE

striae distensae at the time of greatest abdominal distension would seem to suggest that damage to connective tissue due to overstretching may play a central role. Although a previous study found no link with high fetal birth weight [3], this has previously been thought to be an association [5]. The increase of CD1a cells in the inflammatory infiltrate could confirm the theory that previously inert structures develop antigenic character, thus triggering the inflammatory process. Hormonal and immunological changes have not definitively been shown to play a role; nor has an association with increased birth weight or male sex of the newborn been confirmed [3,6]. Serum cortisol levels were found to be low in one study of women with PEP, while human chorionic gonadotrophin (hCG) and oestradiol were normal [6]. Unlike pemphigoid gestationis, there is no HLA association [2]. The phenomenon of peripheral microchimerism in pregnancy, with the deposition of fetal male DNA in the maternal skin, may also play a role in triggering the inflammation [7].

Clinical features

Presentation

Polymorphic eruption of pregnancy typically starts on the abdomen, often within the striae distensae if present, with severely pruritic urticarial papules that coalesce into plaques, spreading to the buttocks and proximal thighs (Figures 115.8 and 115.9). Often the eruption remains on these sites but it can quickly become generalized in severe cases. In contrast to pemphigoid gestationis, umbilical sparing is a characteristic finding. Later on, the morphology becomes more polymorphic; vesicles

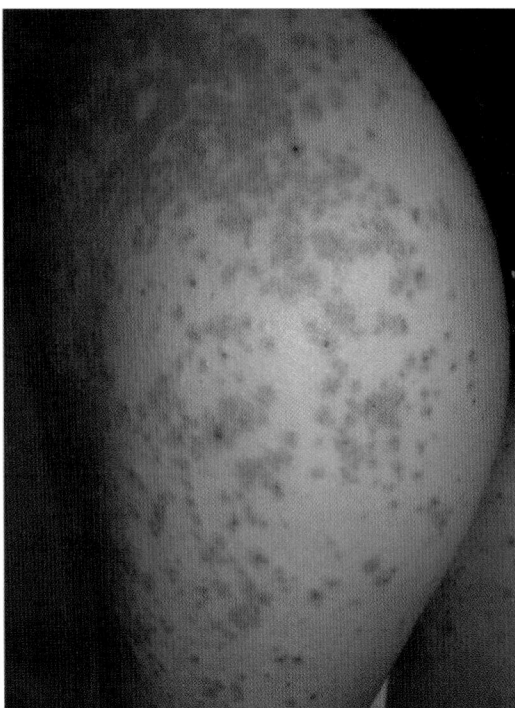

Figure 115.8 Polymorphic eruption of pregnancy showing typical papules and urticarial targetoid lesions on the upper thighs in the third trimester.

(1–2 mm in size; never bullae), widespread non-urticated erythema, and targetoid and eczematous lesions develop in half of patients. The rash usually resolves within 4–6 weeks, independently of delivery [7].

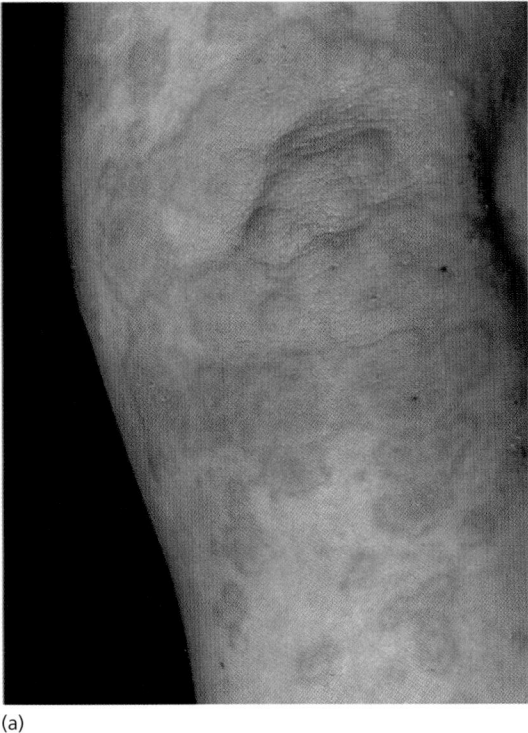

(a)

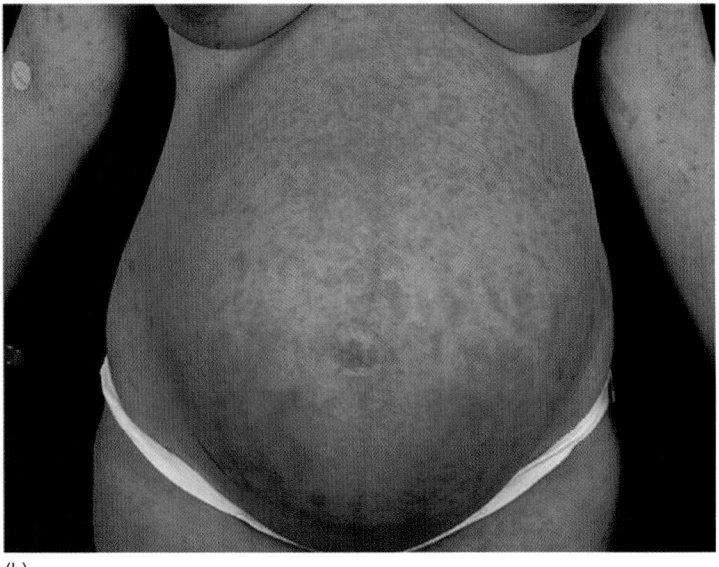

(b)

Figure 115.9 Typical lesions of polymorphic eruption of pregnancy on (a) the arm and (b) the abdomen. (Courtesy of Dr D. A. Burns, Leicester Royal Infirmary, Leicester, UK.)

Disease course and fetal prognosis

Maternal and fetal prognosis is unimpaired and there is no cutaneous involvement of the newborn [7]. Lesions are self-limiting and the disease tends not to recur; the exception being in a multiple pregnancy, when earlier presentation in pregnancy may occur. There is no suggestion that PEP has any adverse effect on the outcome of the pregnancy [4,5].

Investigations

The histopathology of this condition is non-specific and there are many similarities with the early pre-bullous phase of pemphigoid gestationis. Most biopsies show epidermal and upper dermal oedema, with a perivascular infiltrate of lymphocytes and histiocytes. There may be a striking number of eosinophils (as there may be in pemphigoid gestationis). Spongiotic vesicles are also seen, as are hyperkeratosis and patchy parakeratosis [2].

Direct immunofluorescence is generally negative, even by immunoelectron microscopy, and this provides the best means of distinguishing this disorder from pemphigoid gestationis should there be any diagnostic doubt [8]. There are occasional reports of equivocal direct immunofluorescence findings in PEP, including minimal C3 deposition on the basement membrane, in the epidermis and perivascularly [2]. In these rare situations of equivocal immunofluoresence, a BP180 NC16a ELISA has been shown to be highly sensitive and specific in distinguishing pemphigoid gestationis from PEP [9]. Indirect immunofluorescence is also negative [6].

Management

Symptomatic treatment with topical corticosteroids and emollients, with or without antihistamines, is usually sufficient to control pruritus and skin lesions. In severe generalized cases, a short course of systemic corticosteroids (prednisolone starting at 40–60 mg/day and tapering to zero over a few weeks) may be necessary and is usually very effective [4]. Early induction of labour can also be considered if the patient is close to term. Most women are relieved to learn that the condition is not serious, that all should be well with them and their baby and that the rash will disappear at, or soon after, delivery [4,5].

Treatment ladder

First line
- Topical emollients: aqueous cream + 1–2% menthol
- Topical corticosteroids (see section on general treatment guidance)
- Oral antihistamines: loratadine and cetirizine

Second line
- Prednisolone

Consider early induction of labour if patient is close to term

---

Resources

Further information

British Association of Dermatologists, leaflet: http://www.bad.org.uk/for-the-public/patient-information-leaflets/polymorphic-eruption-of-pregnancy?returnlink=http%3a%2f%2fwww.bad.org.uk%2ffor-the-public%2fpatient-information-leaflets%3fl%3d10%26q%3dPOLYMORPHIC+ERUPTION+OF+PREGNANCY#.UKhE1aHeBI (last accessed August 2014).

Pemphigoid gestationis

Synonyms and inclusions
- Herpes gestationis
- Gestational pemphigoid

Introduction and general description

Pemphigoid gestationis (PG) is a rare, autoimmune, bullous disorder that presents mainly in late pregnancy or the immediate postpartum period (see also Chapter 50). It can also occur in association with trophoblastic tumours (choriocarcinoma, hydatidiform mole). Its incidence varies from 1 : 2000 to 1 : 50 000–60 000 pregnancies depending on the prevalence of the HLA haplotypes DR3 and DR4 [1,2]. There is also an increased risk of developing other organ-specific autoimmune diseases, in particular Graves disease.

Pathophysiology

Pathogenetically, circulating complement-fixing IgG antibodies of the subclass IgG1 (formerly known as herpes gestationis factor) bind to a 180 kDa protein, BP-180 or bullous pemphigoid antigen 2, in the hemidesmosomes of the dermo-epidermal junction, leading to tissue damage and blister formation [2]. The immune response is even more highly restricted to the NC16A domain than it is in bullous pemphigoid. Of interest, the primary site of autoimmunity seems not to be the skin, but the placenta, as antibodies bind not only to the basement membrane zone of the epidermis, but also to that of chorionic and amniotic epithelia, both equally of ectodermal origin. Aberrant expression of MHC class II molecules on the chorionic villi suggests an allogenic immune reaction to a placental matrix antigen, thought to be of paternal origin.

Clinical features

Presentation

Pemphigoid gestationis presents with intense pruritus that occasionally may precede skin lesions. Initially, erythematous urticarial papules and plaques typically develop on the abdomen, characteristically involving the periumbilical region, but may spread to the entire skin surface (Fig. 115.10a, b). In the pre-bullous stage, differentiation between PG and PEP is almost impossible, both clinically and histopathologically. Diagnosis becomes clear when lesions progress to tense blisters which resemble those of bullous pemphigoid (Fig. 115.10c). Facial and mucous membranes are usually spared [1].

Disease course and fetal prognosis

The natural course of PG is characterized by exacerbations and remissions during pregnancy, with frequent improvement in late pregnancy followed by a flare-up at the time of delivery (75% of patients). After delivery, the lesions usually resolve within weeks to months but may recur with menstruation and hormonal contraception. Rarely, PG can recur with persistence of skin lesions over several years. Fetal prognosis is generally good but there is an increase in prematurity and small-for-date babies. It has been shown that this risk correlates with disease severity, as represented by early onset and blister formation, and not with corticosteroid treatment, as has been repeatedly speculated before [3]. Due to a passive transfer of antibodies from the mother to the fetus, about 10% of newborns may develop mild skin lesions (neonatal PG) which resolve spontaneously within days to weeks [1]. In all cases, conservative management is all that is required until maternal antibodies are cleared from the fetal circulation.

Pemphgoid gestationis can recur in subsequent pregnancies, and with the use of oral contraceptive therapy. When PG recurs, it often presents at an earlier gestation and with increased severity, so women need to be counselled with this in mind when planning future pregnancies. 'Skip' pregnancies can also occur, and their precise aetiology is still poorly understood.

Investigations

Histopathological findings from lesional skin depend on the stage and severity of the disease. The pre-bullous stage is characterized by oedema of the upper and middle dermis accompanied by a predominantly perivascular inflammatory infiltrate, composed of lymphocytes, histiocytes and a variable number of eosinophils. Histopathology of the bullous stage demonstrates subepidermal blistering that, ultrastructurally, is located at the lamina lucida of the dermo-epidermal junction [1].

Direct immunofluorescence of perilesional skin, the gold standard in the diagnosis of PG, shows linear C3 deposition along the dermo-epidermal junction in 100% of cases and additional IgG deposition in 30% of cases. Depending on the technique used, circulating IgG antibodies in the patient's serum may be detected by indirect immunofluorescence in 30–100% of cases, binding to

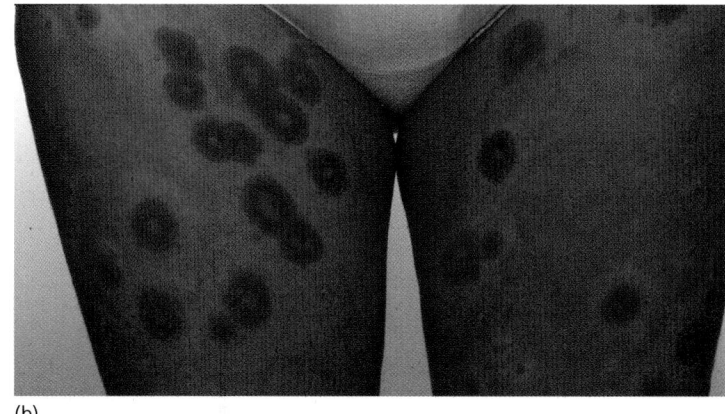

(b)

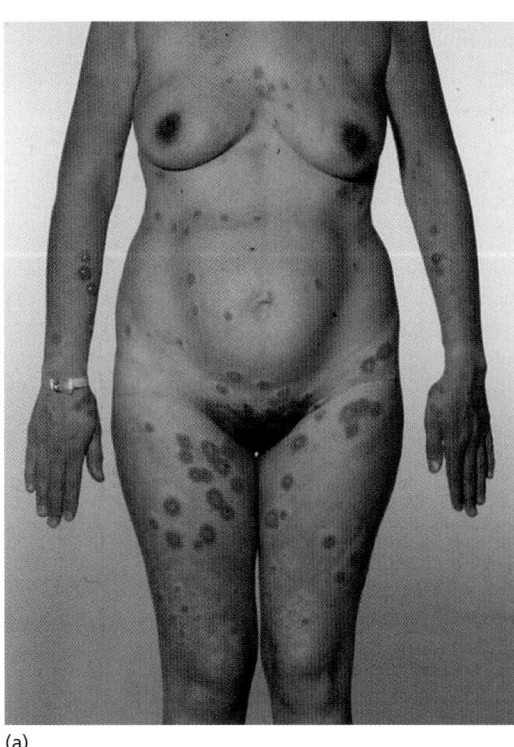

(a)

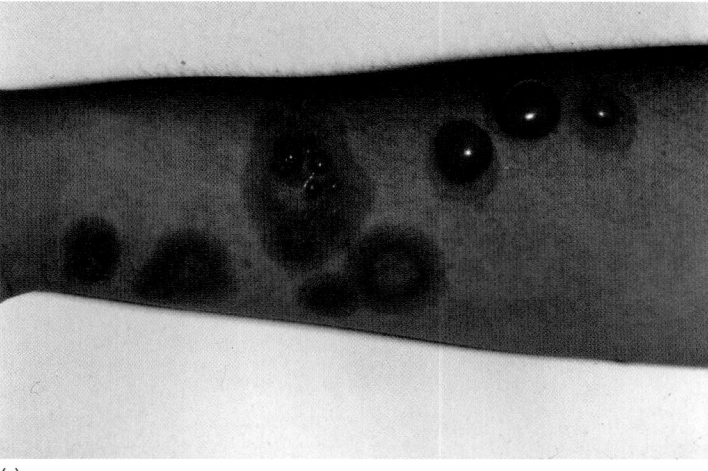

(c)

Figure 115.10 Pemphigoid gestationis that erupted 3 days postpartum showing (a) widespread erythematous urticated plaques on the trunk and limbs with early blistering. (b) Close-up view of urticated targetoid plaques on the upper thighs. (c) Close-up view showing tense intact blisters on the forearms on a background of urticated erythema.

the roof of the artificial split on salt-split skin. Antibody levels may also be monitored using ELISA and immunoblot techniques and show a good correlation with disease activity [1,4].

Management

Treatment depends on the stage and severity of the disease and aims to control pruritus and to prevent blister formation. Topical corticosteroids with or without oral antihistamines may be sufficient in cases of mild pre-bullous pemphigoid [1]. All other cases require systemic corticosteroids (prednisolone, usually started at a dose of 0.5–1 mg/kg/day) [3,5]. When the disease improves, the dose can usually be reduced, but should be increased in time to prevent the flare postpartum. Cases unresponsive to systemic corticosteroid treatment may benefit from third line treatments including azathioprine, intravenous immunoglobulins and plasma exchange [6]. After delivery, if necessary, the full range of immunosuppressive treatment may then be administered.

Treatment ladder

First line
- Topical emollients: aqueous cream + 1–2% menthol
- Potent topical steroids (see section on general treatment guidance)
- Oral antihistamines: loratadine and cetirizine

Second line
- Prednisolone

Third line
- Azathioprine
- Plasma exchange
- Intravenous immunoglobulins

Resources

Further information
British Association of Dermatologists, leaflet: http://www.bad.org.uk/for-the-public/patient-information-leaflets/pemphigoid-gestationis?returnlink=http%3a%2f%2fwww.bad.org.uk%2ffor-the-public%2fpatient-information-leaflets%3fl%3d10%26q%3dPEMPHIGOID+GESTATIONIS#.U-KhdlaHeBI (last accessed August 2014).

Atopic eruption of pregnancy

Synonyms and inclusions
- Early-onset prurigo of pregnancy
- Prurigo of pregnancy
- Prurigo gestationis
- Pruritic folliculitis of pregnancy
- Eczema of pregnancy

Introduction and general description

Atopic eruption of pregnancy (AEP) is a benign pruritic disorder of pregnancy that includes eczematous and/or papular lesions in patients with an atopic diathesis, once the other dermatoses of pregnancy have been excluded (see Chapter 41). It is the most common dermatosis in pregnancy, accounting for 50% of patients. It usually starts early on in pregnancy, with 75% of cases presenting before the third trimester, and a tendency to recur in subsequent pregnancies [1].

Pathophysiology

The pathogenesis of AEP is thought to be triggered by pregnancy-specific immunological changes: a reduced cellular immunity and reduced production of Th1 cytokines (IL-2, interferon-γ, IL-12) in contrast to the dominant humoral immunity and increased secretion of Th2 cytokines (IL-4, IL-10) [2]. Thus the exacerbation of pre-existing atopic eczema and the first manifestation of atopic skin changes can be explained by the dominant Th2 immune response that is typical for pregnancy.

Clinical features

Presentation

Twenty per cent of patients suffer from an exacerbation of pre-existing atopic eczema with a typical clinical picture. The remaining 80% experience atopic skin changes for the first time ever or after a long remission (for example, since childhood). Of these, two-thirds present with widespread eczematous changes (so-called E-type AEP) often affecting typical atopic sites such as the face, neck, décolleté and flexural surfaces of the limbs (Figure 115.11); one-third of patients have papular lesions (P-type AEP) (Figure 115.12) [1]. The latter are characterized by small erythematous papules disseminated on the trunk and limbs as well as typical prurigo nodules, mostly located on the shins and arms. A key feature is severe dryness of the skin and frequent atopic 'minor' features according to Hanifin and Rajka [3].

Disease course and prognosis

Maternal prognosis is good even in severe cases as skin lesions usually respond quickly to therapy. Recurrence in subsequent pregnancies is common. Fetal prognosis is unaffected, but the infant may be at risk of developing atopic skin changes later on.

Investigations

Histopathology is non-specific and varies with the clinical type and stage of the disease. Direct and indirect immunofluorescence are both negative. Laboratory tests may reveal elevated serum IgE levels in 20–70% of patients [1].

Management

Basic treatment with emollients together with topical corticosteroids for several days will usually lead to quick improvement of skin lesions. Severe cases may require a short course of systemic corticosteroids and antihistamines. Phototherapy (UVB) is a safe additional tool, particularly for severe cases in early pregnancy.

PART 10: SITES, SEX, AGE

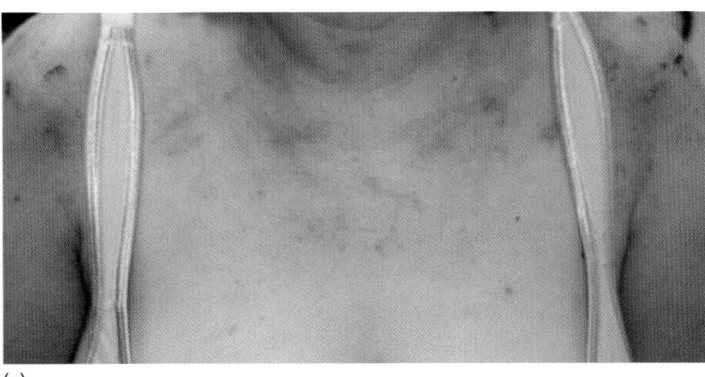

(a)

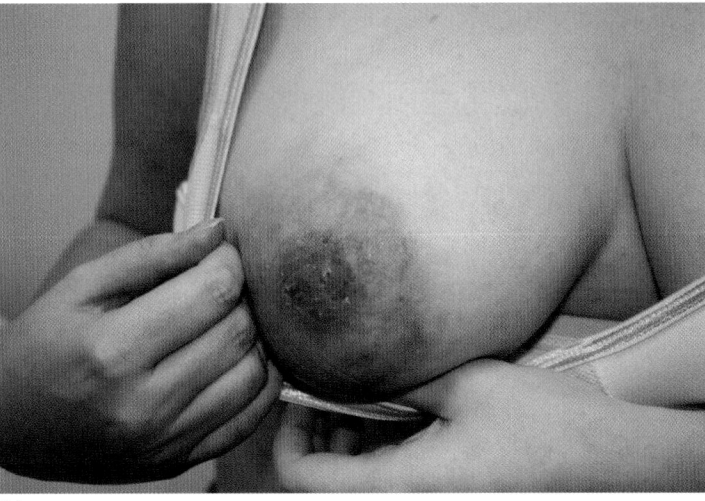

(b)

Figure 115.11 Atopic eruption of pregnancy: (a) on the upper trunk and shoulders in the second trimester and (b) with nipple eczema.

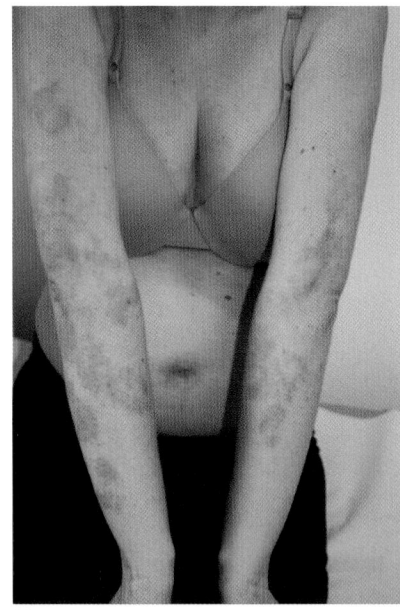

(a)

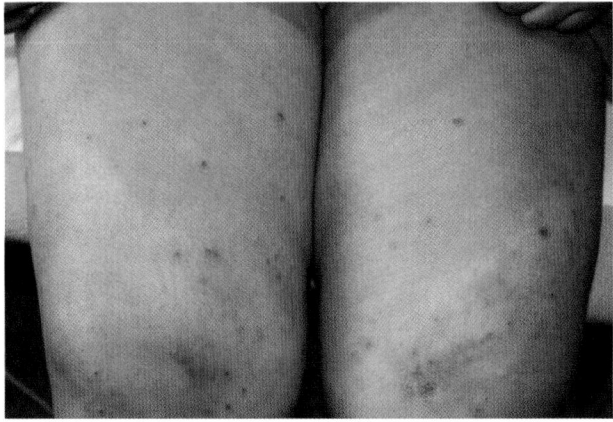

(b)

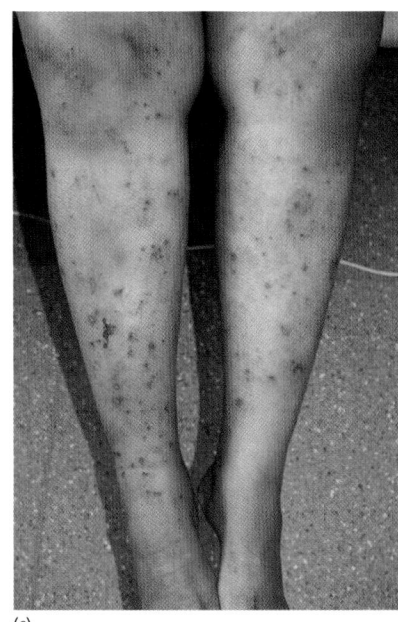

(c)

Figure 115.12 Atopic eruption of pregnancy showing (a) excoriated erythematous patches on the arms, (b) excoriated papules, erythema and dry skin on the upper thighs, and (c) excoriated prurigo lesions on the lower legs (all in the second trimester).

Treatment ladder

First line
- Topical emollients
- Topical corticosteroids (see section on general treatment guidance)
- Oral antihistamines: loratadine and cetirizine

Second line
- Narrow-band UVB phototherapy

Third line
- Prednisolone
- Azathioprine

GENERAL GUIDANCE ON SAFE TREATMENTS IN PREGNANCY

Topical corticosteroids

Recent evidence-based guidelines have been published on the use of topical corticosteroids in pregnancy [1]. This systematic review of topical corticosteroids in pregnancy showed no association between maternal exposure to topical steroids and oro-facial cleft, preterm delivery or fetal death. However, there was a significant association between fetal growth restriction and maternal exposure to potent or super-potent topical corticosteroids. Thus guidance when prescribing topical corticosteroids either in pregnancy or in women of potential child-bearing age should be to use the minimum potency required and for a restricted time period, in order to minimize any potential risk to the fetus.

Systemic treatments

When systemic corticosteroid treatment is necessary in pregnancy non-halogenated corticosteroids should be administered. In the placenta, cortisol, prednisone and prednisolone are inactivated enzymatically, but betamethasone and dexamethasone are not. Prednisolone is the systemic corticosteroid of choice in pregnancy. The usual initial dose is 0.5–2 mg/kg/day depending on the nature and severity of the disease. A maintenance dose should not exceed 10–15 mg/day in the first trimester, as a slightly increased risk for cleft lip or cleft palate cannot be excluded. In treating pregnancy dermatoses, corticosteroids are usually used only as a short-term therapy (<4 weeks) so that side effects are minimized. In rare cases with high-dose therapy over many weeks, fetal growth should be monitored by ultrasound. Should this therapy be continued up to delivery, possible adrenal insufficiency of the newborn must be kept in mind and treated accordingly. If systemic antihistamines are needed during pregnancy, the first generation antihistamine chlorphenamine is preferable due to the greater experience with its use. This is especially valid for the first trimester. If a non-sedating antihistamine is required, then the second generation antihistamines loratadine and cetirizine can be administered in the second and third trimester [2,3].

Key references

The full list of references can be found in the online version at www.rooksdermatology.com.

Physiological changes
8 Vaughan Jones SA. Physiologic skin changes of pregnancy. In: Black MM, Ambros-Rudolph CM, Edwards L, Lynch P, eds. *Obstetric and Gynaecologic Dermatology*, 3rd edn. New York: Mosby, 2008:23–30.

Skin infections
4 De Ruiter A (Chair), Taylor GP, Clayden P, *et al*. British HIV Association guidelines for the management of HIV infection in pregnant women 2012. *HIV Med* 2012;13(2):87–157.

Autoimmune skin diseases
1 Khmashta MA. Systemic lupus erythematosus and pregnancy. *Best Pract Res Clin Rheumatol* 2006;20:685–94.

Skin tumours
7 Khosrotehrani K, Aractingi S, *et al*. Pregnancy promotes melanoma metastasis through enhanced lymphangiogenesis. *Am J Pathol* 2011;178(4):1870–80.

Inflammatory skin diseases
3 Yoon-Soo CB, Van Vorhees AS, Hsu S, *et al*. Review of treatment options for psoriasis in pregnant or lactating women: from the Medical Board of the National Psoriasis Foundation. *J Am Acad Dermatol* 2012;67(3):459–77.

Specific dermatoses
2 Vaughan Jones SA, Hern S, Nelson-Piercy C, *et al*. A prospective study of 200 women with dermatoses of pregnancy correlating clinical findings with hormonal and immunopathological profiles. *Br J Dermatol* 1999;141:71–81.
3 Ambros-Rudolph CM, Müllegger RR, Vaughan-Jones SA, Kerl H, Black MM. The specific dermatoses of pregnancy re- visited and reclassified: results of a retrospective two-center study on 505 pregnant patients. *J Am Acad Dermatol* 2006;54:395–404.

Polymorphic eruption of pregnancy
6 Vaughan Jones SA, Hern S, Nelson-Piercy C, *et al*. A prospective study of 200 women with dermatoses of pregnancy correlating clinical findings with hormonal and immunopathological profiles. *Br J Dermatol* 1999;141:71–81.

Pemphigoid gestationis
1 Jenkins RE, Black MM. Pemphigoid (herpes) gestationis. In: Black MM, Ambros-Rudolph CM, Edwards L, Lynch P, eds. *Obstetric and Gynaecologic Dermatology*, 3rd ed. London: Elsevier, 2008:37–47.
5 Briggs GG, Freeman RK, Yaffe SJ. *Drugs in Pregnancy and Lactation: A Reference Guide to Fetal and Neonatal Risk*, 8th edn. Philadelphia: Lippincot Williams & Wilkins, 2008.

General guidance on safe treatments in pregnancy
1 Chi CC, Wang SH, Kirtschig G, Wojnarowska F. Systematic review of the safety of topical corticosteroids in pregnancy. *J Am Acad Dermatol* 2010;62:694–705.

CHAPTER 116

Dermatoses of the Neonate

David G. Paige

Department of Dermatology, Barts Health NHS Trust, London, UK

INTRODUCTION

Nomenclature

- Neonatal period: first 4 weeks of extrauterine life.
- Infancy: first 1 year of extrauterine life.
- Premature (preterm): born before the 37th week of gestation.
- Full term: born in weeks 37–42 of gestation.
- Post mature: born after the 42nd week of gestation.
- Low birth weight: born under 2500 g.
- Intrauterine growth retardation: birth weight low for gestational age (small for dates).

Skin function in the neonate

Barrier function

Great interest has focused on skin barrier function, both in pre-term and full-term neonates, because of the evidence that both are at high risk of toxicity from topically applied substances [1].

Rook's Textbook of Dermatology, Ninth Edition. Edited by Christopher Griffiths, Jonathan Barker, Tanya Bleiker, Robert Chalmers and Daniel Creamer.
© 2016 John Wiley & Sons, Ltd. Published 2016 by John Wiley & Sons, Ltd.
Companion website: www.rooksdermatology.com

A normal full-term infant has a functional stratum corneum, with an almost fully developed barrier function [2–4,**5**]. Transepidermal water loss is somewhat higher in the first few days of life but this rapidly improves. Toxicity resulting from percutaneous absorption in the full-term neonate is less dependent on impaired barrier function per se and is more often related to one or more of the following:

1 The greatly increased ratio of surface area to volume.
2 The frequent presence of occlusive conditions, such as exist under waterproof nappies.
3 High ambient temperatures and humidity.

There is, in contrast, definite evidence of impaired barrier function in preterm infants, especially those of less than 34 weeks' gestation. Absorption correlates inversely with gestational age, but barrier function appears to improve rapidly after birth in the preterm infant, and will generally be normal by the end of the second or third week after birth [3,4,**6**].

It is clear that nothing should be applied to the skin of any baby without careful consideration of the potential hazards of percutaneous absorption, particularly in those with skin diseases or in small, preterm neonates. The best documented hazards relate to aniline dyes [7], hexachlorophene and related antiseptics [8], alcohol [9–11] and corticosteroids [12]. A number of other substances should never be used in neonates, especially not in preterm neonates; these include neomycin [13], boric acid [14], resorcinol (in Castellani's paint) [15], γ-benzene hexachloride [16], benzyl alcohol [17], urea [18] and salicylic acid [19]. Antiseptics such as chlorhexidine [20] and iodine [21,22] should be used with caution and alcohol-based products should be avoided in view of the risk of 'chemical burns' [23].

However, low-dose (0.25%) aqueous chlorhexidine applied to term babies has been shown to decrease mortality from sepsis in a community-based study of 17 500 low-birth-weight neonates from Nepal but no differences were seen in those with birth weights over 2500 g [24].

Care should also be taken with agents used to launder, sterilize or mark nappies and bed linen [7,25], also with mothballs used in their storage [26].

Even the routine use of topical petrolatum-based emollients in preterms has been challenged recently. Whilst these agents can reduce transepidermal water loss (TEWL), a Cochrane review of four studies showed their use was associated with increased coagulase-negative staphylococcal infection and nosocomial infection [27]. Further studies by Darmstadt *et al.* in Bangladesh confirmed this increase in nosocomial infection in preterm infants with the use of petrolatum emollients, but showed a significant reduction in infections with the use of sunflower oil as an alternative [28,29]. No data yet exist on the use of emollients in preterm infants with severe skin disease, such as Netherton syndrome or harlequin ichthyosis, where nosocomial infection is a common problem and often lethal.

TEWL is greatly increased in preterm compared with full-term babies [3,30]. The resulting outward passage of water can lead to high rates of heat loss by evaporation, which may even exceed the baby's resting rate of heat production. These losses can be reduced by increasing the ambient humidity [29,31] (although this leads to an increased risk of infection) by covering the child with a plastic bubble blanket [32] or a Perspex shield [33], or by applying a lipid barrier [34]. Whilst nursing the child in a relatively high humidity environment helps lessen TEWL in the acute stage, it slows down the maturation and recovery of the skin barrier so that abnormal TEWL takes longer to recover than in those nursed in relatively low humidity environments [35].

It is possible that immaturity of the skin also predisposes the premature neonate to penetration of the skin by microorganisms, leading to systemic infection. This may be the reason that the premature infant with congenital cutaneous candidiasis is at greater risk of disseminated candidiasis [36].

There is very little scientific evidence on which to base recommendations for parents on routine neonatal skin care in terms of cleansing and/or moisturizing, and advice varies considerably between doctors, health visitors and midwives. In view of the risks of percutaneous absorption, it is of concern that a study undertaken in the USA a few years ago revealed that parents had applied over 48 different chemicals in over-the-counter preparations to the skin of their 1-month-old babies [**37**].

A recent study looking at cleansers suggested there was no difference between using plain water and a commercially available wash product for babies, so this at least allows parents some choice. The same group has also shown that olive oil (often used in neonatal units or for baby massage) can damage the skin barrier in adults so probably should be avoided in neonates [38–40]. The sunflower oil used in the study did not show the same deleterious effect but sunflower oils vary considerably in composition and some are indeed harmful. As commercially available sunflower oils are not 'product labelled' they cannot be recommended for neonatal skin. More studies are needed to the answer the most basic of questions about routine neonatal skin care in a term baby.

Eccrine sweating

A full complement of anatomically normal eccrine sweat glands is present by the 28th week of gestation, but these appear to be functionally immature in neonates born before the 36th week in terms of their responses to intradermal injection of acetylcholine and epinephrine (adrenaline), and to thermal stress [**1**,2]. However, responsiveness usually develops in such babies by 2 weeks after birth. Neonates born after the 36th week of gestation sweat in response to thermal stress from birth, although such sweating is initially relatively inefficient as a thermoregulatory mechanism [3]. Care must therefore be taken not to overheat any neonate, particularly the preterm neonate, and although severe overheating leading to hyperpyrexia is probably rare, lesser degrees of iatrogenic overheating appear to be common and may even induce apnoeic attacks [4,5–7].

The forehead appears to be the principal site of thermally induced sweating in the neonate. The palms and soles, however, are sites of 'emotional' sweating, occurring in response to arousal, which appears to be well developed at birth in full-term but not preterm neonates.

Skin conductance measurements (as a measure of increased sweating) may be helpful in assessing pain levels in neonates [**8**].

Sebaceous gland secretion

The secretions of the fetal sebaceous glands make a significant contribution to the vernix caseosa [**1**]. Vernix caseosa acts as a naturally occurring 'barrier cream' that also contains antimicrobial peptides and is formed from week 24 of gestation [2,3]. The presence of vernix at birth is associated with better hydration of the epidermis. One group has even studied it as a 'natural' barrier cream to aid healing in a controlled wound model [4,5]. Sebum secretion rates are high in neonates compared with older pre-adolescent children, and it is assumed that this sebaceous gland activity reflects stimulation by placentally transferred maternal androgen, particularly by dehydroepiandrosterone [6]. Sebaceous gland activity decreases from about the end of the first month to reach a stable level by the end of the first year [6,7].

Appearance of neonatal skin

Full-term neonate

A variety of skin lesions commonly seen in the newborn are regarded as 'physiological'. Their frequency has been studied by several authors, and varies somewhat in different racial groups [1,2,3,4].

Vernix caseosa. At birth the skin is covered with a whitish, greasy film, the vernix caseosa. The vernix may cover the entire skin surface, or it may be present only in body folds such as the groins. It normally dries rapidly and starts to flake off within a few hours of birth. The vernix is comprised of lipids and contains antimicrobial peptides so it may play some role in keeping the skin hydrated and in preventing infection [5,6]. Its colour may reflect intrauterine problems, such as haemolytic disease of the newborn and postmaturity, both of which result in golden yellow staining. Fetal distress *in utero* may lead to staining of the vernix by the bile pigments present in meconium.

Peripheral cyanosis. Peripheral cyanosis (or acrocyanosis) is a feature of the newborn, particularly the full-term newborn, and is usually particularly marked on the palms and soles and around the mouth. In the absence of cyanosis of warm central parts such as the tongue, this may be regarded as normal during the first 48 h or so. It is made more obvious by hypothermia, and is improved by warming [7].

Erythema neonatorum. A few hours after birth, many babies develop a striking, generalized hyperaemia usually known as erythema neonatorum, which fades spontaneously within 24–48 h.

Harlequin colour change. Up to 15% of neonates show a vivid colour difference along the midline at some time during the first week of life. This phenomenon occurs when the baby is lying on its side: the upper half of the body is pale, the lower half a deep red colour [8,9]. The duration of the attack is highly variable, but generally is between 30 s and 20 min. If the baby is turned on the other side, the colour change may reverse. An individual neonate may have only a single episode, or it may recur on several occasions. This curious phenomenon, called harlequin colour change, appears to have no pathological significance in the great majority of cases, and is considered to reflect immaturity of the hypothalamic centres responsible for the control of peripheral vascular tone. If it persists beyond the end of the fourth week, it may be associated with hypoxia due to cardiovascular anomalies [10].

Cutis marmorata. Newborn infants who are subjected to cooling will show distinct marbling of the skin. Although this more or less disappears on rewarming, many normal neonates demonstrate faint marbling, even under optimal environmental conditions. The marbling comprises a reticulate blue vascular pattern, which has often been called cutis marmorata [11]. This response is a physiological one, and may be seen throughout infancy. Cutis marmorata telangiectatica congenita is a distinct vascular developmental disorder, and is easily distinguished as it is fixed (see Chapter 73) and may be associated with a variety of other abnormalities, for example of limb growth or renal anomalies [12,13].

Desquamation (physiological scaling of the newborn). Rather superficial cutaneous desquamation occurs in up to 75% of normal neonates [14]. This usually first appears around the ankles on the first day of life, and is more or less confined to the hands and feet. It may remain localized or may gradually become widespread, usually reaching its maximum extent and intensity by the eighth day. It tends always to be more severe in neonates who are small for dates, whatever their gestational age. Physiological scaling may occasionally be fairly pronounced but not generally sufficient to lead to confusion with any of the more serious types of congenital ichthyosis. Milder varieties of ichthyosis, such as ichthyosis vulgaris, may be difficult to distinguish, and it should be borne in mind that X-linked hypohidrotic ectodermal dysplasia may present with scaling of the skin in the neonatal period [15].

Sucking blisters. One or two solitary blisters or erosions are occasionally present at birth on the fingers, lips or forearms, and are believed to be caused by vigorous sucking *in utero*; hence the term sucking blister. These heal rapidly without sequelae [16].

Neonatal occipital alopecia. The scalp hair is shed synchronously during the fifth month of fetal life, and having regrown enters telogen in a wave from front to back, starting about 12 weeks before term. After shedding of the telogen hairs from the frontal and parietal areas, the roots again enter the anagen phase in a similar wave from front to back [17,18]. The roots in the occipital area do not enter telogen until term, and therefore rather conspicuous alopecia may appear at this site at birth or within the first 2 months (neonatal occipital alopecia). Trauma from lying on this area may also contribute [19].

Hair shedding in infancy. There appear to be two waves of hair loss and regrowth from front to back during early infancy, but by the end of the first year the typical mosaic pattern of hair growth is established [20]. In some babies, there is unusually synchronous hair loss during the neonatal period, resulting in obvious diffuse alopecia (telogen effluvium of the newborn), but, by the end of the first 6 months of life, most babies have a full head of hair. At this stage, the hairline often extends to the lateral ends of the eyebrows, but the terminal hairs comprising this extension gradually convert to vellus hairs during the remainder of the first year of life, causing the hairline to recede to its characteristic childhood position.

Sebaceous gland hypertrophy/milia. Sebaceous gland hyperplasia is a physiological event in the newborn, reflecting the influence of maternal androgens. It is visible to the naked eye in the great majority of infants as multiple, uniform, pinpoint, yellowish papules that are most prominent on the nose, cheeks, upper lip and

PART 10: SITES, SEX, AGE

forehead, but may also be visible on the upper trunk, especially the areolae, genitalia and limbs. The phenomenon is associated in about 40% of infants with milia, which represent minute follicular epidermal cysts [21]. The numbers of milia may vary from one or two to many hundreds. They comprise 1–3 mm diameter, white, globular papules, which occur at the same sites as sebaceous gland hyperplasia. Rather larger and usually single milia, often termed pearls, are seen sometimes on the areolae, scrotum and labia majora. Both the sebaceous gland hyperplasia and the milia tend to disappear spontaneously during the first weeks of life, although a few may persist longer. Milia that are exceptionally extensive or persistent, or whose distribution is atypical, may be features of the oro-facial–digital syndrome type I (see Chapters 67 and 68), Marie–Unna type congenital hypotrichosis (see Chapter 68) or the X-linked Bazex–Dupré–Christol syndrome, which features hypotrichosis and milia (see Chapter 141).

'Miniature puberty'. The influence on the fetus of maternal and placental hormones may give rise to a number of features [22]: an enlarged clitoris; mucoid vaginal discharge; enlarged well-developed genitalia (boys and girls); hypertrophy of the mammary glands (boys and girls), which resolves in 2–4 weeks; desquamation of the hyperplastic vaginal epithelium (few days after birth); frank withdrawal bleeding, which may occur from the uterus on day 3/4, usually lasting for 2 or 3 days; and lactation ('witch's milk') on day2/3 – if persistent this can predispose to mastitis/breast abscess in girls.

Hyperpigmentary disorders. A linea alba occurs in 8% of babies and may persist for 2–3 months. Mongolian blue spots occur in up to 85% of oriental babies [23], are common in black babies but only occur in about 3% of white babies [24]. Hyperpigmentation of the scrotum may occur especially in oriental babies (up to 30%) [23]. Linear/reticulate pigmentary anomalies have been described in black newborns [25].

Oral findings. Epstein's pearls are 1–2 mm diameter, yellowish white, keratinous cysts seen in the mouths of up to 85% of all neonates, along the alveolar ridges and/or in the midline at the junction of the hard and soft palate [26,27]. These generally disappear without treatment within a few weeks. Succulent gums, analogous to the hypertrophic gingivitis often seen in pregnant women, are common in neonates. A whitish hue to the oral mucosa ('leukoedema') is also common. This is probably synonymous with what other authors have called 'suckling pads' [26,27].

Preterm neonate

The skin of the preterm neonate tends to have a rather translucent, gelatinous quality, and the so-called 'miniature puberty' features are much less prominent. Cutaneous vessels are easily visible [1,2]. Preterm infants are often covered in lanugo hairs, which tend to be most dense on the face, limbs and trunk. This hair would normally be shed in utero about 1 month before term, to be replaced by a second coat of shorter lanugo, which is present at birth in full-term infants. Like the terminal scalp hair, this downy lanugo is shed during the first months of life and is itself replaced by vellus hair [1].

Small-for-dates and postmature neonates

The small-for-dates or dysmature neonate presents a characteristic appearance due to relative prenatal malnutrition. The baby is small and, from the dermatological point of view, the most striking feature is the lack of subcutaneous fat, which causes the baby to look thin and wrinkled. Vernix is absent in the extremely immature infant, but may be profuse nearer to term. The skin and vernix are often stained yellowish green by meconium. After birth, the skin dries quickly and becomes 'crazed' with long transverse splits on the trunk. It then peels off to reveal more normal-appearing skin beneath. The fingernails are often long.

The postmature infant is longer but of otherwise similar appearance to the small-for-dates neonate, having also experienced intra-uterine malnutrition due to placental insufficiency. Vernix is often absent [1].

SKIN DISORDERS IN THE NEONATE

Toxic erythema of the newborn

Definition and nomenclature

Toxic erythema of the newborn is a common, transient, blotchy, red macular rash (sometimes with small pustules) seen in the first few days of life. The most widely used term for this condition is inappropriate in view of the complete absence of any evidence of a toxic cause [1].

> **Synonyms and inclusions**
> • Erythema toxicum neonatorum

Epidemiology

Incidence and prevalence

Thirty to 50% of children develop a degree of toxic erythema. The incidence appears to decrease with both prematurity and smallness for dates.

Age

It appears in the first few days of life.

Sex

There is equal prevalence in most studies.

Ethnicity

It occurs in all racial groups.

Associated diseases

Blood eosinophilia is associated.

Pathophysiology

The cause is unknown. There is frequently an associated blood eosinophilia. This probably does not reflect an allergic response as tissue eosinophilia is a non-specific feature of inflammatory responses in neonates [1]. The intrafollicular location of mature pustules has led to the suggestion that the inflammatory response is elicited by some component of sebum [2]. Scanning electron microscopy of neonatal skin shows that colonization of hair follicle epithelium by staphylococci is common in early life. Furthermore, accumulation of tryptase-expressing mast cells around the hair follicles in lesional skin has been recently demonstrated but its relation to the staphylococci and its significance in toxic erythema remains unclear [3,4].

Predisposing factors
No predisposing factors are known.

Pathology
Histologically, the macular erythema shows oedema in the upper dermis, associated with a sparse and largely perivascular inflammatory infiltrate comprising principally of eosinophils. Papular lesions are characterized, in addition, by eosinophil infiltration of the outer root sheath of one or more hair follicles, above the point of entry of the sebaceous duct. Pustular lesions show intrafollicular accumulation of eosinophils immediately below the stratum corneum. Smears of the pustule contents demonstrate inflammatory cells, more than 90% of which are eosinophils [2,5,6–8].

There is an associated blood eosinophilia of up to 20% of the white cell count in around half the cases, and this is generally more marked when there is a prominent pustular element to the eruption.

Causative organisms
No pathogenic bacteria have been isolated from pustules.

Environmental factors
No environmental factors have been demonstrated.

Clinical features

History
Thirty to 50% of full-term infants of all racial types will manifest some degree of toxic erythema during the first few days of life. In most cases, the onset is during the first 48 h after birth, but it may occur at any time until about the fourth day. It very rarely presents at birth [5,8–10].

Presentation
Most commonly, the eruption initially takes the form of a blotchy, macular erythema, the number of individual lesions varying from one or two to several hundred. They are most profuse on the trunk, particularly the anterior trunk, but also commonly appear on the face and proximal parts of the limbs, especially the thighs. Lesions have been recorded, however, at almost any site except the palms and soles. In the mildest cases, these macules fade within a day [11,12–16].

Clinical variants
In more severe cases, urticarial papules arise within the erythematous areas or, occasionally, independently of them (particularly on the back and buttocks). These papules are, in about 10% of cases, surmounted by small pustules 1–2 mm in diameter. Presentation with scrotal pustules present at birth has been reported more recently [17].

Differential diagnosis
Toxic erythema of the newborn has to be distinguished from several other disorders featuring pustular lesions during the neonatal period, particularly miliaria, transient neonatal pustular melanosis, incontinentia pigmenti and, most importantly, herpes simplex virus (HSV) infection, varicella, impetigo neonatorum and *Malassezia furfur* pustulosis. Of these, perhaps pustular miliaria is the one most often confused clinically with toxic erythema.

Classification of severity
No classification exists but more severe cases have papules and pustules.

Complications and co-morbidities
The infant appears well, and unperturbed by the eruption. There are no complications.

Disease course and prognosis
Spontaneous recovery occurs rapidly, usually within 3 days, but recurrences are occasionally seen and have been reported as late as the sixth week of life.

Investigations
Investigations are rarely needed as it is a clinical diagnosis. If there is any diagnostic doubt, toxic erythema can be rapidly diagnosed by microscopic examination of a smear of pustule contents (stained with Giemsa) to show the eosinophils and by negative bacterial and viral cultures.

Management
No treatment is needed.

Resources

Further information
Medscape, toxic eythema of the newborn: emedicine.medscape.com/article/1110731-overview (last accessed December 2014).

Miliaria

Definition and nomenclature
Miliaria is a disorder due to blockage of eccrine sweat ducts (see Chapter 94). It is subdivided into three subtypes dependent on the level of blockage: miliaria crystallina (stratum corneum), miliaria rubra (mid-epidermal) and miliaria profunda (dermal–epidermal junction) [1,2].

Synonyms and inclusions
• Prickly heat (for miliaria rubra)

Epidemiology

Incidence and prevalence
Miliaria occurs in about 3–8% of neonates.

Age
Miliaria may occur at any age but malaria rubra and miliaria crystallina are common in neonates.

Sex
There is an equal sex prevalence.

Ethnicity
It occurs in all racial groups.

Associated diseases
Very rarely hypernatraemia or hyperaldosteronism are associated.

Pathophysiology

Predisposing factors
Immature sweat ducts are an important factor in neonates although high levels of heat and humidity are important at any age. Occlusive clothing is probably more relevant to adults. Hypernatraemia and/or hyperaldosteronism is a very rare underlying factor.

Pathology
Miliaria crystallina is characterized by the presence of intracorneal or subcorneal vesicles in communication with the sweat ducts. In miliaria rubra, focal areas of spongiosis and spongiotic vesicle formation are seen in close proximity to the sweat ducts, which often contain an amorphous, periodic acid–Schiff (PAS) stain-positive plug [3,4,5–7].

Causative organisms
There is a possible link with *Staphylococcus epidermidis* and *S. aureus*.

Environmental factors
Associated factors include heat, humidity, occlusive clothes and plastic sheets.

Clinical features

History
Milaria in the neonate usually presents with a rash in the first few weeks of life.

Presentation
Miliaria crystallina presents as crops of clear, thin-walled, superficial vesicles 1–2 mm in diameter, without associated erythema, resembling drops of water (Figure 116.1). These are exceedingly delicate and generally rupture within 24 h, and are followed by bran-like desquamation. Lesions are asymptomatic. They arise most frequently during the first 2 weeks of life, and are particularly likely to be seen on the forehead, scalp, neck and upper trunk. Though rare during the first 4 days, congenital cases have been reported [7,8,9,10,11].

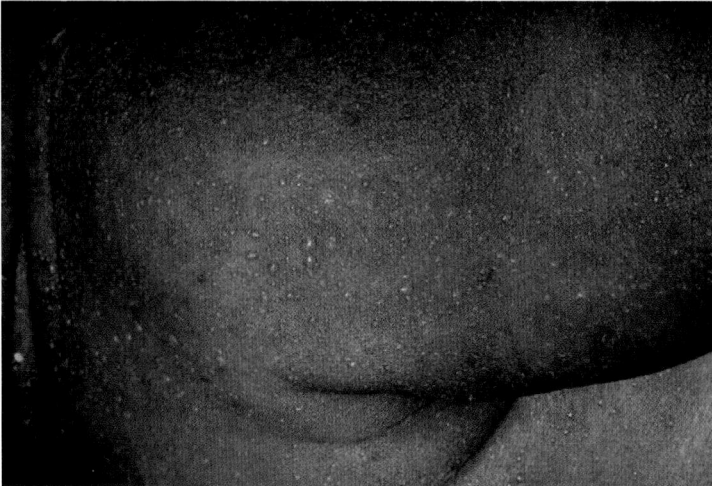

Figure 116.1 Miliaria crystallina on the upper arm of a 7-day-old infant.

Miliaria rubra ('prickly heat') comprises erythematous papules and papulovesicles about 1–4 mm in diameter, on a background of macular erythema. Sometimes, quite large, weal-like lesions occur. Frequently, some of the lesions are pustular (miliaria pustulosa), but this does not necessarily indicate secondary infection. Nevertheless, staphylococcal secondary infection of miliaria (periporitis) is not infrequent, and may lead to sweat gland abscesses.

Miliaria rubra is common and, although it may be seen throughout infancy, it probably occurs most frequently during the neonatal period. Crops of lesions arise fairly symmetrically, most often in flexural areas, especially around the neck and in the groins and axillae. The face, scalp and upper trunk are also frequently affected. It may also occur rather locally at sites that have been occluded, for example where there has been direct contact between the skin and a plastic mattress cover or plastic pants. Lesions can be itchy or sore. Where the eruption is profuse, the child may be restless and distressed. Each crop of lesions will subside within 2–3 days, but recurrences are common unless the provocative environmental conditions are modified.

Recurrent bouts of miliaria pustulosa are a common finding in type 1 pseudohypoaldosteronism [12,13].

Miliaria profunda is very uncommon in neonates as it usually occurs in adults where there have been repeated episodes of miliaria rubra. However, a granulomatous variant of giant centrifugal miliaria profunda was recently described in two 3-month-old babies [14]. This presents with papules and geographical and annular plaques over the extensor aspects of the limbs and the trunk.

Clinical variants
There are three clinical variants: miliaria crystallina, miliaria rubra and miliaria profunda (granulomatous giant centrifugal variant).

Differential diagnosis
Miliaria crystallina is distinguishable from viral infections of the skin (e.g. herpes simplex) by the lack of background erythema, and by the absence of inflammatory cells or giant keratinocytes on

cytological examination of vesicle contents. When it occurs during the first few days of life, miliaria rubra is often confused with toxic erythema, especially if it has become pustular. However, miliaria rubra can generally be distinguished by its flexural predominance, by the frequent presence of vesicular lesions and by its tendency to recur. If in doubt, a smear of a vesicle/pustule will show an absence of eosinophils (large numbers are seen in toxic erythema). Miliaria pustulosa may also be confused with infantile acne or folliculitis, but the lesions are not follicular.

Complications and co-morbidities
Staphylococcal infection and sweat gland abscess rarely occur.

Disease course and prognosis
Miliaria crystallina improves spontaneously as the sweat ducts mature. Milaria rubra improves if the predisposing aetiological factors (high heat/humidity and occlusion) are removed.

Investigations
The diagnosis is usually clinical. Occasionally, a smear from a vesicle or pustule is useful to exclude HSV infection or toxic erythema.

Management
Milaria crystallina spontaneously improves without therapy over a few weeks as the sweat ducts mature.

First line
Miliaria rubra will improve in a few weeks without medical treatment if the child is removed from conditions of high heat/humidity and any occlusive clothing or bedding is removed.

Second line
Antibiotics may be needed if staphylococcal infection occurs but this is rare.

Resources

Further information
Medscape, dermatologic manifestations of miliaria: emedicine.medscape.com/article/1070840-overview (lasat accessed December 2014).

Transient pustular melanosis

Synonyms and inclusions
• Transient neonatal pustular melanosis

Despite having first been described more than 30 years ago [1], the aetiology of transient pustular melanosis remains unknown. It was first reported in black Americans, and appears to be commoner in, but not confined to, black neonates (4.4% in black US neonates against 0.6% in white US neonates). It has been sug-

---

> **Box 116.1 Pustular eruptions in the neonate**
>
> • Congenital or neonatal candidiasis
> • Congenital syphilis
> • Eosinophilic pustulosis
> • Herpes simplex virus infection
> • Impetigo
> • Infantile acne
> • Infantile acropustulosis
> • *Malassezia* pustulosis
> • Miliaria
> • Neonatal listeriosis
> • Neonatal pustulosis of transient myeloproliferative disorder
> • Pustular psoriasis
> • Scabies
> • Toxic erythema of the newborn
> • Transient pustular melanosis

gested that it is merely an early-onset variant of toxic erythema of the newborn [1,2].

Lesions are usually present at birth. The most characteristic component of the eruption is 1–3 mm flaccid, superficial, fragile pustules, with no surrounding erythema. These pustules may occur at any site, but favour the chin, neck, forehead, back and buttocks [3–6,7,8,9]. Sites where they have ruptured are marked initially by a detachable brown crust, and subsequently by a small collarette of scale, which may surmount a pigmented macule. Sometimes, pigmented macules are already present at birth. The pigmented macules are a prominent element in black infants, and are seen more rarely in other races [5]. The pigmentation may persist for about 3 months. Affected infants are otherwise entirely well. Diagnosis can usually be made on clinical grounds without the need for a biopsy or smear.

A skin biopsy of a pustule shows intra- or subcorneal collections of neutrophils and a few eosinophils [1]. The underlying dermis may show no abnormality, or a sparse perivascular and perifollicular inflammatory infiltrate, also mainly of neutrophils with a few eosinophils. The pigmented macules demonstrate basal and suprabasal increases in pigmentation only, apparently without pigmentary incontinence. Smears of pustular contents show predominantly neutrophils, and bacterial culture is negative.

No treatment is needed for this self-resolving condition. The differential diagnosis of neonatal pustular eruptions is given in Box 116.1.

Infantile acropustulosis

Infantile acropustulosis is an uncommon disorder of unknown aetiology. It occurs in all races [1] although it was first described in black infants [2]. It has been suggested that eosinophilic pustular folliculitis and infantile acropustulosis may be different manifestations of the same disease [3]. It has also been suggested that, at least in some cases, infantile acropustulosis occurs following successful treatment of scabies [4,5,6]. It has been reported in siblings [7] and in only one of a pair of identical twins [8].

Infantile acropustulosis presents with recurrent crops of intensely itchy, 1–4 mm vesicopustules that appear principally on the soles and sides of the feet, and on the palms, but may also occur on the dorsa of the feet, hands and fingers, and on the ankles, wrists and forearms. Scattered lesions may also be seen on the face, scalp and trunk, but a predominantly acral distribution is characteristic. Mucosal lesions do not occur [2,7,9,10]. Individual lesions appear to start as tiny, red papules, which evolve into vesicles and then pustules over about 24 h. Excoriation results in erosions and then crusts. Healing is frequently succeeded by macular postinflammatory hyperpigmentation.

In the majority of cases, the onset is in the first year of life, particularly during the first 6 months [7]. Lesions rarely present at birth. Each crop lasts for 7–14 days. They tend to occur at intervals of 2–4 weeks in most cases, often being more frequent and more numerous in the summer months.

The predilection for the palms and soles and the recurrent attacks differentiate this disorder from most other pustular eruptions seen in the neonatal period, particularly toxic erythema, miliaria and transient pustular melanosis. Scabies may initially be extremely difficult to exclude, and where there is any doubt a therapeutic trial of an appropriate acaricide is justified. Diagnosis is usually clinical. Skin biopsy of a pustule will show well-circumscribed subcorneal or intraepidermal aggregations of neutrophils, with a sparse perivascular lymphohistiocytic infiltrate in the underlying papillary dermis [9,11]. Biopsy of a pre-pustular lesion shows focal intraepidermal vesiculation with keratinocyte necrosis. This intraepidermal vesicle is subsequently invaded by neutrophils and/or eosinophils. The pustule starts its life deep in the epidermis, but does not become clinically fully developed until it reaches a subcorneal location. Direct and indirect immunofluorescence studies are negative Stained smears of pustule contents generally show a predominance of neutrophils, but there may be a preponderance of eosinophils early in the course of the disorder. Sometimes peripheral blood eosinophilia is present [12,13,14].

Treatment is with potent topical corticosteroids with or without occlusion [7,9]. Dapsone has been used in a few severe cases [2] as has topical maxacalcitol [15]. The attacks occur with gradually diminishing numbers of lesions, and with decreasing frequency, until they cease altogether, usually within 2 years of the onset.

Neonatal pustulosis of transient myeloproliferative disorder

There have been several reports of neonates with trisomy 21 (and mosaic trisomy 21) developing pustules and vesicles (on an erythematous background), predominantly on the face, as part of congenital leukaemia or transient myeloproliferative disorder (TMD) [1,2,3,4]. They may pustulate at sites of trauma, such as venepuncture sites or under adhesive tape. The patients may also have hepatosplenomegaly. There is an associated high white blood cell count, often with the presence of blasts. Skin biopsy shows intraepidermal pustules with a perivascular dermal infiltrate of neutrophils, eosinophils and atypical mononuclear cells. The lesions often resolve spontaneously over a few weeks paralleled by a decreasing white cell count.

Mutations in the transcription factor GATA1 seem to underlie TMD but a second genetic hit is needed to develop leukaemia [5]. Up to 20% of patients with TMD will go on to develop an acute megakaryoblastic leukaemia within the first 4 years of life so follow-up is mandatory.

Congenital erosive and vesicular dermatosis healing with reticulated supple scarring

Definition and nomenclature
Congenital erosive and vesicular dermatosis healing with reticulated supple scarring is a rare cause of blistering at birth [1–6].

Synonyms and inclusions
- Extensive congenital erosions and vesicles healing with reticulate scarring

Introduction and general description
This is a rare self-limiting blistering disorder of unknown aetiology first described in 1985 by Cohen *et al.* [1].

Epidemiology

Incidence and prevalence
It is very rare. Twenty-eight cases have been reported in the literature up to December 2013.

Age
It occurs at birth and the majority of affected infants have been premature.

Sex
Occurrence is greater in boys than in girls.

Pathophysiology

Pathology
Biopsies of vesicular areas have shown spongiosis or epidermal necrosis with dermal haemorrhage and inflammation [1,2,3–5,6]. In one report, an eroded area showed loss of the epidermis with a superficial and deep dermal inflammatory infiltrate comprising mostly neutrophils [4]. Parakeratotic scale may be present. Scarred areas have shown an increased density of dermal collagen, and absence of eccrine sweat glands. Direct immunofluorescence does not show any specific pattern of deposition of immunoglobulins, C3 or fibrin. Electron microscopy and immunohistochemical mapping of perilesional skin have shown nothing to suggest that this is a variant of epidermolysis bullosa [5].

Clinical features

History
The condition presents at birth with blistering and erosions which heal with soft scars.

Presentation

There are extensive, superficial erosions, with scattered vesicles and bullae, affecting up to 75% of the body surface. These erosions may extend in the first few days. The trunk and limbs tend to be more severely affected than the face and scalp. Hands and feet may be spared [7,8,9]. Patients are prone to infection prior to the skin healing. Bacterial, fungal and HSV infections have been described.

The blisters/erosions heal fairly quickly within the first few weeks of life, leaving rather characteristic soft, reticulated scarring. Following healing of the skin lesions, there may be residual loss of eccrine sweating in scarred areas, with the potential for hyperthermia under appropriate conditions, patchy alopecia, partial loss of eyelashes and the absence or hypoplasia of nails. Teeth are normal. Mild, localized, recurrent vesiculation may occur.

The largest published review of 18 cases revealed the following associations: preterm birth (79%), nail dystrophies (46%), hyperthermia/hypophidrosis (46%), maternal chorioamnionitis (43%), neurological disorders (microcephaly, convulsions, developmental delay) and ophthalmological complications (lacrimal duct obstruction, macular or corneal scars) (36% each) and tongue atrophy (29%) [7].

Differential diagnosis

This includes infective blisters (e.g. herpes simplex), epidermolysis bullosa, bullous ichthyosiform erythroderma, incontinentia pigmenti, aplasia cutis congenita, focal dermal hypoplasia and staphylococcal scalded skin syndrome.

Complications and co-morbidities

Postnatal infection is a risk. It is unclear if the disease associations (see Presentation above) are caused by congenital erosive and vesicular dermatosis itself or by prematurity or an unidentified intrauterine pathology.

Disease course and prognosis

Spontaneous healing occurs within 2 weeks to 3 months.

Investigations

Skin swabs and blood culture are needed to investigate for infections (viral, bacterial and fungal). Skin biopsy may be useful.

Management

The child will need to be nursed on an appropriate neonatal unit for the management of fluid balance, temperature control and any infection if this develops. Non-adhesive dressings (e.g. silicon dressings) will be needed for the first few weeks of life until healing occurs [7,8,9]. There is no specific treatment for this condition.

COMPLICATIONS OF PREMATURITY

Anetoderma of prematurity

Introduction and general description

Anetoderma is due to loss of elastic tissue in the dermis and presents with atrophic lesions that often herniate. Anetoderma may occur in preterm babies appearing at, or soon after, birth [1,2,3]. Its early onset differentiates it from anetoderma of prematurity caused by electrocardiogram (ECG) electrodes [4].

Epidemiology

Incidence and prevalence

Its incidence is unknown but it is very rare.

Age

It is found in extremely premature babies (<29 weeks).

Sex

There is equal sex incidence.

Pathophysiology

The underlying cause is unknown although it is found in premature babies. A skin biopsy of a lesion shows reduced or absent elastic tissue, consistent with anetoderma [1,2,3,4]. There may be an underlying genetic predisposition. Anetoderma has been described in two identical premature twins but all other cases have been sporadic [3].

Clinical features

History

Anetoderma presenting in extremely premature babies was first described by Prizant *et al.* in 1996 [1].

Presentation

Anetoderma of prematurity presents with nummular areas of cutaneous atrophy appearing on the trunk and/or proximal limbs within a few weeks of birth [1,2,3]. All cases have been born between the 24th and 29th weeks of gestation and in almost all cases the lesions first appeared while the child was still in the neonatal intensive care unit. Rarely, anetoderma may be present at birth. Cases that present later at 2–3 months of age are more likely a consequence of trauma from gel ECG electrodes [4].

Differential diagnosis

These include anetoderma from trauma and aplasia cutis congenita type 5.

Complications and co-morbidities

Patients have the co-morbidities of extreme prematurity.

Disease course and prognosis

It is non-progressive and persistent.

Investigations

Skin biopsy should be done.

Management

There is no known treatment for anetoderma.

PART 10: SITES, SEX, AGE

COMPLICATIONS OF MEDICAL PROCEDURES ON THE FETUS AND NEONATE

Antenatal procedures

Antenatal procedures and amniocentesis can lead to a range of problems arising in the fetus (Table 116.1).

Neonatal medical procedures

Adverse consequences of medical procedures on the neonate are more common if the baby was premature (Table 116.2).

Table 116.1 Complications arising from some antenatal procedures.

Procedure	Complication or disorder
Amniocentesis needles Antenatal biopsies (skin, liver, tumours)	Punctate scars and dimples (prevalence decreased with real time ultrasound) [1,**2**,3,4,**5**]
Intrauterine red cell transfusion (used in haemolytic disease/ rhesus incompatibility)	Gangrene abdominal wall [6]
Scalp electrodes (used for monitoring fetal heart rate)	Scarring alopecia/cephalohaematoma [7,8] Neonatal HSV at the site of electrodes (cutaneous blisters/encephalitis) [**9**,10–12]
Scalp blood sampling (monitoring acid–base balance)	Scalp abscess (in 4% of neonates; rarely deep tissue infections) [13–17]
Forceps delivery	Subcutaneous fat necrosis
Scalpel injury during Caesarian section	Lacerations/scars
Ventouse extraction (very rare)	Scarring alopecia (usually after severe caput succedaneum) [18]
Ventouse extraction	Annular blisters scalp ('vesicular eruption of vacuum-assisted delivery') can be traumatic or due to HSV [19]

HSV, herpes simplex virus.

Table 116.2 Complications arising from some neonatal medical procedures.

Procedure	Cutaneous complication
Umbilical artery catheterization [**1**,2–6]	Aortic thrombosis/spasm, arterial embolism (lower limb ischaemia/gangrene)
Transcutaneous oxygen monitoring (heated electrode) [7–10]	Superficial burn (erythema/vesiculation) – less risk with unheated pulse oximetry
Electrocardiograph electrodes [11,12]	Anetoderma secondary to trauma (may be purpuric initially)
Transillumination (more common if infrared filters are switched off) [13]	Blisters: 2–4 mm in diameter, often at acral sites
Extravasation intravenous medication [14–16,**17**]	Cutaneous necrosis
Heel pricks [18–20] Extravasation with calcium-containing solutions [21–23] Scalp electroencephalograph electrodes (calcium chloride-containing paste) [24]	Cutaneous calcification (localized)
Needle insertions (repeated)/chest drain insertions [**17**]	Punctate white scars (speckled scarring)
Chemical burns from antiseptics/alcohol-based cleansers [**25**,26–30]	Cutaneous necrosis (often on the back or buttocks where the cleanser has pooled)

Table 116.3 Phototherapy-induced rashes.

Cutaneous complication	Cause
Erythematous rash	Macular erythematous rash (as bilirubin falls) [1] UV-induced erythema ('burn') [2]
Hyperpigmentation	Skin tanning (especially type 6 skin) [3] Bronze baby syndrome (underlying hepatic disease) [**4**,5–10] (Differential diagnosis: central cyanosis, 'carbon baby' and 'grey baby' syndrome [11,12])
Bullous eruptions	Drug phototoxicity (furosemide, methylene blue) [13,14] Congenital porphyrias [15–17]
Epidermolysis bullosa-like eruptions	Transient porphyrinaemia (after repeated transfusions for severe haemolytic disease of the newborn) [**18**]
Localized purpura on 'exposed' sites	Transient porphyrinaemia (secondary to transfusions) [19,**20**]

Phototherapy

Phototherapy is often used for neonatal jaundice and can lead to various complications (Table 116.3).

ATROPHIC LESIONS OF NEONATES

There are a number of causes of atrophic lesions in neonates (Box 116.2). Some are covered elsewhere in this chapter.

Medallion-like dermal dendrocyte hamartoma

Definition
Medallion-like dermal dendrocyte hamartoma is a benign atrophic lesion presenting at birth amd was first described in 2004 in female neonates [1,2,3,**4**,**5**].

Box 116.2 Causes of atrophic lesions in neonates

- Morphoea
- Atrophic dermatofibrosarcoma protuberans
- Cutis marmorata telangiectatica congenita
- Aplasia cutis congenita
- Anetoderma of prematurity
- Congenital erosive and vesicular dermatosis healing with reticulated supple scarring
- Medallion-like dermal dendrocyte hamartoma
- Congenital infection (HSV and VZV; maybe zosteriform)
- Focal dermal hypoplasia of Goltz
- Neonatal lupus erythematosus

HSV, herpes simplex virus; VZV, varicella zoster virus.

Epidemiology

Incidence and prevalence
It is very rare with less than 15 cases described.

Age
There is congenital presentation.

Sex
It is more common in females.

Pathophysiology
The underlying cause is unknown.

Pathology
It shows epidermal atrophy, spindle cell proliferation in the dermis and to a lesser degree the subcutis, and reduced adnexal structures. Spindle cells stain positive for CD34, factor X111a, vimentin and fascin, suggesting a dermal dendritic origin. Atrophic dermatofibrosarcoma protuberans is also CD34 positive, but is factor X111a negative [1,2,3].

Clinical features

Presentation
This rare condition presents with a reddish brown, congenital, atrophic lesion of the skin often on the side of the neck or on the upper trunk. Lesions are typically round or oval, measure 2–6 cm across and they persist. They may show a slight increase in hair growth and visible underlying blood vessels beneath a wrinkled epidermis [1,2,3,4,5]. Histology and immunohistochemistry help differentiate this disorder from other causes of neonatal cutaneous atrophy.

Differential diagnosis
Differential diagnoses include congenital dermatofibrosarcoma protuberans, aplasia cutis congenita, anetoderma of prematurity, neurofibroma (atrophic blue-red macule variant) and cutis marmorata telangiectatica congenita.

Disease course and prognosis
The course is persistent but there is no recorded case of malignant transformation.

Investigations
Skin biopsy and immunostaining are useful.

Management
There is no known medical therapy. Lesions can be safely left or excised (usually by a plastic surgeon, depending on the size).

DISORDERS CAUSED BY TRANSPLACENTAL TRANSFER/MATERNAL MILK

Transplacental transfer of maternal autoantibodies

Clinical manifestations in the neonate have now been reported in a number of maternal disorders that are believed to be induced by circulating autoantibodies. These include pemphigus vulgaris, pemphigus foliaceus, herpes gestationis and lupus erythematosus.

Because immunoglobulin A (IgA), IgM and IgE antibodies do not cross the placenta in significant amounts, this phenomenon is restricted to diseases caused by autoantibodies of IgG class. Where complement is also involved in pathogenesis, this must be provided by the fetus as it does not pass across the placenta. Complement can be detected in the fetus from about the 11th week of gestation. Maternal IgG is catabolized more or less completely within the first 3–6 months of life, and antibody-mediated transplacental diseases can be expected to remit spontaneously within this period.

Neonatal pemphigus vulgaris
(see also Chapter 50)

Pemphigus vulgaris is unusual in pregnancy because it is largely a disease of an older age group and because affected individuals receiving systemic treatment rarely become pregnant. Nevertheless, several cases of transplacentally transmitted pemphigus vulgaris have been reported [1,2,3–6]. Not all mothers have had clinically apparent disease during pregnancy [7]; in other cases the disease has been mild [8].

Affected infants have had cutaneous and/or mucosal erosions or bullae; several have been stillborn [1,2,3–6]. Direct immunofluorescence has been positive in skin biopsies from all affected infants, and circulating IgG pemphigus antibodies have been found in the majority. No treatment is required; lesions have resolved spontaneously within about 3 weeks, and circulating IgG antibodies have become undetectable by the end of the second month of life.

Transplacental transmission of pemphigus foliaceus has been similarly described [9,10].

Transplacental pemphigoid gestationis

Cutaneous lesions occur in about 10% of infants born to mothers with pemphigoid gestationis, although maternal IgG antibasement membrane autoantibody can be found in all infants of affected mothers [1,2] (see also Chapter 115). The lesions may be present at birth or they may appear at any time up to the third day of life [3]. These lesions may vary from evanescent, non-specific, erythematous or urticarial papules to fully developed bullae [4]. Lesions in the infant may be extensive [5]. Spontaneous regression of lesions within 3 weeks is the rule. Direct immunofluorescence is normal by the end of the first month, and circulating IgG antibasement membrane zone antibody can no longer be found.

Earlier reports of increased fetal and infant morbidity and mortality when mothers have had pemphigoid gestationis [6] have not been confirmed [7,8,9]. However, there does appear to be an increased risk of premature delivery [8,9]. The risk of adrenal insufficiency should be considered in neonates whose mothers have been treated with prednisolone for prolonged periods.

Neonatal lupus erythematosus

Introduction and general description

Neonatal lupus erythematosus (NLE) is a rare syndrome comprising transient skin lesions resembling subacute cutaneous lupus erythematosus (LE) and/or congenital heart block (see also Chapter 51). NLE occurs in the babies of mothers with clinical or subclinical autoimmune connective tissue disease, and is associated with the transplacental passage of maternal autoantibodies to the ribonucleoproteins (RNPs) Ro-SSA (>90%), La-SSB or rarely U_1-RNP [1].

Epidemiology

Incidence and prevalence

Only 1–2% of Ro-positive/La-postive mothers will have babies with NLE but babies from subsequent pregnancies have a 20–25% risk of skin or cardiac disease [2,3].

Age

It occurs in neonates up to 3 months old.

Sex

There is an equal sex incidence.

Ethnicity

It is described in all racial groups.

Associated diseases

The risk of connective tissue disease later in life is increased.

Pathophysiology

It is now accepted that this disease is provoked in the fetus or newborn infant by maternal IgG autoantibodies that have crossed the placenta [4,5]. In 95% of cases, these are of IgG1 class and are directed against the Ro RNP antigen [6–8]. These antibodies are relatively prevalent in young women, and often appear to be compatible with apparently normal health. Anti-La, anti-native DNA, anticardiolipin or antinuclear antibodies, or rheumatoid factor, may be present in addition to Ro antibodies [9]. A small proportion of affected infants do not have detectable Ro antibodies but do have La and U_1-RNP antibodies.

The presence of Ro and La antigens has been demonstrated in fetal skin and cardiac conducting tissue [10,11]. Up to 60% of the mothers of infants with neonatal LE have no clinical evidence of connective tissue disease at the time of birth [5,9,12]. However, there is a substantial risk of a subsequent development of symptoms of autoimmune connective tissue disease. About 40% of mothers have signs or symptoms of systemic LE, subacute cutaneous LE or the sicca syndrome [13,14,15,16], although these may be minimal. More recently, it has been recognized that about 5% of women of child-bearing age who present with leukocytoclastic vasculitis will have Ro antibodies [17], and it is probable that about 5% of babies with neonatal LE have mothers with leukocytoclastic vasculitis [18].

Predisposing factors

There appears to be a genetic predisposition to develop the cardiac complications of neonatal LE.

Pathology

Skin biopsy specimens from infants with cutaneous lesions generally demonstrate the features of LE: epidermal atrophy, liquefaction degeneration of basal keratinocytes, colloid bodies and a perivascular and periappendageal lymphohistiocytic inflammatory infiltrate in the dermis [13,19]. Direct immunofluorescence is positive in about 50% of cases, showing dermal–epidermal junction and perivascular deposition of IgG, IgM and C3.

Environmental factors

Sunlight may induce skin lesions.

Clinical features

Presentation

Most infants with neonatal LE have either skin lesions (90%) or cardiac lesions (1%); approximately 8% have both [2,20,21]. In about two-thirds of those infants who develop cutaneous lesions, these are already present at birth. In the remainder, the lesions appear during the first 2–3 months (sometimes sun-induced), although their appearance may be delayed for as long as 5 months.

The skin lesions of neonatal LE generally take the form of well-defined areas of macular or slightly elevated erythema, frequently annular, occurring predominantly on the face, particularly the forehead, temples and upper cheeks, and on the scalp and neck (Figure 116.2). A 'spectacle-like' distribution of lesions around the eyes is especially characteristic. The chest,

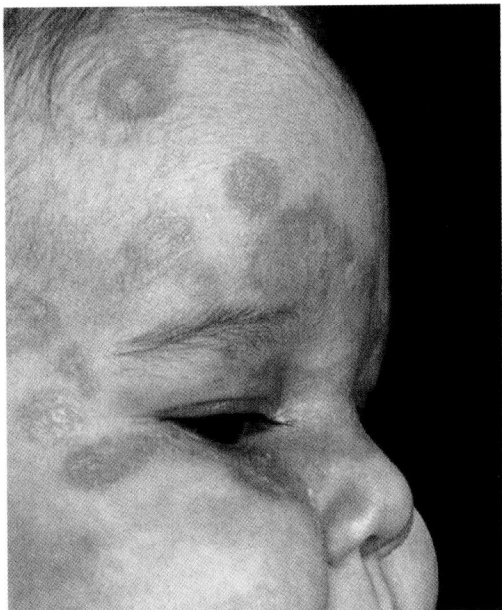

Figure 116.2 Neonatal lupus erythematosus showing fading facial lesions in a characteristic periorbital distribution, with residual atrophy, in a 4-month-old infant.

back or limbs may also be affected [20,21–23]. Provocation or exacerbation of lesions by sun exposure has been reported in some cases.

Follicular plugging is not prominent, but scaling is a common early feature. A degree of atrophy and/or telangiectasia are frequent long-term sequelae. Permanent hair loss may occur.

In most cases, the skin lesions have resolved within the first year, but areas of atrophy and/or telangiectasia may be more persistent [24]. Longstanding depressions have followed subcutaneous lesions. The most frequent sites for such lesions are the temples and scalp [25].

Clinical variants

Less commonly, lesions take the form of annular erythema without an epidermal component; this type of presentation has predominantly been reported in Japanese infants [22]. Subcutaneous lesions have also been described [25].

Occasionally, neonatal LE presents as extensive reticulate erythema with atrophy, closely resembling cutis marmorata telangiectatica congenita [26,27]. Depigmentation may be very prominent in racially pigmented infants [28]. Lesions resembling morphoea have been reported [29].

Differential diagnosis

The lesions of congenital rubella or cytomegalovirus infection may need to be considered, although these are of purplish colour and purpura is generally prominent. Congenital syphilis may also need to be excluded, but whereas mucosal, periorificial and palmar and plantar lesions are common in congenital syphilis, these features are rare in neonatal LE. Confusion may be caused by the false positive antibody tests that are as much a feature of neonatal as of acquired LE.

Atrophy and telangiectasia of the cheeks is seen with photosensitivity in Bloom syndrome (see Chapter 79), and without photosensitivity (in most cases) in the Rothmund–Thomson syndrome (see Chapter 77). In these disorders, skin lesions are not present at birth and generally appear later than in neonatal LE.

Complications and co-morbidities

Systemic features are detectable in over half of all affected infants, of which cardiac involvement is the commonest. Congenital heart block (due to fibrosis of the conducting tissue) occurs in about 1–2% of Ro-positive pregnancies, probably due to genetic susceptibility [2,30–34]. In these families it will recur in 20% of subsequent pregnancies [3]. Anti-Ro antibodies can bind to cardiac conduction cells during mid to late fetal development, leading to altered membrane repolarization and selective damage to the atrioventricular node. Congenital heart block can be detected as early as the 18th week of gestation by ultrasound or electrocardiography [33]. The block is generally permanent, and is not associated with structural cardiac abnormalities such as septal defects. About a half of affected infants require pacemakers [32,33].

A smaller proportion of infants have combinations of hepatomegaly, splenomegaly, lymphadenopathy and pneumonitis, which are generally mild in degree and fairly transient. Autoimmune haemolytic anaemia and thrombocytopenia are seen in a small proportion of affected infants [35].

Central nervous system may be involved in neonatal LE and this can cause an asymptomatic vasculopathy or a more serious cerebral vasculitis [36,37].

Disease course and prognosis

Infants with skin lesions alone, or with skin lesions and systemic features other than heart block, generally show little sign of residual disease after the age of 1 year [38]. However, their long-term prognosis must remain slightly at risk in the light of reports of the later development by some of full-blown connective tissue disease [32,39,40]. Conduction defects of the heart tend to be permanent, and when severe are associated with a significant mortality [2,32,41].

The risk of recurrence in further pregnancies appears to be about 20–25% [2,3]. Spontaneous abortion and stillbirth do not appear to be more frequent in further pregnancies of mothers who have had a previous child with neonatal LE [2].

Neonatal LE antibodies disappear from the infant's serum within about 6 months.

Investigations

A skin biopsy will usually allow an accurate diagnosis of neonatal LE, particularly if combined with direct immunofluorescence studies, and tests for the appropriate circulating autoantibodies in both the mother and the child.

Management

The skin lesions of neonatal LE require no treatment, but sun protection is essential.

Occasionally, thrombocytopenia, haemolytic anaemia or hepatitis may warrant systemic steroid therapy [42]. Up to 50% of infants with cardiac involvement will require a pacemaker [22].

The pregnancy of a woman who has Ro, La or U_1-RNP antibodies should be monitored to detect a slow fetal heart rate [43,44]. Treatment with high-dose systemic steroids may be indicated for fetal bradycardia where there are signs of heart failure [45].

Resources

Further information

Medscape, neonatal and pediatric lupus erythematosus: http://emedicine.medscape.com/article/1006582-overview#aw2aab6b2b4 (last accessed December 2014).

Patient resources

Lupus UK: www.lupusuk.org.uk/ (last accessed December 2014).

Transplacental transfer of maternal malignant disease

Transplacental transfer of maternal malignant disease is fortunately extremely rare, despite the fact that malignancy occurs in one in 1000 pregnancies [1,2], and it is well established that maternal cells regularly reach the fetus.

The malignancy transferred in this way has been melanoma in about 90% of cases, although this particular malignancy accounts for only about 8% of those occurring in pregnant women [3]. Melanoma transmitted in this way may result in the appearance of nodular skin deposits in the neonate. Spontaneous regression of transplacentally transferred melanoma has been reported [4,5].

Transplacental transmission of acute monocytic leukaemia [6], natural killer cell lymphoma [7] and choriocarcinoma [8] have also been reported.

Checking the maternal origin of a tumour in a neonate can be done quickly by a quantitative polymerase chain reaction (PCR) technique [9,10].

Transfer of toxic substances in maternal milk

When considering the cause of any rash in a young infant, the possibility that it reflects exposure of the mother to a toxic substance that has been transferred in her milk needs to be borne in mind. A good example is provided by two reports of bromoderma occurring in neonates whose mothers had taken bromide medicinally [1] or had been accidentally exposed in a photographic laboratory [2].

DISORDERS OF SUBCUTANEOUS FAT

Four separate conditions are described – cold panniculitis, neonatal cold injury, subcutaneous fat necrosis of the newborn and sclerema neonatorum – but there is some clinical and pathological overlap.

Cold panniculitis

Cold panniculitis is a distinctive form of panniculitis provoked directly by cold exposure, to which infants appear particularly predisposed. The fat of the newborn appears to be more highly saturated than that of older children and adults, with the effect that it solidifies at a higher temperature [1,2]. Applying ice for 50 s causes panniculitis in all newborn infants, in only 40% of 6-month-old infants and almost never in 9-month-old infants [3].

Cold panniculitis in infancy has most often followed exposure of the cheeks to: (i) extremely cold air [4]; (ii) ice bags applied as a therapy for supraventricular tachycardia [5,6]; or (iii) frozen lollies (popsicles) [7,8]. Indurated, warm, red, subcutaneous plaques and nodules appear within hours or days of appropriate cold exposure. Skin biopsy is not usually needed but if done early it shows a lymphohistiocytic infiltrate around blood vessels at the junction of the dermis and subcutaneous fat [9]. After a few days, lipocyte rupture leads to the formation of cystic cavities surrounded by areas of marked infiltration by lymphocytes and histiocytes, with a few neutrophils and eosinophils. The induration resolves over a period of a week or so, often leaving some residual postinflammatory hyperpigmentation. No treatment is required.

Neonatal cold injury

Neonatal cold injury is a disorder, now rare in developed countries, in which cold exposure of a small-for-dates neonate causes hypothermia associated with lethargy and generalized pitting oedema of the skin, clinically and pathologically distinct from sclerema neonatorum. A low environmental temperature has been the principal cause of virtually all reported cases of this disorder [1–3,4]. Other factors that appear to have predisposed babies to this complication of cold exposure include intrauterine growth retardation, which results in a relatively thin panniculus, and tight wrappings, which restrict muscular activity.

The infant is usually a full-term neonate, born at home, but small for gestational age. In the great majority of cases, presentation is within the first 4 days of life, and usually during the first 24 h. The most striking features are intense erythema or cyanosis of the face and extremities, and firm, pitting oedema beginning at the extremities and spreading centrally, and becoming progressively more indurated in a proportion of cases [1–3,4]. Petechiae have occasionally been observed. The skin feels cold, and the baby is usually hypothermic with a low core temperature. Associated non-cutaneous features of cold injury are generally present, and may occur in the absence of skin changes. These include immobility, drowsiness, poor feeding, vomiting, oliguria and gastrointestinal bleeding with vomiting of altered blood or melaena.

Skin biopsy shows a thin panniculus; otherwise there is little obvious abnormality apart from dilatation of the dermal blood vessels [5]. Profuse exudation of clear fluid from the cut surface at postmortem suggests that the induration is due to oedema.

The mortality rate of historical cases was about 25% (usually due to massive pulmonary haemorrhage). Fortunately, the condition seems to be much less common in the UK now than it was 40 years ago, probably because of improved heating in homes, reduced frequency of home delivery and abandonment of the previous habit of bathing babies at birth.

Subcutaneous fat necrosis of the newborn

Definition

Subcutaneous fat necrosis of the newborn is an uncommon and transient disorder of neonates in which focal areas of fat necrosis cause nodular skin lesions [1,2].

Epidemiology

Incidence and prevalence
The incidence is unknown but the disease is rare.

Age
Subcutaneous fat necrosis generally occurs in full-term or post-term infants of normal birth weight during the first 6 weeks of life.

Sex
There is an equal sex incidence.

Ethnicity
This is an unknown influence.

Associated diseases
Maternal pre-eclampsia, diabetes, perinatal asphyxia and hypothermia may be associated [1,2,3–7,8,9].

Pathophysiology

Predisposing factors
The precise cause is unestablished, but a variety of insults appear to have contributed in individual cases. These have included birth asphyxia, maternal pre-eclampsia, maternal diabetes, obstetric trauma, hypothermia and hypothermic cardiac surgery [1,2,3–7,8,9]. The most important predisposing factors appear to be the combination of local tissue hypoxia and cold injury. A primary abnormality in brown fat has also been postulated [10].

Pathology
Biopsies of the affected subcutaneous tissue show patchy fat necrosis, with a granulomatous inflammatory reaction of foreign-body type, and fibrosis [1,11,12]. Both the fat cells and the giant cells contain needle-shaped clefts, which may be radially arranged. Fibrotic obliteration of small arterioles has also been observed. Calcium deposits are commonly found in the necrotic fat.

Ultrastructural examination has shown parallel aggregations of electron-lucent, needle-shaped spaces within the adipocytes [11,12]. Similar changes in visceral adipose tissue have been reported in postmortem studies of affected infants [3]. Widespread calcium deposition in internal organs has also been shown in postmortem specimens from hypercalcaemic cases and nephrocalcinosis has been observed in such infants during life [13].

Environmental factors
Hypoxia, cold and trauma all seem to play a role.

Clinical features

Presentation
Infants who develop subcutaneous fat necrosis are generally full-term or post-term neonates of normal weight [1,2,3,7,8,9]. Nodular thickening of the subcutaneous tissues is usually first detected between the second and 21st days of life. Sometimes, the changes are present at birth, and, rarely, they may appear as late as the sixth week. The nodules tend to be symmetrically distributed and show a predilection for the buttocks, thighs, shoulders, back, cheeks and arms. Lesions may be single or multiple, rounded or oval, and pea-sized or many centimetres in diameter. They are initially discrete, but may fuse to form large plaques. The overlying skin is often red or bluish red. The nodules feel rubbery or hard, and are not attached to deeper structures. The lesions may be painful [14]. New nodules may continue to develop for a week or more.

In most cases, the child's health is not substantially impaired, and within a few months the nodules disappear. Where calcium deposition is marked, the lesions may take rather longer to resolve. Usually no trace of the nodules remains but there may be slight atrophy. Rarely, the nodules may ulcerate, discharge their fatty contents and leave scars.

The condition has occasionally been fatal, particularly when visceral fat has been involved [3], or where there has been complicating hypercalcaemia [15–19].

Clinical variants
There have been several reports of the occurrence of lesions analogous to those of subcutaneous fat necrosis of the newborn in children who have had hypothermic cardiac surgery [6,7,8]. The cutaneous application of ice to induce hypothermia, trauma and/or hypoxia may all have contributed. It is noteworthy that these children appear to have developed lesions of subcutaneous fat necrosis rather than cold panniculitis. The ages of the children at the time of surgery varied from 12 days to 20 months. Lesions appeared between 14 and 30 days later, principally at the sites subjected to the greatest cold exposure. The lesions resolve within a few weeks and no treatment is usually required.

Differential diagnosis
Neonates delivered by forceps may develop subcutaneous nodules where the forceps were applied, presumably as a result of traumatic fat necrosis. Subcutaneous fat necrosis of the newborn was in the past frequently confused with sclerema neonatorum. Occasionally, the two conditions may occur simultaneously [20].

Complications and co-morbidities
Subcutaneous fat necrosis of the newborn may be associated with hypercalcaemia, which tends to occur in around a quarter of all cases, appears more frequently in infants with extensive disease, and almost exclusively when the trunk is affected [15–19].

The cause of the hypercalcaemia is unknown. It may be due to increased calcium absorption due to extrarenal production of 1,25-dihydroxyvitamin D [17,18], which has been observed in other granulomatous disorders including sarcoidosis. The finding of increased urinary excretion of prostaglandin E_1 led to the suggestion that increased bone calcium resorption might be responsible [19].

Transient thrombocytopenia has been reported during the period of initial development of the lesions, possibly due to sequestration of platelets [21]. Plasma lipid abnormalities have been reported in a neonate with subcutaneous fat necrosis, but their relevance was unclear [22].

All infants who have experienced subcutaneous fat necrosis should have their serum calcium measured on presentation and every 2–3 weeks for up to 3 months as the increase in calcium can be delayed. If hypercalcaemia is present, its cause requires thorough investigation to exclude disorders such as primary hyperparathyroidism and vitamin D intoxication. Nephrocalcinosis is a common persistent finding even in those children who have undergone treatment for hypercalcaemia, but fortunately renal impairment is very rare.

Disease course and prognosis

The skin condition resolves over several weeks although the hypercalcaemia can persist for a few months.

Investigations

Skin biopsy is required to confirm the diagnosis. Serum calcium needs to be monitored for 3 months.

Management

No treatment is generally required as the condition spontaneously resolves over several weeks.

Analgesia may occasionally be required.

Hypercalcaemia should be treated aggressively to prevent soft-tissue calcification. Treatments include diuretics, dietary restriction of calcium and vitamin D, and sometimes oral corticosteroids [9,15,16]. In resistant cases bisphosphonates can be used [23,24].

Resources

Further information

Medscape, subcutaneous fat necrosis of the newborn: http://emedicine.medscape.com/article/1081910-overview#a0104 (last accessed December 2014).

Sclerema neonatorum

Definition

Sclerema neonatorum is classified as a neonatal panniculitis. It usually affects gravely ill, preterm neonates in the first week of life. It manifests as a hardening of skin and subcutaneous adipose tissue to such an extent that it hinders feeding and respiration, and usually culminates in death [1,2].

Epidemiology

Incidence and prevalence

It is very rare and its prevalence is unknown.

Age

Sclerema neonatorum almost always appears during the first week of life, although it has occasionally been recorded later in infants born preterm.

Sex

There is an equal sex incidence.

Associated diseases

There is underlying severe illness.

Pathophysiology

Predisposing factors

Prematurity and smallness for dates appear to be frequent predisposing factors [2]. It has been recorded as already present at birth in infants subjected to placental insufficiency [3]. The disorder does not seem to occur in otherwise healthy infants, and most characteristically develops during the course of one of a wide variety of severe illnesses, particularly serious infections, congenital heart disease and other major developmental defects [2]. A proportion of these infants have been hypothermic, and occasionally sclerema has been described as a complication of neonatal cold injury [4]. Nevertheless, cold does not appear to be an important aetiological factor in the majority of cases.

Lipolytic mechanisms are poorly developed in the newborn, particularly in those born preterm [5]. The maturation of these enzyme systems might be further compromised by major infection or hypoxia. It has been suggested that sclerema might reflect defective lipolysis within adipose tissue, which would result in failure of fat mobilization, and an impaired capacity to maintain body temperature. It has been reported that the ratio of saturated to unsaturated fatty acids is relatively high in the adipose tissue of all neonates, and that this ratio was even higher in an infant with sclerema [6]. This would lead to a raised melting point, and it is possible that the induration of subcutaneous fat, which is the major clinical feature of sclerema, might reflect its solidification due to a fall in the temperature of the adipose tissue during peripheral circulatory collapse.

Pathology

In most cases the subcutaneous fat layer appears to be thickened due to an increased size of the individual lipocytes and to an increased width of the intersecting bands of connective tissue, probably due to oedema [6,7]. There is very little evidence of fat necrosis and, generally, only the slightest indication of inflammation. The most characteristic histological feature of sclerema neonatorum is the presence of radially arranged, needle-shaped clefts in adipocytes and, occasionally, in multinucleate giant cells, reflecting the presence of crystals prior to processing.

Environmental factors

These are unclear.

Clinical features

History

Sclerema neonatorum was first described by Underwood in 1784 and was called 'skinbound disease' [1]. In 1817, Alibert introduced

Table 116.4 Distinctions between neonatal cold injury, sclerema and subcutaneous fat necrosis.

	Neonatal cold injury	Sclerema	Subcutaneous fat necrosis
Frequency	Previously common, now rare	Rare, usually seen in neonatal intensive care units	Uncommon
Patient	Full-term neonates, often small for dates, born at home	Usually severely ill neonates, often preterm or small for dates or post-term	Healthy infants, usually full term
Onset	During the first week	Almost always during the first week	1–6 weeks
Sites	Extremities, spreading centrally	Lower limbs initially becoming generalized	Trunk, buttocks, thighs, arms, face
Appearance	Pitting oedema initially with erythema or cyanosis of face and extremities	Diffuse, yellow-white, woody induration with immobility of limbs	Firm, reddish violet, subcutaneous nodules
Histology	Thin panniculus	Subtle; thickened connective tissue trabeculae, radial needle-like clefts	Granulomatous inflammation, fat necrosis
Prognosis	Mortality around 25%	Poor; mortality greater than 50% in past	Generally excellent

the term sclerema, derived from the Greek word *skleros*, meaning hard.

Presentation

Sclerema neonatorum is a very rare disorder that almost always appears during the first 1–2 weeks of life [1,2,3]. It has generally been considered a non-specific sign of severe illness, and has been associated with a mortality up to 75%. The affected infant is generally very ill at the time of onset of sclerema. Woody induration of the skin starts on the buttocks, thighs or calves and extends rapidly and symmetrically to involve almost the whole surface, with the exception of the palms, soles and genitalia. This skin is hard and cold to touch, and yellowish white in colour, often with purplish mottling. It will not pit with pressure. Mobility is limited, and as a result the face may take on a mask-like expression.

Differential diagnosis

The main area of diagnostic confusion has been between sclerema and subcutaneous fat necrosis [8,9]. It is now clear that the two disorders are distinct pathologically and clinically, although rarely they can occur together. Table 116.4 outlines their distinguishing features.

Scleredema has been reported in an infant at 2 weeks of age, and was distinguished from sclerema principally on histological grounds [10]. Turner syndrome is often recognizable at birth by the presence in a female of firm, non-pitting lymphoedema of the dorsa of the hands and feet, associated with low birth weight and loose folds of skin around the neck. Where primary lymphoedema occurs in neonates, it will already be clinically evident at birth. The condition may be familial, and generally first affects the legs, particularly the lower legs. The presence of oedema at birth, and its very slow progression in an otherwise healthy neonate, distinguish primary lymphoedema from sclerema.

Complications and co-morbidities

Respiratory insufficiency occurs due to restricted movement of the chest wall.

Disease course and prognosis

The prognosis is poor, and is largely determined by the nature of the underlying disease. In spite of advances in the treatment of

many of the predisposing disorders, particularly sepsis, the mortality probably remains in excess of 50%. In infants who survive, the appearance of the skin returns to normal without long-term complications such as calcification.

Investigations

Skin biopsy is the most useful test.

Management

First line

Treatment of the underlying medical condition(s) in a neonatal unit is the key to survival.

Second line

Systemic corticosteroids [11] are probably not effective but there is evidence that repeated exchange transfusions [12,13] and intravenous immunoglobulin [14] may be helpful in some cases.

Resources

Further information

Medscape, sclerema neonatorum: http://emedicine.medscape.com/article/1112191-overview (last accessed December 2014).

MISCELLANEOUS DISORDERS

Raised linear bands of infancy

Definition and nomenclature

These are raised bands found on the skin, usually of the legs, in the first few months after birth.

Synonyms and inclusions
- Persistent linear bands of infancy
- Acquired raised bands of infancy

Introduction and general description

Raised linear bands of infancy was first described in 2002 in two premature babies [1]. Thirteen cases have since been described in both premature and term babies [2,3–7].

Epidemiology

Incidence and prevalence

It is unknown but very rare.

Age

The onset is usually at 1–2 months of age.

Sex

There is a female to male ratio of 8 : 5.

Associated diseases

In a few cases amniotic band syndrome may be present with potential limb defects obvious from birth.

Pathophysiology

The cause is unknown but various theories have been postulated revolving around the possibility of an abnormal reaction to pressure on the skin [5,6]. In the first four cases described, three of the children were born prematurely (28–31 weeks) and there was documented evidence of amniotic bands or placental abruption/placental tears [1,2,3,4]. Short toes and a club foot were described in two of these children. It was therefore suggested that either amniotic bands or some undetermined prenatal insult was the cause. However of the 13 cases described, nine were in term children with no documented evidence of amniotic bands or limb constriction/defects. Marque *et al.* postulated in their three cases that the lesions arose exactly under where tight socks had been worn and the pressure effect of clothing may be relevant [6]. However, lesions have been described on the trunk, the buttocks and much higher up the leg where it seems less likely that occlusive clothing is an aetiological factor [3,4].

Pathology

Skin biopsy is usually unremarkable. There maybe a little oedema in the dermis and fat, but the collagen and elastin are normal [1,2,3,4]. There are no signs of smooth muscle or lipomatous naevus. One author has described a dermal infiltrate of adipocytes along blood vessels and eccrine ducts in two cases and suggested a similar aetiology to post-traumatic piezogenic pedal papules [5].

Genetics

It is not known if there is an underlying genetic cause. Two familial cases have been described (brother and sister) but no consanguinity has been recorded.

Clinical features

History

The raised bands typically present in the first few months of life. They are often multiple and can be symmetrical. They are common on the legs but may be found on the upper limbs and rarely the trunk. They vary from 1 to 3 mm across.

Presentation

The lesions are palpable and firm but not hard.

Differential diagnosis

This includes amniotic band syndrome/congenital pseudoainhum. Whilst in a few cases, amniotic bands have been suggested as a potential cause for raised linear bands of infancy the amniotic band syndrome is a separate, more severe entity presenting with constrictions at birth. These may lead to limb malformations, lymphoedema and even ischaemia and autoamputation (congenital pseudoainhum). Constriction bands may also occur in other conditions such as Michelin tyre baby syndrome. If the amniotic band syndrome occurs early *in utero* malformations tend to be more extensive and include alopecia, aplasia cutis, neural tube defects, cranio-facial defects as well as limb constriction bands; ultrasound and Doppler are used to assess limbs. Treatment is difficult in this condition and is by fetoscopic surgery when possible [7,8,9].

Classification of severity

It is a benign, non-progressive but persistent condition.

Disease course and prognosis

The condition persisted in all but one case (longest follow-up to date is 18 years [5]).

Investigations

Most cases can be diagnosed clinically but a skin biopsy (which is essentially normal) may occasionally be required to exclude other conditions like Michelin tyre baby syndrome. The finding of adipocyte infiltrates along blood vessels by one author needs to be confirmed in other cases.

Management

Reassurance is usually all that is required and explaining that the lesions will probably persist lifelong. One case failed to respond to oral antihistamines. One case was treated with topical antihistamines and the lesions resolved within 3 months. This case was not biopsied and had some atypical features in that it presented late, at 6 months (much later than the usual 1–3 months) in a child with marked dermographism [10]. Also, the clinical pictures showed more urticated and wider lesions than typical limb bands.

Neonatal adnexal polyp

Solitary, self-healing, polypoid lesions have been observed in some 4% of neonates in a Japanese survey [1,2]; their occurrence in other racial groups has yet to be documented. These lesions are firm, pink, polypoid nodules, about 1 mm in diameter, usually found close and medial to one or other nipple. Histology shows a normal epidermis, a vascular dermis containing prominent hair follicles with vestigial sebaceous glands and well-developed eccrine glands. These lesions generally separate from the skin spontaneously after a few days but they may persist in early life [3,4].

Collodion baby

Definition and nomenclature
This term describes a highly characteristic clinical entity present at birth where a child is born with an 'extra' skin resembling a shiny membrane or collodion.

Synonyms and inclusions
• Lamellar desquamation/exfoliation of the newborn

Introduction and general description
Collodion baby is a distinctive phenotype present at birth. It usually precedes the development of one of a variety of ichthyoses, the commonest of which are the autosomal recessive ichthyoses [1,2].

Epidemiology

Incidence and prevalence
The incidence of collodion baby is approximately one per 100 000 deliveries [3].

Age
It presents at birth.

Sex
There is a slight predominance in males.

Ethnicity
There is an equal distribution.

Associated diseases
Almost 90% of collodion babies will go on to develop a severe form of autosomal recessive ichthyosis in the first few weeks of life: lamellar ichthyosis and non-bullous ichthyosiform erythroderma (syn. congenital ichthyosiform erythroderma) are the most common (see Chapter 65) [1,2]. The collodion baby phenotype is also reported in the rarer autosomal dominant form of lamellar ichthyosis [4] and in bathing suit ichthyosis [5]; it is also characteristic of the trichothiodystrophy–ichthyosis syndrome [6,7].

There are other ichthyoses in which an initial collodion baby phase has occasionally been reported. These include the Netherton syndrome [1], neutral lipid storage disease [8], Loricrin keratoderma (syn. Camisa's keratoderma) [9] and Sjögren–Larsson syndrome [1], but the great majority of neonates with these disorders do not demonstrate the collodion baby phenotype. A transient collodion membrane has also been reported in Gaucher disease [10].

In about 10% of cases, the collodion baby phase is followed by a relatively mild ichthyosis of lamellar type or indeed normal skin (self-healing ichthyosis) [11,12].

Pathophysiology

Predisposing factors
Underlying genetic mutations predispose to this condition.

Pathology
Skin biopsy at birth is rarely done as it is a clinical diagnosis. The pathology does not help predict the outcome of the skin disease. Histologically the membrane is a compact, thickened orthokeratotic stratum corneum: the epidermis and dermis are both relatively normal [1,13,14]. Genetic diagnosis has become increasingly available and affordable.

Genetics
A variety of genotypes can present with the phenotpype of collodion baby.

Clinical features

Presentation
The severely affected infant is bright red and encased in a taut, glistening, yellowish, translucent covering resembling collodion [1,2,15]. The face is immobilized; tension on the skin results in ectropion, eversion of the lips (eclabion), producing a rather fish-like appearance of the mouth, and effacement of the nose and ears. The nostrils may be blocked. The skin over the fingers, hands, toes and feet may result in immobility and may interfere with blood flow, occasionally resulting in the loss of parts of the digits.

Within hours, this membrane dries and cracks, and bleeding may occur along the resulting fissures. Within 1 or 2 days, it starts to peel off, either in extensive sheets or as large, light brown scales, but may reform several times. The shedding will generally be more or less complete within 4 weeks. Subsequently, the typical features of one of several varieties of ichthyosis gradually emerge over a period of weeks or months.

During the first day or two, tightness of the skin on the thorax may interfere with respiration, and very occasionally, respiratory distress may be caused by nasal obstruction.

Clinical variants
Rarely, the collodion phenotype can be confined to acral areas. This usually heals spontaneously ('acral self-healing collodion baby') [12].

Differential diagnosis
The appearance of the collodion baby is unmistakable. However, a baby with a severe collodion phenotype (marked ectropion and eclabium) may be confused with harlequin ichthyosis as the facial appearances can be similar (see Chapter 65). However a child with harlequin ichthyosis has much thicker skin, which typically encases the baby like a suit of armour with deep fissures. Harlequin ichthyosis shows almost fusion of the fingers and toes with thick palmoplantar skin. Finally, the ears are usually bound down to the scalp in harlequin ichthyosis whereas they are normally 'free' in collodion babies.

Restrictive dermopathy also results in a neonate with tight and immobilizing skin, but in this condition the skin appears thin and transparent, with prominent underlying blood vessels. The mouth is also open, but ectropion is not present. The skin does not dry out and come away. Death occurs rapidly as a consequence of respiratory failure.

Neonates with the lethal autosomal recessive Neu–Laxova syndrome may have skin changes closely resembling a collodion membrane. The condition is characterized by intrauterine growth retardation, and central nervous system, skeletal and cranial abnormalities.

Complications and co-morbidities

The collodion baby is at risk, largely because of the consequences of losing the skin barrier function [16]. This results in the following:
- Impaired temperature regulation.
- Increased insensible water loss, hypernatraemic dehydration and acute renal failure [17,18].
- Septicaemia (bacterial, *Candida*).
- Percutaneous toxicity from topical medicaments (increased absorption).
- Respiratory failure. Respiration may be impaired as a result of intrapartum aspiration of squamous debris shed into the amniotic fluid. Immobility of the chest may also compromise respiratory function, and predispose to pneumonia [19].

With good neonatal care mortality figures have fallen from 50% in the 1960s to less than 5% today in the western world.

Disease course and prognosis

The longer term outlook depends on which type of ichthyosis develops, and it is important to be aware that there is no correlation between initial severity in a collodion baby and the gravity of the ichthyosis that follows. Whilst advances in genetics should soon allow routine genetic screening of collodion babies, the genotype does not always correlate well with phenotype so a 'wait and see' policy is still required.

Investigations

Genetic analysis, if available.

Management

The most important element in treatment is an awareness of the possible medical complications from skin barrier failure. The baby should be nursed in an incubator in a high-humidity atmosphere, with careful monitoring of body temperature (overheating can also be an issue). Great attention needs to be given to fluid and electrolyte balance [20]. In severe cases, fluid therapy should be given intravenously, but in less severe cases oral or naso-gastric fluid supplementation will suffice. Peritoneal dialysis may be indicated if renal failure occurs. Fluid loss is significantly reduced by frequent applications of lipid; a 50%/50% mixture of white soft paraffin and liquid paraffin is ideal for this purpose. Frequent oiling of the skin increases mobility and comfort, accelerates healing of fissures and may reduce the risk of infection [21]. Supplemental feeds may be needed via a naso-gastric tube. Avoid topical products that contain active compounds (e.g. urea or salicylic acid) as toxicity is a real risk due to absorption.

Prevention of infection is of the greatest importance in saving these babies. Great attention should be paid to this aspect of care. Skin punctures should be kept to a minimum, and vascular access should be avoided as far as possible. Deeper fissures are more likely to become infected especially if inflamed, so regular swabs should be done for bacteria and *Candida* as septicaemia is a common complication [20].

Bands of tight skin constricting the digits, hands or feet may occasionally require surgical division.

Resources

Further information

Medscape, lamellar ichthyosis: http://emedicine.medscape.com/article/1111300-overview (last accessed December 2014).

Patient resources

Foundation for Ichthyosis and Related Skin Typss: www.firstskinfoundation.org/. Ichthyosis Support Group: www.ichthyosis.org.uk
(Both last accessed December 2014.)

'Blueberry muffin' baby (dermal erythropoiesis)

This term has been used to describe a characteristic eruption in neonates, often present at birth, comprising widespread, purple, erythematous, oval or circular macules, papules and nodules reflecting dermal erythropoiesis. There may be frank petechiae on the surface of some of the lesions. Favoured sites include the trunk, head and neck. The lesions generally fade into light brown macules within a few weeks of birth.

The 'blueberry muffin' type of lesion has been recorded in a number of congenital infections and is also described in a variety of congenital haematological disorders (Table 116.5).

Histologically the lesions show foci of dermal erythropoiesis. The reticular dermis contains aggregates of nucleated and non-nucleated erythrocyte precursors, but generally no cells of myeloid or megakaryocytic type. It is possible that this process represents persistence and exaggeration of the dermal erythropoiesis that is a normal occurrence in early fetal development.

Table 116.5 Causes of blueberry muffin baby.

Underlying disease process	Specific examples
Congenital infections	Rubella, cytomegalovirus, Coxsackie B2, syphilis, toxoplasmosis [1,2,3–6]
Haematological	Hereditary spherocytosis, Rhesus haemolytic anaemia, ABO blood group incompatibility, twin–twin transfusion syndrome [7,8,9]
Drug induced	Erythropoietin [10]
Neoplasia[a]	Congenital leukaemia, neuroblastoma, congenital rhabdomyosarcoma, Langerhan Cell Histiocytosis [11,12,13–17]
Inflammatory[a]	Neonatal lupus erythematosus

[a]Show 'blueberry muffin-like' lesions but dermal erythropoeisis is not always present histologically.

Neonatal purpura fulminans

Neonatal purpura fulminans is a potentially lethal disorder characterized by progressive haemorrhagic necrosis of the skin associated with cutaneous vascular thrombosis. It is usually due to a genetically transmitted thrombophilic disorder: most commonly homozygous deficiency of protein C or, less frequently, protein S [1–6]. Protein C resistance has also been reported, due to mutations in the factor V gene [7,8]. In the older child, purpura fulminans is a highly characteristic feature of meningococcal septicaemia, where it results from acquired deficiency of protein C or S. Rarely, even neonatal purpura fulminans can occur due to infection, such as group B *Streptococcus*, meticillin-resistant *Staphylococcus aureus*, varicella and measles [9,10,11,**12**].

The skin lesions most characteristically appear within the first 12 h of life but their initial development may occasionally be delayed. They generally comprise more or less symmetrical and well-defined 'lakes' of confluent ecchymosis, without petechiae [1–8,**9**,10,11,**12**,**13**]. The lesions occur most often on the limbs, particularly at sites of pressure, but may also appear on the trunk and on the face and scalp. The onset is sudden, and the lesions enlarge rapidly, with coalescence and the development of haemorrhagic bullae and central necrosis. There is surrounding erythema and the lesions are tender. The patient is frequently febrile. These infants are also at risk of thrombosis in the central nervous system and in the retinal vessels. There is a substantial danger of internal haemorrhage, shock and death.

Treatment should be carried out in a specialist neonatal unit [6,**12**,**13**]. Initially, fresh frozen plasma should be given urgently in a dose of 10–15 mL/kg/12 h. If protein C deficiency is confirmed, onward therapy with protein C concentrate should continue until the skin lesions have healed. Longer term treatment is with oral anticoagulants. Liver transplantation can be curative. Any concomitant infection needs to be treated as well.

INFECTIONS

Although infectious diseases affecting the skin are described in detail elsewhere in this book, the clinical features of some of the more important infections affecting the skin during the neonatal period will be briefly considered here because of their importance in the differential diagnosis of other dermatoses.

Viral infections

Neonatal herpes simplex

Herpes simplex virus infection in the newborn is generally a serious disease with a high mortality (see also Chapter 25). The incidence is about 7/100 000 live births and up to 40% of such infants are premature [1]. The majority of such infections result from transmission of HSV type 1 (20%) and HSV type 2 (80%) through the contact with an infected genital tract during delivery [1–3]. However, intrauterine

HSV infection rarely occurs (5% of all neonatal HSV infections) [4], due either to transmission across the placenta or to ascending infection related to prolonged rupture of the fetal membranes. Intrauterine HSV is usually due to HSV type 2 and is more common when the HSV is a primary and/or disseminated infection in the mother. Infection may also occur postnatally by contact with non-genital sites, both maternal and non-maternal [5].

Most infants with neonatal HSV infection are born to mothers who have no previous history of genital HSV and who show no overt clinical signs of herpes at delivery.

Over 70% of all infants with neonatal HSV infection have skin or mucosal lesions [6,**7**], but only in about 10% will the disease be confined to the skin. The skin lesions appear between days 2 and 20, unless intrauterine infection has occurred, in which case they will generally already be present at birth [4,8].

Isolated or grouped vesicles are the most common type of lesion, and the scalp and face are the most commonly affected sites, although lesions can occur at virtually any site (Figure 116.3). Occasionally, the eruption may be generalized and bullous, and widespread erosions may occur without obvious vesicles or bullae, mimicking epidermolysis bullosa [8]. When infection is acquired during birth, the initial lesions have a predilection for the scalp in vertex presentations, and the perianal area in breech presentations. Lesions may also be localized to areas of intrauterine or intrapartum skin damage [9], such as the area in which a fetal scalp electrode was sited. Areas of cutaneous atrophy or scarring are not infrequent in the intrauterine form, and vesicular lesions may continue to appear within or at the periphery of these areas [4,10]. A zosteriform pattern has also been described, and, in some cases [11], localized or generalized non-vesicular erythematous macules. Congenital cutaneous calcification has been reported in a child with intrauterine HSV infection [12].

Oral lesions are also frequent, and take the form of erosions on the tongue, palate, gingivae and buccal mucosa.

A fatal outcome is unusual when infection is limited but mortality is high in disseminated or central nervous system infections even with appropriate therapy. Mortality is also higher with HSV

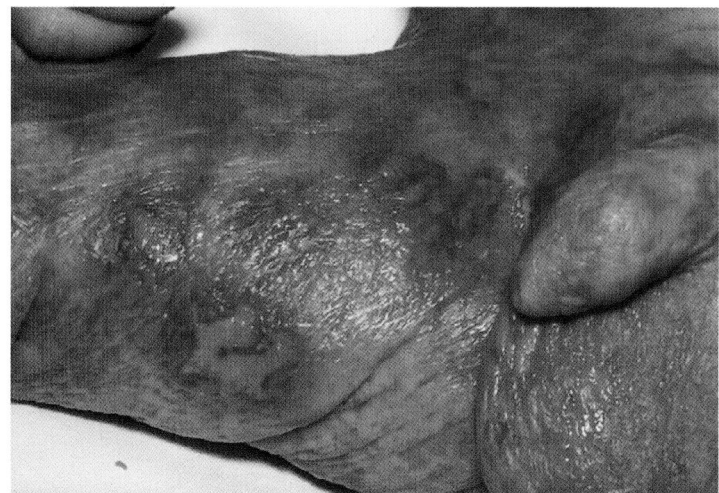

Figure 116.3 Neonatal herpes simplex showing congenital ulceration and scarring at 10 days. This infant responded rapidly to aciclovir therapy and is now entirely healthy apart from residual atrophy.

type 2 infection [2]. Early recognition and adequate early treatment with aciclovir appears to protect infants from dissemination of infection where this is initially confined to the skin [9,10,13].

HSV infection in premature infants is even more severe in terms of clinical outcomes. In one study, nine of 12 infants died and the other three had neurological sequelae [14]. It is also more difficult to diagnose as vesicular lesions are found in less than half of cases. It often presents with respiratory distress and thrombocytopenia. Non-specific signs such as lethargy, hypotension, raised aspartate transaminase and fits have also been observed. Diagnosis is by culture/PCR but treatment with intravenous aciclovir should not be delayed if HSV is suspected.

Ganciclovir (need to monitor for neutropenia) and foscarnet have also occasionally been used in treatment [15]. There is insufficient evidence to suggest that aciclovir prophylaxis in the third trimester of high-risk pregnancies affects the incidence of neonatal HSV although it will lessen the need for Caesarian section [16].

Fetal varicella syndrome

Approximately 90% of adults are seropositive for the varicella-zoster virus (VZV) antibody. If a woman is seronegative, she may develop chickenpox during pregnancy (see also Chapter 25); this occurs in up to 10 per 10 000 pregnancies [1]. The infection may be transmitted to the fetus in about 25% of cases. Such transmission of VZV to the fetus is very rare in mothers who develop herpes zoster (shingles) during pregnancy [2].

When a mother develops varicella between the seventh and 20th week of pregnancy, spontaneous abortion may follow, or the child may be born with a variety of abnormalities considered characteristic of fetal varicella syndrome (FVS) (Box 116.3) [3–5]. This appears to occur most frequently when maternal infection has occurred between weeks 13 and 20 [1]. However, most children of such mothers are born with no detectable abnormality, despite laboratory confirmation of intrauterine infection. FVS therefore appears to be a relatively rare complication of maternal varicella early in pregnancy, with a fetal risk of approximately 2% [2,5,6]. Some authors have argued that occasionally FVS can occur as late as 28 weeks into pregnancy [7].

Localized scarring, presumed to be the sequel to intrauterine ulceration, is the most common cutaneous feature of FVS. The larger single lesions have characteristically occurred on a limb, and have

---

Box 116.3 Principal clinical features of the fetal varicella syndrome

- Low birth weight
- Cutaneous lesions:
  - Localized absence of skin, usually on a limb
  - Scars, often of dermatomal outline
  - Papular lesions resembling connective tissue naevi
- Hypoplasia of one or more limbs (usually the limb affected by localized absence of skin or scarring) and/or malformed digits
- Ocular anomalies, including chorioretinitis, cataracts, microphthalmia, Horner syndrome
- Central nervous system abnormalities, including seizures, mental retardation, hydrocephalus, cortical atrophy, encephalitis, encephalomyelitis, dorsal radiculitis

---

frequently been associated with hypoplasia of that limb; these lesions have generally followed infections occurring in early pregnancy [3,6–12]. Their segmental outline may be a direct consequence of damage to the fetal nervous system [4,8], as VZV is known to be strongly neurotropic, or to fetal herpes zoster [10]. The occurrence of larger numbers of smaller lesions appears to result in the main from varicella later in the pregnancy; their antecedents seem likely to be vesicular lesions, essentially the same as those occurring in postnatal varicella. If fetal infection has occurred in the last trimester, these smaller skin lesions, reflecting fetal varicella, may still be ulcerated at birth [13].

Areas of congenital localized absence of skin, without associated limb hypoplasia or other neurological abnormalities, have been a less well-recognized consequence of intrauterine varicella [14,15], and may reflect fetal herpes zoster infection later in gestation. Skin-coloured papular lesions [16] and more verrucous lesions [17] have also been described in children with FVS.

If a child is born with 'full blown FVS' the mortality is about 25% in the first 3 months of life [1].

Herpes zoster infection in early infancy is likely to indicate that the child has been infected with VZV *in utero* [18].

Pregnant women who are not immune (on the basis of history, and, preferably, serology), and who experience exposure to varicella-zoster, should be given varicella-zoster immune globulin (VZIg) [19,20]. Although this can prevent or modify clinical varicella if given up to 3 days after contact, there is no definite evidence that it prevents fetal infection or damage [2]. Giving VZIg to neonates of mothers who have chickenpox at the time of delivery does not appear to reduce the incidence of clinical infection but may reduce its severity [21]. But, as the risk of fetal damage is small, termination of pregnancy is not indicated. Ultrasound examinations can be performed to detect some of the abnormalities that occur in the cardiovascular system, but several of the important ocular and neurological sequelae cannot be diagnosed in this way.

There are no reports that establish a role for aciclovir therapy in the prevention of FVS. Therefore, the decision whether to treat the mother should be based solely on the severity of her illness [19].

A potentially dangerous situation relates to maternal development of varicella in the 4 days either side of delivery [22]. In this case, neonatal varicella may also occur, but, in the absence of the protection offered by the maternal immune system, mortality may be as high as 30%. Where maternal infection occurs at this time, VZIg is recommended for the newborn. If overt varicella develops in the child, intravenous aciclovir should be added to the VZIg [23].

Congenital rubella

Rubella contracted by the fetus before the 20th week of gestation may result in disseminated infection, causing intrauterine growth retardation, microcephaly, microphthalmia and a wide variety of other abnormalities [1,2] (see also Chapter 25). Cutaneous lesions are among the most prominent clinical features of congenital rubella [3–5]. The typical lesions are present at birth, or make their appearance during the first 48 h. They comprise discrete, rounded, red or purple infiltrated macules, 3–8 mm in diameter. Although such lesions may be seen at any site, they generally occur in the largest numbers on the face, scalp, back of the neck and trunk. Occasionally, the lesions are slightly raised. They tend to fade over a period of weeks. These lesions have often been described as 'purpuric' and have generally been attributed to thrombocytopenia, which is another common feature of congenital rubella [4]. However, histological examination has shown them to comprise foci of dermal erythropoiesis [3,6]. Such lesions have frequently been described as 'blueberry muffin' lesions. Genuine thrombocytopenic purpura is probably rather uncommon.

Other reported skin manifestations of congenital rubella have included cutis marmorata, seborrhoea and hyperpigmentation of the forehead, cheeks and umbilical area [7], and discrete deep dimples over bony prominences, particularly the patellae [8].

Fewer cases are seen today and comprehensive vaccination programmes should allow for eradication of this condition [9].

Human immunodeficiency virus infection

Human immunodeficiency virus (HIV) infection may be transmitted to the infant *in utero*, during delivery or through breastfeeding (see also Chapter 31). Because most infections are probably transmitted around the time of birth, clinical manifestations are not commonly seen for the first few months, and some infected infants will remain asymptomatic for many years before manifestations first appear.

Mucocutaneous manifestations are common in infant HIV infection and frequently have an infective aetiology [1,2,3]. In a recent study in Ethiopia up to 75% of HIV-positive children had one or more mucocutaneous disorders – again showing infection to be more common than inflammatory disorders [4]. Studies in Tanzania [5] and Thailand [6] have shown similar results. Skin disease is more prevalent when there is a higher degree of immuosuppression.

Persistent mucocutaneous candidiasis is the commonest of all. In addition to infection of oral and napkin areas, there may be extensive cutaneous involvement. Dermatophyte fungal infections are also characteristic, and infection with more unusual fungi may occur, including *Aspergillus* [7]. Bacterial infections include unusually severe or recurring impetigo, folliculitis, cellulitis and abscesses. Problems with viruses include atypical chickenpox, herpes zoster, herpes simplex and unusually severe molluscum and human papillomavirus infections. Norwegian scabies may present in infancy.

A wide variety of non-infectious manifestations of HIV infection may also occur. In a study of Ethiopian children [4], 'papular pruritic eruption of HIV' was the most common inflammatory disorder, seen in 30% of cases. Seborrhoeic dermatitis (sometimes severe) was also common, affecting 8% of children.

Drug eruptions are more frequent, especially with trimethoprim–sulfamethoxazole.

Bacterial infections

As in older children and adults, *Staphylococcus aureus* causes a wide variety of cutaneous lesions in neonates. Other bacterial sources are important too, such as streptococci, *Listeria monocytogenes*, *Pseudomonas aeruginosa* and *Neisseria meningitidis*.

Bullous impetigo

The neonate is peculiarly liable to the development of bullous impetigo, which is most often caused by phage group II strains of *S. aureus* [1] (see also Chapter 26). The disorder in neonates differs in no significant way from that in older children and adults, although it was formerly distinguished by the rather confusing term pemphigus neonatorum. Epidemics of bullous impetigo, in which some infants may develop staphylococcal scalded skin syndrome, have occurred in neonates due to transmission of infection in the nursery principally via nursing or medical staff [2,3,4,5,6]. Although the infection is acquired in hospital following delivery, the lesions do not generally appear until the second week of life, when the child will usually have left hospital.

The perineum, periumbilical area and neck creases are predilection sites for the initial lesions. Rapidly enlarging bullae with thin, delicate walls and a narrow, red areola contain clear fluid at first, which may later become turbid or frankly purulent. The condition may remain localized or become widespread. Untreated generalized bullous impetigo in the neonate is associated with a significant mortality; serious complications including lung abscess, staphylococcal pneumonia and osteomyelitis have been reported, even in cases treated with antibiotics [7,8].

The differential diagnoses of bullae and erosions in the neonate are given in Box 116.4.

Box 116.4 Differential diagnoses of bullae and/or erosions in the neonate [9]

More common disorders
- Miliaria crystallina
- Bullous impetigo
- Thermal or chemical burns
- Sucking blisters

Rare disorders
- Mastocytosis
- Infections: neonatal herpes simplex, fetal varicella syndrome, herpes zoster, congenital syphilis
- Passively transferred: pemphigus vulgaris, pemphigoid gestationis
- Bullous pemphigoid
- Porphyrias: congenital erythropoietic porphyria, transient porphyrinaemia
- Transient myeloproliferative disorder (of Down syndrome)
- Congenital absence of skin
- Langerhans cell histiocytosis
- Extensive congenital erosions and vesicles healing with reticulate scarring
- Genodermatoses: epidermolysis bullosa, AEC syndrome, Weary syndrome/Kindler syndrome, ectodermal dysplasia–skin fragility syndrome (plakophilin-1 deficiency), bullous ichthyosiform erythroderma, incontinentia pigmenti

AEC, ankyloblepharon/ectodermal dysplasia/cleft lip and palate.

Staphylococcal scalded skin syndrome

The staphylococcal scalded skin syndrome (SSSS) was first described in neonates by a German, Ritter von Rittershain [1]. It is caused by epidermolytic toxin A and/or B, which are elaborated by certain strains of *S. aureus*, most commonly of phage group II, particularly strains 71 and 55 [2] (see also Chapter 26). These toxins reach the skin via the circulation from a distant focus of infection, usually in the umbilicus, breast, conjunctiva or site of circumcision or herniorrhaphy. Transmission of the causative toxin through human milk has been reported [3]. Both these toxins attack desmoglein 1 (a desmosomal protein), so mucosal involvement does not occur (this is analogous to pemphigus foliaceus, which has the same target antigen) [4,5].

The disorder is most often seen in young children, particularly in neonates. The very much greater incidence of this condition in neonates is believed to reflect less efficient metabolism and excretion of the toxin. Multiple cases can occur in a neonatal unit [5]. Cases occurring in later childhood tend to be associated with underlying disease, especially immunosuppression and renal failure [6].

It does not present at birth, although it may appear within the first few hours thereafter [7]. The first sign of the disease is a faint, macular, orange-red, scarlatiniform eruption [2,3]. The eruption generally becomes more extensive, and over the next 24–48 h turns to a more confluent, deep erythema with oedema. The surface then becomes wrinkled before starting to separate, leaving raw, red erosions. Sites of predilection for the development of erosions are the central part of the face, the axillae and the groins.

Extreme tenderness of the skin is an early feature, and may occur at a stage where cutaneous signs are not yet striking. The child is pyrexial and distressed. These features can lead to a suspicion that the child has arthritis or an acute abdomen. The presence of impetiginous crusting around the nose and mouth can be diagnostically helpful. Recovery is usually rapid, even without antibiotic therapy, although infants occasionally die in spite of such treatment. Healing occurs without scarring.

The scalded appearance of the skin differentiates the disease from bullous impetigo, and the rapid onset with marked cutaneous tenderness distinguishes it from most of the other causes of erythroderma in infancy. The rarity of clinically apparent bullae and the confluent nature of the rash help differentiate it from those bullous disorders likely to be seen in young children.

Milder forms of SSSS have been described where the same toxin-producing *S. aureus* is isolated but where clinically the rash starts as impetigo on the face followed by an exanthem with peeling mostly confined to the skin folds [8]. The children have mild pyrexia but no shock or fluid disturbance.

The main differential diagnosis is toxic epidermal necrolysis but this condition shows mucosal involvement. If there is any doubt, the two conditions may be distinguished by histology; a frozen section provides rapid differentiation. The level of split in toxic epidermal necrolysis is lower at the subepidermal level, but is intraepidermal in SSSS.

Treatment is with either a penicillinase-resistant penicillin analogue, such as co-amoxiclav, or with a cephalosporin or sodium fusidate [9,10]. If the attack is severe, the drug should initially be given intravenously. Systemic corticosteroids are contraindicated as they aggravate the disease [11,12]. Appropriate compensation must be made for heat and fluid losses and hyponatraemia. Pain will also require treatment, and affected infants will generally be much more comfortable if the lesions are dressed rather than left open [13]. In severe cases, it may occasionally be justifiable to ventilate the patient in order to obtain adequate relief of pain. Pneumonia itself can be a complication.

Even with treatment mortality is 2–10% in children but this usually reflects late diagnosis.

Periporitis staphylogenes and sweat gland abscesses

Periporitis staphylogenes is the term applied to pustular lesions appearing in neonatal skin as a result of secondary infection of miliaria by *S. aureus* [1,2,3,4]. Such lesions may progress to sweat gland abscesses, although it is not clear whether sweat gland abscesses are always a complication of miliaria. These disorders have in the past been incorrectly called 'folliculitis and furunculosis of the newborn'. Sweat gland abscesses are distinguished from furuncles clinically by a lack of any tendency to 'point', 'coldness' and the absence of tenderness. Outbreaks caused by medical staff in neonatal units have been described [5].

Periporitis must be distinguished from miliaria pustulosa, which is not an infective disorder, and from bacterial folliculitis, which in the neonate is usually caused by *S. aureus*. *Candida albicans* and *M. furfur* may also cause pustulosis in the neonate, and a number of non-infective conditions may cause confusion, such as eosinophilic pustulosis.

Mastitis and breast abscesses

Infection of the breast is common and is usually associated with *S. aureus*, but a variety of other bacteria may be responsible [1]. It is almost always unilateral; it occurs most commonly in the second or third week of life, more often in girls than boys, and only very rarely in the preterm infant. The affected breast is swollen and often red and hot. Systemic toxicity is usually absent. Fluctuation implies abscess formation, which will require surgical drainage [2]. Colour flow Doppler ultrasound helps distinguish mastitis from an abscess [3]. The development of a breast abscess may lead to the loss of breast tissue in the longer term [2,4].

Neonatal staphylococcal cold abscesses of the large folds

A number of neonates have been described presenting with 'cold' abscesses in the skin folds (groins and axillae) shortly after birth [1]. These children are well with no associated fever or malaise although the lesions may fistulate. Lesions have also been seen in occipital, submandibular and supraclavicular areas. There may be an associated omphalitis. Culture of pus from these lesions grows *S. aureus*. Treatment with oral antibiotics is usually sufficient and leads to rapid resolution of the lesions.

Omphalitis

Omphalitis is rare in the developed world (0.7% of births) but is more of a problem for developing countries (up to 6% of births). It is characterized by redness, oedema and discharge of the 'stump'. Cases can progress to cellulitis and deeper tissue infection. It is more common in protracted labour, non-sterile delivery and cord care, prematurity, low birth weight and some cultural practices such as the application of tobacco ash [1].

The umbilical cord may become colonized by a variety of potentially pathogenic bacteria, and an equally wide variety of topical antiseptics and antibiotics have been used in an attempt to reduce this colonization. The use of hexachlorophane was popular until it became apparent that this could lead to serious neurotoxicity, particularly in the preterm infant [2]. The best substitute may be chlorhexidine, applied as a dusting powder or aqueous solution rather than as an alcoholic solution [3]. In developing countries, 4% chlorhexidine has been shown to reduce omphalitis and to reduce neonatal mortality [4–6].

Occasionally, infection of the umbilical cord becomes disseminated, either by bloodstream invasion or by direct extension via the umbilical vessels to the peritoneal cavity. Tetanus, diphtheria and necrotizing fasciitis [7] may also occur as complications of umbilical infection. Such infections are still responsible for a high proportion of deaths in the neonatal period in developing countries.

Preorbital and orbital cellulitis

Preorbital cellulitis is restricted to the part of the orbit anterior to the orbital septum and is manifest by eyelid swelling. Orbital cellulitis involves the structures deep to the septum and presents with painful proptosis, eyelid oedema and conjunctival erythema [1]. A variety of bacteria can cause these infections, including *S. aureus* and group A and other streptococci. One should always be alert to the possibility of group B *Streptococcus* as a rare cause of periorbital cellulitis or any form of cellulitis in a neonate, in view of the high risk of septicaemia with this organism [2,3]. Treatment is with intravenous antibiotics and occasionally surgery.

Necrotizing fasciitis

This name is given to a distinctive form of cellulitis in which infection tracks along the fascial planes, causing thrombosis of the blood vessels running through the fascia with resulting necrosis of the skin, subcutaneous fat and even muscle [1,2] (see also Chapter 26). In neonates, it may arise spontaneously, but most often is a complication of physical birth trauma, omphalitis, breast abscess or iatrogenic skin

wounds such as result from scalp electrodes [3] or circumcision [4]. The mother's genital tract may also be the source of the infection [5].

Initially, the infant develops what appears to be straightforward cellulitis, usually affecting the abdominal wall. However, the child becomes disproportionately toxic, and the area affected becomes indurated, discoloured and extends progressively [2,6,7,8]. The surface may show a peau d'orange appearance. Purpura and, occasionally bullae, may develop in the centre of the indurated area, often followed quite rapidly by frank necrosis. The destruction of superficial nerves results in local cutaneous anaesthesia. Gas and crepitation may be clinically apparent, or may be seen radiologically. Fever is not invariably present.

A wide variety of bacteria have been associated with necrotizing fasciitis, most commonly group A streptococci, but also group B streptococci, *Staphylococcus aureus* and *Escherichia coli* [6,7,8]. In many cases, a synergistic infection by aerobic and anaerobic organisms appears to be responsible. Occasionally, fungi have been responsible. Antibiotic (and antifungal) therapy appears to be of limited value in this potentially lethal situation. The most important aspect of treatment is early surgical excision of the necrotic tissue [7,8]. This 'gold standard' of treatment has been challenged by some authors who advise a more conservative approach [9,10], but most doctors would still advise early surgical debridement.

Neonatal listeriosis

Listeriosis during the neonatal period is uncommon, but dangerous. The responsible organism, *Listeria monocytogenes*, may be transmitted to humans principally through contaminated foods [1]. In pregnancy, it causes a non-specific, mild, influenza-like illness in the mother [2,3], but it may lead to transplacental infection of the fetus. Maternal HIV infection may predispose to neonatal listeriosis [2]. Adult listeriosis has increased in a number of European countries during the early 21st century, but mostly in the elderly and not as yet in pregnancy-related cases [4]. Attention to food hygiene and recall of contaminated products has reduced the prevalence neonatal listeriosis by 44% in the USA. Products made with unpasteurized milk are a common source of infection.

Clinically, there are early-onset and late-onset forms of neonatal listeriosis [5–8,9,10]. The early-onset form results from the development of miliary granulomas following blood-borne dissemination of infection. Severely affected babies tend to be born prematurely and there is a high mortality. Postmortem studies reveal miliary granulomas in many organs. A few infants will have analogous miliary skin lesions during life, manifest as scattered, discrete, grey or white papules or pustules about 1–2 mm in diameter, with a red margin, which will provide a source of organisms for culture. The back appears to be the site of predilection for such lesions, which are also seen in the mouth and on the conjunctiva. Other cutaneous lesions have been described in such babies, including purpura and morbilliform rashes.

The late form of the disease is commoner, taking the form of meningitis, occurring a week or two after birth.

Diagnosis is by culturing the organism from a variety of sites, including cerebrospinal fluid, blood, urine and from biopsy material, including the skin. Treatment is usually with a combination of parenteral ampicillin with gentamicin or tobramicin, followed by a prolonged 3–4-week course of oral ampicillin.

Ecthyma gangrenosum

Pseudomonas aeruginosa is common in the hospital environment and infections are encouraged by the widespread use of broad-spectrum antibiotics (see also Chapter 26). Most, but not all, neonates who develop the skin lesions of ecthyma gangrenosum have *P. aeruginosa* septicaemia, usually in the context of predisposing factors that include prematurity, renal failure, neutropenia and other immunodeficiencies, necrotizing enterocolitis and bowel surgery [1,2,3]. Occasionally, the lesions develop at the site of direct inoculation of the causative organism. Occasionally, other bacteria have been implicated such as *E. coli* [4].

Histologically, the presence of vasculitis, due to bacterial infiltration of the vessel walls, is characteristic, together with haemorrhage and necrosis [5]. For this reason skin biopsy can be very helpful in diagnosis.

Clinically, lesions initially take the form of painful macular erythema or purple ecchymosis [1,2,3,6,7,8]. The centre then generally develops either vesicles (or less commonly bullae) or pustules, which rapidly ulcerate. Subsequently one or more ulcers occur, each with a depressed, necrotic, often black, crusted centre and a raised edge. The perioral and perianal areas may show grouped lesions.

This infection is potentially dangerous when it occurs in the setting of septicaemia. Appropriate parenterally administered combination antibiotic therapy will be required.

Noma neonatorum (cancrum oris/oro-facial gangrene)

Noma neonatorum is a gangrenous disorder of the nose, lips, mouth, perianal area and, occasionally, the scrotum and eyelids, occurring in low birth weight and/or premature neonates, almost exclusively in underdeveloped parts of the world [1,2,3]. It is frequently caused by *P. aeruginosa* and is almost invariably lethal in the absence of appropriate antibiotic treatment. A similar condition may be seen in older children and adults in the context of poor nutrition, delayed growth and immunodeficiency [4,5]. It was also seen in concentration camp victims in the Second World War.

Treatment is with parentral antibiotics and often requires plastic surgery later to repair large facial defects.

Purpura fulminans

Although in the newborn this condition is most often a reflection of genetically transmitted thrombophilic disorder, it may be caused by acute infections, particularly with endotoxin-associated, Gram-negative bacteria such as *Neisseria meningitidis* [1,2].

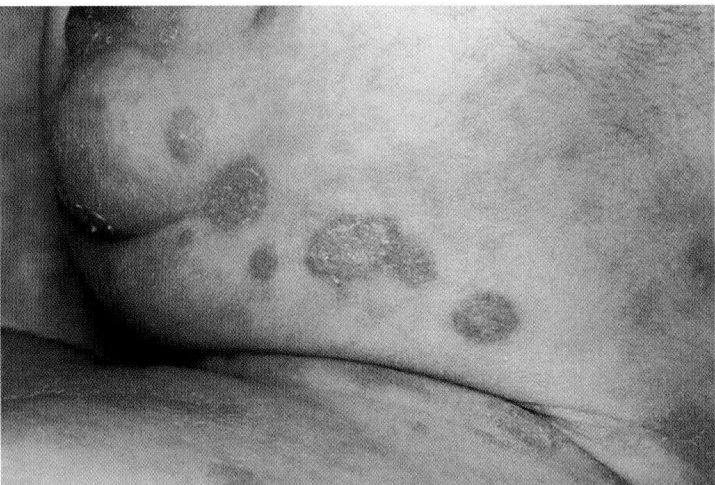

Figure 116.4 Congenital syphilis showing nummular erythematosquamous lesions in a 4-week-old infant.

Congenital syphilis

Congenital syphilis is described in detail in Chapter 29, but its cutaneous manifestations in the neonate will be considered here briefly because of their importance in differential diagnosis [1]. About 15% of children born to mothers with untreated syphilis will contract congenital syphilis, but fetal loss/still birth occurs in about 20% of such pregnancies.

The skin is clinically affected in about 40% of neonates with congenital syphilis [1,2]. In such cases, the skin is usually of normal appearance at birth, the initial lesions occurring between the second and eighth week, and occasionally later. Sites of predilection are the ano-genital area, the face and the palms and soles. The lesions themselves are reddish brown in colour; they may be macular or papular, and tend to be larger and firmer than those seen in acquired secondary syphilis (Figure 116.4). In about 3% of cases the lesions are bullous. Paronychia is commonly present. Small, round, moist, papular lesions, traditionally termed mucous patches, are frequently present in the mouth and on other mucosal surfaces. Condylomata lata may be present in the ano-genital flexures or at other flexural sites, for example between the toes or in the angles of the mouth.

Birth weight is below 2500 g in approximately 50% of affected infants. Apart from the cutaneous features, the most frequent clinical manifestations of congenital syphilis in the newborn are hepatomegaly, splenomegaly, jaundice, pneumonia and rhinitis, often with a blood-stained discharge.

The recent resurgence in the incidence of syphilis in many countries may lead to an increase in cases of congenital disease, especially where antenatal care is poor [2,3,4].

Congenital tuberculosis

Tuberculosis in the newborn due to transmission of infection *in utero* is relatively rare (see also Chapter 27). The lungs and/or liver tend to be the predominant sites of involvement, and skin manifestations are unusual. However, cutaneous lesions have occasionally occurred, in the form of small numbers of discrete, umbilicated, erythematous papules up to 4 mm in diameter [1].

Fungal infections

Both *Candida* and *Malassezia* species can cause neonatal fungal disease. There are two distinct forms of neonatal candidiasis, present at birth or seen in the first weeks of life.

Neonatal candidiasis

This is a relatively common disorder that occurs in the early weeks after birth, in the form of oral candidiasis with or without candidiasis in the napkin area (see also Chapter 32). The rash is usually focused in the perianal area, and is a deep 'beefy' red colour, with a moist appearance, often with pustules at the periphery, which is often scalloped in outline. Just beyond the margin, in as yet unaffected skin, there may be punctate erythematous lesions, sometimes pustular ('satellite' lesions).

It is assumed that the infection is acquired during delivery from the mother's genital tract, and it should be borne in mind that the frequency of vaginal candidiasis at the time of delivery is between 20% and 25% [1].

Occasionally, the rash may become more generalized. The occurrence of localized palmar pustules in an infant with neonatal oral candidiasis was believed to reflect the inoculation of *Candida* from the mouth into the skin as a result of sucking [2].

Treatment is with topical anticandidal creams and oral gels. Systemic neonatal candidiasis is a particular problem for preterm babies on intensive care units where it can cause septicaemia and death. Often there are no associated skin lesions. Treatment is with intravenous antifungal therapy.

Congenital candidiasis

This is a rarer condition, seen at birth, which is generally believed to reflect maternal *Candida* chorioamnionitis resulting from ascending infection from the genital tract [1–4,5,6,7]. It appears that *Candida* is, however, able to find its way into the amniotic fluid without prior rupture of membranes. Foreign bodies in the uterus or the cervix increase the risk, particularly intrauterine contraceptive devices [8]. There is no evidence that maternal antibiotic therapy or immunodeficiency in the infant play a role in predisposition [6,9].

An extensive eruption of scattered pinkish red macules and papules is present at birth or appears within a few hours. The lesions generally progress to a vesicular phase, and then either to a pustular or a bullous phase, over a period of 1–3 days. More or less any part of the skin surface may be affected, including the nails, palms and soles. In fact, palmar and plantar pustules are regarded as a hallmark of congenital cutaneous candidiasis. Paronychia may occur and isolated involvement of the nail plates has been described [10]. Oral involvement is usually absent, and the napkin area tends to be spared, at least initially.

Very-low-birth-weight infants may have a scalded appearance, and are particularly at risk of systemic infection.

When infection is confined to the skin, affected infants are generally well, and the rash clears within a week with appropriate topical antifungal therapy, for example with topical ketoconazole. Usually there is prominent postinflammatory desquamation.

Skin and mucosal involvement may be complicated by systemic candidiasis, particularly in the premature [2,11]. The lungs may be affected [12]; hepatosplenomegaly and abnormal liver function have also been recorded [6]. Candidal meningitis is another potential complication [13]. Criteria have been proposed that indicate a high risk of systemic involvement. Systemic antifungal therapy should be considered in at-risk infants [9]; amphotericin B is probably the drug of choice [8,11].

Studies have shown that intravenous fluconazole prophylaxis in very-low-birth-weight infants can reduce both invasive candidiasis and mortality rates [14,15,16] but a Cochrane review using oral antifungal prophylaxis in preterm infants has not shown a definitive benefit [17].

Malassezia pustulosis

Colonization of the skin by *M. furfur* starts soon after birth and progresses until the age of about 3 months, probably reflecting the activity of the sebaceous glands during this period [1,2]. This yeast has been a cause of systemic infections in infants receiving intravenous lipids, and it is presumed that the source of organisms in such cases was the skin [3].

It is now believed that *M. furfur and M. sympodialis* may be a frequent cause of erythematous papulopustular eruptions occurring on the face and scalp in neonates, a condition now widely termed neonatal cephalic pustulosis [2,4,5] although not all neonates with this clinical presentation had detectable *Malassezia* in the lesions [6]. This type of rash was reported to have a frequency of 10% in neonates seen as out-patients in a paediatric dermatology department [5], with pustule contents showing *M. furfur* yeasts in over half of these. A good therapeutic response to the topical application of 2% ketoconazole cream for 15 days was seen in almost every case. A frequency of 66% was reported in one study, with 62% being culture positive for *Malassezia* [6].

Differential diagnosis includes eosinophilic pustulosis of the scalp, transient pustular melanosis, scabies, neonatal acne and infections with *Candida* or *Staphylococcus aureus* [7].

Key references

The full list of references can be found in the online version at www.rooksdermatology.com.

Skin function in the neonate

Barrier function
5 Raone B, Raboni R, Rizzo N, *et al.* Transepidermal water loss in newborns within the first 24 hours of life: baseline values and comparison with adults. *Pediatr Dermatol* 2014;31:191–5.

6   West DP, Halket JM, Harvey DR, *et al.* Percutaneous absorption in preterm infants. *Pediatr Dermatol* 1987;4:234–7.

37   Cetta F, Lambert GH, Ros SP. Newborn chemical exposure from over-the-counter skin care products. *Clin Pediatr (Phila)* 1991;30:286–9.

Eccrine sweating

1   Szabo G. The number of eccrine sweat glands in human skin. *Adv Biol Skin* 1962;3:1–5.

4   Harpin VA, Rutter N. Sweating in preterm babies. *J Pediatr* 1982;100:614–18.

8   Munsters J, Wallström L, Agren J, *et al.* Skin conductance measurements as pain assessment in newborn infants born at 22–27 weeks gestational age at different postnatal age. *Early Hum Dev* 2012;88:21–6.

Sebaceous gland secretion

1   Rissman R, Groenink HWW, Weerheim AM, *et al.* New insights into ultrastructure, lipid composition and organization of vernix caseosa. *J Invest Dermatol* 2006;126:1823–33.

4   Visscher MO, Utturkar R, Pickens WL, *et al.* Neonatal skin maturation – vernix caseosa and free amino acids. *Pediatr Dermatol* 2011;28:122–32.

6   Agache P, Blanc D, Barrand C, *et al.* Sebum levels during the first year of life. *Br J Dermatol* 1980;103:643–9.

Appearance of neonatal skin

Full-term neonate

1   Hidano A, Purwoko R, Jitsukawa K. Statistical survey of skin changes in Japanese neonates. *Pediatr Dermatol* 1986;3:140–4.

3   Rivers JK, Frederiksen PC, Dibdin C. A prevalence survey of dermatoses in the Australian neonate. *J Am Acad Dermatol* 1990;23:77–81.

20   Barth JH. Normal hair growth in children. *Pediatr Dermatol* 1987;4:173–84.

Toxic erythema of the newborn

3   Marchini G, Nelson A, Edner J, *et al.* Erythema toxicum neonatorum is an innate immune response to commensal microbes penetrated into the skin of the newborn infant. *Pediatr Res* 2005;58:613–16.

5   Levy HL, Cothran F. Erythema toxicum neonatorum present at birth. *Am J Dis Child* 1962;103:617–19.

11   Berg FJ, Solomon LM. Erythema neonatorum toxicum. *Arch Dis Child* 1987;62:327–8.

Miliaria

3   Mowad CM, McGinley KJ, Foglia A, *et al.* The role of extracellular polysaccharide substance produced by *Staphylococcus epidermidis* in miliaria. *J Am Acad Dermatol* 1995;33:729–33.

4   Holzle E, Kligman AM. The pathogenesis of miliaria rubra. Role of the resident flora. *Br J Dermatol* 1978;99:117–37.

9   Engür D, Türkmen MK, Savk E. Widespread miliaria crystallina in a newborn with hypernatremic dehydration. *Pediatr Dermatol* 2013;30:e234–5.

Transient pustular melanosis

2   Ferrándiz C, Coroleu W, Ribera M, *et al.* Sterile transient neonatal pustulosis is a precocious form of erythema toxicum neonatorum. *Dermatology* 1992;185:18–22.

7   Van Praag MC, Van Rooij RW, Folkers E, *et al.* Diagnosis and treatment of pustular disorders in the neonate. *Pediatr Dermatol* 1997;14:131–43.

8   Chia PS, Leung C, Hsu YL, *et al.* An infant with transient neonatal pustular melanosis presenting as pustules. *Pediatr Neonatol* 2010;51:356–8.

Infantile acropustulosis

3   Vicente J, Espana A, Idoate M, *et al.* Are eosinophilic pustular folliculitis of infancy and infantile acropustulosis the same entity? *Br J Dermatol* 1996;135:807–9.

5   Prendiville JS. Infantile acropustulosis: how often is it a sequela of scabies? *Pediatr Dermatol* 1995;12:275–6.

7   Dromy R, Raz A, Metzker A. Infantile acropustulosis. *Pediatr Dermatol* 1991;8:284–7.

Neonatal pustulosis of transient myeloproliferative disorder

1   Burch JM, Weston WL, Rogers M, *et al.* Cutaneous pustular leukemoid reactions in trisomy 21. *Pediatr Dermatol* 2003;20:232–7.

2   Viros A, Garcia-Patos V, Aparicio G, *et al.* Sterile neonatal pustulosis associated with transient myeloproliferative disorder in twins. *Arch Dermatol* 2005;141:1053–4.

5   Groet J, Mc Elwaine S, Spinelli M, *et al.* Acquired mutations in GATA 1 in neonates with Down's syndrome with transient myeloid disorder. *Lancet* 2003;361:1617–20.

Congenital erosive and vesicular dermatosis healing with reticulated supple scarring

2   Gupta AK, Rasmussen JE, Headington JT. Extensive congenital erosions and vesicles healing with reticulate scarring. *J Am Acad Dermatol* 1987;17:369–76.

6   Stein S, Stone S, Paller AS. Ongoing blistering in a boy with congenital erosive and vesicular dermatosis healing with reticulated supple scarring. *J Am Acad Dermatol* 2001;45:946–8.

8   Mashiah J, Wallach D, Leclerc-Mercier S, *et al.* Congenital erosive and vesicular dermatosis: a new case and review of the literature. *Pediatr Dermatol* 2012;29:756–8.

Complications of prematurity

Anetoderma of prematurity

1   Prizant TL, Lucky AW, Frieden IJ, *et al.* Spontaneous atrophic patches in extremely premature infants: anetoderma of pregnancy. *Arch Dermatol* 1996;132:671–4.

2   Wain EM, Mellerio JE, Robson A, *et al.* Congenital anetoderma in a preterm infant. *Pediatr Dermatol* 2008;25:626–9.

4   Goujon E, Beer F, Gay S, *et al.* Anetoderma of prematurity: an iatrogenic consequence of neonatal intensive care. *Arch Dermatol* 2010;146:565–7.

Complications of medical procedures on the fetus and neonate

Antenatal procedures

2   Bruce S, Duffy JO, Wolf JE. Skin dimpling associated with midtrimester amniocentesis. *Pediatr Dermatol* 1984;2:140–2.

5   Cambiaqhi S, Restano L, Cavalli R, *et al.* Skin dimpling as a consequence of amniocentesis. *J Am Acad Dermatol* 1998;39:888–90.

9   Parvey LS, Ch'ien LT. Neonatal herpes simplex virus infection introduced by fetal monitor scalp electrodes. *Pediatrics* 1980;65:1150–3.

Phototherapy

4   Ashley JR, Littler CM, Burgdorf WHC. Bronze baby syndrome. *J Am Acad Dermatol* 1985;12:325–8.

18   Mallon E, Wojnarowska F, Hope P, *et al.* Neonatal bullous eruption as a result of transient porphyrinemia in a premature infant with hemolytic disease of the newborn. *J Am Acad Dermatol* 1995;33:333–6.

20   Paller AS, Eramo LR, Farrell EE, *et al.* Purpuric phototherapy-induced eruption in transfused neonates: relation to transient porphyrinemia. *Pediatrics* 1997;100:360–4.

Neonatal medical procedures

1   Cutler VE, Stretcher GS. Cutaneous complications of central umbilical artery catheterization. *Arch Dermatol* 1977;113:61–3.

17   Cartlidge PH, Fox PE, Rutter N. The scars of newborn intensive care. *Early Hum Dev* 1990;21:1–10.

25   Harpin VA, Rutter N. Percutaneous alcohol absorption and skin necrosis in a premature infant. *Arch Dis Child* 1982;57:477–9.

Atrophic lesions of neonates

Medallion-like dermal dendrocyte hamartoma

1   Rodriguez-Jurado R, Palacios C, Duran-McKinster C, *et al.* Medallion-like dermal dendrocyte hamartoma: a new clinically and histopathologically distinct lesion. *J Am Acad Dermatol* 2004;51:359–63.

4   Cheon M, Jung KE, Kim HS, *et al.* Medallion-like dermal dendrocyte hamartoma: differential diagnosis with congenital atrophic dermatofibrosarcoma protuberans. *Ann Dermatol* 2013;25:382–4.

5   Marque M, Bessis D, Pedeutour F, *et al.* Medallion-like dermal dendrocyte hamartoma: the main diagnostic pitfall is congenital atrophic dermatofibrosarcoma. *Br J Dermatol* 2009;160:190–3.

Disorders caused by transplacental transfer/maternal milk

Transplacental transfer of maternal autoantibodies

Neonatal pemphigus vulgaris
2 Hup JM, Bruinsma RA, Boersma ER, *et al*. Neonatal pemphigus vulgaris: transplacental transmission of antibodies. *Paediatr Dermatol* 1986;3:468–72.
8 Chowdhury MMU, Natarajan S. Neonatal pemphigus vulgaris associated with mild oral pemphigus in the mother during pregnancy. *Br J Dermatol* 1998;139:500–3.
10 Avalos-Diaz E, Olague-Marchan M, Lopez-Swiderski A, *et al*. Transplacental passage of maternal pemphigus foliaceus autoantibodies induces neonatal pemphigus. *J Am Acad Dermatol* 2000;43:1130–4.

Transplacental pemphigoid gestationis
2 Shornick JK. Herpes gestationis. *J Am Acad Dermatol* 1987;17:539–56.
7 Schornick JK, Bangert JL, Freeman RG, *et al*. Herpes gestationis: clinical and histologic features of twenty-eight cases. *J Am Acad Dermatol* 1983;8:214–24.
9 Mascaró JM, Lecha M, Mascaró JM. Fetal morbidity in herpes gestationis. *Arch Dermatol* 1995;131:1209–10.

Neonatal lupus erythematosus
10 Lee LA, Harmon CE, Huff JC, *et al*. The demonstration of SS-A/Ro antigen in human fetal tissues and in neonatal and adult skin. *J Invest Dermatol* 1985;85:143–6.
15 Korkij W, Soltani K. Neonatal lupus erythematosus: a review. *Pediatr Dermatol* 1984;1:189–95.
20 Porcel Chacón R, Tapia Ceballos L, Díaz Cabrera R, *et al*. Neonatal lupus erythematosus: a five-year case review. *Reumatol Clin* 2014;10:170–3.

Transplacental transfer of maternal malignant disease
1 Antonelli NM, Dotters DJ, Katz VL, Kuller JA. Cancer in pregnancy: a review of the literature. *Obstet Gynecol Surv* 1996;51:125–42.
6 Osada S, Horibe K, Oiwa K, *et al*. A case of infantile acute monocytic leukaemia caused by vertical transmission of the mother's leukemic cells. *Cancer* 1990;65:1146–9.
10 Raso A, Mascelli S, Nozza P, *et al*. Detection of transplacental melanoma metastasis using quantitative PCR. *Diagn Mol Pathol* 2010;19:78–82.

Disorders of subcutaneous fat

Cold panniculitis
6 Ter Poorten JC, Hebert AA, Ilkiw R. Cold panniculitis in a neonate. *J Am Acad Dermatol* 1995;33:383–5.
7 Epstein EH, Oren ME. Popsicle panniculitis. *N Engl J Med* 1970;282:966–7.
9 Duncan WC, Freeman RG, Heaton CL. Cold panniculitis. *Arch Dermatol* 1966;94:722–4.

Neonatal cold injury
1 Arneil GC, Kerr MM. Severe hypothermia in Glasgow infants in winter. *Lancet* 1963;ii:756–9.
2 Bower RD, Jones LF, Weeks MM. Cold injury in the newborn: a study of 70 cases. *BMJ* 1960;1:303–9.
3 Mann TP. Hypothermia in the newborn: a new syndrome? *Lancet* 1955;i:613–14.

Subcutaneous fat necrosis of the newborn
2 Burden AD, Krafchik BR. Subcutaneous fat necrosis of the newborn: a review of 11 cases. *Pediatr Dermatol* 1999;16:384–7.
8 Hogeling M, Meddles K, Berk DR, *et al*. Extensive subcutaneous fat necrosis of the newborn associated with therapeutic hypothermia. *Pediatr Dermatol* 2012;29:59–63.
9 Mahe E, Girszyn N, Hadj-Rabia S, *et al*. Subcutaneous fat necrosis of the newborn: a systematic evaluation of risk factors, clinical manifestations, complications and outcome of 16 children. *Br J Dermatol* 2007;156:709–15.

Sclerema neonatorum
1 Zeb A, Darmstadt GL. Sclerema neonatorum: a review of nomenclature, clinical presentation, histological features, differential diagnoses and management. *J Perinatol* 2008;28:453–60.

14 Buster KJ, Burford HN, Stewart FA, *et al*. Sclerema neonatorum treated with intravenous immunoglobulin: a case report and review of treatments. *Cutis* 2013;92:83–7.

Miscellaneous disorders

Raised linear bands of infancy
1 Meggitt SJ, Harper J, Lacour M, *et al*. Raised limb bands developing in infancy. *Br J Dermatol* 2002;147:359–63.
2 Russi DC, Irvine AD, Paller AS. Raised limb bands developing in infancy. *Br J Dermatol* 2003;149:436–7.
8 Rossillon D, Rombouts JJ, Verllen-Dumoulin C, *et al*. Congenital ring-constriction syndrome of the limbs; a report of 19 cases. *Br J Plast Surg* 1988;41:270–7.

Neonatal adnexal polyp
1 Hidano A, Kobayashi T. Adnexal polyp of neonatal skin. *Br J Dermatol* 1975;92:659–62.
2 Hidano A, Purwoko R, Jitsukawa K. Statistical survey of skin changes in Japanese neonates. *Pediatr Dermatol* 1986;3:140–4.
3 Koizumi H, Itoh E, Ohkawara A. Adnexal polyp of neonatal skin observed beyond the neonatal period. *Acta Derm Venereol* 1998;78:391–2.

Collodion baby
1 Larrègue M, Ottavy N, Bressieux JM, *et al*. Collodion baby: 32 new case reports. *Ann Dermatol Vénéréol* 1986;113:773–85.
17 Buyse L, Graves C, Marks R, *et al*. Collodion baby dehydration: the danger of high transepidermal water loss. *Br J Dermatol* 1993;129:86–8.
20 Prado R, Ellis LZ, Gamble R, *et al*. Collodion baby: an update with a focus on practical management. *J Am Acad Dermatol* 2012;67:1362–74.

'Blueberry muffin' baby (dermal erythropoiesis)
2 Bowden JB, Hebert AA, Rapini RP. Dermal hematopoiesis in neonates: report of five cases. *J Am Acad Dermatol* 1989;20:1104–10.
7 Hebert AA, Esterly NB, Gardner TH. Dermal erythropoiesis in Rh hemolytic disease of the newborn. *J Pediatr* 1985;107:799–801.
12 Gottesfeld E, Silverman RA, Coccia PF, *et al*. Transient blueberry muffin appearance of a newborn with congenital monoblastic leukemia. *J Am Acad Dermatol* 1989;21:347–51.

Neonatal purpura fulminans
9 Powars DR, Rogers ZR, Patch MJ, *et al*. Purpura fulminans in meningococcaemia associated with acquired deficiencies of proteins C and S. *N Engl J Med* 1987;317:571–2.
12 Darmstadt GL. Acute infectious purpura fulminans: pathogenesis and medical management. *Pediatr Dermatol* 1998;15:169–83.
13 Price VE, Ledingham DL, Krümpel A, *et al*. Diagnosis and management of neonatal purpura fulminans. *Semin Fetal Neonatal Med* 2011;16:318–22.

Infections

Viral infections

Neonatal herpes simplex
7 Whitley RJ, Corey L, Arvin A, *et al*. Changing presentation of herpes simplex virus infections in neonates. *J Infect Dis* 1988;158:109–16.
15 Wang Y, Smith KP. Safety of alternative antiviral agents for neonatal herpes simplex virus encephalitis and disseminated infection. *J Pediatr Pharmacol Ther* 2014;19:72–82.
16 Hollier LM, Wendel GD. Third trimester antiviral prophylaxis for preventing maternal genital herpes simplex virus (HSV) recurrences and neonatal infection. *Cochrane Database Syst Rev* 2008;Issue 1:CD004946.

Fetal varicella syndrome
1 Sauerbrei A, Wutzler P. Herpes simplex and varicella-zoster virus infections during pregnancy: current concepts of prevention, diagnosis and therapy. Part 2: Varicella-zoster virus infections. *Med Microbiol Immunol* 2007;196:95–102.
2 Enders G, Miller E, Craddock-Watson J, *et al*. Consequences of varicella and herpes zoster in pregnancy: prospective study of 1739 cases. *Lancet* 1994;343:1548–51.
21 Miller E, Cradock-Watson JE, Ridehalgh MK. Outcome in newborn babies given anti-varicella-zoster immunoglobulin after perinatal maternal infection with varicella-zoster virus. *Lancet* 1989;2:371–3.

Congenital rubella

1 Karthikeyan K, Venkatesh C, Soundararajan P. Congenital rubella syndrome: a continuing conundrum. *Lancet* 2012;379:2022.
2 Freij BJ, South MA, Sever JL. Maternal rubella and the congenital rubella syndrome. *Clin Perinatol* 1988;15:247–57.
9 Papania MJ, Wallace GS, Rota PA, *et al.* Elimination of endemic measles, rubella, and congenital rubella syndrome from the Western hemisphere: the US experience. *JAMA Pediatr* 2014;168:148–55.

Human immunodeficiency virus infection

2 Straka BF, Whitaker DL, Morrison SH, *et al.* Cutaneous manifestations of the acquired immunodeficiency syndrome in children. *J Am Acad Dermatol* 1988;18:1089–102.
3 Wananukul S, Deekajorndech T, Panchareon C, *et al.* Mucocutaneous findings in pediatric AIDS related to degree of immunosuppression. *Pediatr Dermatol* 2003;20:289–94.
4 Endayehu Y, Mekasha A, Daba F. The pattern of mucocutaneous disorders in HIV infected children attending care and treatment in Tikur Anbesa specialized hospital, Addis Ababa, Ethiopia. *BMC Dermatol* 2013;13:12.

Bacterial infections

Bullous impetigo

3 Dancer SJ, Simmons NA, Poston SM, *et al.* Outbreak of staphylococcal scalded skin syndrome among neonates. *J Infect* 1988;16:87–103.
5 Koningstein M, Groen L, Geraats-Peters K, *et al.* The use of typing methods and infection prevention measures to control a bullous impetigo outbreak on a neonatal ward. *Antimicrob Resist Infect Control* 2012;1:37.
6 Piechowicz L, Garbacz K, Budzyńska A, *et al.* Outbreak of bullous impetigo caused by *Staphylococcus aureus* strains of phage type 3C/71 in a maternity ward linked to nasal carriage of a healthcare worker. *Eur J Dermatol* 2012;22:252–5.

Staphylococcal scalded skin syndrome

2 Handler MZ, Schwartz RA. Staphylococcal scalded skin syndrome: diagnosis and management in children and adults. *J Eur Acad Dermatol Venereol* 2014;11:1418–23.
8 Hubiche T, Bes M, Roudiere L, *et al.* Mild staphylococcal scalded skin syndrome: an underdiagnosed clinical disorder. *Br J Dermatol* 2012;166:213–15.
9 Braunstein I, Wanat KA, Abuabara K, *et al.* Antibiotic sensitivity and resistance patterns in pediatric staphylococcal scalded skin syndrome. *Pediatr Dermatol* 2014;31:305–8.

Periporitis staphylogenes and sweat gland abscesses

1 Lubowe II, Perlman HH. Periporitis staphylogenes and other complications of miliaria in infants and children. *AMA Arch Dermatol Syphilol* 1954;69:543–53.
2 Maibach HI, Kligman AM. Multiple sweat gland abscesses. *JAMA* 1960;174:140–2.
5 Sylvest B, Eriksen KR. An outbreak of periporitis staphylogenes of complex origin. *Acta Derm Venereol Suppl (Stockh)* 1979;59:181–4.

Mastitis and breast abscesses

2 Panteli C, Arvaniti M, Zavitsanakis A. Long-term consequences of neonatal mastitis. *Arch Dis Child* 2012;97:673–4.
3 Borders H, Mychaliska G, Gebarski KS. Sonographic features of neonatal mastitis and breast abscess. *Pediatr Radiol* 2009;39:955–8.
4 Rudoy RL, Nelson JD. Breast abscess during the neonatal period: a review. *Am J Dis Child* 1975;129:1031–4.

Omphalitis

1 Fraser NIA, Davies BW, Cusack J. Neonatal omphalitis: a review of its serious complications. *Acta Paediatrica* 2006;95:519–22.
4 Imdad A, Mullany LC, Baqui AH, *et al.* The effect of umbilical cord cleansing with chlorhexidine on omphalitis and neonatal mortality in community settings in developing countries: a meta-analysis. *BMC Public Health* 2013;13(Suppl. 3):S15.
6 Imdad A, Bautista RM, Senen KA, *et al.* Umbilical cord antiseptics for preventing sepsis and death among newborns. *Cochrane Database Syst Rev* 2013;Issue 5:CD008635.

Necrotizing fasciitis

2 Hsieh WS, Yang PH, Chao HC, *et al.* Neonatal necrotizing fasciitis: a report of three cases and review of the literature. *Pediatrics* 1999;103:e53.
7 Wilson HD, Haltalin KC. Acute necrotising fasciitis in childhood: report of 11 cases. *Am J Dis Child* 1973;125:591–5.
9 Pandey V, Gangopadhyay AN, Gupta DK, *et al.* Neonatal necrotising fasciitis managed conservatively: an experience from a tertiary centre. *J Wound Care* 2014;23:270–3.

Neonatal listeriosis

1 Schlech WF, Lavigne PM, Bortolussi RA, *et al.* Epidemic listeriosis: evidence for transmission by food. *N Engl J Med* 1983;203:203–6.
3 Lamont RF, Sobel J, Mazaki-Tovi S, *et al.* Listeriosis in human pregnancy: a systematic review. *J Perinat Med* 2011;39:227–36.
9 Smith K, Yeager J, Skelton H, *et al.* Diffuse petechial pustular lesions in a newborn: disseminated *Listeria monocytogenes*. *Arch Dermatol* 1994;130:245–8.

Ecthyma gangrenosum

1 Boisseau AM, Sarlangue J, Perel Y, *et al.* Perineal ecthyma gangrenosum in infancy and early childhood: septicemic and nonsepticemic forms. *J Am Acad Dermatol* 1992;27:415–18.
6 Prindaville B, Nopper AJ, Lawrence H, *et al.* Chronic granulomatous disease presenting with ecthyma gangrenosum in a neonate. *J Am Acad Dermatol* 2014;71:e44–5.
8 Yan W, Li W, Mu C, Wang L. Ecthyma gangrenosum and multiple nodules: cutaneous manifestations of *Pseudomonas aeruginosa* sepsis in a previously healthy infant. *Pediatr Dermatol* 2011;28:204–5.

Noma neonatorum (cancrum oris/oro-facial gangrene)

3 Enwonwu CO, Falkler WA, Jr, Phillips RS. Noma (cancrum oris). *Lancet* 2006;368:147–56.
4 Rotbart HA, Levin MJ, Jones J, *et al.* Noma in children with severe combined immunodeficiency. *J Pediatr* 1986;109:596–600.
5 Enwonwu CO. Noma – the ulcer of extreme poverty. *N Engl J Med* 2006;354:221–4.

Congenital syphilis

1 Chawla V, Pandit P, Nkrumah FK. Congenital syphilis in the newborn. *Arch Dis Child* 1988;63:1393–4.
3 Gomez GB, Kamb ML, Newman LM, *et al.* Untreated maternal syphilis and adverse outcomes of pregnancy: a systematic review and meta-analysis. *Bull World Health Organ* 2013;91:217–26.
4 Hawkes S, Matin N, Broutet N, *et al.* Effectiveness of interventions to improve screening for syphilis in pregnancy: a systematic review and meta-analysis. *Lancet Infect Dis* 2011;11:684–91.

Fungal infections

Congenital candidiasis

5 Darmstadt GL, Dinulos JG, Miller Z. Congenital cutaneous candidiasis: clinical presentation, pathogenesis and management guidelines. *Pediatrics* 2000;105:438–44.
6 Cosgrove BF, Reeves K, Mullins D, *et al.* Congenital cutaneous candidiasis associated with respiratory distress and elevation of liver function tests: a case report and review of the literature. *J Am Acad Dermatol* 1997;37:817–23.
14 McGuire W, Clerihew L, Austin N. Prophylactic intravenous antifungal agents to prevent mortality and morbidity in very low birth weight infants. *Cochrane Database Syst Rev* 2004;Issue 1:CD003850.

Malassezia pustulosis

2 Niamba P, Weill FX, Sarlangue J, *et al.* Is common neonatal cephalic pustulosis (neonatal acne) triggered by *Malassezia sympodialis*? *Arch Dermatol* 1998;134:995–8.
4 Ayhan M, Sancak B, Karaduman A, *et al.* Colonization of neonate skin by *Malassezia* species: relationship with neonatal cephalic pustulosis. *J Am Acad Dermatol* 2007;57:1012–18.
6 Bernier V, Weill FX, Hirigoyen V, *et al.* Skin colonisation by *Malassezia* species in neonates: a prospective study and relationship with neonatal cephalic pustulosis (neonatal acne). *Arch Dermatol* 2002;138:215–18.

CHAPTER 117

Dermatoses and Haemangiomas of Infancy

Elisabeth M. Higgins[1] and Mary T. Glover[2]

[1]King's College Hospital, London, UK
[2]Great Ormond Street Hospital for Children NHS Foundation Trust, London, UK

Introduction

No hard and fast definition of infancy exists, so for the purposes of this chapter the infant period is regarded as from 4 weeks to 18 months, with emphasis on the first year of life. An overview of the most common or important dermatoses presenting in this age group is discussed, as well as infant and congenital haemangiomas, but the list is not exhaustive.

INFANTILE DERMATOSES

INFLAMMATORY CONDITIONS

Cradle cap

Although cradle cap may be seen in the neonate, the condition is most common between the ages of 4 and 16 weeks, and is estimated to affect up to 41.7% of infants [1]. It can occur in isolation or in association with seborrhoeic dermatitis (see the next disorder).

Large flakes of yellowish scale are seen on the scalp, especially over the vertex and frontal regions (Figure 117.1a), and may become matted into large plaques of crust. There is usually minimal inflammation, but the eyebrows may be involved (Figure 117.1b). Mild cases are very common, but the condition can become quite extensive. The condition is asymptomatic and the infant is always well, however the disorder may be a source of concern to parents. In extensive cases, Langerhans cell histiocytosis (LCH) should be considered, but in LCH the lesional skin tends to ooze, and systemic features may be apparent.

Most cases of cradle cap resolve spontaneously after a few weeks. An emollient will help lift the scale, and should be used in combination with an appropriate shampoo. A recent trial has indicated that a topical non-steroidal cream may be therapeutically beneficial [2].

Rook's Textbook of Dermatology, Ninth Edition. Edited by Christopher Griffiths, Jonathan Barker, Tanya Bleiker, Robert Chalmers and Daniel Creamer.
© 2016 John Wiley & Sons, Ltd. Published 2016 by John Wiley & Sons, Ltd.
Companion website: www.rooksdermatology.com

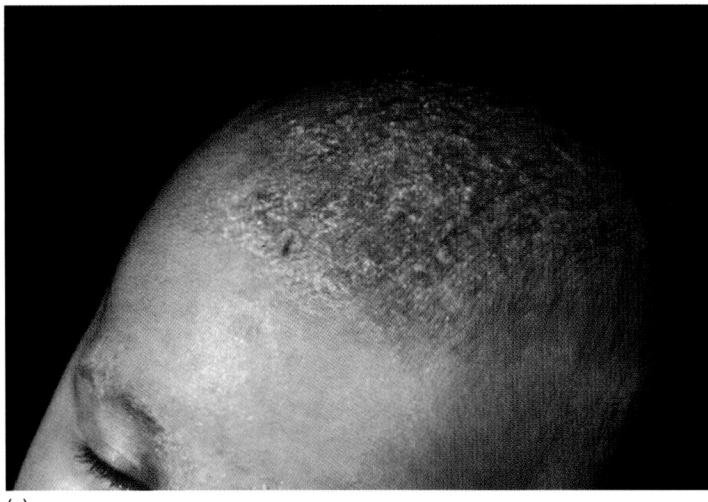

(a)

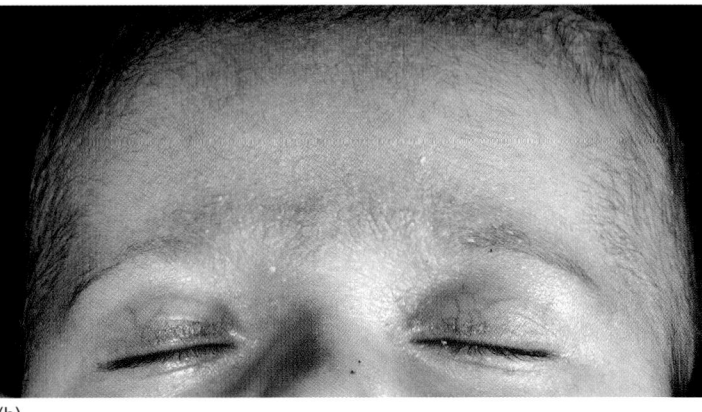

(b)

Figure 117.1 Cradle cap. (a) Scale over the vertex and frontal regions in a 6-week-old infant. (b) Adherent yellow scale in the eyebrows and on the forehead of an 8-week-old infant.

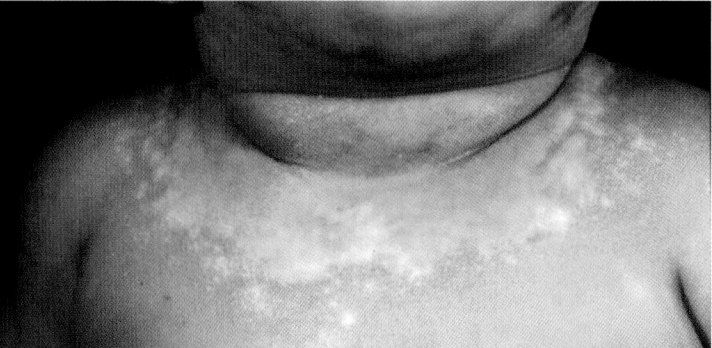

Figure 117.2 Seborrhoeic dermatitis showing macerated erythema in the neck folds of a 3-month-old girl, associated with some post-inflammatory hypopigmentation.

Seborrhoeic dermatitis

Infantile seborrhoeic dermatitis (ISD) is distinct from seborrhoeic dermatitis in later life (see also Chapter 40). Typically, ISD occurs between the ages of 4 and 12 weeks, but most commonly before the age of 2 months (64%) with 28 % occurring later, between 2 and 4 months [1]. Characteristically, in addition to erythema and scale on the scalp and eyebrows (see the section on cradle cap), more macerated erythema occurs in the skin folds, especially the neck (Figure 117.2) and the inguinal regions. Yeasts, particularly *Malassezia* species, may be isolated from intertriginous areas and colonization with yeasts is significantly greater in infants with ISD than in their healthy counterparts [2].

The child is healthy and often well above the median centile for weight. ISD is rarely symptomatic, but may cause great parental concern. Typically the inflammation resolves with transient hypopigmentation, which can be very pronounced in children with darker skin colour. However, this is a post-inflammatory phenomenon, and always recovers within a few weeks, and is not due to the treatments applied.

Differential diagnosis includes irritant napkin dermatitis, atopic eczema, and LCH. If the onset is very acute, the infant is febrile or there is significant desquamation, Kawasaki disease should be considered.

In mild cases, treatment with emollient alone has been shown to be as effective as a weak topical steroid [3]. Combination steroid–antifungal creams are often employed in cases where inflammation is marked, but should only be used for short periods.

Some infants may go on to develop atopic eczema and the two conditions can merge. It is estimated that 34% of infants with ISD go on to develop infantile eczema at an average time interval of 6 months [4].

Atopic eczema

Atopic eczema (AE) is very common in developed countries and is the most frequent reason for infants to be referred to a dermatologist (see also Chapter 41). Mutations in the filaggrin encoding gene (*FLG*) have been shown to be a major factor in susceptibility to AE, through the disruption of the epidermal barrier function [1]. A European cohort study has estimated that the cumulative prevalence of AE in the first 2 years of life is 21.5% [2], but prevalence peaks at 10% at 18 months [3], and slightly earlier for boys than girls [4]. Epidemiological studies have shown that the prevalence of AE amongst black children born in the UK or USA is significantly higher than in their white peers [5,6], and that being born abroad appears to confer protection from atopic disease for at least a decade after migration [6].

In infants, AE characteristically begins on the face in a balaclava-like distribution (Figure 117.3) [4], with subsequent spread to involve the torso and limbs, depending on severity. In some children, a more nummular (discoid) pattern occurs, particularly on the back and legs, especially in toddlers, which may be mistaken for tinea corporis. However, evidence of flexural involvement in infancy has the highest predictive value of AE persisting at age 3 years [4]. Although secondary infection is a common component of AE, early colonization with *Staphylococcus aureus* is not associated with persistence of AE [7].

Infantile eczema present at 1 month of age is associated with a cord blood eosinophilia and a higher rate of wheezing and

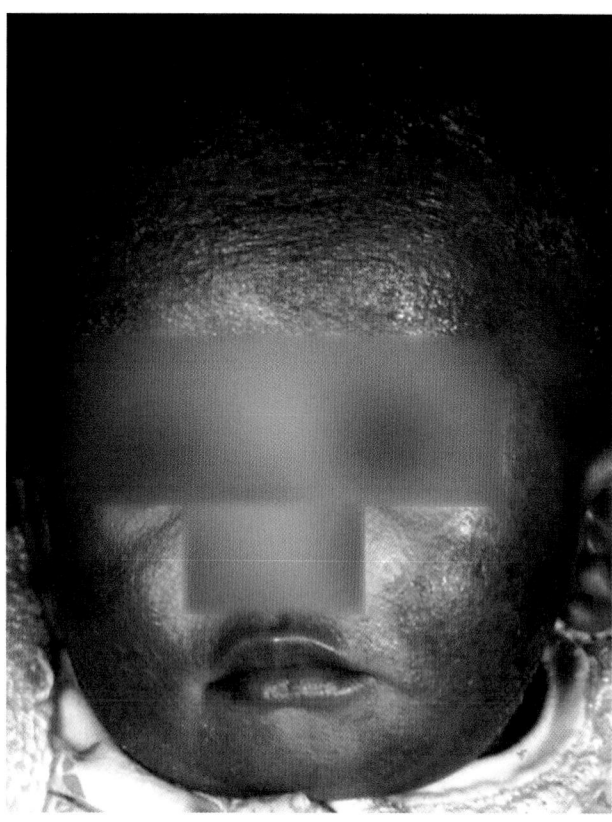

Figure 117.3 Atopic eczema showing facial involvement in the characteristic 'balaclava 'pattern in a 5-month-old.

subsequent AE [8]. Infants with AE who are exclusively breast-fed are also significantly more likely to be sensitized to common foodstuffs, particularly if the disease is severe, possibly through epidermal barrier dysfunction [9]. However, there is a lower incidence of AE in infants who were born extremely prematurely (<29 weeks' gestation) [10].

AE in the majority of infants clears over time: 43.2% of children with early AE are in complete remission by age 3 years [2]; 38.3 % have intermittent disease, but 18.7% have evidence of symptoms every year [2]. A history of early AE is associated with asthma at school age [2]. However, estimates of total IgE at 6 months is the best predictor of the persistence of AE [11]. Certain *FLG* mutations have also been found to predict persistent symptoms [12].

The management of infantile atopic eczema for the most part is topical and primarily aimed at restoring skin barrier function [13,14], reducing inflammation, treating secondary infection and providing parental education and support.

Food allergy is reported in 10–30% of children with AE. In infants it is cow's milk, egg, peanut and soy that are the most prevalent [15]. Although exclusive breastfeeding for the first 6 months appears protective [16], prolonged breastfeeding beyond this time does not appear to confer an advantage. Breastfeeding has a clear benefit over intact cow's milk formula [16,17], and the use of hydrolysed formula is preferred in infants with cow's milk sensitization [17]. However there appears to be no benefit in delaying weaning onto solids beyond 4 months of age [18,19].

There is some disparity in the approach to the initial management of infants with AE, with paediatricians favouring dietary

interventions, while dermatologists are more likely to recommend an initial trial of topical therapy [20]. Although dietary manipulation is common and popular with parents, it needs to be undertaken in an informed and evidence-based manner to ensure it is appropriate and that the essential nutrition, growth and development of the infant is maintained.

Napkin dermatitis

Napkin (diaper) dermatitis is seen far less frequently in the UK since the advent of modern disposable nappies, which are much more absorbent than their terry-towelling predecessors and promote preservation of the normal skin barrier [1]. However, traditional cloth nappies are still in widespread use in other parts of the world; estimates of napkin dermatitis in areas of China are as high as 50–70% [2]. Prolonged contact with urine induces an irritant erythema, which may break down to form erosions if untreated. Transepidermal water loss and pH are higher in infants with napkin dermatitis than those without [2], emphasizing the importance of skin barrier function in the pathogenesis.

Involved areas are those in contact with the irritant (e.g. the buttocks), while the skin folds may be spared (Figure 117.4) – in contrast to seborrhoeic dermatitis or infantile psoriasis.

Treatment is aimed at keeping the skin dry and using barrier creams or emollients to restore normal epidermis. Topical steroids should only be used in the short term, and only if inflammation is severe; secondary infection should be treated appropriately.

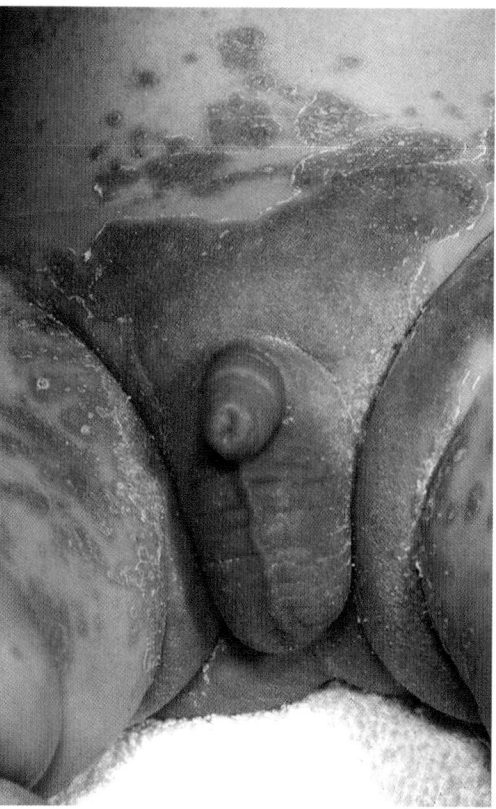

Figure 117.4 Napkin dermatitis showing erythema and scale in the groin region, with sparing of the skin folds.

Jacquet dermatitis

Punched-out ulcers may be seen in persistent cases of napkin dermatitis. They are thought to be due to the irritant effect of urine compounded by secondary infection, and are considered to be part of the spectrum of presentation of napkin dermatitis, along with infantile gluteal granuloma [1]. However, Jacquet dermatitis is rare nowadays due to the technological advances in absorbency of modern nappies.

Infantile gluteal granuloma

Overuse of potent, especially fluorinated, steroids under occlusion in infants with napkin dermatitis has been thought to lead to the formation of a granulomatous inflammatory reaction, characterized by reddish brown nodules on the buttocks [1]. Treatment is avoidance of further topical steroids and the use of appropriate emollients to restore the epidermal barrier.

Although rarely seen now, a similar eruption has been described in the elderly who wear cloth nappies for incontinence [2].

Infantile psoriasis

One-third of individuals with psoriasis develop the disease in childhood (before the age of 15 years), although infantile psoriasis is less common [1] (see also Chapter 35). Estimates of the frequency of psoriasis in children are 3–4% [2,3], but the prevalence appears to be increasing over time [2], and 27% of children affected present before the age of 2 years [4]. Napkin psoriasis with dissemination is the most common pattern in infants (Figure 117.5) [4].

Although some authors consider infantile psoriasis to be a self-limiting disease [5], it may be a prelude to more typical chronic plaque psoriasis in later life [6]. All patterns of psoriasis have been described in children: guttate, chronic plaque, pustular and

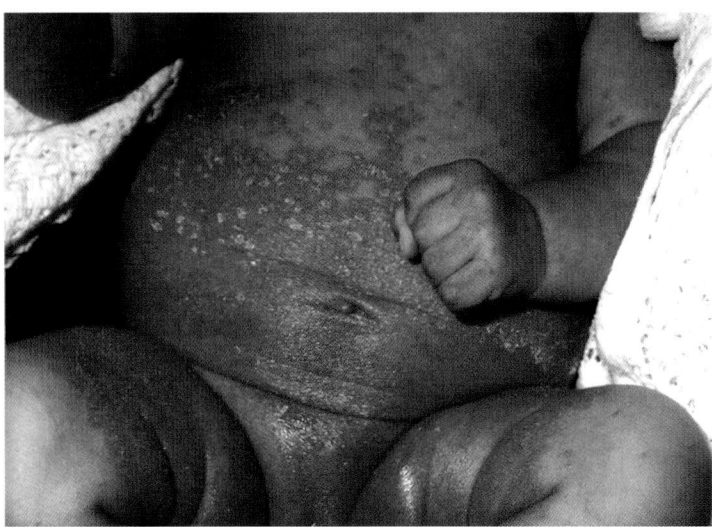

Figure 117.5 Infantile psoriasis.

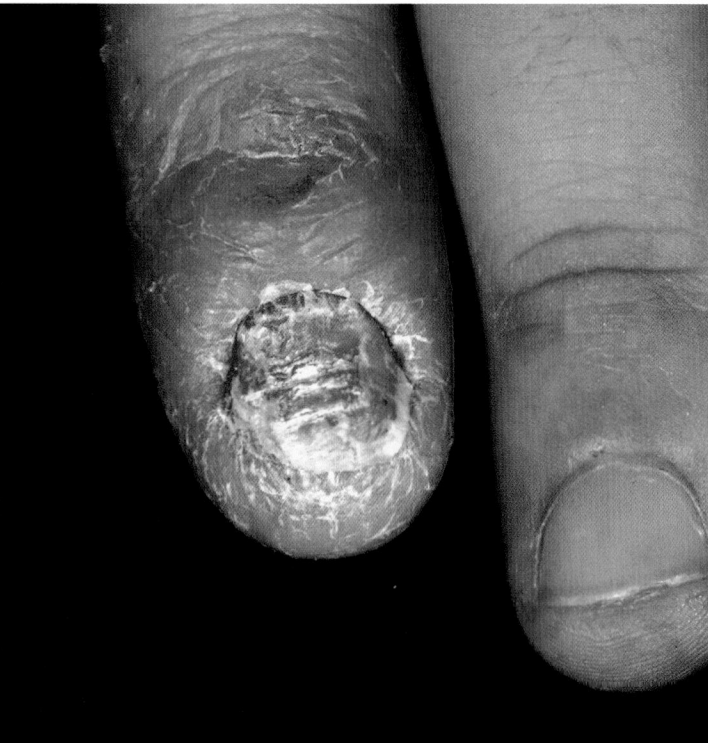

Figure 117.6 Parakeratosis pustulosa showing erythema of the index finger with associated nail dystrophy.

erythrodermic [3,5], but severe disease and joint involvement are relatively rare [1].

Treatment is determined by the extent and severity of disease. In the majority of infants, mild topical steroids, often in combination with an anticandidal agent, and emollients usually suffice [6].

Parakeratosis pustulosa

Parakeratosis pustulosa is a localized inflammatory condition involving the distal phalanx. Usually a solitary digit is involved – fingers more frequently than toes. Characteristically, the thumb, index finger or great toe is affected. The skin signs are very characteristic [1,2], with sharply demarcated erythema and scale of the skin adjacent to the nail fold, with accompanying nail dystrophy, resembling the changes seen in Hallopeau psoriasis (Figure 117.6). Pustulation is seen in 25% [1], but swabs are sterile and mycology is negative. The nail may be shed.

The condition is fairly resistant to treatment, but usually resolves over the course of 12–18 months. Combination topical preparations of potent steroids and antibiotics are usually used.

There may be a family history of psoriasis, and the condition is thought to predispose to psoriasis in later life [1].

Infantile acropustulosis

Synonyms and inclusions
• Acrodermatitis pustulosa

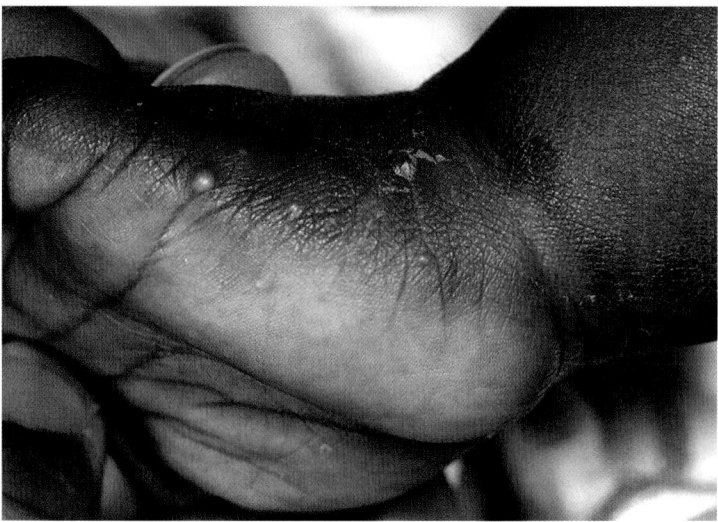

Figure 117.7 Infantile acropustulosis showing discrete pustules along medial border of the foot of an 11-month-old boy.

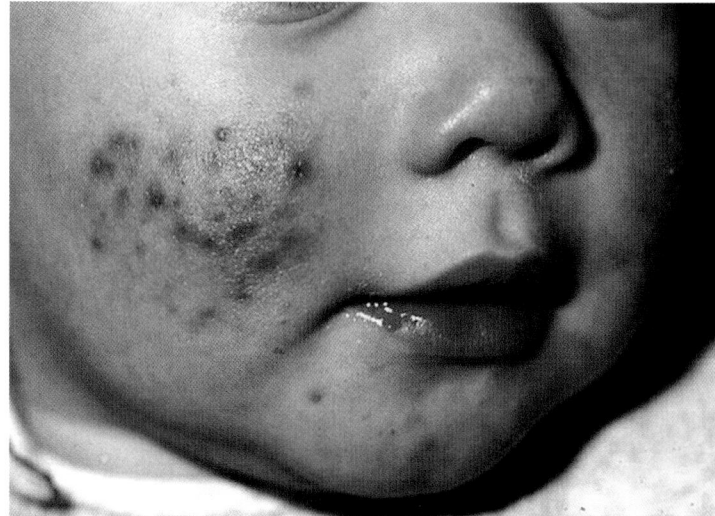

Figure 117.8 Infantile acne showing papules, pustules and comedones in a 6-month-old boy.

Infantile acropustulosis is a rare disorder characteristically affecting children between the ages of 1 and 2 years [1]. It appears more frequent in boys. Crops of itchy vesicopustules, 2–4 mm in diameter, appear along the borders of the feet, particularly around the heel (Figure 117.7). Occasionally, similar changes occur on the palm.

The pathogenesis is not well understood. The differential diagnosis is scabies infestation, and sometimes the condition is seen to follow a genuine scabies infection, as a persistent, reactive, post-inflammatory phenomenon.

Topical steroids are usually employed, but often have little impact. The condition tends to resolve spontaneously over 6–12 months.

Pityriasis alba

Transient, hypopigmented areas on the face, associated in some cases with fine scale, are not uncommon in childhood but are usually seen in slightly older children rather than infants. When pityriasis alba does occur in infants, it may be more extensive [1]. It is more common in boys [2]. It is most frequent on the lower cheeks, and lesions are ovoid in shape, with indistinct margins. Although entirely asymptomatic, the condition is most noticeable in children with darker skin types [1], and may be a source of great concern to parents.

Individual lesions resolve over a few weeks, but can be recurrent. The condition is considered to be part of the atopic spectrum [2,3] (85% have an atopic history [3]), but no specific treatment is required. Emollients can help reduce the scale, but topical steroids should be avoided. Calcineurin inhibitors may speed resolution [1], but are rarely required.

Infantile acne

Infantile acne is rare, but should be easily distinguished from the transient sebaceous gland hyperplasia/milk spots seen in the neonate (see also Chapter 90). In a 25-year period, only 29 cases were seen in a large specialist centre [1]. The majority of infants affected

(75%) are male, and most do not have a family history of acne [1]. The mean age of onset is 6 months (range 0–21 months), and the cheeks are predominantly affected [2].

Most infants have mild or moderate disease with inflammatory papules (Figure 117.8), but 17% have comedones and in 14% the disease is classified as severe [1]. No underlying endocrinopathy was found in infants [1,3], in contrast to older children presenting with preadolescent acne in whom more detailed investigation may be merited.

Treatment may be topical (benzoyl peroxide, erythromycin or retinoids) in mild cases [1]. In more extensive disease, the majority of children will clear with oral erythromycin , but trimethoprim can also be used if there is erythromycin resistance [1]. Prolonged treatment may be required (for 18–24 months) [1]. In severe disease, oral isotretinoin has been shown to be safe and effective in infants [2]. Scarring is estimated to occur in 17% of infants with acne [1], reflecting the proportion with more severe disease.

Urticaria

Uricaria in infancy differs from urticaria in adults in that it presents with haemorrhagic lesions in approximately 50% cases, and angio-oedema in 60% [1] (see also Chapter 42). Anaphylactic shock is very rare in the first year of life but incidence increases with age, particularly in industrialized societies [2,3]. Approximately half of infants presenting with urticaria have a personal or family history of atopy [1].

Infection, usually viral, with or without drug intake, appears to be the cause of urticaria in the majority of cases [1]. Foods appear to be responsible in approximately 10% of cases. In the first year of life cow's milk, hen's eggs and wheat are the most common allergens. In the second and third year of life the top three food allergens were hen's eggs, cow's milk and peanuts [4].

Chronic or recurrent urticaria is reported to occur in 30% of cases [1]. Physical factors are more likely to be implicated in chronic urticaria [5]. Cholinergic urticaria, precipitated by exercise, emotion and heat, is common. Cold may be a trigger in up to 8% of cases [6].

Urticaria in infancy may be a feature of systemic disease including systemic lupus erythematosus, juvenile rheumatoid arthritis, mastocytosis and Kawasaki disease [7], but is rarely the only presenting feature. Urticaria is associated with attacks of fever, musculoskeletal and sensorineural inflammation and high levels of acute-phase reactants in the cryopyrin-associated periodic syndromes including the Muckle–Wells syndrome and NOMID/CINCA (neonatal-onset multisystem inflammatory disease/chronic infantile neurological, cutaneous and articular syndrome). These conditions arise from gain-of-function mutations in the *NLRP3* gene leading to excessive interleukin 1 (IL-1) signalling [8–10].

INFECTIVE CONDITIONS

Viral exanthems

Many viral infections are associated with a transient rash, which may be macular, maculopapular (with or without petechiae), urticarial or vesicular [1,2]. Often this is non-specific and harmless [1], but some viral infections have very characteristic features that allow a diagnosis to be made. Atypical exanthems present more of a challenge [2]. A detailed account of viral infections appears in Chapter 25, but the most frequent or important infections seen in children are highlighted here. Viral exanthems account for the most common presentation to a paediatric emergency department [3]. However, differentiation from exanthems due to other causes (drugs, bacterial toxins, autoimmune disease) must be made [1,2]. Overall, petechial changes are much more likely to occur in exanthems associated with infections, particularly of viral origin (although meningococcal septicaemia should always be considered) [2]. Viral exanthems have a seasonal prevalence (spring and summer) [2]. Newer polymerase chain reaction (PCR) based laboratory screening methods can help in the diagnosis of viral exanthems [4].

Roseola

Synonyms and inclusions
• Exanthem subitum

Although initially associated with human herpesvirus 6 (HHV-6) infection [1], cases due to HHV-7 are now also reported [2]. The disease is common, with a male preponderance reported in infants in Japan, but a higher incidence of female infection in the USA [2]. Forty per cent of children have evidence of HHV-6 infection by 12 months of age, and 90% by 2 years [3].

A high fever develops that lasts for 3 days and may rarely be associated with febrile convulsions [4]. As the pyrexia subsides a fine, lacy, macular erythema appears, which may be accompanied by occipital lymphadenopathy. The rash fades over 48 h without desquamation. The incubation period is 5–14 days.

Fifth disease

Synonyms and inclusions
• Exanthem infantum

Infection is due to parvovirus B19 [1] and the incubation period is 7–14 days. Infection occurs in epidemics, predominantly in the spring. The sudden onset of a rash on the face, with hot, bright red cheeks, gives rise to the typical 'slapped cheek' appearance. A more reticulate rash then appears on the limbs and body, and palmoplantar erythema is common. The eruption fades over 7 days, but recrudescences are not infrequent, particularly if the child gets hot (e.g. in sunlight, after a bath or exertion).

European studies estimate seroprevalence to be 20% in children aged 1–3 years, and rising with age [2]. Older individuals may develop a papulopruritic eruption in a glove and stocking distribution with parvovirus B19 infection [3], but this pattern is rarely seen in infants. The virus may lead to serious cytopenia in children with leukaemia [4].

Hand, foot and mouth disease

This is a common infection in young children, affecting the oral cavity and extremities. Vesicles, which may be very painful, develop in the mouth and may ulcerate. Small, tense blisters, with a surrounding rim of erythema occur on the palms (Figure 117.9)

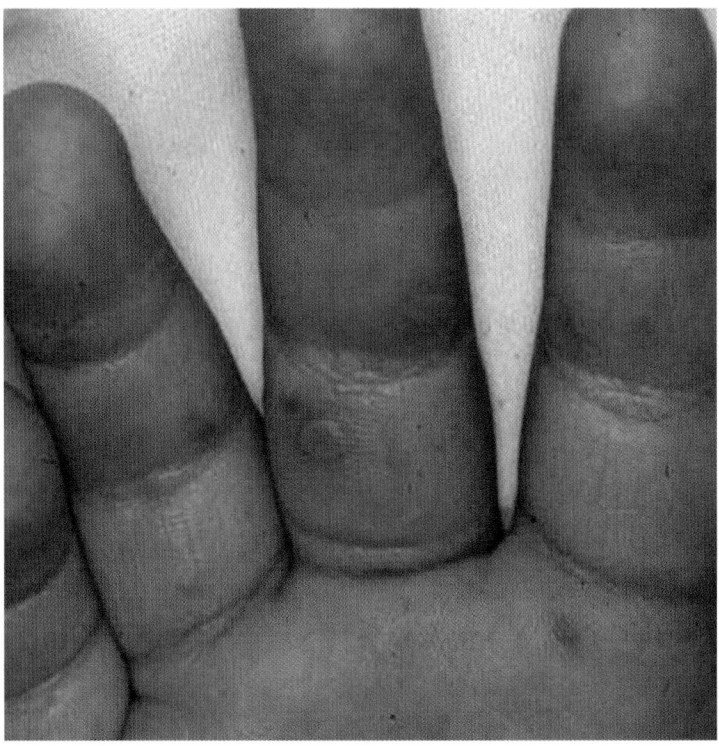

Figure 117.9 Hand foot and mouth disease showing small vesicles with surrounding erythema on the palmar aspect of the fingers.

and soles and fade within 3 days. It is most commonly associated with Coxsackie A viral infection, most usually A16 [1], but infection with A6 [2], Coxsackie B [1] and enterovirus 71 [1] have also been described. Spread is by droplets or faecal contamination and the incubation period is 7 days. However, virus may be present in the faeces for several weeks after infection, making isolation impractical [1]. Symptomatic treatment only is required, but it is highly contagious and widespread outbreaks are common.

Varicella

Synonyms and inclusions
- Chickenpox

Varicella is still common in the UK, where vaccination is not routine. The incubation period is 14–21 days. Small erythematous papules appear on the trunk, scalp or genital regions. The onset of the rash may be preceded by 1–2 days of malaise and fever. Lesions occur in crops, crusting over as they resolve, and lesions in different stages of evolution are evident. The eruption may become widespread but retains a centripetal pattern. The child should be isolated until the lesions have crusted over. The majority of cases are self-limiting and can be managed in the community. Severe cases, or chickenpox occurring in immunosuppressed children, should be treated with aciclovir. Encephalitis may occur, but is rare in infants aged less than 12 months. The prevalence of complications in infants is inversely proportional to the level of antivaricella zoster virus maternal antibodies and varicella severity [1]. Passively acquired maternal immunity persists for about 4 months, but then rapidly declines after the neonatal period [2]. The incidence of complications from varicella amongst infants with severe disease hospitalized for infection rises from 10% in babies less than 1 month of age to over 70% at 5 months [1].

Measles

The decline in uptake of MMR vaccination in the UK over recent years has been associated with a resurgence of measles infections due to loss of herd immunity. In a recent outbreak in northwest England, 22% of cases were aged <13 months [1]. At this age, children would not usually have received their initial vaccination in this county, but herd immunity would have conferred protection. Encouragingly, recent public health campaigns and immunization programmes in schools seem to be increasing uptake again [2].

Measles is caused by an RNA paramyxovirus. The infection is spread by droplets and the incubation period is 7–14 days. An initial prodrome of fever and coryzal symptoms is followed after 3 days by the development of small, white Koplik spots on the buccal mucosa. On the fourth day of the illness the rash appears, initially on the forehead, spreading caudally down the face onto the trunk and limbs. Complications can be serious and include bronchiolitis, otitis media and encephalitis. Treatment is supportive, but children remain infectious for 7 days after the onset of the rash.

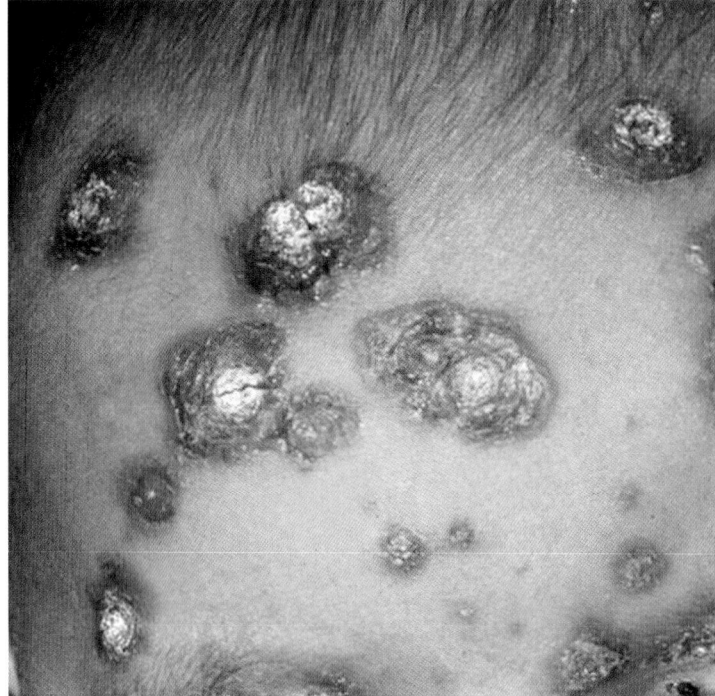

Figure 117.10 Impetigo showing multiple crusted lesions on the forehead of a 9-month-old.

Impetigo

Impetigo is a highly contagious cutaneous infection and the commonest overall infection in children worldwide [1]. The usual causal organism is *Staphylococcus aureus*, but less frequently *Strepococcus pyogenes* may also be implicated (see also Chapter 26). Honey-coloured crusts appear on a background of erythema. The child is usually well. Most frequently, children aged 2–5 years are affected, but as the condition is so highly infectious, spread within families, including to infants, is common.

Bullous and non-bullous forms exist. Non-bullous impetigo most typically occurs on the face (Figure 117.10), whereas bullous impetigo is more often seen in intertriginous areas such as the napkin area, axilla or neck folds. In bullous impetigo, the *Staphylococcus* produces exotoxins specific for desmoglein 1 [2], and affected areas are painful and become eroded. The bullous form is more frequent in the autumn, possibly because viral co-infection predisposes the skin to staphylococcal colonization [2]. Minor non-bullous cases may be self-limiting, but treatment is usually required. Topical or oral antibiotics are given depending on severity, but antibiotic resistance is emerging [3]. Topical disinfectants can help reduce colonization [3].

Other infections and infestations

Staphylococcal scalded skin syndrome

The estimated incidence of staphylococcal scalded skin syndrome (SSSS) is 0.56 cases/million population per year, with a median age of 2 years and an equal sex incidence [1] (see also Chapter 26).

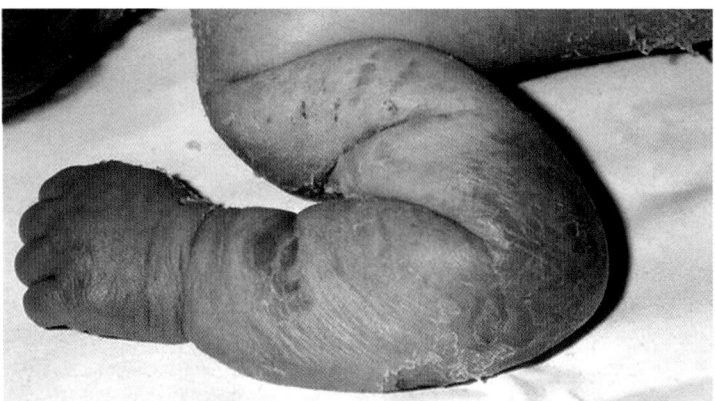

Figure 117.11 Staphylococcal scalded skin syndrome showing widespread peeling and erosion in a 3-month-old.

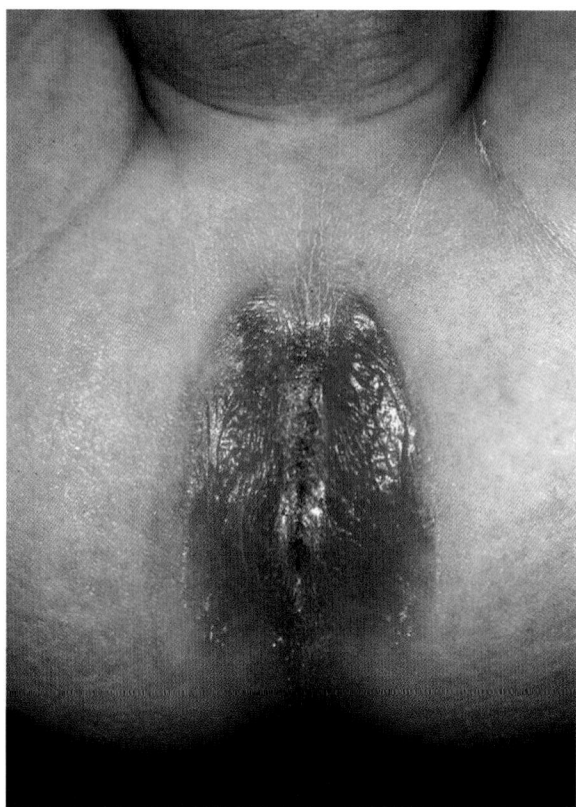

Figure 117.12 Perianal dermatitis showing well-circumscribed erythema and oedema in an 8-week-old.

There is a seasonal peak in the autumn [1]. Several exfoliative toxins have been identified [1], but exfoliative toxin B is more likely to be associated with SSSS and exfoliative toxin A with bullous impetigo [2]. Isolating the causal organism can be difficult.

Following a prodrome of fever, irritability and malaise, tender erythema appears with subsequent development of superficial flaccid blisters, typically around the flexures and perioral region, progressing to peeling and erosion (Figure 117.11). Pain is a prominent feature and affected infants resist movement or touch.

Management is with intravenous antibiotics and supportive care with liberal emollients, attention to fluid balance and adequate analgesia. Differentiation from Stevens–Johnson syndrome/toxic epidermal necrolysis should be made clinically, due to sparing of the mucous membranes. Resolution over 2–3 weeks is usual and mortality is low in otherwise healthy infants.

Blistering distal dactylitis

Typically, large acral bullae, oval in shape and up to 1–3 cm in diameter, develop on the finger pulps, but may also occur more proximally on the digits and even occasionally on the palms. The condition is due to infection with a Gram-positive bacteria, most frequently *Staphylococcus aureus* [1], but occasionally a β-haemolytic *Streptococcus* may be implicated. When multiple bullae are present, *Staphylococcus* is the more likely culprit organism, and the condition is considered to be a localized bullous impetigo.

Infants should be swabbed for coexistence of bacterial colonization of the nares, conjunctiva and anus [1]. The differential diagnosis includes epidermolysis bullosa simplex and sucking blisters, but the clinical signs are fairly diagnostic and swabs are confirmatory. Management is by deflating the blisters, dressing eroded areas and using appropriate antibiotics. Resolution is usually fairly rapid.

Perianal dermatitis

A beefy erythema with oedema is seen in a circumferential and well-demarcated distribution 2–3 cm around the anal margin in young infants (Figure 117.12) [1]. Pain can be severe and blood may be seen in the stool. The condition is due to β-haemolytic streptococcal infection and should be easily distinguished from napkin dermatitis, although the two can coexist. It responds rapidly to appropriate oral antibiotics and rarely recurs unless an intrafamilial reservoir of *Streptococcus* is responsible for its transmission.

Cutaneous *Candida* infection

Candidiasis is a yeast infection and transient oral candidiasis is not infrequent in infants. Infection may have been acquired during delivery [1]. Secondary colonization of eroded or macerated skin in intertriginous areas, especially the napkin region [2], may occur, but is much less common since the decline in diaper dermatitis generally. Satellite pustules are characteristic.

Topical treatment will usually suffice and resistance is rare [2], but oral *Candida* requires treatment with an anti-yeast antimicrobial suspension. Recurrent, persistent or extensive infections should prompt investigation for an underlying immunodeficiency.

Tinea corporis

Tinea infections have been reported in children less than 1 year of age and are nearly always acquired from an older child [1] (see also Chapter 32). However, the infection remains rare in infants, but when it does occur the diagnosis may be missed. In

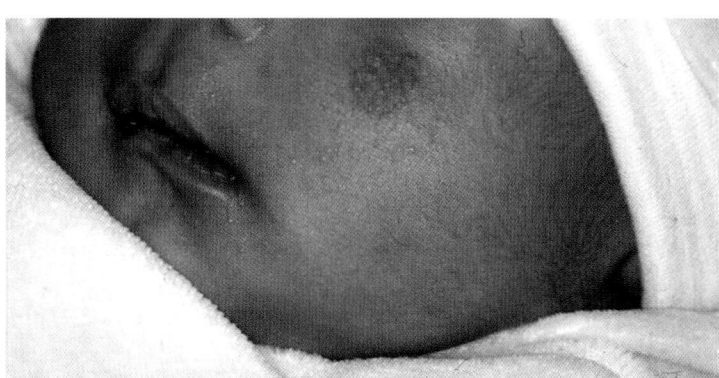

Figure 117.13 Tinea facei in a 4-week-old baby innoculated from an older sibling with tinea capitis.

very young infants, the face is the most common site of inoculation (Figure 117.13) [1]. In the UK, infection with *Trichophyton tonsurans* now predominates, especially in urban areas and amongst children of Afro-Caribbean heritage, but occasional sporadic cases of *Microsporum canis* or M. audouinii may occur. In cases of *T. tonsurans* tinea corporis, the reservoir of infection is always an infected scalp, so if an infant is seen with tinea faceii their own scalp, but particularly those of their older siblings, should be screened for tinea capitis.

Annular, inflammatory lesions, which clear from the centre, occur on the face and body but most usually the cheek in infants. Lesions may be vesicular and often resolve with post-inflammatory hyperpigmentation. Treatment for purely cutaneous lesions is a topical antifungal agent for 2 weeks, but if scalp involvement is suspected or proven, oral therapy will be required.

Tinea capitis

Scalp ringworm due to *T. tonsurans* has reached epidemic proportions in urban areas of the UK and USA over the past two decades (see also Chapter 32). Spread through nurseries and day care facilities is common, and in the UK the highest prevalence is in pre-school children. However, the infection remains rare in infants [1,2], but when it does occur, the diagnosis may be missed [1] and mistaken for seborrhoeic dermatitis. In rural areas, sporadic cases of animal ringworm may occasionally occur, but are exceedingly rare in this age group. In Europe, *M. canis* still predominates, but patterns of infection are changing with wider migration [3].

The presentation and clinical signs vary and include patchy or localized alopecia, diffuse scale and black dots due to swollen, broken-off hairs. Pustules, or a focal inflammatory kerion, may also occur. Cervical lymphadenopathy is common. Mycological confirmation is always recommended as treatment schedules vary depending on the causal fungus [1]. Oral therapy is the gold standard [1], and although griseofulvin remains the only licensed treatment for tinea capitis in children in the UK, worldwide practice has demonstrated that in cases of *T. tonsurans*, oral terbinifine or itraconazole are preferred for their greater efficacy and are well tolerated in young children. Itraconazole has the advantage of being available in a liquid formulation, so is preferred in infants. All family contacts should be screened to try and minimize reinfection [3].

Scabies

Extreme pruritus characterizes infestation with the mite *Sarcoptes scabei*. The condition is highly contagious. Estimates of prevalence in children range from 4.8% in parts of Europe [1] to 21.5% in India [2], but worldwide it is very common and has a significant impact on global health [3] (see also Chapter 34). In infants, burrows may be seen on the palms and soles more characteristically than in the finger webs, and the wrists are also commonly involved. Burrows can appear quite inflammatory with surrounding secondary eczematous changes. Nodular lesions develop in the axillae and genital region if the infection is untreated.

Eradication requires treatment of the individual and all close contacts using a topical scabecidal lotion or cream, in two applications 7 days apart. In recalcitrant cases, ivermectin has been shown to be safe and well tolerated in infants [4]. Post-scabetic pruritus may be prolonged and symptomatic treatment is usually required.

Molluscum contagiosum

This is an extremely common cutaneous viral infection, and is characterized by discrete, pearly, umbilicated papules 2–5 mm in diameter. Lesions usually occur in the axilla or groin, but may be widespread, especially in children with atopic eczema [1]. Spread between siblings is frequent and the condition is more prevalent in tropical climates [2]. The eruption is usually self-limiting, but is often a source of great parental concern [2]. Ablative treatment with cryotherapy (if tolerated) or topical treatment with either hydrogen peroxide creams or commercially available potassium hydroxide solutions can speed resolution.

REACTIVE CONDITIONS

Acute haemorrhagic oedema in infancy

Acute haemorrhagic oedema is a benign, cutaneous, leucocytoclastic vasculitis, arising after respiratory infection, medication administration or immunization in approximately 75% of cases [1]. It is thought likely to be an immune complex-mediated vasculitis.

Although histopathology typically shows leucocytoclastic vasculitis with fibrinoid necrosis and erythrocyte extravasation [2], in some cases fibrinoid necrosis is not evident [1]. Perivascular IgA deposits have been found in about one-third of cases [2].

The condition affects children between the ages of 4 months and 2 years, with males being affected twice as frequently as females. Fever is mild and systemic disturbance is minor. The limbs and face are the most commonly affected areas. Lesions are discrete

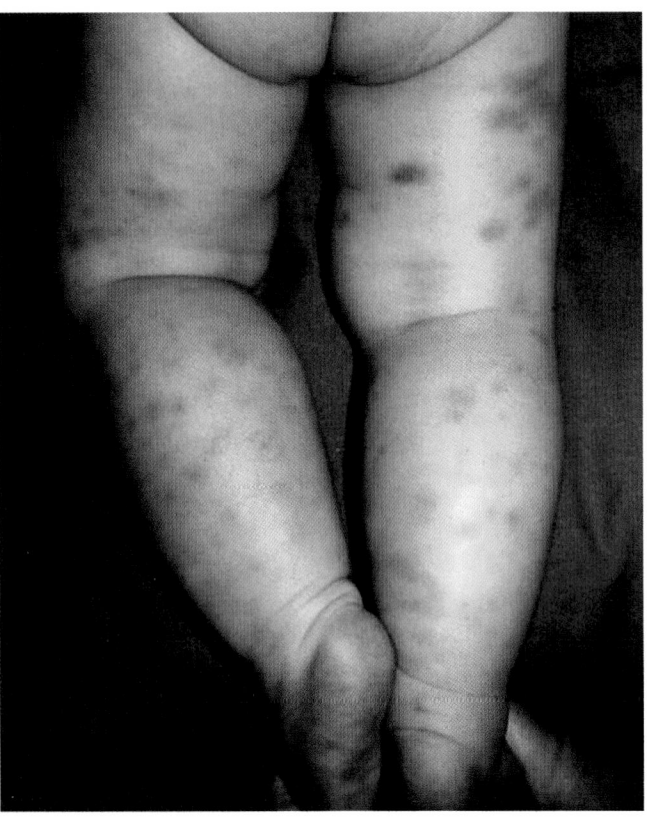

Figure 117.14 Multiple eccymotic and purpuric areas on the legs of a 10-month-old with acute haemorrhagic oedema in infancy.

or confluent with purpura often appearing in a targetoid or cockade pattern (Figure 117.14). Oedema mainly affects the eyelids, face and extremities. Visceral and joint involvement is not typical. Some cases may show features of Henoch–Schönlein purpura [1]. The differential diagnosis includes purpura fulminans, erythema multiforme, urticarial disease and Kawasaki disease. Resolution occurs within 3 weeks, and recurrences are not a feature.

Kawasaki disease

Kawasaki disease is a febrile illness with systemic vasculitis, first described in Japan four decades ago, but now recognized worldwide [1] (see also Chapter 102). It typically affects children aged 3–6 years, but can be seen in infants. It is estimated that about 17% of cases occur in children under 1 year of age, with a median age of 7 months [2].

Recognition of the clinical signs is imperative, as early diagnosis and treatment are central to preventing complications, such as coronary artery aneurysms. Kawasaki disease in infants is more likely to be atypical (the rash and conjunctivitis may be much less prominent), and treatment instituted late, resulting in a higher risk of complications and poorer outcome [2,3]. Kawasaki disease should be considered in all infants less than 6 months of age with unexplained, persistent fever, as presentation is often 'incomplete' [1].

High fever lasting up to 8 days, associated with conjunctival injection and red, cracked lips, is followed by the development of a generalized maculopapular rash with prominent swelling and erythema of the hands and feet, which then desquamate. Cervical lymphadenopathy may be pronounced. Leucocytosis, thrombocytosis and high erythrocyte sedimentation rate are characteristic. Echocardiography may contribute diagnostically in infants with atypical presentation [2]. Management comprises the early administration of intravenous immunoglobulin, as soon as the diagnosis is suspected, plus supportive measures.

Chronic bullous disease of childhood

Chronic bullous disease of childhood (CBDC) (see also Chapter 50) is a non-familial, autoimmune, blistering disease that occurs in pre-pubertal children and is characterized by linear IgA staining of the basement membrane zone on direct immunofluorescence [1]. The disease is often idiopathic but may be triggered by infections, drugs, vaccinations, ultraviolet radiation or malignancy [2]. The production of an IgA autoantibody suggests either that a cross-reacting antigen enters via the mucosa or that an IgA diathesis exists in affected patients [3]. Autoantibodies are most often directed against proteolytic fragments of collagen XVII.

CBDC is often initially diagnosed as bullous impetigo and may even temporarily improve with a course of antibiotics. Children present with the abrupt onset of tense, clear or hemorrhagic vesicles and bullae on normal or erythematous skin. New lesions often arise around resolving lesions, and these arciform or annular bullae surrounding a central crust have been described as being in a string of pearls, cluster of jewels or rosette pattern (Figure 117.15). The eruption occurs on the face, trunk and extremities. There is a predilection for the lower trunk, genital area and medial thighs; disease onset in the perineum has been mistaken for sexual abuse [4]. On the face, lesions tend to occur in a perioral pattern. Younger children more often have the classic distribution of facial and perineal lesions.

The disease is associated with significant morbidity and usually requires systemic therapy. Treatment is aimed at controlling blistering while avoiding adverse reactions. There are several

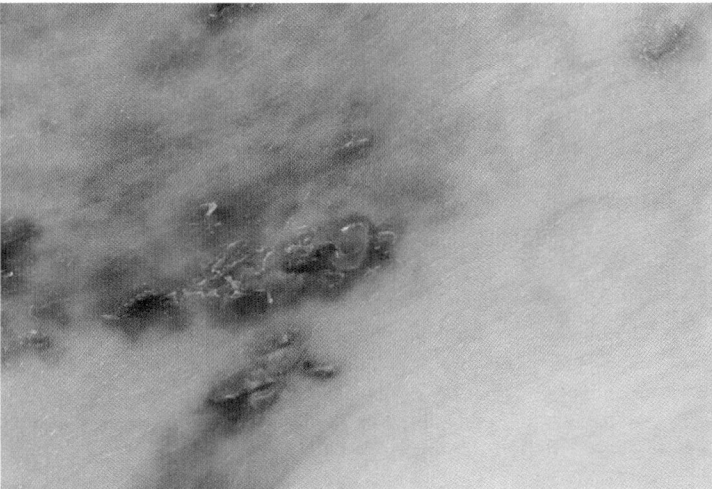

Figure 117.15 Clusters of small bullae in the groin of a child with chronic bullous disease of childhood.

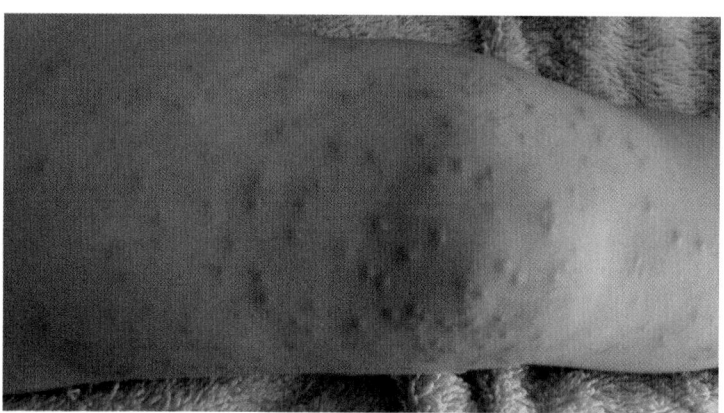

Figure 117.16 Gianotti–Crosti syndrome. Multiple monomorphic papules over the knees developed 2 weeks after an upper respiratory tract infection in this 1-year-old.

anecdotal reports of treatment options, but controlled or comparative studies are lacking [5]. Spontaneous resolution usually occurs in a matter of months or years.

Gianotti–Crosti syndrome

Synonyms and inclusions
- Papular acrodermatitis
- Infantile papular acrodermatitis

Early reports of this distinctive erythematous papular eruption on the face, buttocks and extremities showed a strong association with hepatitis B infection [1]. However, since the introduction of vaccination against hepatitis B this is now rare as a cause and it has become clear that the eruption may be associated with a variety of viruses [2], including Epstein–Barr virus [3], herpesvirus 6 [4] and Coxsackie virus [5], as well as with immunization [6,7].

The rash appears as monomorphic, flat-topped, pink to red-brown papules or papulovesicles in a symmetrical distribution favouring the cheeks and extensor surfaces of the limbs and buttocks, often preceded by a minor illness (Figure 117.16). Lesions may sometimes be found on the trunk and flexor surfaces [8,9]. Particularly in infancy, lesions may be oedematous. Constitutional symptoms are usually mild. The presence of lymphadenopathy and hepatitis are no longer required to make the diagnosis [10]. The rash lasts for a minimum of 10 days and may persist for up to 8 weeks. Recurrences are unusual.

Histopathology is not specific [11] and there is no specific treatment.

Papular urticaria

Papular urticaria arises as a result of a hypersensitivity reaction to insect bites, usually appearing as crops of more-or-less symmetrically distributed, itchy papules and papulovesicles,

most frequently on exposed areas of the extremities. They are often heavily excoriated, and secondary bacterial infection is common.

It tends to occur more in the summer months, when blood-feeding insects are most plentiful [1], but can occur at any time of year, particularly if caused by insects that breed in a domestic environment, such as cat fleas and bedbugs. The elapsed time between an insect bite and the formation of a firm, intensely itching papule begins to lengthen as children have increased exposure to these allergens. This delay can make it hard for parents to accept that insects are the cause of the eruption [2]. Diagnosis may also be complicated by reactivation of old lesions by new bites at a different site [2], thought to arise from circulating insect antigen-stimulating cutaneous T cells in previously sensitized sites [3].

Histopathological findings in papular urticaria vary with the particular insect, age of the lesion and sensitivity of the patient. The characteristic urticarial lesions will demonstrate prominent papillary dermal oedema and perivascular lymphocytes, eosinophils and mast cells; there may be superficial and deep perivascular and interstitial infiltrate with a variable density of lymphocytes and eosinophils. Chronic lesions may demonstrate pseudoepitheliomatous hyperplasia and atypical dermal infiltrates [2,4].

The treatment of papular urticaria includes topical steroids and systemic antihistamines, but response is usually limited, and the condition will only be controlled if insect bites can be avoided. Children eventually outgrow this disease, probably through desensitization after multiple arthropod exposures [5].

Eosinophilic pustular folliculitis

Synonyms and inclusions
- Eosinophilic pustulosis

Eosinophilic pustular folliculitis in infants is an uncommon condition, which appears to be distinct from the condition encountered in adults and older children [1,2]. As lesions are not always truly follicular [3], the term eosinophilic pustulosis is sometimes preferred. It is more common in males than females (4 : 1), and usually presents before the age of 14 months and clears by the age of 3 years [4]. The cause is unknown. Theories include a hypersensitivity response to microorganisms or dust mites [5], and a possible role for neuronal nitric oxide synthetase [6].

Histopathology of scalp lesions usually shows a perifollicular and periapendigeal infiltrate in the upper and mid dermis composed mainly of eosinophils, with neutrophils and mononuclear cells. Interstitial eosinophilic flame figures may be seen between collagen bundles [2,7]. There are some histopathological similarities to erythema toxicum neonatorum, which has led to the suggestion that they may be related conditions [7].

The condition is characterized by recurrent outbreaks of groups of very itchy papulopustules on an erythematous base, most commonly on the scalp, but also on the trunk and limbs, including

PART 10: SITES, SEX, AGE

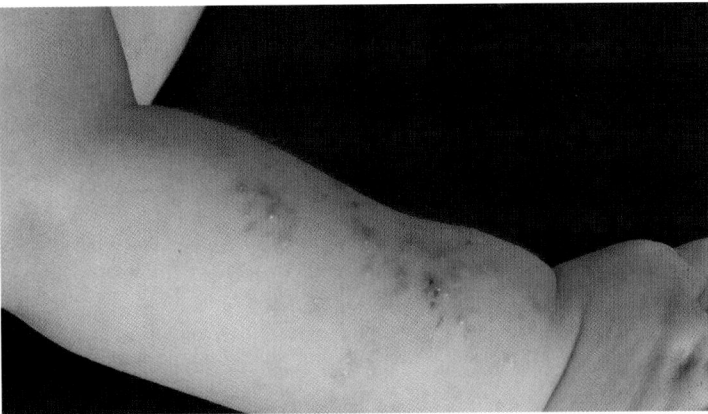

Figure 117.17 Eosinophilic pustulosis showing crops of small itchy pustules on the arm of a male infant.

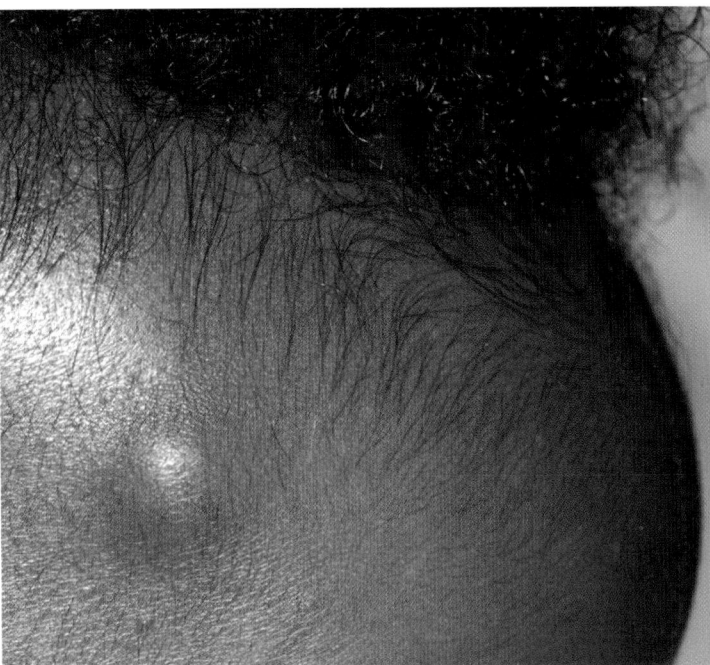

Figure 117.18 A dermoid cyst.

the hands and feet (Figure 117.17) [7]. These may resolve in 1 or 2 weeks, to be followed by further crops every few weeks. Spontaneous resolution usually occurs by 3 years of age. Affected infants are well.

During exacerbations there is peripheral blood eosinophilia and leukocytosis. Abundant eosinophils can be seen on Wright's stained smear of pustular contents. The differential diagnosis includes staphylococcal folliculitis, scabies, herpes simplex, infantile acropustulosis and Langerhans cell histiocytosis.

Because of the self-limiting nature of the condition, and lack of controlled trials, it is difficult to make specific recommendations for treatment. Benefit has been reported with cetirizine dihydrochloride [8], mid- to high-potency topical steroids [1,7] and topical calcineurin inhibitors [9].

DEVELOPMENTAL/GENETIC CONDITIONS

Dermoid cysts

Dermoid cysts arise from skin trapped within embryonic fusion lines. They may contain adnexal structures such as hair or eccrine glands, and very rarely bone and teeth. They occur most commonly on the head, presenting as firm subcutaneous nodules (Figure 117.18), particularly in the area of the anterolateral frontozygomatic suture [1], but also the parieto-occipital scalp and nose. They may connect to underlying structures, including the central nervous system if lying over the midline [2].

Preauricular cysts and sinuses

Preauricular cysts and sinuses are thought to arise from a failure of fusion of the auditory component or the first two branchial arches. They usually present as very small pits just anterior to the upper anterior helix. When bilateral they may be transmitted as an autosomal dominant trait. They may be associated with deafness and with other anomalies, as in branchio-oto-renal syndrome and branchio-otic syndrome [1,2]. Auditory testing and renal ultrasound are

indicated if a preauricular pit is associated with dysmorphic features or another anomaly, or with a family history of deafness [3].

Preauricular sinuses are usually asymptomatic in infancy, but may occasionally become infected. Surgery requires complete excision of the sinus tract and associated cysts [4].

Pigmentary mosaicism

Pigmentary mosaicism is a general term used to describe a wide range of phenotypes that include genetically determined variation of skin pigmentation [1]. It often presents as streaks and whorls of hypo- or hyperpigmentation following Blaschko's lines (Figure 117.19), with midline demarcation, determined by the embryonal migration paths from the neural crest of clones with different pigment-producing potential [2]. Pigmentary mosaicism may also manifest as patches, flag-like, leaf-like (phylloid) [3] or chequerboard shapes, or as patchy variation without midline demarcation. It may arise from a very wide variety of cytogenetic abnormalities [4], and may therefore be found in association with a broad range of associated clinical features, most frequently neurological and musculoskeletal. Infants with pigmentary mosaicism should be thoroughly assessed with particular attention to development, the internal organs and skeletal and ophthalmological abnormalities.

Linear morphoea

Morphoea develops less commonly in infancy than in early-school-aged children [1], and most commonly presents in the linear form [1,2] (see also Chapter 57). The cause remains unknown. Triggers may include vaccination [3], infections, including with Epstein–Barr virus [4] and *Borrelia burgdorferi* [5], autoimmune processes [2] and

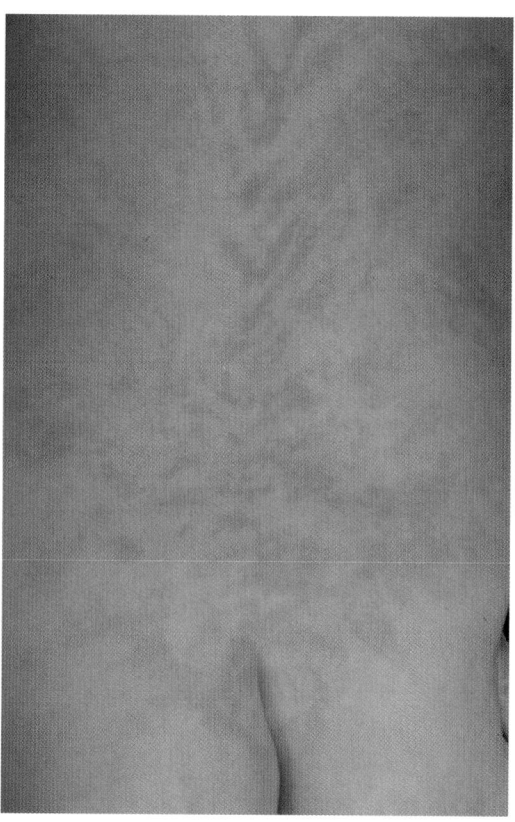

Figure 117.19 Whorls of hyperpigmentation following Blashko's lines.

genetic factors [6]. Linear morphoea follows Blaschko's lines, suggesting that susceptible cells may be present in a mosaic state [7].

Linear morphoea tends to progress faster than plaque-type morphoea, and is more likely to involve muscle and bone [8], which may lead to facial hemiatrophy [9]. It may present with macular erythema, sometimes leading to misdiagnosis as a vascular malformation [10]. When on the head (so called 'en coup de sabre'), scarring alopecia and partial loss of the brow or lashes is characteristic. Up to 13% of children with linear morphoea en coup de sabre have seizures [11].

Proposed minimum standards of care for children with linear morphoea on the face or scalp include brain magnetic resonance imaging (MRI), screening for uveitis and dental assessment [12]. Disease activity is difficult to determine clinically. Scanning laser Doppler imaging may be useful in predicting disease progression [13].

There is lack of consensus on optimal treatment [14], but first line treatment is usually with combined systemic steroids and methotrexate, and maintenance with methotrexate alone for at least 3 years [15].

MISCELLANEOUS CONDITIONS

Milia

Small, firm, white papules, predominantly occurring on the face of newborn babies and infants, are common and harmless. Lesions should not be confused with milk spots or the more florid milia associated with bullous disorders. Infantile milia may occasionally be associated with oral lesions on the gingivae or palate. The estimated prevalence is 16%, and the majority of lesions occur on the cheeks, forehead or chin [1]. Milia are more common in white children, but less frequent in children born prematurely or of low gestational weight [1].

Koilonychia

The nail plate of infants is very soft and malleable. Transient concavity of the nail plate is not uncommon [1] and not usually a manifestation of iron deficiency. The condition is self-resolving, growing out normally over time.

Non-accidental injury

Sadly, non-accidental injury (NAI) is still a widespread problem, especially amongst infants and toddlers. Injuries can take many forms [1] but all health care professionals, nursery workers and social service agencies should be fully aware of possible signs of NAI and the mechanisms for reporting and safeguarding children at risk.

Subconjunctival haemorrhages in an infant should arouse suspicion that the child is a victim of shaken baby syndrome. Toddlers and older children frequently have genuine accidents, but these are less likely in infants who are not yet mobile [1,2]. In children with multiple attendances at A&E, delayed attendance after an injury or unexplained injuries, the concern of NAI should be raised, and investigating clinicians must consider undertaking a skeletal survey. Bites, burns, signs of neglect or sexual abuse may all form part of the spectrum [1,2]. Emotional abuse may coexist or occur in isolation. A young child becoming withdrawn, or wary of adults, should arouse suspicion and appropriate measures to investigate taken.

Bite injuries

Bite injuries in infants are not infrequent. Establishing the source of the bite is imperative. Animal bites are usually clear-cut, in that they present rapidly to A&E with a clear history, but the wounds can be deep and ragged and usually require antibiotics to treat infection and expert plastic surgery to minimize scarring.

Human bites may simply leave bruising or purpura, rather than puncture marks. However, it is essential to establish whether the injury has been inflicted by an adult or another child by assessing the size of the dentition from the marks on the skin. Bites inflicted by adults are indicative of NAI and need to be managed accordingly. Bites perpetrated by children may reflect sibling rivalry/jealousy over a new arrival in the home (Figure 117.20) [1], and can usually be managed with temporary support for the family.

PART 10: SITES, SEX, AGE

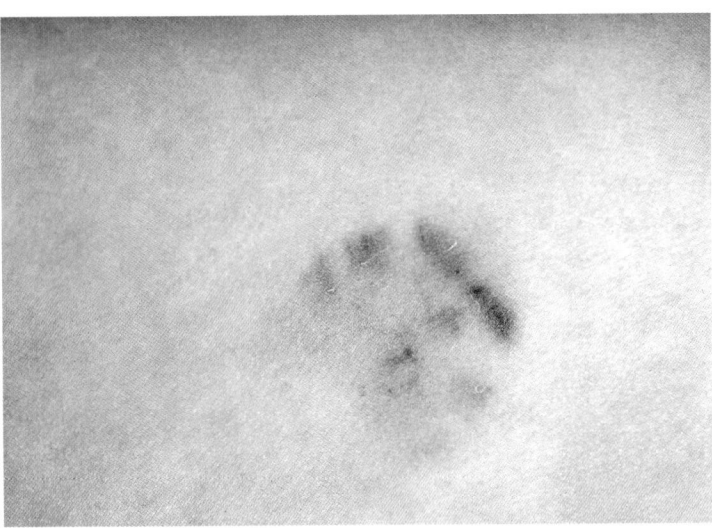

Figure 117.20 A bite mark on the upper limb of a 10-month-old (inflicted by his 4-year-old brother).

Pedal papules of infancy

Symmetrical, painless, flesh-coloured nodules, characteristically on the medial aspect of the heels in infants, may be present at birth, but are usually not apparent until infancy [1]. Although once thought to be uncommon, recent surveys suggest that they may occur in up to 40% of infants [1]. They may be solitary (Figure 117.21), but unlike piezogenic papules in adults, tend to be larger and asymptomatic [2].

Calcified cutaneous nodules of the heels

Small firm, calcified dermal lesions have been described on the heels of infants who have been on neonatal intensive care units and subjected to multiple heel pricks for venesection [1]. Histologically, the lesions appear to have features of epidermal cysts and so are believed to arise from epidermal implantation through trauma,

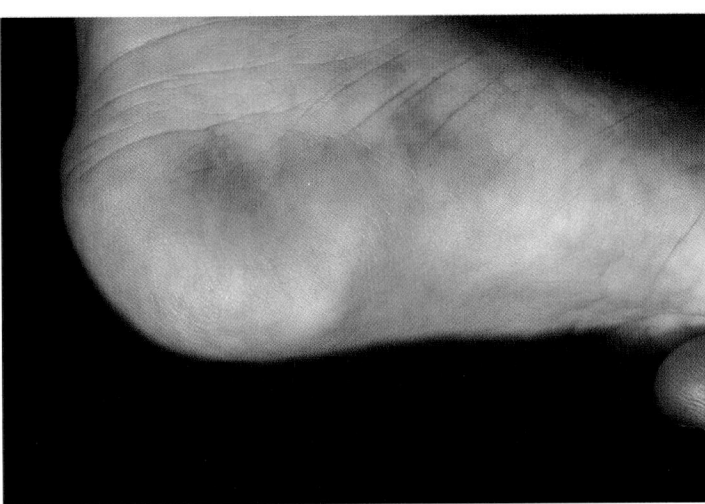

Figure 117.21 Pedal papule of infancy showing a soft swelling on the medial aspect of the heel.

with subsequent calcification of the cyst, rather than dystrophic calcification per se [2]. Natural resolution over the course of 18 months is the norm, but if slow to resolve they may cause pain on pressure when walking in older children [1].

Hair loss in infancy

Shedding of hair occurs during the seventh to eighth month *in utero* in all areas except the occiput, where shedding is delayed until 2–3 months postpartum [1], leading to the normal occipital alopecia in this age group.

Absent or diffusely sparse hair in infancy can arise from abnormalities of initiation of growth, hair shaft abnormalities and abnormal cycling.

Alopecia areata is relatively rare in the first year of life [2] and early onset tends to indicate a poor prognosis. It is important to distinguish rarer causes of extensive hair loss in infancy, including vitamin D-resistant rickets [3].

Telogen effluvium is less common in infants than in adults, and is more likely to be related to a sudden and transient illness than to drugs or hormonal fluctuations.

Loose anagen syndrome refers to a condition seen in children, usually girls, who have sparse hair with easily extracted anagen hairs, with misshapen bulbs, absent root sheaths and ruffled cuticles [4].

Juvenile xanthogranuloma

Juvenile xanthogranuloma (JXG) often presents in the first year of life, and is more common in boys than girls [1]. Lesions generally start as red-brown papules, that become orange (Figure 117.22), occurring

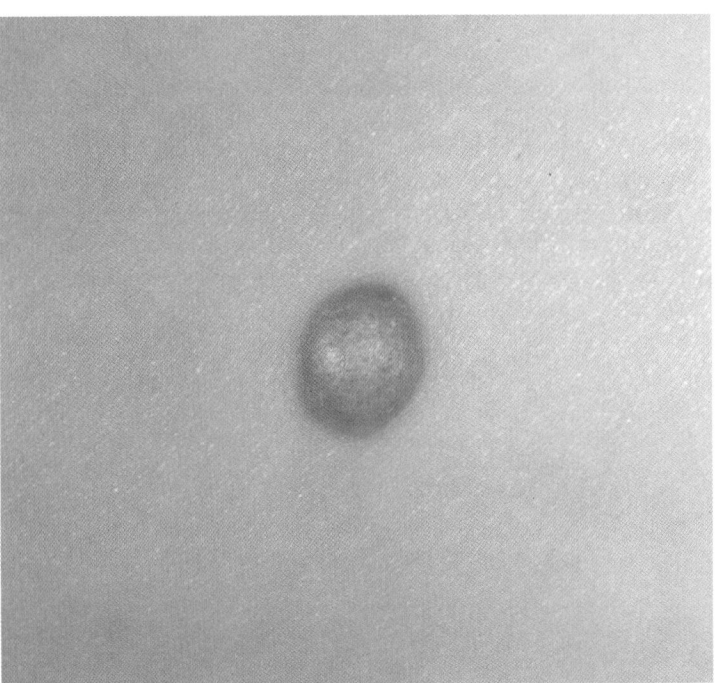

Figure 117.22 Juvenile xanthogranuloma showing a well-circumscribed yellowish nodule with an erythematous margin on the upper back of a 6-month-old.

most frequently on the face and scalp and upper torso. The eye is involved in 0.4% of cases under the age of 2 years [2], and may lead to spontaneous hyphema, glaucoma, cataract and uveitis [3]. Localized cutaneous JXG heals spontaneously, sometimes leaving atrophic scars.

Benign cephalic histiocytosis has many similarities to JXG and may be the same disease [4]. It usually presents in the first or second year of life, as multiple, small, yellow-red macules and papules, initially on the head, but sometimes spreading to other sites [5]. The lesions heal spontaneously without scarring.

Langerhans cell histiocytosis

Langerhans cell histiocytosis is the commonest of the histiocytic disorders in childhood, most frequently presenting in infants under the age of 1 year [1], with boys affected twice as often as girls [2] (see also Chapter 136). The cause of LCH is unknown. *BRAF V600E* mutations have been demonstrated in a number of cases [3], but the clinical significance of this mutation is unclear [4].

LCH can be divided into: (i) an acute, disseminated form (formerly Letterer–Siwe disease); (ii) a chronic, localized form (eosinophilic granuloma); (iii) a progressive, multifocal, chronic form (Hand–Schüller–Christian disease); and (iv) a benign, self-healing form (congenital self-healing reticulohistiocytosis or Hashimoto–Pritzker disease). In practice these tend to overlap and are therefore best regarded as a continuum.

Because the cutaneous features are very variable, including seborrhoeic dermatitis-like erythema and scaling (Figure 117.23), papules, pustules, vesicles, nodules, petechiae and ulceration, the diagnosis is often delayed [5]. The prognosis depends on the extent of the disease. Truly single-system disease has almost 100% survival [6], but up to 56% infants presenting with skin-only disease may progress to multisystem disease [7].

Non-Langerhans cell histiocytoses are rare in infancy, and may be related predominantly to the dendritic cell line (the juvenile xanthogranuloma group) or to the macrophage line (reticulohistiocytoma, cutaneous Rosai–Dorfman disease, multicentric reticulohistiocytosis and sinus histiocytosis) [8].

Mastocytosis

Mastocytosis in infancy is usually limited to the skin, with three distinct clinical presentations: maculopapular (formerly urticaria pigmentosa) (Figure 117.24a), diffuse cutaneous mastocytosis (Figure 117.24b) and solitary mastocytoma (Figure 117.25).

Activating c-kit mutations can be demonstrated in a proportion of patients, but mutational status appears insufficient to explain the divergent biology of childhood and adult-onset disease [1]. Serum tryptase is the best marker for mast cell burden in infants, and, at baseline, correlates well with the severity of symptoms [2]. Whilst in adults mastocytosis is considered systemic until proved otherwise, in infants this is not the case [3] as systemic mastocytosis is extremely rare in children and is usually indolent [4].

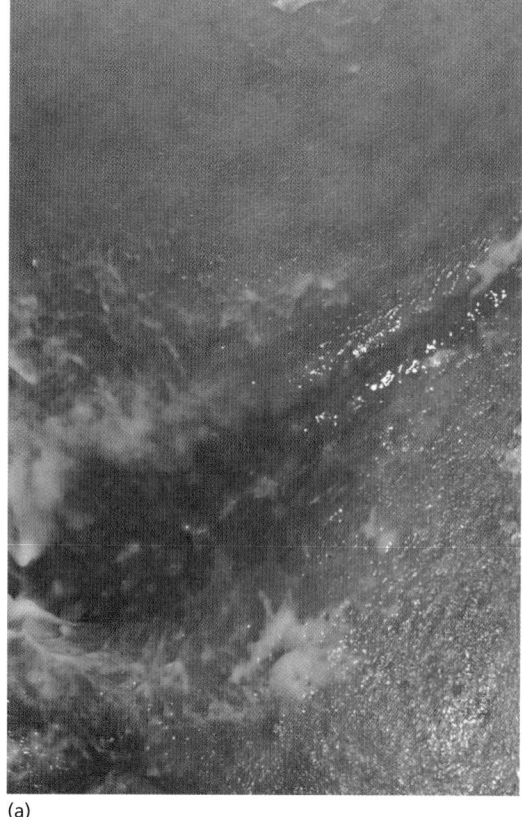

(a)

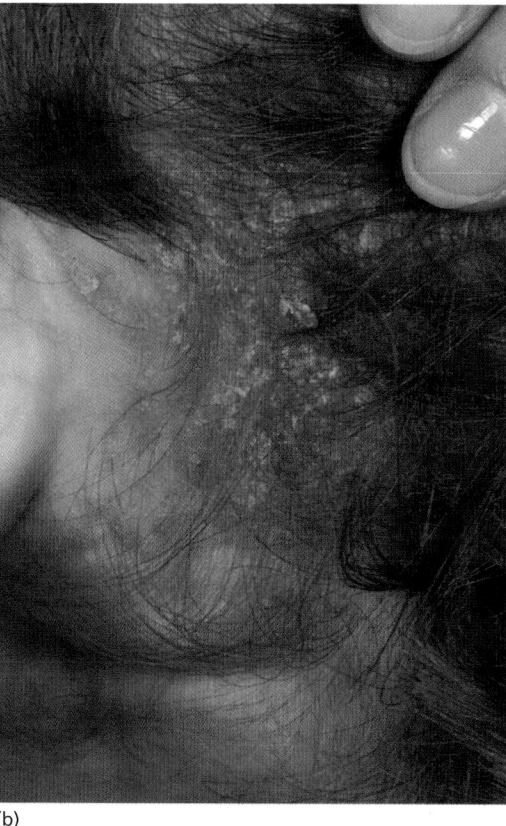

(b)

Figure 117.23 Langerhans cell histiocytosis. (a) Macerated and eroded erythema in the groin. (b) Crusted papules and erythema on the scalp.

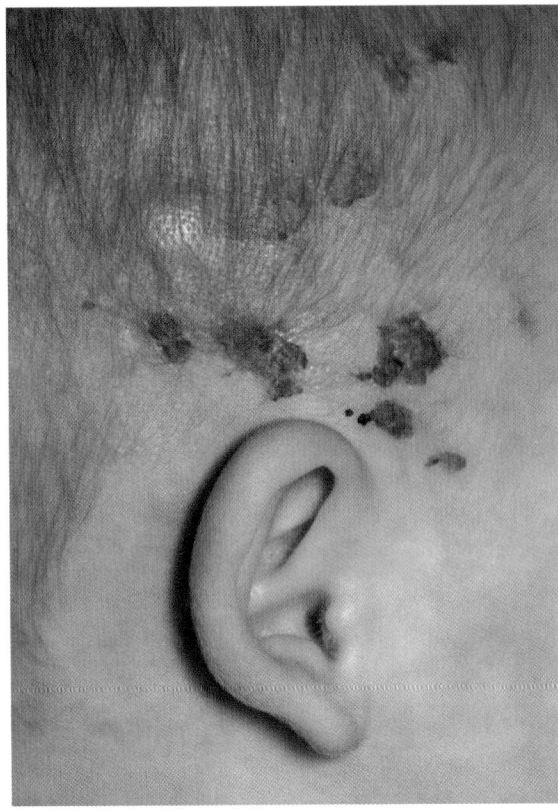

(a)

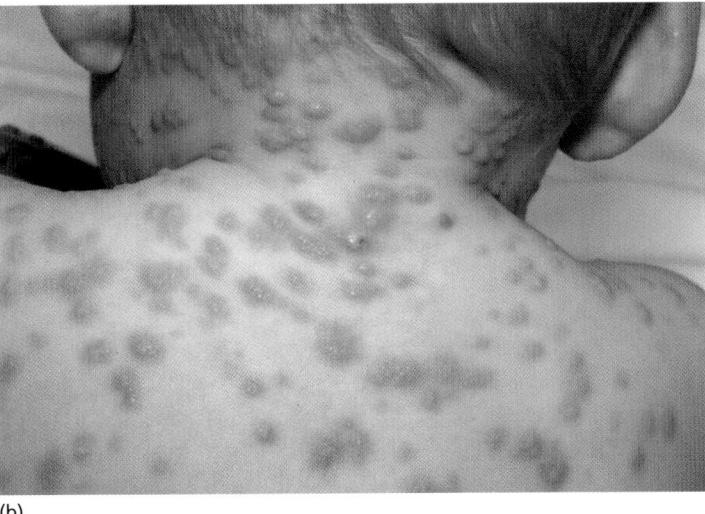

(b)

Figure 117.24 Mastocytosis. (a) Mast cell degranulation causing erythematous papules and crusts on the scalp. (b) Papules and plaques on the back of an infant with diffuse cutaneous mastocytosis.

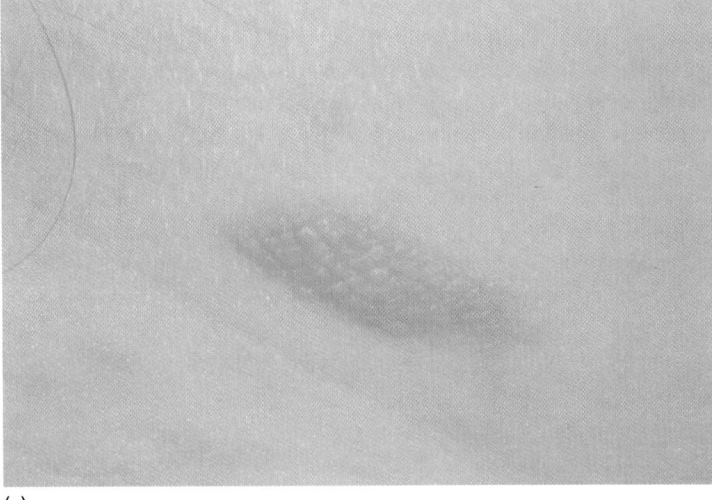

(a)

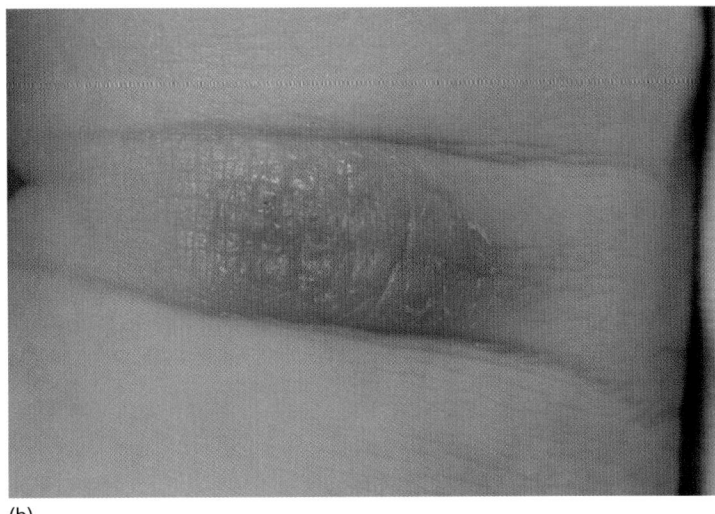

(b)

Figure 117.25 Solitary mastocytoma: (a) before rubbing; (b) urticated after rubbing.

H_2 blocker if there are symptoms of hyperacidity or ulceration [7], with or without oral sodium cromoglycate for diarrhoea [8,9]. Children with a history of anaphylaxis should be supplied with an adrenaline autoinjector.

INFANTILE AND CONGENITAL HAEMANGIOMAS

Infantile haemangiomas

Definition and nomenclature

Infantile haemangiomas are common, benign, vascular tumours that develop in early infancy and undergo spontaneous involution thereafter.

Parents of infants with extensive skin involvement should be given advice on the avoidance of factors known to stimulate mast cell degranulation, including aspirin, non-steroidal anti-inflammatory drugs, codeine, opiates, polymyxin B and intravenous radiograph contrast fluids and MRI contrast media [5]. Symptomatic therapy, usually consisting of an H_1 receptor blocker, may help control itch, blistering, flushing and urtication [6], plus an

Synonyms and inclusions
- Haemangioma of infancy
- Terms such as strawberry naevus, capillary haemangioma and cavernous haemangioma have contributed to the diagnostic confusion in the field of vascular anomalies, and are best avoided

Introduction and general description

Infantile haemangiomas are by far the most common benign vascular tumours encountered in infancy. The natural history is of proliferation in the first few months of life, and involution over a matter of years. Most resolve spontaneously without sequelae, but treatment is indicated for those causing, or likely to cause, impairment of function, disfigurement or ulceration.

Segmental or plaque-like infantile haemangiomas of the head and neck and of the lumbo-sacral region may be associated with structural anomalies. Multifocal infantile haemangiomas are usually asymptomatic but may occasionally be associated with extensive visceral involvement. Rapidly involuting congenital haemangiomas (RICH), non-involuting congenital haemangiomas (NICH) and partially involuting congenital haemangiomas (PICH) are clinically distinct from infantile haemangiomas, and appear to have completed their proliferative phase *in utero*.

The classification approved at the April 2014 General Assembly of the International Society for the Study of Vascular Anomalies (ISSVA) divides vascular anomalies into tumours (including infantile haemangiomas and congenital haemangiomas) and malformations (Table 117.1) [1]. The distinction between infantile haemangiomas and vascular malformations is often straightforward on the basis of history and examination, but occasionally investigations such as ultrasound, histopathology and immunohistochemistry are required (Table 117.2).

Infantile haemangiomas can be classified morphologically as different types:
- Superficial.
- Deep.
- Mixed (superficial and deep).
- Reticular, abortive or minimal growth.
  These can exist in different patterns:
- Focal.

Table 117.1 Benign vascular tumours and vascular malformations: simplified classification.

Benign vascular tumours	Vascular malformations
Infantile haemangioma (IH):	High flow:
Hepatic haemangioma (HH)	Arteriovenous
Multifocal IH	Low flow:
Without systemic involvement	Capillary
With systemic involvement	Venous
Congenital haemangiomas:	Lymphatic
Rapidly involuting (RICH)	Mixed
Non-involuting (NICH)	For example:
Partially involuting (PICH)	Capillary venous
Tufted angioma	Capillary lymphatic venous
Spindle cell haemangioma	Capillary arteriovenous
Epithelioid haemangioma	
Pyogenic granuloma	

- Multifocal.
- Segmental.
- Indeterminate.

Infantile haemangiomas can also occur with or without associated lesions (Table 117.3) [1].

Epidemiology

Infantile haemangiomas are the most common tumours of infancy, occurring in up to 10% of infants, more commonly in girls than boys [2]. Most cases are sporadic. Amniocentesis, *in vitro* fertilization, breech presentation, being first born and low birth weight (<2500 g) appear to be independently associated with the development of infantile haemangioma [2].

Pathophysiology

Pathogenesis

The aetiology of infantile haemangioma remains unclear. Endothelial cells are characterized by the surface marker GLUT-1, an erythrocyte-type glucose transporter protein, which is also expressed on the placental vasculature. It has been proposed that this placental phenotype may be the result of embolization of placental endothelial cells to the fetal circulation [3]. Against this theory is the lack of evidence of maternal–fetal chimerism [4].

Table 117.2 Distinction between infantile haemangiomas and vascular malformations.

	Infantile haemangioma	Vascular malformation
Clinical features	Usually evident within the first week of life	Usually present at birth
	Proliferate rapidly	Proportionate growth
	Involute over years	Do not involute
Epidemiology	More common in girls and low birth weight infants	No gender or birth-weight bias
Immunohistochemistry	GLUT-1 positive	GLUT-1 negative

Table 117.3 Anomalies associated with segmental or plaque-type infantile haemangiomas.

Facial segmental haemangioma	Lower body segmental haemangioma
Posterior fossa malformations, haemangiomas, arterial anomalies, cardiac anomalies, eye abnormalities, sternal pit/supraumbilical raphe (PHACES association)	Lower body IH, uro-genital anomalies, ulceration, myelopathy, bony deformities, ano-rectal malformations, arterial anomalies and renal anomalies (LUMBAR association)
	Spinal dysraphism, ano-genital anomalies, cutaneous anomalies, renal and urological anomalies, lumbosacral IH (SACRAL association)
	Perineal IH, external genitalia, malformations, lipomyelomeningocele, vesico-renal abnormalities, imperforate anus (PELVIS association)

From International Society for the Study of Vascular Anomalies (ISSVA) 2014 [1].
© 2014 ISSVA. Available at http://issva.org/ (last accessed April 2015).
IH, infantile haemangioma.

An autosomal dominant inheritance pattern and a linkage to 5q have been reported in a small number of families [5] and a two-fold increased relative risk for the disorder among siblings of an affected proband has been reported [6]. Somatic mutations leading to uncontrolled proliferation of haemangioma cells have been proposed. In support of this theory, clonality of endothelial cells from haemangioma lesions has been shown in a small subset of infantile haemangiomas [6]. Mutations in the integrin-like receptor tumour endothelial marker 8, and in *VEGFR2*, have been identified in a subpopulation of haemangioma-derived endothelial cells and corresponding blood samples from patients with infantile haemangioma [7].

Pathology

The diagnosis is nearly always clinical, and biopsy is rarely required to distinguish infantile haemangioma from other vascular anomalies. During the early phase of growth the haemangiomas consist of solid groups of cells with few lumina. The endothelial cells flatten out as the lumina develop. The cells are surrounded by a thickened basement membrane. During the process of involution a more lobular appearance develops, with islands of fibrous and fatty tissue between the lobules. Mast cells are evident at all phases. Immunohistochemistry is positive for factor VIII, CD31 and von Willebrand factor. Glucose 1 transporter protein (GLUT-1) positivity can be useful in differentiating infantile haemangiomas from other vascular lesions, such as congenital haemangiomas, but it may also be positive in verrucous vascular malformations.

Clinical features

Haemangiomas may be evident shortly after birth as a faint telangiectatic patch or an area of pallor (Figure 117.26), or as a flat pink mark which rapidly becomes red and raised (Figure 117.27). Superficial types of infantile haemangioma show their most rapid growth between 5.5 and 7.5 weeks of age [8] (Figure 117.28). Deep haemangiomas, which develop in the lower dermis and subcutis,

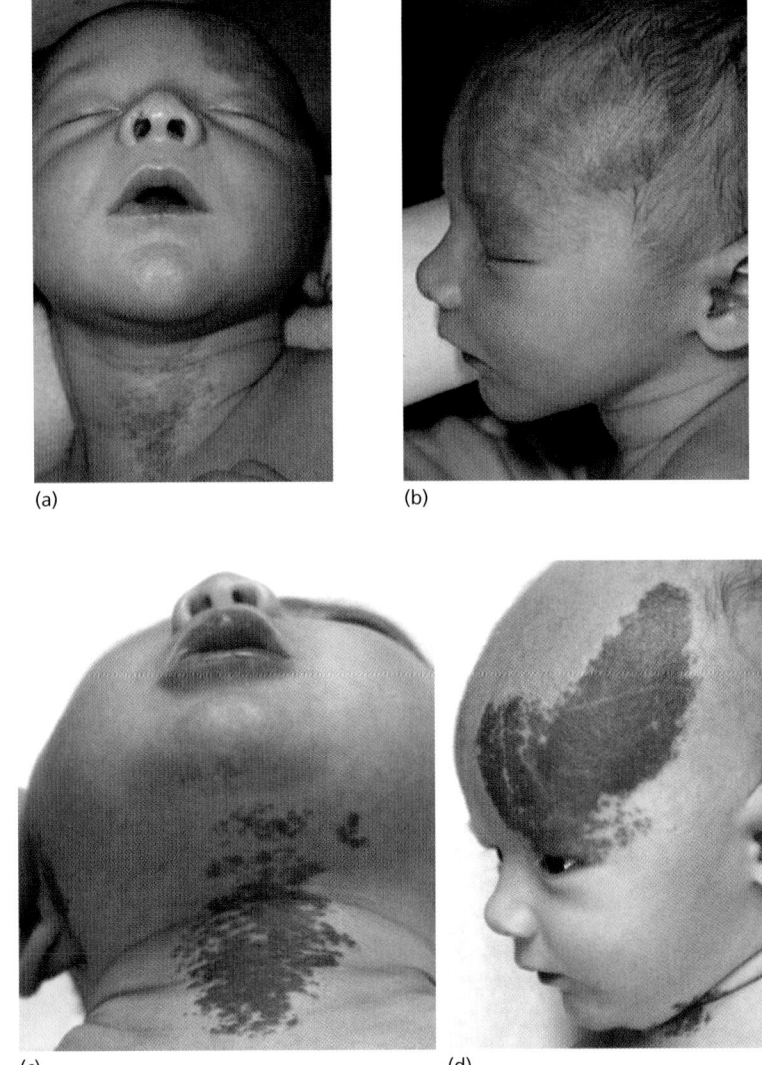

(a) (b)

(c) (d)

Figure 117.27 Evolution of facial and neck plaque-type haemangiomas from day 1 (a, b) to day 10 (c, d).

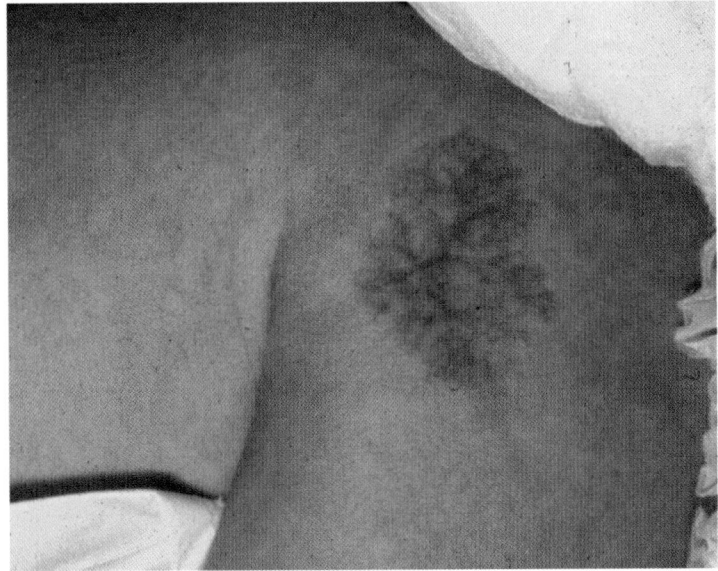

Figure 117.26 Haemangioma precursor.

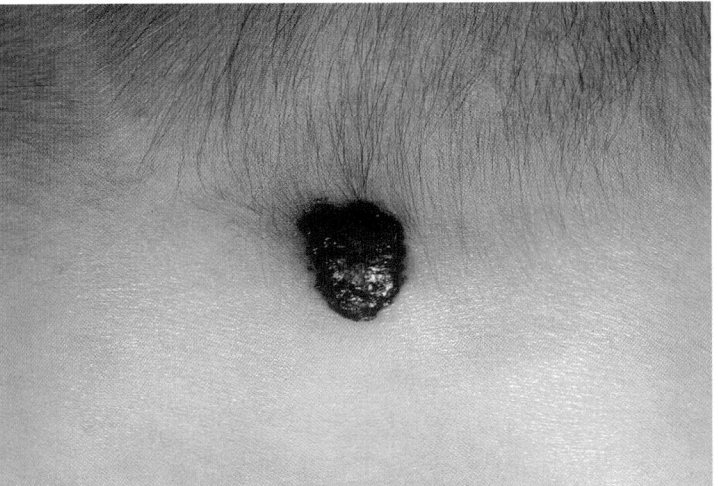

Figure 117.28 A small capillary haemangioma in the proliferative phase on the forehead of a 3-month old infant.

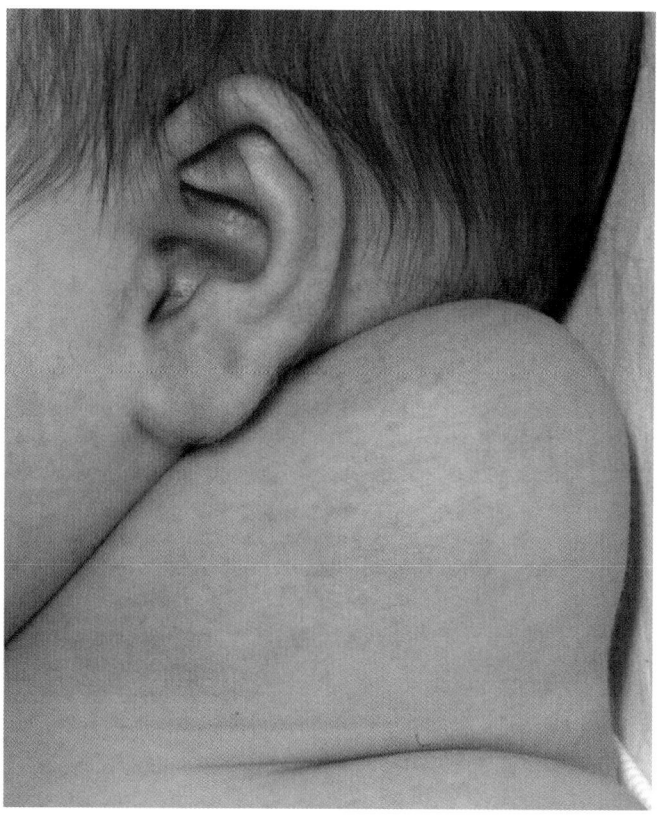

Figure 117.29 An 8-week-old infant with a deep infantile haemangioma involving the lateral neck.

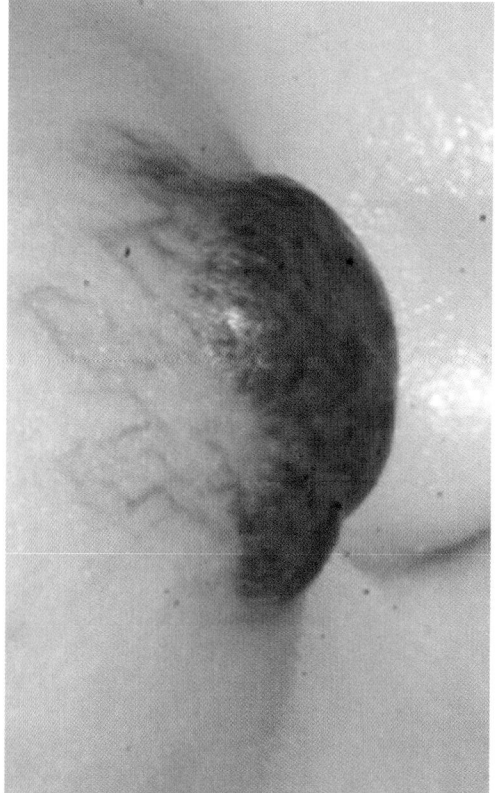

Figure 117.31 Lateral view of an infantile haemangioma on the face of a 7-week-old infant showing both superficial and deep components (mixed form).

tend to appear blue or purple, may have no overlying skin changes (Figure 117.29), often present later and continue to grow for longer than superficial haemangiomas. Irrespective of subtype or depth, most infantile haemangiomas reach 80% of their final size by 3 months of age [9]. Mixed infantile haemangiomas, sharing features of both the superficial and deep types, are common (Figures 117.30 and 117.31). A minority of infantile haemangiomas, sometimes

referred to as abortive infantile haemangioma, show relatively little proliferation, remaining as a patch of telangiectatic vessels.

During the proliferative phase, infantile haemangiomas are firm. With involution they become softer. Superficial haemangiomas develop islands of greying within the redness, with some flattening of the surface. In untreated lesions, involution is complete at a median age of 3 years, and most cases cease to

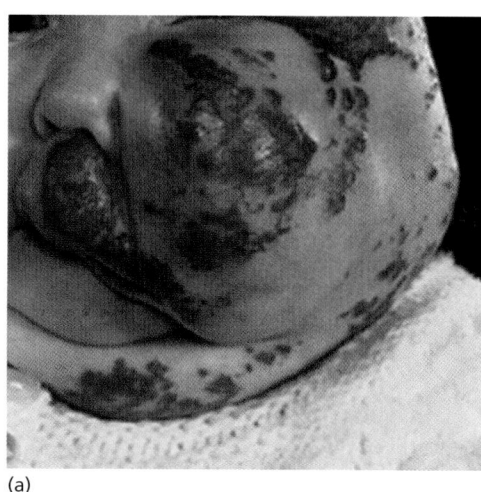

(a)

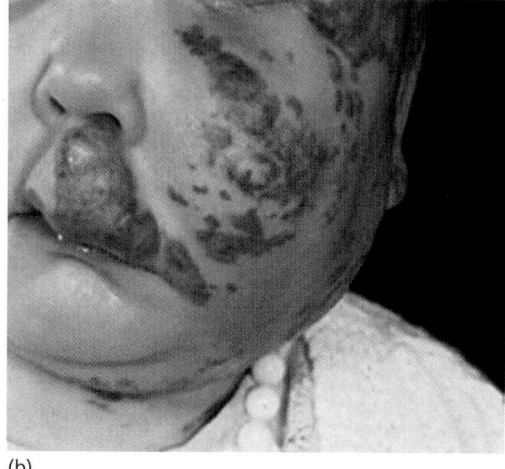

(b)

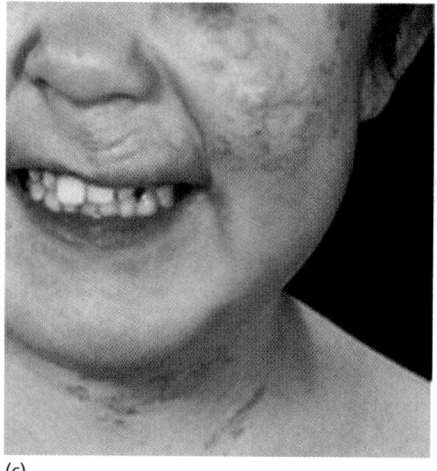

(c)

Figure 117.30 Large, mixed infantile haemangioma at (a) 3 months, (b) 16 months and (c) 3 years. A course of oral prednisolone was given at 3 months.

improve significantly after 3.5 years of age [10]. Therefore, surgical reconstruction, if indicated, may be best undertaken at this age, as further aesthetically beneficial, spontaneous improvement is unlikely to occur. Permanent changes – most frequently telangiectases, atrophy and residual bulk in the form of fibrofatty tissue (Figure 117.30c) – have been reported to remain in up to 69% of untreated haemangiomas [11]. Atrophic scars frequently follow ulceration.

Clinical variants

Segmental infantile haemangioma. A proportion of infantile haemangiomas, referred to as segmental or plaque-like, involve a broad anatomical region, thought to reflect embryological metameres [12]. Segmental infantile haemangioma of the face (Figure 117.32) and of the lumbo-sacral region (Figure 117.33) may be associated with underlying structural anomalies (see Table 117.3). Up to 30% of large segmental facial infantile haemangiomas are associated with the PHACES syndrome (*p*osterior fossa malformations, *h*aemangiomas, *a*rterial anomalies, *c*ardiac anomalies, *e*ye abnormalities and *s*ternal pit/*s*upraumbilical raphe) [**13**]. Segmental infantile haemangiomas of the frontotemporal or mandibular regions are at the highest risk, but rare cases of PHACES have been reported without facial involvement [14]. Abnormalities of the cerebral vasculature and

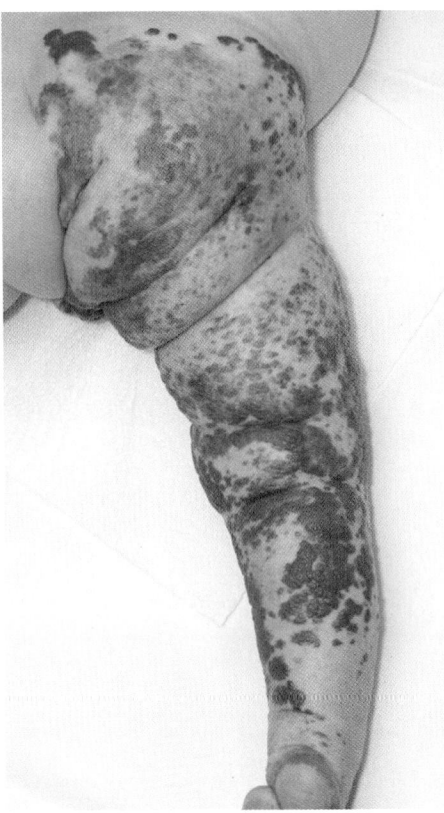

Figure 117.33 Male infant aged 6 weeks with segmental infantile haemangioma associated with complex spinal dysraphism.

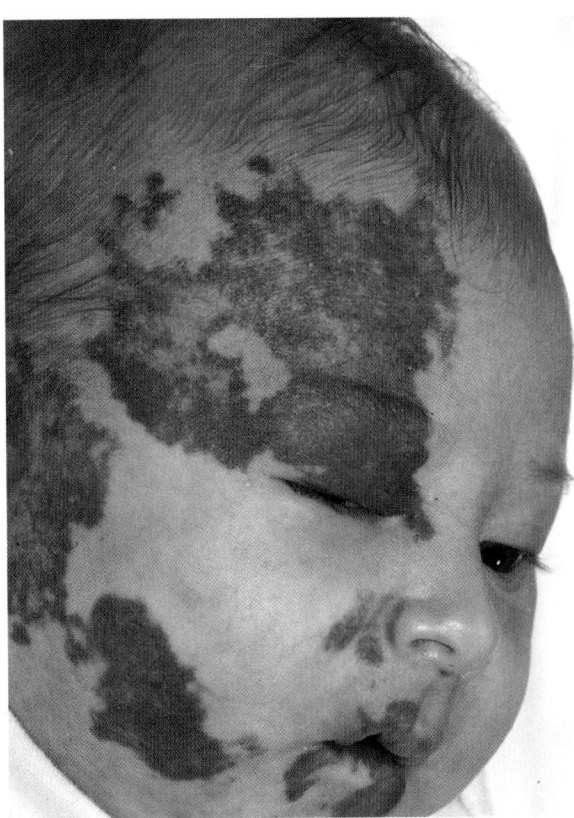

Figure 117.32 Female infant aged 4 weeks with facial segmental infantile haemangioma associated with dilatation of the right internal carotid, proximal middle cerebral and posterior communicating arteries, right III nerve palsy, and vascular ring arising from a right-sided aortic arch, retro-oesophageal left subclavian artery and patent left ductus arteriosus.

coarctation of the aorta are the most common extracutaneous findings [15]. Head and neck magnetic resonance angiography (MRA), echocardiogram and ophthalmological examination are recommended for patients with large segmental facial infantile haemangiomas.

Segmental infantile haemangiomas in the beard region, especially if bilateral, may be associated with airway haemangiomas. Otolaryngological advice should be sought for such infants, even in the absence of overt respiratory symptoms.

Segmental infantile haemangioma in the lumbo-sacral and perineal regions may be associated with spinal dysraphism, uro-genital abnormalities, ano-rectal malformations, arterial anomalies and renal abnormalities [16]. For infants under the age of 3 months, spinal ultrasound may be useful for the initial assessment, but spinal MRI with contrast is advisable.

Multifocal cutaneous infantile haemangioma with and without extracutaneous involvement. Historically the term haemangiomatosis – qualified variously as diffuse, miliary or disseminated – has been used to refer to multiple haemangiomas, with or without visceral involvement. Further confusion has arisen from inclusion under this term of GLUT-1-negative conditions such as multifocal lymphangioendotheliomatosis. In this text the terms multifocal infantile haemangioma, with or without extracutaneous involvement, will be used.

Multifocal haemangiomas may range in number from a few to hundreds, and are usually small (Figure 117.34). They are

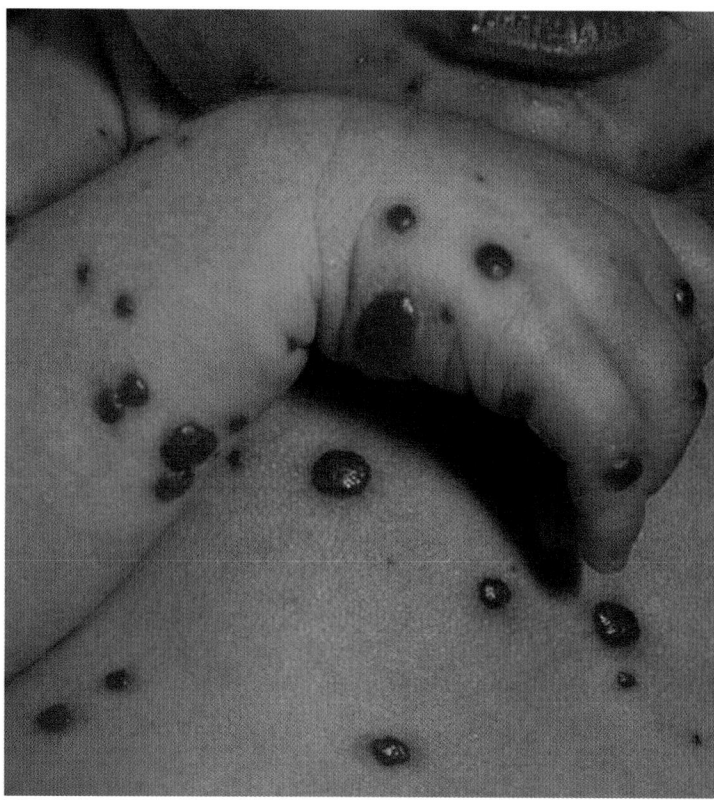

Figure 117.34 Multifocal cutaneous infantile haemangioma.

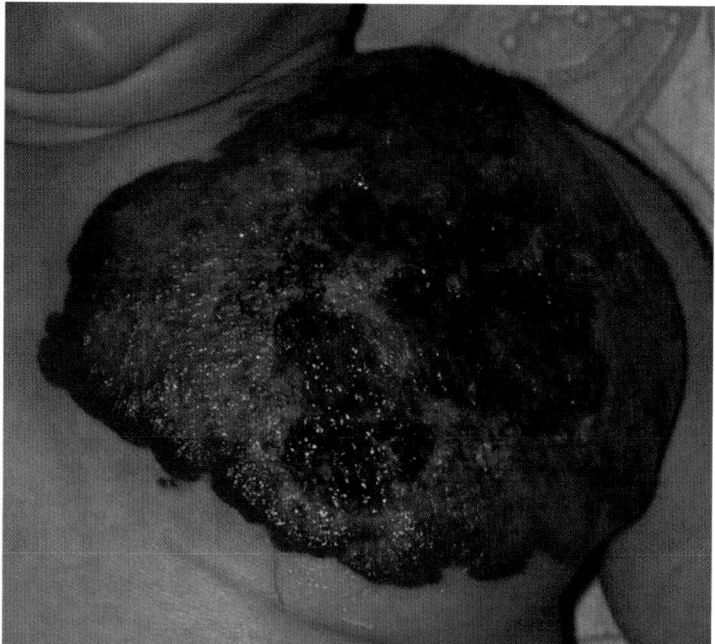

Figure 117.35 Large segmental ulcerated infantile haemangioma.

histologically and immunohistochemically identical to solitary cutaneous infantile haemangiomas. Most affected infants follow an uncomplicated course, but some have symptomatic visceral lesions, with liver involvement being the most common.

Hepatic haemangioma. Hepatic haemangioma (HH) may occur with or without cutaneous infantile haemangioma. Many HH are asymptomatic, and those that become symptomatic usually do so within the first 3 months of life [17], presenting with hepatomegaly and high-output cardiac failure. HH may be focal, multifocal or diffuse [18]. Focal HH may be evident on antenatal ultrasound, are usually GLUT-1-negative, occur without cutaneous lesions, regress rapidly and probably represent RICH of the liver.

Multifocal HH are usually associated with multiple, small, cutaneous infantile haemangiomas, and are GLUT-1 positive [19]. Most HH in this group are asymptomatic and do not require treatment [20].

Diffuse HH is a term that has been used to describe massive involvement of the liver, often with symptomatic arteriovenous shunting and high-output cardiac failure. It is possible that historically the morbidity of HH may have been overestimated as a result of the misinterpretation of multifocal lymphangioendotheliomatosis and multifocal kaposiform haemangioendothelioma as HH.

Complications and co-morbidities

The main complications of infantile haemangiomas are ulceration, disfigurement and functional impairment.

- Ulceration is common, the risk being greatest between 4 and 6 months of age. Ulceration is more likely in large infantile haemangiomas (Figure 117.35), segmental morphology and location on the neck, ano-genital area or lip, where there is exposure to friction and moisture. Ulceration can occur in up to 20% cases, is painful, may be associated with bleeding and infection, and almost always results in scarring [21].
- The risk of disfigurement depends on the location, morphological subtype and size. Even relatively small infantile haemangiomas on the central face, lips and nose (Figure 117.36), particularly those with a dermal component, can lead to permanent distortion [22].

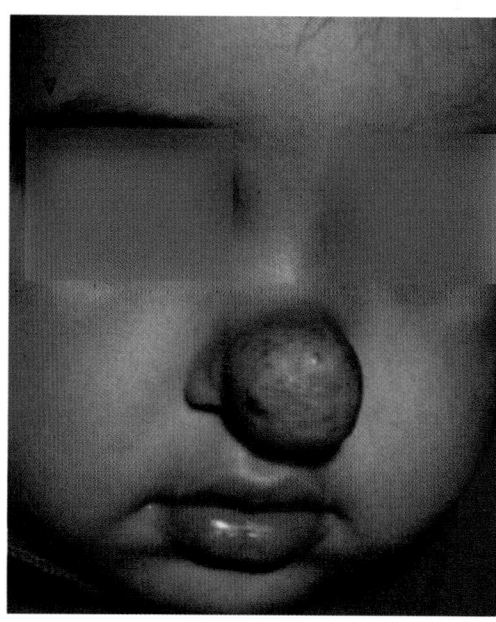

Figure 117.36 Residuum from a nasal tip haemangioma.

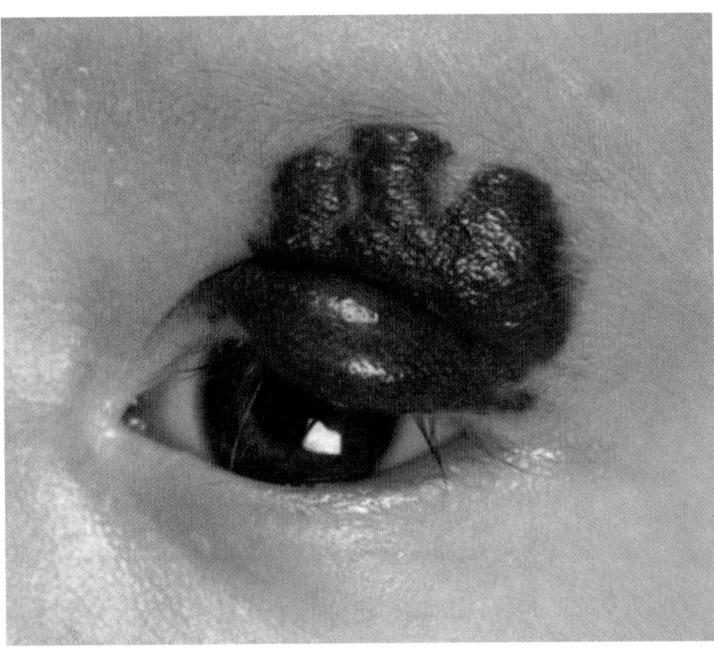

Figure 117.37 Eyelid haemangioma in the line of vision.

- Impairment of function is most commonly encountered with peri-ocular infantile haemangiomas (Figure 117.37), which may cause astigmatism, visual axis obstruction and strabismus, which in turn can lead to amblyopia and the risk of permanent visual loss [23]. Haemangiomas involving the airway and the nose can endanger breathing, and those on the lip may interfere with feeding.

Disease course and prognosis

Most infantile haemangiomas follow a predictable course, appearing shortly after birth, usually achieving 80% of their growth by 3 months, and completion of growth by about 9 months. Approximately 3% of infantile haemangiomas, mainly deep ones, may show growth for longer. Involution occurs over a matter of years, leaving evident residual skin changes in between 25% and 60% of untreated cases.

The prognosis is excellent without treatment for small infantile haemangiomas. Prognosis is also excellent for larger haemangiomas if there is no functional impairment, and if it is not at an aesthetically important site. If appropriate treatment is started in a timely fashion prognosis is also good for infantile haemangiomas causing (or likely to cause) functional or aesthetic impairment.

Investigations

Investigation is rarely required as the diagnosis is usually clinical. Occasionally ultrasound may be required to distinguish infantile haemangiomas from other soft tissues masses or vascular malformations. Investigation may also be indicated for plaque-type infantile haemangiomas on the face and lower trunk and before treatment with β-blockers.

Management

Treatment will depend on the location, morphology and stage of evolution, impact on function, risk of disfigurement and co-morbidities. Active non-intervention is appropriate if there is no impairment of function, no ulceration and it is considered that spontaneous regression will produce an excellent outcome. In the early stages parents are often very concerned about aesthetic issues, and require detailed explanation of the natural history of infantile haemangioma, supported with serial photography illustrating examples from the time of maximum proliferation until complete resolution.

Until 2008, treatment for infantile haemangiomas causing, or likely to cause, impairment of function or permanent disfigurement included systemic and intralesional corticosteroids and α-interferon. All of these treatments were associated with significant adverse effects. In 2008 the first report of the successful use of propranolol radically changed the therapeutic approach to infantile haemangioma, and propranolol is now the first line treatment (Appendix 117.1) [24]. Propranolol has been shown to induce a better and faster response than systemic steroids, and is associated with fewer and less concerning adverse effects [25–29].

Recommendations for pre-treatment investigation, dosage and monitoring schedules have varied, but most protocols emphasize particular care when treating very small infants and those with co-morbidities [29,30,31] (Appendix 117.1). Relapse appears to be less likely if treatment is continued for at least 12 months [32].

Although the efficacy of topical propranolol 1% twice daily for superficial infantile haemangioma has been reported [33], there is far greater experience with timolol maleate, usually as a gel-forming solution (GFS), with benefit reported particularly for very small superficial lesions [34]. Despite widespread use there are few data on percutaneous absorption, with estimates of equivalence with oral propranolol varying widely [35,36]. The use of one drop of timolol maleate 0.5% GFS up to three times a day to non-ulcerated, non-mucosal lesions appears to be safe.

Although β-blockers may be helpful for the treatment of ulcerated infantile haemangioma, worsening of ulceration can occur, perhaps reflecting reduced blood flow. Most ulcerated infantile haemangiomas respond well to protective non-adherent dressings, and topical or systemic antimicrobial treatment based on sensitivities on culture of swabs. The specific mechanism of action of β-blockers remains largely unknown, but it appears that clinical improvement may occur through the induction of vasoconstriction and the decreased expression of pro-angiogenic factors [37].

Pulsed dye laser (PDL) can be helpful for the treatment of ulcerations [38], and may be required for telangiectases and erythema post-involution. Use of PDL in the early proliferative phase of non-ulcerated infantile haemangioma does not appear to improve long-term outcomes, the evidence indicating that treated lesions are more likely to show atrophy or hypopigmentation [39,40–43].

Surgery may very occasionally be required for infantile haemangioma in the proliferative phase if functional impairment or ulceration cannot be managed medically. In the involuting phase, surgery may be indicated provided the size and appearance of the scar is likely to be superior to the result from surgery when involution has ceased. In the involuted phase, indications for surgery include abnormal contour due to a fibrofatty residuum and distortion of an important anatomical structure [44,45].

Embolization may have a role for life-threatening haemangiomas, particularly those leading to congestive cardiac failure that have not responded to medical therapy.

Congenital haemangiomas

Congenital haemangiomas are benign vascular tumours that proliferate *in utero*, and do not show further proliferation postnatally [1]. They may be evident as early as 12 weeks of gestation by prenatal ultrasound studies [2]. They either regress within 1–2 years (rapidly involuting congenital haemangioma, RICH) or not at all (non-involuting congenital haemangioma, NICH). An uncommon intermediate type is also recognized, presenting with early features similar to a RICH, but showing only partial involution, and referred to as partially involuting congenital haemangioma (PICH) [3]. All three types are GLUT-1 negative.

Congenital haemangiomas occur equally in male and female infants, and usually arise on the head or the extremities. The pathogenesis is unknown.

RICH typically present as blue or purple tumours, often with telangiectases and peripheral pallor (Figure 117.38), and sometimes with a central ulcer, scar or depression. The rapid regression may leave pronounced atrophy. Ultrasonography demonstrates a uniform hypoechoic mass with centrilobular draining channels [4]. Histology shows small lobules of capillaries with plump endothelium peripherally, and more thin-walled vessels with surrounding fibrous tissue centrally [5]. RICH may be associated with transient

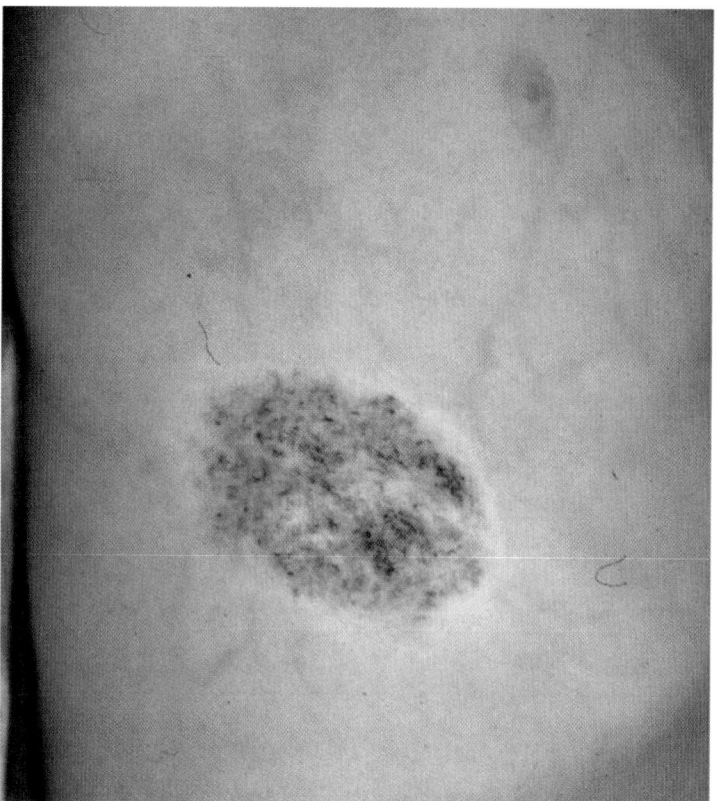

Figure 117.39 Non-involuting congenital haemangioma in an 11-year-old child.

thrombocytopenia, which usually resolves spontaneously [6]. Large lesions may cause haemodynamic instability.

Embolization or excision may need to be considered for RICHs that are ulcerated, bleeding or causing haemodynamic instability. There is no convincing evidence that β-blockers accelerate involution of RICH. Sclerotherapy may be indicated for prominent veins in areas of atrophy following involution.

NICH present as violaceous plaques or tumours with coarse telangiectases and peripheral pallor (Figure 117.39), and may be warm to touch. They grow in proportion with the affected individual, but never regress. On ultrasound, NICH often show prominent arterial flow. Histology shows large lobules of small vessels in a stroma of fibrous tissue containing abnormal appearing arteries and veins [5].

For NICH requiring treatment, surgery is the preferred option [7].

Resources

Patient resources

Birth Mark Support Group: www.birthmarksupportgroup.org.uk.
Changing Faces: https://www.changingfaces.org.uk.
Great Ormond Street Hospital, haemangioma information: http://www.gosh. nhs.uk/medical-information/search-for-medical-conditions/haemangioma/ haemangioma-information/.
(All last accessed August 2015.)

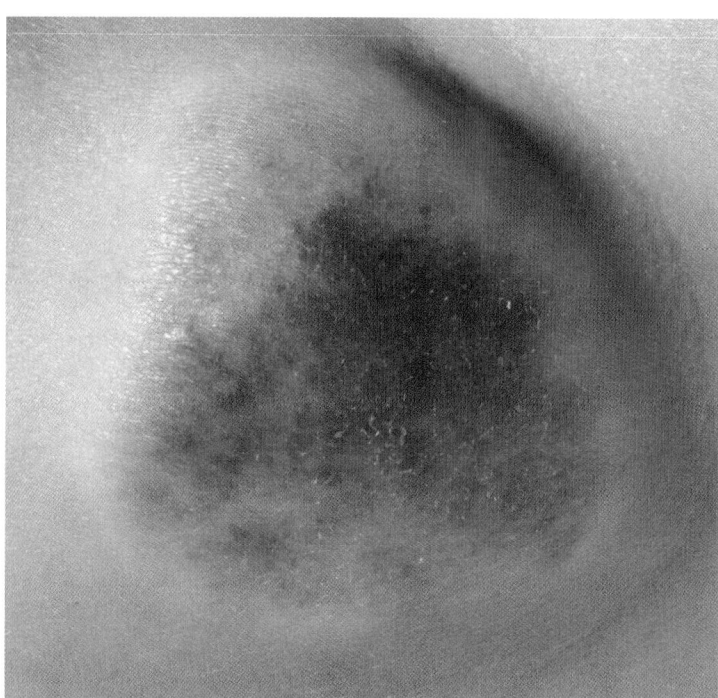

Figure 117.38 Rapidly involuting congenital haemangioma on the leg of a 6-week-old male, showing peripheral pallor.

PART 10: SITES, SEX, AGE

Appendix 117.1 Protocol for the use of propranolol in treating infantile haemangiomas

Before starting propranolol
- Full clinical history and examination including HR, BP and oxygen saturation
- Treatment explanation plus written information given to parents
- Clinical photography
- ECHO and ECG in selected patients (please see table below)

ECG	ECG and ECHO
If the HR is below normal for age	Patients with history, symptoms or signs of cardiovascular disease, including patients with suspected high-output heart failure
History of arrhythmia or arrhythmia on examination	
Family history of congenital heart condition, arrhythmia or maternal history of connective tissue disease	Patients with large segmental haemangioma of the face and neck and suspected PHACE syndrome

Dosage regimen

Week 1	1 mg/kg/day divided into three equal doses
Week 2	2 mg/kg/day divided into three equal doses
Patients with suspected PHACE syndrome	0.5 mg/kg/day and very cautious increase of the dose in small increments until MRA excludes clinically significant arterial anomalies of head and neck

Observation and monitoring

Weight >3.5 kg and no co-morbidities	BP and HR immediately before first dose and every 30 min for 2 h
Weight <3.5 kg and/or co-morbidities	BP and HR immediately before the dose and every 30 min for 4 h or longer

Other investigations[a]

Investigations	Group of patients
Thyroid function test	Liver haemangioma
	Parotid haemangioma
	PHACE syndrome
Liver function tests	Liver haemangioma
Full blood count	Bleeding haemangioma
Abdominal ultrasound	More than 10 cutaneous haemangiomas
	Perianal and perineal haemangioma crossing the midline and/or extending into the gluteal cleft
MRA brain and neck	Large segmental haemangioma of head and neck with suspected PHACE syndrome
MRI spine	Plaque haemangioma in lumbosacral area crossing the midline or perianal/perineal haemangioma extending into gluteal cleft

Referrals

ENT	Suspected airway haemangioma
Ophthalmology	Periocular haemangioma

Continuation of the treatment

Reviews	4–6 weeks after starting treatment, then 3–4 monthly
Increments	Increments greater than 0.5 mg/kg/day should include 2 h post dose monitoring of HR and BP
Treatment stopping	Usually at 12–14 months of age but can be later Gradual dose reduction over 2–4 weeks

From Solman 2014 [30]. Reproduced with permission of BMJ Publishing Group Ltd.

[a] Propranolol can be commenced while the investigations/results are pending.

BP, blood pressure; ECG, electrocardiogram; ECHO, echocardiogram; ENT, ear, nose and throat; HR, heart rate; MRA, magnetic resonance angiography; MRI, magnetic resonance imaging; PHACE, posterior fossa malformations, haemangiomas, arterial anomalies, cardiac anomalies, eye abnormalities and sternal pit/supraumbilical raphe.

Key references

The full list of references can be found in the online version at www.rooksdermatology.com.

Infantile dermatoses

Seborrhoeic dermatitis
4 Alexopoulos A, Kakourou T, Orfanou I, Xaidara A, Chrousos G. Retrospective analysis of the relationship between infantile seborrhoeic dermatitis and atopic dermatitis. *Pediatr Dermatol* 2014;31(2):125–30.

Atopic eczema
11 Kawamoto N, Fukao T, Hirayama K, *et al.* Total IgE at 6 months predicts the persistence of atopic dermatitis at 14 months. *Allergy Asthma Proc* 2013;34:362–9.

Napkin dermatitis
2 Liu N, Wang X, Odio M. Frequency and severity of diaper dermatitis with use of traditional Chinese cloth diapers: observations in 3–9 month old chidren. *Pediatr Dermatol* 2011;28:380–6.

Infantile psoriasis
2 Tollefson MM, Crowson CS, McEvoy MT, Maradit Kremers H. Incidence of psoriasis in children: a population-based study. *J Am Acad Dermatol* 2010:62:979–87.

Infantile acne
1 Cunliffe WJ, Baron SE, Coulson IH. A clinical and therapeutic study of 29 patients with infantile acne. *Br J Dermatol* 2001;145:463–6.

Urticaria
1 Mortureux P, Leaute-Labreze C, Legrain-Lifermann V, *et al.* Acute urticaria in infancy and early childhood: a prospective study. *Arch Dermatol* 1998;134(3): 319–23.

Viral exanthems
2 Drago F, Paolino S, Rebora A, *et al.* The challenge of diagnosing atypical exanthems: a clinico-laboratory study. *J Am Acad Dermatol* 2012;67:1282–8.

Varicella
1 Pinquier D, Lécuyer A, Levy C, *et al.* Inverse correlation between varicella severity and level of anti-varicella zoster virus maternal antibodies in infants below one year of age. *Hum Vaccin* 2011;7:534–8.

Staphylococcal scalded skin syndrome
1 Lamand V, Dauwalder O, Tristan A, *et al.* Epidemiological data of staphylococcal scalded skin syndrome in France from 1997 to 2007 and microbiological characteristics of Staphylococcus aureus associated strains. *Clin Microbiol Infect* 2012;12:514–21.

Tinea capitis

1 Michaels BD, Del Rosso JQ. Tinea capitis in infants: recognition, evaluation and management suggestions. *J Clin Aesthet Dermatol* 2012;5:49–59.

Acute haemorrhagic oedema in infancy

1 Legrain V, Lejean S, Taieb A, *et al.* Infantile acute hemorrhagic edema of the skin: study of ten cases. *J Am Acad Dermatol* 1991;24(1):17–22.

Kawasaki disease

3 Chang FY, Hwang B, Chen SJ, *et al.* Characteristics of Kawasaki disease in infants younger than 6 months of age. *Pediatr Infect Dis J* 2006;25:241–4.

Chronic bullous disease of childhood

1 Mintz EM, Morel KD. Clinical features, diagnosis, and pathogenesis of chronic bullous disease of childhood. *Dermatol Clin* 2011;29(3):459–62, ix.

Gianotti–Crosti syndrome

10 Chuh A, Zawar V. The epidemiology, etiology and Chuh and Zawar's diagnostic criteria of Gianotti-Crosti syndrome. *Exp Rev Dermatol* 2013;8.1:57–64.

Eosinophilic pustular folliculitis

4 Hernandez-Martin A, Nuno-Gonzalez A, Colmenero I, *et al.* Eosinophilic pustular folliculitis of infancy: a series of 15 cases and review of the literature. *J Am Acad Dermatol* 2013;68(1):150–5.

Pigmentary mosaicism

4 Taibjee SM, Bennett DC, Moss C. Abnormal pigmentation in hypomelanosis of Ito and pigmentary mosaicism: the role of pigmentary genes. *Br J Dermatol* 2004;151(2):269–82.

Non-accidental injury

1 Maguire S. *Which injuries may indicate child abuse? Arch Dis Child Educ Pract Ed* 2010;95:170–7.

Langerhans cell histiocytosis

7 Lau L, Krafchik B, Trebo MM, *et al.* Cutaneous Langerhans cell histiocytosis in children under one year. *Pediatr Blood Cancer* 2006;46(1):66–71.

Mastocytosis

2 Torrelo A, Alvarez-Twose I, Escribano L. Childhood mastocytosis. *Curr Opin Pediatr* 2012;24(4):480–6.

Infantile and congenital haemangiomas

Infantile haemangiomas

1 International Society for the Study of Vascular Anomalies (ISSVA). *ISSVA classificaiton for vascular anomalies 2014.* http://www.issva.org (last accessed May 2015)

13 Metry D, Heyer G, Hess C, *et al.* Consensus statement on diagnostic criteria for PHACE syndrome. *Pediatrics* 2009;124(5):1447–56.

16 Luu M, Frieden IJ. Haemangioma: clinical course, complications and management. *Br J Dermatol* 2013;169(1):20–30.

17 Dickie B, Dasgupta R, Nair R, *et al.* Spectrum of hepatic hemangiomas: management and outcome. *J Pediatr Surg* 2009;44(1):125–33.

19 Vredenborg AD, Janmohamed SR, de Laat PC, *et al.* Multiple cutaneous infantile haemangiomas and the risk of internal haemangioma. *Br J Dermatol* 2013;169(1):188–91.

30 Solman L, Murabit A, Gnarra M, *et al.* Propranolol for infantile haemangiomas: single centre experience of 250 cases and proposed therapeutic protocol. *Arch Dis Child* 2014.

31 Drolet BA, Frommelt PC, Chamlin SL, *et al.* Initiation and use of propranolol for infantile hemangioma: report of a consensus conference. *Pediatrics* 2013;131(1):128–40.

34 Chakkittakandiyil A, Phillips R, Frieden IJ, *et al.* Timolol maleate 0.5% or 0.1% gel-forming solution for infantile hemangiomas: a retrospective, multicenter, cohort study. *Pediatr Dermatol* 2012;29(1):28–31.

39 Batta K, Goodyear HM, Moss C, *et al.* Randomised controlled study of early pulsed dye laser treatment of uncomplicated childhood haemangiomas: results of a 1-year analysis. *Lancet* 2002;360(9332):521–7.

Congenital haemangiomas

3 Nasseri E, Piram M, McCuaig CC, *et al.* Partially involuting congenital hemangiomas: a report of 8 cases and review of the literature. *J Am Acad Dermatol* 2014;70(1):75–9.

PART 10: SITES, SEX, AGE

Index

Note: Page numbers in *italics* refer to figures, those in **bold** refer to tables and boxes. References are to pages within chapters, thus 58.10 is page 10 of Chapter 58.

Rook's Textbook of Dermatology, Ninth Edition. Edited by Christopher Griffiths, Jonathan Barker, Tanya Bleiker, Robert Chalmers and Daniel Creamer.
© 2016 John Wiley & Sons, Ltd. Published 2016 by John Wiley & Sons, Ltd.
Companion website: www.rooksdermatology.com